Thrall's Textbook of

VETERINARY DIAGNOSTIC RADIOLOGY

EIGHTH EDITION

Thrall's Textbook of VETERINARY DIAGNOSTIC RADIOLOGY

Gabriela S. Seiler Dr.Med.Vet., DECVDI, DACVR
Professor of Radiology
Molecular Biomedical Sciences
North Carolina State University
Raleigh, North Carolina

Donald E. Thrall, DVM, PHD
Emeritus Professor
College of Veterinary Medicine
North Carolina State University
Raleigh, North Carolina
Radiologist
IDEXX Telemedicine Consultants
Clackamas, Oregon

ELSEVIER

Elsevier
3251 Riverport Lane
St. Louis, Missouri 63043

THRALL'S TEXTBOOK OF VETERINARY DIAGNOSTIC RADIOLOGY,
EIGHTH EDITION ISBN: 978-0-323-93235-6

Executive Content Strategist: Lauren Willis
Content Development Specialist: Casey Potter
Publishing Services Manager: Deepthi Unni
Project Manager: Gayathri S
Design Direction: Ryan Cook

Printed in the United States of America

Last digit is the print number: 9 8 7 6 5 4 3 2 1

List of Contributors

Graeme Allan, DVSc, MVSc, FACVS, DACVR
Veterinary Radiologist
Veterinary Imaging Associates
St Leonards, Sydney
NSW, Australia

Melanie Anderson, DVM, DACVR
Radiologist
Radiology
University of Missouri
Columbia, Missouri

Ryan Appleby, DVM, DACVR
Assistant Professor
Clinical Studies
Ontario Veterinary College
Guelph, Ontario, Canada

Fabrice Audigié, DVM, PhD, HDR, Ass. LA-ECVDI
Professor in Equine Imaging and Locomotor Pathology
Cirale
Ecole Nationale Vétérinaire d'Alfort
Goustranville, France

Myra F. Barrett, DVM, MS, DACVR, DACVR-EDI
Professor of Radiology
Environmental and Radiological Health Sciences
Colorado State University
Fort Collins, Colorado

Clifford Berry III, DVM, DACVR
Associate Clinical Professor
Department of Molecular Biomedical Sciences
North Carolina State University
Apex, North Carolina

Kathryn W. Bills, VMD, DACVR, DACVR-EDI
Associate Professor
Department of Clinical Studies, New Bolton Center
University of Pennsylvania, School of Veterinary Medicine
Kennett Square, Pennsylvania

Elizabeth Biscoe, DVM, DACVR, DACVR-EDI
Equine Veterinary Radiologist
Equine Diagnostic Imaging
Archer, Florida
Veterinary Teleradiologist
VetRad
Worthington, Ohio

Valeria Busoni, DVM, PhD, DECVDI
Associate Professor
Service d'Imagerie Médicale—Clinique Vétérinaire Universitaire
Faculté de Médecine Vétérinaire
Université de Liège
Liège, Belgium

Eli B. Cohen, DVM, DACVR
Founder-Radiologist
Dragonfly Imaging, PLLC
Cary, North Carolina
Adjunct Clinical Professor
Molecular & Biomedical Sciences
NC State College of Veterinary Medicine
Raleigh, North Carolina

Marc-Andre d'Anjou, DMV, DACVR
Veterinary Radiologist
Diagnostic Imaging
Animages Inc.
Longueuil, Québec, Canada

Sarah Davies, BVSc, MS, DACVR
Veterinary Radiologist
Department of Radiology
The Pet Specialists
Terrey Hills, NSW, Australia

Randi Drees, Dr. Med. Vet., PhD, DACVR (Radiology & Radiation Oncology), DipECVDI (add Rad Oncol), MRCVS, CertAVP
Associate Professor
Department of Clinical Science and Services
The Royal Veterinary College
Hatfield, United Kingdom

Wm Tod Drost, DVM, DACVR
Radiologist
Telemedicine
IDEXX
Keswick, Virginia
Executive Director
American College of Veterinary Medicine
Harrisburg, Pennsylvania

Lisa J. Forrest, VMD, DACR, DACVR-RO
Professor
Surgical Sciences
University of Wisconsin-Madison
Madison, Wisconsin
Professor
Carbone Cancer Center
University of Wisconsin-Madison
Madison, Wisconsin

Lorrie Gaschen, DVM, PhD, Dr.Med.Vet, DECVDI
Adjunct Professor of Diagnostic Imaging
Veterinary Clinical Sciences
Louisiana State University
Baton Rouge, Louisiana
Radiologist
VetCT
Cambridge, United Kingdom

Lindsey J. Gilmour, DVM, DACVR, DACVR-EDI
Clinical Associate Professor
Department of Veterinary Large Animal Clinical Sciences
Texas A&M University
College of Veterinary Medicine
College Station, Texas

Christine L. Gremillion, DVM, DACVR, DACVR-EDI
Clinical Assistant Professor
Department of Large Animal Clinical Sciences
Texas A&M University College of Veterinary Medicine and Biomedical Sciences
College Station, Texas

Hock Gan Heng, DMV, MVS, MS, DACVR, DECVDI
Radiologist
VetCT
Cambridge, United Kingdom
Department of Veterinary Clinical Sciences,
Purdue University College of Veterinary
West Lafayette, Indiana

Elodie Huguet, DVM, DACVR
Assistant Professor of Diagnostic Imaging
Small Animal Clinical Sciences
The University of Florida
Micanopy, Florida
IDEXX Teleradiologist
IDEXX Telemedicine Consultants
Clackamas, Oregon

Martha Moon Larson, DVM, MS, DACVR
Professor, Radiology
Department of Small Animal Clinical Sciences
Va-MD College of Veterinary Medicine
Va Tech
Blacksburg, Virginia

Jimmy C. Lattimer, DVM, MS, DACVR, DACVR-RO
Associate Professor
Department of Veterinary Medicine and Surgery
University of Missouri
Columbia, Missouri

Jody E. Lawver, DVM, DACVR, DACVR-EDI
Assistant Professor
Department of Large Animal Clinical Sciences
Michigan State University
East Lansing, Michigan

Wilfried Mai, DVM, MS, PhD, DACVR, DECVDI
Professor
Department of Clinical Sciences and Advanced Medicine
University of Pennsylvania School of Veterinary Medicine
Philadelphia, Pennsylvania

Angela Marolf, DVM, DACVR
Professor and Chair
Department of Veterinary Clinical Sciences
The Ohio State University
Columbus, Ohio

Isabelle Masseau, DVM, PhD, DACVR
Associate Professor
Sciences Cliniques
Université de Montréal
Saint-Hyacinthe, Québec, Canada
Adjunct Professor
Veterinary Medicine & Surgery
University of Missouri
Columbia, Missouri

Federica Morandi, DVM, MS, DECVDI, DACVR
Professor of Radiology
Small Animal Clinical Sciences
University of Tennessee
Knoxville, Tennessee

Dana A. Neelis, DVM, MS, DACVR, DACVR-EDI
Radiologist
Radiology
Neelis Veterinary Imaging
Emmett, Idaho

Nathan C. Nelson, DVM, MS, DACVR, DACVR-EDI
Clinical Professor
Department of Molecular Biomedical Sciences
North Carolina State University
Raleigh, North Carolina

Stephanie G. Nykamp, DVM, MSc, DACVR
Veterinary Radiologist
Vet's Choice Radiology
Northbrook, Illinois

Kathryn L. Phillips, DVM, DACVR, DACVR-EDI
Associate Professor
Veterinary Surgical and Radiological Sciences
UC Davis
Davis, California

Rachel E. Pollard, DVM, PhD, DACVR
Professor Emerita of Diagnostic Imaging
Surgical and Radiological Sciences
University of California, Davis School of Veterinary Medicine
Davis, California

Erin G. Porter, DVM, DACVR, DACVR-EDI
Clinical Associate Professor
Large Animal Clinical Sciences
University of Florida College of Veterinary Medicine
Gainesville, Florida

Elissa K. Randall, DVM, MS, DACVR
Professor Diagnostic Imaging
Environmental and Radiological Health Sciences
Colorado State University
Fort Collins, Colorado

Jennifer A. Reetz, DVM, DACVIM (LA), DACVR
Veterinary Radiologist
Department of Clinical Sciences and Advanced Medicine
School of Veterinary Medicine
University of Pennsylvania
Philadelphia, Pennsylvania

Elizabeth A. Riedesel, DVM, DACVR
Emeritus Professor Retired
Veterinary Clinical Sciences
Iowa State University
Ames, Iowa
Consulting Radiologist
eImaging
Fort Worth, Texas

Ian Robertson, BVSc, DACVR
Emeritus Clinical Professor
Department of Molecular Biomedical Sciences
NC State University
Raleigh, North Carolina
Radiologist
Dragonfly Imaging PLLC
Cary, North Carolina

Federica Rossi, DVM, SRV, DECVDI
Veterinary Radiologist
Diagnostic Imaging
Anicura Clinica Veterinaria dell'Orologio
Sasso Marconi, Italy

Gabriela S. Seiler, Dr.Med.Vet., DECVDI, DACVR
Professor of Radiology
Molecular Biomedical Sciences
North Carolina State University
Raleigh, North Carolina

Kathy A. Spaulding, DVM, DACVR
Clinical Professor Radiology Emeritus—Retired
Department of Veterinary Large Animal Clinical Sciences
Texas A&M University
College Station, Texas

Susanne M. Stieger-Vanegas, Dr. Med. Vet., PhD, DECVDI
Professor, Diagnostic Imaging
Clinical Sciences
Carlson College of Veterinary Medicine
Oregon State University
Corvallis, Oregon

Donald E. Thrall, DVM, PhD, DACVR
Emeritus Professor
College of Veterinary Medicine
North Carolina State University
Raleigh, North Carolina
Radiologist
IDEXX Telemedicine Consultants
Clackamas, Oregon

Elizabeth Acutt, BVSc, MS, DACVR-EDI
Assistant Professor
Department of Large Animal Diagnostic Imaging
School of Veterinary Medicine
University of Pennsylvania
Philadelphia, Pennsylvania

Lenin Arturo Villamizar Martinez, DVM, MS, PhD, DAVDC
Assistant Professor of Veterinary Dentistry and Oral Surgery
Department of Clinical Sciences
North Carolina State University College of Veterinary Medicine
Holly Springs, North Carolina

Andra K. Voges, DVM, DACVR
Clinical Professor
Large Animal Clinical Sciences, Radiology
Texas A&M College of Veterinary Medicine
College Station, Texas

William R. Widmer, DVM, MS, DACVR
Emeritus Professor College of Veterinary Medicine
Veterinary Clinical Sciences
Purdue University
West Lafayette, Indiana
Adjunct Professor, Diagnostic Imaging
College of Veterinary Medicine
Lincoln Memorial University
Harrogate, Tennessee

Preface

The first edition of this text was published in 1986…over 37 years ago. I'm guessing this predates the birth year of some of the authors contributing to this eighth edition. I clearly remember celebrating the release of the first edition with my then Department Head, Arthur Aronson, and a nice bottle of champagne. His support was so critical regarding many of my accomplishments, including this text. Art is no longer with us, but I think of him often. I doubt he would have predicted that this book would survive so many revisions; I know I did not.

I became involved with the first edition solely by chance. It was not something I sought. But, having been presented with the opportunity, I was intrigued and decided to give it a go. I had been involved with an earlier veterinary radiology book, *Carlson's Veterinary Radiology*, along with Drs. Edward Gillette and Jacques Lebel. This was at a time when I thought I knew much more than I did. That book, at least my part, was largely unsuccessful so the opportunity to have a leadership role with another radiology text was a chance at redemption.

When writing this preface for the eighth edition, I looked at my copy of the first edition. What struck me immediately was the extremely poor quality of the illustrations. I remember being reminded of that on numerous occasions and I was quite surprised that a second edition was even requested by the publisher. Fortunately, this problem of poor radiographic reproduction into the print medium has been solved by the greatly increased quality of digital image capture compared to film cassettes. All the images in this text were acquired initially in a digital format, making for the highest quality of reproduction, and select digital images are also available directly on the textbook website.

While numerous things about this book have changed along the way, such as inclusion of CT and MRI concepts and images, normal anatomy, and web-based ancillary materials, the core principles of the book have not. The basis of interpretation used in this textbook remains centered upon description of radiographic abnormalities in terms of roentgen signs—changes in size, shape, location, number, margination, and opacity. Having a firm understanding of roentgen sign description makes one less inclined to make errors by jumping immediately to a diagnosis rather than thoroughly considering radiographic changes in an orderly and efficient manner. The audience also remains the same, with content aimed toward students of imaging at all levels, private practitioners, and to some extent specialists in other fields. Chapters covering the basic principles of interpretation of images of the axial and appendicular skeleton in small and large animals, and the thorax and abdomen in small animals, should be of value to beginning interpreters. These basic chapters offer a framework upon which to base an understanding of more detailed chapters dealing with specific abnormalities. And, as in the second through seventh editions, all chapters in this eighth edition have been either completely rewritten by a new author or thoroughly revised. No chapter has escaped in-depth scrutiny, ensuring that the latest and most accurate information is included.

From the first edition onward, I have always believed that is impossible for one person to prepare a meaningful, comprehensive textbook of veterinary imaging. Thus, as in all previous editions, a group of highly trained specialists in imaging have come together to produce what I think is a magnificent complication of veterinary imaging from the basic to the advanced. I would like to extend my heartfelt thanks to this group of radiologists for taking time from their busy schedules to help create this product.

Nothing lasts forever, including my tenure as Editor of this book. One of my most significant accomplishments while at North Carolina State University was to convince Dr. Gabriela (Gabi) Seiler to join our radiology faculty. Gabi is one of the brightest radiologists that I know, and a wonderful person. She has been extremely productive at North Carolina State University and quickly rose to the rank of Professor. When I was presented with the opportunity of preparing an eighth edition of this book, I knew immediately that I no longer had the stamina for such an immense undertaking. When thinking about a successor, Gabi was the first person who came to mind. I discussed the possibility of assuming Editorship with Gabi and after earnest consideration she agreed to take it on, which was a big relief and a source of great joy for me. As a result, the work you have before you is really a product of Dr. Gabi Seiler and not me. She developed the content for the eighth edition, recruited a cadre of new accomplished authors, and edited much of the text. Although she and I are listed at coeditors, this is Dr. Seiler's book.

From here forward, my involvement with this work will be in name only…*Thrall's Textbook of Veterinary Diagnostic Radiology*. I am honored to have been charged with stewardship of this book for all these years. I trust this eighth edition will be well received and I anticipate many more successful editions under the guidance of Dr. Seiler.

Donald E. Thrall

Acknowledgement

I am deeply honored to be selected as the new editor of the Thrall Textbook of Veterinary Diagnostic Radiology—a truly iconic resource that has profoundly enhanced student learning and remains indispensable for both students and clinicians. I want to acknowledge Dr. Don Thrall's extraordinary achievement in creating and advancing this book to its current 8th edition. I genuinely believe that no one else could have accomplished this, and generations of veterinarians have and will benefit from it. I also deeply appreciate the invaluable contributions of the current and previous authors. Thank you all so much.

Gabriela S. Seiler

Contents

Video Table of Contents

SECTION I

Physics and Principles of Interpretation

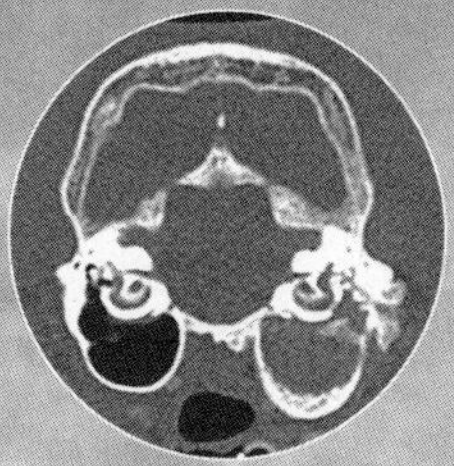
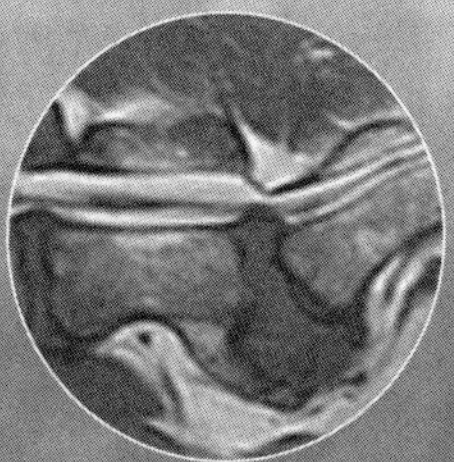
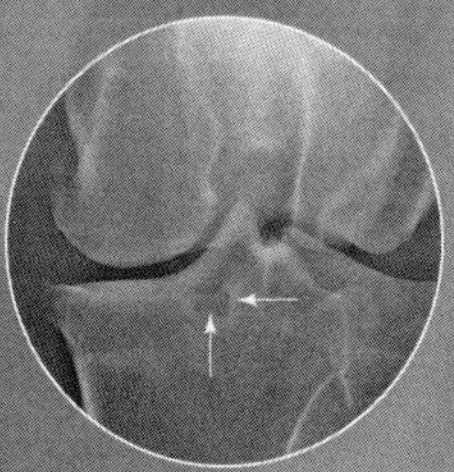
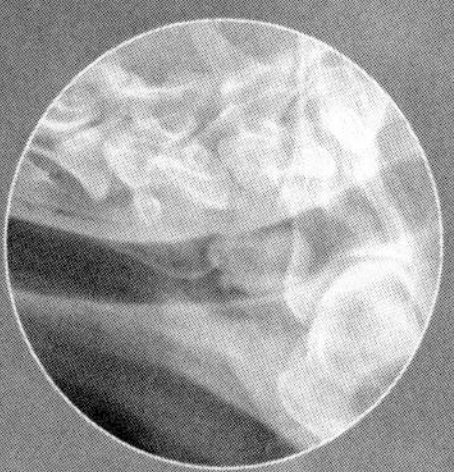
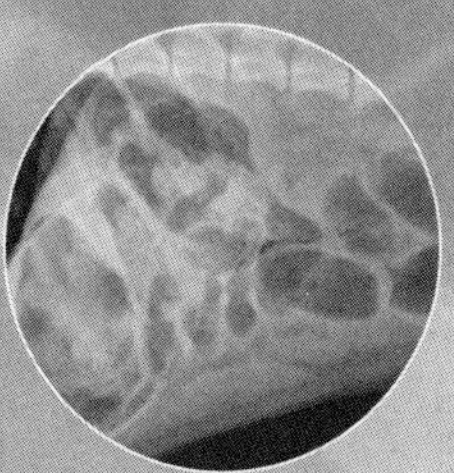

CHAPTER 1

Radiation Protection and Physics of Diagnostic Radiology

William R. Widmer • Donald E. Thrall

X-rays were discovered on November 8, 1895, by Wilhelm Conrad Roentgen, a German physicist (Fig. 1.1).[1] X-rays were immediately used for medical purposes, and many sophisticated applications were soon devised. For example, angiography was described in 1896, only 1 year after the initial discovery of x-rays. Roentgen's finding revolutionized the diagnosis and treatment of disease, and in recognition he was awarded the first Nobel Prize for Physics in 1901. More than 125 years after their discovery, imaging using x-rays is one of the most important and widely used diagnostic tests in people and animals. Despite the advances afforded by diagnostic ultrasound, computed tomography, and magnetic resonance imaging, conventional radiography remains the "workhorse" of veterinary imaging.

BASIC PROPERTIES OF X-RAYS

X-rays and gamma rays are part of the spectrum of electromagnetic (EM) radiation. The only distinction between x-rays and gamma rays is their source; x-rays are produced by electron interactions outside the nucleus, and gamma rays are released from inside the nucleus of unstable atoms having excess energy. There is a false impression that gamma rays are more energetic than x-rays, but this is not universally true. The energy of a gamma ray depends on the amount of energy released by the unstable atom, and the energy of an x-ray depends on the energy of the electron that interacts with the atom. Radiopharmaceuticals used in nuclear imaging generally emit gamma rays with energy similar to x-rays used for diagnostic imaging.

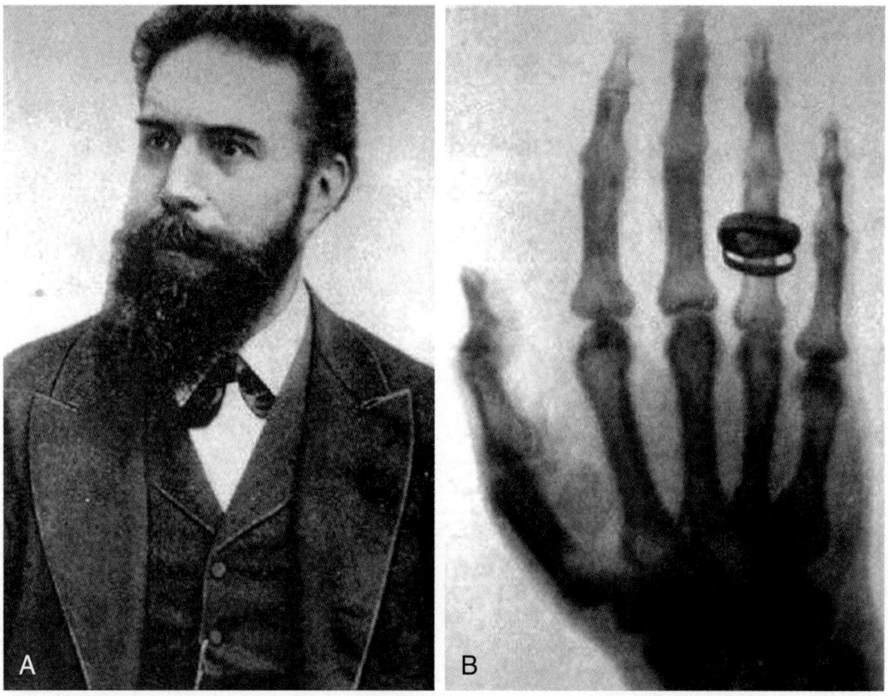

Fig. 1.1 **A,** Wilhelm Conrad Roentgen accidentally discovered x-rays while working with a cathode ray tube containing an inert gas. Roentgen noted that high voltage applied to the tube caused fluorescence of a photographic plate. Roentgen deduced that an unknown, invisible "x" radiation must be produced by the cathode ray tube. **B,** The first known radiograph was made of his wife's hand. (Images in the public domain.)

Table • 1.1

Wavelength and Origin of Common Types of Electromagnetic Radiation.

TYPE OF ELECTROMAGNETIC RADIATION	WAVELENGTH	ORIGIN
Radio waves	1 mm–100 km	Oscillating electrons in antennae
Microwaves	1 mm–1 m	Oscillating electrons in antennae
Infrared	780 nm–1 mm	Electron energy level transition
Visible light	380 nm–700 nm	Electron energy level transition
Ultraviolet	100 nm–400 nm	Electron energy level transition
X-rays	0.1 nm–10 nm	Bremsstrahlung, characteristic
Gamma Rays	1×10^{-6} nm	Nuclear decay

From Bushberg JT, Seibert JA, Leidholdt EM, Jr, et al. *The Essential Physics of Medical Imaging*. 2nd ed. Lippincott Williams & Wilkins; 2012.

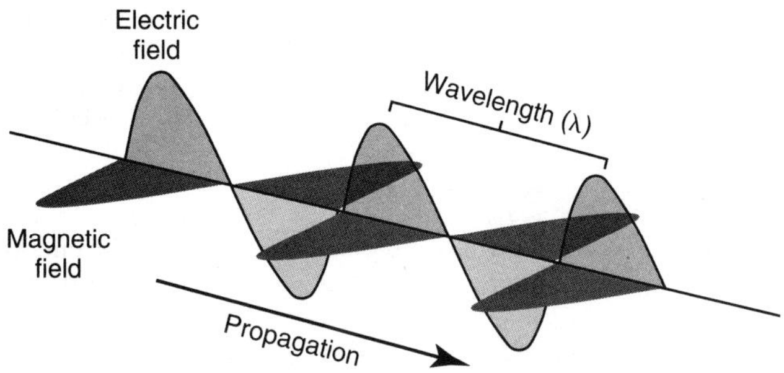

Fig. 1.2 All forms of electromagnetic radiation are characterized by oscillating electric and magnetic fields that move in planes at right angles to each other. Any form of electromagnetic radiation is described by the wavelength, λ, which is the distance between crests, and the frequency, f, which is the number of crests per unit time. The frequency and wavelength determine the specific characteristics of that form of radiation. The velocity (c) of all forms of electromagnetic radiation is the same—the speed of light. The product of wavelength and frequency equals the velocity: $c = f \times \lambda$. Therefore, because velocity is constant, as frequency increases, the wavelength must decrease, and vice versa.

Familiar types of EM radiation other than x-rays and gamma rays include radio waves, radar, microwaves, and visible light (Table 1.1).

EM radiation is a combination of electric and magnetic fields that travel together, oscillating in orthogonal planes in sine-wave fashion (Fig. 1.2). Sine waves are characterized by two related parameters—frequency and wavelength. The velocity of EM radiation is constant, the speed of light, resulting in an inverse relationship between frequency and velocity according to the formula:

$$V = f\lambda$$

- V = speed of light (m/s)
- f = frequency in Hz
- λ = wavelength in m

Properties of x-rays and gamma rays are given in Box 1.1. Some properties of EM radiation cannot be explained adequately by the theories of wave propagation illustrated in Fig. 1.2. Therefore, the *photon* concept was developed to explain the apparent particulate behavior of x-rays and gamma rays. A photon can be considered as a discrete bundle of EM radiation as opposed to a wave. This makes it easier to understand how x-rays create an image or cause radiation damage. In this book, the terms *x-ray* and *photon* are used interchangeably.

Box • 1.1

Properties of X-Rays and Gamma Rays

Have no charge
Have no mass
Travel at the speed of light
Are invisible
Cannot be felt
Travel in a straight line
Cannot be deflected by magnetic fields
Penetrate all matter to some degree
Cause certain substances to fluoresce
Can expose photographic emulsions
Can ionize atoms

The ***energy*** of EM radiation is described according to the formula:

$$\text{Energy} = \text{Planck's constant} \times \frac{\text{speed of light}}{\text{wavelength}}$$

Planck's constant is a proportionality constant between the energy of a photon and its wavelength, and the speed of light is also a constant. Therefore, the energy of EM radiation is inversely proportional to wavelength. The biologic effects of EM radiation are a function of the energy.

The unit of energy for EM radiation is the *electron volt* (eV). One electron volt is the energy gained by one electron as it is accelerated through a potential difference of 1V. On an absolute scale, this is a very small amount of energy. However, x-rays with energy of only 15 eV* can produce ionization of atoms. Ionization occurs when an electron is ejected from the atom, in radiography by an x-ray. This creates an ion pair consisting of the negatively charged electron and the positively charged atom (Fig. 1.3). When x-rays strike a person, they can result in ionizations of DNA, leading to (1) mutations, (2) abortion or fetal abnormalities, (3) susceptibility to disease and shortened life span, (4) carcinogenesis, and (5) cataracts.[2] Therefore, minimizing exposure of personnel working in a radiation environment is critical. Radiation also causes ionizations in patients undergoing medical imaging procedures, but the risk of

*The electron volt (eV) should not be confused with the concept of kilovoltage peak (kVp) applied in an x-ray tube during an exposure; kVp is discussed later in the Production of X-rays section.

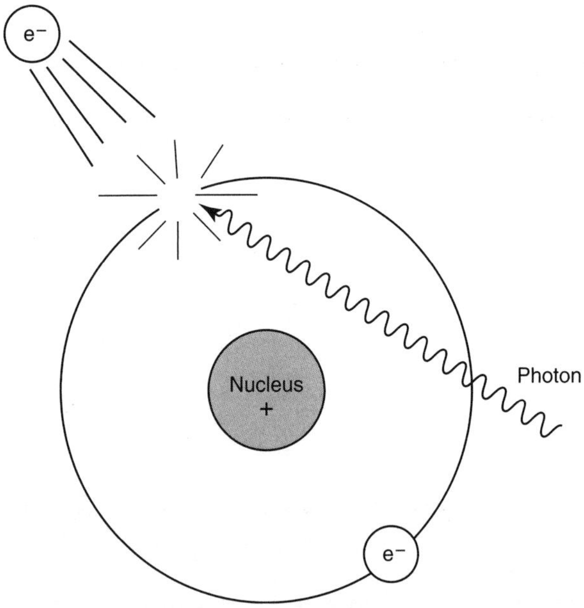

Fig. 1.3 The principle of ionization. A photon ejects an electron from an atom, causing ionization and forming an ion pair, consisting of a negatively charged electron and a positively charged atom. After this ionization event, the photon, depending on its energy, may be completely absorbed, or it may interact with other atoms to produce more ionization. The ejected electron can also interact with biologic molecules, such as DNA, and produce damage. The relative size of the nucleus, electrons, and orbital shells in this figure is not to scale. The "+" symbol in the nucleus designates the normal nuclear positivity created by the presence of positively charged protons. In a neutral atom, this positive charge in the nucleus is balanced by an equal negative charge of orbital electrons.

radiation injury from an imaging procedure is offset by the diagnostic value of the procedure. Radiation workers, on the other hand, are subject to repeated potential low-level exposure and the risk for damage is increased. Also important is the fact that radiation damage to DNA can be amplified biologically because DNA controls cellular processes that extend into subsequent generations of daughter cells. Although only 15 eV of energy is required for ionization of biologic molecules, the energy of x-rays used for medical imaging is much greater. Therefore, each x-ray photon can lead to multiple ionizations in tissue.

The relative risk of biologic injury from x-rays or gamma rays is greater than from other types of EM radiation. For example, the wavelength of visible light is 10,000 times longer than the wavelength of x-rays, and the wavelength of radio waves is even longer (see Table 1.1). Therefore, the energy of light waves and radio waves is many orders of magnitude lower than the energy of x-rays, meaning that light and radio waves do not produce tissue ionization or DNA damage. Other forms of EM radiation, such as microwaves, can lead to biologic damage such as tissue heating but do not lead to molecular ionization.

RADIATION PROTECTION

A goal in diagnostic radiology is to obtain maximum diagnostic information with minimal radiation exposure of the patient, radiology personnel, and general public. This is achievable if guidelines for safe practice are followed and personal protective equipment (PPE) is used. However, because x-rays cannot be seen or felt, it is easy to disregard the danger associated with occupational x-ray exposure (Fig. 1.4). Many veterinarians and technologists have developed a cavalier attitude regarding the hazards associated with ionizing radiation and put themselves at risk, from both medical and legal perspectives. While the use of digital radiograph has vastly improved radiographic quality in veterinary imaging, it has also in many instances led to further disregard for safe radiation practices since the cost and time investment in retakes are minimal.

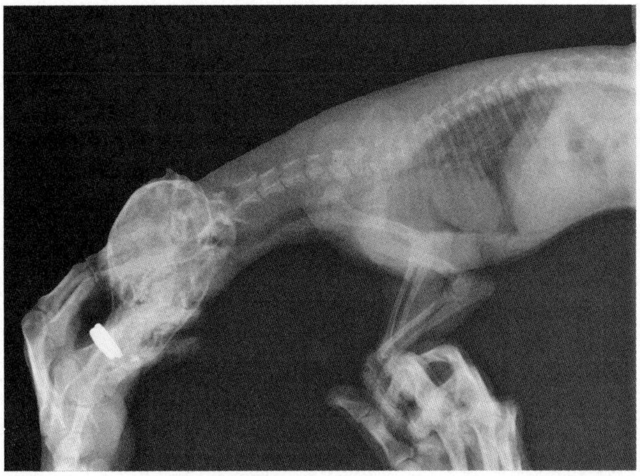

Fig. 1.4 Careless and unacceptable approach to radiography. The technologist's hands are in the primary x-ray beam. Careless habits such as this are perpetuated because of the stealthy properties of x-rays and lead to unnecessary personnel exposure that could become biologically significant.

Table • 1.2

Radiation Weighting Factor (Quality Factor) for Various Radiation Types.

TYPE OF RADIATION	WEIGHTING FACTOR
X-rays	1
Gamma rays	1
Beta particle (electron)	1
Neutrons	
<10 keV	5
10–100 keV	10
100 keV–2 MeV	20
Alpha particles	20

General principles of radiation protection that can form the basis of a safe workplace are discussed in this chapter. Any specific recommendations regarding radiation safety or protection made in this chapter are subject to overrule by local, state, and/or federal regulations.

Radiation Units

Two related concepts must be understood before radiation units are considered. First, radiation *exposure* and radiation *absorption* are not the same. Some tissues absorb radiation more effectively than others, meaning that exposure to the same amount of radiation will result in different absorbed doses in these tissues. Second, the biologic effect of the same absorbed dose can also be different, being a function of both radiation type and energy. A numeric *weighting factor* or *quality factor* has been derived to estimate the difference in biologic effectiveness of various types of radiation (Table 1.2).

Radiation exposure, radiation absorption, and dose equivalent each have their own unit of measure that was defined originally in the centimeter-gram-second (CGS) system of measures. In 1977, the International System of Units (SI units) was developed in keeping with the trend toward universal adoption

Table • 1.3

Radiation Units.

QUANTITY	CGS[a] UNIT	VALUE	SI[b] UNIT	VALUE
Exposure dose	roentgen	One electrostatic unit of electricity in 1 cubic centimeter of dry air at 0°C and standard atmospheric pressure	roentgen[c]	$2.58 \times 10 - 4$ C/kg
Absorbed dose	rad	100 ergs/g of tissue	gray (Gy)	1 Gy = 1 joule/kg (1 Gy = 100 rads)
Equivalent biologic dose	rem	Dose in rads times weighting factor[d]	sievert (Sv)	Dose in Gy times weighting factor (1 rem = 10 mSv)

[a]CGS, centimeter-gram-second system of units.
[b]International System of Units.
[c]Although the use of roentgen is allowable under the SI system, it is not itself an SI unit, and continued use is strongly discouraged by the National Institute of Standards and Technology.
[d]Weighting factor is a radiation type-specific quantity that compares the ionization density of various types of radiation; see Table 1.2.

of the metric system[3] (Table 1.3). In general, the system of SI units has not been universally adopted in the United States,[4,5] and CGS radiation units are still used, which can be a source of confusion.

Exposure

Radiation exposure is based on the amount of ionization in air that the radiation produces and is quantified by the amount of electrical charge resulting from the ionization. Radiation exposure is expressed in the SI system as coulombs[†] per kilogram of air (C/kg) (see Table 1.3). This SI unit of exposure is cumbersome; thus, an older term of exposure, the roentgen, is still used. One roentgen equals a charge of 2.58 C/kg in air.

Absorbed Dose

The efficiency of x-ray absorption in different materials can vary widely. For example, lead is a much more efficient absorber than water. Therefore, the radiation dose in tissues with different absorption efficiencies will be different when exposed to the same amount of radiation (Fig. 1.5). The SI unit for absorbed dose is the *gray* (Gy). One gray is the amount of radiation leading to absorption of 1 joule[‡]/kg of tissue. Before SI units were accepted, the unit of absorbed dose was the rad, which is equal to 100 ergs[§]/g of tissue (see Table 1.3). The term *rad* is obsolete, but it is so engrained in the radiology lexicon that it has not been replaced universally by the Gy. One gray is equal to 100 rad.

In soft tissue such as muscle, exposure to 1 roentgen amounts to an absorbed dose of approximately 0.9 centigray (cGy) or 0.9 rad. In comparison, bone is a more efficient absorber of x-rays than soft tissue, and exposure to bone of 1 roentgen results in a higher bone-absorbed dose. This difference in absorption between bone and soft tissue may be as great as a factor of 4–5 with low-energy radiation. Differential x-ray absorption between various tissues is the basis of radiographic contrast, and without this difference making a meaningful radiograph would not be possible. As discussed later, the magnitude of the difference between exposure and absorbed dose is the greatest for low energy photons and decreases as photon energy increases.

[†] A coulomb is the unit of electric charge in the SI units. It is the charge transferred by a constant current of 1 ampere in 1 second.
[‡] The joule is the unit of energy in the SI units. It is the energy exerted by the force of one newton acting to move an object through a distance of 1 m.
[§] The erg is the unit of energy in the CGS system of units. It is the energy exerted by the force of one dyne acting to move an object through a distance of 1 cm.

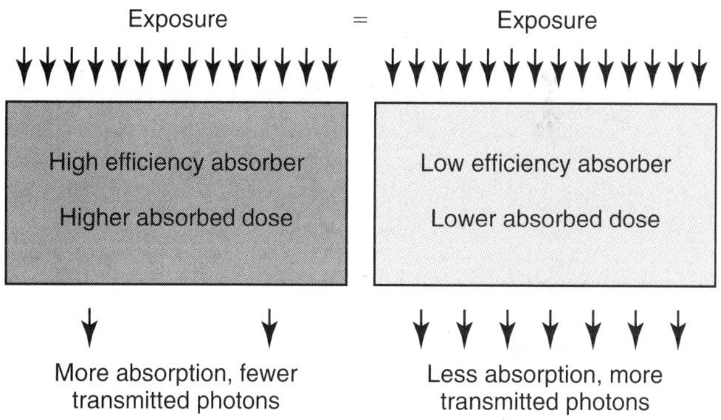

Fig. 1.5 Two materials are exposed to the same number of x-ray photons, represented by the *arrows* at the top. Thus, the exposure dose, in roentgens, or in coulombs per kilogram, is the same for both materials. However, the efficiency of x-ray absorption for the two materials is different. The material on the left is more efficient in absorbing x-rays than the material on the *right*. Therefore, the absorbed dose will be higher in the material on the left even though the exposure dose is the same. One real-life example of this phenomenon is a limb, where bone would be the high-efficiency absorber and fat or muscle the low-efficiency absorber.

Dose Equivalent

As noted earlier, the same absorbed dose, in Gy, from different types of radiation may not produce the same biologic effect. For example, damage from particulate radiation, such as an alpha particle[**] is greater on a Gy-for-Gy basis than damage from the same dose of x-rays (see Table 1.2). This is related to differences in *ionization density* for different types of radiation. A large, heavily charged particle, such as an alpha particle, creates many ionizations that are close together compared to a small lightly charged particle, such as an electron, where ionizations are more widely spaced (Fig. 1.6). The closer the ionizations are to each other, i.e., greater ionization density, the more biologic

[**] An alpha particle is a helium nucleus, containing two protons and two neutrons, without orbital electrons. An alpha particle has an electrical charge of 2+ and a mass more than 7000 times larger than that of an electron.

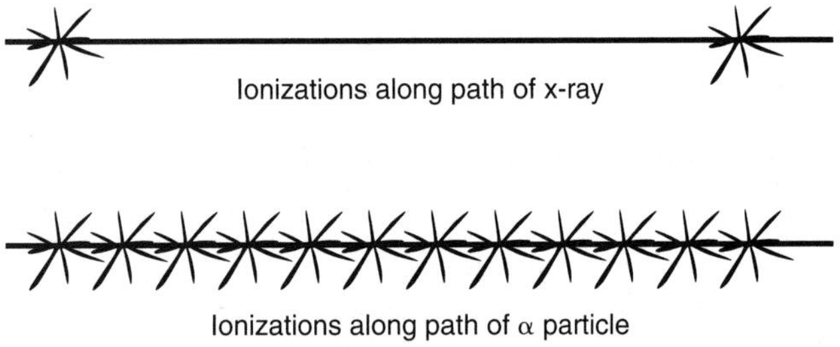

Fig. 1.6 Representation of the ionization density along the paths of an x-ray and an alpha particle. The ionization density along the path of the alpha particle is much higher because of its large mass and 2+ charge. This will lead to greater biologic damage on a Gy-per-Gy basis, and a correction factor will be needed to compare the biologic damage resulting from equal absorbed doses of x-rays versus alpha particles.

damage results from a given dose. Therefore, deposition of 1 Gy from an alpha particle does more biologic damage than deposition of 1 Gy from an x-ray because the ionizations are more clustered. The difference in biologic damage from the same absorbed dose of various radiation types is estimated by the weighting factor, as described earlier (see Table 1.2).

In the SI system, the unit of dose equivalency is the sievert (Sv); the Sv is derived from the product of the absorbed dose in Gy and the weighting factor. Before SI units were accepted, the unit of dose equivalency was the *radiation equivalent in man*, or *rem* (see Table 1.3). The rem was derived from the product of the absorbed dose in rads and the weighting factor, because 1 Gy = 100 rads, 1 Sv = 100 rem.

Radiation Safety

Principles of radiation safety are based on establishment of guidelines to prevent unnecessary exposure of radiation workers and the general public to ionizing radiation. The premise of radiation protection is that some low level of radiation exposure to radiation workers is permissible and will not lead to significant abnormalities or disease. Adverse effects can be classified as either *deterministic* or *stochastic*. Deterministic effects have a threshold. In other words, below some dose there is no effect, but above the threshold dose the severity of the effect is dose related. Radiation-induced cataracts are an example of a deterministic effect. Conversely, stochastic (random) effects have no dose threshold, and the severity of the effect is independent of dose. Radiation-induced cancer is an example of a stochastic effect.[6]

Maximum permissible dose (MPD) is the maximal amount of absorbed radiation that can be delivered to an individual as a whole-body dose or a dose to a specific organ and still be considered safe. The term *safe* in this context means that there is no conclusive evidence that the MPD will lead to harmful immediate or long-term effects to the body as a whole or to any individual structure or organ. Although the effect of very low doses of radiation is not known with certainty, it is safe to assume that any amount of radiation will have some effect and keeping one's dose below the MPD is important. An analogy could be made to smoking a cigarette once a month. There is no evidence that physical damage results from this frequency of smoking, but with increased smoking the probability of physical damage escalates by virtue of a cumulative effect. Unfortunately, an absolute threshold below which damage will definitely not occur has not been established for either cigarette smoking or radiation exposure.

There are multiple levels of bureaucracy regarding the establishment of guidelines for radiation exposure, aimed at avoiding deterministic and stochastic effects. Understanding the mission of all involved organizations can be confusing. Furthermore, different exposure limits are defined for radiation workers versus the general public. These exposure limits vary according to risk versus benefit. For example, the small risk to a member of the general public from being subjected to a radiographic study is outweighed by the benefit of a diagnosis. Likewise, the slightly higher exposure limits allowed for radiation workers are considered acceptable with respect to the missions of the occupation.

The International Commission on Radiological Protection (ICRP) is the primary international body focusing on protection against ionizing radiation. The ICRP is an independent, international, nongovernmental organization. The ICRP provides recommendations and guidance on protection against the risks associated with ionizing radiation. Their recommendations are published approximately four times each year as the journal *Annals of the ICRP.* The whole-body limit for radiation workers set by the ICRP for avoiding stochastic effects is 20 millisievert (mSv) per year, averaged over 5 years, with the provision that dose in any one year should not exceed 50 mSv.[7] The ICRP maintains exposure per quarter should not exceed 12.5 mSv.

In the United States, the National Council on Radiation Protection (NCRP) was chartered by Congress in 1964. Some of the objectives of the NCRP are to develop recommendations about radiation protection and to cooperate with the ICRP. The whole-body limit set for radiation workers by the NCRP for avoiding stochastic effects is 50 mSv per year with a lifetime accumulation not to exceed 10 mSv × age in years.[8] The NCRP also recommends that no occupational exposure occur until the age of 18 years.

The Nuclear Regulatory Commission (NRC) is the agency officially responsible for defining federal exposure standards in the United States. The NRC has adopted the annual radiation dose to adult radiation workers as recommended by the NCRP, a maximum of 50 mSv (5 rem) per year.[9] However, the NRC has not established an upper limit for cumulative exposure because of the uncertainty of such predictions.

The difference in opinion between the NRC and the NCRP regarding the limits for cumulative exposure can be confusing. However, rather than focusing on a specific number for cumulative or annual exposure, the goal should be to minimize any exposure. This is the basis of the ALARA approach, discussed later.

The allowable limit for radiation workers who become pregnant is lower than for nonpregnant radiation workers but ideally should be zero. The monthly exposure limit for the embryo or fetus should not exceed 0.5 mSv (0.05 rem). It is the responsibility of the pregnant radiation worker to notify the supervisor of the pregnancy ***in writing*** so that any change in work habits needed to stay within the recommended dose limit can be implemented.

For the general public, radiation exposure, excluding that related to medical use such as diagnostic imaging and radiation therapy, should not exceed 1 mSv (0.1 rem) per year.

In addition to occupational exposure of radiation workers, the entire population is exposed continually to very low levels of natural and man-made radiation. A revised breakdown of relative exposure of the U.S. public to radiation by various sources was published by the NCRP in 2015 (Fig. 1.7).[10] Revised estimates were needed because in 2006, Americans were exposed to more than seven times as much ionizing radiation from medical procedures as in the early 1980s, mainly due to increases in CT imaging. The number of CT studies performed in human patients doubled between 1997 and 2006.[11] In 2006, medical exposure constituted nearly half of the total radiation exposure of the U.S. population from all sources. The next largest contributor to population exposure was background radiation, mainly from radon gas. The relative level of background radiation varies with geographic location. For

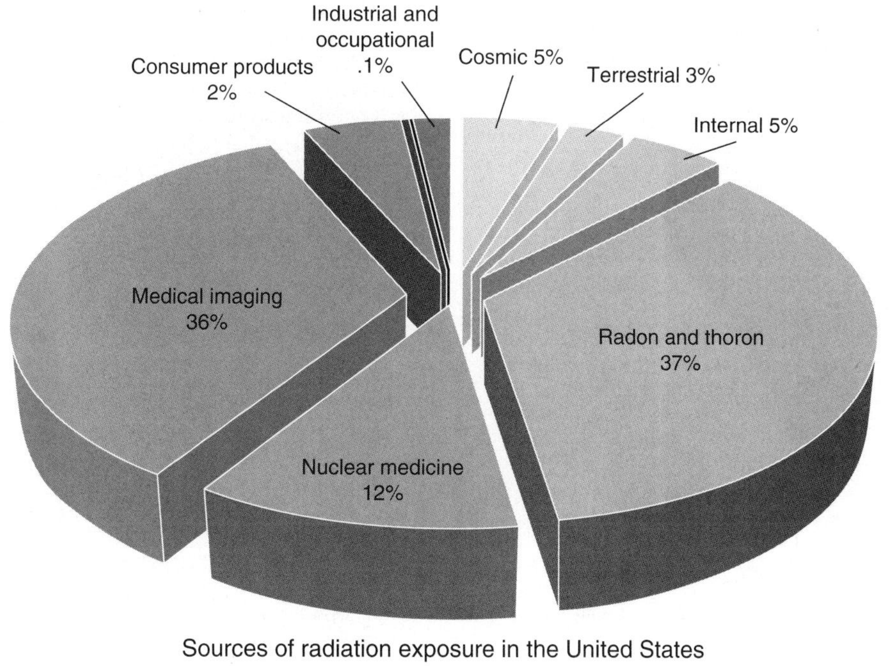

Fig. 1.7 An estimate of sources of exposure dose from ionizing radiation in the United States. (With permission of the National Council on Radiation Protection and Measurements, http://NCRPonline.org.)

example, exposure to cosmic radiation increases at higher elevations, and household radon exposure is greater in the eastern United States. In general, these types of radiation exposures are not considered harmful, providing the use of medical imaging is monitored. The United States Environmental Protection Agency (EPA) provides a calculator that allows estimation of your yearly dose from the most significant sources of ionizing radiation.[††]

Practical Considerations

Technologists assuming the role of radiation workers in veterinary practices must be aware of the risks of radiation. They should be trained in patient positioning for radiography and should be proficient in equipment operation. Technologists should be instructed on the proper use and care of PPE such as lead-impregnated aprons and gloves, and how to adhere to the ALARA (**a**s **l**ow **a**s **r**easonably **a**chievable) principle.[12] The variables used in adhering to ALARA are distance, time, and shielding.

Distance

The distance between personnel in the room and the x-ray tube should be as great as possible because distance is one of the most effective ways of reducing dose. Exposure dose does not change linearly with distance but is dependent on the square of the distance. For example, doubling the distance reduces exposure by a factor of 4, not by a factor of 2. Holding cassettes by hand for equine radiography is discouraged because this can place the employee in the primary beam. Handholding of portable x-ray machines for radiography of the equine distal limb is safe, as long as the machine is adequately shielded.[13] Handholding of companion animals for radiography is permissible, but body parts should be as far from the primary x-ray beam as possible and no part of the body should ever be in the primary beam, regardless of whether protective aprons and gloves are used. With the use of chemical restraint, tape, and sandbags for positioning, it is often possible for the technologist to exit the room during the exposure. Some state veterinary practice acts stipulate that the technologist cannot be in the room during the exposure.

Effective use of beam collimation is another component of distance as this further increases the distance of the technologist from the primary x-ray beam, and also reduces scattered radiation. However, failure to properly collimate the primary x-ray beam is a major error in veterinary radiology. Digital software also allows the visibility of unprotected hands in an image to be cropped out of view (Fig. 1.8).

Time

Time is directly related to the number of images created. Time can be minimized by using sedation or anesthesia for uncooperative patients, or for complicated examinations such as spine or skull studies. Rotation of the technical staff through the radiology service will also dilute any exposure over a larger pool, leading to reduction in individual exposure levels.

Retake examinations also increase personnel dose, and these have likely increased with the increase in digital imaging as retakes are less labor intensive.

Shielding

State building codes require structural shielding to protect personnel and the general public, such as clients in the waiting or examination rooms, from unnecessary radiation exposure. The specific details regarding requisite structural shielding can be obtained from the state radiation protection office.

The most effective PPE for radiation workers is lead-impregnated aprons, gloves, thyroid shields, and eyeglasses. Protective aprons and gloves designed for use in the x-ray room are usually 0.5 mm Pb equivalent. Unfortunately, this equipment is not used consistently. When apron and glove use was monitored in a university setting with video cameras, gloves were used properly in only 46.3% of the studies and leaded eyeglasses were worn only 1.7% of the time.[14] PPE use was also

[††] https://www.epa.gov/radiation/calculate-your-radiation-dose

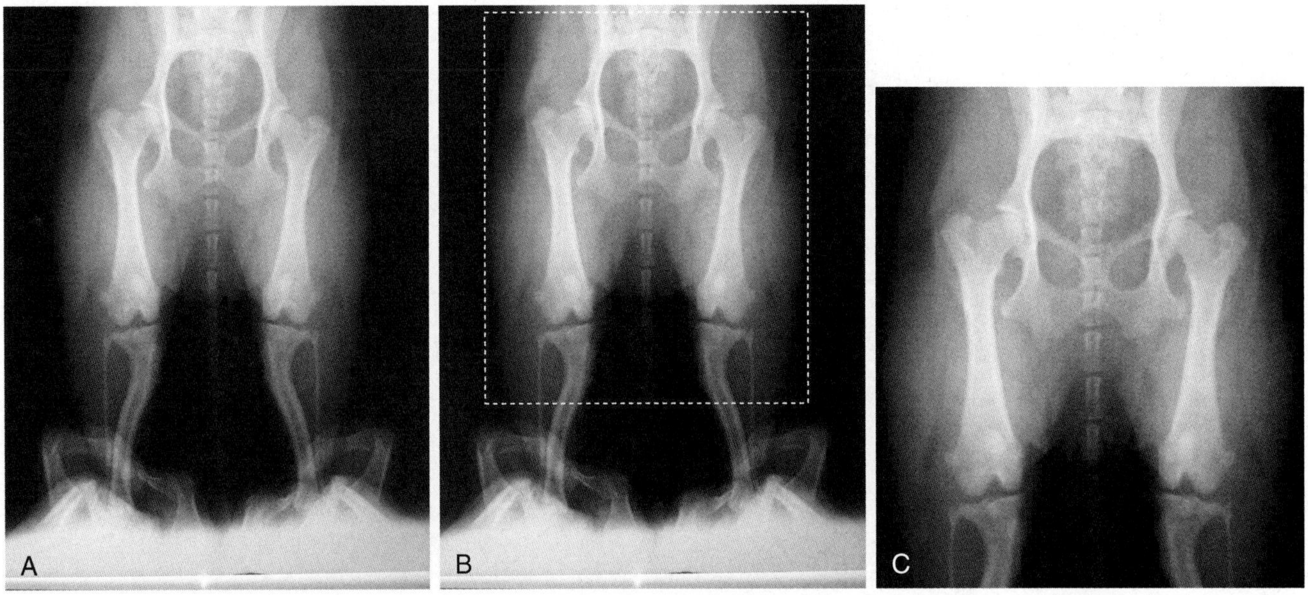

Fig. 1.8 **A,** Ventrodorsal view of a canine pelvis with worker's ungloved hand holding patient's pelvic limbs. **B,** *Dashed line* shows application of software cropping tool. **C,** Cropped image is ready to send to workstation. Daily repetition of this hazardous practice leads to continued overexposure of the hands and wrists, increasing the risk for squamous cell or basal cell carcinomas.

found to be deficient in equine practice.[15] Although not documented, glove use is almost certainly inadequate in private small animal practice (Fig. 1.9A; see Fig. 1.4).

More commonly, when lead gloves are not used, the technologist attempts to keep the unshielded hands outside of the primary beam, thinking that the collimator eliminates radiation exposure in this area. This is not true. There is always enough scattered radiation outside the primary beam to capture an image of parts of the patient or technologist in that area, and this also leads to unnecessary personnel exposure (see Fig. 1.9B). Additionally, the hand will frequently end up in the periphery of the primary beam, leading to even higher exposure. In fact, in Fig. 1.9B the tip of a finger (white arrowhead) is in the edge of the primary beam, but the fingertip is not visible because of overexposure.

Another common mistake is the belief that because lead aprons and gloves are very heavy, they can be used to shield body parts within the primary beam (see Fig. 1.9A). This is also not true. Lead aprons and gloves are designed solely for protecting against scattered radiation and must never be placed in the primary beam because they do not entirely attenuate the x-ray beam. Covering a hand in the primary x-ray beam with an apron or glove is not adequate protection, and the hand will receive unnecessary, excessive radiation (see Fig. 1.9C). The effects of scattered photons from the floor of the x-ray room, or x-ray table, are also usually ignored, but these are important sources of scattered radiation (see Fig. 1.9D). Lastly, radiation protection mittens with a slit in the palm are available. Extending the fingers through the slit facilitates positioning but reduces the amount of overlying protective lead material and leads to excessive extremity dose whether the hand receives primary or secondary radiation.

Aprons and gloves should be placed on racks when not in use. This decreases the risk of creasing and folding that lead to cracking or separation of the protective lead layering. Use of a glove rack also facilitates the evaporation of perspiration that reduces odor. Aprons and gloves should be inspected visually on an annual basis, and any portion that appears physically damaged should be evaluated radiographically for evidence of a crack.

Radiation Supervisor

Identifying a member of the technical staff as a radiation supervisor will optimize the quality of images produced and minimize occupational radiation dose. Having a dedicated radiation protection supervisor provides the technologist with ownership in the process, which will increase quality. The continuity of supervision will contribute to a steady stream of high-quality images and low personnel exposure readings.

The following are some reasonable responsibilities of a radiation supervisor:

- Establish and supervise the implementation of written operating procedures for all employees involved with radiography.
- Periodically review procedures to ensure conformity with local regulations.
- Instruct all personnel in proper radiation protection practices and in efficient and safe equipment operation.
- Oversee conduction of required radiation surveys and keep records of such surveys and tests, including summaries of corrective measures recommended or instituted.
- Routinely observe and periodically test interlock switches and warning signals.
- Ensure that warning signs and signals are properly located.
- Ensure that all equipment is maintained in top-notch working order. Perform annual evaluation of radiation protection equipment.
- Determine the cause of each known or suspected case of excessive abnormal exposure and take steps to prevent its recurrence.
- Train staff in proper radiographic positioning and restraint procedures.
- Radiation safety seminars should be held on a yearly basis to ensure compliance and to educate new personnel.

Personnel Dose Monitoring

Personnel dose monitoring is used to check the adequacy of the radiation safety program, disclose improper radiation protection practices, and detect potentially serious radiation exposure situations. A radiation dosimetry badge is the most commonly used personnel monitoring device. A radiation badge consists of

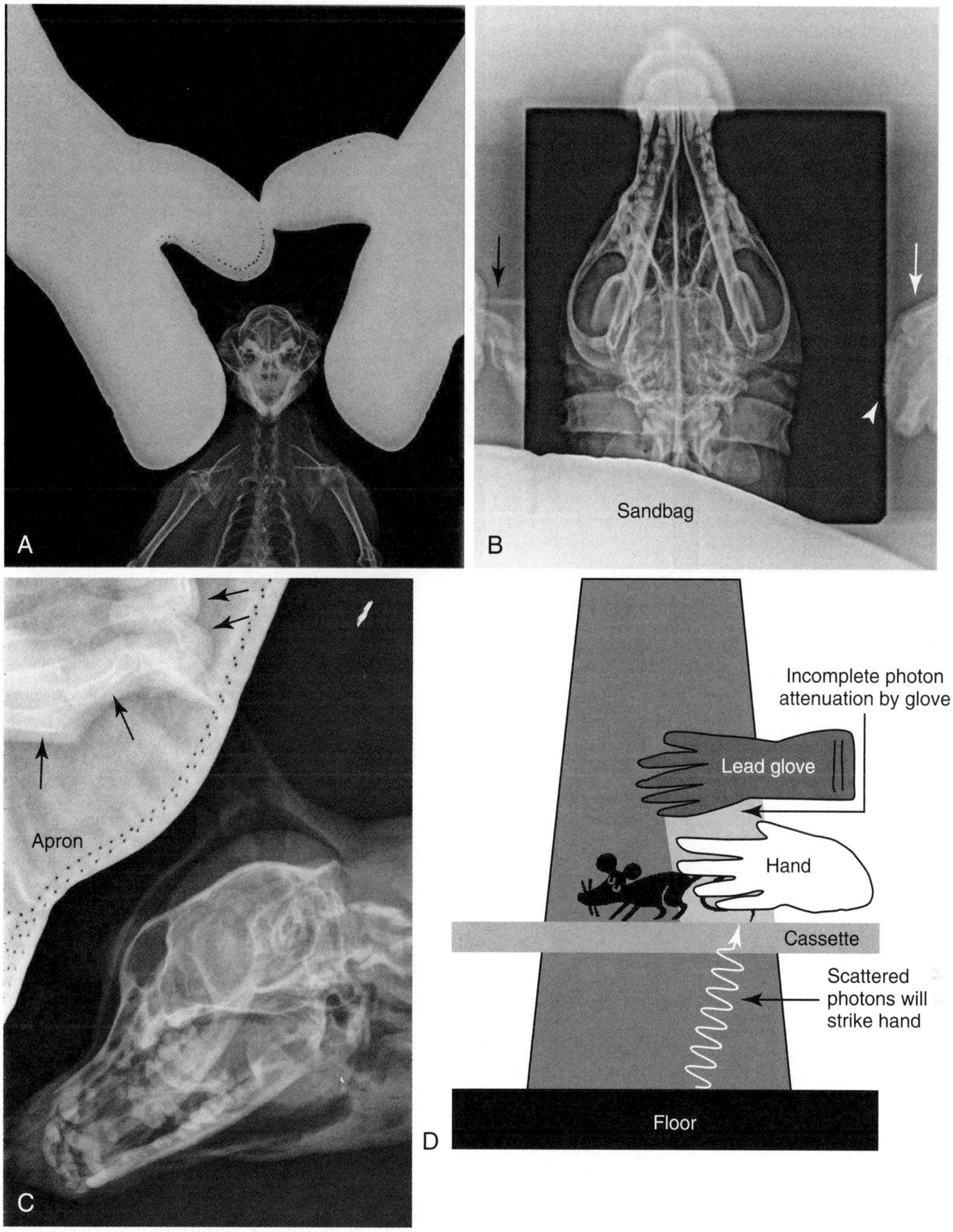

Fig. 1.9 Examples of poor radiation safety practice. **A,** Hands were placed in the primary beam to position this small patient. Although gloves were used, they are not adequate for shielding against the primary x-ray beam and the hands will receive an unacceptable dose. **B,** Dorsoventral skull radiograph of a dog. A sandbag is being used to secure the neck. The technologist is not wearing lead gloves and has grasped the ears of the dog, which are outside of the primary beam, to keep the head in the proper position. The dog's right ear can be seen (*black arrow*). On the left side, the technologist's fingers can also be seen (*white arrow*), because of exposure from radiation outside of the primary beam. The tip of a finger is also in the primary beam (*white arrowhead*). A portion of the technologist's hand can also be seen on the dog's right side, peripheral to the dog's ear but not to the extent that it is identifiable as a hand. The most rostral portion of the dog's nose is also visible outside of the primary beam. **C,** A lateral radiograph of a canine skull was being made. The technologist held the ears in the primary beam with an unprotected hand and then covered their hand with a lead apron, thinking the apron would attenuate the x-rays. It did not. The bones in the technologist's hand are clearly visible (*black arrows*) because of x-rays penetrating the apron. **D,** A small patient is being restrained by an unprotected hand but a lead glove is placed on top of the hand, similar to the situation illustrated in part **C** of this figure. As already stated, this is ineffective because many of the oncoming high-energy photons will penetrate the glove and strike the hand. Also, photons penetrating the cassette and table will strike the floor and be scattered back, also striking the hand. Radiation backscatter is also a reason that the technologist should not sit on the edge of the x-ray table while restraining a patient for radiography. In that instance the scattered photons are going to strike a body part or parts that are more revered than a hand.

a plastic holder, measuring approximately 2 to 3 cm on a side, which has a clip allowing it to be secured to clothing. Modern radiation badges contain either radiation-sensitive aluminum oxide or lithium fluoride crystals. These compounds trap electrons energized by oncoming radiation, and the number of trapped electrons can be quantified and related to the amount of exposure. Radiation badges should be analyzed at least quarterly, but a monthly analysis is preferable so that exposure problems are detected sooner. Badges for declared pregnant workers should be analyzed monthly.

Personnel dose monitoring should be performed in controlled areas for each occupationally exposed individual who has a reasonable possibility of receiving a dose exceeding 10% of the applicable MPD. The radiation badge must be worn only in the workplace and never when the person is exposed to ionizing radiation as part of his or her own medical or dental examinations. The badge is intended to monitor occupational radiation exposure and not medical exposure. If the badge is worn outside of the workplace erroneous readings can result. The radiation badge should be worn on the upper or lower torso. When a protective apron is worn, the radiation badge should be on the outside of the apron for monitoring the radiation environment, but a second radiation badge may also be worn inside the apron when an estimate of body exposure is desired. Anyone occupationally exposed to radiation should have their own badge and radiation badges should never be shared.

Basic Radiation Safety Rules for Diagnostic Radiology

The basic radiation safety rules for diagnostic radiology are:

- Only personnel necessary to complete the procedure should be in the x-ray room at the time of exposure.
- Persons younger than 18 years and pregnant women must not be in the x-ray room during the examination.
- Personnel who assist with radiographic examinations should have a rotating duty roster to minimize exposure to any one person.
- Sandbags, sponges, tape, or other restraining devices should be used for positioning the patient rather than manual restraint.
- Anesthesia or sedation should be used, when possible, to facilitate patient restraint.
- No part of the technologist should be in the primary beam, whether or not protected by gloves or aprons.
- Protective aprons should always be worn when positioning an animal.
- Protective gloves should be worn if hands are near the primary beam.
- Protective glasses should be worn if the work level is heavy or when radiographing large animals. These glasses provide 0.25 mm Pb equivalent protection to the lens.
- Thyroid shields should always be worn. These are "mini-aprons" that are worn around the neck to protect the thyroid gland.
- The primary beam should be collimated so each image has an unexposed border, proving that the primary beam does not exceed the size of the cassette or imaging plate.
- All personnel involved with patient radiography should wear a radiation badge during working hours.
- The radiographic procedure should be planned carefully, and the machine settings double-checked prior to exposure.

PRODUCTION OF X-RAYS

X-rays are produced when high-speed electrons strike metal. For radiography, this occurs in the controlled environment of

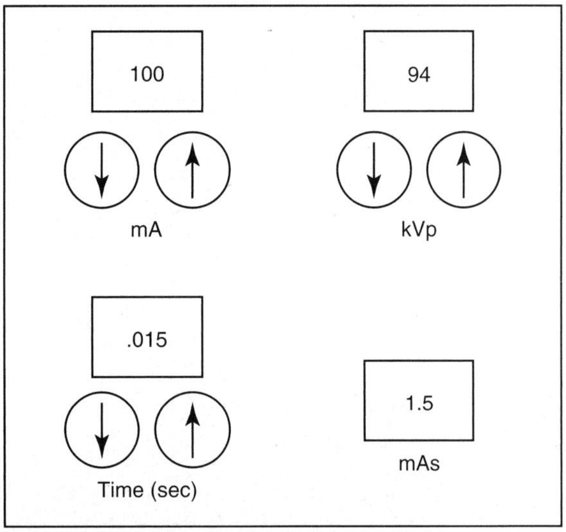

Fig. 1.10 Typical x-ray machine control panel. The time (in seconds), the mA (milliamperes), and the kVp (in kilovolts) are indicated by digital displays and are adjustable individually. As mA and/or time change, the resulting mAs is calculated and displayed automatically.

an x-ray tube. An x-ray tube contains a positively charged target, the anode, and a negatively charged filament, the cathode, within a glass envelope. X-ray tubes provide for acceleration of electrons from their source at the filament to the metal target where x-rays are produced. To create a source of electrons, electric current is passed through the x-ray tube filament raising its temperature in much the same way that an electric current is used to heat the filament of an incandescent lightbulb. The heating allows electrons to "boil" off the surface of the filament, forming a cloud of free, negatively charged, electrons. The number of electrons in the cloud is directly related to the amount of electric current passing through the filament, which is regulated by the milliamperage (mA) control on the x-ray machine control panel (Fig. 1.10). Increasing the mA is analogous to increasing the wattage of a lightbulb. A 100 W bulb has a hotter filament and emits more light rays instantaneously than does a 60 W bulb because more current flows through the filament of a 100 W bulb.

Electrons produced at the filament are accelerated to the metallic target by applying a voltage differential between the filament and target. As electrons are negatively charged, they will be attracted to the target when the target is positively charged with respect to the filament (opposite charges attract). The energy of the x-rays produced is dependent on the energy of the electrons striking the target. The voltage difference between the filament and target is adjusted with the kilovoltage peak (kVp) control on the x-ray machine control panel (see Fig. 1.10). Increasing kVp increases the voltage difference between the filament and target, and electrons are accelerated to higher velocities and have more kinetic energy when striking the target (Fig. 1.11). Higher energy electrons can produce higher energy x-rays.

X-rays are produced by two mechanisms when electrons strike the target: collisional and radiative interactions. Collisional interactions occur when the oncoming electron hits an orbital electron and ejects it from the target atom. Energy is subsequently released as an x-ray (Fig. 1.12). The energy required to eject an orbital electron is specific to the atom and the shell the orbital electron resides in, and this is called the *binding energy*. Because the binding energy is specific, the x-rays produced by collisional interactions also have specific energies and are termed *characteristic x-rays*—a unique characteristic of the atom, the shell from which they are ejected, and the source of electron that fills the shell vacancy. X-rays created by collisional interactions account for only a small fraction of the total number of x-rays produced in a diagnostic x-ray tube.

In a radiative interaction (Fig. 1.13), the oncoming electron passes close to the nucleus of the tungsten target atom, attracted by the opposite charge. The oncoming electron does not hit or eject another electron or interact with the target atom in any way, but instead the oncoming electron slows (brakes) as it bends around the nucleus and releases energy in the form of an x-ray. The nucleus of the tungsten atom has a high positive charge due to the presence of 74 positively charged protons. The much smaller electron, with a charge of only −1, is therefore attracted strongly to the nucleus causing the electron to decelerate, or "brake." X-rays generated by a radiative interaction are called *bremsstrahlung* (from the German, translated as *braking radiation*). Braking radiation has a broad spectrum of energies, depending on the energy of the oncoming electron and how much it slows as it bends around the nucleus. The closer to the nucleus the electron travels, the more it curves, the slower it becomes, the more energy it loses, and the more energetic the x-ray produced. Most oncoming electrons undergo multiple braking interactions with the target atoms, and thus a single electron can lead to the production of multiple braking x-rays.

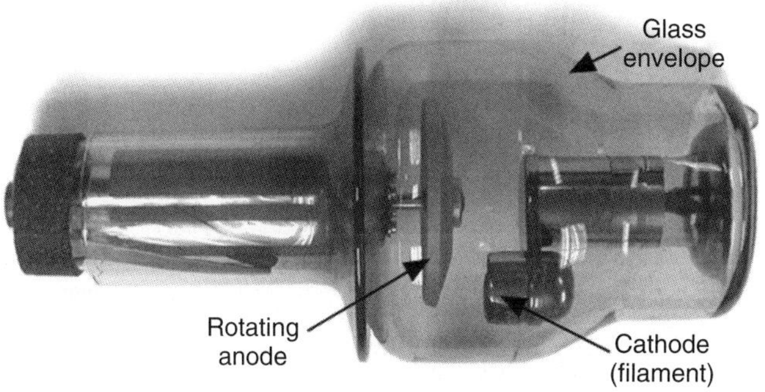

Fig. 1.11 Photograph of an x-ray tube with a rotating anode. The target (anode) rotates at high speed, dissipating heat over a large surface area. Electrons emanate from the filament (cathode). The x-ray tube is encased in a glass envelope from which air has been evacuated. This vacuum prevents electrons from interacting with air molecules when the electrons are accelerated to the target. In the x-ray machine, the x-ray tube is encased in a steel cylinder to control the direction in which x-rays are emitted. (Courtesy of Oak Ridge Associated Universities.)

Collisional and radiative processes both contribute to the overall energy spectrum of an x-ray beam (Fig. 1.14), but most x-rays arise from radiative processes. The most energetic x-ray possible in the spectrum will have an energy, in kiloelectron volts (keV), equal to the kVp that was set at the control panel. For a photon to have this maximal energy, an electron must be accelerated from the filament at maximal velocity. This occurs when the voltage between the target and filament is at its maximum (the pattern of voltage fluctuation in the x-ray tube is discussed in the next paragraph). This electron must then lose all of its energy in one radiative interaction. The number of x-ray photons in the spectrum with energy equal to the kVp is very small (see Fig. 1.10). The additional x-rays coming from collisional interactions have specific energies and therefore create peaks at specific points on the curve (see Fig. 1.14).

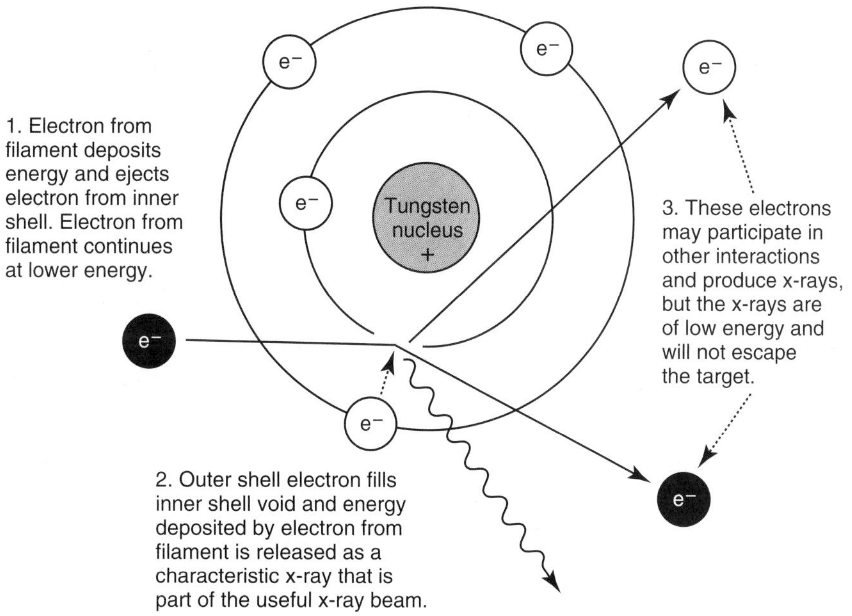

Fig. 1.12 The collisional method of x-ray production. An electron from the filament (shown here in *black* for illustrative purposes) strikes a tungsten atom in the target after being accelerated to high speed through a voltage difference. The oncoming electron deposits energy and ejects an inner shell electron from the target atom. The electron from the filament continues at a different angle, with reduced energy. Atoms with vacancies in electron shells are unstable, and the vacancy is quickly filled by a more peripheral electron. When the electron shell vacancy is filled, the energy deposited by the electron from the filament required to eject the target electron, called the binding energy, is released in the form of a *characteristic* x-ray. The electron ejected from the inner shell and the electron from the filament may continue on and be involved in other interactions and produce additional x-rays, but these x-rays are of low energy and usually do not escape the target. The relative size of the nucleus, electrons, and orbital shells is not to scale. The "+" symbol in the nucleus designates the normal nuclear positivity created by the presence of positively charged protons.

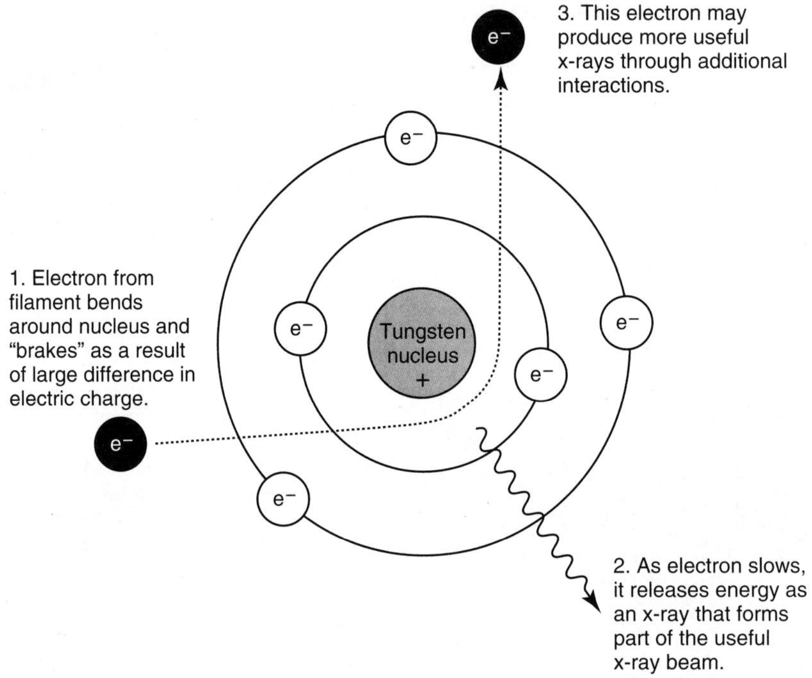

Fig. 1.13 The radiative, or braking, model of x-ray production. An electron from the filament (shown here in *black* for illustrative purposes) changes direction as it nears the nucleus because of the attraction of differing charges. The deflected electron decelerates (brakes) and releases energy in the form of an x-ray. As the deflected electron may pass within various distances of the nucleus, braking radiation has a spectrum of energies. The deflected electron may be involved with additional interactions and produce additional x-rays that contribute to the useful x-ray beam. The relative size of the nucleus, electrons, and orbital shells is not to scale. The "+" symbol in the nucleus designates the normal nuclear positivity created by the presence of positively charged protons.

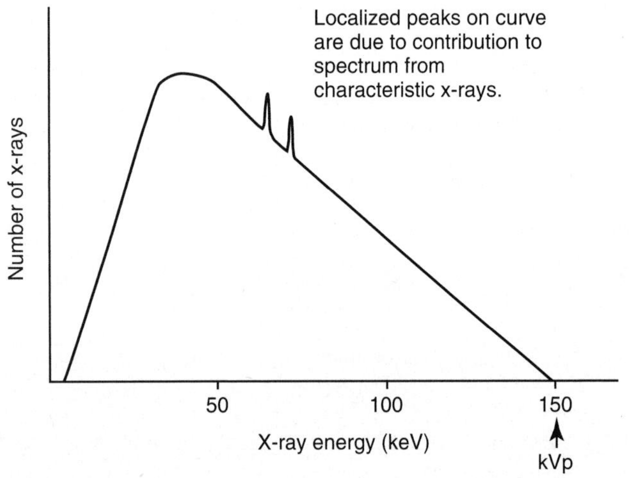

Fig. 1.14 The spectrum of x-ray energies produced by braking and characteristic radiation. The maximum x-ray energy achievable is equal to the kVp (kVp = 150 in this example). For this to occur, an electron must be accelerated at the time when the voltage differential between the filament and target is at the maximum value and then the electron must lose all of its energy in one interaction at the target. As illustrated, the number of x-rays with energy equal to the kVp is very small.

It is important to understand the difference between kVp and keV.[‡‡] The kVp is the maximum voltage applied across the target-filament gap. In the United States, electric current is alternating at 60 Hz (60 cycles per second). Current coming into the x-ray machine is either at 120V or 240V, but this is increased to the selected kVp in a transformer. At a kVp of 80 for example, the 120V or 240V current is increased to 80,000V. The alternating nature of the incoming current results in the voltage difference between the filament and target fluctuating between +kVp and −kVp every 1/60 of a second unless the waveform of the current is modified (Fig. 1.15). The kilo-electron volt (keV), on the other hand, is a unit of energy that describes the energy of either electrons or photons. If the kVp is 100 (100,000V maximum voltage difference between the target and filament), electrons traveling from filament to the target have energies equal to or less than 100 keV (100,000 eV). There are very few electrons having an energy of 100 keV because of the fluctuating nature of the voltage differential as shown in Fig. 1.15; the voltage differential is at the peak value of 100,000V for only an instant in each cycle. So, if an electron is accelerated exactly when the voltage difference between the filament and target is 100,000V, the electron will have, by definition, an energy of 100 keV. If this electron loses all its energy in one single radiative (bremsstrahlung) event, the x-ray created will also have an energy of 100 keV, the same energy as the kVp in the x-ray tube. However, this is very uncommon. Most electrons are accelerated at a voltage lower than the kVp, and most also do not lose all their energy in one braking reaction. This is what leads to the wide spectrum of energies of x-rays present in beam (see Fig. 1.14).

If alternating current (AC) (see Fig. 1.15, *top panel*) is used for x-ray production, the target is positive with respect to the filament only 50% of the time. During the other 50%, the target would be negative with respect to the filament and any free electrons at the surface of the target that might be present because of the high temperature of the target would be attracted to the filament and damage it. To avoid this, the negative phase of the AC is eliminated by a process called *rectification* (see Fig. 1.15, *second* and *third panels*). An in-depth discussion of rectification is beyond the scope of this

[‡‡] An electron volt (eV) is the amount of energy an electron gains as it is accelerated by a potential difference of 1V. 1 keV = 1000 eV.

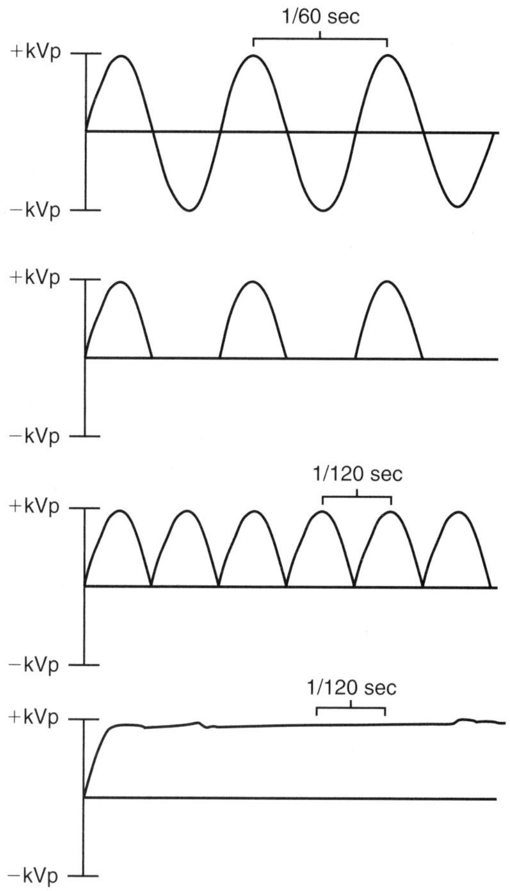

Fig. 1.15 The concept of rectification and the ripple factor. The *upper panel* shows the typical waveform of alternating current in the United States. One complete cycle occurs each 1/60 sec. If this current were used to apply the kVp in the x-ray tube, the target would be positive with respect to the filament, which is desired, only 50% of the time. The other 50% of the time, the filament would be positive with respect to the target. This is a waste of time because electrons are not attracted to the target to produce x-rays when the filament is positive. Also, any free electrons at the target created by heat buildup would travel to the filament, causing damage. The *second panel* illustrates the waveform obtained when current is not allowed to flow during the negative phase of the cycle; this is termed *half-wave rectification*. In this instance, the filament is never positive with respect to the target, but half of each cycle is wasted. Fortunately, there are electronic methods to reverse the polarity of current flow in the negative portion of the cycle leading to the waveform shown in the *third panel*. This is called *full-wave rectification* and results in one useful pulse of current every 1/120 sec. This increases the efficiency of x-ray production by 100%. Now, with what is termed a *high-frequency generator,* electronic circuitry is used to convert alternating current to nearly direct current with little voltage fluctuation during the cycle. The waveform of this current is shown in the *bottom panel*. The target is always positive with respect to the filament and the voltage difference between the filament and target approximates the kVp at all times. Thus, the voltage fluctuation, or the ripple factor, is the lowest with current from a high-frequency generator, and this increases the efficiency of x-ray production significantly.

chapter. What must be understood here is that rectification results in the target always being positive with respect to the filament, despite the use of AC. Thus, electrons travel only from the filament to the target.

X-ray production is a very inefficient process with more than 90% of the energy of the electrons striking the target being converted to heat, not x-rays. Therefore, the target becomes very hot and must be constructed of material with a high melting point. Targets are often made of tungsten, which has a melting point of 3422° C (6192° F). Even with this high melting point, the target in high-output x-ray tubes is designed to rotate

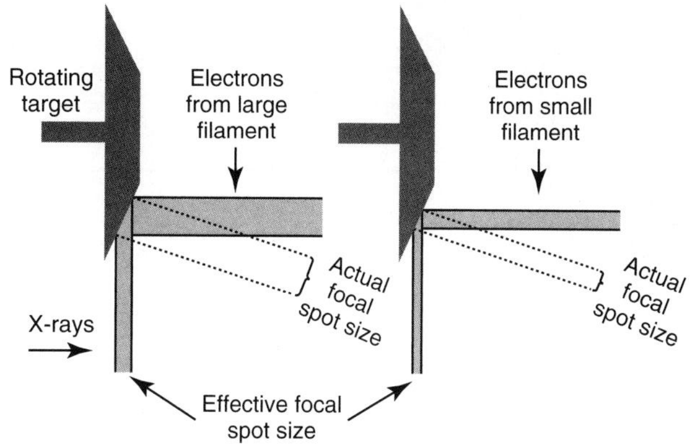

Fig. 1.16 Illustration of the principle of effective focal spot size in an x-ray tube. By angling the edge of the rotating anode, the size of the focal spot from the perspective of the patient appears smaller than it actually is. This facilitates heat distribution. On the *left*, the electrons have emanated from the large filament in the x-ray tube. Although the size of the effective focal spot is reduced compared to the size of the electron stream, the effective focal spot can be reduced even further to improve radiographic detail, as shown on the *right*, by having the electrons emanate from a smaller filament.

to increase the surface area struck by the oncoming electrons. Rotation of the target prevents the target from melting or becoming "pitted," as would happen if electrons struck the same region of a stationary target continually. Tungsten also has a high atomic number (74), which increases the efficiency of x-ray production. The high positive charge of the nucleus of tungsten target atoms leads to more effective braking and bending of electrons from the filament that pass nearby.

The focal spot is the location on the target struck by electrons and is the site of x-ray production. The smaller the focal spot, the better the detail on the radiograph. A practical example of this principle is the sharpness of a shadow cast by a small versus a large light source. A shadow of an object cast by a small light source will be sharper than the shadow cast by a large light source. Therefore, radiographs produced using a small focal spot will have more detail than radiographs produced with a large focal spot. Angling the target is one way to make the focal spot function as being smaller than it really is, creating a small *effective* focal spot, while at the same time maintaining a larger area being struck by electrons to facilitate heat distribution (Fig. 1.16).

Some x-ray tubes have two filaments of different sizes, allowing the technologist to select the size of the filament from which the electrons originate. A smaller filament leads to a smaller effective focal spot. This is illustrated in the right side of Fig. 1.16, where the width of the electron path from the filament has been reduced by 50% by using a smaller filament. As a result, the size of the effective focal spot is also reduced. Reducing focal spot size is useful theoretically when enhanced image detail is necessary, as for radiographing a small bird or reptile. A disadvantage of using the small filament is that higher mA values are not allowed by the electronics, which prevents the filament from overheating and burning out or melting.

As already stated, the number of electrons, and thus the number of x-rays, produced is directly related to the mA setting on the x-ray machine control panel. The number of x-rays produced can also be controlled by the length of time that current is allowed to pass through the filament. The timer on the x-ray machine panel (see Fig. 1.10) controls the length of time current is applied to the filament and is also the time that voltage is applied across the gap between the filament and target of the x-ray tube. X-rays are produced only when a source of electrons and a voltage differential are present across the filament-target gap.

Table • 1.4

Sample of mA and Time Combinations That Result in 5 mAs.

mA	TIME (sec)	mAs
50	0.1	5
100	0.05	5
500	0.01	5
1000	0.005	5

The milliampere second (mAs) is the unit that quantifies the amount of radiation produced and is analogous to leaving a 60 W lightbulb burning twice as long as a 120 W lightbulb. In both instances, the total number of light rays emitted would be roughly the same, although the intensity at any one time would be twice as great for the 120-W bulb. The mAs is the product of mA and time in seconds. A variety of combinations of milliamperage and time can be used to produce the same mAs value and thus the same number of x-rays (Table 1.4).

The x-ray tube is one of the two major components of the x-ray machine, the other being the x-ray generator. The generator has a high-voltage circuit that increases the voltage of the incoming current to provide the large potential voltage difference between the filament and target. The generator also has a low-voltage circuit to provide current to heat the filament. The generator contains a timer to control the time that the filament is hot and the time that the voltage difference is applied between the filament and the target, that is, the *exposure time*. Finally, the generator configures the nature of the cyclic current used in the high-voltage circuit. As already mentioned, one manipulation that is done to increase the efficiency of x-ray production is to reverse the polarity of the negative phase of the 60 Hz AC so that the target is always positive with respect to the filament—that is, full-wave rectification (see Fig. 1.15, *third panel*). This increases the efficiency of x-ray production, but there is still a large amount of time during each phase of the cycle when the voltage is relatively low; in fact, the voltage is at zero every 1/120 second (see Fig. 1.15, *third panel*). Therefore, if the cyclic nature of each cycle could be minimized, there is great opportunity to increase the efficiency of x-ray production. For example, one type of x-ray generator uses a three-phase AC line source (e.g., three voltage sources).[16] Through rectification and staggering of each AC pulse over a 120-degree AC cycle, 2 pulses for each line are produced. Therefore, six electrical pulses are produced over one AC cycle. Despite this improvement, these six pulse generators have largely been replaced by high-frequency generators.

High-frequency generators are the state-of-the-art power source for x-ray tubes. These generators produce nearly constant voltage output (see Fig. 1.15, *bottom panel*). The elimination of the valleys of the voltage waveform increases the efficiency of x-ray output significantly. In a direct comparison of a conventional generator with a high-frequency generator, the high-frequency generator was approximately two times more efficient with a better reproducibility.[17] High-frequency generators are compact, relatively inexpensive, and easily maintained. Therefore, they are the most desired type of x-ray generator and are commonly used in x-ray machines that are manufactured for permanent installation in veterinary practices. Portable units used in the field have voltage waveforms more typical of that shown in the second or third panels of Fig. 1.15. Although conventional generators can be used with digital radiography platforms, high frequency x-ray generators are preferred.

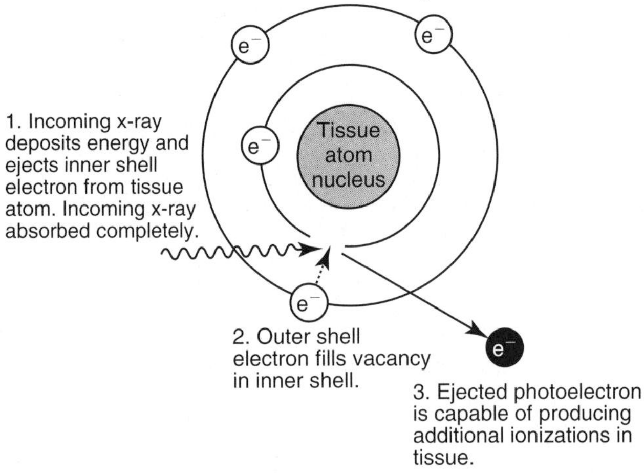

Fig. 1.17 The photoelectric absorption process. An x-ray from the x-ray tube ejects a tissue electron, usually from an inner shell (K shell) of a tissue atom. The incoming x-ray is absorbed completely. The ejected electron, the photoelectron, has sufficient energy to create additional ionizations in tissue but does not contribute in any way to image formation.

INTERACTION OF RADIATION WITH MATTER

To understand how radiographs are produced, it is necessary to understand how photons interact with matter. Photons can interact with matter in one of five possible mechanisms: (1) coherent scattering, (2) photoelectric effect, (3) Compton scattering, (4) pair production, and (5) photodisintegration. Pair production and photodisintegration have no relevance to diagnostic radiology and are not discussed. A basic description of coherent, photoelectric, and Compton processes is given herein; sources for more detailed reading are available.[16]

Coherent Scattering

A photon interacts with an object and the direction of the photon is changed, but the object does not absorb the photon, and the energy of the photon does not change. The fraction of x-rays striking a patient that undergoes coherent scattering is small, approximately 5%. Not only is coherent scattering not useful in the production of the radiograph, but also it is disadvantageous because the scattered photons may strike the x-ray film and degrade image quality, or they may strike the technologist and increase personnel exposure.

Photoelectric Effect

The photoelectric effect is the most important type of radiation interaction with reference to producing a radiograph; this is what results in formation of an image. In a photoelectric interaction, the x-ray striking the patient is absorbed completely (Fig. 1.17), and therefore there are no scattered x-rays to contend with. The complete absorption of the oncoming x-ray leads to reduced exposure of the film or imaging plate under that part of the patient. The absorbed x-ray photon ejects an electron, called a ***photoelectron***, from an inner shell of a tissue atom. The photoelectron is eventually absorbed in the patient.

When the vacancy created by ejection of the photoelectron is filled by a peripheral shell electron, a characteristic x-ray is given off.[§§] The energy of characteristic radiation is a function of the atomic number of the atom from which it arises. Because tissue atoms have a low effective atomic number, the energy of characteristic x-rays produced in tissue is very low, and they are

[§§] This is similar in principle to the characteristic x-ray given off in the target of an x-ray tube when the oncoming electron from the filament creates a vacancy in a target atom.

absorbed locally where they contribute to the absorbed dose in the patient being radiographed, but not to production of the radiographic image. This low-energy characteristic x-ray production is not shown in Fig. 1.17.

The probability of a photoelectric interaction increases proportionally to the third power of the atomic number (proportional to Z^3) and decreases proportionally to the third power of the photon energy (proportional to $1/E^3$). The third-power relationship between the photoelectric process and atomic number is very important because it amplifies differences in absorption between various tissues, such as bone versus soft tissue and soft tissue versus fat. If it were not for the third-power atomic number dependence of the photoelectric effect, there would be insufficient differential absorption of x-rays between tissues for the image to have any contrast. That is, all tissues would be of similar radiographic opacity and the radiograph would be useless. The complete absorption of the x-ray in the photoelectric effect, rather than having a scattered photon, is also advantageous because there are no scattered photons to result in fogging of the x-ray film and increased personnel exposure.

The photoelectric effect occurring in the patient should not be confused with collisional x-ray production in the x-ray tube. A characteristic x-ray is produced in both instances because an electron is ejected from an atom in each process, and the void created by the ejected electron being filled by another electron leads to characteristic x-ray production. However, in the photoelectric effect, a photon from the target ejects an electron from an atom in tissue, while in collisional x-ray production, it is a high-energy electron from the filament that ejects the electron from an atom in the target of the x-ray tube. When the vacancy created by the electron ejection is filled, a characteristic x-ray is emitted in both processes. In the case of the photoelectric effect, this x-ray has very low energy because of the low binding energy of inner shell electrons in tissue versus x-ray production where the characteristic x-ray is of much higher energy because of the much higher inner shell binding energy of elections in tungsten, the target material in an x-ray tube.

Compton Scattering

All significant scattered radiation encountered in diagnostic radiology results from Compton scattering. In Compton scattering, an incoming x-ray photon interacts with a peripheral shell electron of a tissue atom. The peripheral shell electron is ejected, and the original photon is scattered at a different angle and at a lower energy (Fig. 1.18). The scattered electron is called either a *Compton electron* or a *recoil electron*. The probability of a Compton reaction is independent of atomic number and depends mainly on the physical density (grams per cubic centimeter) of the tissue. The probability of a Compton interaction increases with increasing photon energy and then decreases at photon energies over 1.02 megaelectron volt (MeV). The independence of Compton scattering on atomic number is disadvantageous with reference to producing a radiograph because all tissues tend to absorb x-rays similarly. For example, the atomic number dependence of photoelectric absorption results in great differences in absorption between tissues such as bone and muscle, and thus good tissue contrast. With Compton absorption being independent of atomic number, differential absorption by different tissue types is diminished, and image contrast is reduced. Thus, if the Compton absorption predominates, the image will have very poor contrast. In good radiographic technique, x-ray beams have an energy in which photoelectric absorption predominates. This maximizes differential x-ray absorption between tissues and image contrast. The photon scattering that occurs with Compton interactions is also disadvantageous because the scattered photons are radiation safety considerations for technologists, and they also degrade the image by producing fog.

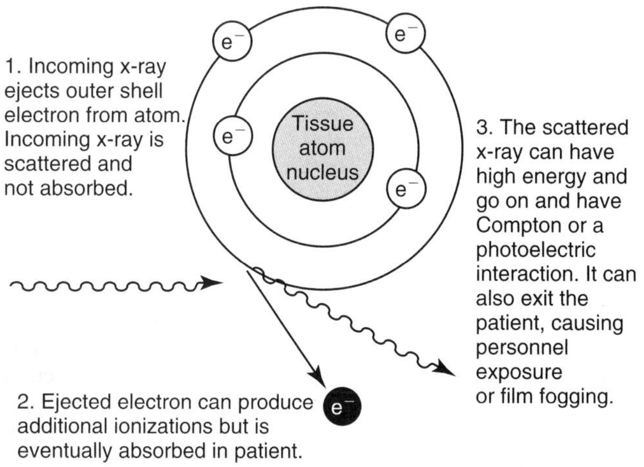

Fig. 1.18 The Compton absorption process. An x-ray produced in the x-ray tube ejects an electron, usually from an outer shell, of a tissue atom. The incoming photon is scattered at an angle and with lower energy but is not absorbed as in the photoelectric process. The energy of the scattered photon is always lower than that of the original photon. The ejected electron and scattered photon may produce additional ionizations and the scattered photon may exit the patient and fog the film or strike personnel.

BASIC CONCEPT OF MAKING A RADIOGRAPH

To make a radiograph, the patient is placed between the x-ray tube and the film cassette or imaging plate (Fig. 1.19). As noted earlier, x-rays produced in a diagnostic x-ray tube have a broad spectrum of energies. Very low-energy x-rays serve no useful purpose because they are all absorbed by the patient and make no useful contribution to the image. Therefore, filters are placed in the x-ray tube housing to remove these very low-energy x-rays from the x-ray beam before they ever strike the patient. The geometric shape of the x-ray beam striking the patient is configured to the size needed by the beam-shaping collimator. In Fig. 1.19, three x-rays pass through the collimator opening. The left x-ray penetrates the patient and will be

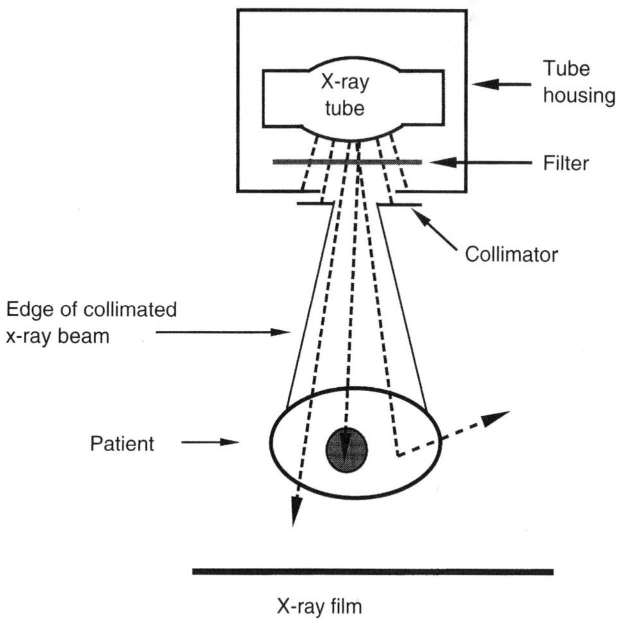

Fig. 1.19 The geometric relation between the x-ray tube, patient, and cassette or imaging plate. A filter in the tube housing removes low-energy x-rays that serve only to increase patient dose. The shape of the beam is configured with a collimator. The fate of three x-rays that pass through the collimator opening and strike the patient is shown. The x-ray on the *left* penetrates the patient and strikes the cassette. The x-ray in the *center* is absorbed by the patient. The x-ray on the *right* is scattered by the patient and could fog the film or contribute to personnel exposure dose.

recorded on the x-ray film. Some fraction of the oncoming x-rays must penetrate the patient and strike the cassette or imaging plate, or no information would be recorded. The middle x-ray hits a structure within the patient and is absorbed. Absorption of some of the x-rays is necessary for the image to have contrast. The x-ray on the right strikes the patient and is scattered. At this direction of scatter, the x-ray may strike a technologist. If the technologist is not wearing a lead apron, lead gloves, or a thyroid shield, they will receive unnecessary radiation dose. If the angle of scatter had been different, the scattered x-ray may have struck the cassette or imaging plate, causing fog and degrading the image.

A radiograph is the image of the internal makeup of an object based on the spatial distribution of x-rays transmitted through the patient. For decades, radiographic images have been recorded on film but as technology has advanced, the pattern of x-rays transmission through a patient is recorded in a digital format. The digital radiograph can then be viewed and manipulated on a computer monitor. The basis of film-based (analog) imaging is discussed briefly in this chapter, and digital radiographic imaging is discussed in Chapter 2.

Film Blackness and Opacity

X-ray film is a photographic film with a light-sensitive emulsion containing silver halide. After exposure to either x-rays or visible light, and film processing, silver halide crystals precipitate and form neutral silver deposits. These deposits are black on processed film. Unexposed crystals are removed during processing, leaving clear areas on the film. Thus, the distribution of precipitated silver determines how black, gray, or clear that part of the film appears. The degree of film blackness is directly related to the number of x-rays striking the film, controlled in part by the mAs (Fig. 1.20).

Film blackness is also affected by the energy of the x-ray beam, which is controlled by the kVp setting. As x-ray energy increases, a greater proportion of the x-rays will penetrate the patient, increasing film blackness (Fig. 1.21).

The distance from the x-ray tube to the film, referred to as the focal spot—film distance (FFD), also affects film blackness. As FFD increases the film blackness decreases because the intensity of x-rays in the x-ray beam (x-rays/unit area) decreases (Fig. 1.22). In most x-ray machines used in small animal practices, the FFD is relatively fixed (~40 inches). However, when using a portable x-ray machine, as in many large animal radiographic settings, the FFD can vary. An incorrect FFD will lead to either overexposure (FFD too short) or underexposure (FFD too long). Changes in FFD are not as important in digital imaging due to the great inherent exposure latitude (see Chapter 2), but a few inches difference in FFD will lead to a marked difference in film blackness, magnified because of the inverse square law:

$$\frac{I_1}{I_2} = \frac{(d_2)^2}{(d_1)^2}$$

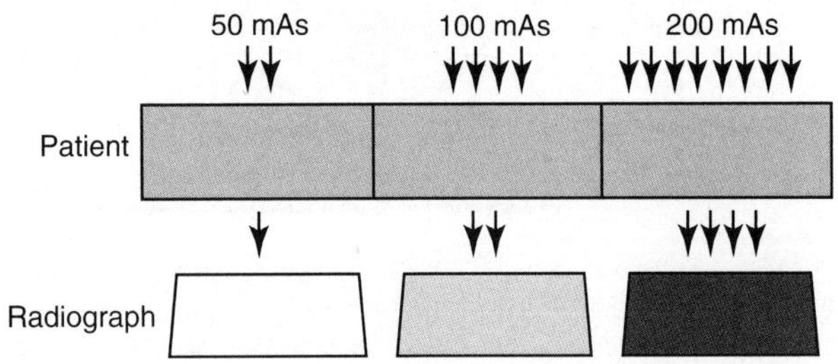

Fig. 1.20 The effect of mAs on the number of x-rays reaching the film, and thus the film blackness. Increasing mAs while keeping the kVp constant will result in more x-rays striking the patient, and then proportionally more will pass through the patient, increasing the blackness of the radiograph. Thus, as mAs is increased, film blackness also increases.

where I is intensity in terms of number of x-rays/unit area, and d is distance. In the equation, I_1 is the intensity at d_1, and I_2 is the intensity at d_2 (Fig. 1.23). For example, if the FFD decreases from 40 to 32 inches, a difference of only 8 inches, exposure increases by slightly over 50% which will result in excessive film blackness (calculation shown online).

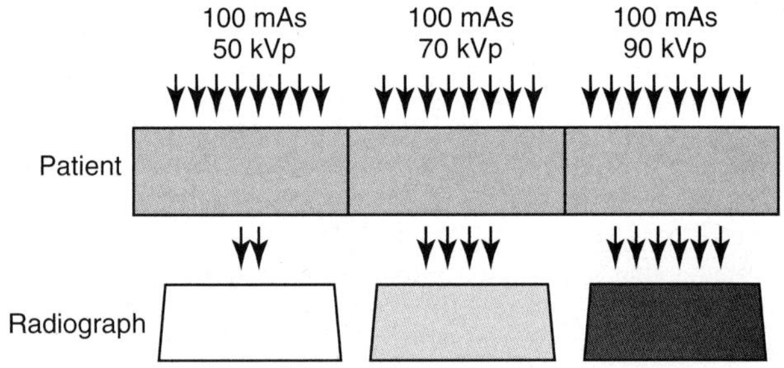

Fig. 1.21 The effect of kVp on the number of x-rays reaching the film, and thus the film blackness. Increasing kVp while keeping mAs constant results in the same number of x-rays being produced, but at higher kVp settings the x-rays have more energy, and a larger fraction will penetrate the patient. This will result in more x-rays hitting the film and an increase in film blackness.

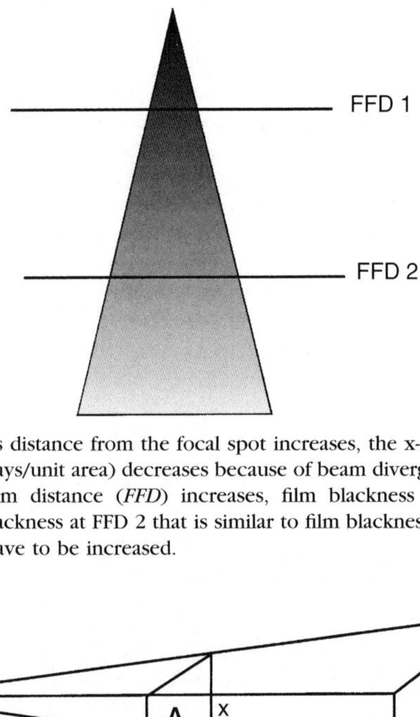

Fig. 1.22 As distance from the focal spot increases, the x-ray intensity in the beam (x-rays/unit area) decreases because of beam divergence. Thus, as focal spot—film distance (*FFD*) increases, film blackness decreases. To obtain film blackness at FFD 2 that is similar to film blackness at FFD 1, the mAs would have to be increased.

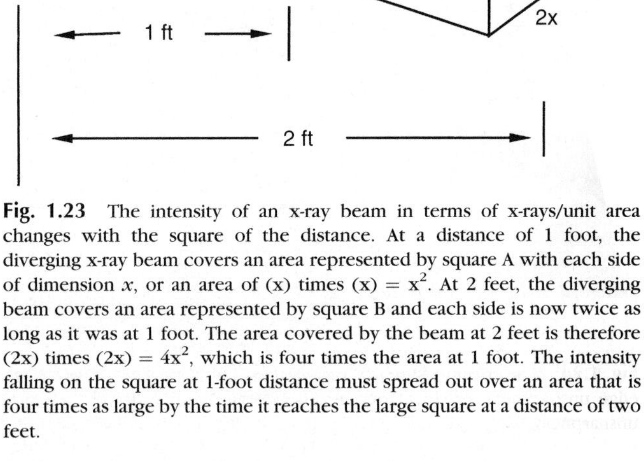

Fig. 1.23 The intensity of an x-ray beam in terms of x-rays/unit area changes with the square of the distance. At a distance of 1 foot, the diverging x-ray beam covers an area represented by square A with each side of dimension x, or an area of (x) times (x) = x^2. At 2 feet, the diverging beam covers an area represented by square B and each side is now twice as long as it was at 1 foot. The area covered by the beam at 2 feet is therefore (2x) times (2x) = $4x^2$, which is four times the area at 1 foot. The intensity falling on the square at 1-foot distance must spread out over an area that is four times as large by the time it reaches the large square at a distance of two feet.

As an example, assume that when an equine limb is radiographed the FFD should be 40 inches, but instead the machine is held too close, at a distance of 32 inches. If we arbitrarily define the x-ray intensity at 40 inches as 100, what change in intensity will result from the error of having the x-ray machine at 32 inches rather than at 40? Thus, in the equation $I_1 = 100$, $d_1 = 40$ inches, $I_2 = ?$, $d_2 = 32$ inches. Substituting, the equation becomes:

$$100/I_2 = (32)^2/(40)^2$$
$$100/I_2 = 1024/2500$$
$$100/I_2 = 0.64$$
$$I_2 = 1.56$$

Therefore, by being 8 inches too close, the exposure to the film is increased by 56%, which leads to observable overexposure.

FACTORS AFFECTING IMAGE DETAIL

Motion

Motion, which leads to image unsharpness, is the biggest enemy of detail in veterinary radiology. Short exposure times are used to minimize the effect of motion. Some x-ray machines are capable of millisecond exposures. When exposure time is very short, the mA must be large; otherwise, the mAs will be too low. Milliampere values up to 1500 can be obtained in some x-ray machines. In private veterinary practices, however, a typical maximum mA value is 300, meaning that exposure time must be longer to obtain suitable film blackness, and motion can become more of a problem.

Focal Spot Size

Some x-ray tubes have an operator selectable focal spot size (see Fig. 1.16). Use of the small focal spot results in improved detail (Fig. 1.24). The disadvantage of the small focal spot is that lower mAs values must be used to prevent the filament from overheating. With a large focal spot, edges of anatomic structures are projected more unsharply than with the small focal spot. This edge unsharpness is termed *penumbra* (see Fig. 1.24). In practice, small focal spots are used rarely because of the associated mAs limitations to prevent filament burn out or melting, as mentioned earlier.

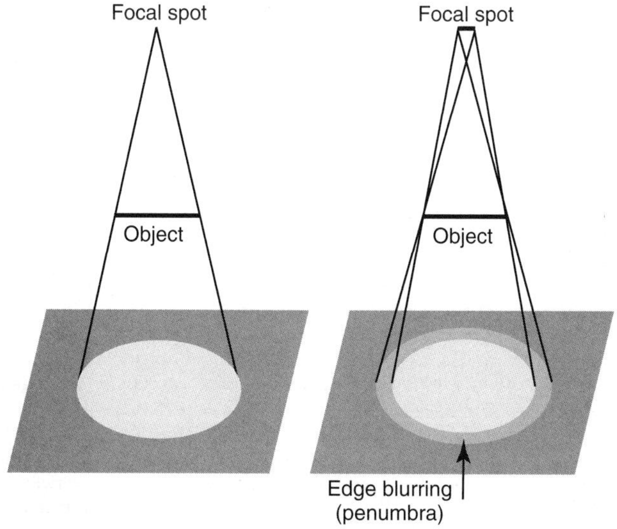

Fig. 1.24 The effect of focal spot size on detail. With a large focal spot, the edge unsharpness, or the penumbra, is larger. This contributes to image unsharpness.

Intensifying Screens

In reality, the x-ray film emulsion is much more sensitive to visible light than to x-rays. Therefore, converting the x-ray energy into visible light via an intensifying screen and then using the visible light to expose the film and create the image is a convenient way to increase the efficiency of radiographic production. For example, it may require 100 mAs to obtain a suitable radiograph when using x-rays to expose film directly, but 1 to 2 mAs might be suitable when an intensifying screen intermediary is used.

Intensifying screens contain phosphorescent crystals that emit light when struck by x-rays (Fig. 1.25). The thicker the crystal layer, the greater the chance of an x-ray being absorbed in the screen and thus more light is produced at any given mAs. But with a thicker layer, there is more light diffusion before hitting the film and degradation in image quality (Figs. 1.26 and 1.27).

Grids

Many digital radiographic systems have processing software that will eliminate the effect of scattered radiation from the patient. However, software may not eliminate enough scattered radiation and scatter must be removed by a *grid*. Grids are also necessary when using film and the patient thickness exceeds 10 cm.

A grid is a flat, rectangular plate with alternating strips of an x-ray absorbent material, such as lead, and an x-ray transparent material, such as fiber, plastic, or aluminum (Fig. 1.28). Some x-rays passing through the patient will be aligned with the transparent material and reach the plate/film (see Fig. 1.28, *photon 2*). Some x-rays interacting with the patient will be scattered at an angle that does not allow them to pass cleanly through the space between the lead strips and they will be absorbed by the lead and not reach the plate/film (see Fig. 1.28, *photon 4*). These scattered x-rays serve only to fog the film. Some primary x-rays also are absorbed by the lead if they strike the lead strips head on (see Fig. 1.28, *photon 1*). Therefore, the mAs must be increased when grids are used to compensate for the portion of the primary x-ray beam absorbed by the lead

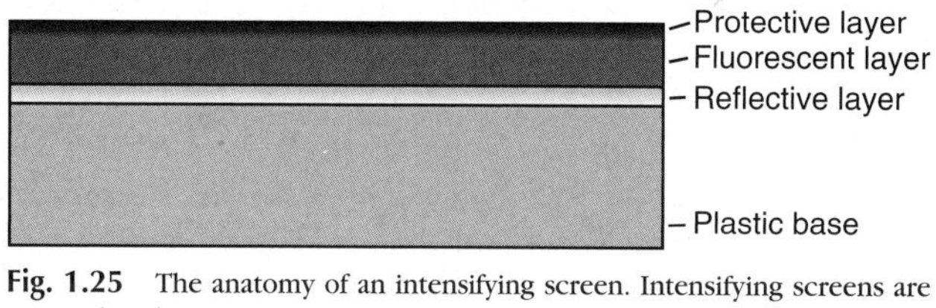

Fig. 1.25 The anatomy of an intensifying screen. Intensifying screens are covered with a protective layer. Beneath this is the fluorescent layer, which emits visible light when struck by x-rays. A reflective layer, which lies deep beneath the fluorescent layer, reflects light back in the direction of the x-ray film. The plastic base provides support for the intensifying screen. In the cassette, the x-ray film is in contact with the protective layer, and the protective base is glued to the cassette.

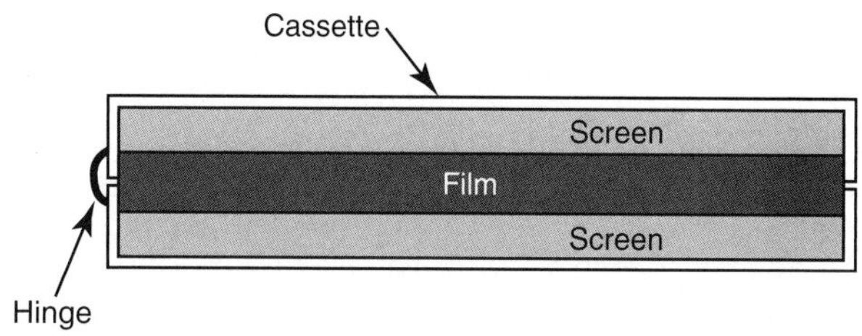

Fig. 1.26 The anatomy of a film-screen cassette. X-ray film is placed in a cassette, sandwiched between two intensifying screens. The use of two intensifying screens increases the efficiency of image production compared to using only one screen. The tradeoff of using two intensifying screens rather than one is a slight loss of detail compared with only one screen. The relative thickness of the film versus intensifying screen is not to scale in this image; in reality the film is much thinner than shown here.

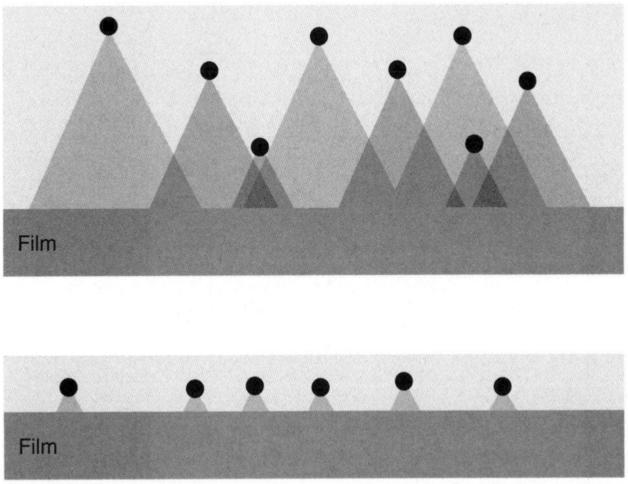

Fig. 1.27 Effect of thickness of the fluorescent layer in an intensifying screen on light diffusion. The fluorescent layer in the top intensifying screen is thicker than in the intensifying screen at the bottom. Phosphorescent crystals are shown in each screen as *small black circles*; there are many more crystals in the thicker fluorescent layer than in the thin layer. In the thicker fluorescent layer, there is more light diffusion from each crystal before striking the film. This will lead to some slight blurring of the image compared with the thinner fluorescent layer at the bottom where there is less light diffusion from each crystal before striking the film. There is also more overlapping of the light emitted from each crystal in the thicker fluorescent layer, which will also contribute to degradation in detail. However, the thicker fluorescent layer requires less radiation (lower mAs) to produce the radiograph than the thinner fluorescent layer, but the detail of the radiograph made using the thicker fluorescent layer will be reduced.

strips. The increase in mAs needed to use a grid is offset by the marked increase in contrast resulting from removal of scattered photons.

The size of each lead strip in Fig. 1.28 has been exaggerated greatly. Typically, a grid contains 80 to 160 lead strips per linear inch. Thus, the lead strips are very thin. Grids with more lead strips per linear inch are preferable because if the lead strips become too thick, they will be visible in the radiograph as radiolucent lines. The radiolucent lines created by the lead strips in a grid can be obscured by causing the grid to oscillate during the radiographic exposure. This blurs the radiolucent lines, rendering them invisible. The device in the x-ray table that causes the grid to oscillate is called the *Bucky,* after its inventor.

Besides the number of lead lines per inch, the grid ratio is another parameter used to describe a grid. The grid ratio describes the relationship of the height of the lead strips (typically up to 5 mm) to the distance between them (typically 0.4 mm or less). That is, if lead strips are five times as high as the space between them, the grid ratio is 5:1 (Fig. 1.29). The higher the grid ratio, the more effective the grid is in absorbing scattered radiation, but the more difficult it will be for primary x-rays to pass through it. This should be apparent by comparing the 5:1 and 8:1 grids in Fig. 1.29. Thus, the higher the grid ratio, the more mAs needed to produce acceptable film blackness. The grid ratio is independent of the number of grid lines per inch. For example, in a 5:1 grid having the same number of lines per inch as an 8:1 grid, the height of the lead strips would have to be lower. In Fig. 1.29, there are more grid lines per inch for the 8:1 grid than for the 5:1 grid. The number of lines per inch determines how conspicuous the lead grid lines will be in a radiograph, assuming that the Bucky is not used. The grid ratio determines the effectiveness of scatter removal. A summary of the relationship of grid lines per inch versus grid ratio is given in Table 1.5.

Note that in Fig. 1.28 the lead and aluminum strips are angled more steeply toward the periphery of the grid. This is

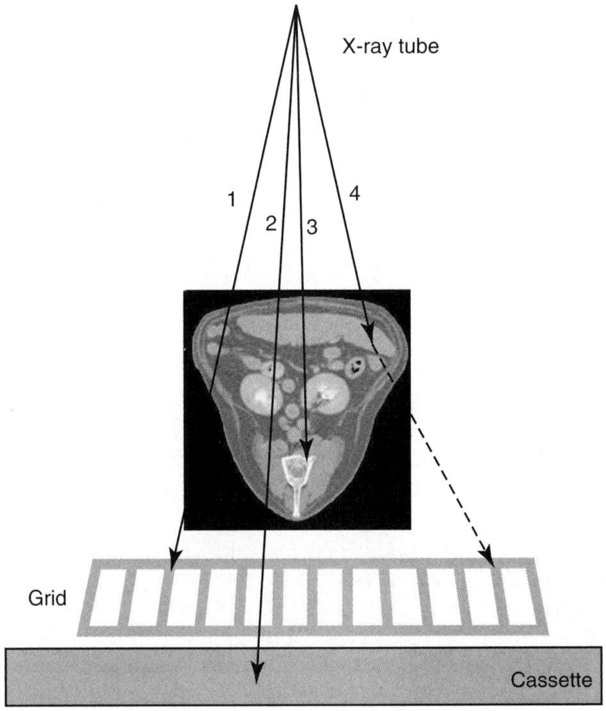

Fig. 1.28 A grid is composed of alternating strips of an x-ray absorbing material, such as lead, and an x-ray transparent material, such as aluminum. The grid is positioned between the patient and the film, usually fixed in the x-ray table, to intercept scattered radiation before it reaches the cassette or imaging plate. The lead strips in this illustration are shown as *gray* regions, and the interposed aluminum strips are shown as the interposed *white* regions. The size of these strips is exaggerated greatly in this drawing. The aluminum absorbs very little radiation, but the lead absorbs nearly all of the x-rays that strike it. Photon 1 penetrates the patient, carrying useful information, but does not reach the cassette because it hits a lead strip and is absorbed. Therefore, a grid does remove useful information, meaning that the mAs must be increased when a grid is used to ensure that adequate numbers of x-rays reach the cassette. Usually, the mAs must be increased by a factor of 2–3. Photon 2 penetrates the patient, carrying useful information, hits an aluminum strip, and is not absorbed so it reaches the cassette. Photon 3 is absorbed in the patient. Differential x-ray absorption, with some x-rays being absorbed and others penetrating the patient, is necessary to create an image. Photon 4 is scattered but strikes a lead strip and is removed by the grid before it hits the cassette. If the grid were not present, this photon would have degraded the image by fogging.

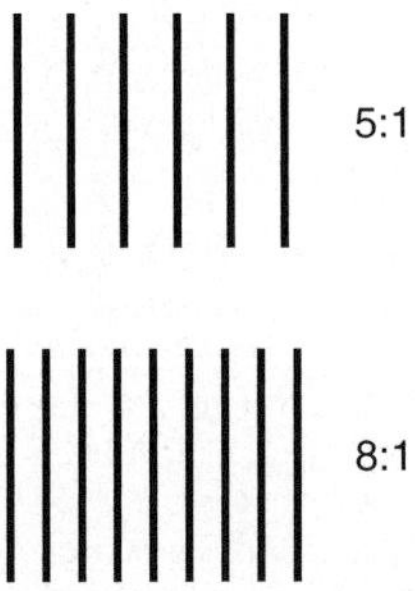

Fig. 1.29 The grid ratio is the ratio of the height of the lead strips, shown here in *black*, to the distance between them. Two grids are shown here. One has a ratio of 5:1 and the other a ratio of 8:1. It is easy to see that more oncoming radiation will be absorbed in the 8:1 grid because the space between the lead strips is thinner. This increases the chance that an incident x-ray will hit a lead strip.

necessary because the divergence of the grid lines must match the divergence of the primary x-ray beam from center to periphery so that the grid does not *cut off* excessive x-rays from the primary beam (Fig. 1.30). Grids constructed with peripheral angulation of the lead strips are called *focused grids*. Focused

Table • 1.5

Criteria Characterizing Grid Efficacy.

CRITERION	DEFINITION	TYPICAL VALUES	INFLUENCE ON RADIOGRAPHIC TECHNIQUE
Lines per inch	Number of lead strips per linear inch of grid	80 lines per inch 100 lines per inch 140 lines per inch	Has no effect on mAs required
Grid ratio	Ratio of height of lead strips to distance between them	5:1 8:1 10:1	Higher grid ratio requires more mAs for comparable film blackness

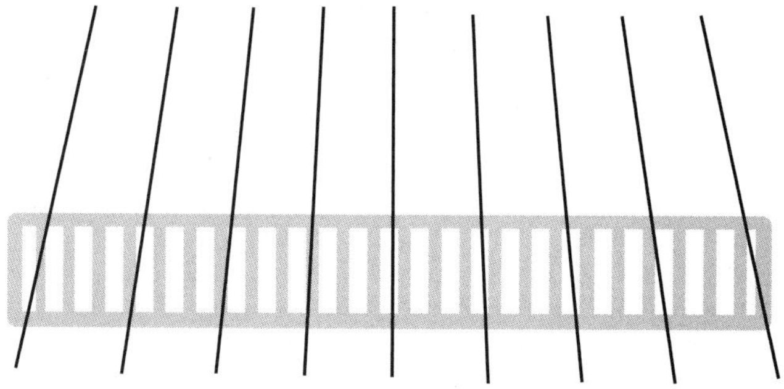

Fig. 1.30 Cutoff of useful radiation because of malalignment of the grid lines to the pattern of x-ray beam divergence. In this example, the lead and aluminum strips in the grid are all vertical. This would be called an *unfocused grid*. The diverging nature of the primary x-ray beam does not match the verticality of the lead and aluminum strips, and many oncoming x-rays are absorbed in the grid, particularly at the edge where the divergence of the x-ray beam is maximal. An unfocused grid would only be functional if the oncoming primary x-ray beam had little or no divergence. This example illustrates the importance of having the geometry of the x-ray beam match the geometry of the grid.

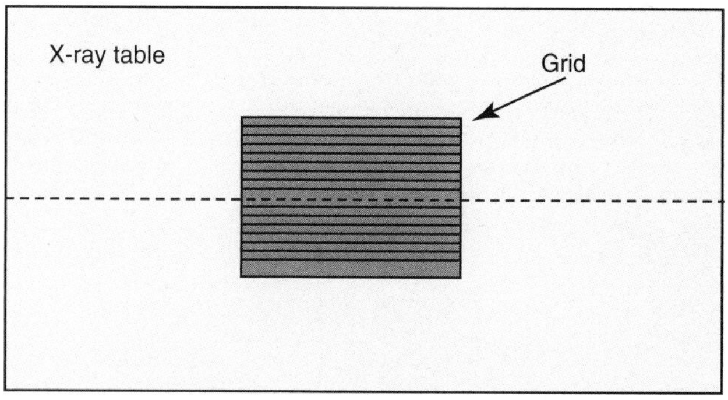

Fig. 1.31 Illustration of proper orientation of the grid with the x-ray table. The grid is centered in the table, and the lead and aluminum strips run parallel with the long axis of the table. If the grid is a focused grid, with angled lead strips, the center of the primary x-ray beam can be positioned anywhere along the dotted line. But if the center of the primary x-ray beam is peripheral to the dotted line, there will be grid cutoff because the divergence of the x-ray beam no longer matches the divergence of the lead strips.

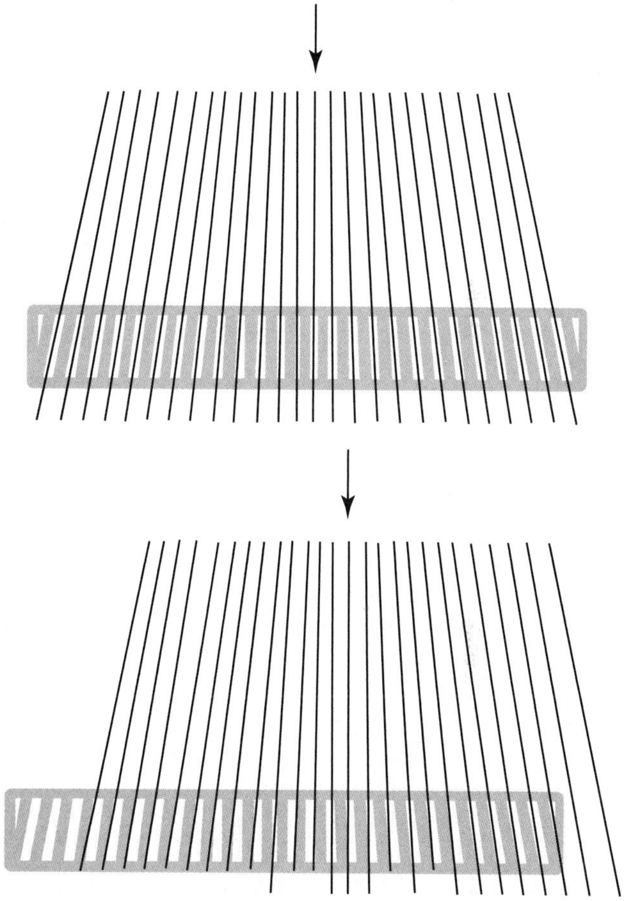

Fig. 1.32 Lateral decentering. When the central ray is centered over a focused grid, the divergence of the x-ray beam matches the divergence of the lead and aluminum strips and a high percentage of the oncoming primary photons pass through the grid. When the central ray is laterally decentered, the divergence of the beam no longer matches the divergence of the lead and aluminum strips in the grid, and the lead strips will absorb more of the primary beam, reducing film blackness. Lateral decentering is the most common grid-induced artifact.

grids must be used within a defined range of FFDs to maintain a parallel relationship between the oncoming x-ray beam and the radiolucent strips.

When a grid is installed into the x-ray table, the grid must be oriented such that the lead strips run parallel with the long axis of the x-ray table (Fig. 1.31). The center of the primary x-ray beam must always be aligned with the centerline of the grid or cutoff will occur because the diverging pattern of the x-ray beam does not match the diverging pattern of the grid lines (Fig. 1.32). The excessive loss of the primary beam caused by positioning the center of the primary x-ray beam peripheral to the center line is called *lateral decentering*.

FACTORS AFFECTING CONTRAST

Radiographic contrast refers to the difference in film blackness between structures in the image. If no contrast were present, all parts of the patient would be of the same opacity and individual structures would not be visible. Radiographic contrast in a film image depends mainly on the relationship between kVp and mAs, and the amount of film fogging by scattered x-rays. In a digital system, the contrast is highly dependent on software parameters applied for image processing.

Radiographic Technique

Radiographic contrast refers to the distribution of gray shades in the image and is caused by differential x-ray absorption in

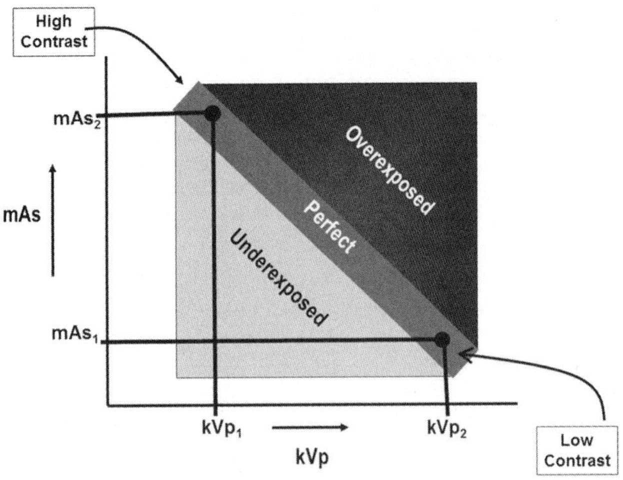

Fig. 1.33 Many combinations of mAs and kVp will produce a perfect radiograph. The term *perfect* is used here to mean a radiograph that is neither underexposed nor overexposed. With low numbers of x-rays, the energy must be high (mAs_1 and kVp_2) so that sufficient numbers reach the film. With many numbers of x-rays, their energy must be low (mAs_2 and kVp_1) or too many will reach the film. Although both of the mAs and kVp combinations shown here will produce adequate film blackness, the contrast of the image will be different. A low mAs and high kVp technique will result in a lower contrast image than one made with a high mAs and low kVp.

various body parts. Radiographic contrast is affected by differences in thickness, physical density, atomic number, and x-ray beam energy. The effects of thickness, physical density, and atomic number on x-ray absorption were covered earlier. The effect of x-ray beam energy (kVp) on contrast is covered in this section.

The ability of an x-ray to penetrate tissue depends on its energy (see Fig. 1.21). X-rays generated at higher kVp values have higher energy. Selecting the kVp setting is one of the most important factors to consider in choosing the exposure factors.[11] For a constant mAs, if the kVp is too low, too few x-rays penetrate the patient, and the radiograph is underexposed (too white), whereas if the kVp is too high, too many x-rays penetrate the patient, and the radiograph is overexposed (too black). The kVp also influences subject contrast. If high mAs values are used (many x-rays generated), then low kVp values must be used to prevent too many of the x-rays from penetrating the patient and reaching the film. If low mAs values are used, then high kVp values must be used so that more of the x-rays penetrate the patient and reach the film (Fig. 1.33).

Even though multiple combinations of mAs and kVp can result in a satisfactory radiograph in terms of film blackness, the contrast of the image will depend on the specific kVp-to-mAs combination selected (Fig. 1.33). In a high-contrast radiograph, also referred to as having a *short scale* of contrast, mostly black and white opacities and very few shades of gray are present. Low-contrast radiographs have a *long scale* of contrast with few blacks and whites but many shades of gray (Fig. 1.34).

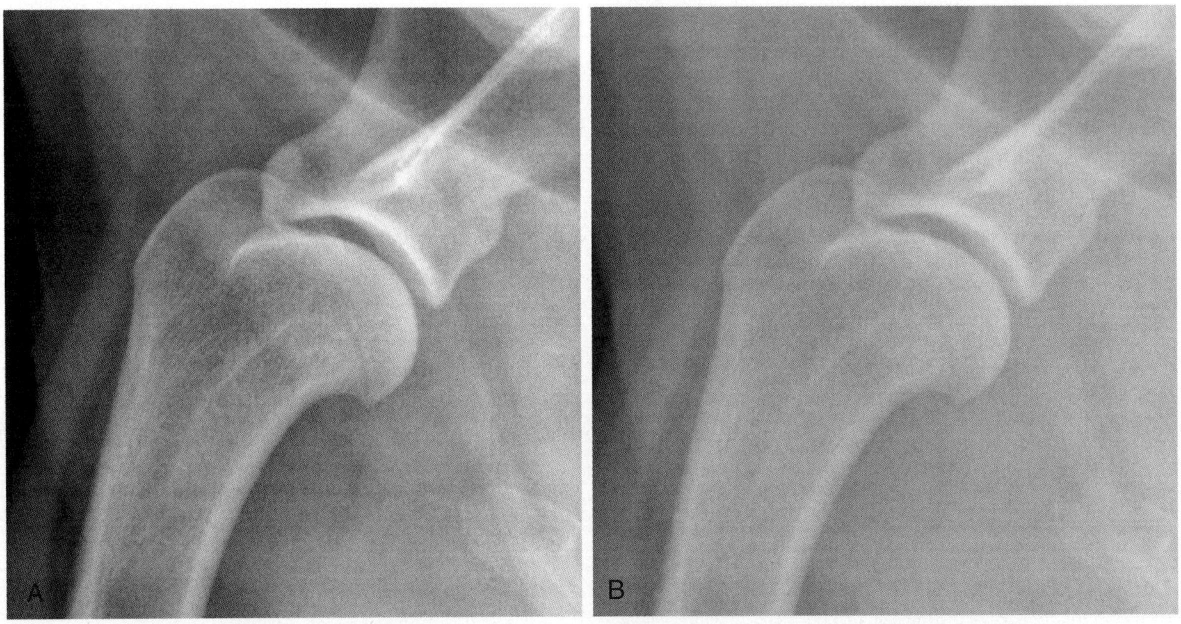

Fig. 1.34 A high-contrast (**A**) and low-contrast (**B**) radiograph of the same canine shoulder. The high-contrast radiograph would be made using a low kVp and high mAs technique, whereas the low-contrast radiograph would be made with a high kVp and low mAs technique. Both radiographs are of acceptable overall film blackness, but the high-contrast image is more useful for assessment of bone architecture. In areas of the body with high inherent contrast, such as the thorax, it would be desirable to use a high kVp—low mAs technique to prevent the radiograph from having too much contrast. Conversely, in areas of the body with low inherent contrast, such as the abdomen, where only fat provides contrast, it would be desirable to use a low kVp—high mAs technique to maximize contrast, and therefore organ discrimination, in the radiograph.

[11] The selection of exposure factors is less critical if one is using a digital radiographic system compared with a film-screen system; this is discussed in detail in Chapter 2.

In general terms, the reason that high mAs—low kVp techniques result in greater radiographic contrast than low mAs—high kVp techniques relates to the relative energies of the x-ray beams produced using these techniques. With the high mAs—low kVp technique, the energy of the x-ray beam is relatively low, and this predisposes to x-rays either being absorbed or not. Using a high mAs—low kVp technique also means that the photoelectric absorption predominates, which is highly dependent on atomic number. Thus, bone will absorb many x-rays whereas soft tissue will absorb fewer, and there will be high contrast between these tissues. This technique is appropriate for abdominal radiography where contrast between soft tissue and fat should be maximized. Conversely, with the low mAs—high kVp technique, the energy of the x-ray beam is higher, and all tissues become less efficient absorbers of x-rays. More photons are absorbed by the Compton process, which is independent of atomic number. Therefore, the differential absorption between bone and soft tissue is minimized, and their radiographic opacity becomes more similar; that is, the radiograph has less contrast. This technique is used for thoracic radiography to decrease the contrast between the ribs and the underlying lung tissue.

REFERENCES

1. Roentgen W. On a new kind of rays. *Vet Radiol Ultrasound.* 1995;36:371—374.
2. Hall E, Giaccia A. *Radiobiology for the Radiologist.* 7th ed. Philadelphia: Lippincott Williams & Wilkins; 2011.
3. NCRP: National Council on Radiation Protection and Measurements. *NCRP Report No. 82—SI Units in Radiation protection and Measurements.* Bethesda: NCRP Publications; 1985.
4. Campion EW. A retreat from SI units. *N Engl J Med.* 1992;327(1):49.
5. Clark DE, Laeseke PF. Systeme international in the ICU in the United States. *Chest.* 2010;137(4):932—937.
6. Hall E, Giaccia A. Radiation carcinogenesis. In: Hall E, Giaccia A, eds. *Radiobiology for the Radiologist.* 7th ed. Philadelphia: Lippincott Williams & Wilkins; 2011.
7. ICRP. Chapters 5 and 6. *Ann ICRP.* 2007;37(2—4):81—123.
8. NCRP: National Council on Radiation Protection and Measurements. *NCRP Report No. 116—limitation of Exposure to Ionizing Radiation.* Bethesda: NCRP Publications; 1993.
9. NRC, Title 10. Chapter 1, Code of federal regulations—energy. Part 20, standards for protection against radiation. In: *United States Nuclear Regulatory Commission Rules and Regulations.* Washington: U.S. Government Printing Office; 1995:20—27.
10. NCRP: National Council on Radiation Protection and Measurements. *NCRP Report No. 160—ionizing Radiation Exposure of the Population of the United States (2009).* NCRP Publications; 2015.
11. Smth-Bindman R, Miglioritti DL, Larson EB. Rising use of diagnostic medical imaging in a large integrated health system: the use of imaging has skyrocketed in the past decade, but no one patient population or medical condition is responsible. *Health Aff.* 2008;27:1491.
12. NCRP: National Council on Radiation Protection and Measurements. *NCRP Report No. 107—implementation of the Principle of as Low as Reasonably Achievable (ALARA) for Medical and Dental Personnel.* Bethesda: NCRP Publications; 1990.
13. Tyson R, Smiley DC, Pleasant RS, et al. Estimated operator exposure for hand holding portable x-ray units during imaging of the equine distal extremity. *Vet Radiol Ultrasound.* 2011;52:121.
14. Mayer MN, Koehncke NK, Belotta AF, Cheveldae IT, et al. Use of personal protective equipment in a radiology room at a veterinary teaching hospital. *Vet Radiol Ultrasound.* 2018;59:137—146. https://doi.org/10.1111/vru.12583.
15. Belotta A, Mayer MN, Koehncke NK, et al. Survey of self-reported radiation safety practices among North American veterinary technicians involved in equine radiography using portable x-ray equipment. *J Am Vet Med Assoc.* 2021;259:919. —926.
16. Bushberg JT, Seibert JA, Leidholdt Jr EM, et al. *The Essential Physics of Medical Imaging.* 2nd ed. Lippincott Williams & Wilkins; 2012.
17. Barthez PY, et al. Comparison of single-phase and high-frequency generators for x-ray units. *Vet Radiol Ultrasound.* 2002;43(2):118—122.

ELECTRONIC RESOURCES

Additional information related to the content in Chapter 1 can be found online at eBooks.Health.Elsevier.com

- Chapter Quiz

CHAPTER 2

Digital Radiographic Imaging

Ian Robertson • Donald E. Thrall • Nathan C. Nelson

WHAT IS DIGITAL RADIOGRAPHIC IMAGING?

Digital radiographic imaging involves the following steps: (1) electronic measurement of the pattern of x-ray transmission through the patient, (2) conversion of the electronic measurement into a digital computer file, and (3) viewing the digital file on a computer monitor. This process is analogous to acquiring a photograph with a digital camera where the camera records the pattern of colors and intensities irradiating from an object and converts that information to a picture. Digital radiographic imaging is *not* photographing a radiographic film image with a digital camera, nor is it running an analog radiograph through a film scanner to convert the hard copy image into a digital file.

Conventional x-ray machines are used for digital radiography. Thus, to transition from analog to digital imaging, for example, the purchase of a new x-ray machine is usually not necessary. A new x-ray machine purchase could be considered if the existing unit is substandard, or if the hardware associated with the new digital-imaging system is actually housed in the x-ray table. In veterinary medicine, the transition from analog (film-to-screen) radiographic imaging to digital radiographic imaging is nearly complete, with the vast majority of veterinary practices relying on digital rather than analog radiography systems.

Although the price of digital radiography systems has fallen since their initial entry into the veterinary market, there remains substantial capital outlay required in their purchase. Selecting the correct system requires significant time, energy, and planning. All digital systems are not equal, and low-end, less expensive systems may not deliver optimal quality. In the end, the full range of advantages of the digital radiographic environment will not be realized. The old saying "you get what you pay for" is relevant. Unless one is thoroughly versed in digital technology, it is worth hiring a consultant to assist with equipment purchase.

Radiation protection and patient positioning are just as important in digital radiography as they were in analog imaging. Overall, however, the digital transition has improved the quality of radiographic studies acquired in veterinary medicine appreciably. It is critical that those working with or considering the purchase of a digital radiographic system have a thorough understanding of all aspects of this modality.

THE DIGITAL IMAGE FILE

The basis of a digital image is a computer file that contains information relating to a signal that has been measured. In diagnostic medical imaging, the signal can be the pattern of x-ray emission from a patient (radiography), quantification of fan-beam x-ray attenuation by the patient (computed tomography [CT]), the pattern of sound waves reflected by the patient (ultrasound), or the pattern of radiofrequency emission from the patient (magnetic resonance imaging [MRI]).

In diagnostic medical imaging, the computer file is a Digital Imaging and Communications in Medicine (DICOM) format. A DICOM file is a computer file format of the same basic type as .jpeg and .tiff files, and is listed with a .dcm file extension.[1] In addition to the actual image information, every DICOM file contains a large amount of ancillary information stored in what are called *metadata tags*. These tags contain other related information about the image, including the manufacturer of the device that generated the image; the date and time of image acquisition; patient demographic information; acquisition parameters; referrer, practitioner, and operator identifiers; and various other image parameters.[1]

The DICOM file format was derived mainly for consistency to ensure interconnectivity between imaging devices.[2] Without seamless interconnectivity, such as would occur if every vendor encoded the digital radiographic image into a proprietary file format, the convenience of having images in a digital format is reduced greatly. For example, without a standard DICOM file format, images acquired on a digital plate from vendor "A" could be viewed only on software provided by vendor "A." This is a disadvantage because the purchaser might like the features of the hardware but not the features of the software. With the DICOM standard, images created on equipment from vendor "A" can be viewed on a variety of platforms, not only on those from vendor "A." Compliance with formatting digital image files in DICOM format is voluntary. Most reputable vendors realize the advantages of total DICOM compliance, and the DICOM format has become the universal standard in medical imaging, across vendors, modalities, and computer operating systems. It is important that vendor adherence to the DICOM standard be verified before the digital system is purchased, otherwise this tremendous flexibility in viewing and file transmission is lost. The DICOM standard provides for the transmission of medical images from one device to another, such as from the x-ray machine to the server or server to workstation, using a network protocol that runs on top of the existing Internet standard protocol. DICOM images can also be transferred using browser-based technology, and this enhances image portability, particularly when accessing images beyond the local area network.

THE COMPONENTS OF A DIGITAL IMAGE

When the digital file is viewed using appropriate software, discussed later, the digital image comprises individual *pic*ture *el*ements termed *pixels*. The pixels are arranged in a row-by-column matrix. In radiographic, ultrasound, CT, and MRIs, each pixel has a specified shade of gray. The more pixels in a digital file, the greater the matrix size and the larger the file size. Uncompressed digital radiographic image DICOM files are typically in the order of 4 to 12 MB per image, compared to approximately 0.1 MB for a 30-page document (.doc) file and

0.5 MB to 2.0 MB for a high-resolution, color, digital photographic (.jpg) file.

The size of each pixel in a digital image determines the *spatial resolution* of the image, that is, how small of an object can be detected (Fig. 2.1). The hardware provided by the vendor determines the size of the pixel array in a digital radiographic image. In general, more pixels are better, but for any imaging system, there is a point at which more pixels do not result in a superior image. Pixel size (also termed pixel pitch) may be measured in microns or line pairs per mm; guidelines for minimum recommended standards for spatial resolution are available.[3] Although pixel size is important, there are many other hardware and technical factors that ultimately affect the "clinically useful" spatial resolution. Also, detailed later, software manipulation of the raw image file to optimize the displayed image is, within limits, more important than pixel density.

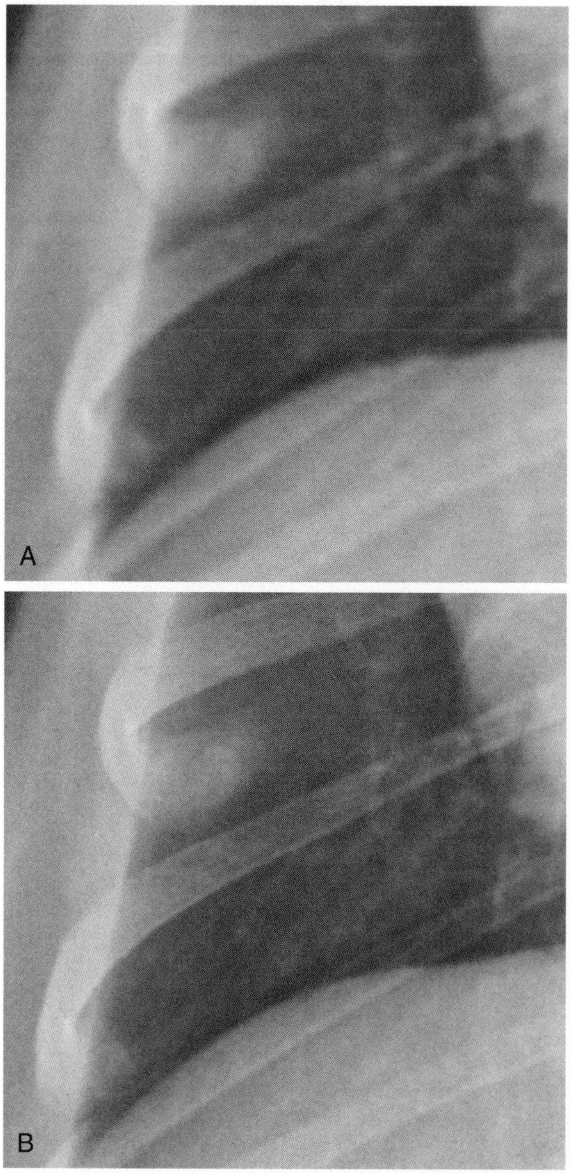

Fig. 2.1 Close-up view of the caudal thorax of a dog. **A,** The resolution of the image is 72 pixels per inch. **B,** The resolution is 300 pixels per inch. The effect of pixel size on image detail is clear with improved resolution due to smaller pixel size in **B**. The requirement for a small pixel size is one reason that digital radiographic image files are very large.

As noted before, in medical digital images, each pixel is assigned a shade of gray. The number of available gray shades for each pixel will influence the contrast of the image. If a pixel can have only a few gray shades, the image can only have a very short scale of contrast (high contrast) because there will be only black pixels, white pixels, and pixels of a few gray shades. If, conversely, there are many gray shade options for each pixel, the scale of contrast can be long. Computer files use binary notation to assign a gray shade to a pixel. In binary notation, the only digits used are 0 and 1. For grayscale assignment, a 0 is assigned black, and a 1 is assigned white; combinations of zeros and ones can be used for various intermediate gray shades. If n equals the number of allowable number of zeroes and ones per pixel, then 2^n is the number of combinations of zeroes and ones, and consequently the number of gray shades that are possible. The more combinations of zeroes and ones, the more gray shades there are possible in each pixel. The number of possible gray shades is referred to as the *bit depth* of the image (Fig. 2.2). Image file size and bit depth are directly related. Without the ability to assign multiple gray shades to each pixel, the image would have no diagnostic value (Fig. 2.3).

DIGITAL RADIOGRAPHY ACQUISITION HARDWARE

There are two main types of digital radiography acquisition hardware: computed radiography (CR) and direct digital radiography (DDR).[4]

As noted, a conventional x-ray tube and x-ray table are used for both CR and DDR applications. The difference between analog and digital imaging is that the film cassette, used for analog imaging, is replaced with a digital recording device to record the distribution of x-rays transmitted through the patient. In CR systems the digital recording device is a cassette that contains a flexible imaging plate, and in DDR systems the digital recording device is a rigid imaging plate or imaging chip (no cassette). Charge-coupled device (CCD) systems, which are a special type of DDR, may require purchase of a new x-ray

Bit depth	Possible pixel values	Number of shades of gray
1	0,1	2
2	00,01,10,11	4
4	0000,0001,0010, 0011,0100,0101 0110,0111,1000, 1001,1010,1011, 1100,1101,1110, 1111	16
8	00000000, 00000001, etc. to 11111111	256
12	000000000000, 000000000001, etc. to 111111111111	4096

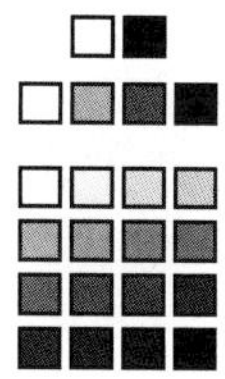

Fig. 2.2 The concept of bit depth. The number of gray shades possible in an image depends on bit depth, which is the range of binary values that can be assigned to a pixel. If only 0 or 1 is possible (bit depth = 1), the pixel can be only black or white. If both 0 and 1 are possible (bit depth = 2), the possible pixel values are 00, 01, 10, and 11, and the pixel can have one of four gray shades. Other possible pixel values can be seen in this figure, along with a representation of the possible grayscale values for bit depths of 1, 2, and 4. The sheer number of possibilities prevents illustrating all grayscale shades for a bit depth greater than 4.

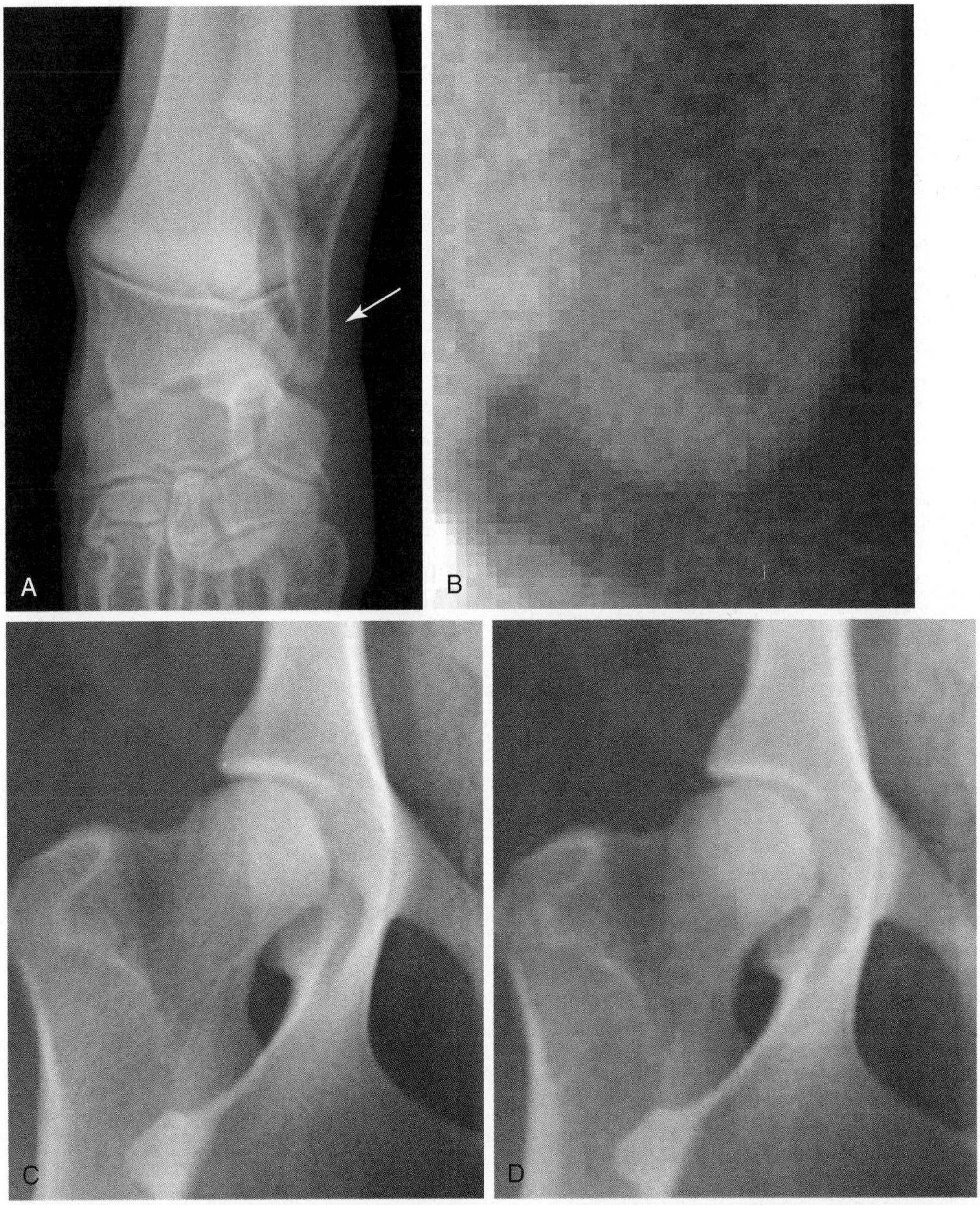

Fig. 2.3 **A,** Craniocaudal radiograph of the distal antebrachium of a dog with a bit depth of 12, meaning that 4096 shades of gray are available for pixel assignment. **B,** Close-up of the styloid process of the ulna (region of *arrow* in **A**). At this magnification, individual pixels are visible, and the large number of gray shades used to create the image can be appreciated. It is easy to see how if the number of gray shades were reduced the contrast in the image would have a very short scale with many blacks and whites but few intermediate gray tones. **C,** The image was acquired at a bit depth of 10. Image **D** was acquired at a bit depth of 8. The inadequate range of gray tones is readily apparent in the 8-bit image.

table because the hardware components are housed in the x-ray table, and it may not be possible to retrofit the new equipment into an existing x-ray table adequately.

Computed Radiography

CR was the earliest digital radiographic system to come on the market. In CR, a cassette that appears outwardly similar to a film cassette is used. The CR cassette does not contain an intensifying screen or x-ray film but instead contains a flexible imaging plate coated with a photostimulable phosphor ([PSP]; Fig. 2.4). In CR, the x-ray attenuation pattern of the patient is temporarily stored as a latent image in the PSP. The latent image is created by changes in electron energy bands that result from x-rays striking the PSP. The latent image is read out optically as photostimulated luminescence when the PSP plate is subsequently stimulated using a scanning laser (Fig. 2.5).[5,6] Therefore, the CR plate must be processed in a plate reader following radiographic exposure (see Fig. 2.4). The processing steps in the CR radiography process are summarized as follows:

- After exposure, the CR cassette is removed from the x-ray table and inserted into the reader.
- The reader automatically removes the PSP plate from the CR cassette.
- The PSP plate is illuminated in the reader by a laser.
- Laser illumination causes visible light to be emitted from the PSP plate.

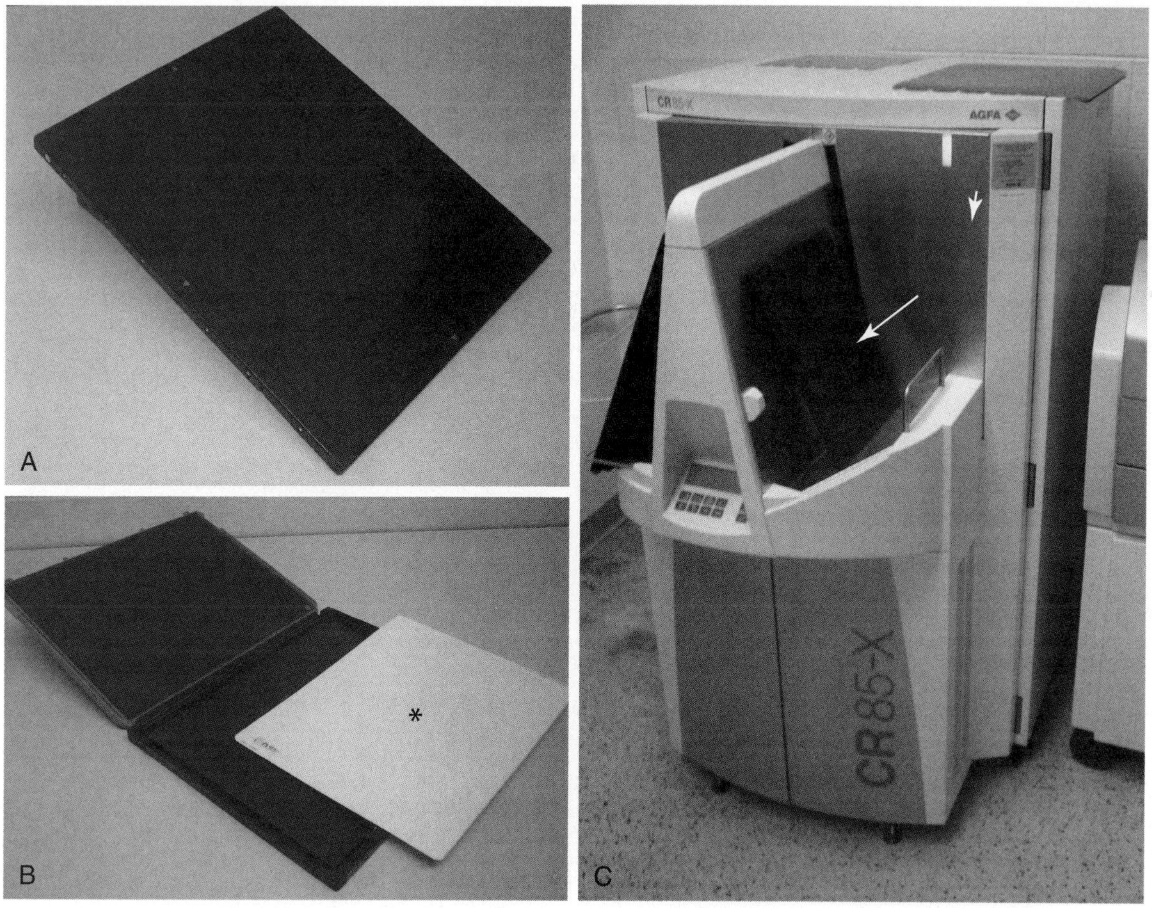

Fig. 2.4 **A,** Computed radiography (CR) cassette. On external examination, the CR cassette appears similar to a traditional film cassette. **B,** Opened CR cassette. When opened, the photostimulable phosphor (PSP) plate (*asterisk*) is apparent within the CR cassette. **C,** CR reader. The CR cassette (*arrow*) is placed on the reader, which internalizes it and acquires the digital image stored on the PSP. This particular reader is a high-volume, rapid reader suitable for a large facility with high caseload. Smaller footprint, less expensive CR readers are available.

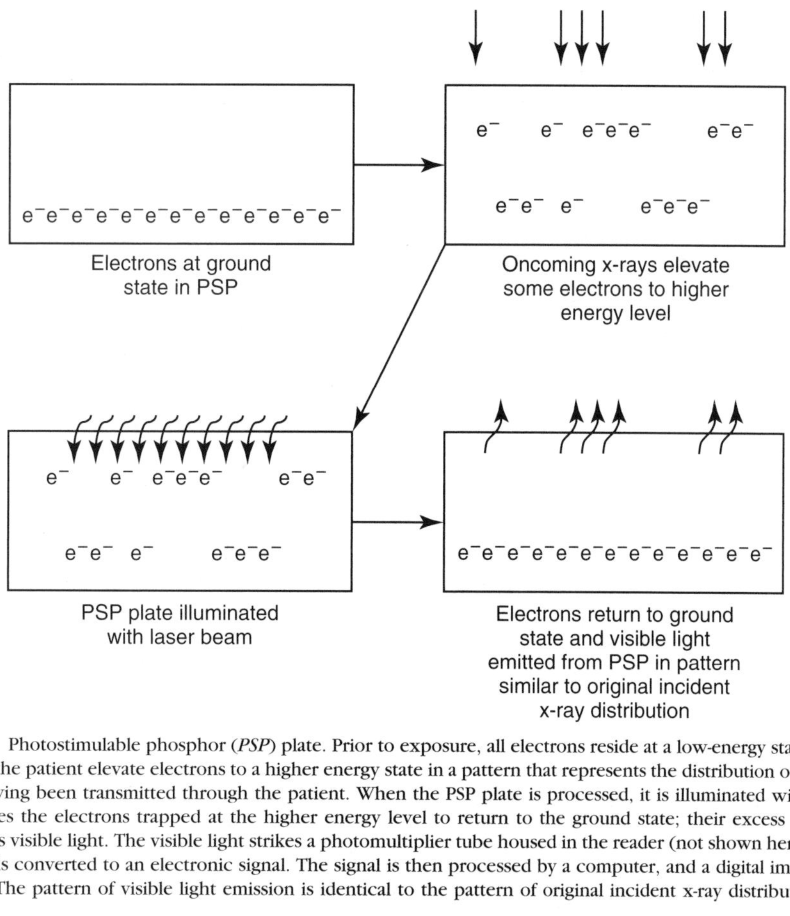

Fig. 2.5 Photostimulable phosphor (*PSP*) plate. Prior to exposure, all electrons reside at a low-energy state. X-rays that exit the patient elevate electrons to a higher energy state in a pattern that represents the distribution of incident x-rays having been transmitted through the patient. When the PSP plate is processed, it is illuminated with a laser that causes the electrons trapped at the higher energy level to return to the ground state; their excess energy is emitted as visible light. The visible light strikes a photomultiplier tube housed in the reader (not shown here) where the light is converted to an electronic signal. The signal is then processed by a computer, and a digital image file is created. The pattern of visible light emission is identical to the pattern of original incident x-ray distribution.

- Emitted visible light strikes a photomultiplier tube where it is converted into electronic signal.
- The electronic signal is digitized and stored as a digital file.
- The PSP plate is exposed to bright white light to make sure all electrons are at ground state in preparation for the next exposure.
- The PSP plate is automatically returned to the cassette in the reader.
- The cassette is ejected from the reader for use on the next patient.

CR remains in widespread use in human imaging but is not as popular in veterinary imaging. There is nothing inherently wrong with CR imaging, and the reason for this relative lack of market penetration is multifactorial. Because the CR plate is handled and manipulated much the same way as an analog film cassette, it may take 1 to 2 minutes for the digital plate to be processed completely in the plate reader, whereas with DDR systems the image is available almost immediately. Because of this, CR does not increase workflow compared with analog imaging. For example, a CR plate reader that can read only one plate at a time is actually slower than a modern automatic x-ray film processor on a per-image basis. While CR cassettes are portable, the reader is typically not mobile and is permanently housed in the veterinary practice. In an ambulatory situation, where x-ray exposures are performed off-site (such as in a horse barn), exposed CR cassettes must be returned to the veterinary practice for processing, preventing rapid evaluation of radiographs in the field. This is a similar workflow as film radiography, so when throughput is not an issue, a good-quality CR system can be perfectly adequate as a replacement for an analog system. One advantage of a CR system is that damaged cassettes can be replaced relatively inexpensively, whereas the cost of replacing a damaged DDR plate, discussed in the next section, is considerably more expensive. Another advantage of CR is that the cassette is not tethered to a computer by a cable as nonwireless digital-imaging plates are. This provides more flexibility and reduces constraints in obtaining nonstandard views, such as images made with a horizontally directed x-ray beam, because the geometric relationship between the x-ray tube and CR plate can be adjusted easily.

Direct Digital Radiography

There are three distinct types of DDR: (1) indirect flat-panel detector system, (2) direct flat-panel detector system, and (3) CCD system. In DDR, the detector replaces the film cassette, and within a few seconds after the radiographic exposure, the digital radiographic image is ready for quality-control evaluation.

Indirect Flat-Panel Detectors

Indirect flat-panel detectors are termed *indirect* because they produce visible light as an intermediate step in image formation. An x-ray intensifying screen, identical in principle to those mentioned in Chapter 1, is used to convert x-ray energy emerging from the patient into visible light.[6,7] The intensifying screen may be comprised of gadolinium oxysulfide or cesium iodide. Cesium iodide innately possess higher efficiency of x-ray detection compared to gadolinium oxysulfide, allowing lower radiation dose and thinner flat-panel device, but comes at a price premium.[8] Regardless of composition, the intensifying screen is layered onto a panel containing an array of tiny photodiodes. Much as with the PSP found in the CR plate, the photodiodes convert visible light emitted from the intensifying screen into an electronic signal that is then read out by a thin-film transistor array and transformed into an electronic file (Fig. 2.6). To have good spatial resolution, the size of each detector element is very small, and a full-size imaging plate measuring approximately 43 cm × 43 cm may have a photodiode matrix of 2600 × 2600. Thus, an indirect flat-panel

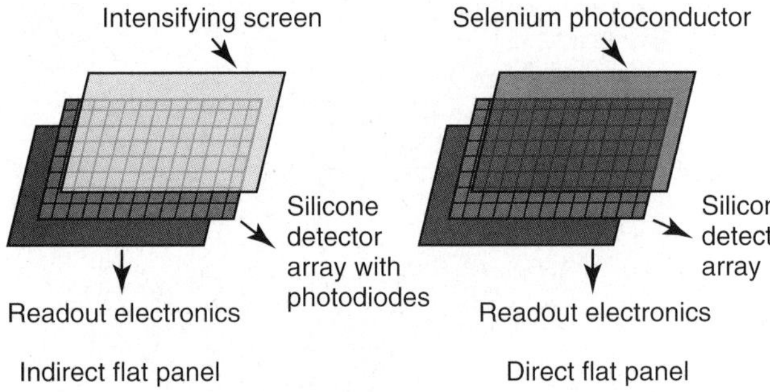

Fig. 2.6 Comparison of the makeup of indirect versus direct flat-panel detectors. With the indirect detector, an x-ray intensifying screen converts oncoming x-ray energy to visible light. The visible light interacts with the detector array, which is composed of small elements that each contain a photodiode and an amorphous selenium detector. The light from the intensifying screen is converted to an electronic signal by the photodiode and then readout by the amorphous selenium detector. Readout electronics maintain spatial resolution and transmit the information to the computer, where it is converted to an electronic file. With the direct detector, there is no light intermediary. The oncoming x-rays strike a selenium photodetector, where the energy is converted to an electronic signal that is collected by the amorphous silicon detector array directly, with subsequent processing by the readout electronics and formation of an electronic file.

detector can have 6 to 7 million photodiodes or more. As can be imagined, the electronics needed to record and spatially localize the signal from each photodiode, or pixel, and to also incorporate the photodiode into each detector element is quite complicated. This contributes to the relatively high cost of flat-panel detectors compared with a film-screen cassette system. Indirect flat-panel detectors are commonly capable of a bit depth of 14, meaning there is a grayscale resolution of 16,384 gray shades per pixel.[5] Most digital radiographic systems range in bit depth from 10 to 16 (1024–65,536 shades of gray). Because the human eye can register only 50 to 100 simultaneous shades of gray, even with extreme manipulation of image contrast (postprocessing—see later), there is probably little benefit in generating images with more than 14- to 16-bit depth.

Direct Flat-Panel Detectors

In a direct flat-panel detector, there is no visible light intermediary. Oncoming x-rays strike a photoconductor, typically composed of amorphous selenium, which has high efficiency x-ray absorption. Electrons liberated in the selenium layer by the oncoming x-ray beam are collected to form a charge. This charge is then read out directly by the thin-film transistor array, processed by the readout electronics and converted to an electronic file (see Fig. 2.6).[6,7] As with indirect flat-panel detectors, there are millions of detectors in the array, and the pixel matrix is of comparable size, also with a bit depth of 14. Thus, the main difference between indirect and direct flat-panel detectors is the intermediate step of light production from the intensifying screen in indirect systems.

As discussed in Chapter 1, there is some light diffusion within an x-ray intensifying screen. This light diffusion, which can potentially lead to blurring, is a purported disadvantage of indirect flat-panel detectors versus direct flat-panel detectors. However, with modern engineering techniques, and the structure of the crystals in the intensifying screen, the amount of light diffusion that actually occurs in the intensifying screen is minimal and not clinically significant. For all practical purposes, the functionality of modern-day indirect and direct flat-panel detectors is comparable.

Flat-panel systems are increasingly replacing CR systems as the preferred digital radiograph technology in veterinary medicine, given their higher throughput and recent decreases in price. Flat-panel systems can produce diagnostic images with

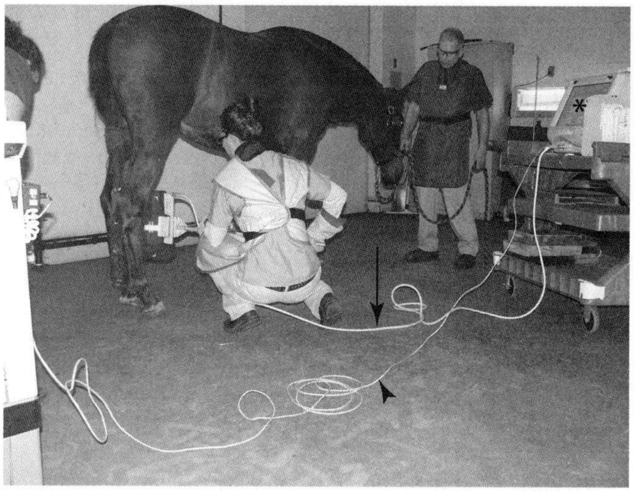

Fig. 2.7 Use of a flat-panel detector during radiography in a horse. Note that a cable (*arrow*) connects the flat-panel detector to an acquisition computer (*asterisk*). A second cable (*arrowhead*) extends from the x-ray tube to the acquisition computer; this cable carries the signal to activate the flat-panel detector when an exposure is made (wireless flat-panel systems and x-ray tubes have eliminated the need for these cables). (Modified with permission from Nelson NC, Zekas LJ, Reese DJ. Digital radiography for the equine practitioner: basic principles and recent advances. *Vet Clin North Am Equine Pract*. 2012;28(3):483–495. https://doi.org/10.1016/j.cveq.2012.08.003. Epub Oct. 18, 2012. PMID: 23177127.)

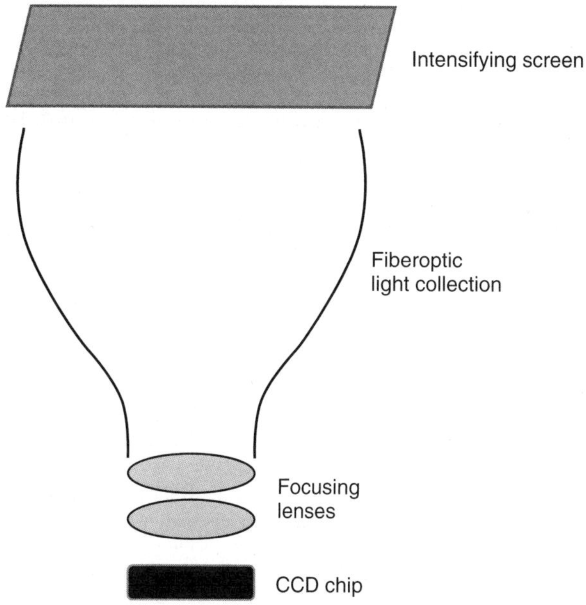

Fig. 2.8 A charge-coupled device (*CCD*) radiography system. X-rays from the patient strike a conventional intensifying screen where the spatial distribution of x-rays is converted to a comparable spatial distribution of visible light. The light is collected using fiberoptics and strikes focusing lenses that direct it onto the light-sensitive CCD chip. Overall image quality is determined mainly by the efficiency of light collection and the quality of the focusing lenses. All of these components are encased in a housing that must be incorporated into the x-ray table. The housing is fixed, which means that the x-ray tube must always be perpendicular to the face of the housing.

lower radiation doses (up to 30% less than CR systems), providing radiation safety benefit to personnel working in the x-ray suite.[9,10] While direct and indirect flat-panel detectors are commonly tethered to a processing computer by a cable, wireless DDR plates are becoming more affordable and widely available (Fig. 2.7). Wireless DDR plates provide particular benefit in the equine setting, where additional cables are a tripping hazard. The recent advent of battery-powered, portable x-ray devices combined with a wireless flat-panel display provides the ultimate in portability and convenience for the equine clinician working in the field.

Additionally, although CR is largely a fully developed technology, material improvements in flat-panel systems continue. Newer flat-panel detectors use a flexible plastic film as the base substrate for the thin-film transistor array, rather than the traditional silicone-based glass substrates currently in use, promising better durability and improved x-ray detection.[11] Newer flat-panel detectors may also allow dynamic digital radiography, allowing rapid capture of multiple sequential images at once.

Charged-Coupled Device

CCD chips are used routinely in video camcorders and digital cameras, but their use in radiographic imaging is less common than either CR or flat-panel DDR radiography. However, some vendors continue to market veterinary radiography systems based on the CCD chip. CCD systems are included in the discussion of DDR because no equipment manipulation is needed between radiographic exposure and image visualization, such as is required in processing a CR cassette.

CCD chips are relatively small compared with a flat-panel detector, being only a few centimeters on each side, compared with up to 43 cm for flat-panel detectors. Although small, there may be millions of pixel elements on the surface of a CCD chip. The CCD chip is sensitive to visible light, not x-rays; this is the basis for their use in camcorders and digital cameras. Thus, for radiography based on CCD technology, a light intermediary is necessary, and this is accomplished by integration of a relatively standard x-ray intensifying screen between the patient and CCD chip. When the CCD chip is exposed to visible light that has been collected and focused from the intensifying screen, the pixels in the CCD chip accumulate electronic charge, which is read out and converted to an electronic file.[6]

The geometry of the CCD system deserves special consideration. Given the small size of the CCD chip, the visible light output from the intensifying screen needs to be focused onto the chip, whereas in an indirect flat-panel detector, the intensifying screen is layered directly onto the detector. Focusing of light from the intensifying screen onto the CCD chip is usually accomplished by integration of fiberoptic light collection and a focusing lens between the intensifying screen and CCD chip (Fig. 2.8). Thus, the quality of the image depends more on the quality of light collection and focusing than on the quality of the CCD chip. Also, there is some loss of light and potentially much light distortion between the intensifying screen and CCD chip, leading to image degradation.

In general, CCD radiography in humans has been reserved for situations where the part being imaged is relatively small (e.g., dental radiography and mammography) and there is less need for light focusing. In veterinary medicine, the parts being radiographed are larger and requirements for focusing more stringent; this can lead to poorer images than obtained with flat-panel detectors, and image quality from CCD systems is considered by many to be inferior to both flat-panel and CR systems. Also, the distance required for collecting and focusing the light from the intensifying screen means that the physical device is large compared with a flat-panel detector. As a result, CCD detectors are housed within the x-ray table. This hardware cannot be retrofitted easily and purchase of a new x-ray machine may be necessary if CCD technology is chosen. The size of the device also limits portability, and there is a requirement for a constant vertical relationship between the x-ray tube and CCD camera. Both of these factors eliminate the possibility of using CCD technology for portable imaging and horizontal

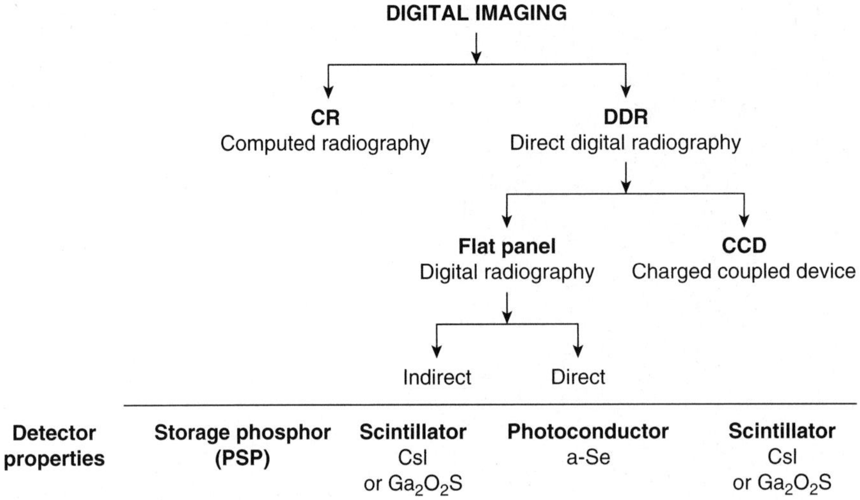

Fig. 2.9 Chart showing the image capture hardware options available in digital imaging. From Lanca L, Silva A. *Digital Imaging Systems for Plain Radiography*. New York: Springer; 2013:9–19.

beam radiography. CCD systems are typically less expensive than flat-panel imaging systems or high-quality CR systems, but image quality is usually inferior. A summary of the various hardware options is shown in Fig. 2.9.[12]

IMAGE PROCESSING AND VIEWING

Regardless of the type of digital radiographic hardware selected, the electronic data are processed by a computer before the final image file is created and displayed. Image file processing and modification occur at a number of points and can be broken down into preprocessing, processing, and postprocessing steps.[13]

Preprocessing of the image is usually beyond the control of the user. Manufacturers apply various corrections to the raw image data to accommodate such things as inhomogeneity in light collection, image distortion by focusing lenses in CCD systems, nonfunctional or dead pixels in the detector, and variation in efficiency between individual detector elements. These preprocessing steps are aimed at eliminating artifacts created by the imaging system itself[13] and are critical to image quality optimization.

The *processing* step is aimed at converting the corrected raw image data to a usable radiographic image. These manipulations, also done on the raw image data, can be controlled to some extent by the user and are aimed at optimizing image contrast, edge enhancement, minimizing image noise, and optimizing other aspects of image presentation.[6,13] These settings are usually configured by the vendor as "presets" or factory default settings, such as *thorax*, *abdomen*, and *extremity*. However, most systems allow customization by the user. Most commonly, the raw data file is not permanently overwritten, and additional image processing can be performed later, if necessary, provided the raw data files have not been deleted. Assessing image quality when the digital image first appears at the QC workstation at the x-ray machine, and making adjustments to optimize image presentation, is part of the "processing" step. Preprocessing and, most importantly, effective image processing are critical, and this functionality is often what sets good vendors and products apart. Progress in digital technology in recent years has centered around improvement in the processing step. Improved algorithms limit the impact of scatter and image noise on the final image, in some case allowing up to 50% reduction in radiation dose necessary to create a diagnostic image.[8,14] The various algorithms and processing techniques are typically proprietary and may vary greatly between products. Once the preprocessing and processing adjustments have been completed, the image is ready for viewing and interpretation. The processed image file is in DICOM format; it may have been converted from another file type. Appropriate header information is inserted, and the study is distributed through the local network to the viewing computer(s) and an appropriate archive. DICOM files, although a graphics file, cannot be viewed directly in programs such as Adobe Photoshop or Microsoft Paint. Rather, they must be viewed with dedicated DICOM file-viewing software. Licenses for this software are typically sold by the hardware vendor and are part of the original purchase package, but some free DICOM viewers are available. The most popular viewers for Apple computers are OsiriX (http://www.osirix-viewer.com) and freeware Horos (https://www.horosproject.org). RadiAnt DICOM viewer (https://www.radiantviewer.com) is a capable, small footprint PC-based viewer with a free trial period, but thereafter requires a paid subscription. ClearCanvas Open Source Project (https://clearcanvas.github.io) is a freeware, open-source PC-based viewer. Which viewing software will be adequate for any particular practice should be considered carefully, and consultation with an expert may be needed to make the best selection.

The functionality of DICOM viewing software represents one of the major advantages of digital radiography. This is the *postprocessing* step of image manipulation, and this is 100% user controlled. DICOM viewers allow images to be magnified and rotated, and the image blackness and contrast can be adjusted independently (Fig. 2.10). Other features are also available, such as viewing multiple images simultaneously and obtaining quantitative measures of area and length. The myriad of image adjustments that can be accomplished is a tremendous advancement over viewing film-based radiographs, which cannot be manipulated at all following their creation. Postprocessing image manipulation does not permanently alter the original image in any way.

Ambient lighting and monitor quality are two important considerations when optimizing image viewing. As ambient light increases, the perceived difference between light and dark on a monitor decreases, and this can affect image interpretation negatively.[15,16] Interestingly, viewing of digital radiographs in a completely dark room with no light other than the monitor light also reduces accuracy.[17] For this reason, computers used

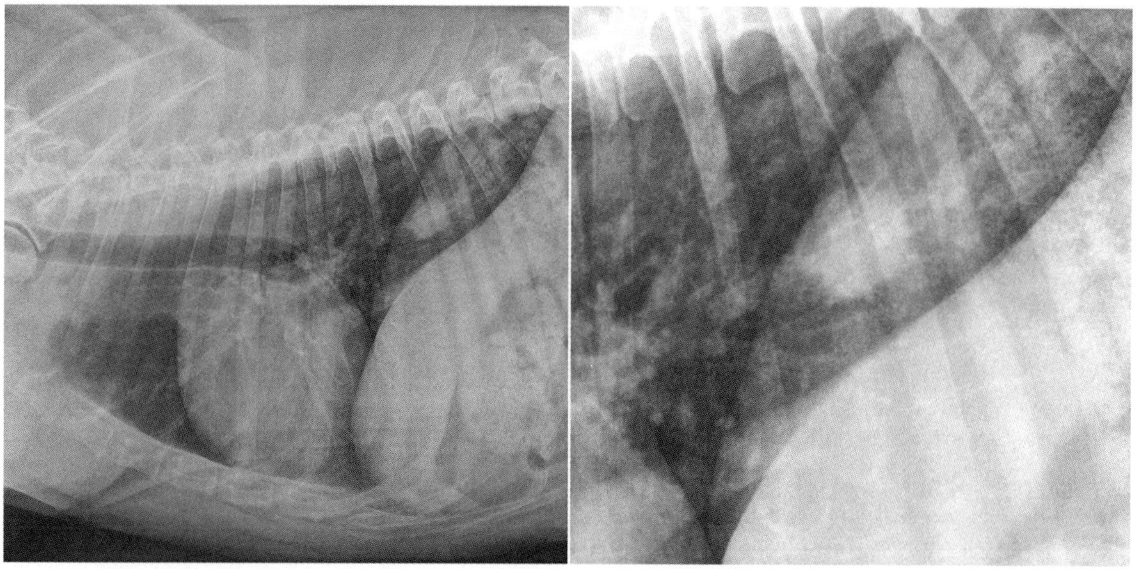

Fig. 2.10 Screen capture from a DICOM viewing program. A left lateral thoracic radiograph is displayed in the *left panel*. In the *right panel*, the same radiograph has been enlarged and the contrast adjusted to increase the conspicuity of a nodule in the caudal lung field.

for primary image interpretation should be in a room with adjustable, or permanently dimmed, lighting but not in total darkness.

Monitor quality is another factor that influences the accuracy of interpretation of digital radiographic images. Both monochrome (black and white) and color liquid-crystal display (LCD) monitors are available, and their technical specifications are highly variable, leading to a wide range of image display quality. Ideally, radiographic images are best viewed on a dedicated medical-grade monochrome LCD monitor.[18] Such monitors are characterized by superior brightness, contrast ratio, and resolution. Monitor brightness relates to how bright a white screen is, and a brighter display enables the user to resolve more shades of gray. Contrast ratio is a measure of the monitor's ability to display true black as black and true white as white. Because LCD technology relies on backlighting, displaying true black is technically challenging, and as a result, LCD monitors with a high contrast ratio are more expensive. Monitor resolution also affects how well digitally captured images appear on the screen. Medical-grade monochrome LCD monitors typically have 3 megapixel resolution or higher. For example, a typical display for such a monitor is 2048 pixels × 1536 pixels, yielding a 3.1-megapixel display. This level of resolution approximates the average resolution of most digital radiographs, which means there is no image downsizing by the graphics card during initial image display. For the user, this means there is no need to routinely magnify images to ensure all the digital information available is evaluated. Unfortunately, medical-grade monochrome LCD monitors are expensive, and their routine use throughout the veterinary imaging environment cannot be justified financially. Consumer-grade color LCD monitors are improving continuously, eroding the diagnostic advantage of more expensive monochrome monitors. However, given the substantial investment that occurs when deploying a digital radiography system, an additional investment to acquire at least one medical-grade monochrome monitor for the primary interpretation of digital radiographic images is justifiable.

Whatever viewing system is chosen, it is important to ensure that monitors are calibrated correctly. Test patterns to assist in monitor calibration are available through the Internet. Medical-grade monochrome LCD monitors should be calibrated using the DICOM grayscale display function standard. LCD monitors lose brightness over time, with consumer-grade monitors affected more rapidly than medical-grade monitors, so brightness should be periodically measured.

DIGITAL VERSUS ANALOG IMAGING

The advantages of digital imaging are quite far reaching, and some have been alluded to in prior sections. It is noteworthy to outline specifically what these advantages are and to expand on those that have not been covered in adequate detail. Advantages of digital radiography are (1) reduced expendable supply cost and elimination of darkroom maintenance; (2) contrast optimization and exposure latitude; (3) image postprocessing, ability to adjust image blackness and contrast after exposure; (4) improved image accessibility and consolidated image storage; (5) enhanced portability enables consultation; (6) use of artificial intelligence, and (7) an opportunity to change the imaging paradigm.

Reduced Expendable Supply Cost and Elimination of Darkroom

In a digital imaging environment, the requirement for purchasing x-ray film, film-filing envelopes, darkroom chemistry, and other related supplies is eliminated. Although these items are not inherently expensive, their use over time as well as the time and effort required for maintenance amount to a considerable sum, which is eliminated in digital imaging. Darkroom errors, such as outdated chemicals, incorrect temperature settings, chemical spills and splashes, and safelight fog or other light leaks, make up a substantial fraction of errors that compromise analog image quality. Additionally, there are increasingly more stringent local government requirements in ensuring personnel safety with respect to darkroom chemicals and fumes and also in the safe disposal of exhausted darkroom chemicals.

Contrast Optimization and Exposure Latitude

When one begins to evaluate digital radiographic images, the initial impression may be that of improved detail when compared with analog film radiographic images. This is a misconception created by the excellent contrast optimization that characterizes digital radiographs. The detail of an image relates to how small of a structure can be discriminated in the image; this is termed *spatial resolution*. The spatial resolution in a digital or analog radiographic image depends on many factors, some of which apply equally to both analog and digital imaging, but there are a few differences (Box 2.1). In the end, it is the collective effect of these factors that determines the final spatial resolution. The relative inherent spatial resolution from various medical-imaging techniques is provided in Table 2.1.[19] From Table 2.1, it can be seen that the inherent spatial resolution of digital radiographs is roughly half that of analog radiographs; this is the end result of all factors listed in Box 2.1. Although there is a factor of two difference in spatial resolution between analog and digital radiography, this difference is not relevant clinically because the spatial resolution of both analog and digital radiography is excellent. Thus, it is not spatial resolution that sets digital radiography apart. The major factors contributing to the superior image quality of digital radiographs are contrast optimization and exposure latitude.

Because an antiscatter grid can improve both spatial resolution and image contrast, it is worth commenting specifically on their use in digital radiography. Although antiscatter grids can be used in digital radiography, some manufacturers have incorporated a scatter-correction algorithm into the image-processing software that makes grid use unnecessary (Fig. 2.11).[20] Implementation of an antiscatter algorithm avoids the higher milliampere second (mAs) values that are needed to compensate for the presence of an actual grid in the x-ray beam (see Fig. 2.11). The possibility of a grid artifact is also eliminated when grids are not used. Whether or not the end user will be satisfied with the quality of the antiscatter image-processing algorithm will be a matter of individual preference, and the functionality of this feature should be evaluated in any digital system prior to purchase.

Box • 2.1

Factors Contributing to Inherent Spatial Resolution in Digital Versus Analog Radiographs

Digital Radiograph
Focal spot size
Patient scatter
Grid efficiency, if used
Size of crystals in intensifying screen*
Size of detector element in digital plate

Analog Radiograph
Focal spot size
Patient scatter
Grid efficiency, if used
Size of crystals in intensifying screen
Size of light-sensitive crystal in x-ray film emulsion

*For digital radiography, an intensifying screen is used only in indirect flat panels and in CCD systems.

Table • 2.1

Inherent Spatial Resolution of Various Imaging Modalities.

MODALITY	RESOLUTION (mm)
Screen film radiography	0.08
Digital radiography	0.17
Ultrasound imaging (5 megahertz [MHz])	0.30
Computed tomography	0.40
Magnetic resonance imaging	1.00

Modified from Bushberg JT, Seibert JA, Leidholdt Jr. EM, et al. Introduction to medical imaging. In: Bushberg JT, Seibert A, Leidholdt EM, Boone JM, eds. *The Essential Physics of Medical Imaging*. 3rd ed. Philadelphia: Lippincott Williams & Wilkins; 2011:60–68.

Contrast Optimization

Contrast optimization, also termed *contrast resolution*, is a feature of digital radiography that is related to the bit depth of each pixel and the processing software that accompanies the digital-imaging system. The processing software can assign a gray shade to a pixel in a digital image that would have been either black or white in an analog image. This results in more of the image having interpretable gray shades and not appearing over- or underexposed.

With radiographic film, radiographic contrast is associated rigidly with the relationship between kilovoltage peak (kVp) and mAs, as discussed in Chapter 1. Consider the film radiography of a patient where the thickness of various parts of the patient within the primary x-ray beam varies considerably; one example of this would be a lateral radiograph encompassing the caudal abdomen, pelvis, and femurs and stifle joints of a dog. The lumbosacral region of the pelvis is very thick and primarily bone. The caudal abdomen is somewhat thinner and primarily soft tissue. The distal femur and stifle joints are much thinner. When the radiographic technique that is suitable for the average thickness and physical density is selected (e.g., caudal abdomen), the lumbosacral region in the film image will be underexposed and the thinner parts in the film image overexposed because of excessive x-ray transmission. One can think of this result as being caused by the film having a bit depth that is too low to capture all the needed gray shades. The region of the film in the lumbosacral region can only be white, and the region of film in the stifle region can only be black.

With digital radiography, however, the computer can compensate for the wide range of thickness of the patient by assigning a suitable gray shade to pixels in the thick lumbosacral and thin stifle regions, as well as in the caudal abdomen. What this means in practical terms is that in digital imaging, opacity differences associated with variation in thickness are much lower than in analog radiographs (Fig. 2.12). This same principle applies to structures of similar thickness but containing parts that have markedly different physical density, such as massive bones (Fig. 2.13) or air-filled lung (Fig. 2.14). The result is a more pleasing image with more gray shades, with no regions that cannot be assessed because of being over- or underexposed. Making a lateral view of the pelvis of a medium-to-large dog with the pelvic limbs displaced cranially and caudally, as illustrated in Fig. 2.12, is a good field test for contrast optimization software which varies from vendor to vendor.

The terminology used to describe this contrast optimization feature of digital radiographic systems can be confusing. Some have used the term *dynamic range* to mean the same thing as contrast resolution, but there are, in fact, many differing definitions of dynamic range, depending on the system being discussed. The term *dynamic range* has also been used to describe the low dependence of digital-imaging plates on absolute x-ray exposure (kVp and mAs), which in this chapter we call *exposure latitude*.[21] To avoid this confusion, we recommend use of *contrast resolution* or *contrast optimization* to define the ability of an imaging system to display thick and thin regions, and regions of low and high atomic number, suitably in one image, and the term *exposure latitude* to define the ability

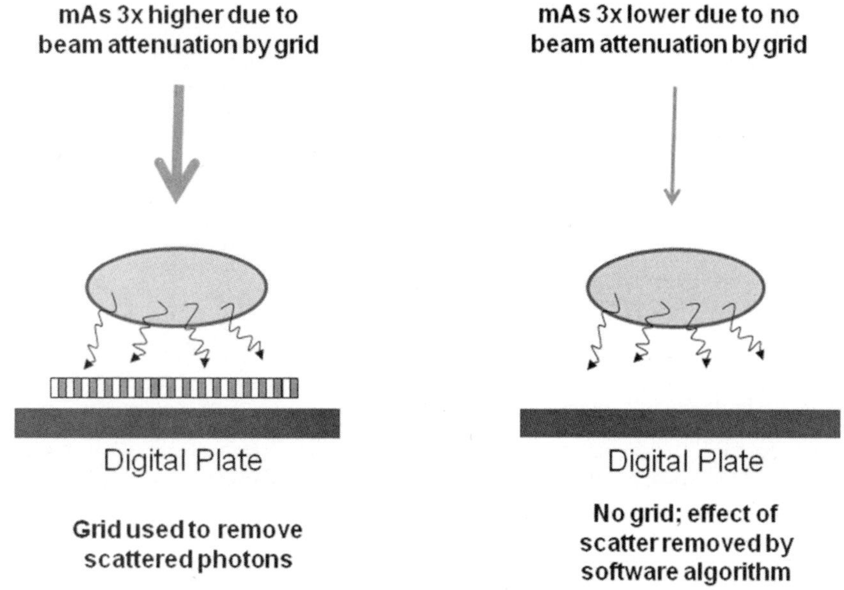

Fig. 2.11 Diagram illustrating the principle of scatter removal by a grid versus a scatter-correction software algorithm. On the *left*, the scattered photons are removed by a grid. This is standard practice in analog radiography and can also be used with computed radiography (CR), direct digital radiography (DDR), and charge-coupled device (CCD) systems. On the *right*, there is no grid, and the effect of the scattered photons has been corrected by a software scatter-correction algorithm. The mAs can be lower on the right because there is no attenuation of the primary beam by the grid. Whether the efficacy of any scatter-correction software will be adequate is subjective and should be field-tested prior to purchase.

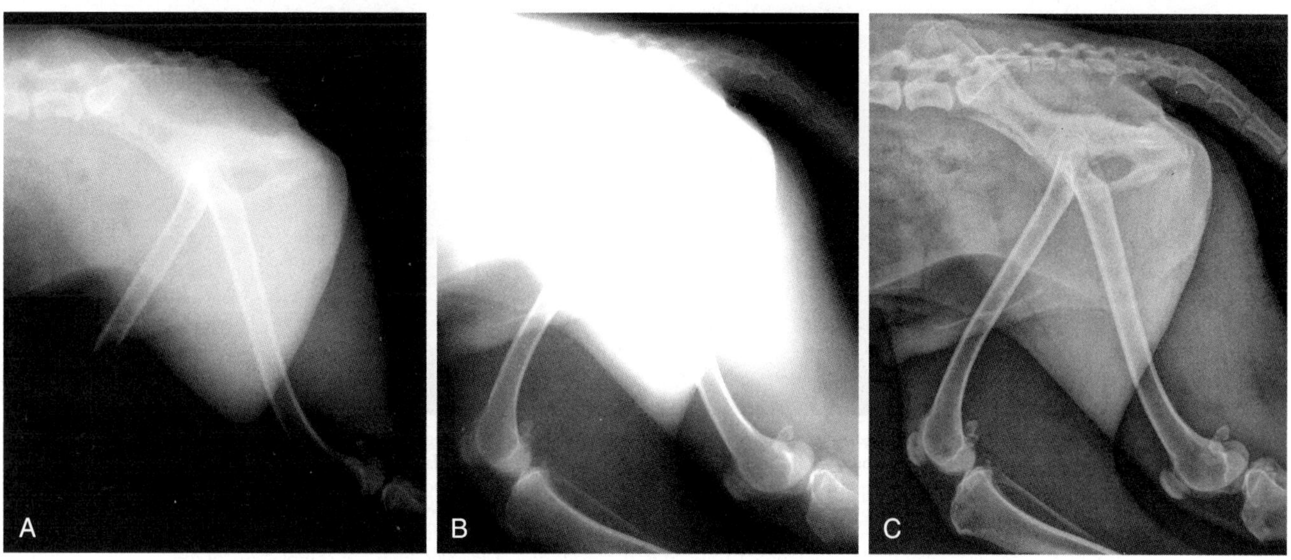

Fig. 2.12 Radiographs illustrating the contrast resolution of digital radiographs versus analog radiographs. **A,** Film radiograph made with exposure factors appropriate for the lumbar spine. The distal aspect of the femurs and the stifles are overexposed because they are thinner and cannot be adequately evaluated. **B,** Film radiograph made with exposure factors appropriate for the stifles. The spine and pelvis are underexposed because they are thicker. **C,** Digital radiograph where both the thick and thin aspects of the patient can be assessed. This wide range of gray shades characterizes the wide contrast resolution of digital radiographs. The ability to assign a gray shade to a pixel is the basis of this wide range of gray shades; this is a feature of the processing software provided by the hardware vendor.

of digital plates to compensate for either high or low kVp-to-mAs combinations that would result in overexposure or underexposure, respectively, in an analog system.

In analog imaging for any given anatomy, image contrast was controlled primarily by kVp, with some contribution from film type and use of an antiscatter grid. If a high contrast image was desired, a low kVp was used, necessitating an increase in mAs to ensure appropriate film blackness. In digital imaging, image contrast is controlled largely by algorithms (and can also be manipulated by the viewer) and as a result, is for the most part, independent of kVp. Therefore, when creating a digital technique chart, the kVp range selected for any given anatomy can be higher than would typically be used for analog imaging. This means a corresponding reduction in mAs. Reducing mAs is always desirable as it reduces the potential for motion artifact, an everyday issue in veterinary radiography.

Improved Image Accessibility and Consolidated Image Storage

The full advantages of digital imaging are best realized when digital imaging is incorporated into the global practice environment. This means integrating image acquisition and management with the hospital's electronic medical record. In a fully integrated system, radiographic studies are ordered in the electronic medical record. The order appears seamlessly at the x-ray machine computer using functionality known as *DICOM modality worklist*. Selecting the study to be performed from a list of the examinations requested for the day eliminates data entry errors that might result from having to reenter all patient information de novo and improves workflow. When the study has been acquired, appropriate charges are posted automatically in the medical record, and the images are sent to a local server for distribution and archiving. Distribution might include transmission of the images to an off-site radiologist for interpretation, with the radiographic report being entered seamlessly into the patient record after it is completed. The images are viewable through the electronic medical record using either DICOM viewing software, as described previously, or through an Internet browser.

Picture archiving and communication system (PACS) refers to the host of technologies that contribute to the creation, distribution, and archiving of digital images. The basic components of a PACS that might be found in a private veterinary practice are (1) the device, that is, the x-ray machine and the CR or DDR radiography system; (2) a server that acts as the local image archive; (3) workstations that can retrieve images from the server for remote viewing, in the examination room or surgery for example; (4) a local area network for data transfer; (5) an image communication protocol (the DICOM standard); and (6) off-site or cloud-based secure image storage (Fig. 2.21). When purchasing a digital-imaging system, there is often little attention paid to integration of the radiographic hardware and software into the overall hospital environment. This is a mistake and can result in functionality problems that compromise the advantages of transitioning to digital imaging.

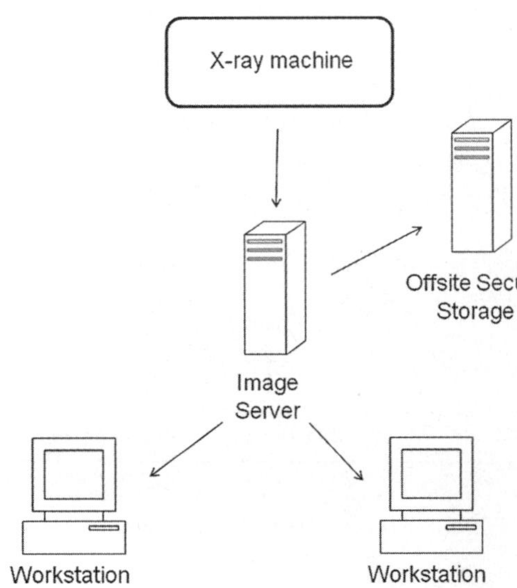

Fig. 2.21 Components of a rudimentary picture archiving and communication system (PACS) system. Images in Digital Imaging and Communications in Medicine (DICOM) format are transferred from the acquisition device, an x-ray machine in this example, to the central server. Images have been assessed by the technical staff for quality prior to being transmitted to the server. The central server must not be relied on as the sole image storage device. Secure off-site image archiving is needed. Clinicians at remote locations, such as the examination room, the intensive care unit (ICU), or surgery, can retrieve images from the server for interpretation and consultation. Images can also be sent from the server to remote locations for additional consultation.

Traditionally, DICOM images have been viewed on a DICOM workstation software that is loaded on the client computer. The images are "downloaded" to the workstation using software that is installed onto the local device, whether it is a MAC or PC operating system.

As discussed previously, the DICOM standard provides for the transmission of medical images from an imaging device or server to a DICOM workstation, using a network protocol that runs on top of the existing Internet standard protocol. There are three important aspects to this connectivity, namely, the application entity (AE) title, port, and internet protocol (IP) address or full registered host name of the computer. Typically, the "DICOM" address of the destination to which you wish to send images can be configured in modality, server, and workstation software. The DICOM transfer protocol uses nonstandard computer ports (usually 104, 4006, and 11112, depending on software). This can make receipt of images using this system problematic if firewall and other security measures are not appropriately configured. Web access to DICOM objects (WADO) is an image transmission protocol that uses http/https to transfer image data, negating some of the network configuration issues inherent in the traditional DICOM connection. DICOM images can also be transferred using browser-based technology, and this enhances image portability, particularly when accessing images beyond the local area network.[27]

The demand for enhanced image portability with minimal delays in transmission is increasing. Clinicians would like to be able to view images on mobile devices, show images to clients in consultation rooms, and provide clients with web links to images and patient data.[28,29] Two significant changes have occurred in medical image management in the last few years that have significantly enhanced image viewing. With the development of the hypertext markup language 5 (HTML5) standard for web browsers has come a tremendous opportunity to develop browser-based medical image viewers that do not require complex browser plug-ins or programs that need to be installed locally on the client computer (so called *thick client configuration*). These new viewers, known as *zero footprint viewers*, require only an HTML5-compatible browser, and many of these viewers have all the functionality of dedicated DICOM workstation software that would otherwise need to be loaded on the client computer. These viewers are browser and operating system agnostic, meaning that they work equally as well in any of the modern browses (Google Chrome, Safari, Microsoft Edge, Mozilla Firefox), running on modern Windows or Apple operating systems and also on iOS and Android devices. In addition to being browser based, they may also be a mobile device "app." There are many advantages to this technology. First, some browser plug-ins pose an increased security risk. As a result of the enhanced functionality of HTML5 and potential security issues associated with Java, browser-based viewers that use Java as a plug-in are losing popularity. Second, DICOM workstations and older browser-based viewers require the images to be downloaded; this takes time, particularly if the study is large and there is poor bandwidth. Third, most older, browser-based viewers are OS and browser specific and DICOM workstations are usually OS specific; this reduces convenience. The programs require downloading and installing (many are not free), and there is always some degree of program upkeep required. These complexities are eliminated by HTML5 zero footprint viewers.

Whereas historically, medical image archives have been limited to the DICOM file format, modern medical archives are designed to archive all types of file formats in addition to DICOM. Many other medical services in addition to diagnostic imaging generate images which should be archived in the medical record. Ophthalmologic, dermatologic, endoscopic, and arthroscopic photographs and movies are such examples. Additionally, scanned hard copy documents can be an integral part of the patient's medical record and need to be archived. Typical file formats for such medical data include .tiff, .jpeg, .pdf, and .mp4. With the advent of vendor neutral archives (VNAs), all images related to a medical record can be archived in one resource whether they were acquired by diagnostic imaging, or any other service. The term *vendor neutral archive* is somewhat of a misnomer, the important point is not that the archive is vendor neutral, but rather it is file format agnostic. Some modern HTML5 medical image viewers can display these non-DICOM format files as readily as those in DICOM format, meaning that only one interface is needed to view a variety of patient data. In human imaging the deployment of an "enterprise viewer" (defined as a thin-client or zero-client application used on any off-the-shelf device to distribute, display, and manipulate multi-specialty image, video, audio, and scanned documents stored in separate centralized archives) is becoming increasingly popular.[28]

With digital radiography, space costs for filing cabinets and cost of film envelopes and film cataloging are eliminated. Also eliminated is the problem of lost or destroyed radiographs. Digital radiographs are stored as digital files on an image server, an integral part of the PACS. A common mistake, however, is relying on only one primary storage device to archive the collection of digital radiographic files. Storing digital files on a single archive, typically on a single hard disk drive on one server, is not adequate because the hard drive can fail. Also, any other component of the server can also fail and lead to corrupt data, or the server can be destroyed during a physical disaster such as fire or flood. Storage using a redundant array of independent disks (RAID), where data are distributed over multiple disks such that if one disk fails, data integrity is preserved, is an absolute minimum for hardware redundancy. Data storage using RAID is much safer than relying on a single hard disk drive. However, although a RAID configuration does protect against individual hard drive failure, it does not protect against other hardware failures, including RAID controllers and other critical components of a server. Additionally, the data are still subject to loss through server damage during a physical disaster, an unprotected power surge, or corruption through a computer virus. The best solution is redundant off-site duplication and storage where digital radiographic data are duplicated and transferred to an off-site computer on a regular basis, preferably daily, for safe storage.

Cloud storage is commonplace in today's environment and while it is common to have a small image archive in the house, most PACS are configured such that either the primary archive is cloud-based or all studies are sent to the cloud for backup and disaster recovery.

Enhanced Portability Enables Consultation

It is difficult for most practicing veterinarians to become totally competent in radiographic interpretation. The volume of information and the nearly endless variation in how disease manifests radiographically is simply too much. Getting a second opinion on radiographic studies has been employed for decades. Analog film images were either hand-carried to a specialist, if one was lucky enough to be sufficiently close, or sent to the expert by mail or courier. The expert would interpret these images, usually telephone the veterinarian with the results, and prepare a written report that would be returned to the veterinarian along with the radiographs.

With the explosion of digital radiography in veterinary medicine, veterinary teleradiology was born. Teleradiology is a type of telemedicine that involves the electronic transmission of radiological images from one location to another for the purposes of interpretation and/or consultation with a specialist.[30] Veterinary teleradiology was first introduced commercially in the early 1990s with limited success, mostly influenced by slow Internet speeds and large file sizes, but has grown dramatically in recent years, reflecting the recent growth of the broader veterinary telemedicine market.[30–33] It is worth noting that while telemedicine is a valuable tool that augments patient care, it does not replace the patient-client relationship, and should be viewed as a supplemental service.[32]

DICOM files are large, and transmission as an email attachment can be problematic. For teleradiology consultation to work smoothly, a method of direct DICOM transfer needs to be established; this is why it is so important to ensure that the vendor of the digital radiography equipment has configured its DICOM file format appropriately. Currently, the practice of teleradiology in veterinary medicine is widespread because of the availability of broadband Internet connections, image compression, and economically priced PACS and DICOM software.[31] Also, there are many teleradiology service providers throughout the world who have teleradiographic interpretation as their primary mission. These advancements have made turnaround time very short and STAT interpretations possible.

Artificial Intelligence

Artificial intelligence (AI) is a broad term that describes a situation where a computer system performs tasks that mimic human intelligence or serves an analytical role typically satisfied by humans.[34] The field of AI has rapidly progressed in the last 20 years and has now entered the veterinary market, with vendors actively advertising AI systems that provide interpretation input on radiographs in dogs and cats.[34] In human medicine, AI imaging interpretation is bound by FDA regulations, and implementation must include strict proof of design and accuracy.[35] As a result, AI imaging interpretation tends to be narrow-focus and task specific, and often provides computer-aided diagnosis or computer-aided detection tools, rather than all-encompassing or definitive image interpretation.

In comparison, there is no regulatory framework limiting AI in veterinary medicine. Proof of efficacy is not required before a veterinary vendor can offer an AI tool. Whereas AI provides great promise and likely will result in eventual improvements in veterinary practice, the benefits of AI and proof of efficacy are not currently known. The quality of an AI model is heavily influenced by the quality of AI training and validation data used to build the AI model.[36] This type of information is not readily available for commercially available veterinary AI products. The individual veterinary practitioner who implements these tools should be aware of these limitations when evaluating a potential AI interpretation tool. This is a rapidly developing market; individual research publications evaluating AI tools in veterinary medicine have begun to appear, but more are necessary before evidence of efficacy is available.[34–39]

An Opportunity to Change the Imaging Paradigm

Veterinary medicine can be a competitive enterprise, especially in times of economic downturn. Also, pet owners are highly educated and have a wealth of information at their fingertips that they use to help make decisions regarding medical care for their pet. Being perceived as having a modern contemporary practice environment can help maintain and increase a healthy client base regardless of economic and client-education factors. Having digital radiography is one way that practices are viewed as being progressive, and being able to provide high-quality radiographic services can bolster one's professional persona.

The transition to digital radiography can help alleviate problems with radiographic exposure, and darkroom errors are also eliminated. Positioning and selecting the correct radiographic views will not be solved automatically by the transition to digital radiography, but with a digital system, the economic cost of making these modifications is insignificant. For example, with film imaging, many veterinarians were reluctant to obtain all needed views routinely, three projections of the thorax for example, because of the increased cost of expendable supplies required to do so. Radiographic studies should be priced on an examination basis, not on a per-image or per-view basis. The fee should be set such that the practice makes a profit, all necessary views are included, and the quality standards are acceptable.

Similarly, offering teleradiology consultation signals that a veterinary practice has adopted modern medical technology services. Telemedicine benefits all parties; the improved diagnostic ability improves quality of care for the owner and pet and is an additional service that can be advertised and charged by the veterinarian. The benefits of teleradiology can only be realized if high-quality, well-positioned radiographs are submitted for evaluation. Even the most experienced radiologist cannot provide meaningful consultation if the radiographs are marred by artifact, are poorly positioned, or do not focus on the area of interest.

ARTIFACTS

As with all medical-imaging modalities, there is potential for digital radiographic imaging artifacts. An artifact is an unwanted, usually non-patient-related anomaly in the image that may or may not compromise image interpretation. These occur in both CR and DDR systems and are unique from those encountered in analog film radiography. Overexposure and underexposure and how these differ in appearance from exposure errors in analog radiography were described previously. The discussion of other imaging artifacts that are observed in digital radiography is beyond the scope of this chapter, but excellent references are available.[26,40]

REFERENCES

1. Graham RN, Perriss RW, Scarsbrook AF. DICOM demystified: a review of digital file formats and their use in radiological practice. *Clin Radiol*. 2005;60:1133–1140.
2. Wright MA, Ballance D, Robertson ID, et al. Introduction to DICOM for the practicing veterinarian. *Vet Radiol Ultrasound*. 2008;49:S14–S18.
3. ACVR. Image resolution & DICOM guidelines. https://acvr.org/dashboard/resources/image-resolution-dicom-guidelines/. Accessed 9/1/2022.
4. Widmer WR. Acquisition hardware for digital imaging. *Vet Radiol Ultrasound*. 2008;49:S2–S8.
5. Watt KN, Yan K, DeCrescenzo G, et al. The physics of computed radiography: measurements of pulse height spectra of photostimulable phosphor screens using prompt luminescence. *Med Phys*. 2005;32:3589–3598.
6. Bushberg JT, Selbert JA, Leidholdt Jr EM. *The Essential Physics of Medical Imaging*. Philadelphia: Lippincott Williams & Wilkins; 2002.
7. Cowen AR, Kengyelics SM, Davies AG. Solid-state, flat-panel, digital radiography detectors and their physical imaging characteristics. *Clin Radiol*. 2008;63:487–498.
8. Knight SP. Contemporary research in digital radiography. *J Med Radiat Sci*. 2020;67:254–256.
9. Roch P, Celier D, Dessaud C, et al. Using diagnostic reference levels to evaluate the improvement of patient dose optimisation and the influence of recent technologies in radiography and computed radiography. *Eur J Radiol*. 2018;98:68–74.
10. DeMaio DN, Herrmann T, Noble LB, et al. Best practices in digital radiography. *Radiol Technol*. 2019;91:198–201.
11. Fornell D. *Advances in DR X-ray Technology at RSNA 2019*; 2020. https://www.itnonline.com/article/advances-dr-x-ray-technology-rsna-2019. Accessed 9/1/2022, 2022.
12. Lanca L, Silva A. *Digital Imaging Systems for Plain Radiography*. New York: Springer; 2013:9–19.
13. Lo WY, Puchalski SM. Digital image processing. *Vet Radiol Ultrasound*. 2008;49:S42–47.
14. Feghali JA, Chambers G, Delepierre J, et al. New image quality and dose reduction technique for pediatric digital radiography. *Diagn Interv Imaging*. 2021;102:463–470.
15. Goo JM, Choi JY, Im JG, et al. Effect of monitor luminance and ambient light on observer performance in soft-copy reading of digital chest radiographs. *Radiology*. 2004;232:762–766.
16. Pollard BJ, Samei E, Chawla AS, et al. The effects of ambient lighting in chest radiology reading rooms. *J Digit Imaging*. 2012;25:520–526.
17. Brennan PC, McEntee M, Evanoff M, et al. Ambient lighting: effect of illumination on soft-copy viewing of radiographs of the wrist. *AJR Am J Roentgenol*. 2007;188:W177–W180.
18. Krupinski EA, Kallergi M. Choosing a radiology workstation: technical and clinical considerations. *Radiology*. 2007;242:671–682.
19. Bushberg JT, Seibert JA, Leidholdt Jr EM. *Essential Physical Medical Imaging*. 2nd ed. Philadelphia: Lippincott Williams & Wilkins; 2002.
20. Lo WY, Hornof WJ, Zwingenberger AL, et al. Multiscale image processing and antiscatter grids in digital radiography. *Vet Radiol Ultrasound*. 2009;50:569–576.
21. Korner M, Weber CH, Wirth S, et al. Advances in digital radiography: physical principles and system overview. *Radiographics*. 2007;27:675–686.
22. Shepard SJ, Wang J, Flynn M, et al. An exposure indicator for digital radiography: AAPM Task Group 116 (executive summary). *Med Phys*. 2009;36:2898–2914.
23. Butler ML, Rainford L, Last J, et al. Are exposure index values consistent in clinical practice? A multi-manufacturer investigation. *Radiat Prot Dosimetry*. 2010;139:371–374.
24. Don S, Whiting BR, Rutz LJ, et al. New exposure indicators for digital radiography simplified for radiologists and technologists. *AJR Am J Roentgenol*. 2012;199:1337–1341.
25. Akhtar W, Aslam M, Ali A, et al. Film retakes in digital and conventional radiography. *J Coll Physicians Surg Pak*. 2008;18:151–153.
26. Drost WT, Reese DJ, Hornof WJ. Digital radiography artifacts. *Vet Radiol Ultrasound*. 2008;49:S48–S56.
27. Lipton P, Nagy P, Sevinc G. Leveraging internet technologies with DICOM WADO. *J Digit Imaging*. 2012;25:646–652.
28. Roth CJ, Lannum LM, Dennison DK, et al. The current state and path forward for enterprise image viewing: HIMSS-SIIM Collaborative White Paper. *J Digit Imaging*. 2016;29:567–573.
29. Roth CJ, Lannum LM, Joseph CL. Enterprise imaging governance: HIMSS-SIIM collaborative white paper. *J Digit Imaging*. 2016;29:539–546.
30. AVMA. *Veterinary Telehealth: The Basics*; 2022. https://www.avma.org/resources-tools/animal-health-and-welfare/telehealth-telemedicine-veterinary-practice/veterinary-telehealth-basics. Accessed 9/1/2022.
31. Poteet BA. Veterinary teleradiology. *Vet Radiol Ultrasound*. 2008;49:S33–S36.
32. Drummond A. *Regarding Veterinary-Client-Patient Relationship and Telemedicine*. California Veterinary Medical Board; 2019. https://www.vmb.ca.gov/meetings/materials/072019item11c.pdf.
33. AVMA. *Telehealth & Telemedicine in Veterinary Practice*; 2022. https://www.avma.org/resources-tools/animal-health-and-welfare/telehealth-telemedicine-veterinary-practice. Accessed 9/1/2022.
34. Appleby RB, Basran PS. Artificial intelligence in veterinary medicine. *J Am Vet Med Assoc*. 2022;260:819–824.

35. Hosny A, Parmar C, Quackenbush J, et al. Artificial intelligence in radiology. *Nat Rev Cancer*. 2018;18:500–510.
36. Basran PS, Appleby RB. The unmet potential of artificial intelligence in veterinary medicine. *Am J Vet Res*. 2022;83:385–392.
37. Hur B, Hardefeldt LY, Verspoor K, et al. Overcoming challenges in extracting prescribing habits from veterinary clinics using big data and deep learning. *Aust Vet J*. 2022;100:220–222.
38. Awaysheh A, Wilcke J, Elvinger F, et al. Identifying free-text features to improve automated classification of structured histopathology reports for feline small intestinal disease. *J Vet Diagn Invest*. 2018;30:211–217.
39. Kim E, Fischetti AJ, Sreetharan P, et al. Comparison of artificial intelligence to the veterinary radiologist's diagnosis of canine cardiogenic pulmonary edema. *Vet Radiol Ultrasound*. 2022;63:292–297.
40. Jimenez DA, Armbrust LJ, O'Brien RT, et al. Artifacts in digital radiography. *Vet Radiol Ultrasound*. 2008;49:321–332.

ELECTRONIC RESOURCES

Additional information related to the content in Chapter 2 can be found online at eBooks.Health.Elsevier.com

- Chapter Quiz

CHAPTER 3

Physics of Ultrasound Imaging

Hock Gan Heng • Wm Tod Drost

Diagnostic ultrasound is a widely used, indispensable diagnostic imaging modality that does not use electromagnetic radiation. An understanding of the physics of ultrasound is important because it helps explain some of the limitations of the modality and the artifacts encountered. In this chapter, the physical principles of ultrasound waves, the interactions of ultrasound waves with matter, transducers, Doppler techniques, and ultrasound artifacts are discussed.

PHYSICAL PRINCIPLES OF ULTRASOUND WAVES

Sound travels in waves and transmits energy by alternating regions of low pressure (rarefaction) and high pressure (compression).[1-3] Unlike light and radio waves, sound waves require a medium through which to travel.[4,5] Frequency, wavelength, and velocity are parameters used to describe sound waves; these terms are also used in reference to electromagnetic radiation.

Frequency is the number of times a wave is repeated per second. One wave or cycle occurs when pressure starts at a normal value, increases to a high value, decreases (passing the normal value) to a low value, and then returns to normal. A cycle may also be defined as the combination of compression and successive rarefaction.[3] Frequency is expressed in hertz (Hz), where 1 Hz equals one cycle per second. Sound greater than 20,000 Hz (0.02 MHz) is defined as ultrasound.[3,4] In diagnostic ultrasound, the frequencies are typically between 2 megahertz (MHz) and 15 MHz (1 MHz = 1,000,000 Hz).

Wavelength is the distance traveled by a sound wave in one cycle. In ultrasonography, wavelength is expressed in millimeters (mm). Wavelength is important for image resolution.

Velocity is the rate at which sound travels through an acoustic medium; it is determined by the physical density (mass per unit volume) and stiffness (hardness) of the acoustic medium.[1,3] As a rule, velocity is highest in solids, lower in liquids, and the lowest in gases. Within soft tissue, the average velocity of sound is 1.54 mm/μs (1540 m/s).[1-4] The velocity of sound in soft tissue is important because ultrasound machines use this constant velocity for all calculations.

Velocity is related to frequency and wavelength of a sound wave in the following equation:

$$\text{Velocity (mm}/\mu\text{s)} = \text{Frequency (MHz)} \times \text{Wavelength (mm)}$$

ULTRASOUND WAVE INTERACTION WITH MATTER

Acoustic impedance of a tissue is the product of the tissue's physical density and sound velocity within the tissue.[3] Changes in acoustic impedance from one tissue to another determine how much of the sound wave is reflected and how much is transmitted into the second tissue. The amplitude of the returning echo, which is what is used to make the image, is proportional to the difference in acoustic impedance in two adjacent tissues or substances. If two tissues have the same acoustic impedance, then no echo is created. If a large difference in acoustic impedance exists between two tissues, then almost all the sound is reflected in an echo.[1,3] Almost all sound is reflected at soft tissue/gas and soft tissue/bone interfaces. Thus, little or no sound passes these boundaries. Hence, the speed of sound in bone and gas-filled lung is not important clinically. This nearly total sound reflection creates an acoustic void, or *shadow*, deep to the tissue interface. Without placement of acoustic coupling gel between the patient and transducer, the soft tissue/gas interface created by gas trapped between the skin and transducer would prevent imaging because of reflection of all sound waves and no transmission of sound waves into the body.

Angle of incidence is the angle at which a sound wave encounters a medium. If the angle of incidence is perpendicular (90 degrees) to the reflector, the reflected portion of the sound wave travels 180 degrees opposite to the direction of the initial sound wave, returning to the transducer, and the transmitted portion of the sound wave continues in the same direction as the initial sound wave. If the angle of incidence is not perpendicular, then the angle of reflectance equals the angle of incidence. Any sound wave that is not reflected toward the transducer will not be recorded. A key fact is that the amount of reflected and transmitted sound depends on the *difference in acoustic impedance* of the two media.

An ultrasound beam is attenuated (loses strength), as it travels through a medium. The amount of attenuation is determined by the distance traveled and the frequency of the sound wave. High-frequency sound waves are attenuated more than low-frequency sound waves. Attenuation of the sound wave involves three components: absorption, reflection, and scattering.[1-3]

Absorption is the conversion of the mechanical energy of sound waves to heat.[2,3] Absorption is the dominant component of attenuation of sound in soft tissue.[2,3] However, the relative amount of sound absorbed is quite low, and the temperature change is insignificant and imperceptible.

Reflection of the sound beam contributes to attenuation. As the sound wave encounters tissue interfaces of different acoustic impedance, a reflection is generated. Only reflections that return to the transducer are used for image formation.

Scattering is independent of frequency and occurs when sound waves encounter small, irregular surfaces. This occurs mainly within the parenchyma of organs and is responsible for the echotexture of internal organs.[2,3]

TRANSDUCERS

In ultrasound imaging, transducers contain piezoelectric crystals that convert electric current into sound waves.[2,6] As an electric charge is applied to a piezoelectric crystal, the material deforms and creates a sound wave. Conversely, when sound waves are applied to piezoelectric crystals, they produce an electric signal. Therefore, the same crystal is used to send and receive sound waves.[3] For typical ultrasound imaging, the transducer emits sound waves less than 1% of the time and receives sound waves more than 99% of the time.[7] The pulse repetition frequency (PRF) is the number of times this pattern of sending and receiving is repeated within 1 second.[3] The length of space in one pulse of ultrasound is called the spatial pulse length (SPL). If a sound wave has a wavelength of 0.5 mm and three pulses are sent each time, the SPL is 1.5 mm. SPL is important for axial resolution, with shorter SPL resulting in better axial resolution.

Ultrasound transducers come in many shapes and sizes. The selection of a transducer depends on the physical properties of the transducer and the anatomic region to be imaged.

Electronic transducers, also called *array transducers*, are composed of several small elements in various arrangements. The elements may be arranged in a line or rectangle (linear array), in a curved line (convex array), or in concentric ring fashion (annular array).[8] The elements that compose these transducers are electronically fired in various sequences to create different-shaped fields of view (e.g., rectangular, wedge) and to focus the sound beam at specific depths.

Images made using a sector transducer are pie shaped (Fig. 3.1A), and images made using a linear transducer are rectangular (see Fig. 3.1B). The *footprint* of a transducer is the amount of the transducer that contacts the patient and linear transducers usually have larger footprints than sector transducer. For thoracic imaging, sector-shaped transducers are preferable because images must be acquired intercostally. For abdominal imaging, the use of sector or linear transducers is often dictated by the anatomic structure being imaged and the size of the patient. In most instances, more than one transducer is used during a single examination.

Resolution is the ability of an ultrasound machine to distinguish echoes based on space, time, and strength.[6] Axial resolution is the ability to distinguish two separate reflectors along the direction in which the sound wave is traveling and is equal to half the SPL. When two reflectors are separated by a distance that is greater than half the SPL, the echoes from these two reflectors do not overlap as they return to the transducer and are displayed as separate echoes. If the distance between the reflectors is less than half the SPL, the returning echoes overlap and are displayed as a single echo. Because transducers with higher frequency have a shorter SPL, axial resolution is improved.

Lateral resolution is the ability to distinguish two separate reflectors perpendicular to the direction in which the sound wave is traveling.[6] This is determined by the width of the ultrasound beam.[6] To recognize the objects discretely, the ultrasound beam must be narrower than the distance between the objects. The width of an ultrasound beam decreases with increasing frequency. In a focused ultrasound beam, where the width of the beam is restricted, the lateral resolution is best at the focal point of the ultrasound beam because this is the narrowest part of the beam.[6]

Depth of sound-wave penetration into the body varies inversely with sound wave frequency. Higher-frequency transducers are best for structures that are close to the surface while lower-frequency transducers are best for deeper structures. As a guide, one can begin with a higher-frequency transducer because it has better resolution (higher image quality) and then

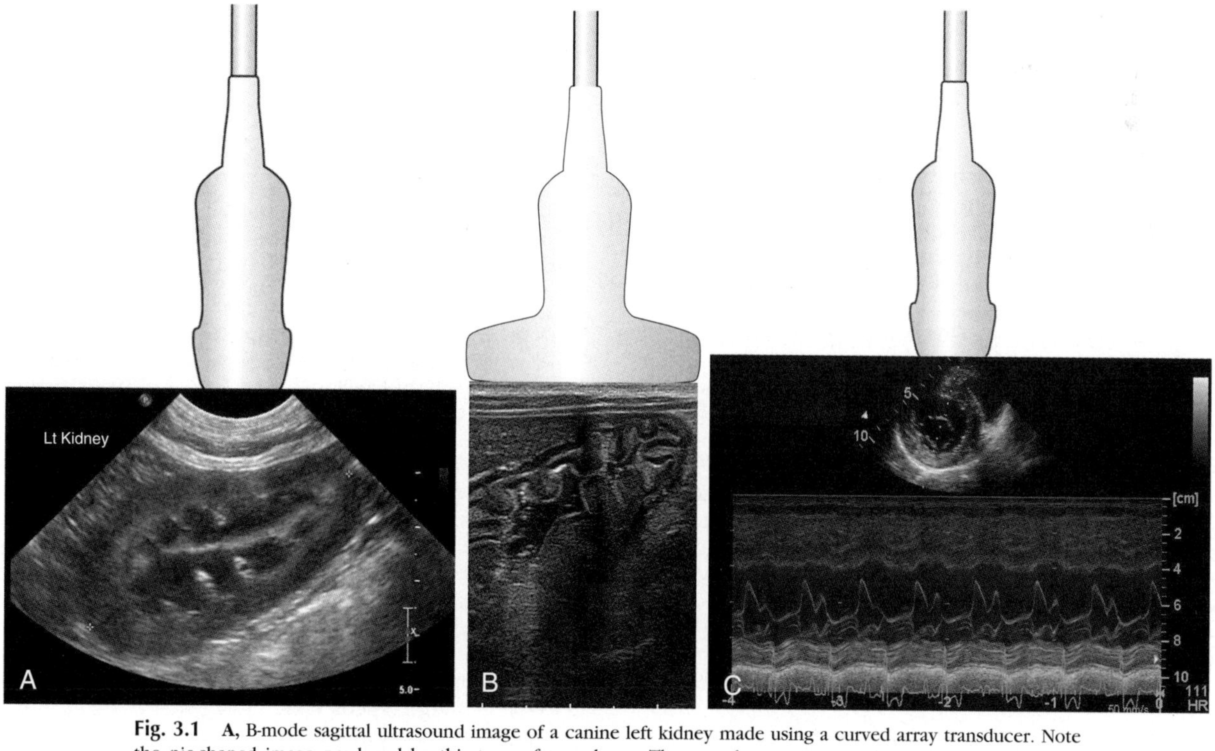

Fig. 3.1 **A,** B-mode sagittal ultrasound image of a canine left kidney made using a curved array transducer. Note the pie-shaped image produced by this type of transducer. The transducer points to the cranial of the patient (indicated by the ■ symbol at the *left* side of the screen). Thus, the cranial pole of the kidney is at the *left* side of the screen and the caudal pole of the kidney is at the right side of the screen. **B,** Image of a feline stomach made using a linear array transducer. Note the rectangular image. **C,** M-mode image depicting movement of the mitral valve. At the top of the image is a B-mode, short-axis image of the left ventricle at the level of the mitral valve. The *dotted line* in the middle of the B-mode image marks the location of the M-mode tracing on the bottom of the image. The M-mode tracing depicts the movement of the mitral valve and left ventricle over time. An electrocardiograph tracing is superimposed in the bottom of the image.

switch to a lower-frequency transducer if deeper structures are not imaged well.

New Technologies in Ultrasound

These technologies are incorporated in most of the newer ultrasound machines and influence the image quality greatly. Thus, knowing the basics and adjusting these features when scanning patients will help improve lesion conspicuity.

Broad bandwidth technology allows for transducers to emit a wide range of frequencies. This allows the user to select various frequencies from the same transducer.[6] A modern broadband 4 MHz transducer can emit frequencies between 1 and 7 MHz.[9] The broadband frequency transducers improve near-field resolution by using the higher frequency of the spectrum and far-field resolution by using the lower frequency of the spectrum. Additionally, axial resolution is improved because these transducers use shorter SPLs.[9]

Harmonic imaging improves normal organ and lesion conspicuity.[9] Harmonics are integer multiples of the frequency of the transmitted ultrasound pulse.[10] If the transmitted frequency (the fundamental frequency or first harmonic) is 4 MHz (F), then the second harmonic is 8 MHz (2F), and the third harmonic is 12 MHz (3F), and so forth.[2,3,9,10] During the interaction of sound waves and tissue, weak echoes are generated at harmonic frequencies.[4] When the echoes return to the ultrasound machine operating in harmonic mode, bandpass filters are applied to reject frequencies that are outside of the specific range.[4,11] For harmonic imaging, the bandpass filter can remove the fundamental frequency allowing the second harmonic frequencies to pass.[10] This results in improved image quality because of three fundamental factors.[11] First, the primary beam is much narrower, improving lateral resolution. Second, some artifacts (discussed later) are reduced or eliminated because the extra beams are not sufficiently strong to generate harmonics. Third, the harmonic beam is generated at a depth beyond where some of the artifactual problems occur, thus reducing image degradation and reducing noise in the near field of the image.

Spatial compounding is a composite image generated by combining multiple frames from ultrasound beams that are angled in different directions.[2,4,11-13] The sound waves from electronic transducers can be steered in multiple directions without moving the transducer. The multiple angles increase the probability of the sound wave encountering a reflector at a 90-degree angle.[5,11] The frames from different angles are compounded and displayed as a single image. Compound images were perceived to have improved contrast resolution, border definition, and/or increased signal-to-noise ratio compared with noncompounded images.[2,13] The number of frames for spatial compounding are an odd number, 3, 5, 7, 9, and so on. The higher the number of frames, the better the spatial resolution and image quality. Generally, a linear transducer has a higher number of frames for spatial compounding. This control is important as spatial compound imaging reduces shadowing artifact, which is used to recognize high attenuating structures such as renal calculi. Turning off spatial compound imaging may help the operator identify the renal calculi (see Fig. 3.7B,D)[2,4]

DISPLAY

Image formation is based on the pulse echo principle.[2,14] The electric signals generated from the returning echoes are amplified to form the final image. When the initial burst of sound is sent into the tissue, a timer is started to determine the amount of time it takes to receive echoes. The elapsed time from sending to receiving is directly related to the distance traveled by the sound wave.[14] The ultrasound machine assumes a constant rate for the velocity of sound (1.54 mm/μs), and because time is recorded, distance can easily be calculated.

Two modes of echo display are used commonly in ultrasonography: brightness mode (B-mode, B scan, or grayscale) and motion mode (M-mode). B-mode is used commonly in both abdominal and cardiac imaging. M-mode is used only for echocardiography.[3]

B-mode images are composed of a collection of dots that correspond to the amplitude or strength of the returning echo.[11] These dots are displayed on a black background, and the brightness or grayscale of the dot is highest (whitest) for the strongest returning echoes. The depth of the structure returning the echoes determines the position of the dots. Multiple thin scan lines make up a complete image so that B-mode images look like a slice of tissue (see Fig. 3.1A,B).[1]

M-mode records a thin section of an ultrasound image over time (see Fig. 3.1C). The region for M-mode imaging is chosen using a B-mode image; the selected M-mode region is usually represented on the screen as a line. Once the M-mode cursor is in the desired location, M-mode is activated. On an M-mode image, the depth of the image is displayed on the vertical axis, and time is displayed on the horizontal axis. The brightness of the dots is proportional to the strength of the returning echoes, as in B-mode. When holding the transducer stationary, the examiner can evaluate how structures move over time. M-mode imaging is used most commonly in echocardiography to evaluate the function of the ventricles and heart valves.

In B-mode imaging, the displayed organs vary with the orientation of the structures being imaged and the position of the transducer. Generally, the transducer should point to cranial with the left side of the screen representing cranial in longitudinal and sagittal orientation (see Fig. 3.1A) and to the right of the patient in transverse orientation. For cardiac imaging, the right side of the screen is cranial in long-axis images. The portion of the image closest to the transducer, the top of the screen, is called the *near field* and the opposite side is called the *far field*.

BASIC SCANNER CONTROLS

Gain affects the amplification of the returning echoes within the receiver. There are two types of gain: general gain and time gain compensation (TGC) that could be adjusted.

General gain: Increasing or decreasing the gain increases or decreases the overall brightness of the image; this should be adjusted at the beginning of each scan. If the gain is too low, the subtle parenchymal detail of tissue is lost. If the gain is too high, contrast resolution is lost due to overall bright image.[11]

Time gain compensation (TGC): Because sound waves lose intensity (attenuation) as they travel in tissue, echoes returning from deeper tissues are weaker than echoes returning from tissues closer to the transducer. To make an image uniform in brightness, amplification of the echoes from deeper tissues to a greater degree than echoes from shallow tissues is helpful. TGC controls allow the user to adjust the gain in selected regions/depth of the image.[11] Typically, an ultrasound machine has a series of slider-bars that control gain to echoes that emanate from various depths. The top sliders control gain for structures in the near field and bottom sliders for gain in the far field (Fig. 3.2). Overall, gain should be adjusted first, then specific regions of the image using the TGC.[11]

Frequency: The highest frequency available to penetrate to the depth of interest should be used because this helps to increase the axial resolution of the image. Thus, using a linear transducer with higher frequency for superficial

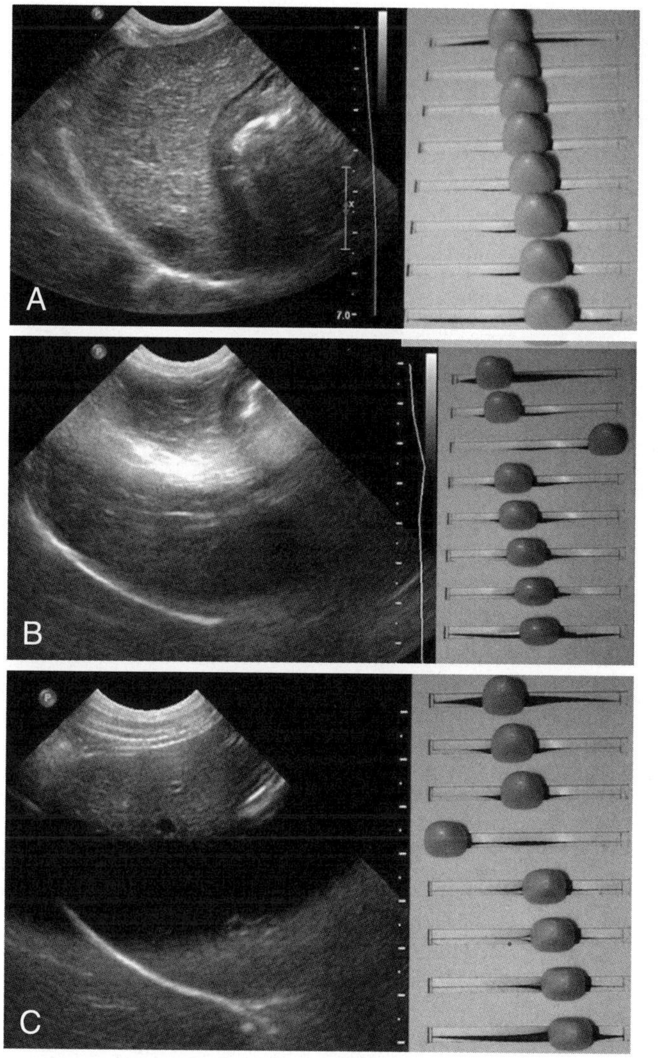

Fig. 3.2 **A,** Ultrasound image of a canine liver using a correct time gain compensation. **B,** The time gain compensation at the third zone was incorrectly overcompensated causing a hyperechoic band in the region. **C,** The time gain compensation at the fourth zone was undercompensated causing hypoechoic band in the region.

structures, such as the gastrointestinal tract, will provide a study with better imaging quality.

Focal point or region: The focal point or region should be adjusted to the region of interest as this will help to increase the lateral resolution. This will also make the identification of abnormality easier. In most ultrasound machines, a single or multiple focal points can be selected. However, the frame rate will be slower when the number of focal points increases. Thus, the use of a single focal point is encouraged. In some ultrasound machines, there is no focal point, and a region/range of focus is present.

Depth of field: The depth of field will determine the displayed size of the organs examined. As a norm, the depth of field should be adjusted so the image of organ is as large as possible to fill the monitor once the structure is identified.

PRINCIPLES OF INTERPRETATION

Echogenicity relates to the relative brightness of a structure. Anechoic structures have no echoes and appear black. When the echogenicity of two structures is compared, the darker structure is hypoechoic, and the brighter structure is hyperechoic. If the structures have the same degree of brightness, they are isoechoic to each other. Because tissue derangements result in changes in echogenicity, it is important to know the relative echogenicity of each abdominal organ. Box 3.1 lists abdominal organs in order of relative echogenicity; however, there is some variability of normal particularly in renal cortex echogenicity.[15] Detecting diffuse changes in echogenicity of a whole organ is difficult, and accurate detection is related to the experience of the sonographer. Machine settings and transducer selection may alter the echogenicity of an organ. Thus, internal organ auto referencing, or multiple abdominal organs, may be compared to determine organ echogenicity.[16] Focal changes in echogenicity are easier to detect because the adjacent normal parenchyma can be compared (Fig. 3.3).

Box 3.1

General Guidelines of Relative Echogenicity of Commonly Encountered Structures in Order of Decreasing Echogenicity

Bone, gas, organ boundaries
Structural fat, vessel walls
Renal sinus
Prostate (intact male)
Spleen
Storage fat
Liver
Renal cortex
Muscle
Renal medulla
Prostate (neutered male)
Bile, urine

From Park RD, Nyland TG, Lattimer JC, et al. B-Mode Gray-scale ultrasound — imaging artifacts and interpretation principles. Vet Radiol. 1981;22:204–210.

DOPPLER TECHNIQUES

The Doppler technique is used in the investigation of blood flow direction and velocity. There are a few different techniques that are based on the Doppler principles.[17]

Doppler Principle

The pitch of a train whistle or a siren changes as the source of the sound approaches or moves away from the listener. The change in pitch, or sound-wave frequency, is called the *Doppler shift*. This principle has been applied to medical sonography, allowing imaging of the direction and velocity of blood flow. The Doppler effect is named for Johann Christian Andreas Doppler, an Austrian mathematician and physicist, who first proposed the effect in 1842.

In ultrasonography, the change in sound frequency is caused by a moving reflector, most commonly red blood cells. The Doppler shift is the frequency difference between the incident sound waves and the reflected sound waves and is described by the following formula[17]:

$$f_D = (2 \times f_O \times U_{RBC})/c \qquad \text{(Eq. 3.1)}$$

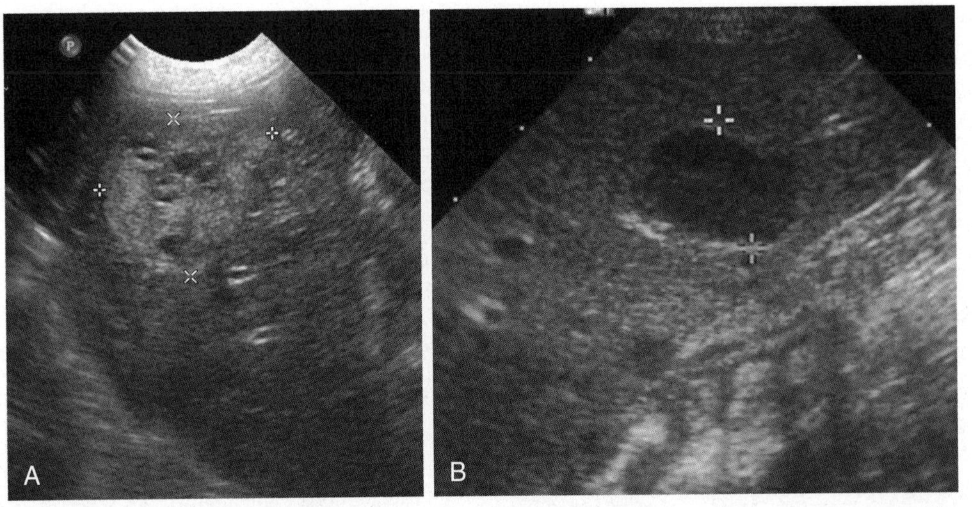

Fig. 3.3 Long-axis ultrasound images of the liver. **A,** A hyperechoic nodule in the liver of a dog indicated by calipers. **B,** A hypoechoic nodule in the liver of a dog, indicated by calipers.

where f_D is the frequency of Doppler shift, f_O is the original frequency; U_{RBC} is the velocity of red blood cells; and c is the speed of sound in soft tissue. The frequency of Doppler shift, recorded in Hz (versus MHz used for sonographic imaging), is in the audible range. Hence, ultrasound machines emit sound related to the Doppler shift.

It is assumed in Eq. 3.1 that the sound waves are parallel to the direction of blood flow. Realistically, when sound waves strike blood vessels, the sound waves are rarely parallel to the direction of flow. The Doppler angle is the angle between the blood-flow direction and the sound wave direction.[18] Without accounting for the Doppler angle, the Doppler shift is underestimated.[18] This is very important for quantification of blood flow. Accounting for the Doppler angle, the velocity of blood flow is calculated by the following formula[19]:

$$U_{RBC} = (f_D \times c)/(2 \times f_O \times \cos\theta)$$

where U_{RBC} is the velocity of red blood cells, f_D is the frequency of Doppler shift, c is the speed of sound in soft tissue, f_O is the original frequency, *cos* is cosine, and θ is the Doppler angle.

Doppler shift cannot be measured if the Doppler angle is 90 degrees because the cosine of a 90-degree angle is 0, and division by 0 is not possible. The Doppler angle θ should be less than 60 degrees for the velocity to be considered accurate,[20] with angles between 30 and 60 degrees being easiest to image.[17]

DOPPLER MODES

Four Doppler modes are discussed: (1) continuous-wave Doppler, (2) pulsed-wave Doppler, (3) color Doppler, and (4) power Doppler.

Continuous-wave Doppler is performed by using two separate crystals housed in one transducer.[17] One crystal emits sound continuously, and the second receives echoes continuously. Continuous-wave Doppler is highly accurate for measuring the Doppler shift. Compared with pulsed-wave Doppler, much higher velocities can be recorded with continuous-wave Doppler because of the continuous signal sampling. The crystal emitting the sound does not have to wait to receive echoes because the second crystal handles the echo-receiving task. However, with continuous-wave Doppler, all Doppler shifts along the path of the sound wave are measured, making differentiation of blood-flow velocity from two blood vessels in the path of the sound wave impossible. This mode is commonly used in echocardiography.

Pulsed-wave Doppler is performed by using the same crystal for sending and receiving sound.[21] Pulsed-wave Doppler is used in combination with B-mode imaging; this is termed *duplex Doppler* (Fig. 3.4A).[17] A blood vessel is selected in the B-mode image for Doppler interrogation, and an electronic region of frequency sampling, called the *gate*, is positioned in the blood vessel. In Fig. 3.4A, the gate, the two parallel lines, is in the aorta. The electronic gate is the only area from which echoes are accepted for flow quantification. Being able to select a blood vessel for interrogation visually is a benefit of pulsed-wave Doppler. This is commonly used in measuring portal vein velocity.

A spectral tracing is produced with both continuous- and pulsed-wave Doppler. The tracing records the velocity and direction of blood flow as a function of time (see Fig. 3.4A). Tracing above the baseline represents blood flow toward the transducer, and tracing below the baseline represents blood flow away from the transducer.[20] If the blood-flow velocity within the sample area is homogenous, the spectral tracing will be thin (see Fig. 3.4A) with an empty area under the curve. Spectral broadening is caused by turbulence or variable speed blood flow and refers to the thickness of the spectral tracing.[17] If a large range of blood-flow velocity is present within the sample area, the spectral tracing will be broad and the area under the curve is filled in. Alternatively, spectral broadening can occur if the transducer is close to the blood vessel, resulting in multiple ultrasound beam angles between the transducer and blood vessel.[17] Spectral tracing is routinely performed in echocardiography to assess blood flow direction and measure velocity.

Color Doppler is a variation of pulsed-wave Doppler.[17] Blood-flow velocity is recorded in multiple regions within an image, and the mean velocities are color-coded. The user determines the size and location of the color Doppler region of interest, which can be much larger than the sample gate used for pulsed-wave Doppler. Color-coded

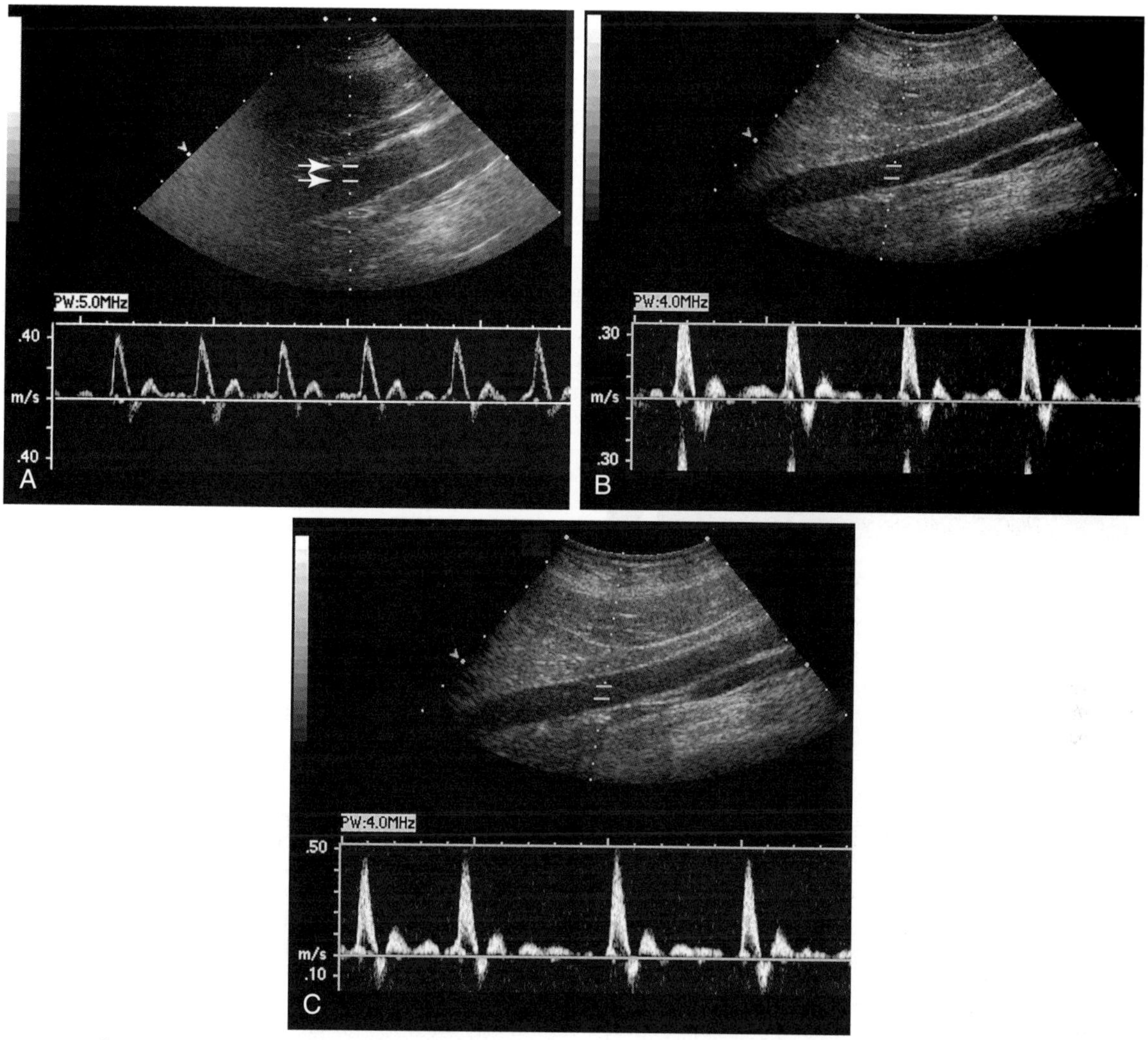

Fig. 3.4 **A,** Duplex Doppler ultrasound image illustrating pulsed-wave Doppler interrogation of a canine aorta. The B-mode image, in the near field, shows placement of the pulsed-wave Doppler gate (*parallel lines, white arrows*) in the central aspect of the aorta. This is the region in which blood-flow velocity is measured. The pulsed-wave Doppler spectral tracing is in the far field. The *solid white line* in the center of the spectral tracing represents the baseline where blood flow = 0 m/s. Signal above baseline represents flow toward the transducer, whereas signal below the baseline represents flow away from the transducer. The velocity scale on the *left* ranges from 0 to 0.40 m/s toward the transducer and 0 to 0.40 m/s away from the transducer. The pulsatile velocity tracing is typical of an artery. **B,** Aliasing of the spectral tracing is noted by the peaks of the "tall spike" being displayed on the bottom of the spectral tracing. The scale indicates that the highest velocity is 0.30 m/s. Because the peak velocity of blood flow within the aorta is greater than 0.30 m/s, the computer displays the tracing on the other end of the scale. Aliasing is corrected (see **A**) by increasing the scale, which increases the pulse repetition frequency (PRF). Note that the width of the spectral tracing in **B** is wider than in **A**. This is caused by more homogeneous velocity of blood flow within the pulsed-wave Doppler gate in part **A**. **C,** Aliasing is corrected by changing the range of velocities displayed; this is also called adjusting the baseline. The velocity range displayed is now from 0.20 m/s away from the transducer to 0.50 m/s toward the transducer compared with part **B**, and aliasing has been eliminated.

information is superimposed on the grayscale B-mode image within the region of interest (Fig. 3.5). Red and blue hues are used commonly for color Doppler. One color indicates net blood flow toward the transducer (most commonly red), and the other color in the reference scale indicates net blood flow away from the transducer (most commonly blue). Velocity of flow is indicated by the intensity or hue of the color. Limitations of color Doppler include that only mean velocity is displayed and that the maximum velocity that can be displayed is limited. Color Doppler is angle dependent so that no Doppler shift is recorded when blood flow is 90 degrees to the transducer. Color Doppler is useful to determine the presence or absence, direction, speed, and/or character of blood flow.[19]

Power Doppler is a signal-processing method that analyzes the total strength of the Doppler signal. This could be related to the direction of the blood flow (directional power Doppler) or ignoring direction of blow flood (nondirectional power Doppler).[17,21,22] This is determined by the concentration of the moving red blood cells. With power Doppler, a color map of the Doppler shift will be created, where the hue and brightness of the color represent the power of the Doppler signal. Power Doppler information

9. Ziegler L, O'Brien RT. Harmonic ultrasound: a review. *Vet Radiol Ultrasound*. 2002;43:501–509.
10. Anvari A, Forsberg F, Samir AE. A primer on the physical principles of tissue harmonic imaging. *Radiographics*. 2015;35:1955–1964.
11. Kremkau FW. Instruments. In: Kremkau FW, ed. *Sonography: Principles and Instruments*. St. Louis: Elsevier Saunders; 2011:69–124.
12. O'Brien RT, Holmes SP. Recent advances in ultrasound technology. *Clin Tech Small Anim Pract*. 2007;22:93–103.
13. Whatmough C, Guitian J, Baines E, et al. Ultrasound image compounding: effect on perceived image quality. *Vet Radiol Ultrasound*. 2007;48:141–145.
14. Kremkau FW. Introduction. In: Kremkau FW, ed. *Sonography: Principles and Instruments*. St. Louis: Elsevier Saunders; 2011:1–12.
15. Park RD, Nyland TG, Lattimer JC, et al. B-Mode Gray-scale ultrasound – imaging artifacts and interpretation principles. *Vet Radiol*. 1981;22:204–210.
16. Chou PH, Gan HH, Lin FJ, et al. Absence of renal cortical anisotrophic backscattering artifact in feline chronic kidney disease. *Vet Q*. 2021;41, 210-116.
17. Boote EJ. AAPM/RSNA physics tutorial for residents: topics in US: Doppler US techniques: concepts of blood flow detection and flow dynamics. *Radiographics*. 2003;23: 1315–1327.
18. Prabhu SJ, Kanal K, Bhargava P, et al. Ultrasound artifacts: classification, applied physics with illustrations, and imaging appearances. *Ultrasound Q*. 2014;30:145–157.
19. Kremkau FW. Doppler principles. In: Kremkau FW, ed. *Sonography: Principles and Instruments*. St. Louis: Elsevier Saunders; 2011:125–175.
20. Wood MM, Romine LE, Lee YK, et al. Spectral Doppler signature waveforms in ultrasonography: a review of normal and abnormal waveforms. *Ultrasound Q*. 2010;26: 83–99.
21. Kremkau FW. Artifacts. In: Kremkau FW, ed. *Sonography: Principles and Instruments*. St. Louis: Elsevier Saunders; 2011:176–210.
22. Bude RO, Rubin JM. Power Doppler sonography. *Radiology*. 1996;200:21–23.
23. Nikolina L, Pascaline P, Marco BT, et al. Contrast-enhanced ultrasonography in dogs with inflammatory bowel disease. *J Vet Intern Med*. 2021;35:2167–2176.
24. Banzato T, Rubini G, Orlandi R, et al. Contrast-enhanced ultrasound features of hepatocellular carcinoma in dogs. *Vet Rec*. 2020;186:187.
25. Tamura M, Ohta H, Shimbo G, et al. Usefulness of noninvasive shear wave elastography for the assessment of hepatic fibrosis in dogs with hepatic disease. *J Vet Intern Med*. 2019;33:2067–2074.
26. Seiler GS, Griffith E. Comparisons between elastography stiffness scores for benign versus malignant lymph nodes in dogs and cats. *Vet Radiol Ultrasound*. 2018;59:79–88.
27. Feldman MK, Katyal S, Blackwood MS. US artifacts. *Radiographics*. 2009;29:1179–1189.
28. Shriki J. Ultrasound physics. *Crit Care Clin*. 2014;30:1–24. v.
29. Kirberger RM. Imaging artifacts in diagnostic ultrasound – a review. *Vet Radiol Ultrasound*. 1995;36:297–306.
30. Heng HG, Widmer WR. Appearance of common ultrasound artifacts in conventional vs. spatial compound imaging. *Vet Radiol Ultrasound*. 2010;51:621–627.
31. Barthez PY, Leveille R, Scrivani PV. Side lobes and grating lobes artifacts in ultrasound imaging. *Vet Radiol Ultrasound*. 1997;38:387–393.
32. Ruth JD, Gan HH, Miller MA, et al. Effect of anisotropy and spatial compound imaging on renal cortical echogenicity in dogs. *Vet Radiol Ultrasound*. 2013;54:659–665.
33. Louvet A. Twinkling artifact in small animal color – Doppler sonography. *Vet Radio Ultrasound*. 2006;47:384–390.
34. O'Brien RT, Zagzebski JA, Delaney FA. Ultrasound corner: range ambiguity artifact. *Vet Radiol Ultrasound*. 2001;42: 542–545.

ELECTRONIC RESOURCES

Additional information related to the content in Chapter 3 can be found online at eBooks.Health. Elsevier.com.

- Chapter Quiz

CHAPTER 4

Principles of Computed Tomography and Magnetic Resonance Imaging

Marc-André d'Anjou

Computed tomography (CT) and magnetic resonance (MR) imaging have become essential assets to veterinarians in the pursuit of many diagnoses. A general understanding of the physical principles inherent to both modalities is important not only to optimize their use in practice but also to recognize their limitations.

THE ROLE OF COMPUTED TOMOGRAPHY AND MAGNETIC RESONANCE IMAGING IN VETERINARY PRACTICE

CT and MR imaging offer superior diagnostic possibilities over conventional radiography because of two primary advantages, which are their *tomographic nature* and *increased contrast resolution*. Indeed, as opposed to radiographs that represent two-dimensional, or flat, projections of three-dimensional (3D) structures, tissues are examined with CT and MR in thin sections, or slices, thereby eliminating superimposition. Organs and other structures can then be identified more easily and differentiated (Figs. 4.1 and 4.2). Moreover, CT and MR volume datasets can be reformatted in any imaging plane, or as 3D projections (eFig. 4.1), allowing better representation of structural anatomic relationships.

Contrast resolution is the capacity of a system to accurately represent differences in tissue, physical, and/or biochemical characteristics, which are intrinsically linked to x-ray attenuation on CT, or signal intensity on MR imaging. The better the contrast resolution, the more likely subtle variations in tissue components will be displayed as pixels of different shades of gray (Fig. 4.3A). For example, much smaller differences in x-ray attenuation can be detected in CT images when compared to a radiograph.[1,2] This difference is explained by the elimination of scatter that reduces image contrast on radiography and by the use of more sensitive x-ray detectors in CT. As with ultrasonography, pure liquids can be differentiated from soft tissues with CT, which cannot be done with radiographs. MR imaging is recognized even more for its great contrast resolution (see Fig. 4.3B), which can be enhanced by the combined use of different imaging sequences.

Conversely, *spatial resolution*, which corresponds to the minimum resolvable separation between high-contrast objects (see Fig. 4.3A), is more limited with CT and MR imaging, as compared to radiography. The spatial resolution of CT and MR imaging, which is typically linked to the slice thickness, is approximately 0.3 and 1.0 mm,[3] respectively, although technical advances and increased magnetic field strength have contributed to reducing this value for MR imaging. In

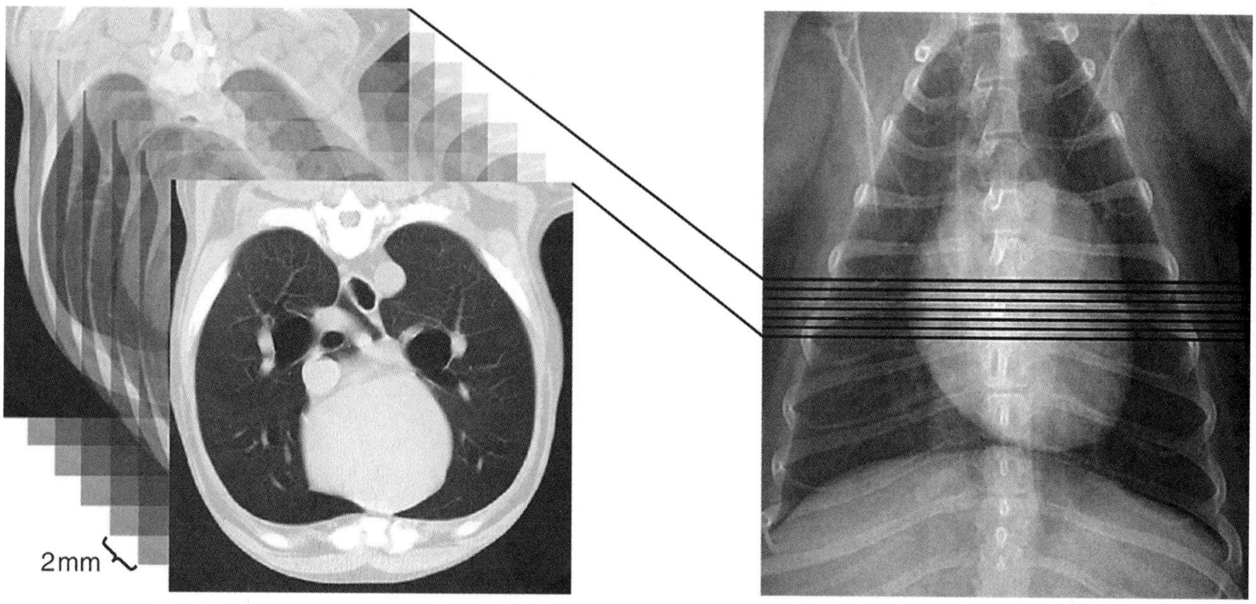

Fig. 4.1 In a computed tomography (CT) study, images are acquired and displayed as sections, or slices, of the body, allowing visualization of structures without superimposition. This fundamental characteristic of tomographic imaging is evident on these contiguous 2-mm-thick images of the thorax of this dog.

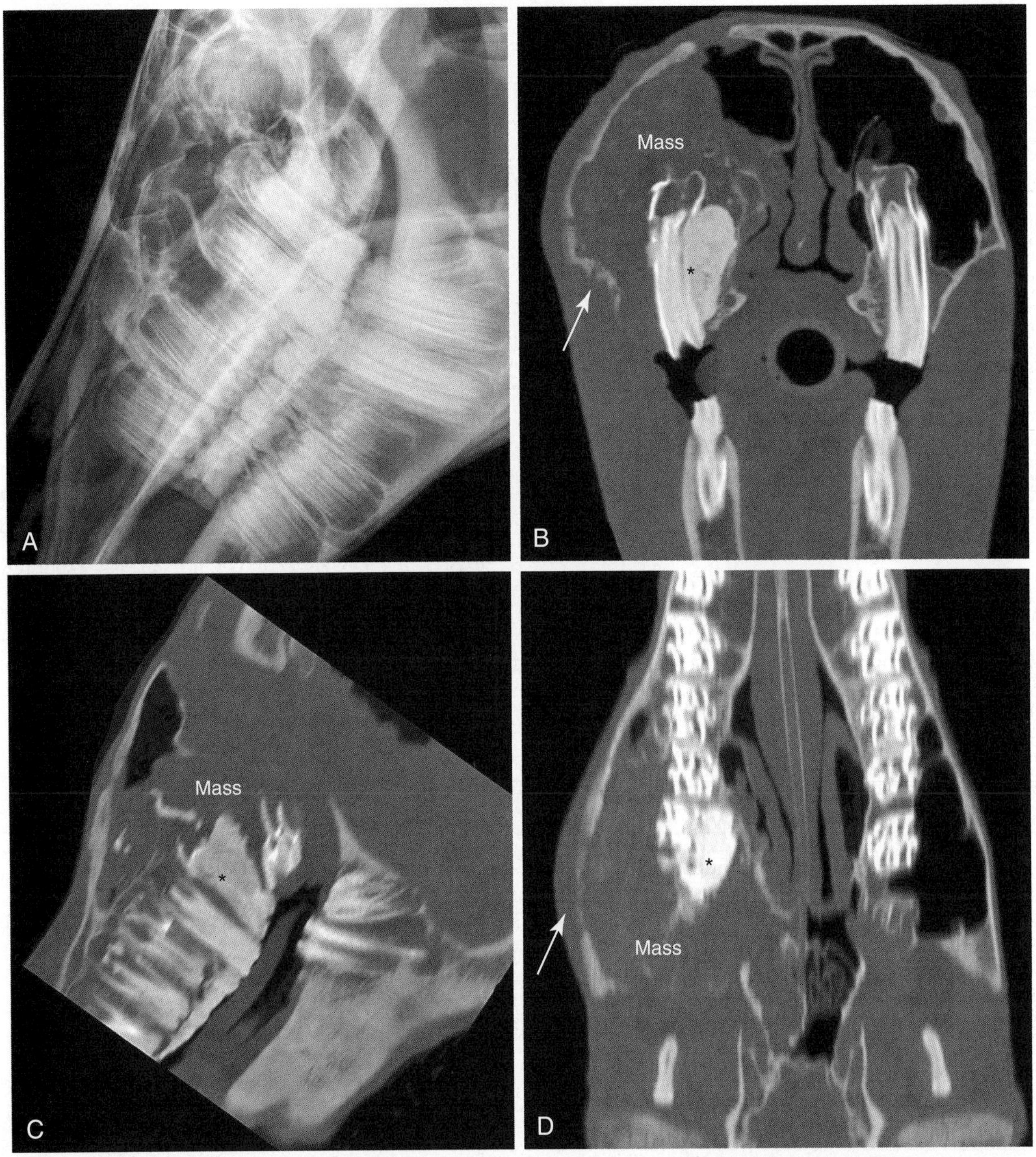

Fig. 4.2 The equine head is anatomically complex with several superimposed structures of variable opacity, making radiographic (**A**) interpretation challenging. In this horse, a large mass associated with maxillary sinus enlargement and bone lysis (*arrows*) is more easily evaluated on transverse (**B**) and reformatted sagittal (**C**) and dorsal (**D**) computed tomography (CT) images. The mass is mainly comprised of soft tissue with a well-defined mineral component attached to the last molar alveolar bone. An odontoma was confirmed histologically.

comparison, screen-film and digital radiography are associated with a spatial resolution of approximately 0.08 to 0.17 mm,[3] which allows smaller details to be depicted. However, the elimination of superimposition and the superior contrast resolution inherent to CT and MR imaging more than compensate for this limitation in spatial resolution.

IMAGE FORMATION: GENERAL CONCEPTS

CT and MR imaging share several characteristics regarding image formation. Each CT or MR image represents a thin section, or slice, of the body, composed of a matrix filled with small cubical sections, known as *voxels*, or *vo*lume *el*ements. The image is displayed on a flat monitor as a matrix of *pixels*, or *pi*cture *el*ements (Fig. 4.4). A voxel associated with greater tissue signal intensity on MR or x-ray attenuation on CT will be displayed as a brighter, or whiter, pixel, whereas lack of signal or x-ray attenuation, such as with air, will appear dark. Although several different values can coexist in each voxel, especially if the voxel is large and if composed of heterogeneous tissue components, only the mean value is expressed and converted to pixel brightness (Fig. 4.5). Hence, both normal and abnormal tissue elements may be combined in a voxel, limiting the resolving capabilities of the modality. Generally, the limiting factor with CT and MR imaging is the slice thickness, which is typically the largest dimension of each voxel. Technical advances in scanners have aimed to reach isotropic resolution, that is, to image sections of tissue with perfectly cubical voxels—the *x*, *y*, and *z* dimensions are the same.[2] Near isotropic resolution has been achieved in multidetector row scanners allowing submillimeter slice generation, which greatly

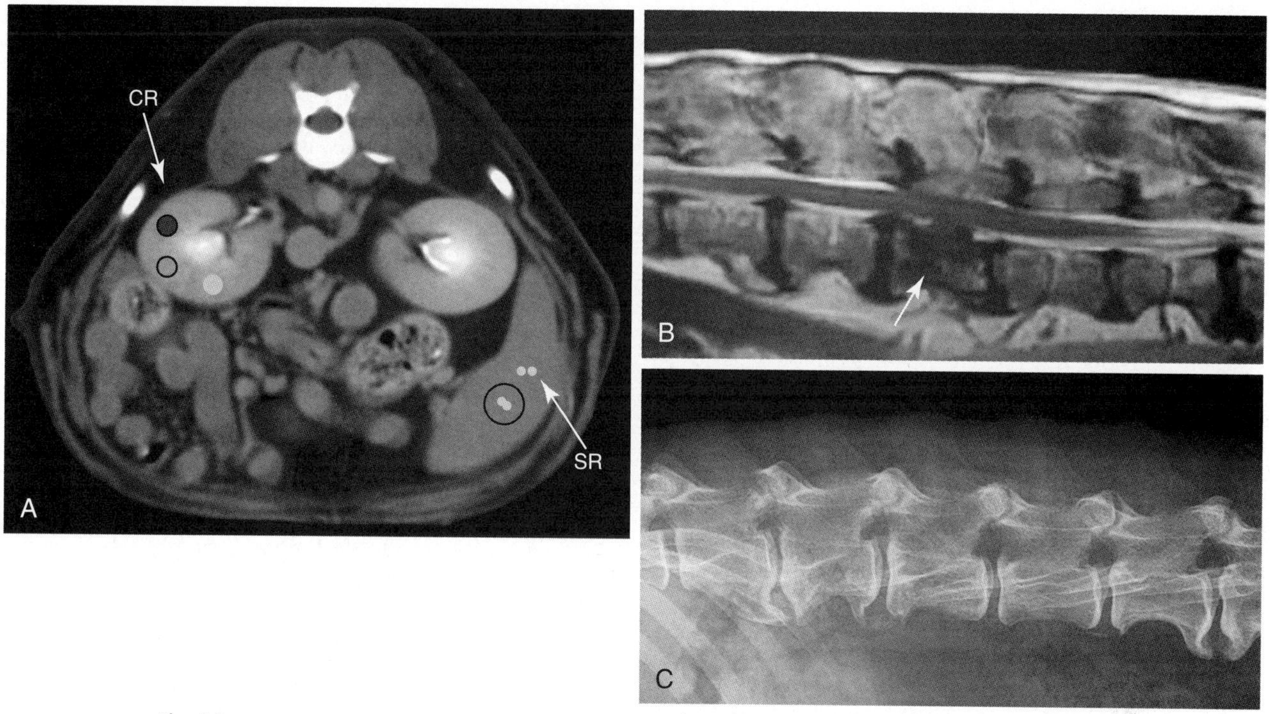

Fig. 4.3 **A,** Schematization of contrast resolution (*CR*) and spatial resolution (*SR*) using a transverse computed tomography (CT) image through the level of the kidneys. Simulated nodules in the right kidney are more easily detected due to the high contrast resolution because their x-ray attenuation characteristics (physical density) differ from the rest of the renal parenchyma. CT offers superior contrast resolution over radiography. In the spleen, the two most dorsal simulated nodules (*arrow*) are visible as independent structures, whereas the more ventral simulated nodules (*circle*) are not visible independently and appear as a single lesion, highlighting the limit of spatial resolution in this image. **B** and **C,** magnetic resonance (MR) imaging is recognized for its outstanding contrast resolution. In this dog with back pain, a malignant neoplasm involving the third lumbar vertebra (*arrow*) is clearly detected with MR imaging (**B**) but was not conspicuous radiographically (**C**).

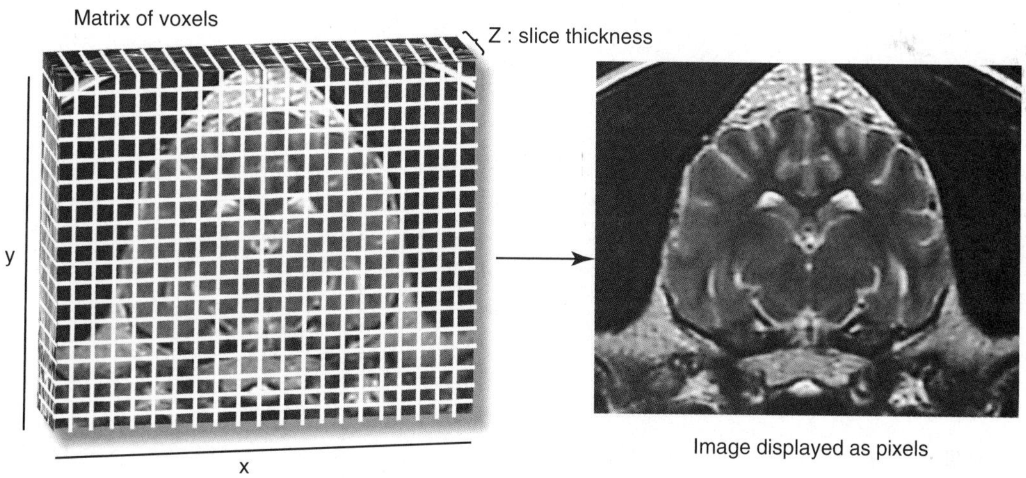

Fig. 4.4 Concept of "voxel-to-pixel" translation in tomographic imaging. The information contained in individual cubes (voxels) of the imaged matrix is displayed as pixels on the computer monitor. Hence, the two-dimensional image is a representation a three-dimensional slab or slice of tissue.

enhances image detail in all planes. Fig. 4.6 illustrates the impact of voxel dimension on image detail.

Among the differences between CT and MR imaging, an important aspect is that image sections can be acquired in any *plane* with MR imaging, including oblique planes (Fig. 4.7). Conversely, with CT, images can be acquired only parallel to the system gantry. Thus, CT images are typically transverse to body parts lying on the table. Fortunately, CT sections are scanned contiguously, forming a volume dataset of millions of tiny cubes, each associated with an attenuation value. It is therefore possible to rearrange, or *reformat*, CT images so that voxels along a plane different than the transverse plane are now displayed as a new matrix of pixels (Fig. 4.8, Video 4.1). This process is known as *multiplanar reformatting*, or *MPR*. These new images can assist in structure recognition, especially for tubular or tortuous structures, and allow more complete assessment (measurements, etc.) of normal and abnormal tissues. Moreover, imaging software can be used to generate 3D representations through volume or surface rendering methods, helping clinicians, especially those less familiar with tomographic imaging, better understand morphologic changes and plan surgery.

COMPUTED TOMOGRAPHY

In 1979, G. N. Hounsfield and A. M. Cormack were awarded the Nobel Prize in medicine for the development of CT imaging,[1] which was considered by many to be the greatest advance in medicine since the discovery of x-rays. Individual CT images that took several minutes to acquire and reconstruct back then can now be generated in fractions of a second, significantly expanding the range of diagnostic applications while improving patient comfort and reducing motion artifact.

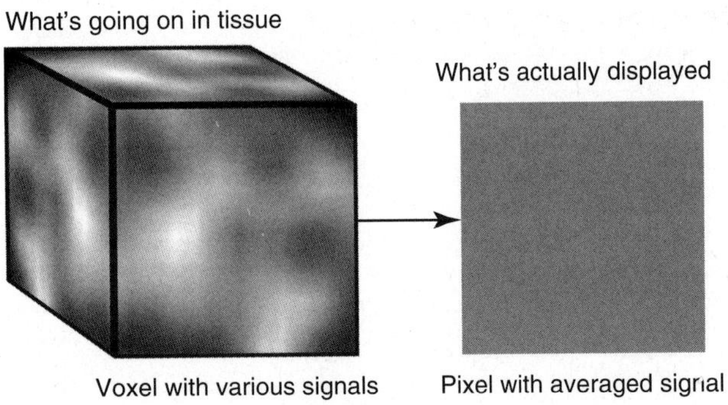

Fig. 4.5 Signal averaging. Although a single voxel may contain tissue of heterogeneous signal intensity, only the average is displayed as a pixel of uniform brightness. More signal in a magnetic resonance image, or increased x-ray attenuation in a computed tomography study, would translate to brighter pixel, whereas lack of signal would be displayed as a dark pixel.

CT technology was based on Radon's mathematic principles developed in 1917, which proved that an image of an object could be produced using an infinite number of projections through that object.[1] With conventional radiographs, orthogonal projections are used to mentally reconstruct anatomic structures in 3D based on the visualization of their shape on perpendicular projections. This process is reliable for simple shapes, but to represent structures with irregular contours accurately, many more radiographic projections are necessary. Now, if thousands of projections could be performed at precise angles, and if x-ray transmission through tissues could be quantified for each of these projections, a sophisticated computer would be able to geometrically *reconstruct* these data and assign specific x-ray transmission values to individual regions of the body. By using a thinly collimated x-ray beam rotating around a patient, slices of tissues can then be computer-generated, each with its own matrix of voxels associated with definite attenuation values. This is the fundamental concept of CT.

Computed Tomography System Geometry

A CT system is mainly composed of a scanning unit (i.e., the *gantry*) with a rotating x-ray emitting tube and a detector system, a patient table, and a console equipped with a sophisticated computer that allows adjusting acquisition parameters and image reconstruction (Fig. 4.9). The rotating x-ray tube is

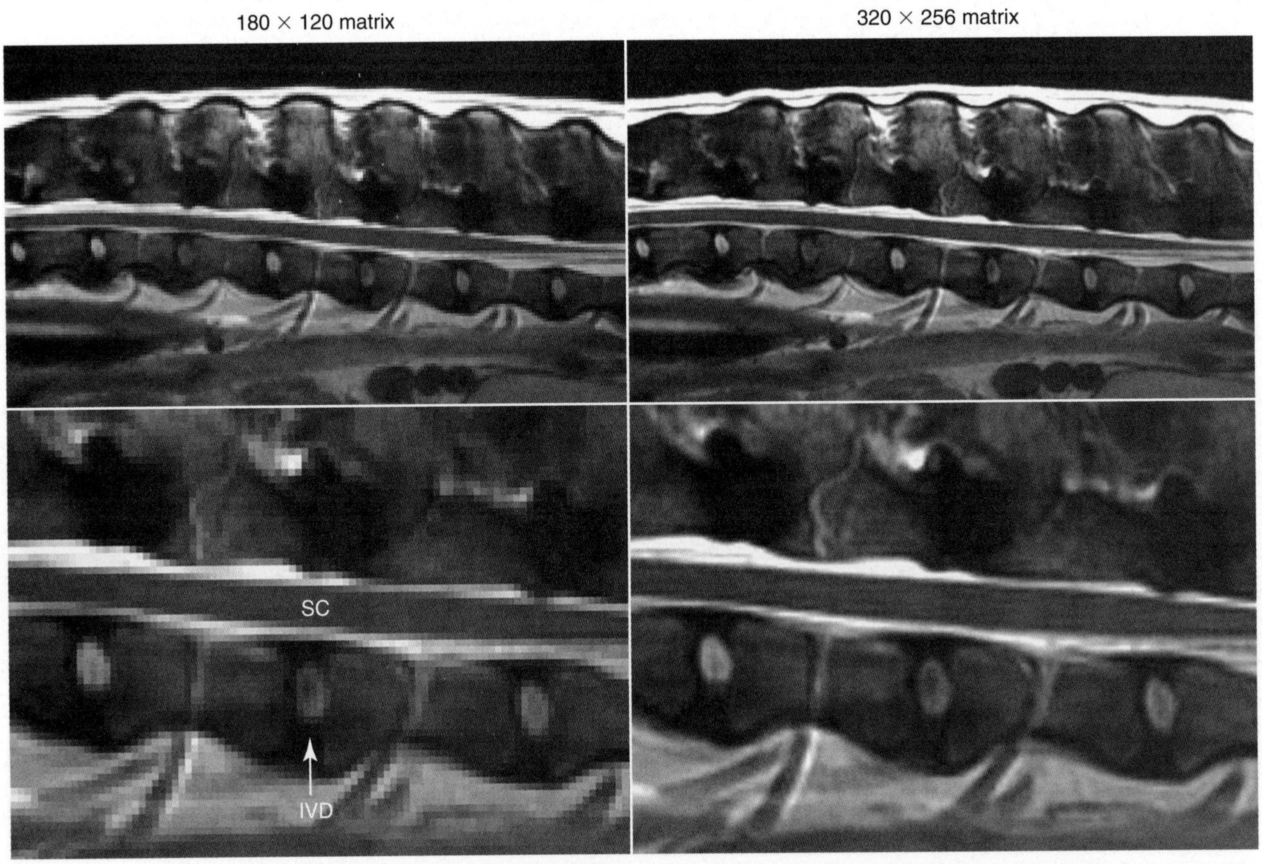

Fig. 4.6 Image matrix and spatial resolution. With a given field of view, a small matrix (180 × 120) contains larger pixels that result in step-like contours. The spinal cord (*SC*) in this dog is smoother in contour when a larger matrix (320 × 256) (i.e., smaller pixels) is used. This superior spatial resolution increases diagnostic accuracy. *IVD*, Intervertebral disc.

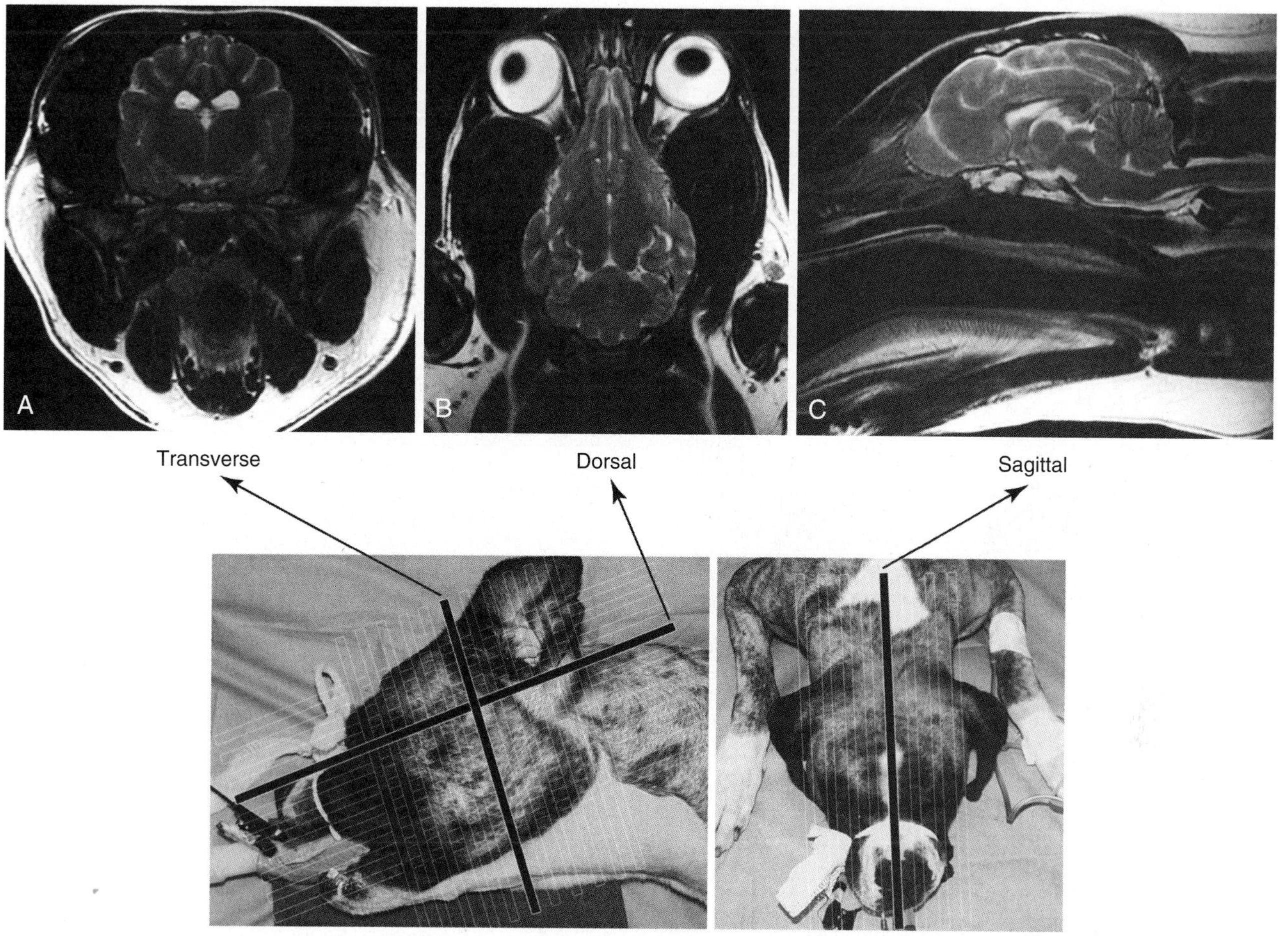

Fig. 4.7 MR images can be acquired in any plane. Transverse (**A**), dorsal (**B**), and sagittal (**C**) planes are typically obtained in most patients, allowing better three-dimensional representation. Image localization is illustrated in the bottom images. Note that all planes can be obtained without having to move the patient.

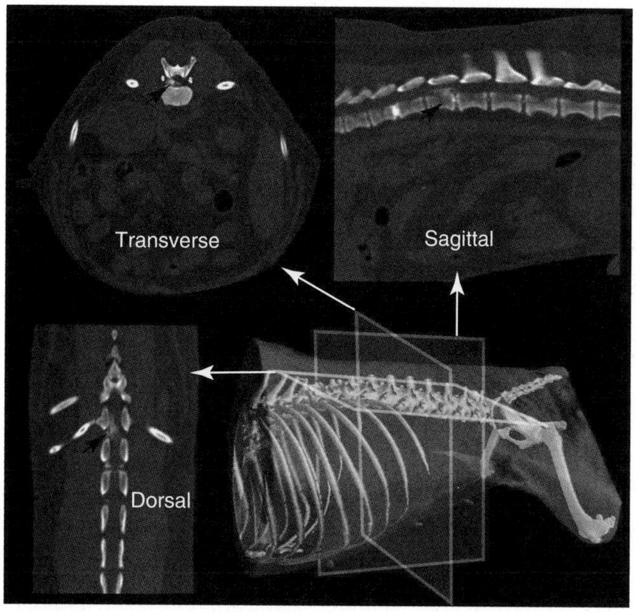

Fig. 4.8 Multiplanar reformatting with computed tomography (CT). Transverse images are obtained initially, but can be reformatted in any plane to help better understand the anatomy. With multidetector CT, thinner sections can be acquired more rapidly, resulting in smoother images with reduced step-like artifacts. The three-dimensional extent of the extruded mineralized disc material is well depicted in all planes (*arrows*).

powerful enough to operate for long periods of time without overheating, thus permitting acquisition of large volumes of data. Modern systems use helical scanning that can rapidly image a large body region without interruption (Fig. 4.10). Rapid tube rotation around the table that simultaneously advances inside the gantry traces a helical path around the patient body, producing a data volume rather than a single slice. Using interpolation methods, flat slices of cubical voxels can be reconstructed from any part of the dataset. Fast scanners reduce motion artifact and allow more precise angiographic procedures with contrast-medium bolus tracking. Advanced scanners that can rapidly acquire sub-millimeter slices generate much smoother images in multiplanar (MP) and 3D reformatting.

The *detector system* also plays an important role in image quality. It converts the incident x-rays that traverse tissue into electronic signals. Ceramic, solid-state detectors have better x-ray absorption and are used in current scanners.[1,4] Each detector is composed of a scintillation crystal that reacts with the incident x-ray and, through an amplification process, generates light that is converted into digital pulses (Fig. 4.11). Detectors are aligned over a semicircular (generally 60 degrees) or annular (360 degrees) array, depending on the system geometry. Annular arrays are stationary, whereas semicircular arrays move synchronously with the opposing x-ray tube (see Fig. 4.9B). CT scanners with multidetector row configurations have become the standard in veterinary hospitals (Fig. 4.12). Such units allow multiple thin contiguous slices to be acquired at a time, an important advantage over previous single-row

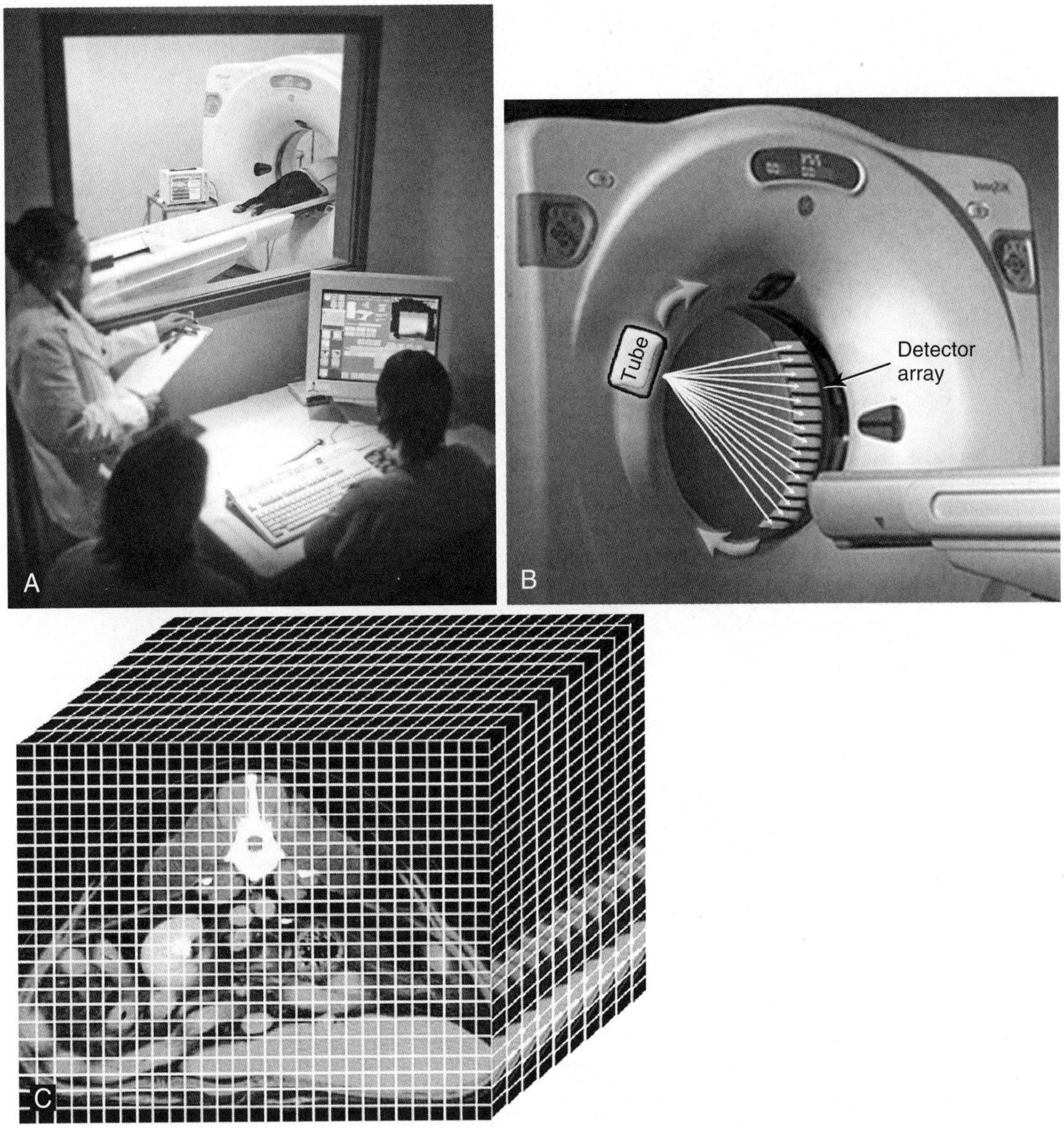

Fig. 4.9 **A,** Typical components of computed tomography (CT). Using a dedicated computer, a technician controls image acquisition and reconstruction. A dog under general anesthesia is observed through a leaded glass window as the CT table advances into the CT gantry. **B,** Most CT scanners are now constructed with a curved array of detectors that rotates around the patient synchronously with the x-ray tube. **C,** The dataset reaching the computer is reconstructed to represent contiguous slices of voxels forming a volume. This volume can then be displayed slice by slice (i.e., transverse images) or reformatted in any plane.

systems. For example, 1-mm-thick slices of a 30-cm-long thorax may require a few seconds to image with a 64-slice scanner, as opposed to a few minutes with a single-row scanner. Images are also more rapidly reconstructed and available for review on the monitor with more recent systems equipped with faster computers. Apart from this significant gain in *temporal resolution* that reduces motion artifacts and tissue misregistration, multidetector row detectors use radiation delivered from x-ray tube more efficiently than single-row detectors.[2] Interscan delays required for tube cooling are significantly reduced with multidetector row systems, allowing for angiographic procedures with multiple series in a short period of time such as those used for portosystemic shunt detection.

Image Formation

The mechanism by which the system reconstructs the data measured by each detector into images as the tube rotates around the patient is sophisticated, yet relatively simple. It starts with the concept of x-ray attenuation, which mainly depends on the electron density of the medium. X-ray attenuation is quantified by measuring the fraction of radiation removed in passing through a given thickness of a specific material, which is based on the *linear attenuation coefficient* (μ) of this material. For image display purposes, x-ray attenuation values calculated by the computer during scanning are expressed as Hounsfield units (HU), normalized to the x-ray attenuation value of water (HU = zero). Any structure or tissue causing more x-ray attenuation than water will have a HU value above zero, whereas any structure or tissue causing less x-ray attenuation than water will have a HU value less than zero (negative). Fig. 4.13 illustrates the range of HU among normal and abnormal tissues. The fact that liquids and soft tissues can be discriminated based on their HU values confirms the greater contrast resolution of CT over radiography.

Other important parameters that are set before image reconstruction include *slice reconstruction interval*, which

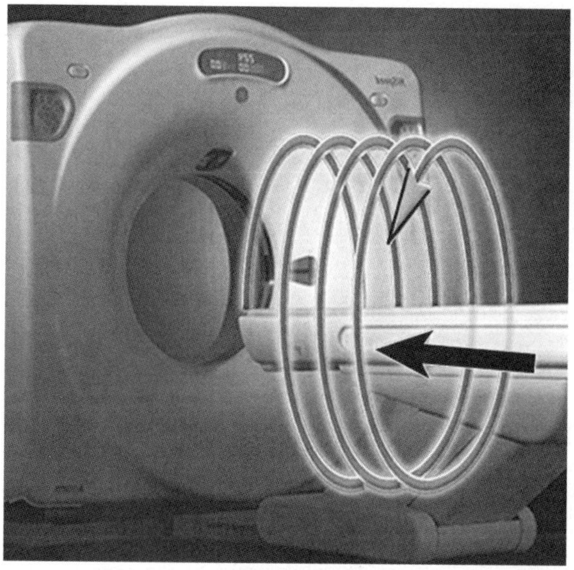

Fig. 4.10 Helical computed tomography (CT). scanning. The table incursion into the gantry as the tube rotates around it results in helicoidal, or spiral, body scanning. This type of acquisition allows images of contiguous sections of tissue, preventing gaps and allowing much faster image acquisition than previous CT generations.

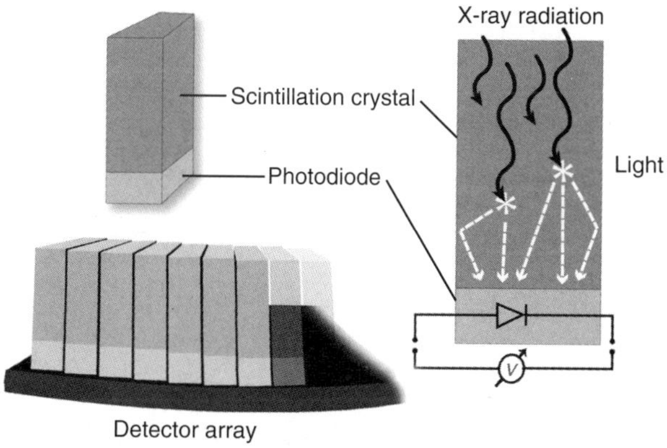

Fig. 4.11 Solid state computed tomography (CT) detectors. X-rays reaching the scintillation crystal generate light photons that are converted to electric current in the photodiode, which is then converted to attenuation values that are used to form the image.

adjusts the proportion of overlap between adjacent slices of tissues used for image reconstruction, and *reconstruction filter*, which determines the level of edge reinforcement applied while processing raw data. These parameters must be set carefully according to the region of interest (ROI). For example, a low-pass filter, commonly known as "standard or soft tissue filter," is recommended when soft tissue contrast must be emphasized, such as in brain imaging, with the downside of creating a blurrier image (Fig. 4.14). "Bone filters," conversely, maximize spatial resolution, but introduce more noise, thus reducing contrast resolution. Such images are sharper but grainier. Intermediate pass filtration may also be used for the reconstruction of smaller soft tissue areas to prevent excessive blurring. Hence, reconstruction filter(s) must be selected according to the size of the body part to be imaged and the content to be highlighted (e.g., soft tissue and/or bone).

Image Display

HU values that can be measured with typical scanners range from approximately −1000 to +3095 HU, for a total of 4096

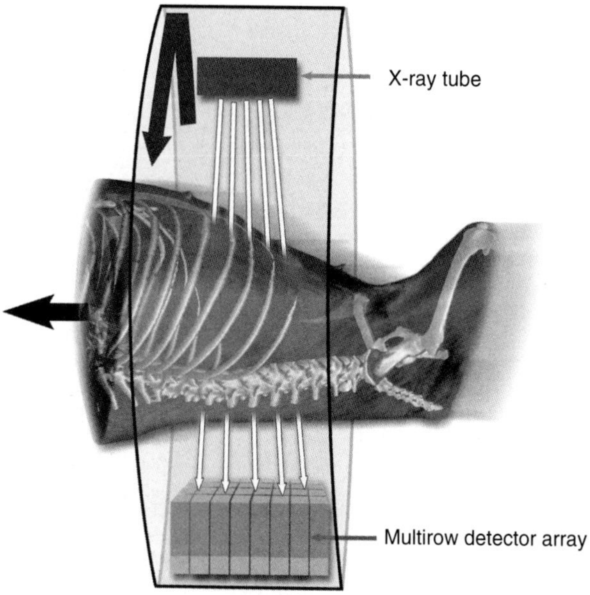

Fig. 4.12 Multidetector (or multislice) computed tomography (CT) scanning. When using more than one row of detectors, larger areas of the body can be imaged during a single tube rotation, allowing faster table advancement, and thus faster scanning. In this illustration there are 8 rows of detectors but newer scanners can contain up to 256 rows, which significantly increases the volume of tissue that can be imaged during one rotation of the x-ray tube.

shades of gray (12 bits of grayscale*). This range of values cannot be resolved by the human eye, which cannot differentiate more than 40 shades of gray.[5] To display and appreciate all tissues composed of variable HU, the *window width* (W) and *level* (L) of the image grayscale can be adjusted, according to the median and range of HU composing the area of interest. The Digital Imaging and Communications in Medicine (DICOM) viewing software allows adjustment of the extent (maximum-to-minimum) of gray shades (W) displayed (i.e., the image *contrast*) and the HU at the center of the window (L) (Fig. 4.15, Video 4.2). W/L must be adapted to the tissues being evaluated and usually requires several adjustments during evaluation of a CT study for all tissues to be evaluated completely.

Interpretation of CT images requires an appropriate understanding of radiographic opacities and anatomy. The attenuation characteristics of tissues can be assessed qualitatively, but also quantitatively. With the DICOM viewing software, HU values are determined precisely after defining a ROI over a selected number of pixels (Fig. 4.16). This can help in distinguishing subtle differences in HU that might not be initially perceived, thus increasing contrast resolution.

Contrast-Enhanced Procedures

The use of iodinated contrast medium has become standard for many CT procedures in veterinary medicine.[6] See Chapter 5 for more information about contrast media used for medical imaging. After an intravenous bolus injection, the distribution of hyperattenuating contrast medium provides information on the perfusion of tissues and integrity of natural barriers, such as the blood–brain barrier. Typically, for nonangiographic procedures, postcontrast scans are performed a few minutes following a bolus injection, to allow contrast medium to pass into the extravascular space. Hence, the HU of a tissue will increase in proportion to the concentration of the contrast medium, the volume of its blood space, and the permeability of its capillary

*See Chapter 2 for a discussion of bit depth.

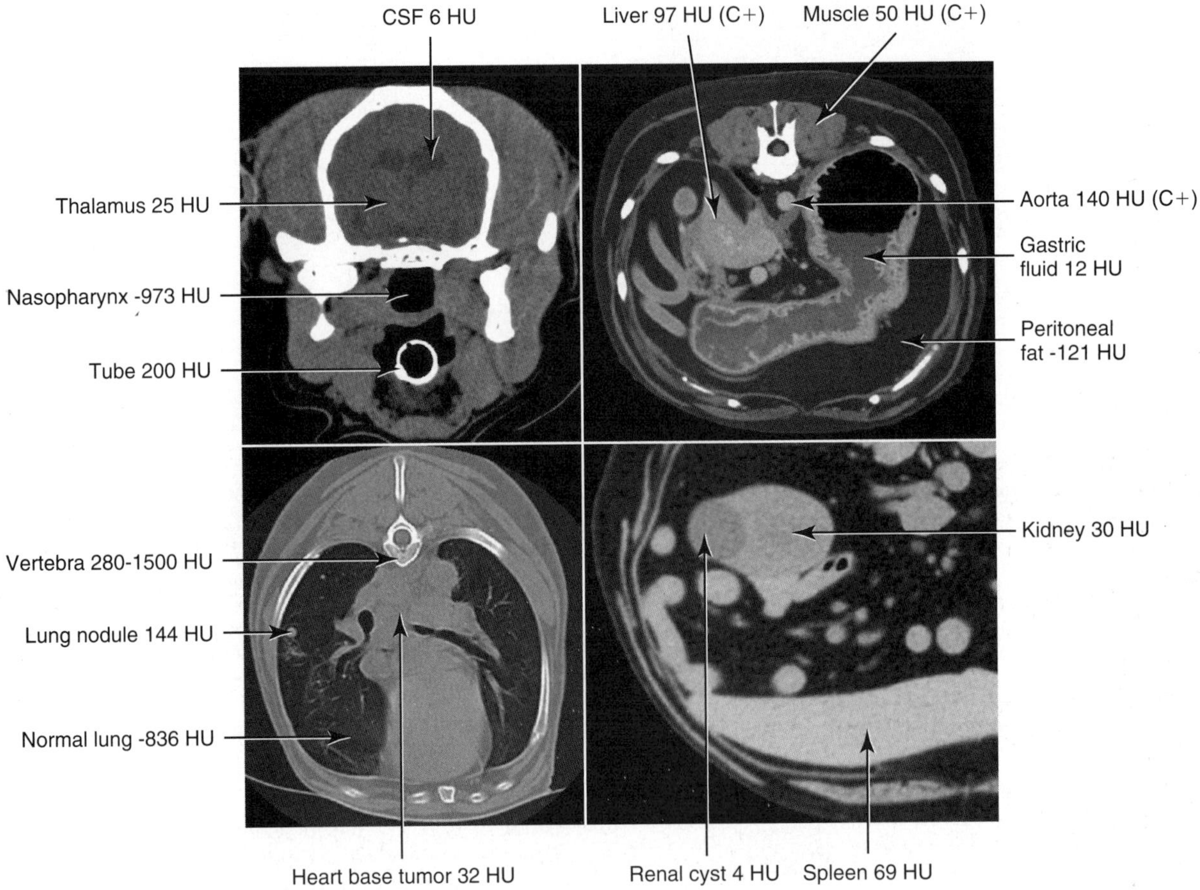

Fig. 4.13 Tissue attenuation (determined as Hounsfield units [*HU*]) can be quantified precisely based on values measured by the CT computer. More subtle differences in attenuation (HU values) are perceived with computed tomography (CT) than radiography, leading to the increasing contrast resolution of CT. For example, the fluid contained in a renal cyst or in the cerebral ventricles can be differentiated from surrounding soft tissue; this is not possible radiographically. Intravenous injection of iodinated contrast medium (C+) increases the HU of vascularized tissues, further increasing the contrast resolution of CT. *CSF,* Cerebrospinal fluid.

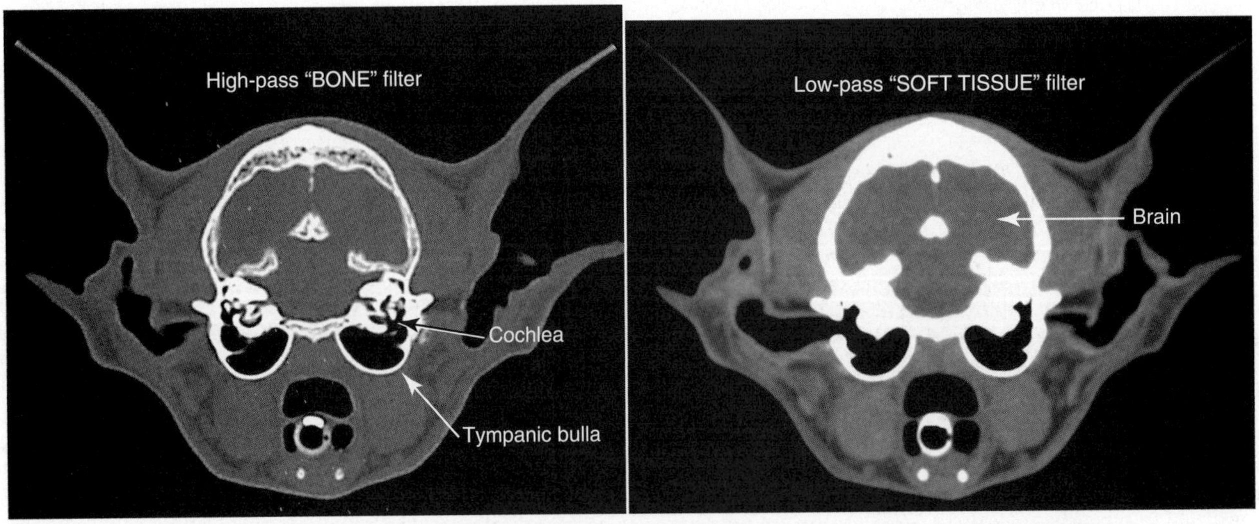

Fig. 4.14 Image reconstruction algorithm. High-pass filtering, also known as "bone filtering," results in sharper images, whereas images reconstructed with low-pass "soft tissue" filter are smoother (or blurrier). The inner ear cochlea is better defined, and the tympanic bulla is thinner with bone filtering, but the brain and other soft tissues of the head are grainier (i.e., noisier) with the same filter. Such filtering is an important part of the image reconstruction steps and requires raw data.

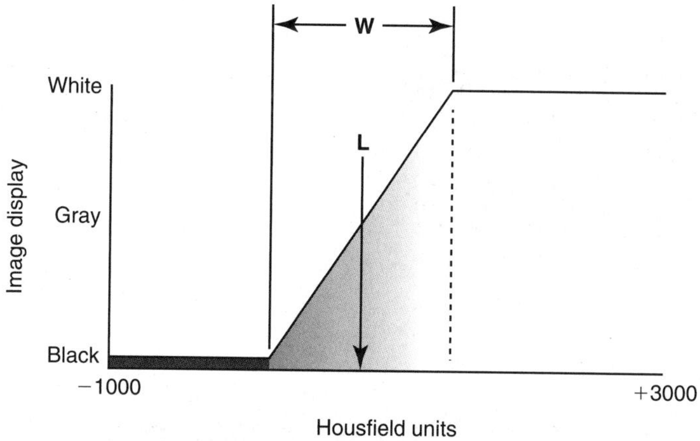

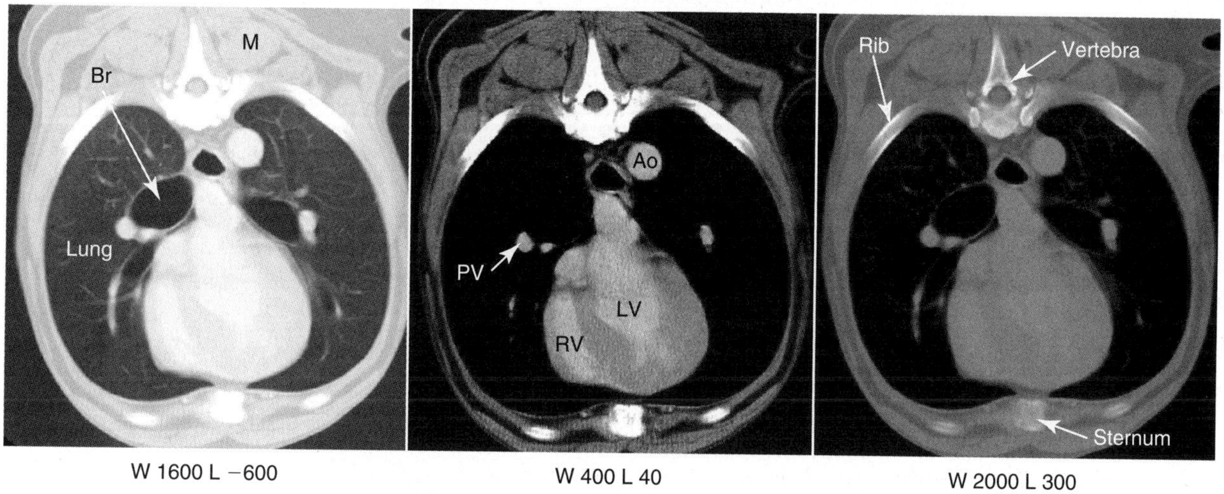

Fig. 4.15 Window width and level adjustments. Because of the limited capacity of the human eye to distinguish different shades of gray, the range of computed tomography (CT) numbers (or Hounsfield units [HU]) composing the image, from approximately −1000 to +3000, cannot all be displayed at once. With the Digital Imaging and Communications in Medicine (DICOM) viewing software, the window level (*L*) is set at the mean HU of the region of interest, and the window width (*W*) is set to include the range of values to be represented. Practically, L controls the image brightness, and W, the image contrast. A small W, such as 400, will result in a high contrast image. Setting the L to 40 allows better distinction of cardiac chambers filled with diluted contrast medium. Conversely, with these settings, lungs and bone exceed the lower and upper limits of the grayscale and are thus represented with totally black or white pixels, respectively. To assess lung tissue, the W must be widened (1600) and the L must be centered on its mean HU of lung (−600 to −800), whereas bone assessment requires even larger W (2000) and higher L (300). These values must be adapted to the patient. *Ao,* Aorta; *Br,* bronchus; *LV,* left ventricle; *M,* muscle; *PV,* pulmonary vein; *RV,* right ventricle.

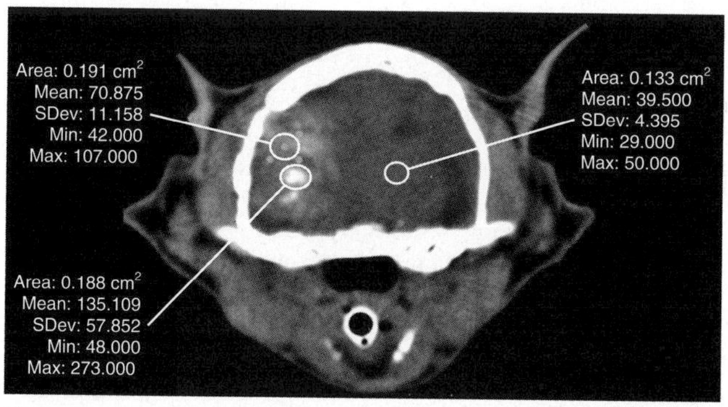

Fig. 4.16 Hounsfield unit (HU) measurements. Differences in HU among normal and pathologic tissues can be determined with the computed tomography (CT) viewing software in specific regions of interest (ROI). Information such as ROI surface area and mean, maximal, and minimal HU is provided. This method allows detection of more subtle differences in HU than what the eye can perceive. In this cat, a mineralized meningioma was identified.

bed.[7] When comparing postcontrast to precontrast CT images, the degree of enhancement can be assessed qualitatively (Fig. 4.17) and quantitatively (see Figs. 4.13 and 4.16). Enhancement characteristics can be used to complement other morphologic observations and increase both sensitivity and specificity of CT examinations.

Angiography represents another important application of CT imaging. CT angiography requires helical scanning and is optimized with multidetector scanners and automated contrast-medium injectors. Scans are performed rapidly after the injection of a contrast-medium bolus and timed according to the vascular phase being examined and its enhancement peak. For example, when injecting into a cephalic vein, contrast medium sequentially reaches the cranial vena cava, right atrium, right ventricle, pulmonary arteries and veins, left atrium and ventricle, aorta and peripheral arteries, before returning to the heart through the vena cava, and to the liver through the portal vein. Precise acquisition timing is required to isolate a group of vessels, which is important when, for example, looking for portosystemic shunts (eFig. 4.2).

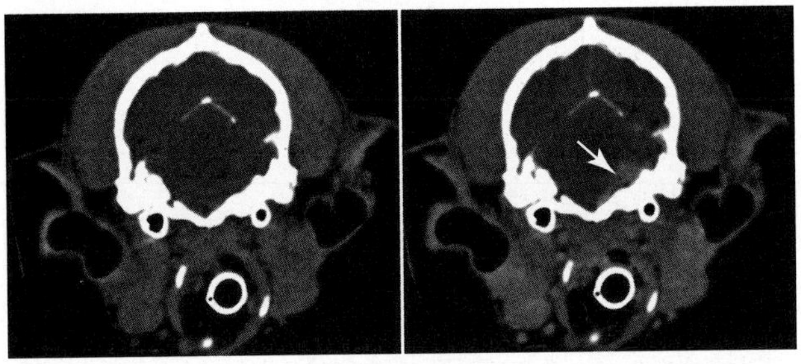

Fig. 4.17 Intravenous injection of iodinated contrast medium increases contrast resolution of computed tomography (CT). In this dog, a contrast-enhancing meningioma (*arrow*), with a broad base along the left temporal bone, was detected only after contrast-medium injection.

Because iodinated contrast medium is eliminated essentially by glomerular filtration, contrast-enhanced CT can also be used to estimate the rate at which this occurs, as well as to assess the renal collecting system.[8]

Risks associated with contrast medium injection are discussed in Chapter 5.

CONE-BEAM COMPUTED TOMOGRAPHY

Cone-beam CT is gaining in popularity in veterinary medicine due to the lower cost of the equipment and installation. Like conventional CT, cone-beam CT consists of an x-ray source, an image detector, a computer, and an image, but uses a cone-shaped x-ray beam as opposed to a collimated fan beam. Use of a cone-beam has the advantage of reducing patient radiation dose, but also leads to increased scatter radiation and reduced contrast-to-noise ratio, which affects image quality. Instead of detectors aligned in row(s), flat panels or image intensifiers are used in cone beam CT technology and these rotate synchronously around the patient through 360 degrees (eFig. 4.3). Cone-beam CT is valuable for the assessment of small head parts and particularly dental structures in dogs and cats as it offers high *spatial resolution*,[9] but its usefulness for larger body regions remains to be determined.

MAGNETIC RESONANCE IMAGING

MR imaging has become an important diagnostic tool in veterinary medicine because of its inherent high-contrast resolution that allows soft tissues to be characterized more sensitively than with CT. The high contrast resolution of MR imaging fundamentally revolves around the electromagnetic properties of hydrogen nuclei (protons), which are abundant in body tissues. Energy transfer to and from these protons can be localized spatially (i.e., in individual voxels) and is the source of image formation. MR imaging can therefore be compared, in a clinical setting, to mapping the distribution of H^+ protons in the water (H_2O) and lipid (CH_2/CH_3) component of tissues. Equipment sophistication and pulse-sequence development are responsible for the growing applicability and accuracy of MR imaging. Although MR imaging is used mainly to investigate neurologic conditions, several other body parts of small and large animals, especially the horse, can be imaged satisfactorily with MR imaging.

Instrumentation

MR systems constitute the most sophisticated equipment in diagnostic imaging, combining electronics, radiofrequency (RF) generators, coils, and gradients that interact with a computer. This combination is necessary for proper tissue excitation and reception and localization of tissue signals. The magnet

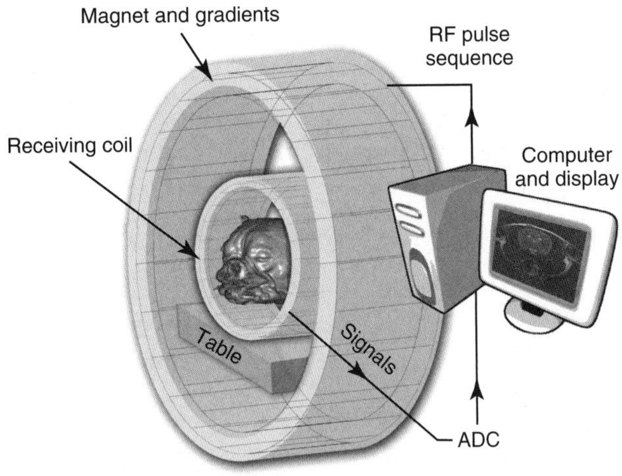

Fig. 4.18 Components of a magnetic resonance (MR) imaging system. The region of the patient to be imaged is placed in the center of the gantry (i.e., maximal magnetic field) and a coil (of variable shape) is placed around or very close to this region. The computer is manipulated to prepare radiofrequency (*RF*) pulse sequences that cause tissue magnetization before signals can be detected as echoes. Different gradients inside the gantry allow localization of individual echoes and are used for gradient-recalled pulse sequences. Analog signals are converted into digital pulses that are transformed into interpretable images. *ADC*, Analog-to-digital converter.

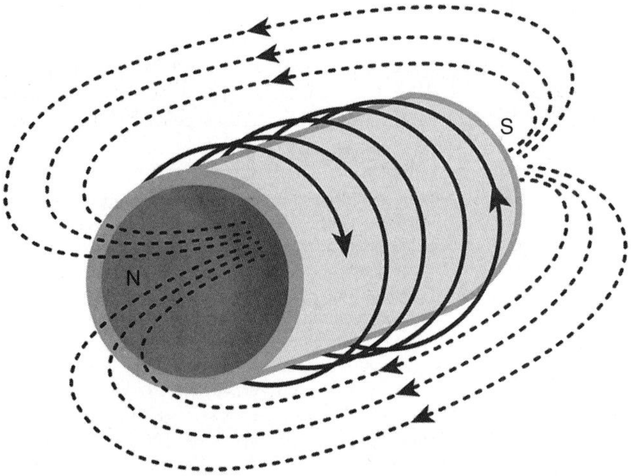

Fig. 4.19 According to Faraday's law of induction, when electronic current travels through a loop of wire, a magnetic field is generated perpendicularly in proportion to the strength of the current. The magnetic field—illustrated here as *curved dashed lines*—is oriented from north (*N*) to south (*S*).

provides the external magnetic field in which the patient is placed, and its performance is influenced by its field strength, stability, and uniformity. Several types of systems are available, and some of their characteristics will be discussed later. Fig. 4.18 illustrates the main components of the typical MR system.

Main Magnetic Field and Radiofrequency Energy

According to Faraday's law of induction, when electronic current travels along a loop of wire, a magnetic field is generated perpendicularly in proportion to the strength of the current (Fig. 4.19).[10] Fundamentally, this is how most MR scanners work, particularly high field-strength systems (magnetic field strength >1 tesla [T]). To generate and maintain such high magnetic fields, superconducting wires are immersed in liquid helium, which serves as cooling agent.

Spins, Excitation, and Relaxation

Each hydrogen proton is positively charged (H^+) and rotates about its axis, like a spinning top. These spinning protons, or *spins*, each act like tiny magnets whose individual magnetization vectors are oriented randomly and cancel out under normal circumstances (Fig. 4.20).

When placed in a strong external magnetic field, spinning protons are forced to align along the axis of this field (B_0), either in the same direction (parallel) or opposite (antiparallel). The magnetic fields of most of these spinning protons cancel out, but a slight excess of protons, which is proportional to the strength of the magnetic field, will be parallel to B_0, producing a *net magnetization* along that axis (see Fig. 4.20). The size of this equilibrium magnetization also depends on the photon density (PD) of tissues present in the field.[10,11]

Influenced by the external B_0 in which they are placed, protons wobble about their axis, a behavior called *precession* (Fig. 4.21).[10,11] This wobbling motion is controlled by application of an external force. The frequency of this precession, also called resonance or *Larmor frequency* (ω_0), is proportional to the main magnetic field strength: $\omega_0 = \gamma B_0$. The constant γ, or *gyromagnetic ratio*, is specific to each type of nuclei. For hydrogen protons, this constant equals 42.6 MHz/T (megahertz per tesla).[10,11]

The phenomenon of precession implies that the magnetization moment of each spinning proton can be broken down into two vector components: one aligned or longitudinal to B_0—the *z*-axis—and one transverse to it, lying on the *xy*-plane (see Fig. 4.21). Although a positive net magnetization is present along the *z*-axis in the equilibrium state, *xy* vector components of spinning protons that precess out of phase cancel out.

By applying a RF pulse that matches the Larmor frequency of the spinning protons, energy can be transferred through a process known as *resonance*. The absorption of this energy by the proton, called *excitation*, causes a state of imbalance. The excited protons jump to a higher energy state during excitation (from parallel to antiparallel), and the macroscopic net magnetization vector flips away from the *z*-axis, toward the *xy*-plane, following a spiral path caused by the precession phenomenon.[10,11] The angle that the net magnetization vector flips away from the *z*-axis is called the *flip angle*, which depends on the strength and duration of the RF pulse. As soon as the RF pulse is stopped, protons will return to their original state of equilibrium in a recovery process called *relaxation* and release and transmit their excess energy.

Whereas the change in longitudinal magnetization is caused by a difference in the number of protons in parallel as opposed to antiparallel states, the transverse magnetization vector growth is caused by protons getting into phase coherence.[10,11] That is, these tiny magnets become globally aligned and precess synchronously. Once the RF current is turned off and relaxation

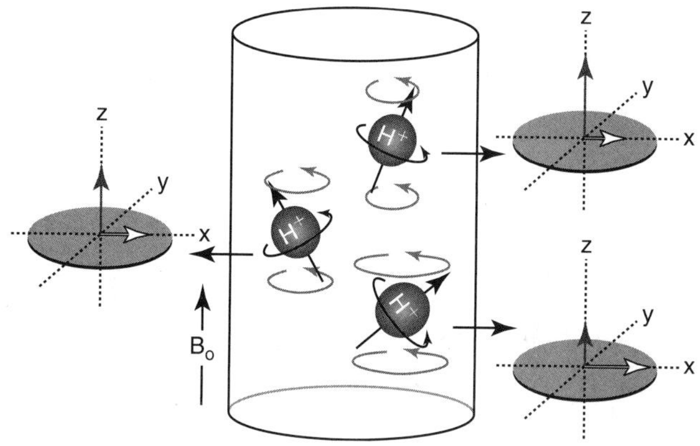

Fig. 4.21 Spin precession. Influenced by the strong external magnetic field, spinning protons wobble about its linear axis, a process called *precession*. The magnetization moment of each spinning proton can be broken down into two vector components: one aligned or longitudinal to B_0—the *z*-axis—and one transverse to it, lying on the *xy*-plane. The relative magnitude of each of these vectors depends on the orientation of the spinning protons in regard to B_0 during the MR imaging sequence process. Notice that as the proton becomes progressively out of alignment with the main magnetic field (B_0), the size of the magnetization vector in the *z*-axis decreases and the size of the magnetization vector in the *xy*-axis increases.

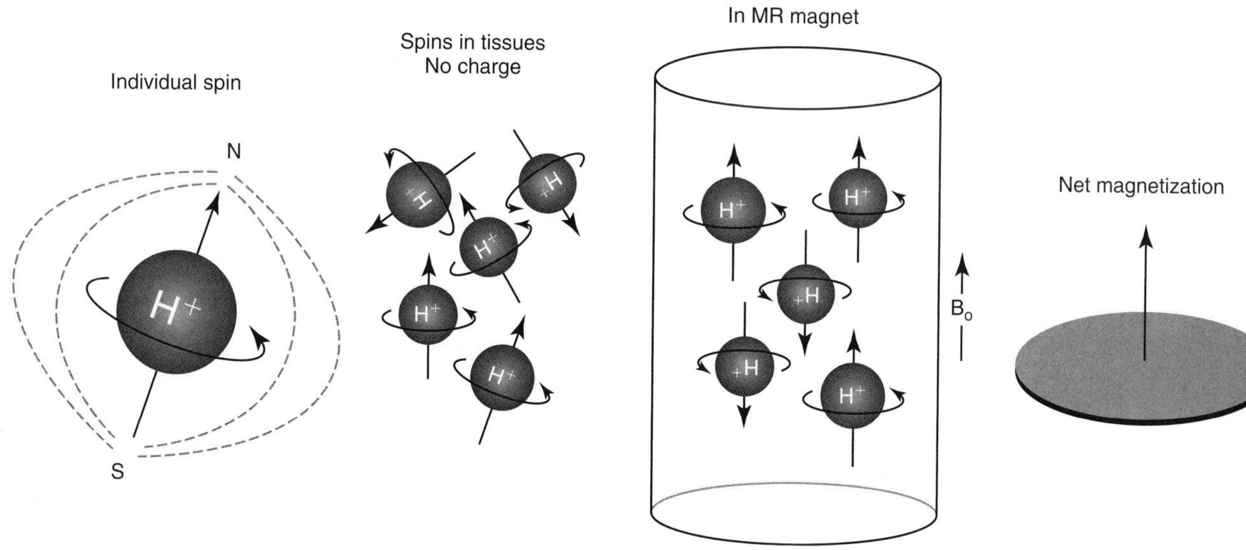

Fig. 4.20 Hydrogen protons (H^+) are used for magnetic resonance (*MR*) imaging because of their abundance in soft tissues and their magnetic characteristics. The positively charged nucleus spins about its axis, generating a very small, local magnetic field, and thus acting as tiny magnet. These protons, or spins, are oriented randomly in tissues under normal conditions so that their magnetic fields cancel out. When placed inside a strong external magnetic field with linear orientation (B_0), these spins are realigned and orient themselves either parallel or antiparallel to this field. A small excess of these spins (proportional to the strength of B_0) are oriented in the parallel direction, thus generating a net magnetization of the tissue. This net magnetization, which at equilibrium is oriented longitudinally, is targeted during imaging sequences.

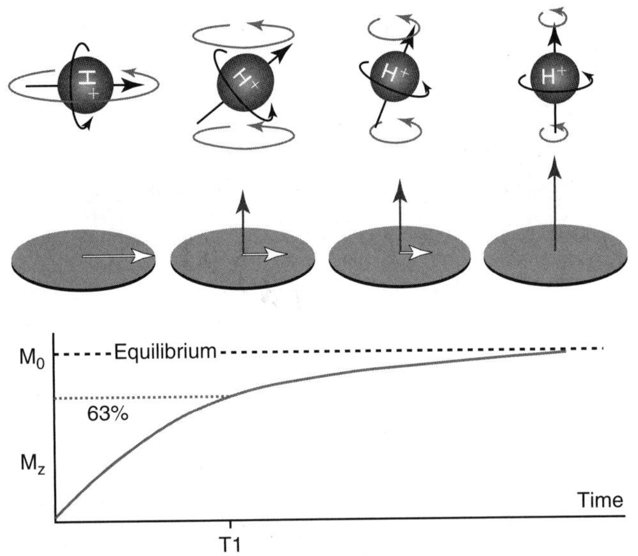

Fig. 4.22 Once the radiofrequency pulse is stopped, the spinning protons immediately start to realign with the main magnetic resonance (MR) magnetic field in the *z*-axis direction transferring their absorbed energy to their molecular environment, also called the lattice. This is T1 relaxation. During this process, the transverse vector component of magnetization (M_z) decreases while the longitudinal component increases to reach an equilibrium (i.e., low-energy state). The T1 time required for the longitudinal magnetization to recover approximately 63% of its original value is called the T1-relaxation time, and is tissue specific. M_0, Longitudinal magnetization at equilibrium state.

begins, two distinct processes occur simultaneously: longitudinal, *T1*, and transverse, *T2*, relaxations. The release of energy from the relaxing protons into their molecular environment, also called the *lattice*, results in more protons returning to the low-energy state, that is, realigned with B_0 (T1 relaxation; Fig. 4.22). At the same time, in-phase spinning protons start interacting with each other, rapidly causing dephasing, and thus eliminating the transverse magnetization vector (T2 relaxation; Fig. 4.23). The rate at which T1 and T2 relaxation occurs is tissue specific and exploitation of these differences is the fundamental source of tissue contrast in MR imaging.

Spin-Echo Sequences

MR images are created once signals arising from excited tissues are detected as echoes by receiving coils, localized spatially, and processed. Because of the differences in T1- and T2-relaxation time between tissues, several technical methods, or *sequences*, can be used to excite and receive signals using RF and gradient pulses, with variable timing and duration. Sequences are divided into two main groups—*spin-echo* and *gradient recalled* sequences. Image interpretation is then based on the evaluation of all sequences obtained in a single examination.

As previously discussed, RF pulses energize tissue protons, which then start to process synchronously, leading to strong transverse magnetization. This process of "flipping" the magnetization away from the *z*-axis is essential to measuring a signal. By placing one or several loops of wire (i.e., *receiving coil*) around the patient, in a plane perpendicular to the transverse axis, the strength of the electronic current induced in the coil is proportional to the transverse magnetic field (Fig. 4.24).

Once the RF pulse is stopped, protons in the *xy*-plane dephase rapidly because of their molecular interactions (i.e., T2 relaxation). In the body, T2 relaxation is accelerated further by the fact that the magnetic field is not perfectly uniform in tissues. Indeed, the magnetic field is slightly stronger in some areas because of the presence of metallic objects, air, or calcium or because of the imperfections of the MR system, for example, 1.505 T for a 1.5 T magnet, and weaker in other parts, for example, 1.495 T.[12] Such inhomogeneities cause protons to rotate at different speeds once the RF pulse is stopped (i.e., some slower than the average and some faster), leading to very rapid dephasing. Thus, instead of decaying according to the specific T2-relaxation time of the tissue, the transverse magnetization decays at a more rapid rate, called *T2** (see Fig. 4.23).

Spin-echo sequences have been developed specifically to eliminate the effect of T2*, the effect caused by magnet inhomogeneities and tissue substances such as calcium. The rationale is simple: By adding a 180-degree RF pulse after the initial 90-degree pulse, protons start rotating effectively in the opposite direction. This effective change in direction allows slow protons, still affected by the same environment inhomogeneities, to become relocated "in front of" faster protons. Shortly thereafter, all protons become coherent again, exponentially increasing transverse magnetization, which peaks at a time called *time of echo* or *TE* (Fig. 4.25; see Fig. 4.23). TE then represents the time between this peak of echo and the initial 90-degree RF pulse. The time it takes for this sequence to be run one time is called the *time to repetition* or *TR* (see Fig. 4.25). For basic pulse sequences, one row of image data is acquired during each TR. Thus, the time required for acquisition of an MR image with a matrix of 256 by 256 pixels (i.e., voxels) takes 256 times TR. With such matrix, a T1-weighted spin-echo image (at 1.5 T) with a TR of 500 ms would take 128 seconds to acquire.

Tissue Contrast

The great diagnostic potential of MR imaging comes from the fact that tissue contrast can be manipulated to enhance anatomy and/or lesion conspicuity. Indeed, by adjusting TE and TR, differences in T1 and T2 relaxation characteristics among tissues can be detected in images (Fig. 4.26).[10,12,13]

Recall that the MR signal that is measured is at its maximum when the transverse magnetization of tissues is completely in phase. When transverse magnetization begins to dephase, the measured MR signal also begins to decrease and becomes null when the transverse magnetization is completely dephased. To detect T2 differences between tissues, time must be allowed for short-T2 tissues to decay enough so that long-T2 tissues are highlighted—that is, high signal at the time of the echo (i.e., at TE). Conversely, maximizing T1 differences requires that the time between subsequent 90-degree RF pulses (i.e., TR) is relatively shorter so that longitudinal recovery of tissues in the *z* direction of short and long T1 is separated. Finally, because T1 and T2 effects occur at the same time, optimizing one necessitates that the other one is inhibited. Hence, *T1-weighting* requires short TR (and short TE), and *T2-weighting* requires long TE (and long TR). If both T1 and T2 effects are inhibited by using long TR and short TE, signal intensities mainly depend on tissue PD, called *proton-density (PD) weighting*. These manipulations result in varying signal intensity (or pixel brightness) levels for the same tissue (Fig. 4.27). Although some tissues can appear similar in one given sequence, they can become quite distinct in another. MR imaging of a body part includes multiple sequences to highlight these tissue differences, but new sequences are developed every day to improve the capacity to identify even more subtle differences.

Magnetic Resonance Signal Localization

Now that the processes of tissue magnetization and echo detection have been discussed, one important feature of MR imaging relates to the ability to determine the precise anatomic location of the signals coming out of tissues. This process is performed by intermittently using three orthogonal linear magnetic gradients that generate short-term variations in

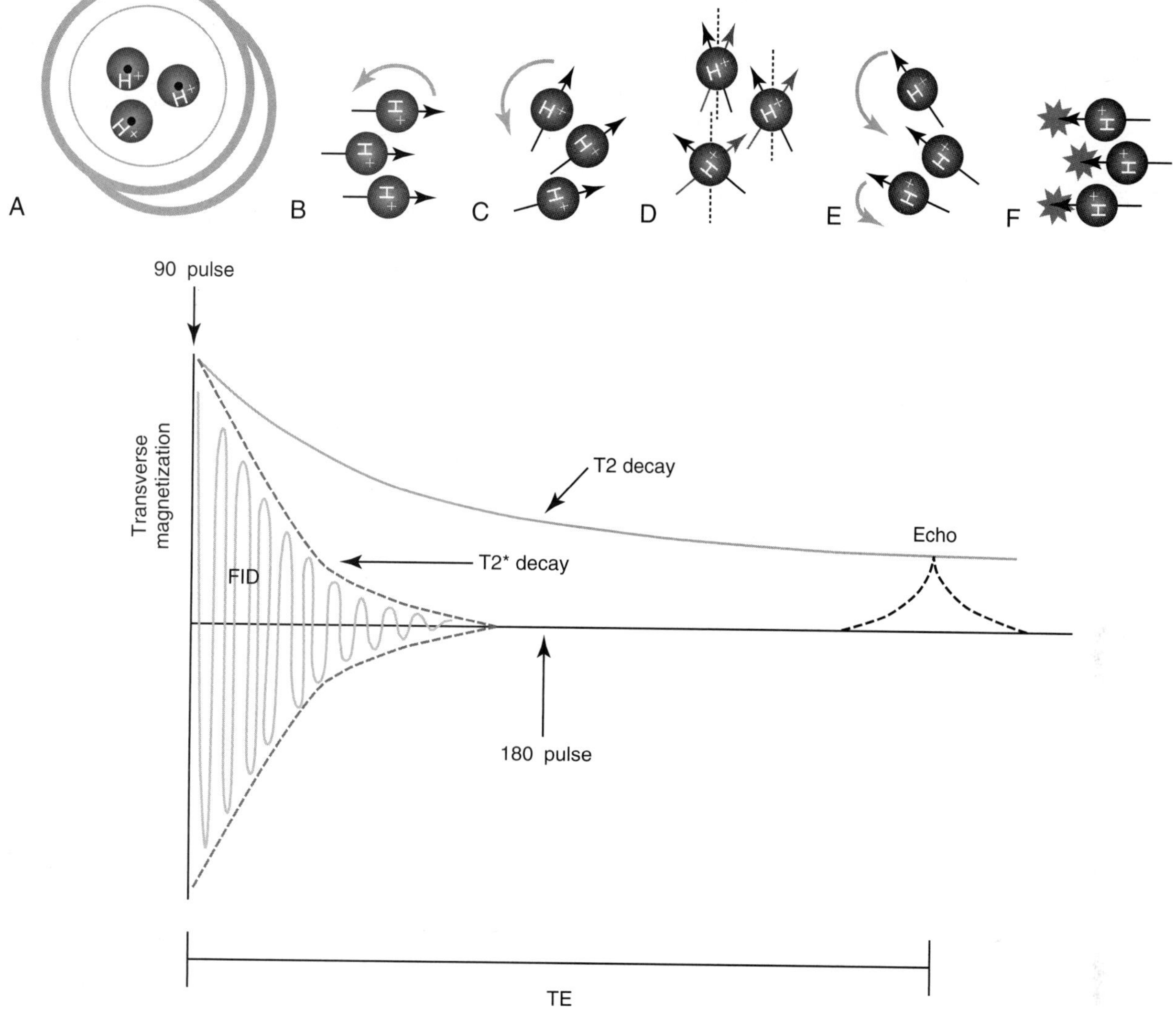

Fig. 4.23 T2 and T2*-relaxation. **A,** When placed in the magnetic resonance (MR) magnet (cylindrical in this case), protons align longitudinally along the axis of its magnetic field. **B,** The first step of a spin-echo sequence consists of a radiofrequency (RF) pulse that flips the magnetization moment of protons toward the transverse plane. This pulse is sometimes referred to as a 90-degree pulse. At this point, protons precess in coherence (i.e., synchronously), which causes strong transverse magnetization in the *xy*-axis. **C,** As soon as the RF pulse is terminated, protons start to dephase because of imperfections in the magnetic field, which is never completely uniform. These slight changes in field uniformity, or field strength, cause protons to precess either more rapidly or less rapidly. This results in rapid loss of transverse net magnetization—called T2* (T2-star) decay, or relaxation. **D,** To counteract the proton dephasing caused by the inhomogeneous magnetic field, another RF pulse is applied to flip back the protons 180 degrees. **E,** Spins rotating more rapidly are then behind slower spins, and as the protons regain coherence the transverse *xy* magnetization regrows (**F**), and ultimately peaks at a time called time *between excitation and echo (TE)*. The rate at which the protons diphase and then rephrase is called the T2-relaxation time, and the amount of signal present at the TE is also tissue dependent. *FID,* Free induction decay.

magnetic field strength across the patient, and therefore the Larmor frequencies of protons.[13] These gradients are produced by additional coiled wires placed in the bore of the magnet, linked to electronic circuitry that is adjusted constantly and precisely through additional *pulses* in the imaging sequence. These gradients are responsible for the tapping or clicking sounds heard during scanning, and the gradient strength influences the anatomic details (i.e., spatial resolution) that can be achieved as well as the speed of image acquisition.

Selection of Spin-Echo Sequences

Several types of spin-echo sequences are available, some used more consistently and others used in more specific circumstances (Fig. 4.28). T1-weighted and T2-weighted sequences are acquired in most patients. In both sequences, multiple 180-degree rephasing pulses are usually applied after the single 90-degree RF pulse during the same TR. This allows more signals to be localized during each TR and speeds up the acquisition process.[12] Spin-echo sequences with more than one 180-degree rephrasing pulse are called *fast spin-echo* or *turbo spin-echo* sequences.

Inversion recovery sequences are used to null the signal from specific tissues or substances, which can help confirm the presence of such components, or improve the conspicuity of nearby tissues with similar signal characteristics. A short inversion time recovery (STIR) sequence is commonly used to

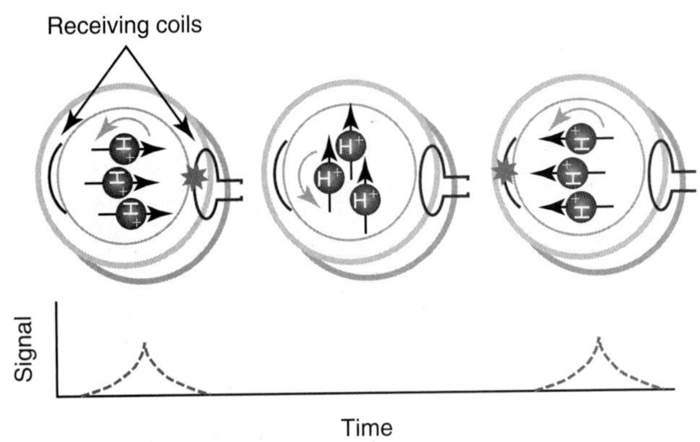

Fig. 4.24 Signal reception. When protons are flipped 90 degrees and precess in phase, they generate a strong transverse magnetization vector, which in turn induces an electric current in loops of wire placed perpendicularly around the body part being imaged. Signals peak when the transverse magnetization vector from the spinning protons is fully perpendicular to each of the wire loop coils and the signal in the coil decreases when the magnetic vector rotates away. Using more loops around the patient increases signal intensity.

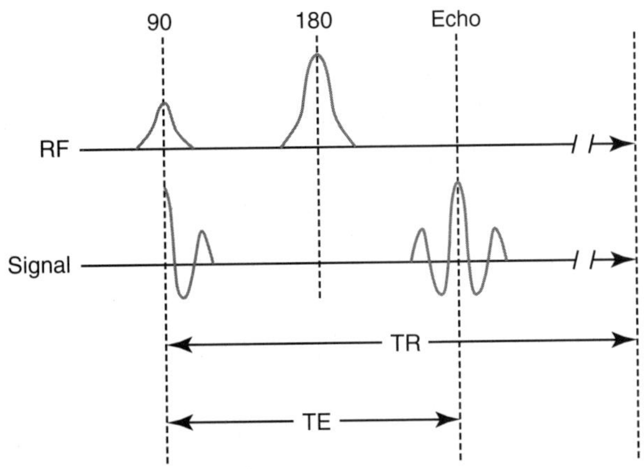

Fig. 4.25 Configuration of a standard spin-echo pulse sequence. Radiofrequency (*RF*) pulses consist of an initial 90-degree pulse followed by a 180-degree pulse. Signals associated with magnetized tissues echo exactly at a time twice that of the 180-degree pulse. The time it takes for this sequence to be run one time is called the *time to repetition (TR)*. *TE,* Time of echo.

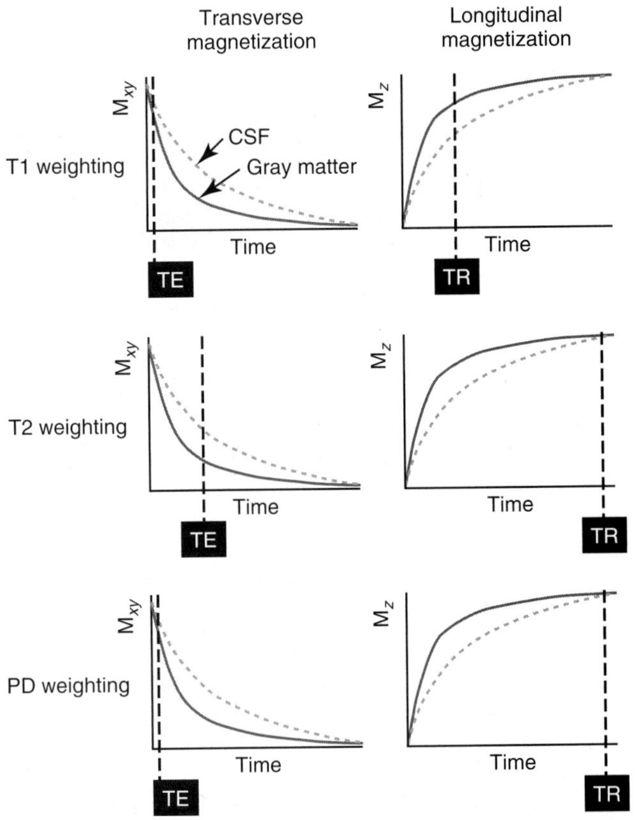

Fig. 4.26 Impact of time of echo (*TE*) and time to repetition (*TR*) on tissue contrast. By adjusting TE and TR, differences in T1- and T2-relaxation characteristics among tissues can be highlighted. By using short TE and short TR, signal echoes from cerebrospinal fluid *(CSF)* and gray matter mainly depend on differences in time for magnetization to regrow in the *z* direction, or longitudinal magnetization (T1 relaxation), as differences in transverse magnetization (T2 relaxation) of CSF and gray matter are negligible. This type of sequence is said to be T1-weighted. If, however, differences in T2 need to be highlighted and differences in T1 inhibited—i.e., T2-weighting—both TE and TR must be prolonged. Finally, using short TE and long TR inhibits both T1 and T2 effects. In that case, T1 and T2 contrast is reduced between CSF and gray matter, and signal intensity is predominantly associated with the density of protons in these tissues. These images have proton-density (*PD*) weighting.

suppress the signal from fat, and because this sequence has T2-weighting, it increases the conspicuity of soft tissue lesions, most of which have prolonged T2 (Fig. 4.29). Unlike chemical fat-signal suppression (discussed later), STIR sequences are not affected by magnetic-field inhomogeneities and therefore result in more uniform fat suppression.[10,11]

Inversion recovery can also be used to null the signal of fluids, such as cerebrospinal fluid (CSF). Such a fluid-attenuated inversion recovery (FLAIR) sequence helps differentiate brain parenchymal lesions from CSF (Fig. 4.30; see Fig. 4.28).[14] For example, a region of increased signal adjacent to a lateral ventricle may not be seen in the T2-weighted spin-echo sequence because of the similar signal characteristics of CSF and tissue water. However, in the FLAIR image, the periventricular lesion may be much more conspicuous because the signal from the free fluid in the ventricle has been nulled (see Fig. 4.30). The FLAIR sequence also aids in confirming a cystic component and the nature of the fluid present. FLAIR sequences are typically used for the brain and can be T2-weighted or T1-weighted and then referred as T2-FLAIR and T1-FLAIR, respectively.[15]

Gradient Recalled Sequences

As opposed to spin-echo sequences, gradient echo sequences use smaller flip angles[†] (i.e., <90 degrees) to start and the 180-degree refocusing RF pulse is not used. Instead, gradients are used to diphase (negative gradient) and rephase (positive gradient) transverse magnetization to generate echoes from tissues. Gradient echo sequences use a shorter TR along with smaller flip angles (i.e., shorter RF pulses), allowing rapid studies with reduced motion artifact, which can be convenient for procedures such as angiography. Gradient echo sequences are also used typically for initial anatomic orientation at the beginning of an examination, so called localizer images.

Although changing the orientation of the gradient allows spinning protons to rephase, field inhomogeneities are not compensated for. Thus, gradient echo sequences with long TEs are T2*-weighted rather than T2-weighted, such as in spin-echo sequences. This also means that gradient echo sequences are more sensitive to magnetic-field inhomogeneity secondary to magnetic susceptibility differences between tissues. Magnetic susceptibility is the property that describes the degree to which

[†]Remember, the flip angle quantifies the amount of deviation of the resting net magnetic vector from the *z*-axis by the first RF pulse.

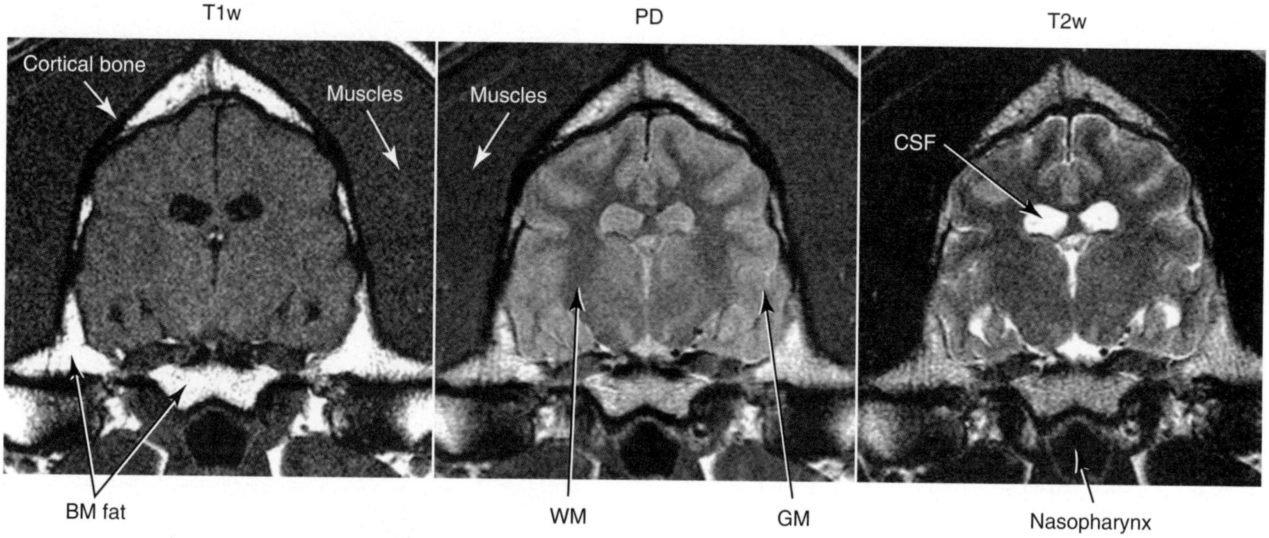

Fig. 4.27 Tissues are associated with variable signal intensity according to the type of weighting. Indeed, cerebrospinal fluid (*CSF*) appears hypointense (dark) in T1-weighting (*T1W*), moderately intense (midgray) in proton-density (*PD*) weighting, and hyperintense (bright) in T2-weighting (*T2W*). Other soft tissue structures also vary in signal intensity between sequences. Normal cortical bone and air are not magnetized enough to generate a signal on any sequence. *BM,* Bone marrow; *GM,* gray matter; *WM,* white matter.

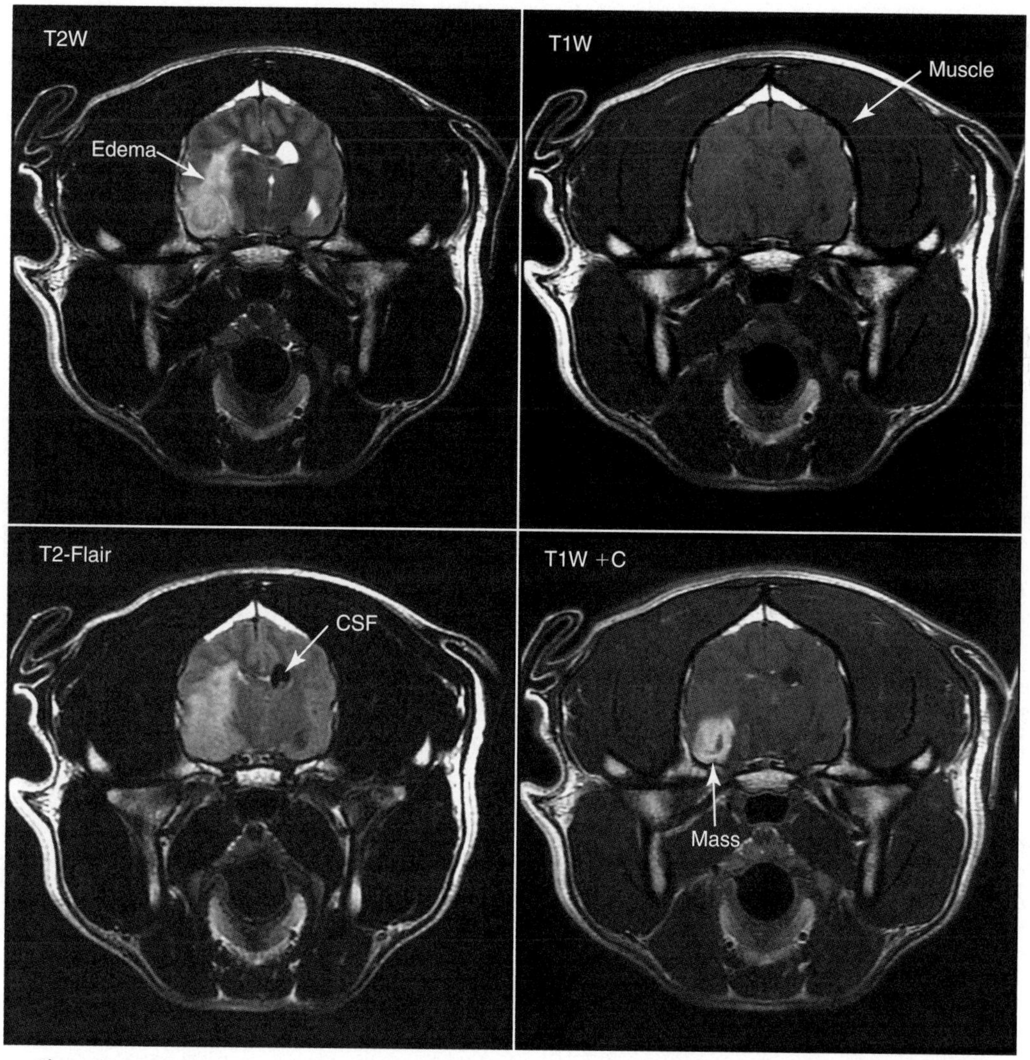

Fig. 4.28 Meningioma in the piriform lobe of a dog. In T2-weighted (*T2W*) images, the mass is hyperintense and also confluent with hyperintense regional vasogenic edema, whereas both the tumor and edema are isointense to the rest of the brain in precontrast T1-weighted (*T1W*) images. Following contrast-medium (gadolinium) injection (*T1W+C*), the mass enhances becoming very hyperintense, except for a central fusiform hypointense area. In a T2W fluid-attenuated inversion recovery (*T2-FLAIR*) sequence (designed to decrease signal coming from pure fluid), the signal from the pure cerebrospinal fluid (*CSF*) is attenuated.

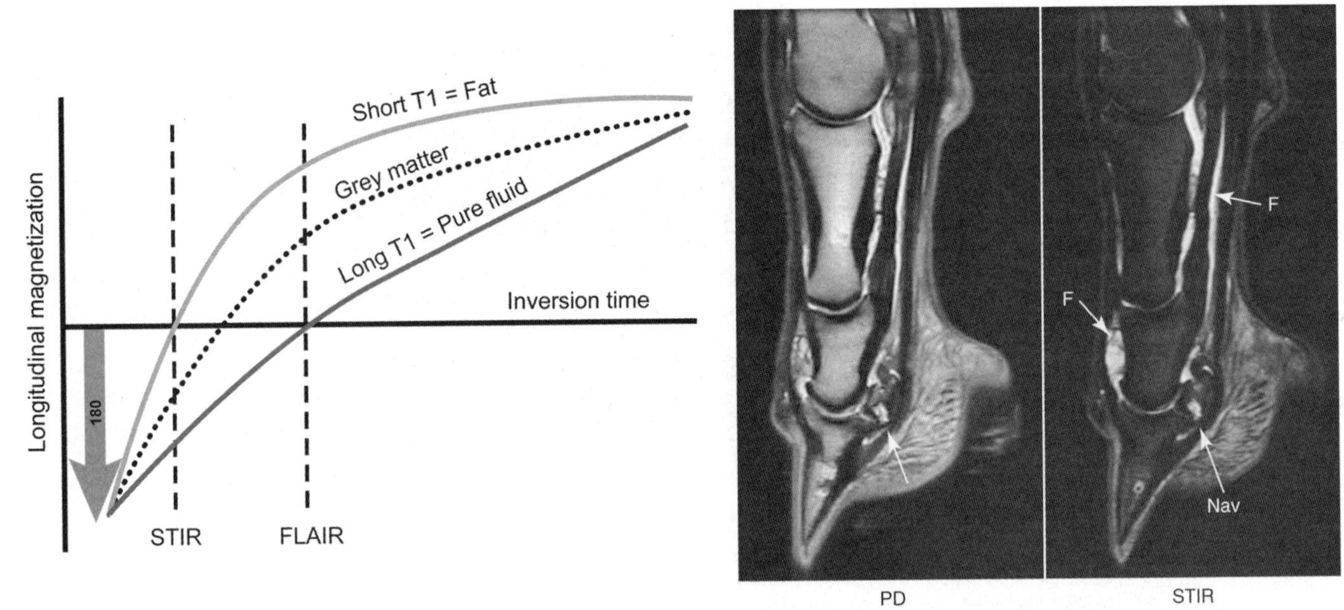

Fig. 4.29 Inversion recovery sequences are used to null the signal from fluids or fat and therefore improve the conspicuity of nearby tissues of similar signal characteristics. This graph illustrates the differences in longitudinal magnetization (T1) recovery rate after a 180-degree pulse is produced, before a regular spin-echo sequence is initiated. The time between the 180-degree pulse and the beginning of the spin-echo sequence is called the inversion time. Fat has very rapid T1-relaxation; therefore, with a short inversion time, the magnetization vector from fat will be in the *xy*-plane and no signal will be recorded in the spin-echo sequence. Sequences with a short inversion time are called ***short tau inversion recovery***, or ***STIR*** sequences. Images on the ***right*** demonstrate the clinical application of a STIR sequence. By suppressing the signal of fat in the bone marrow, the fluid-filled navicular cyst (*arrow*) becomes more apparent than in the proton-density (*PD*) sequence. Other fluid-filled structures such as synovial fluid (*F*) are also better delineated than on the PD sequence. Because free fluid has a longer T1-relaxation time, the use of a longer inversion time will result in the magnification vector from fluid being in the *xy*-plane and if the spin-echo sequence is initiated now there will be no signal measured from free fluid. Sequences with a longer inversion time are called fluid-attenuated inversion recovery (FLAIR) sequences. FLAIR sequences are mainly used for brain imaging, allowing parenchymal lesions to be better distinguished from normal cerebrospinal fluid (CSF) by eliminating the signal from CSF. See Figs. 4.28 and 4.30.

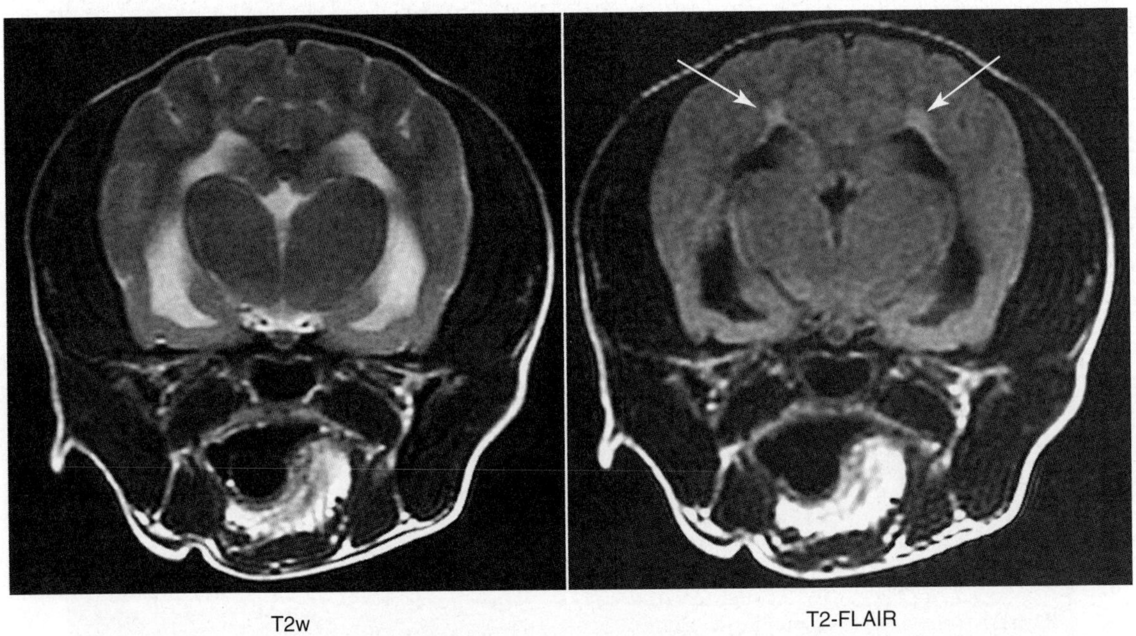

Fig. 4.30 A T2-weighted fluid-attenuated inversion recovery (*T2-FLAIR*) sequence can allow periventricular hyperintensities (*arrows*) to be depicted better than with regular spin-echo T2-weighting (*T2W*) by eliminating the signal from cerebrospinal fluid (CSF). Here, periventricular edema is more evident on T2-FLAIR in this dog with necrotizing encephalitis.

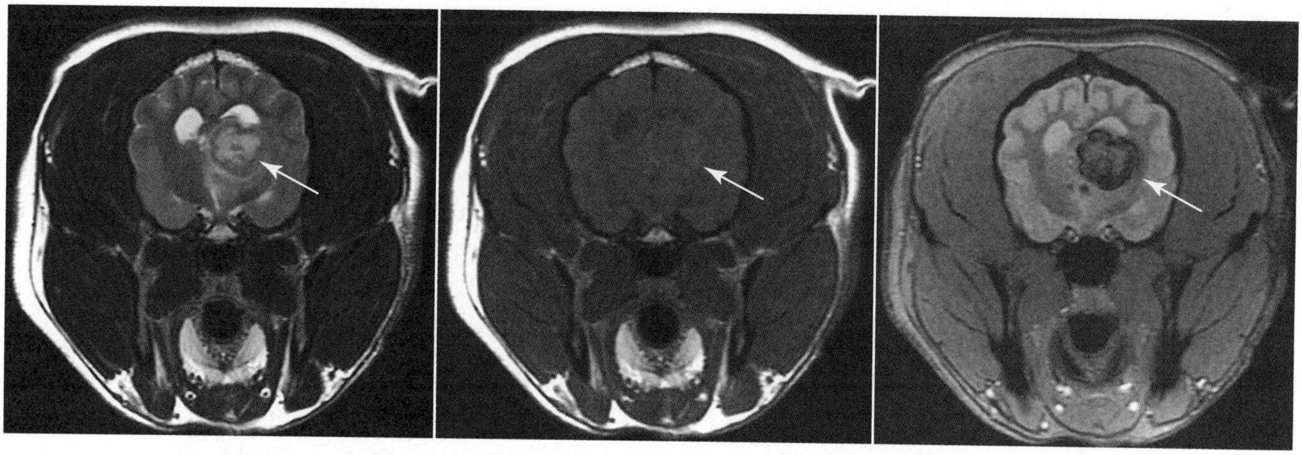

Fig. 4.31 T2* gradient echo (*GRE*) sequences are sensitive to magnetic susceptibility. In this dog with spontaneous brain hemorrhage, the mass lesion (*arrow*) with annular signal void on T2*-GRE in the thalamus corresponds with a susceptibility artifact. The peripheral portion of this lesion appears hyperintense on precontrast T1-weighted fast spin-echo (*T1W-FSE*) and hypointense on T2-weighted FSE (*T2W-FSE*), further confirming the presence of subacute hemorrhage.

these tissues are magnetized when exposed to a magnetic field.[16] Substances can increase (paramagnetic, ferromagnetic) or decrease (diamagnetic) local magnetic field strength and thus exert an effect on nearby spinning protons. Tissues with protons affected by local field inhomogeneity dephase more rapidly, causing signal loss and/or signal misregistration. This phenomenon is even more evident when using a high-field magnet and long TE (e.g., T2*-weighted gradient echo sequence). This concept is exploited for the detection of hemorrhage. Indeed, the iron contained in the hemoglobin increases the local magnetic field substantially, leading to local signal loss and misregistration.[12] T2*-weighted sequences are thus sensitive for detecting hemorrhage (Fig. 4.31).

Several other gradient echo sequences exist, some with more specific application. For example, a spoiled gradient recalled (SPGR) echo sequence highlights articular cartilage (eFig. 4.4),[17] whereas steady state free precession techniques can help depict cranial nerves.[18] It must be pointed out that gradient sequences have specific names that vary among MR imaging system vendors, which can lead to some confusion.[12,19]

Contrast Media

As with CT, contrast media can be injected intravenously for MR imaging to assess the vascular network and tissue perfusion, helping to better detect and characterize pathologic tissues. As opposed to iodinated contrast medium used in CT that increases x-ray attenuation, contrast media commonly used in MR imaging are not meant to be directly visible. Rather, they exert a strong paramagnetic effect that decreases the T2- and T1-relaxation time of protons in vicinity of the contrast medium molecule. Gadolinium-based agents chelated to protective ligands are typically used. At low concentration, such as used in clinical practice, the predominant effect is a shortening of the T1-relaxation time.[10] Thus, tissues accumulating this substance generate greater signal—*contrast-enhance*—on a T1-weighted pulse sequence (Fig. 4.32; see Fig. 4.28). At high gadolinium concentration, T2 shortening may result in a significant decrease in signal intensity noticeable on both T1- and T2-weighted images. This effect can be observed in the bladder as a triple-layer intensity pattern, or pseudolayering.[20]

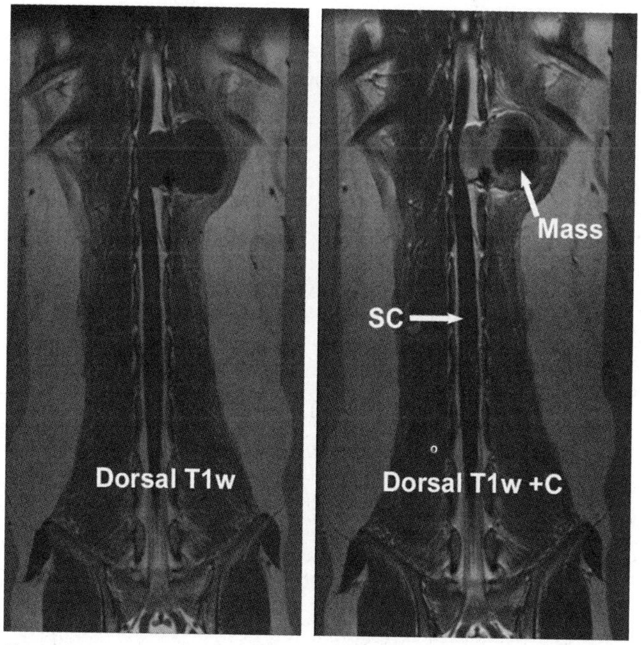

Fig. 4.32 As for computed tomography (CT) imaging, the addition of contrast medium in magnetic resonance (MR) imaging (e.g., gadolinium) increases the contrast resolution of this modality. In this ataxic dog, a large mass is seen in dorsal T1-weighted (*T1W*) images to the *left* of the spine, markedly compressing the spinal cord (*SC*). The periphery of this mass enhances intensity after gadolinium injection (*+C*), as opposed to its central part. An undifferentiated sarcoma with a large cavitary component was diagnosed.

Fat Saturation Sequences

The high signal intensity of adipose tissue on several sequences can limit the visibility of nearby tissues or substances with prolonged T2 relaxation (on T2-weighted sequences) or short T1 relaxation (on T1-weighted sequences). As seen previously, a STIR inversion recovery sequence can be used to attenuate fat signal intensity. Alternatively, fat can be selectively attenuated by exploiting the inherent difference of precessional frequency,

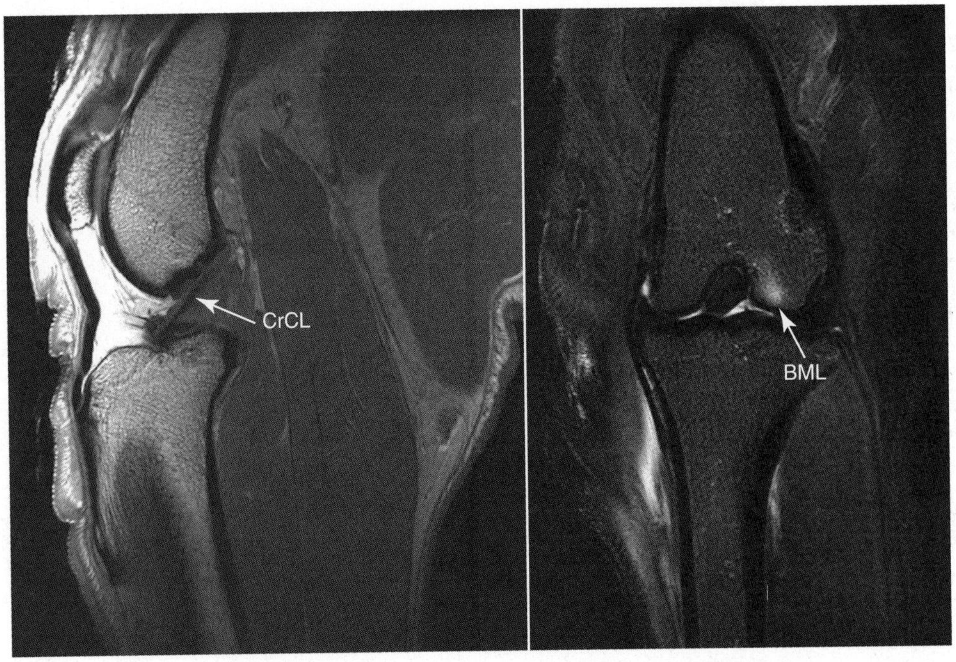

Fig. 4.33 Like short TI inversion recovery (STIR) sequences, chemical fat saturation (*FS*) used with T2-weighting (*T2W*) increases the conspicuity of lesions with prolonged T2 relaxation. A hyperintense bone marrow lesion (*BML*) is identified in the fat suppressed sequence in the lateral femoral condyle of this dog with intact cranial cruciate ligament (*CrCL*). *PD,* Proton density.

or *chemical shift*, that exists between fat and water protons. The magnitude of this difference is 220 Hz at a field strength of 1.5 T. The difference in precessional frequency becomes smaller at lower field strengths; therefore, chemical fat suppression is limited to field strengths of 1.0 Tesla or greater.

As opposed to the 90-degree and 180-degree pulses that have a frequency range large enough to excite both water and lipid protons, *chemical fat saturation* uses a frequency-specific preparation pulse to selectively excite lipid protons, followed by a spoiling gradient pulse that dephases the fat signal. Once the initial fat-specific pulse is produced, the signal generated by the subsequent pulse sequence (spin echo or gradient echo) arises only from nonfatty tissues. If a T2-weighted sequence is employed, tissues with prolonged T2, typically pathologic tissues, become more conspicuous (Fig. 4.33). In combination with gadolinium injection, fat-suppressed T1-weighted sequences maximize the visibility of contrast-enhancing lesions. This can be beneficial for detecting lesions embedded in fat, such as within the epidural or retro-orbital spaces, and in bone marrow, for example.[21] Spinal lesions and abnormal nerves are better recognized (eFig. 4.5).

Other Magnetic Resonance Sequences

Several other imaging sequences can provide important information on the characteristics of tissues. As for chemical fat saturation pulses, most of these sequences are only available with high-field units (>1.0 T).

Diffusion-weighted imaging is very sensitive to cytotoxic edema in the early hours of ischemia. Tissue contrast on diffusion-weighted imaging reflects Brownian motion or microscopic movement of water, which is restricted in ischemic tissue.[22] Such technique helps in discriminating early stroke events from structural lesions, such as neoplasia, which can be difficult to differentiate on conventional sequences (Fig. 4.34). *Perfusion-weighted* imaging is another technique that can support a diagnosis of brain infarct.[22] It uses a particular T2*-weighted pulse sequence following a bolus injection of contrast medium such as gadolinium. Images are obtained during the first pass of contrast medium through the capillary beds, which results in susceptibility-induced signal loss that resolves over time. Relative blood flow can then be semiquantified.

Image Quality and Imaging Time

The challenge of imaging animals under anesthesia is to balance image quality and acquisition time. That is, to achieve the most diagnostic examination as quickly as possible. Several parameters are interconnected, making this balance very complex.[23] As discussed earlier, *spatial resolution* dictates the amount of image detail, which influences the ability to clearly see and distinguish anatomic and pathologic structures. Spatial resolution is determined by adjusting slice thickness (voxel depth), field of view (FOV), and matrix size (number of voxels). The height and width of each voxel is determined by the number of rows and columns in the matrix, respectively, divided by the image FOV. The smaller the voxels are, the better the spatial resolution. Conversely, image quality also greatly depends on the amount of signal arising from protons forming each voxel, often described as the signal-to-noise ratio (SNR) of an image. High spatial resolution images, those with small voxels, are then subject to poor SNR. Although it can be tempting to reduce slice thickness or increase matrix size to improve tissue definition, image quality can suffer greatly. SNR can be improved by averaging signal from sequential excitations, which unfortunately increases acquisition time. Technical improvements in software and hardware (high-field magnets, stronger gradients, more sensitive receiving coils, parallel imaging, etc.) have allowed an increase in SNR and spatial resolution at the same time, which is beneficial in small patients (Fig. 4.35).[15,24]

MR Image Artifacts

As with any modality, artifacts can degrade image quality or lead to misdiagnosis. Acknowledgment and comprehension of these artifacts are essential for interpreters.

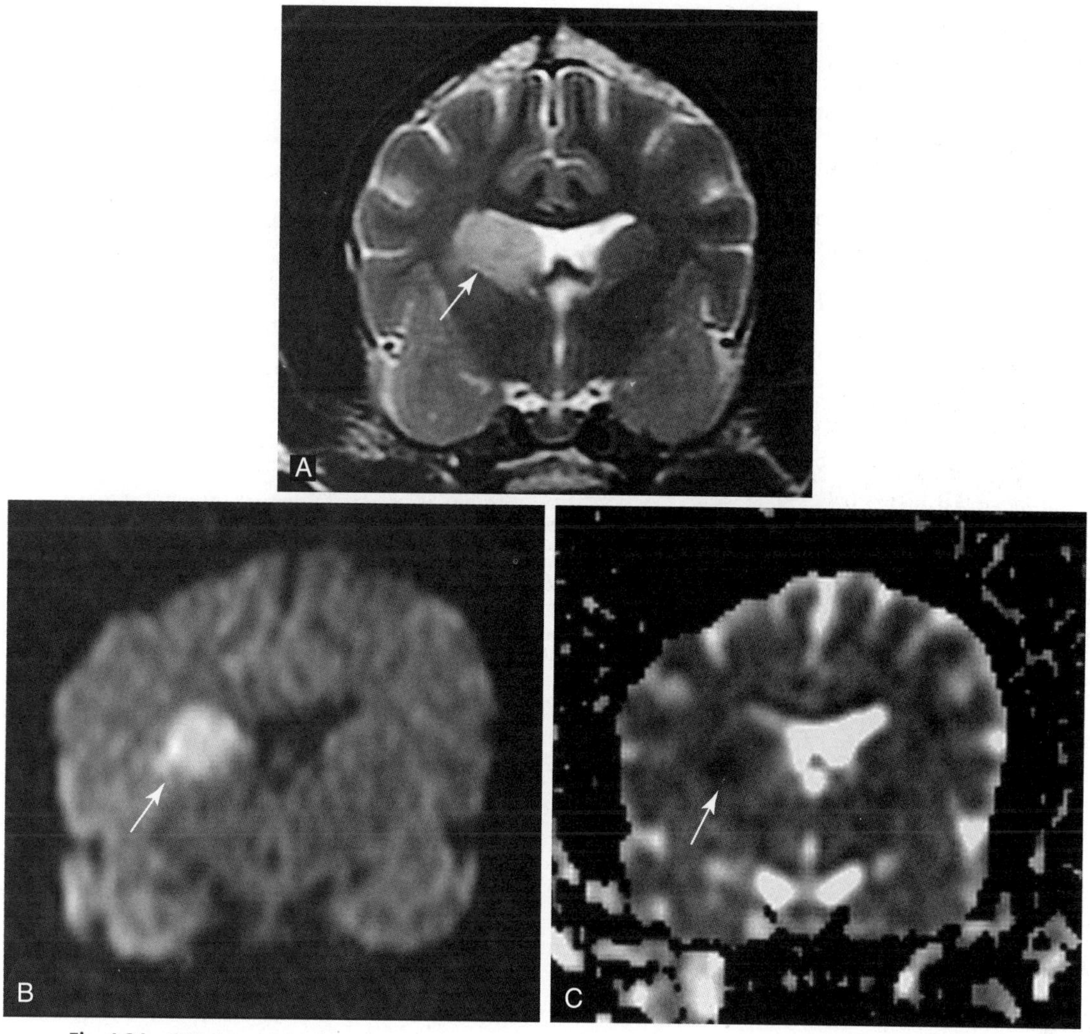

Fig. 4.34 Diffusion-weighted imaging (DWI) is used to confirm early ischemic stroke (*arrow*). The right caudate nucleus is enlarged and hyperintense in transverse T2-weighted fast spin-echo (**A**) and in a diffusion-weighted image (**B**). **C**, In an image of the apparent diffusion coefficient (ADC) the lesion becomes hypointense, indicating restricted water diffusion.

Besides those that can be controlled to a certain degree (e.g., ghosting and aliasing artifacts),[25] artifacts are often related to magnetic susceptibility and are predominant with gradient echo sequences, as discussed previously. Magnetic susceptibility artifacts occur because of local magnetic field inhomogeneity. Structures that substantially affect this homogeneity, such as metallic objects, whether ferrous or not, have strong magnetic susceptibility effects that lead to field distortion.[26] These artifacts appear as geometric image distortion with progressive or abrupt signal void and sharply defined hyperintense boundaries (Fig. 4.36). In veterinary practice, microchips (eFig. 4.6) and orthopedic devices are most often the source of these artifacts, hampering assessment of nearby structures. It may also occur when microscopic metal fragments are left in place when some devices are used during surgery (e.g., drill bits).[16] Other ballistic or gastrointestinal foreign bodies may cause magnetic susceptibility artifacts that can limit the use of MR imaging in these patients significantly, particularly if these objects are ferromagnetic and can therefore migrate because of magnetic attraction. Magnetic susceptibility can also occur at soft tissue/air interfaces. This is typically observed on T2* transverse images obtained at the junction of the frontal sinuses and rostral brain.[26] The magic angle effect is another important MR artifact that can alter the signal intensity of tendons and ligaments in both low- and high-field MR units, mainly described in the distal equine limb.[27] This artifact appears when tendons or ligaments are positioned at specific angles in the magnetic field.

Impact of Magnetic Field Strength

Although high-field (>1.0 T) MR systems are associated with superior SNR and spatial resolution, and offer more advanced imaging protocols, low-field (0.2–0.4 T) units are installed in many veterinary practices, mainly because of lower purchase and maintenance costs.[19] Units can be dedicated veterinary units or produced originally for human use. The limited SNR with these low-field systems is associated with longer scan times and reduced spatial resolution. Also, FOV is generally reduced, which may necessitate moving the patient in the magnet for complete anatomic coverage. Low-field MR imaging is, however, associated with reduced susceptibility artifact, and its open design allows easy access to patients. Also, because of the lower magnetic field strength, accidents associated with the attraction or migration of ferromagnetic objects, located outside or inside the patient, can be prevented more easily. Extremities of horses can also be imaged while the animal is standing using dedicated MR units, which is beneficial.

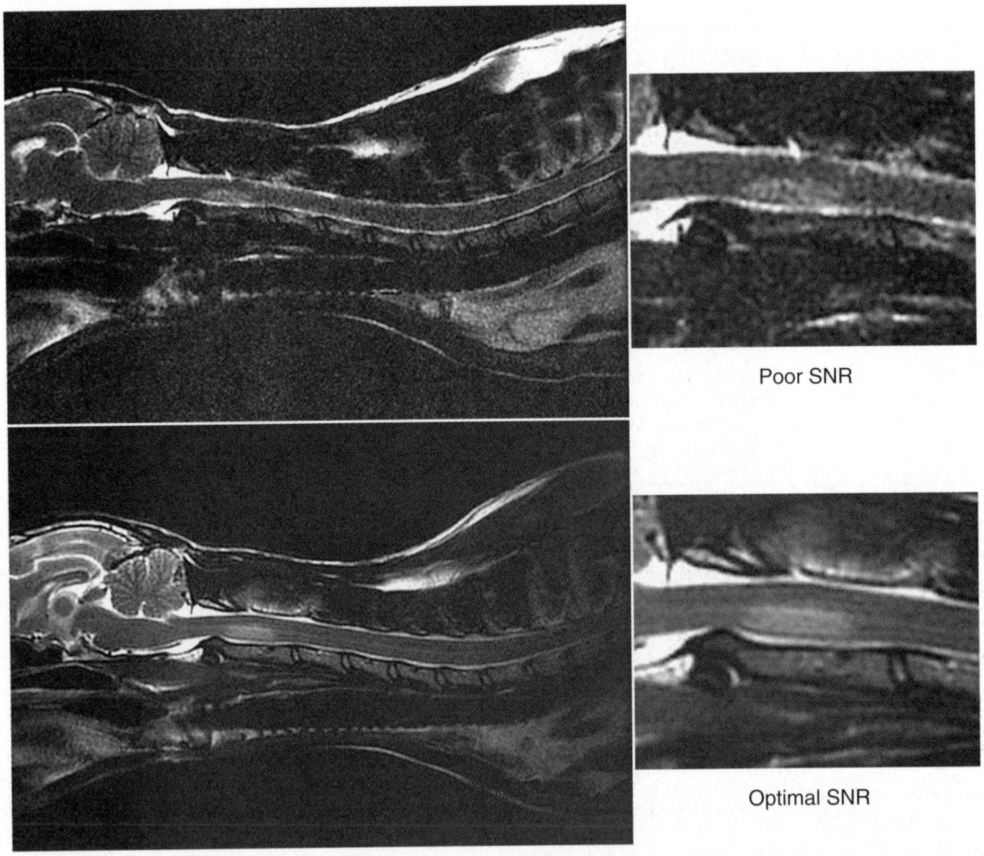

Fig. 4.35 Several factors can influence signal-to-noise (*SNR*) ratio in magnetic resonance (MR) imaging. In this dog, optimal SNR of the cervical spine was obtained after replacing the receiving coil with a more sensitive one (*bottom images*). The initial image with poor SNR is grainier. The ventral spinal cord hyperintensity is better delineated in the bottom image.

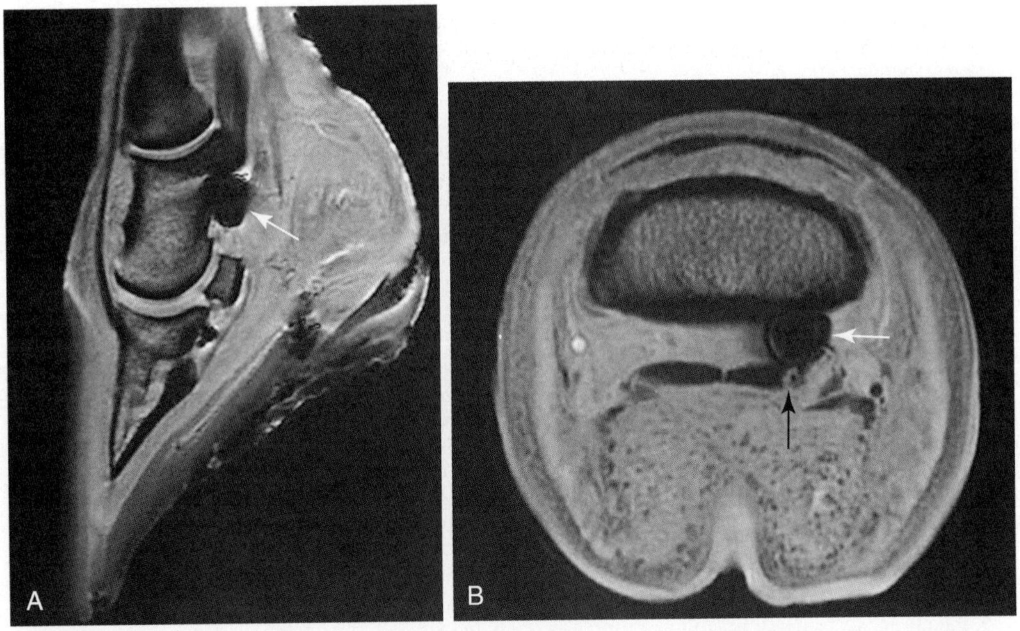

Fig. 4.36 Susceptibility artifact in gradient recalled echo (GRE) sequences. In this equine foot imaged with T1-weighted GRE sequences in sagittal (**A**) and transverse (**B**) planes, there is a sharply demarcated round signal void (*white arrow*), which was the result of a microscopic metallic fragment left in place after a street nail was removed. Note also the damage to the medial lobe of the deep digital flexor tendon (*black arrow*).

REFERENCES

1. Euclid Seeram E. Computed tomography: an overview. In: Euclid Seeram E, ed. *Computed Tomography: Physical Principles, Clinical Applications, and Quality Control*. 4th ed. Burnaby: Elsevier Canada; 2015:1–30.
2. Bushberg J, Seibert J, Leidholdt Jr E, et al. Computed tomography. In: Bushberg J, Seibert J, Leidholdt Jr E, et al., eds. *The Essential Physics of Medical Imaging*. 3rd ed. Philadelphia: Lippincott Williams & Wilkins; 2011:312–374.
3. Bushberg J, Seibert J, Leidholdt Jr E, et al. Introduction to medical imaging. In: Bushberg J, Seibert J, Leidholdt Jr E, et al., eds. *The Essential Physics of Medical Imaging*. 3rd ed. Philadelphia: Lippincott Williams & Wilkins; 2011:3–17.
4. Saunders J, Ohlerth S. CT physics and instrumentation. In: Schwarz T, Saunders J, eds. *Veterinary Computed Tomography*. 1st ed. Oxford: Wiley-Blackwell; 2011.
5. Euclid Seeram E. Physical principles of CT. In: Euclid Seeram E, ed. *Computed Tomography: Physical Principles, Clinical Applications, and Quality Control*. 4th ed. Burnaby: Elsevier Canada; 2015:60.
6. Pollard R, Puchalski S. CT contrast media and applications. In: Schwarz T, Saunders J, eds. *Veterinary Computed Tomography*. 1st ed. Oxford: Wiley-Blackwell; 2011.
7. Miles KA. Tumour angiogenesis and its relation to contrast enhancement on computed tomography: a review. *Eur J Radiol*. 1999;30:198–205.
8. Alexander K, Dunn M, Carmel EN, et al. Clinical application of Patlak plot CT-GFR in animals with upper urinary tract disease. *Vet Radiol Ultrasound*. 2010;51:421–427.
9. Soukup JW, Drees R, Koenig LJ, et al. Comparison of the diagnostic image quality of the canine maxillary dentoalveolar structures obtained by cone beam computed tomography and 64-multidetector row computed tomography. *J Vet Dent*. 2015;32:80–86.
10. McRobbie DW, Moore EA, Graves MJ, et al. In: *MRI from Pictures to Protons*. ed 1. Cambridge: Cambridge University Press; 2003.
11. Mitchell DG, Cohen MS. In: *MRI Principles*. 2nd ed. Philadelphia: Saunders; 2004.
12. Bitar R, Leung G, Perng R, et al. MR pulse sequences: what every radiologist wants to know but is afraid to ask. *Radiographics*. 2006;26:513–537.
13. Balter S. An introduction to the physics of magnetic resonance imaging. *Radiographics*. 1987;7:371–383.
14. Benigni L, Lamb CR. Comparison of fluid-attenuated inversion recovery and T2-weighted magnetic resonance images in dogs and cats with suspected brain disease. *Vet Radiol Ultrasound*. 2005;46:287–292.
15. Robertson ID. Optimal magnetic resonance imaging of the brain. *Vet Radiol Ultrasound*. 2011;52:S15–S22.
16. Freer SR, Scrivani PV. Postoperative susceptibility artifact during magnetic resonance imaging of the vertebral column in two dogs and a cat. *Vet Radiol Ultrasound*. 2008;49:30–34.
17. Olive J, d'Anjou MA, Girard C, et al. Fat-suppressed spoiled gradient-recalled imaging of equine metacarpophalangeal articular cartilage. *Vet Radiol Ultrasound*. 2010;51: 107–115.
18. Parry AT, Volk HA. Imaging the cranial nerves. *Vet Radiol Ultrasound*. 2011;52:S32–S41.
19. Konar M, Lang J. Pros and cons of low-field magnetic resonance imaging in veterinary medicine. *Vet Radiol Ultrasound*. 2011;52:S5–S14.
20. Mai W. Pseudolayering artefact on postcontrast magnetic resonance images of the bladder of 18 dogs and three cats. *Vet Rec*. 2008;163:117.
21. d'Anjou MA, Carmel EN, Tidwell AS. Value of fat suppression in gadolinium-enhanced magnetic resonance neuroimaging. *Vet Radiol Ultrasound*. 2011;52:S85–S90.
22. Tidwell AS, Robertson ID. Magnetic resonance imaging of normal and abnormal brain perfusion. *Vet Radiol Ultrasound*. 2011;52:S62–S71.
23. Gavin P, Bagley RS. In: Ames IA, ed. *Practical Small Animal MRI*. 2nd ed. Wiley-Blackwell; 2009.
24. Glockner HU. Parallel MR imaging: a user's guide. *Radiographics*. 2005;25:1279–1297.
25. Cooper JJ, Young BD, Hoffman A, et al. Intracranial magnetic resonance imaging artifacts and pseudolesions in dogs and cats. *Vet Radiol Ultrasound*. 2010;51:587–595.
26. Hecht S, Adams WH, Narak JN, et al. Magnetic resonance imaging susceptibility artifacts due to metallic foreign bodies. *Vet Radiol Ultrasound*. 2011;52(4):409–414 [Epub March 7, 2011].
27. Werpy NM, Ho CP, Kawcak CE. Magic angle effect in normal collateral ligaments of the distal interphalangeal joint in horses imaged with a high-field magnetic resonance imaging system. *Vet Radiol Ultrasound*. 2010;51:2–10.

ELECTRONIC RESOURCES

Additional information related to the content in Chapter 4 can be found online at eBooks.Health.Elsevier.com.

- Chapter Quiz
- Videos

CHAPTER 5

Contrast Media in Diagnostic Imaging

Jennifer A. Reetz

INTRODUCTION

A contrast medium (plural media) is a substance used in medical imaging to change the opacity of a tissue, organ or cavity. By changing the opacity, contrast is increased thereby making tissues, organs, or cavities more conspicuous. Contrast media have applications in radiography, fluoroscopy, ultrasonography, computed tomography (CT), and magnetic resonance imaging (MRI).

RADIOGRAPHIC CONTRAST MEDIA

Radiographic contrast media are characterized as either positive or negative. Positive contrast media (e.g., barium sulfate and iodinated media) result in an increase in radiographic opacity due to increased absorption of x-ray photons (Fig. 5.1). The effective atomic number (Z) of barium (Z = 56) and iodine (Z = 53) is higher than that for soft tissue (Z = 7), which means that there is greater x-ray absorption by barium and iodine through the photoelectric effect and this increases the contrast of the tissues or fluids that contain them. X-ray absorption by barium and iodine is also enhanced by the K-absorption edge (K-edge) effect. The K-edge describes an abrupt increase in photoelectric absorption that occurs when the x-ray beam energy is just beyond the binding energy of inner k-shell electrons. The K-edges of barium (37.4 keV) and iodine (33.2 keV) are near the mean energy of the typical x-ray emission spectrum.[1] Low kVp settings in CT imaging closer to the k-edge of iodine can be used to increase the contrast between enhanced and non-enhanced regions for low dose or delayed postcontrast series.

Negative contrast media, on the other hand, result in a decrease in radiographic opacity due to lower absorption of x-ray photons, rendering the area of interest less radiopaque (more radiolucent) (Fig. 5.2). Typical negative contrast media include room air, CO_2, or NO_2. Sometimes studies combine both positive and negative contrast media and are termed *double-contrast studies*.

When using contrast media in CT (usually iodinated), the concepts are similar in that positive and negative contrast media increase and decrease x-ray beam absorption, respectively, but in CT, grayscale changes are described in terms of attenuation as opposed to opacity because CT images are computed based on quantification of x-ray attenuation. The attenuation values in the acquired voxels are translated into Hounsfield units (HU), which then allows for objective measurements of attenuation changes associated with contrast media (Fig. 5.3).

BARIUM CONTRAST MEDIA

General Information

Barium sulfate ($BaSO_4$) is an insoluble, inert, mineral salt commonly used in gastrointestinal contrast studies. Micropulverized liquid barium preparations are the most common

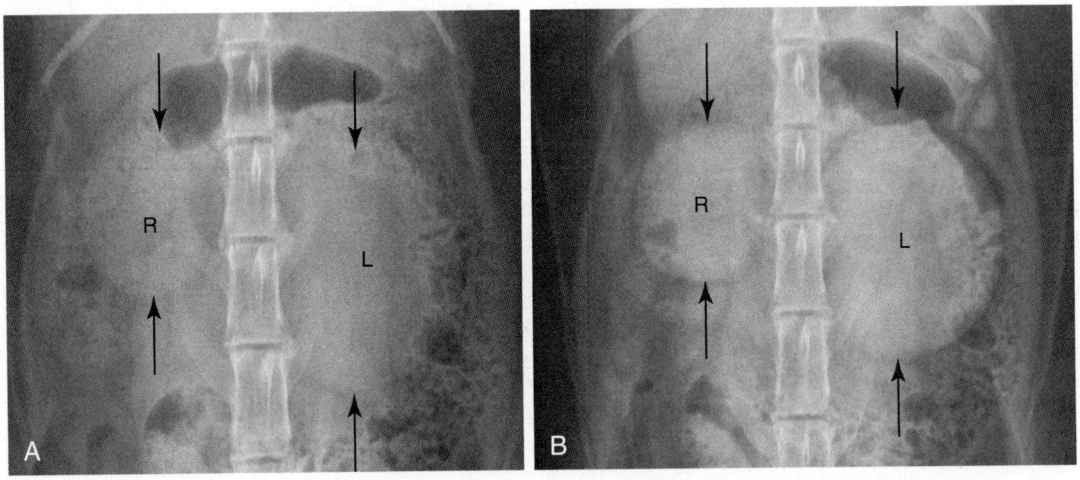

Fig. 5.1 Example of a radiographic positive contrast medium (intravenous excretory urography or IVU). **A**, Survey radiograph of the right (*R*) and left (*L*) kidneys (between *black arrows*) in a cat. Some of the soft tissue opaque renal margins are visible due to contrast provided by fat in the retroperitoneal space, but some portions are indistinct. **B**, Iodinated contrast medium was administered intravenously, and a repeat radiograph obtained almost immediately. Due to the high atomic number of iodine in the contrast medium, there is increased renal radiopacity, which provides additional radiographic contrast such that the renal margins are now clearly visible in their entirety.

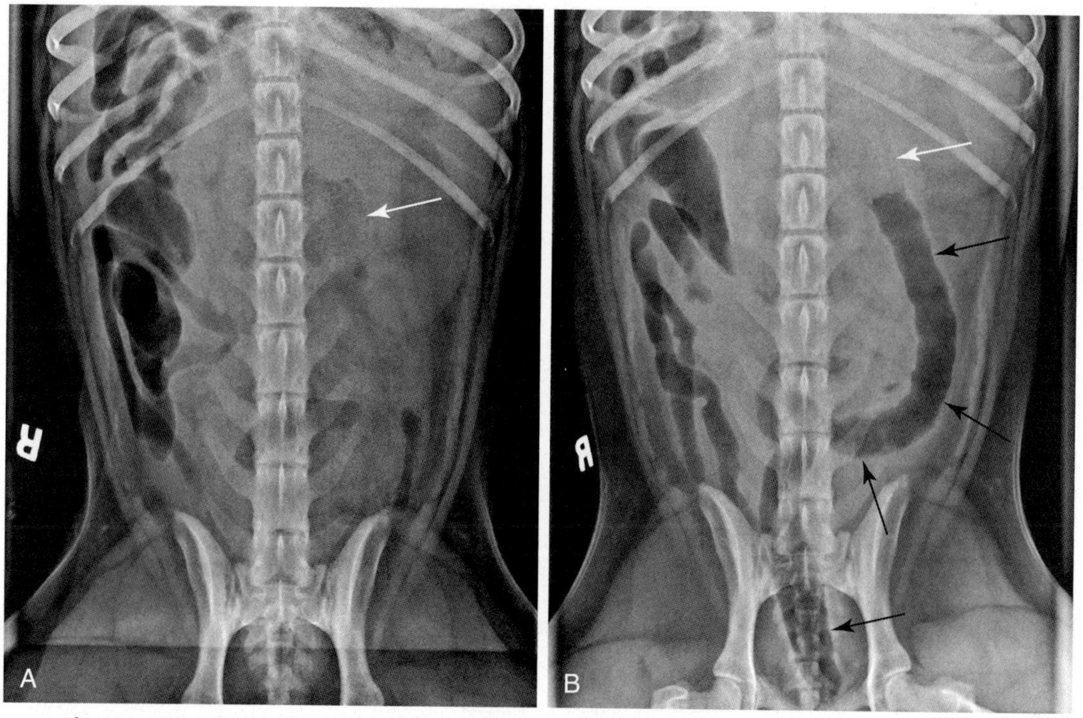

Fig. 5.2 Example of a radiographic negative contrast medium (pneumocolonography performed with room air). **A**, A corn cob foreign body is present within an intestinal segment in the left mid abdomen (*white arrow*) on this ventrodorsal view. Localization of the foreign body to the descending colon vs. jejunum was not possible on this view or the orthogonal view (not shown). **B**, Room air was instilled into the rectum via a red rubber catheter, to delineate the colon. Now that the rectum and descending colon (*black arrows*) contain air, the foreign body can be clearly localized to the colon. The decreased radiopacity (increased radiolucency) of the air-filled colonic lumen provides additional radiographic contrast such that the margins of the foreign body are more readily visible.

formulations used in veterinary medicine. Given the insoluble nature of barium, emulsifiers, stabilizers, and dispersants are added to the barium-water suspension to maintain the barium in suspension (Fig. 5.4).[2] Other barium formulations used in veterinary medicine include barium sulfate powder, barium sulfate paste and barium impregnated polyethylene spheres (BIPS). Barium sulfate powder manually mixed with water can be problematic as the barium particles may sediment and lead to poor quality studies (see Fig. 5.4).[3]

Liquid barium sulfate is the preferred contrast medium for gastrointestinal studies where perforation is not a concern. It allows for a more detailed evaluation of the mucosal surface compared to iodinated water soluble contrast media,[4] and is more resistant to dilution by fluid in the gastrointestinal tract.[5] Double-contrast studies using barium sulfate and room air, as with double-contrast gastrography, allow for more precise mucosal assessment.[6] Interestingly, liquid barium sulfate is sometimes used as a therapeutic agent in patients with acute gastroenteritis to cathartically coat intestinal mucosa and bind bacterial toxins.[7]

The concentration of barium sulfate suspensions is expressed in terms of either weight/volume (w/v) or weight/weight (w/w), which is the percentage of the weight of barium sulfate (grams) relative to the volume (100 mL) or weight (100 g) of the final product, respectively. For example, a liquid barium sulfate suspension labeled as 105% w/v and 58% w/w indicates: 105 g of barium sulfate in 100 mL of the final product (105% w/v) and 58 g of barium sulfate in 100 g of the product (58% w/w). Different concentrations of barium may be used for contrast studies and depending on the baseline concentration of the available barium suspension (e.g., 105% w/v vs. 60% w/v), dilution with water may be needed to achieve the desired concentration.

Adverse Effects

The most serious complication of barium studies is leakage of barium into the mediastinum or abdominal cavity from an esophageal or gastrointestinal perforation.[8] Barium sulfate alone can lead to peritonitis and adhesions,[9] but in association with a gastrointestinal perforation, it may further complicate septic peritonitis through the formation of granulomatous nodules on visceral and parietal surfaces that trap spilled intestinal content and bacteria, thereby contributing to fibrinous adhesions.[10] As with any septic peritonitis, this can be life-threatening and immediate aggressive therapy including surgery is recommended.[10] Similarly, leakage of barium sulfate associated with esophageal perforation can lead to mediastinitis.[8] If a positive contrast study of the gastrointestinal tract is indicated and perforation is of concern, the use of an iodinated, nonionic, water-soluble contrast medium is recommended.

Aspiration of barium following oral administration is another potential complication. Based on knowledge acquired from use of barium sulfate for bronchography, small volumes of barium sulfate aspiration are not problematic owing to its inert nature, and the barium can be cleared from the airways through coughing and the mucociliary apparatus.[5,11] Barium sulfate also undergoes phagocytosis by macrophages and some aspirated barium can remain in the pulmonary interstitium or be translocated to regional lymph nodes.[12] Aspiration of large volumes of barium, however, can result in pneumonia and acute respiratory distress, and ultimately death.[8,13] Other side effects of barium sulfate reported in human beings include allergic reactions, nausea, vomiting, abdominal pain, barolith formation resulting from barium sulfate remaining in the intestine too long, vasovagal reflex (e.g., during colonography), bacteremia (e.g., from barium enema), and intravasation.[5]

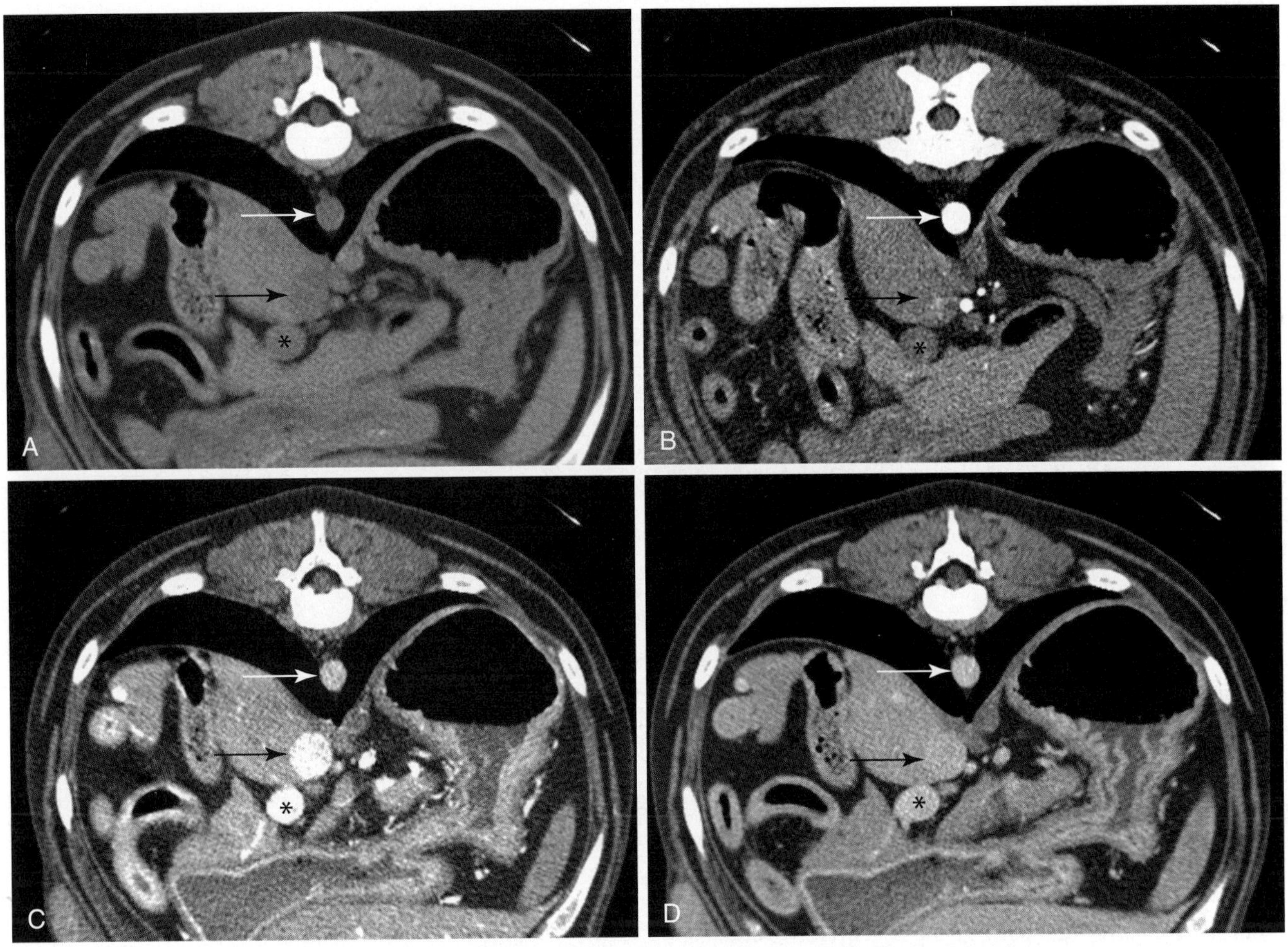

Fig. 5.3 Example of a triple-phase CT angiography to demonstrate changes in vascular attenuation over time after an intravenous bolus of an iodinated contrast medium (iohexol 350 mgI/mL). **A,** Precontrast image of the cranial abdomen. **B,** Arterial phase, with images acquired ~15 seconds after contrast medium injection. The aorta is markedly hyperattenuating relative to the other great vessels, as the contrast medium has not yet reached the venous system. **C,** Venous phase, with images acquired ~80 seconds after contrast injection. The contrast is decreasing in the arterial system and is peaked in the venous system, so that the aorta is less attenuating while the caudal vena cava and portal vein are markedly hyperattenuating. **D,** Delayed phase, with images acquired approximately 120 seconds after contrast medium injection. While all the great vessels are hyperattenuating relative to precontrast images, there is overall less attenuation compared to the arterial and venous phases, as the iodine content in the bloodstream is decreasing. For an objective example, the Hounsfield units (HU) of the aorta over time are: precontrast = 22.8, arterial phase = 829.00, venous phase 191.60, delayed phase = 160.76. *White arrow,* aorta; *black arrow,* caudal vena cava; *black asterisk,* portal vein.

IODINE-BASED CONTRAST MEDIA

General Information

Iodine-based contrast media are based upon a tri-iodinated benzene ring (Fig. 5.5). There are water-soluble and water-insoluble contrast media, with water-soluble media being the primary ones used in clinical practice. Water-soluble contrast media can be classified based on charge (ionic, nonionic), number of benzene rings (monomer, dimer) and osmolality (high, low, iso-osmolar). Contrast ratio (iodine to solute particle ratio), viscosity, and hydrophilicity (vs. lipophilicity) are other important factors when considering iodinated contrast media. Iodinated contrast media are used in a wide variety of clinical applications in diagnostic imaging, including radiography, fluoroscopy, and CT. Intravascular (IV) administration is the most common route of administration, but other routes exist, such as oral or rectal administration, injection into the urinary system, or intrathecal injection.

Iodinated contrast media normally undergo glomerular filtration and rapid renal excretion after IV administration. Extrarenal excretion pathways exist, most notably biliary excretion. In human beings, extrarenal excretion can occur in patients with renal dysfunction or obstruction, but it can also be seen in normal patients on delayed CT scans (e.g., 24 hours later).[14] Binding of contrast media to serum proteins plays a role in excretion, and with higher protein binding, there is longer plasma retention, which leads to less renal and more biliary excretion.[15] For example, meglumine iotroxate (Biliscopin) has high protein binding; therefore, it can be used for cholecystography after IV administration.[16] Occasionally, renal excretion is seen after oral or rectal contrast administration, as described in normal patients and in those with intestinal mucosal disease, obstruction, or perforation.[17,18]

Properties of Iodinated Contrast Media

Ionic vs. nonionic—Ionic media undergo dissociation into positive and negative ions, whereas nonionic media do not undergo dissociation owing to hydrophilic polar hydroxyl (OH) groups that increase solubility.[19] Ionic media contain

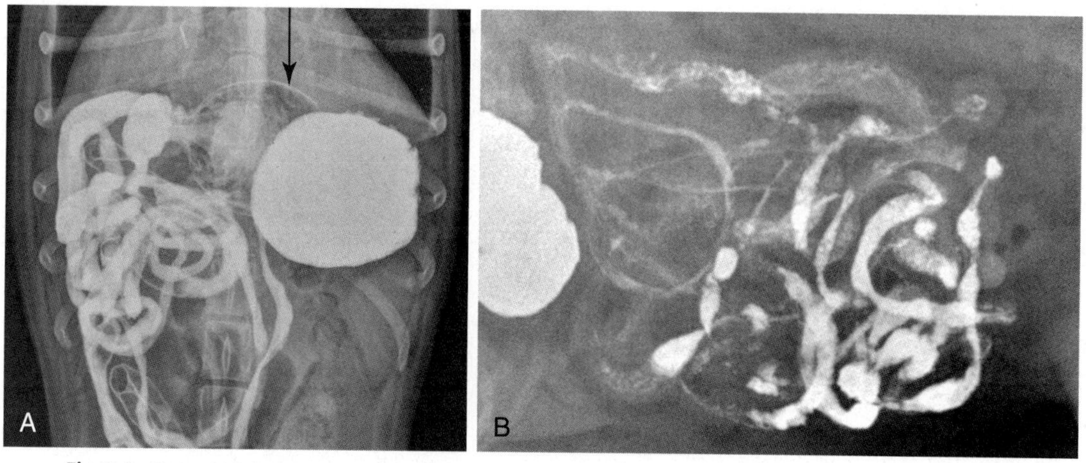

Fig. 5.4 Examples of gastrointestinal studies using liquid barium sulfate. **A**, Upper gastrointestinal study in a dog using commercially available liquid barium sulfate, which is filling part of the stomach and multiple small intestinal segments. There is excellent mucosal coating, which is particularly evident in the gastric body (*black arrow*) where luminal gas highlights the wall. **B**, Upper gastrointestinal study in a dog using barium sulfate powder where the barium in the small intestinal lumen has clumped and come out of suspension. This is termed flocculation and results in very poor mucosal coating.

substances (e.g., sodium, meglumine) that are necessary for improving the solubility of iodine and obtaining physiological pH, but these substances contribute to the higher osmolality of these media as compared to nonionic media (see Fig. 5.5).[19]

Monomers vs. dimers—Monomer contrast media have one tri-iodinated benzene ring whereas dimer contrast media have two rings joined together (see Fig. 5.5). Dimers have a higher concentration of iodine atoms per particles in solution and lower osmolality compared to monomers.

Osmolality—Osmolality is expressed as milliosmole per kilogram of water (mOsm/kg water) and is largely determined by the number of independent particles (molecules, ions) in solution. The dissociative properties of ionic media increase osmolality. Higher iodine concentrations (milligrams of iodine/milliliter of solution, mgI/mL) in any contrast medium (ionic or nonionic) also increases osmolality.[19,20] Ionic monomers are high-osmolality contrast media (Table 5.1), with a much higher osmolality compared to blood (e.g., diatrizoate = 2100 mOsm/kg, blood = 290 mOsm/kg).[21] Nonionic monomers are low-osmolality contrast media, but their osmolality is still two to three times higher than blood (e.g., iohexol 350 mgI/mL = 844 mOsm/kg). The only currently available nonionic dimer contrast medium is iso-osmolar to blood. Osmolality is the main issue related to side effects, with high-osmolality media being associated with more adverse reactions. Osmolality can also affect study quality. For example, fluid will be drawn into the bowel if using a high-osmolar contrast medium for a gastrointestinal contrast study. This will dilute the contrast medium, which then decreases radiographic opacity and lessens the contrast and quality of the study, in addition to potentially leading to dehydration of the patient.

Contrast ratio—This is the number of iodine atoms per number of particles in solution (I/P ratio). Owing to the dissociation of ionic media, there are 2 particles per aliquot of solution as compared to 1 particle for the nonionic media. Therefore, nonionic monomer contrast media have a higher contrast ratio (I/P ratio = 3) compared to ionic monomers (I/P ratio of 1.5). A nonionic dimer has an even higher ratio (I/P ratio = 6) since it contains 6 iodine atoms per 1 solute particle. A higher I/P ratio implies greater opacity, meaning there could be similar contrast enhancement even in the face of a lower contrast medium dose.

Viscosity—Viscosity is the ability of a solution to flow, measured as millipascal × second (mPa·s). High viscosity can make injection of the contrast medium difficult, especially with small-bore IV catheters. The factors that contribute to improving solubility, osmolality, and hydrophilicity inversely affect the viscosity; for example, an iso-osmolar dimer has a higher viscosity compared to a low-osmolar monomer.[20] Viscosity also increases with increasing iodine concentrations and decreases with higher temperatures. Warming contrast media (up to 37°C) prior to administration will decrease viscosity and facilitate injection.[19]

Hydrophilicity vs. lipophilicity—Tri-iodinated benzene rings have an inherent degree of lipophilicity associated with the iodine atoms.[19] On the other hand, hydroxyl groups and nitrogen atoms, which are high in nonionic media, help shield the iodine atoms thereby increasing hydrophilicity (see Fig. 5.5).[22] There is a correlation between lipophilicity and side effects, especially regarding neurotoxicity after intrathecal contrast medium administration.[22,23]

Water-insoluble contrast media—The only available contrast medium in this category is an ethiodized oil medium (Lipiodol), which is commonly added to embolization solutions during interventional radiology procedures, such as thoracic duct embolization in dogs with idiopathic chylothorax.[24]

Adverse Reactions

Adverse reactions associated with water-soluble iodinated contrast media can be acute (occurring within 1 hour of IV injection) or delayed (occurring within hours for up to 1 week).[25] They can be classified by their cause: (1) hypersensitivity reactions (also known as allergic-like, pseudoallergic, or anaphylactic-like reactions), which are dose independent, idiosyncratic, and unpredictable; and (2) physiologic, dose-dependent, nonallergic reactions, which are usually associated with the pharmacological properties of the medium.[18,25]

Hypersensitivity reactions—These reactions are usually acute and range from mild to severe and life-threatening. Most reactions in people are mild and include nausea, vomiting,

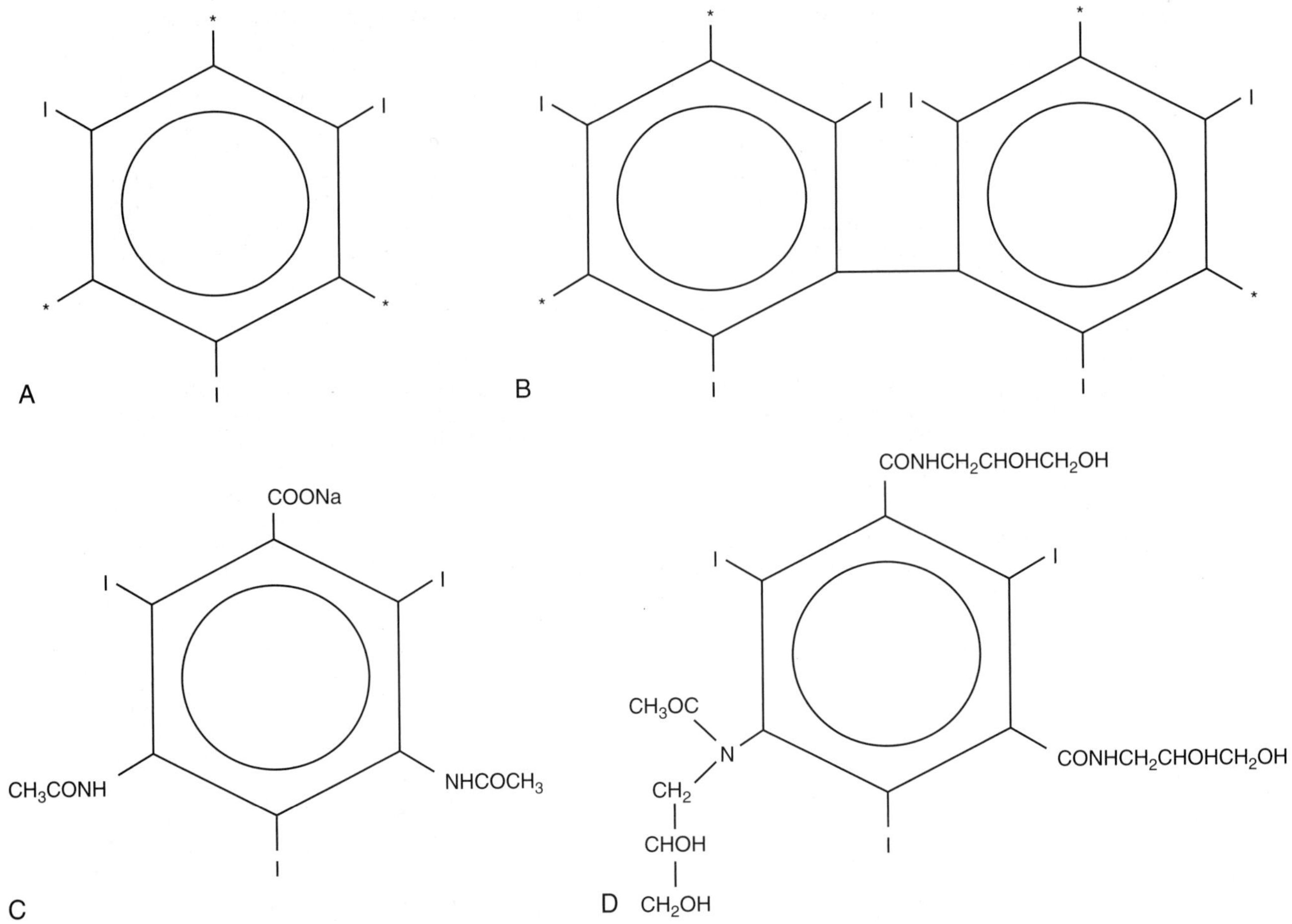

Fig. 5.5 Chemical composition of iodinated contrast media. **A** and **B,** Basic composition of a tri-iodinated monomer (**A**) and dimer (**B**). The *asterisks* (*) indicate the side chains occupied by various contrast media that act to increase solubility (e.g., polar OH groups and sodium or meglumine cations). **C,** Example of an ionic contrast medium (diatrizoate sodium). The sodium ion (COONa) contributes to the high osmolality and the methyl groups (CH_3) contribute to the lipophilicity of ionic contrast media. **D,** Example of a nonionic contrast media (iohexol). The polar OH groups contribute to the hydrophilicity of nonionic contrast media.

or urticaria. More severe reactions, such as bronchospasm, laryngeal edema, hypotensive shock, pulmonary edema, seizures, and cardiopulmonary arrest, can occur. The pathophysiologic mechanisms of these reactions may include histamine release, triggering of the complement cascade, and immune mediated reactions. Many of the reactions are not necessarily a true allergy.[18] The frequency of these reactions is lower with nonionic media;

Table • 5.1

Currently Available Water-Soluble Iodinated Contrast Media and Their Properties.

CONTRAST MEDIUM	TRADE NAME[a]	STRUCTURE	CHARGE	OSMOLALITY @ 37°C (MOSM/KG WATER)	IODINE CONCENTRATION (MG I/ML)[a]	VISCOSITY @ 37° C (MPA · S)
Diatrizoate	Gastrografin	Monomer	Ionic	High—2100	370	8.4
Iothalamate	Conray	Monomer	Ionic	High—1400	282	4.0
Iohexol	Omnipaque	Monomer	Nonionic	Low—844	350	10.7
Iopamidol	Isovue	Monomer	Nonionic	Low—796	370	9.4
Ioversol	Optiray	Monomer	Nonionic	Low—792	350	9.0
Iopromide	Ultravist	Monomer	Nonionic	Low—774	370	10.0
Ioxilan	Oxilan	Monomer	Nonionic	Low—721	350	8.1
Iomeprol	Iomeron	Monomer	Nonionic	Low—618	350	7.5
Iodixanol	Visipaque	Dimer	Nonionic	Iso-osmolar—290	320	11.8

[a]The list is not all inclusive and various additional formulations (e.g., varied iodine concentrations, different trade names) exist.
From the U.S. Food and Drug Administration and Andreucci M, Faga T, Pisani A. The choice of the iodinated radiographic contrast media to prevent contrast-induced nephropathy. *Adv Nephrol*. 2014. https://doi.org/10.1155/2014/691623.

for example, the prevalence of severe reactions in human beings ranges from 0.05% to 0.22% with ionic media and 0.01% to 0.04% with nonionic media.[25]

Severe, acute hypersensitivity reactions to both ionic and nonionic media have been reported in veterinary medicine. In dogs, reported reactions have included hypotension, hypertension, tachycardia, ventricular premature contractions, bronchospasm, erythema, twitching, periocular edema, and diarrhea.[26–28] Cardiopulmonary arrest has been documented in a cat.[29] Reactions in horses have included bronchospasm, hypotension, sweating, urticaria, and edema.[30,31] A high mortality rate in small birds (45.5%) after CT with contrast medium administration has been reported, although it was not possible to determine whether the birds died because of a contrast medium reaction or because of their underlying illness or anesthesia; regardless, the authors advised cautious use of iodinated contrast media in ill, small birds.[32]

In people, two risk factors for hypersensitivity reactions are a previous reaction to iodinated contrast medium and having asthma or other severe allergies.[18] One study in cats, which included three cats with asthma/chronic bronchitis, did not document any hypersensitivity reactions, but the small number of patients precluded identification of any increased risk of a hypersensitivity reaction with possible predisposing conditions.[33] While almost all acute reactions occur with intravascular use, hypersensitivity reactions in people with extravascular use (e.g., cystography) have been reported.[34] There is potential advantage to premedication with steroids +/- antihistamines in people at higher risk for a hypersensitivity reaction, but breakthrough reactions can still occur and there is no proof that it will reduce the chances of a moderate-to-severe reaction or death.[18,35] Note that given the dose-independent nature of these reactions, a test dose of contrast medium to assess for any possible reactions prior to a full contrast medium dose is not useful.

Delayed adverse reactions in people are predominantly T-cell mediated skin reactions.[18] To date, no delayed reactions have been described in veterinary medicine.

Fatality following iodinated contrast medium use is rare, with an estimation in human beings of 1 in 170,000.[36] In animals, the fatality rate in one source has been estimated at 1 in 80 cases[37]; however, this is an old estimate based on ionic contrast media, and therefore, this number is presumably much lower with the now widespread use of nonionic media. All veterinarians performing contrast studies, though, should be aware of the associated risks and be prepared to provide emergency treatment as required (e.g., IV fluids, epinephrine, atropine, oxygen, diphenhydramine).

Dose-dependent physiologic reactions—Dose-dependent reactions can also range from mild to severe and are related to contrast medium type, concentration, and volume. Since these reactions are generally associated with osmolality and ionicity, low- or iso-osmolar, nonionic media are less likely to induce these reactions compared to high-osmolar, ionic media. Chemotoxicity, associated with lipophilicity and cations (sodium, meglumine), is also worse with ionic media.

Cardiovascular effects—The most common reported effects in veterinary medicine are mild to moderate bradycardia, tachycardia, hypertension, or hypotension, reported in up to 37% of cases.[27,31,33,38–40] Arrhythmias are also possible, especially during coronary arteriography.[41] More severe cardiovascular reactions and arrhythmias have been reported in two dogs, including supraventricular tachycardia and severe tachycardia with isolated ventricular premature contractions.[27]

Cellular and vascular effects—Contrast media can reduce erythrocyte plasticity, which could lead to capillary obstruction and local tissue anoxia, and affect leukocyte migration into tissues, which could dampen immune response, but this of minimal clinical significance.[42,43] Both prothrombotic and anticoagulant effects have been noted after local administration (coronary angiography).[44,45]

Respiratory effects—The most commonly reported effect is either increased or decreased respiratory rate in dogs and decreased respiratory rate in cats.[27] Aspiration of hyperosmolar ionic contrast medium into the lungs can lead to pulmonary edema and severe airway irritation, whereas iso- and low-osmolar contrast medium aspiration is generally tolerated by the lungs.[46,47]

Neurologic effects—Ionic contrast media are no longer approved for use in myelography owing to the higher rate of seizures associated with their chemotoxicity. While there are fewer side effects with nonionic contrast media, they do still occur; for example, the incidence of seizures after myelography in dogs ranges from 3% to 21.4%.[22,23,48–51] Higher total contrast medium dose may lead to a higher incidence of seizures,[49,50] and the authors in one study stated that a maximum contrast medium dose in large dogs should be considered.[49] The rate of seizures is also higher with cerebellomedullary cistern injection compared to lumbar injection in dogs.[48,49] Although osmolality is not the primary reason for neurologic side effects, nonionic media with lower iodine concentration, and therefore lower osmolality, should be used in myelography.[23,52] Note that the dimeric contrast medium iodixanol has been shown to be safe for use in myelography in experimental studies in dogs and cats,[53,54] but it is not approved for intrathecal use in human beings in the United States.

Contrast-induced acute kidney injury (CI-AKI)—Contrast-induced nephropathy (CIN) in human beings is now known as contrast-induced acute kidney injury (CI-AKI). This is a subgroup of contrast-medium-associated acute kidney injury (CA-AKI), which is the broad term for a sudden decrease in kidney function within 48 hours of an IV injection of iodinated contrast medium, whether from direct renal injury due to the contrast medium itself (considered rare) or from causes coincident to contrast medium administration (more common).[35] CI-AKI is likely multifactorial, with possible pathophysiologic mechanisms including (1) direct toxicity to renal tubular cells, (2) alterations in renal microvasculature leading to decreased renal blood flow, (3) reperfusion and subsequent oxidative stress, (4) parenchymal toxicity associated with complement cascade activation and inflammatory cytokines, and (5) toxicity from obstruction of renal tubules by precipitating proteins.[55] These effects are related to osmolality, viscosity, and ionicity. In human beings, the biggest risk factor for CI-AKI is pre-existing severe renal impairment.[56] Other risk factors include but are not limited to dehydration, diabetes, cardiovascular disease, older age, diuretic use, hypertension, and anemia.[35,55] Another potential risk factor is receiving multiple doses of contrast medium in a short time period, and as such, dosing intervals should probably be at least 24 hours apart.[35] High-osmolar, ionic contrast media are associated with higher nephrotoxicity in human beings with underlying renal impairment, but not in those with normal renal function. Contrast medium retention in the kidney (slower transit time of contrast medium through the nephrons) is a risk factor for the development of CI-AKI in human beings.[57] Contrast medium retention was reported in a cat undergoing excretory urography, where a persistent nephrogram phase was noted and then oliguria developed, which resolved after treatment.[58] See Fig. 5.6 for a CT example of contrast medium retention.

Table • 5.3

Currently Available Ultrasound Microbubble Contrast Media and Their Properties.[a]

CONTRAST MEDIUM	GAS TYPE	SHELL TYPE	DISTRIBUTION
Definity	Octofluoropropane	Phospholipid	Blood pool only
Luminity	Octofluoropropane	Phospholipid	Blood pool only
Lumason	Sulfur hexafluoride	Phospholipid	Blood pool only
SonoVue	Sulfur hexafluoride	Phospholipid	Blood pool only
Optison	Perfluoropropane	Albumin	Blood pool only
Sonazoid	Perfluorobutane	Phospholipid	Intravascular + delayed liver/spleen
Visphere[b]	Perfluorocarbon	Phospholipid	Intravascular + delayed liver[†]

[a]Not all contrast media are available in all countries.[b]Contrast medium only available in Taiwan. [†]One exploratory study utilizing this contrast medium did not include imaging of the spleen (Lin LS, Chung CS. Novel contrast medium Visphere™ is feasible for contrast-enhanced ultrasonography in dogs. *Vet Radiol Ultrasound.* 202:61(4):461–470).

assesses signals of the nonlinear oscillation of the bubbles, or the signals produced from their destruction. Harmonic ultrasound techniques can separate the fundamental from the secondary harmonic frequencies and can eliminate background tissue echoes, to enable the usage of only the contrast medium echoes in image formation. This allows for greater evaluation of organ perfusion and their afferent vessels. Harmonic imaging requires specific capabilities of the ultrasound machine and appropriate image analysis programs.

Adverse Reactions

Ultrasound contrast media are generally considered safe and there are no organ-specific toxicities. In human beings, most reactions are mild, such as a warm sensation, itching, nausea, and vomiting. In one study, the incidence of any reaction was 0.125%, with much less frequent serious hypersensitivity reactions at 0.009%.[97] In a multicenter retrospective case study of 488 animals imaged using either SonoVue or Definity, adverse reactions (vomiting, syncope) were reported in about 1% of dogs (4/411) and no cats (0/77).[98] In two of these dogs, however, there were confounding factors that could have caused the clinical signs. Severe hypersensitivity reactions were reported in 2/26 dogs with use of the contrast medium Optison, which was thought to be associated with the human albumin contained within the shell.[99] Based on this study, contrast media containing human albumin should probably be avoided in animals. Overall, when compared to the use of iodinated contrast media, ultrasound contrast media are considered very safe.

Acknowledgment

With special thanks to prior authors of this chapter for their contributions.

REFERENCES

1. Bushberg JT, Seiber JA, Leidholdt EM, Boone JM. *Essential Physics of Medical Imaging.* 4th ed. Philadelphia: Lippincott Williams & Wilkins; 2021.
2. Sireci S. Clinical utility of barium sulfate products. Formulation determines appropriate use. *Appl Radiol.* 2021.
3. Gelfand DW, Ott DJ. Barium sulfate suspensions: an evaluation of available products. *Am J Roentgenol.* 1982;138:935–941.
4. Agut A, Sanchez-Valverde MA, Lasaosa JM, et al. Use of iohexol as a gastrointestinal contrast medium in the dog. *Vet Radiol Ultrasound.* 1993;34:171–177.
5. Saylisoy S, Erturk SM. Gastrointestinal iodinated contrast agents. In: Erturk SM, Ros PR, Ichikawa T, Saylisoy S, eds. *Medical Imaging Contrast Agents: A Clinical Manual.* Switzerland: Springer; 2021.
6. Evans SM, Laufer I. Double gastrography in the normal dog. *Vet Radiol Ultrasound.* 1981;22:2–9.
7. Simpson KW. Diseases of the stomach. In: Ettinger SJ, Feldman EC, eds. *Textbook of Veterinary Internal Medicine.* 7th ed. St Louis Missouri: Saunders; 2010.
8. Beckett KR, Moriarity AK, Langer JM. Safe use of contrast media. What the radiologist needs to know. *Radiographics.* 2015;35:738–750.
9. Westfall RH, Nelson RH, Musselman MM. Barium peritonitis. *Am J Surg.* 1966;112:760–763.
10. Ko JJ, Mann FA. Barium peritonitis in small animals. *J Vet Med Sci.* 2014;76:621–628.
11. Thompson IM, Whittlesey GC, Slovis TL, et al. Evaluation of contrast media for bronchography. *Pediatr Radiol.* 1997;27:598–605.
12. McAlister WH, Askin FB. The effect of some contrast agents in the lung. An experimental study in the rat and dog. *Am J Roentgenol.* 1983;40:245–251.
13. Meola SD, Mazzaferro EM, Wheeler JL, McKiernan B. Medical and surgical management of severe barium aspiration in a dog. *J Vet Emerg Crit Care.* 2008;18:639–645.
14. Yamazaki H, Oi H, Matsushita M, et al. Gallbladder opacification 12–24 h after angiography by CT examination: a multivariate analysis. *Abdom Imaging.* 1996;21:507–511.
15. Lasser EC, Farr RS, Fujimagari T, et al. The significance of protein binding of contrast media in roentgen diagnosis. *Am J Roentgenol.* 1962;87:338–360.
16. Fujita M, Orima A. Effect and safety of meglumine iotroxate for cholangiocystography in normal cats. *Vet Radiol Ultrasound.* 1994;35:79–82.
17. O'Brien T. *Radiographic Diagnosis of Abdominal Disorders of the Dog and Cat: Radiographic Interpretation, Clinical Signs, Pathophysiology.* Philadelphia: Saunders; 1978.
18. Saylisoy S, Erturk SM. Adverse reactions to iodinated contrast agents. In: Erturk SM, Ros PR, Ichikawa T, Saylisoy S, eds. *Medical Imaging Contrast Agents. A Clinical Manual.* Switzerland: Springer; 2021.
19. Speck U. Physicochemical properties of water-soluble contrast media. In: Speck U, ed. *X-Ray Contrast media. Overview, Use and Pharmaceutical Aspects.* Berlin: Springer; 2018.
20. Erol K, Yigitaslan S. Chemistry, physicochemical, properties and pharmacokinetics of iodinated contrast agents. In: Erturk SM, Ros PR, Ichikawa T, Saylisoy S, eds. *Medical*

Imaging Contrast Agents. A Clinical Manual. Switzerland: Springer; 2021.

21. Windberger U, Bartholovitsch A, Plasenzotti R, et al. Whole blood viscosity, plasma viscosity and erythrocyte aggregation in nine mammalian species: reference values and comparison of data. *Exp Physiol*. 2003;88:431.
22. Widmer WR. Iohexol and iopamidol. New contrast media for veterinary myelography. *J Am Vet Med Assoc*. 1989;194: 1714–1716.
23. Widmer WR, Blevins WE. Veterinary myelography. A review of contrast media, adverse effects, and technique. *J Am Anim Hosp Assoc*. 1991;27:163–176.
24. Carvajal JL, Case JB, Grosso FRV, et al. Prospective evaluation of lymphatic embolization as part of the treatment in dogs with presumptive idiopathic chylothorax. *Vet Surg*. 2022;51:O128–O137.
25. Speck U. Risks of contrast media use. In: Speck U, ed. *X-Ray Contrast Media. Overview, Use and Pharmaceutical Aspects*. Berlin: Springer; 2018.
26. Basher KL, Porter IR, Martin-Flores M. Severe (grade IV) hypersensitivity to iodinated contrast agent in an anesthetized dog. *Can Vet J*. 2019;60:766–769.
27. Scarabelli S, Cripps P, Rioja E, Alderson B. Adverse reactions following administration of contrast media for diagnostic imaging in anaesthetized dogs and cats. A retrospective study. *Vet Anaesth Analg*. 2016;43:502–510.
28. Pollard RE, Pascoe PJ. Severe reaction to intravenous administration of an ionic iodinated contrast agent in two anaesthetized dogs. *J Am Vet Med Assoc*. 2008;233:274–278.
29. Rodrigo-Mocholi D, Willems A, Schauvliege S, et al. Cardiopulmonary arrest in a cat as a result of a suspected anaphylactic reaction to an intravenously administered iodinated contrast agent. *Vet Anaesth Analg*. 2015;42: 554–555.
30. Gunkel CI, Valverde A, Robertson SA, et al. Treatment for a severe reaction to intravenous administration of diatrizoate in an anaesthetized horse. *J Am Vet Med Assoc*. 2004;224: 1143–1146.
31. Pollard RE, Puchalski SM. Reaction to intra-arterial iodinated contrast medium administration in anaesthetized horses. *Vet Radiol Ultrasound*. 2011;52:441–443.
32. McCready JE, Gardhouse SM, Appleby R, Beaufrère H. Mortality rate of birds following intravenous administration of iodinated contrast medium for computed tomography. *J Am Vet Med Assoc*. 2021;259:77–83.
33. Pollard RE, Puchalski SM, Pascoe PJ. Hemodynamic and serum biochemical alterations associated with intravenous administration of three types of contrast media in anaesthetized cats. *Am J Vet Res*. 2008;69:1274–1278.
34. Davis PL. Anaphylactoid reactions to the nonvascular administration of water-soluble iodinated contrast media. *Am J Roentgenol*. 2015;204, 1140–114.
35. *ACR Committee on Drugs and Contrast Media. ACR Manual on Contrast Media*. Reston: American College of Radiology; 2023. https://www.acr.org/-/media/ACR/files/clinical-resources/contrast_media.pdf.
36. Morcos SK, Thomsen HS. Adverse reactions to iodinated contrast media. *Eur Radiol*. 2001;11:1267–1275.
37. Walter PA, Feeney DA, Johnston GR. *Current Veterinary Therapy IX Small Animal Practice*. Philadelphia: Saunders; 1986.
38. Pollard RE, Puchalski SM, Pascoe PJ. Hemodynamic and serum biochemical alterations associated with intravenous administration of three types of contrast media in anaesthetized dogs. *Am J Vet Res*. 2008;69:1268–1273.
39. Vance A, Nelson M, Hofmeister EH. Adverse reactions following administration of an ionic iodinated contrast media in anesthetized dogs. *J Am Anim Hosp Assoc*. 2012;48:172–175.
40. Kan J, Milne M, Tyrrell D, Mansfield C. Lean body weight-adjusted intravenous iodinated contrast dose for abdominal CT in dogs reduces interpatient enhancement variability while providing diagnostic quality organ enhancement. *Vet Radiol Ultrasound*. 2022;63:719–728.
41. Kløw NE, Tande PM, Hevrøy O, Refsum H. Mechanism of ECG changes and arrhythmogenic properties of low osmolality contrast media during coronary arteriography in dog. *Cardiovasc Res*. 1990;24:303–308.
42. Grainger RG. Osmolality of intravascular radiological contrast media. *Br J Radiol*. 1980;53:739.
43. O'Donnell DH, Moloney MA, Bouchier-Hayes DJ, Lee MJ. Iodinated contrast media alter immune responses in proinflammatory states. *Acta Radiol*. 2010;51:635–640.
44. Gabelman A, Haberstroh J, Weyrich G. Ionic and non-ionic contrast agent-mediated endothelial injury. *Acta Radiol*. 2001;42:422.
45. Husted SE, Kanstrup H. Thrombotic complications in coronary angioplasty-ionic versus non-ionic low osmolar contrast media. *Acta Radiol*. 1998;39:340–343.
46. Morcos SK. Effects of radiographic contrast media on the lung. *Br J Radiol*. 2003;76:290–295.
47. Davenport D, Cohen MD, Hanna MP, et al. Studies of iodixanol in the rabbit lung and peritoneum. *Pediatr Radiol*. 1999;29:724–730.
48. Barone G, Ziemer LS, Shofer FS, Steinberg SA. Risk factors associated with development of seizures after use of iohexol for myelography in dogs. 182 cases. *J Am Vet Med Assoc*. 2002;220:1499–1502.
49. da Costa RC, Parent JM, Dobson H. Incidence of and risk factors for seizures after myelography performed with iohexol in dogs. 503 cases (2002–2004). *J Am Vet Med Assoc*. 2011;238:1296–1300.
50. Mullen KR, Furness MC, Johnson AL, et al. Adverse reactions in horses that underwent general anesthesia and cervical myelography. *J Vet Intern Med*. 2015;29:954–960.
51. Lexmaulova L, Zatloukal J, Proks P, et al. Incidence of seizures associated with iopamidol or iomeprol myelography in dogs with intervertebral disk disease: 161 cases (2000-2002). *J Vet Emerg Crit Care*. 2009;19:611–616.
52. Fatone G, Lamagna F, Pasolini MP, et al. Myelography in the dog with non-ionic contrast media at different iodine concentrations. *J Small Anim Pract*. 1997;38:292–294.
53. Larsen LE, Heglund IF, Fabian R, et al. Neural tolerability of iodixanol in mice and dogs after single and repeated intracisternal administration. *Acta Radiol Supplementum*. 1995;399:238–243.
54. Ghadiri A, Avizeh R, Faramarzi G. Comparison between iodixanol and iohexol for cervical myelography in cat. *IJVS*. 2015;10:23–29.
55. Perrin T, Descombes e, Cook S. Contrast-induced nephropathy in invasive cardiology. Incidence, pathophysiology, diagnosis, prevention and prognosis. *Swiss Med Wkly*. 2012;142:w13608.
56. Andreucci M, Faga T, Pisani A. The choice of the iodinated radiographic contrast media to prevent contrast-induced nephropathy. *Adv Nephrol*. 2014. https://doi.org/10.1155/2014/691623.
57. Ariyoshi S, Tanabe M, Ito K. Evaluation of the renal parenchymal retention of iodinated contrast agent during follow-up computed tomography performed one day after undergoing contrast-enhanced computed tomography. *Euro J Radiol*. 2020;132:109335.
58. Carr A, Reed A, Pope E. Persistent nephrogram in a cat after intravenous urography. *Vet Radiol Ultrasound*. 1994;35(5):350–354.
59. Goic JB, Koenigshof AM, McGuire LD, et al. A retrospective evaluation of contrast-induced kidney injury in dogs (2006–2012). *J Vet Emerg Crit Care*. 2016;26(5):713–719.

60. Griffin MA, Culp WTN, Palm CA, Poppenga RH. Suspected contrast-induced nephropathy in three sequential patients undergoing computed tomography angiography and transarterial embolization for nonresectable neoplasia. *J Am Vet Med Assoc*. 2021;259:1163–1170.
61. Ihle S, Kostolich M. Acute renal failure associated with contrast medium administration in a dog. *J Am Vet Med Assoc*. 1991;199(7):899–901.
62. Kirberger RM, Cassel N, Carstens A, et al. The effects of repeated intravenous iohexol on renal function in healthy beagles – a preliminary report. *Acta Vet Scand*. 2012;54(1):47.
63. Prüllage ML, Schwendenwein I, Eberspächer-Schweda KS. Does intravenous contrast medium administration result in altered renal biomarkers? A study in clinically stable cats with and without azotemia. *J Feline Med Surg*. 2022;24(6):565–579.
64. Cagnasso F, Bruno B, Bellino C, et al. Alterations of serum biochemical and urinary parameters in a canine population before and after intravenous contrast administration. *Vet Sci*. 2021;8:146.
65. Pasternak JJ, Williamson EE. Clinical pharmacology, uses, and adverse reactions of iodinated contrast agents. A primer for the non-radiologist. *Mayo Clin Proc*. 2012;87:390–402.
66. Devriendt N, van de Velde N, Stock E, et al. Suspected haemorrhagic cystitis in a dog as delayed complication after contrast-enhanced computed tomography. *Vet Rec Case Rep*. 2020. https://doi.org/10.1136/vetreccr-2019-001011.
67. Johnston GR, Stevens JB, Jessen CR, Osborne CA. Complications of retrograde contrast urethrography in dogs and cats. *Am J Vet Res*. 1983;44:1248–1256.
68. Lee WR, Pease AP, Berry CR. The effects of iohexol administration on technetium thyroid scintigraphy in normal cats. *Vet Radiol Ultrasound*. 2010;51:182–185.
69. Peremans K, Vandermeulen E, van Hoek I, et al. Interference of iohexol with radioiodine thyroid uptake in the hyperthyroid cat. *J Feline Med Surg*. 2008;10:460–465.
70. Pollard R, Puchalski S. CT contrast media and applications. In: Schwarz T, Saunders J, eds. *Veterinary Computed Tomography*. West Sussex: John Wiley & Sons; 2011.
71. Ackerman N, Wingfield WE, Corley EA. Fatal air embolism associated with pneumo-urethrography and pneumocystography in a dog. *J Am Vet Med Assoc*. 1972;160:1616–1618.
72. Zontine WJ, Andrews LK. Fatal air embolism as a complication of pneumocystography in two cats. *J Am Vet Rad Soc*. 1978;19:8–11.
73. Yigitaslan S, Erol K. Chemistry, physicochemical properties and pharmacokinetics of gadolinium-based contrast agents. In: Erturk SM, Ros PR, Ichikawa T, Saylisoy S, eds. *Medical Imaging Contrast Agents. A Clinical Manual*. Switzerland: Springer; 2021.
74. Rogosnitzky M, Branch S. Gadolinium-based contrast agent toxicity. a review of known and proposed mechanisms. *Biometals*. 2016;29:365–376.
75. Port M, Idée JM, Medina C, et al. Efficiency, thermodynamic and kinetic stability of marketed gadolinium chelates and their possible clinical consequences. A critical review. *Biometals*. 2008;21:469–490.
76. Lohrke J, Frenzel T, Endrikat J, et al. 25 Years of contrast-enhanced MRI. Developments, current challenges and future perspectives. *Adv Ther*. 2016;33:1–28.
77. Bendszus M, Roberts D, Kolumban B, et al. Dose finding study of gadopiclenol, a new macrocyclic contrast agent, in MRI of central nervous system. *Invest Radiol*. 2020;55:129–137.
78. Marks AL, Hecht S, Stokes JE, et al. Effects of gadoxetate (Eovist) contrast on magnetic resonance imaging characteristics of the liver in clinically healthy dogs. *Vet Radiol Ultrasound*. 2014;55:286–291.
79. Yonetomi D, Kadosawa T, Miyoshi K, et al. Contrast agent Gd-EOB-DTPA (EOB·Primovist®) for low-field magnetic resonance imaging of canine focal liver lesions. *Vet Radiol Ultrasound*. 2012;53:371–380.
80. Constant C, Hecht S, Craig LE, et al. Gadoxetate disodium (GD-EOB-DTPA) on contrast enhanced magnetic resonance imaging characteristics of hepatocellular carcinoma in dogs. *Vet Radiol Ultrasound*. 2016;57:594–600.
81. Muñoz A, Mateo I, Lorenzo V, Martínez J. Imaging diagnosis: traumatic dural tear diagnosed using intrathecal gadopentate dimeglumine. *Vet Radiol Ultrasound*. 2009;50:502–505.
82. Agnello KA, Puchalski SM, Wisner ER, et al. Effect of positioning, scan plane, and arthrography on visibility of periarticular canine shoulder soft tissue structures on magnetic resonance images. *Vet Radiol Ultrasound*. 2008;49:529–539.
83. Schaefer SL, Baumel CA, Gerbig JR, Forrest LJ. Direct magnetic resonance arthrography of the canine shoulder. *Vet Radiol Ultrasound*. 2010;51:391–396.
84. Prince MR, Arnoldus C, Frisoli JK. Nephrotoxicity of high-dose gadolinium compared with iodinated contrast. *J Magn Reson Imaging*. 1996;1:162–166.
85. Heinrich MC, Kuhlmann MK, Kohlbacher S, et al. Cytotoxicity of iodinated and gadolinium-based contrast agents in renal tubular cells at angiographic concentrations: in vitro study. *Radiology*. 2007;242:425–434.
86. Forsting M, Palkowitsch P. Prevalence of acute adverse reactions to gadobutrol—a highly concentrated macrocyclic gadolinium chelate: review of 14,299 patients from observational trials. *Eur J Radiol*. 2010;74(3):e186–e192.
87. Ichikawa S. Gadolinium-based contrast agent toxicity and accumulation. In: Erturk SM, Ros PR, Ichikawa T, Saylisoy S, eds. *Medical Imaging Contrast Agents: A Clinical Manual*. Switzerland: Springer; 2021.
88. Mair AR, Woodley J, Martinez M. Cardiovascular effects of intravenous gadolinium administration to anesthetized dogs undergoing magnetic resonance imaging. *Vet Anaesth Analg*. 2010;37:337–341.
89. Girard NM, Leece EA. Suspected anaphylactoid reaction following intravenous administration of a gadolinium-based contrast agent in three dogs undergoing magnetic resonance imaging. *Vet Anaesth Analg*. 2010;37:352–356.
90. Tucker PK, MacFarlane P. Severe bronchoconstriction as part of a suspected anaphylactic reaction in a dog following administration of gadobutrol. *Vet Record Case Reports*. 2020;8:e001051.
91. Argano M, Hewetson M, Kiviranta AM, Menzies MPL. Seizure-like activity after gadolinium administration in an anaesthetised foal undergoing magnetic resonance imaging. *Vet Record Case Reports*. 2018;6:e000636.
92. Thomsen HS, Morcos SK, Dawson P. Is there a causal relation between the administration of gadolinium based contrast media and the development of nephrogenic systemic fibrosis (NSF)? *Clin Radiol*. 2006;61:905–906.
93. Kanda T, Ishii K, Kawaguchi H, et al. High signal intensity in the dentate nucleus and globus pallidus on unenhanced T1-weighted MR images: relationship with increasing cumulative dose of a gadolinium-based contrast material. *Radiology*. 2014;270:834–841.
94. Richter H, Bücker P, Dunker C, et al. Gadolinium deposition in the brain of dogs after multiple intravenous administrations of linear gadolinium based contrast agents. *PLoS One*. 2020;15:e0227649.

95. Haers H, Saunders J. Review of clinical characteristics and applications of contrast-enhanced ultrasonography in dogs. *J Am Vet Med Assoc.* 2009;234(4):460–470.
96. Correas JM, Bridal L, Lesavre A, et al. Ultrasound contrast agents: properties, principles of action, tolerance, and artifacts. *Eur Radiol.* 2001;11:1316–1328.
97. Piscaglia F, Bolondi L. The safety of Sonovue in abdominal applications: retrospective analysis of 23188 investigations. *Ultrasound Med Biol.* 2006;32:1369–1375.
98. Seiler GS, Brown JC, Reetz JA, et al. Safety of contrast-enhanced ultrasonography in dogs and cats: 488 cases (2002-2011). *J Am Vet Med Assoc.* 2013;242(9):1255–1259.
99. Yamaya Y, Niizeki K, Kim J, et al. Anaphylactoid response to Optison and its effects on pulmonary function in two dogs. 2004. *J Vet Med Sci.* 2004;66:1429–1432.

ELECTRONIC RESOURCES

Additional information related to the content in Chapter 5 can be found online at eBooks.Health.Elsevier.com.

- Chapter Quiz

CHAPTER 6

Radiographic Interpretation

Donald E. Thrall

WHAT IS A RADIOGRAPH?

A radiograph is an image of the distribution of x-rays* that emerge from the patient. When struck by the primary x-ray beam, which is spatially uniform, there is differential absorption of x-rays by the different tissues in the body. This creates nonuniformity in the distribution of x-rays leaving the patient. The character of the nonuniformity is specific to the makeup of the tissue (Fig. 6.1). In normal subjects, the distribution of x-rays exiting the patient has a repeatable pattern, which is recognized as the normal appearance. When looking at radiographs of diseased patients, the examiner is looking for alterations in the distribution of the exiting x-rays that have been created by disease, and also by normal variations in anatomy. Artifacts will also influence the appearance of the final image. With experience, normal appearance and the effects of artifacts are recognized with more confidence, and different appearances of the distribution of exiting x-rays come to be associated with certain diseases. Many sources of normal radiographic anatomy are available to assist with interpretation, including this text, other published material,[1] and online.[2]

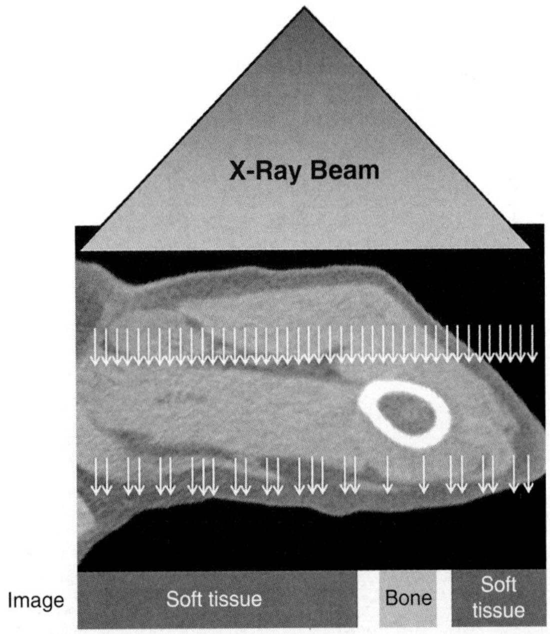

Fig. 6.1 The structure in the image is a transverse computed tomography (CT) image of a canine thigh, which represents a limb being radiographed. The white ring structure is the femur surrounded by muscle with fat in the fascial planes. The primary x-ray beam, represented by the *triangle*, is diverging and uniform. As x-rays (*arrows*) pass through the tissue, some are absorbed and some pass through. X-ray absorption will be relatively homogeneous in the soft tissues but increased in the femur, especially where the x-ray beam strikes the cortex tangentially. This creates a distribution of exiting x-rays that corresponds to the makeup of the thigh. The exiting x-rays are used to create a radiograph.

HOW X-RAY EXPOSURE IS REPRESENTED IN THE IMAGE

Crucial to proper interpretation of radiographs, and in comprehending radiology reports, is an understanding of the fundamental relationship of x-ray exposure with the degree of blackness or whiteness in the image. Areas of the radiograph that are *black* or *dark gray* are highly exposed regions where many x-rays pass through the patient and strike the imaging plate. Areas of the radiograph that are *white* or *light gray* are less-exposed regions where more x-rays were absorbed by the patient and fewer pass through and fewer strike the plate. Descriptions of blackness and whiteness in a radiograph are described in terms or lucency vs. opacity, respectively. Unfortunately, multiple synonyms are used to describe lucency and opacity (Table 6.1). The term *density or radiographic density* has also been used to describe film blackness and whiteness, i.e., dense = white. However, use of density has fallen out of favor and descriptions based on opacity are preferred.

RADIOGRAPHIC INTERPRETATION

The ability of x-rays to allow us to "see" inside of the body is taken for granted, perhaps because there are many other sophisticated technical advances that are commonplace. But the relatively simple process of using differential x-ray absorption in

Table • 6.1

Terms Used to Describe the Degree of Blackness or Whiteness in a Radiograph.

HIGHLY EXPOSED OR MORE EXPOSED (BLACKER) AREAS	UNEXPOSED OR LESS EXPOSED (WHITER) AREAS
Decreased opacity	Increased opacity
Less opaque	More opaque
Lucent	Opaque
Radiolucent	Radiopaque
Increased radiolucency	Decreased radiolucency

*Sometimes, the term *x-ray* is used incorrectly as a substitute term for radiograph. The term *x-ray* describes the energy used to create the image, not the radiographic image itself.

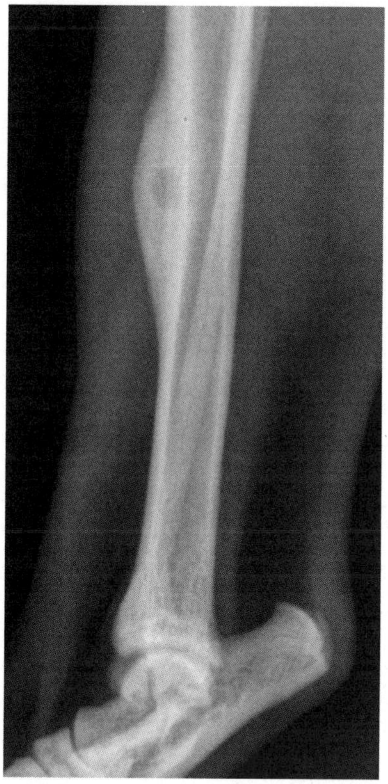

Fig. 6.2 Lateral view of the tibia of a cat. The history specified a lameness of 2 days' duration. The changes on the tibia are extensive, and it is highly unlikely that this extent of new bone formation could have developed over a 2-day interval. This is an example of a history that does not match the radiographic findings. This makes it difficult to assess the significance of the radiographic changes.

the patient to create a radiograph remains a mainstay of diagnostic medicine in both general and specialty practices. Maximizing the potential value of this relatively simple technique still requires constant and ardent attention to detail.

Many factors influence the accuracy of radiographic interpretation. The interpreter must have access to information pertaining to the patient.[3] This includes the signalment, medical history, and the physical abnormalities that are present. The history provided by the owner is often helpful in guiding radiographic interpretation, but the history may also be misleading. Recognizing that radiographic findings may not always agree with the history is a critical step in formulating a correct radiographic assessment (Fig. 6.2).

The physical examination is also very important regarding the identification of the region(s) that should be radiographed and in formulating a preliminary list of rule-outs. Radiographs should never be a substitute for a good physical examination. Also, one might expect radiographs to provide a definitive diagnosis, but more often they lead to a ranking of differential diagnoses, and provide direction for further patient evaluation with other tests or additional imaging.

When obtaining radiographs, it is critical that accurate positioning and proper radiographic technique be used. When compared to film (analog) imaging systems, the extreme exposure latitude that characterizes digital imaging has reduced the number of errors that occur as a result of incorrect kVp and/or mAs settings. However, overexposure and underexposure are still problems, along with poor positioning and lack of proper views. When an owner agrees to have radiographs of their animal made, a contract has been established between the client and veterinarian and implicit in that is the production of adequate images. Unfortunately, many substandard radiographs of animal patients are produced each day. Submission of poor images to a teleradiology service for interpretation by a specialist cannot compensate for errors in radiographic acquisition.

Positioning is not discussed in detail in this book, but the standard views recommended for various areas are outlined in other chapters. One aspect of positioning is important to mention here. It has become common for practices to include the whole body of cats and small dogs in one image, i.e., cat-o-gram and dog-o-gram, respectively. This should be avoided as the anatomy at the cranial and caudal edge of the image will be distorted because these regions are struck by very diverging x-rays. Also, a single radiographic exposure technique will not be optimal for the very different makeup of the thorax vs. abdomen. There is no reason to avoid getting individual studies of both the thorax and abdomen in all patients.

Once suitable radiographs of the patient have been produced, interpretation should be done in a quiet, relatively isolated, environment. This seems obvious, but taking the time to make sure the viewing environment is suitable will pay off with increased accuracy. Concentration and thoroughness are the major determinants of accurate interpretation.

Many of us never receive any instruction in actually how to examine a radiograph. Some people develop a highly accurate examination method whereas others are never able to accomplish this. Everyone will look at radiographs differently. Some look from the periphery to the center, others from the center to the periphery and some haphazardly. Regardless of the examination method, the most important aspect of viewing is to make sure that the entire image is examined. Not finding a lesion is often linked to not looking rather than not seeing. Having a checklist of the regions/structures to be examined will also help in making sure that the entire image is examined. Examples of checklists are included in Chapters 9, 17, 28, and 38.

In addition to examining the overall "real estate" of the image, there is an ancillary examination method that can be useful in evaluating juvenile bone disease. This is called *targeted viewing*. Certain bone diseases have a propensity for certain areas of the skeleton, e.g., osteochondrosis in the caudal humeral head, metaphyseal osteopathy/hypertrophic osteodystrophy (HOD) in the distal radius and ulna, and canine panosteitis in the diaphysis of long bones. Therefore, if during the clinical examination of a young, lame dog, a specific disease is suspected, the commonly affected area should be examined closely in the radiograph. This targeted viewing is ancillary to the general overview and will reduce the incidence of subtle lesions being overlooked.

NAMING AND VIEWING RADIOGRAPHS

There is a systematic naming system for radiographic views that employs standardized terminology (Fig. 6.3). Standardized naming of views allows correct interpretation of radiology reports and implementation of recommendations for additional images. Radiographic views are named according to the location that the central ray of the primary x-ray beam traverses the body part of interest, from point-of-entrance to point-of-exit.[4] For example, an abdominal radiograph made with the dog in dorsal recumbency and an overhead, vertically directed, x-ray beam is a ventrodorsal view. With the dog in ventral recumbency, it is a dorsoventral view. The same method is used for other body parts, with the appropriate directional term applied.

An exception to this system of image nomenclature is that lateral radiographs of the head, neck, thorax, abdomen, and pelvis are usually abbreviated according to side of the body that the patient is lying on, rather than using the more accurate

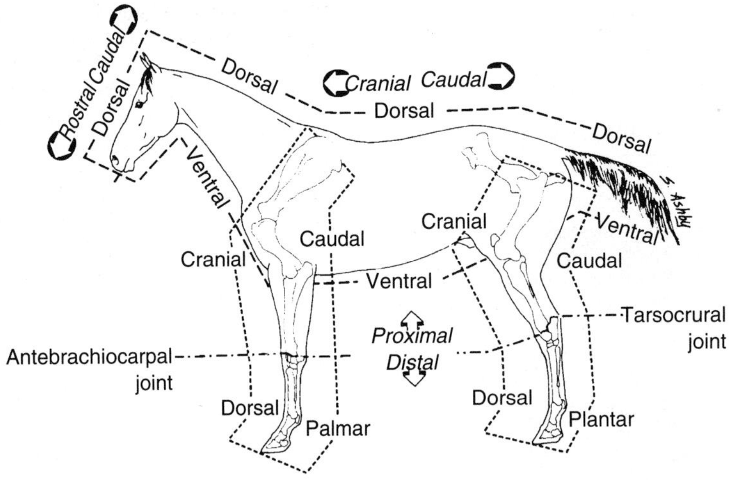

Fig. 6.3 Proper anatomic directional terms as they apply to various parts of the body. (Courtesy Dr. J. E. Smallwood.)

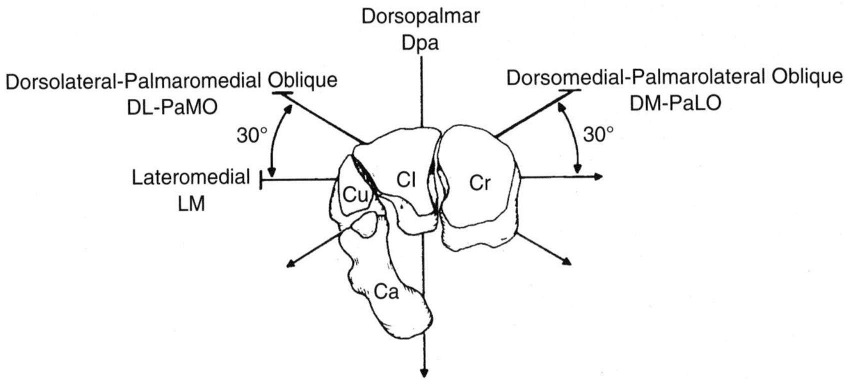

Fig. 6.4 Transverse plane view of the proximal row of equine carpal bones illustrating the principle of naming radiographic projections by the direction of the primary x-ray beam from the point of entrance to the point of exit. (Courtesy Dr. J. E. Smallwood.)

point-of-entrance to point-of-exit method. For example, an abdominal radiograph with the patient lying on the left side is referred to as a left lateral rather than the more correct right-left lateral.

Oblique views are also named by designating the points of entrance and exit (Fig. 6.4). Angles of obliquity can be specified by inserting the number of degrees of obliquity between the directional terms involved. For example, if the dorsolateral palmaromedial oblique (DLPaMO) view in Fig. 6.4 was made by positioning the x-ray tube 60 degrees laterally with respect to dorsal, the designation would be D60LPaMO.

Standardizing the orientation of images for viewing is also important. The brain learns what to expect a certain part to look like when oriented a certain way. Therefore, images should be oriented on the monitor in a predetermined orientation, not randomly. The following has become the standard for image orientation:

- Lateral views of any part are oriented with the cranial (rostral) aspect of the animal pointing to the interpreter's left.
- Ventrodorsal or dorsoventral radiographs of the head, neck, or trunk are oriented with the cranial (rostral) part of the animal pointing up and with the left side of the animal to the interpreter's right.
- Lateromedial or mediolateral radiographs of the extremities, including oblique projections, are oriented with the proximal aspect of the limb pointing up and the cranial or dorsal aspect of the limb to the interpreter's left.
- Caudocranial (plantarodorsal, palmarodorsal) or craniocaudal (dorsopalmar, dorsoplantar) radiographs of the extremities are oriented with the proximal end of the extremity at the top. No convention exists regarding whether the medial or lateral side of the extremity is oriented to the interpreter's right or left.

RADIOGRAPHIC OPACITIES

Various body parts and lesions appear differently in radiographs because a change in the makeup of a tissue will change the x-ray absorption pattern. The extent that a radiograph is able to display differences in blackness or whiteness between various structures is termed *contrast resolution*. Radiographs have poorer contrast resolution than either computed tomography or magnetic resonance images. Therefore, many normal structures and pathologic states that differ only slightly in x-ray absorption will not be able to be identified in radiographs. It takes a relatively large difference in x-ray absorption for a difference in radiographic opacity to be created. As a result, there are only a few distinct differences in radiographic opacity. These opacities are described according to the appearance of only five tissues or objects—*air* (or *gas*), *fat*, *water* (or *fluid* or *soft tissue*), *bone* (or *mineral*), and *metal* (Figs. 6.5 and 6.6). Importantly, a radiographic opacity is not specific for any particular tissue or substance, but only indicates a group of tissues or substances

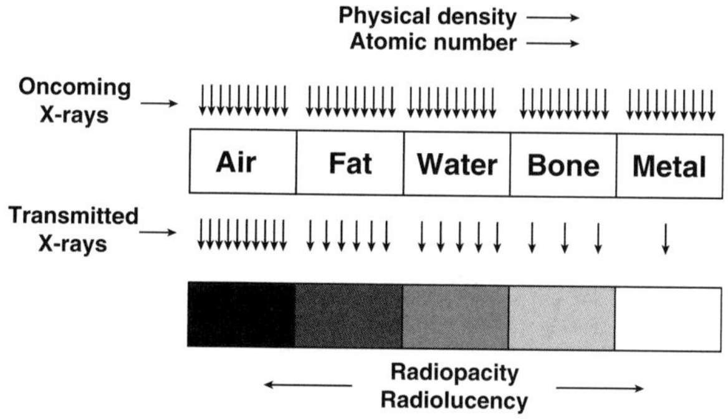

Fig. 6.5 Identical thicknesses of air, fat, water, bone, and metal are struck by an equal number of x-rays. Each material absorbs x-rays differently (differential absorption), depending on the physical density and effective atomic number of the material. This results in five distinct opacities.

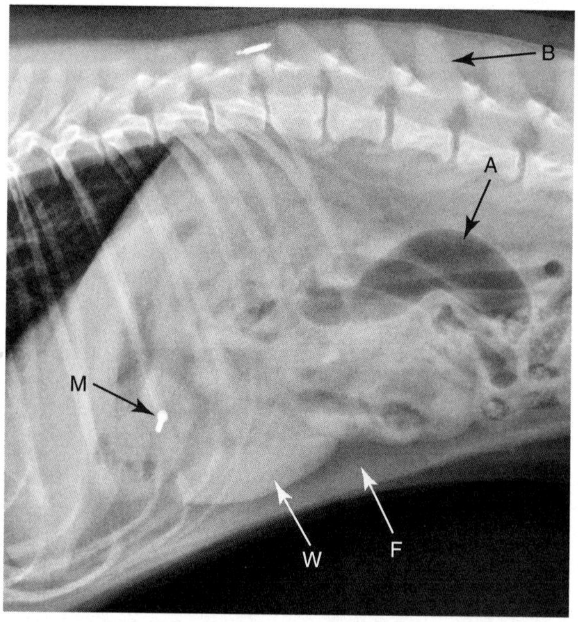

Fig. 6.6 Lateral radiograph of the cranial aspect of the abdomen of a dog. All five radiographic opacities are visible. For example: Air (*A*)—gas in the lumen of the bowel; Fat (*F*)—fat in the omentum; Water (*W*)—the spleen; Bone (*B*)—the spinous process of a vertebra; Metal (*M*)—a foreign body in the stomach. The slightly more radiolucent nature of fat vs. soft tissue is critical in abdominal radiography, as the contrast provided by fat is the reason why most abdominal organs are visible radiographically. Water opacity is a generalization and is also called fluid or soft tissue opacity. Most organs and fluids have this opacity.

that have a similar x-ray attenuation properties (Table 6.2). These five descriptive terms (the five opacities) are used regularly in radiology reports and in conversation to describe radiographic findings.

Thickness also affects radiographic opacity. As thickness increases, the radiopacity will increase (Fig. 6.7). Thus, the five basic opacities are relative, assuming a similar thickness.

RADIOGRAPHIC CONTRAST

An individual structure will not be visible in a radiograph unless there is another structure of a different radiographic opacity that is in contact with it to provide *contrast*. Examples are liver margin visible due to adjacent fat, bone margin visible due to adjacent muscle, and pulmonary vessel margin visible due to adjacent air in the alveoli. Images can have varying degrees of contrast. A *high-contrast* image is one that has mostly blacks and whites and few gray shades, whereas a *low-contrast* image is one that has many gray shades and few blacks and whites (Fig. 6.8). To some extent, this depends on the relative values of kVp vs. mAs, but in digital imaging systems the contrast of the image is affected mainly by the processing algorithm the computer applies to the image data (see Fig. 6.8).

Table • 6.2

Examples of Various Tissues and Substances Having the Same Radiographic Opacity.

RADIOGRAPHIC OPACITY	SUBSTANCES HAVING THAT OPACITY
Air (gas)	Any gas collection present in the body • Air in lung or bowel • Gas in the colon from performing a pneumocolonogram • Nitrogen in a joint from the vacuum phenomenon • Gas from bacterial fermentation • Gas pockets from an injury • Free gas in abdomen after laparotomy • Tissue gas after fracture or joint surgery
Fat	Any tissue composed mainly of fat • Omentum • Mediastinal fat • Intrafascial fat • Falciform fat • Retroperitoneal fat • A lipoma
Water (soft tissue)	Any fluid or soft tissue • Parenchymal organs • Fibrous connective tissue • Muscle • Ligaments • Tendons • Cartilage • Blood • Bile • Cerebrospinal fluid • Urine • Transudate • Exudate • Hematoma • A soft tissue tumor
Bone (mineral)	Any mineralized region • Normal skeletal components • Ingested bone (before digestion) • Periosteal reaction • Dystrophic calcification, as from a calcifying hematoma • Metastatic calcification, as from renal failure
Metal	Anything containing metal • Metallic internal fixation devices • Identification microchip • Bullets or bullet fragments • Ingested foreign material • Horseshoe nails

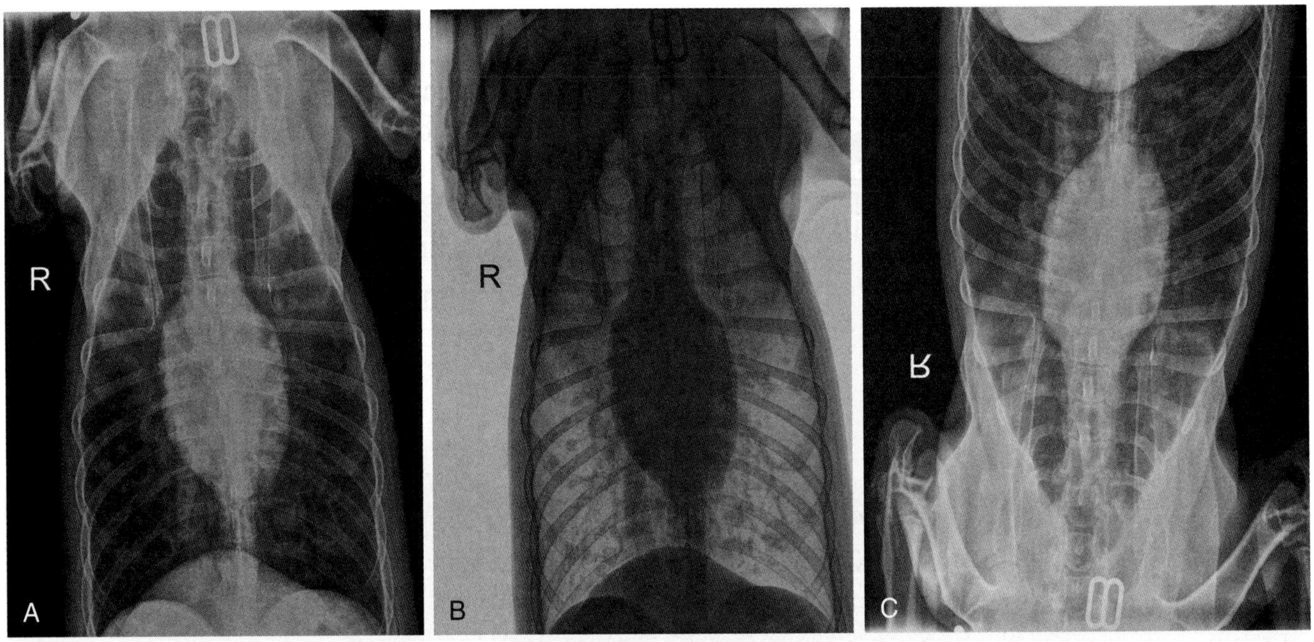

Fig. 7.5 There are tricks one can employ to revert back to a novice brain and break out of pattern recognition. **A, B,** and **C** are the same radiograph, but the grayscale has been inverted in **B**, and the image flipped vertically in **C**. The patient has pulmonary nodules; do you find it easier to see them in one image vs. another? While these tricks may work in the short-term, used enough, our brains will create a new schema of inverted ventrodorsal radiograph or upside down ventrodorsal radiograph, and we will be subject to the same search errors again. A better method is to develop a robust method for searching and interpreting images.

2. Reporting errors encompass errors committed by the reader during assessment, and can be further classified into the following categories:
   a. A search error is one in which we simply "don't see" the lesion, meaning we never physically foveate on it. It is the inability to discriminate embedded targets or a lesion from normal anatomy. Multiple factors lead to search errors.
      i. This can include physical/environmental factors including individual eye anatomy and health, workstation setup (proper monitor resolution and luminance, ambient light, veiling glare, uncluttered interfaces which do not distract attention), image quality (resolution, contrast, motion, positioning), and fatigue (time of day, image volume). Simply having proper/higher luminance monitors results in shorter search time, time to fixate on targets, and dwell time before reaching a decision. Reading performance will also wane later in the day as visual fatigue increases.[1,3,10,11,17]
      ii. Behavioral or systematic factors can also lead to search errors, including inadequate time to search an image, not searching the whole image, and having inadequate target knowledge. Being rushed when reading an image can decrease performance because it can prevent a systematic search. Target knowledge, or knowing what we are looking for, will physically change how we view an image. This highlights the importance of clinical history when interpreting an image.[1–3,11] It can be useful to interpret images without the history first (to limit bias), with a subsequent read after reading the history in order to provide target knowledge.
   b. A fixation error is one in which we "see" the lesion, meaning our eye physically foveates or fixates on a target, but we do not perceive or recognize it consciously. This type of error is directly impacted by training and experience. This is evident when you "see" a lesion only after someone else points it out even though you may have "looked" at it before. You will be better able to recognize that type of lesion on future radiographs.
      i. Fixation errors can also occur secondary to inadequate or incorrect target knowledge, as we are more apt to find what we are looking for. This concept is called inattentive blindness. In a prior study, a series of computed tomography (CT) lung images were provided to expert readers (radiologists) and naïve observers with no medical training. The images had lung nodules, but experimenters also inserted an image of a gorilla 48× larger than a typical nodule into the study. Both groups were asked to count nodules, but were not told to look for gorillas. Some 83% (20/24) of the radiologists did not report seeing the gorilla, even though 60% (12/20) did foveate on it identified with eye tracking (Fig. 7.6). None (0/24) of the naïve observers saw the gorilla. The results show that while expert readers may be less affected by inattentive blindness, both naïve and expert readers are affected by inadequate target knowledge even when a lesion is physically visible. The study also showed the radiologists outperformed the naïve observers in nodule detection (55% vs. 12%), which is the relevant clinical task for a radiologist.[18]
   c. A decision error is one in which we "see" the lesion, fixate, and perceive the lesion, but we do not reach the correct choice (poor judgment).[3] Reaching the correct decision about an image or lesion is directly related to prior training and experience. To reach a decision that pulmonary nodules indicate metastatic neoplasia, one first has to know that neoplasms can metastasize (including to the lung), and ideally there is a clinical history and target knowledge that support

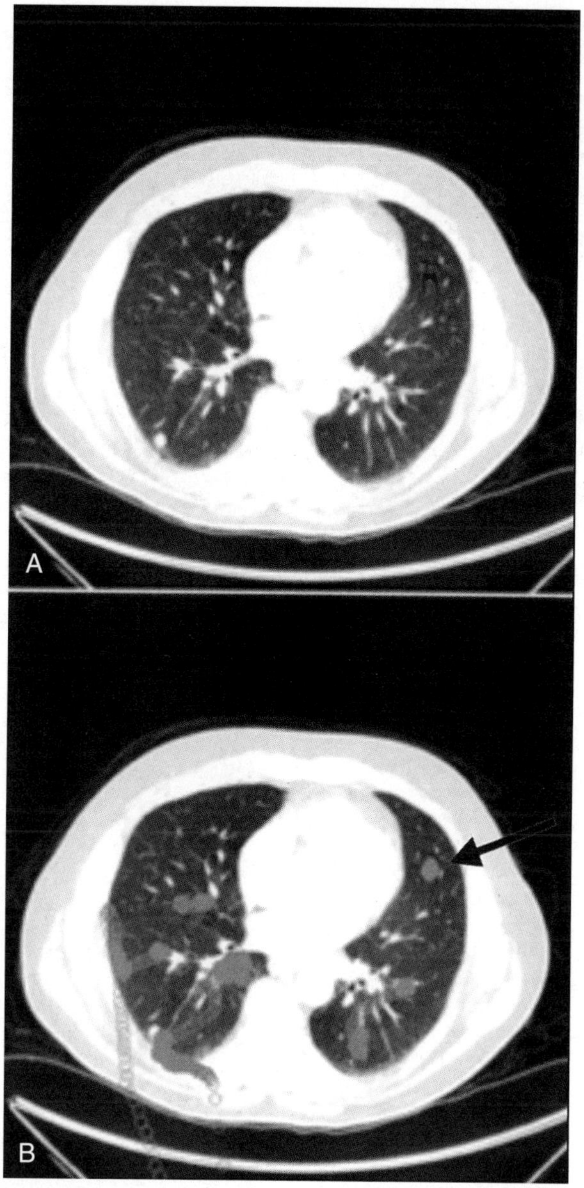

Fig. 7.6 Inattentional blindness is the tendency to miss something you were not looking for or expecting to find. The figure demonstrates this phenomenon, where expert readers (human radiologists), and nonexpert readers were given computed tomography (CT) lung studies to examine and report on pulmonary nodules, but were not told that a small gorilla much larger than a typical nodule would be present in some portions of the studies. Examples **A** and **B** are the same CT lung slice, as presented to the readers (**A**), and with the overlay of where they fixated on using eye tracking (**B**). In **B** it can be seen that the reader looked directly at the gorilla (*light gray dot with black arrow*), but never reported seeing it. In other words, the gorilla was "seen," but not "recognized." Since this is not a real pathology, it was ignored by expert readers even though it was technically "seen." This highlights the importance of target knowledge (knowing what you are looking for). (From Drew T, Vo MLH, Wolfe JM. The invisible gorilla strikes again: sustained inattentional blindness in expert observers. *Psychol Sci.* 2013;24(9):1848-1853.)

that as the correct diagnosis (e.g., the patient is a 12-year-old dog with known splenic hemangiosarcoma). It also requires knowledge and consideration of other differential diagnoses that could result in pulmonary nodules (parasitic granulomas, abscesses, immune mediated granulomas such as eosinophilic bronchopneumopathy), and cognitively filtering what is most likely based not only on the radiographic appearance, but the patient's signalment and clinical history.

d. A thorough list of types of cognitive errors and biases are listed in eTable 7.1, but a few that relate directly to decision error include pattern recognition, prevalence effect, premature closure, satisfaction of search, diagnostic momentum, and automation bias.[19]
   i. Pattern recognition is a tool of system 1 thinking, which is an efficient (although not always accurate) way to recognize a lesion as something you have seen before. Pattern recognition is only accurate under typical circumstances. For example, a cranioventrally distributed alveolar pattern is a common finding in bronchopneumonia/aspiration pneumonia and would be a common diagnosis for a patient

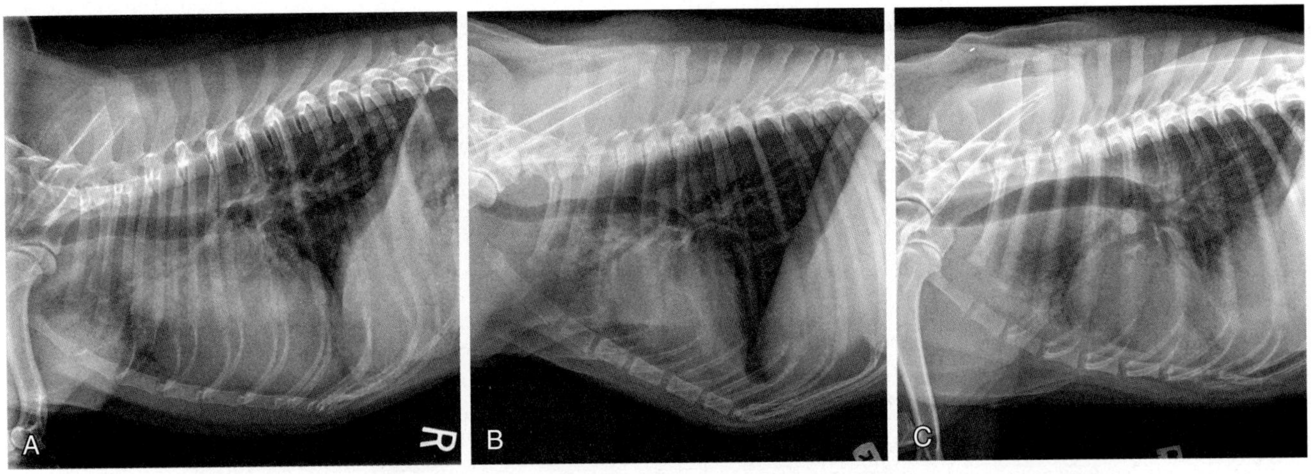

Fig. 7.7 Pattern recognition may work in usual reproducible circumstances but will not work in all situations. Examples **A, B,** and **C** are right lateral thoracic radiographs of patients who all have a ventrally distributed alveolar pattern. This pattern and distribution are commonly seen in bronchopneumonia, which is also a common condition. However, not every ventral alveolar pattern will be pneumonia. There are some other features on these radiographs that may offer clues to other diagnoses. Have a look and decide how you would diagnose these patients on these single views, then read on for the final diagnoses. **A,** Pulmonary infiltrates secondary to pulmonary hypertension. **B,** Bronchopneumonia/aspiration pneumonia. **C,** Bronchopneumonia and pulmonary lymphoma.

with respiratory signs. However, other disease processes can also result in a cranioventral alveolar pattern (Fig. 7.7), and may also result in respiratory signs. While the frequency of other diseases may be less common, they must still be considered.

ii. Frequency of disease also impacts decision making with regard to prevalence effect, whereby lesions you have seen/diagnosed before or are more common are more likely to be diagnosed for subsequent patients. Cranial cruciate ligament rupture is a common diagnosis, and results in increased soft tissue opacity and distention of the stifle joint. While cruciate rupture is much more common than a joint centric neoplasm or septic arthritis in a dog, these other conditions do occur, and other features of an aggressive process may be unconsidered (if they are seen) and a false-positive diagnosis of cruciate rupture may be made.[19]

iii. Premature closure and satisfaction of search can both be considered types of tunnel vision. Premature closure is making a diagnosis such as identifying a lung tumor on thoracic radiographs for a large ovoid soft tissue opacity, but not considering that the patient was recently hit by a car, has a rib fractures, and the "tumor" has a fluid line making a hematocele a more likely diagnosis. This is the cessation of thinking once a diagnosis is made.[19] Satisfaction of search is making a diagnosis (such as esophageal distention consistent with megaesophagus on thoracic radiographs) but discontinuing the search and not identifying that the patient also has pneumonia.[19] This can be thought of as only identifying the tip of the iceberg. An example of these types of errors is demonstrated in Fig. 7.8.

iv. Diagnostic momentum and automation bias can be thought of as types of peer pressure. Diagnostic momentum is peer pressure from human to human and can take the form of another clinician labeling a patient with a certain diagnosis, or that label being present in prior records. There is often reluctance to challenge the correctness of what has been repeated, and a tendency to carry it forward even if the clinical picture no longer fits.[19] An example could be a well-respected radiologist has diagnosed a pathologic bone lesion on prior radiographs, but you think the lesion is more consistent with degenerative change. You may defer to the prior diagnosis instead of asserting what you really think is correct. Automation bias is peer pressure from machine to human, trusting a machine or computer output in replacement of your own

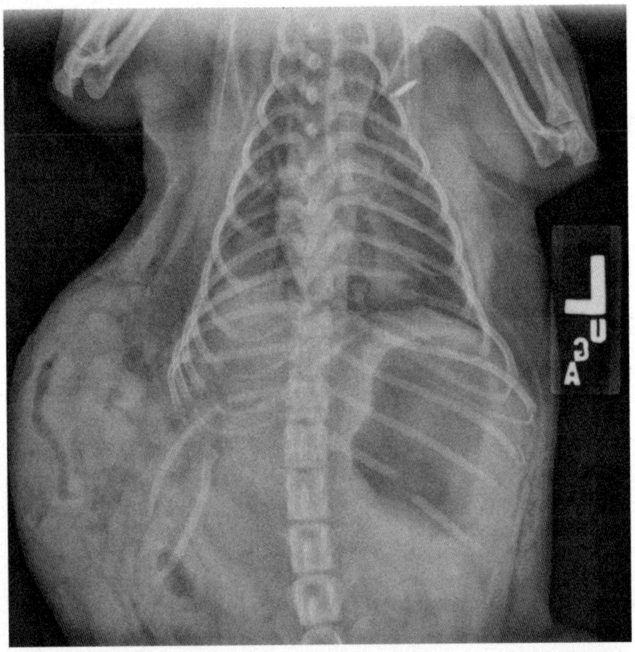

Fig. 7.8 Premature closure and satisfaction of search are types of errors similar to having tunnel vision. A lesion or diagnosis may be seen, and accepted as the full answer, missing other lesions and diagnoses. The ventrodorsal radiograph shown is from a dog who was hit by a car with severe trauma. There is obvious swelling of the right lateral extrathoracic and abdominal soft tissues with gas and intestinal segments indicative of body wall hernia, and there are some right-sided rib luxations and fractures. The swelling certainly draws the eye. However, did you catch/identify all of the left-sided rib fractures?

thought process. This could be accepting a diagnosis provided by artificial intelligence (AI) regardless of the evidence. The result is errors of commission (AI diagnoses pulmonary nodules and you agree even though you do not see nodules) and errors of omission (AI does not identify pulmonary nodules even though present on radiographs, and you do not report them).[20] Studies have shown that we all our susceptible to automation bias regardless of our level of expertise, but there is a protective effect of expertise (experts are less affected by automation bias vs. novices).[21]

e. Intraobserver variability is the variation/accuracy of search, recognition, and decision making by the same person over multiple times points and interobserver variability is the variation/accuracy between separate observers. As humans all the factors mentioned earlier impact accuracy and performance, which is unlikely to be completely consistent and uniform over time (even when evaluating the same images).
   i. Human studies have shown that intraobserver variability can be as high as 20% and interobserver variability as high as 30% to 50%.[22,23] Reader training, experience, and skill directly affect performance, as do physical and environmental factors. You may be less likely to identify pulmonary nodules at the end of the day when you are fatigued or if there are increasing distractions. Even if a nodule or lesion is identified, there could be variation in reporting of size over time, which affects treatment decisions (stable disease, remission, progression).
   ii. In human radiology, studies have shown false-negative rates of 20% to 30%, and false-positive rates of 2% to 15%.[1,3,17,22] More experienced observers will typically have more efficient visual search/fixation/dwell patterns, find lesions faster, process more information, and be more accurate than novice observers.[17,24]

3. Post reporting errors occur during the communication after image interpretation, be it from clinician to clinician, clinician to technician, or clinician to client. These can range from typos or mistakes in the imaging report, particularly if reports generated using voice dictation are not proofread, format or reporting style, lack of or inappropriate recommendations, delayed reporting, or simply misunderstanding between people when the clinical information is exchanged.[16]

ERROR REDUCTION

As humans, we are not infallible, and even the most competent and experienced clinician will occasionally commit an error. While no one is accurate 100% of the time, we can employ strategies to reduce errors, and control variables. As has been related in legal writing surrounding medical errors, this includes reaching and maintaining competence, developing habits of practice, and using proper techniques.[25]

1. Physical factors and limiting distractors/stressors
   a. Having a proper workstation, including high-resolution monitors with appropriate luminance.
   b. Acquiring studies with impeccable technique and positioning whenever possible.
   c. Limiting ambient noise and light (quiet and dark reading room).
   d. Managing fatigue
      i. Taking regular breaks.
      ii. Allow your eyes to accommodate to different distances during breaks.
      iii. Maintaining a manageable workload.
2. Accurate and complete clinical history/target knowledge
   a. Performing a blind read without the clinical history to avoid clinical bias.
   b. Performing an unblinded read with signalment and clinical history for appropriate context and to avoid inattentional blindness.
   c. Availability of prior reports and imaging for comparison when possible.
3. Structured reporting/checklists
   a. Checklists are a way to build system 2 thinking into your practice, providing prompts to ensure the reader has assessed all parts of the imaging study. Checklists have been shown to reduce error, particularly task-focused checklists.[26–28]
4. Double reads/second opinions
   a. Leverage the visual and cognitive resources of more than one person.
   b. Independent second reads can reduce false-negatives but may increase false-positives and interobserver variability. One study showed optimal balance between accuracy and agreement was four independent readings with a reviewer of composite results.[14,20,22,23]
5. Metacognition
   a. Metacognition is thinking about thinking.
   b. Being familiar with the types of errors and biases that can occur allows for error reduction (consciously switching from system 1 to system 2 thinking).[16]
   c. In practice, this could be stopping after interpretation of a set of images, to check that all anatomic regions and parts of the image assessed, the signalment and clinical history considered, and questioning whether the imaging findings fit with the clinical picture.
6. Follow-up/communication
   a. There should be open and effective communication with all members of the medical team, and between the medical team and pet owner.[16]
   b. Clear communication ensures that what was perceived and interpreted is relayed accurately so that treatment steps can reflect those diagnoses.
   c. Communication also allows for feedback and learning from both accurate and inaccurate interpretations.
7. Error assessment
   a. When errors occur, a root cause analysis should be performed.
   b. This allows determination of how/why an error occurred, and whether it was a human or systems error.[14,16]

REFERENCES

1. Krupinski EA. The role of perception in imaging: past and future. *Semin Nucl Med*. 2011;41:392–400.
2. Tuddenham WJ, Calvert WP. Visual search patterns in Roentgen diagnosis. *Radiology*. 1961;76(2):225–226.
3. Tuddenham WJ. Visual search, imaging organization, and reader error in Roentgen diagnosis. *Radiology*. 1962;78(4):694–704.
4. Anderson BL, Winawer J. Image segmentation and lightness perception. *Nature*. 2005;434:3.
5. Papageorges M, Sande R. The Mach phenomenon. *Vet Radiol Ultrasound*. 1990;31(6):274–280.
6. Papageorges M. How the Mach phenomenon and shape affect the radiographic appearance of skeletal structures. *Vet Radiol Ultrasound*. 1991;32(4):191–195.
7. Eckstein MP. Visual search: a retrospective. *J Vis*. 2011;11(5):1–36, 14.
8. Manning D, Ethell SC, Donovan T. Time-dependent observer errors in pulmonary nodule detection. *Br J Radiol*. 2006;79:342–346.

9. Yang GZ, Depmere-Marco L, Hu XP, Rowe A. Visual search: psychophysical models and practical applications. *Image Vis Comput*. 2002;20:291–305.
10. Krupinski EA, Kallergi M. Choosing a radiology workstation: technical and clinical considerations. *Radiology*. 2007;242(3).
11. Kundel HL, Nodine CF, Toto L. Searching for lung nodules: the guidance of visual scanning. *Invest Radiol*. 1991;26(9):777–781.
12. Sowden P, Pringle A, Gabora L. The shifting sands of creative thinking: connections to dual process theory. *Think Reas*. 2015;21(1):4060.
13. McVee MB, Dunsmore K, Gavelek JR. Schema theory revisited. *Rev Educ Res*. 2005;75(4):531–566.
14. Brady A, Laoide RO, McCarthy P. Discrepancy and error in radiology: concepts, causes, consequences. *Ulster Med J*. 2012;81(1):3–9.
15. Goddard P, Leslie A, Jones A, Wakeley C, Kabala J. Error in radiology. *Br J Radiol*. 2001;74:949–951.
16. Onder O, Yarasir Y, Azizova A, Durham G, Onur MR, Ariyurek OM. Errors, discrepancies and underlying bias in radiology with case examples: a pictorial review. *Insights Imaging*. 2021;12:51.
17. Krupinski EA. The importance of perception research in medical imaging. *Radiat Med*. 2000;18(6):329–334.
18. Drew T, Vo MLH, Wolfe JM. The invisible gorilla strikes again: sustained inattentional blindness in expert observers. *Psychol Sci*. 2013, September;24(9):1848–1853.
19. Croskerry P. The importance of cognitive errors in diagnosis and strategies to minimize them. *Acad Med*. 2003;78(8):775–780.
20. Goddard K, Roudsari A, Wyatt JC. Automation Bias: a systematic review of frequency, effect mediators, and mitigators. *J Am Med Assoc*. 2012;19:121–127.
21. Dratsch T, Chen X, Mehrizi MR, et al. Automation bias in mammography: the impact of artificial intelligence BI-RADS suggestions on reader performance. *Radiology*. 2023;307(4):e222176.
22. Yerushalmy J. The statistical assessment of the variability in observer perception and description of roentgenographic pulmonary shadows. *Radiol Clin North Am*. 1969;7:381–392.
23. Kulberg NS, Reshetnikov RV, Novik VP, et al. Inter-observer variability between readers of CT images: all for one and one for all. *Digital Diagnostics*. 2021;2(2):105–118.
24. Nodine CF, Krupinski EA. Perceptual skill, radiology expertise, and visual test performance with NINA and WALDO. *Acad Radiol*. 1998;5:603–612.
25. Caldwell C, Seamone ER. Excusable neglect in malpractice suits against radiologists: a proposed jury introduction to recognize the human condition. *Ann Health Law*. 2007;16:43–77.
26. Al-Khafaji J, Townshend RF, Townsend W, Chopra V, Gupta A. Checklists to reduce diagnostic error: a systematic review of the literature using a human factors framework. *BMJ Open*. 2022;12:e058219.
27. Pronovost P, Needham D, Berenholtz S, et al. An intervention to decrease catheter-related bloodstream infections in the ICU. *N Engl J Med*. 2006;355:2725–2732.
28. Haynes AB, Weiser TG, Berry WR, et al. A surgical safety checklist to reduce morbidity and mortality in a global population. *N Engl J Med*. 2009;360:491–499.

ELECTRONIC RESOURCES

Additional information related to the content in Chapter 7 can be found online at eBooks.Health.Elsevier.com.

- Chapter Quiz

SECTION II

The Axial Skeleton: Canine, Feline, and Equine

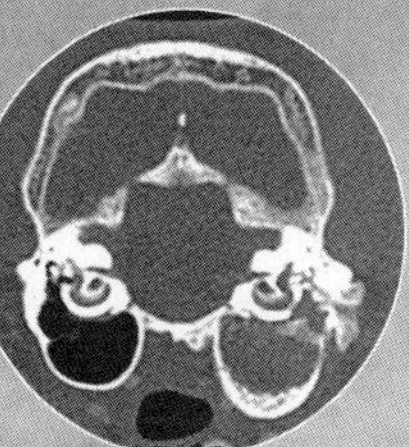

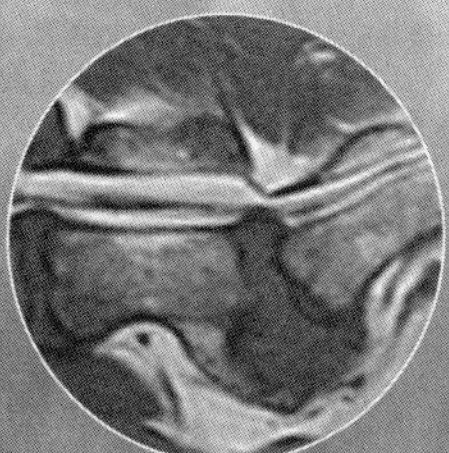

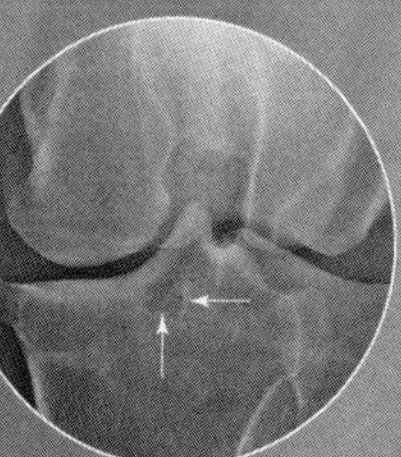

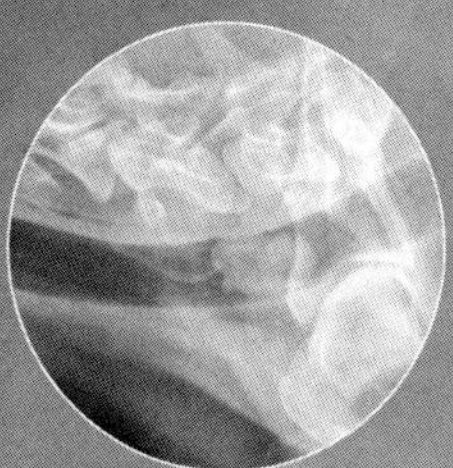

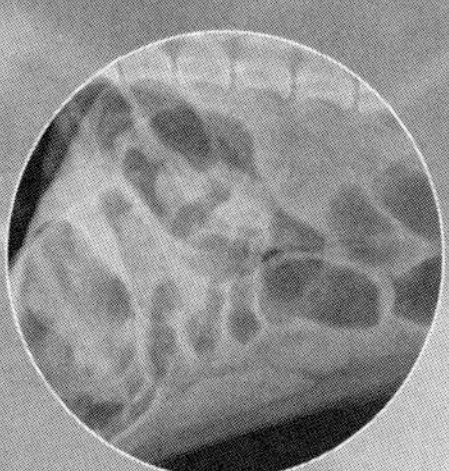

CHAPTER 8

Radiographic Anatomy of the Axial Skeleton

Andra K. Voges • Kathy A. Spaulding

To use the roentgen sign method of recognizing abnormal radiographic findings effectively, an understanding of normal radiographic anatomy for the specific area of interest is necessary. Within the space constraints of a comprehensive veterinary radiology text, this chapter provides a limited reference for the radiographic anatomy of the axial skeleton (Figs. 8.1–8.21). For more detailed information, readers are referred to comprehensive texts on radiographic anatomy.[1–5]

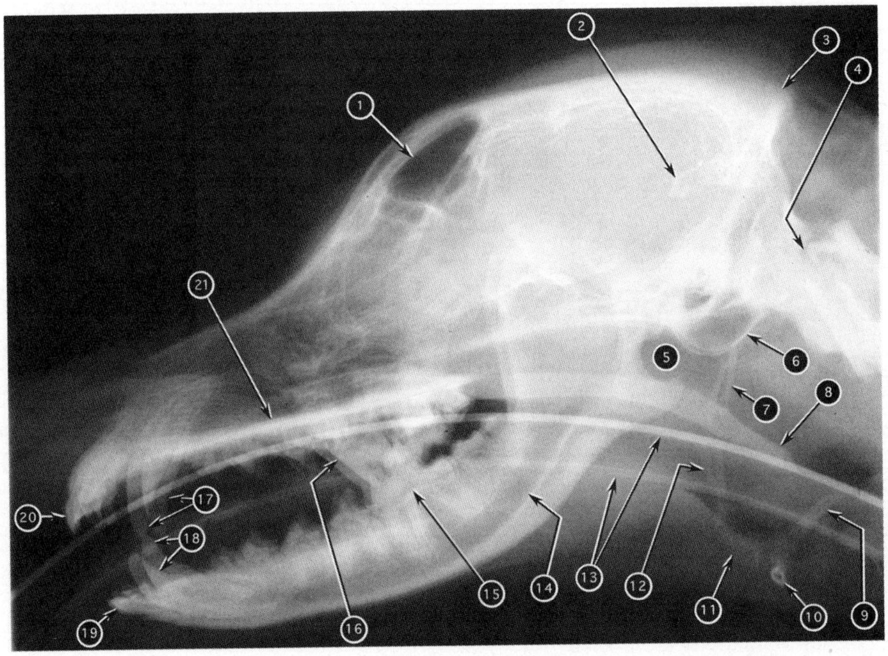

Fig. 8.1 Left–right lateral radiograph of canine head.
1. Frontal sinuses
2. Tentorium osseum cerebelli
3. External occipital protuberance
4. Atlantooccipital joints
5. Air in nasopharynx
6. Tympanic bullae
7. Stylohyoid bones
8. Soft palate
9. Thyrohyoid bones
10. Basihyoid bone
11. Ceratohyoid bones
12. Epihyoid bones
13. Endotracheal tube
14. Inferior alveolar canals of mandibles
15. Inferior first molar teeth (superimposed 309 left/409 right)
16. Superior fourth premolar teeth (superimposed 208 left/108 right)
17. Superior canine teeth (superimposed 204 left/104 right)
18. Inferior canine teeth (superimposed 304 left/404 right)
19. Inferior incisor teeth (superimposed 301, 302, 303 left/401, 402, 403 right)
20. Superior incisor teeth (superimposed 201, 202, 203 left/101, 102, 103 right)
21. Hard palate

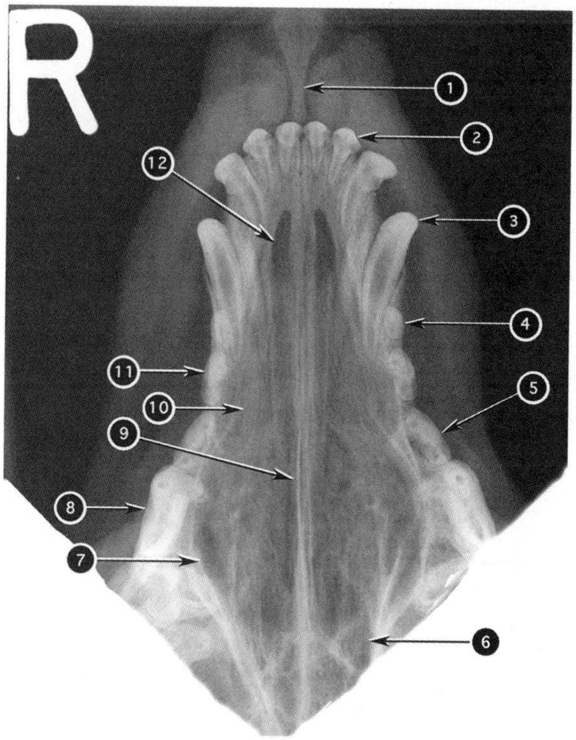

Fig. 8.2 Intraoral dorsoventral radiograph of canine nasal cavity.
1. Cartilaginous nasal septum
2. Superior incisor 2 (202)
3. Superior canine tooth (204)
4. Superior premolar 1 (205)
5. Superior premolar 3 (207)
6. Ethmoidal conchae
7. Maxillary recess
8. Superior premolar 4 (108)
9. Nasal septum
10. Dorsal and ventral nasal conchae
11. Superior premolar 2 (106)
12. Palatine fissure

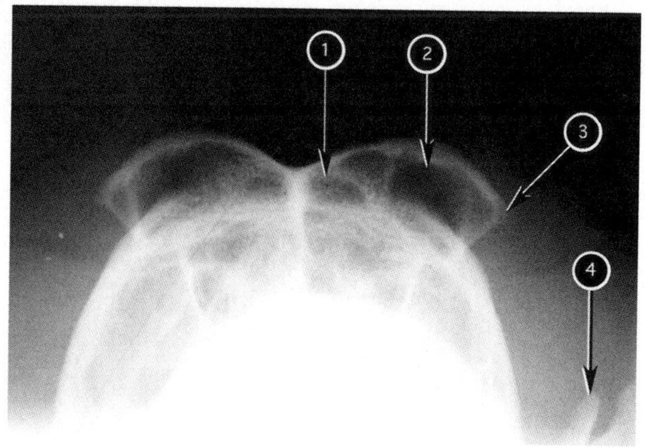

Fig. 8.3 Rostrodorsal-caudodorsal oblique radiograph of canine frontal sinuses.
1. Medial frontal sinus
2. Lateral frontal sinus
3. Zygomatic process of frontal bone
4. Coronoid process of mandible

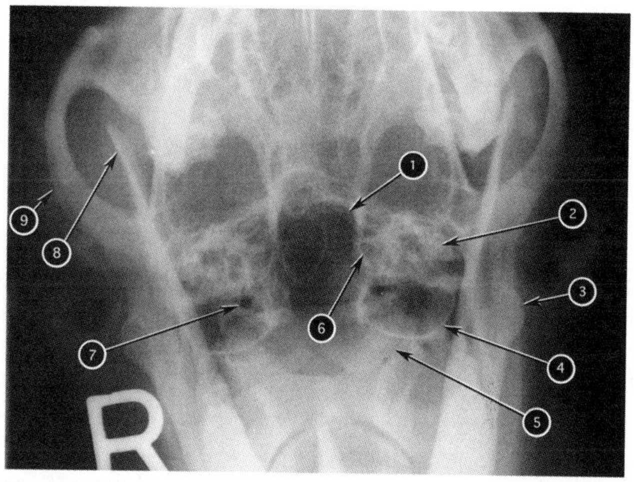

Fig. 8.4 Rostroventral-caudodorsal oblique (open-mouth) radiograph of canine tympanic bullae.
1. Nasopharynx
2. Petrous temporal bone
3. Angular process of mandible
4. Tympanic bulla
5. Atlantooccipital joint
6. Foramen lacerum
7. Jugular foramen
8. Coronoid process of mandible
9. Zygomatic arch

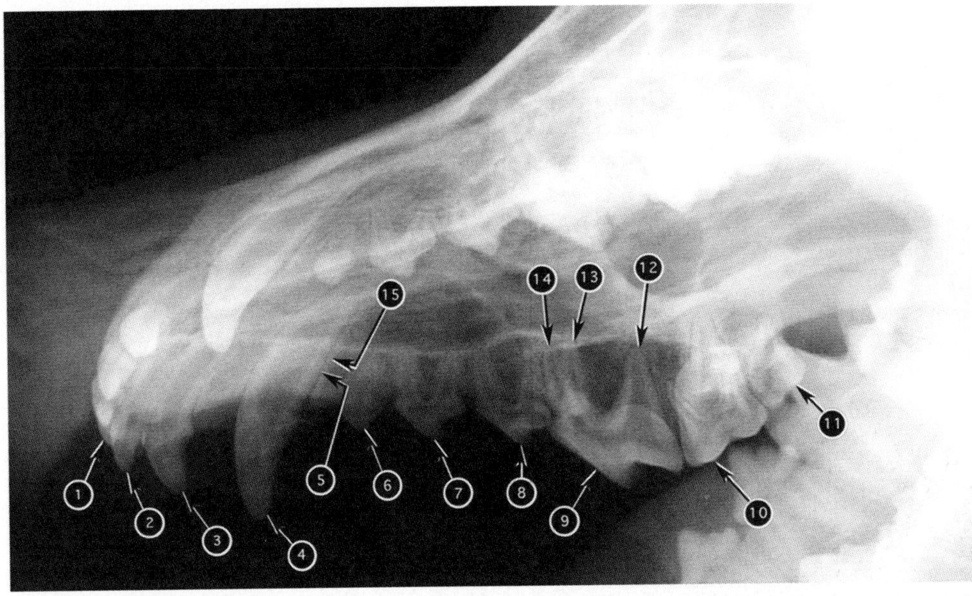

Fig. 8.5 Caudal left ventral/rostral right dorsal oblique radiograph of canine maxillary teeth (right maxilla projected ventrally).

1. Maxillary incisor 1 (101)
2. Maxillary incisor 2 (102)
3. Maxillary incisor 3 (103)
4. Maxillary canine tooth (104)
5. Periodontal ligament
6. Maxillary premolar 1 (105)
7. Maxillary premolar 2 (106)
8. Maxillary premolar 3 (107)
9. Maxillary premolar 4 (108)
10. Maxillary molar 1 (109)
11. Maxillary molar 2 (110)
12. Distal root of maxillary premolar 4 (108)
13. Mesiobuccal root of maxillary premolar 4 (108)
14. Mesiopalatal root of maxillary premolar 4 (108)
15. Cortical bone forming wall of alveolus

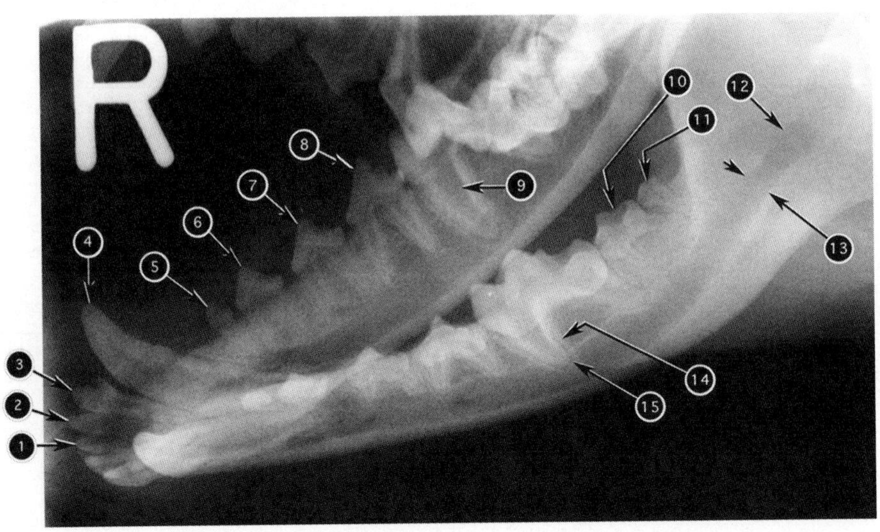

Fig. 8.6 Left ventral/right dorsal oblique radiograph of canine mandibular teeth.

1. Right mandibular incisor 1 (401)
2. Right mandibular incisor 2 (402)
3. Right mandibular incisor 3 (403)
4. Right mandibular canine tooth (404)
5. Right mandibular premolar 1 (405)
6. Right mandibular premolar 2 (406)
7. Right mandibular premolar 3 (407)
8. Right mandibular premolar 4 (408)
9. Dental cavity of right mandibular molar 1 (409)
10. Left mandibular molar 2 (310)
11. Left mandibular molar 3 (311)
12. Left mandibular foramen
13. Left mandibular canal
14. Lamina dura (cortical bone forming wall of alveolus) of mesial root of left mandibular molar 1 (309)
15. Periodontal ligament of mesial root of left mandibular molar 1 (309)

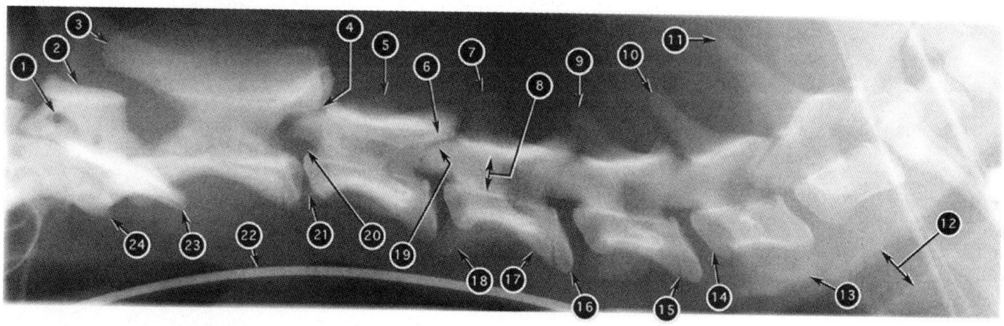

Fig. 8.7 Left-right lateral radiograph of canine cervical vertebrae.

1. Lateral vertebral foramina (left and right) of atlas; emergence of cervical nerve 1
2. Dorsal arch of atlas (C1)
3. Spinous process of axis (C2)
4. Synovial joints between articular processes of C2 and C3
5. Spinous process of C3
6. Caudal articular processes of C3
7. Spinous process of C4
8. Vertebral canal of C4
9. Spinous process of C5
10. Spinous process of C6
11. Spinous process of C7
12. Trachea
13. Expanded ventral laminae of transverse processes of C6
14. Cranial extremity (head) of C6
15. Caudal physis of C5
16. Caudal extremity (fossa) of C4
17. Body of C4
18. Transverse processes of C4
19. Cranial articular processes of C4
20. Intervertebral foramina between C2 and C3
21. Intervertebral disk space between C2 and C3
22. Endotracheal tube
23. Wings (transverse processes) of atlas
24. Ventral tubercle of atlas

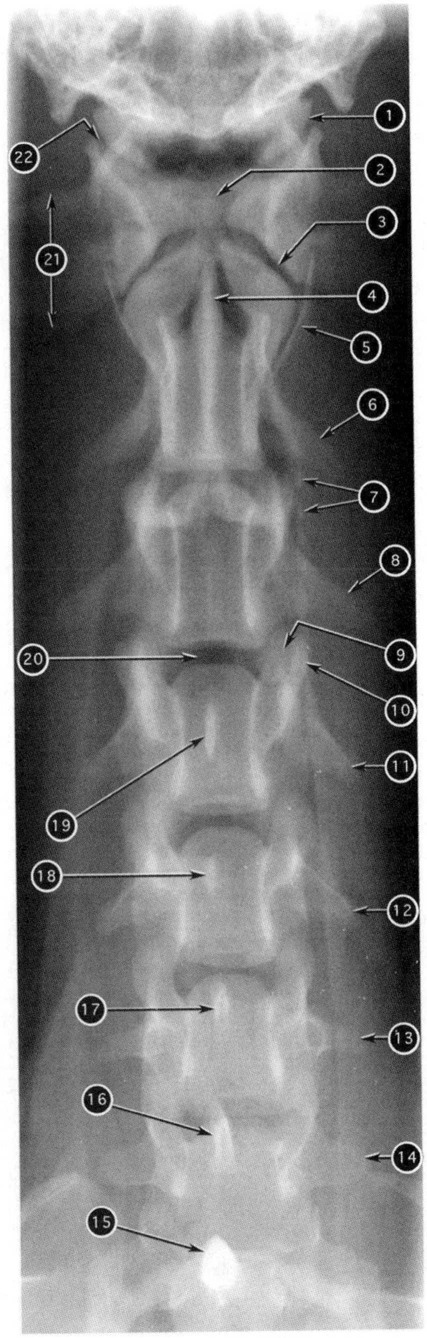

Fig. 8.8 Ventrodorsal radiograph of canine cervical vertebrae.
1. Left occipital condyle
2. Dens of axis
3. Atlantoaxial joint
4. Spinous process of axis
5. Left thyrohyoid bone
6. Left transverse process of axis
7. Tracheal cartilages
8. Left transverse process of C3
9. Left caudal articular process of C3
10. Left cranial articular process of C4
11. Left transverse process of C4
12. Left transverse process of C5
13. Left transverse process of C6
14. Left transverse process of C7
15. Spinous process of T1
16. Spinous process of C7
17. Spinous process of C6
18. Spinous process of C5
19. Spinous process of C4
20. Intervertebral disk space between C3 and C4
21. Right wing of atlas
22. Right atlantooccipital joint

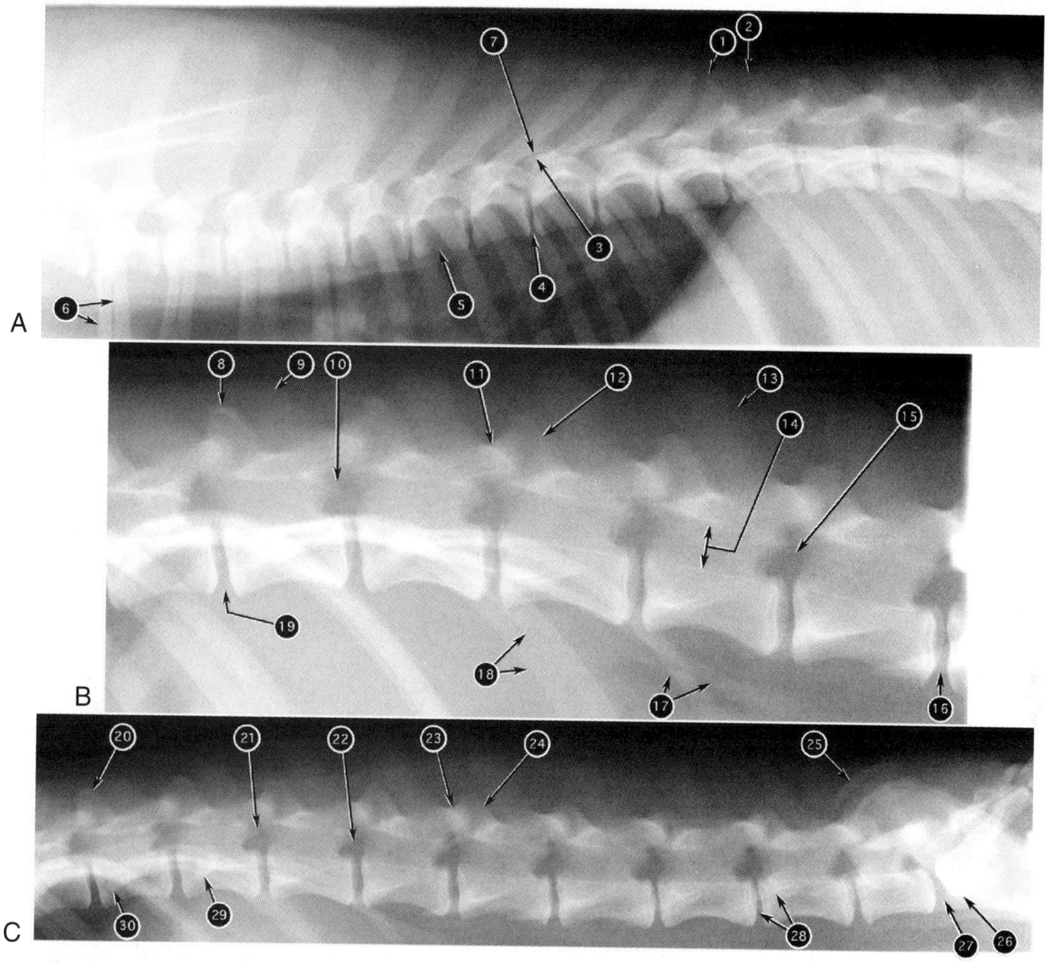

Fig. 8.9 Left-right lateral radiographs of canine thoracic and lumbar vertebrae.

A, Left–right (right) lateral radiograph of thoracic spine.
1. Spinous process of T10
2. Spinous process of T11 (anticlinal vertebra)
3. Cranial articular processes of T8
4. Intervertebral disk space between T7 and T8
5. Body of T6
6. First pair of ribs
7. Caudal articular processes of T7

B, Left–right (right) lateral radiograph of thoracolumbar spine.
8. Mammillary processes atop cranial articular processes of T12
9. Spinous process of T12
10. Accessory processes of T12
11. Caudal articular processes of T13
12. Cranial articular processes of L1
13. Spinous process of L2
14. Vertebral canal of L2
15. Intervertebral foramina between L2 and L3
16. Transverse processes of L4 superimposed over L3–4 intervertebral disk space
17. Thirteenth pair of ribs
18. Twelfth pair of ribs
19. Intervertebral disk space between T11 and T12

C, Left–right (right) lateral radiograph of lumbar spine.
20. Mammillary processes atop cranial articular processes of T12
21. Accessory processes of T13
22. Intervertebral foramina between L1 and L2
23. Caudal articular processes of L2
24. Cranial articular processes of L3
25. Secondary ossification center for crest of ilium
26. Promontory of sacrum
27. Intervertebral disk space between L7 and S1
28. Transverse processes of L6
29. Heads of 13th ribs superimposed on body of T13
30. Heads of 12th ribs superimposed on body of T12

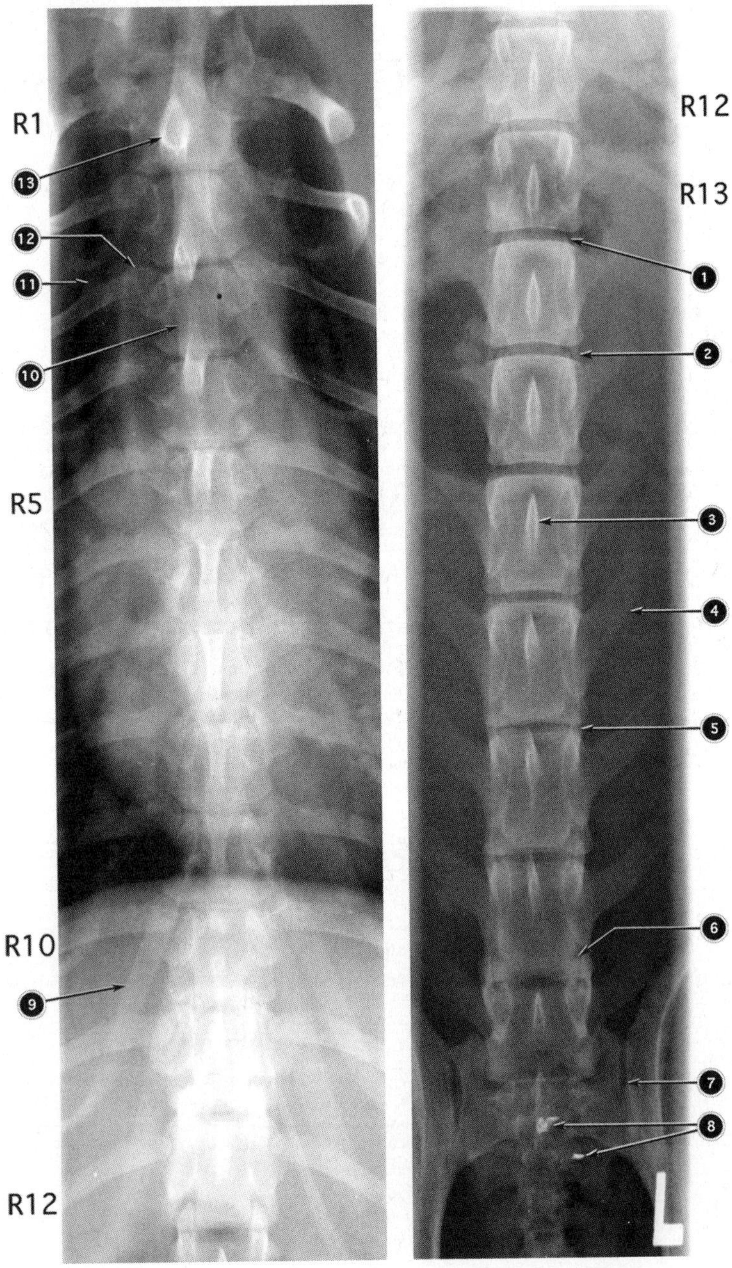

Fig. 8.10 Ventrodorsal radiographs of canine thoracic and lumbar vertebrae. *R,* Rib.

1. Intervertebral disk space between T13 and L1
2. Left accessory process of L2
3. Spinous process of L3
4. Left transverse process of L4
5. Left cranial articular process of L5
6. Left caudal articular process of L6
7. Left sacroiliac joint
8. Metallic foreign bodies in descending colon
9. Costal cartilage of right rib 11
10. Sternum superimposed over vertebrae
11. Tubercle of right rib 3
12. Head of right rib 3, articulating with bodies of vertebrae T2 and T3
13. Spinous process of T1

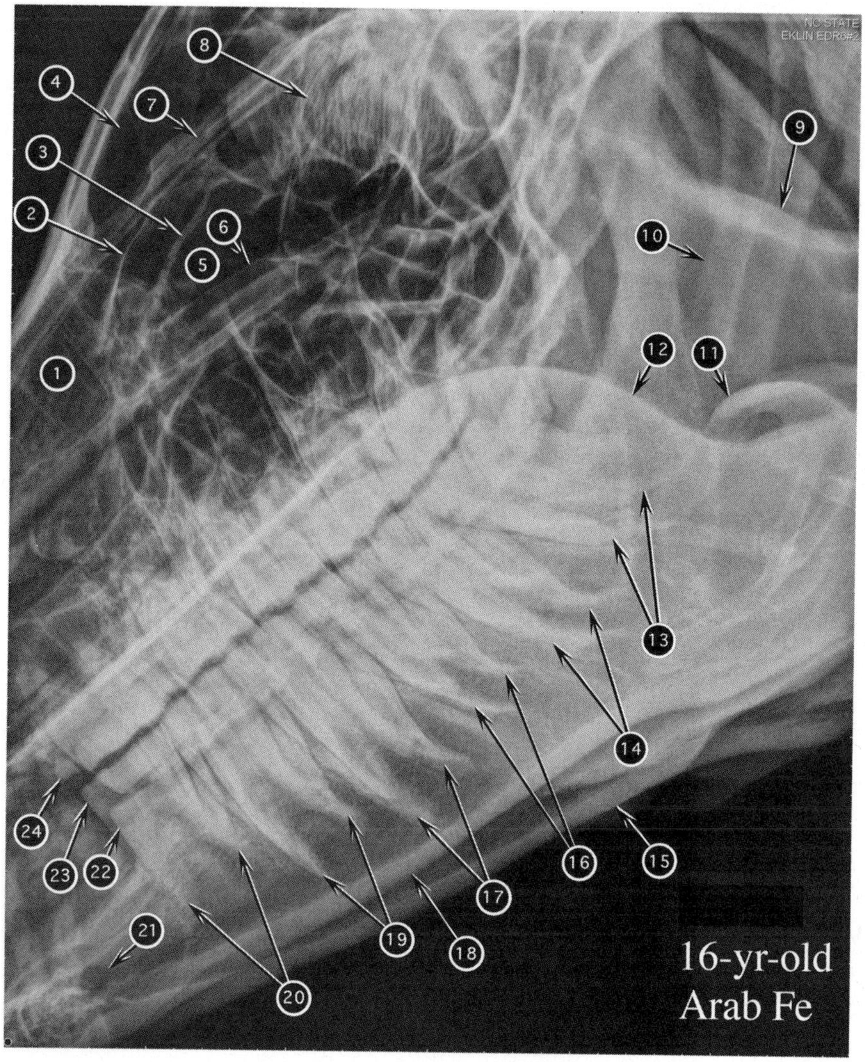

Fig. 8.11 Right-left (left) lateral radiograph of middle region of equine head (16 years old).

1. Dorsal conchal sinuses
2. Septum between left rostral and caudal maxillary sinuses
3. Septum between right rostral and caudal maxillary sinuses
4. Frontal sinuses (communicate with 1)
5. Caudal maxillary sinuses
6. Left infraorbital canal
7. Nasolacrimal ducts
8. Ethmoidal labyrinth
9. Dorsal wall of nasopharynx
10. Left stylohyoid bone
11. Epiglottic cartilage
12. Soft palate resting on root of tongue
13. Roots of right mandibular molar 3 (tooth 411)
14. Roots of right mandibular molar 2 (tooth 410)
15. Ventral border of right mandible
16. Roots of right mandibular molar 1 (tooth 409)
17. Roots of right mandibular premolar 4 (tooth 408)
18. Ventral border of left mandible
19. Roots of right mandibular premolar 3 (tooth 407)
20. Roots of right mandibular premolar 2 (tooth 406)
21. Left mental foramen
22. Right mandibular premolar 2 (tooth 406)
23. Left mandibular premolar 2 (tooth 306)
24. Left and right maxillary premolar 1 (teeth 205 and 105 superimposed)

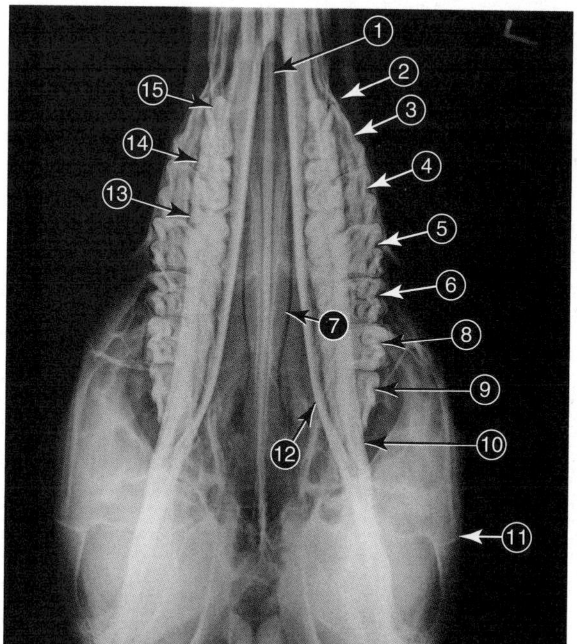

Fig. 8.12 Dorsoventral radiograph of middle region of equine head (16 years old).

1. Cartilaginous nasal septum superimposed on vomer
2. Left maxillary premolar 1 (tooth 205)
3. Left maxillary premolar 2 (tooth 206)
4. Left maxillary premolar 3 (tooth 207)
5. Left maxillary premolar 4 (tooth 208)
6. Left maxillary molar 1 (tooth 209)
7. Mucosa covering left side of nasal septum
8. Left maxillary molar 2 (tooth 210)
9. Left maxillary molar 3 (tooth 211)
10. Lateral surface of left mandible
11. Zygomatic arch
12. Medial surface of left mandible
13. Right mandibular premolar 4 (tooth 408)
14. Right mandibular premolar 3 (tooth 407)
15. Right mandibular premolar 2 (tooth 406)

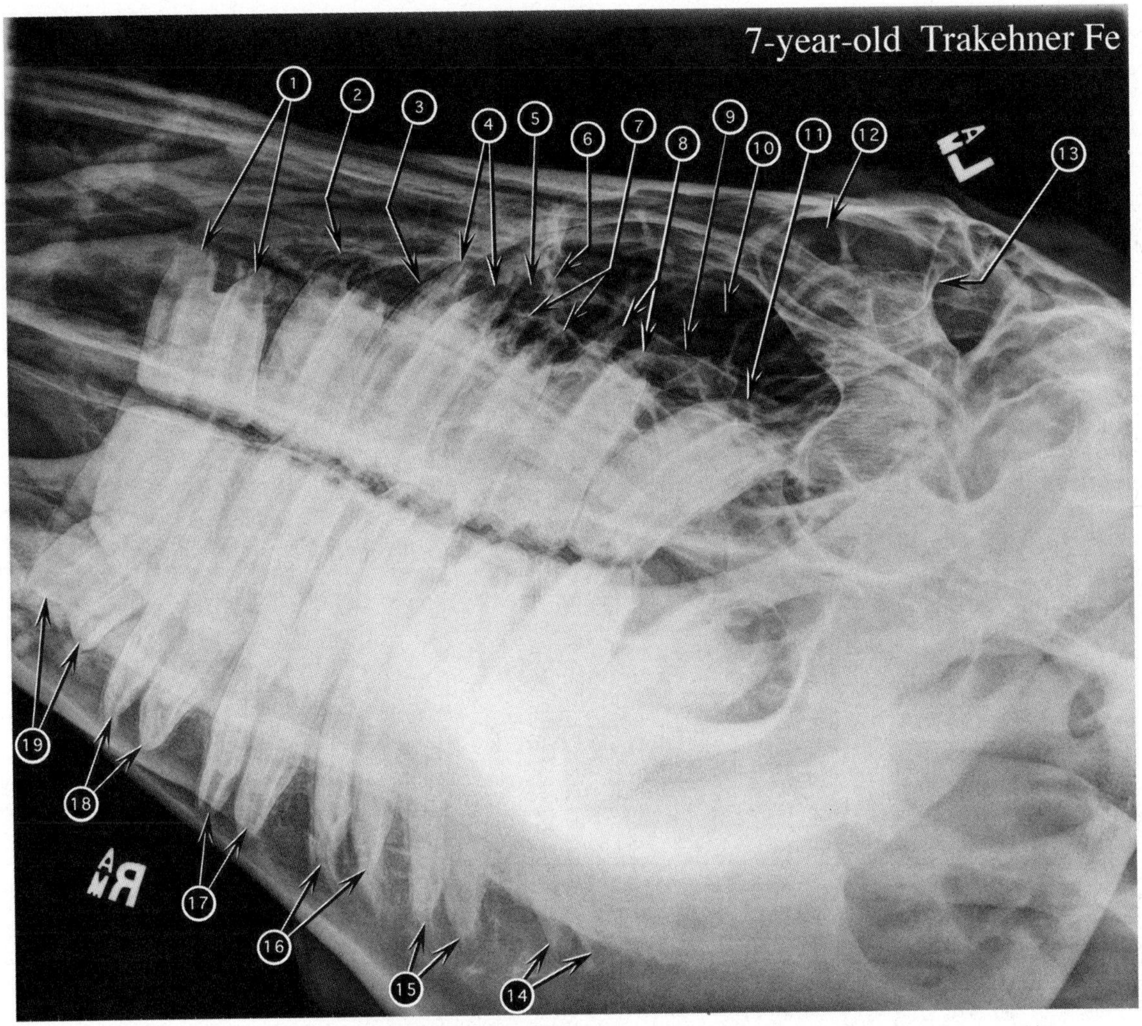

Fig. 8.13 Left ventral-right dorsal oblique (LeV-RtDO) radiograph of middle region of equine head (7 years old).

1. Roots of left maxillary premolar 2 (tooth 206)
2. Roots of left maxillary premolar 3 (tooth 207)
3. Wall of alveolus (*lamina dura dentes*)
4. Roots of left maxillary premolar 4 (tooth 208)
5. Left rostral maxillary sinus
6. Osseous septum separating 5 from 10
7. Roots of left maxillary molar 1 (tooth 209)
8. Roots of left maxillary molar 2 (tooth 210)
9. Left infraorbital canal
10. Left caudal maxillary sinus
11. Roots of left maxillary molar 3 (tooth 211)
12. Left conchofrontal sinus
13. Zygomatic process of left frontal bone
14. Roots of right mandibular molar 3 (tooth 411)
15. Roots of right mandibular molar 2 (tooth 410)
16. Roots of right mandibular molar 1 (tooth 409)
17. Roots of right mandibular premolar 4 (tooth 408)
18. Roots of right mandibular premolar 3 (tooth 407)
19. Roots of right mandibular premolar 2 (tooth 406)

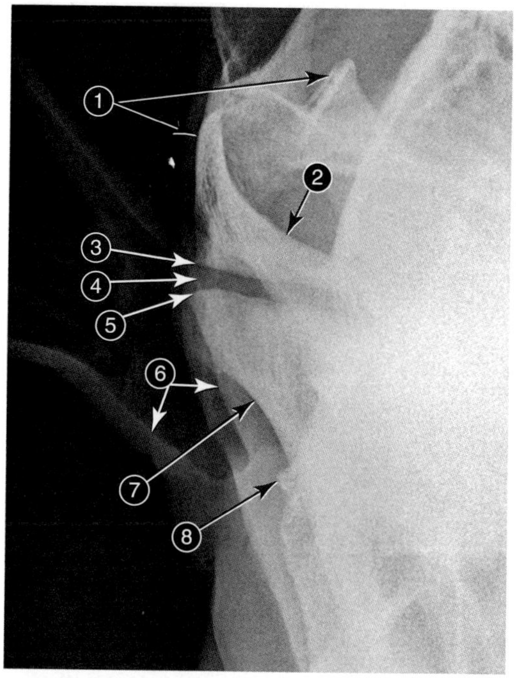

Fig. 8.14 Rostrodorsal-caudoventral oblique (RD-CdVO) radiograph of right equine temporomandibular joint (11 years old).

1. Zygomatic arch
2. Zygomatic process of frontal bone
3. Articular surface of squamous temporal bone
4. Articular disc, which completely divides temporomandibular joint into upper (temporal) and lower (mandibular) compartments
5. Head of mandible
6. Air in cartilaginous part of external acoustic meatus
7. Neck of mandible
8. Caudal lacrimal process projecting from rostromedial edge of orbit

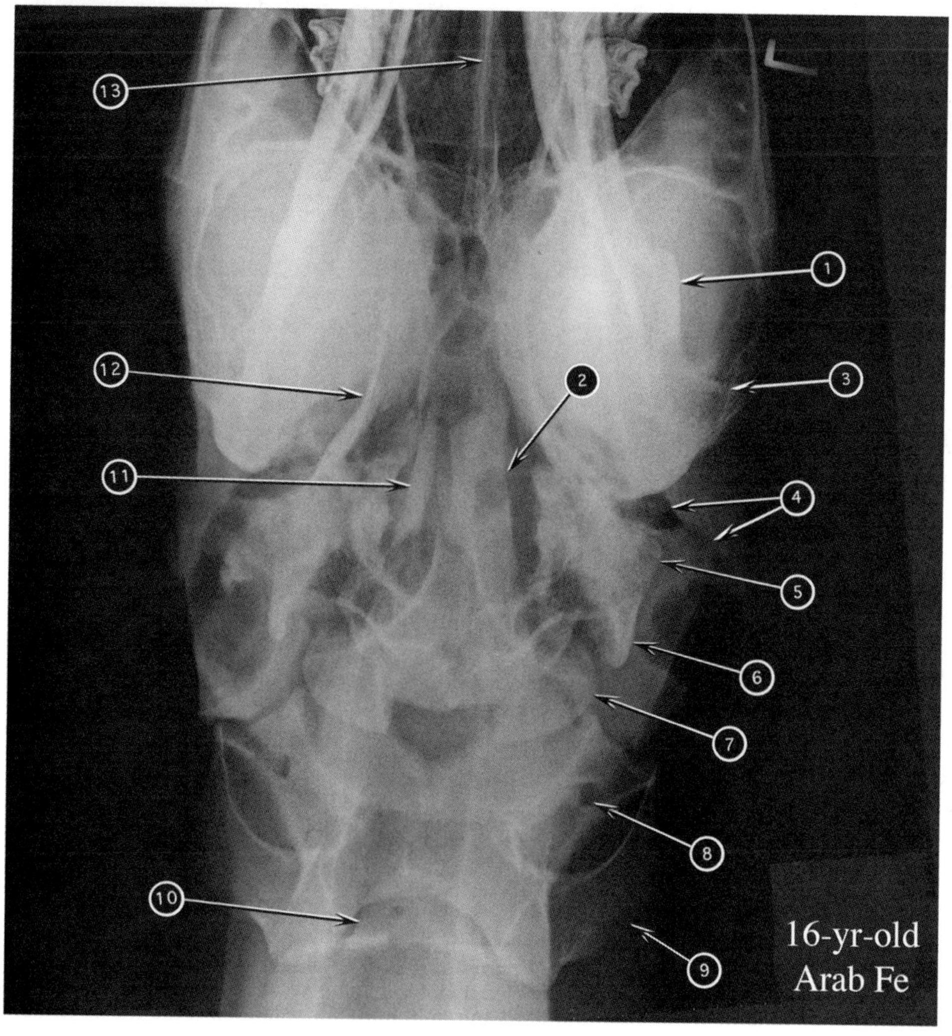

Fig. 8.15 Dorsoventral radiograph of caudal region of equine head (16 years old).

1. Coronoid process of left mandible
2. Left laryngeal ventricle
3. Left temporomandibular joint
4. External ear canal
5. Mastoid process of temporal bone
6. Paracondylar process of occipital bone
7. Occipital condyle
8. Alar foramen of atlas (C1)
9. Wing of atlas (C1)
10. Dens of axis (C2)
11. Right arytenoid cartilage of larynx
12. Right stylohyoid bone
13. Nasal septum

Table • 9.1

Ancillary Radiographic Projections of the Canine or Feline Skull.

VIEW NO.	PART OF INTEREST	NAME OF PROJECTION	BRIEF DESCRIPTION
1	Frontal sinuses	Rostrocaudal projection of frontal sinuses	Subject in dorsal recumbency. Head flexed 90 degrees to spine such that nose points directly at x-ray tube. Center x-ray beam on frontal sinuses.
2	Right maxillary dental arcade or right tympanic bulla	Open-mouth left 20-degree ventral–right dorsal[a]	Subject in right recumbency. Secure mouth open with speculum. Elevate mandibles 20 degrees with sponge wedge. Center x-ray beam on right maxillary arcade or tympanic bulla.
3	Left maxillary dental arcade or left tympanic bulla	Open-mouth right 20-degree ventral–left dorsal	Subject in left recumbency. Secure mouth open with speculum. Elevate mandibles 20 degrees with sponge wedge. Center x-ray beam on left maxillary arcade or tympanic bulla.
4	Right mandibular dental arcade	Open-mouth left 20-degree dorsal–right ventral	Subject in right recumbency. Secure mouth open with speculum. Elevate maxilla 20 degrees with sponge wedge. Center x-ray beam on right mandibular arcade.
5	Left mandibular dental arcade	Open-mouth right 20-degree dorsal–left ventral	Subject in left recumbency. Secure mouth open with speculum. Elevate maxilla 20 degrees with sponge wedge. Center x-ray beam on left mandibular arcade.
6	Nasal cavity	Open-mouth ventral 20-degree rostral–dorsocaudal	Subject in dorsal recumbency. Secure maxilla against x-ray table such that hard palate is parallel to tabletop. Open mouth widely with speculum or gauze traction on mandible. Angle x-ray beam 20 degrees rostrally and center x-ray beam on hard palate.
7	Nasal cavity	Intraoral dorsoventral	Subject in ventral recumbency. Slide cassette into mouth. Center x-ray beam on dorsal aspect of maxilla.
8	Tympanic bullae	Open-mouth rostrocaudal	Subject in dorsal recumbency. Head flexed 90 degrees to spine such that nose points directly at x-ray tube. Open mouth by retracting maxilla and mandible equally with gauze or tape. Center x-ray beam in back of mouth.
9	Tympanic bullae (cats and brachycephalic dogs)	Rostral 10 degrees ventral –caudodorsal	Subject in dorsal recumbency. Head flexed 90 degrees to spine such that nose points directly at x-ray tube. Angle head/neck 10 degrees caudally, keeping mouth closed. Center x-ray beam at base of skull.
10	Right tympanic bulla/right temporomandibular joint	Left 20 degrees rostral–right caudal	Subject in right recumbency. Elevate nose 20 –30 degrees with sponge. Center x-ray beam on region of temporomandibular joint.
11	Left tympanic bulla/left temporomandibular joint	Right 20 degrees rostral–left caudal	Subject in left recumbency. Elevate nose 20–30 degrees with sponge. Center x-ray beam on region of temporomandibular joint.

[a]Any angle specified in this table for this or any other ancillary skull radiograph is an estimate. This will vary among dogs and should be selected based on visual determination of the angle that results in optimal isolation of the area of interest.

views of the skull require changing the position of the patient while a few require that the x-ray beam be angled (Fig. 9.10). The use of an antiscatter grid will improve image quality in larger patients where the thickness of the skull exceeds approximately 10 cm.

An external marking system must be used to label oblique radiographs of the skull so that the left side can be distinguished reliably from the right side. Both "L" and "R" markers are needed to designate which structures are being projected (Fig. 9.11). If only one marker is used, it is not possible to differentiate left-sided from right-sided structures (Fig. 9.12).

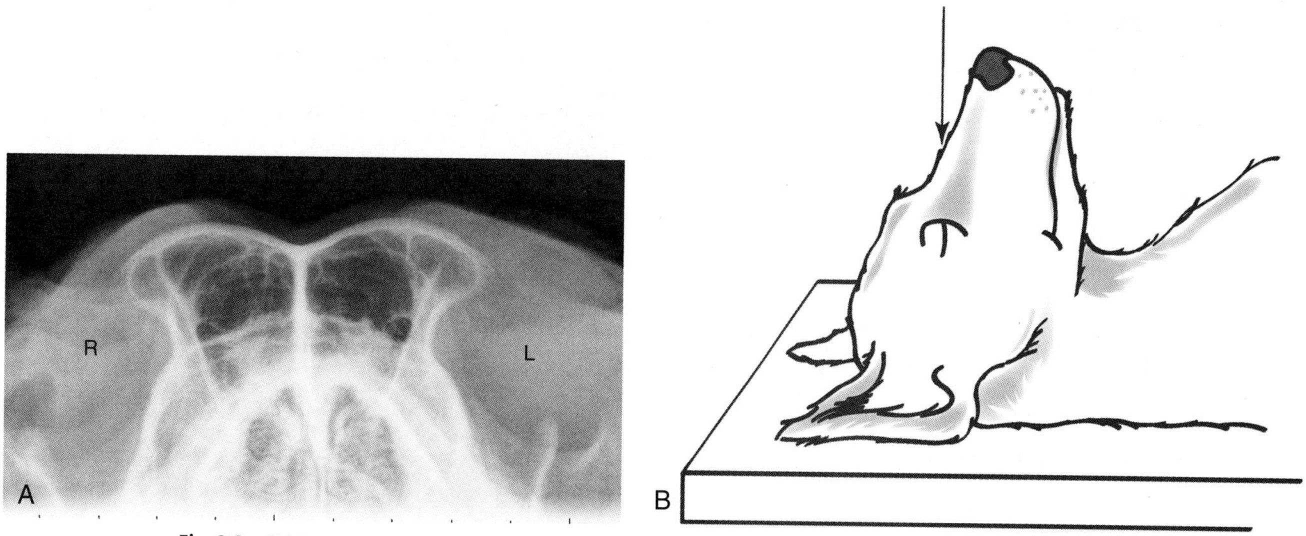

Fig. 9.3 **(A)** Rostrocaudal frontal sinus view in a dog and **(B)** diagram of positioning (see Table 9.1, View No. 1). The patient is in dorsal recumbency with the nose pointing at the x-ray tube. This view provides an unobstructed view of each frontal sinus. It should be kept in mind that brachycephalic dogs and some cats have incompletely developed frontal sinuses. In those patients, the main value of this projection would be to assess the frontal bone itself. *L,* Left side; *R,* right side. (**B,** From Owens JM, Biery DN. *Radiographic Interpretation for the Small Animal Clinician*. Baltimore: Williams & Wilkins; 1999.)

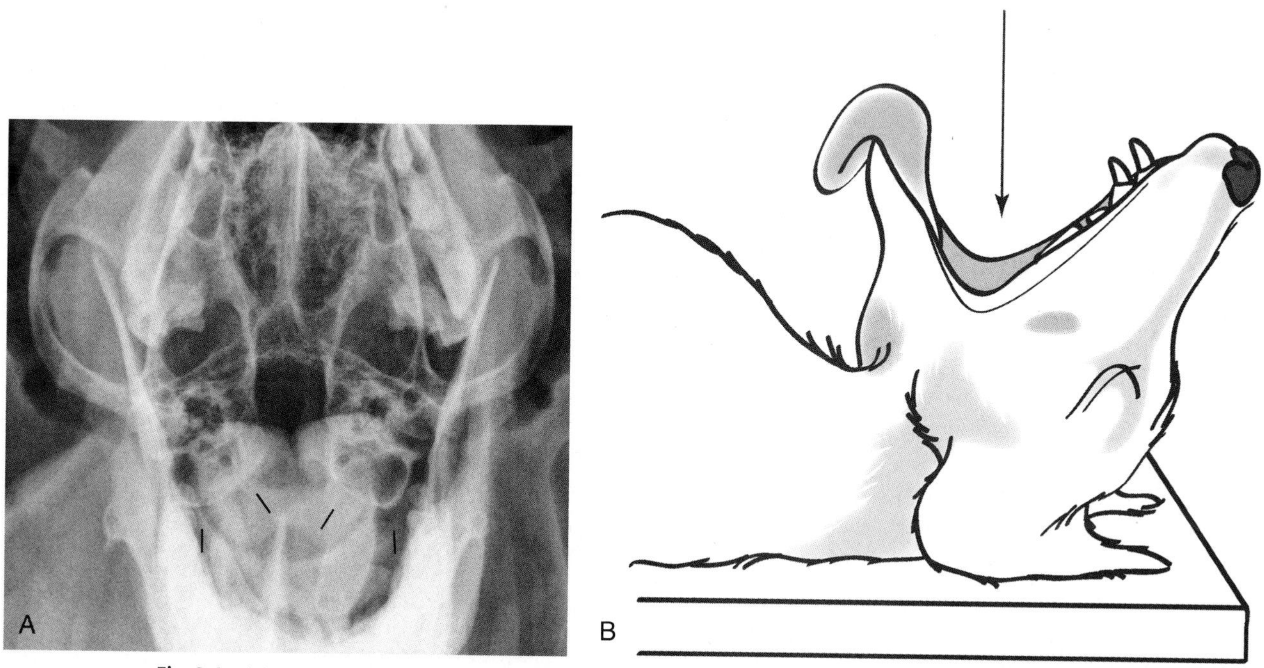

Fig. 9.4 **(A)** Open-mouth rostrocaudal view of the tympanic bullae in a dog and **(B)** diagram of positioning (see Table 9.1, View No. 8 and Fig. 9.10). The patient is in dorsal recumbency with the nose pointing at the x-ray tube. The mouth is held open by retracting the mandible and maxilla with gauze. Centering the x-ray beam in the back of the mouth provides a relatively unobstructed view of the tympanic bullae (*black arrow*). (**B,** From Owens JM, Biery DN. *Radiographic Interpretation for the Small Animal Clinician*. Baltimore: Williams & Wilkins; 1999.)

Positioning: Horse

Sedation is not required for equine skull radiography, but it is recommended to facilitate positioning, especially for the DV view, where the dropped position of the head will make it easier to position the x-ray tube dorsally. Skull radiographs of adult horses are typically acquired with the horse standing.

For the lateral view, the cassette is positioned against the head of the standing horse and a horizontal x-ray beam directed from the opposite side (Fig. 9.13A). The thickness of the equine head leads to radiographic magnification being more pronounced than in the dog or cat. Magnification of a lesion on the side of the head closest to the x-ray tube may result in the lesion not being visible because of blurring. Thus, if the laterality of a lesion is known, the plate should be positioned against that side of the head and the x-ray beam directed from the opposite side. If the laterality of the lesion is not known, it is good practice to obtain both left-right and right-left radiographs to make sure that a lesion is not overlooked because of magnification.

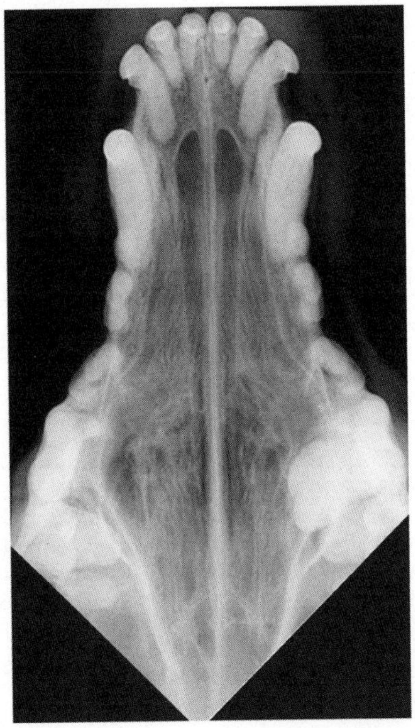

Fig. 9.5 Intraoral dorsoventral (DV) radiograph of maxilla in a dog (see Table 9.1, View No. 7). The patient is in sternal recumbency with the plate inserted into the mouth and the x-ray beam directed onto the dorsal surface of the maxilla. This projection provides an unobstructed view of the nasal cavity. With the increase in digital imaging, this view is used infrequently as the large size of the plate, or computed radiography (CR) cassette, limits the extent that it can be inserted into the mouth. Also, many digital plates are permanently mounted in the x-ray table. The view illustrated in Fig. 9.10 is a more practical substitute.

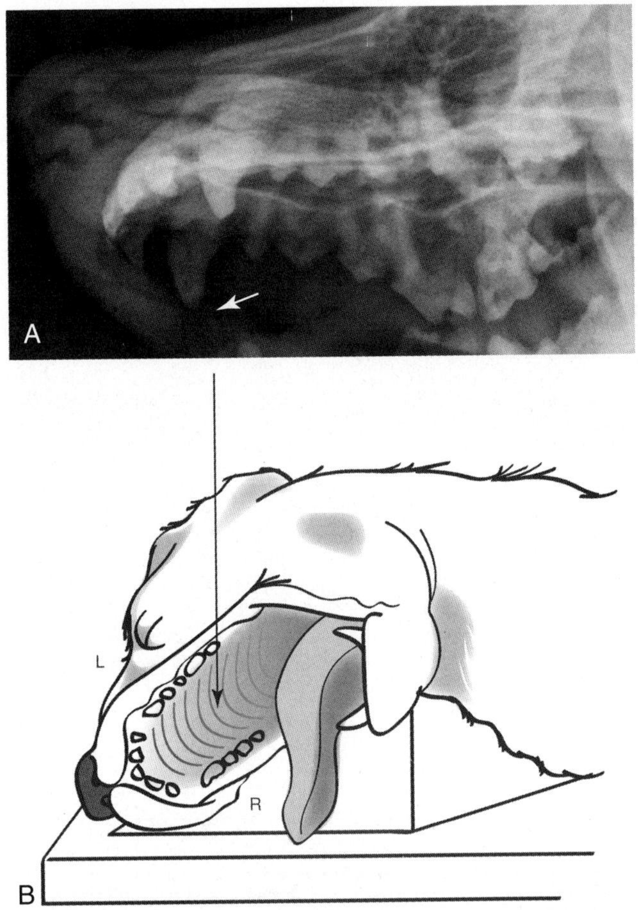

Fig. 9.6 **(A)** Open-mouth, left 20-degree ventral–right dorsal projection of the right maxillary dental arcade in a dog and **(B)** diagram of positioning (see Table 9.1, View No. 2). The patient is in right recumbency and the mouth held open with a speculum. A portion of the plastic speculum is visible in **A** (*white arrow*). The mandibles are elevated 20 degrees from the tabletop with a positioning sponge. This projects the left side of the maxilla dorsal to the right. The x-ray beam, which is vertical to the tabletop, is centered on the right maxillary arcade. This view is mainly used to evaluate bone lesions. For evaluation of teeth, a full mouth dental radiographic study with a small intra-oral plate is preferred. *L,* Left side; *R,* right side. (**B,** From Owens JM, Biery DN. *Radiographic Interpretation for the Small Animal Clinician*. Baltimore: Williams & Wilkins; 1999.)

For the DV view, the plate is ventral to the mandibles and the x-ray beam directed onto the dorsal aspect of the head (see Fig. 9.13B). It is important to keep the x-ray beam perpendicular to the plate. As already noted, sedation is helpful for the DV view because as the horse lowers its head in response to the sedative, dorsal positioning of the x-ray tube is facilitated. Without sedation, one might be able to acquire a DV view of the nasal passage, but a DV view of the calvarium or brain case will usually not be possible. VD views of the skull are not made in the standing horse.

Radiation safety becomes paramount when radiographing the equine head. Positioning the plate by placing it in a plate holder with an extension handle is impractical because of the weight of the plate. This commonly results in motion and blurring of the image. In many practices, equine skull radiographs are acquired by handholding the plate. If this is done, a lead apron, lead gloves, a lead thyroid shield, and lead-impregnated glasses should be worn. The x-ray beam must also be collimated such that the gloved hands, or any other part of the body, are never in the primary x-ray beam.

As in the dog and cat, ancillary oblique views of the equine skull are often needed because of the anatomic complexity. Oblique views are commonly used in the horse to evaluate a nasal passage or a dental arcade (Fig. 9.14). As in the dog and cat, use of properly placed L and R markers is critical to ensure that the structures being projected are identified accurately (Fig. 9.15).

Radiographic Technique

The wide exposure latitude of digital imaging systems means that selecting kVp and mAs values for skull radiography is much less critical than when film-screen technology was used. In digital imaging, many more kVp/mAs combinations will result in a diagnostic image than with film. Exposure latitude also results in the ability to evaluate both the thicker and thinner parts of the skull in the same image; for example, proper exposure of a thicker part does not result in overexposure of a thinner part, and vice versa.

Despite the exposure latitude of digital systems, an inherent problem associated with equine skull radiography is the tendency to overexpose the image (Fig. 9.16). This probably occurs because of a concern that the thick bony components require massive exposure factors for proper imaging.

Ancillary Factors

Although use of an antiscatter grid would be very useful in equine skull radiography, the necessary increase in mAs needed to compensate for the grid may not be possible. Also, a cassette that contains a grid is heavy and difficult to hold steadily by hand, leading to motion and/or grid-line artifacts. A wall-mounted plate holder, discussed subsequently for equine cervical radiographs, is one method to incorporate the use of a grid for equine skull radiography without increasing the risk of motion artifact. A wall-mounted plate holder will also lead to reduced personnel exposure.

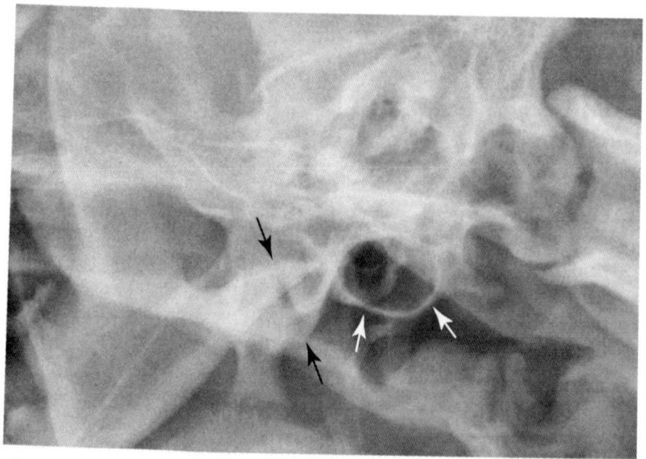

Fig. 9.7 Open-mouth, left 20-degree ventral–right dorsal projection of the right tympanic bulla and temporomandibular joint in a dog (see Table 9.1, View No. 2). This view is identical to that in Fig. 9.6, except the x-ray beam is centered on the middle ear. This allows assessment of the right (dependent) tympanic bulla (*white arrows*) and right temporomandibular joint (*black arrows*). The left (nondependent) tympanic bulla and left temporomandibular joint are projected more dorsally and are superimposed on the skull. Only the right tympanic bulla and temporomandibular joint can be assessed using this positioning. If the left-sided structures are of interest, then the view described in Table 9.1, View No. 3, should be used.

Interpretation Paradigm

The following is a reasonable step-by-step process for interpreting skull radiographs.

- Have adequate radiographic views been obtained according to the clinical problem being assessed? If not, what additional views would help?
- Are there positioning problems that will interfere with interpretation?
- Are the images overexposed or underexposed?
- Has sedation or anesthesia been used? If not, did this affect the usefulness of the radiographs?
- What species or breed characteristics should be considered?
- Are external markers adequate to distinguish between left and right sides?

After these variables have been considered, the images can be scrutinized for abnormalities. The Roentgen sign and DAMNITV (degenerative, anomalous, metabolic, neoplastic, infectious [inflammatory, immune], traumatic, and vascular) methods described in Chapter 6 should be used. In many patients, the cause of the clinical signs will not be found in skull radiographs, or the lesion will be incompletely characterized, and other modalities, such as CT or MRI, will be needed.[3–5] And, even when the lesion is identified, aspiration or biopsy is commonly necessary to obtain a definitive diagnosis.

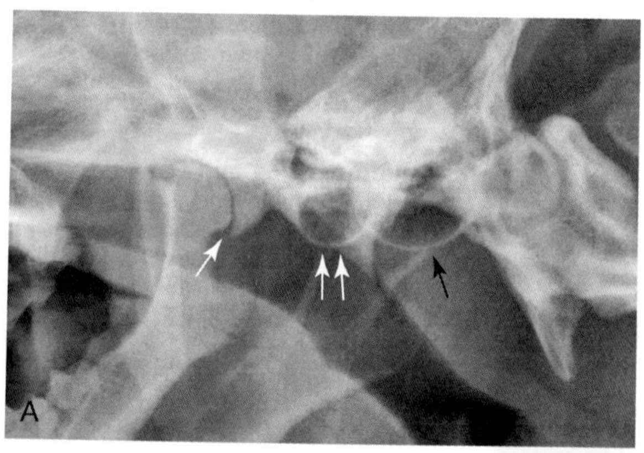

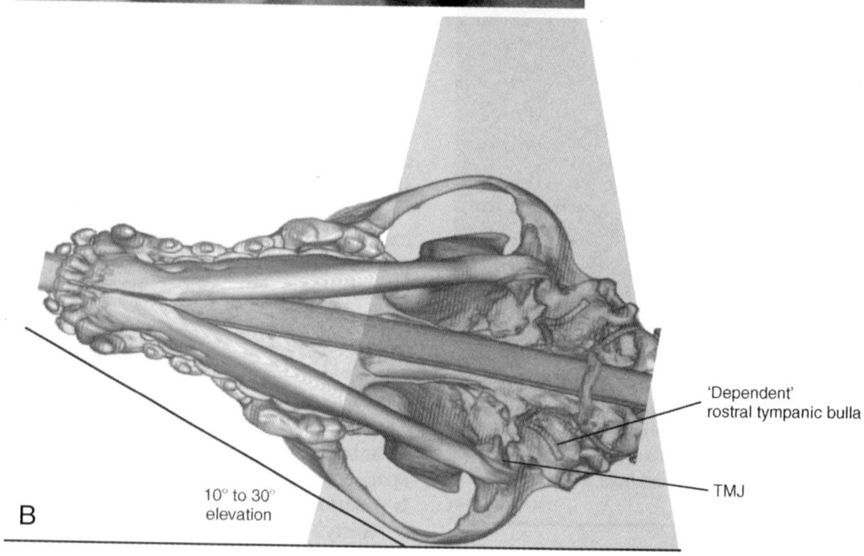

Fig. 9.8 **(A)** Left 20-degree rostral–right caudal projection of the right temporomandibular joint (*single white arrow*) and right tympanic bulla (*double white arrows*) in a dog and **(B)** positioning diagram (see Table 9.1, View No. 10). The patient is in right recumbency, and the tip of the nose is elevated 20 degrees from the tabletop. The x-ray beam is perpendicular to the tabletop and centered on the tympanic bulla. Elevating the nose projects the upper, left, nondependent tympanic bulla (*single black arrow*), caudal to the lower, right, dependent tympanic bulla (*double white arrows*). Compared with Fig. 9.7, the contralateral, nondependent, left tympanic bulla (*black arrow*) is caudal to the one of interest rather than being dorsal. Note that the nondependent, left tympanic bulla is larger because of radiographic magnification. In this view, the nondependent, left temporomandibular joint is superimposed on the region where the tympanic bullae overlap. *TMJ*, Temporomandibular joint. (From Thrall D, Robertson I, eds. *Atlas of Radiographic Anatomy and Normal Anatomic Variants in the Dog and Cat*. 3rd ed. St. Louis: Elsevier; 2023.)

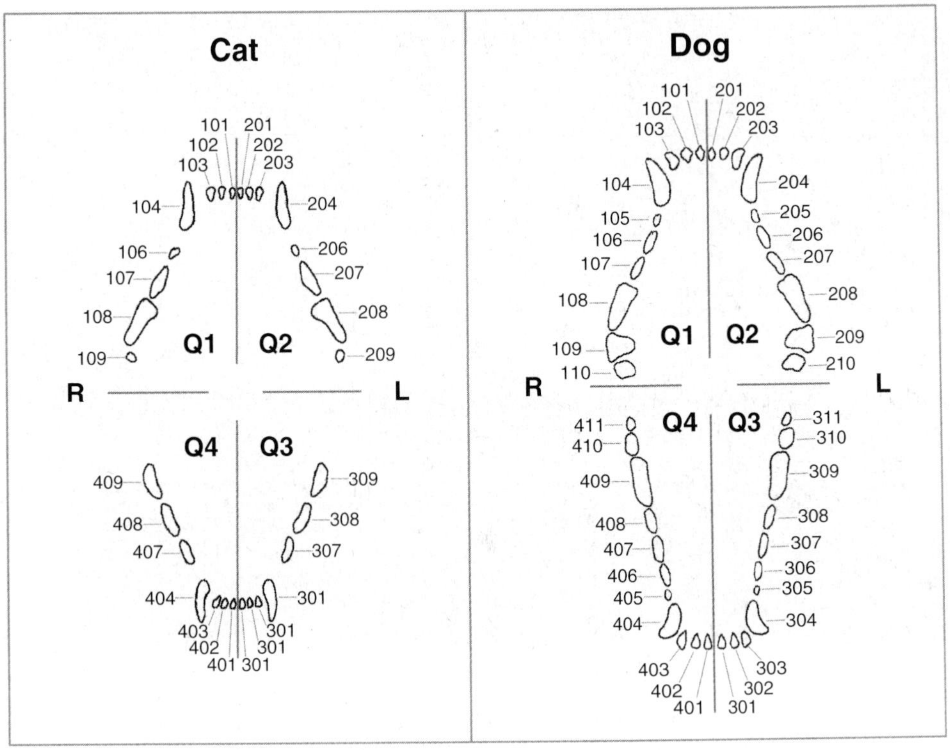

Fig. 10.9 Modified Triadan system in adult cat and dog. The mouth is divided into four quadrants (Q1–Q4) in a clockwise direction where each tooth is numbered with a three-digit number. The first number is associated with the quadrant, and the second and third numbers refer to the tooth position. For deciduous teeth numbering, the first digit for the right maxilla corresponds to "5," the left maxilla to "6," the left mandible to "7," and the right mandible to "8" (e.g., tooth 804: right mandibular deciduous canine tooth).

The intra- and extraoral structures in dogs and cats may be affected by inflammatory, neoplastic, traumatic, developmental, metabolic, congenital, or hereditary disorders. The anatomic complexity of the skull poses a challenge during radiographic interpretation when two-dimensional images of three-dimensional structures are evaluated.[26,27] Knowledge of the dentoalveolar anatomy is critical for understanding alterations of the normal radiographic appearance.

The maxillofacial structures, including the dentoalveolar complex, consist of soft and hard tissues. Depending on the structural chemical composition, each tissue type has a different capacity to attenuate the x-ray beam during a radiographic exam. In this way, highly mineralized structures, such as the enamel, dentin, and alveolar bone, are the most radiopaque areas in the radiograph. At the same time, regions like the pulp cavity, the periodontal ligament space, the gums, and the nasal cavities are less radiopaque (Fig. 10.10).[26–28]

The radiographic assessment of patients undergoing professional dental cleaning includes full-mouth intraoral dental radiographs (Fig. 10.11). However, intraoral views of a specific area may be required if the primary concern and the reason for the consultation are a specific dental structure or region of the oral cavity (e.g., dental fracture). Orthogonal views may be necessary when the dental and maxillofacial structures are superimposed, which can make it challenging to identify a radiographic alteration.[26,27]

Radiographic interpretation of dental radiographs should be systematic. The anatomical structures may be approached from the most general to the most specific to ensure that all relevant information is evaluated. Thus, a general view of the radiopacity and integrity of the maxillary or mandibular bone that supports the teeth, areas of bone lysis or proliferation, and bone morphologic alterations that may be associated with current or past pathologic events should be recorded.[7]

The initial general evaluation can be followed by a more specific assessment of the periodontal structures. This assessment may include[7,12]:

- Identification of alveolar bone loss at the alveolar margin, the periapical and furcation regions
- Widening or absence of the periodontal ligament space
- Loss of the lamina dura, which is the radiographic term for the cribriform plate of the alveolar socket
- Radiopaque or radiolucent areas next to the dental roots

The dental element and its endodontic system can finally be evaluated. Tooth assessment includes[7,29–31]:

- Identification of morphological alterations of the crown and root, unerupted teeth, external tooth resorption, and excessive or missing number of teeth.
- Evaluation of the endodontic system includes comparing the pulp cavity size between permanent teeth in the same patient (e.g., maxillary left vs. right canine), internal tooth resorption, increased radiopacity of the pulp cavity, and periapical lesions associated with tooth fractures or tooth discoloration.

PERIODONTAL DISEASE

Periodontal disease is the most prevalent oral disease in dogs and cats, and is caused by the destructive action of bacterial plaque and its inflammatory effect on the periodontium.[32,33] The periodontium consists of both hard and soft tissue components that support the teeth in the mandibular or maxillary bone. These structures are the alveolar bone, the periodontal ligament, the gums, and the cementum. Teeth suffering from periodontal disease can be associated with gingival bleeding, either spontaneous or during periodontal probing, gingival recession, periodontal pockets, or tooth mobility.[24,32]

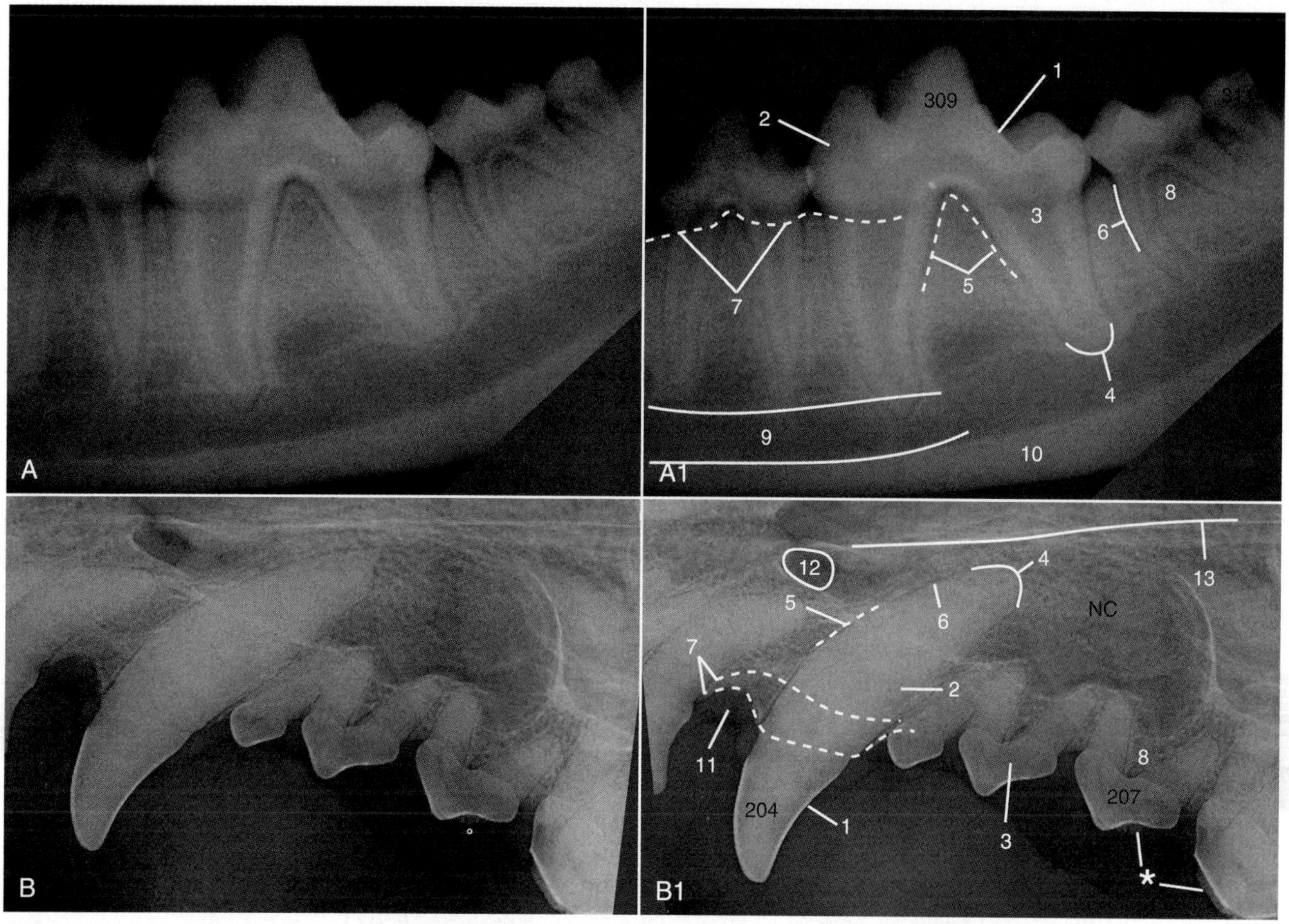

Fig. 10.10 Intraoral parallel technique view of the left mandibular molar teeth region **(A–A1)** and bisecting angle technique view of the left maxillary teeth **(B–B1)** of adult dogs showing the dental, periodontal, and surrounding structures: (1) enamel, (2) dentin, (3) pulp cavity, (4) apex, (5) lamina dura, (6) periodontal ligament space, (7) alveolar margin, (8) interradicular bone, (9) mandibular canal, (10) ventral cortex of the mandible, (11) gingiva, (12) palatine fissure, (13) vomer. Note the *double interrupted lines* in **B1** that correspond to moderate horizontal bone loss at the lingual alveolar margin of the left maxillary canine tooth. *NC,* Nasal cavity; *asterisk,* dental calculus. (Courtesy Lenin A. Villamizar.)

Identifying the radiographic changes in the periodontium associated with periodontal disease is extremely valuable for determining the treatment plan and prognosis. At the initial stage of the disease, the gingival tissue appears edematous due to the presence of bacterial plaque at the gingival sulcus.[34] At this moment, radiographic alterations on the periodontium are not present, as the inflammatory process is limited to soft tissue.

If dental plaque is not removed, the subsequent inflammatory reaction can cause, depending on the stage of the disease, mild, moderate, or advanced alveolar bone loss with destruction of the lamina dura and the periodontal ligament. Radiographic findings associated with periodontal disease may include (Fig. 10.12, eFigs. 10.1–10.3):

- Mild reduction of the alveolar margin height
- Horizontal, oblique, or vertical alveolar bone loss
- Furcation bone loss

Although the cementum can be reabsorbed due to the inflammatory response triggered by periodontitis, this is generally not seen in the radiograph due to the thin nature of the cementum and its similar opacity to dentin.

In cats, chronic periodontitis may lead to alveolar bone expansion or alveolar osteitis besides provoking bone loss. This condition is characterized by thickening of the buccal alveolar bone along areas of severe periodontitis.[35,36] Tooth resorption, tooth extrusion, and osteomyelitis of the jaws have also been linked to alveolar bone expansion. Although this can affect any tooth in the cat's mouth, the maxillary canine teeth seem more affected. Clinically, areas with alveolar bone expansion show gingivitis, gum recession, tooth extrusion, tooth mobility, and periodontal infrabony (vertical) pocket formation.[35,37] On dental radiography, the affected area can have a rarifying osseous proliferation or a mottled pattern with prominent trabeculae (Fig. 10.13). In severe cases where the bone lesion has extended beyond the alveolar bone and osteomyelitis is suspected, biopsies should be obtained to rule out a neoplastic process.[35,38,39]

ENDODONTIC DISEASE

Endodontic disease pertains to any pathologic event affecting the pulp of the tooth. The pulp is an unmineralized dental tissue located in the pulp cavity and is mainly composed of connective tissue, blood vessels, nerves, and dentin-producing cells named odontoblasts.[40,41] The pulp cavity is topographically divided into two areas, the pulp chamber that corresponds to the pulp cavity located in the crown and the root canal that corresponds to the portion of the pulp cavity situated in the root. In multirooted teeth, the most coronal portion of the pulp may slightly protrude into the dentin forming the pulp horns (Fig. 10.14).[7,40]

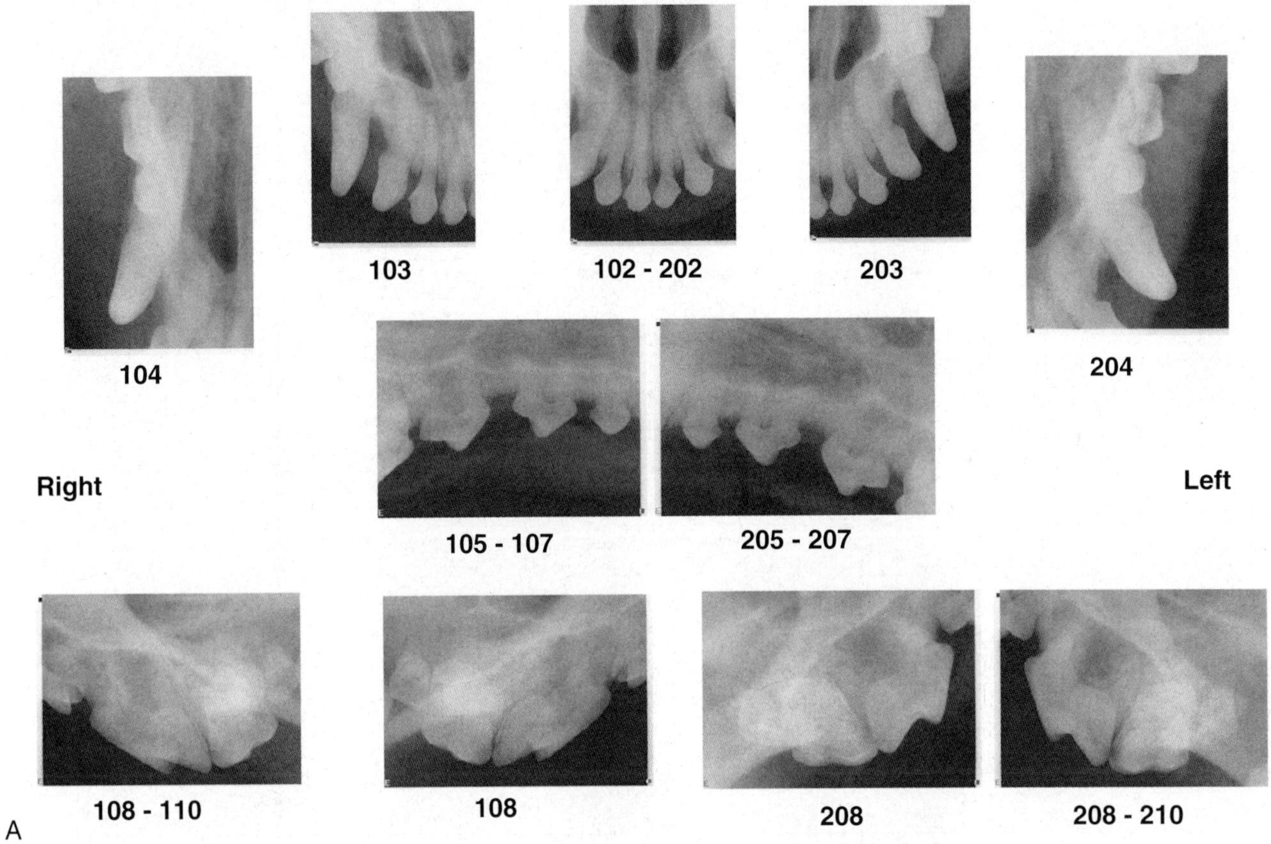

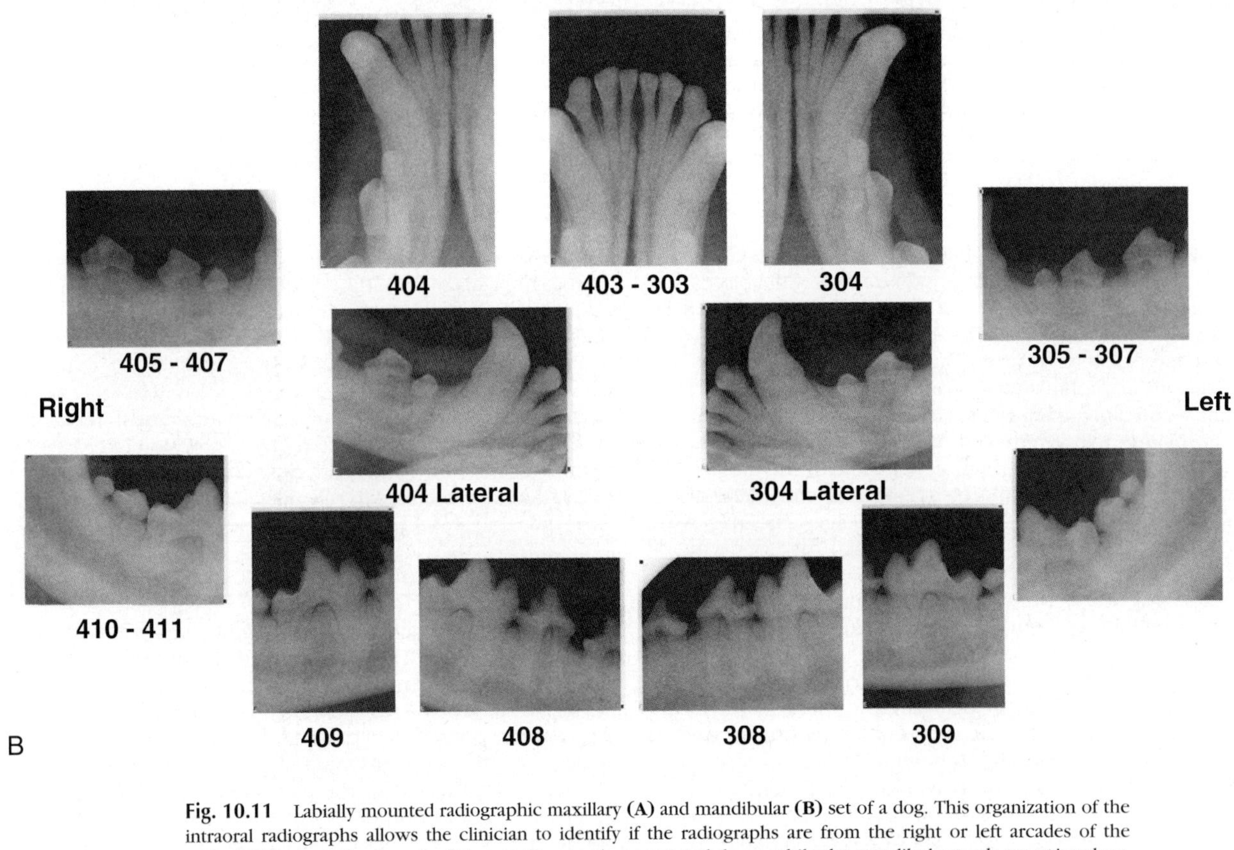

Fig. 10.11 Labially mounted radiographic maxillary **(A)** and mandibular **(B)** set of a dog. This organization of the intraoral radiographs allows the clinician to identify if the radiographs are from the right or left arcades of the patient. Note how the images of the maxillary teeth are pointed down while the mandibular teeth are pointed up.

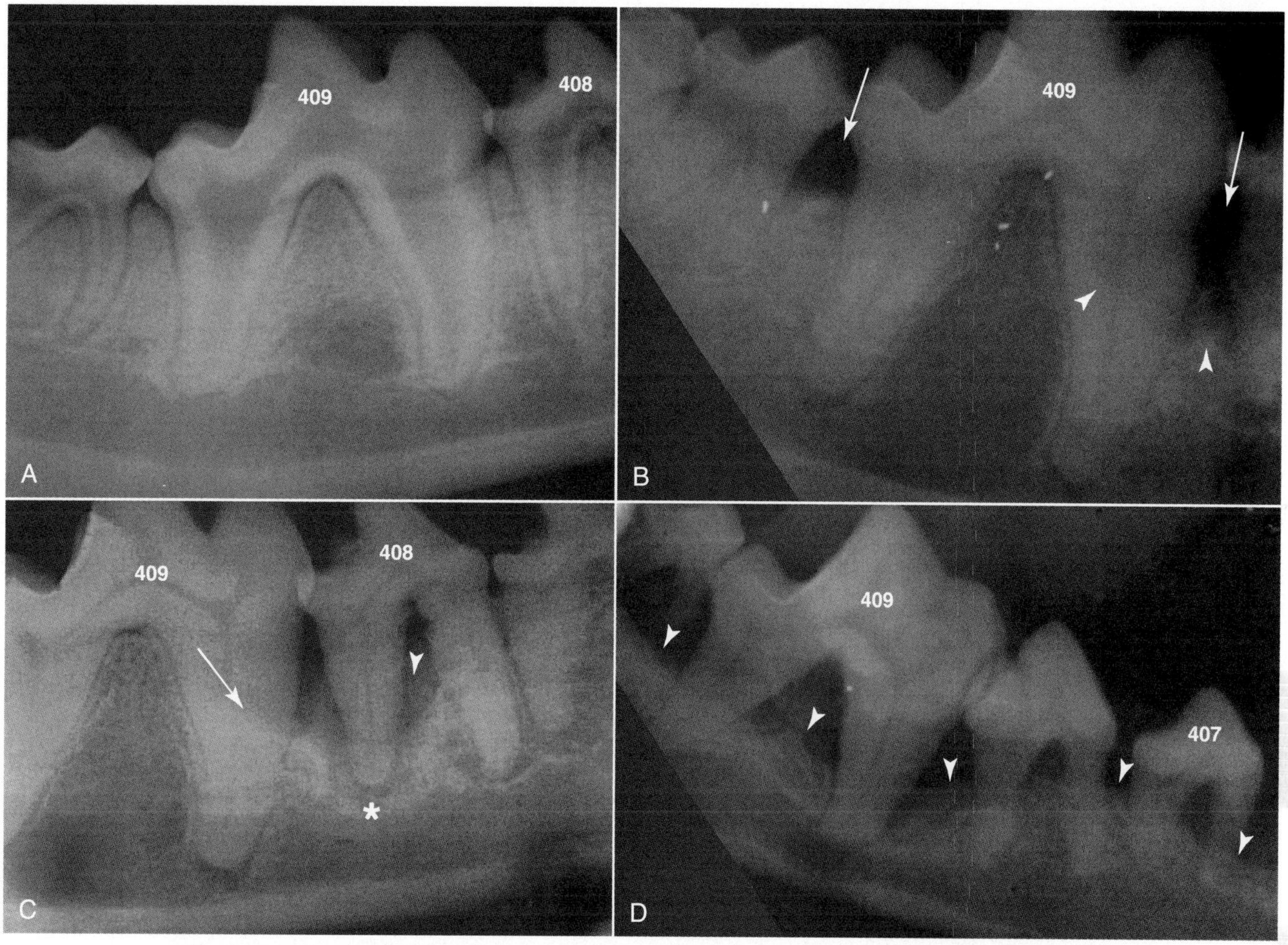

Fig. 10.12 Intraoral parallel technique of the right mandibular teeth in four different adult dogs with normal periodontium **(A)** and several stages of periodontitis: **(B)** mild (*arrows*) and moderate alveolar bone loss between the right mandibular first molar (*409*) and fourth premolar teeth (*arrowheads*). **C,** Severe oblique and vertical (*arrowhead*) alveolar bone loss between 409 and 408. Note the condensing osteitis (*asterisk*) associated with a chronic inflammatory condition. **D,** Severe horizontal bone loss (*arrowheads*) and condensing osteitis.

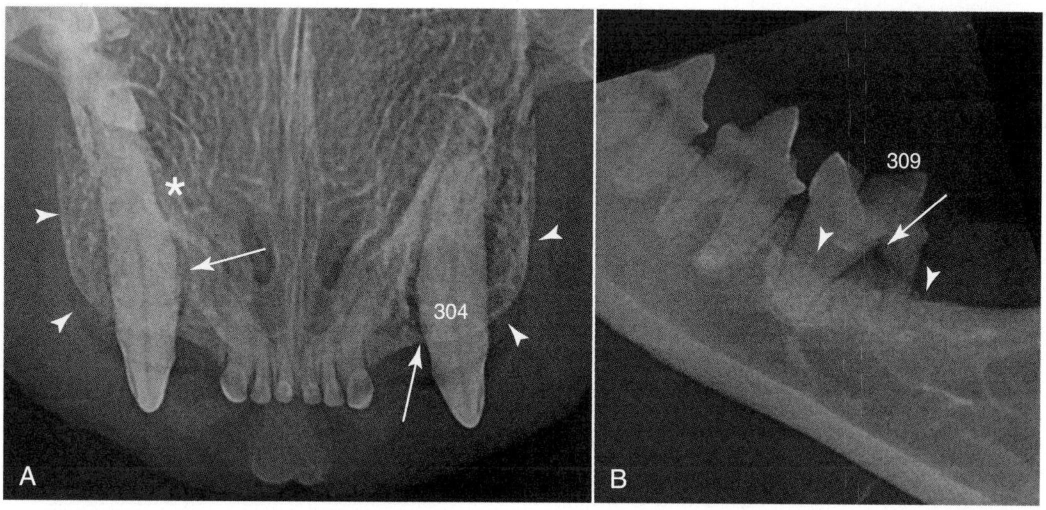

Fig. 10.13 Intraoral bisecting-angle technique occlusal view of the maxilla and parallel technique of the left mandible of an adult cat showing **(A)** bilateral alveolar bone expansion (*arrowheads*), vertical bone loss (*arrows*), and moderate root resorption (*asterisk*). Note the mottled pattern with prominent trabeculae at the buccal aspect of the maxillary canine teeth. **B,** Severe horizontal alveolar bone loss (*arrowheads*) and exposure of the furcation of 309 (*arrow*).

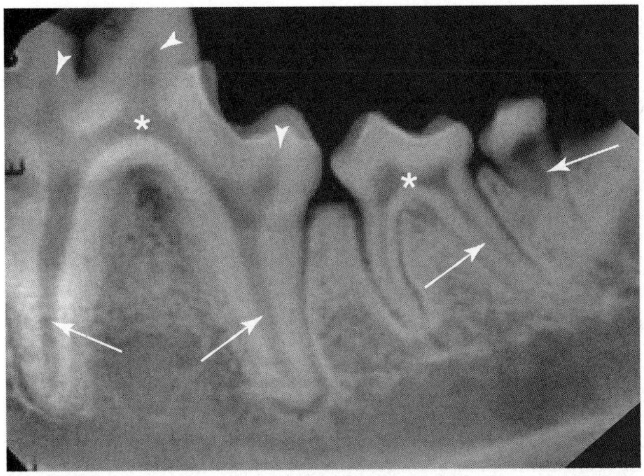

Fig. 10.14 Intraoral radiographs of the right mandibular molar teeth showing the regions of the pulp cavity: pulp chamber (*asterisk*), root canal (*arrows*). In multirooted teeth, the extension of the pulp chamber into the cusp corresponds to the pulp horns (*arrowheads*).

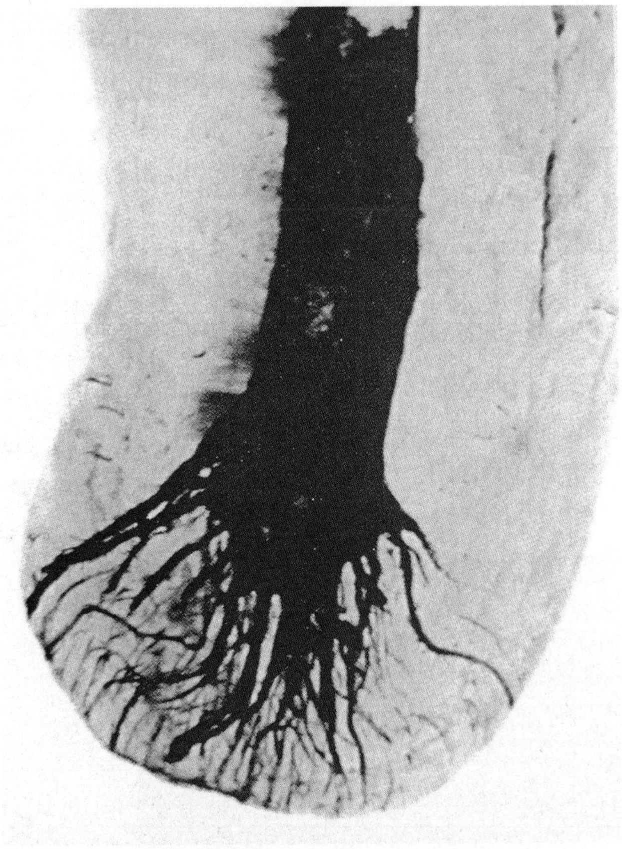

Fig. 10.15 Photomicrograph of the apical delta in a canine tooth. (From Hernandez SZ, Negro VB, Maresca BM. Morphology features of the root canal system of the maxillary fourth premolar and the mandibular first molar in dogs. *J Vet Dent*. 2001;18:9–13.)

The pulp has sensory and nourishment functions that keep the tooth alive, allowing the odontoblasts located at the most outer region of the pulp tissue to build up dentin during the normal development of the tooth. The pulp, and hence the viability of the odontoblast, is supported by arterioles that enter the pulp cavity through the apical delta (Fig. 10.15).[22] The intraoral radiographic approach of the endodontic system includes assessing the size and shape of the pulp cavity and radiographic appearance of the periapical region. Dental radiography allows visibility of the pulp cavity as a narrow radiolucent band in the center of the tooth. In young animals, the pulp cavity is still wide; as the animal ages, this space narrows due to dentin deposition. Asymmetry of the pulp cavity between adjacent or contralateral teeth may indicate pulp necrosis and lack of dentin deposition by odontoblasts (Fig. 10.16).[30,42]

Dentoalveolar injuries such as tooth concussion, subluxation, luxation, or alveolar fracture along the apical portion of the root may also lead to tooth devitalization due to severe pulpitis or disruption of blood supply. Tooth discoloration is the most frequent clinical finding (87%–92%) in teeth suffering from pulp necrosis.[30,42]

Periapical inflammatory lesions associated with endodontic disease may be acute or chronic depending on the host autoimmune response and virulence of the bacteria in the necrotic pulp. During the early stage of the inflammatory lesion, the microflora from the affected pulp triggers an inflammatory response at the apical periodontal ligament and surrounding alveolar bone, known as acute apical periodontitis. Depending on the autoimmune response, pus may form at this stage of the inflammatory process, leading to an apical abscess.[43,44]

Acute apical periodontitis is histologically characterized by the presence of lymphocytes and neutrophils, along with vascular congestion, hyperemia, and edema of the periodontal ligament. Since it is possible that destruction of the mineralized tissues (dentin, cementum, and bone) has not occurred during acute apical periodontitis, the radiographic changes can be limited to widening of the periodontal ligament space only, and radiographic identification can be challenging or underestimated.[44–46]

If the initial inflammatory injury is not resolved, a more chronic inflammatory response occurs with the formation of a periapical granuloma. Radiographically, a periapical granuloma is characterized by ill or well-defined circumscribed radiolucent or radiopaque areas around the tooth apex. During this stage of the inflammatory process, in an attempt to heal, the periapical region is infiltrated by granulation tissue and inflammatory cells such as plasma cells, lymphocytes, and histiocytes.[46,47]

The effect of inflammatory byproducts of a nonvital tooth on the epithelial cells of Malassez located in the periodontal ligament may result in a radicular or periapical cyst formation.[47] Radiographically, a radicular cyst generally corresponds to a single round radiolucent cavitary lesion with a well-defined cortical wall. During the early stage of the periapical cyst, it is challenging to differentiate it from the periapical abscess or granuloma due to its similar osteolytic appearance on dental radiography.[47] Although the radiographic examination may aid in localizing apical periodontitis, histopathology remains the method of choice to identify the type of inflammatory lesion. Histologically, a periapical cyst is associated with an epithelium-lined cavity with an inflamed fibrovascular connective tissue wall.[48,49] Fig. 10.17 depicts the radiographic features of some inflammatory periapical lesions in different patients.

Dental radiography can help identify the origin of the endodontic pathologic condition. In an endo-perio lesion, the endodontic injury from dental trauma leads to the destruction of the periapical periodontal structures. In contrast, in a perio-endo lesion, the endodontic disease results from the invasion of the tooth apex by periodontal microflora from deep periodontal pockets in patients suffering from severe periodontitis (Fig. 10.18).[50,51]

The chevron sign, a nonpathologic radiolucent area that resembles periapical inflammatory lesions, can be observed in

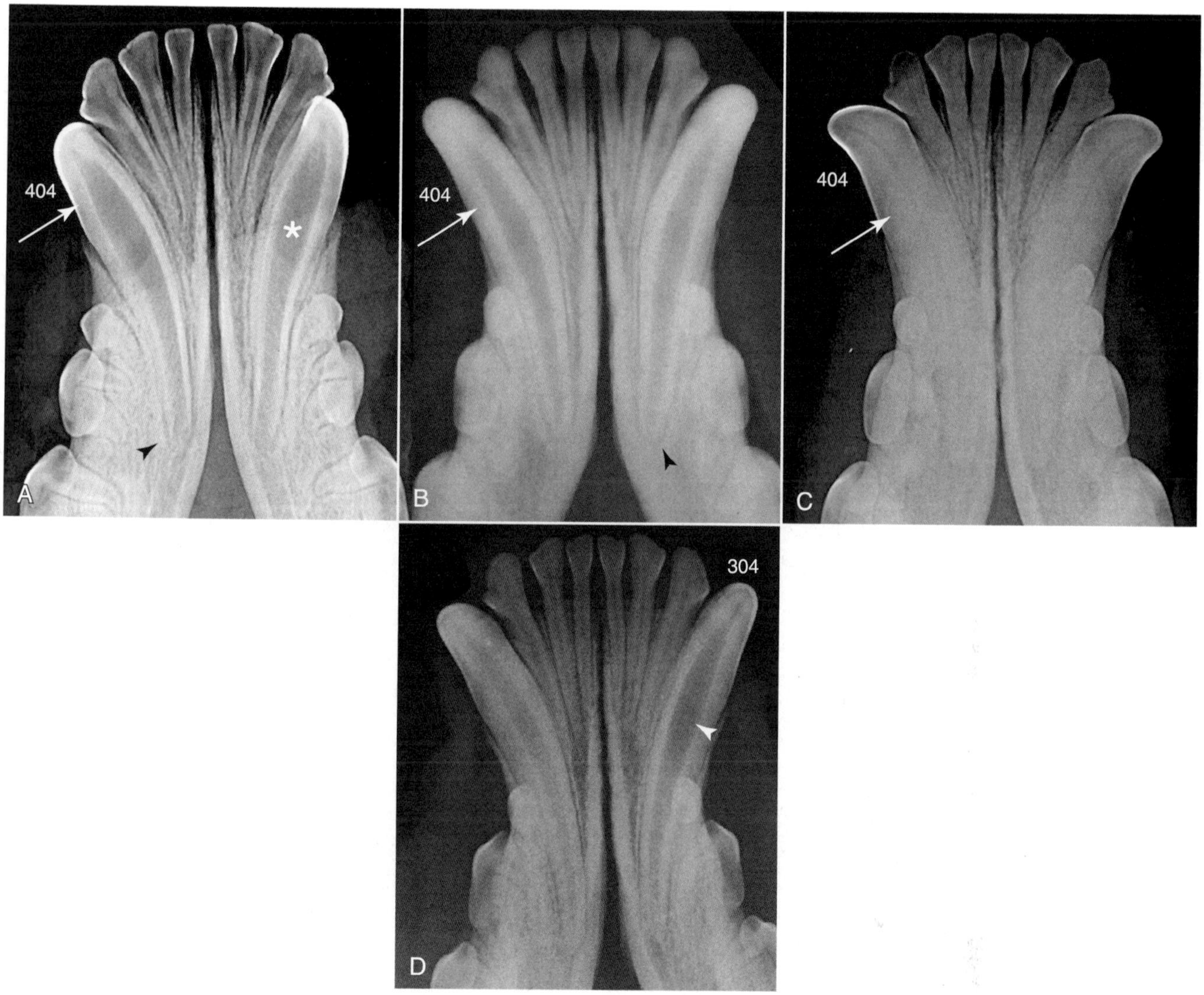

Fig. 10.16 Intraoral occlusal views of the mandibular incisors and canine teeth showing dentin deposition in different age dogs. **A,** 8-month-old Border Collie. Note the open apex (*arrowhead*), the wide pulp cavity (*asterisk*), and the low dentin build-up (*arrow*). **B,** 19-month-old German Shepherd. Note that there is more dentin build-up (*arrow*), and the apex is closed (*arrowhead*). **C,** 11-year mix-breed dog. The pulp cavity appears as a thin radiolucent band with thick dentin walls (*arrow*). **D,** Nonvital *304*. Note the asymmetry between the pulp cavity of the mandibular canine teeth. *304* displays a wider pulp cavity due to a lack of dentin deposition due to pulp necrosis (*arrowhead*).

healthy clinical teeth.[52] Radiographically, this lucency sign may appear as a chevron or V-shape area of decreased radiodensity at the apex of the canine, incisor, and mandibular first molar teeth, as well as the distal root of the maxillary premolar teeth. The chevron sign corresponds to normal trabecular bone and vascular canals projected at the tooth's periapical area (Figs. 10.19 and 10.20).[52] True periapical inflammatory lesions are displayed as more rounded radiolucent areas associated with fractured and discolored teeth or affected by severe periodontal disease.[53]

Internal inflammatory resorption of the inner surface of the pulp cavity is also associated with endodontic disease. As in humans, internal inflammatory resorption is uncommon in dogs. In 224 dogs, only 4.0% had tooth resorption affecting the middle third of the root canal.[31] Although it is unknown why odontoclasts start reabsorbing the dentin, it is suggested that the inflammatory response in a tooth suffering from pulpitis or necrosis leads to self-limiting continuous intraradicular dentin resorption. On dental radiographs, the teeth affected by internal inflammatory resorption display a focal circumscribed, oval, or elongated radiolucent area at the middle third of the root canal.[31,54]

TOOTH RESORPTION

Resorption can affect dogs and cats, ranging from 43% to 53% and 29% to 85%, respectively. This condition is characterized by the progressive destruction of the mineralized components of the tooth, resulting in pulp exposure, dental pain, tooth fracture, and, eventually, tooth loss.[31] Although in dogs and cats, this dental disorder has been associated with inflammatory or neoplastic processes, age, breed, and body weight, and more specifically with chronic excess dietary vitamin D intake in the cat, tooth resorption etiology remains unknown.[35,55,56]

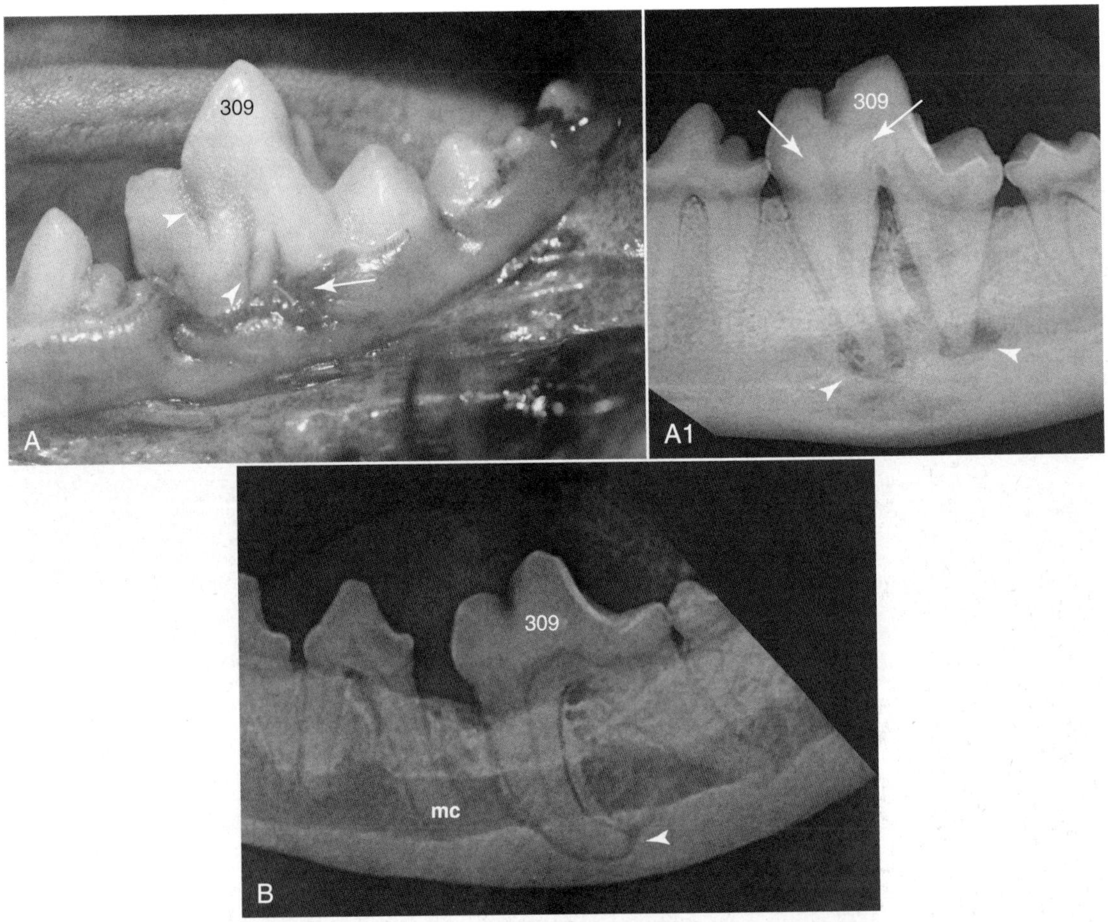

Fig. 10.33 **A, A1,** Clinical photograph and radiograph of dens-in-dente in a Maltese dog (*309*). **A,** Observe the crown malformation (*arrowheads*) and severe gingivitis of *309* (*arrow*). **A1,** Convergent roots of *309*, severe periodontitis, and periapical lucencies (*arrowheads*). Note the radiopaque material at the pulp chamber, resembling a tooth within a tooth (*arrows*). **B,** Dilaceration of the mesial root of *309* (*arrowhead*) in a Chihuahua dog. The dilacerated root extends into the mandible's ventral cortex, overlapping with the mandibular canal (*mc*).

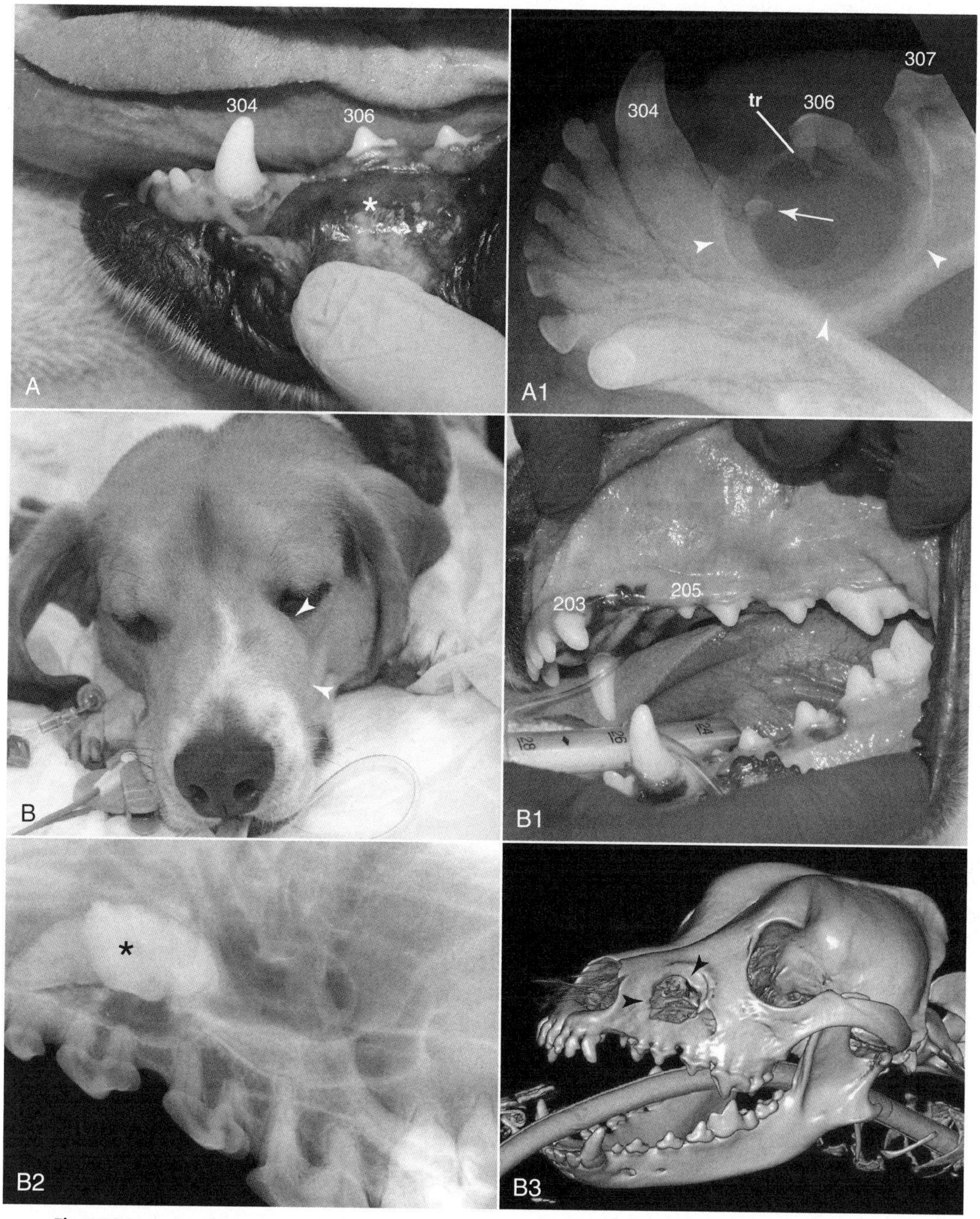

Fig. 10.34 **A, A1,** Clinical photograph and radiograph showing a dentigerous cyst lesion in an adult Boxer dog. **A,** Missing left mandibular first premolar tooth and fluctuant swelling at the adjacent oral mucosa (*asterisk*). **A1,** Nonerupted partially reabsorbed *305* (*arrow*) and locular radiolucent lesion with the presence of a well-defined cortical boundary (*arrowheads*). Note the root resorption of *303* and the bone loss at the mesial root of *307*. **(B, B1)** Extraoral and intraoral clinical photographs, **(B2)** dental radiograph, and **(B3)** three-dimensional (3D) rendering from a cone-beam CT (CBCT) examination in an adult dog affected by a nonerupted canine tooth. **B,** Swelling at the maxillary region (*arrowheads*). **B1,** Missing *204*. **B2,** Nonerupted *204* (*asterisk*) located in the nasal cavity at the level of the second maxillary premolar tooth. **B3,** 3D rendering showing the bone destruction at the maxillary bone (*arrowheads*). (Reproduced with permission from Lenin A. Villamizar.)

Acknowledgment

With special thanks to prior authors of this chapter for their contributions.

REFERENCES

1. Thatcher G. Performing dental procedures in dogs and cats without dental radiographs: malpractice? *Can Vet J.* 2020;61(2):197–200. (Accessed November 8, 2022). /pmc/articles/PMC6973222/.
2. Verstraete FJM, Kass PH, Terpak CH. Diagnostic value of full-mouth radiography in dogs. *Am J Vet Res.* 1998;59(6):686–691. (Accessed August 20, 2020). https://pubmed.ncbi.nlm.nih.gov/9622735/.
3. Heney CM, Arzi B, Kass PH, Hatcher DC, Verstraete FJM. Diagnostic yield of dental radiography and cone-beam computed tomography for the identification of anatomic structures in cats. *Front Vet Sci.* 2019;6(FEB):58. https://doi.org/10.3389/fvets.2019.00058.
4. Roza MR, Silva LAF, Barriviera M, Januário AL, Bezerra ACB, Fioravanti MCS. Cone beam computed tomography and intraoral radiography for diagnosis of dental abnormalities in dogs and cats. *J Vet Sci.* 2011;12(4):387–392. https://doi.org/10.4142/jvs.2011.12.4.387.
5. Villamizar-Martinez LA, Villegas CM, Duailibi E, et al. Morphometry and morphology of the articular surfaces of the medial region of the temporomandibular joint in the Felis catus (domestic cat) - a cone beam computed tomography study. *J Vet Dent.* 2023;40(2):134–142. https://doi.org/10.1177/08987564221141985. In press.
6. Macready DM, Hecht S, Craig LE, Conklin GA. Magnetic resonance imaging features of the temporomandibular joint in normal dogs. *Vet Radiol Ultrasound.* 2010;51(4):436–440. https://doi.org/10.1111/j.1740-8261.2010.01680.x.
7. Villamizar-Martinez LA, Tsugawa AJ. Diagnostic imaging of oral and maxillofacial anatomy and pathology. *Vet Clin North Am – Small Anim Pract.* 2022;52(1):67–105. https://doi.org/10.1016/j.cvsm.2021.08.003.
8. Coffman CR, Brigden GM. Oral and dental imaging equipment and techniques for small animals. *Vet Clin North Am – Small Anim Pract.* 2013;43(3):489–506. https://doi.org/10.1016/j.cvsm.2013.02.007.
9. Lee H, Badal A. A review of doses for dental imaging in 2010–2020 and development of a web dose calculator. *Radiol Res Pract.* 2021;2021:1–18. https://doi.org/10.1155/2021/6924314.
10. National Council on Radiation Protection and Measurements. In: O'Brien C, ed. *NCRP Report No. 177 - Radiation Protection in Dentistry and Oral Maxillofacial Imaging: Recommendations of the National Council on Radiation Protection and Measurements*. Bethesda, MD: NCRP 2020; 2019:18–26. (Accessed November 8, 2022). https://ncrponline.org/shop/reports/report-no-177/.
11. ARIBEX. *Aribex Nomad Pro2 X Ray Operator Manual.* Aribex; Published online 2020:9–12. (Accessed April 25, 2024.) https://archive.org/details/manual_Aribex_Nomad_Pro2_X-Ray_Operator_Manual/page/12/mode/2up.
12. Harvey CE, Emily PP. Oral examination and diagnostic techniques. In: *Small Animal Dentistry*. Mosby-Year Book, Inc.; 1993:29–41.
13. Dental radiology. In: Holmstrom SE, Fitch PF, Eisner ER, eds. *Veterinary Dental Techniques for the Small Animal Practitioner*. 3rd ed. Saunders, Elsevier; 2004:131–174.
14. Villamizar-Martinez LA, Villegas CM, Gioso MA, et al. Radiographic assessment of the feline temporomandibular joint with oblique projections: a preliminary ex vivo study. *J Vet Dent.* 2021;38(4):199–207. https://doi.org/10.1177/08987564211066571.
15. Hammond G, King A, Lapaglia J. Assessment of five oblique radiographic projections of the canine temporomandibular joint. *Vet Radiol Ultrasound*. 2012;53(5):501–506. https://doi.org/10.1111/j.1740-8261.2012.01956.x.
16. Schwarz T, Weller R, Dickie AM, Konar M, Sullivan M. Imaging of the canine and feline temporomandibular joint: a review. *Vet Radiol Ultrasound*. 2002;43(2):85–97. https://doi.org/10.1111/J.1740-8261.2002.TB01656.X.
17. Niemiec BA. Digital dental radiography. *J Vet Dent.* 2007;24(3):192–197. https://doi.org/10.1177/089875640702400311.
18. Villamizar LA, Burgese L, Carvalho VG, Brandão AC, Gioso MA. Uso da radiografia digital na odontologiaveterinária. *Rev Cient Med.* 2010;8(26):447–452. Accessed November 8, 2022 https://pesquisa.bvsalud.org/portal/resource/pt/vti-1578.
19. Bedard A, Davis TD, Angelopoulos C. Storage phosphor plates: how durable are they as a digital dental radiographic system? *J Contemp Dent Pract.* 2004;5(2):057–069. https://doi.org/10.5005/jcdp-5-2-57.
20. Verstraete FJM, Kass PH, Terpak CH. Diagnostic value of full-mouth radiography in cats. *Am J Vet Res.* 1998;59(6):692–695.
21. The skeleton. In: Hermanson JW, de LAEHE, eds. *Miller and Evans' Anatomy of the Dog*. 5th ed. Elsevier; 2020:91–125.
22. Wiggs RB, Lobprise HB. Oral anatomy and physiology. In: Wiggs RB, Lobprise HB, eds. *Veterinary Dentistry Principles & Practice*. 1st ed. Lippincott-Raven; 1997:55–85.
23. Hale FA. Juvenile veterinary dentistry. *Vet Clin North Am – Small Anim Pract.* 2005;35(4 Spec. Iss.):789–817. https://doi.org/10.1016/j.cvsm.2005.02.003.
24. Harvey CE, Emily PP. Function, formation, and anatomy of oral structures in carnivores. In: Harvey CE, Emily PP, eds. *Small Animal Dentistry. Mosby-Year Book.* Inc.; 1993:1–18.
25. Nomenclature. *American Veterinary Dental College*. Published; 2022. (Accessed August 11, 2022). https://avdc.org/avdc-nomenclature/.
26. Gracis M, Harvey CE. Radiographic study of the maxillary canine tooth in mesaticephalic dogs. *J Vet Dent.* 1998;15(2):73–78. https://doi.org/10.1177/089875649801500202.
27. Gracis M. Radiographic study of the maxillary canine tooth of four mesaticephalic cats. *J Vet Dent.* 1999;16(3):115–125. https://doi.org/10.1177/089875649901600303.
28. DuPont GA, DeBowes LJ. Introduction. In: DuPont GA, DeBowes LJ, eds. *Atlas of Dental Radiography in Dogs and Cats*. Saunders, Elsevier; 2009:1–4.
29. Farhadi F, Ruhani MR, Zarandi A. Frequency and pattern of idiopathic osteosclerosis and condensing osteitis lesions in panoramic radiography of Iranian patients. *Dent Res J.* 2016;13(4):322–326. https://doi.org/10.4103/1735-3327.187880.
30. Hale FA. Localized intrinsic staining of teeth due to pulpitis and pulp necrosis in dogs. *J Vet Dent.* 2001;18(1):14–20. https://doi.org/10.1177/089875640101800102.
31. Peralta S, Verstraete FJM, Kass PH. Radiographic evaluation of the types of tooth resorption in dogs. *Am J Vet Res.* 2010;71(7):784–793. https://doi.org/10.2460/ajvr.71.7.784.
32. Harvey CE. Periodontal disease in dogs. Etiopathogenesis, prevalence, and significance. *Vet Clin North Am Small Anim Pract.* 1998;28(5):1111–1128. https://doi.org/10.1016/S0195-5616(98)50105-2.

33. Stella JL, Bauer AE, Croney CC. A cross-sectional study to estimate prevalence of periodontal disease in a population of dogs (*Canis familiaris*) in commercial breeding facilities in Indiana and Illinois. *PLoS One*. 2018;13(1):e0191395. https://doi.org/10.1371/journal.pone.0191395.
34. Harvey CE, Laster L, Shofer F, Miller B. Scoring the full extent of periodontal disease in the dog: development of a Total Mouth Periodontal Score (TMPS) system. *J Vet Dent*. 2008;25(3):176–180. https://doi.org/10.1177/089875640802500303.
35. Bell CM, Soukup JW. Histologic, clinical, and radiologic findings of alveolar bone expansion and osteomyelitis of the jaws in cats. *Vet Pathol*. 2015;52(5):910–918. https://doi.org/10.1177/0300985815591079.
36. D'Astous J. Periodontology: an overview of alveolar bone expansion. *Can Vet J*. 2015;56(3):295–299. (Accessed November 8, 2022). https://www.ncbi.nlm.nih.gov/pmc/articles/PMC4327146/pdf/cvj_03_295.pdf.
37. Lewis JR, Okuda A, Shofer FS, Pachtinger G, Harvey CE, Reiter AM. Significant association between tooth extrusion and tooth resorption in domestic cats. *J Vet Dent*. 2008;25(2):86–95. https://doi.org/10.1177/089875640802500209.
38. Kapatkin AS, Marretta SM, Patnaik AK, Burk RLMR. Mandibular swellings in cats: prospective study of 24 cats. *Am Anim Hosp Assoc*. 1991;27(6):575–580. (Accessed November 14, 2022). https://www.webofscience.com/wos/woscc/full-record/WOS:A1991GV01000001?UT=A1991GV01000001&SID=USW2EC0B12VwAUd6D92ToG9ZBLMIF.
39. Arzi B, Fiani N, Pritchard WB. Diagnostic imaging in veterinary dental practice. *J Am Vet Med Assoc*. 2009;235(10):1149–1151. https://doi.org/10.2460/javma.235.10.1149.
40. Fristad I, Berggreen E. Structure and function of the dentin-pulp complex. In: Hargreaves K, Berman LH, eds. *Cohen's Pathways of the Pulp*. 11th ed. Elsevier; 2016:532–572.
41. Ghannam MG, Bordoni B. *Anatomy, Head and Neck, Pulp (Tooth)*. StatPearls Publishing; 2019. Accessed November 14, 2022 https://www.ncbi.nlm.nih.gov/books/NBK537112/.
42. Feigin K, Bell C, Shope B, Henzel S, Snyder C. Analysis and assessment of pulp vitality of 102 intrinsically stained teeth in dogs. *J Vet Dent*. 2022;39(1):21–33. https://doi.org/10.1177/08987564211060387.
43. Menzies RA, Reiter AM, Lewis JR. Assessment of apical periodontitis in dogs and humans: a review. *J Vet Dent*. 2014;31(1):8–21. https://doi.org/10.1177/089875641403100101.
44. Kovačević M, Tamarut T, Jonjić N, Braut A, Kovačević M. The transition from pulpitis to periapical periodontitis in dogs' teeth. *Aust Endod J*. 2008;34(1):12–18. https://doi.org/10.1111/j.1747-4477.2008.00120.x.
45. Tanomaru-Filho M, Jorge EG, Duarte MAH, Gonçalves M, Guerreiro-Tanomaru JM. Comparative radiographic and histological analyses of periapical lesion development. *Oral Surg Oral Med Oral Pathol Oral Radiol Endod*. 2009;107(3):442–447. https://doi.org/10.1016/J.TRIPLEO.2008.12.009.
46. Marmary Y, Kutiner G. A radiographic survey of periapical jawbone lesions. *Oral Surgery, Oral Med Oral Pathol*. 1986;61(4):405–408. https://doi.org/10.1016/0030-4220(86)90427-5.
47. Lee L. Inflammatory lesions of the jaws. In: White SC, Pharoah M, eds. *Oral Radiology Principles and Interpretation*. 6th ed. 2009:325–342.
48. Verstraete FJM, Zin BP, Kass PH, Cox DP, Jordan RC. Clinical signs and histologic findings in dogs with odontogenic cysts: 41 cases (1995-2010). *J Am Vet Med Assoc*. 2011;239(11):1470–1476. https://doi.org/10.2460/javma.239.11.1470.
49. Murphy B, Bell CM, Soukup JW. Odontogenic cysts. In: Murphy B, Bell CM, Soukup JW, eds. *Veterinary Oral and Maxillofacial Pathology*. 1st ed. John Wiley & Sons, Inc.; 2020:207–215.
50. Al-Fouzan KS. A new classification of endodontic-periodontal lesions. *Int J Dent*. 2014;2014:1–5. https://doi.org/10.1155/2014/919173.
51. Kerns DG, Glickman GN. Endodontic and periodontal interrelationships. In: Cohen S, Hargreaves KM, eds. *Pathways of the Pulp*. 9th ed. Mosby Elsevier; 2006:650–667.
52. Hale FA. The chevron sign. Published 2008. Accessed November 9, 2022. http://www.toothvet.ca/PDFfiles/Chevron.pdf.
53. DuPont GA, DeBowes LJ. Intraoral radiographic anatomy of the dog. In: DuPont GA, DeBowes LJ, eds. *Atlas of Dental Radiography in Dogs and Cats*. Saunders, Elsevier; 2009:6–80.
54. Mittal S, Kumar T, Mittal S, Sharma J. "Internal root resorption: an endodontic challenge": a case series. *J Conserv Dent*. 2014;17(6):590–593. https://doi.org/10.4103/0972-0707.144612.
55. Reiter AM, Lyon KF, Nachreiner RF, Shofer FS. Evaluation of calciotropic hormones in cats with odontoclastic resorptive lesions. *Am J Vet Res*. 2005;66(8):1446–1452. https://doi.org/10.2460/AJVR.2005.66.1446.
56. Nemec A, Arzi B, Murphy B, Kass PH, Verstraete FJM. Prevalence and types of tooth resorption in dogs with oral tumors. *Am J Vet Res*. 2012;73(7):1057–1066. https://doi.org/10.2460/ajvr.73.7.1057.
57. Reiter AM, Lewis JR, Okuda A. Update on the etiology of tooth resorption in domestic cats. *Vet Clin North Am – Small Anim Pract*. 2005;35(4 Spec. Iss.):913–942. https://doi.org/10.1016/j.cvsm.2005.03.006.
58. Vapalahti K, Neittaanmäki H, Lohi H, Virtala A-M. Feline tooth resorption findings from a questionnaire survey on 8115 Finnish cats and a case-control study for a more defined population drawn from the survey. Published online *bioRxiv*. July 14, 2021. https://doi.org/10.1101/2021.01.22.427753, 2021.01.22.427753.
59. Önem E, Baksi BG, Şen BH, Söğüt Ö, Mert A. Diagnostic accuracy of proximal enamel subsurface demineralization and its relationship with calcium loss and lesion depth. *Dentomaxillofac Radiol*. 2012;41(4):285–293. https://doi.org/10.1259/dmfr/55879293.
60. Soltero-Rivera M, Elliott MI, Hast MW, et al. Fracture limits of maxillary fourth premolar teeth in domestic dogs under applied forces. *Front Vet Sci*. 2019;5(JAN):339. https://doi.org/10.3389/fvets.2018.00339.
61. Soukup JW, Hetzel S, Paul A. Classification and epidemiology of traumatic dentoalveolar injuries in dogs and cats: 959 injuries in 660 patient visits (2004–2012). *J Vet Dent*. 2015;32(1):6–14. https://doi.org/10.1177/089875641503200101.
62. Lopes FM, Gioso MA, Ferro DG, Leon-Roman MA, Venturini MAFA, Correa HL. Oral fractures in dogs of Brazil – a retrospective study. *J Vet Dent*. 2005;22(2):86–90. https://doi.org/10.1177/089875640502200202.
63. Lee S, Lee K, Kim H, et al. Comparison of dental radiography and computed tomography: measurement of dentoalveolar structures in healthy, small-sized dogs and cats. *J Vet Sci*. 2020;21(5):e75. https://doi.org/10.4142/JVS.2020.21.E75.
64. Chia H, Taney K, Hoover D, Robertson JB, Villamizar-Martinez LA. Localization of the first mandibular molar roots in relationship to the mandibular canal in small breed dogs—a tomography imaging study. *Front Vet Sci*. 2021;8:684763. https://doi.org/10.3389/fvets.2021.684763.
65. Carvalho CM, Rahal SC, Dos Reis Mesquita L, Castilho MS, Kano WT, Mamprim MJ. Mandibulectomy for treatment of

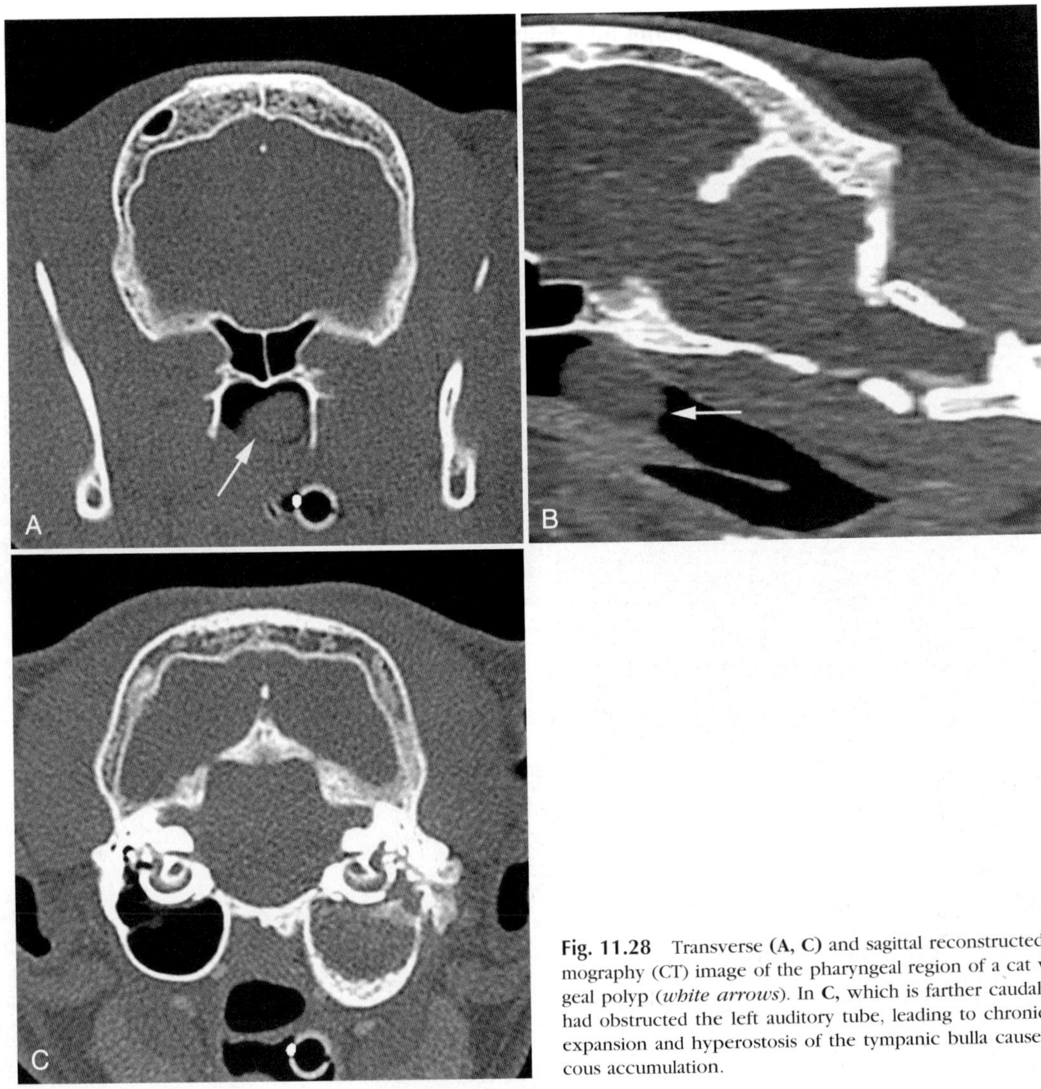

Fig. 11.28 Transverse **(A, C)** and sagittal reconstructed **(B)** computed tomography (CT) image of the pharyngeal region of a cat with a nasopharyngeal polyp (*white arrows*). In **C,** which is farther caudal than **A,** the polyp had obstructed the left auditory tube, leading to chronic otitis media with expansion and hyperostosis of the tympanic bulla caused by fluid and mucous accumulation.

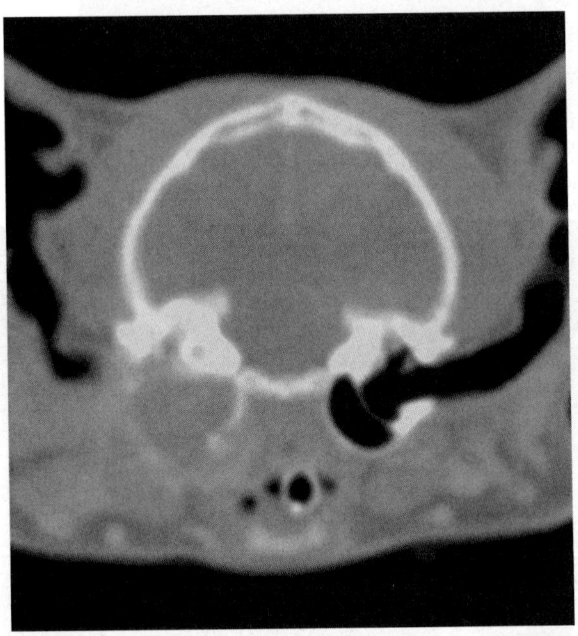

Fig. 11.29 Computed tomography (CT) image of the tympanic bulla region of a cat with a malignant tumor of the left middle ear. Increased tissue or fluid is present in the left tympanic bulla, and there has been expansion of the lateral and ventral aspects of the left tympanic bulla along with bone lysis. This aggressive appearance is typical of a malignant process and should not occur as a result of infection.

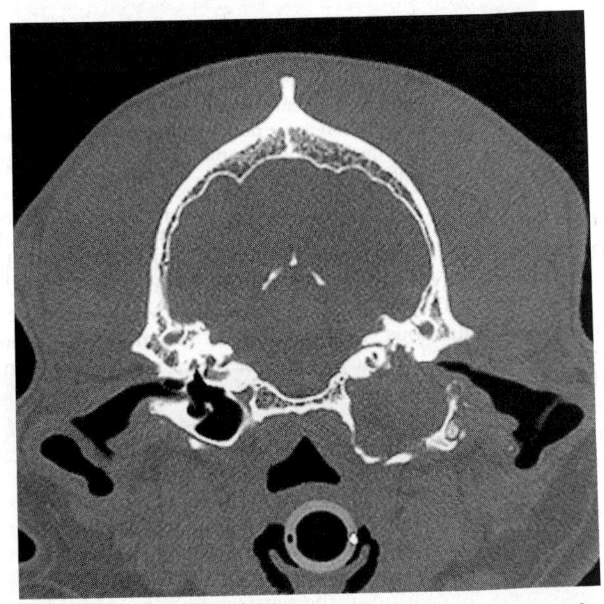

Fig. 11.30 Computed tomography (CT) image of a dog with a left tympanic bulla cholesteatoma. The lesion causes expansion and pressure necrosis of the tympanic bulla.

Masticatory Muscle Myositis

Masticatory muscle myositis is an immune-mediated inflammatory disease where antibodies are formed against type 2M muscle fibers that are present in the temporalis, masseter, and pterygoid muscles. Dogs with this condition often present with a history of lethargy, fever, regional lymphadenopathy, reluctance to eat, and swelling and/or atrophy of the masticatory muscles. The diagnosis is made by detection of antibodies against type 2M fibers in the serum or with histopathology. Cross-sectional imaging can be useful in identifying typical changes and guiding further diagnostics. Typical findings include change in size of the masticatory muscles, and heterogeneous appearance of the musculature with multifocal strong contrast enhancement (Fig. 11.31). The digastric muscle is not affected by the changes. Regional lymphadenopathy is usually present.[154]

TRAUMATIC INJURIES

TMJ luxation can occur in both dogs and cats after external trauma. In the cat, TMJ luxation often occurs after the cat has jumped from a height, and in both dogs and cats, dislocation can occur secondary to vehicular trauma.[155] The TMJ is capable of luxation without fracture because it has considerable lateral sliding movement, and the synchondrosis of the mandibular symphysis allows independent movement of the mandibular rami.[4] Dislocation of the TMJ tends to be in the rostrodorsal direction (Figs. 11.32 and 11.33, eFig. 11.9), because ventrocaudal luxation is prevented by the retroarticular process of the temporal bone.[4] Dogs and cats with TMJ dislocation are unable to close the mouth completely, have dental malocclusion with the mandible displaced to one side, and display excessive salivation.[4] Luxation is most often unilateral; it may

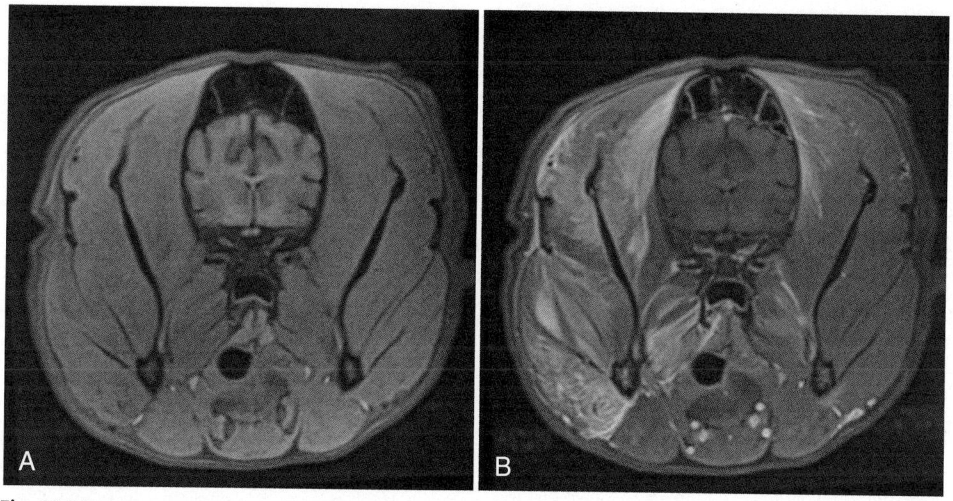

Fig. 11.31 T1-weighted precontrast **(A)** and postcontrast **(B)** transverse MR images of a dog with masticatory muscle myositis. There is marked heterogeneous contrast enhancement of the temporalis, masseter, and pterygoid muscles, worse on the right side. Note that the digastric muscles are not affected.

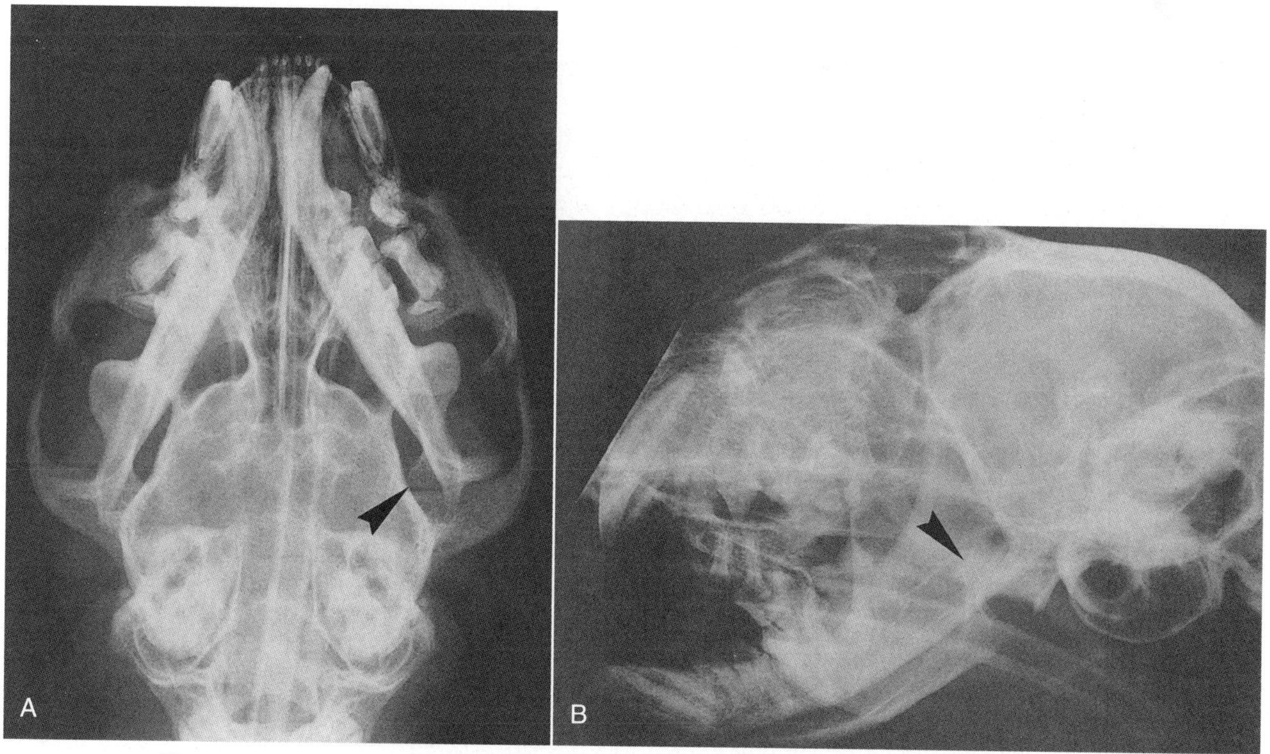

Fig. 11.32 Ventrodorsal **(A)** and right dorsal-left ventral oblique **(B)** radiographs of a 1-year-old domestic shorthair cat with a left temporomandibular luxation. Note the rostral location of the left mandibular condylar process (*arrowhead*) in the ventrodorsal radiograph **(A)**. In the lateral oblique radiograph **(B)**, note the rostral and dorsal luxation of the mandibular condylar process (*arrowhead*).

occur alone or with concomitant fractures of the retroarticular process, mandibular fossa, and zygomatic process of the squamous temporal bone or with the condyloid process of the mandible.[4,156]

Radiographic views necessary for evaluating the TMJ include ventrodorsal and 20-degree lateral oblique views in the cat.[4] These views are useful in the dog, but the angle of rotation varies depending on head conformation.[2] A sagittal oblique radiograph, in which the nose is elevated with a foam wedge so that the head is at a 20-degree angle to the cassette from a lateral position, is advocated in dogs as an alternative to lateral oblique views.[2,4] CT imaging provides for more accurate assessment of the TMJ, and it is helpful in diagnosing osteoarthritis, dysplasia, and other disorders.[4,156]

Skull trauma can occur after vehicular collision in dogs and cats. Currently, CT is used most often to image these patients for surgical planning. The ability to perform 3D reconstructions of the region enhances this planning (Fig. 11.34).

MISCELLANEOUS DISEASES

Craniomandibular Osteopathy

Craniomandibular osteopathy (CMO) is a proliferative bone disease that occurs mainly in young West Highland White, Scottish, Cairn, Boston, and other terriers.[4] CMO is occasionally seen in nonterrier breeds. There is a known autosomal recessive inheritance in West Highland White terriers.[157,158] CMO is usually seen in young dogs aged 3 to 8 months; affected dogs have mandibular swelling, prehension difficulties, pain on opening the mouth or with mastication, pyrexia, or combinations of these clinical signs.[4] Bone proliferation can extend to the bullae, mandibular ramus, TMJ, and calvarium occasionally leading to complications.[159]

Radiographically, there is irregular new bone formation in affected areas, primarily the mandible, the tympanic bulla, and the petrous temporal bone (Fig. 11.35). Bone proliferation is often bilateral and may be asymmetric,

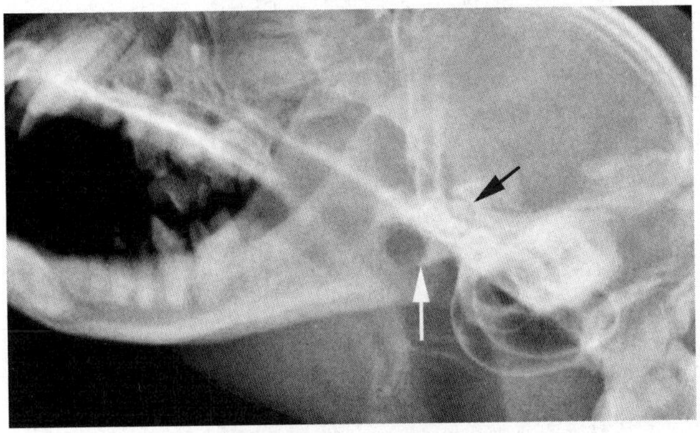

Fig. 11.33 Lateral radiograph of a cat with a unilateral temporomandibular luxation. In the affected joint the articular portion of the mandible is displaced dorsally, leaving an empty appearance to the articular portion of the temporal bone (*white arrow*). In the normal joint, there is good congruity between the articular portions of the mandible and temporal bone (*black arrow*).

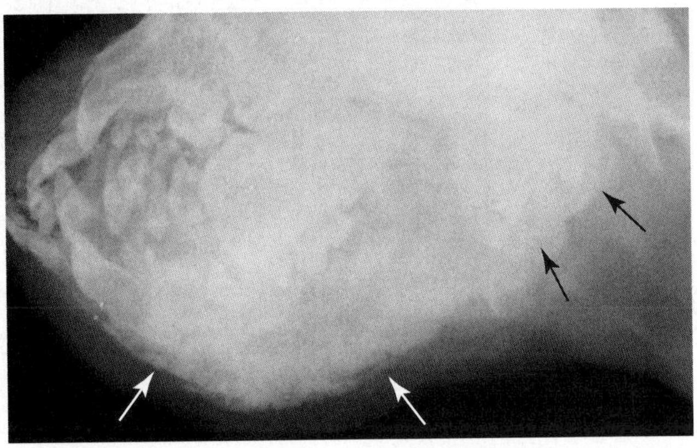

Fig. 11.35 Oblique skull radiograph of a Boston terrier with craniomandibular osteopathy (CMO). There is extensive bone proliferation on the mandibular ramus (*white arrows*), as well as the tympanic bulla (*black arrows*).

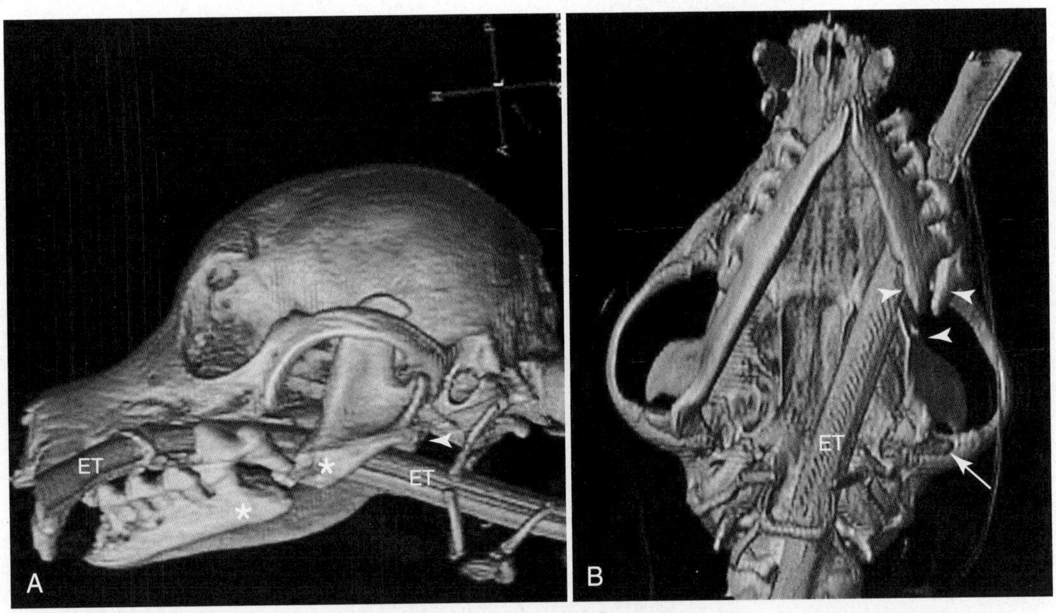

Fig. 11.34 Three-dimensional reconstructed volume rendering of the skull of a dog that sustained a left mandibular fracture. **A,** Left view. Note the obvious fracture fragments of the left mandible (*asterisks*) and that the caudal root of mandibular first molar is no longer embedded in bone. The angular and articular processes of the ramus are ill defined and displaced (*white arrowhead*), indicating probable temporomandibular joint (TMJ) subluxation and possible fracture. **B,** Ventral view. Note three fragments of the fractured left mandible (*white arrowheads*), deviation of the rostral mandible to the left, and caudal displacement of the left mandibular articular process (*white arrow*) indicating TMJ subluxation. *ET,* Endotracheal tube.

although unilateral disease can occur. Bone proliferation can involve the TMJ and can affect jaw movement. Diagnosis is based on signalment and on radiographic findings. Concurrent metaphyseal long-bone changes similar to metaphyseal osteopathy (hypertrophic osteodystrophy [HOD]) have been seen in dogs with CMO, but this is uncommon.[160,161] CMO is a self-limiting disease with unknown etiology. Bone proliferation generally ceases with skeletal maturation (Fig. 11.36).

Calvarial Hyperostosis

Calvarial hyperostotic syndrome resembles canine CMO but is characterized mainly by progressive and often asymmetric skull-bone involvement. The disease affects young male and female Bullmastiff dogs.[161,162] Radiographic findings are smooth thickening of various bones of the calvaria, to various degrees (Fig. 11.37). The smooth bone thickening is dissimilar from the irregular thickening seen in CMO. The etiology of calvarial hyperostosis is unknown.

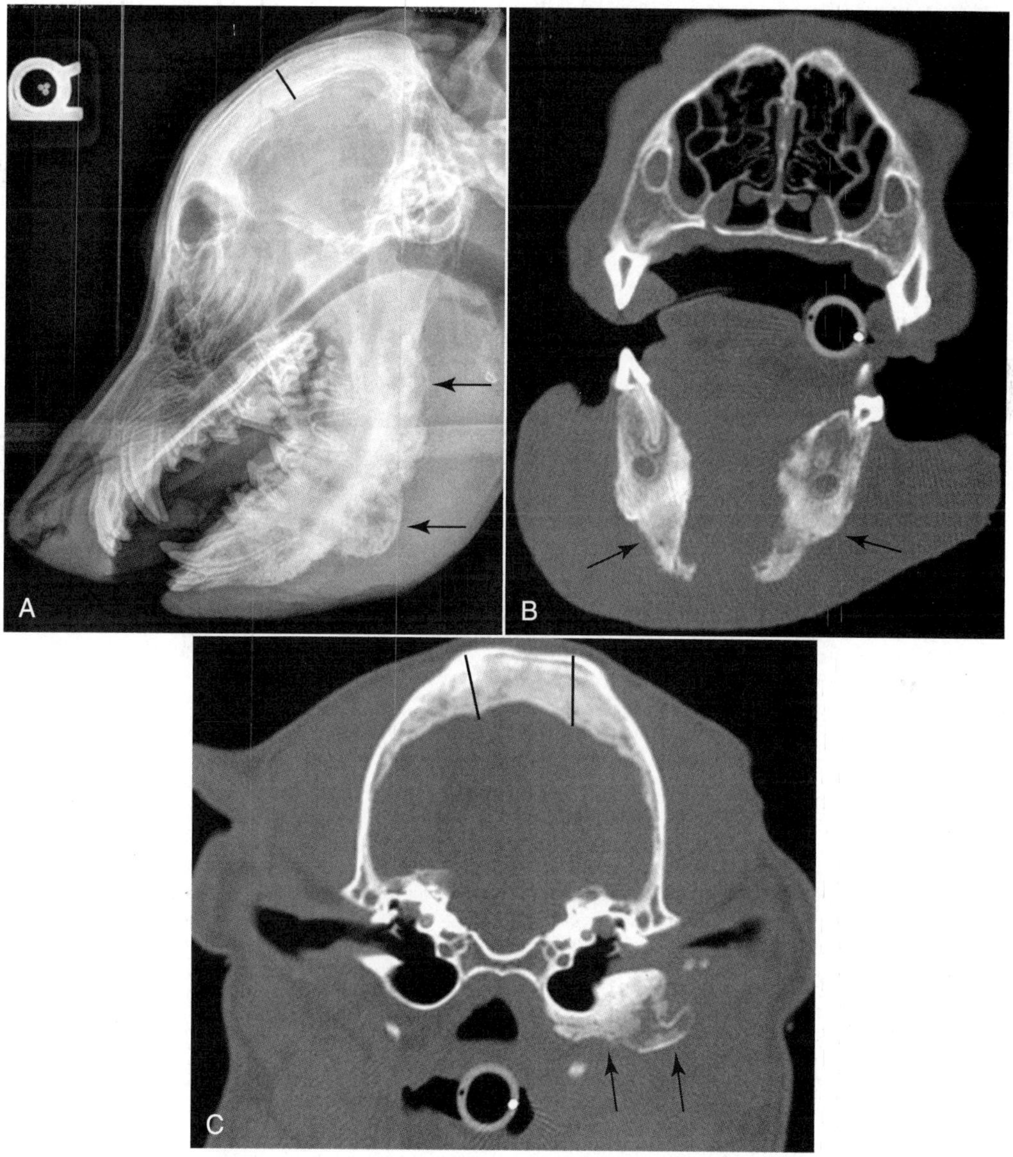

Fig. 11.36 Referral lateral radiograph and CT images of a 6-month-old female Labrador retriever cross with thickened, painful mandible, fever, and chronic hyporexia progressing to anorexia. Clinical signs and bone biopsy consistent with craniomandibular osteopathy (CMO). Right lateral skull image **(A)** and CT images **(B, C)**. In **(A)**, note the proliferative bone thickening of the mandible and the calvarium (*black arrows* and *black line*). In **(B)**, rostral aspect of skull at level of mandibles, note the smooth bordered and thickened bone attenuation of the mandibles (*black arrows*) and associated soft tissue attenuation. In **(C)**, caudal aspect of skull at level of tympanic bullae, note the smooth bordered and thickened bone attenuation of the left bulla, as compared to normal right side (*black arrows*) along with soft tissue attenuation with narrowing of left external ear canal. Note smooth bordered and thickened bone attenuation of dorsal calvarium (*black lines*).

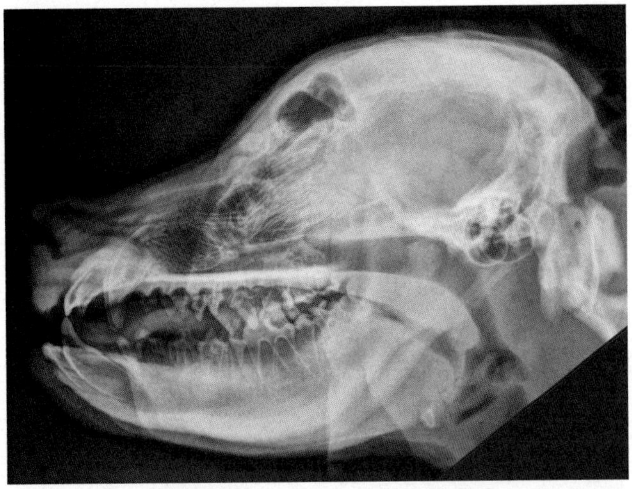

Fig. 11.37 Lateral radiograph of a 6-month-old mastiff. There is smooth thickening of the mandibular, dorsal nasal, and calvarial cortices. Note the small size of the frontal sinuses caused by the peripheral hyperostosis.

REFERENCES

1. Hermanson JW, de Lahunta A, Evans HE. *Miller and Evans' Anatomy of the Dog*. 5th ed. St. Louis: Elsevier; 2020.
2. Dickie AM, Sullivan M. The effect of obliquity on the radiographic appearance of the temporomandibular joint in dogs. *Vet Radiol Ultrasound*. 2001;42(3):205–217.
3. Hammond G, King A, Lapaglia J. Assessment of five oblique radiographic projections of the canine temporomandibular joint. *Vet Radiol Ultrasound*. 2012;53(5):501–506.
4. Schwarz T, Weller R, Dickie AM, Konar M, Sullivan M. Imaging of the canine and feline temporomandibular joint: a review. *Vet Radiol Ultrasound*. 2002;43(2):85–97.
5. Arzi B, Cissell DD, Verstraete FJ, Kass PH, DuRaine GD, Athanasiou KA. Computed tomographic findings in dogs and cats with temporomandibular joint disorders: 58 cases (2006–2011). *J Am Vet Med Assoc*. 2013;242(1):69–75.
6. Macready DM, Hecht S, Craig LE, Conklin GA. Magnetic resonance imaging features of the temporomandibular joint in normal dogs. *Vet Radiol Ultrasound*. 2010;51(4): 436–440.
7. De Rycke LMS JH, Gielen IM, et al. Magnetic resonance imaging, computed tomography, and cross-sectional views of the anatomy of normal nasal cavities and paranasal sinuses in mesaticephalic dogs. *Am J Vet Res*. 2003;64: 1093–1098.
8. Couturier LD C, Ruel Y, Dennis R, Begon D. Anatomical study of cranial nerve emergence and skull foramina in the dog using magnetic resonance imaging and computed tomography. *Vet Radiol Ultrasound*. 2005;46(5):375–383.
9. Gomes E, Degueurce C, Ruel Y, Dennis R, Begon D. Anatomic study of cranial nerve emergence and associated skull foramina in cats using CT and MRI. *Vet Radiol Ultrasound*. 2009;50(4):398–403.
10. Kneissl SP A, Konar M. Low-field magnetic resonance imaging of the canine middle and inner ear. *Vet Radiol Ultrasound*. 2004;45(6):520–552.
11. Lefebvre J, Kuehn NF, Wortinger A. Computed tomography as an aid in the diagnosis of chronic nasal disease in dogs. *J Small Anim Pract*. 2005;46(6):280–285.
12. Schwarz TSJ. *Veterinary Computed Tomography*. West Sussex: UK: Wiley Blackwell; 2011.
13. Wisner ERZ A. *Atlas of Small Animal CT and MRI*. Ames, IA: Wiley Blackwell; 2015.
14. Estey CM. Congenital hydrocephalus. *Vet Clin North Am Small Anim Pract*. 2016;46(2):217–229.
15. Hecht S, Adams WH. MRI of brain disease in veterinary patients part 1: basic principles and congenital brain disorders. *Vet Clin North Am Small Anim Pract*. 2010;40(1):21–38.
16. Thomas WB. Hydrocephalus in dogs and cats. *Vet Clin North Am Small Anim Pract*. 2010;40(1):143–159.
17. Thomas WB. Nonneoplastic disorders of the brain. *Clin Tech Small Anim Pract*. 1999;14(3):125–147.
18. Cerda-Gonzalez S, Dewey CW. Congenital diseases of the craniocervical junction in the dog. *Vet Clin North Am Small Anim Pract*. 2010;40(1):121–141.
19. De Haan CEK SL, Gavin PR, Wendling LR, Griebenow ML. Normal variation in size of the lateral ventricles of the Labrador retriever dog as assessed by magnetic resonance imaging. *Vet Radiol Ultrasound*. 1994;35(2):83–86.
20. Cerda-Gonzalez S, Dewey CW, Scrivani PV, Kline KL. Imaging features of atlanto-occipital overlapping in dogs. *Vet Radiol Ultrasound*. 2009;50(3):264–268.
21. Parry AT, Upjohn MM, Schlegl K, Kneissl S, Lamb CR. Computed tomography variations in morphology of the canine atlas in dogs with and without atlantoaxial subluxation. *Vet Radiol Ultrasound*. 2010;51(6):596–600.
22. Cerda-Gonzalez S, Olby NJ, McCullough S, Pease AP, Broadstone R, Osborne JA. Morphology of the caudal fossa in cavalier king Charles spaniels. *Vet Radiol Ultrasound*. 2009;50(1):37–46.
23. Rusbridge C. Neurological diseases of the cavalier king Charles spaniel. *J Small Anim Pract*. 2005;46(6):265–272.
24. Rusbridge C, Knowler SP. Hereditary aspects of occipital bone hypoplasia and syringomyelia (Chiari type I malformation) in cavalier King Charles spaniels. *Vet Rec*. 2003;153(4):107–112.
25. Rusbridge C, Knowler SP. Inheritance of occipital bone hypoplasia (Chiari type I malformation) in cavalier king Charles spaniels. *J Vet Intern Med*. 2004;18(5):673–678.
26. Freeman AC, Platt SR, Kent M, Huguet E, Rusbridge C, Holmes S. Chiari-like malformation and syringomyelia in American Brussels Griffon dogs. *J Vet Intern Med*. 2014;28(5):1551–1559.
27. Gatineau M, El-Warrak AO, Marretta SM, Kamiya D, Moreau M. Locked jaw syndrome in dogs and cats: 37 cases (1998–2005). *J Vet Dent*. 2008;25(1):16–22.
28. Dickie AM, Schwarz T, Sullivan M. Temporomandibular joint morphology in cavalier king Charles spaniels. *Vet Radiol Ultrasound*. 2002;43(3):260–266.
29. Nutt AE, Anderson T, Gracis M, Doran I, Warren-Smith C, Langley-Hobbs SJ. Open-mouth jaw locking in cats: a literature review and use of CT in three cases. *J Feline Med Surg*. 2018;20(12):1180–1191.
30. Reiter AM. Symphysiotomy, symphysiectomy, and intermandibular arthrodesis in a cat with open-mouth jaw locking—case report and literature review. *J Vet Dent*. 2004;21(3):147–158.
31. Beam RC, Kunz DA, Cook CR, Carson RL, Briscoe P, Cook JL. Use of three-dimensional computed tomography for diagnosis and treatment planning for open-mouth jaw locking in a cat. *J Am Vet Med Assoc*. 2007;230(1):59–63.
32. Crawley AC, Muntz FH, Haskins ME, Jones BR, Hopwood JJ. Prevalence of mucopolysaccharidosis type VI mutations in Siamese cats. *J Vet Intern Med*. 2003;17(4):495–498.
33. Haskins M, Casal M, Ellinwood NM, et al. Animal models for mucopolysaccharidoses and their clinical relevance. *Acta Paediatr Suppl*. 2002;91(439):88–97.
34. Haskins ME. Animal models for mucopolysaccharidosis disorders and their clinical relevance. *Acta Paediatr*. 2007;96(455):56–62.
35. Konde LJT MA, Gaser P, Dial SM, McBiles K, Colgan S, Haskins M. Radiographically visualized skeletal changes associated with mucopolysaccharidosis VI in cats. *Vet Radiol*. 1987;28(6):223–228.

36. Cotugno G, Annunziata P, Tessitore A, et al. Long-term amelioration of feline Mucopolysaccharidosis VI after AAV-mediated liver gene transfer. *Mol Ther*. 2011;19(3): 461–469.
37. Bonczynski J. Primary hyperparathyroidism in dogs and cats. *Clin Tech Small Anim Pract*. 2007;22(2):70–74.
38. Feldman EC, Hoar B, Pollard R, Nelson RW. Pretreatment clinical and laboratory findings in dogs with primary hyperparathyroidism: 210 cases (1987–2004). *J Am Vet Med Assoc*. 2005;227(5):756–761.
39. Kumar R, Thompson JR. The regulation of parathyroid hormone secretion and synthesis. *J Am Soc Nephrol*. 2011;22(2):216–224. Epub 2010-12-16.
40. Parker VJ, Harjes LM, Dembek K, Young GS, Chew DJ, Toribio RE. Association of vitamin D metabolites with parathyroid hormone, fibroblast growth factor-23, calcium, and phosphorus in dogs with various stages of chronic kidney disease. *J Vet Intern Med*. 2017;31(3): 791–798.
41. Krook LW JP. Nutritional secondary hyperparathyroidism in the animal kingdom: report of two cases. *Clin Imaging*. 2010;34(6):458–461.
42. Wisner ER, Nyland TG. Ultrasonography of the thyroid and parathyroid glands. *Vet Clin North Am Small Anim Pract*. 1998;28(4):973–991.
43. Lautscham E, von Klopmann C, Schaub S, Stengel C, Hartmann A. CT imaging features of the normal parathyroid gland in the dog. *Tierarztl Prax Ausg K Kleintiere Heimtiere*. 2020;48(5):313–320. Epub 2020-10-21.
44. Liles SR, Linder KE, Cain B, Pease AP. Ultrasonography of histologically normal parathyroid glands and thyroid lobules in normocalcemic dogs. *Vet Radiol Ultrasound*. 2010;51(4):447–452.
45. Taeymans O, Dennis R, Saunders JH. Magnetic resonance imaging of the normal canine thyroid gland. *Vet Radiol Ultrasound*. 2008;49(3):238–242.
46. Taeymans O, Schwarz T, Duchateau L, et al. Computed tomographic features of the normal canine thyroid gland. *Vet Radiol Ultrasound*. 2008;49(1):13–19.
47. Thompson D, Skelly B. Prevalence of canine primary hyperparathyroidism recurrence in Keeshond and non-Keeshond dogs after curative parathyroidectomy. *Vet Rec*. 2020;187(11):e93.
48. Amorós O, Espada Y, Vila A, Jiménez A, Novellas R. Precontrast CT attenuation of the thyroid gland is lower in brachycephalic dogs versus non-brachycephalic dogs. *Vet Radiol Ultrasound*. 2021;62(1):54–60.
49. Fischetti AJ, Gisselman K, Peterson ME. CT and MRI evaluation of skull bones and soft tissues in six cats with presumed acromegaly versus 12 unaffected cats. *Vet Radiol Ultrasound*. 2012;53(5):535–539.
50. Lamb CR, Ciasca TC, Mantis P, et al. Computed tomographic signs of acromegaly in 68 diabetic cats with hypersomatotropism. *J Feline Med Surg*. 2014;16(2): 99–108.
51. Niessen SJ. Feline acromegaly: an essential differential diagnosis for the difficult diabetic. *J Feline Med Surg*. 2010;12(1):15–23.
52. Malinowski C. Canine and feline nasal neoplasia. *Clin Tech Small Anim Pract*. 2006;21(2):89–94.
53. Ferguson S, Smith KC, Welsh CE, Dobromylskyj MJ. A retrospective study of more than 400 feline nasal biopsy samples in the UK (2006–2013). *J Feline Med Surg*. 2020;22(8):736–743.
54. Nakazawa M, Tomiyasu H, Suzuki K, et al. Efficacy of chemotherapy and palliative hypofractionated radiotherapy for cats with nasal lymphoma. *J Vet Med Sci*. 2021;83(3):456–460.
55. Reczynska AI, LaRue SM, Boss MK, et al. Outcome of stereotactic body radiation for treatment of nasal and nasopharyngeal lymphoma in 32 cats. *J Vet Intern Med*. 2022;36(2):733–742.
56. Giuliano A, Dobson J. Clinical response and survival time of cats with carcinoma of the nasal cavity treated with palliative coarse fractionated radiotherapy. *J Feline Med Surg*. 2020;22(10):922–927.
57. Haney SM, Beaver L, Turrel J, et al. Survival analysis of 97 cats with nasal lymphoma: a multi-institutional retrospective study (1986–2006). *J Vet Intern Med*. 2009;23(2): 287–294.
58. Mayer MN, DeWalt JO, Sidhu N, Mauldin GN, Waldner CL. Outcomes and adverse effects associated with stereotactic body radiation therapy in dogs with nasal tumors: 28 cases (2011–2016). *J Am Vet Med Assoc*. 2019;254(5):602–612.
59. Mortier JR, Blackwood L. Treatment of nasal tumours in dogs: a review. *J Small Anim Pract*. 2020;61(7):404–415.
60. Poirier VJ, Koh ESY, Darko J, Fleck A, Pinard C, Vail DM. Patterns of local residual disease and local failure after intensity modulated/image guided radiation therapy for sinonasal tumors in dogs. *J Vet Intern Med*. 2021;35(2): 1062–1072.
61. Lawrence JA, Forrest LJ, Turek MM, et al. Proof of principle of ocular sparing in dogs with sinonasal tumors treated with intensity-modulated radiation therapy. *Vet Radiol Ultrasound*. 2010;51(5):561–570.
62. Kubicek L, Milner R, An Q, et al. Outcomes and prognostic factors associated with canine sinonasal tumors treated with curative intent cone-based stereotactic radiosurgery (1999–2013). *Vet Radiol Ultrasound*. 2016;57(3): 331–340.
63. Stevens A, Turek M, Vail D, Christensen N, Forrest L. Definitive-intent intensity modulated radiotherapy for modified-Adams' stage 4 canine sinonasal cancer: a retrospective study of 29 cases (2011–2017). *Vet Radiol Ultrasound*. 2020;61(6):718–725.
64. Stiborova K, Meier VS, Takada M, et al. Definitive-intent radiotherapy for sinonasal carcinoma in cats: a multicenter retrospective assessment. *Vet Comp Oncol*. 2020;18(4):626–633.
65. Russo M, Lamb CR, Jakovljevic S. Distinguishing rhinitis and nasal neoplasia by radiography. *Vet Radiol Ultrasound*. 2000;41(2):118–124.
66. Kirberger RM, Fourie SL. An investigation into the usefulness of a rostrocaudal nasal radiographic view in the dog. *J S Afr Vet Assoc*. 2002;73(4):171–176.
67. Ciekot PA, Powers BE, Withrow SJ, Straw RC, Ogilvie GK, LaRue SM. Histologically low-grade, yet biologically high-grade, fibrosarcomas of the mandible and maxilla in dogs: 25 cases (1982–1991). *J Am Vet Med Assoc*. 1994;204(4):610–615.
68. Morris JS, Dunn KJ, Dobson JM, White RA. Radiological assessment of severity of canine nasal tumours and relationship with survival. *J Small Anim Pract*. 1996;37(1): 1–6.
69. Adams WM, Kleiter MM, Thrall DE, et al. Prognostic significance of tumor histology and computed tomographic staging for radiation treatment response of canine nasal tumors. *Vet Radiol Ultrasound*. 2009;50(3):330–335.
70. Drees R, Forrest LJ, Chappell R. Comparison of computed tomography and magnetic resonance imaging for the evaluation of canine intranasal neoplasia. *J Small Anim Pract*. 2009;50(7):334–340.
71. Miles MS, Dhaliwal RS, Moore MP, Reed AL. Association of magnetic resonance imaging findings and histologic diagnosis in dogs with nasal disease: 78 cases (2001–2004). *J Am Vet Med Assoc*. 2008;232(12):1844–1849.

72. Miles S, Schwarz T. Canine nasal septum deviation can be a normal variation and correlates with increasing skull indices. *Vet Radiol Ultrasound*. 2020;61(3):279–284.
73. Schwarz T, Sullivan M, Hartung K. Radiographic detection of defects of the nasal boundaries. *Vet Radiol Ultrasound*. 2000;41(3):226–230.
74. Bouyssou S, Hammond GJ, Eivers C. Comparison of CT features of 79 cats with intranasal mass lesions. *J Feline Med Surg*. 2021;23(10):987–995.
75. Tromblee TC, Jones JC, Etue AE, Forrester SD. Association between clinical characteristics, computed tomography characteristics, and histologic diagnosis for cats with sinonasal disease. *Vet Radiol Ultrasound*. 2006;47(3): 241–248.
76. Avner A, Dobson JM, Sales JI, Herrtage ME. Retrospective review of 50 canine nasal tumours evaluated by low-field magnetic resonance imaging. *J Small Anim Pract*. 2008;49(5):233–239.
77. Bradshaw T, Fu R, Bowen S, Zhu J, Forrest L, Jeraj R. Predicting location of recurrence using FDG, FLT, and Cu-ATSM PET in canine sinonasal tumors treated with radiotherapy. *Phys Med Biol*. 2015;60(13):5211–5224.
78. Bradshaw TJ, Bowen SR, Jallow N, Forrest LJ, Jeraj R. Heterogeneity in intratumor correlations of 18F-FDG, 18F-FLT, and 61Cu-ATSM PET in canine sinonasal tumors. *J Nucl Med*. 2013;54(11):1931–1937.
79. Liptak JM. Cancer of the gastrointestinal tract. In: Vail DMT,DH, Liptak JM, eds. *Withrow and MacEwen's Small Animal Clinical Oncology*. 6th ed. St. Louis, MO: Elsevier; 2020:432–491.
80. Mikiewicz M, Paździor-Czapula K, Gesek M, Lemishevskyi V, Otrocka-Domagała I. Canine and feline oral cavity tumours and tumour-like lesions: a retrospective study of 486 cases (2015–2017). *J Comp Pathol*. 2019;172:80–87.
81. Liptak JMC, Christensen NI. Soft tissue sarcomas. In: Vail DMT DH, Liptak JM, eds. *Withrow and MacEwen's Small Animal Clinical Oncology*. 6th ed. St. Louis, MO: Elsevier; 2020:404–431.
82. Bergman PJ, Selmic LE, Kent MS. Melanoma. In: Vail DMT,DH, Liptak JM, eds. *Withrow and MacEwen's Small Animal Clinical Oncology*. 6th ed. St. Louis, MO: Elsevier; 2020:367–381.
83. Forrest LJ, Chun R, Adams WM, Cooley AJ, Vail DM. Postoperative radiotherapy for canine soft tissue sarcoma. *J Vet Intern Med*. 2000;14(6):578–582.
84. Camerino M, Giacobino D, Manassero L, et al. Prognostic impact of bone invasion in canine oral malignant melanoma treated by surgery and anti-CSPG4 vaccination: a retrospective study on 68 cases (2010–2020). *Vet Comp Oncol*. 2022;20(1):189–197.
85. Soltero-Rivera MM, Krick EL, Reiter AM, Brown DC, Lewis JR. Prevalence of regional and distant metastasis in cats with advanced oral squamous cell carcinoma: 49 cases (2005–2011). *J Feline Med Surg*. 2014;16(2):164–169.
86. Gendler A, Lewis JR, Reetz JA, Schwarz T. CT features of oral squamous cell carcinoma in cats: 18 cases (2002–2008). *J Am Vet Med Assoc*. 2010;236(3):319–325.
87. Giacobino D, Camerino M, Riccardo F, et al. Difference in outcome between curative intent vs marginal excision as a first treatment in dogs with oral malignant melanoma and the impact of adjuvant CSPG4-DNA electrovaccination: a retrospective study on 155 cases. *Vet Comp Oncol*. 2021;19(4):651–660.
88. Bertone ER, Snyder LA, Moore AS. Environmental and lifestyle risk factors for oral squamous cell carcinoma in domestic cats. *J Vet Intern Med*. 2003;17(4):557–562.
89. Zaccone R, Renzi A, Chalfon C, et al. Environmental risk factors for the development of oral squamous cell carcinoma in cats. *J Vet Intern Med*. 2022;36(4):1398–1408.
90. Bilgic O, Duda L, Sánchez MD, Lewis JR. Feline oral squamous cell carcinoma: clinical manifestations and literature review. *J Vet Dent*. 2015;32(1):30–40.
91. Poirier VJ, Kaser-Hotz B, Vail DM, Straw RC. Efficacy and toxicity of an accelerated hypofractionated radiation therapy protocol in cats with oral squamous cell carcinoma. *Vet Radiol Ultrasound*. 2013;54(1):81–88.
92. Lee S, Jang Y, Lee G, Jeon S, Kim D, Choi J. CT features of malignant and benign oral tumors in 28 dogs. *Vet Radiol Ultrasound*. 2021;62(5):549–556.
93. Randall EK, Kraft SL, Yoshikawa H, LaRue SM. Evaluation of 18F-FDG PET/CT as a diagnostic imaging and staging tool for feline oral squamous cell carcinoma. *Vet Comp Oncol*. 2016;14(1):28–38.
94. Kawabe M, Mori T, Ito Y, et al. Outcomes of dogs undergoing radiotherapy for treatment of oral malignant melanoma: 111 cases (2006–2012). *J Am Vet Med Assoc*. 2015;247(10):1146–1153.
95. Murphy S, Hayes AM, Blackwood L, Maglennon G, Pattinson H, Sparkes AH. Oral malignant melanoma – the effect of coarse fractionation radiotherapy alone or with adjuvant carboplatin therapy. *Vet Comp Oncol*. 2005;3(4):222–229.
96. McCaw DL, Pope ER, Payne JT, West MK, Tompson RV, Tate D. Treatment of canine oral squamous cell carcinomas with photodynamic therapy. *Br J Cancer*. 2000;82(7):1297–1299.
97. Baja AJ, Kelsey KL, Ruslander DM, Gieger TL, Nolan MW. A retrospective study of 101 dogs with oral melanoma treated with a weekly or biweekly 6 Gy × 6 radiotherapy protocol. *Vet Comp Oncol*. 2022;20(3):623–631.
98. Boston SE, Lu X, Culp WT, et al. Efficacy of systemic adjuvant therapies administered to dogs after excision of oral malignant melanomas: 151 cases (2001–2012). *J Am Vet Med Assoc*. 2014;245(4):401–407.
99. Ottnod JM, Smedley RC, Walshaw R, Hauptman JG, Kiupel M, Obradovich JE. A retrospective analysis of the efficacy of Oncept vaccine for the adjunct treatment of canine oral malignant melanoma. *Vet Comp Oncol*. 2013;11(3):219–229.
100. Proulx DR, Ruslander DM, Dodge RK, et al. A retrospective analysis of 140 dogs with oral melanoma treated with external beam radiation. *Vet Radiol Ultrasound*. 2003;44(3):352–359.
101. Tarone L, Giacobino D, Camerino M, et al. Canine melanoma immunology and immunotherapy: relevance of translational research. *Front Vet Sci*. 2022;9:1–11.
102. Soukup JW, Snyder CJ, Simmons BT, Pinkerton ME, Chun R. Clinical, histologic, and computed tomographic features of oral papillary squamous cell carcinoma in dogs: 9 cases (2008–2011). *J Vet Dent*. 2013;30(1):18–24.
103. Gardner H, Fidel J, Haldorson G, Dernell W, Wheeler B. Canine oral fibrosarcomas: a retrospective analysis of 65 cases (1998–2010). *Vet Comp Oncol*. 2015;13(1):40–47.
104. Riggs J, Adams VJ, Hermer JV, Dobson JM, Murphy S, Ladlow JF. Outcomes following surgical excision or surgical excision combined with adjunctive, hypofractionated radiotherapy in dogs with oral squamous cell carcinoma or fibrosarcoma. *J Am Vet Med Assoc*. 2018;253(1):73–83.
105. Selmic LE, Lafferty MH, Kamstock DA, et al. Outcome and prognostic factors for osteosarcoma of the maxilla, mandible, or calvarium in dogs: 183 cases (1986–2012). *J Am Vet Med Assoc*. 2014;245(8):930–938.

106. Dernell WS, Straw RC, Cooper MF, Powers BE, LaRue SM, Withrow SJ. Multilobular osteochondrosarcoma in 39 dogs: 1979–1993. *J Am Anim Hosp Assoc.* 1998;34(1): 11–18.
107. Ehrhart NP, Christensen NI, Fan TM. Tumors of the skeletal system. In: Vail DMT,DH, Liptak JM, eds. *Withrow and MacEwen's Small Animal Clinical Oncology*. 6th ed. St. Louis, MO: Elsevier; 2020:524–564.
108. Banks TA, Straw RC. Multilobular osteochondrosarcoma of the hard palate in a dog. *Aust Vet J.* 2004;82(7):409–412.
109. Hathcock JT, Newton JC. Computed tomographic characteristics of multilobular tumor of bone involving the cranium in 7 dogs and zygomatic arch in 2 dogs. *Vet Radiol Ultrasound.* 2000;41(3):214–217.
110. Gallegos J, Schwarz T, McAnulty JF. Massive midline occipitotemporal resection of the skull for treatment of multilobular osteochondrosarcoma in two dogs. *J Am Vet Med Assoc.* 2008;233(5):752–757.
111. Lipsitz D, Levitski RE, Berry WL. Magnetic resonance imaging features of multilobular osteochondrosarcoma in 3 dogs. *Vet Radiol Ultrasound.* 2001;42(1):14–19.
112. Volker MK, Luskin IR. Oral osteoma in 6 dogs. *J Vet Dent.* 2014;31(2):88–91.
113. Grozdanic S, Riedesel EA, Ackermann MR. Successful medical treatment of an orbital osteoma in a dog. *Vet Ophthalmol.* 2013;16(2):135–139.
114. Polizopoulou ZS, Koutinas AF, Souftas VD, Kaldrymidou E, Kazakos G, Papadopoulos G. Diagnostic correlation of CT-MRI and histopathology in 10 dogs with brain neoplasms. *J Vet Med A Physiol Pathol Clin Med.* 2004;51(5): 226–231.
115. Motta L, Mandara MT, Skerritt GC. Canine and feline intracranial meningiomas: an updated review. *Vet J.* 2012;192(2):153–165.
116. Sharman MJ, Mansfield CS. Sinonasal aspergillosis in dogs: a review. *J Small Anim Pract.* 2012;53(8):434–444.
117. Cooley S, Galustanian G, Moon A, Summers S. CT findings of nasal cryptococcosis in cats and dogs: a case series. *Vet Radiol Ultrasound.* 2022;63(4):422–429.
118. Trivedi SR, Sykes JE, Cannon MS, et al. Clinical features and epidemiology of cryptococcosis in cats and dogs in California: 93 cases (1988–2010). *J Am Vet Med Assoc.* 2011;239(3):357–369.
119. Saunders JH, Clercx C, Snaps FR, et al. Radiographic, magnetic resonance imaging, computed tomographic, and rhinoscopic features of nasal aspergillosis in dogs. *J Am Vet Med Assoc.* 2004;225(11):1703–1712.
120. Saunders JH, van Bree H. Comparison of radiography and computed tomography for the diagnosis of canine nasal aspergillosis. *Vet Radiol Ultrasound.* 2003;44(4): 414–419.
121. Barrs VR, Beatty JA, Dhand NK, et al. Computed tomographic features of feline sino-nasal and sino-orbital aspergillosis. *Vet J.* 2014;201(2):215–222.
122. Barrs VR, Talbot JJ. Feline aspergillosis. *Vet Clin North Am Small Anim Pract.* 2014;44(1):51–73.
123. Cormack CA, Donahoe SL, Talbot JJ, Beatty JA, Barrs VR. Disseminated invasive aspergillosis caused by *Aspergillus felis* in a cat. *J Vet Intern Med.* 2021;35(5):2395–2400.
124. Karnik K, Reichle JK, Fischetti AJ, Goggin JM. Computed tomographic findings of fungal rhinitis and sinusitis in cats. *Vet Radiol Ultrasound.* 2009;50(1):65–68.
125. Furtado AR, Caine A, Herrtage ME. Diagnostic value of MRI in dogs with inflammatory nasal disease. *J Small Anim Pract.* 2014;55(7):359–363.
126. Roccabianca P, Turchetto S, Ferrari N, et al. Feline lymphoplasmacytic rhinitis (FLPCR): severity of inflammation correlates with reduced mucosal IgA expression. *Vet Immunol Immunopathol.* 2021;234:1–11.
127. Windsor RC, Johnson LR, Herrgesell EJ, De Cock HE. Idiopathic lymphoplasmacytic rhinitis in dogs: 37 cases (1997–2002). *J Am Vet Med Assoc.* 2004;224(12): 1952–1957.
128. Dias MJ, Mouro S, Englar RE, Leal RO. Nasal foreign bodies identified by rhinoscopy in dogs: 42 cases. *J Small Anim Pract.* 2020;61(12):752–756.
129. Fischer MC, Busse C, Adrian AM. Magnetic resonance imaging findings in dogs with orbital inflammation. *J Small Anim Pract.* 2019;60(2):107–115.
130. Lafuma F, Baudin Tréhiou C, Bernardin F, Blond L. Computed tomography may be helpful in discriminating grass awn foreign body rhinitis from non-foreign body rhinitis in dogs. *Vet Radiol Ultrasound.* 2021;62(5):533–540.
131. Moreno-Aguado B, Carrera I, Holdsworth A, Agthe P, Maddox TW, Trevail T. CT findings in 20 dogs and six cats with confirmed nasal foreign bodies. *Vet Radiol Ultrasound.* 2020;61(4):417–426.
132. Belmudes A, Pressanti C, Barthez PY, Castilla-Castaño E, Fabries L, Cadiergues MC. Computed tomographic findings in 205 dogs with clinical signs compatible with middle ear disease: a retrospective study. *Vet Dermatol.* 2018;29(1):45-e20.
133. Bischoff MG, Kneller SK. Diagnostic imaging of the canine and feline ear. *Vet Clin North Am Small Anim Pract.* 2004;34(2):437–458.
134. Rohleder JJ, Jones JC, Duncan RB, Larson MM, Waldron DL, Tromblee T. Comparative performance of radiography and computed tomography in the diagnosis of middle ear disease in 31 dogs. *Vet Radiol Ultrasound.* 2006;47(1):45–52.
135. Owen MC, Lamb CR, Lu D, Targett MP. Material in the middle ear of dogs having magnetic resonance imaging for investigation of neurologic signs. *Vet Radiol Ultrasound.* 2004;45(2):149–155.
136. Shanaman M, Seiler G, Holt DE. Prevalence of clinical and subclinical middle ear disease in cats undergoing computed tomographic scans of the head. *Vet Radiol Ultrasound.* 2012;53(1):76–79.
137. Lorek A, Dennis R, van Dijk J, Bannoehr J. Occult otitis media in dogs with chronic otitis externa – magnetic resonance imaging and association with otoscopic and cytological findings. *Vet Dermatol.* 2020;31(2):146–153.
138. Detweiler DA, Johnson LR, Kass PH, Wisner ER. Computed tomographic evidence of bulla effusion in cats with sinonasal disease: 2001–2004. *J Vet Intern Med.* 2006;20(5):1080–1084.
139. Goodale EC, Outerbridge CA, White SD. Aspergillus otitis in small animals—a retrospective study of 17 cases. *Vet Dermatol.* 2016;27(1):3-e2.
140. Cole LK. Primary secretory otitis media in Cavalier King Charles spaniels. *Vet Clin North Am Small Anim Pract.* 2012;42(6):1137–1142.
141. Kent M, Glass EN, de Lahunta A, Platt SR, Haley A. Prevalence of effusion in the tympanic cavity in dogs with dysfunction of the trigeminal nerve: 18 cases (2004–2013). *J Vet Intern Med.* 2013;27(5):1153–1158.
142. Wessmann A, Hennessey A, Goncalves R, Benigni L, Hammond G, Volk HA. The association of middle ear effusion with trigeminal nerve mass lesions in dogs. *Vet Rec.* 2013;173(18):449.
143. Parzefall B, Rieger A, Volk HA, Maierl J, Brühschwein A, Blutke A. Prevalence and characterization of small tympanic bone spicules and drumstick-like hyperostotic tympanic bone spicules in the middle ear cavity of dogs. *Vet Radiol Ultrasound.* 2015;56(1):25–32.
144. Beck T, Brühschwein A, Meyer-Lindenberg A. Occurrence of tympanic bone spicules and bone crests in domestic cats. *Anat Histol Embryol.* 2020;49(2):216–221.

145. Greci V, Mortellaro CM. Management of otic and nasopharyngeal, and nasal polyps in cats and dogs. *Vet Clin North Am Small Anim Pract*. 2016;46(4):643–661.
146. Swales N, Foster A, Barnard N. Retrospective study of the presentation, diagnosis and management of 16 cats with otitis media not due to nasopharyngeal polyp. *J Feline Med Surg*. 2018;20(12):1082–1086.
147. MacPhail CM, Innocenti CM, Kudnig ST, Veir JK, Lappin MR. Atypical manifestations of feline inflammatory polyps in three cats. *J Feline Med Surg*. 2007;9(3): 219–225.
148. Lamb CR, Sibbing K, Priestnall SL. Pathologic basis for rim enhancement observed in computed tomographic images of feline nasopharyngeal polyps. *Vet Radiol Ultrasound*. 2016;57(2):130–136.
149. Tanaka T, Akiyoshi H, Mie K, Nishida H. MRI findings, including diffusion-weighted imaging and apparent diffusion coefficient value, in two cats with nasopharyngeal polyps and one cat with lymphoma. *JFMS Open Rep*. 2018;4(2):1–7.
150. Hauck ML. Tumors of the skin and subcutaneous tissues. In: Vail DM, Thamm DH, Liptak JM, eds. *Withrow and MacEwen's Small Animal Clinical Oncology*. 6th ed. St. Louis, MO: Elsevier; 2020:360–361.
151. Herberger A, Hammond J, Miller A, Olson B. *MRI of a Middle Ear Cholesteatoma in a Cat*. Vet Radiol Ultrasound; 2022.
152. Risselada M. Diagnosis and management of cholesteatomas in dogs. *Vet Clin North Am Small Anim Pract*. 2016;46(4):623–634.
153. Travetti O, Giudice C, Greci V, Lombardo R, Mortellaro CM, Di Giancamillo M. Computed tomography features of middle ear cholesteatoma in dogs. *Vet Radiol Ultrasound*. 2010;51(4):374–379.
154. Reiter AM, Schwarz T. Computed tomographic appearance of masticatory myositis in dogs: 7 cases (1999–2006). *J Am Vet Med Assoc* 2007;231(6).
155. Hecht S, Anderson KM, Castel A, et al. Agreement of magnetic resonance imaging with computed tomography in the assessment for acute skull fractures in a canine and feline cadaver model. *Front Vet Sci*. 2021;8:1–9.
156. Maas CP, Theyse LF. Temporomandibular joint ankylosis in cats and dogs. A report of 10 cases. *Vet Comp Orthop Traumatol.* 2007;20(3):192–197.
157. Padgett GA, Mostosky UV. The mode of inheritance of craniomandibular osteopathy in West Highland White terrier dogs. *Am J Med Genet*. 1986;25(1):9–13.
158. Letko A, Leuthard F, Jagannathan V, et al. Whole genome sequencing indicates heterogeneity of hyperostotic disorders in dogs. *Genes*. 2020;11(2).
159. Beever L, Swinbourne F, Priestnall SL, Ter Haar G, Brockman DJ. Surgical management of chronic otitis secondary to craniomandibular osteopathy in three West Highland white terriers. *J Small Anim Pract*. 2019;60(4):254–260.
160. Matiasovic M, Caine A, Scarpante E, Cherubini GB. Imaging diagnosis-magnetic resonance imaging features of craniomandibular osteopathy in an Airedale Terrier. *Vet Radiol Ultrasound*. 2016;57(3):E27–E29.
161. McConnell JF, Hayes A, Platt SR, Smith KC. Calvarial hyperostosis syndrome in two bullmastiffs. *Vet Radiol Ultrasound*. 2006;47(1):72–77.
162. Pastor KF, Boulay JP, Schelling SH, Carpenter JL. Idiopathic hyperostosis of the calvaria in five young bullmastiffs. *J Am Anim Hosp Assoc*. 2000;36(5):439–445.

ELECTRONIC RESOURCES

Additional information related to the content in Chapter 11 can be found online at eBooks.Health.Elsevier.com.

- Chapter Quiz

CHAPTER 12

Magnetic Resonance Imaging and Computed Tomographic Features of Brain Disease in Small Animals

Ian Robertson • Gabriela S. Seiler

The superior soft tissue contrast of magnetic resonance imaging (MRI) makes it the preferred modality for imaging almost all aspects of intracranial disease, whereas computed tomography (CT) is less sensitive. CT is suitable for brain imaging in trauma cases, as outlined later, and if magnetic resonance (MR) is not available. This chapter is a basic overview of the MR and CT characteristics of common small animal intracranial disorders. A review of the technical details associated with brain imaging in small animals and a more comprehensive review of uncommon disorders is available elsewhere.[1,2]

BASIC MAGNETIC RESONANCE EXAMINATION OF THE BRAIN

A standard MR examination of the canine or feline brain involves the acquisition of multiple pulse sequences in different anatomic planes (Table 12.1). In MR, it is the tissue chemical characteristics that determine the signal intensity in the various sequences. Pulse sequences are selected to assess anatomy and to maximize lesion conspicuity. Images are usually acquired in transverse, sagittal, and dorsal planes (Fig. 12.1).

Rationale for Sequence Selection

In T2-weighted sequences, free fluid (e.g., cerebrospinal fluid [CSF]) is extremely bright/T2 hyperintense. Bright/T2-hyperintense tissues have a longer T2 relaxation (see Chapter 4 for a discussion of T1 and T2 relaxation). Most common pathologic processes, whether neoplastic or inflammatory, result in increased fluid within tissues, and this results in an increase in brightness of the abnormal tissue relative to surrounding normal tissue; the term *increased T2-signal intensity* is commonly used to describe this.

Sometimes it is difficult to identify a T2-hyperintense lesion when it is adjacent to a normal region of high signal, such as adjacent to CSF within the ventricles. With respect to T2-weighted sequences, the signal from free fluid can be eliminated using a fluid-attenuated inversion recovery (FLAIR) sequence. In T2-weighted FLAIR images, free fluid has very low signal, while other hydrated lesions remain bright (Fig. 12.2).[3] Proteinaceous or inflammatory fluid will have less or no signal reduction. The term *nulling* or *null* is used to describe the signal change produced when using an inversion recovery sequence like FLAIR (e.g., the T2 hyperintensity nulls in the FLAIR sequence). A FLAIR sequence may also provide additional information about T2-hyperintense lesions that must be distinguished from CSF, such as cystic meningioma, dermoid and epidermoid cysts, and arachnoid cysts.[4]

In T1-weighted spin-echo sequences, high signal arises from tissues having rapid T1 relaxation, such as fat and methemoglobin. Conversely, fluid and hydrated lesions have reduced signal intensity in T1-weighted images, appearing dark or hypointense. A T1-weighted image is excellent for evaluation of extracranial anatomy, but on its own has poor sensitivity for detection of most intracranial lesions because of their hydrated nature, which leads to low T1 signal. However, blood-brain barrier disruption and regions of altered perfusion can be detected in T1-weighted sequences acquired after the administration of MR contrast medium. The most common MR contrast media are chelated forms of gadolinium, a transitional compound with paramagnetic properties that shorten the T1 relaxation time of tissue in which the material accumulates.[5] Therefore, regions of higher gadolinium concentration will have increased signal (bright) in T1-weighted sequences.

Many pathologic processes in the brain result in some disruption to the blood-brain barrier, often allowing an accumulation of contrast medium after intravenous injection, and thereby increased signal intensity in postcontrast T1-weighted images. Contrast medium should be administered after all other imaging sequences have been acquired, because contrast medium can sometimes affect the appearance of tissues/organs in other sequences.

Certain abnormalities are easier to detect in a specific scan plane, and ensuring these scan planes are part of the routine examination is imperative. For example, a T2-weighted sagittal sequence should be performed routinely to allow better evaluation of the morphology of the midbrain, cerebellum, and caudal brainstem. This is particularly important in the assessment of increased intracranial pressure and caudal fossa crowding.[6]

Table • 12.1

Standard Sequences for Brain Magnetic Resonance Imaging.

SEQUENCE	IMAGE PLANE
T2-weighted spin echo	Transverse and sagittal
T2-FLAIR	Transverse
T1-weighted spin-echo sequence	At least one plane, usually transverse
T2-weighted GRE to assess for hemorrhage	Transverse
T1-weighted spin-echo sequence after administration of contrast medium	Same image plane and acquisition parameters as precontrast, may add image planes
Additional specialized sequences as indicated and available	Depends on indication

FLAIR, Fluid-attenuated inversion recovery; *GRE,* gradient recall echo.

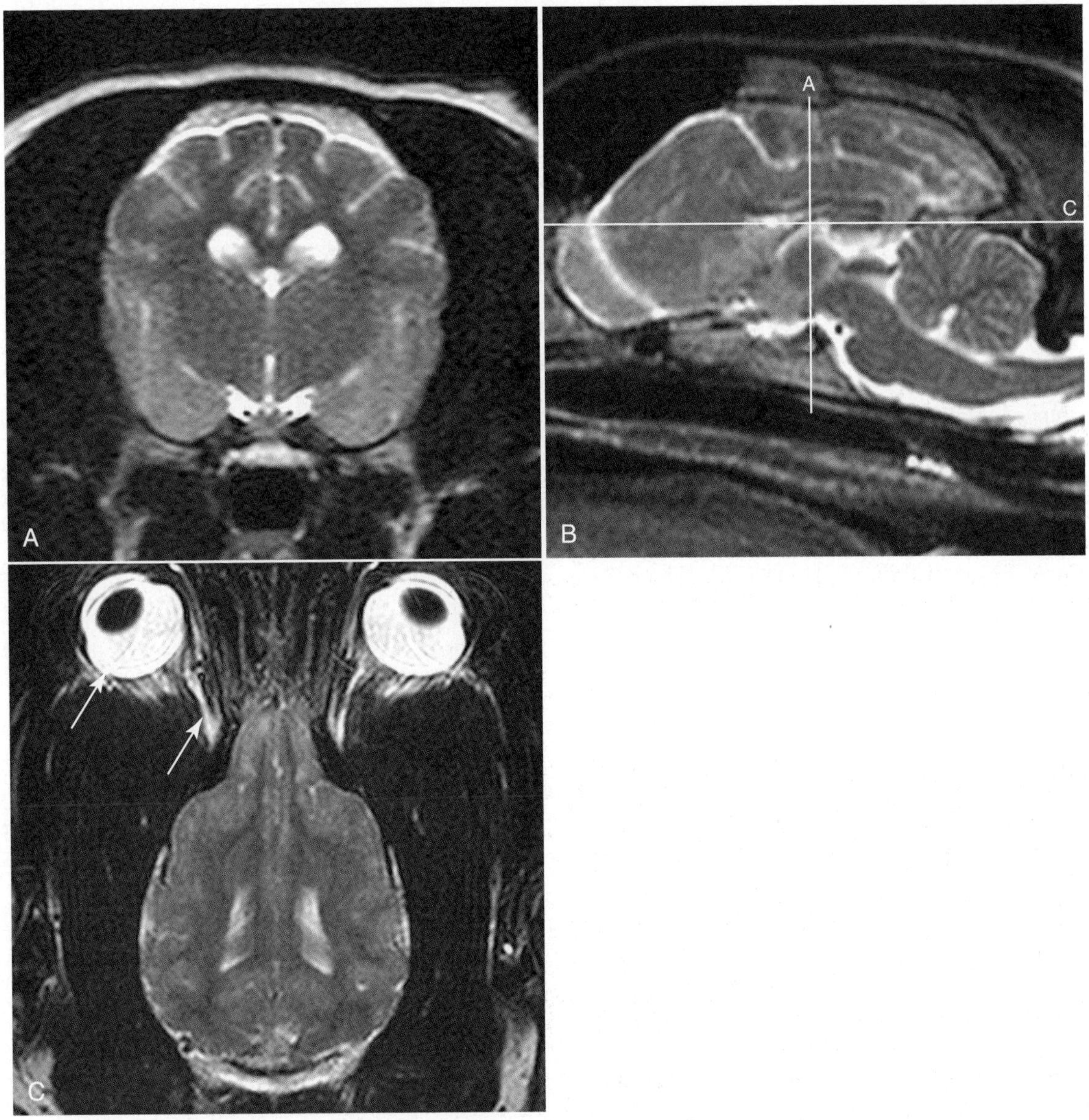

Fig. 12.1 T2-weighted magnetic resonance (MR) images acquired in transverse **(A)**, sagittal **(B)**, and dorsal planes **(C)**. (Unless specified, "images" refers to conventional spin-echo images.) The sagittal plane image is midline. The locations of the transverse and dorsal plane image are shown in the sagittal plane image. In these T2-weighted images of a normal canine brain, cerebrospinal fluid (CSF) within the ventricles is bright (i.e., has high signal). In **C**, retrobulbar fat and the vitreous humor also have high signal (*white arrows*).

As discussed in Chapter 4, images can be acquired using spin-echo or gradient recall echo (GRE) pulse sequences. GRE images are more susceptible to magnetic field inhomogeneity, and this is exploited when assessing the brain for evidence of chronic hemorrhage (longer than 2–3 days). As hemorrhage is broken down, the magnetic properties of the ferric/ferrous ions in hemoglobin metabolites cause a local field distortion that destroys the MR signal. This appears as a signal void (a black, so-called susceptibility artifact). This is an extremely sensitive indicator of chronic hemorrhage as might occur in patients with intracranial trauma, hemorrhagic tumors, hemorrhagic infarcts, coagulopathies, or hemorrhagic metastasis. The image void is typically much larger than the actual lesion because of blooming (see Hemorrhagic Infarct section).

Putting It All Together

The imaging characteristics of a lesion need to be evaluated in various sequences, so that an accurate assessment of the underlying disease process can be established. For example, a T2-hyperintense region in the brain may represent free fluid such as CSF or brain edema and the two conditions can be differentiated with a T2 FLAIR sequence (see Fig. 12.2). T2 hyperintensity may also represent pathology such as neoplasia which may be contrast enhancing, or necrosis which does not enhance and does not null in a T2-weighted FLAIR sequence (Fig. 12.3). All pulse sequences must be interpreted together to reach the correct conclusion.

Secondary Effects of Focal Intracranial Disease

In addition to altering local signal intensity, brain masses and swelling can also cause major changes to brain morphology. Many masses and the secondary perilesional edema result in brain compression, with a contralateral midline shift, ventricular compression and obstruction, and ultimately either transtentorial and/or cerebellar herniation at the foramen magnum (Fig. 12.4). Herniation of the cingulate gyrus across midline is

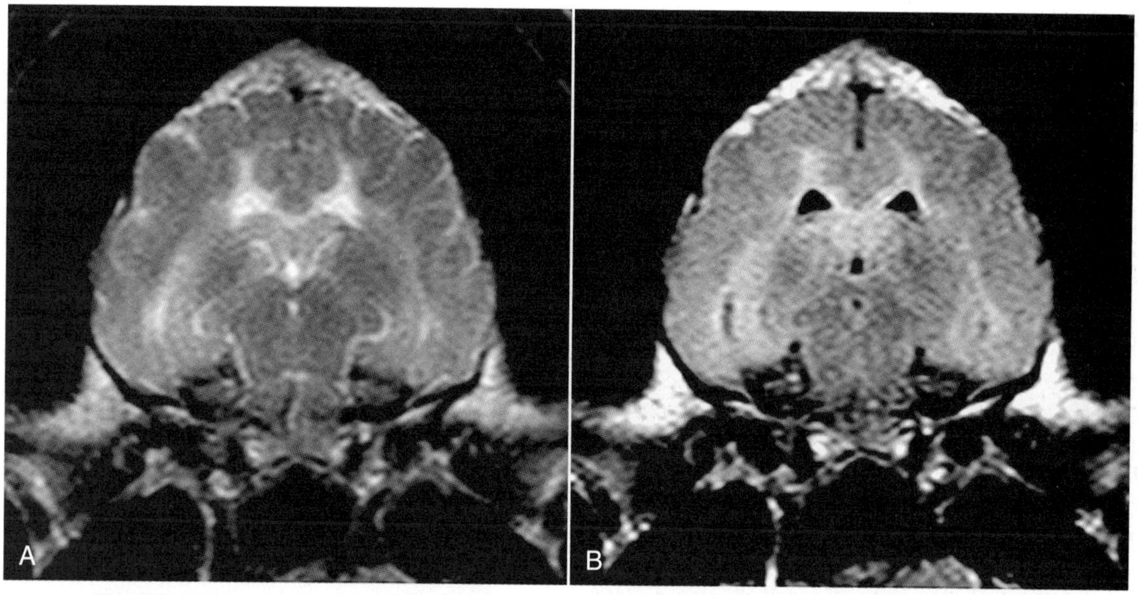

Fig. 12.2 Comparison of T2-weighted spin-echo **(A)** and T2-weighted fluid-attenuated inversion recovery (FLAIR) **(B)** MR images in a dog with leukoencephalitis. In the T2-weighted spin-echo image **(A)**, there is considerable T2-hyperintensity in the ventricular region, but it is impossible to determine whether this is caused by signal from cerebrospinal fluid (CSF) or brain edema or both. Obvious periventricular T2 signal is more conspicuous in the FLAIR image **(B)** as a result of nulling, or elimination, of the high signal from the CSF. Note the lack of signal from CSF in the lateral ventricles in the T2-weighted FLAIR image, as expected.

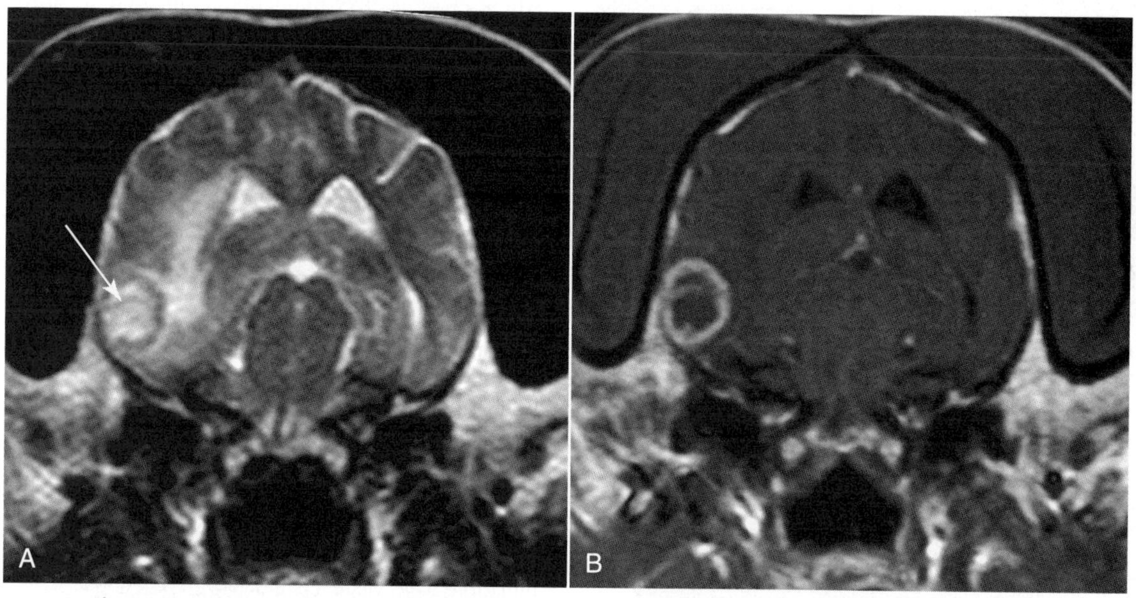

Fig. 12.3 **A,** T2-weighted magnetic resonance (MR) image. There is a focal T2-hyperintense mass (*white arrow*) with a T2-hypointense border surrounded by adjacent wispy regions of T2-hyperintensity consistent with perilesional white matter edema. **B,** Postcontrast T1-weighted image. The T2-hypointense border is now characterized by marked peripheral contrast enhancement, often called *ring enhancement*. The center of the mass does not enhance. In both images, there is a contralateral midline shift as a result of the mass and perilesional edema. Final diagnosis was metastatic hemangiosarcoma, but these signs are not specific for this.

called subfalcine herniation. It is critical not to overlook the signs of cerebellar herniation (Fig. 12.5).

BASIC COMPUTED TOMOGRAPHIC EXAMINATION OF THE BRAIN

CT examination of the brain typically includes acquisition of images in a transverse plane, followed by dorsal and sagittal image reconstructions which do not require acquisition of additional image sequences. The basic principles of CT imaging are outlined in Chapter 4. In most instances, intravenous administration of iodinated contrast medium is required for optimal delineation of normal anatomy outside the blood-brain barrier such as the pituitary gland, choroid plexus, and vasculature. The brain parenchyma itself does not enhance. Differentiation of the gray matter, white matter, and cerebrospinal fluid is possible due to their different attenuation

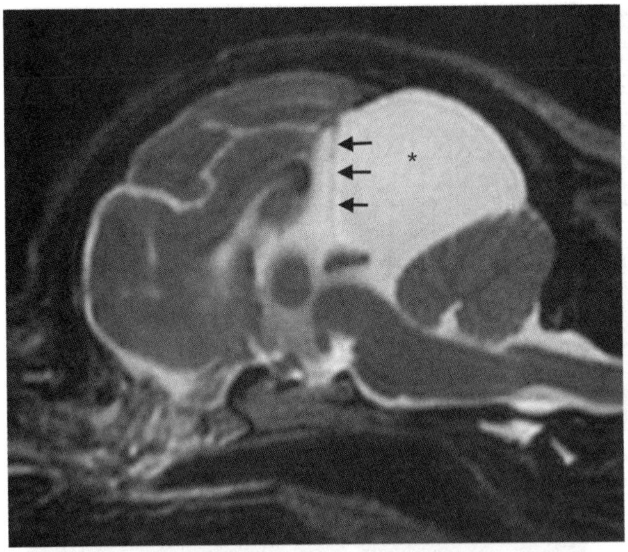

Fig. 12.10 Sagittal T2-weighted magnetic resonance (MR) image of a 13-year-old Pekingese with an acute onset of seizures. There is marked enlargement of the quadrigeminal cistern (*black asterisk*) resulting in flattening of the rostrodorsal aspect of the cerebellum. Despite this, there is no evidence of caudal fossa herniation. This was a pre-existing condition and unrelated to the adult-onset seizures. The membrane between the caudodorsal aspect of the third ventricle and the quadrigeminal cistern is readily evident and is displaced rostrally (*arrows*).

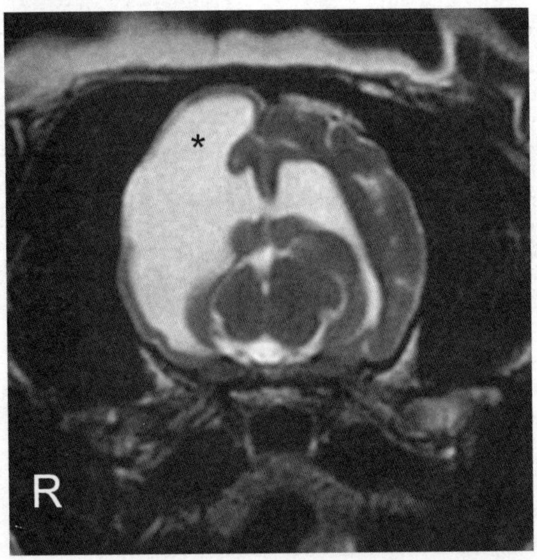

Fig. 12.11 Transverse T2-weighted magnetic resonance (MR) image of an 8-year-old pug with an acute onset of neck pain due to a cervical disc. An incidental finding was right encephaloclastic porencephaly of undetermined etiology. There is expansion of the right lateral ventricle extending to the subarachnoid space (*black asterisk*).

There are a number of uncommon cystic structures that can occur within the cranial vault as a result of incomplete or aberrant separation of the neuroectoderm from the overlying ectodermal tissue. Intracranial epidermoid cysts, intracranial dermoid cysts, Rathke cleft cysts, and craniopharyngiomas originate during gestation from remnants of ectodermal tissue due to defects of neural tube closure.[16] Intracranial epidermoid or dermoid cysts are most commonly located in the fourth ventricle or the cerebellopontine angle (Fig. 12.13). Cystic structures are hypoattenuating in CT images. Signal intensity is variable and dependent on cyst content in MRIs. Cysts with a high lipid content appear hyperintense in T1-weighted and T2-weighed images, whereas cysts with lower lipid content appear T1 hypointense and T2 hyperintense.[17] Dermoid cysts containing adnexa (e.g., hair) may have suspended low intensity foci in all sequences.[18] Cysts often contain protein and keratin and, therefore, do not null in FLAIR sequences. Typically, these complex cysts do not enhance, although ring enhancement may occasionally be present. Rathke cleft cysts and craniopharyngiomas occur in the region of the sella turcica and are typically associated with anomalous development of the pituitary gland.

Other Developmental Morphologic Anomalies

Chiari-like malformation, also called *caudal occipital malformation syndrome (COMS)*, is an all-encompassing term that describes anomalies in the development and morphology of the caudal fossa. This commonly results in crowding of the cerebellum and varying degrees of protrusion of the cerebellum into and through the foramen magnum (Fig. 12.14). The Cavalier King Charles spaniel is the most affected breed, wherein the condition is inherited and thought to affect as much as 95% of the population.[19–22] However, COMS is observed in many other small breeds. MR is commonly used as a screening tool to assist breeding programs in reducing the incidence and severity of COMS. Crowding of the caudal fossa results in protrusion of the caudal cerebellar vermis against or through the foramen magnum. This can result in disruption to CSF flow and an increase in pressure within the spinal cord, leading to the development of fluid-filled cavities within the central and dorsocentral aspect of the spinal cord, termed *syringohydromyelia*. In some patients, syringohydromyelia extends to the thoracic and lumbar spinal cord. There is some association between Chiari-like malformation syndrome and the development of dorsal atlanto-axial bands.[23] While CT is a valuable tool to assess bone pathology, evaluation of the soft tissues of the caudal fossa is limited due to lower contrast resolution and beam hardening artifact. With CT, sagittal reconstructions are most valuable to identify presence of caudal fossa crowding or cerebellar herniation. The accuracy and interobserver agreement for identification of cerebellar herniation and presence of syringomyelia were shown to be higher using high-field MRI compared to multislice CT.[24]

Holoprosencephaly is the failure of the forebrain to bifurcate normally into two discrete cerebral hemispheres. Holoprosencephaly exists in three forms depending on the severity of the malformation, alobar, semilobar, and lobar. Lobar holoprosencephaly has been described in dogs,[25] and dysgenesis/agenesis of the corpus callosum is a feature of this condition. Dogs with developmental abnormalities of the corpus callosum may have hypodipsic hypernatremia. Miniature schnauzers appear to be overrepresented for both dysgenesis of the corpus callosum and lobar holoprosencephaly (Fig. 12.15).

Lissencephaly is an extremely rare condition whereby there is an absence or severe lack of normal gyral formation resulting in a smooth outer surface to the brain (Fig. 12.16). It results from failure of normal neural migration during fetal development. In dogs, the Lhasa Apso is overrepresented, and there may be a genetic predisposition in this breed.[26]

Inherent Disorders in Brain Metabolism

There are many developmental, often breed-specific, inborn errors of brain metabolism that result in MR changes. These conditions, collectively known as *storage diseases*, can result in changes to both brain morphology and signal characteristics due to the abnormal accumulation of one or more products of interrupted metabolic pathways. Mucopolysaccharidosis, neuronal cell lipofuscinosis, cerebellar abiotrophy, and globoid cell leukodystrophy are the most common—albeit rare. There is

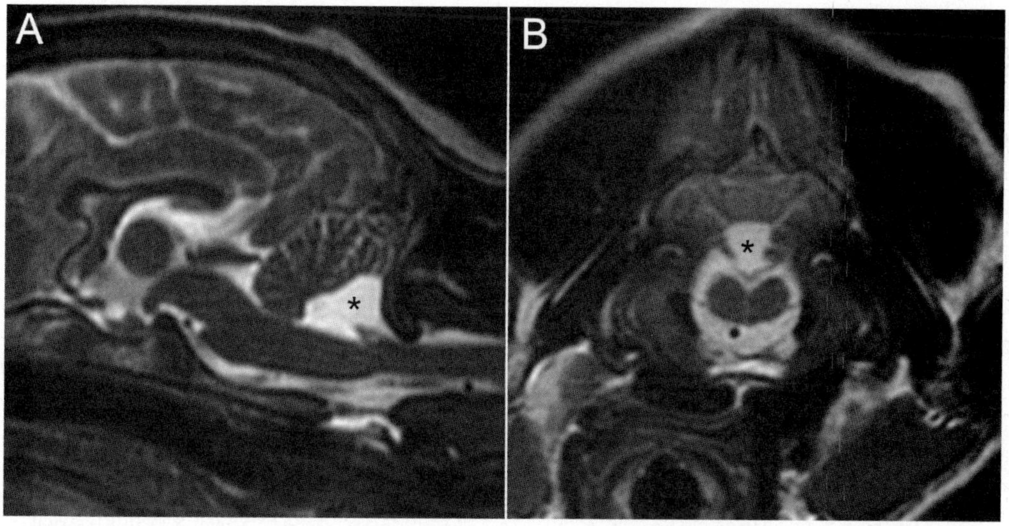

Fig. 12.12 Dandy Walker variant. Sagittal T2-weighted **(A)** and transverse **(B)** magnetic resonance (MR) images of a 4-month-old Labrador retriever puppy with signs of central vestibular disease. Failure of development of the caudoventral aspect of the cerebellar vermis has resulted in an accumulation of fluid, denoted by the *black asterisk.*

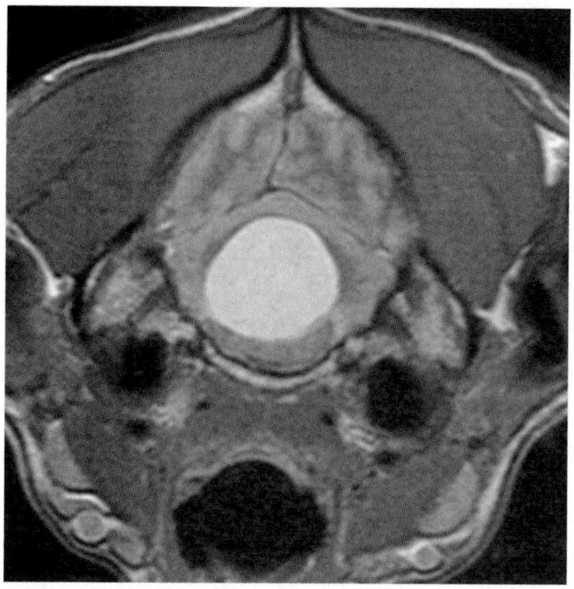

Fig. 12.13 A proton-density (PD)–weighted transverse magnetic resonance (MR) image at the level of the mid aspect of the cerebellum of a 4-year-old mix breed dog. A large spherical cystic mass is present in the fourth ventricle resulting in marked compression and deformation of both the cerebellum and medulla. Histology confirmed an epidermoid cyst.

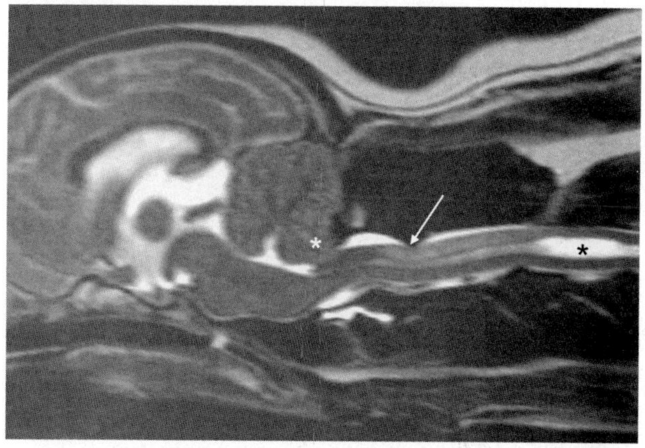

Fig. 12.14 Sagittal T2-weighted magnetic resonance (MR) image of a 4-year-old Cavalier King Charles spaniel. There is crowding of the caudal cerebellar vermis at the foramen magnum (*white asterisk*) and cranial cervical syringohydromyelia (*black asterisk*). There is focal attenuation of the dorsal aspect of the subarachnoid space and a mild indentation in the dorsal aspect of the spinal cord at the caudal aspect of arch of C1 (*white arrow*). This morphology is thought to reflect a dorsal atlanto-axial band and is commonly associated with caudal occipital malformation syndrome. There is mild enlargement of the caudodorsal aspect of the third ventricle.

considerable variation in the appearance of such disorders. Mucopolysaccharidosis and neuronal cell lipofuscinosis typically result in progressive juvenile cortical atrophy and hydrocephalus and an abnormally small corpus callosum, and in the latter, there is often severe peripheral meningeal thickening and enhancement[27] (Fig. 12.17). Cerebellar abiotrophy results in progressive cerebellar atrophy, manifesting as increased conspicuity of the cerebellar folia[28] (Fig. 12.18). Globoid cell leukodystrophy typically results in symmetrical white matter disease, mild hydrocephalus, and symmetrical contrast enhancement of the corpus callosum, internal capsule, and corona radiata.

Nutritional, Metabolic, and Toxic Disorders

There are a number of nutritional disorders that result in morphological signal change within the brain that are detectable with MR. Most commonly, nutritional, toxic, and metabolic disturbances are bilaterally symmetrical. There is considerable overlap in the MR features of many nutritional, metabolic, and toxic disorders, and this confounds the MR assessment. Generally, the presence of lesion symmetry should alert the reader to the possibility of such disorders. Subtle changes in attenuation may be visible with CT imaging; however, in a majority of cases, CT imaging is not sensitive enough and the study will be normal.

Thiamine deficiency results in bilaterally symmetric multifocal abnormalities affecting nuclei of brain and brainstem,

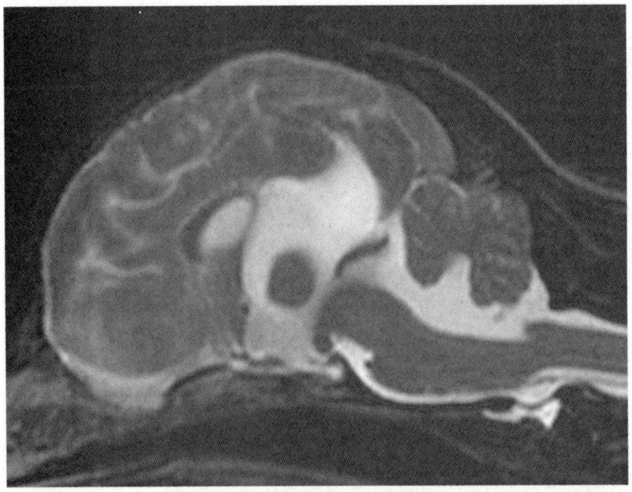

Fig. 12.15 Sagittal T2-weighted magnetic resonance (MR) image of a 2-year-old Chinese Crested dog. There is dysplasia of the caudal aspect of the corpus callosum and with subsequent enlargement of the third ventricle.

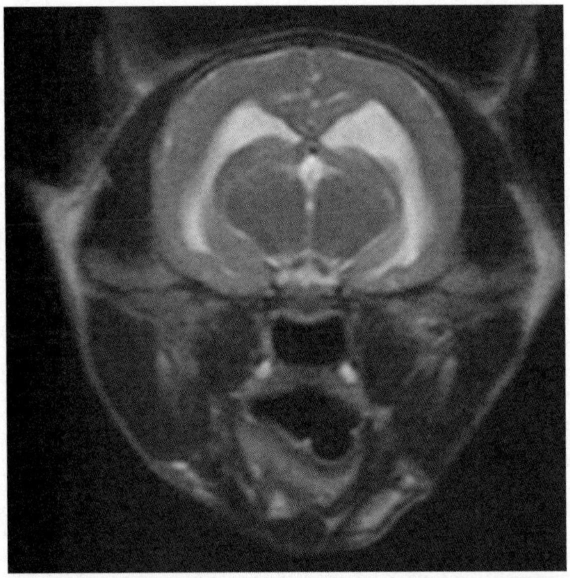

Fig. 12.16 T2 transverse magnetic resonance (MR) image of a 5-month-old domestic medium hair cat with seizures. The surface of the brain is excessively smooth, and there is a paucity of the normal sulci and gyri, which are changes commonly associated with lissencephaly.

including the lateral geniculate nuclei, caudal colliculi, vestibular nuclei, and others[29,30] (Fig. 12.19).

Bilaterally symmetrical T1 hyperintensity in the basal ganglia, specifically the lentiform nuclei, has been observed in human patients with hepatic insufficiency and those receiving total parenteral nutrition and specifically in cats and dogs with hepatic insufficiency associated with portosystemic shunts. The increase in T1 signal is thought due to a buildup of manganese, which is paramagnetic[31] (Fig. 12.20).

There are a number of metabolic disorders that result in intracranial changes that can be detected with MR. A full description of these is beyond the scope of this chapter. One example is subacute necrotizing encephalopathy, which has been documented in the Alaskan husky. This condition closely resembles Leigh syndrome in people and is an incapacitating, ultimately fatal neurodegenerative disorder.[32] The condition has been reported in the Bull terrier[33] and also the Yorkshire terrier. The disorder is characterized by degeneration and necrosis that manifests as bilaterally symmetrical regions of T2 and FLAIR hyperintensity within the central aspect of the thalamus. Additionally, focal T2 hyperintensity has been documented within the midbrain and medulla (Fig. 12.21).

Severe electrolyte disturbances in otherwise normal patients (unrelated to holoprosencephaly) can result in parenchymal changes that manifest with MR detectable changes. Severe hypernatremia can result in a number of symmetrical signal changes, most commonly a bilaterally symmetrical increase in T2 signal in signal at the junction of the internal capsule and lateral margin of the thalamus (Fig. 12.22). In people, this is an uncommon but important postpartum complication.[34]

Inflammatory Conditions

Encephalitis and meningoencephalitis can often be detected using MR, whereas changes may or may not be detectable with CT. Most commonly, cytologic and immunologic analysis of CSF is required to help establish a definitive diagnosis. Meningoencephalitis is typically either infectious or due to dysregulation of the patient's immune system—so-called *immune mediated.* The group of idiopathic noninfectious meningoencephalomyelitides (NIME) includes several subtypes, including steroid responsive meningitis-arteritis (SRMA), eosinophilic meningoencephalitis (EME), granulomatous meningoencephalomyelitis (GME), necrotizing meningoencephalomyelitis (NME), and necrotizing leucoencephalitis (NLE). As SRMA and EME have fairly distinct diagnostic characteristics, the term *meningitis of unknown etiology* (MUE) is used to describe the three specific subtypes that can only be confirmed based on histopathology. These include GME, NME, and NLE.[35]

Generally, immune-mediated brain disease is more common than infectious brain disease.[36] Small breed dogs are more likely to have an immune-mediated etiology and large breed dogs could have either infectious or immune-mediated disease. While there are some breed-specific predispositions and some disorders affect different regions of the brain more commonly, overall, the lesions are patchy or diffuse, T2 and FLAIR hyperintense, T1 iso or hypointense and have variable enhancement—ranging from no enhancement to intense enhancement (Fig. 12.23). The T2 and FLAIR hyperintensity could reflect focal pathology or perilesional edema. In chronic cases, regions of brain necrosis from any etiology may be present, sometimes manifesting as compensatory hydrocephalus, depending on the maturity of the lesion (Fig. 12.24). Encephalitis is often accompanied by meningitis, where there is increased meningeal contrast enhancement.[37] Contrast enhancement is best detected by comparing T1-weighted images acquired before and after contrast medium administration. Not acquiring the precontrast sequence or using different acquisition parameters will invalidate objective assessment of meningeal enhancement. Increased meningeal contrast enhancement and/or multifocal poorly delineated hypoattenuation of the brain tissue with no or mild contrast enhancement may be seen in CT imaging (Fig. 12.25).

Idiopathic hypertrophic pachymeningitis is an uncommon condition whereby there is marked nonspecific thickening and fibrosis of the pachymeninges without extension into the sulci. The Greyhound breed appears overrepresented, and the condition appears to have an immune etiology. The condition should be considered as a possible differential diagnosis for dogs with pachymeningeal thickening and marked enhancement with no identified underlying cause[37] (Fig. 12.26).

Infectious meningoencephalitis includes diseases caused by bacterial, viral, protozoal, rickettsial, fungal, parasitic, and algal agents.[36] Bacterial meningoencephalitis is uncommon and

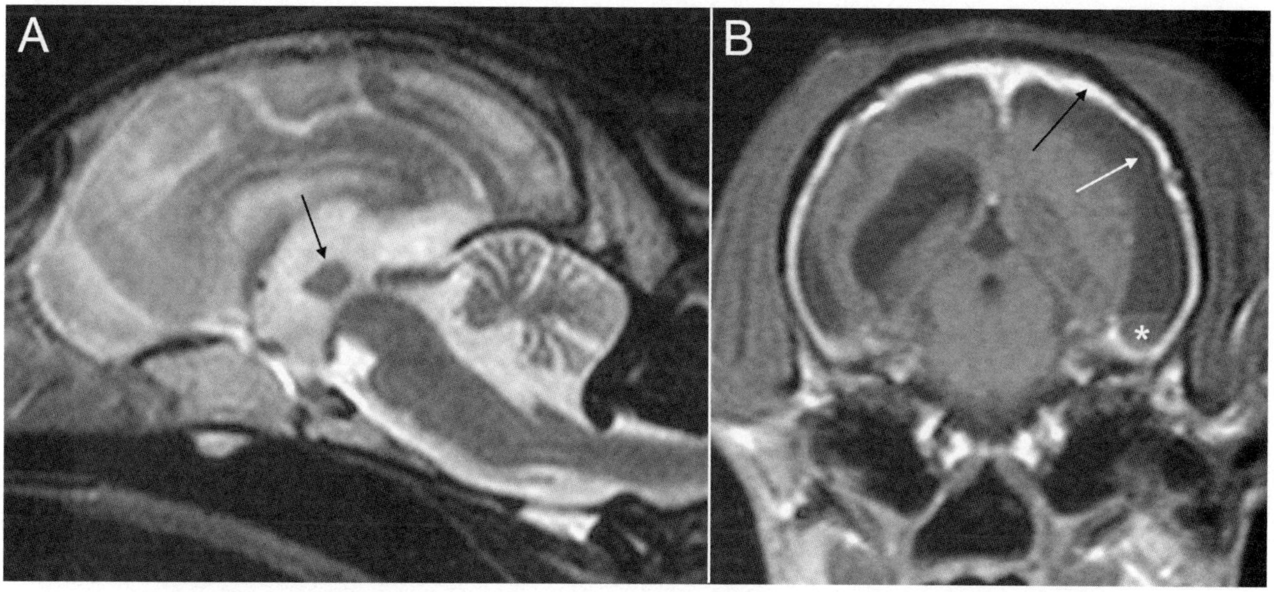

Fig. 12.17 Sagittal T2-weighted image **(A)** and T1-weighted postcontrast magnetic resonance (MR) image **(B)** of an 11-month-old Dachshund with cerebellar and vestibular signs since 6 months of age. Marked atrophy of the interthalamic adhesion is present in **A** (*black arrow*). Atrophy of the cerebellum is also readily evident. In **B**, there is marked pachymeningeal enhancement (*black arrow*) and a large accumulation of peripheral cerebrospinal fluid (CSF) (*white arrow*). A fluid line is evident in the peripheral fluid on the left (*asterisk*). In a gradient echo sequence, the debris in the ventral aspect of the peripheral fluid accumulation had a susceptibility artifact confirming it was hemorrhage. In these instances, hemorrhage is thought to be due to meningeal tearing with progressive brain atrophy.

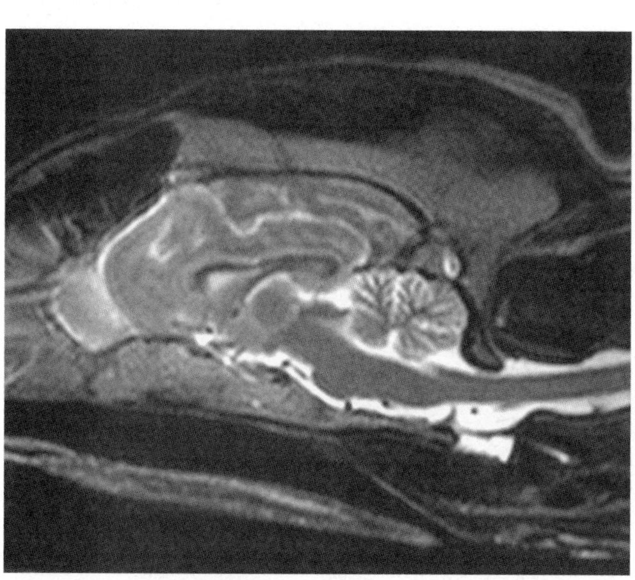

Fig. 12.18 Sagittal T2-weighted magnetic resonance (MR) image of a 4-year-old American bulldog with occasional tremors. Cerebrospinal fluid (CSF) surrounding the atrophic cerebellar folia makes the folia more conspicuous.

when present usually results from extension of a chronic middle ear infection, or chronic sinusitis, or hematogenously (Fig. 12.27). Intracranial feline infectious peritonitis usually causes ependymitis, resulting in marked contrast enhancement of the lining of the ventricular system (Fig. 12.28). Toxoplasmosis and *Neospora* are important infectious disease differentials. Feline ischemic encephalopathy is caused by seasonal transnasal aberrant migration of a *Cuterebra* larva[38,39] (Fig. 12.29). Fungal infections can be region specific and most commonly involve *Cryptococcus neoformans* (feline), *Blastomyces dermatitidis*, and *Coccidioides immitis* and usually manifest as solitary or multifocal T2 hyperintense lesions with variable enhancement.

A normal MR or CT study does not rule out the possibility of inflammatory disease, and evaluation of CSF is required. In 25 patients with CSF alterations consistent with inflammatory brain disease, 24% of the MR studies were normal.[37]

MISCELLANEOUS DISORDERS

Reversible seizure-associated brain edema is typically characterized by nonenhancing T2 and FLAIR hyperintensity with negligible mass effect in patients with a recent history of extensive seizures. The regions most commonly affected are the piriform and temporal lobes.[40] Typically, the changes are bilateral, but changes can also be unilateral and occur elsewhere, including the region of the cingulate gyrus (Fig. 12.30).

Otitis media and interna are important differentials for nystagmus and head tilt. The assessment of inner ear disease is a practical application of using signal differences between T2 and FLAIR sequences to establish a diagnosis.[41] Normal inner ear fluid is T2 hyperintense and should null completely in the T2 FLAIR sequence, similar to CSF. Incomplete nulling suggests altered inner ear fluid content, as occurs with otitis interna (Fig. 12.31). As with all patients with aural disease, close interrogation of the osseous structures and neuroparenchyma is important.

BRAIN NEOPLASIA

Extra-Axial Tumors

Meningiomas are extra-axial tumors of dural origin. They are the most common intracranial tumor in cats and one of the most common in dogs. Meningiomas are usually benign and

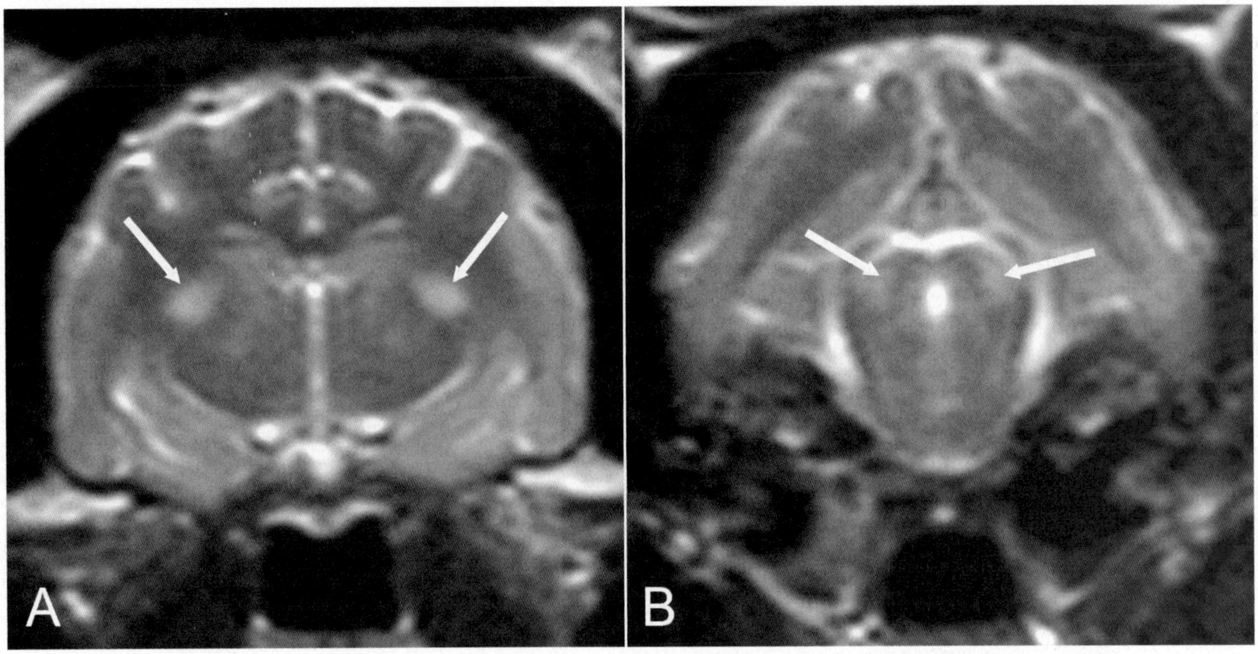

Fig. 12.19 T2-weighted transverse magnetic resonance (MR) images of a 6-year-old domestic short hair cat presenting with a recent history of seizures, ataxia, and vestibular signs. There is bilaterally symmetrical T2 hyperintensity at the level of the thalamus (**A,** *white arrows*) and also in the colliculi (**B,** *white arrows*) due to thiamine deficiency.

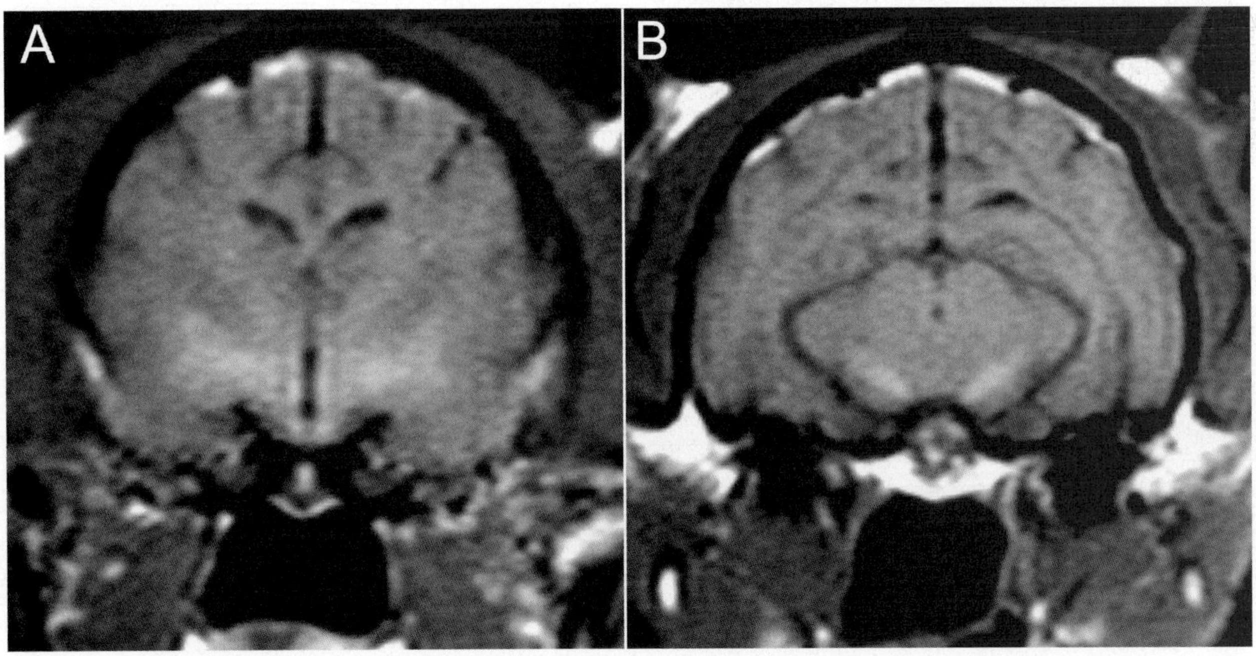

Fig. 12.20 T1-weighted transverse magnetic resonance (MR) images of a 5-year-old domestic short hair cat, at the level of the basal ganglia **(A)** and **(B)** lentiform nuclei. The T1 hyperintensity is thought due to manganese deposition secondary to a portosystemic shunt.

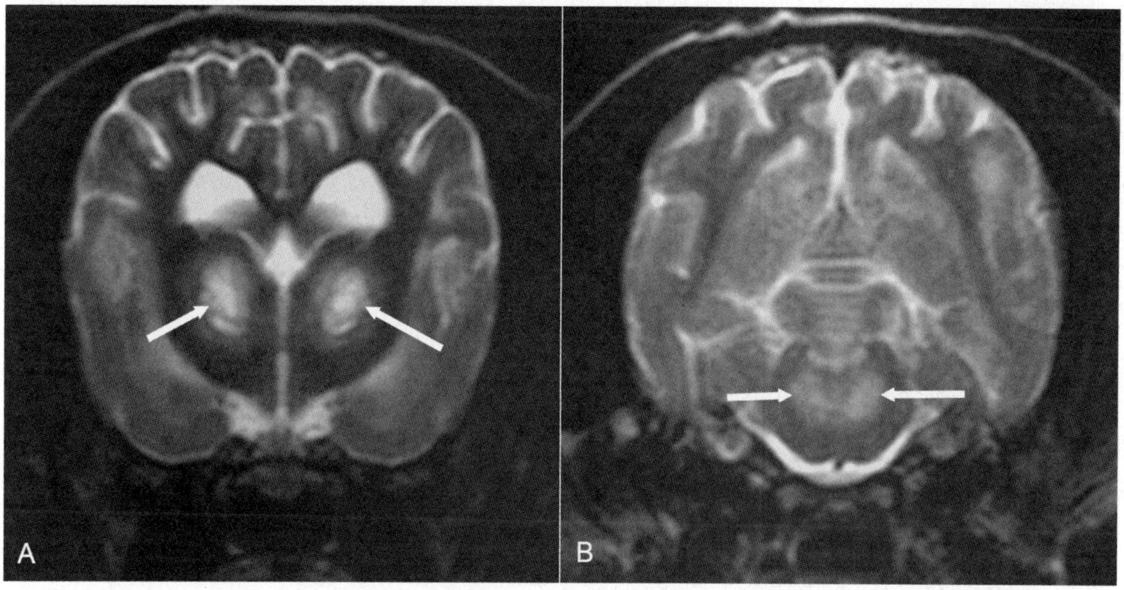

Fig. 12.21 T2-weighted transverse magnetic resonance (MR) image at the level of the thalamus **(A)** and the level of the medulla **(B)** in a 1-year-old Yorkshire terrier. There is bilaterally symmetrical T2 hyperintensity within the central aspect of the thalamus bilaterally (**A**, *white arrows*). There is a bilaterally symmetrical increase in T2 signal intensity within the brainstem at the level of the rostral aspect of the cerebellum (**B**, *white arrows*). Final diagnosis was subacute necrotizing encephalopathy.

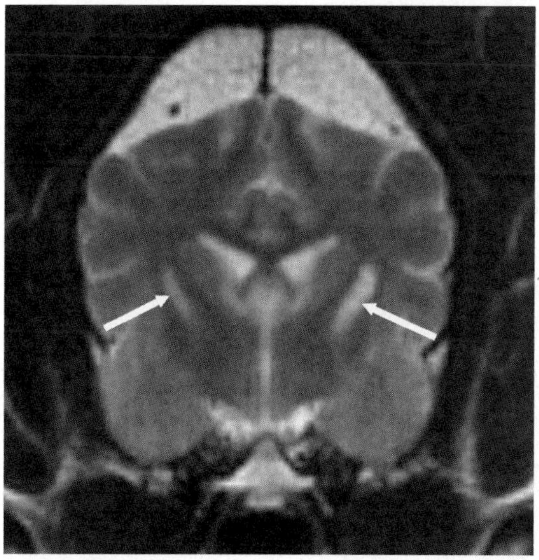

Fig. 12.22 T2-weighed transverse magnetic resonance (MR) image of a 7-year-old mixed-breed dog presenting comatose. The patient was reportedly normal 3 hours earlier. This patient has marked hypernatremia of unknown etiology and responded to fluid therapy. There is bilaterally symmetrical T2 hyperintensity in the white matter tracks adjacent to the thalamus (*white arrow*). The serum sodium in this patient on presentation was more than 180 mEq/L. The changes present in this patient are similar to those reported in people and are sometimes referred to as the *wine glass sign*. (Courtesy Jeff Clarke, DVM, DACVIM [neurology].)

grow slowly. They are variable in size and shape and may be irregular, nodular, ovoid, lobulated, or plaque-like (Fig. 12.31), ranging from a few millimeters to several centimeters in diameter. Meningiomas are often firm and encapsulated, are usually discrete, and may contain mineralization or pockets of fluid (Fig. 12.32). Basal and plaque-like meningiomas are common in the floor of the cranial cavity, especially in the optic chiasm and suprasellar regions. They also occur commonly over the cerebral hemispheres, less commonly in the cerebello-pontomedullary region, and rarely in the retrobulbar space, arising from the optic nerve. Multiple meningiomas can occur; this is more common in cats than in dogs. Thickening of bone adjacent to meningiomas, termed *hyperostosis*, may occur, especially in cats (Fig. 12.33). Meningiomas can usually be distinguished from intra-axial tumors because meningiomas are usually peripherally located, or falx-associated broad-based masses that enhance following contrast-medium administration in both CT and MR imaging (see Fig. 12.33). Meningiomas are also often associated with linear contrast enhancement of thickened dura mater adjacent to an extra-axial mass, termed a *dural tail*. In one study, the predictive value of the dural tail sign for meningioma was 94%.[6] It is uncertain whether the dural tail represents neoplastic infiltration beyond the margins of the meningioma or a manifestation of associated inflammation. The amount of disruption to adjacent parenchyma is variable, depending on tumor size and location. Some meningiomas have minimal peripheral edema, although others may have extensive peripheral edema that can result in ventricular compression and brain herniation. An important differential for meningeal enhancement/masses is round cell neoplasia (histiocytic sarcoma and lymphoma).

Choroid Plexus Tumors and Ependymomas

Choroid plexus tumors most commonly occur in the third ventricle and in the lateral recess of the fourth ventricle. The choroid plexus epithelium originates from differentiation of the primitive medullary epithelium and is embryologically related to ependymal cells. Choroid plexus tumors have a tendency to bleed, and exfoliation of choroid plexus cells, from both benign and malignant variants, may occur with subsequent tumor seeding to other areas of the brain or spinal cord through the CSF.[42] Because of the intraventricular location of choroid plexus tumors, obstructive hydrocephalus is common and may be life-threatening. Additionally, some choroid plexus tumors will cause an overproduction of CSF, which exacerbates any

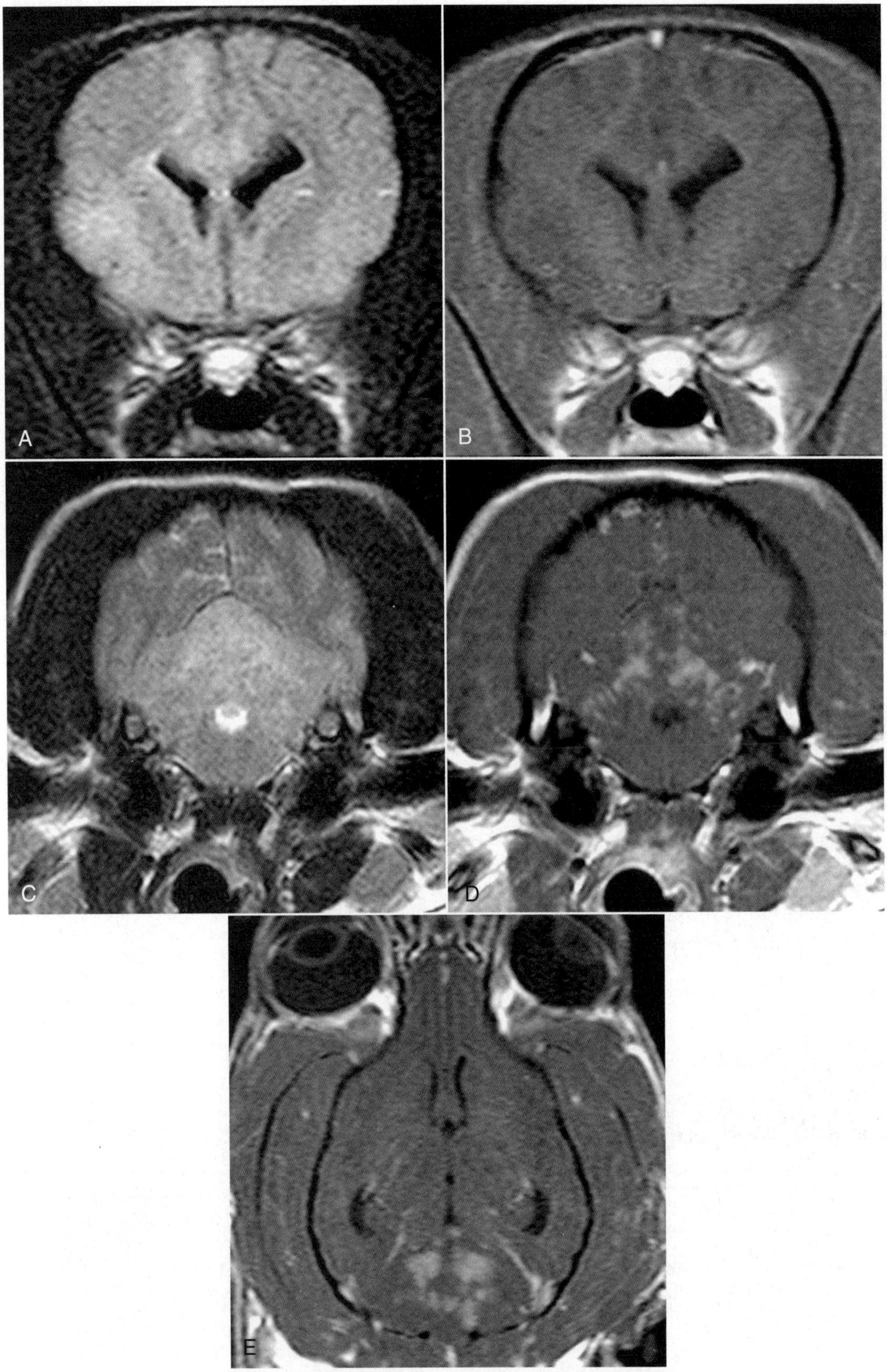

Fig. 12.23 A T2–fluid-attenuated inversion recovery (FLAIR) **(A)** and postcontrast T1-weighted magnetic resonance (MR) image **(B)** of a 4-year-old pug with a history of seizures of progressing severity over a 4-day period. Patchy, ill-defined regions of T2 hyperintensity are present in the right cerebral cortex, most severe in the temporal and parietal lobes. There is minimal mass effect. These regions are mildly T1 hypointense and do not enhance. The most common considerations for these findings are encephalitis, necrotizing encephalitis, and cerebral infarct. On the basis of breed, progressive clinical signs, multifocal distribution of lesions, cerebrospinal fluid (CSF) analysis, and MR findings, necrotizing encephalitis is the most likely diagnosis. **C,** A T2-weighted transverse MR image at the level of the cerebellum, a T1-weighted postcontrast transverse image **(D)** made at the same level as **C,** and a dorsal T1-weighted postcontrast image **(E).** This is a 9-year-old miniature poodle with confirmed granulomatous meningoencephalitis (GME). An ill-defined region of T2-hyperintensity is present in the central aspect of the cerebellum. Multiple patchy regions of contrast enhancement are visible within the cerebellum, as are additional multifocal regions of contrast enhancement, primarily within the corona radiata. The MR findings with GME are variable, and some lesions have minimal contrast enhancement.

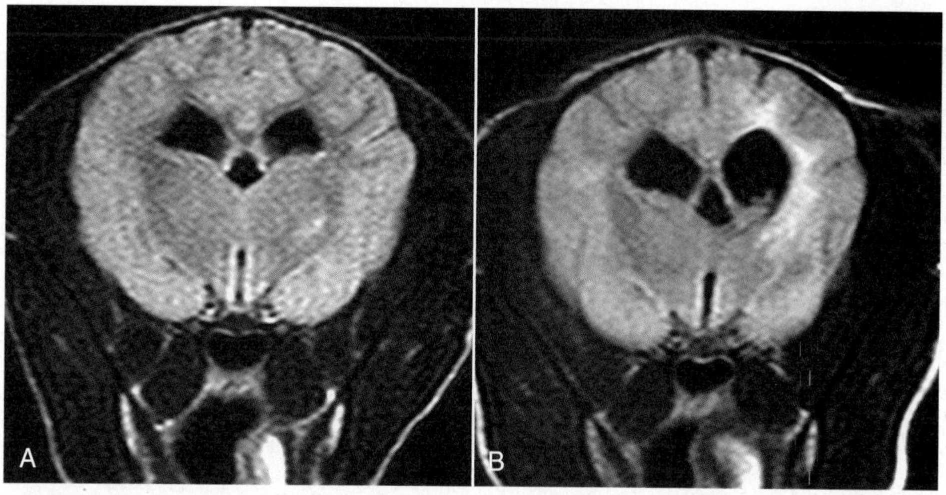

Fig. 12.24 Transverse T2–fluid-attenuated inversion recovery (FLAIR) magnetic resonance (MR) image **(A)** of a 2-year-old Yorkshire terrier and a follow-up image **(B)** at the same level acquired 18 months later. **A,** At presentation, a diagnosis of necrotizing encephalitis was made based on signalment, clinical findings, MR findings, and cerebrospinal fluid (CSF) analysis. In **A**, the ventricular system is mildly enlarged but symmetric. In the later study **B,** the lateral ventricles are larger, asymmetric, and there is a midline shift to the left, toward the side of the larger ventricle. T2 hyperintensity is present in the white matter lateral to the left lateral ventricle. It is likely the ventricular enlargement and midline shift are secondary to parenchymal necrosis; this is often referred to as *compensatory hydrocephalus*. The T2 hyperintensity in **B** did not enhance and, in this patient, reflects unresolved neuropil inflammation.

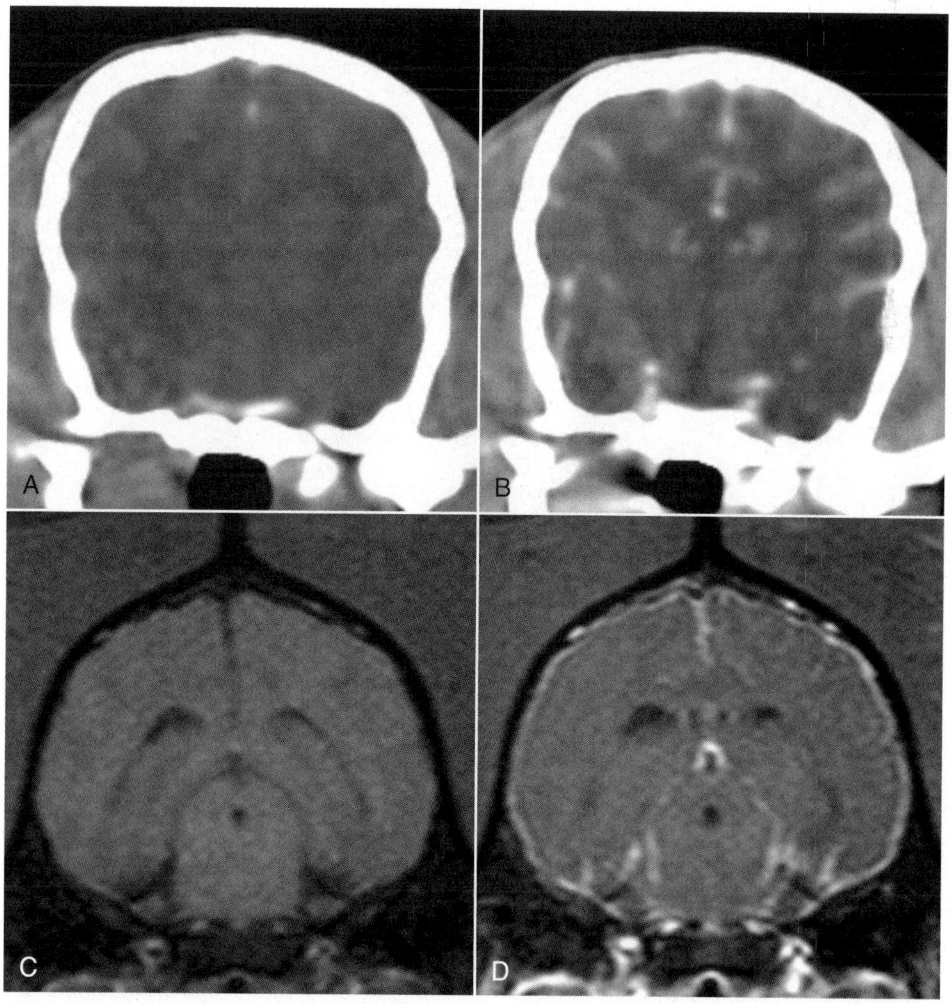

Fig. 12.25 Pre **(A)** and **(B)** postcontrast medium administration transverse computed tomography (CT) images of a 7-year-old Maltese dog with severe meningitis. The meningeal enhancement is readily evident in post-contrast images **(B)**. Pre **(C)** and **(D)** postcontrast medium transverse fat saturation magnetic resonance (MR) images of a 5-year-old Labrador with a 4 day history of lethargy, inappetence, ataxia, and dull mentation. There is severe meningeal enhancement. The final (necropsy) diagnosis was immune-mediated lymphoplasmocytic meningoencephalitis.

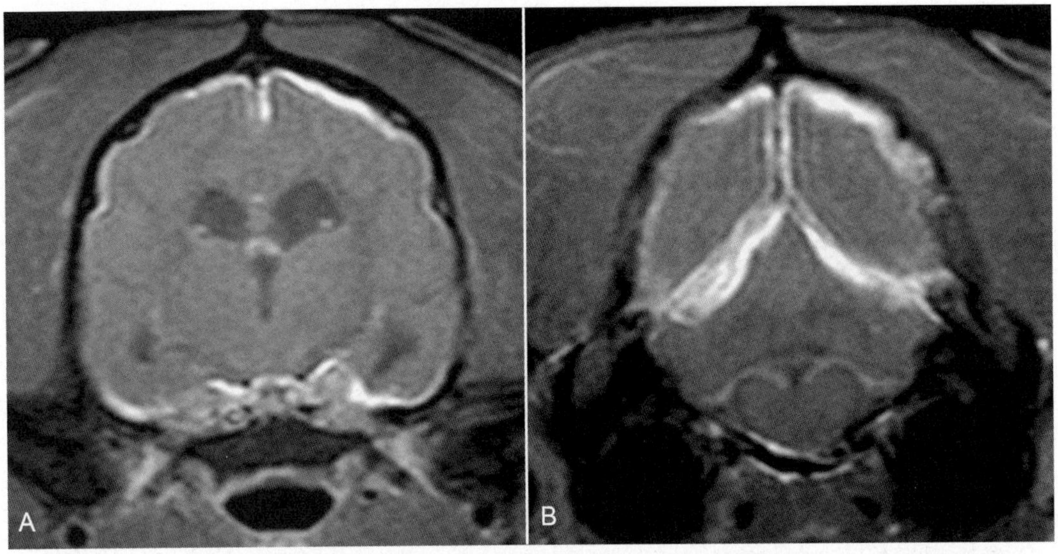

Fig. 12.26 T1-weighted transverse image at level of caudal aspect of the pituitary fossa **(A)** and lateral aperture of the fourth ventricle **(B)** acquired post intravenous contrast medium administration of a 5-year-old Greyhound with a history of progressive cervical pain over many months. There is marked enhancement of the pachymeninges/dura but not of the sulci. The final diagnosis was idiopathic hypertrophic pachymeningitis.

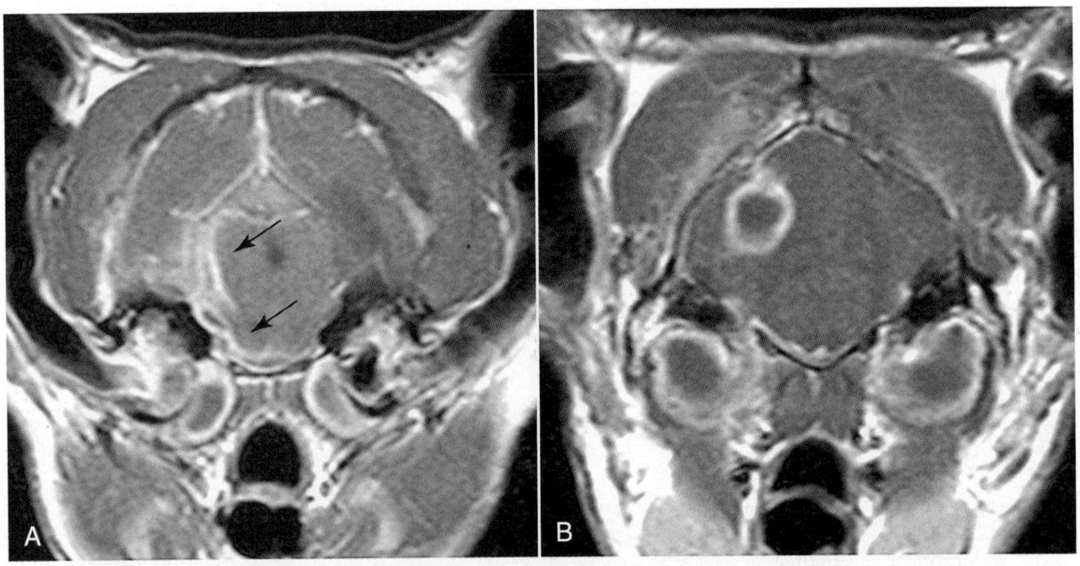

Fig. 12.27 Adjacent transverse T1-weighted postcontrast magnetic resonance (MR) images in a 5-year-old cat with a head tilt and otitis externa. Increased signal intensity in both tympanic bullae is visible. The lining of the bullae is enhanced, but material within either bulla does not enhance. This is consistent with inflammation (exudate in bullae). The meninges adjacent to the right tympanic bulla are characterized by marked contrast enhancement (*arrows* in **A**), and a ring-enhancing mass is present in the right aspect of the cerebellum **(B).** The imaging findings are attributable to otitis media and otitis interna that has progressed to meningoencephalitis and cerebellar abscess.

obstructive process. CSF overproduction can result in massive dilation of the downstream central canal. An important distinguishing feature of choroid plexus tumors is that they are located within a ventricle (Fig. 12.34). Like meningiomas, choroid plexus tumors usually have marked contrast enhancement and sometimes have evidence of hemorrhage and/or dystrophic mineralization. The MR characteristics of intraventricular ependymomas are similar to choroid plexus tumors, but ependymomas are much less common.

Pituitary Tumors

Pituitary tumors are common in dogs but uncommon in cats. They may be nonfunctional or functional. Functional pituitary tumors are typically characterized by pituitary-dependent hyperadrenocorticism (PDH). Up to 60% of dogs with PDH but without neurologic signs have a pituitary tumor 4 to 12 mm in diameter at greatest vertical height.[42] Most pituitary tumors tend to grow dorsocaudally, leading to compression and obliteration of the infundibulum, ventral aspect of the third

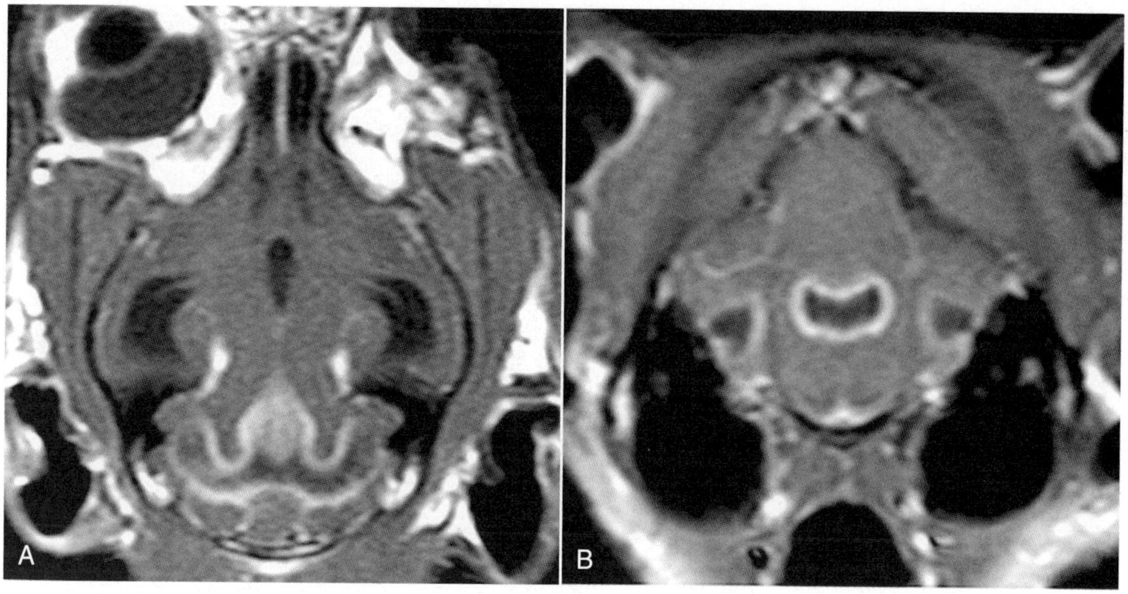

Fig. 12.28 Dorsal **(A)** and transverse **(B)** T1-weighted postcontrast magnetic resonance (MR) images of a cat with feline infectious peritonitis. Intense contrast enhancement of the lining of the ventricular system is present. This is consistent with ependymitis, a common finding in feline infectious peritonitis. The left eye is absent, removed previously as a result of trauma.

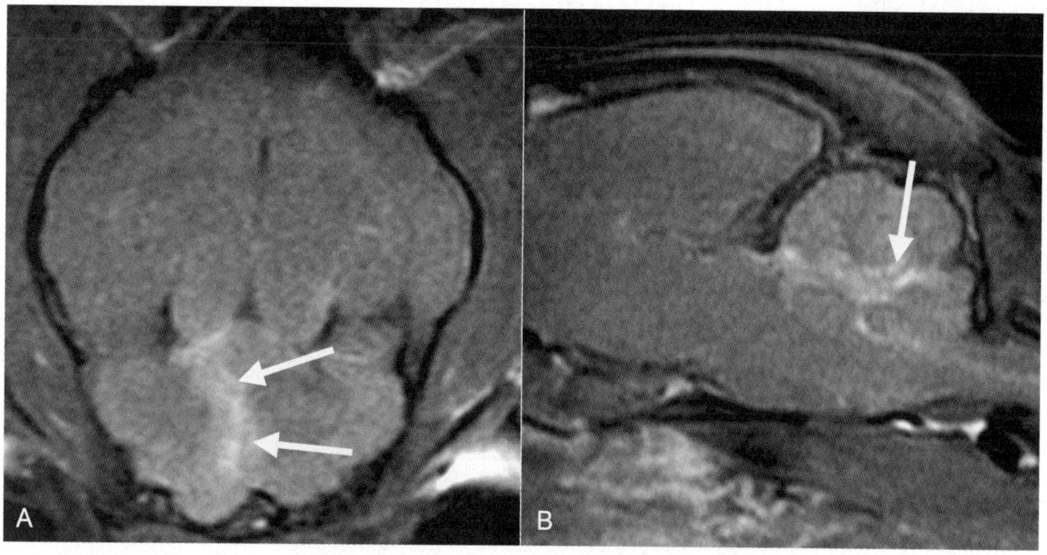

Fig. 12.29 T1-weighted postcontrast dorsal **(A)** and sagittal **(B)** magnetic resonance (MR) images of a 5-year-old indoor/outdoor cat with a recent history of being missing for some days. She was ataxic, anorexic, and depressed. A presumptive diagnosis of feline ischemic encephalopathy (Cuterebra larval migration) was made based on numerous tests, the MR imaging findings and clinical course. There was a curvilinear enhancing region in the frontal lobe (not shown) and a somewhat linear tract of enhancement in the cerebellum (*white arrows*). (Courtesy Heather Jones DVM, DACVIM [neurology].)

ventricle, hypothalamus, and thalamus. They eventually impinge on the internal capsule and optic tracts. MR is useful for visualizing the presence of both microtumors (3–10 mm in diameter) and macrotumors (>10 mm) in dogs with PDH, with or without neurologic signs, especially when endocrine test results are equivocal. Pituitary tumors are always better visualized after contrast medium administration. Usually these tumors have minimal peritumoral edema, uniform contrast enhancement, and well-defined margins (Fig. 12.35). Cystic regions, or evidence of chronic or recent hemorrhage, sometimes extensive, may be present. Pituitary tumors less than 3 mm in diameter may not be visible with MR.

Intra-Axial Tumors: Glioma

Gliomas arise from the neuropil and include astrocytomas, oligodendrogliomas, and glioblastoma multiforme and are particularly common in brachycephalic breeds, such as the Boxer, Boston terrier, and bulldog. Gliomas range in malignancy from

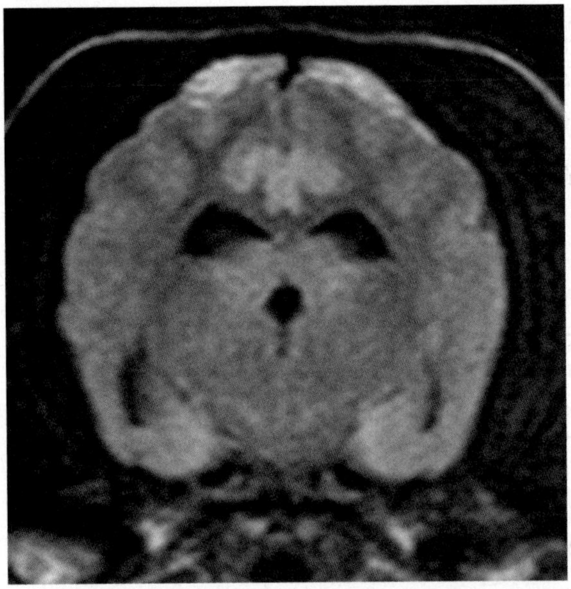

Fig. 12.30 Transverse fluid-attenuated inversion recovery (FLAIR) magnetic resonance (MR) sequence of an 8-year-old beagle with a recent onset of severe cluster seizures. There is FLAIR hyperintensity in the region of the cingulate gyrus, hippocampus, and piriform lobe, bilaterally. The final diagnosis was cryptogenic epilepsy.

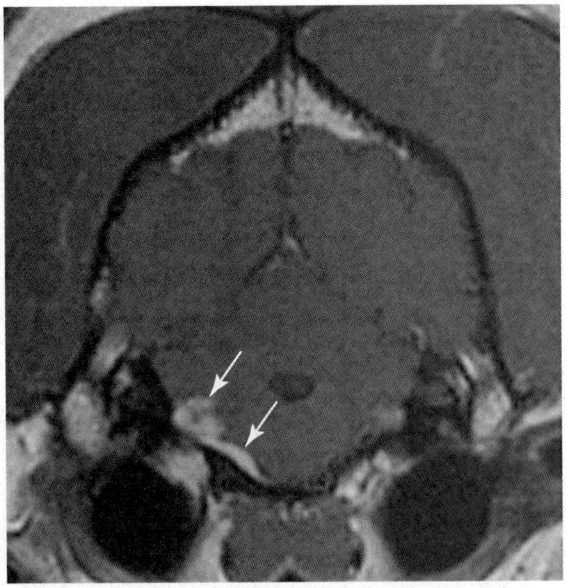

Fig. 12.32 Transverse T1-weighted postcontrast magnetic resonance (MR) image of an 11-year-old Golden retriever. The linear meningeal enhancement (*white arrows*) is a plaque meningioma. Mild ipsilateral temporal muscle atrophy is present, caused by disruption to the adjacent trigeminal nerve nucleus.

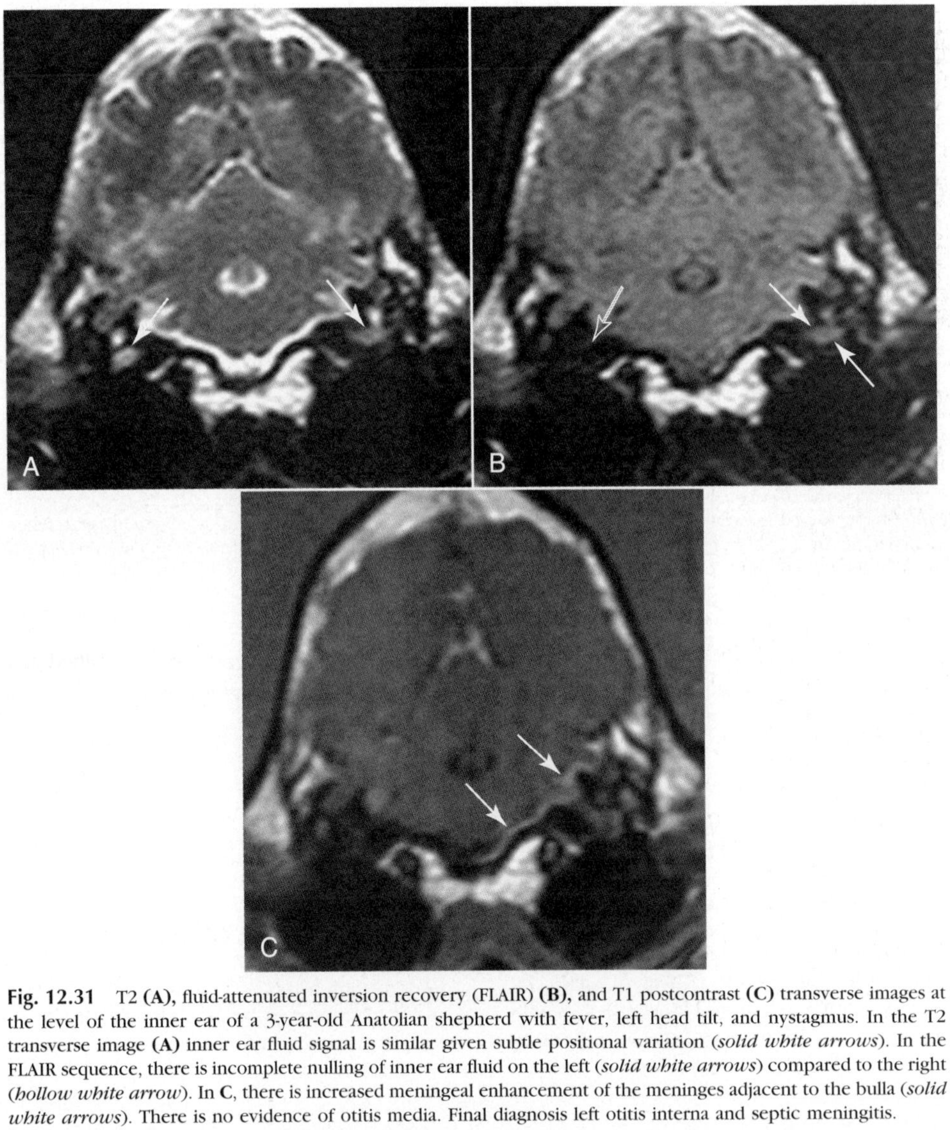

Fig. 12.31 T2 **(A)**, fluid-attenuated inversion recovery (FLAIR) **(B)**, and T1 postcontrast **(C)** transverse images at the level of the inner ear of a 3-year-old Anatolian shepherd with fever, left head tilt, and nystagmus. In the T2 transverse image **(A)** inner ear fluid signal is similar given subtle positional variation (*solid white arrows*). In the FLAIR sequence, there is incomplete nulling of inner ear fluid on the left (*solid white arrows*) compared to the right (*hollow white arrow*). In **C**, there is increased meningeal enhancement of the meninges adjacent to the bulla (*solid white arrows*). There is no evidence of otitis media. Final diagnosis left otitis interna and septic meningitis.

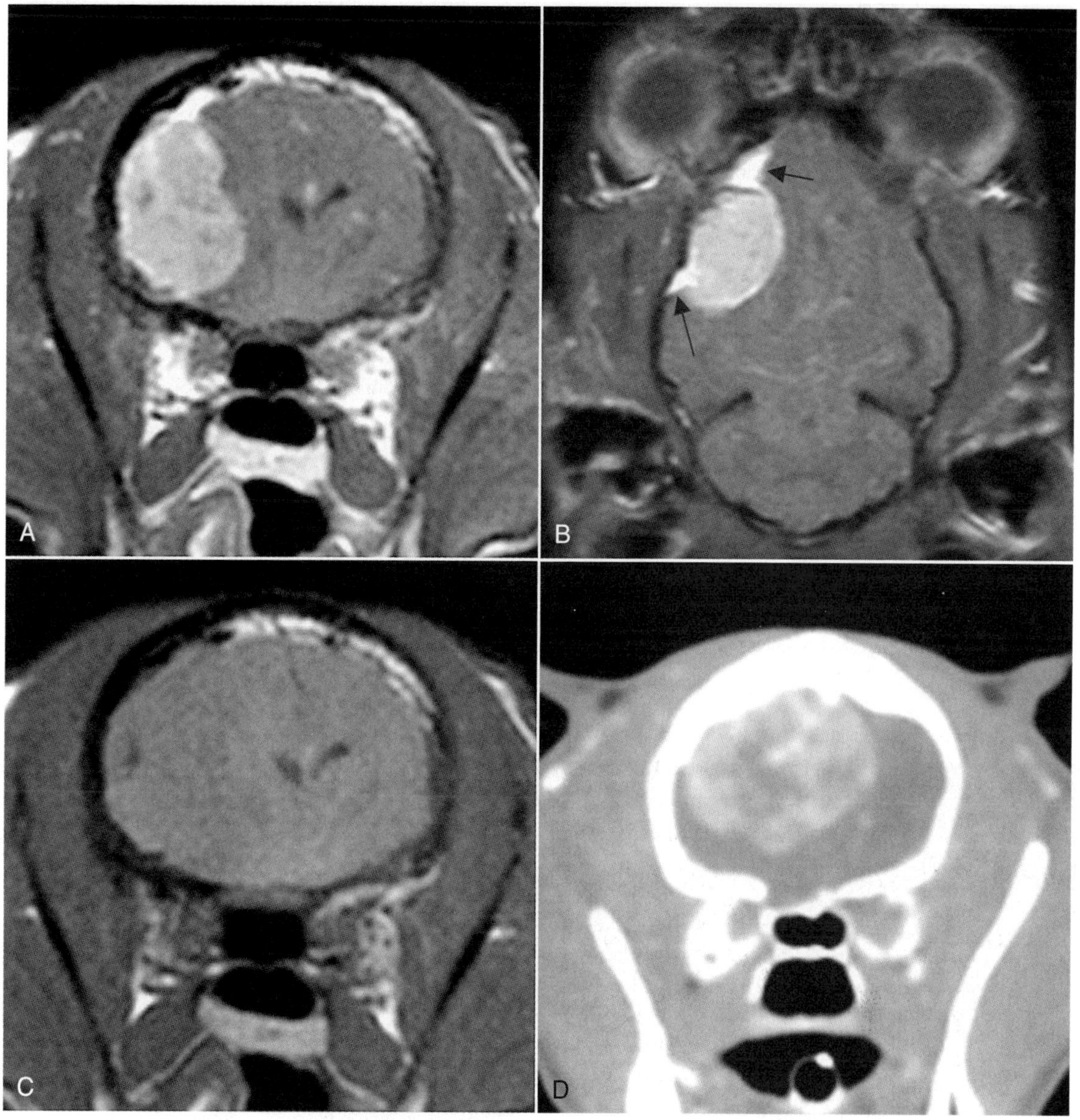

Fig. 12.33 Transverse **(A)** and dorsal **(B)** postcontrast T1-weighted magnetic resonance (MR) images of a feline meningioma. A broad peripheral base and contrast enhancement of the adjacent meninges (*arrows* in **B**) are visible. Dural enhancement in this pattern is termed the *dural tail sign*. **C,** A precontrast T1-weighted transverse image. A midline shift to the left has occurred, and the calvarium on the right is thickened, with replacement of the T1-hyperintense marrow fat with T1-hypointense bone. Calvarial hyperostosis is seen commonly with feline meningioma. **D,** transverse postcontrast computed tomography (CT) image of a feline meningioma. The mass is heterogeneously contrast enhancing and causes a severe midline shift.

low grade and slow growing, to high grade, poorly differentiated highly malignant tumors.

Gliomas vary widely in their MR features. They are often difficult to detect using contrast-enhanced CT imaging of the brain because, unlike meningiomas, many gliomas do not enhance, or enhance only minimally, are often ill-defined, and have varying degrees of perilesional edema (Fig. 12.36). Occasionally, contrast enhancement is not present. A glioma can be difficult to differentiate from a brain abscess and other focal inflammatory conditions of the brain parenchyma,[6] or even from massive infarction.

Gliomatosis cerebri is a rare neoplasm characterized by diffuse and widespread infiltration of the central nervous system by neoplastic glial cells with relative preservation of the neural tissue architecture. It is classified as a malignant (grade III) neuroepithelial tumor of astrocytic origin.[43,44] The MR findings are nonspecific, mimicking many more common conditions, including encephalitis, leukodystrophies, and metabolic encephalopathies. Typically, there may be a diffuse increase in T2 and FLAIR signal throughout regions of the cerebrum with some mass effect but overall relative preservation of the neural morphology and minimal contrast enhancement (Fig. 12.37).

Cranial Nerve Tumors

The terminology given to cranial and spinal nerve and nerve root tumors is confusing because of differing opinions regarding their cell of origin. Although schwannoma, neurilemmoma, and neurofibroma are used interchangeably, the

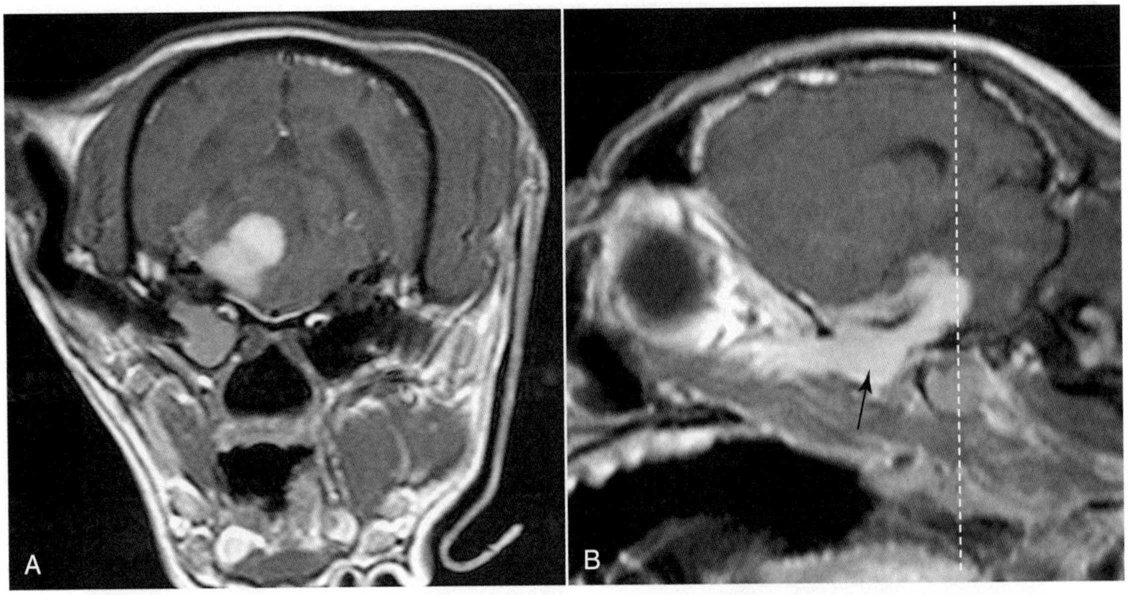

Fig. 12.38 Transverse **(A)** and sagittal **(B)** T1-weighted postcontrast magnetic resonance (MR) images. There is marked atrophy of the temporal musculature on the right side, and an intensely contrast-enhancing tubular mass emanates from the right ventral aspect of the pons and courses rostrally through an enlarged orbital fissure (*arrow* in **B**) to the retrobulbar region. The *vertical dashed line* in **B** designates the location of the transverse image seen in **A.** Final diagnosis was trigeminal nerve sheath tumor. Incidentally, fluid is present in the right tympanic cavity.

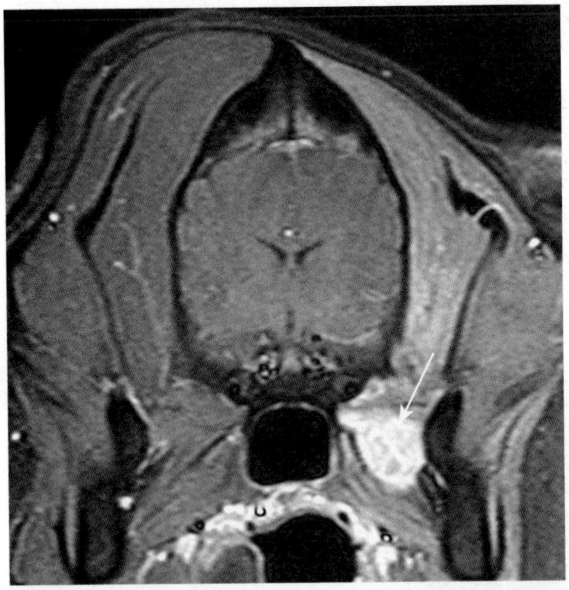

Fig. 12.39 Transverse T1-weighted postcontrast magnetic resonance (MR) image of a 10-year-old mixed-breed dog with left temporal muscle atrophy. In this image, the inherent bright signal from fat has been suppressed, and this increases the conspicuity of the extracranial trigeminal nerve tumor (*arrow*) in this patient. There is increased enhancement of the atrophic left temporal muscles compared to the right. This is commonly seen in muscles affected by neurogenic atrophy and thought to be associated with alterations in autonomic control of vascular and capillary bed secondary to denervation.

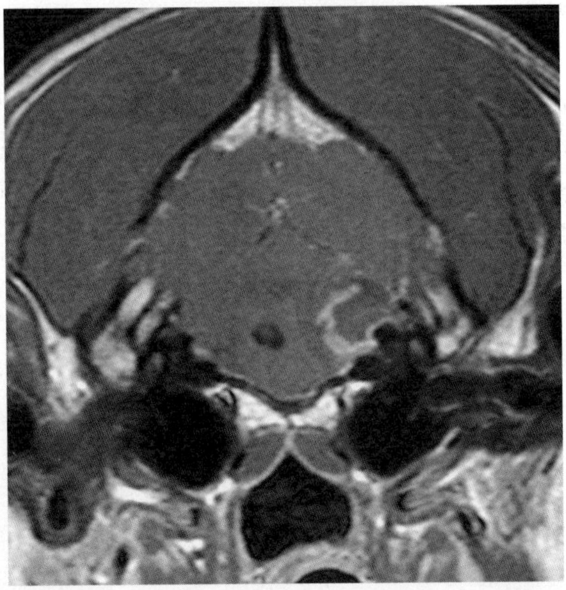

Fig. 12.40 Transverse T1-weighted postcontrast magnetic resonance (MR) image of a 7-year-old Golden retriever. There is a peripherally contrast-enhancing mass at the cerebellopontine angle that appears similar to a cystic meningioma. Extensive peripheral edema and brainstem compression was evident on other sequences. The final diagnosis was histiocytic sarcoma.

noninfectious middle ear effusion, thought due to neurogenic dysfunction of the eustachian tube.[47]

Other Primary Tumors and Metastatic Tumors

A complete review of brain tumors reported in dogs and cats is beyond the scope of this text, and excellent reviews are available.[42,48] Histiocytic sarcoma is an uncommon extra-axial tumor that has imaging characteristics similar to meningioma, including a dural tail[49] (Fig. 12.40); histiocytic sarcoma can also be intra-axial.[50] Meningeal enhancement remote from the tumor epicenter is not an uncommon finding (Fig. 12.41).

Lymphoma is a common tumor both in dogs and cats, manifesting in many ways. With respect to intracranial

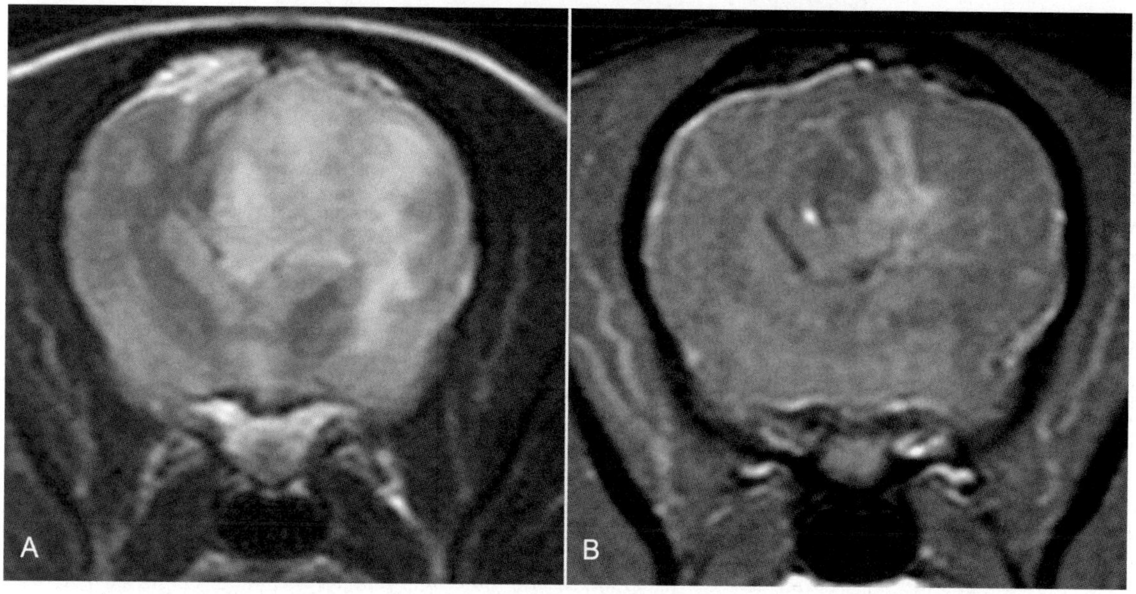

Fig. 12.41 Transverse fluid-attenuated inversion recovery (FLAIR) **(A)** and T1-weighted postcontrast magnetic resonance (MR) image **(B)** at the level of the pituitary gland. The patient is a 12-year-old Schipperke with a recent onset of seizures, depression, and syncope. There is extensive primarily left parietal lobe white matter edema with ventricular compression and a paradoxical midline shift. There is amorphous regional parenchymal enhancement in the region of the presumed mass. The final diagnosis was histiocytic sarcoma. Meningeal enhancement remote from the lesion (in this case right dorsolateral) is not an uncommon finding with histiocytic sarcoma.

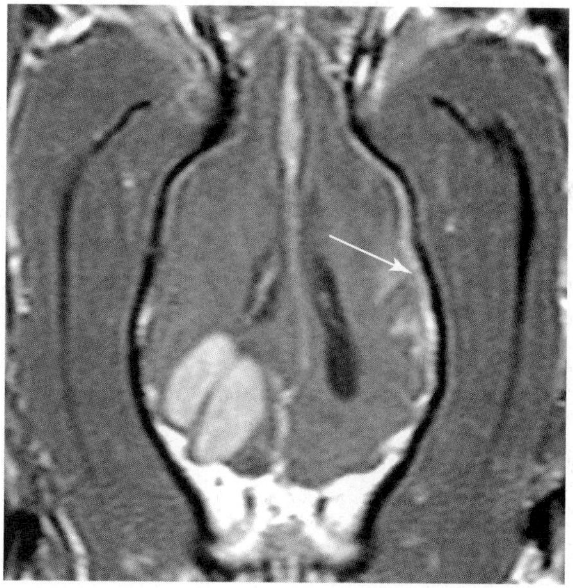

Fig. 12.42 Dorsal T1-weighted postcontrast magnetic resonance (MR) image of a 4-year-old Labrador retriever with lymphoma. There is a lobulated intensely contrasting mass in the occipital lobe that is causing ventricular compression and a leftward shift of midline structures. There is thickening of both the peripheral meninges (particularly on the left, *arrow*) and the falx (rostrally). Mass lesions and meningeal infiltration are common manifestations of intracranial lymphoma in both cats and dogs.

lymphoma, it can be solitary or present in multiple other organs. Typically, lymphoma has at least moderate enhancement and can be asymmetric in distribution (Fig. 12.42) or bilaterally symmetrical (Fig. 12.43).

In one study,[29] brain metastases were as common as primary intracranial tumors, with hemangiosarcoma being the most common metastatic lesion (Fig. 12.44). The brain is not immune to metastases, and secondary intracranial neoplasia is common.

Invasive Extracranial Tumors

Aggressive nasal tumors can extend through the cribriform plate, caudal nasal region, or frontal sinus into the cranial vault, and it is important to include the caudal aspect of the nasal

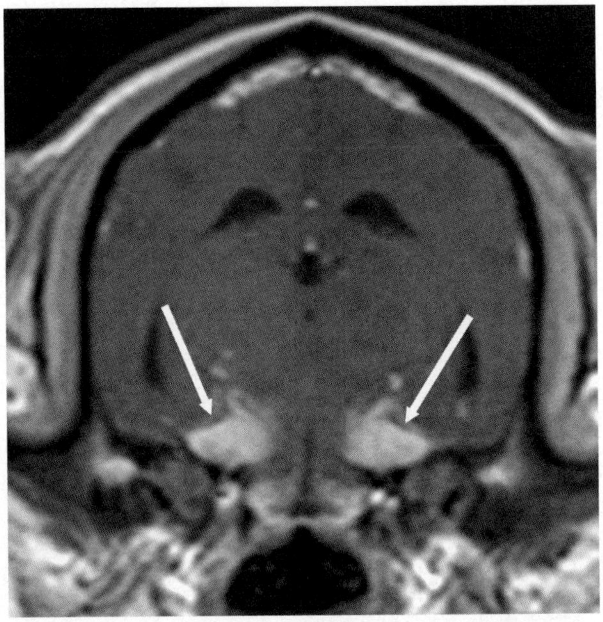

Fig. 12.43 Transverse T1-weighted postcontrast magnetic resonance (MR) image (fat saturation not applied) of a 6-year-old Jack Russell terrier with bilateral temporal muscle wasting and multiple cranial nerve deficits. The image is at the level of the midbrain. There was marked enhancement extending along the floor of the calvarium bilaterally (*white arrows*). Temporalis muscle wasting and enhancement are evident. Bilateral otitis media is also present, likely secondary to dysfunction of the levator veli palatini muscle. The final diagnosis was lymphoma.

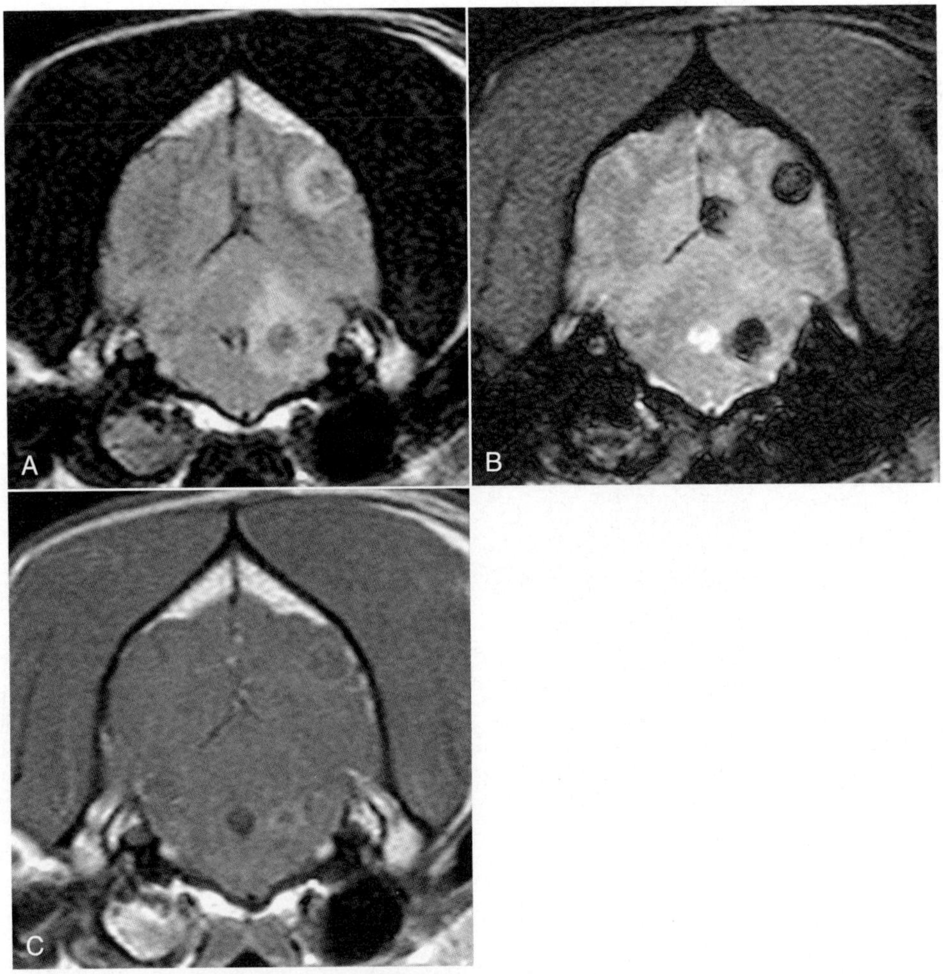

Fig. 12.44 Transverse T2–fluid-attenuated inversion recovery (FLAIR) **(A)**, gradient recalled echo (GRE) **(B)**, and T1-weighted postcontrast **(C)** magnetic resonance (MR) images of a 9-year-old Golden retriever with metastatic hemangiosarcoma. In **A**, there are two focal hypointense regions with surrounding T2 hyperintensity, presumably edema, in the left occipital lobe and left ventral cerebellum. Minimal mass effect is present. Both lesions have mild peripheral contrast enhancement **(C)** and a susceptibility artifact **(B)** indicating hemorrhage. In **B**, a susceptibility artifact is also present adjacent to the osseous tentorium. This is the border of a similar "out-of-plane" lesion. The imaging characteristics are consistent with both hemorrhagic infarction of some days' duration (approximately >3) and hemorrhagic tumor foci but in this dog were proven to be metastasis. Incidentally, there is right otitis media.

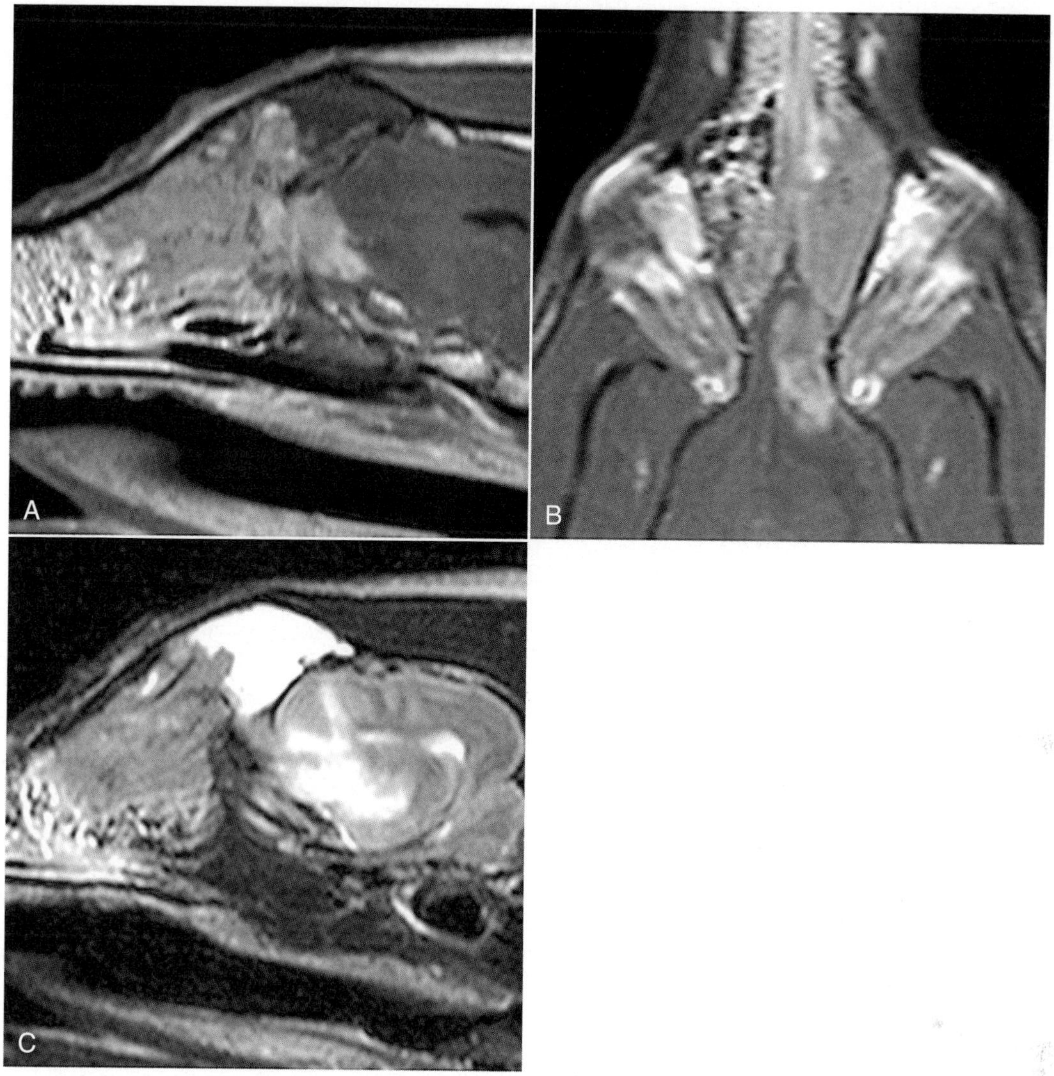

Fig. 12.45 T1-weighted sagittal **(A)**, dorsal **(B)**, and a T2-weighted sagittal magnetic resonance (MR) image **(C)** of an elderly dog with intermittent epistaxis. A mass is present in the caudal aspect of the left nasal cavity, which extends into the right nasal cavity and also into the rostral fossa. The material in the left frontal sinus is T2 hyperintense **(C)** and T1 isointense **(A)** and does not enhance. On the basis of these signal characteristics, the frontal sinus lesion is more likely to be trapped fluid rather than tumor. Distinguishing mass from trapped fluid cannot be made as easily with contrast-enhanced computed tomography (CT). In the T2-weighted image, extensive white-matter edema is visible as a result of the intracranial extension. The histologic diagnosis was carcinoma.

cavity when imaging the brain (Fig. 12.45). Brain tumors do not commonly extend rostrally through the cribriform plate into the nasal cavity. A rare neural tumor that does traverse the cribriform plate is an olfactory neuroblastoma (esthesioneuroblastoma).[51]

VASCULAR DISRUPTIONS

Occlusive Infarcts

Occlusive brain infarcts are being diagnosed with increasing frequency with MRI but are rarely detectable with CT imaging.[30–32] Infarcts occur most commonly in the cerebellum but also occur in the brainstem and forebrain.

Patients with brain infarction are typically older and present with acute nonprogressive focal neurologic signs. When the brainstem or cerebellum is involved, an important clinical differential is idiopathic peripheral vestibular disease, in which no abnormal MR findings are present. The typical MR characteristics of an acute cerebellar infarct include a triangular or segmental region of T2 hyperintensity that persists in the FLAIR sequence. The shape of the signal change usually closely reflects the territory of the affected artery (Fig. 12.46).

With cerebral infarction, the MR findings may overlap with those of a glioma or focal encephalitis; there is usually ill-defined T2 hyperintensity, T1 hypointensity, no mass effect, and little to no initial contrast enhancement (Fig. 12.47). Typically, after 3 days, regional vascularity increases, particularly at

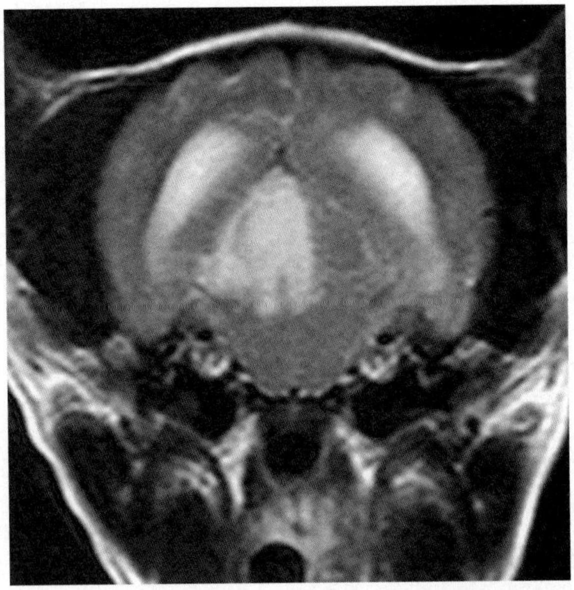

Fig. 12.46 Transverse T2-weighted magnetic resonance (MR) image at the level of the rostral aspect of the cerebellum of an 8-year-old Papillon that developed acute tetraplegia, a right head tilt, and positional vertical nystagmus less than 24 hours previously. The large triangular region of T2 hyperintensity in the right rostral aspect of the cerebellum was mildly T1 hypointense and had no discernible contrast enhancement. The clinical presentation, lesion location, shape, and imaging characteristics are typical of an infarct. This is a particularly large lesion. Diffusion-weighted imaging confirmed restricted water movement, also supporting acute infarction.

the periphery of the lesion.[33] One differentiating feature between infarction and glioma is the initial lack of a mass effect with an infarct. Later, however, a mass effect may develop 3 to 5 days post infarct due to vasogenic edema. Differentiating a cerebral infarct and glioma may not be possible in some patients, and diffusion-weighted MR or follow-up imaging may be necessary. Diffusion imaging quantifies the rate of Brownian motion of water molecules in brain tissue. *Brownian motion* refers to the random movement of molecules. Water molecules are in constant motion, and the rate of movement or diffusion depends on the kinetic energy of the molecules and temperature. In acute infarction, brain cells become overhydrated from failure of the adenosine triphosphate pump, resulting in restricted movement of water (Fig. 12.48). In tumors, water movement is usually less restricted, and tumors will have less evidence of restricted water diffusion. However, restricted water diffusion in an infarct typically only lasts up to 3 to 5 days post infarct, so after this time the ability of diffusion-weighted imaging to distinguish infarct from glioma is lost.

When an occlusive infarct is suspected, the patient should be evaluated for conditions resulting in a hypercoagulable state (e.g., Cushing disease) and loss of antithrombin III.

Hemorrhagic Infarcts

Hemorrhagic infarcts are most commonly associated with hypertension, thrombocytopenia, or other coagulopathies. The MR characteristics may be similar to those for an occlusive infarct (Fig. 12.49). However, the presence of hemorrhage typically results in more signal heterogeneity and larger size of the lesion. The appearance of cerebral hemorrhage changes as the hematoma matures (Table 12.2). The use of standard spin-echo sequences sometimes allows one to estimate the age of a hemorrhagic lesion, based roughly on the signal characteristics. The change in appearance of a hematoma in different sequences over time is related to the magnetic properties of iron within hemoglobin as it transitions through intracellular deoxyhemoglobin to methemoglobin and finally extracellular hemosiderin (Fig. 12.50).

As discussed previously, in comparison to fast (turbo) spin-echo sequences, GRE sequences are more susceptible to magnetic field inhomogeneity created by hemoglobin degradation. Chronic hemorrhage acts like ferromagnetic material, causing pronounced local distortion of the local magnetic field resulting in a signal void (Fig. 12.51; see Figs. 12.44 and 12.49), and for this reason, a GRE sequence should be acquired routinely, even though hemorrhage may not be suspected. Low signal in T2-weighted spin-echo and GRE images is, however, not specific for hemorrhage and may also be seen with mineralization, gas, fibrous tissue, or iron deposits.[33] Susceptibility artifacts in GRE images must be interpreted in light of information gained from all other sequences in the study and the available clinical information.

Trauma

Both MRI and CT can be used to assess patients with head trauma; however, CT is often preferred due to faster acquisition time and excellent ability to detect skull fractures and intracranial hemorrhage in the acute stage. Acute hemorrhage is hyperattenuating to brain tissue in precontrast CT imaging due to the high hemoglobin content. The average Hounsfield units (HUs) of hemorrhage is between 60 and 100, whereas those of gray and white matter are in the range of 30 to 40 and 20 to 30, respectively. Edema may be present as a hypoattenuating halo around the hemorrhagic focus.[52,53] Viewing the CT images in a narrow window is essential to detect subtle changes in attenuation and small foci of hemorrhage (Fig. 12.52).

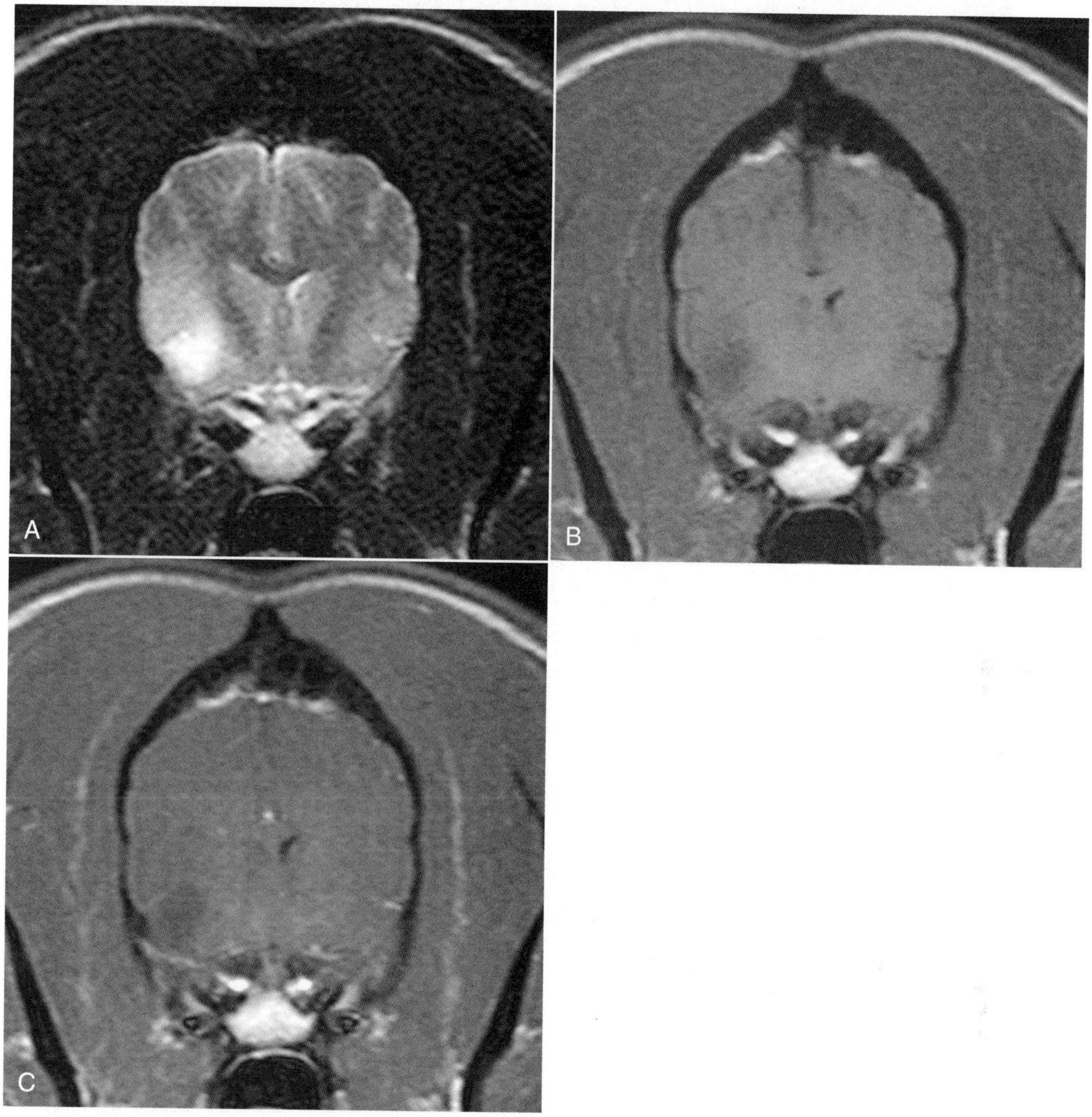

Fig. 12.47 Transverse T2-weighted **(A)** and T1-weighted magnetic resonance (MR) images made before **(B)** and after **(C)** contrast-medium administration in a 10-year-old Labrador retriever with an acute onset of seizures that began 5 days previously. An ill-defined region of T2 hyperintensity is present in the right piriform lobe. The region is T1 hypointense; there is no associated mass effect, and only scant peripheral contrast enhancement. The two most likely differentials are an infarct or a nonenhancing glial cell tumor. The sudden onset of nonprogressive signs is important collaborating history in these patients and helps decide the likelihood of infarction versus glioma. Other considerations for the findings in this patient include necrotizing encephalitis and granulomatous meningoencephalitis (GME), which sometimes has minimal contrast enhancement. Diffusion-weighted imaging can be used to help differentiate these conditions more accurately in the first 1 to 3 days.

25. Shimokawa MT, Iwamoto E, Umeki S, et al. Magnetic resonance imaging and clinical findings in a miniature schnauzer with hypodipsic hypernatremia. *J Vet Med Sci*. 2009;71(10):1387–1391.
26. Lee KI, Lim CY, Kang BT, et al. Clinical and MRI findings of lissencephaly in a mixed breed dog. *J Vet Med Sci*. 2011;73(10):1385–1388.
27. Asakawa MG, Mackillop E, Olby NJ, et al. Imaging diagnosis-neuronal ceroid lipofuscinosis with a chronic subdural hematoma. *Vet Radiol Ultrasound*. 2010;51(2):155–158.
28. Urkasemsin G, Olby NJ. C. hereditary ataxia. *Vet Clin North Am Small Anim Pract*. 2014;44:1075–1089.
29. Snyder M, Lipitz L, Skorupski KA, et al. Secondary intracranial neoplasia in the dog: 177 cases (1986-2003). *J Vet Intern Med*. 2008;22:172–177.
30. Garosi L, McConnell JF, Platt SR, et al. Clinical and topographic magnetic resonance characteristics of suspected brain infarction in 40 dogs. *J Vet Intern Med*. 2006;20:311–321.
31. Rossmeisl JH, Rohleder JJ, Pickett JP, et al. Presumed and confirmed striatocapsular brain infarctions in six dogs. *Vet Ophthalmol*. 2007;10:23–36.
32. Tidwell AS, Robertson ID. Magnetic resonance imaging of normal and abnormal brain perfusion. *Vet Radiol Ultrasound*. 2011;52:62–71.
33. Mulkern RV. Fast imaging techniques. In: Atlas SW, ed. *Magnetic Resonance Imaging Brain Spine*. ed 3. Philadelphia: Lippincott Williams & Wilkins; 2002:178.
34. Sood S, Gupta R, Sharma J, et al. *MRI Spectrum in Acute Toxic and Metabolic Encephalopathies*. Vienna, Austria: European Congress of Radiology; 2014. https://doi.org/10.1594/ecr2014/C-0492.
35. Cornelis I, Van Ham L, Gielen I, De Decker S, Bhatti SFM. Clinical presentation, diagnostic findings, prognostic factors, treatment and outcome in dogs with meningoencephalomyelitis of unknown origin: a review. *Vet J*. 2019;244:37–44.
36. Gonçalves R, De Decker S, Walmsley G, Butterfield S, Maddox TW. Inflammatory disease affecting the central nervous system in dogs: a retrospective study in England (2010–2019). *Frontiers in Veterinary Medicine 27*. 2022. https://doi.org/10.3389/fvets.2021.819945.
37. Lamb CR, Croson PJ, Cappello R, et al. Magnetic resonance imaging findings in 25 dogs with inflammatory cerebrospinal fluid. *Vet Radiol Ultrasound*. 2005;46:17–22.
38. Glass EN, Cornetta AM, Kent M. Clinical and clinicopathologic features in 11 cats with *Cuterebra larvae* myiasis of the central nervous system. *J Vet Intern Med*. 1998;12(5):365–368.
39. Cline JL, Lockaby SB. Pathology in practice: *Aspergillus flavus* mycosis. *J Am Vet Med Assoc*. 2012;241(10):1297–1299.
40. Mellema LM, Koblik PD, Kortz GD, et al. Reversible magnetic resonance imaging abnormalities in dogs following seizures. *Vet Radiol Ultrasound*. 1999;40(6):588–595.
41. Russo M, Covelli EM, Meomartino L, et al. Computed tomographic anatomy of the canine inner and middle ear. *Vet Radiol Ultrasound*. 2005;43(1):22–26.
42. Braund CH, Vite KG: Braund's clinical neurology in small animals: localization, diagnosis and treatment, developmental disorders, *International Veterinary Information Service* (website): http://www.ivis.org/advances/Vite/toc.asp.
43. Martin-Vaquero P, Da Costa RC, Wolk KE, et al. MRI features of gliomatosis cerebri in a dog. *Vet Radiol Ultrasound*. 2012;53:189–192.
44. Porter B, de Lahunta A, Summers B. Gliomatosis cerebri in six dogs. *Vet Pathol*. 2003;40:97–102.
45. Bagley R, Wheeler S, Klopp L, et al. Clinical features of trigeminal nerve-sheath tumor in 10 dogs. *J Am Anim Hosp Assoc*. 1998;34:19–25.
46. Katz ML, Coates JR, Sibigtroth CM, et al. Enzyme replacement therapy attenuates disease progression in a canine model of late-infantile neuronal ceroid lipofuscinosis (CLN2 disease). *J Neurosci Res*. 2014;92:1591–1598.
47. Musso C, Le Boedec K, Gomes E, et al. Diagnostic values of clinical and magnetic resonance findings in presumptive trigeminal Neuropathy: 49 dogs. *J Am Anim Hosp Assoc*. 2020;56:106–113. https://doi.org/10.5326/JAAHA-MS-6997.
48. Wisner ER, Dickinson PJ, Higgins RJ. Magnetic resonance imaging features of canine intracranial neoplasia. *Vet Radiol Ultrasound*. 2011;52:52–61.
49. Tamura S, Tamura Y, Nakamoto Y, et al. MR imaging of histiocytic sarcoma of the canine brain. *Vet Radiol Ultrasound*. 2009;50:178–181.
50. Snyder JM, Shofer FS, Van Winkle TJ, et al. Canine intracranial primary neoplasia: 173 cases (1986-2003). *J Vet Intern Med*. 2006;20:669–675.
51. Söffler C, Hartman A, Gorgas D, et al. Magnetic resonance imaging features of esthesioneuroblastoma in three dogs and one cat. *Tierarztl Prax Ausg K Kleintiere Heimtiere*. 2016;44(5):333–340. https://doi.org/10.15654/TPK-150963. Epub 2016 Jul 7.
52. Platt SR, Radaelli S, McDonnell JJ. Computed tomography after mild head trauma in dogs. *Vet Rec*. 2002;151:243.
53. Chai O, Peery D, Bdolah-Abram T, et al. Computed tomographic findings in dogs with head trauma and development of a novel prognostic computed tomography-based scoring system. *Am J Vet Res*. 2016;78(9):1085–1090.

ELECTRONIC RESOURCES

Additional information related to the content in Chapter 12 can be found online at eBooks.Health.Elsevier.com.

- Chapter Quiz

CHAPTER 13

The Equine Head

Nathan C. Nelson

RADIOLOGY VERSUS OTHER IMAGING MODALITIES

The equine head is composed of numerous overlying structures and complex anatomy, and can be difficult to evaluate completely with radiography. Despite the inherent challenges, radiography remains the mainstay of imaging the equine head due to its widespread availability, low cost, and ability to perform while the patient is standing. The large size of the equine head (which is larger than radiography plates) dictates that projections must be centered over the area of interest. Lateral and dorsoventral (DV) projections are standard, but additional oblique projections may be necessary to optimally evaluate the included anatomy.

The recent advent of standing computed tomography (CT) is revolutionizing imaging of the equine head. The cross-sectional nature of CT removes anatomic superimposition, making it ideally suited to evaluate the complex structures of the equine head. Up until recently, CT examination of the head required anesthesia and dorsal or lateral recumbency, using a special table designed to support the weight of the horse (Fig. 13.1). A number of CT systems now allow standing examinations of the head under sedation alone (see Fig. 13.1). These solutions generally require either a pit with a hydraulic lift to lower the horse to the height of the CT gantry or a lift to elevate the CT scanner.

Magnetic resonance imaging (MRI) of the equine head is rarely performed as it requires general anesthesia and other modalities satisfy most indications for head imaging. The exception is disease of the central nervous system (brain, cranial nerves, and cranial spinal cord), where MRI is the gold standard imaging test. Indications for MRI include imaging the brain, cranial nerves, or inner/middle ear when standing CT is not available or otherwise displays normal structures.

DISEASES OF THE NASAL CAVITY/PARANASAL SINUSES

Radiographic Projections

Maxillary/nasal anatomy is complex (Fig. 13.2). To fully characterize pathology, a minimum of four standard radiographic projections, centered on the sinuses, should be performed in horses with suspected sinus or nasal disease: lateral projection, DV projection, right 30-degree dorsal to left ventral, and left 30-degree dorsal to right ventral obliques.

Sinusitis

Sinusitis is the most common disease of the paranasal sinuses, caused by infection (usually bacterial) within the paranasal sinuses. Affected horses have purulent nasal discharge with a fetid odor and may have facial swelling. In roughly a quarter of horses with sinus disease, there is no history of trauma, dental disease, or other underlying cause for sinusitis, and these are considered cases of *primary sinusitis. Secondary sinusitis* occurs when there is a predisposing factor resulting in bacterial infection. Dental disease is the most common cause of secondary sinusitis, although prior facial fractures, cysts, or other masses affecting the nasal cavity may also result in sinusitis. Radiographs or CT are indicated to confirm the presence of sinus fluid, and screen for possible underlying causes of secondary sinusitis. In some cases, CT can discriminate soft tissue masses that might be obscured by fluid on radiography.

Sinusitis causes distinct fluid lines on radiography which are horizontal to the ground (Fig. 13.3, eFig. 13.1). There are two bullae within the nasal conchae rostral to the maxillary sinus: the dorsal and ventral nasal conchal bullae. These bullae may become infected in cases of sinusitis. Chronic empyema of these bullae may serve as a source of chronic, recurrent sinusitis if not treated (Fig. 13.3).[1]

Cysts

Paranasal sinus cysts are the second most common cause of equine secondary sinusitis after dental disease.[2] Their cause is unknown, although there may be an association with ethmoid hematomas given the presence of hemorrhage in cyst walls on histopathologic examination.[3] On radiographs, cysts cause a soft tissue opaque mass within the paranasal sinuses, although it may be gas opaque if internal fluid drains. Cysts can cause mild pressure resorption of regional bones, but rarely cause severe regional lysis. On CT, cysts often have a discrete hyperattenuating wall at their periphery which discriminates cysts from other sinus masses (Fig. 13.4, eFig. 13.2).[4]

Progressive Ethmoid Hematoma (PEH)

PEH is an expansile mass typically arising from the submucosa of the ethmoidal labyrinth, but can occur anywhere within the nasal cavity or paranasal sinuses. The cause is unknown but presumably due to repeated hemorrhage into the submucosa. The result is a mass comprised of blood and fibrous tissue, encapsulated by respiratory epithelium. Radiographs reveal a mass in the area of the ethmoid turbinates (Fig. 13.5, eFig. 13.3). Most PEHs have a characteristic appearance on CT with internal hyperattenuating "swirling" heterogeneity attributable to the presence of hemorrhage or early mineralization in the mass (Fig. 13.6). Unlike radiographs, CT and MR readily identify cribriform plate lysis caused by the PEH, which may preclude some forms of therapy.[5]

Neoplasia

Sinonasal neoplasms are an uncommon cause of sinusitis. Various tumor types are reported, including epithelial tumors (carcinomas of various types), sarcomas such as osteosarcoma and hemangiosarcoma, neuroendocrine tumors/neuroblastoma, hemangiosarcoma, and lymphoid tumors.[6,7] The radiographic appearance of sinonasal neoplasia overlaps with other

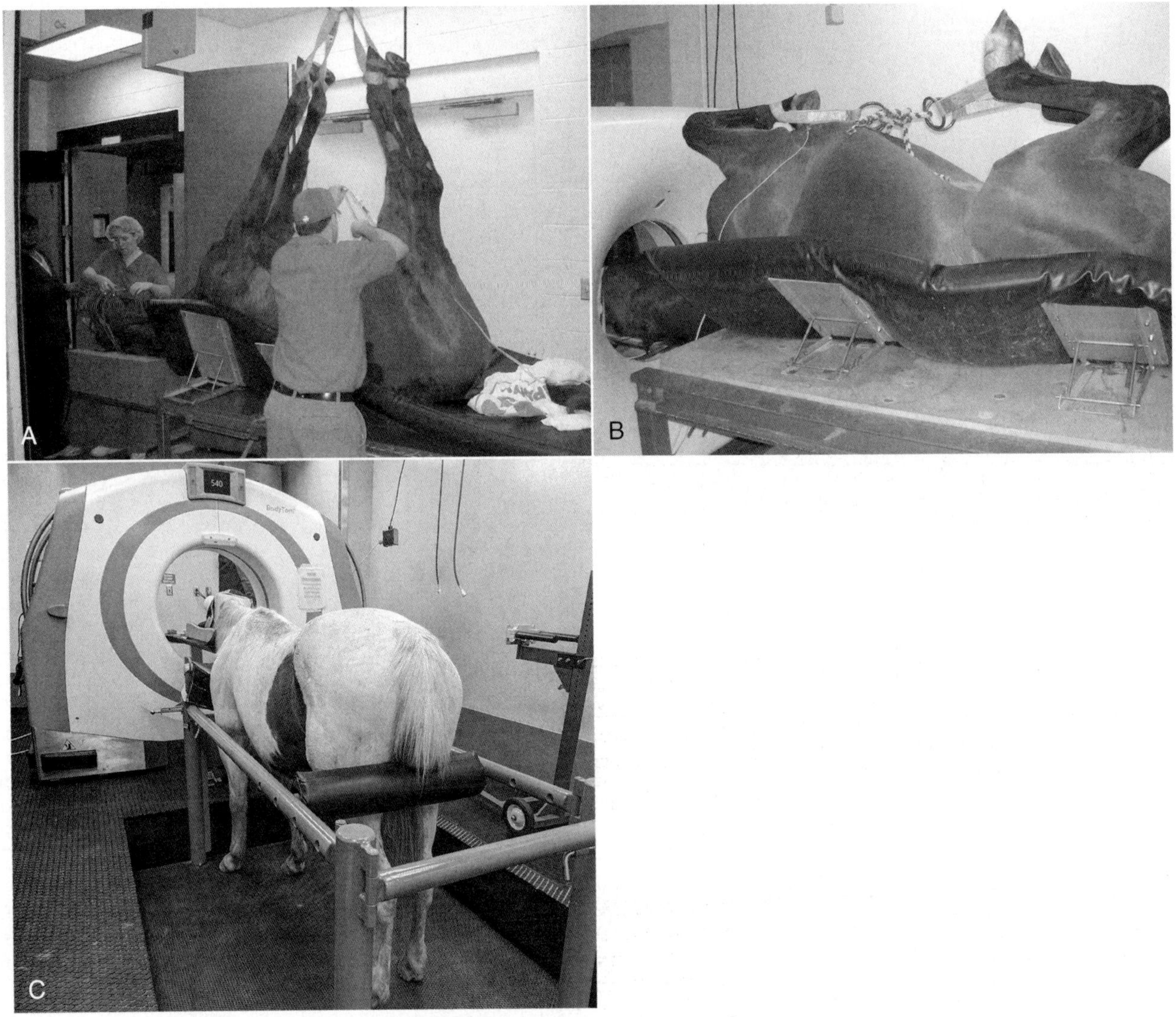

Fig. 13.1 **A,** Anesthetized horse lifted into dorsal recumbency with a hoist and then positioned (**B**) for computed tomography (CT) of the head. **C,** A horse positioned for a standing CT of the head, with the lift lowered below the floor level.

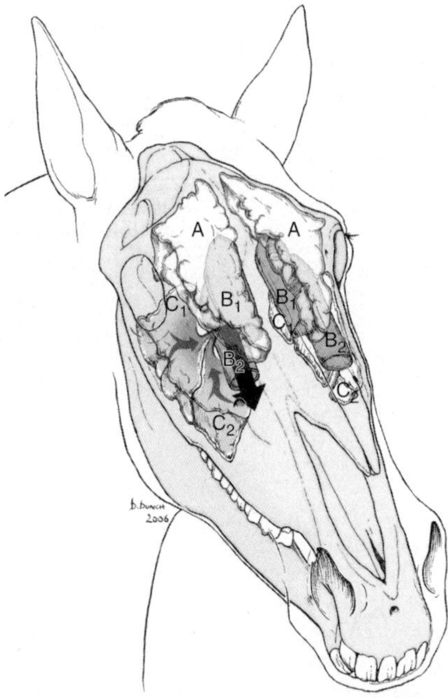

Fig. 13.2 A schematic representation of the equine nasal sinuses and their communications. *A,* Conchofrontal sinus; B_1, dorsal nasal meatus; B_2, middle nasal meatus; C_1, caudal maxillary sinus; C_2, rostral maxillary sinus.

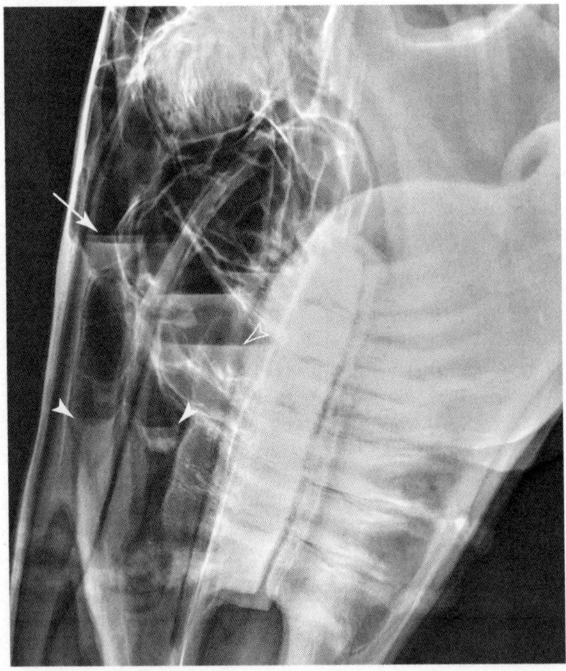

Fig. 13.3 Lateral radiograph showing fluid in the conchofrontal sinus (*arrow*), rostral maxillary sinus (*open arrowhead*), and dorsal and ventral conchal bullae (*closed arrowheads*).

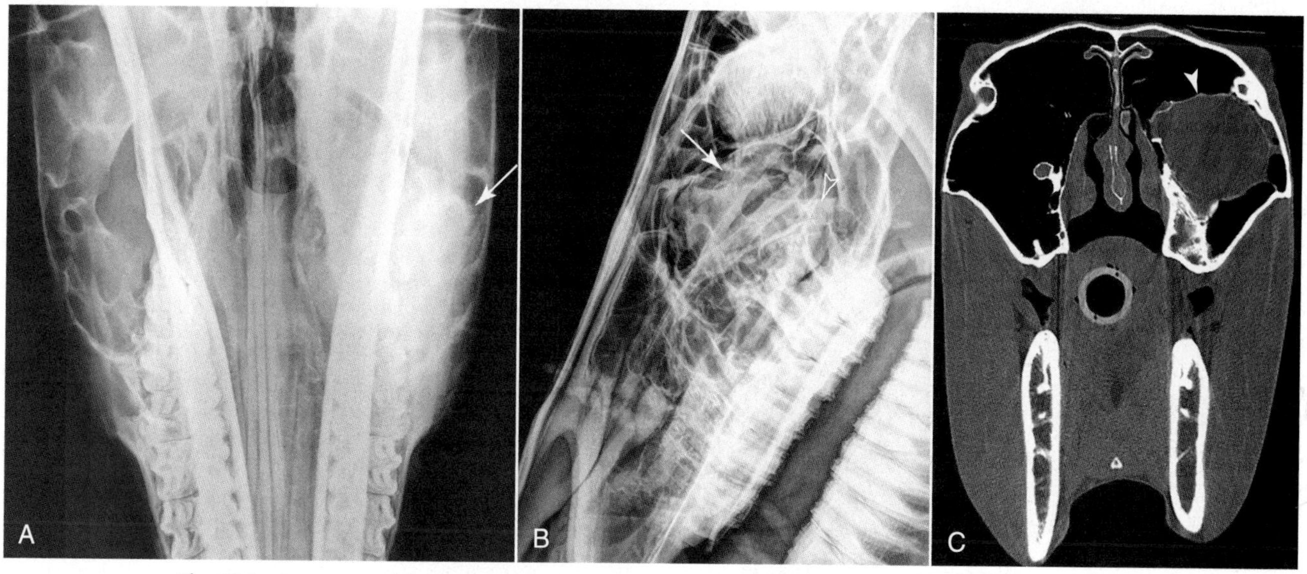

Fig. 13.4 Dorsoventral **(A)** and lateral **(B)** radiographs of a horse with a left paranasal sinus cyst (*arrow*) with effusion in the sinuses (*open arrowhead*). **(C)** Computed tomography (CT) of the same horse showing the mineralized rim of the sinus cyst (*closed arrowhead*).

sinonasal disease such as hematomas or cysts, and radiographs underestimate potential features of malignancy such as bone lysis.[6] Historical and physical examination findings may help prioritize neoplasia as a cause of sinusitis; firm facial swellings or lysis/extension into the hard palate are seen more commonly with neoplastic disease than other causes of paranasal pathology (Fig. 13.7, eFig. 13.4).[8] CT clearly determines regions of bone lysis and MRI best determines invasion of soft tissue structures such as the brain (Fig. 13.8). Extensive regional bone lysis, contrast enhancement of the mass, and extensive osseous production make a neoplastic mass more likely.

Polyps

Polyps are uncommon, benign soft tissue proliferations that occur within the nasal passage or sinuses and likely represent polyploid epithelial proliferation as a response to regional chronic inflammation.[9] On radiographs (Fig. 13.9), polyps are soft tissue masses that have a nonaggressive appearance. They generally do not cause significant bone lysis or production though may cause bone pressure resorption (Fig. 13.10).

DENTAL DISEASE

Normal Dentition

Discussions of equine dentition employ the modified Triadan system, which assigns each tooth a specific number depending on its anatomic quadrant in the mouth (Fig. 13.11). The term "cheek teeth" informally refers to the premolar and molar teeth. The hypsodont (continually erupting) nature of equine teeth means younger horses will have a long reserve crown, which extends further into the sinuses and nasal cavity compared to older horses. Horses between 2 and 4 years of age develop "eruption bumps," sometimes incorrectly referred to as "eruption cysts," over the premolar teeth of the maxilla and mandible. The periapical area of these teeth appears relatively lucent compared to older horses and should not be confused with periapical abscessation (Fig. 13.12). Young horses will have "caps" (retained deciduous teeth) over their mandibular and maxillary teeth when they are between 3 and 5 years of age. The Triadan 05s are small brachydont teeth referred to as "wolf teeth" (Fig. 13.13) that may be retained. Wolf teeth typically do not directly cause clinical signs, but can cause discomfort particularly if they interfere with a bit in the mouth.

Equine teeth are subjected to high abrasive forces and continual wear, which shapes the occlusal surface of the tooth and ultimately affects the rate of dental attrition. A complete description of equine dental anatomy is beyond the scope of this text. Like brachydont teeth, the equine tooth is constructed of cementum, dentin, and enamel, but unlike the brachydont tooth, the grinding surface is continually worn. The common pulp chamber resides in the apex of the tooth and the pulp horns extend towards the occlusal surface. Deposition of secondary dentin closes these pulp horns as the tooth undergoes normal wear, but there is risk for pulp exposure, infection, and apical abscessation if there is failure of this process. The periodontal space surrounding the tooth should be thin and well defined, and can be difficult to see radiographically compared to CT.

Dental Radiographic Projections

Maxillary cheek teeth: If maxillary premolar/molar dental disease is suspected, the standard projections listed for the maxillary sinuses may be employed, although opening the mouth with a gag during image acquisition facilitates evaluation of the occlusal surfaces. Additional oblique projections are available that better isolate the apices of the maxillary cheek teeth, projecting the palatal root dorsal to the buccal roots: open-mouth right 60-degree ventral to left dorsal oblique and open-mouth left 60-degree ventral to right dorsal oblique (Fig. 13.14). A shallow lateral oblique projection is ideal for evaluation of occlusal abnormalities (wavemouth) (see Fig. 13.14). An offset DV projection (when the mandible is distracted to one side relative to the maxilla) prevents superimposition of the mandibular and maxillary arcades on the DV projection (Fig. 13.15).

Mandibular dental disease: Projections to isolate the mandibular dental apices are similar to those for the maxillary arcade, but centered on the mandible and steeper angles may be necessary to prevent superimposition of the contralateral side.

Maxillary/mandibular incisor disease: Open mouth, intraoral projections allow evaluation of incisor teeth without superimposition of the opposite dental arcade. To acquire these

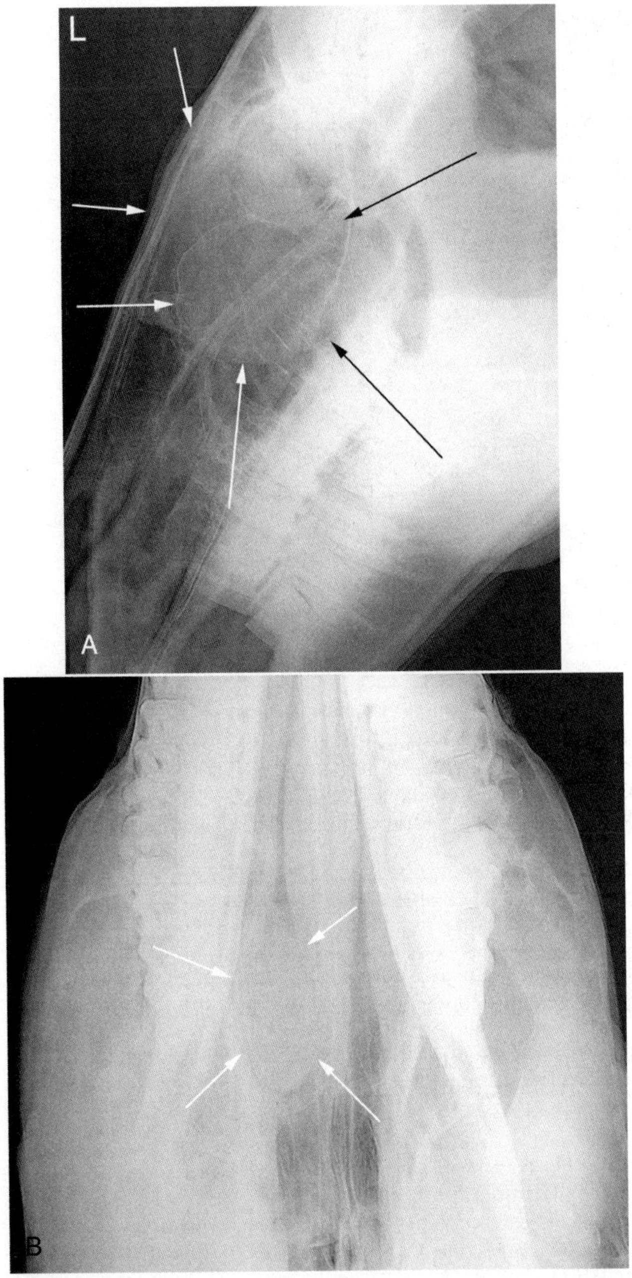

Fig. 13.5 **A,** Lateral radiograph of the head. The ethmoid hematoma (*white* and *black arrows*) is visible in the region of the ethmoid labyrinth. **B,** Dorsoventral radiograph. The lateralized mass (*white arrows*) is in a typical location of an ethmoid hematoma.

projections, a gag is placed in the mouth, and DV and oblique projections acquired (Fig. 13.16).

The complex nature of dental anatomy and pathology precludes an exhaustive review of equine dental disease in this chapter; however, the most common diseases will be discussed later.

Conformational Defects

The occlusal surface may wear in an abnormal pattern. In some cases, the harder enamel folds of the teeth will protrude from the occlusal surface due to differential wear between the enamel and the softer cementum and dentin. These "enamel points" are the most common equine dental disease and cause discomfort during chewing by impinging on regional soft tissues. Enamel points are typically diagnosed on oral examination, but may be apparent on CT imaging or radiographs.

Overwear or fracturing of the occlusal surface of a tooth allows compensatory overgrowth of the opposite tooth, due to loss of the normal rasping that occurs during mastication. In older horses, there can be generalized overgrowth of some teeth of one arcade and undergrowth of the opposing arcade. This results in an occlusal conformation referred to as "wavemouth" (Fig. 13.17).[10]

Cheek Teeth Fractures

Cheek teeth fractures are common, with the 109/209 most commonly affected (see Fig. 13.15). Fractures are most often sagittal in their orientation, and usually extend centrally through the infundibula or more peripherally through the pulp horns. These may lead to pulp exposure and periapical infection if left untreated.

Apical Infections of Cheek Teeth

Periapical cheek tooth infection is a common disorder. Most are caused by blood or lymphatic borne bacterial infection. Pulp exposure, due to imbalance between cheek tooth wear and the formation of secondary dentin or due to dental trauma/fractures, can also lead to infection which ascends to the apical region of the tooth.[10] Regardless of cause, infected teeth are recognized radiographically by surrounding alveolar sclerosis, blunting of tooth roots, and widening of the periodontal space (Fig. 13.18, eFig. 13.5). The interpretation of dental radiographs is challenging; CT greatly improves the specificity when determining which teeth have apical or pulpal infection. The caudal maxillary cheek teeth extend into the paranasal sinuses, so periapical infection can lead to sinusitis. The mandibular and rostral maxillary check teeth do not extend into the sinuses; infection of these teeth can eventually cause fistula formation and a draining tract (Fig. 13.19). Fistulas are more easily identified on CT compared to radiographs (Fig. 13.20).

Odontogenic Tumors

Odontogenic tumors are uncommon and arise from embryonic remnants of the dental lamina.[11] Multiple tumor types occur, including ameloblastoma, ameloblastic carcinomas, and odontomas. There is overlap in the imaging appearance of different tumor types, but all result in an expansile, aggressive lesion centered on the teeth (Fig. 13.21).[11]

Equine Odontoclastic Tooth Resorption and Hypercementosis (EOTRH)

EOTRH is a common dental disorder predominantly affecting the incisors and canine teeth. It causes various degrees of progressive internal and external root resorption and excessive cemental deposition (Fig. 13.22). EOTRH is recognized most commonly in middle aged and geriatric (<15 years of age) horses, although younger horses can also be affected.[12,13] In one study of horses 10 years and older, 94% of horses had at least minor and 62% had moderate to severe radiographic changes from EOTRH.[14] The etiology is likely multifactorial, and represents a response to periodontal disease or infection, ischemic necrosis, mechanical stress, or genetics.[12] Radiographic findings mimic those on histopathology, with some teeth primarily showing resorptive or proliferative change, but most commonly a mix of both.[12] Hypercementosis results in root and reserve crown enlagement.[13] With the advent of high resolution digital images and increased use of standing CT examination of the head, earlier lesions are being recognized.

NONDENTAL DISEASES OF THE MANDIBLE AND MAXILLA

Bone Cysts

Aneurysmal bone cysts are caused by increased venous pressure and dilatation/rupture of vascular networks, leading to

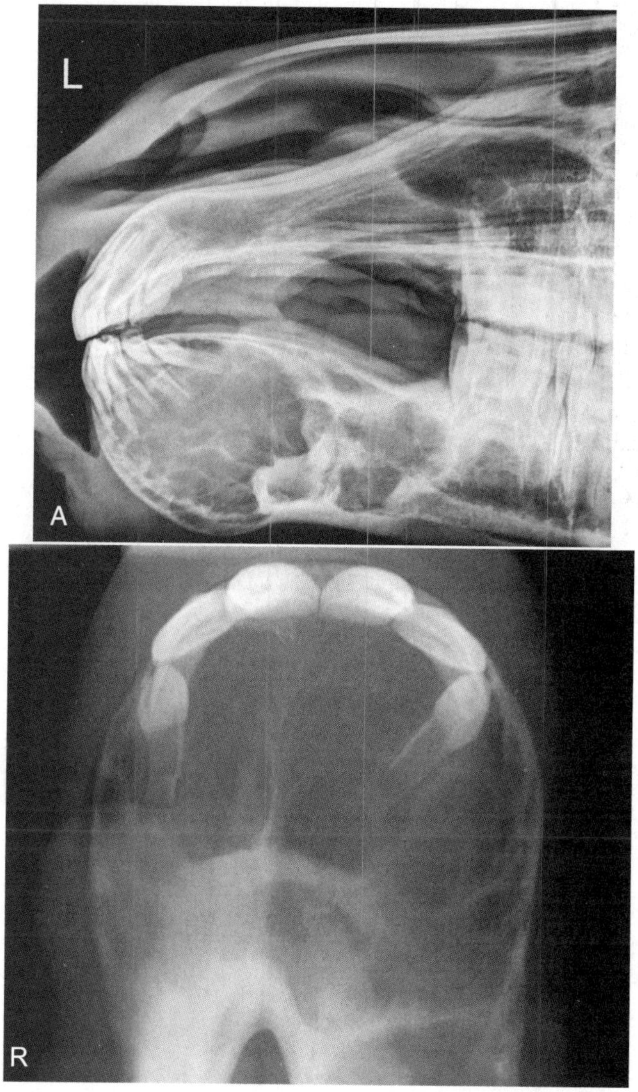

B

Fig. 13.23 Lateral (A) and ventrodorsal (B) intraoral radiographs of the rostral aspect of the mandible in a 7-month-old thoroughbred with an expansile, relatively nonaggressive appearing lesion caused by an aneurysmal bone cyst.

plexus, most commonly in the lateral ventricles, though the fourth ventricles may also be involved. Their exact etiology is unknown, but likely result from chronic/intermittent vascular congestion and secondary hemorrhage. This releases cholesterol from erythrocytes which acts as a foreign body inciting a granulomatous, mineralizing response.[53] They are very common, being present in up to 20% of older horses, and rarely cause clinical signs, although can cause ataxia, blindness, depression, and somnolence when large.[53,54] They have a characteristic appearance on CT, being relatively hyperattenuating to adjacent parenchyma with Hounsfield units (HU) values that indicate the presence of mineralization (Fig. 13.47).

Traumatic Brain Injury

Traumatic brain injury (TBI) in horses is usually due to blunt force trauma or occasionally penetrating injuries.[55] Blunt force trauma from rearing and falling over backwards is the most common cause of injury (especially common in younger horses) but TBI also occurs from struggling after being cast, kick injuries, and injuries during anesthetic recovery.[55,56] The choice of imaging modality in cases of head trauma depends on cost and availability, as well as the capability of the patient to stand or recover from anesthesia. Radiographs are less sensitive for skull fractures compared to MRI/CT, and do not directly image the brain. CT is particularly useful in detecting hematoma formation, as the high proteinaceous and hemoglobin content of acute hemorrhage renders it hyperattenuating on precontrast images (Fig. 13.48).

OTHER CONDITIONS OF THE HEAD

Other Fractures

Due to the uncertain nature of head trauma, fractures may occur anywhere in the head, beyond those previously discussed in this chapter. Horses have a complete bony orbit, comprised of the frontal, lacrimal, zygomatic, and temporal bones.[57] Radiographs or CTs are indicated in horses with orbital fractures to determine whether there is sinus or nasal involvement, with most fractures in this area requiring a combination of medical and surgical therapy.[57] Multiple oblique radiographs at varied, steep angles may be necessary to better characterize fractures in this location (Fig. 13.49).

The paracondylar processes are bilateral, long osseous structures caudal to the bulla extending ventrally from the occipital region. Multiple muscles involved with deglutition and opening

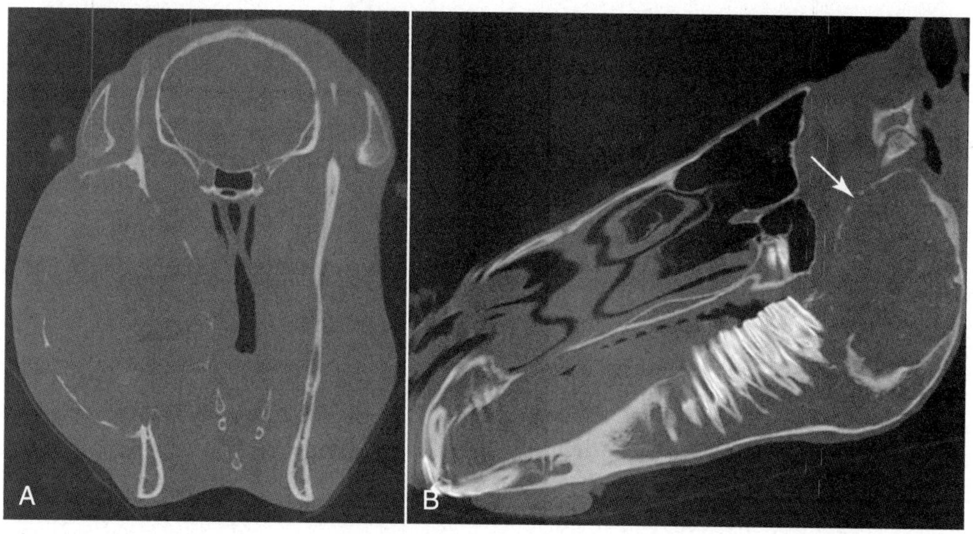

Fig. 13.24 Transverse (A) and sagittal (B) computed tomography (CT) image of a horse with mandibular fibrosarcoma (*arrows*) causing marked expansion and lysis of the right mandibular ramus.

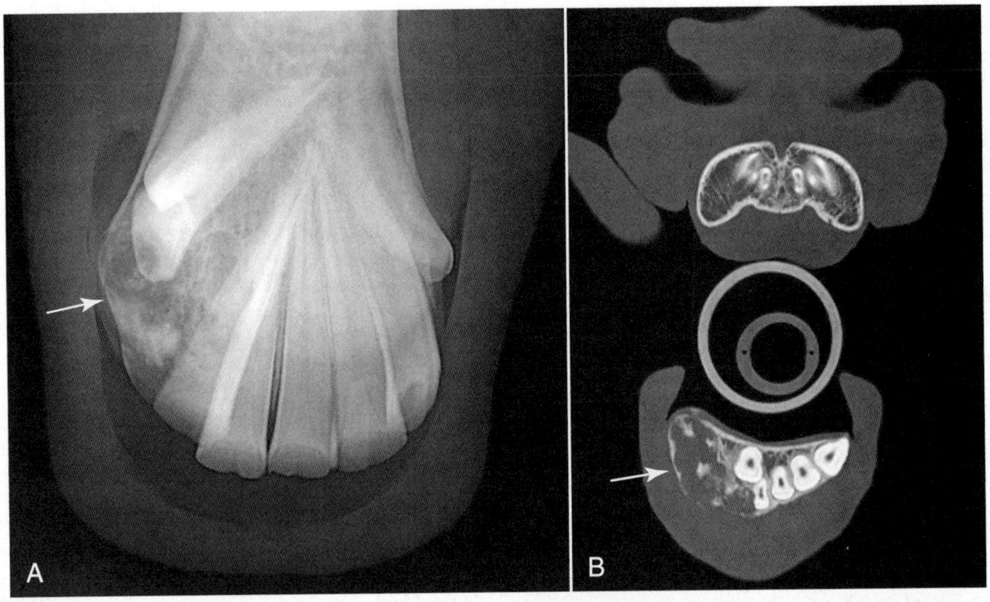

Fig. 13.25 Intraoral mandibular radiograph **(A)** and transverse computed tomography (CT) image **(B)** of an ossifying fibroma (*arrows*). The lesion causes expansion and mixed bone loss and proliferation of the rostral mandible.

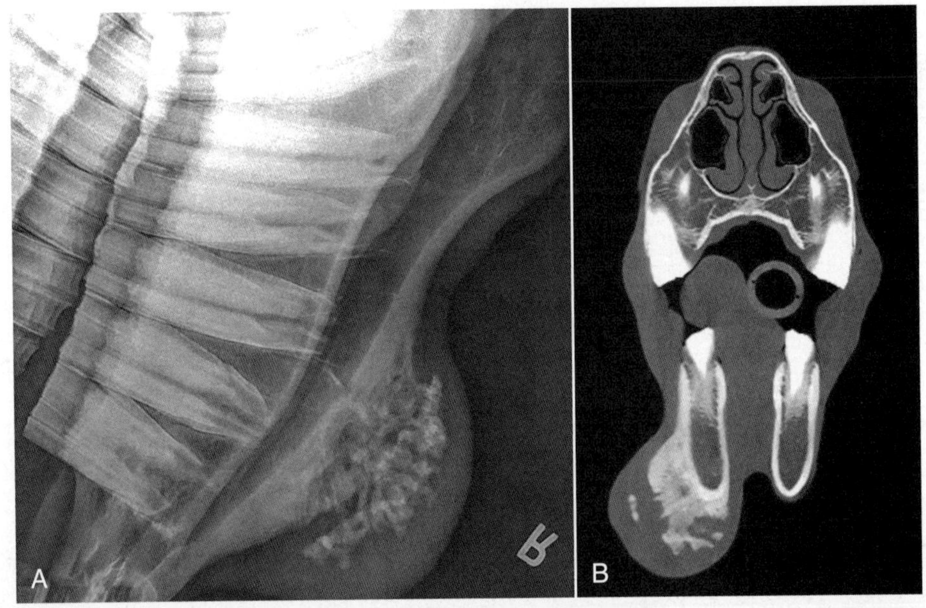

Fig. 13.26 **A,** Oblique radiograph of the right mandible showing a proliferative lesion and thickening of the mandibular cortex that was biopsied as an osteoma. The computed tomography (CT) image **(B)** more clearly shows the lack of medullary involvement.

the mouth arise on these processes.[58] Trauma to the base of the skull can fracture the paracondylar processes. There may be neurological signs (such as facial nerve paralysis given the proximity to the paracondylar process of the facial canal and stylomastoid foramen where the facial nerve emerges), but these fractures may also be seen incidentally in clinically normal horses, presumably from prior healed or unrecognized trauma. Paracondylar process fractures may be difficult to recognize as they superimpose with the complex anatomy of the skull base, and often easiest seen on the DV projection by comparing the fractured process to the contralateral side. CT provides more sensitive detection of small or nondisplaced fractures (Fig. 13.50).

Melanomas

Melanomas are common neoplasms in horses (representing up to 15% of equine neoplasms) with a known genetic predisposition to the gray horse.[30] While they occur in multiple locations, including the perineal/tail base region, they are also frequently seen on the head. They may be superficial in nature, and affect the eyelids and ears, but also occur deeper within the head and can affect lymph nodes, sinuses, guttural pouch, and salivary tissue. Most melanomas are pigmented due to a high concentration of melanin. The presence of melanin results in characteristic high attenuation values on CT compared to adjacent soft tissue structures (Fig. 13.51).[30]

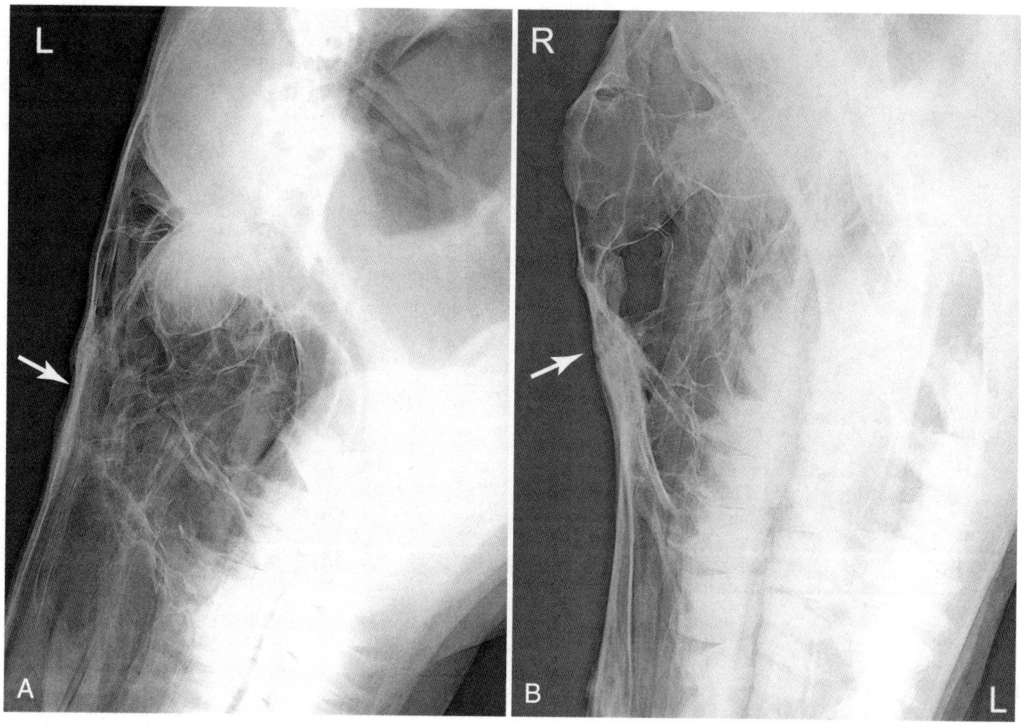

Fig. 13.27 Right-left **(A)** and left rostrodorsal-right caudoventral oblique **(B)** radiographs. There is nasofrontal suture separation at the rostral aspect of the frontal bone causing increased bone opacity (*arrows*).

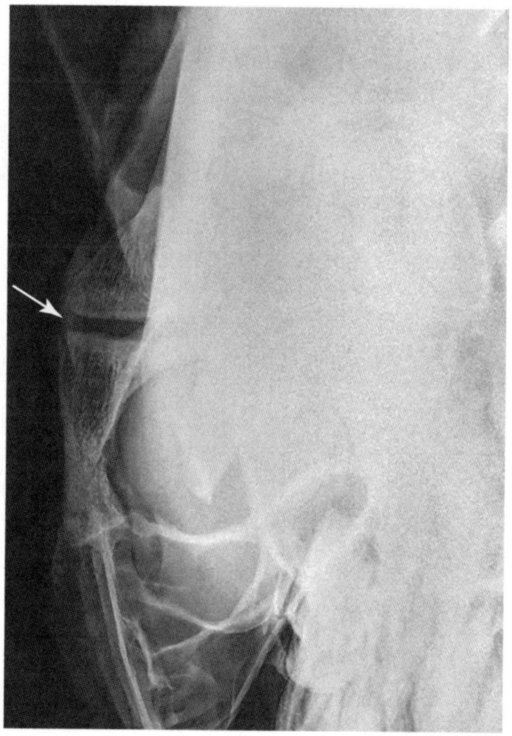

Fig. 13.28 Rostral 45-degree ventral 30-degree lateral-caudodorsolateral oblique radiograph of a normal temporomandibular joint (*arrow*).

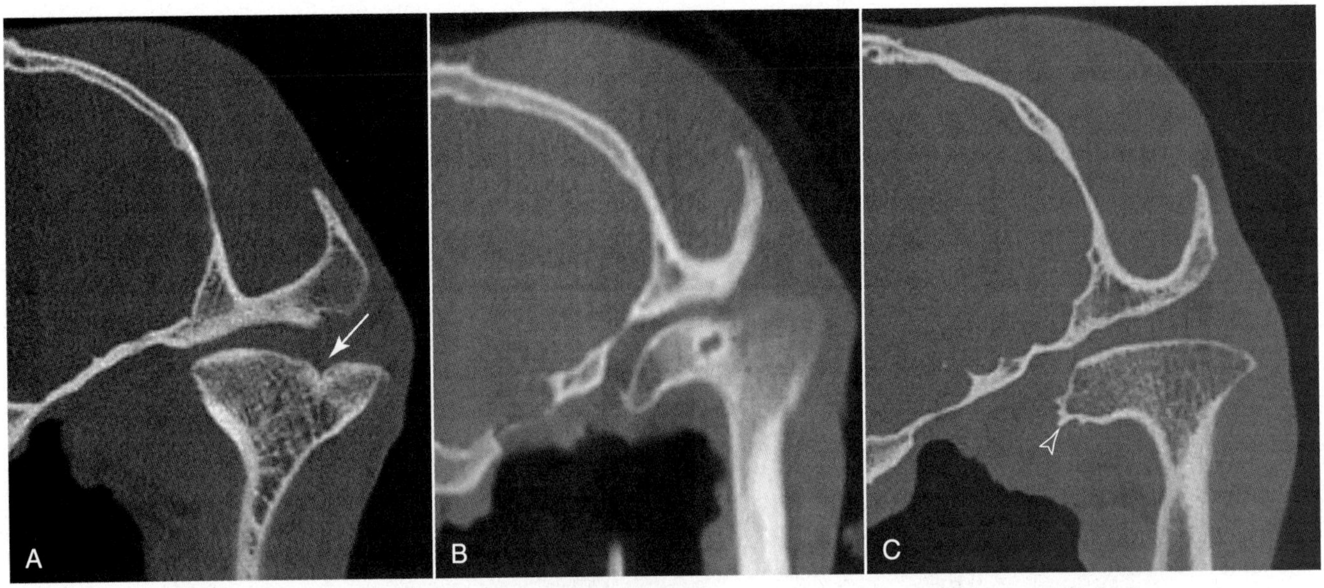

Fig. 13.29 Transverse computed tomography (CT) images showing variations of the mandibular condyle. **A,** Small indentation on the condylar articular surface (*arrow*). **B,** A cyst-like lesion in the mandibular condyle. **C,** Small irregularities along the medial condylar margin (*open arrowhead*).

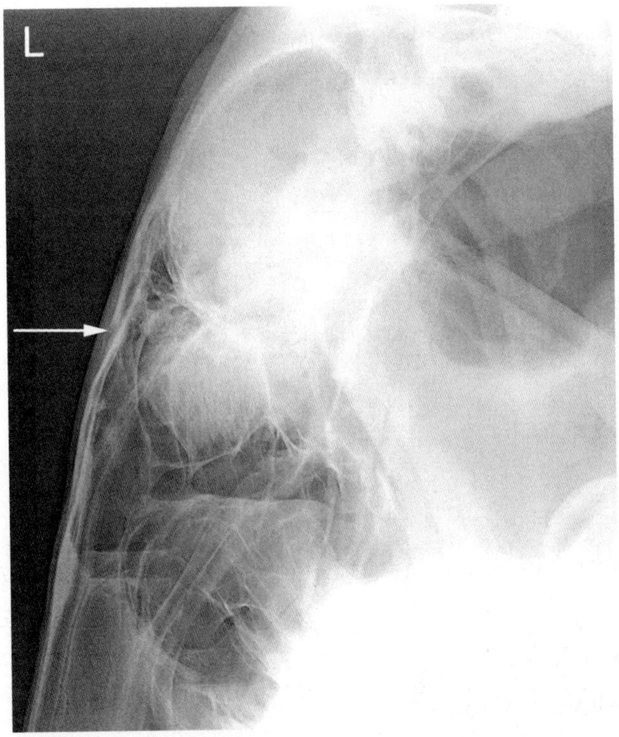

Fig. 13.30 Lateral radiograph of a depression fracture of the frontal bone (*arrow*). Fluid lines due to hemorrhage are also present in the conchofrontal, caudal maxillary, and rostral maxillary sinuses.

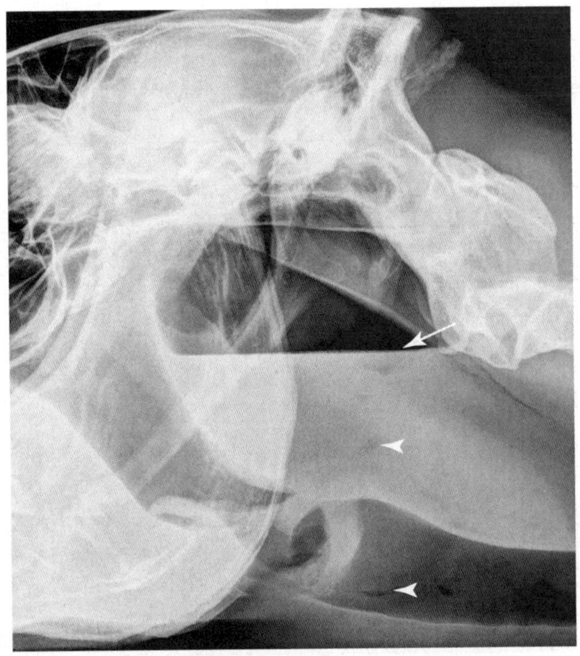

Fig. 13.31 Lateral radiograph of guttural pouch empyema with a distinct fluid line (*arrow*). Small superimposed gas bubbles (*arrowheads*) represent abscesses within adjacent soft tissues.

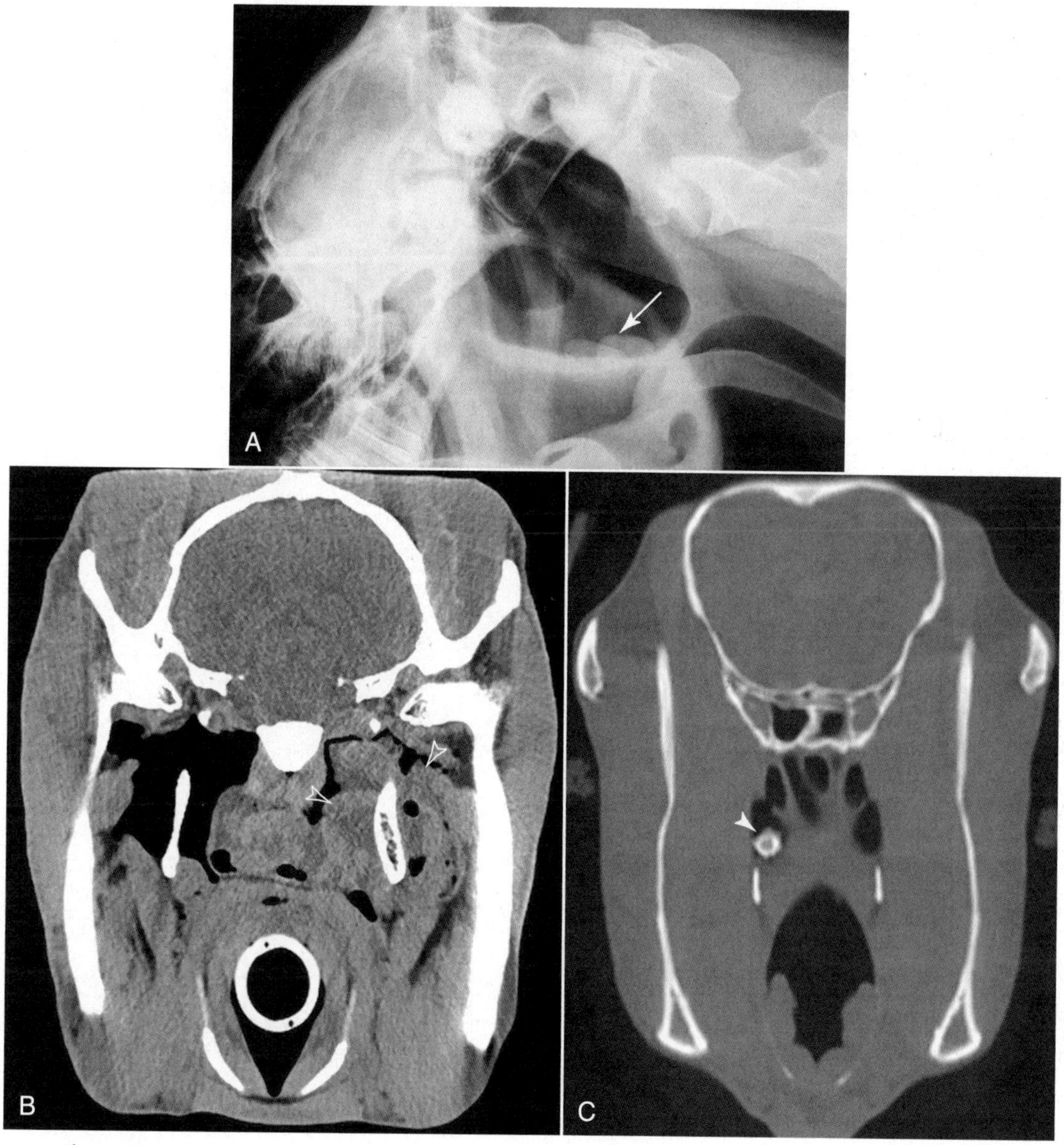

Fig. 13.32 **A,** Lateral radiograph showing two chondroids (*arrow*) in the guttural pouches. **B,** Transverse computed tomography (CT) showing inspissated pus (*open arrowheads*) of a horse with strangles, representing early chondroid formation. **C,** Transverse CT showing a chronic, mineralized chondroid in the guttural pouch (*closed arrowhead*).

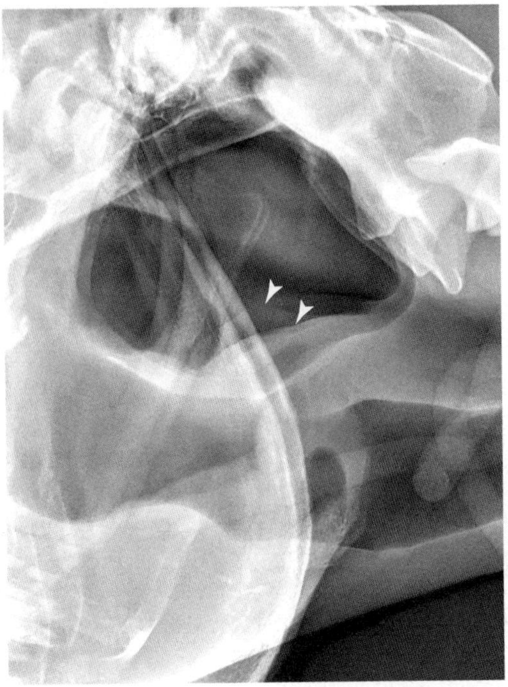

Fig. 13.33 Lateral radiograph showing enlarged medial retropharyngeal lymph nodes (*arrowheads*) causing a broad-based soft tissue bulge into the guttural pouches.

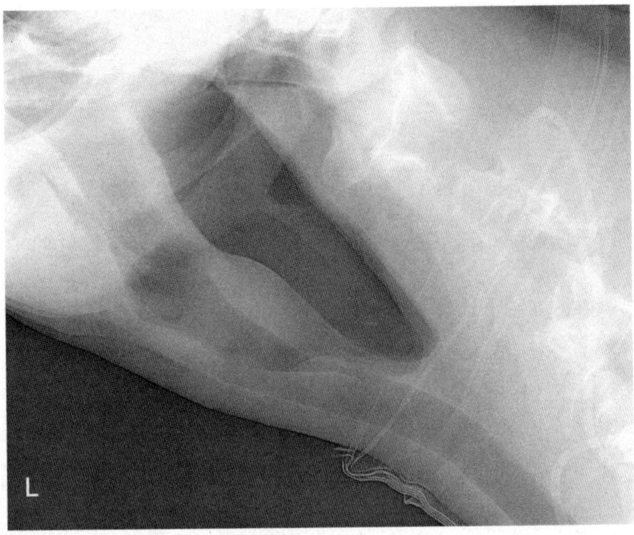

Fig. 13.34 Lateral radiograph of the cranial cervical region in a 2-month-old quarter horse with guttural pouch tympany. Note the elongated appearance of the guttural pouch that extends beyond its normal anatomic limit of the caudal margin of the first cervical vertebra.

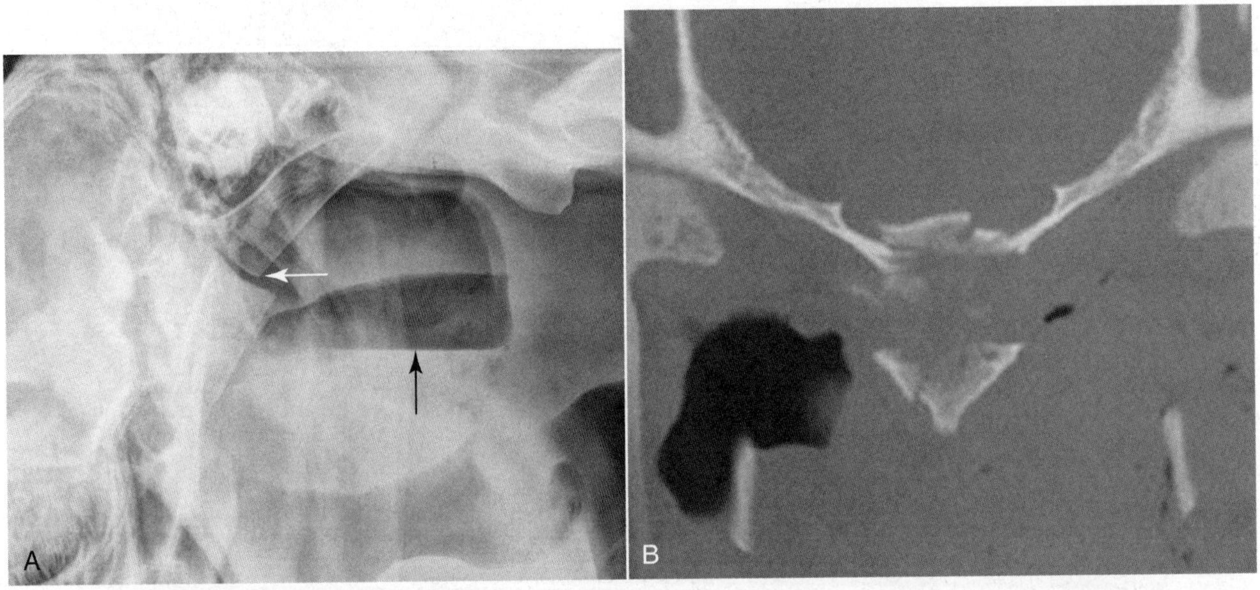

Fig. 13.35 **A,** Lateral radiograph of the head in an 8-month-old Hanoverian that sustained a fall. The basioccipital bone (*white arrow*) is displaced dorsally in relation to the basisphenoid bone. The guttural pouch is partially filled with a soft tissue-fluid opacity that compresses the nasopharynx. A gas/fluid interface is also present (*black arrow*), caused by hemorrhage, a result of avulsion of the ventral skull muscles and fracture of the skull base. Small gas bubbles are visible just caudal to the *black arrow*; this suggests an avulsion of the ventral aspect of the sphenoid sinus with release of air. **B,** Computed tomography (CT) examination thorough the basisphenoid region in another horse with a comminuted basisphenoid-basioccipital fracture.

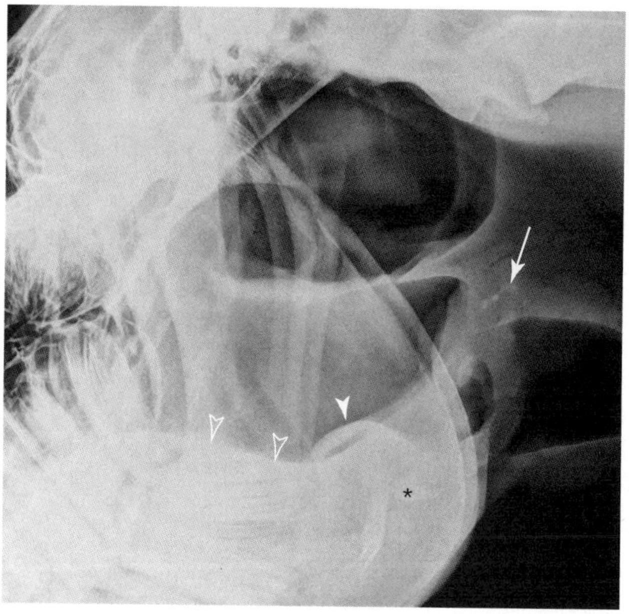

Fig. 13.36 Lateral radiograph showing the tip of the epiglottis (*closed arrowhead*) appropriately dorsal to the soft palate (*open arrowheads*). There is mineralization of the dorsal arytenoid region (*arrow*) and base of the laryngeal cartilages (*asterisk*).

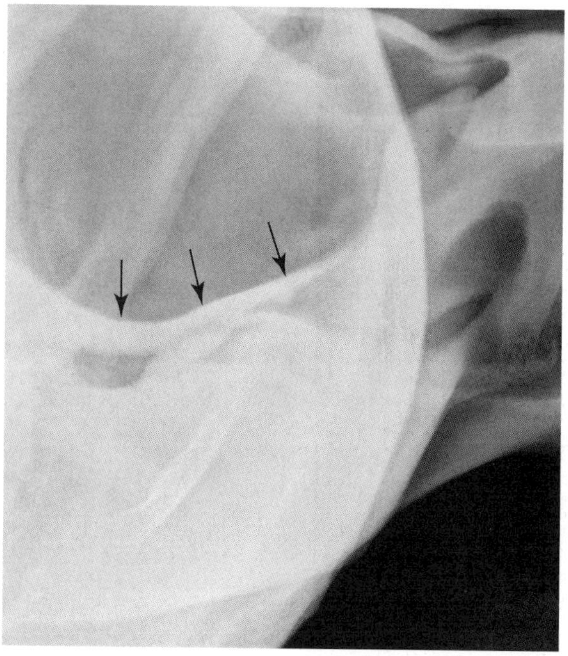

Fig. 13.37 Lateral radiograph of the laryngeal region. The epiglottis is ventral to the soft palate (*black arrows*), indicating a dorsally displaced soft palate.

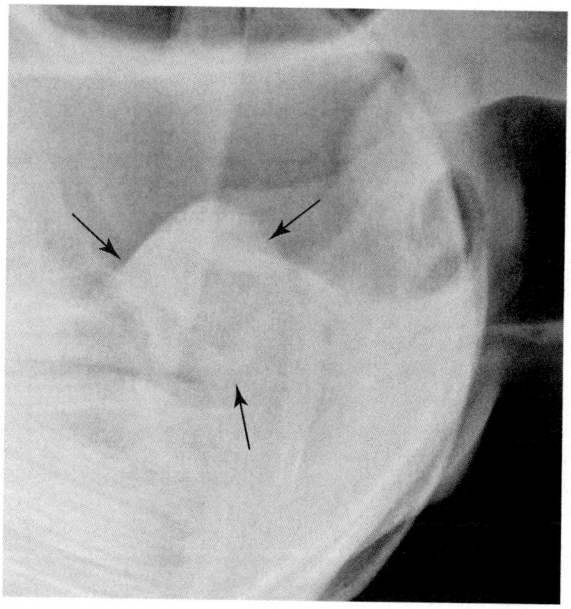

Fig. 13.38 Lateral radiograph of the laryngeal region of a subepiglottic mass (*black arrows*) displacing the epiglottis dorsally; this was a cyst.

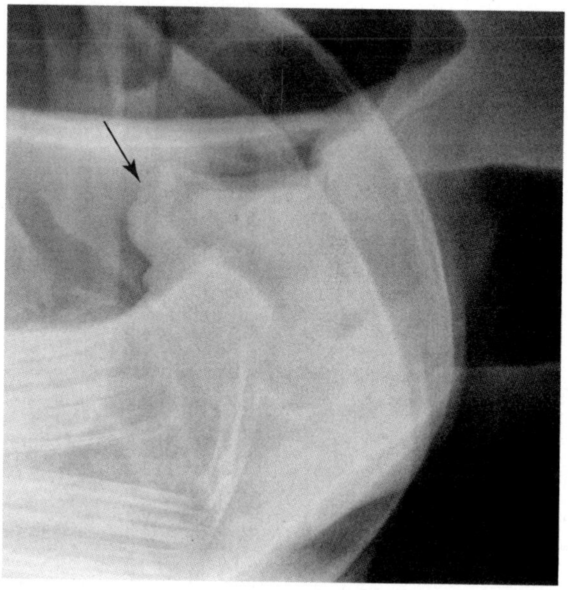

Fig. 13.39 Lateral radiograph of the laryngeal region of a horse with epiglottic entrapment. Note the blunt appearance of the epiglottis (*black arrow*) and the conspicuous aryepiglottic fold.

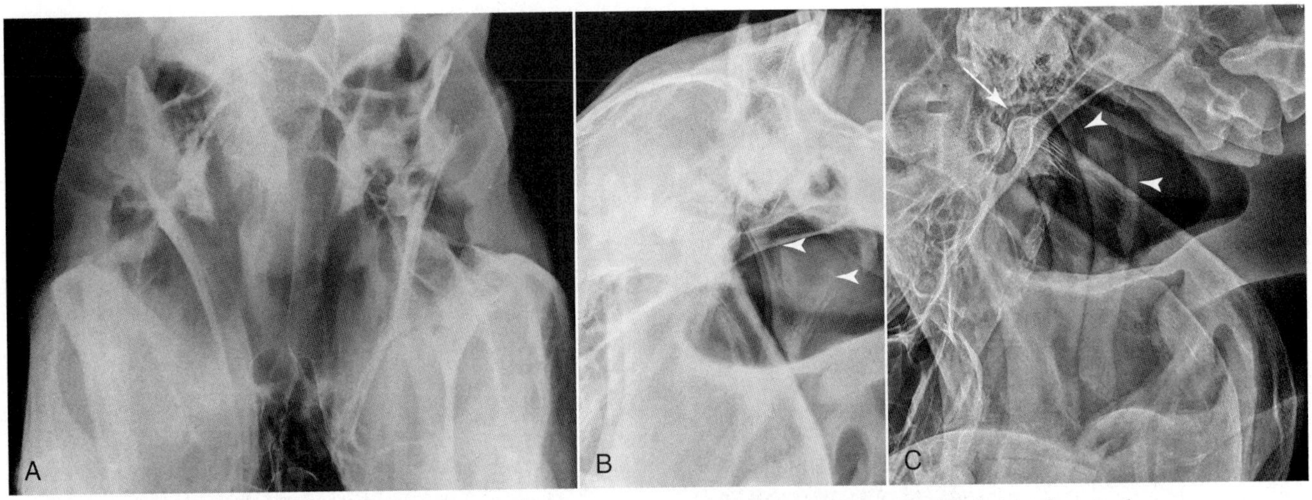

Fig. 13.40 Dorsoventral **(A)**, lateral **(B)**, and lateral 10-degree rostral-laterocaudal oblique **(C)** showing the normal temporomandibular joint (*arrow*) and proximal stylohyoid bone (*arrowheads*). On the lateral projection, the left and right stylohyoid bones are superimposed.

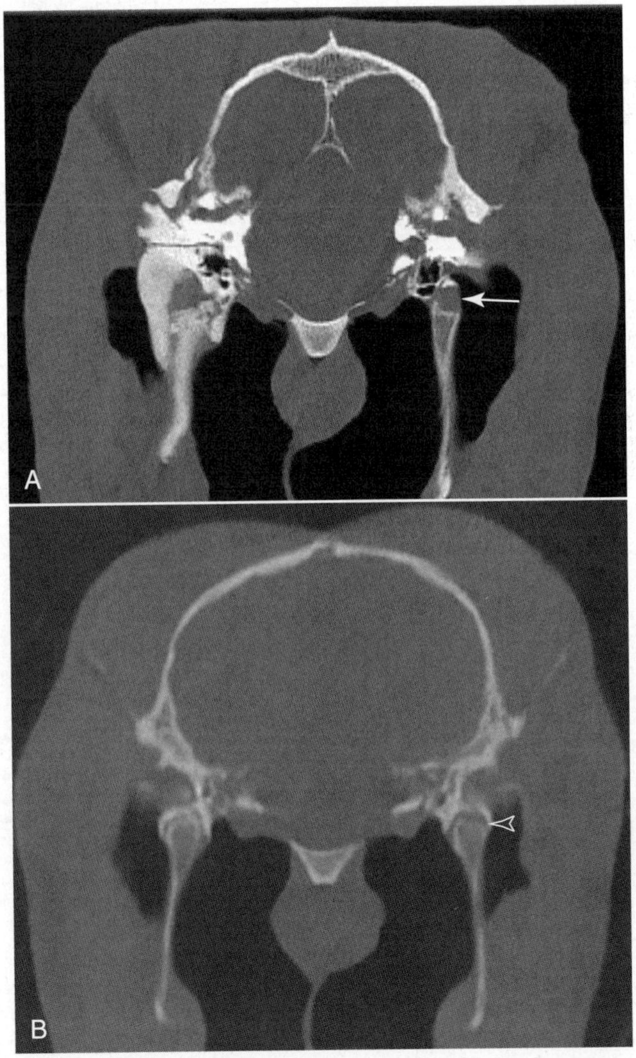

Fig. 13.41 Computed tomography (CT) images of a horse with unilateral severe temporohyoid osteoarthropathy (THO) **(A)** and mild bilateral THO **(B)**. The normal temporohyoid joint (*arrow*) has nonmineralized tympanohyoid cartilage (*arrow*) between the bulla and stylohyoid bone. The contralateral temporohyoid joint in **A** has severe bridging proliferation characteristic of severe THO. The other affected horse **(B)** has mild bilateral mineralization of the tympanohyoid cartilage (*arrowhead*).

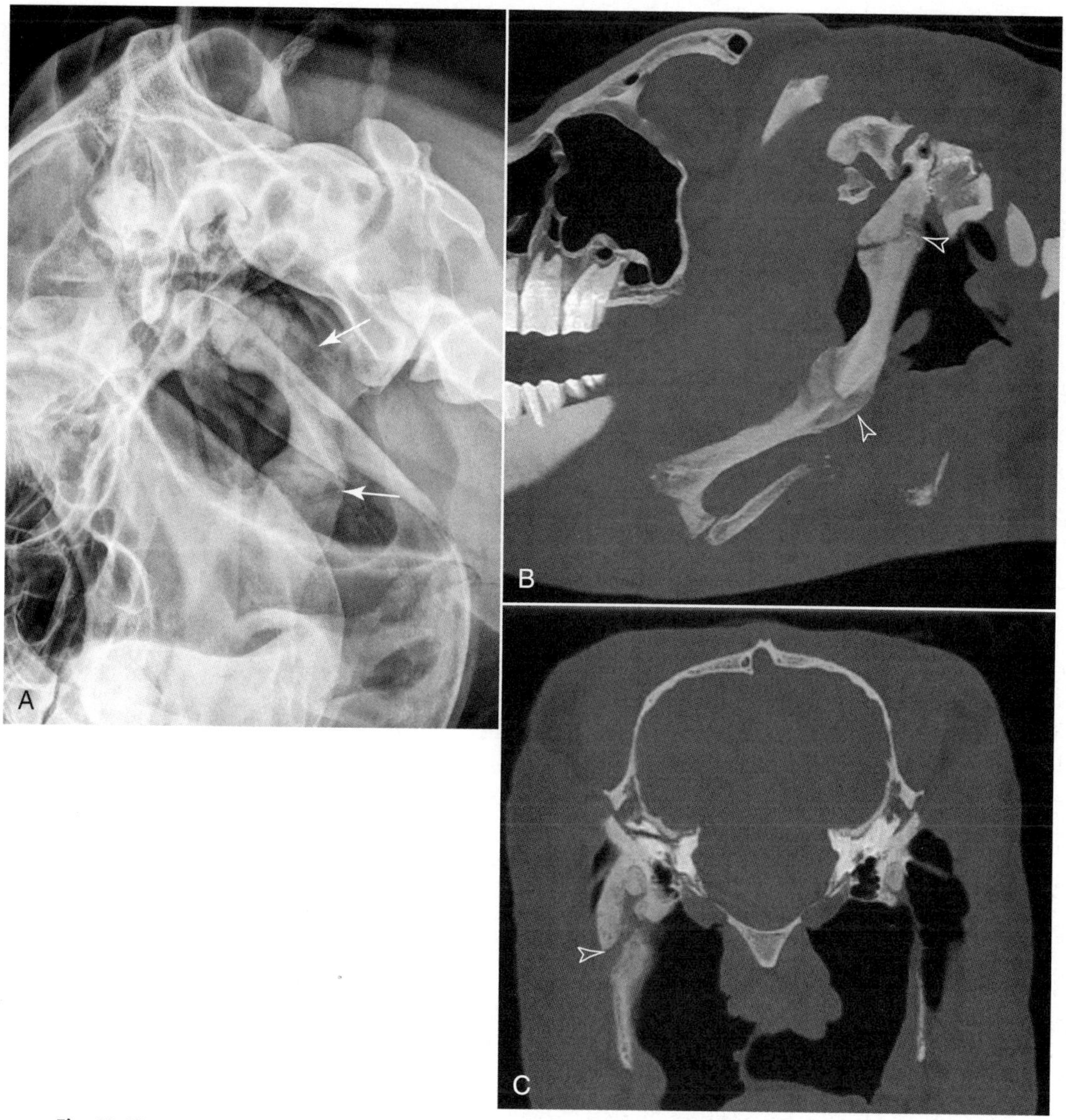

Fig. 13.42 Radiograph **(A)**, sagittal **(B)**, and transverse **(C)** computed tomography (CT) images of a horse with severe temporohyoid osteoarthropathy resulting in stylohyoid diffuse thickening (*arrows*) and chronic fractures (*open arrowheads*). CT better demonstrates the presence of fractures.

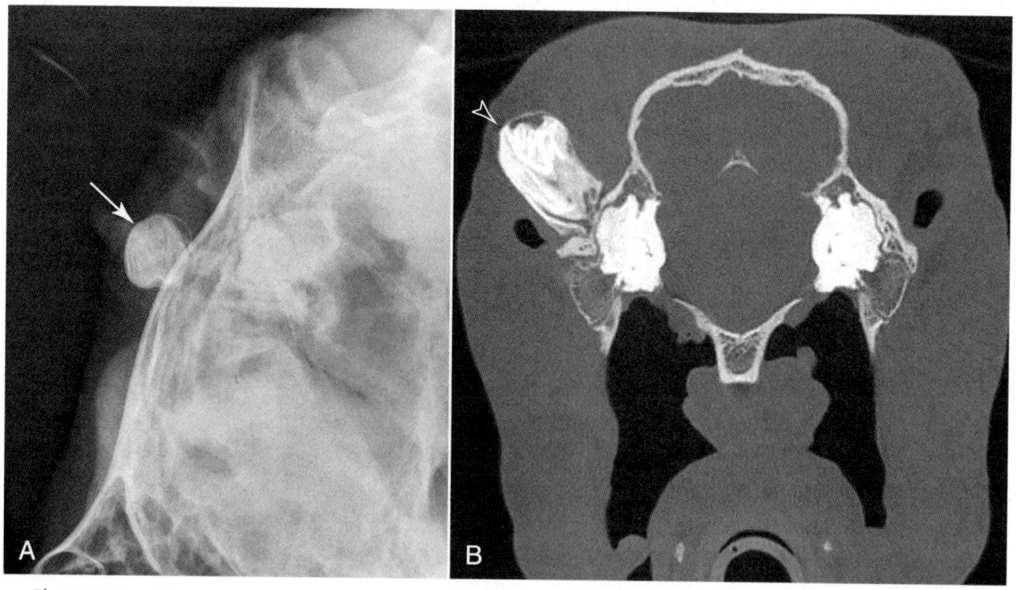

Fig. 13.43 Oblique radiograph of the right ear **(A)** and computed tomography (CT) **(B)** showing a dentigerous cyst. On the radiograph the dentigerous cyst is superimposed with the pinna (*arrow*) with the inner tooth-like structure more apparent on the CT (*open arrowhead*).

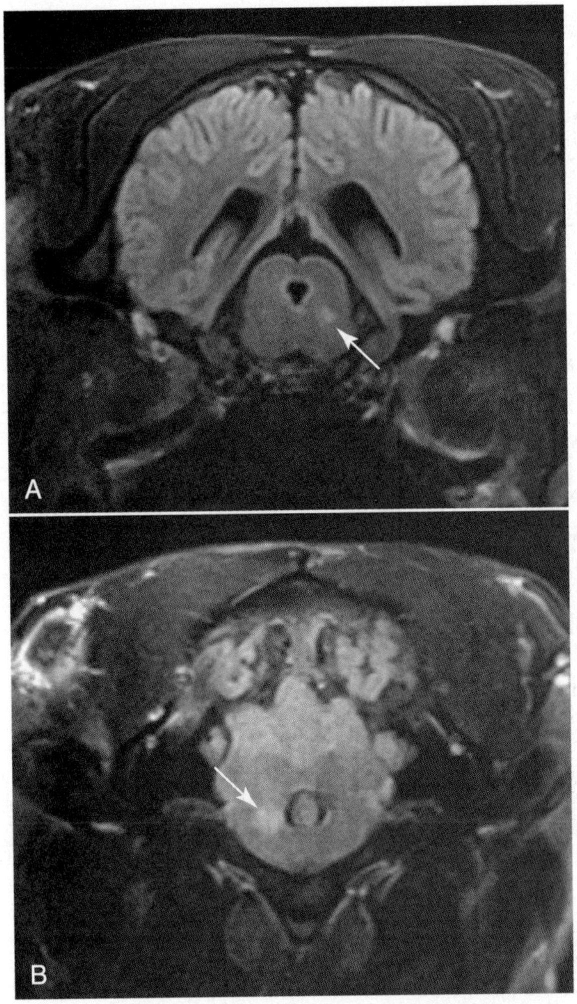

Fig. 13.44 A and B, Transverse fluid-attenuated inversion recovery (FLAIR) images of a horse with equine protozoal myeloencephalitis showing multifocal hyperintensities within the brainstem (*arrows*).

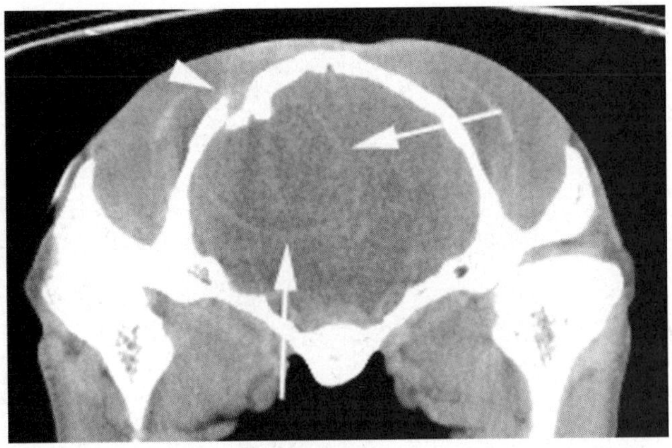

Fig. 13.45 Contrast-enhanced transverse computed tomography (CT) image of the brain. There is a depression fracture of the right parietal bone (*white arrowhead*) and a ring-enhancing lesion within the brain (*white arrows*). The ring-enhancing lesion is the vascular capsule of a brain abscess caused by penetrating trauma.

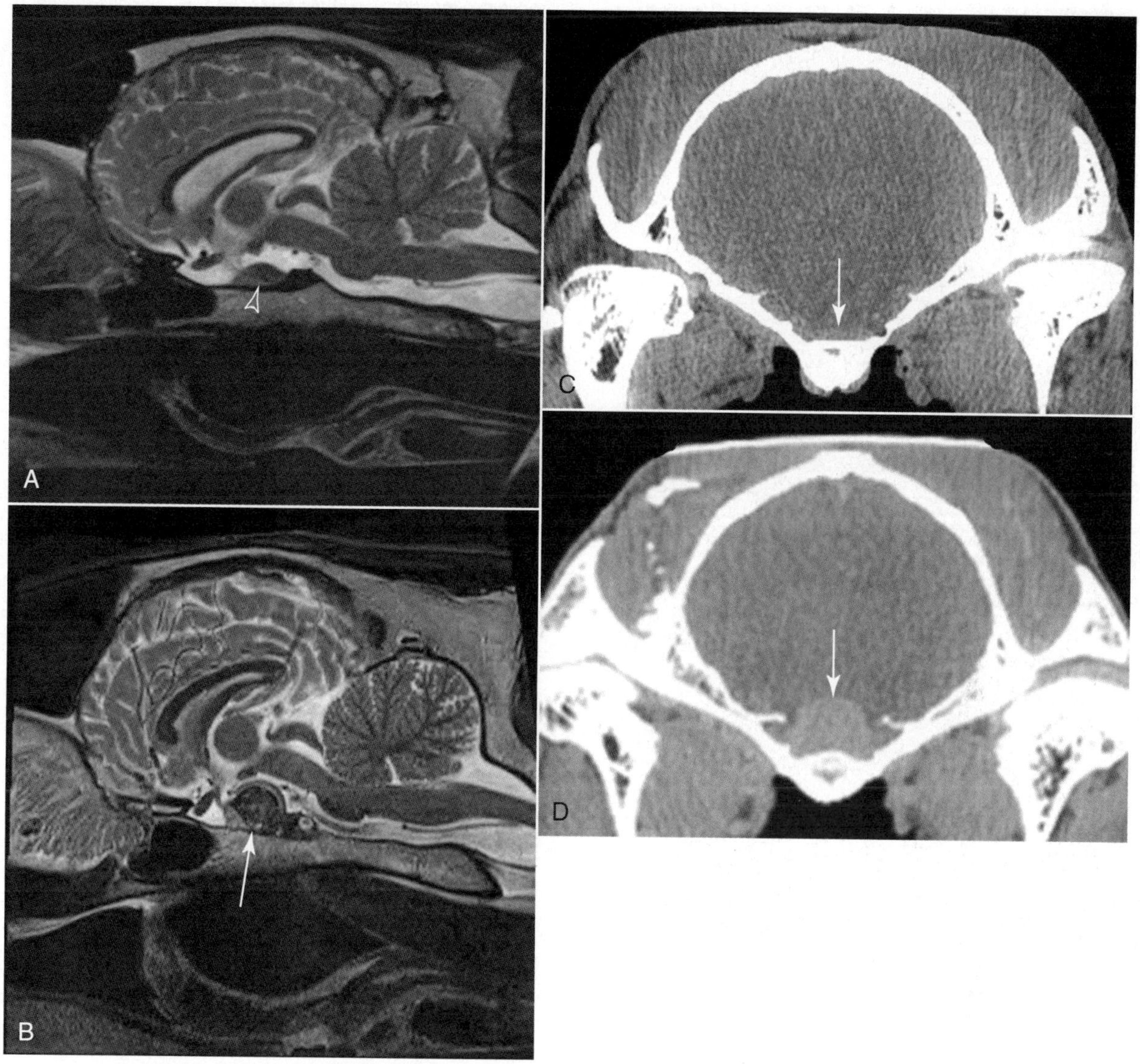

Fig. 13.46 Sagittal T2-weighted magnetic resonance imaging (MRI) image of the brain in a normal horse **(A)** and a horse with hyperadrenocorticism **(B)**. The normal pituitary gland (*arrowhead*) is homogenously hypointense. The affected pituitary gland (*arrow*) is enlarged and hypointense. The low-signal area is likely secondary to increased dopamine, which is paramagnetic and causes a susceptibility artifact on gradient recalled echo sequences. No evidence of hemorrhage was found histopathologically. Transverse postcontrast computed tomography (CT) image of the brain in a normal horse **(C)** and a horse with hyperadrenocorticism **(D)**. There is diffuse enlargement of the pituitary gland in the affected horse (*arrows*).

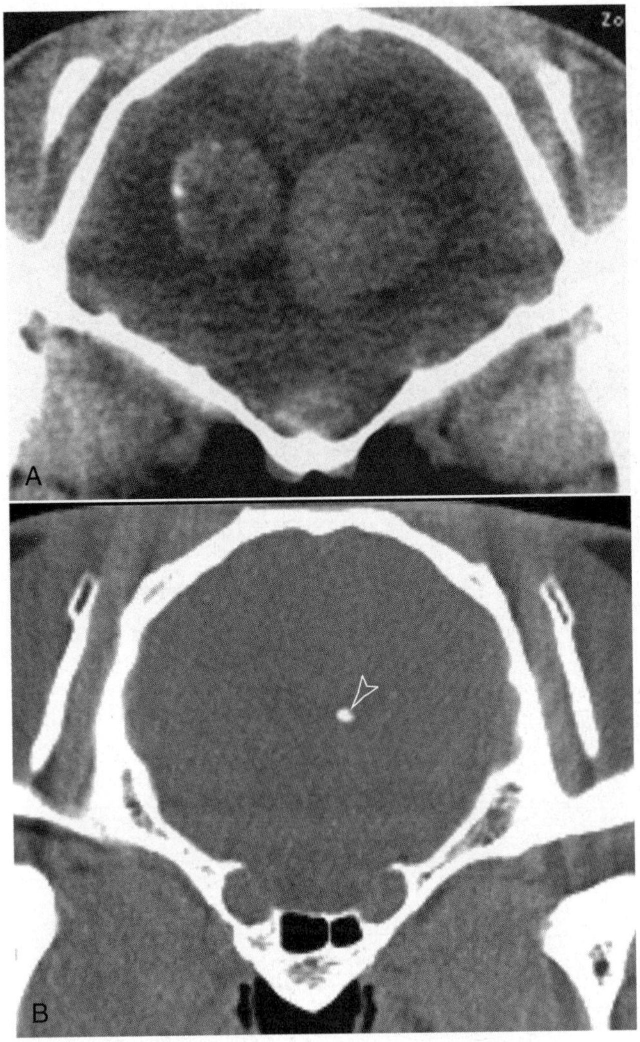

Fig. 13.47 Transverse computed tomography (CT) images of a horse with bilateral very large cholesterol granulomas **(A)** and a horse with a small unilateral granuloma (**B**, *open arrowhead*). The small granulomas are much more commonly seen.

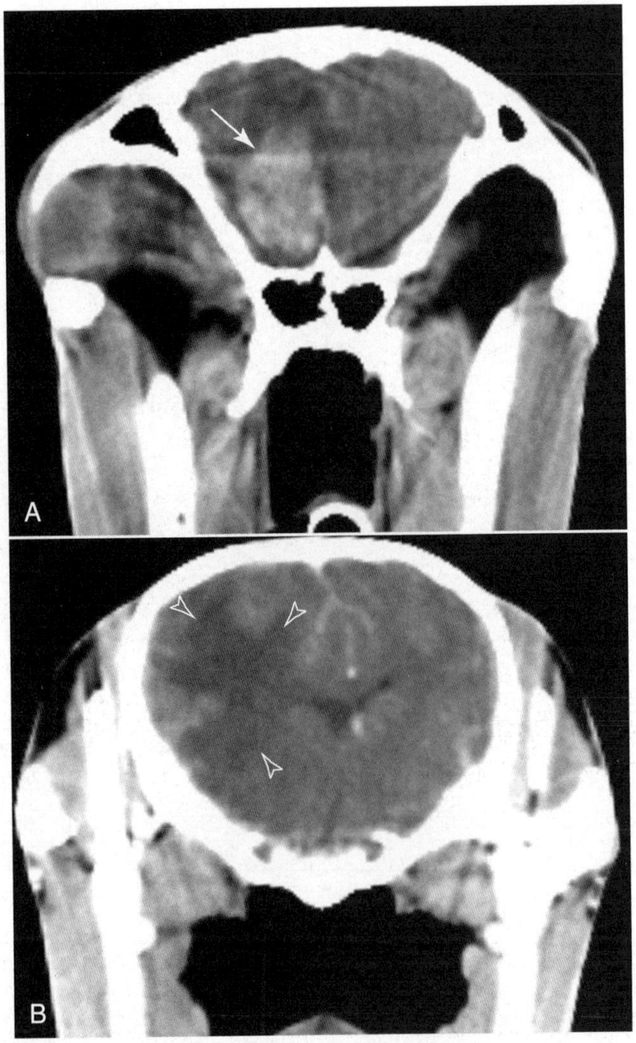

Fig. 13.48 Transverse computed tomography (CT) images of a horse with head trauma showing a large hyperattenuating hematoma in the right forebrain (**A**, *arrow*). There is extensive vasogenic edema caudal to this (**B**, *open arrowheads*) characterized by hypoattenuation and expansion of the white matter tracts.

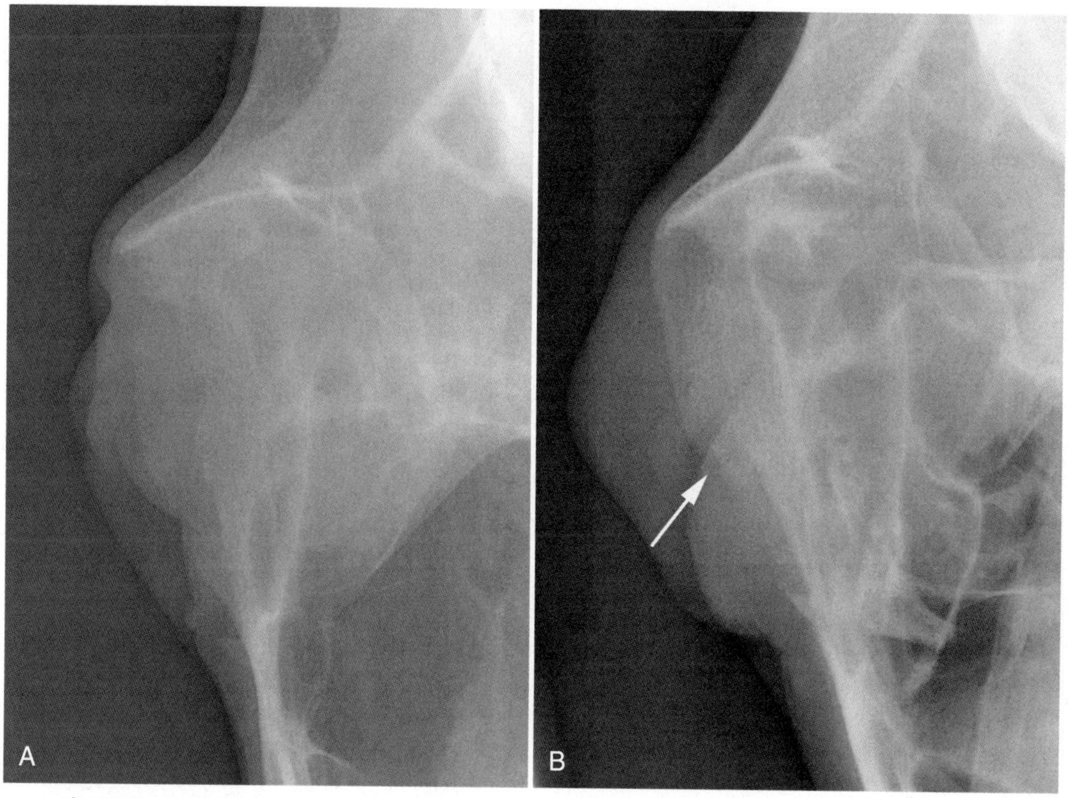

Fig. 13.49 Oblique radiographs of a normal left supraorbital process **(A)** and a right **(B)** supraorbital process with multiple fractures (*arrow*). These images are from the same horse.

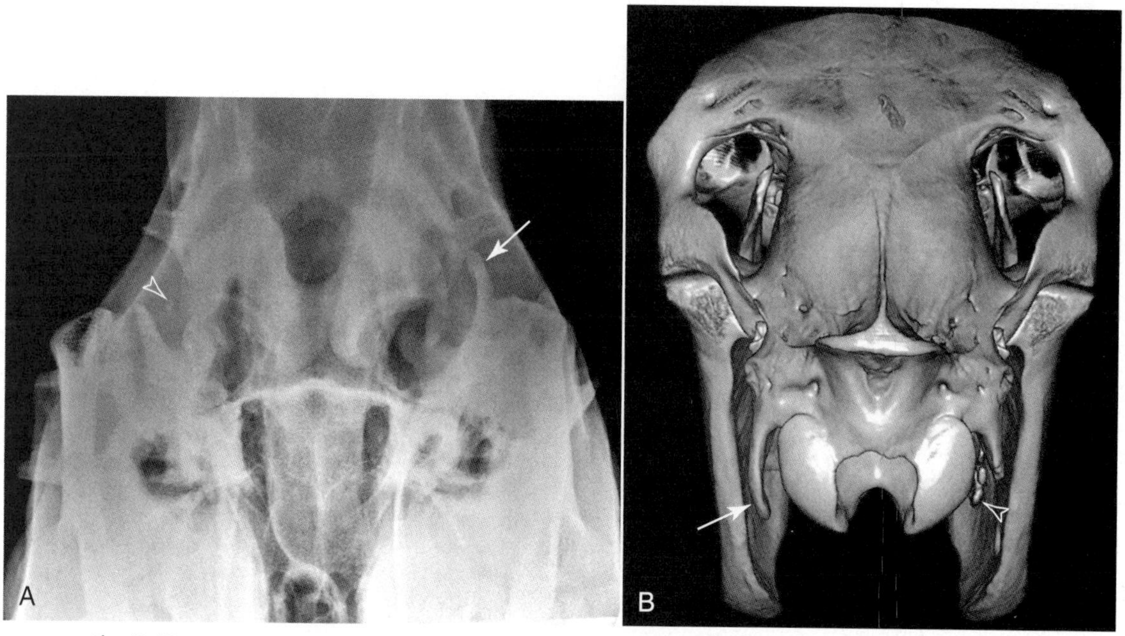

Fig. 13.50 Dorsoventral radiograph **(A)** and three-dimensional, computed tomography (CT) image **(B)** of a horse with a paracondylar process fracture (*open arrowheads*) made most apparent when compared to the normal side (*arrows*). The fracture is more readily identified on the CT image.

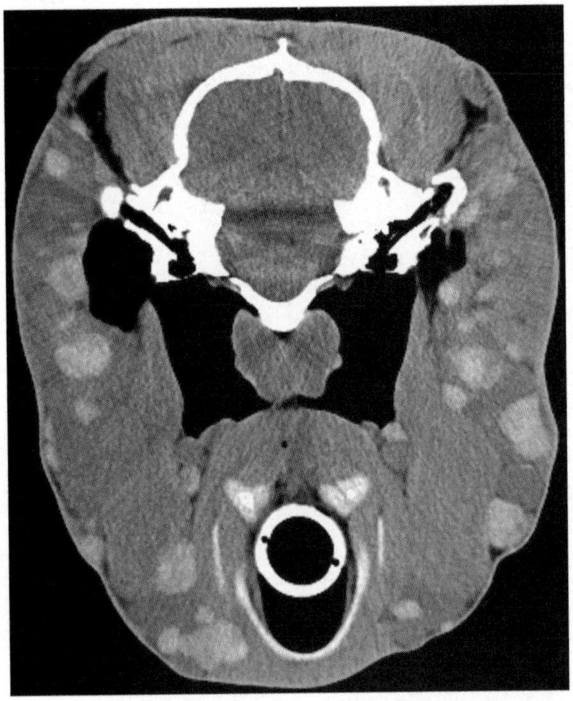

Fig. 13.51 Computed tomography (CT) image without intravenous contrast agent showing numerous hyperattenuating nodules throughout the soft tissues of the head, consistent with melanomas.

Acknowledgment

With special thanks to prior authors of this chapter for their contributions.

REFERENCES

1. Dixon PM, Froydenlund T, Luiti T, et al. Empyema of the nasal conchal bulla as a cause of chronic unilateral nasal discharge in the horse: 10 cases (2013–2014). *Equine Vet J*. 2015;47:445–449.
2. Fenner MF, Verwilghen D, Townsend N, et al. Paranasal sinus cysts in the horse: complications related to their presence and surgical treatment in 37 cases. *Equine Vet J*. 2019;51:57–63.
3. Woodford NS, Lane JG. Long-term retrospective study of 52 horses with sinunasal cysts. *Equine Vet J*. 2006;38:198–202.
4. Ostrowska J, Lindstrom L, Toth T, et al. Computed tomography characteristics of equine paranasal sinus cysts. *Equine Vet J*. 2020;52:538–546.
5. Textor JA, Puchalski SM, Affolter VK, et al. Results of computed tomography in horses with ethmoid hematoma: 16 cases (1993-2005). *JAVMA-J Am Vet Med A*. 2012;240:1338–1344.
6. Cissell DD, Wisner ER, Textor J, et al. Computed tomographic appearance of equine sinonasal neoplasia. *Vet Radiol Ultrasound*. 2012;53:245–251.
7. Head KW, Dixon PM. Equine nasal and paranasal sinus tumours. Part 1: review of the literature and tumour classification. *Vet J*. 1999;157:261–278.
8. Dixon PM, Parkin TD, Collins N, et al. Historical and clinical features of 200 cases of equine sinus disease. *Vet Rec*. 2011;169:439.
9. Tremaine WH, Clarke CJ, Dixon PM. Histopathological findings in equine sinonasal disorders. *Equine Vet J*. 1999;31:296–303.
10. Dixon PM, Dacre I. A review of equine dental disorders. *Vet J*. 2005;169:165–187.
11. Morgan RE, Fiske-Jackson AR, Hellige M, et al. Equine odontogenic tumors: clinical presentation, CT findings, and outcome in 11 horses. *Vet Radiol Ultrasoun*. 2019;60:502–512.
12. Limone LE. Update on equine odontoclastic tooth resorption and hypercementosis. *Vet Clin North Am Equine Pract*. 2020;36:671–689.
13. James O. Equine odontoclastic tooth resorption and hypercementosis. *J Vet Dent*. 2022;39:346–357.
14. Rehrl S, Schroder W, Muller C, et al. Radiological prevalence of equine odontoclastic tooth resorption and hypercementosis. *Equine Vet J*. 2018;50:481–487.
15. David F, Levingstone TJ, Schneeweiss W, et al. Enhanced bone healing using collagen-hydroxyapatite scaffold implantation in the treatment of a large multiloculated mandibular aneurysmal bone cyst in a thoroughbred filly. *J Tissue Eng Regen Med*. 2015;9:1193–1199.
16. Lamb CR, Schelling SH. Congenital aneurysmal bone cyst in the mandible of a foal. *Equine Vet J*. 1989;21:130–132.
17. Mendoza FJ, Toribio RE, Perez-Ecija A. Nutritional secondary hyperparathyroidism in equids: overview and new insights. *Equine Vet Educ*. 2017;29:558–563.
18. Leitzen E, Stumpf S, Zimmermann C, et al. A rare case of vascular proliferation in the mandible of a juvenile horse. *Front Vet Sci*. 2020;7:573540.
19. Nottle BF, Tatarniuk DM, Caldwell FJ, et al. Fibro-osseous lesions of the craniofacial complex in horses: 30 cases (2001–2019). *Vet Surg*. 2021;50:383–392.
20. Sponseller BA, Caston SS, Winter MD, et al. What is your diagnosis? Chronic juvenile ossifying fibroma. *J Am Vet Med Assoc*. 2006;229:1727–1728.
21. Bonilla AG, Wilson K, Santschi EM. Suture exostosis with concurrent nasal septum chondrosarcoma in a horse. *Equine Vet Educ*. 2015;27:579–584.
22. Verwilghen D, Easley J, Zwick T, et al. Equine suture exostosis: a review of cases from a multicenter retrospective study. *Vet Sci*. 2022;9.
23. Ebling AJ, McKnight AL, Seiler G, et al. A complementary radiographic projection of the equine temporomandibular joint. *Vet Radiol Ultrasound*. 2009;50:385–391.
24. Townsend NB, Cotton JC, Barakzai SZ. A tangential radiographic projection for investigation of the equine temporomandibular joint. *Vet Surg*. 2009;38:601–606.
25. Ramzan PH, Marr CM, Meehan J, et al. Novel oblique radiographic projection of the temporomandibular articulation of horses. *Vet Rec*. 2008;162:714–716.
26. Carmalt JL, Kneissl S, Rawlinson JE, et al. Computed tomographic appearance of the temporomandibular joint in 1018 asymptomatic horses: a multi-institution study. *Vet Radiol Ultrasound*. 2016;57:237–245.
27. Rizk A, Hamed M. The use of cerclage wire for surgical repair of unilateral rostral mandibular fracture in horses. *Iran J Vet Res*. 2018;19:123–127.
28. Huggons NA, Bell RJW, Puchalski SM. Radiography and computed tomography in the diagnosis of nonneoplastic equine mandibular disease. *Vet Radiol Ultrasoun*. 2011;52:53–60.
29. Freeman DE. Update on disorders and treatment of the guttural pouch. *Vet Clin N Am-Equine*. 2015;31:63–89.
30. Dixon J, Smith K, Perkins J, et al. Computed tomographic appearance of melanomas in the equine head: 13 cases. *Vet Radiol Ultrasoun*. 2016;57:246–252.
31. Hance SR, Bertone AL. Neoplasia. *Vet Clin N Am-Equine*. 1993;9:213–234.
32. McCarrel TM, Woodie JB. Update on laryngeal disorders and treatment. *Vet Clin North Am Equine Pract*. 2015;31:13–26.

33. Virgin JE, Holcombe SJ, Caron JP, et al. Laryngeal advancement surgery improves swallowing function in a reversible equine dysphagia model. *Equine Vet J*. 2016;48:362–367.
34. Bowkett-Pritchard C, Morgan RE. Laryngeal dysplasia: computed tomographic findings in an Oldenburg mare. *Equine Vet Educ*. 2023;35:26–30.
35. Orsini PG, Raker CW, Reid CF, et al. Xeroradiographic evaluation of the equine larynx. *Am J Vet Res*. 1989;50: 845–849.
36. Garrett KS, Embertson RM, Woodie JB, et al. Ultrasound features of arytenoid chondritis in Thoroughbred horses. *Equine Vet J*. 2013;45:598–603.
37. Barakzai SZ, Hawkes CS. Dorsal displacement of the soft palate and palatal instability. *Equine Vet Educ*. 2010;22:253–264.
38. Aitken MR, Parente EJ. Epiglottic abnormalities in mature nonracehorses: 23 cases (1990–2009). *Javma-J Am Vet Med A*. 2011;238:1634–1638.
39. Hawkins JF, Tulleners EP. Epiglottitis in horses: 20 cases (1988-1993). *J Am Vet Med Assoc*. 1994;205:1577–1580.
40. Saulez MN, Gummow B. Prevalence of pharyngeal, laryngeal and tracheal disorders in thoroughbred racehorses, and effect on performance. *Vet Rec*. 2009;165: 431–435.
41. Ducharme NG, Rossignol F. Larynx In: Auer JA, Stick JG, eds. *Equine Surgery*. 5th ed. St. Louis: Elsevier; 759.
42. Naylor RJ, Perkins JD, Allen S, et al. Histopathology and computed tomography of age-associated degeneration of the equine temporohyoid joint. *Equine Vet J*. 2010;42: 425–430.
43. Walker AM, Sellon DC, Cornelisse CJ, et al. Temporohyoid osteoarthropathy in 33 horses (1993–2000). *J Vet Intern Med*. 2002;16:697–703.
44. Pownder S, Scrivani PV, Bezuidenhout A, et al. Computed tomography of temporal bone fractures and temporal region anatomy in horses. *J Vet Intern Med*. 2010;24: 398–406.
45. Ruby JL, Scrivani PV, Thompson MS. What is your diagnosis? *Javma-J Am Vet Med A*. 2015;247:1097–1099.
46. Garrett KS. Special diagnostic techniques in equine neurology (radiography, ultrasonography, computed tomography, and magnetic resonance imaging). *Vet Clin North Am Equine Pract*. 2022;38:171–188.
47. Scrivani PV. Advanced imaging of the nervous system in the horse. *Vet Clin North Am Equine Pract*. 2011;27:439–453.
48. Cavasin JP, Miller AD, Duhamel GE. Intracerebral astrocytoma in a horse. *J Comp Pathol*. 2020;177:1–4.
49. van der Kolk JH, Heinrichs M, van Amerongen JD, et al. Evaluation of pituitary gland anatomy and histopathologic findings in clinically normal horses and horses and ponies with pituitary pars intermedia adenoma. *Am J Vet Res*. 2004;65:1701–1707.
50. Hobbs KJ, Porter E, Wait C, et al. Magnetic resonance imaging of the normal equine pituitary gland. *Vet Radiol Ultrasound*. 2022;63:450–455.
51. McKlveen TL, Jones JC, Sponenberg DP, et al. Assessment of the accuracy of computed tomography for measurement of normal equine pituitary glands. *Am J Vet Res*. 2003;64:1387–1394.
52. Pease AP, Schott 2nd HC, Howey EB, et al. Computed tomographic findings in the pituitary gland and brain of horses with pituitary pars intermedia dysfunction. *J Vet Intern Med*. 2011;25:1144–1151.
53. Tofflemire KL, Whitley RD, Wong DM, et al. Episodic blindness and ataxia in a horse with cholesterinic granulomas. *Vet Ophthalmol*. 2013;16:149–152.
54. Jackson CA, deLahunta A, Dykes NL, et al. Neurological manifestation of cholesterinic granulomas in three horses. *Vet Rec*. 1994;135:228–230.
55. Nout-Lomas YS. Traumatic nervous system injury. *Vet Clin North Am Equine Pract*. 2022;38:363–377.
56. Feary DJ, Magdesian KG, Aleman MA, et al. Traumatic brain injury in horses: 34 cases (1994–2004). *J Am Vet Med Assoc*. 2007;231:259–266.
57. Gerding JC, Clode A, Gilger BC, et al. Equine orbital fractures: a review of 18 cases (2006–2013). *Vet Ophthalmol*. 2014;1:97–106, 17 Suppl.
58. Lischer CJ, Walliser U, Witzmann P, et al. Fracture of the paracondylar process in four horses: advantages of CT imaging. *Equine Vet J*. 2005;37:483–487.

ELECTRONIC RESOURCES

Additional information related to the content in Chapter 13 can be found online at eBooks.Health.Elsevier.com.

- Chapter Quiz

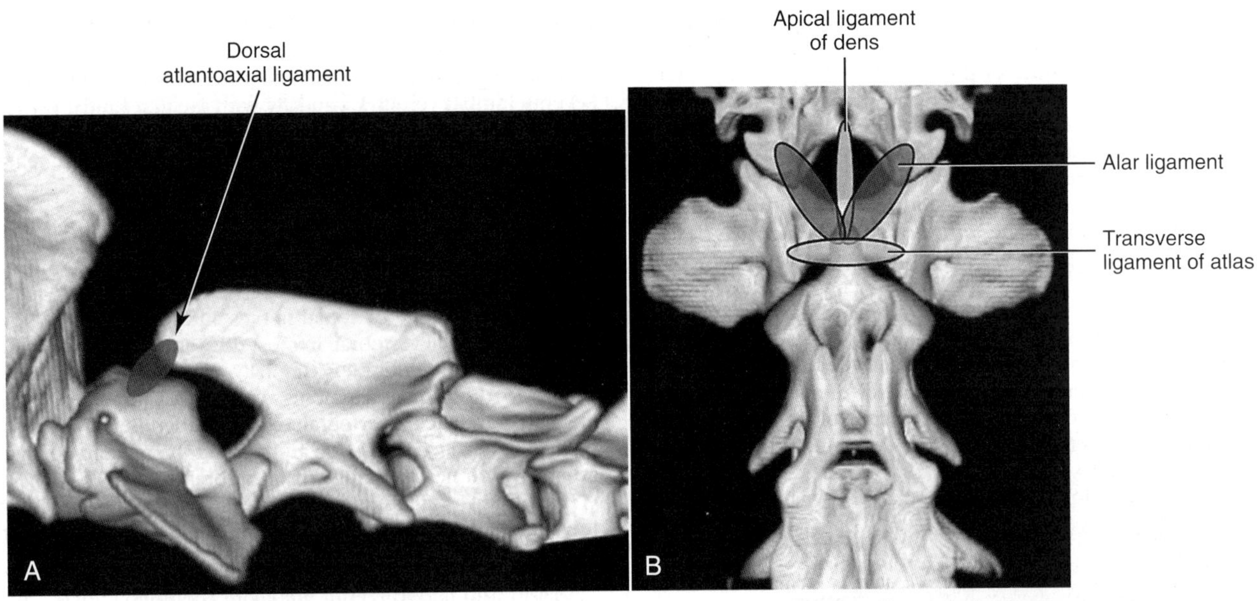

Fig. 14.4 **A,** Lateral view of a three-dimensional rendering of the cranial aspect of the cervical spine in a dog. Note the position of the dorsal atlantoaxial ligament. **B,** Dorsal view of a three-dimensional rendering of the cranial aspect of the cervical spine in a dog. The dorsal lamina of C1 and C2 has been removed to allow visualization of the ligaments on the floor of the vertebral canal. Note how the apical ligament of the dens along with its alar branches and the transverse ligament of the atlas provide stabilization of the atlantoaxial joint.

retinaculum of the articular process joints.[7] Maintaining stability of the atlantoaxial joint is particularly important given the potential for the dens to damage the spinal cord if displaced dorsally. This stabilization is provided by the short, dorsal atlantoaxial ligament, the apical ligament of the dens with its alar branches, and the transverse ligament of the atlas (Fig. 14.4).

In the dog, the nuchal ligament extends from the spinous process of the axis to the spinous processes of the first three thoracic vertebrae and is continued caudally as the supraspinous ligament. It prevents abnormal separation of the spinous processes during flexion. Short interspinous ligaments join each spinous process, adding additional support to the vertebral column. There are also short interarcuate ligaments that contain yellow elastic fibers, which bridge each vertebral arch dorsally. Collectively, these short ligaments have been referred to as the *ligamentum flavum.* These ligaments are difficult to visualize with drawings; thus, see multiplanar MR images in eFig. 14.1A for a better anatomical understanding. There is no nuchal ligament in the cat.

The dorsal longitudinal ligament lies on the floor of the vertebral canal and extends from the dens to the sacrum (Fig. 14.5). The *intercapital* ligaments are short, transverse fibrous bands that lie ventral to the dorsal longitudinal ligament, joining contralateral rib heads between T2 and T11. These ligaments buttress the dorsal part of the annulus cranial to T11 and lead to a reduced incidence of disc herniation between T1 and T11.[7,8]

The ventral longitudinal ligament is smaller than the dorsal longitudinal ligament and spans the ventral surface of the vertebral column (see Fig. 14.5). The annulus fibrosus of each intervertebral disc has oblique fibers that course from one endplate to the next, serving as ligaments.

The intervertebral disc is composed of a tough outer annulus fibrosus, which contains the gelatinous, inner nucleus pulposus (see Fig. 14.5).[7,8] The disc forms a cartilaginous joint between vertebral segments (except at C1–C2 and the sacrum where intervertebral discs are not present) and thus functions as a hydraulic shock absorber. Shock absorption is dependent on a hydrated, deformable nucleus and an intact, elastic annulus.[7]

Compared to canine vertebral, feline vertebra have a shorter body (centrum), narrower intervertebral disc spaces, and more prominent lumbar transverse processes (eFig. 14.2).

A summary of the most important anatomic considerations of the canine and feline vertebrae relative to radiographic interpretation is provided in Box 14.1.[9–11]

ANOMALIES OF THE VERTEBRAL COLUMN

Anomalies of the vertebral column are common and include congenital and developmental malformations.[12,13] Many of these abnormalities are normal variants and have no clinical importance. Additional information on normal variants can be found in Thrall and Robertson.[1]

Block Vertebrae

A block vertebra results from fusion of two or more adjacent vertebral bodies. The vertebral arches may also be fused, or they may be unaffected (Fig. 14.6, eFig. 14.3).[1] The disc space between a block vertebra often appears radiographically as a thin radiolucent line but may not be visible at all if the fusion is complete. Block vertebrae are most common in the cervical region, but they also occur in the lumbar spine. Biomechanically, block vertebrae may act as a fulcrum, leading to altered and increased loading immediately adjacent to the fusion. This has been hypothesized to increase the risk of disc disease at adjacent sites (see eFig. 14.3) and has also been implicated in leading to atlantoaxial subluxation.[14] The fused sacral vertebrae are a normal type of block vertebra.

Hemivertebrae

Hemivertebrae are the result of failure of the development and eventual ossification of part of a vertebra, usually the body.[1,12,15] The shape of a hemivertebra depends on the area that fails to develop. A wedge-shaped vertebra is seen on the lateral projection when the ventral aspect of the vertebral body is developed incompletely (Fig. 14.7). When this occurs, the vertebral column often acquires a kyphotic configuration that can lead to extradural compression of the spinal cord. Not all

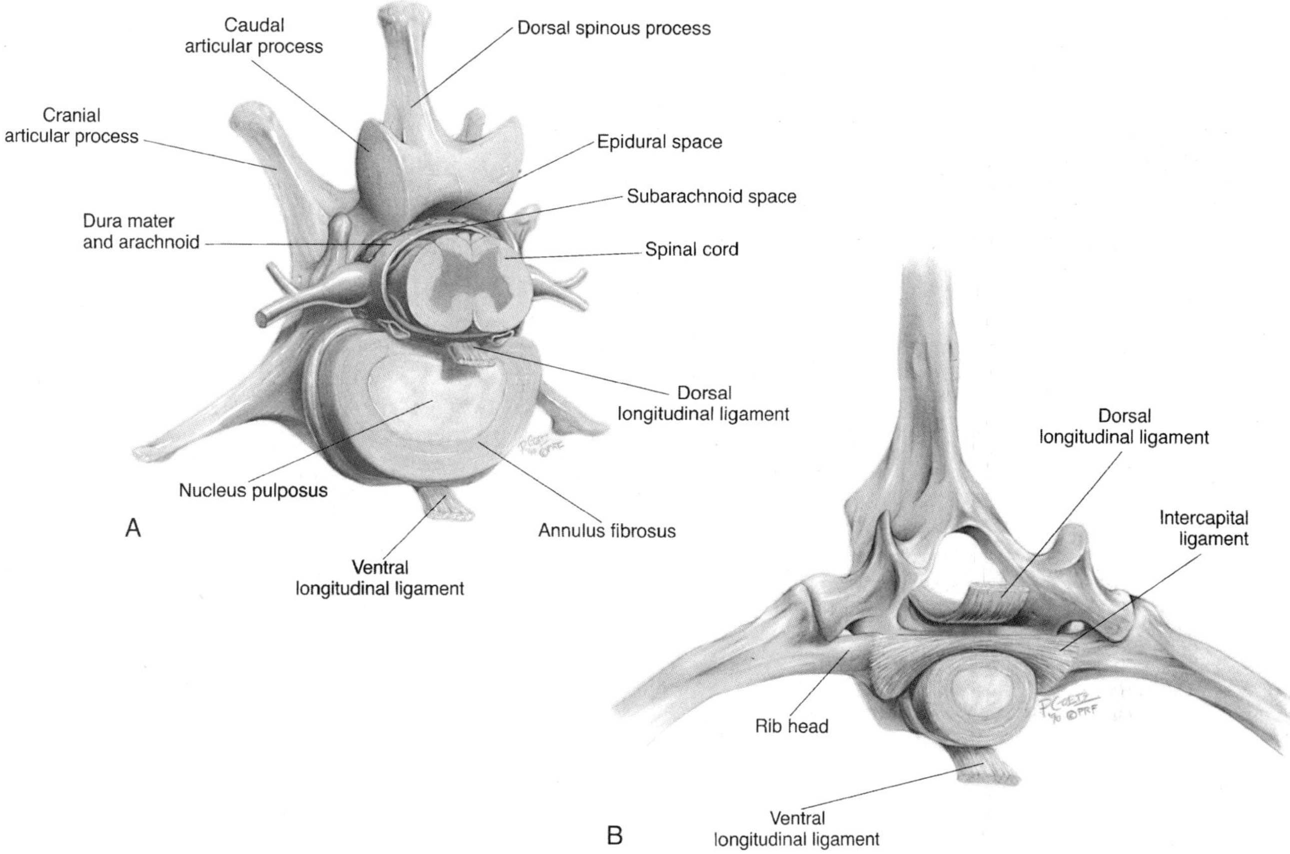

Fig. 14.5 Anatomic components of a typical lumbar vertebra **(A)** and a typical thoracic vertebra and articulation with ribs **(B)**. (Modified from Evans HE, Christensen, JC. *Miller's Anatomy of the Dog*. 2nd ed. Philadelphia: Saunders; 1979.)

Box 14.1

Summary of Important Anatomic Features of the Vertebral Column in Small Animals

- Vertebral formulae
  - Dog: C7 T13 L7 S3 Cd6-Cd23
  - Cat: C7 T13 L7 S3 Cd18-Cd21
- The articular processes of adjacent vertebrae overlap, with the cranial articular process lying ventral to the caudal articular process of an adjacent vertebra.
  - In the cervical region, the articular processes are oriented in an oblique plane, summating the intervertebral foramina and vertebral canal.
  - In the lumbar region, the articular processes lie in a dorsal plane and do not summate the foramina and canal.
- C1–C2 does not have an intervertebral disc.
- The dens is usually masked on a true lateral projection but is easily recognized on a lateral view made with slight axial rotation (obliquity).
- The spinous processes of C1 and C2 normally are in close proximity, and the dorsal laminae are nearly parallel, on the lateral projection. This normal relationship is important in recognizing atlantoaxial subluxation.
- C6 is distinguished by large transverse process.
- The intervertebral disc spaces of the cervical vertebrae become progressively wider between C2–C3 and C6–C7.
- T1 has a pronounced spinous process compared with C7.
- T11 is the anticlinal vertebra in most dogs; however, T10 may also be designated the anticlinal vertebra.
- The T10–T11 intervertebral disc space is narrower than adjacent disc spaces in most dogs.
- The ventral aspect of the bodies of L3 and L4 are entheses for the diaphragmatic crura and may be indistinct, especially in large dogs.

From Walker MA. The vertebrae—canine and feline. In: Thrall DE, ed. Textbook of Veterinary Diagnostic Radiology. 4th ed. St. Louis: Saunders; 2002:98–109; Baines EQ, Grandage J, Herritage ME, et al. Radiographic definition of the anticlinal vertebra in the dog. Vet Radiol Ultrasound. 2009;50:69–73.

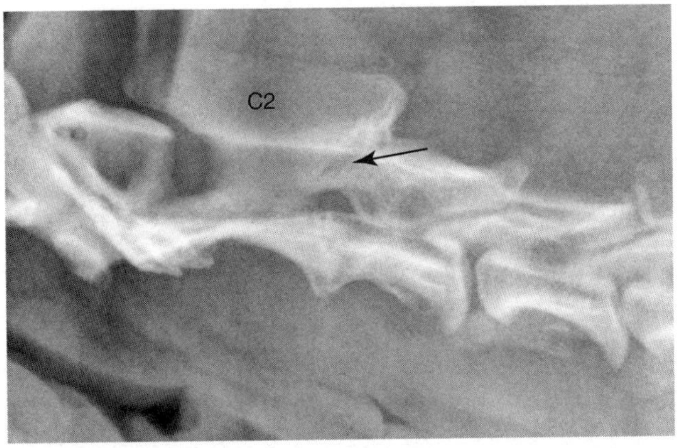

Fig. 14.6 Lateral radiograph of a dog with a block vertebra affecting C2–C3. The intervertebral disc space appears as a thin vertical radiolucent line. A radiolucent line is also visible dorsally at the dorsal articular process joint (*arrow*). These lines signify that complete fusion has not occurred in this dog although there is still increased risk of altered loading of the intervertebral disc at C3–C4, immediately caudal to the fusion.

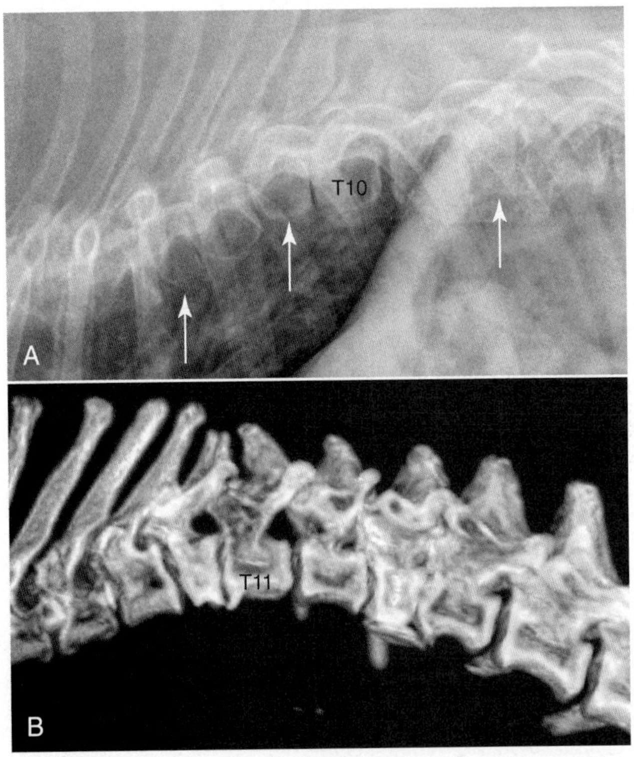

Fig. 14.7 **A,** Lateral thoracic radiograph of a bulldog with multiple hemivertebrae (*white arrows*). **B,** Lateral view of a three-dimensional rendering of the spine of another bulldog. There are hemivertebrae at T10 and T13. *T10,* Tenth thoracic vertebral body; *T11,* eleventh thoracic vertebral body.

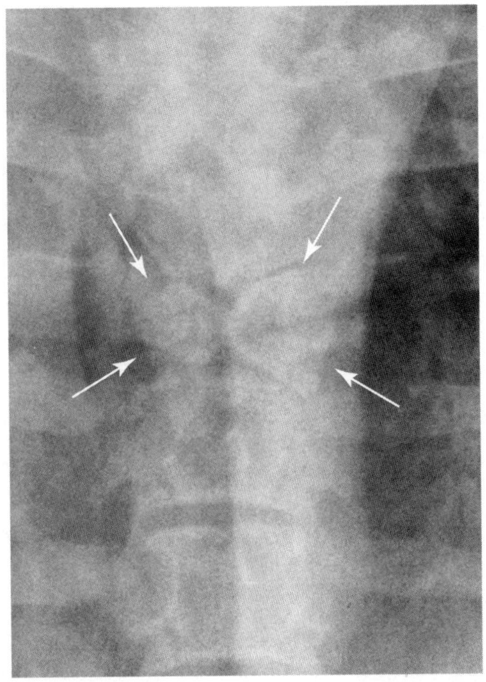

Fig. 14.8 Ventrodorsal (VD) radiograph of the caudal aspect for the thoracic spine in a bulldog. A butterfly anomaly is present (*arrows*).

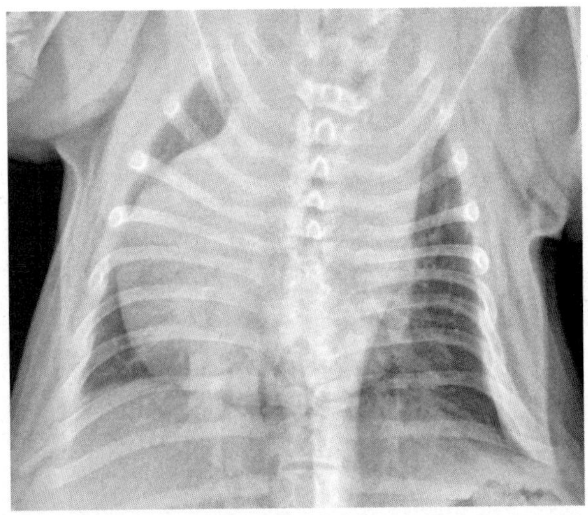

Fig. 14.9 Ventrodorsal (VD) radiograph of a bulldog with multiple thoracic hemivertebrae. The abnormal vertebrae have resulted in thoracic spine foreshortening with secondary crowding of the ribs. This is most noticeable in the left hemithorax.

hemivertebrae are significant clinically, and MRI is required to determine if hemivertebrae are the cause of a spinal neuropathy. A butterfly-shaped vertebra occurs when the midaspect of the body fails to develop, this is best seen on the ventrodorsal (VD) projection[16] (Fig. 14.8). Decreased rib spacing on the VD projection is an important clue that hemivertebrae are present (Fig. 14.9). A hemivertebra should not be confused with a compression fracture; their multiplicity and occurrence in a brachycephalic breed are helpful in this distinction. Also, hemivertebrae have a smoothly marginated cortex, whereas vertebrae affected with a compression fracture have a disrupted margin. The bulldog, French bulldog, Boston terrier, pug and other screw-tail breeds are most affected with hemivertebrae.[12,13]

Transitional Vertebrae

Vertebrae that have characteristics of two different anatomic divisions are known as *transitional vertebrae*.[1,12,17] These anomalies usually involve the vertebral arch rather than the body and occur at cervicothoracic, thoracolumbar, and lumbosacral junctions. The main clinical significance of transitional vertebral anomalies relates to the use of the most caudal ribs as a landmark to identify a site of spinal decompressive surgery. T13 may have malformed, hypoplastic, or absent ribs. L1 may also have ribs, and they may be symmetric or asymmetric. If the most caudal ribs are asymmetric, then surgery can be performed at the incorrect site unless the asymmetry is

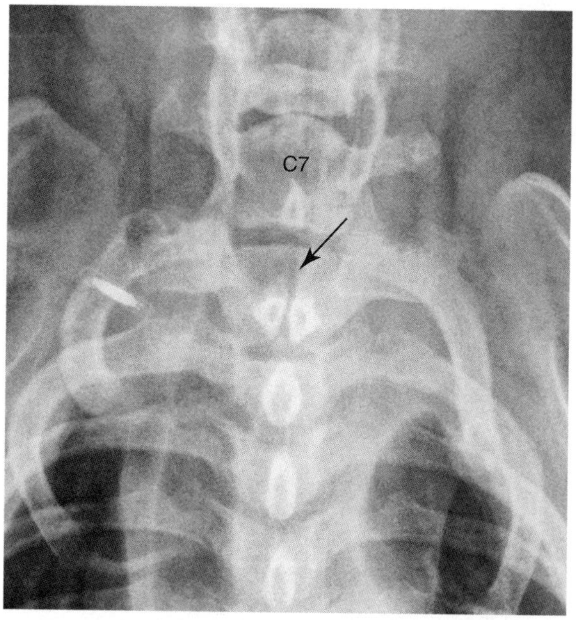

Fig. 14.10 Ventrodorsal (VD) thoracic radiograph of a dog with spina bifida. T1 is characterized by a split spinous process (*arrow*). *C7,* Seventh cervical vertebral body.

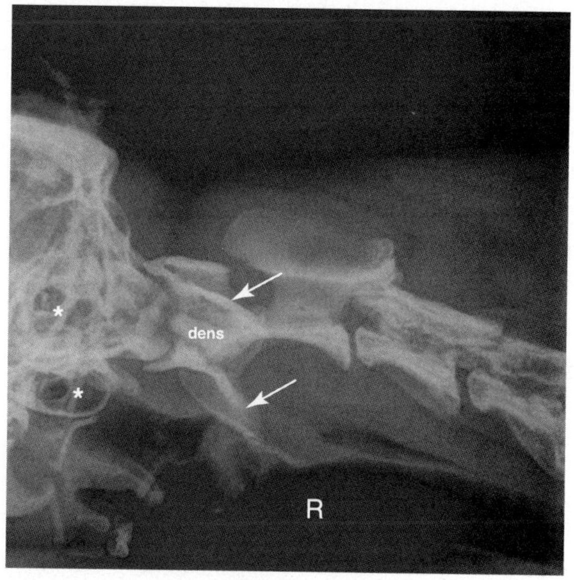

Fig. 14.11 Lateral cervical radiograph of a normal dog. The patient was placed in lateral recumbency and the head and neck were allowed to fall into a natural position on the table; e.g., the head was not rotated into true lateral positioning with the bulla and atlas wings superimposed. *Asterisks* mark the tympanic bullae and the wings of the atlas are denoted by *arrows*. This projection allows good visualization of the dens compared to the standard lateral view where the dens is summated by the lateral masses of the atlas.

recognized. Therefore, the entire spine should be radiographed, or included in CT or MR images, to be certain the thoracolumbar vertebrae are enumerated correctly prior to surgery. Another significant feature of transitional anomalies is the increased incidence of lumbosacral disc disease and nerve root compression that occurs in dogs with a lumbosacral transitional malformation.[18] This relates to the altered, asymmetrical lumbosacral loading that leads to disc degeneration, instability, spondylosis, and nerve root compression. Lumbosacral transitional vertebrae have been established as a risk factor for lumbosacral stenosis in cats.[19] Cats with nontraumatic lumbosacral abnormalities, including absence of L7, transitional vertebra, and L7-S1 degeneration, were at increased risk for constipation and megacolon.[20]

Spina Bifida

Spina bifida results from the lack of development of the vertebral arch and may be associated with neural tube defects—that is, meningocele or meningomyelocele.[1] Typically, there is a cleft in the dorsal part of the vertebral arch and absence or splitting of the spinous process. If the defect in the neural arch is large, a meningocele or meningomyelocele may develop. The most common radiographic manifestation of spina bifida is a split spinous process (Fig. 14.10). There is rarely a neural tube defect in dogs with thoracic spina bifida. At the lumbosacral junction, however, the morphologic derangements are often more severe with absent spinous process, laminar defect, and neural tube defect (eFig. 14.4). MRI is preferred for characterizing the presence and extent of any neural tube defect (see eFig. 14.4). Spina bifida is most common in bulldogs and Manx cats.[13,21]

Atlantoaxial Subluxation

In atlantoaxial subluxation, the axis (C2) is displaced dorsally with respect to the atlas (C1), causing extradural compression of the spinal cord. Atlantoaxial subluxation can be a result of either congenital malformation or trauma.[13,21,22] With congenital malformation, the dens is often absent or incompletely ossified,[23] and there may be deficiencies in the ligaments that support the atlantoaxial joint and prevent flexion (see Fig. 14.4). The clinical signs may be acute with trauma or chronic with congenital malformation and are characterized mainly by pain and cervical neuropathy.

A variety of lesions may occur in association with atlantoaxial subluxation, and a working knowledge of the components of the atlantoaxial region is needed for radiographic interpretation.[1,2] Malformation or rupture of the transverse ligament of the atlas frequently leads to atlantoaxial subluxation. This ligament bridges the ventral aspect of the vertebral arch and stabilizes the dens, preventing the rostral aspect of the axis from impinging on the spinal cord (see Fig. 14.4B). A short apical ligament connects the tip of the dens with the occiput along with the alar ligaments (see Fig. 14.4B). A short, dorsal atlantoaxial ligament is also present dorsally (see Fig. 14.4A). Atlantoaxial subluxation caused by congenital predisposition is most common in toy breed dogs, such as the Yorkshire terrier, but acquired atlantoaxial subluxation can occur in any breed.

Atlantoaxial subluxation is best diagnosed radiographically on a lateral projection of the cranial aspect of the cervical spine. When subluxation is suspected, the patient should be handled carefully, especially when tetraparetic, and the head and neck should not be flexed, because this could exacerbate spinal cord damage, especially if the dens is present. On a routine lateral radiograph, the dens is masked by the sheer mass of the atlas. Making a left 15- to 30-degree ventral/right dorsal radiograph will reduce osseous superimposition on the dens and help identify fractures and malformations. A similar radiographic projection can often be made if there is no attempt to obtain a true lateral projection, for example, allowing the axial rotation of the head and neck ventrally (Fig. 14.11). Even with this projection, small fractures may not be apparent. VD projections can also be made, but there is the risk of exacerbating the spinal cord compression, especially in anesthetized patients. The VD projection is unnecessary to confirm atlantoaxial subluxation. The lateral radiographic view is usually diagnostic and two typical findings should be identified:

- If subluxation is present, the axis is displaced dorsally, widening the distance between the vertebral arch of the atlas and the spinous process of the axis. Atlantoaxial instability is characterized by a decreased C1–C2 overlap.[24]

- Most important, the normal linear relationship between the dorsal lamina of the atlas and the dorsal lamina of the axis becomes angular (Fig. 14.12).

Multiple indices to evaluate the relationship between the lamina of C1 and C2 have been described.[24] CT is useful for assessing the morphology of the atlantoaxial junction if surgical stabilization is contemplated (see Fig. 14.12).

Incomplete Ossification of the Atlas

Three centers of ossification fuse to form the atlas and this process is normally complete by approximately 4 months of age. Incomplete ossification can lead to osseous defects at the junction of the centers of ossification and may lead to instability and atlantoaxial subluxation. Surgical stabilization may be necessary in dogs with clinical signs (Fig. 14.13).[25]

Cervical Spondylomyelopathy

Cervical spondylomyelopathy is included under anomalies because anomalous development of vertebrae or inadequate soft tissue stabilization is likely to play a role in manifestation of clinical signs. Cervical spondylomyelopathy encompasses a variety of pathologic changes that are not all seen in every affected animal.[21,26–30] Abnormalities include malformation of the vertebral body and articular processes, malarticulation, instability and malalignment, and stenosis of the vertebral canal. Secondary changes involve dorsal longitudinal ligament and ligamentum flavum hypertrophy and Hansen type II disc protrusion and/or herniation. The end result and cause of clinical signs are static or dynamic extradural cervical spinal cord compression.

The pathophysiology of canine spondylopathy is complex and understood incompletely.[26–28,31] There is debate as to whether vertebral changes are caused by strict malformation of

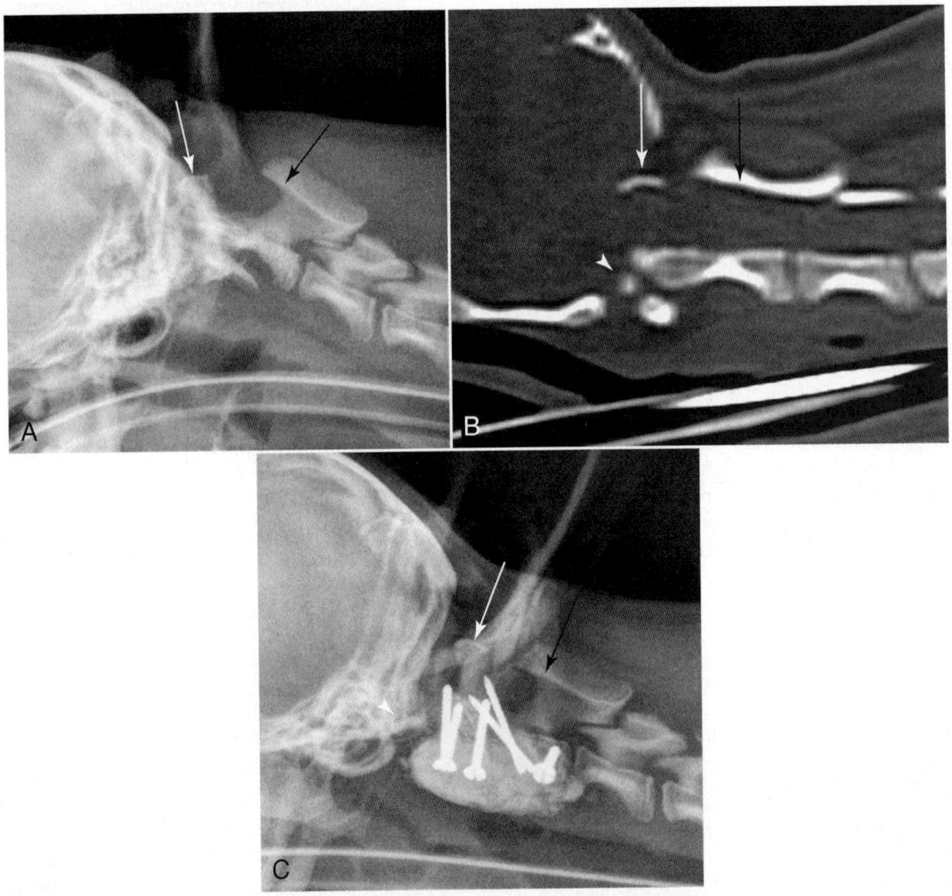

Fig. 14.12 **A,** Lateral radiograph of the cranial aspect of the cervical spine of a dog with an atlantoaxial subluxation. The key to diagnosing atlantoaxial subluxation radiographically is to assess the angular relationship between the lamina of these two vertebrae. Clearly in this dog, the lamina of the atlas (*white arrow*) is not parallel with the lamina of the axis (*black arrow*). A parallel, or nearly parallel, relationship between these structures is normal, whereas a nonparallel relationship indicates malalignment. **B,** Sagittally reformatted computed tomography (CT) image of the cranial aspect of the cervical spine of the dog in **A.** The atlantoaxial subluxation has been reduced spontaneously during positioning of the dog for the CT study. The dorsal lamina of the atlas (*white arrow*) and dorsal lamina of the axis (*black arrow*) are parallel, although there may be some cranial displacement of C2. There is a small avulsion fracture of the apical aspect of the dens (*white arrowhead*) that likely contributed to the instability and subluxation. **C,** Postoperative radiograph of the dog in **A.** Screws and pins have been inserted into the body and transverse processes of C1 and the body of C2 and embedded in methylmethacrylate. The dorsal laminae of the atlas (*white arrow*) and axis (*black arrow*) are nearly parallel. This is a normal angular relationship of these laminae.

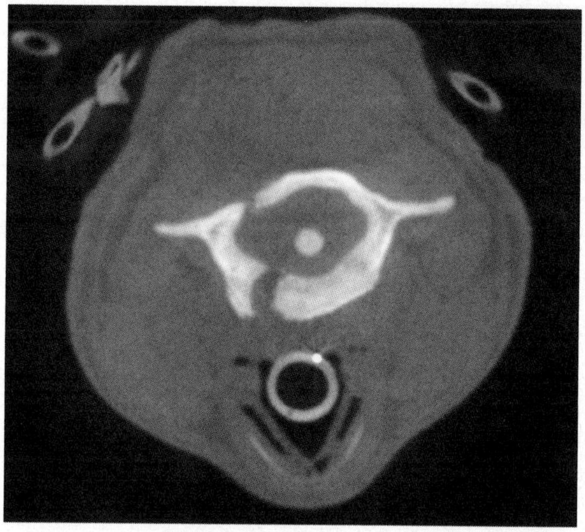

Fig. 14.13 Transverse computed tomography (CT) image of the atlas of a dog with incomplete ossification. There is a focal defect in the body and lamina of the C1 vertebra with mild dislocation of the separated segment. The dens is visible as a round osseous structure in the ventral aspect of the vertebral canal.

the vertebrae or result from remodeling due to underlying instability of the vertebral column. Because of the uncertain etiology, there are multiple synonyms for this condition, including cervical spondylomyelopathy, cervical spondylopathy, cervical vertebral malformation-malarticulation, cervical vertebral stenotic myelopathy, and wobbler syndrome, with the latter arising from the fact that affected animals are often ataxic with a wobbling or swaying gait. No term is accepted universally.[21,28] *Cervical spondylomyelopathy* is used in this discussion.

Cervical spondylomyelopathy is common in young Great Danes and mature Doberman pinschers, but there are many other large breeds that can be affected.[26–28] In the Doberman pinscher, vertebral canal stenosis, Hansen type II disc protrusion and/or herniation, and dorsal annulus fibrosus and dorsal longitudinal ligament hypertrophy are common.[27–30] Affected vertebrae sometimes have cranioventral flattening because of abnormal formation or remodeling. There can also be stenosis of the vertebral canal that results from underdevelopment of the pedicles (Fig. 14.14). This can result in the vertebral canal appearing cone shaped over the length of a vertebra, with it being narrower at the cranial aspect of the vertebra.[26,28]

Cervical spondylomyelopathy in the Great Dane is characterized primarily by articular process malformation and hyperostosis. The hyperostotic articular processes commonly extend medially and ventrally into the vertebral canal and cause extradural spinal cord compression (Fig. 14.15, eFig. 14.5). Vertebral measurements made from the mediolateral projection have been used to assess cervical spondylomyelopathy in Doberman pinschers.[32] Because the pathologic changes between Doberman pinschers and Great Danes often differ, a new method of vertebral mensuration has been proposed in Great Danes, using the VD projection.[33] This method uses the ratio of the distance between the articular process joints versus vertebral body width to screen for suspected cervical spondylomyelopathy. The rationale for this method is that hypertrophy of the articular process joints resulting in dorsolateral canal stenosis is a fundamental change in the Great Dane and is best recognized on the VD projection.

Although the differences in the manifestation of cervical spondylomyelopathy in the Doberman pinscher versus the Great Dane have been described,[27–30] it is important to realize that any individual dog of these breeds or others can have any combination of the changes described.

As should be apparent from Figs. 14.14 and 14.15, survey radiographic changes of cervical spondylomyelopathy may be sufficient to suggest the diagnosis, but conventional myelography, CT, CT myelography, and MRI are necessary to evaluate the location and severity of compressive extradural lesions. MRI is the modality of choice, because it allows assessment of the integrity of the spinal cord in addition to providing for identification of the osseous changes, disc herniation or protrusion, ligamentous hypertrophy, and synovial cyst formation (see Figs. 14.14 and 14.15).[34,35] Although controversial, obtaining myelographic projections with linear traction, flexion, and extension of the cervical spine, in addition to conventional projections, has been advocated to identify the presence of dynamic compression.[26,30] Although these maneuvers might provide insight for surgical decision making, flexion and extension place the anesthetized patient at risk for exacerbation of spinal cord damage. Linear traction, as illustrated in Fig. 14.14, is not likely to be harmful, but its clinical value is questionable. Table 14.1 provides a summary of imaging signs of cervical spondylomyelopathy.

FRACTURE AND LUXATION

Vertebral fracture is usually a result of being hit by a motor vehicle, falling, or gunshot injury.[36] Many vertebral fractures and luxations occur at regional junctions, for example, atlantooccipital, atlantoaxial, cervicothoracic, thoracolumbar, and so forth.[37–39] These junctions may be more subject to flexion-extension and torsion and axial loading compared with the vertebrae within a region. Radiographic features of vertebral fractures include asymmetry, specifically of the articular processes and endplates; displacement of a vertebra with respect to adjoining vertebrae (malalignment); and comminution of the endplate or body. Any fracture has the potential to cause narrowing of the vertebral canal and spinal cord contusion and/or compression. Shortening of the vertebral body and spinal malignment are often seen with compression fractures of the thoracic vertebrae and L7 (Fig. 14.16).[40]

Radiographic evaluation of patients with suspected vertebral fractures is limited by summation and failure to obtain accurate positioning or an adequate number of projections. Patients with vertebral column trauma are frequently unstable and medically unable to receive chemical restraint. In addition, maneuvers to obtain correct positioning may be detrimental to existing spinal trauma, especially VD projections. Flexion, extension, and traction should never be used in animals with spinal trauma. One approach is first to obtain only lateral projections of the spine of patients with a suspected vertebral fracture without or with minimal sedation to avoid further instability after muscle relaxation. If a suspected fracture is seen, a horizontally directed x-ray beam can be used to obtain VD projections. This principle was discussed and illustrated in Chapter 9.

Because of its tomographic nature, CT is superior to radiography for identifying and characterizing vertebral fractures (Fig. 14.17, eFigs. 14.6 and 14.7). In 30 dogs with acute spinal trauma, radiographic sensitivity for fractures and luxations was only 72% and 77%, respectively, and fracture fragments within the vertebral canal and narrowing of the vertebral canal were often unrecognized.[41]

A three-compartment approach has been advocated for evaluating the severity and instability of vertebral fractures and luxations.[36,41] The vertebra is divided into three areas: dorsal, middle, and ventral. The dorsal compartment contains the

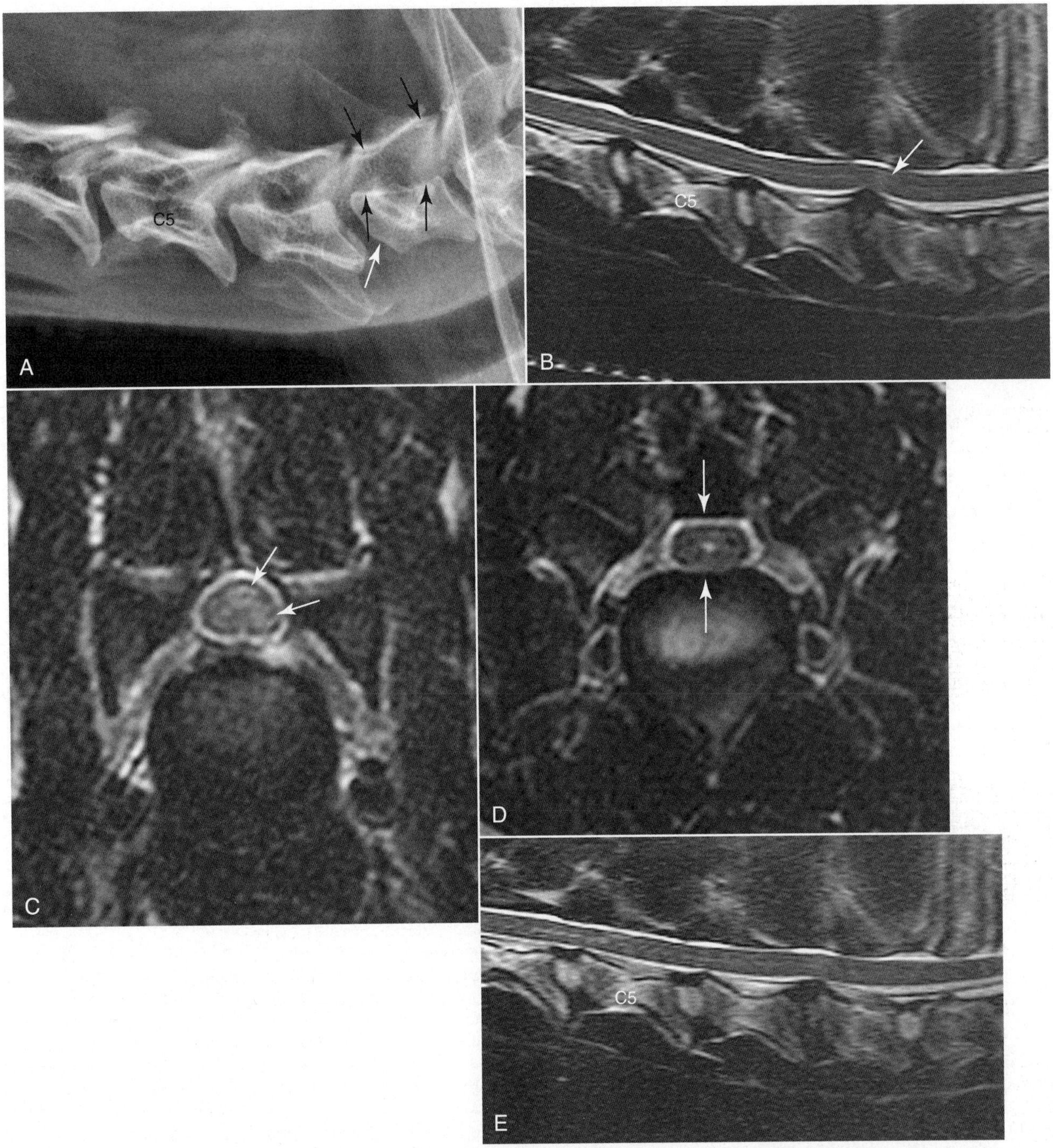

Fig. 14.14 Images from a 6-year-old Doberman pinscher with clinical signs of cervical spondylomyelopathy. **A,** Lateral cervical radiograph. The cranioventral aspect of C7 is flat (*white arrow*). The diameter of the vertebral canal is narrower, or cone shaped, at the cranial aspect of C7 than at the caudal aspect of C7 (*black arrows*). **B,** Sagittal T2-weighted image. There is a hypointense mass in the ventral aspect of the vertebral canal at C6–C7 that is causing extradural spinal cord compression; this is consistent with disc protrusion and/or hypertrophy of the dorsal longitudinal ligament as a result of chronic instability. The spinal cord has a faint area of T2 hyperintensity (*white arrow*) consistent with bruising from the chronic compression. There also is narrowing of the spinal cord at C4–C5. **C,** Transverse T2-weighted image of the spinal cord at C6–C7. There is only mild spinal cord compression, but the intramedullary T2 hyperintensity caused by chronic compression is obvious (*white arrows*). For comparison, the signal of the spinal cord in **D** is normal. **D,** Transverse T2-weighted images of the spinal cord at C4–C5. There is extradural compression of the spinal cord (*white arrows*) because of laminar malformation with secondary vertebral canal stenosis. The signal of the spinal cord is normal; compare this spinal cord signal to the bruised spinal cord in **C**. This compression at C4–C5 was not detected radiographically. **E,** T2-weighted sagittal image acquired with traction placed on the head. The amount of extradural spinal cord compression at C6–C7 is reduced compared with that present in **A,** which was made without traction. In cervical spondylomyelopathy, traction-responsive compression is attributed to hypertrophy of the dorsal longitudinal ligament rather than disc herniation. This has implications for the type of corrective surgery to be done. *C5,* Fifth cervical vertebral body.

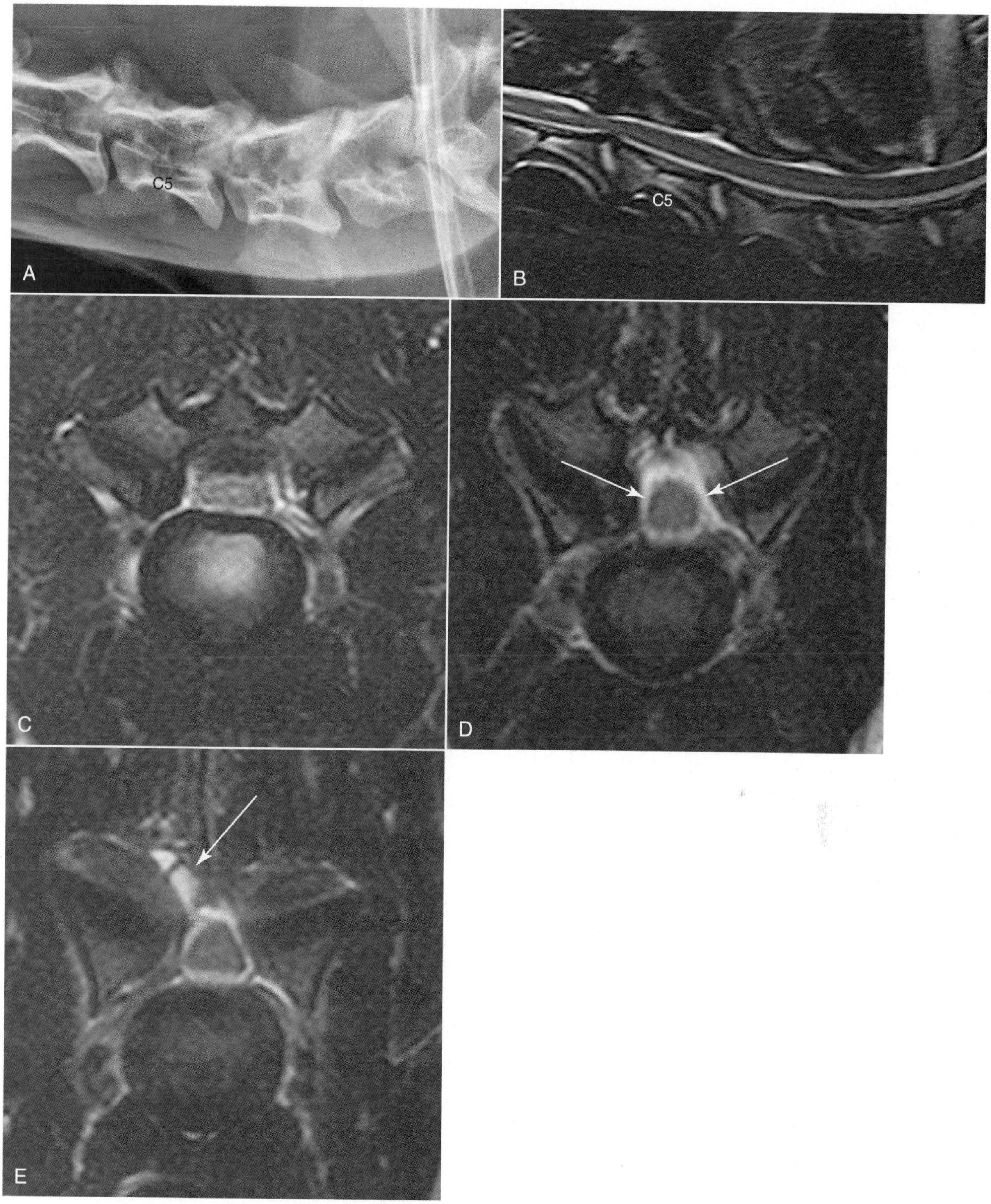

Fig. 14.15 Images from a 2-year-old Great Dane with clinical signs of cervical spondylomyelopathy. **A,** Lateral cervical radiograph. There is moderate to pronounced articular process degenerative joint disease at C4–C5, C5–C6, C6–C7, and C7–T1. These changes occur commonly as a consequence of articular process malformation or instability, or both. What cannot be determined from cervical radiographs is whether the articular process malformation is impinging on the vertebral canal. **B,** T2-weighted sagittal image of the cervical spine. There is mild ventral and marked dorsal extradural compression of the spinal cord at C4–C5. The dorsal compression is typical of laminar malformation leading to vertebral canal narrowing. **C,** Transverse T2-weighted image at C4–C5. The dorsal compression from the laminar malformation is obvious. **D,** Transverse T2-weighted image at C5–C6. At this site, there is bilateral vertebral canal narrowing with extradural spinal cord compression (*white arrows*) that results from the hyperostotic malformed articular processes extending into the vertebral canal. **E,** Transverse T2-weighted image at C6–C7. As at C5–C6, there is articular process malformation and hyperostosis that extends into the vertebral canal and causes extradural spinal cord compression. There is also an articular process synovial cyst (*white arrow*). Synovial cysts develop secondary to the degenerative joint disease and, if large enough, they can extend into the vertebral canal and contribute to the extradural spinal cord compression; in this dog, this cyst is not causing neural compression. The lateral vertebral canal narrowing seen at C5–C6 and C6–C7 was not apparent radiographically. *C5,* Fifth cervical vertebral body.

Table • 14.1

Summary of Typical Imaging Signs of Cervical Spondylomyelopathy.

ABNORMALITY	RADIOGRAPHY	MYELOGRAPHY	COMPUTED TOMOGRAPHY[A]	MAGNETIC RESONANCE[B]
Vertebral body malformation	√	√	√	√
Vertebral canal stenosis	√	√	√	√
Vertebral malalignment	√	√	√	√
Vertebral tipping	√	√	√	√
Articular process remodeling	√	√	√	√
Disc degeneration/prolapse	—	√	√	√
Extradural spinal cord compression	—	√	√	√
Ligamentum flavum, interarcuate ligament, or joint capsule hypertrophy	—	—	—	√

[a]Identifying vertebral malformation, tipping and malignant, is dependent on obtaining sagittal MR images or high-quality sagittally reformatted computed tomography images. Stenosis is apparent on transverse images.
[b]Magnetic resonance is true multiplanar imaging, and it is assumed that dorsal and sagittal, as well as transverse, images are acquired.

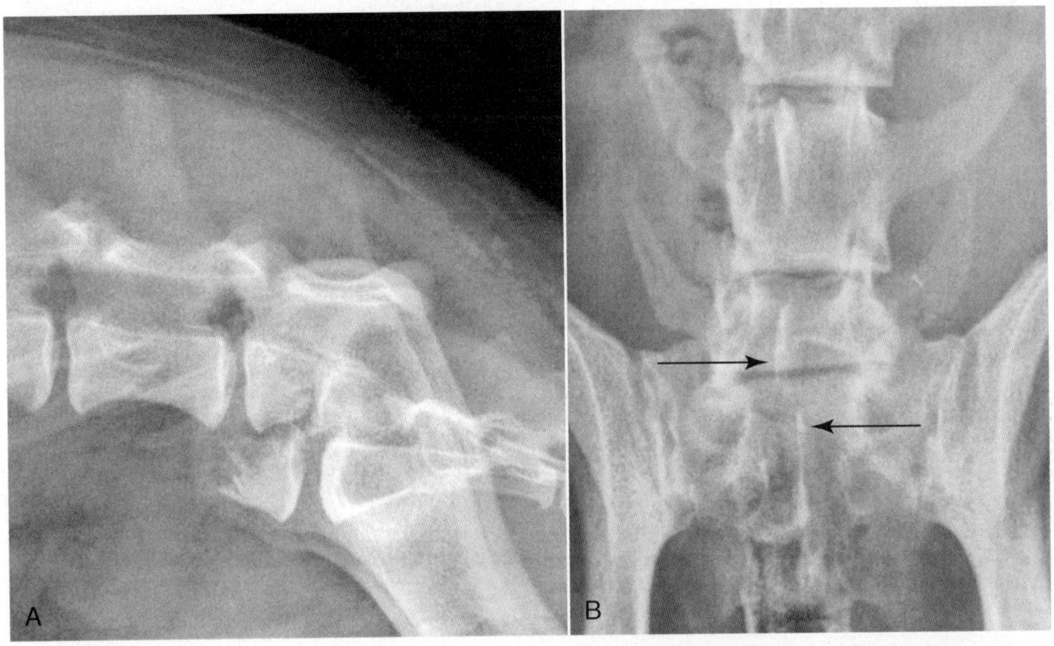

Fig. 14.16 Lateral **(A)** and ventrodorsal (VD) **(B)** radiographs of a dog with a comminuted L7 fracture. In **A**, the caudal fragment is displaced ventrally and cranially because of contraction of the spinal hypaxial muscles. The fracture is obvious in the lateral view. In **B**, L7 is foreshortened; and unless this is recognized, the fracture would be missed if the lateral view were not available. There is slight sagittal malalignment of the spinous processes of L7 and S1 (*black arrows*) because of axial rotation of the caudal fragment, but this is subtle.

vertebral arch, articular processes, and supportive ligaments; the middle compartment contains spinal cord, dorsal longitudinal ligament, annulus fibrosus, and the dorsal margin of the body; and the ventral compartment includes the remainder of the vertebral body, the annulus, and the ventral longitudinal ligament. If more than one compartment is involved, the fracture-luxation is likely unstable and requires stabilization.[36]

With vertebral fractures and luxations, soft-tissue injury is invariably present and may involve the spinal cord, intervertebral discs, ligaments, and joint capsules. Blunt trauma-induced supraphysiologic forces can result in herniation of the nucleus pulposus of a normal disc (so-called *acute nonprogressive nucleus pulposus extrusion* [ANNPE]). CT, or preferably MRI, should be considered in all animals with vertebral injury, especially if spinal cord impingement is suspected clinically.

INTERVERTEBRAL DISC DISEASE

Clinical signs of intervertebral disc disease result from extension of disc material into the vertebral canal, compressing the spinal cord or spinal nerve roots.[42,43] Descriptive terms used relative to disc lesions are overlapping and include *protrusion, hernia, extrusion, expulsion,* and *prolapse*. The distinction among these lesions cannot be made with conventional radiography and can be difficult even with CT and MRI or at

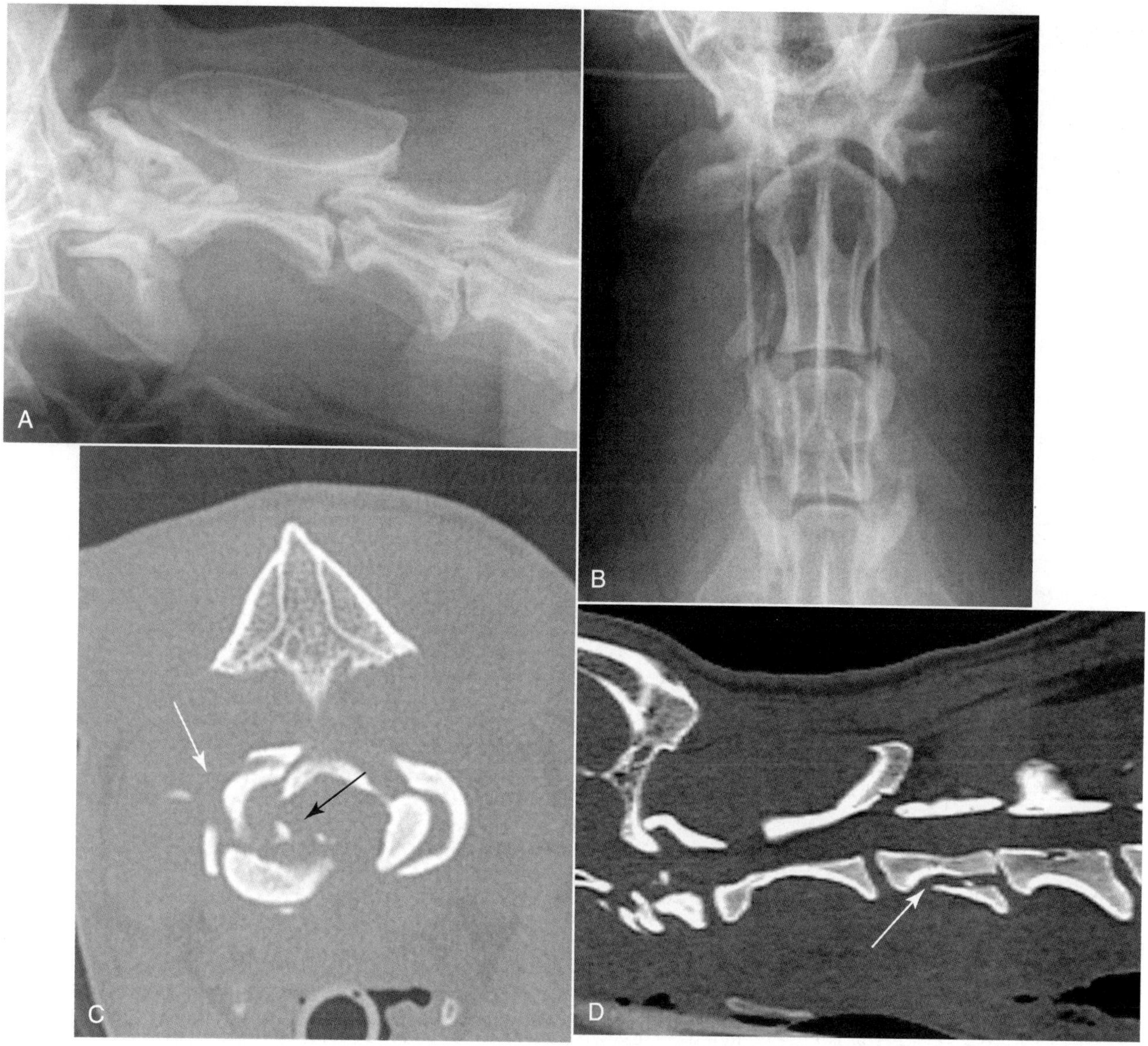

Fig. 14.17 Lateral **(A)** and ventrodorsal (VD) **(B)** radiographs of a dog that was hit by a car. There are severe neurologic signs pointing to a cervical spinal cord injury. In the lateral view, there is narrowing of the C3–C4 disc space and mild subluxation with mild dorsal displacement of the cranial aspect of C4 with respect to C3. The atlas looks very abnormal, but this region is rotated and cannot be assessed. Misdiagnosis of a C1 fracture is common in malpositioned cervical radiographs. In the VD view, there is angulation at the atlanto-occipital articulation, but specific injuries cannot be identified. In a transverse computed tomography (CT) image of the atlanto-occipital junction **(C)**, there are obvious fractures of the occipital bone (*black arrow*) and C1 (*white arrow*). In a sagittally reconstructed cervical image **(D)**, there is also an obvious fracture of C3 (*white arrow*). CT was needed in this dog to identify the traumatic bone injuries accurately.

surgery. *Herniation* will be used here to describe any discal mass that is impinging on the spinal cord or spinal nerve roots. Up-to-date classification schemes and nomenclature for intervertebral disc disease are afforded by cross-sectional imaging with CT and MRI, and discussed in Chapter 15. An extensive review of various imaging methods used for intervertebral disc disease has been recently published.[44]

Chondrodystrophic breeds are most commonly affected,[45] but intervertebral disc disease can occur in any breed, including Doberman pinschers with cervical spondylomyelopathy and German shepherds with cauda equina syndrome. Common sites of disc herniation are C2–C3, C3–C4, T12–T13, and T13–L1. Although clinical signs of intervertebral disc disease are uncommon in cats, cervical disc degeneration frequently occurs in cats older than 6 years old.[43]

The sensitivity and specificity of survey radiography to determine the site and severity of disc herniation are poor compared with CT and MRI. Currently, the most important use of survey radiography in animals with signs of intervertebral disc disease is ruling out other conditions, such as a fracture, luxation, or aggressive bone lesions.

Radiographic signs consistent with intervertebral disc disease include one or more of the following[46]:

- Narrowing of the intervertebral disc space
- Narrowing of the intervertebral articular process joint space
- A small intervertebral foramen
- Increased opacity within the intervertebral foramen
- Mineralized disc material within the vertebral canal (Fig. 14.18, eFig. 14.8).

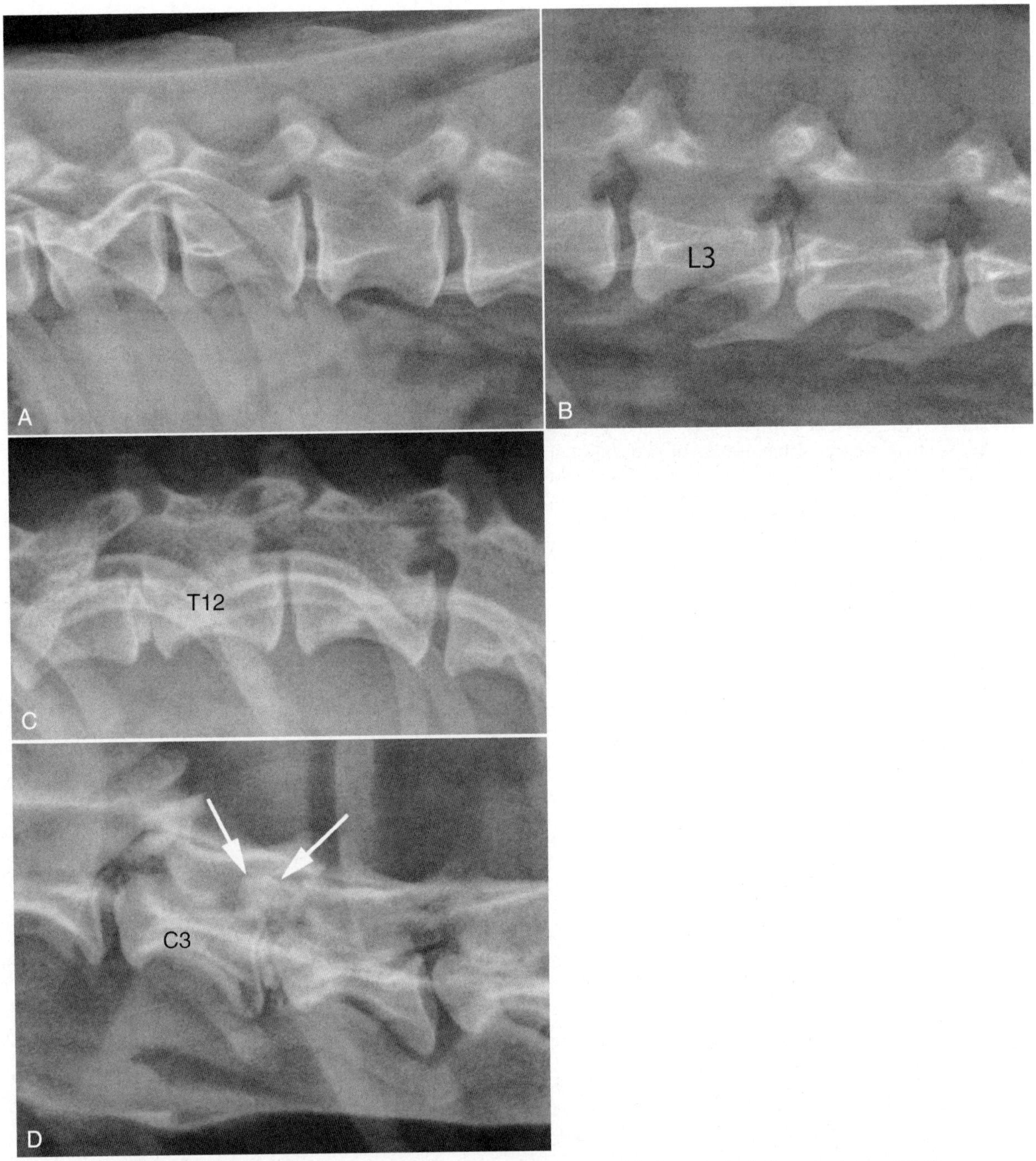

Fig. 14.18 Survey radiographic signs of intervertebral disc disease. **A,** The intervertebral disc space, intervertebral foramen, and dorsal articular process joint space at L1–L2 are all decreased in size compared with adjacent vertebrae. These signs result from vertebrae adjacent to the disc herniation moving closer together. Mild spondylosis deformans is present at L1–L2. **B,** Mineralization of the disc at L3–L4 and mineralized material superimposed over the intervertebral foramen, consistent with mineralized disc material in the vertebral canal. The disc at L3–L4 has not herniated completely; some residual disc material remains between the vertebral endplates. The intervertebral foramen at L3–L4 is slightly smaller than the foramen at L4–L5. **C,** The intervertebral disc space, intervertebral foramen, and dorsal articular process joint space at T12–T13 are all decreased in size compared with adjacent vertebrae. As in **A,** these signs are caused by vertebrae adjacent to the affected disc moving closer together. There is in situ mineralization of the disc at T11–T12. This is not important clinically and signifies only degeneration of the disc. **D,** Mineralization of the disc at C3–C4, with a narrow disc space. The cervical articular processes are larger than in the thoracic or lumbar region and are typically superimposed on the intervertebral foramina, making assessment of cervical foramina more difficult. However, a large mineralized opacity is visible in a position consistent with it being in the vertebral canal (*white arrows*). Confirmation that this opacity is within the vertebral canal requires additional images or modalities. *C3,* Third cervical vertebral body; *L3,* third lumbar vertebral body; *T12,* twelfth thoracic vertebral body.

Careful radiographic technique is critical for interpretation of these changes, keeping in mind that some patients presenting with clinical signs of disc disease may not have any radiographic changes.[47] While narrowing of disc spaces is the most reliable survey sign of disc herniation, false-positives are common.[48] For example, in normalcy, disc spaces at T10–T11 and L5–L6 are usually narrower than adjacent disc spaces. Following hemilaminectomy or fenestration, disc spaces may be narrow in asymptomatic animals. Midsize to large-breed dogs with chronic intervertebral disc disease may have multiple narrowed disc spaces that do not correlate with the neurologic examination. Small intervertebral foramina and narrowed articular process joint spaces are merely a result of partial collapse of the space between two vertebrae and may not be associated with disc hernation. Increased opacity of the intervertebral foramen is caused by either extruded disc material in the vertebral canal or local inflammation of epidural fat at the site of extrusion. This change is evident only on a true lateral projection with exact superimposition of both lateral margins of both intervertebral foramina. Discal mineralization within the intervertebral disc space, so-called *mineralization in situ*, is indicative of intervertebral disc degeneration but does not confirm that this particular disc is causing a clinical problem. Most herniated disc material is nonmineralized or lacks sufficient mineral content to be detected on survey radiographs, whereas the superior contrast resolution of CT allows detection of both nonmineralized and low-mineral-content herniated disc material.[49] Myelographic technique and interpretative principles for the diagnosis of disc herniation are described later.

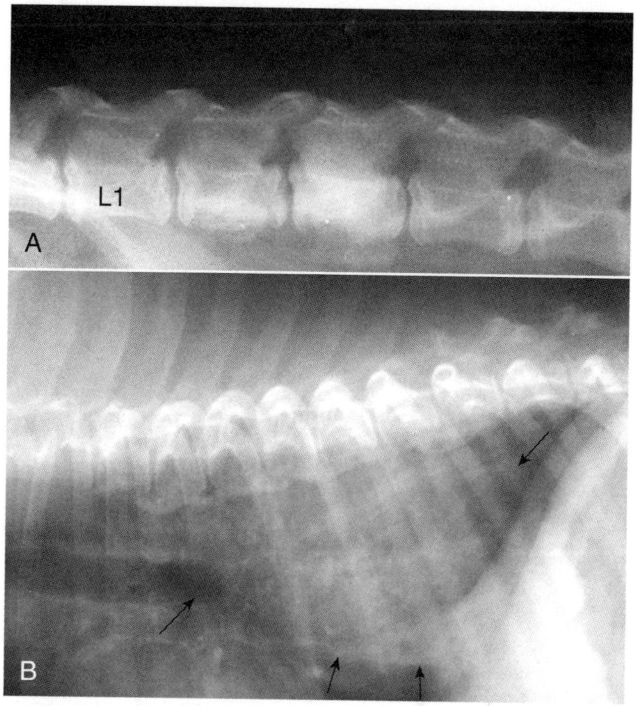

Fig. 14.19 Radiographic signs of spondylitis. **A,** Radiograph of patient with plant awn-induced spondylitis; note increased opacity of the vertebral bodies of L2 and L3 and periosteal reaction. **B,** Lateral radiograph of a dog with *Spirocerca lupi* infection. There is an irregular periosteal response along ventral borders of the thoracic vertebra. Note that the new bone is not centered at the ventral aspect of the disc space, as would be expected in spondylosis. An indistinct soft tissue esophageal mass is present ventral to this area (*arrows*). *L1,* First lumbar vertebral body. (**B,** Courtesy Dr. R. M. Kirberger, University of Pretoria, South Africa.)

INFLAMMATORY CONDITIONS

Spondylitis, Vertebral Osteomyelitis, and Vertebral Physitis

Spondylitis is a nonspecific term referring to inflammation of the vertebrae. *Vertebral osteomyelitis* has also been used synonymously with spondylitis when osteomyelitis of the vertebral body is present. Spondylitis should not be confused with *spondylosis*, or *spondylosis deformans*, a degenerative condition of the vertebral column. Common causes of spondylitis include microbial infection, plant awn migration, and infection with *Spirocerca lupi*.[50–58] Paraspinal abscesses may extend to the spine and cause spondylitis.[59] Radiographic changes are mainly those of increased opacity of the vertebral body with an irregular periosteal reaction. With osteomyelitis, radiographic features include an aggressive bone response with patchy lysis of the vertebral bodies and an irregular periosteal response[51–53] (Fig. 14.19). Parasite-induced spondylitis caused by *S. lupi* infection results in osseous proliferation of the ventral aspect of the vertebral bodies of T8–T11.[56] Metastatic neoplasia can cause similar periosteal lesions.[50]

Vertebral physitis occurs in young dogs, and initial radiographic signs include osteolysis of the physeal zone of the affected vertebrae with sparing of the endplates.[60] With progression, there is collapse of the cranial or caudal aspect of the vertebral body and endplate sclerosis. Sepsis is the proposed cause because of hematogenous localization in the slow-flowing capillaries of the vertebral physis. *Acinetobacter* and *Enterococci* species have been isolated from vertebral biopsy material.[60]

Discospondylitis

Discospondylitis is inflammation of an intervertebral disc and its adjacent vertebral endplates.[57,58,61,62] There is also paraspinal soft tissue infection, but this is not detected radiographically. The etiology involves hematogenous spread of microorganisms from distant sites, frequently associated with genitourinary infections and occasionally paraspinal abscess or foreign body migration.[57,62,63] Middle-aged, large-breed dogs are affected commonly, and single or multiple intervertebral discs and adjacent endplates may be involved. Common isolates include *Staphylococcus, Streptococcus, Brucella* species, and *Escherichia coli*, although numerous other bacterial species and yeasts have been isolated.[57,58,62,63] Discospondylitis caused by aspergillosis is mainly seen in German shepherd dogs, possibly associated with the breed's documented immunoglobulin A (IgA) immunodeficiencies.[64] Discospondylitis is less common in cats but has a similar etiopathogenesis.[61] Initial radiographic features include irregular endplate lysis with extension into the vertebral body (Fig. 14.20, eFigs. 14.9 and 14.10). Later, there is collapse of the intervertebral disc space, sclerosis peripheral to the endplate lysis, ventral enthesophyte production, and in some instances subluxation (see Fig. 14.20B). Resolved discospondylitis may have the same appearance as spondylosis deformans (discussed later); usually, the disc space is collapsed at this point. Clinical features of discospondylitis can include fever, leukocytosis, paresthesia, paresis, and rarely paralysis.[57–59,62,63] Meningitis is possible if the inflammatory process extends into the vertebral canal and enters the subarachnoid space.[62] Diagnosis is based on clinical signs and presence of lysis of the vertebral endplates. Radiographic changes of discospondylitis lag behind changes that are apparent in MR images; thus, negative radiographs do not rule out a diagnosis of discospondylitis.[62,65] In a study of juvenile dogs with discospondylitis, CT and ultrasonography were used to identify abnormal discs prior to the onset of typical radiographic changes. The earliest radiographic sign of discospondylitis in juvenile dogs was disc space narrowing.[66]

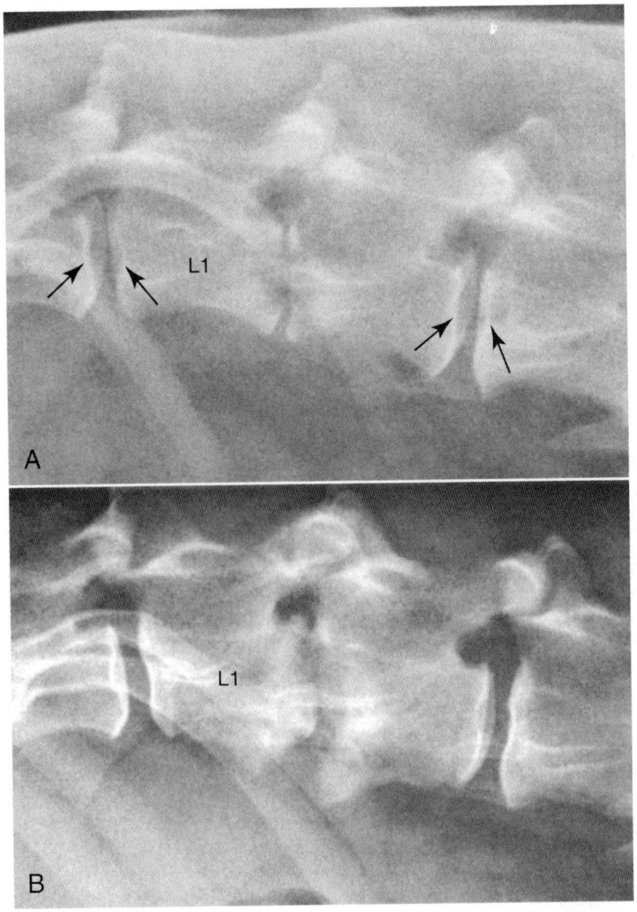

Fig. 14.20 **A,** Lateral radiograph of a dog with acute discospondylitis at L1–L2. There is endplate lysis but no evidence of new bone formation. The disc space at L1–L2 is also narrow, signifying that the disc is herniated, although the location of the disc material cannot be determined. The disc material may be in the vertebral canal, lateral to the disc, or even within the vertebral body as a result of herniation through the diseased endplate. Note the discrete linear opacity associated with a normal endplate (*arrows*). These discrete opacities are absent at L1–L2, and this absence is a clue that the endplates at this site have been effaced. **B,** Lateral radiograph of the same patient made 6 weeks later is characterized by more extensive lysis of the vertebral endplates and sclerosis of the vertebral body adjacent to the endplates. Early changes of spondylosis deformans are also present, and ventral enthesophytes are developing. There is mild subluxation at L1–L2, with L2 being displaced slightly ventrally. The intervertebral foramen at L1–L2 is small because of the disc being herniated and the vertebrae moving closer together.

DEGENERATIVE CONDITIONS

Spondylosis Deformans

Spondylosis is defined as ankylosis of a vertebral joint.[67] The term *spondylosis deformans* is preferred, because it addresses the spectrum of changes associated with this degenerative condition more completely. Spondylosis deformans is common in dogs, especially boxers and large-breed dogs, and it tends to be most prevalent in the thoracolumbar and lumbosacral region.[68–71] Most dogs will eventually develop radiographic criteria of spondylosis deformans. Clinicians should be aware that spondylosis deformans is not an inflammatory process but rather a disease of the attachments of the vertebral joints, which involves the fibers joining the intervertebral discs to the vertebral endplates.[71,72] The outer rim of the annulus fibrosus has strong circumferential attachments to the vertebral endplate with Sharpey's fibers, which are enmeshed in cortical bone (Fig. 14.21). The annulus fibrosus is also anchored to the dorsal longitudinal ligaments by short fibers, adding stability to the vertebral column. The intervertebral disc acts as a thick-walled pressure vessel that is subject to dynamic loading and deformation during locomotion.[73] The exact cause of spondylosis deformans is unknown, but etiopathogenesis might include repetitive trauma, instability, normal aging and wear and tear, and hereditary predisposition.[70,71] However, convincing evidence of a hereditary component was not found in studies of boxer dogs.[74,75] Presently accepted theory states that disruption of Sharpey's fibers is the initiator, leading to radiographically evident osseous proliferation or *enthesopathy* of the margins of the endplate (see Fig. 14.21).[72,73] Eventually, ventral vertebral enthesophytes can bridge the intervertebral disc space at single or multiple sites, leading to fusion. In the thoracolumbar column, fusion leads to increased stress and strain of adjacent vertebral junctions and may result in disc herniation. Radiographic findings may also include endplate thickening and narrowing of the intervertebral disc space, which is possibly related to concurrent disc degeneration and loss of elasticity of the disc[70,71] (Fig. 14.22). It should be noted that dorsal and dorsolateral enthesophytes can form, but these may not be seen on conventional orthogonal radiographic studies because of superimposition on adjacent structures.[76]

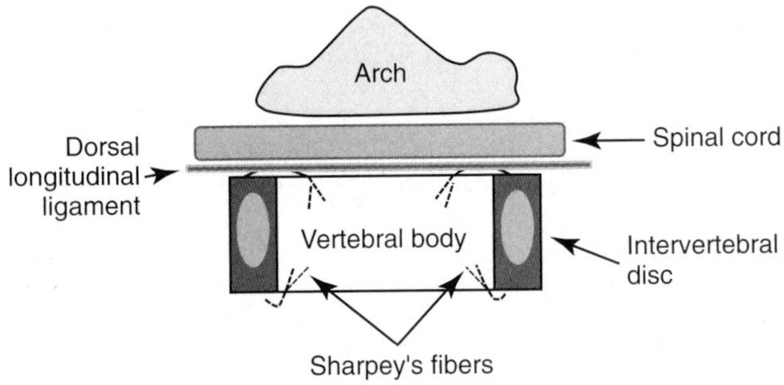

Fig. 14.21 Graphic of the lateral aspect of a typical vertebra and attachments (entheses) of the annulus fibrosis to the vertebral endplate and dorsal longitudinal ligament. Sharpey's fibers are a continuation of annular collagen fibers originating in the annulus and are firmly anchored in the cortical bone of the vertebral endplate. Stimuli of these attachments have been postulated to initiate osseous proliferation at the ventral and lateral margins of endplates in animals with spondylosis deformans.

Whether or not disc degeneration is a factor in the development of spondylosis deformans is unclear. In dogs, type II intervertebral disc disease may be part of the pathogenesis of spondylosis deformans (Fig. 14.23).[77] Tears of the annulus may occur in dogs with spondylosis deformans, predisposing to type II-disc protrusion. Most clinicians and radiologists agree that spondylosis deformans is clinically insignificant, unless a concurrent herniated disc is present, or if there is impingement on the spinal cord or spinal nerve roots. Nerve root compression from spondylosis is rare except in lumbosacral instability where foraminal impingement results from dorsal extension of the enthesophytes.

Osteoarthritis of the Dorsal Intervertebral Articular Process Joints

The synovial joints of the vertebral column are composed of the articular processes of adjoining vertebrae and are subject to degeneration or osteoarthritis as is any other synovial joint.[1] Typical radiographic changes include remodeling of the articular processes, osteophytosis, and thinning of the joint space. These changes are best seen on lateral radiographs (Fig. 14.24). Although osteoarthritis of the articular process joints can be seen concomitantly with spondylosis deformans, these are separate entities. No specific clinical signs have been attributed

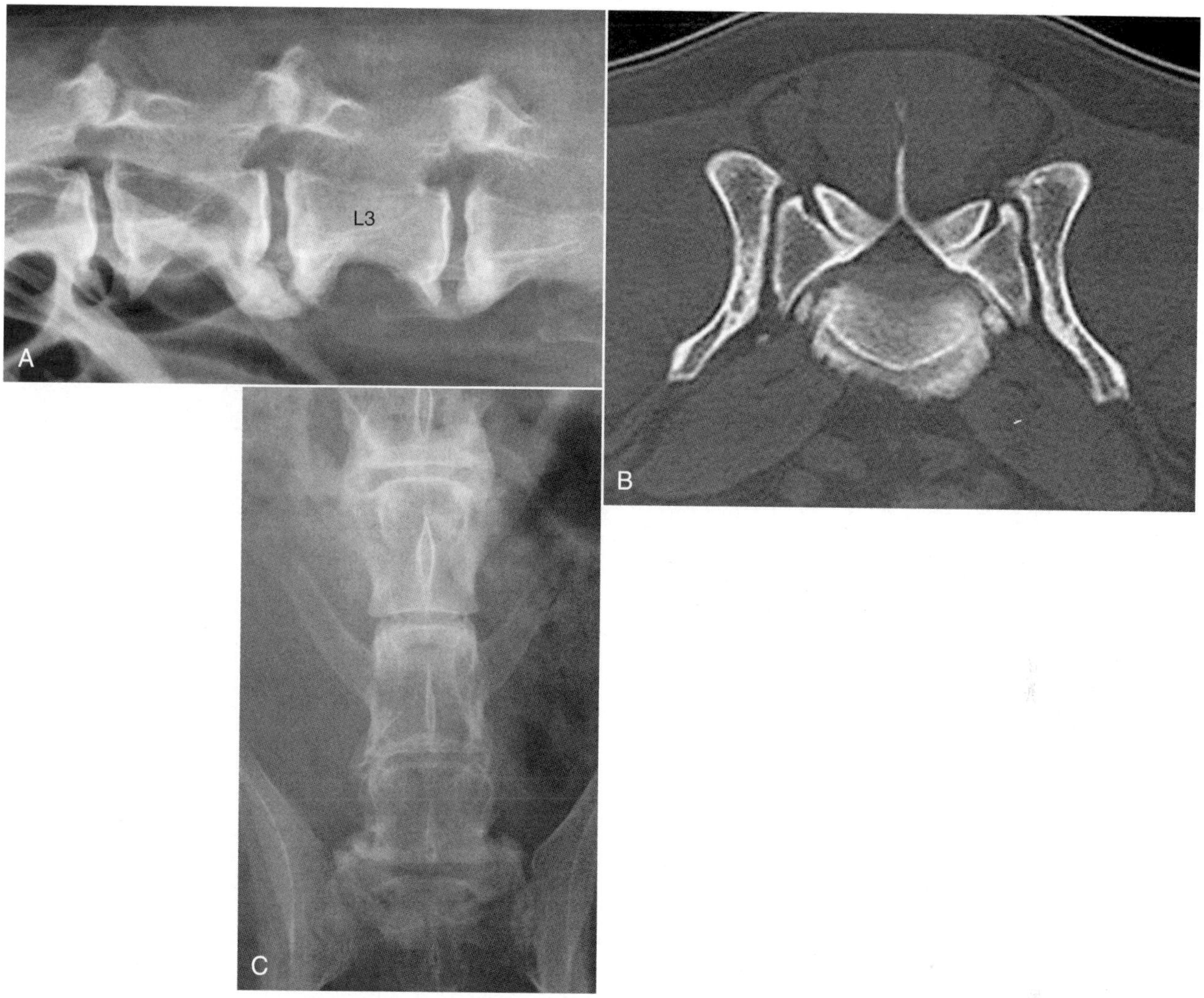

Fig. 14.22 **A,** Lateral radiograph of the lumbar spine. There are ventral enthesophytes at L1–L2, L2–L3, and L3–L4. There is endplate sclerosis of the cranial aspect of L4. The radiolucent region between the ventral enthesophytes at L2–L3 is often confused with a fracture, but this is only a region where the enthesophytes are approaching each other and have not fused. This gap may eventually fuse completely. **B,** Transverse computed tomography (CT) image of a dog with spondylosis. There is ventral osseous proliferation without impingement of the vertebral canal. Note that the dorsal intervertebral articular process joints are unaffected. **C,** Ventrodorsal (VD) radiograph of a dog with spondylosis that has resulted in lateral enthesophytes at L4–L5, L6–L7, and L7–S1. Lateral enthesophytes are rarely of clinical importance because their location is ventral to the spinal cord and nerve roots. *L3,* Third lumbar vertebral body.

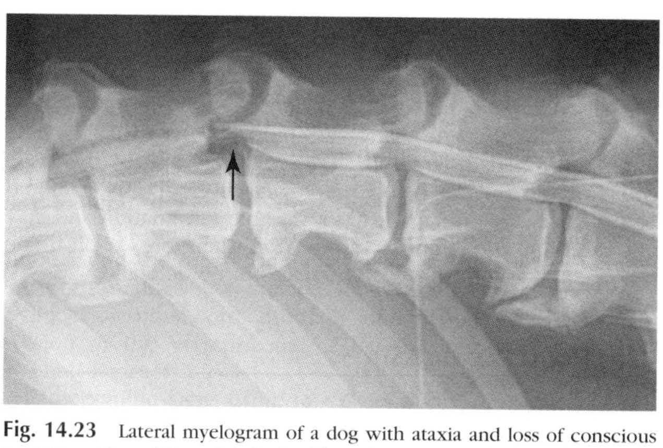

Fig. 14.23 Lateral myelogram of a dog with ataxia and loss of conscious proprioception of the pelvic limbs. There is extensive ventral enthesophyte formation at multiple sites. There is dorsal displacement of the contrast medium in the ventral aspect of the subarachnoid space (*arrow*) at T13–L1, and extradural spinal cord compression secondary to a type II intervertebral disc protrusion. The disc herniation, and not the advanced spondylosis deformans, was responsible for clinical signs.

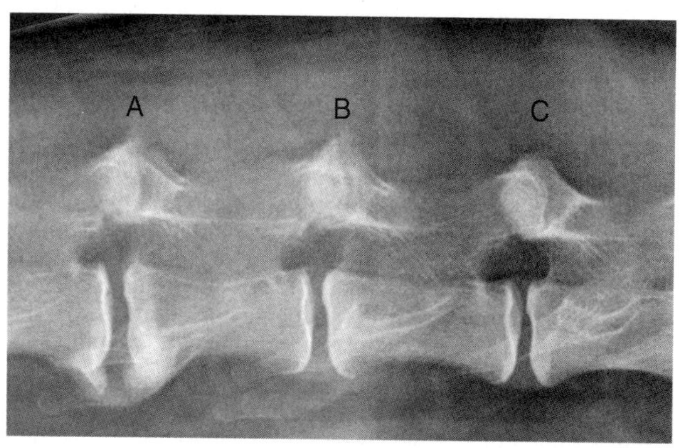

Fig. 14.24 Lateral radiograph of a dog with articular process degenerative joint disease. The joint *C* is normal. The joint *A* has subchondral sclerosis and mild osteophyte formation. The joint *B* is narrow with large osteophytes. Because of the limited motion of these joints, clinical signs of degenerative joint disease are rarely present; however, in some instances, enlarged articular processes may impinge the spinal cord dorsally, causing neurologic signs. Synovial cysts may also impinge the spinal cord laterally as previously discussed.

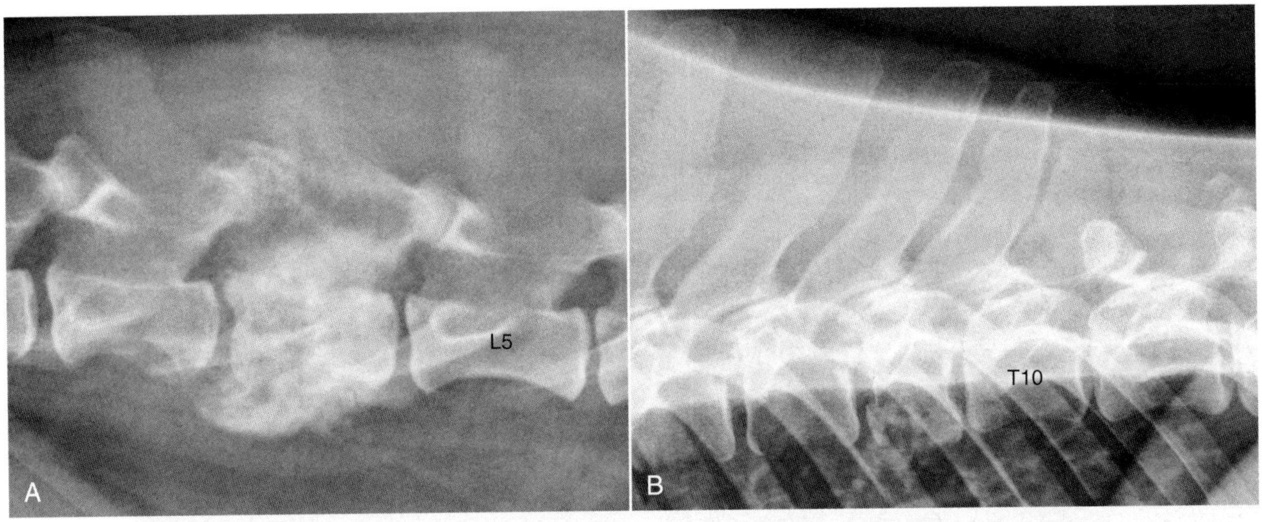

Fig. 14.27 **A,** Lateral radiograph of a dog with a tumor of L4. There are regions of lysis in the vertebral arch and the body, and there is also active new bone formation on the ventral aspect of the body. **B,** Lateral radiograph of a dog with a compression fracture of T9 caused by metastatic cancer. The body is heterogeneously lytic and foreshortened with multiple areas of cortical effacement. Each of these lesions is characterized as aggressive radiographically. *L5*, Fifth lumbar vertebral body; *T10*, tenth thoracic vertebral body.

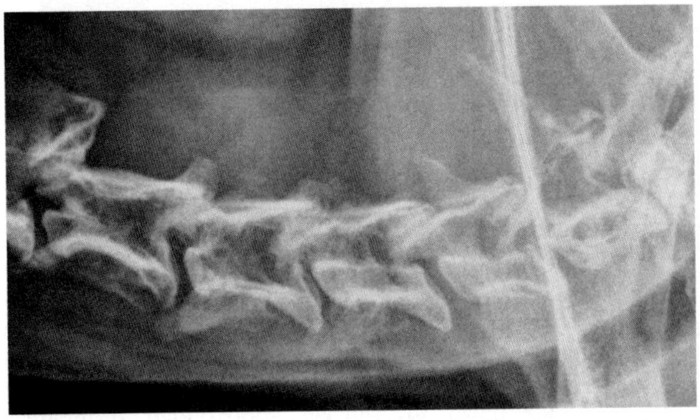

Fig. 14.28 Lateral cervical radiograph of a dog with multiple myeloma. There are numerous regions of bone lysis in the cervical spine, affecting C2–C5.

METABOLIC AND UNCLASSIFIED CONDITIONS

Disseminated Idiopathic Skeletal Hyperostosis

Disseminated idiopathic skeletal hyperostosis (DISH) is recognized infrequently in dogs and has been reported in a cat.[96] Principal radiographic features include extensive linear new bone formation along the ventrolateral aspect of the vertebral column and ankylosis (Fig. 14.29). Although these changes appear similar to advanced spondylosis deformans, DISH is likely a separate entity; the predominant excessive ventral distribution supports this contention. In the dog, seven criteria have been proposed to help distinguish DISH from spondylosis deformans.[97]

1. Bridging ossification along ventral and lateral aspects of three contiguous vertebral bodies
2. Relative preservation of disc-space width within involved areas and absence of changes of degenerative disc disease,

Table • 14.2

Radiographic Features of Inflammatory Conditions of the Vertebral Column.

CONDITION	OSSEOUS PRODUCTION	OSTEOLYSIS	NARROWED DISC SPACE
Spondylitis	+; vertebral body	–	–
Vertebral osteomyelitis	+; vertebral body	+; vertebral body	–
Vertebral physitis	+; vertebral endplate	+; vertebral physis	–
Discospondylitis	+; vertebral body and endplate	+; endplate erosion	+

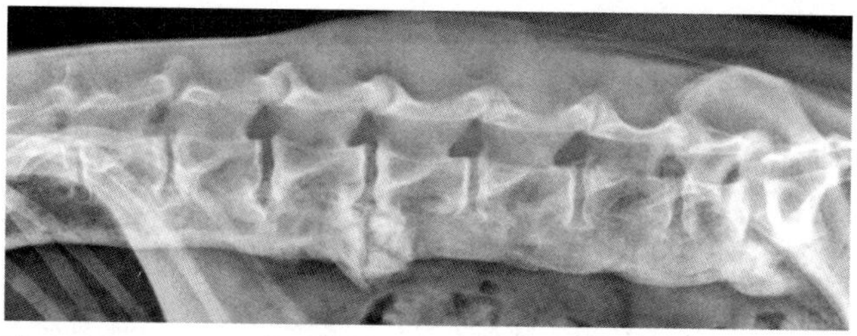

Fig. 14.29 Lateral radiograph of a dog with extensive bridging ventral spondylosis that is consistent with disseminated idiopathic skeletal hyperostosis.

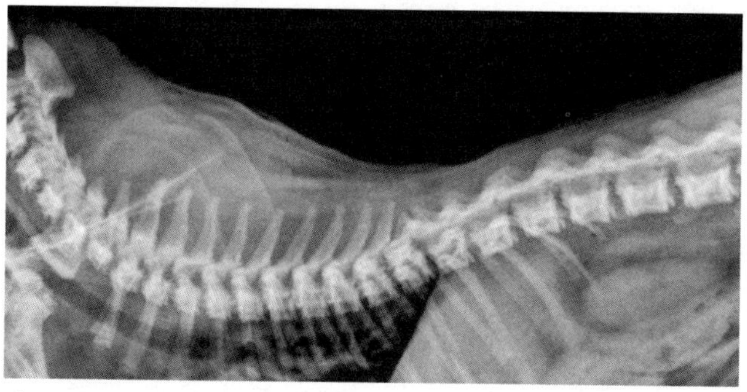

Fig. 14.30 Lateral radiograph of a cat with mucopolysaccharidosis. There is extensive remodeling and shape change of the cervical and thoracic vertebrae. Note the small and irregularly mineralized vertebral epiphyses, typical of this condition.

such as endplate sclerosis, nuclear calcification, or localized spondylosis deformans

3. Osteoarthritis of the dorsal intervertebral process joints
4. Pseudoarthrosis of the spinous processes
5. Enthesopathy of soft tissue attachments in both axial and appendicular skeleton
6. Osteophytes, sclerosis, and ankylosis of the sacroiliac joints
7. Ankylosis of the symphysis pubis

It is suggested that at least four of the seven criteria be present for confirmation of DISH in dogs.[97]

Mucopolysaccharidosis

Radiographic changes of mucopolysaccharidosis type VI in cats include multiple skeletal abnormalities.[98] In the vertebral column, principal changes are remodeling, and shape change of the vertebra, spondylosis deformans, and abnormal development of the dens. These changes are primarily a manifestation of vertebral epiphyseal dysplasia (Fig. 14.30). Changes in the appendicular skeleton include epiphyseal dysplasia of long bones, abnormal nasal conchal development, and coxofemoral subluxation.

Osteopenia

Nutritional secondary hyperparathyroidism can result in generalized bone loss with cortical and trabecular thinning of the vertebra and pathologic fracture (Fig. 14.31). As with radiographically evident metastatic lesions, considerable bone loss must be present to recognize osteopenic conditions. In humans, 30% to 60% of bone matrix must be lost for radiographic detection in metabolic bone diseases.[99] Although senile osteopenia and osteopenia secondary to other endocrinopathies have been described,[9] the degree of bone loss is usually insufficient for detection on survey radiographs of the vertebral column.

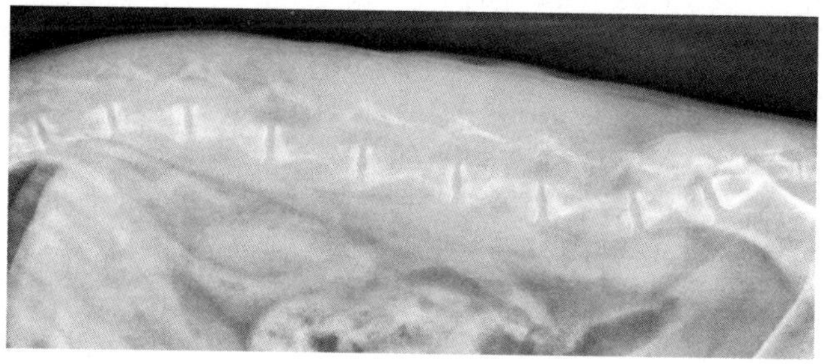

Fig. 14.31 Lateral radiograph of a cat with nutritional secondary hyperparathyroidism. There is marked generalized osteopenia with reduction in bone opacity. The normal high contrast between bone and soft tissue has been lost.

MYELOGRAPHY

Myelography is valuable for identifying extradural compressive lesions but rarely provides meaningful information about the condition of the spinal cord. For this reason, it has largely been replaced by CT and MRI. MRI is noninvasive, and intrathecal injection of contrast medium is unnecessary. However, MRI is not universally available for veterinary patients and may be too expensive for some pet owners. Therefore, conventional myelography and CT-myelography are still viable modalities for use in high-quality practices and referral centers without access to MRI.[44,49]

Common indications for myelography include (1) confirming and localizing spinal cord compression due to intervertebral disc herniation, (2) defining the extent of spinal cord impingement from fractures and luxations, (3) identifying a suspected extradural compressive or intramedullary spinal cord lesion when survey radiographs are normal.

Technique

Myelographic technique is well described[48,100–103]; therefore, a summary is presented here. Myelography is always performed under aseptic conditions, and with the animal under general anesthesia. An accurate survey radiographic or CT study serves as a baseline and should always precede myelography. Nonionic iodinated contrast media such as iohexol (Omnipaque, 240 mgI/mL) are safe and efficacious, and are the contrast media of choice for small animal myelography. Under no circumstances should ionic iodinated benzoic acid derivatives such as diatrizoate or iothalamate salts be used for myelography. Serious side effects with ionic media include seizures, intensification of preexisting neurologic signs, or even death. Nonionic contrast media are relatively safe for myelography if solutions are near iso-osmolal, and careful technique is used. Maintenance intravenous fluid administration during and after myelography speeds contrast medium elimination by the kidneys, helping reduce side effects.

The full-spine dosage is approximately 0.45 mL/kg and the regional dosage is approximately 0.30 mL/kg.[100] These dosages are only guidelines and it is important to administer sufficient contrast medium to fill the subarachnoid space in the region of interest. Contrast medium can be diluted for CT-myelography. A 22-gauge spinal needle with stylet is preferred for myelography because it has a short bevel, which increases the likelihood that the needle will be positioned in the thin subarachnoid space. The stylet is kept in place during subarachnoid puncture to minimize damage if the spinal cord is pierced and to prevent tissue from clogging the needle lumen.

Lumbar myelography is routinely performed because lumbar punctures are relatively safe compared to cervical punctures. The subarachnoid space ends blindly; therefore; the lumbar

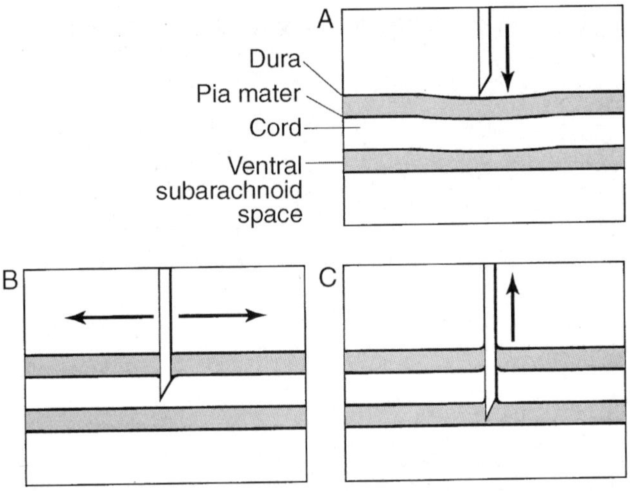

Fig. 14.32 Lumbar puncture may cause mechanical damage to the neural tissue. **A,** Compression of the spinal cord by resistance of the tough dura. **B,** Compression is released as the needle tip passes through the dura, entering the spinal cord. Horizontal movement must be minimized to avoid spinal cord damage. **C,** The needle is retracted slightly (1–2 mm) after it has reached the ventral aspect of the vertebral canal, reducing the chance of epidural injection. (Reproduced with permission from Widmer WR, Blevins WE. Veterinary myelography: a review of contrast media, adverse effects, and technique. *J Am Anim Hosp Assoc.* 1991;19:755.)

injection usually allows contrast medium to be forced cranially past extradural lesions and intramedullary swellings. With a cervical injection, contrast medium tends to flow rostrally into the ventricular system rather than flowing past extradural lesions and cord swellings.[35] Therefore, only the cranial aspect of a compressive lesion is identified with cervical injection myelography. Even in normalcy, full-spine myelograms are rarely achieved with cervical punctures and limited to the cervical vertebral region. Flow of contrast medium into the ventricular system can enhance neurotoxic effects, an additional disadvantage of cervical myelography.

Lumbar myelography is performed by puncture of the ventral subarachnoid space, preferably at L5–6 or L6–7, but L4–5 can be used if injection at these sites cannot be made successfully. Injection at L4–5 should be avoided because of the greater chance for injury to the lumbar intumescence of the spinal cord by the needle. Transneural passage of the needle is necessary for needle placement on the ventral aspect of the subarachnoid space and invariably damages the spinal cord or nerve roots. This can be minimized by keeping the stylet in place and avoiding horizontal movement of the needle during puncture. However, the dorsal aspect of the spinal cord is compressed 2 to 3 mm ventrally as the needle tip is resisted by the tough dura (Fig. 14.32).[103] The animal is placed in lateral recumbency and either of two methods can be used to puncture the subarachnoid space.[100] With the paramedian approach, the needle is inserted slightly caudolateral to the spinous process of L6 or L7 and is directed cranioventrally at a 45-degree angle, through the interarcuate space. The median approach requires insertion of the needle just cranial to the spinous process of L5 or L6, at a 90-degree angle to the vertebral column. When performing lumbar myelography, it can be advantageous to obtain a first lateral radiograph during injection to maximize contrast medium flow past a compressive lesion. Once the needle is removed, lateral VD and oblique VD radiographs should be obtained immediately to again maximize contrast medium volume near a compressive lesion.

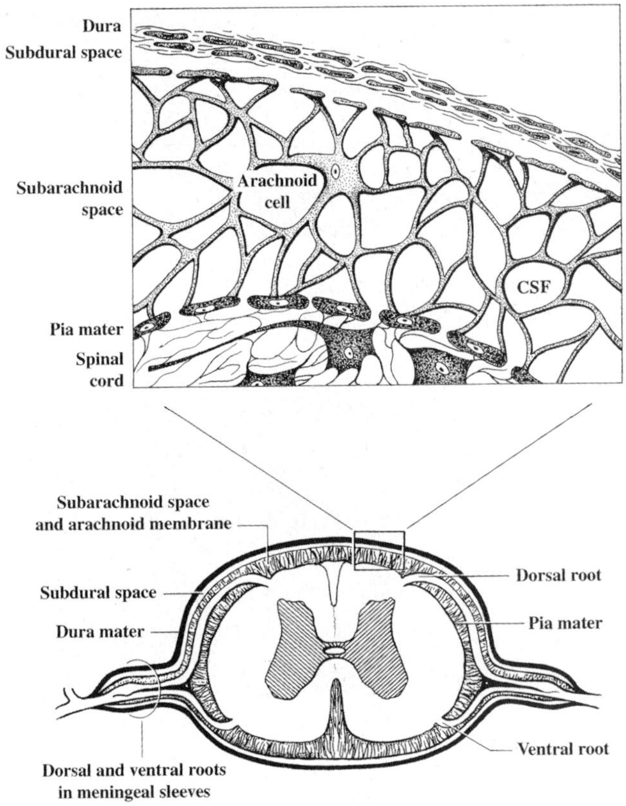

Fig. 14.33 Anatomic relationship (*transverse plane*) of spinal cord, meningeal layers, and subarachnoid space. *Inset* shows microscopic structure of a segment of the meninges and cord. *CSF,* Cerebrospinal fluid. (Modified from Hoerlein BF. *Canine Neurology: Diagnosis and Treatment.* 3rd ed. Philadelphia: WB Saunders; 1978. This figure was redrawn by the Medical Illustration Unit at the Purdue University College of Veterinary Medicine with credits to B.F. Hoerlein.)

Interpretive Principles

Knowing the relationship of the spinal cord to the meninges, epidural space, and vertebral canal is essential for accurate myelography interpretation (Fig. 14.33). This relationship is important for proper localization of vertebral canal mass lesions with respect to the dura, whether interpreting a myelogram or CT/MR images. CT myelography is advantageous over standard myelography because transverse plane images are acquired, thus summation is not a problem. If needed, sagittal and dorsal plane reconstructions can be made, increasing diagnostic information.

The normal conventional myelogram is typified by a sharply marginated, thin line of contrast medium in the subarachnoid space (Figs. 14.34 and 14.35). Small-breed dogs and cats tend to have relatively large spinal cords, and as a result, a thin subarachnoid space[24] (see Fig. 14.34C,D). The ventral aspect of the epidural (extradural) space is normally wide in the caudal cervical region, giving the false impression of spinal cord displacement. The dorsal aspect of the subarachnoid space is widest at the C1–C2 level and tends to be wider than the corresponding ventral aspect of the subarachnoid space in the thoracolumbar region. Small filling defects often seen dorsal to the cervical discs are caused by hypertrophy of the dorsal longitudinal ligament or the annulus fibrosus (see Fig. 14.34) but are not indicative of spinal cord compression if the dorsal subarachnoid space is normal. Clinically significant subarachnoid space filling defects should be accompanied by thinning of the opposite aspect of the contrast medium column or

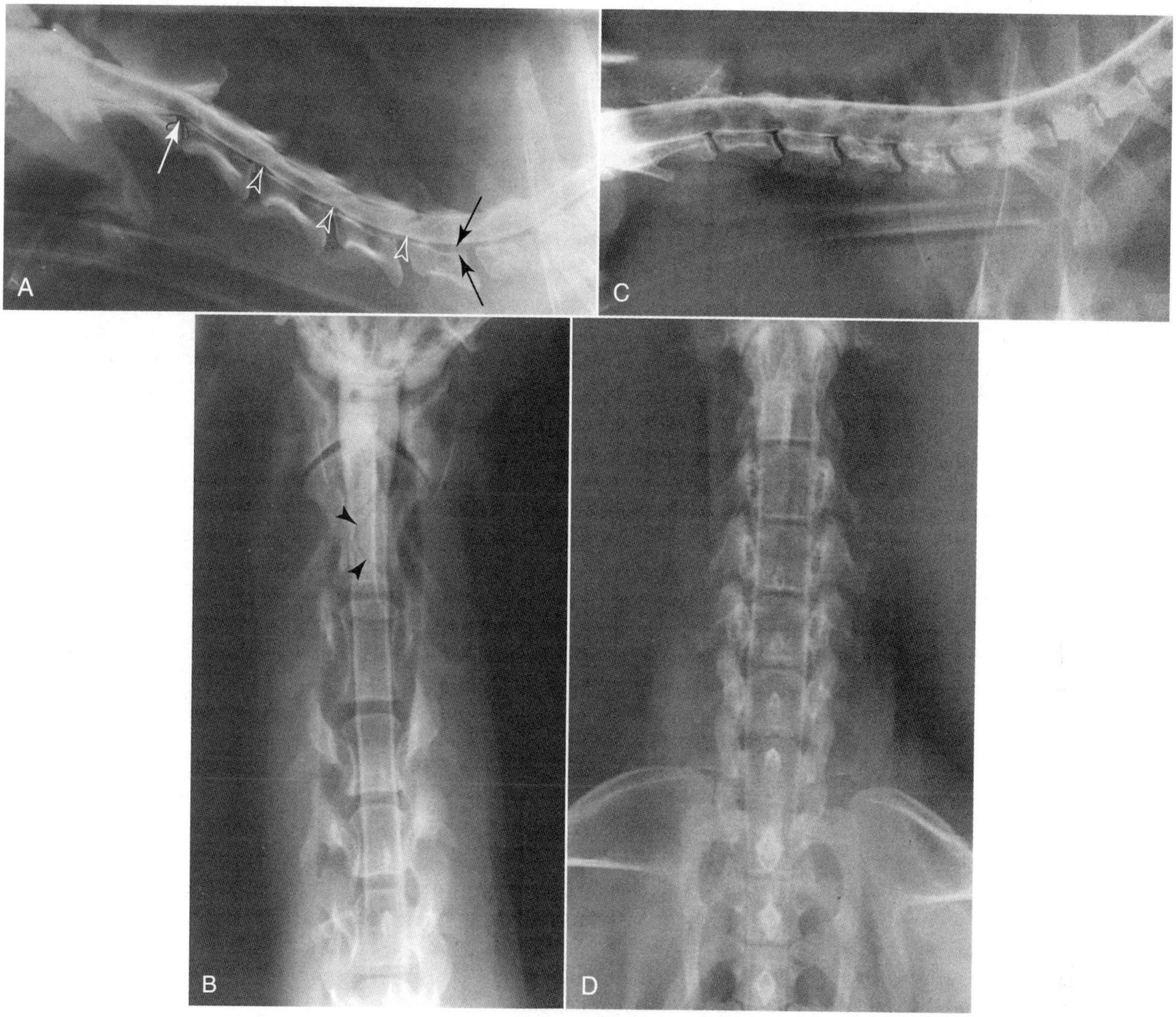

Fig. 14.34 Normal cervical myelogram. **A,** In a dog, on the lateral radiograph the subarachnoid space is wide cranially and thin caudally. Soft tissues (dorsal longitudinal ligament or annulus) normally cause thinning of the ventral aspect of the subarachnoid space C2–C3 (*large white arrow*) and should not be confused with disc herniation. Smaller indentations (*small white arrows*) are also seen in normal dogs. The epidural space is widest dorsal to C6–C7 (*closed black arrows*). **B,** In a dog, on the ventrodorsal radiograph, a serpentine subarachnoid filling defect (*black arrowheads*) is caused by the basilar artery. The subarachnoid space is also wider cranially. Note poor filling of the subarachnoid space in the caudal cervical region, which is caused by the effect of dependency. **C and D,** In the cat, the spinal cord is relatively wide and occupies a large percentage of the vertebral canal. As a result, the subarachnoid space is thin and conforms closely to the margins of the vertebral canal; this can give a false impression of cord swelling.

evidence of spinal cord compression. The thoracic spinal cord lacks an intumescence and is smaller than the cervical and lumbosacral regions of the spinal cord. Although the canine spinal cord typically terminates at L5–6, the contrast medium-filled dural sac often extends beyond the lumbosacral junction (see Fig. 14.35).[102] CT myelograms are typified by an opaque symmetrical ring surrounding the spinal cord (Fig. 14.36). The epidural space is well seen and easily distinguished due to the superior contrast resolution of CT. CT myelograms are excellent for determining the laterality of an extradural lesion such as a herniated disc, aiding the surgeon's decision on right versus left hemilaminectomy.

The abnormal myelogram is characterized by changes in the size and location of the opacified subarachnoid space, and in the width and opacity of the spinal cord. Myelographic lesions can be grouped into the following patterns: extradural lesions, intradural-extramedullary lesions, intramedullary swelling, and intramedullary opacification (Fig. 14.37 and Table 14.3).[102]

Several technical factors affecting myelographic quality and interpretation have been previously detailed (Fig. 14.38).[104] However, two issues are worthy of mention. (1) Epidural injection is problematic with lumbar punctures because contrast medium may leak around the needle punctures in the dura and can obscure the subarachnoid space, limiting interpretation. While this may render a conventional myelogram useless, a follow-up CT study can distinguish between the epidural spill versus and the subarachnoid space, salvaging the procedure. (2) Occasionally, the central canal of the spinal cord is visible after injecting contrast medium vial lumbar puncture. Presence of contrast medium in the central canal occurs when the needle shaft is placed in the central canal or when the central canal communicates with the subarachnoid space at the level of the conus medullaris.[105] In the former instance, contrast medium is presumed to leak back along the needle, especially during rapid injection.[105] "Canalograms" are most likely to occur when puncture is made at L4–5, where the spinal cord–to–vertebral

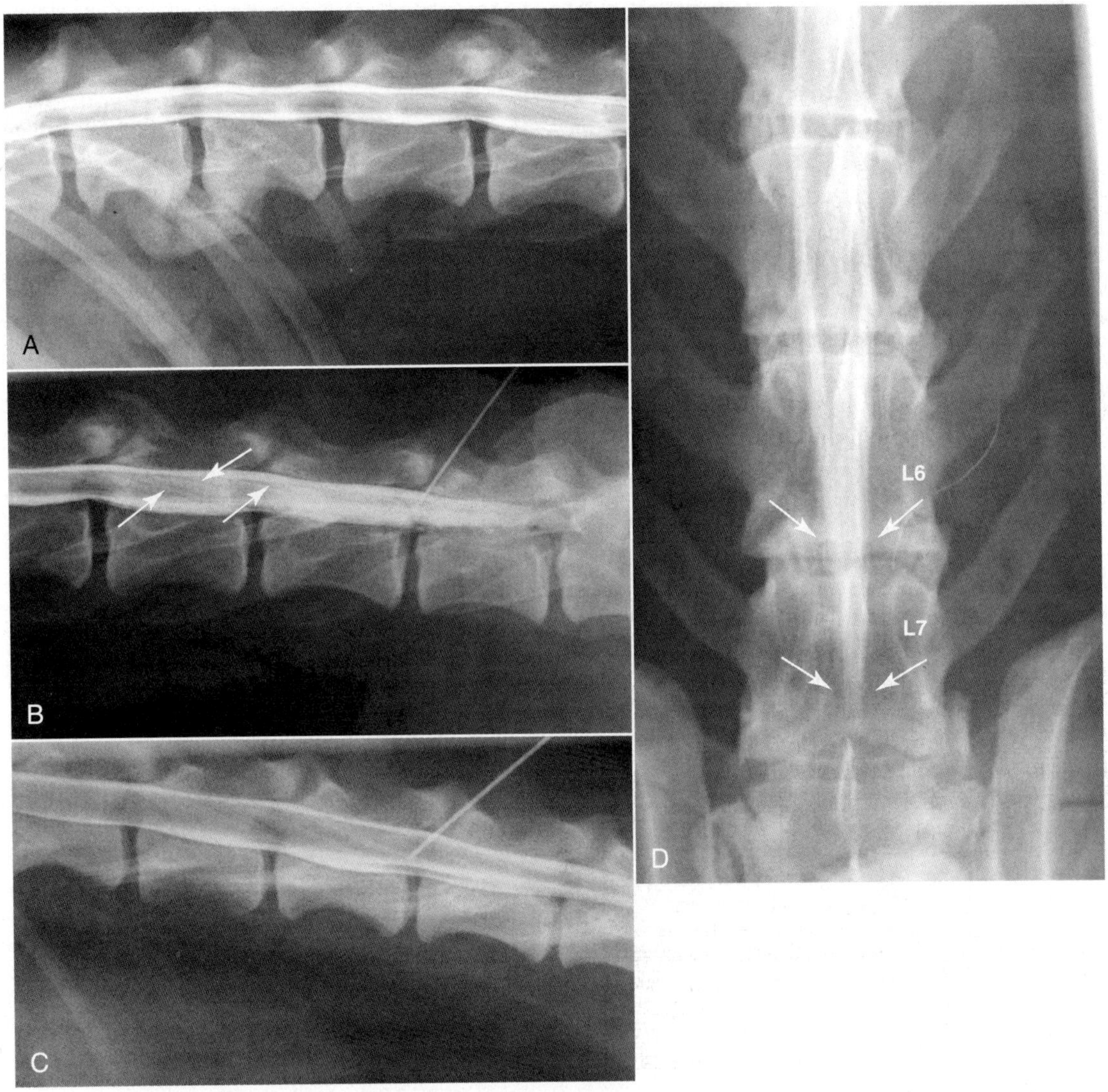

Fig. 14.35 Normal lumbar myelogram. **A,** Lateral myelogram centered at the cranial lumbar area. The dorsal and ventral subarachnoid space is well-filled with contrast medium and there is no epidural opacification. **B,** Lateral myelogram centered at the caudal lumbar area with a puncture at L5–L6. The subarachnoid space terminates at L6–L7. A puncture at L6–L7 would likely have placed the tip of the needle ventral to the thin terminal subarachnoid space and resulted in epidural leakage of contrast medium. Linear filling defects (*arrows*) are due to spinal nerves exiting the spinal cord, a normal finding in good quality study. **C,** Ventrodorsal myelogram centered at the caudal lumbar area with a L4–L5 puncture. Puncture should not be attempted cranial to this area and may cause significant cord injury. **D,** Ventrodorsal myelogram of the same dog as in **C.** The terminal subarachnoid space is thin (*arrows*) and would be difficult to puncture at L6–L7 or L7–S1.

canal ratio is large. The presence of contrast medium in a normal appearing central canal should not be confused with focal, indistinct opacification of the cord typical of myelomalacia. Enlargement of the central canal is associated with hydromyelia. The central canal may also become opacified when severe trauma or neoplasia disrupts the spinal cord parenchyma.

Intervertebral Disc Herniation

An extradural, and in some instances an intramedullary, pattern may result from disc herniation (Box 14.2).[102,106]

Disc herniation typically causes an extradural lesion characterized by thinning and dorsal deviation of the ventral aspect of the subarachnoid space in the lateral radiograph and compensatory widening of the spinal cord in the VD radiograph if the disc material is located in the ventral vertebral canal (Fig. 14.39).[104] On the lateral radiograph, the spinal cord is compressed and is deviated away from the site of disc herniation. The aspect of the contrast medium column adjacent to the herniation tends to be dome shaped, and the opposite side of the contrast medium column is narrowed by the displaced spinal cord. When herniated disc material is slightly lateral to the midline, a split, or forked, appearance to the contrast medium column may be seen on the lateral projection (see Fig. 14.39C). This finding should not be confused with an intradural-extramedullary lesion (see eFig. 14.14).[104,107]

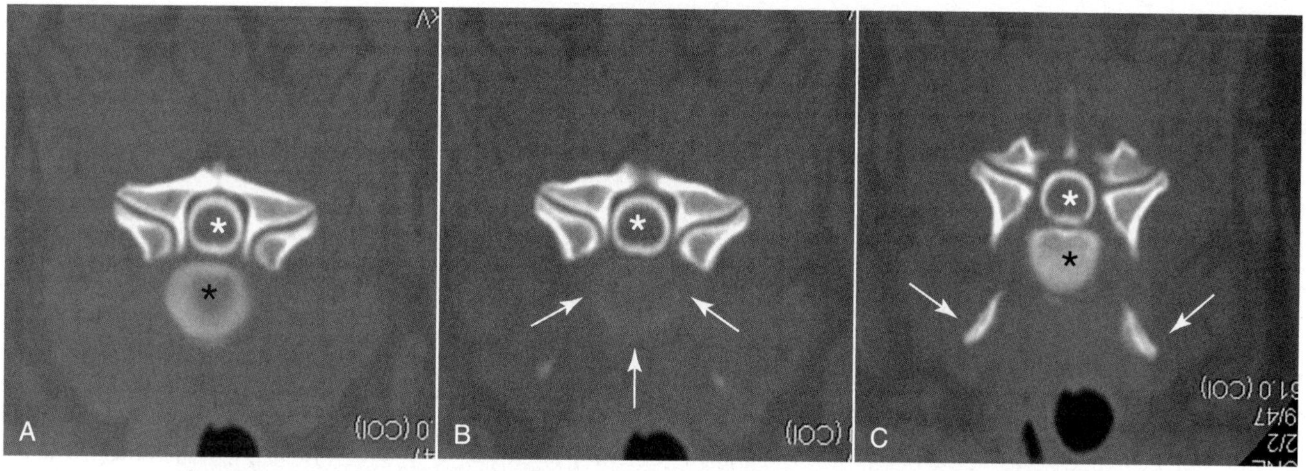

Fig. 14.36 Normal canine postmyelographic computed tomography (CT) transverse images made with a bone algorithm and 3-mm slice thickness. **A,** C2–C3 junction showing caudal endplate of C2 (*black asterisk*) and spinal cord (*white asterisk*) surrounded by contrast medium in the subarachnoid space. The epidural space is the circumferential area between opacified subarachnoid space and the vertebral canal. **B,** CT images made at the C2–C3 intervertebral disc space. *Arrows* delineate normal intervertebral disc, which has similar attenuation of surrounding soft tissue. Spinal cord (*white asterisk*) is surrounded by contrast medium in the subarachnoid space. **C,** CT images made at the C2–C3 junction showing cranial end-plate of C3 (*black asterisk*) and spinal cord (*white asterisk*) surrounded by contrast medium in the subarachnoid space. *Arrows* identify transverse processes of C3.

In type I herniation, an intramedullary pattern may be present due to severe spinal cord swelling. Swelling due to edema may obscure the classic extradural appearance of an extruded disc. Displacement of the subarachnoid space due to intramedullary swelling differs from that of extradural compression. With intramedullary swelling, the subarachnoid space is thin and displaced abaxially in all projections (Fig. 14.40). In some instances, severe spinal cord swelling may completely obliterate the subarachnoid space (see Fig. 14.40C).

If intramedullary swelling is present, slight axial deviation of the subarachnoid space somewhere within the region of spinal cord swelling suggests the site of an extradural discal mass (see Fig. 14.40B). This important clue is often found on only one radiographic projection but can help determine the site for surgical exploration and decompression. If CT is available, postmyelographic imaging can routinely depict the exact site of extradural compression when severe intramedullary swelling is present. It should be kept in mind that hemorrhage from rupture of the ventral vertebral veins is a complication of acute disc extrusion and the resultant hematoma may cause an extradural mass lesion.

Oblique radiographic projections should be obtained during every myelographic study because they frequently provide useful information. If disc material is located lateral to midline, the lateral and VD radiographs will be characterized by only a widened appearance to the spinal cord, whereas in oblique radiographic projections (VL-DR [ventral 25-degree left—dorsal right oblique] and VR-DL [ventral-25 degree right—dorsal left oblique]), an extradural pattern will be seen (Fig. 14.41). In some instances, both left and right lateral radiographic projections are needed for accurate identification of an extradural lesion.[108]

The gradual onset of type II disc protrusion tends to minimize spinal cord swelling, resulting in an extradural myelographic pattern (Fig. 14.42). Chronic changes, including hypertrophy of the annulus fibrosus, ligamentum flavum, and joint capsule of the dorsal intervertebral articular process joint, cause circumferential compression of the spinal cord ("hourglass appearance"). Type II protrusion is part of the cervical vertebral malformation-instability (wobbler) and lumbosacral stenosis-instability (cauda equina) syndromes of large-breed dogs.[82,109]

Acute noncompressive nucleus pulposus extrusion (ANNPE) is typified by an intramedullary myelographic pattern. Contrast medium uptake in the spinal cord can be a sign of cord penetration by the extruded disc material (Fig. 14.43).

Arachnoid Diverticula

Arachnoid diverticula are benign cyst-like areas in the subarachnoid space that may cause extramedullary compression and neural signs.[110–112] Histologically, these are not true cysts because they are not lined with epithelial cells. The cause of arachnoid diverticula is unknown, but a congenital or acquired etiology is possible. Resistance to cerebrospinal fluid (CSF)

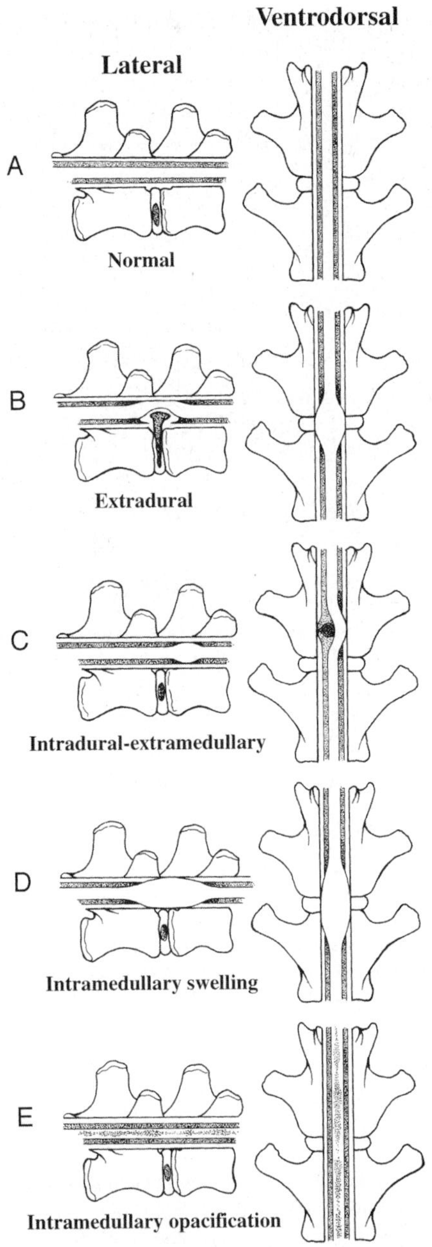

Fig. 14.37 Classification of myelographic lesions. **A,** Normal. **B,** Extradural. An aspect of the contrast medium column is displaced toward the center of the vertebral canal and often thinned or obliterated on one radiographic projection. On the orthogonal projection, the spinal cord may appear widened with peripheral displacement of the subarachnoid space because of an increase in spinal cord diameter caused by the compression. **C,** Intradural-extramedullary mass lesion within the subarachnoid space causes a filling defect in at least one projection. On the orthogonal projection, spinal cord swelling may be present depending on the size of the mass. As the contrast medium abuts the mass in the subarachnoid space, it flares around the mass and has been described as having the appearance of a *golf tee*. **D,** Intramedullary swelling. The spinal cord is swollen, causing thinning and obliteration of the subarachnoid space on both myelographic projections. **E,** Intramedullary opacification. Opacification of the spinal cord parenchyma is caused by the presence of contrast medium. This may be secondary to myelomalacia, which allows intramedullary diffusion of contrast medium. Opacification of the central canal differs and should not be confused with myelomalacia.

Table • 14.3

Diagnostic Possibilities Associated With Myelographic Patterns.

PATTERN	DIAGNOSIS
Extradural	Intervertebral disc herniation Ligamentous hypertrophy Hematoma/hemorrhage Neoplasia (vertebral or epidural soft tissue) Vertebral fracture/dislocation
Intradural-extramedullary	Neoplasia (nerve sheath tumors, meningioma) Lateralized extradural masses, such as discs, may give the appearance of an intradural-extramedullary lesion Arachnoid diverticulum
Intramedullary swelling	Spinal cord edema or hemorrhage Neoplasia (neural, metastatic discrete cell, e.g., granulomatous meningoencephalitis) Ischemic myelopathy
Intramedullary opacification	Myelomalacia Hematomyelia, spinal cord perforation by high-velocity disc extrusion
Normal	Degenerative myelopathy[a] Ischemic myelopathy Myelitis Meningitis

[a]It is the author's opinion that cord size may be decreased in some dogs with degenerative myelopathy. However, this evidence based studies are lacking, thus this is an anecdotal observation.

flow, possibly induced by trauma, resulting in back pressure and dilation of the subarachnoid space, has been implicated as a cause in older animals. With arachnoid diverticula, survey radiographic examination is usually normal. After myelography, contrast medium fills the "cystic" area, defining abrupt dilation of the subarachnoid contrast medium and compression of the adjacent spinal cord (Fig. 14.44) Recognition of the intradural-extramedullary location of arachnoid cysts is important so that they can be differentiated from nonsurgical intramedullary lesions such as hydromyelia or syringomyelia. The intradural-extramedullary sign in this instance differs from that of a mass lesion (e.g., neurofibroma) in which a filling defect is present as well as subarachnoid dilation. Arachnoid diverticula that arise from causes other than previous trauma or surgery are commonly located in the dorsal aspect of the cervical subarachnoid space.[113]

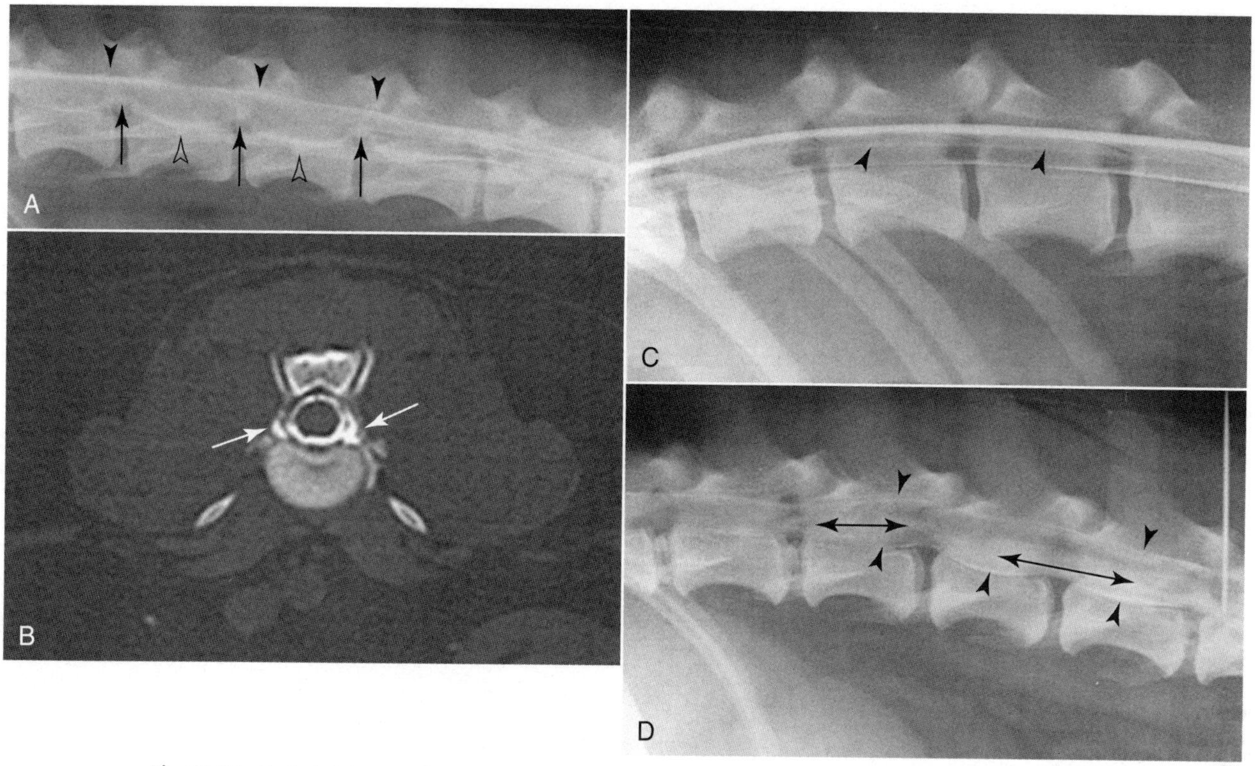

Fig. 14.38 Technical factors affecting myelographic quality. **A,** Moderate epidural leakage after lumbar myelography at L5–L6. Epidural contrast medium is recognized ventrally by the appearance of opacified vertebral venous sinuses (*large closed arrows*) and dorsally by opacification dorsal to the subarachnoid space (*small closed arrows*). Opacified depressions in the vertebral bodies contain the basivertebral veins (*open black arrows*). Epidural contrast medium summates with the subarachnoid space limiting interpretation. **B,** Follow-up computed tomography (CT) study reduces the effect of summation from epidural leakage (*arrows*). Due to the cross-sectional nature of CT, the subarachnoid space is still visualized and interpretation is possible. **C,** Opacification of the central canal (*arrows*) occurs when communication exists between the central canal and the subarachnoid space. **D,** Myelomalacia is typified by diffusion of contrast medium into the spinal cord parenchyma (*double-headed arrows*). Intramedullary swelling is also present, and the subarachnoid space is thin (*arrowheads*).

Box • 14.2

Myelographic Signs of Intervertebral Disc Disease

Extradural Pattern

- Deviation and thinning of subarachnoid contrast medium at intervertebral disc space (ventral, dorsal, or lateral)
- Forked subarachnoid contrast medium (false intradural-extramedually sign) if disc is lateralized
- Spinal cord displacement
- Spinal cord compression (compensatory displacement flattens cord owing to extradural mass, mimics cord swelling)
- "Hourglass" subarachnoid space filling defect

Intramedullary Pattern

- Uniform spinal cord swelling caused by edema; subarachnoid contrast medium displaced, thin, or absent
- Opacification of spinal cord parenchyma

Synovial Cysts

Synovial cysts secondary to osteoarthritis of the dorsal intervertebral process joints may cause extradural signs and are most frequently seen in the cervical and lumbar areas (Fig. 14.45). Protrusion of the synovial membrane may cause the formation of a para-articular cavity filled with synovial fluid, leading to extradural compression of the cord and nerve roots.[112,113]

Neoplasia

Neoplasms of the meninges may cause intradural/extramedullary myelographic patterns, including meningiomas and nerve sheath tumors (neurofibromas, neurofibrosarcomas, and Schwannomas and nephroblastomas) (Fig. 14.46). Other tumors are possible, including metastatic tumors. Lymphomas and histiocytic sarcoma may cause any type of myelographic pattern, including an extradural pattern (Fig. 14.47). Tumors of the spinal cord usually cause cord swelling and an intramedullary myelographic pattern.

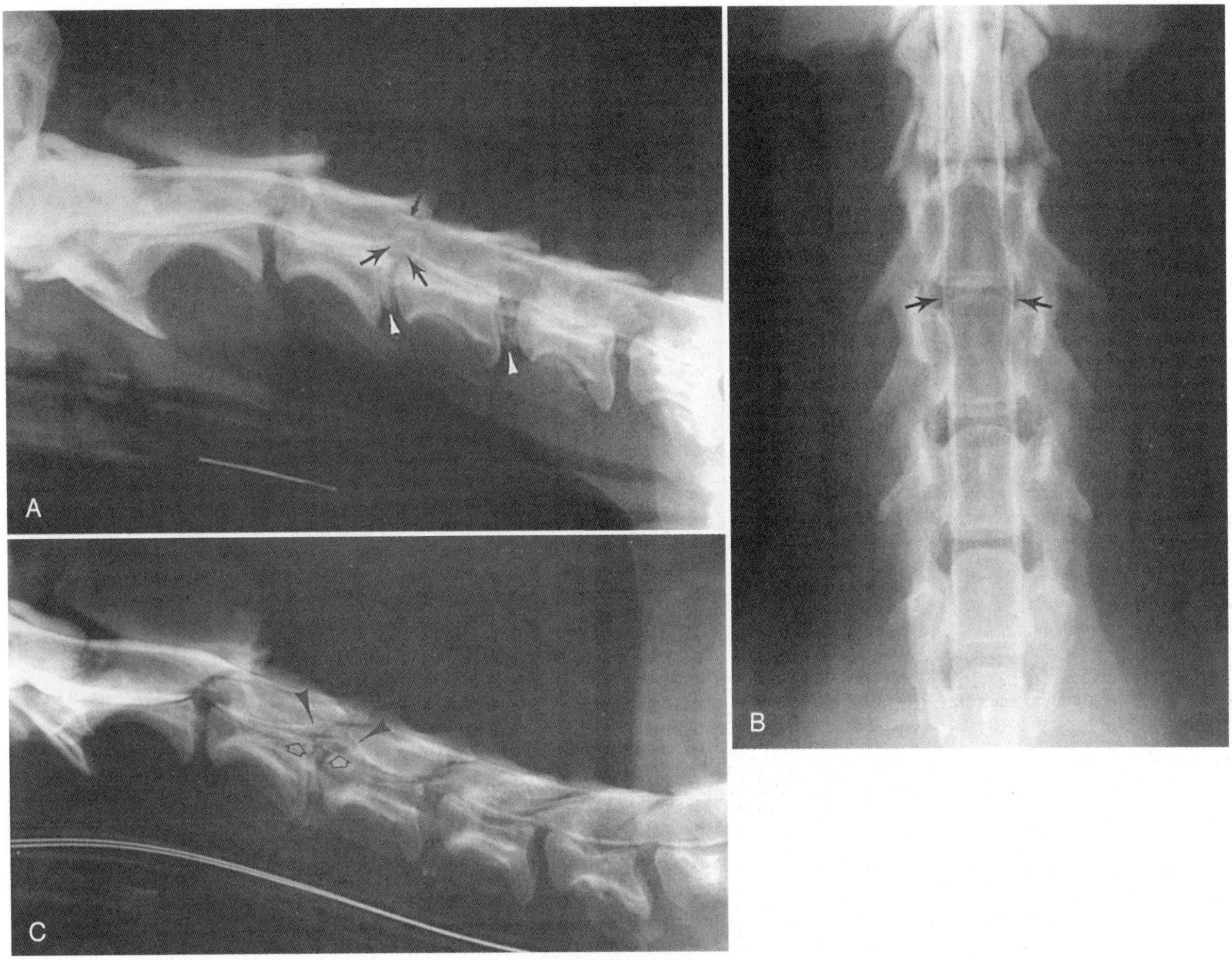

Fig. 14.39 Extradural lesions caused by a type I intervertebral disc herniation at C3–C4 are visible. **A,** Lateral myelogram. Dorsal deviation of the ventral aspect of the subarachnoid space is visible (*large arrows*). The dorsal aspect of the subarachnoid space is thin owing to displacement of the spinal cord (*small arrow*). Note mineralized disc material remaining in situ (*white arrowheads*). **B,** Ventrodorsal myelogram. Spinal cord swelling is typified by thinning and peripheral deviation of the subarachnoid space at C3–C4 (*arrows*). **C,** Forked appearance of the ventral aspect of the subarachnoid space is caused by the x-ray beam striking two tangents of the subarachnoid space. The extruded disc material is located lateral to the midline, causing the ventral aspect of the contrast medium column to appear as a *double line* on the lateral radiograph (*open arrows*). The double line is not seen in **A** because of a slight difference in patient positioning.

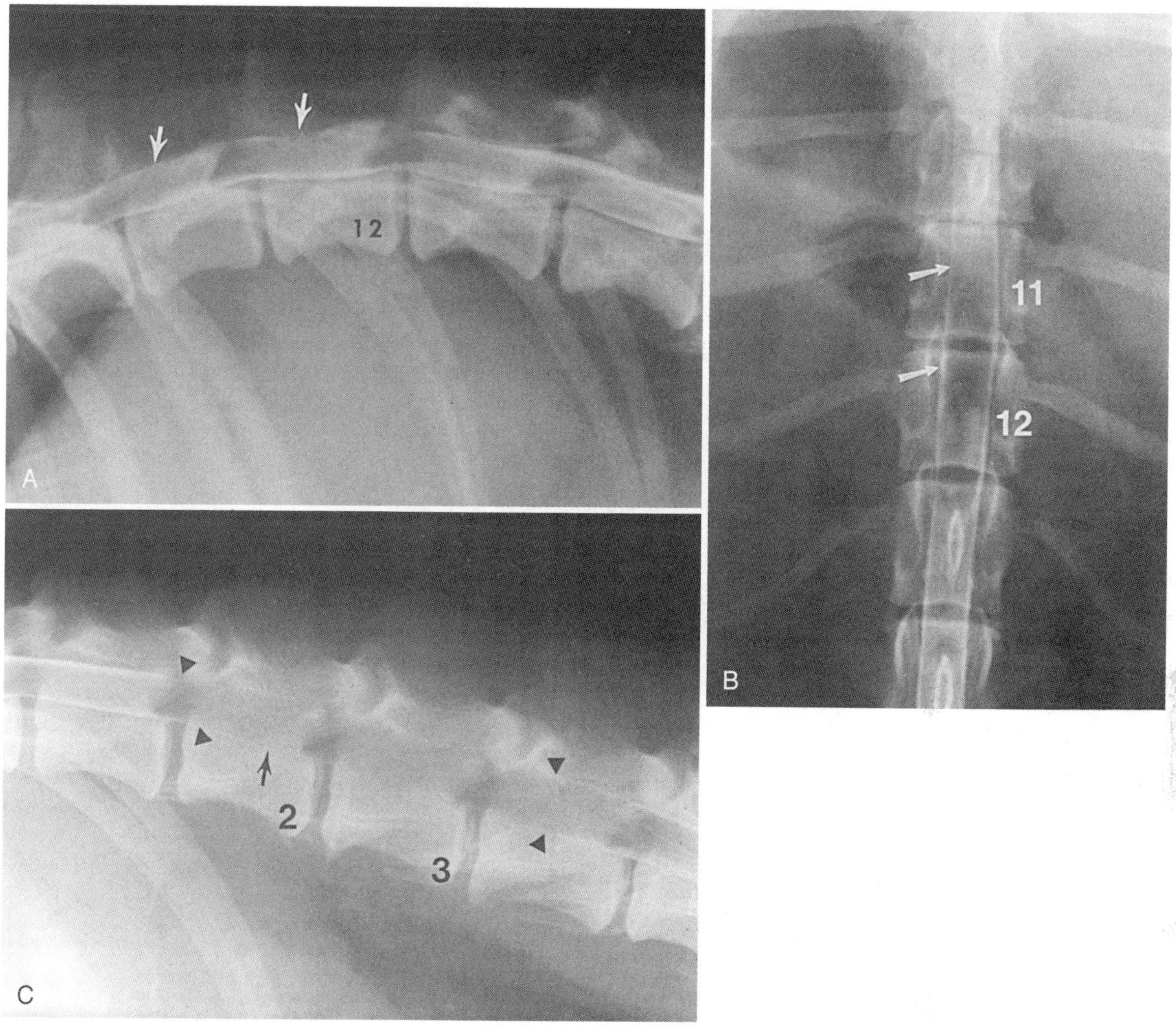

Fig. 14.40 Type I disc prolapse with intramedullary pattern. **A,** Lateral myelogram. Intramedullary swelling and a thin subarachnoid space (*arrows*) at T11–T12 are visible. **B,** Ventrodorsal myelogram of the dog in **A**. The spinal cord is wide at T11–T12; note the central shift of the right aspect of the contrast medium column (*arrows*), which indicates lateralization of the prolapse. In this instance, the surgeon may elect to perform a right hemilaminectomy. Intervertebral disc herniation at T11–T12 was confirmed at surgery. **C,** With severe intramedullary swelling, the contrast medium column may be totally obliterated (*arrowheads*), masking the extradural component of the lesion on all myelographic views. Intervertebral disc herniation at L2–L3 was confirmed at surgery.

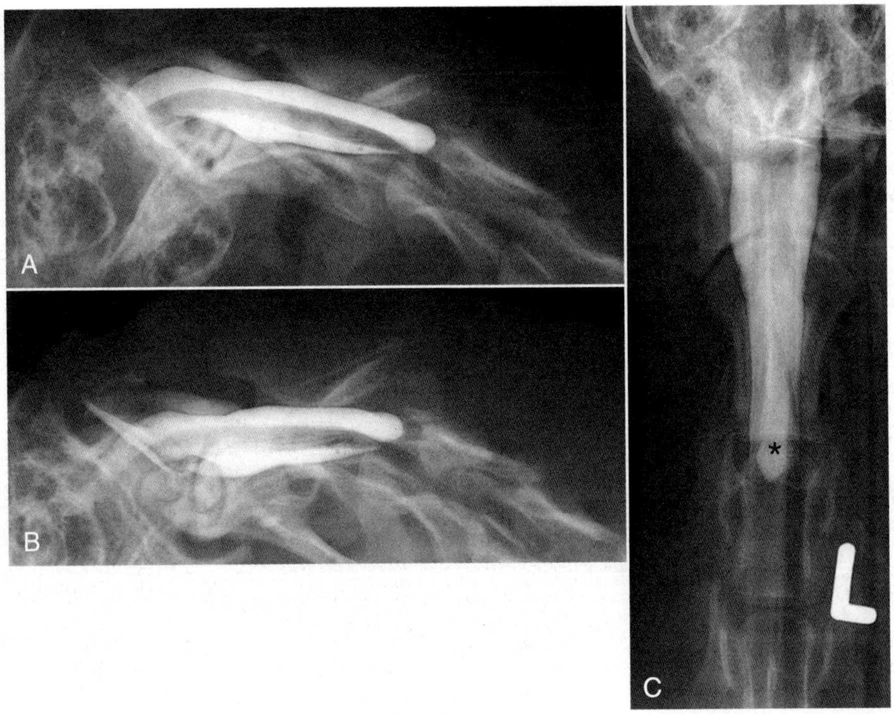

Fig. 14.44 Arachnoid diverticulum in a 3-year-old Rottweiler with cervical pain. **A and B,** 90-degree orthogonal oblique positioned myelograms of the atlantoaxial area following cervical myelography. These images are approximately 15 degrees from true lateral positioning and were made to maximize the diverticulum. An intradural extramedullary pattern is present. The opacified subarachnoid diverticulum is identified by *asterisks*. Note narrowing of cervical spinal cord at C2–C3. **C,** Ventrodorsal myelogram. Note blunted subarachnoid diverticulum (*asterisk*). The spinal cord is summated by the wide dorsal contrast column seen in **A**. (Images courtesy Gabriela Seiler, DVM, PhD, North Carolina State University College of Veterinary Medicine, with permission.)

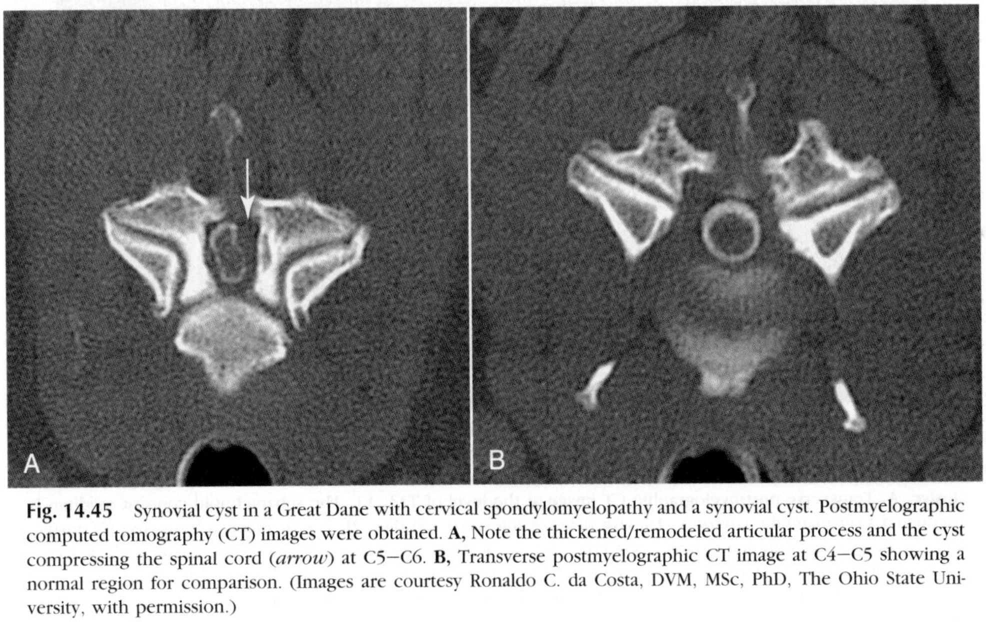

Fig. 14.45 Synovial cyst in a Great Dane with cervical spondylomyelopathy and a synovial cyst. Postmyelographic computed tomography (CT) images were obtained. **A,** Note the thickened/remodeled articular process and the cyst compressing the spinal cord (*arrow*) at C5–C6. **B,** Transverse postmyelographic CT image at C4–C5 showing a normal region for comparison. (Images are courtesy Ronaldo C. da Costa, DVM, MSc, PhD, The Ohio State University, with permission.)

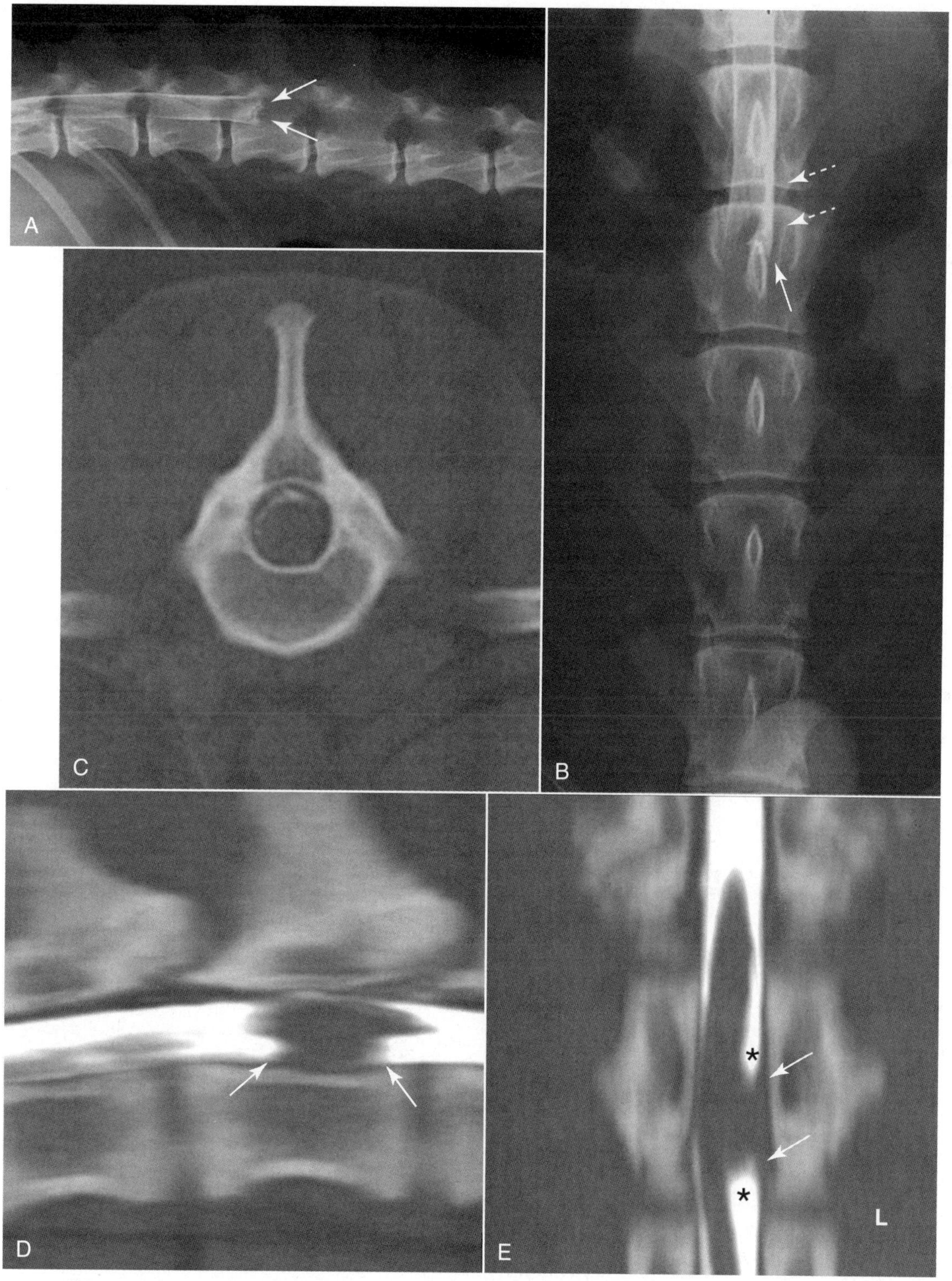

Fig. 14.46 Extraskeletal osteosarcoma in a 3-year-old mixed-breed dog with left pelvic limb monoparesis and decreased patellar reflex. Lateral **(A)** and ventrodorsal **(B)** myelograms are typified by an intradural extramedullary pattern. **A,** There is abrupt cessation of flow of contrast medium caudally at L3 (*arrows*). **B,** The spinal cord has undergone slight axial shift (*dotted arrows*) and the left subarachnoid space is widened as it ends in a blunted appearance. This blunted appearance has been referred to as a "golf tee" pattern as it suggests an intradural mass has caused a filling defect in the subarachnoid space. However, this pattern is not uniformly present with intradural lesions. Transverse **(A)**, sagittal **(D)** and dorsal **(E)** postmyelographic CT images of a dog with an intradural lesion. **C,** Transverse CT slice through L3 showing poor contrast medium filling of the subarachnoid space. **D,** Sagittal reformat at L3. *Arrows* show blunting of contrast medium. **E,** *Asterisks* indicate the widening of the subarachnoid space before it ends bluntly in the dorsal reformatted image.

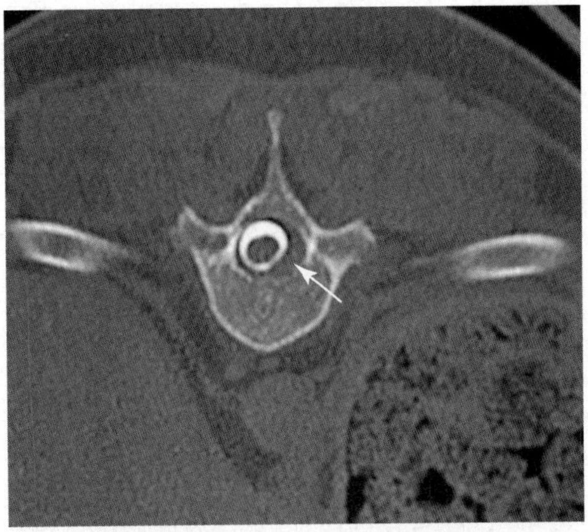

Fig. 14.47 Spinal lymphoma in an old mixed-breed dog with a 3-month history of slowly progressive intermittent cervical pain with a thoracic limb root signature sign. Transverse postmyelographic computed tomography (CT) image of a thoracic vertebra. The *arrow* denotes an extradural hypoattenuating mass displacing the subarachnoid contrast medium and the spinal cord. Additional extradural lesions were found in the cervical region.

Acknowledgment

With special thanks to prior authors of this chapter for their contributions.

REFERENCES

1. Thrall DE, Robertson ID. The spine. In: *Atlas of Normal Radiographic Anatomy and Anatomic Variants of the Dog and Cat*. 3rd ed. St Louis: Saunders; 2023.
2. Evans HE. Chapter 4. The skeleton. In: *Miller's Anatomy of the Dog*. 3rd ed. Philadelphia: Saunders; 1993:166–180.
3. Watson AG. *Phylogeny and Development of the Atlas-Axis Complex in the Dog, Master's Thesis*. Ithaca, NY: Cornell University; 1981.
4. Watson AG. Prenatal development of the composite occipito-atlanto-axial synovial joint cavity in the dog. *Anat Rec*. 1986;216:423–433.
5. Watson AG, Evans HE, DeLahunta A. Ossification of the atlas-axis complex in the dog. *Anat Histol Embryol*. 1986;15:122–138.
6. Evans HE. Chapter 4. The skeleton. In: *Miller's Anatomy of the Dog*. 3rd ed. Philadelphia: Saunders; 1993:178.
7. Evans HE. Chapter 4. The skeleton. In: *Miller's Anatomy of the Dog*. 3rd ed. Philadelphia: Saunders; 1993:225–231.
8. Shores A. Intervertebral disc syndrome in the dog. Part I. Pathophysiology and management. *Compend Contin Educ Pract Vet*. 1981;7:639.
9. Walker MA. The vertebrae—canine and feline. In: Thrall DE, ed. *Textbook of Veterinary Diagnostic Radiology*. ed 4. St Louis: Saunders; 2002:98–109.
10. Macpherson J, Ye Y. The cat vertebral column: stance configuration and range of motion. *Exp Brain Res*. 1998;119:324–332. https://doi.org/10.1007/s002210050348.
11. Baines EQ, Grandage J, Herritage ME, et al. Radiographic definition of the anticlinal vertebra in the dog. *Vet Radiol Ultrasound*. 2009;50:69–73.
12. Morgan JP. Congenital anomalies of the vertebral column of the dog: a study of the incidence and significance based on a radiographic and morphologic study. *J Am Vet Radiol Soc*. 1968;9:21–29.
13. Bailey CS, Morgan JP. Congenital spinal malformations. *Vet Clin North Am Small Anim Pract*. 1992;72:985–1015.
14. Lin JL, Coolman BR. Atlantoaxial subluxation in two dogs with cervical block vertebrae. *J Am Anim Hosp Assoc*. 2009;45:305–310.
15. Done SH, Drew RA, Robins GM, et al. Hemivertebra in the dog: clinical and pathological observations. *Vet Rec*. 1975;14:313–317.
16. Muller F, O'Rahilly R, Benson DR. The early origin of vertebral anomalies, as illustrated by a "butterfly" vertebra. *J Anat*. 1986;149:157–169.
17. Damur-Djuric N, Steffen F, Hassig M, et al. Lumbosacral transitional vertebrae in dogs: classification, prevalence and association with sacroiliac morphology. *Vet Radiol Ultrasound*. 2006;47:32–38.
18. Fluckiger M, Damur-Djuric N, Hassig M, et al. A lumbosacral transitional vertebra in the dog predisposes to caudal equina syndrome. *Vet Radiol Ultrasound*. 2006;47:39–44.
19. Harris G, Ball J, De Decker S. Lumbosacral transitional vertebrae in cats and its relationship to lumbosacral vertebral canal stenosis. *J Feline Med Surg*. 2019;21(4):286–292.
20. Thanaboonnipat C, Kumjumroon K, Boonkwang K, Tangsutthichai N, Sukserm W, Choisunirachon N. Radiographic lumbosacral vertebral abnormalities and constipation in cats. *Vet World*. 2021;14(2):492–498.
21. Lorenz MD, Kornegay JN. *Handbook of Veterinary Neurology*. 4th ed. St Louis: Saunders; 2004:164–189.
22. Cook JR, Oliver JE. Atlantoaxial luxation in the dog. *Compend Contin Educ Pract Vet*. 1981;3:242–252.
23. Watson AG, DeLahunta A. Atlantoaxial subluxation and absence of a transverse ligament of the atlas in dog. *J Am Vet Med Assoc*. 1989;195:235–237.
24. Cummings KR, Vilaplana Grosso F, Moore GE, et al. Radiographic indices for the diagnosis of atlantoaxial instability in toy breed dogs. *Vet Radiol Ultrasound*. 2018;59(6):667–676.
25. Warren-Smith C, Kneissl S, Benigni L, et al. Incomplete ossification of the atlas in dogs with cervical signs. *Vet Radiol Ultrasound*. 2009;50(6):635–638.
26. Lincoln JD. Cervical vertebral malformation/malarticulation syndrome in large dogs. *Vet Clin North Am Small Anim Pract*. 1992;22:923–935.
27. Seim HB, Withrow SJ. Pathophysiology and diagnosis of caudal cervical spondylo-myelopathy with emphasis on the Doberman pinscher. *J Am Anim Hosp Assoc*. 1982;18:241.
28. Van Gundy T. Canine wobbler syndrome. Part I: pathophysiology and diagnosis. *Compend Contin Educ Pract Vet*. 1989;11:269.
29. Selcer B, Oliver J. Cervical spondylopathy: wobbler syndrome in dogs. *J Am Anim Hosp Assoc*. 1975;11:175–179.
30. Seim H. Diagnosis and treatment of cervical vertebral instability-malformation syndromes. In: Bonagura JD, ed. *Kirk's Current Veterinary Therapy XIII: Small Animal Practice*. Philadelphia: Saunders; 2000:992–1000.
31. Headhammer A, Wu F, Krook L, et al. Over nutrition and skeletal disease. An experimental study in growing Great Dane dogs. *Cornell Vet*. 1974;64(suppl 5):58.
32. Drost WT, Lehenbauer TW, Reeves J. Mensuration of cervical vertebral ratios in Doberman pinschers and Great Danes. *Vet Radiol Ultrasound*. 2002;43:124–231.
33. Martin-Valuero P, Da Costa R. Evaluation of traditional and novel radiographic vertebral ratios in Great Danes with versus without cervical spondylomyelopathy. *Vet Radiol Ultrasound*. 2014;55:448–495.
34. Lipsitz D, Levitski RE, Chauvet AE, et al. Magnetic resonance features of cervical stenotic myelopathy in 21 dogs. *Vet Radiol Ultrasound*. 2001;42:20–27.

35. Da Costa RC, Parent J, Dobson H. Comparison of magnetic resonance imaging and myelography in 18 Doberman pinscher dogs with cervical spondylo-myelopathy. *Vet Radiol Ultrasound*. 2006;47:523–531.
36. Shores A. Spinal trauma. Pathophysiology and management of traumatic spinal injuries. *Vet Clin North Am Small Anim Pract*. 1992;22:859–867.
37. Matthiesen DT. Thoracolumbar spinal fractures and luxations: surgical management. *Compend Cont Educ Pract Vet*. 1983;5:867.
38. Walker TL, Tomlinson J, Sorjonen DC, et al. Diseases of the spinal column. In: Slatter DH, ed. *Textbook of Small Animal Surgery*. Philadelphia: Saunders; 1985:1367.
39. Watters DH, Blevins WE, Wallace LJ. Cervical vertebral fractures in 56 dogs: a retrospective study. *J Am Anim Hosp Assoc*. 1999;35:135–146.
40. Slocum B, Rudy RL. Fractures of the seventh lumbar vertebra in the dog. *J Am Anim Hosp Assoc*. 1975;11:67.
41. Kinns J, Mai W, Seiler G, et al. Radiographic sensitivity and negative predictive value for acute canine spinal trauma. *Vet Radiol Ultrasound*. 2006;47:563–570.
42. Hoerlein BF. *Philadelphia*. *Canine Neurology: Diagnosis and Treatment*. 3rd ed. Saunders; 1978:470–560.
43. DeLahunta A, ed. *Veterinary Neuroanatomy and Clinical Neurology*. 2nd ed. Philadelphia: Saunders; 1983:186–188.
44. da Costa RC, De Decker S, Lewis MJ, Volk H. Canine Spinal Cord Injury Consortium (CANSORT-SCI): diagnostic imaging in intervertebral disc disease. *Front Vet Sci*. 2020;7:588338. https://doi.org/10.3389/fvets.2020.588338.
45. Priester W. Canine intervertebral disc disease—occurrence by age, breed, and sex among 8,117 cases. *Theriogenology*. 1976;6:93–303.
46. Chang Y, Dennis R, Platt SR, et al. Magnetic resonance imaging of traumatic intervertebral disc extension in dogs. *Vet Rec*. 2007;160:795–799.
47. Fen J. Olby NJ and the canine spinal cord injury consortium (CANSORT-SCI): classification of intervertebral disc disease. *Front Vet Sci*. 2020;7:579025.
48. Lamb CN, Nichols A, Targett P, Mannion P. Accuracy of survey radiographic diagnosis of intervertebral disc protrusion in dogs. *Vet Rad Ultrasound*. 2002;43:222–228.
49. Robertson ID, Thrall DE. Imaging dogs with suspected disc herniation: pros and cons of myelography, computed tomography and magnetic resonance, Vet Radiol Ultrasound. 2011;52(suppl 1):S81–S84.
50. Owens JM, Biery DN. Spine. In: Owens JM, Biery DN, eds. *Radiographic Interpretation for the Small Animal Clinician*. 2nd ed. Philadelphia: Williams & Wilkins; 1999: 143–144.
51. Hugnet C, Marrou B, Dally C, et al. Osteomyelitis and discospondylitis due to *Scedosporium apiospermum* in a dog. *J Vet Diagn Invest*. 2009;21:120–123.
52. Csébi P, Jakab C, Jánoski K. Vertebral osteomyelitis and meningitis caused by *Pasteurella canis* in a dog—clinicopathological case report. *Acta Vet Hung*. 2010;58:13–21.
53. La Croix JA. Vertebral body osteomyelitis: case report. *J Am Vet Rad Soc*. 1973;14:17–21.
54. Kuwamura M, Ide M, Yamate J, et al. Systemic candidiasis in a dog, developing spondylitis. *J Vet Med Sci*. 2006;68:1117–1119.
55. Johnston DE, Summers BA. Osteomyelitis of the lumbar vertebrae in dogs caused by grass-seed-foreign bodies. *Aust Vet J*. 1971;47:289.
56. van der Merwe L, Kirberger RM, Clift S, et al. *Spirocerca lupi* infection in the dog: a review. *Vet J*. 2008;176:294–309.
57. Thomas WB. Discospondylitis and other vertebral infections. *Vet Clin North Am Small Anim Pract*. 2000;30:169–182.
58. DeLahunta A. Small animal spinal cord disease. In: DeLahunta A, ed. *Veterinary Neuroanatomy and Clinical Neurology*. 2nd ed. Philadelphia: Saunders; 1983:190.
59. Naughton JF, Tucker R, Bagley RS. Radiographic diagnosis-paraspinal abscess in a dog. *Vet Radiol Ultrasound*. 2005;46:23–26.
60. Jimenez MM, O'Callaghan MW. Vertebral physitis: a radiographic diagnosis to be separated from discospondylitis, a preliminary report. *Vet Radiol Ultrasound*. 1995;36:188–195.
61. Packer RA, Coates JR, Cook CR, et al. Sublumbar abscess and discospondylitis in a cat. *Vet Radiol Ultrasound*. 2005;46:396–399.
62. Tipold A, Stein VM. Inflammatory diseases of the small animal spine. *Vet Clin North Am Small Anim Pract*. 2010;40:871–879.
63. Moore MP. Discospondylitis. *Vet Clin North Am Small Anim Pract*. 1992;22:1027–1033.
64. Schultz RM, Johnson EG, Wisner ER, et al. Clinicopathologic and diagnostic imaging characteristics of systemic aspergillosis in 30 dogs. *J Vet Intern Med*. 2008;22(4): 851–859.
65. Carrera I, Sullivan M, McConnell F, et al. Magnetic resonance features of discospondylitis in dogs. *Vet Radiol Ultrasound*. 2011;52:125–131.
66. Kirberger RM. Early diagnostic imaging findings in juvenile dogs with presumed diskospondylitis: 10 cases (2008–2014). *J Am Vet Med Assoc*. 2016;249:539–546.
67. *Dorland's Illustrated Medical Dictionary*. 28th ed. Philadelphia: Saunders; 1994:1564.
68. Morgan JP. Spondylosis deformans in the dog. *Acta Orthop Scand Suppl*. 1967;96:7–87.
69. Morgan JP, Biery DN. Spondylosis deformans. In: Newton CD, ed. *Textbook of Small Animal Orthopaedics*. Philadelphia: Lippincott Williams & Wilkins; 1985: 733–738.
70. Morgan JP. Spondylosis deformans in the dog: its radiographic appearance. *J Am Vet Radiol Soc*. 1967;8:17.
71. Morgan JP, Miyabayashi T. Degenerative changes in the vertebral column of the dog: common radiographic findings. *Vet Radiol Ultrasound*. 1988;29:72–77.
72. Resnick D. Degenerative disease of the spine. In: Resnick D, ed. *Bone and Joint Imaging*. 2nd ed. Philadelphia: Saunders; 1996:355.
73. Hulkins DW, Meakin JR. Relationship between structure and mechanical function of the tissues of the intervertebral joint. *Am Zool*. 2000;40:42–52.
74. Carnier P, Gallo L, Sturaro E, et al. Prevalence of spondylosis deformans and estimates of genetic parameters for the degree of osteophytes development in Italian boxer dogs. *J Anim Sci*. 2004;82:85–92.
75. Langeland M, Lingaas F. Spondylosis deformans in the boxer: estimates of heritability. *J Small Anim Pract*. 1995;36:166–169.
76. Breit S, Kunzel W. The position and shape of osteophyte formations at canine vertebral endplates and its influence on radiographic diagnosis. *Anat Histol Embryol*. 2001;30:179–184.
77. Levine GJ, Levine JM, Walker MA, et al. Evaluation of the association between spondylosis deformans and clinical signs of intervertebral disc disease in dogs: 172 cases (1999–2000). *J Am Vet Med Assoc*. 2006;228:96–100.
78. Fletcher TF. Chapter 16. Spinal cord and meninges. In: Evans HE, ed. *Miller's Anatomy of the Dog*. ed 3. Philadelphia: Saunders; 1993:804–806.
79. Morgan JP, Atilola M, Bailey CS. Vertebral canal and spinal cord mensuration. A comparative study and its effect on lumbosacral myelography in the dachshund and German shepherd dog. *J Am Vet Med Assoc*. 1987;191:951–957.

80. Pardo AD, Morgan JP. Myelography in the cat: a comparison of cisternal versus lumbar puncture, using metrizamide. *Vet Radiol*. 1988;29:89–95.
81. *Dorland's Illustrated Medical Dictionary*. 28th ed. Philadelphia: Saunders; 1994:280.
82. Wheeler SJ. Lumbosacral disease. *Vet Clin North Am small Anim Pract*. 1992;22:937–950.
83. Lenehan TM. Canine caudal equina syndrome. *Comp Cont Educ Pract Vet*. 1983;5:941–950.
84. Ramirez O, Thrall DE. A review of imaging techniques for canine cauda equina syndrome. *Vet Radiol Ultrasound*. 1998;39:283–296.
85. Jones JC, Sorjonen DC, Simpson ST, et al. Comparison between computed tomographic and surgical finding in 9 large breed dogs with lumbosacral stenosis. *Vet Radiol Ultrasound*. 1996;37:247–256.
86. Lang J, Hani H, Schwalder P. A sacral lesion resembling osteochondrosis in the German shepherd dog. *Vet Radiol Ultrasound*. 1992;33:69–76.
87. Adams WH, Daniel GB, Pardo AD, et al. Magnetic resonance imaging of the caudal lumbar and lumbosacral spine in 13 dogs (1990–1993). *Vet Radiol Ultrasound*. 1995;36:3–13.
88. Seiler GS, Hani H, Busato AR, et al. Facet joint geometry and intervertebral disk degeneration in the L5-S1 region of the vertebral column in German shepherd dogs. *Am J Vet Res*. 2002;63:86–90.
89. Lang J. Flexion-extension myelography canine caudal equina. *Vet Radiol Ultrasound*. 1988;29:242–257.
90. Widmer WR, Thrall DE. Canine and feline intervertebral disc disease, myelography, and spinal cord disease. In: Thrall DE, ed. *Textbook of Veterinary Diagnostic Radiology*. 5th ed. St Louis: Saunders; 2007:194–219.
91. Roberts RE, Selcer BA. Myelography and epidurography. *Vet Clin North Am small Anim Pract*. 1993;23:307–329.
92. Barthez PY, Morgan JP, Lipstiz D. Discography and epidurography for evaluation of the lumbosacral junction in dogs with cauda equina syndrome. *Vet Radiol Ultrasound*. 1994;35:152–157.
93. Morgan JP, Ackerman N, Bailey CS. Vertebral tumors in the dog: a clinical radiologic and pathologic study of 61 primary and secondary lesions. *Vet Radiol Ultrasound*. 1980;21:197–212.
94. Luttgen PL. Neoplasms of the spine. *Vet Clin North Am Small Anim Pract*. 1992;22:973–984.
95. Edelstyn GA, Gillespie PJ, Grebbel FS. The radiological demonstration of osseous metastasis: experimental observations. *Clin Radiol*. 1967;18:158.
96. Bossens K, Bhatti S, Van Soens I, et al. Diffuse idiopathic skeletal hyperostosis of the spine in a nine-year-old cat. *J Small Anim Pract*. 2016;57:33–35.
97. Morgan JP, Stavenborn M. Disseminated idiopathic skeletal hyperostosis (DISH) in a dog. *Vet Radiol Ultrasound*. 1991;32:65–70.
98. Konde LJ, Thrall MA, Gasper P, et al. Radiographically visualized skeletal changes associated with mucopolysaccharidosis VI in cats. *Vet Radiol Ultrasound*. 1987;28:223–228.
99. Harris WH, Heaney RP. Skeletal renewal and metabolic bone disease. *N Engl J Med*. 1969;280(4):193–202.
100. Widmer WR, Blevins WE. Veterinary myelography: a review of contrast media, adverse effects and technique. *J Am Anim Hosp Assoc*. 1991;27:163–177.
101. Olby NJ, Dyce J, Houlton JEF. Correlation of plain radiographic and lumbar myelographic findings in thoracolumbar disc disease. *J Small Anim Pract*. 1994;35:345–350.
102. Roberts RE, Selcer BA. Myelography and epidurography. *Vet Clin North Am Small Anim Pract*. 1993;23:307–329.
103. Tilmant L, Ackerman N, Spencer CP. Mechanical aspects of subarachnoid space puncture in the dog. *Vet Radiol*. 1984;25:227–232.
104. Lamb CR. Common difficulties with myelographic diagnosis of acute intervertebral disc disease in the. dog. *J Small Anim Pract*. 1994;35:549–558.
105. Kirberger RM, Wrigley R. Myelography in the dog: a review of patients with contrast medium in the central canal. *Vet Radiol*. 1993;3:253–258.
106. Burk RL. Problems in the radiographic interpretation of intervertebral disc disease in the dog. *Probl Vet Med Intervert Disc Dis*. 1989;1:381–481.
107. Kirberger RM, Roos CJ, Lubbe AM. The radiological diagnosis of thoracolumbar disc disease in the dachshund. *Vet Radiol Ultrasound*. 1992;33:255–261.
108. Matteucci ML, Ramirez 3rd O, Thrall DE. Radiographic diagnosis: effect of right vs. left lateral recumbency on myelographic appearance of a lateralized extradural mass. *Vet Radiol Ultrasound*. 1999;40:351–352.
109. Mattoon JS, Koblik PD. Quantitative survey radiographic evaluation of the lumbosacral spine of normal dogs and dogs with degenerative lumbosacral stenosis. *Vet Radiol Ultrasound*. 1993;34:194–206.
110. Cambridge AJ, Bagley RS, Britt LG, et al. Radiographic diagnosis: arachnoid cyst in a dog. *Vet Radiol Ultrasound*. 1997;38:434.
111. Bentley JF, Simpson ST, Hathcock JT. Spinal arachnoid cyst in a dog. *J Am Anim Hosp Assoc*. 1991;27:549.
112. da Costa RC, Cook LB. Cystic abnormalities of the spinal cord and vertebral column. *Vet Clin Small Anim*. 2016;46:277–293.
113. Lowrie ML, Platt SR, Garosi LS. Extramedullary spinal cysts in dogs. *Vet Surg*. 2014;43:650–662.

ELECTRONIC RESOURCES

Additional information related to the content in Chapter 14 can be found online at eBooks.Health.Elsevier.com.

- Chapter Quiz

CHAPTER 15

Magnetic Resonance Imaging and Computed Tomography Features of Canine and Feline Spinal Cord Disease

Wilfried Mai

Computed tomography (CT) and magnetic resonance imaging (MRI) are used routinely in the investigation of spinal diseases in the dog and cat.[1,2] They are both superior to radiography in the diagnosis of most spinal conditions. MRI has a better overall diagnostic sensitivity than CT and can be used to diagnose virtually all conditions of the spine. However, there are patients in which CT is still the preferred method, for example, vertebral trauma caused by a gunshot wherein metallic foreign material is present that would cause considerable artifact in magnetic resonance (MR) images, or for the diagnosis of subtle bone lesions, such as vertebral subluxation or fractures. Although a number of spinal conditions can be diagnosed with radiographs (e.g., discospondylitis), CT and MRI may still be warranted to better assess the extent of the condition, which may be important for diagnostic or therapeutic purposes. Earlier diagnosis of some conditions may also be permitted by CT or MRI.

NORMAL APPEARANCE OF THE SPINE ON COMPUTED TOMOGRAPHY AND MAGNETIC RESONANCE IMAGING

Normal Anatomy

A schematic representation of the components of the vertebrae and main ligaments of the spine is shown in Fig. 15.1. The longitudinal ligaments of the vertebral column provide dorsal and ventral support for the intervertebral discs.[3] The dorsal longitudinal ligament lies on the floor of the vertebral canal. In the cervical region, it is wide and thick, which explains why lateral disc extrusion leading to radiculopathy, or root signature, is more common in the cervical region than other spinal regions. In the thoracolumbar area, the dorsal longitudinal ligament is thinner and centered on the midline allowing dorsal protrusion of disc material leading to spinal cord compression. The intercapital ligaments are short, transverse fibrous bands that lie ventral to the dorsal longitudinal ligament, joining left-to-right rib heads between T2 and T11.[3] They, therefore, buttress the dorsal part of the annulus fibrosus cranial to T11, reducing the probability of dorsal disc protrusion in this region. The ventral longitudinal ligament spans the ventral surface of the vertebral column.[3] The yellow ligaments *(ligamentum flavum)*, also called *interarcuate ligaments*, are loose, thin, elastic sheets that bridge the space between the arches of adjacent vertebrae.[3] Another ligament of interest, recently described, is the meningovertebral ligament, which forms a continuous attachment between the ventral surface of the dura mater and dorsal aspect of the vertebral bodies and intervertebral discs, attaching to the dorsal longitudinal ligament. This ligament creates an anatomic barrier which can cause some pathological lesions in the ventral epidural space to have a bilobed shape on cross-sectional imaging.[4]

The spinal cord and spinal nerve roots lie in the vertebral canal, which is formed by the juxtaposition of all the individual vertebral foramina of the spine. The spinal cord begins at the foramen magnum and terminates caudally at the *conus medullaris*, around L6. The actual termination is caudal to L6 in smaller breeds of dogs and cats, whereas it is cranial to L6 in larger canine breeds.[5] Normal segmental widening of the spinal cord is present at the cervical and lumbar intumescences, and this should not be mistaken for pathologic cord swelling.[3] Spinal cord segments and vertebrae have the same numeric designation, with the exception of spinal cord segment C8, but the location of each spinal cord segment is usually cranial to the corresponding vertebral segment.[3] The ratio between the diameter of the spinal cord and the diameter of the vertebral canal varies between dog breeds, being higher in dachshunds and in other chondrodystrophic breeds in general versus non-chondrodystrophic breeds.[6]

The spinal cord is surrounded by the meninges (see Fig. 15.2). The pia mater is the innermost meningeal layer; it is firmly attached to the spinal cord and highly vascular.[7] The arachnoid membrane is next, and the dura mater is the outermost meningeal layer. The arachnoid and dura are attached closely to each other by a layer of dural border cells.[7] The subarachnoid space lies between the arachnoid and pia mater and contains cerebrospinal fluid (CSF) and arachnoid trabeculae that attach the arachnoid to the pia mater. The epidural space is peripheral to the dura mater and contains fat and the internal vertebral venous plexus.[7] The nerve roots exit through the intervertebral foramina. The collection of spinal nerve roots in the lumbosacral area is known as the *cauda equina.* CSF is found in the spinal subarachnoid space, which begins at the foramen magnum, where it communicates with the intracranial subarachnoid space, and ends caudally at the *filum terminale* near the lumbosacral junction. CSF is also found in the central canal of the spinal cord, which communicates with the fourth ventricle cranially and terminates caudally blindly at the *conus medullaris* or in some subjects is continuous with the lumbar subarachnoid space (see Figs. 15.1 and 15.2).[3]

Computed Tomography

On CT, cortical bone is thin and of uniformly high attenuation with smooth margins. Cancellous bone has a lacy or honeycomb appearance (Fig. 15.3). All components of the vertebra (laminae, pedicles, body, foramina, basivertebral venous canal, bony processes) are well visualized with CT. At the midportion of the body, the basivertebral venous canal is visible as a Y-shaped lucency, and a small dorsally projecting ridge of bone is present within the ventral floor of the vertebral foramen at this site (see Fig. 15.3; see also Fig. 15.10).[8] The articular process joints are diarthrodial joints with a thin, smooth subchondral bone; the articular processes are separated by a hypoattenuating space corresponding to synovial fluid and

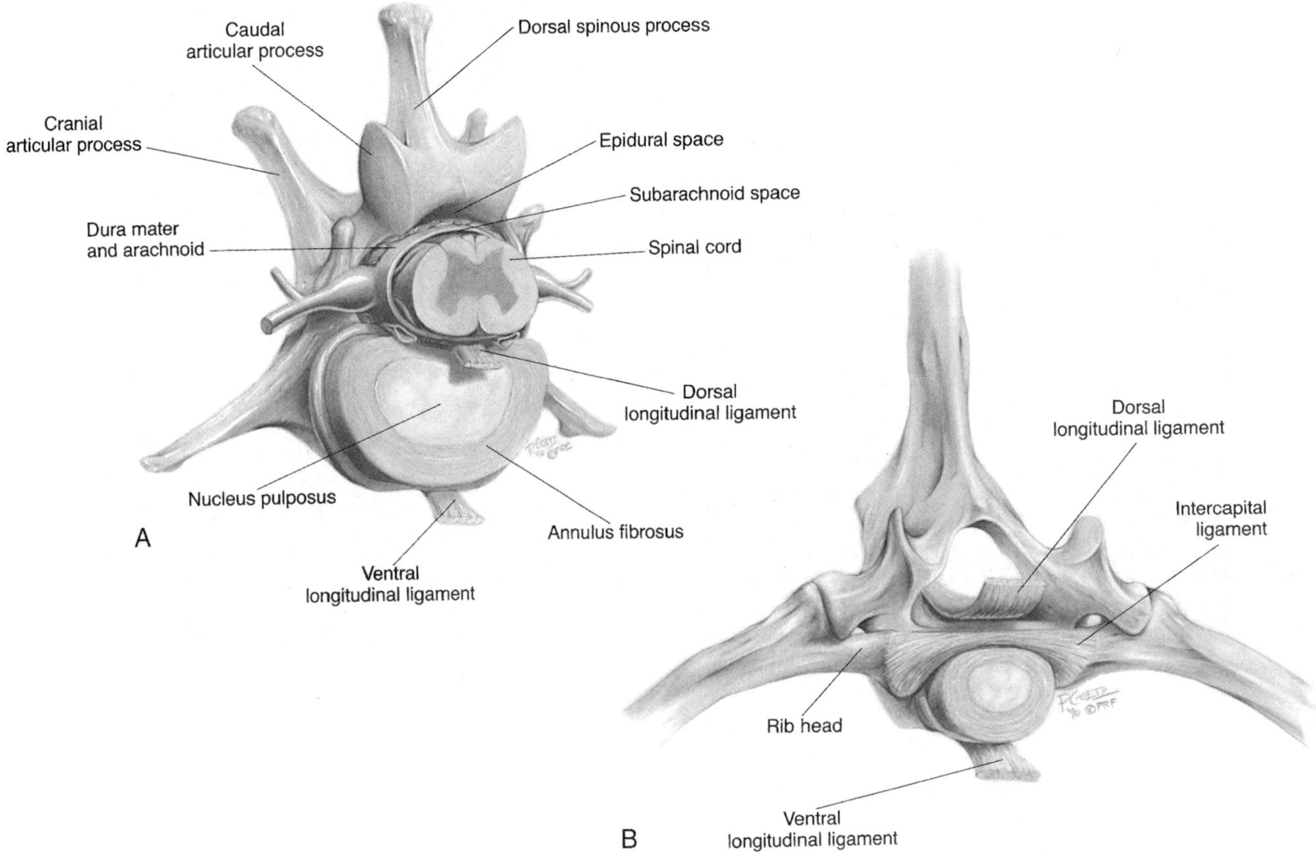

Fig. 15.1 Anatomic components of a typical lumbar vertebra **(A)** and a typical thoracic vertebra and articulation with ribs **(B)**. (Modified from Evans HE, Christensen JC. *Miller's Anatomy of the Dog*. 2nd ed. Philadelphia: Saunders; 1979.)

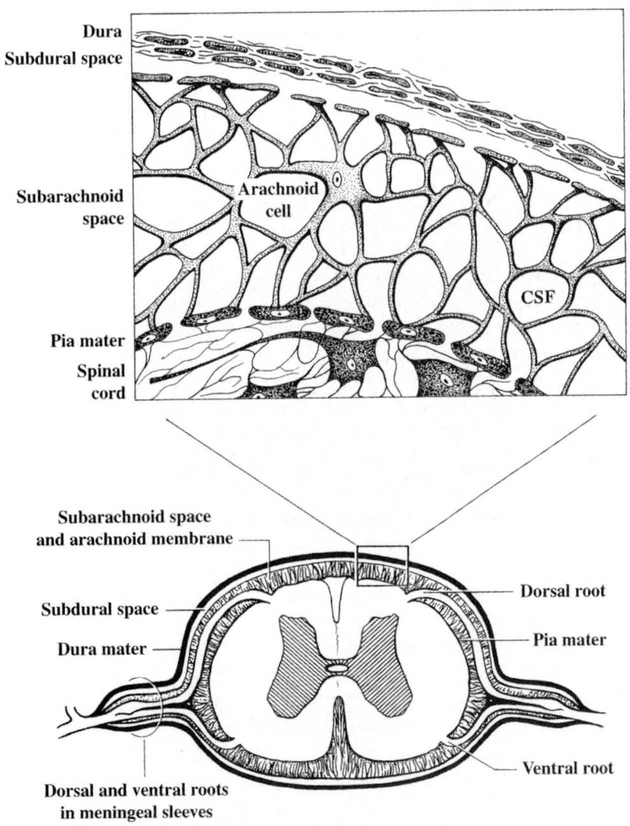

Fig. 15.2 Anatomic relation (transverse plane) of spinal cord, meningeal layers, and subarachnoid space. *Inset* shows microscopic structure of a segment of the meninges and spinal cord. *CSF*, Cerebrospinal fluid. (Modified from Hoerlein BF. *Canine Neurology: Diagnosis and Treatment*. 3rd ed. Philadelphia: Saunders; 1978.)

articular cartilage. On transverse images centered at the disc spaces, the combined margins of the dorsal aspect of the annulus of the intervertebral disc and dorsal longitudinal ligament and ventral aspect of the annulus and ventral longitudinal ligament appear as elliptical soft tissue attenuating structures. Occasionally, the interarcuate ligament *(ligamentum flavum)* is seen as a curvilinear opacity spanning the dorsal laminae and blending with the joint capsule of the articular process joints. The ventral, dorsal, interspinous, and intertransverse ligaments are not resolved from surrounding structures. Epidural fat is hypoattenuating with respect to the soft tissue structures of the vertebral canal. The combination of the spinal cord, blood vessels, subarachnoid space with CSF, and meninges forms a round to oval soft tissue attenuating structure in the middle of the vertebral canal that is surrounded by a rim of hypoattenuating epidural fat (see Fig. 15.3). Nerve roots can be seen as circular or linear soft tissue attenuating structures, depending on their orientation in the scan plane.

When CT is performed after myelography, the thecal sac is hyperattenuating, allowing for more accurate differentiation among intramedullary, intradural, and extradural conditions. CT myelography can be achieved by injecting iodinated contrast medium in the subarachnoid space at 25% of the regular myelographic dose.[9] This allows excellent delineation of the spinal cord and is useful in characterizing compressive lesions or spinal cord atrophy. The normal cross-section of the cervical spinal cord is kidney shaped and slightly larger at C6 to C7. In the thoracic area, there is a dramatic reduction of the spinal cord diameter, and it is also more round.[9]

Magnetic Resonance Imaging

On MRI, cortical bone appears as a black shell around the vertebra on all pulse sequences.[10]

On T1-weighted (T1W) images, epidural fat and paraspinal fat are hyperintense to the spinal cord, whereas the intervertebral discs have medium signal intensity (Fig. 15.4).[10] The

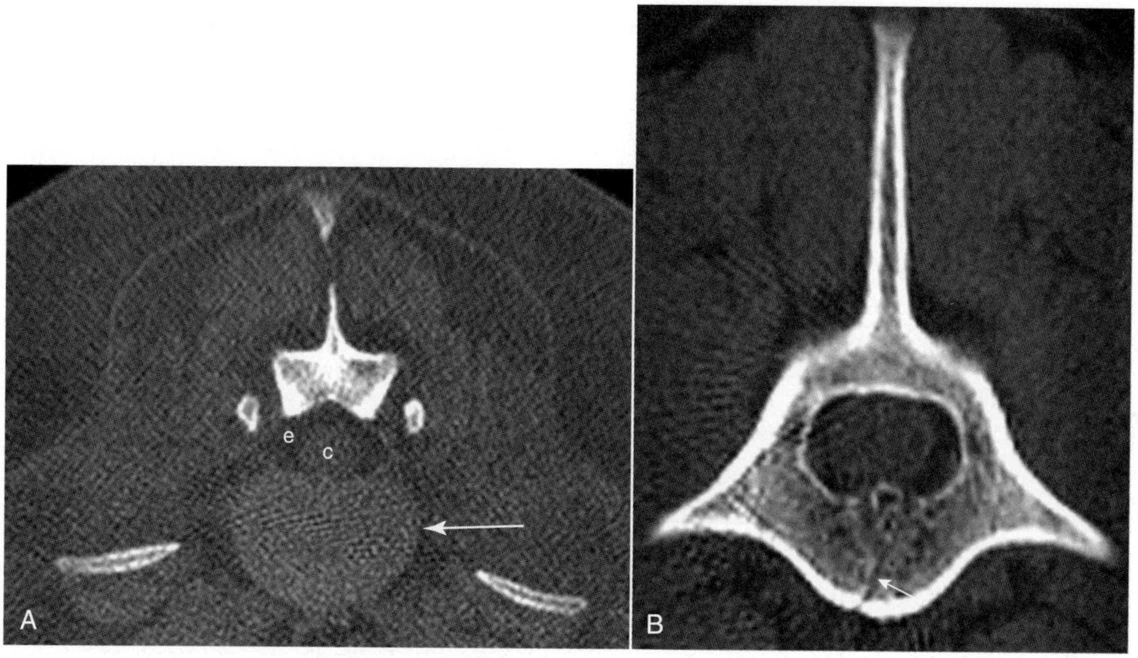

Fig. 15.3 **A,** Transverse computed tomography (CT) image at the level of a lumbar intervertebral disc space: the intervertebral disc is indicated by the *white arrow*. The spinal cord together with the meninges and subarachnoid space form an oval soft tissue attenuating structure in the middle of the vertebral canal (*c*). The epidural fat (*e*) is hypoattenuating and surrounds the spinal cord and meninges. **B,** Transverse CT image in the midportion of the vertebral body. Note the basivertebral venous canal (*white arrow*). The cortical bone forms a homogeneous hyperattenuating boundary around the vertebra, whereas the cancellous bone has a lacy appearance.

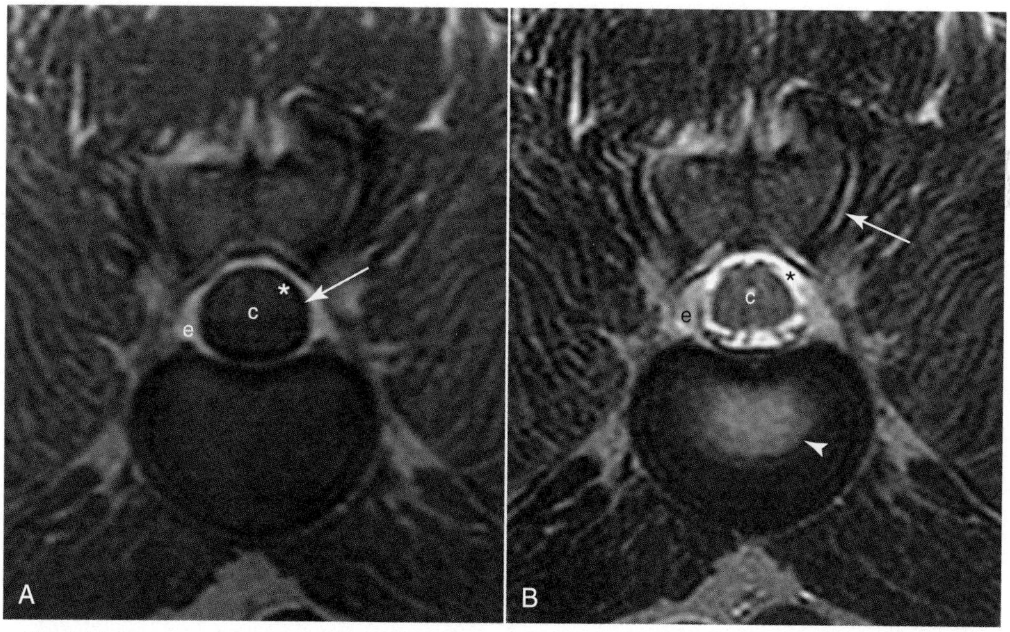

Fig. 15.4 Transverse T1-weighted **(A)** and T2-weighted image **(B)** centered at the L3–L4 intervertebral disc space in a normal dog. The spinal cord (*c*) is in the middle of the vertebral canal. The epidural fat (*e*) is hyperintense on both images. In the T1-weighted image **(A)**, the cerebrospinal fluid (CSF) signal (*asterisk*) is barely distinguished from the spinal cord. A hypointense rim around the spinal cord and CSF represents a combination of the meninges and chemical shift artifact (*white arrow*). In the T2-weighted image **(B)**, the hyperintense CSF forms a bright ring around the spinal cord (*asterisk*). Synovial fluid in the articular process joints forms a thin linear hyperintense signal between the articular processes (*white arrow*). The cortical bone of the articular processes forms a black linear curved structure. The *nucleus pulposus* is the hyperintense signal in the middle of the disc (*white arrowhead*).

hyperintense epidural fat provides contrast for other spinal structures. The spinal cord, nerve roots, and bone marrow are isointense or slightly hypointense to the intervertebral discs. A low-signal shell around the spinal cord represents a combination of CSF in the subarachnoid space, chemical shift artifact, and meningeal structures.[10] The dorsal and ventral longitudinal ligaments, as well as the *ligamentum flavum*, are visible only in the intervertebral areas where they are separated

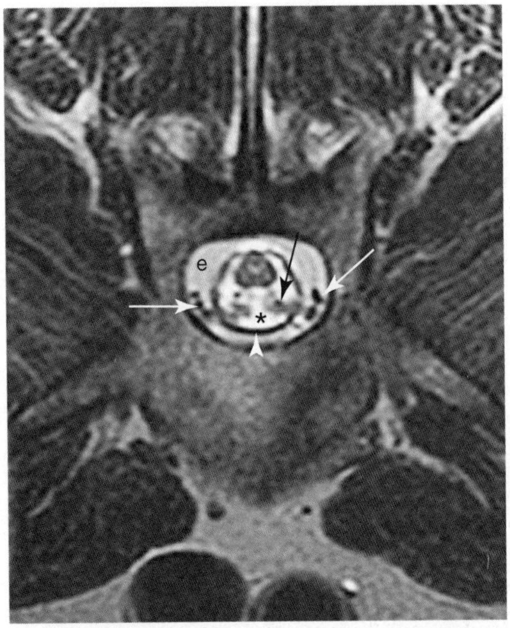

Fig. 15.5 T2-weighted image centered at L5 in a normal dog. The hyperintense cerebrospinal fluid (CSF) within the dural sac is indicated by (*asterisk*). The extremity of the spinal cord and intradural nerve roots are visible (*black arrow*) in the dural sac, which forms a hypointense rim around the CSF (*white arrowhead*). The epidural fat around the dural sac (*e*) is less hyperintense than CSF. Extradural nerve roots are visible as focal hypointensities *(white arrows)* in the epidural space.

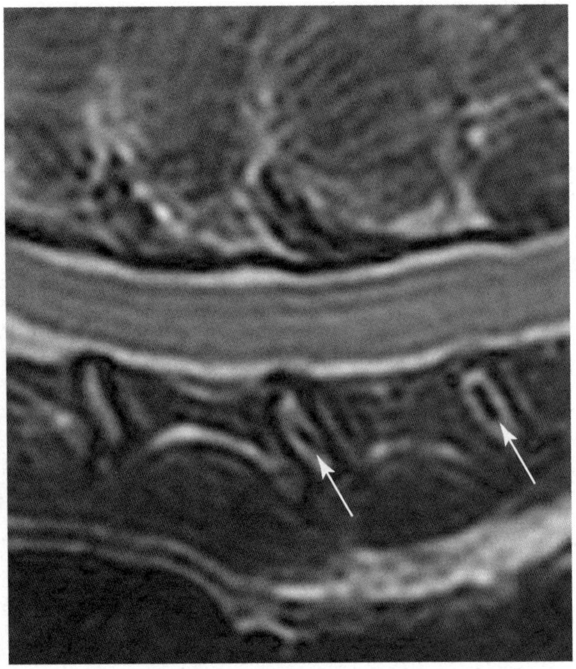

Fig. 15.6 Sagittal T2-weighted image of the caudal aspect of the cervical spine in a dog. Formation of hypointense clefts in the *nucleus pulposus* (*white arrows*) are signs of intervertebral disc degeneration, with reduced water content.

from the bone; they are of low signal intensity.[10] The joint capsule and synovial fluid of the articular process joints are not visible. The internal vertebral venous plexus consists of two symmetric hypointense oval structures, sharply marginated, located ventral to the spinal cord in the midbody regions and diverging slightly from the ventral location at the level of the intervertebral disc spaces.

On T2-weighted (T2W) images, normal intervertebral discs have a high signal because of high water content in the *nucleus pulposus* and inner portion of the *annulus fibrosus* (see Fig. 15.4).[10,11] The epidural fat and paraspinal fat are still hyperintense, and the spinal cord and nerve roots are hypointense (Fig. 15.5). The bone marrow is hypointense compared with fat and is isointense or hypointense to the spinal cord. Depending on the amount of T2 weighting, the CSF in the subarachnoid space forms a thin hyperintense shell around the cord.[10] Sequences with a very heavy T2 weighting, such as single-shot fast spin echo (SSFSE) or half-Fourier acquisition single-shot turbo spin-echo (HASTE), enhance the signal from CSF while suppressing the signal from background tissue, giving a natural myelographic effect.[12,13]

INTERVERTEBRAL DISC DISEASE

The Normal Intervertebral Disc

Intervertebral discs are made of a peripheral *annulus fibrosus* and a central *nucleus pulposus*.[11] The disc lies in close contact with the cartilaginous vertebral endplates with fibers from the *nucleus pulposus* and *annulus fibrosus* being interwoven with the collagen fibers of the cartilaginous endplates and bony trabeculae.[10]

Both the annulus and the nucleus are made of fibrocartilage but differ in the amount of collagen and ground substance.[14] There is more collagen and less ground substance in the annulus than in the nucleus. The ground substance is composed of hyaluronic acid and glycosaminoglycans that hold water because of their strong negative charge.[14] A normal *nucleus pulposus* has a gelatinous consistency. Water, bound to large proteoglycan molecules, is the principal component of the *nucleus pulposus* (80%–88%).[15] The normally very bright signal of the *nucleus pulposus* on T2W images is caused by the long T2 relaxation time of water (see Fig. 15.4).[11]

Classification of Intervertebral Disc Disease

Apart from trauma causing extrusion of nondegenerated (hydrated) disc material (see section on Compressive and Noncompressive Hydrated Nucleus Pulposus Extrusion), degeneration of the intervertebral disc occurs before clinically significant intervertebral disc disease (IVDD).[11] Degenerative IVDD was first classified by Hansen.[16] Hansen type I IVDD is herniation of the *nucleus pulposus* through annular fibers with subsequent extrusion of nuclear material into the vertebral canal. Type I IVDD is more common in chondrodystrophic dogs. The degenerative process leading to type I herniation involves shifting concentrations of glycosaminoglycan, loss of water and proteoglycan content, and increased collagen content. The disc becomes more cartilaginous, and its nucleus becomes more granular, often mineralizes, and loses its hydroelastic shock-absorbing qualities (Fig. 15.6). The degenerative process starts early in life, and herniation is observed in younger animals (2–7 years old, with a peak incidence at 4–5 years old).

Hansen type II IVDD is an annular protrusion caused by shifting of the central nuclear material and is commonly associated with fibroid degeneration. Type II herniation is usually observed in nonchondrodystrophic dogs, and the degenerative process starts later in life, with herniation usually observed at approximately 8 to 10 years old.

With more detailed imaging of the patterns of disc herniation that can be appreciated with MRI, IVDD can be divided into several categories based on appearance more than physiopathology.[17–19] Classification systems have evolved over the years as we learned more about the variable imaging features of disc disease.[20] Fig. 15.7 describes a proposed classification of IVDD. General features include:

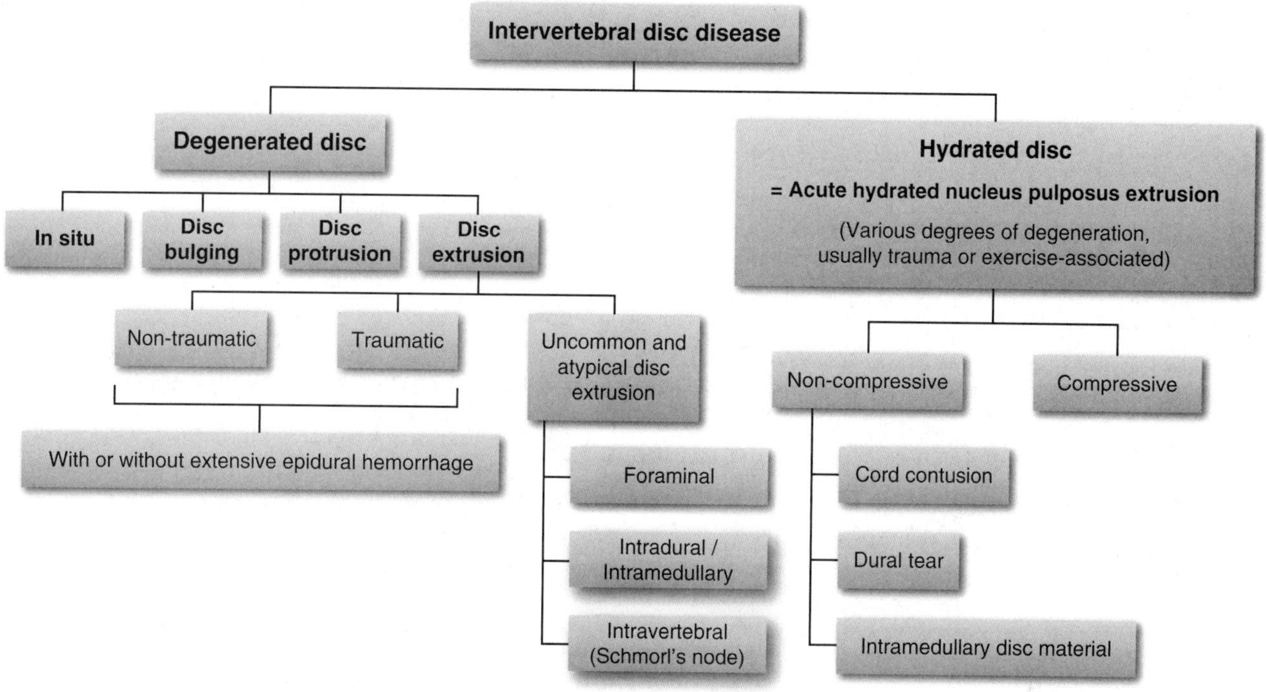

Fig. 15.7 Diagram of a proposed classification for intervertebral disc disease (IVDD) in dogs and cats.

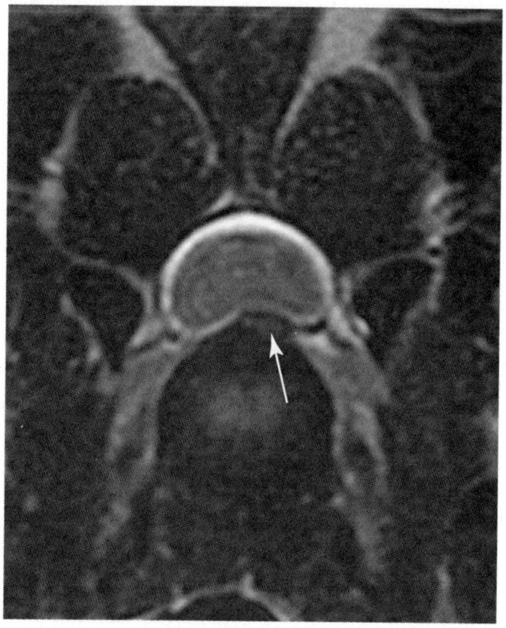

Fig. 15.8 Transverse T2-weighted image of a cervical intervertebral disc space in a dog. There is a Hansen type II disc herniation with protruding hypointense disc material (*white arrow*) causing mild left ventral spinal cord compression.

- A bulging disc corresponds to circumferential extension of the disc beyond the margins of the vertebral endplates.
- A protruding disc is the partial extension of the nucleus and inner annulus through disrupted fibers of the outer annulus but without complete rupture of the outer annulus (Hansen type II). The presence of partial rather than complete intervertebral disc degeneration, midline herniation, and/or multiple herniations makes protrusion more likely than extrusion (Fig. 15.8, eFig. 15.1).[18,19]
- An extruded disc represents true herniation (Hansen type I), where portions of the nucleus and inner annulus traverse through all the layers of the outer annulus and form a focal extradural mass deviating epidural fat and, depending on the size of the herniation, the subarachnoid space and spinal cord (Fig. 15.9, eFig. 15.2). This herniated disc material can detach completely from the disc where it originates and form a free extradural mass, with various degrees of dispersion.[17] The presence of a single intervertebral disc herniation, complete disc degeneration, lateralized herniation, and/or dispersion of the intervertebral disc material makes disc extrusion more likely than protrusion.[18,19] In some animals, the extruded material can lacerate the internal vertebral venous plexus resulting in disc-associated extensive epidural hemorrhage.[21,22]
- Hydrated traumatic disc herniation: If a disc with a normally hydrated *nucleus pulposus* is placed under extreme stress, the dorsal *annulus fibrosus* may rupture, and some of the normal jelly-like *nucleus pulposus* may explode into the vertebral canal and cause spinal cord contusion or dural tears.[23] Because the nucleus material is normally hydrated (although possibly with some degree of degeneration), it diffuses in the peridural fat, leaving only the secondary changes attributable to acute spinal cord contusion with little or no spinal cord compression.[15] In some patients, the herniated disc material can penetrate the spinal cord parenchyma.[24–26] Several terms have been used to describe this syndrome, including *traumatic disc prolapse, traumatic disc herniation, disc explosion, noncompressive nucleus pulposus extrusion, Hansen type III disc disease, high-velocity-low-volume disc disease, traumatic intervertebral disc extrusion, missile disc,* and *acute noncompressive nucleus pulposus extrusion.*[15,27] The term *Hansen type III disc disease* is discouraged because this type of herniation was never described by Hansen. Such herniations are associated most commonly with trauma (such as a road traffic accident or running into an obstacle) but can also be associated with vigorous exercise.[28] In some patients, the herniated hydrated disc

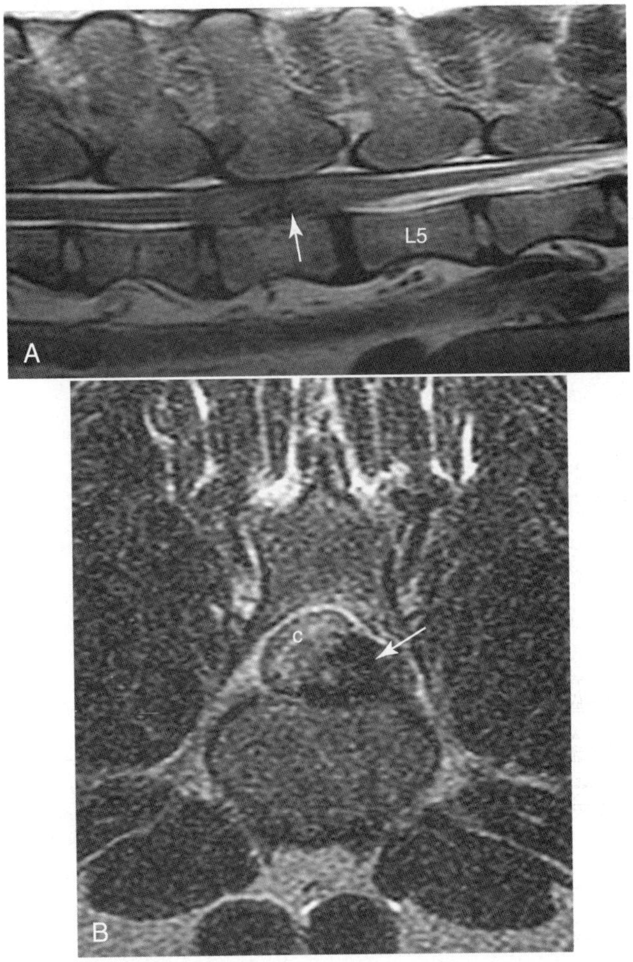

Fig. 15.9 Sagittal **(A)** and transverse **(B)** T2-weighted images in a dog with Hansen type I disc herniation at L4 to L5. The longitudinal extent of the hypointense extruded disc material *(white arrow)* is apparent on the sagittal image. The L4 to L5 disc is markedly hypointense, consistent with degeneration. On the transverse image **(B)**, the hypointense extruded disc material (*white arrow*) causes marked left ventral compression of the spinal cord (*c*).

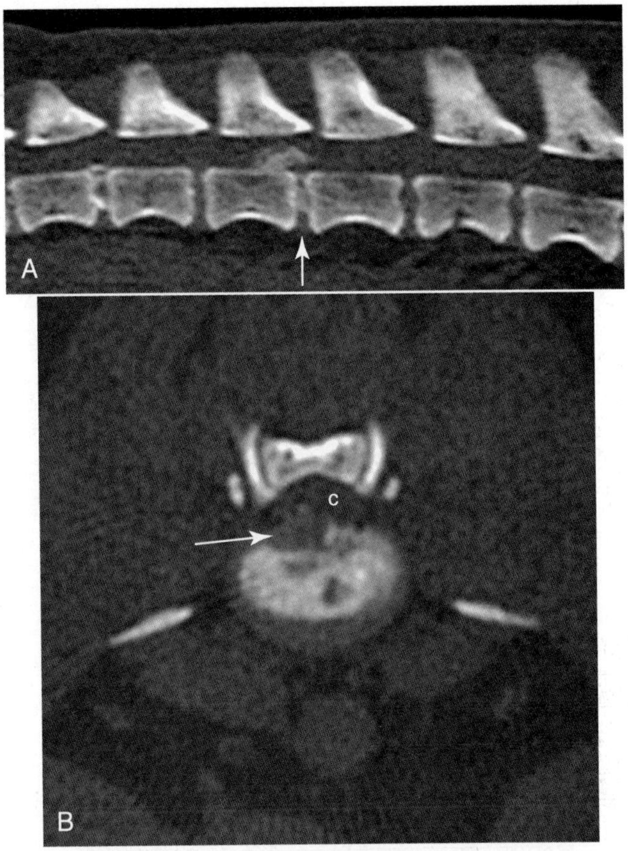

Fig. 15.10 Computed tomography (CT) without intrathecal contrast medium in a dachshund with acute intervertebral disc herniation. **A,** Sagittal reformatted image. Note the hyperattenuating disc material dorsal to the affected narrowed disc space (*white arrow*). Extruded disc material extends cranial to the affected disc space. Mineralized disc material is seen in this space and at two intervertebral disc spaces cranial to this. **B,** Transverse image centered on the affected disc space. There is hyperattenuating material (*white arrow*) in the vertebral canal that causes ventral right-sided spinal cord (*c*) compression.

material may cause focal extradural compression of the spinal cord,[29–31] a condition that may have previously been erroneously referred to as *discal cyst.*[32–34]

Computed Tomography of Intervertebral Disc Disease

CT of the spine for assessing the intervertebral disc should be obtained using thin slices (1–2 mm), low pitch (<2), and a medium-frequency image-reconstruction algorithm.[35] When CT is used in the assessment of the spinal cord, subarachnoid injection of iodinated contrast medium is often performed concurrently, because the spinal cord is often not clearly visible on CT images. Obviously, the use of CT with subarachnoid contrast medium invalidates the potential advantage of diagnosing disc herniation without the side effects associated with myelography, although the dose of contrast medium for CT myelography is less than that for myelography.

CT without intrathecal injection of iodinated contrast medium for detection of IVDD has been evaluated in chondrodystrophic dogs, which are likely to have some degree of mineralization of the herniated material.[36] On CT, vertebrae can be identified as thoracic or lumbar without difficulty based on the presence of ribs or transverse processes. The location of any particular image, therefore, can be identified by counting sequential vertebrae or by using scout images depicting slice location. Acquiring lateral and ventrodorsal scout images reduces the risk of missing a vertebral malformation that could affect accurate localization of individual disc spaces at surgery. This is important, because 10% of dachshunds have transitional anomalies that lead to deranged vertebral anatomy.[37] If the scout images are not of sufficient quality to identify vertebral abnormalities, it may be useful to obtain a routine survey radiograph before performing the CT scan. In chondrodystrophic breeds, CT is excellent at identifying herniated disc material and provides accurate information as far as location, laterality, and extent of spinal cord compression (Fig. 15.10). In chondrodystrophic dogs, acute herniation leads to either a large focal amount of markedly hyperattenuating material (~200 Hounsfield units [HU]) compressing the spinal cord or to more diffuse and less hyperattenuating material (~60 HU) causing less severe spinal cord compression. In the latter instance, the material in the vertebral canal corresponds to areas of epidural hemorrhage. In chronic disc herniation, the attenuation of the herniated material is higher than that of acutely herniated disc material (~700 HU) because the herniated material continues to mineralize after acute herniation.[36] Some pitfalls exist when interpreting CT images. For example, a round focus of mineralization is seen occasionally on transverse images dorsal to the vertebral bodies. This focus has been thought to represent mineralization of the dorsal longitudinal ligament,[36] which fans out to a thin sheet over the intervertebral disc space but narrows to a circular midline structure over the vertebral body. However, this focal hyperattenuation is more likely a transverse image of the small bony ridge between the dorsal vertebral foramina (Fig. 15.11). This hyperattenuation can be mistaken for disc material.

Although conventional CT is adequate for the diagnosis and localization of mineralized disc extrusions in chondrodystrophic breeds, CT myelography is often necessary for diagnosis if no lesion is identified in a chondrodystrophic dog, if paraplegia is present because of concurrent extradural compression and spinal cord swelling, or if the dog is nonchondrodystrophic.[38]

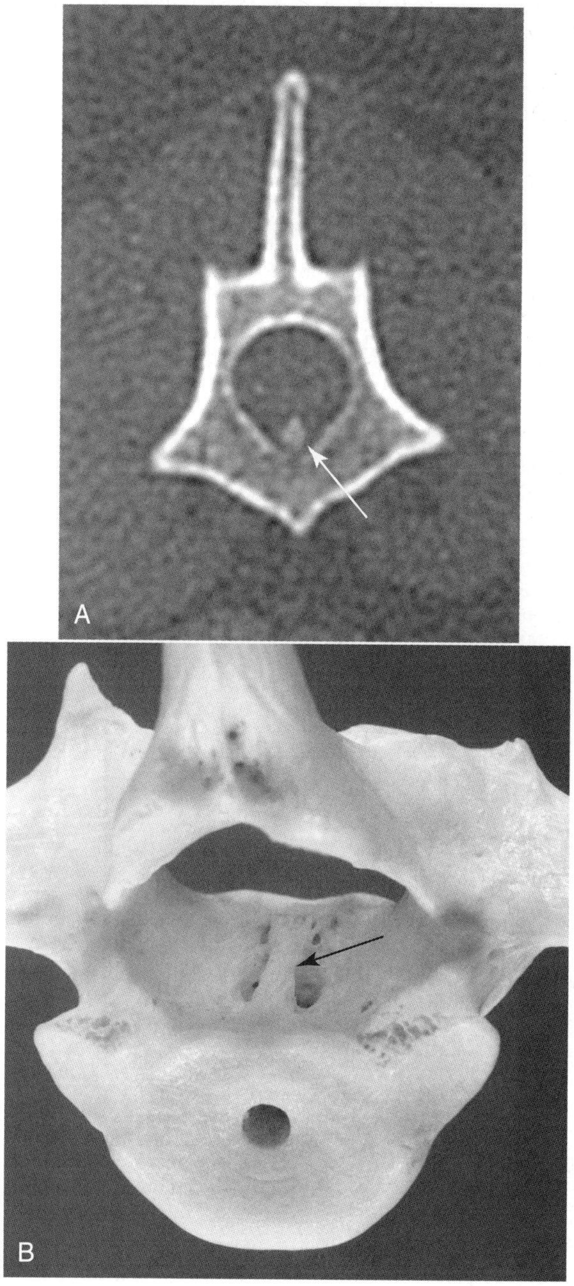

Fig. 15.11 Transverse computed tomography (CT) image **(A)** and photograph **(B)** of a canine vertebra. There is a focal hyperattenuation dorsal to the vertebral body (*white arrow* in **A**) that is created by the bony bridge covering a portion of the dorsal foramina (*black arrow* in **B**). This hyperattenuation is confused with mineralization of the dorsal longitudinal ligament and herniated disc material but is a normal finding. The hole in the end-plate in **B** is a drill hole; this drilling did not disturb the normal appearance of the dorsal foramina.

Magnetic Resonance Imaging of Intervertebral Disc Disease

Although there may be no improvement in patient outcome when using MRI for the diagnosis of IVDD,[39] it is the method of choice for presurgical diagnosis, because it is noninvasive and provides superior anatomic detail, as well as potential prognostic indicators (e.g., myelomalacia). MRI is also more accurate than conventional CT in differentiating disc extrusion from protrusion and also has overall higher sensitivity.[40] Differences in surgical planning based on MRI versus CT were reported in chondrodystrophic dogs with thoracolumbar disc extrusion, with variations in site (but not side) of approach and size of laminectomy. Surgeries planned based on MRI images may result in larger laminectomy windows than when planned with CT, although the clinical implication of this is unknown at this time.[41]

Diagnosis of IVDD is made from magnetic resonance (MR) images when the following signs are seen:

- Extradural compression of the spinal cord centered at the level of an intervertebral disc (Fig. 15.12; see also Fig. 15.9): This is recognized by a loss of signal from the epidural fat and a change in the shape of the spinal cord, as well as a change in the normal ovoid shape of the disc, and is best appreciated on transverse images (see Fig. 15.8).
- Degeneration of the disc (loss of T2-hyperintense signal from the disc).
- Narrowing of the intervertebral disc space: This is usually best evaluated on sagittal T1W images.[42]

MRI is accurate in determining the location and craniocaudal length of extruded intervertebral disc material. T2W images are more reliable in determining the extent of the compressive material.[43] Heavily T2W sequences, such as SSFSE, provide a myelographic effect by enhancing the signal of the CSF and

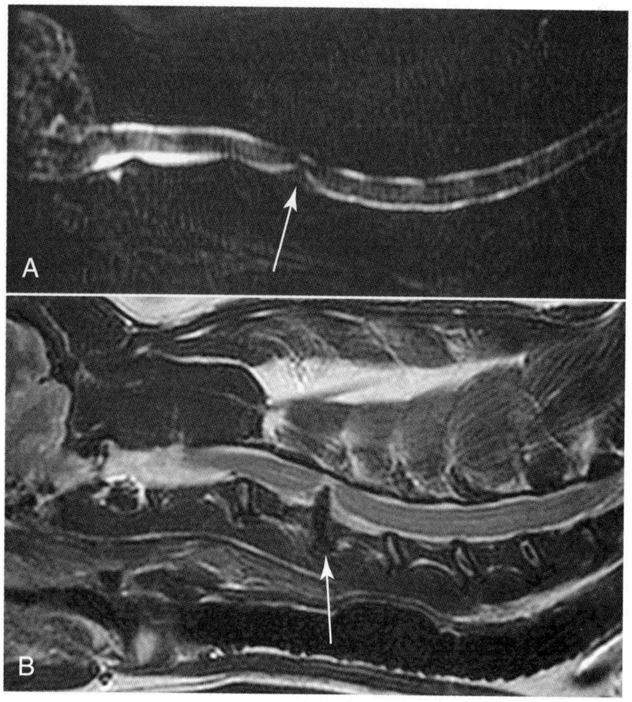

Fig. 15.12 Sagittal single-shot fast spin echo (SSFSE) slab (T2 myelogram) **(A)** and sagittal T2-weighted image **(B)** in a dog with disc herniation at C3–C4. The area of spinal cord compression is obvious on the T2 myelogram (*white arrow*). On the sagittal T2-weighted image, hypointense material is seen extruded from the disc at C3–C4, causing marked ventral spinal cord compression. The disc has lost its normal hyperintense signal (*white arrow*).

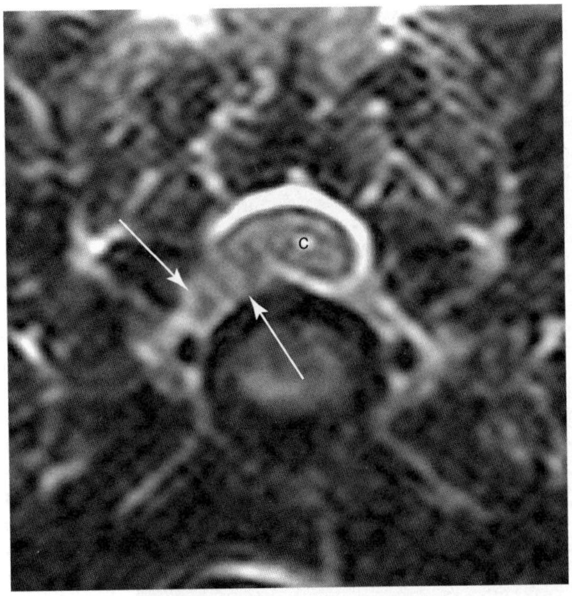

Fig. 15.16 Transverse T2-weighted image of a dog with a foraminal disc herniation at C5–C6. There is disc material in the right ventral aspect of the vertebral canal and in the right foramen (*white arrows*). The disc material is also compressing the spinal cord (*c*).

compression with root signature and cervical pain (Fig. 15.16, eFig. 15.3). Also, some studies found that the cervical spinal cord occupies a smaller proportion of the vertebral canal so that the degree of compression caused by an equal volume of herniated disc material is less than in the thoracolumbar area.[53] A recent study in French bulldogs, however, found an inverse relationship, with a smaller epidural space in the cervical compared to the thoracolumbar region.[56] In the cervical area, there may be a correlation between the degree of spinal cord compression caused by disc herniation and the neurologic grade at time of imaging; however, there is no correlation with outcome after surgery.[53]

Thoracolumbar Intervertebral Disc Disease

The most commonly affected discs in the thoracolumbar region are T12–T13 and T13–L1.[57] Cranial thoracic disc herniation causing spinal cord compression has been reported to be more common in German shepherd dogs compared to other large-breed dogs, especially at T2–T3, T3–T4, and T4–T5.[58–60] Therefore, it is important to include the cranial thoracic spine (including T2–T3) when imaging dogs of this breed with T3–L3 myelopathy.

In dogs with neurologic deficits caused by thoracolumbar disc extrusion (Hansen type I), there is no definitive association between the degree of spinal cord compression as defined on T2W transverse images and the neurologic grade at presentation or outcome after surgery.[57,61] However, the length over which the spinal cord is compressed is associated with the neurologic grade at presentation but not with outcome.[62] In dogs with paraplegia because of acute thoracolumbar disc extrusion, areas of spinal cord hyperintensity on T2W series are often present (Fig. 15.17). The development of intramedullary T2 hyperintensity following disc herniation is associated with more severe neurologic deficits at presentation.[44,47,62] Areas of intramedullary T2 hyperintensity that exceed the length of L2 on sagittal images have been associated with a poor outcome in approximately 50% of patients.[63] This feature has been reported to be a better predictor of poor outcome than loss of deep pain perception,[63,64] and it is independent from the severity of neurologic signs at presentation.[62] However, more recent studies at higher field strength (3 Tesla) did not find an association between length of T2W hyperintensity and recovery of motor function.[65]

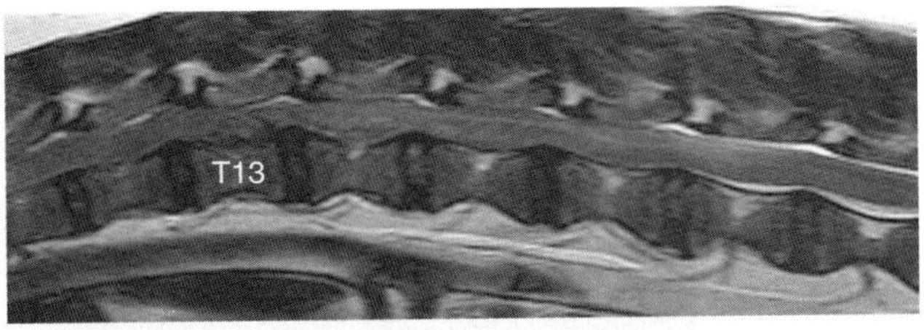

Fig. 15.17 Sagittal T2-weighted image of a dog with disc herniation at T12–T13. There is a heterogeneous mass dorsal to T13 that represents migrated disc material and hemorrhage. Caudal to this lesion, there is diffuse intramedullary T2 hyperintensity consistent with edema and inflammation.

Sacrocaudal Disc Herniation

There has been an anecdotal report of sacrocaudal disc extrusion causing tail pain and problems with defecation, with resolution of these clinical signs after surgical correction. MRI and CT can be useful in confirming the presence of extruded disc material in the sacrocaudal canal.[66,67]

Lumbosacral Stenosis

Degenerative lumbosacral stenosis is an abnormal narrowing of the L5–S3 vertebral canal or intervertebral foramina, with compression of the cauda equina and/or its blood supply.[68] Degenerative lumbosacral stenosis is characterized by intervertebral disc degeneration, intervertebral disc protrusion, bone proliferation on the vertebral endplates and articular processes, vertebral subluxation, and hypertrophy of the articular process joint capsule and interarcuate ligament *(ligamentum flavum)*.[68] Acute lumbosacral disc extrusion is much less common but carries an excellent postsurgical prognosis.[69] CT and MRI are both excellent for characterizing degenerative lumbosacral stenosis in dogs.[8,10,68,70–75] In dogs with clinical signs of cauda equina syndrome, CT changes include loss of epidural fat, increased soft tissue opacity in the intervertebral foramen, bulging of the intervertebral disc, spondylosis, thecal sac displacement, narrowed intervertebral foramen, narrowed vertebral canal, thickened articular processes, articular process subluxation, and articular process osteophytosis. On sagittal images, a step between the floor of the vertebral foramen of L7 and the floor of the vertebral foramen of S1 is often seen (Figs. 15.18 and 15.19, eFig. 15.4).[75] Enhancement of the soft tissue compressive material is often observed after injection of contrast medium, and this feature should not be interpreted as evidence of a tumor.[68] Compression should be suspected in sites where there is increased perineural soft tissue material with absence of epidural fat.[70,74] Interpretation of CT changes in the lumbosacral area must be made with caution, because some changes can be present in dogs free of clinical signs and, therefore, insignificant clinically. In particular, idiopathic lumbosacral stenosis and loss of perineural fat have been reported in dogs with no clinical signs.[71] In addition, only slight to fair agreement was found when comparing the results of CT or MRI of the lumbosacral spine to surgery.[75]

For both CT and MRI, there does not appear to be an association between imaging findings and clinical outcome after surgery in working dogs with clinical signs of degenerative lumbosacral stenosis.[68] Late postsurgical CT and MRI changes are common in dogs that underwent dorsal laminectomy for treatment of lumbosacral stenosis, importantly even in dogs with improved clinical status: such changes include ongoing nerve compression, enhancement of the L7 nerves, lumbosacral intervertebral joints, and paraspinal soft tissues.[76]

Foraminal and Far Lateral Disc Extrusion

With the increasing availability of MRI, clinical foraminal disc extrusion has been recognized more often.[77–79] In the cervical spine, the most common affected sites are C6–C7 and C5–C6.[77] There are also reports of foraminal or extraforaminal

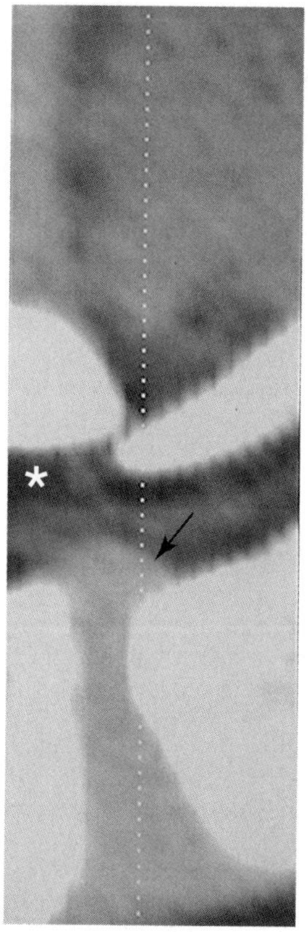

Fig. 15.18 Sagittal reformatted computed tomography (CT) image of the L7 to S1 junction in a dog with clinical signs of lumbosacral disease. There is bulging of the intervertebral disc (*black arrow*) causing mild nerve root compression. Peridural fat is still present in the area indicated by the hypoattenuating material (*asterisk*) around the nerves. There is a slight step between the floor of the vertebral canal of L7 and that of S1, indicating lumbosacral subluxation and/or instability.

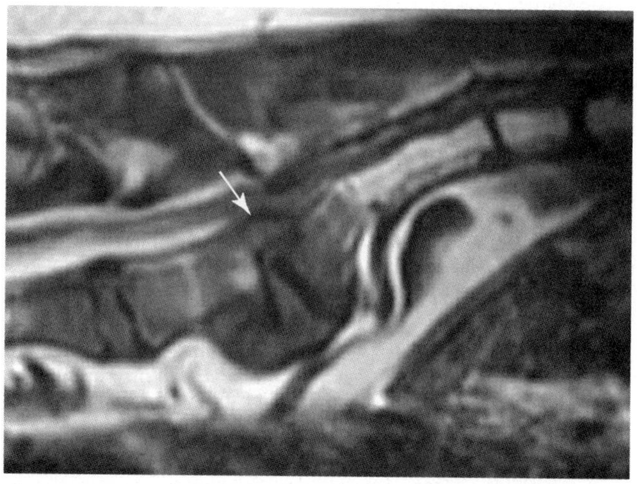

Fig. 15.19 Sagittal T1-weighted image of the caudal lumbar area in a German shepherd with clinical signs of lumbosacral disease. There is a step between the floor of the vertebral canal of L7 and that of S1 indicating lumbosacral subluxation and/or instability. Bulging disc material (*white arrow*) is present dorsal to the lumbosacral disc space causing attenuation of the hyperintense epidural fat. The combined effects of the subluxation and bulging disc are causing stenosis of the vertebral canal with nerve root compression. Ventral spondylosis is present at L7 to S1.

("far lateral") disc herniation in the thoracolumbar or lumbosacral segments, with the most common affected sites being L5–L6 and L6–L7.[78–80] MRI is a more appropriate tool for this diagnosis, due to its excellent soft tissue contrast. Careful examination of transverse images across the disc space and intervertebral foramina is important for correct identification of this condition. Gradient echo images can be useful, because they allow better contrast between the venous sinus and intervertebral disc. On sagittal images, the affected disc has often decreased signal intensity on T2W images. In the cervical spine, differentiation between foraminal stenosis due to foraminal disc extrusion and overgrowth of the articular process can prove challenging.[77] Transverse images show T2-hypointense material associated with the affected disc extruded in a dorsolateral direction and causing impingement of the nerve roots in the foramen or lateral to it. Contrast enhancement of the nerve roots as well as around the compressive lesion is reported.[79,80] Occasionally, foraminal disc extrusion can cause ganglioneuritis,[81] when disc fragments extruded in the foramen induce mechanical and chemical damage to the perineurium of the nerve sheath, and/or penetrate into the nerve root leading to inflammatory changes. These changes can cause thickening of the nerve root and ganglion, with the disc material possibly contributing to the impression of a soft tissue mass in the area. At MRI, these changes appear as a tubular space-occupying lesion in the intervertebral foramen, which is T1-isointense, T2-hyperintense compared to the contralateral nerve, with strong contrast enhancement.[81] Such lesions can easily be mistaken for a peripheral nerve sheath tumor.

Noncompressive Hydrated Nucleus Pulposus Extrusion

Occasionally, disc extrusion occurs without significant preexisting degenerative disc disease when a relatively healthy disc is subjected to a brief excessive force. Such extrusions occur typically during performance of strenuous exercise or following trauma. Names applied to this syndrome were outlined previously in the Classification of Intervertebral Disc Disease section.[15,23,26–28,82–85] Typically, the condition is characterized by an acute, often asymmetric myelopathy that is nonprogressive after the first 24 hours.[27,86] In the majority of cases, this type of herniation is noncompressive, and spinal cord lesions result from contusion rather than compression, with a clinical presentation very similar to primary ischemic myelopathy.[27,86,87]

On MRI, acute noncompressive intervertebral disc extrusion is characterized by the following[15,27,86,88]:

- Focal intramedullary T2 hyperintensity overlying an intervertebral disc: The area of maximal hyperintensity is usually just dorsal to the affected intervertebral disc but can sometimes be seen just cranial or caudal to the disc space. The longitudinal extension of the intramedullary hyperintensity is usually more focal than with ischemic myelopathy, which has a similar clinical presentation (Fig. 15.20).[15,27,86]
- This intramedullary lesion is usually isointense on T1W images and does not enhance after gadolinium injection, although occasional focal precontrast T1W hyper- or hypointensity and mild postcontrast enhancement may be present.[15,27,86]
- There is reduction in volume and signal intensity of the *nucleus pulposus* of the corresponding disc on T2W images (see Fig. 15.20).
- A narrowed intervertebral disc space is seen on sagittal images.
- There is extraneous material or heterogeneous signal changes within the epidural space dorsal to the affected disc space with absence of or minimal spinal cord compression.
- A communicating T2-hyperintense and/or T1-hypointense tract can occasionally be seen traversing the dorsal annulus between the residual *nucleus pulposus* and the vertebral canal.[15]

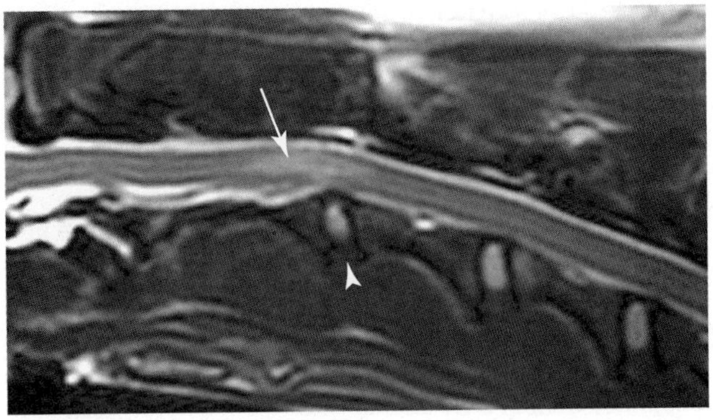

Fig. 15.20 Sagittal T2-weighted image of a dog that ran into a tree and sustained acute noncompressive intervertebral disc extrusion. There is mild loss of volume of the *nucleus pulposus* at C2–C3 (*white arrowhead*) and ill-defined intramedullary T2 hyperintensity (*white arrow*) overlying this space consistent with edema caused by spinal cord contusion. There is no spinal cord compression.

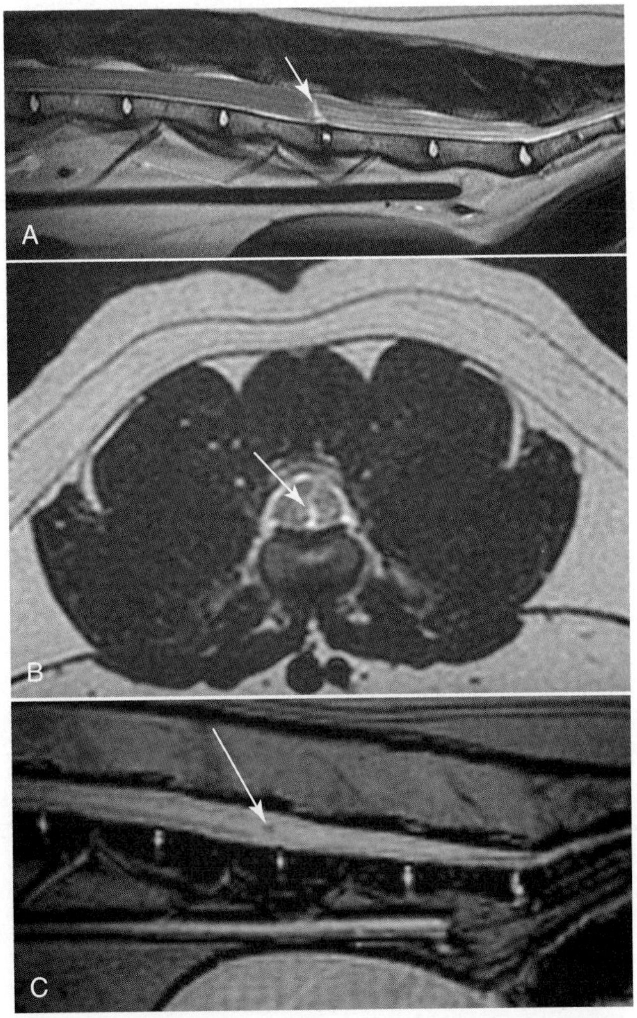

Fig. 15.21 Acute noncompressive intervertebral disc extrusion at L5–L6 in a cat. **A,** T2-weighted sagittal image. **B,** Transverse T2-weighted image centered at L5–L6. **C,** Sagittal gradient recalled echo image matching the location in **A**. A hyperintense intramedullary linear tract extends from the disc space in **A** and **B** (*white arrows*) consistent with intramedullary extrusion of disc material after perforation of the dura mater. Note the loss of volume of the *nucleus pulposus* at L5–L6. A hypointense intramedullary lesion consistent with hemorrhage (*white arrow*) is present in the gradient recalled echo image.

The acutely extruded disc material most commonly damages the spinal cord through contusion without penetrating the dura, but occasionally it can cause a dural tear and penetrate the spinal cord.[23,26,82,84,85] In these instances, a vertical intramedullary linear T2-hyperintense lesion crosses the spinal cord and is contiguous ventrally with the intervertebral disc space (Fig. 15.21, eFig. 15.5). Areas of hypointensity can be seen associated with that tract in gradient recalled echo images because of hemorrhage.[26,85]

Up to 33% of affected patients with acute noncompressive hydrated *nucleus pulposus* extrusion have an unsuccessful outcome.[27] Prognostic factors of unsuccessful outcome include severity of neurologic signs at presentation, percentage of cross-sectional area of the intramedullary lesion on transverse T2W images, and presence of intramedullary hemorrhage. An intramedullary cross-sectional area of the T2-hyperintense lesion exceeding 90% of the spinal cord area is associated with a 92% chance of an unsuccessful outcome.[27]

On CT myelography, acute traumatic or exercise-induced disc extrusion can be associated with narrowing of the affected disc space, seen on sagittal or dorsal reformatted images, with evidence of a small amount of minimally compressive extradural material at the level of the disc with spinal cord swelling adjacent to these areas. When the extruded disc material causes rupture of the dura, small leaks of iodinated contrast medium can be seen extending from the subarachnoid space into the epidural space.[89] Leakage of contrast medium into the intervertebral disc in patients with disc-associated dural rupture can be seen with application of spinal traction during conventional myelography.[84] On CT performed after myelography, presence of intramedullary contrast medium can also be seen in patients with intramedullary extrusion.[24]

Compressive Hydrated Nucleus Pulposus Extrusion

In some cases, the extruded hydrated disc material accumulates focally in the epidural space and causes spinal cord compression.[29–31] In this case, the neurological deficits are more severe, and the pain less severe than with other compressive myelopathies.[30]

The MRI features of the compressive form of the disease include the following (Fig. 15.22)[29–31,33,34,90]:

- Space-occupying T2-hyperintense material ventral to the spinal cord, on midline and centered immediately dorsal to a slightly narrowed intervertebral disc space (most commonly C4–C5, C3–C4, C5–C6), causing ventral compression and dorsal displacement of the spinal cord centered at the intervertebral disc space.
- On sagittal T2W images, this extruded material has an elongated shape and is difficult to distinguish from the hyperintense epidural fat and CSF, because it has similar signal intensity. On transverse T2W images centered on the affected disc space, the extruded material lies symmetrically on the midline, ventral to the spinal cord, and often has a characteristic "seagull" shape. That shape is presumed to be due to the presence of the meningovertebral ligament, which creates a midline longitudinal anatomic barrier that confers the gelatinous extruded material that bilobed shape.[4]
- On T2-fluid-attenuated inversion recovery (FLAIR) images, the extruded material typically retains a hyperintense signal,[33,34] but sometimes it is suppressed.[34,90]
- Focal intramedullary T2W hyperintensity dorsal to the affected disc, which is T1W isointense and nonenhancing after gadolinium injection.
- This focal intramedullary T2W hyperintensity is usually iso- to hyperintense on T2*W images, consistent with spinal cord contusion.
- There is inconstant mild diffuse[29] or peripheral[33,34] contrast enhancement of the extruded material.

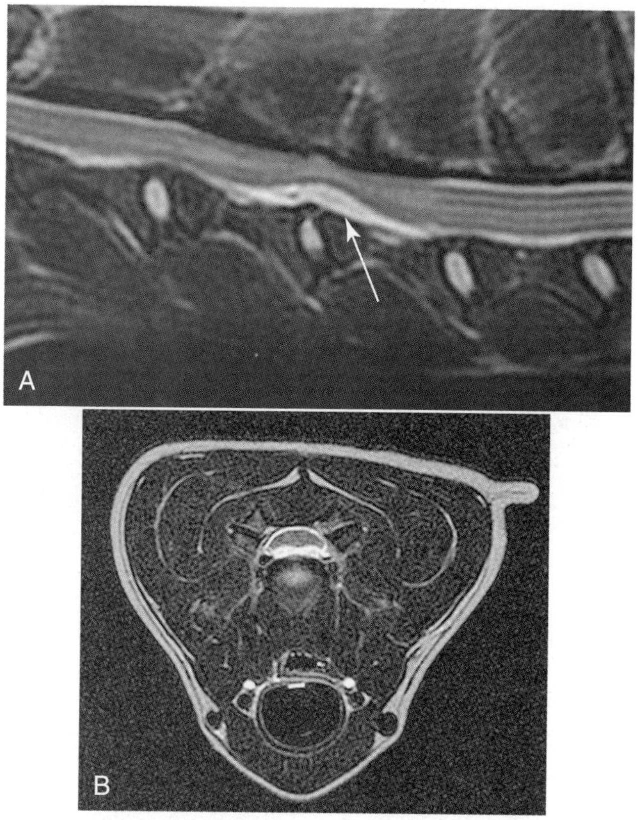

Fig. 15.22 **A,** Sagittal T2-weighted image in a dog with an acute compressive hydrated *nucleus pulposus* extrusion at C4–C5. Note the mild degenerative changes in the disc at C4–C5 with reduced size and signal of the *nucleus pulposus*. The compressive hydrated disc material appears as a broad-based T2-hyperintense structure (*white arrow*) present dorsal to the C4–C5 space that causes ventral spinal cord compression. Intramedullary T2 hyperintensity at that level is consistent with edema. A fluid-filled cystic structure was found during surgery in the ventral epidural space associated with the C4–C5 disc. **B,** Transverse T2-weighted image of the cervical spine in another dog with an acute compressive hydrated *nucleus pulposus* extrusion at C3–C4. Note the seagull pattern caused by the extruded disc material in the ventral epidural space causing marked ventral spinal cord compression.

Intradural And Intramedullary Disc Herniation

Occasionally, extruded disc material can cause laceration of the dura mater and end up in the intradural/extramedullary compartment or in the intramedullary compartment.[26,91–93] During CT myelography, leakage of iodinated contrast material in the epidural space can be seen, and in cases of intradural location of the extruded disc material, focal expansion of the subarachnoid space with a filling defect can be observed.[93] At MRI, in cases of intramedullary disc extrusion, one may observe a linear tract in the spinal cord parenchyma dorsal to the disc space, which is T2-hyperintense, T1-hypointense and with susceptibility artifacts on T2*W images due to parenchymal hemorrhage, often with enhancement on postcontrast T1W images. A thin cleft in the dorsal annulus of the affected disc may also be noted on transverse images.[92] In cases of intradural but extramedullary disc extrusion, a characteristic "Y-sign" has been reported on T2W sagittal images appearing as a hyperintense horizontal Y pattern along the cranial and/or caudal edge of the hypointense compressive disc material; it is thought that this pattern is due to a cleft forming between the dura mater and arachnoid membrane expanding the subdural space.[91] A "beak sign" is also reported, although less commonly, and seen as a triangular hypointense lesion dorsal to the disc and causing cord compression, with occasionally peripheral enhancement on postcontrast T1W series.[91]

CERVICAL SPONDYLOMYELOPATHY

Cervical spondylomyelopathy refers to a collection of disorders of the caudal cervical spine in large-breed dogs resulting in progressive and chronic spinal cord compression. Other terminology used for this condition includes *wobbler disease, cervical vertebral instability, cervical spondylopathy, cervical spondylolisthesis,* and *cervical vertebral malformation-malarticulation*.[94] The clinical signs range from cervical hyperesthesia to tetraplegia, with the most common being a gait disturbance.[94–101]

Pathologic changes observed with cervical spondylomyelopathy include the following[94]:

- Stenosis of the vertebral canal because of malaligned or misshapen vertebral bodies and/or abnormal, hypertrophied articular processes
- Hansen type II disc protrusion alone or in combination with hypertrophy of the dorsal longitudinal ligament resulting in ventral compression of the spinal cord
- Hypertrophy of the interarcuate ligament *(ligamentum flavum)* and the joint capsule of the articular process joints, resulting in dorsal and dorsolateral spinal cord compression
- Osteoarthrosis of the articular processes with excessive soft tissue proliferation and synovial cyst formation also potentially causing dorsolateral spinal cord compression.

Cervical spondylomyelopathy is seen most commonly in Great Danes and Doberman pinschers but also occurs in other large and giant breeds. In middle-aged to older Doberman pinschers, the most common lesion is Hansen type II disc protrusion and hypertrophy of the ligamentum flavum (interarcuate ligament); this condition is often referred to as "disc-associated cervical spondylomyelopathy."[102] In young Doberman pinschers, Great Danes, and other large-breed dogs (such as older German shepherds[103] or Bernese mountain dogs[104]), the disease is more of the stenotic type myelopathy, caused by hypertrophy and degenerative changes of the articular processes and *ligamentum flavum* hypertrophy, which, combined, cause reduction in the size of the vertebral canal; this condition is often referred to as "osseous-associated cervical spondylomyelopathy."[103,105–107] Clinical signs associated with these conditions usually develop at around 2 to 3 years of age, although juvenile presentation is occasionally seen and mostly of the osseous-associated type.[108]

Both CT, with or without myelography, and MRI provide useful information for diagnosis of this condition; however, there is considerable intermethod and interobserver variability in the information gathered from these imaging modalities, and they may be considered as complementary to each other for a thorough evaluation in a given patient.[95,100,109]

Intermethod and interobserver variability is less pronounced for disc-associated cervical spondylomyelopathy as opposed to the stenotic-type myelopathy.[95,100,109]

Computed Tomography of Cervical Spondylomyelopathy

Noncontrast CT is not very useful in the diagnosis of cervical spondylomyelopathy. It allows assessment of the bone abnormalities, such as articular process hypertrophy, malalignment, and spondylosis, but performs poorly in identifying and grade the location of spinal cord compression correctly and does not

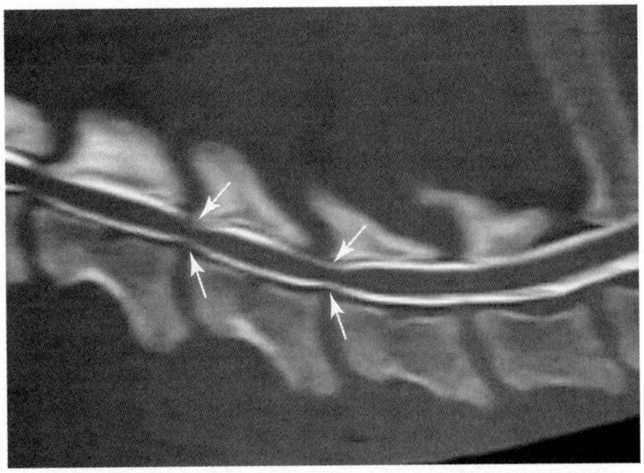

Fig. 15.23 Sagittal reformatted computed tomography (CT) myelogram in a dog with caudal cervical spondylomyelopathy. Note the dorsal and ventral spinal cord compression at C4–C5 and C5–C6 (*white arrows*) because of a combination of ligamentum flavum hypertrophy and dorsal longitudinal ligament hypertrophy with disc bulging. (Image courtesy Dr. Paul Barthez, Clinique Vétérinaire des Halles, Strasbourg, France.)

allow identification of spinal cord atrophy that may be of prognostic value. With CT myelography, conversely, there is excellent delineation of the spinal cord and characterization of the areas of compression (Figs. 15.23 and 15.24). CT myelography provides more information than conventional myelography on the exact location and degree of spinal cord compression. In particular, spinal cord atrophy can be distinguished with CT from reversible spinal cord compression. A further advantage of CT myelography is the superior contrast resolution, which can provide diagnostic images with very little contrast medium in the subarachnoid space.[9] In the Doberman pinscher, several patterns of spinal cord compression have been described on CT[9]:

- Central spinal cord deformity occurs, which most of the time is caused by bulging of the *annulus fibrosus* and occasionally by *nucleus pulposus* extrusion.
- Asymmetric spinal cord compression with intervertebral foramen impingement is caused by unilateral disc protrusion.
- Spinal cord atrophy is characterized by a reduction in the cross-sectional area of the spinal cord, together with relative widening of the subarachnoid space. The atrophic spinal cord can assume an abnormal shape, from a flattened appearance to triangular. It is unclear if spinal cord atrophy is a prognostic indicator of poor outcome, although there are reports of histologic damage, which is likely irreversible, in spinal cords with such a pattern on CT myelography.[9]

The use of traction can provide information on the dynamic nature of spinal cord compression when comparing images in neutral versus stressed positions; sagittal reformatted images are especially useful for this purpose (Fig. 15.25).

Magnetic Resonance Imaging of Cervical Spondylomyelopathy

MRI is accurate in imaging the changes associated with cervical spondylomyelopathy.[95–97,99–101,109–111] Compared with conventional myelography, MRI is more accurate in predicting the site, severity, and nature of the spinal cord compression. Using myelography can lead to an underestimate in the severity of spinal cord compression.[95] MRI is also better than myelography in locating the sites of compressive lesions.[95]

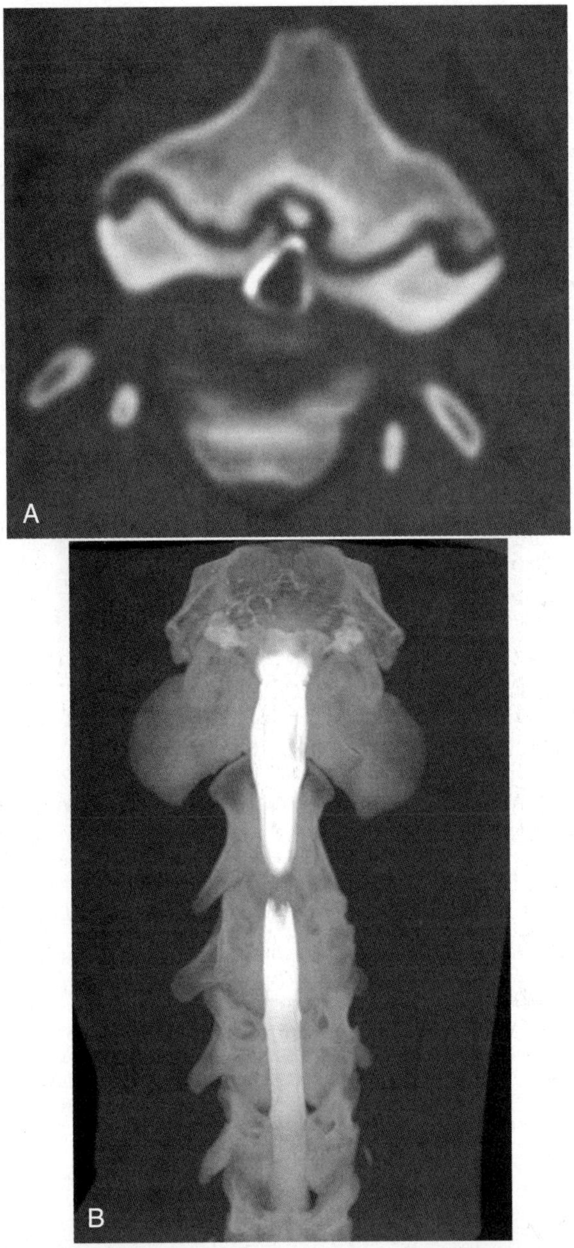

Fig. 15.24 Computed tomography (CT) myelography in a 7-month-old Great Dane with osseous-associated cervical spondylomyelopathy. **A,** Transverse image centered at C2–C3. **B,** Dorsal subvolume maximum intensity projection. There is severe hypertrophy of the articular processes causing marked dorsolateral spinal cord compression at C2–C3. (Image courtesy Dr. Paul Barthez, Dierenkliniek Causus, Oudenburg, Belgium.)

With disc-associated cervical spondylomyelopathy, seen in middle-aged or older Doberman pinschers, the disease is characterized by:

- Disc degeneration, disc bulging, and/or herniation causing spinal cord compression
- *Ligamentum flavum* hypertrophy causing dorsal spinal cord compression
- Alterations in spinal cord signal intensity
- Vertebral body abnormalities and spondylosis

The presence of alterations in spinal cord signal intensity is a reliable indicator of clinically relevant spinal cord compression,[95,97] although this has occasionally been reported in the caudal cervical spine of clinically normal dogs.[110] However, such T2 hyperintensities do not seem to correlate to prognosis.[96] What is causing the T2 hyperintensity of the gray matter in the spinal cord of affected dogs is not clearly established, but possible reasons include loss of nerve cells, gliosis, and edema. White matter T2 hyperintensity can be caused by demyelination, edema, and Wallerian degeneration. When areas of corresponding T1 hypointensity are present, more severe changes, such as necrosis, myelomalacia, and spongiform changes, may be suspected.[96] There may be a positive correlation between severity of cord compression and neurologic grade; however, multilevel compression is not associated with worse deficits.[102] Dynamic studies with traction MRI have questionable accuracy in identifying the static or dynamic nature of the compression.[95,112]

With osseous-associated cervical spondylomyelopathy, seen in younger Doberman pinschers and giant-breed dogs such as Great Danes, there appears to be a weak correlation between neurologic grade and severity of spinal cord compression, number of affected sites, and presence of T2W spinal cord hyperintensity.[105] The MRI abnormalities seen with this condition include the following[94,99–101]:

- Degenerative changes of the intervertebral discs are seen as decreased signal intensity on T2W images, especially at C6–C7 and C5–C6.
- Hypertrophy of the dorsal longitudinal ligament and osteoarthrosis of the articular process from C3–C4 to C7–T1 is seen, with the most common sites being C4–C5, C5–C6, and C6–C7. These compressive structures appear T1 and T2 hypointense, and spinal cord deformity can be seen on sagittal/parasagittal and transverse images. These abnormalities can cause unilateral or bilateral dorsolateral spinal cord compression, which is best identified on transverse images (Fig. 15.26).

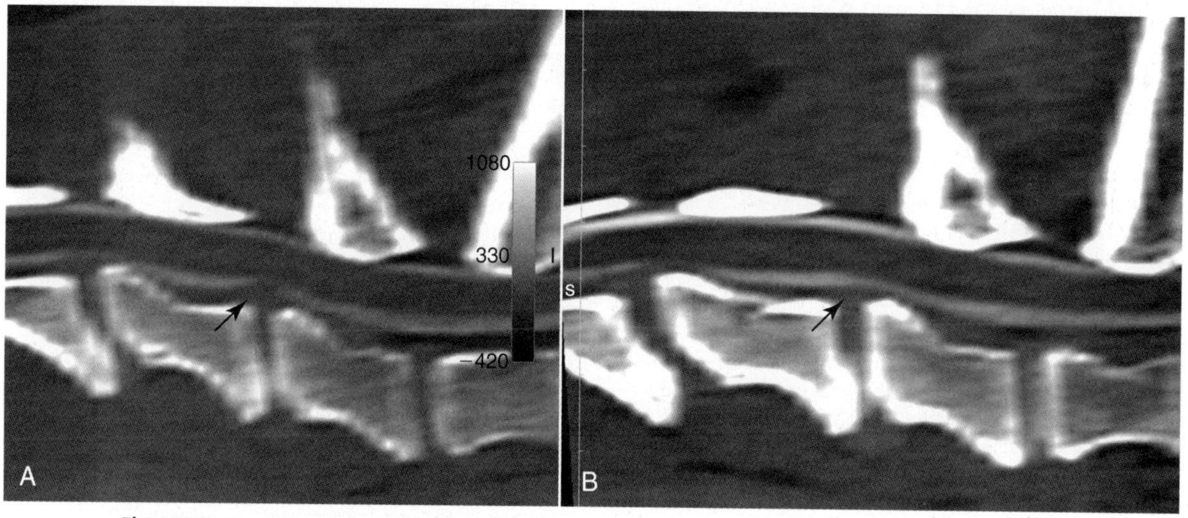

Fig. 15.25 Sagittal reformatted computed tomography (CT)-myelographic images of the caudal cervical spine of a middle-aged Doberman pinscher with disc-associated cervical spondylomyelopathy. **A** shows neutral position, and there is ventral spinal cord compression caused by a bulging disc and/or dorsal longitudinal ligament hypertrophy (*black arrow*). **B** was obtained during cervical traction, and there is reduction in spinal cord compression (*black arrow*), thereby characterizing the dynamic nature of the compression. (Image courtesy Dr. Laurent Couturier, Azur Vet, Cagnes sur Mer, France.)

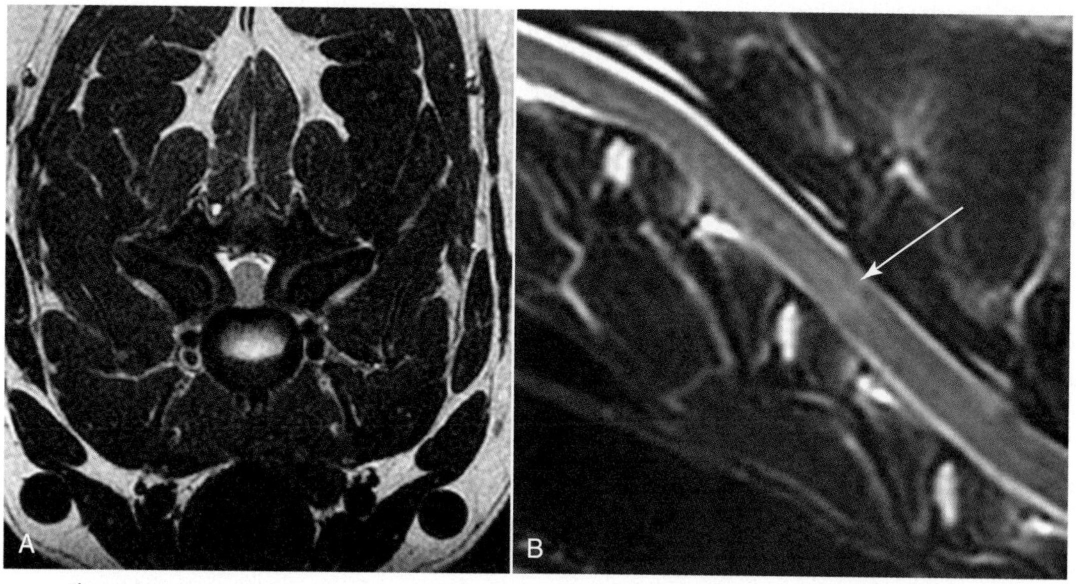

Fig. 15.26 Transverse **(A)** and sagittal **(B)** T2-weighted images in a Great Dane with osseous-associated cervical spondylomyelopathy at C3 to C4. There is marked hypertrophy of the articular processes causing lateral spinal cord compression. There is intramedullary T2 hyperintensity in the sagittal image (*white arrow*). This hyperintensity can help determine the clinical significance of the cervical anomalies.

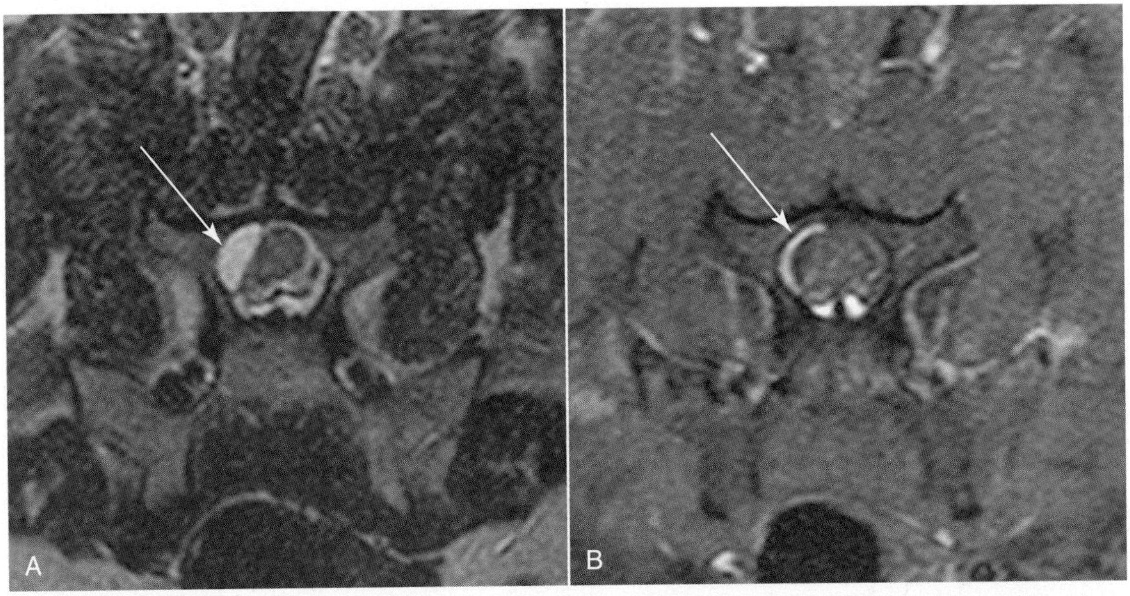

Fig. 15.27 T2-weighted **(A)** and postcontrast, fat-suppressed, T1-weighted **(B)** transverse images of a dog with cervical spondylomyelopathy. There is a large synovial cyst (*white arrow* in **A**) arising from a degenerate articular process joint that is causing moderate spinal cord compression. The joint itself is caudal to this image plane because the cyst has bulged cranially. Following contrast medium administration, there is enhancement of the wall of the cyst (*white arrow* in **B**).

- Intramedullary T2 hyperintensity is associated with areas of spinal cord compression (see Fig. 15.26).
- Synovial cysts are identified as T1-hypointense, T2-hyperintense structures associated with the articular processes and sometimes contributing to dorsolateral spinal cord compression (Fig. 15.27). The wall of these cysts occasionally enhances after gadolinium injection.
- Occasional disc protrusion (Hansen type II) contributes to ventral spinal cord compression, especially at C6–C7.
- Kinematic MRI may reveal an increased number of compressive lesions and changes in site of the most compressive lesion on images obtained in extension vs. neutral positioning.[113]

There is a high incidence of MRI abnormalities of the cervical vertebral column in clinically normal large-breed dogs; these have been documented in Doberman pinschers and foxhounds and include complete disc degeneration, spinal cord compression, vertebral body abnormalities, and even intramedullary T2 hyperintensity.[110] In clinically normal Great Danes, foraminal stenosis (sometimes severe), and less commonly spinal cord compression have been reported.[99] Therefore, caution should be exercised when attributing clinical signs to structural abnormalities seen on MR images. Also, there can be significant variability in the assessment and interpretation of MRI abnormalities across observers in dogs with disc-associated wobbler syndrome so that interpretation of imaging results must be made with caution.[110]

CYSTIC CHANGES OF THE SPINE

Several types of intraspinal cyst-like changes occur in dogs; the most common being arachnoid diverticula, epidermoid/dermoid cysts, articular process synovial, and ganglion cysts. Uncommon cystic changes include perineurial or perineural cysts, also called *Tarlov cysts*, which originate from the dorsal nerve root and ganglion sheath, close to the point where the pia and arachnoid membrane differentiate into endoneurium and perineurium, respectively. Unlike arachnoid diverticula, they are extradural lesions filled with CSF and contain neural structures pertaining to the nerve root and ganglion.[114,115] Cysts of ligamentous or discal origin are extremely rare. Cyst-like changes associated with the intervertebral disc, similar to the "discal cysts" seen in humans, are rarely described in the thoracolumbar spine of dogs and are called "discal pseudocysts."[116,117]

Spinal Arachnoid Diverticula

Spinal arachnoid diverticula are a rare cause of spinal cord compression in dogs and rarely reported in cats.[13,118–138] In dogs, they are located in the subarachnoid space, lined by arachnoid and pia mater, and communicate freely with CSF in the subarachnoid space. Because no true epithelial lining is present, the term *arachnoid diverticula* is used here. These lesions are often congenital but can be associated with spinal cord trauma, IVDD, or previous arachnoiditis.

The most common location is in the cranial cervical or caudal thoracic region. These lesions are usually single but can be multiple. They are most commonly dorsal or dorsolateral to the spinal cord but can be ventral occasionally. Rottweilers are likely to be predisposed to cervical arachnoid diverticula, and pug dogs seem to have a high incidence of thoracolumbar arachnoid diverticula. In pugs, there may be an association between development of arachnoid diverticula and aplasia of the caudal articular processes in the caudal thoracic spine. In addition, in this breed,[139] a familial form of the condition has been reported in the cervical spine.[132]

In CT without contrast medium, there is a hypoattenuating lesion causing spinal cord compression. Diagnosis is established after subarachnoid injection of contrast medium leads to pooling of contrast medium in the diverticulum. Sagittal reformatted images allow recognition of the typical teardrop shape of the lesion.

On MRI, a discrete T1-hypointense region contiguous with the subarachnoid space is present adjacent to the spinal cord (usually dorsal). This lesion is T2 hyperintense and usually suppressed with FLAIR techniques, although a lack of suppression on T2-FLAIR has been reported,[127] and may reflect that occasionally the fluid in the diverticulum is of different chemical composition than CSF, as has been described in intracranial arachnoid cysts in people.[140] Heavily T2W pulse sequences such as HASTE or SSFSE, which highlight fluid-filled spaces while suppressing background signal, have been reported to increase the sensitivity of MRI for the identification of arachnoid diverticula in dogs.[13]

The diagnosis is usually most obvious on sagittal images where the typical teardrop shape of these lesions is apparent (Fig. 15.28). The spinal cord is compressed to various degrees at the level of the diverticulum. CSF pulsation within the diverticulum can lead to spinal cord edema from the repetitive concussion, or there may be syrinx formation because of altered CSF flow in the region of the diverticulum (Fig. 15.29, eFig. 15.6). MRI is superior to CT myelography for the diagnosis of spinal arachnoid diverticula in the rare instance where the diverticulum does not communicate with the subarachnoid space.

Epidermoid and Dermoid Cysts or Sinuses

Epidermoid and dermoid cysts and sinuses are caused by failure of separation of the surface ectoderm (forming the epidermis) and neuroectoderm (forming the nervous system) during embryogenesis. They have a complex wall and contain both epidermoid tissue and adnexa. They can be associated with the dermal, ocular, and central nervous system (CNS), and the most common CNS manifestation is of a sinus connection with the skin surface that may extend into the vertebral canal to affect the spinal cord ("dermoid sinus").[141] As opposed to sinuses, epidermoid and dermoid cysts do not have an opening onto the midline surface of the skin.[142] With epidermoid cysts or sinuses, the wall of the lesion consists of stratified squamous epithelium, supported by connective tissue stroma. Keratin squames are found within the lesion along with a few inflammatory cells. Dermoid cysts and sinuses differ from epidermoid cysts because the dermoid cyst contains other features of skin, such as sweat glands, hair follicles, and sebaceous glands.

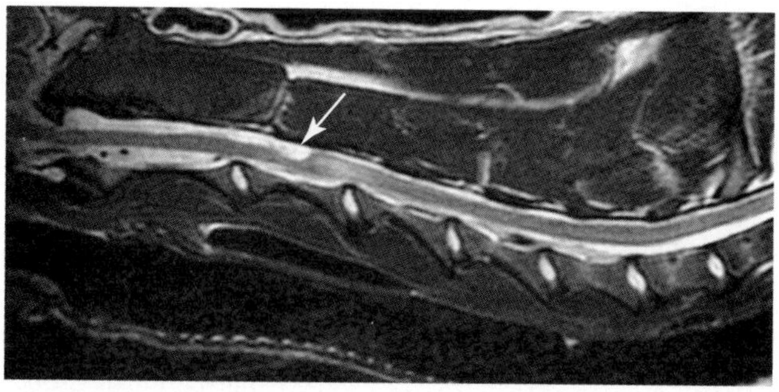

Fig. 15.28 T2-weighted sagittal image in a dog several months after diagnosis of meningitis caused by *Cryptococcus* infection. There is a spinal arachnoid diverticulum (*white arrow*) dorsal to C3 forming a typical teardrop-shaped hyperintense structure dorsal to the spinal cord.

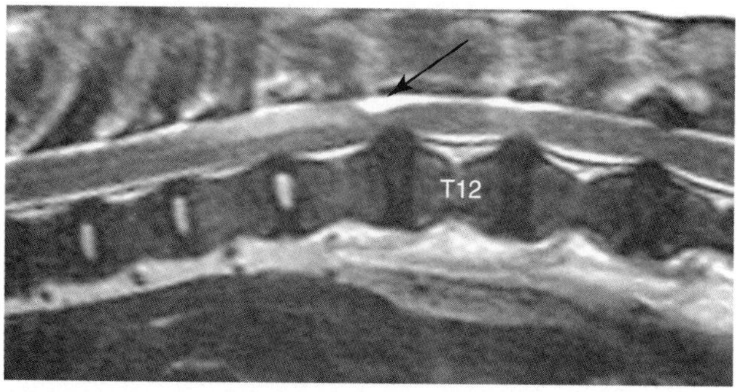

Fig. 15.29 Sagittal T2-weighted image of a dog with a dorsal arachnoid diverticulum (*arrow*) at T11 to T12. There is a region of intramedullary T2 hyperintensity just cranial to the diverticulum that likely represents early syringomyelia because of altered cerebrospinal fluid (CSF) flow.

Epidermoid and dermoid cysts confined strictly to the CNS without a cutaneous or subcutaneous tract develop from skin-determining ectoderm, which remains attached to mesoderm and as the neural tube closes becomes surrounded by the meninges.[143] In such instances, no tract or sinus is present in the dorsal paraspinal soft tissue or skin.[143]

Spinal dermoid sinuses fall into one of six categories, depending on how deep the connecting tract penetrates[144]:

- Type I: Tubular sac extending from the skin to the supraspinous or nuchal ligament
- Type II: More superficial tract, with a deep fibrous strand connecting to the supraspinous or nuchal ligament
- Type III: Superficial tract with no connection to the supraspinous or nuchal ligament
- Type IV: Deep tract that communicates with the vertebral canal and is attached to the dura mater
- Type V: True dermoid "cyst," with a closed capsule and no deeper connection or opening to the skin
- Type VI: Deep tract that extends to the supraspinous or nuchal ligament and continues deeper as a fibrous strand that connects to the dura mater

Only types IV and VI may be associated with neurologic signs, due to their relationship with the dura mater; in these cases, neurologic signs can be the result of infection (abscessation, meningitis, meningomyelitis, and so on), compression of the spinal cord due to progressive enlargement of the deeper portion of the tract with accumulated debris (hair follicles, sebum, keratin, desquamated epithelial cells), tethering of the spinal cord,[144] and syringomyelia.[144]

There are only a few reports on the use of CT and MRI in the diagnosis and presurgical assessment of epidermoid and dermoid cysts in dogs. CT imaging can allow detection of a communication with the vertebral canal through a defect in the vertebral arch, with subsequent spinal cord compression and displacement.[145,146]

The MRI abnormalities reported with spinal dermoid sinus include a focal invagination of the cutaneous tissues toward the spinous processes corresponding to the clinically palpable lesion (Fig. 15.30). Deep to that area, there may be a focal rounded or lenticular subcutaneous lesion, corresponding to the main cavity of the sinus, followed by a tubular tract extending ventrally to a variable depth, depending on the type of dermoid sinus. The lumen of the sinus and its tract is often filled with sebum, keratin debris, and hair, resulting in a variable and unpredictable MR signal. Compared to muscles, the lesions tend to be T2-hyperintense to muscles, whereas T1W signal is more variable (hypo-, iso-, hyperintense).[147–149] Areas that are hyperintense on both T1W and T2W images may correspond to lipid lining.[147] In a report where gadolinium contrast medium was administered intravenously, only minimal enhancement was seen.[147] In a patient where the sinus was abscessed, the lesion was markedly T2-hyperintense and T1-hypointense with a hypointense wall on both T1W and T2W images, suggestive of a thick capsule.[142] In types IV and VI, which have a dural connection, additional signs may include a linear, somewhat tortuous tract of variable signal intensity, extending deep to the skin toward the spine and entering the vertebral canal, connecting with the dura mater, usually through an interarcuate space, and in some instances through a defect of the dorsal arch (schisis).[147,149–151] Concurrent vertebral malformations may be present, such as *spina bifida*, vertebral blocks, partial fusion of adjacent spinous processes, and incomplete dorsal lamina.[144,147,149–151] Such anomalies seem to be more commonly associated with dermoid sinuses that have connection with the dura mater, and therefore their identification should trigger a careful examination of the meninges, subarachnoid space, and spinal cord in that general area. Focal dorsal tenting of the meninges of the spinal cord, due to the dural connection pulling the dura dorsally, may be

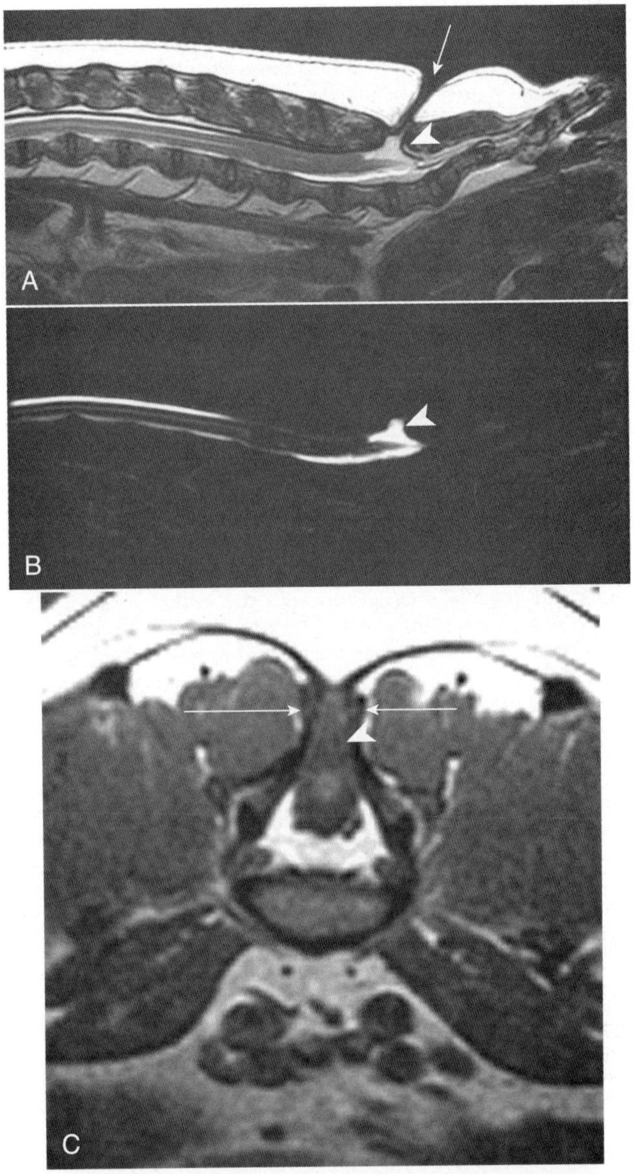

Fig. 15.30 Dermoid sinus and meningocele in a 1-year-old French bulldog. This was an incidental finding as the dog was imaged with MRI because of acute paraplegia due to an intervertebral disc extrusion at L5–L6 (causing the cord swelling seen in the caudal lumbar area). Sagittal T2-weighted **(A)**, sagittal single-shot fast spin echo (SSFSE) "T2-myelogram" **(B)**, and transverse T2-weighted **(C)** images are presented. On the T2-weighted sagittal image, a focal invagination of the cutaneous surface is seen at the level of the lumbosacral region (**A,** *white arrow*) extending towards a split spinous process as seen on the transverse image (**B,** *black arrows*) consistent with spina bifida. A flame-like dorsal expansion of the subarachnoid space is seen on all images (*arrowheads*) directed towards the dermoid sinus consistent with a concurrent meningocele.

seen. In instances of tenting, the dorsal subarachnoid space is focally widened and assumes a characteristic triangular shape on transverse images.[147,150] In instances of tethering, there is dorsal displacement of the spinal cord at the level of the sinus.[144] There may be syringomyelia adjacent to the dural connection, likely associated with focal alterations of the CSF flow dynamics caused by the dural connection or concurrent adhesions or vertebral anomalies.[144] In rare instances, extension of the distal end of the sinus through the dura mater forms a progressively enlarging, debris-filled blind-ended cystic component that appears as an intradural-extramedullary T2-hyperintense mass lesion compressing/displacing the spinal cord.[149]

The MR or CT appearance of strictly intramedullary epidermoid and dermoid cysts has not been reported in dogs or cats, although there is a report of a dermoid cyst in the medulla oblongata of a dog. That lesion was heterogeneous but predominantly hyperintense on both T1W and T2W images with no contrast enhancement.[141]

Articular Process Cysts

Cysts associated with the articular process are extradural fluid-filled round or oval well-defined structures that develop as a result of degeneration of the articular process joint.[115,152–155] They are divided histologically into (1) synovial cysts lined by synovium-like epithelial cells resulting from outpouching of synovial membrane through weakened capsular tissue and (2) ganglion cysts, which are the result of mucinous degeneration of periarticular connective tissue and which do not have a synovial lining. From clinical and imaging perspectives, the two entities are indistinguishable and can therefore be grouped under the terminology *articular process cyst*.[154]

Clinical signs associated with articular process cysts vary from pain to ataxia and tetra- or paraparesis, although in a number of instances, the clinical signs are not attributable to the cyst, but to other causes of spinal cord compression, such as disc herniation, articular process hypertrophy, and vertebral instability. These articular process cysts appear to be more common in large- to giant-breed dogs.[115,152–155] In giant-breed dogs, the cysts tend to be multiple and located in the cervical spine and more common in young dogs.[153] In large-breed dogs, cysts are more commonly found in the thoracolumbar or lumbosacral area in young adults and older dogs.[115,152–155] The cysts can be single or multiple and present at one or several locations.

On MRI, these lesions have the characteristic signal of a fluid-filled lesion appearing as well-defined round lesions associated with the articular processes and are T1 hypointense and T2 hyperintense (Fig. 15.31).[115,152,154,155]

Discal Pseudocyst

Although initial reports of compressive myelopathy due to so-called "discal cysts"[33,34] were deemed to more likely represent compressive forms of hydrated *nucleus pulposus* extrusions in subsequent studies,[32] a rare condition resembling discal cysts seen in humans has been reported.[116,117] These are seen in the thoracolumbar region of medium- to large-breed dogs presenting with acute to subacute neurologic deficits. At MRI, they form rounded to oval-shaped, ventral to ventrolateral extradural compressive lesions arising from the dorsal aspect of the intervertebral disc; they are iso-/hypointense on T1W images, mostly hyperintense on T2W images, with a thin enhancing capsule on postcontrast images and occasional enhancement of the content of the cyst-like lesion. Histologically, the wall of the lesions consists of dense fibrous connective tissue containing clusters of chondroid cells accompanied by notochordal cells with no nerve tissue or disc material; due to the lack of an epithelial lining, discal pseudocyst is a preferred terminology for these lesions.

SPINAL TUMORS

Spinal tumors can be classified on the basis of their location relative to the dura mater and can be described as intramedullary, intradural-extramedullary, or extradural.[156] Most extradural tumors are malignant tumors of constituents of the vertebral column, such as the vertebrae or the soft tissues within or surrounding the vertebral column. Intradural-extramedullary tumors are mostly nerve sheath tumors and meningiomas. Intramedullary neoplasms are usually of glial cell origin, such as astrocytomas or ependymomas, but multicentric

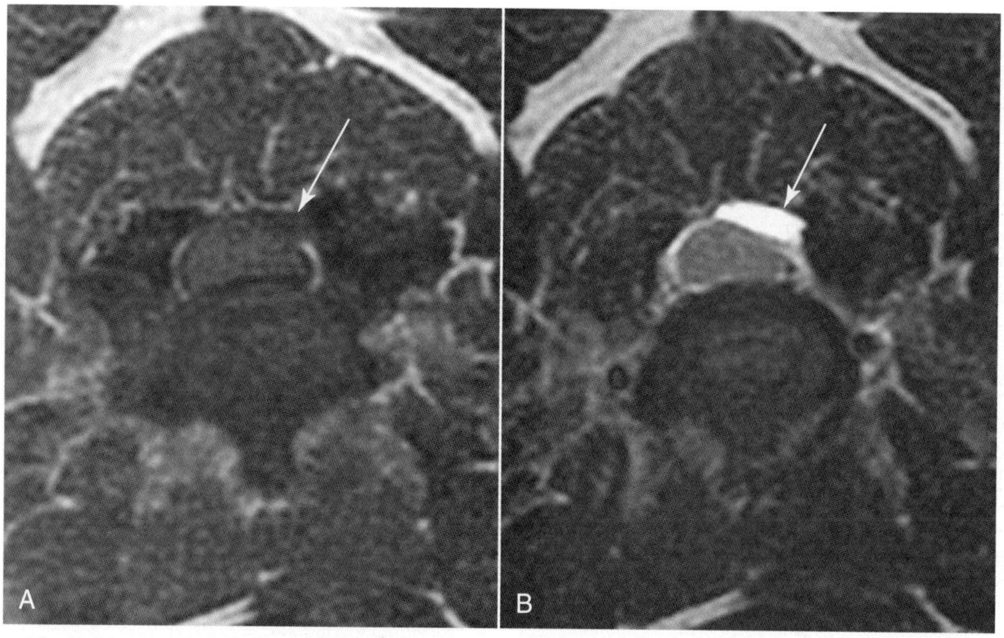

Fig. 15.31 Transverse T1-weighted **(A)** and T2-weighted **(B)** images at C3 to C4 in a dog with a left-sided articular process cyst. The cyst (*white arrows*) is T1 hypointense and markedly T2 hyperintense because of its fluid content. In this dog, the cyst caused mild left dorsolateral spinal cord compression.

non-neural neoplasia (such as, lymphoma) or metastatic lesions (such as, hemangiosarcoma) also occur.

Extradural Tumors

The most common extradural spinal cord tumors in dogs include osteosarcoma and chondrosarcoma.[157] In cats, extradural lymphosarcoma is also frequent.[158,159] Solitary or disseminated histiocytic sarcoma can also affect the vertebrae and cause spinal cord compression.[160] Other disseminated canine tumors with possible vertebral involvement include lymphosarcoma and multiple myeloma.[157] Metastatic vertebral tumors are also common, in particular prostatic carcinoma or transitional cell carcinoma of the bladder and urethra in dogs.[157] Tumors of the paravertebral soft tissues or extradural soft tissue components of the vertebral canal are also possible, and local invasion can cause spinal cord compression. Examples include soft tissue sarcoma, infiltrative lipoma,[161–165] extradural lymphosarcoma, mast cell tumor (primary or metastatic), and hemangiosarcoma.[166–171]

Both MRI and CT are more sensitive than radiography in detecting vertebral lesions and in particular bone lysis that is not apparent radiographically can be demonstrated readily using CT. Vertebral canal tumors can be difficult to localize to the intradural, extradural, or intramedullary compartments on noncontrast CT images.[172] Injection of intravenous contrast medium and, more important, CT myelography are more precise for determining the location of masses in the vertebral canal with respect to the dura. MRI is also good for localizing these lesions; however, with MRI, it is more difficult to localize vertebral canal masses with respect to the dura because of lower spatial resolution.[173] There are no specific CT or MRI features that are associated with a specific tumor type.[172,173]

Vertebral tumors produce variable degrees of bone lysis or proliferation, which is detected easily on CT images (Fig. 15.32, eFig. 15.7). On MR images, alteration of the shape of the affected vertebra can be seen, as well as disruption of the normally hypointense vertebral cortex (Fig. 15.33). In MR images, periosteal reaction appears as hypointense material surrounding the lesion in the affected vertebra. The signal intensity of the lesion itself varies between patients and depends on tumor type. For example, vertebral osteosarcoma has been

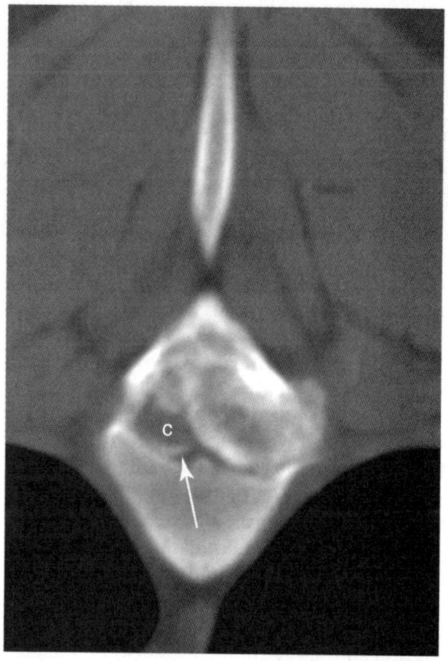

Fig. 15.32 Transverse computed tomography (CT)-myelographic image of the thoracic spine in a dog with a vertebral osteochondroma. There is a large proliferative lesion arising from the vertebral arch that causes marked stenosis of the vertebral canal and left dorsolateral compression of the spinal cord (*c*). The subarachnoid space filled with iodinated contrast medium is indicated by the *white arrow*.

reported to have T2W heterogeneous signal, with heterogeneous contrast enhancement and osteolysis.[166,174] However, relevant conclusions cannot be drawn as to what the signal intensity of a specific tumor type would be. Most vertebral tumors are monostotic; however, polyostotic lesions are possible in cases of metastatic neoplasia (e.g., from prostatic carcinoma or bladder urothelial carcinoma, metastatic mast cell neoplasia[170]), as well as in cases of bone marrow neoplasia such as multiple myeloma.[175] With multiple myeloma, multiple

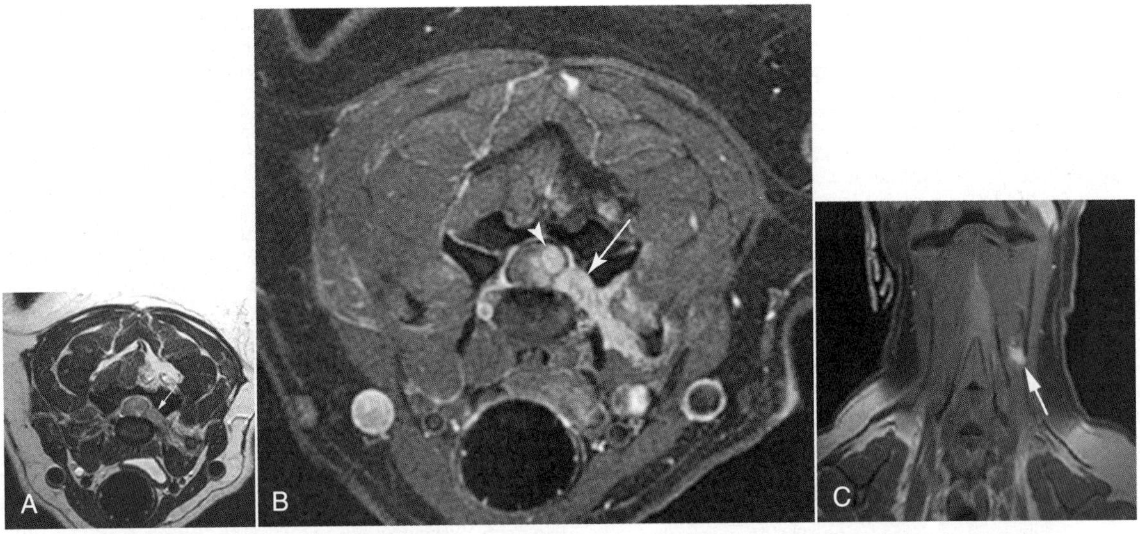

Fig. 15.37 Transverse T2-weighted **(A)**, transverse fat-saturated postcontrast T1-weighted **(B)**, and dorsal fat-saturated postcontrast T1-weighted **(C)** images in a dog with a nerve sheath tumor in the left C3–C4 intervertebral foramen. There is a soft tissue tumor obliterating the left intervertebral foramen at C3–C4 (**A,** *white arrow*). The tumor is nearly isointense to spinal cord and extends peripheral to the foramen in the form of an elongated mass. There is marked diffuse contrast enhancement of the tumor (**B,** *white arrow*). The tumor tracks along the nerve path in the paraspinal muscles (**C,** *white arrow*). An intradural component was apparent on the postcontrast images (*white arrowhead,* **B**).

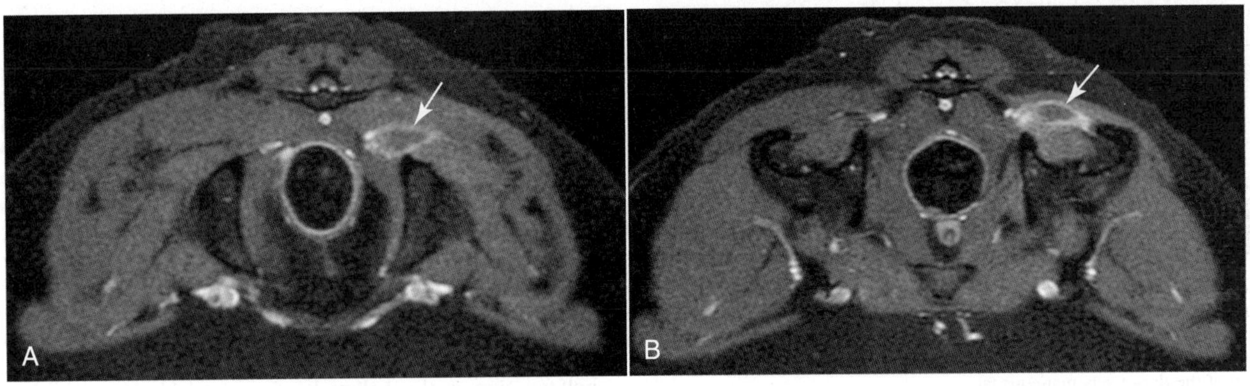

Fig. 15.38 **A and B,** Transverse fat-saturated postcontrast T1-weighted images in a cat with a large extradural sciatic nerve tumor. There is muscle atrophy on the left side. The tumor is slightly hypointense with strong peripheral contrast enhancement (*white arrow*) and follows the path of the sciatic nerve. Fat saturation facilitates the recognition of the abnormal enhancing tissue on postcontrast series.

lesion and is appreciated best on CT when reformatted sagittal and dorsal images are obtained. If iodinated contrast medium is injected intravenously, there may be enhancement of the mass.[193]

On MRI, meningiomas appear as focal masses that are usually hyperintense to the spinal cord on T2W images, and isointense to hypointense to the spinal cord on precontrast T1W images. However, T2 hypointensity and T1 hyperintensity have also been reported.[173,192,193] After gadolinium injection, meningiomas usually have moderate to strong well-defined contrast enhancement.[192,193] Features that help in determining the intradural/extramedullary location include the following[192]:

- The broad-based dural margin is seen on at least one of the imaging planes (Fig. 15.39, eFig. 15.10).
- The gradual expansion of the subarachnoid space cranial and caudal to the mass that can be detected on T2W images, especially in the dorsal plane, creates a golf-tee sign similar to that observed with conventional myelography or CT myelography. Heavily T2W MR pulse sequences (T2-myelograms) can be useful in recognizing this sign.[12,173]

An MRI feature often associated with spinal meningiomas is the dural tail sign, which is seen as strong linear enhancement of the border of the tumor confluent with the adjacent meninges (see Fig. 15.39).[192] Confusion with a nerve sheath tumor is possible when the meningioma is located within or exits the intervertebral foramen.[192]

Nephroblastoma

This is a rare tumor typically occurring in young dogs (<3 years old), with German shepherd dogs possibly predisposed.[179–186] The tumor is intradural/extramedullary and located consistently between T10 and L2. It is thought that the tumor arises from ectopic embryonic remnants of renal tissue. A single mass is usually present, although there are rare reports of intraspinal metastases.[186]

On noncontrast CT, swelling of the spinal cord with obliteration of the epidural fat is observed in the affected area; however, the intradural nature of the lesion can only be determined with CT myelography. Even then, it can be difficult to tell if the tumor is intradural/extramedullary or intramedullary, especially because the tumor can invade the spinal cord.

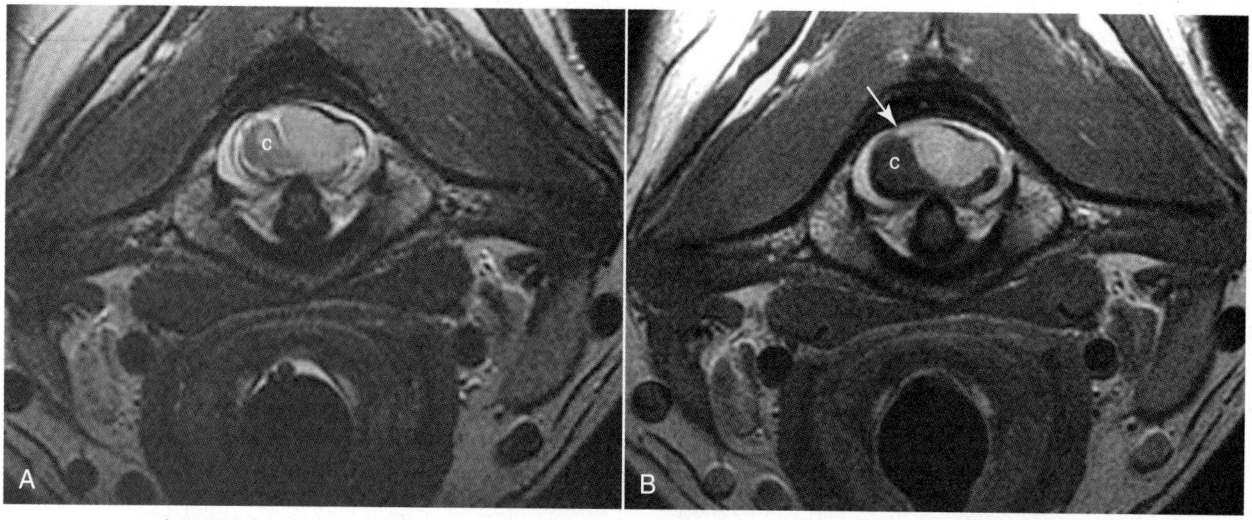

Fig. 15.39 Transverse T2-weighted **(A)** and postcontrast T1-weighted **(B)** images at the level of C1 in a dog with a meningioma. There is an intradural mass in the left dorsal aspect of the subarachnoid space that is broad-based toward the dura and is causing severe spinal cord *(c)* compression. After contrast medium injection **(B)** the mass is markedly and homogeneously contrast enhancing, and a dural tail (*white arrow*) is present on the dorsal right margin of the mass.

On MRI, the tumor is isointense to the spinal cord in T2W images, but it may have heterogeneous signal.[181,183–185] The mass is also usually isointense to the spinal cord on T1W images, but there is moderate to strong contrast enhancement.[181,183–185] Transverse and dorsal images allow the peripheral location of the mass in the dural sac to be detected, often with a broad base toward the meninges. Widening of the subarachnoid space cranial or caudal to the mass (golf-tee sign) can be present and help determine its intradural location. However, this sign is not present consistently, and, as with CT, it can be difficult to determine the intradural/extramedullary origin of the mass, especially when the tumor invades the spinal cord (Fig. 15.40).[185]

Intramedullary Tumors

Intramedullary tumors are rare in dogs and cats, and they can be primary or metastatic.[156] In a retrospective study, the most common canine primary intramedullary tumor was ependymoma, followed by astrocytoma, and less commonly nephroblastoma, chordoma, oligodendroglioma, and teratoma.[196] The most common metastatic lesions were transitional cell carcinoma and hemangiosarcoma, with less common metastatic lesions including pheochromocytoma, mammary/pancreatic/prostatic carcinoma, and sarcoma of unknown etiology.[196] Intramedullary neoplasia is even less common in cats, and most are glial cell tumors (most commonly astrocytomas, but also ependymomas and oligodendrogliomas).[158,197,198] They seem to be more common in the cervical spinal cord.[158,197,198]

CT is poorly sensitive for diagnosis of intramedullary tumors; focal cord swelling may be seen, with variable degrees of parenchymal enhancement on postcontrast series. Reports of the MRI appearance of intramedullary neoplasms are scarce in the veterinary literature. Astrocytomas and oligodendrogliomas form ovoid to elliptical mass lesions that are well marginated, located eccentrically in the spinal cord causing variable degrees of spinal cord swelling; the lesions are T1 iso- to hypointense, T2 and STIR hyperintense, and moderately contrast enhancing.[196] Ependymomas appear as elongated fusiform to ellipsoid lesions with a central location in the spinal cord, and sometimes a multifocal distribution along the neuraxis; they are T1 isointense, T2 hyperintense and strongly contrast enhancing; on sagittal T2W or T2*W images, a hypointense curved area may be seen along the cranial and caudal margins of the lesion due to chronic hemorrhage, and has been referred to as a "cap sign."[196,199]

Tumors With Variable Spinal Distribution

Some types of spinal tumors may have variable distributions and can involve several compartments simultaneously (extradural, intradural/extramedullary, and intramedullary). The most common tumors with this behavior are histiocytic sarcoma, lymphoma, and hemangiosarcoma.

Histiocytic Sarcoma

Histiocytes are a category of leukocytes that occur in many tissues throughout the body. They are derived from stem cell precursors and differentiate into cells of the monocyte/macrophage lineage or dendritic cell lineage.[200] Histiocytic sarcoma is due to neoplastic transformation of interstitial dendritic cells, with the exception of a hematophagocytic variant, which occurs within the splenic red pulp and arises from macrophages.[201] Histiocytic sarcoma can be localized (most commonly as a soft tissue mass along the limbs), or disseminated, affecting multiple organ systems, including the spleen, liver, lungs, lymph nodes, bone marrow, and CNS.[201] The spinal cord can be secondarily affected in histiocytic sarcoma arising from a vertebra. This has been reported more commonly in the disseminated form than the localized form.[160] Such lesions can cause extradural spinal cord compression when they invade into the vertebral canal. They may arise from the soft tissues around the bone and invade bone secondarily, or they may grow initially within the bone marrow and extend to the cortex and adjacent soft tissues. The appearance is similar to that of other aggressive vertebral neoplasm, with bone lysis and soft tissue proliferation.

Direct involvement of the CNS can occur both in the disseminated form of histiocytic sarcoma and as an entity isolated to the CNS ("primary CNS histiocytic sarcoma"). In both cases, all parts of the neuraxis can be affected.[200–203] Retrievers and Pembroke Welsh corgis may be predisposed to CNS involvement with histiocytic sarcoma, with corgis possibly predisposed to the primary CNS form.[201] Histopathologically, neoplastic infiltration in the subarachnoid space and leptomeninges with infiltration into the white matter of the spinal cord and nerve roots is commonly found. Meningeal infiltration is consistently seen; even lesions that appear intramedullary on

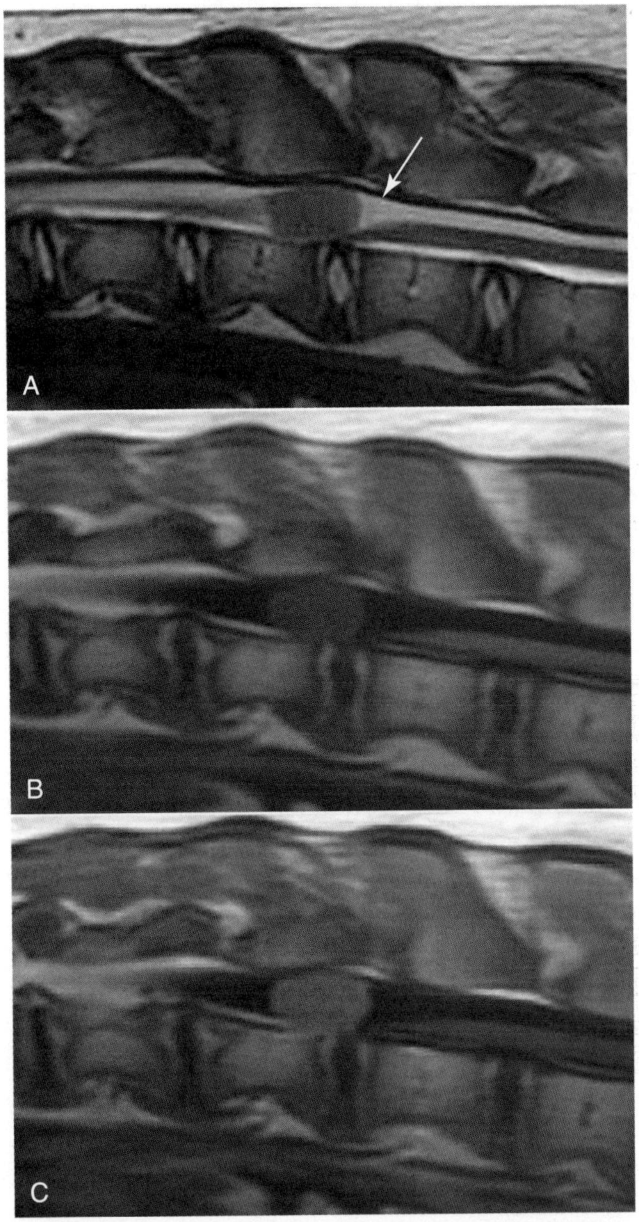

Fig. 15.40 Sagittal T2-weighted **(A)**, T1-weighted with fluid-attenuated inversion recovery (FLAIR) **(B)**, and postcontrast T1-weighted FLAIR **(C)** images of a young dog with a nephroblastoma. There is an ovoid intradural mass at the level of L1. It is isointense to the spinal cord on precontrast images, and there is strong contrast enhancement. Focal widening of the subarachnoid space is present caudal and cranial to the mass, forming a golf-tee sign (*white arrow* in **A**); the cerebrospinal fluid (CSF) in the subarachnoid space is T2 hyperintense and T1 hypointense. (Images courtesy Dr. Shannon Holmes, University of Georgia.)

MRI typically have some form of meningeal association histopathologically.[201–203]

Various MRI features of CNS histiocytic sarcoma can be seen,[200–202] including focal or multifocal intramedullary and/or intradural/extramedullary mass(es) lesion(s), most commonly isointense (less commonly hypo- or hyperintense) on T1W images, hyperintense or of mixed signal intensity on T2W images, hyperintense on STIR, with moderate to marked contrast enhancement after gadolinium injection. Ill-defined diffuse intramedullary T2 hyperintensity with loss of the epidural fat and gray/white matter definition may also be seen, with moderate parenchymal contrast enhancement after gadolinium injection and mild diffuse meningeal enhancement. Meningeal enhancement in the vicinity of focal mass lesions, sometimes with a dural tail sign, may also be seen; this meningeal enhancement often extends over long distances from the mass lesion, and isolated areas of meningeal enhancement away and separate from the mass lesion is also possible, suggestive metastatic spread of the condition through the subarachnoid space. In some cases, the only abnormality can be meningeal enhancement without a mass lesion (leptomeningeal histiocytic sarcoma). MRI features of spinal histiocytic sarcoma, such as focal mass lesions, meningeal thickening, and enhancement, can also be seen with other neoplasms (such as, lymphoma) or rare tumors (such as, meningeal oligodendrogliomatosis) and are therefore nonspecific. Intradural/extramedullary masses with dural tail can also be seen with meningioma.

Lymphoma

In both dogs and cats, lymphoma may involve many tissues outside of the lymphatic system, including the CNS. Spinal lymphoma can be secondary or primary, based on whether neoplastic lymphocytes are or not identified in other organ systems, respectively. Clinical signs depend on the distribution of the lesions in the CNS and on the presence and extent of other organ systems involvement.

In cats, lymphoma is the most common tumor affecting the spinal cord.[158,159] Affected cats are typically young, with short duration of clinical signs.[158,204,205] In that species, the most common location of spinal lymphoma is extradural, or mixed extra- and intradural (affecting the leptomeninges and/or the spinal cord).[158,205] Exclusive intradural location is rare.[158] Extramedullary hematopoietic tissue has been cited as the possible anlage for the development of primary lymphoma of the spine.[205] Involvement of other organ systems is common in cats with spinal lymphoma, with bone marrow and kidneys being more commonly affected.[158,204,205] In some case series, affected cats had lesions in multiple regions of the CNS, including the brain,[158] whereas in other series, single epidural lesions were more common.[205] At MRI, feline spinal lymphoma manifests as both intradural and extradural lesions, often affecting multiple compartments including the paraspinal tissues; the lumbar and lumbosacral regions are more commonly affected.[167,168,206] Lesions are ill-defined, hypointense on T1W images, hyperintense on T2W images, with homogeneous, often strong enhancement on postcontrast T1W images.[167,168,206] Another study where MRI was used reports intramedullary location of lymphoma in less than half the cases of spinal lymphoma, although it does not describe details on their MRI appearance.[207] Pathologic studies are in agreement with these imaging reports, reporting involvement of both extra- and intradural structures, including the spinal cord parenchyma and nerve roots.[159] There are also reports on specific infiltration of the nerves of the brachial plexus, forming mass-like lesions of the affected plexus, resembling a peripheral nerve sheath tumor, and extending into the subarachnoid space and spinal cord parenchyma proximally.[188,205] The MRI appearance of these lesions has not been reported, but one should keep this in mind when identifying mass-like lesions infiltrating the brachial plexus and extending into the vertebral canal in cats.

In dogs, lymphoma is one of the most common neoplasms, and the multicentric form accounts for about 80% of cases. In this species, lymphoma can affect the epidural tissues of the vertebral canal, vertebrae, nerve roots, paraspinal soft tissues, and less commonly the spinal cord (although the spinal cord is commonly affected secondary to compression by extradural neoplastic infiltrates).[173,206,208–214] At MRI, canine spinal lymphoma causes multifocal disease more commonly than focal disease.[208] There is common simultaneous regional involvement of multiple spinal compartments (vertebrae, paraspinal soft tissues, epidural space).[208,210,213,214] The paraspinal lesions are often ill defined. The vertebral canal and paraspinal components can be seen to communicate through the intervertebral foramens. There are variable degrees of spinal cord compression by the epidural component of the neoplasm.[208,213,214] Signal characteristics are similar for the lesions in the paraspinal and vertebral canal areas, being T1 iso- to hypointense, T2 and STIR hyperintense, moderately to strongly contrast enhancing.[208] In some cases, the lesions can be hyperintense on T1W precontrast images.[173,214] Heterogeneous signal on T2W images, with hypo- and hyperintense areas, is also reported,[213] as well as isointensity to surrounding muscles.[173] Visible vertebral lesions may involve none, one, several, or all vertebrae, and consist of patchy hyperintense areas on T2W images, which unlike fat, remain hyperintense on STIR images. In one case series, vertebral cortical involvement was not observed, even when paravertebral and epidural infiltration around the affected vertebrae was present[208]; however, other reports have described changes in shape of the affected vertebra with cortical involvement, seen as T2W and STIR hyperintense signal with enhancement on T1W postcontrast images, disrupting the normal hypointense signal of the cortex.[210] Cortical involvement has also been reported in pathologic studies.[211] Visible vertebral bone marrow involvement on MRI is not necessarily present, even in cases of simultaneous paravertebral and epidural infiltration.[213,214] Depending on the cellularity of the infiltrate, vertebral bone marrow involvement with lymphoma may be present even in the absence of changes in MRI signal, including on fat-suppressed images.[215] Leptomeningeal involvement with enhancement on postcontrast images is also reported,[206] as well as involvement of the nerve roots and spinal cord parenchyma.[212] Due to the multicentric nature of this tumor, additional lesions may be seen in the field of view, including lymphadenopathy, hepatomegaly, splenomegaly, and splenic nodules.

Hemangiosarcoma

Hemangiosarcoma is a malignant neoplasm of vascular endothelial origin and can arise from any vascular tissue. Spinal hemangiosarcoma has been reported in dogs, either in the intramedullary location,[173,196,216] or extradural location. The extradural form can arise from the vertebrae,[217,218] accounting for about 2% to 3% of primary bone tumors of the vertebral column in dogs. Rarely, hemangiosarcoma can affect the epidural space.[171,219] Intramedullary hemangiosarcoma is usually metastatic,[196,216] while the vertebral and the rare epidural forms are typically primary tumors.[166,169,220] Intradural/extramedullary hemangiosarcoma has only been reported once.[221]

MRI features of primary vertebral hemangiosarcoma include monostotic or segmental polyostotic lesions affecting several consecutive vertebrae. Signal intensity is variable and heterogeneous and signal voids due to susceptibility artifacts may be seen on T2*W images. Signal enhancement is usually strong and heterogeneous, and cortical lysis with extension into the vertebral canal and paraspinal tissues is common.[166,169,220]

At MRI, epidural or intramedullary hemangiosarcoma typically shows a focal mass lesion, usually well defined, that is either in the epidural location causing spinal cord compression, or intramedullary.[171,173,196,216,219] Epidural lesions are isolated (primary tumor),[169,171] whereas intramedullary lesions, being metastatic, can be multifocal.[196] The signal of the mass is typically hyperintense to normal spinal cord parenchyma on T2W images (homogeneous or heterogeneous), hyperintense on STIR images, isointense to hyperintense on T1W precontrast images, and moderately to strongly contrast enhancing (sometimes rim-like).[169,171] Signal voids associated with hemorrhage can be seen within the lesion on T2*W gradient echo images or susceptibility weighted imaging.[216] The spontaneous hyperintensity on T1W images may also reflect the presence of blood degradation products.

MYELOMALACIA

Myelomalacia corresponds to gross softening of the spinal cord resulting from hemorrhagic necrosis.[222,223] It can occur following acute spinal cord injury and is caused by extensive damage to intramedullary vasculature. A core of necrosis may extend cranially and caudally from the level of the spinal cord injury, typically in the base of the dorsal funiculi. A small proportion of dogs with acute disc extrusion will have diffuse myelomalacia, often called *ascending* or *descending myelomalacia.*[223] Myelomalacia can affect up to 10% of dogs with acute disc extrusion that exhibit paraplegia and loss of deep pain perception.[223] The prognosis for patients with myelomalacia is usually poor, but improvement is possible in focal disease. Therefore, MRI is useful in determining prognosis by providing information about the extent of involvement.

On MRI, myelomalacia is characterized by diffuse swelling of the spinal cord that is recognized by loss of visualization of the hyperintense signal from CSF and fat around the spinal cord on T2W images. There is diffuse patchy T2 hyperintensity of the spinal cord (Fig. 15.41) that extends over the length of several vertebral bodies. The affected spinal cord parenchyma is isointense to normal spinal cord on T1W images.[222] Areas of hypointensity associated with spinal cord hemorrhage may be visible in T2*W gradient recalled echo images.[223] In addition to the areas of T2 hyperintensity, areas of T2 hypointensity may be detected at high field strengths because of deoxyhemoglobin in hemorrhagic spinal cord foci.[222,223] Studies have suggested that in dogs with thoracolumbar disc herniation, a longitudinal extent of spinal cord parenchyma T2W hyperintensity higher than 4.5 to 6 times the length of L2 vertebral body could be a predictor of developing ascending/descending myelomalacia.[222,224] A length of CSF signal attenuation on HASTE/SSFSE pulse sequences ("T2-myelogram") >7.4 times the length of L2 vertebral body has also been reported as a predictive MRI criterion,[225] and some studies have found this criterion as more reliable than the length of parenchymal T2W hyperintensity.[226] Another recent study found that the length of parenchymal T2 hyperintensity was not a useful predictor for future development of myelomalacia in dogs with severe neurologic deficits who are not exhibiting clinical signs of myelomalacia.[227] Absence of T2W spinal cord hyperintensity, however, does not rule out future development of myelomalacia particularly if imaging occurs less than 24 hours after onset of paraplegia.[224,226,228,229]

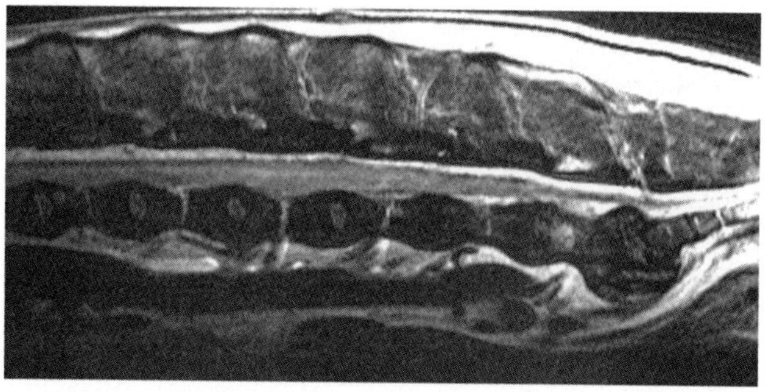

Fig. 15.41 Sagittal T2-weighted image of the lumbar spine in a dog with acute disc herniation at L5–L6 and secondary ascending myelomalacia. There is an ill-defined patchy intramedullary T2 hyperintensity in visible segments of the lumbar spinal cord.

VASCULAR PATHOLOGY

Ischemic Myelopathy

The most common cause of spinal cord ischemia and infarction in dogs and cats is fibrocartilaginous embolism from the *nucleus pulposus* of the intervertebral disc.[86,87,230–235] In cats, hyaline degeneration of the ventral spinal artery has also been reported as a predisposing factor.[233] In dogs other causes include thromboembolism; a hypercoagulable state; vasculopathy; and parasitic, septic, or neoplastic embolization.[230]

The typical clinical presentation is a sudden, frequently asymmetric, mono-, hemi-, or tetraparesis or tetraplegia.[236] Spinal cord thromboembolism is usually nonpainful and nonprogressive after the first 24 hours.[86,230–232] MRI is useful in recognizing changes associated with ischemic myelopathy and differentiating it from other conditions with similar clinical presentations, such as spinal trauma or intervertebral disc herniation.

Typically, there is a focal T2-hyperintense intramedullary lesion that is either T1 hypointense or T1 isointense. On transverse images, the lesion is usually asymmetric (Fig. 15.42, eFig. 15.11). The infarct can sometimes have variable contrast enhancement during the first week.[86,230,231] The lesion involves mostly gray matter, although a large number of dogs also have some white matter involvement. Focal areas of hypointensity suggestive of hemorrhage are identified occasionally on T2*W gradient recalled echo images or susceptibility-weighted imaging. Reduced field-of-view diffusion weighted imaging can help detect areas of restricted diffusion due to cytotoxic edema secondary to ischemia: these appear bright on diffusion-weighted images and dark on apparent diffusion coefficient maps.[237]

The imaging appearance of ischemic myelopathy can be somewhat similar to that seen with acute non-compressive hydrated nucleus pulposus extrusion, however with ischemic myelopathy the T2W hyperintense parenchymal lesions are typically not directly dorsal to an intervertebral disc, and have a more pronounced longitudinal extent; in addition, the epidural space is normal with ischemic myelopathy, whereas heterogeneous signal is often seen in the epidural space adjacent to the lesion with hydrated disc extrusion, due to diffusion of the extruded disc material mixed with the epidural fat. No abnormalities are seen on MR images in approximately 20% of patients. This usually happens when dogs are imaged less than 72 hours after onset of clinical signs.[231] The incidence of abnormal MRI findings is higher in nonambulatory dogs with higher neurologic scores than mildly affected dogs.[231] Dogs with clinically suspected ischemic myelopathy and no MRI changes have a good clinical outcome.[231]

On average, the length of the spinal cord T2 hyperintensity observed on sagittal MR images in dogs with ischemic myelopathy is approximately 1.8 times the length of C6 for cervical or cervicothoracic lesions and 2.2 times the length of L2 for thoracolumbar and lumbosacral lesions. There is an association between the length of spinal cord affected and severity of clinical signs.[231] A lesion-length–to–vertebral-length ratio greater than 2.0 has a sensitivity of 100% in predicting a poor clinical outcome.[231] The percentage cross-sectional area of the spinal cord with T2 hyperintensity is also associated with the severity of the clinical signs.[231] A percentage cross-sectional area of the lesion of more than 67% has a sensitivity of 100% in predicting poor clinical outcome.[231]

Vertebral Venous Plexus Pathology

Enlargement of the cervical vertebral venous system, including of the internal vertebral plexus causing spinal cord compression, has been reported in dogs, particularly sighthounds, although the etiology is unknown.[238] Enlargement of the internal vertebral plexus due to thrombosis or neoplastic infiltration with lymphoma and causing spinal cord compression has also been reported.[239,240]

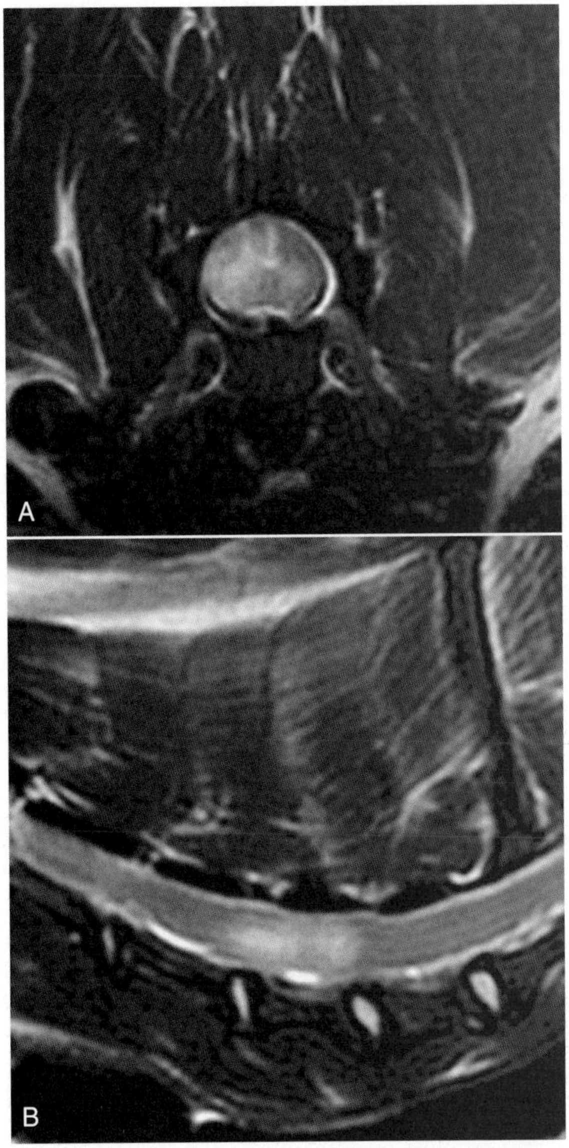

Fig. 15.42 Presumed fibrocartilaginous embolism in a dog. Transverse **(A)** and sagittal **(B)** T2-weighted images. There is a hazy focal hyperintense signal in the spinal cord that is asymmetric on the transverse image, involving both gray and white matter on the right and the ventral gray matter on the left. The intervertebral discs in the vicinity were normal, and there is no compression of the spinal cord. Clinical signs were acute and nonprogressive.

Spinal Hemorrhage

Intraparenchymal spinal cord hemorrhage most commonly occurs secondary to underlying pathology such as ischemic myelopathy, cord contusion such as secondary to disc herniation or trauma, coagulopathy, or neoplasia, particularly hemangiosarcoma.[169,216] Spontaneous intraparenchymal hemorrhage (primary hematomyelia) has been rarely reported in dogs.[241] Spinal cord hemorrhage may be difficult to identify at CT; however, areas of hyperattenuation in the spinal cord may be detected, particularly when using relatively narrow windows. MRI is more sensitive to detect spinal cord hemorrhage, especially when using pulse-sequences sensitive to such changes such as T2*W or susceptibility-weighted imaging (SWI).[216] On these pulse sequences, the byproducts of hemoglobin cause susceptibility artifacts that show up as areas of signal void with various degrees of blooming.[216]

Extraparenchymal hemorrhage can have an extradural (epidural) or more rarely intradural location. Focal hyperacute

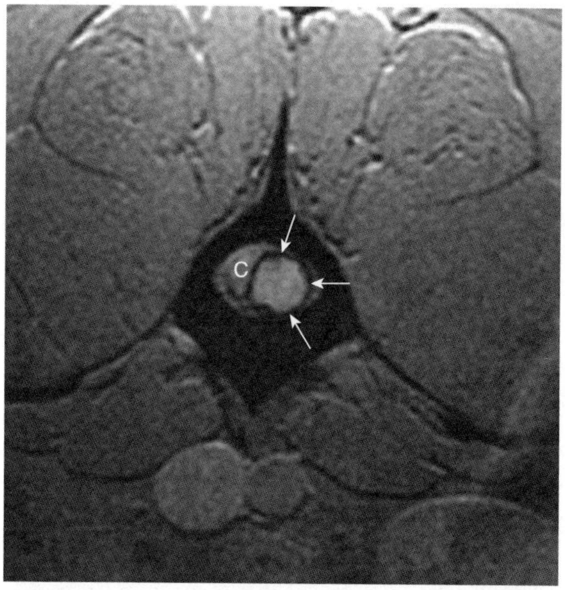

Fig. 15.43 Spontaneous epidural hematoma in a 4-year-old mixed-breed female dog presenting with acute paraplegia with no history of trauma. On this T2*-weighted gradient echo transverse image at the level of L4 vertebral body, there is a rounded extradural lesion (*arrows*) that is causing severe compression of the spinal cord (*c*). A rim of signal void is seen around the lesion consistent with hemorrhage.

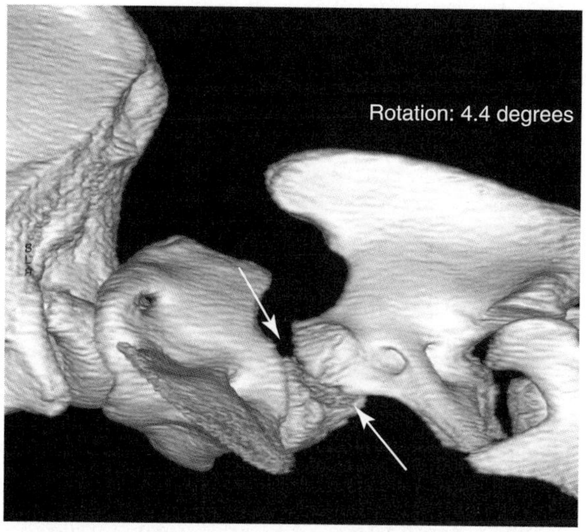

Fig. 15.44 Fracture of the cranial extremity of C2 in a dog. Three-dimensional volume rendering of the cranial cervical spine where the mildly displaced complete transverse fracture of the cranial apex of C2 (*white arrows*) can be seen.

intradural extramedullary hemorrhage causing cord compression has been reported in a dog with presumed steroid-responsive meningitis arteritis; the lesion was rounded, iso- to slightly T1W hyperintense and hyperintense on T2W, gradient echo, and T2-FLAIR, with strong homogeneous enhancement on postcontrast T1W images; the hyperintense signal on gradient echo was attributed to peracute arterial bleeding, characterized by high concentration of diamagnetic oxyhemoglobin in the erythrocytes (as opposed to the paramagnetic byproducts of hemoglobin degradation seen in later stages of hemorrhage).[242] Spontaneous extraparenchymal hematomas causing spinal cord compression have been reported in dogs.[243] They are most commonly extradural, rarely intradural. They present as compressive, variably shaped lesions that are T2W-hyperintense, iso- to mildly T1W-hyperintense, with susceptibility artifacts on T2*W images and rare contrast enhancement (Fig. 15.43). Laceration of the internal vertebral plexus secondary to disc extrusion can also cause epidural hemorrhage and contribute to spinal cord compression and inflammatory changes; these were described in the paragraph covering disc herniation.[22,44,45]

SPINAL TRAUMA

Acute spinal trauma can cause unstable spinal injuries that have the potential to lead to failure of the vertebral column to protect the spinal cord and nerve roots from severe insult. Resultant myelopathy and radiculopathy can lead to temporary or permanent paralysis. Rapid and accurate evaluation of the vertebral column and the status of the spinal cord facilitate appropriate treatment and a better-informed prognosis. Radiography is inadequate to rule out acute vertebral fractures and subluxations and is a poor diagnostic tool to assess the stability of spinal fractures. Survey radiography also cannot be used reliably to detect compressive lesions. CT is recommended in patients with a high clinical suspicion of acute fracture and is superior to radiography in the traumatized patient.[244] Multidetector scanners now provide the ability to obtain 1 mm or submillimeter CT images in a short time, and to perform high-quality multiplanar reformatted images with surface and volume rendering (Fig. 15.44). This enables depiction of complex fractures in a three-dimensional format that can assist in surgical planning.[2] The short acquisition time makes it possible to perform a CT study with the anesthetized or sedated patient strapped to a spinal board, thus protecting against further damage.[244]

In canine spinal trauma, MRI can provide helpful information on the location and extent of damage to supportive soft tissue structures and can enable assessment of spinal cord injury in dogs with suspected vertebral instability associated with fracture or subluxation.[245] However, comparative studies between MRI and CT found limited agreement between the two techniques for vertebral fractures, with up to 79% of fractures missed at MRI. Therefore, MRI and CT may be seen as complementary techniques to assess spinal trauma.[246]

INFLAMMATORY/INFECTIOUS CONDITIONS

Discospondylitis

Discospondylitis is infection of two adjacent vertebral endplates and the associated intervertebral disc; *Staphylococcus* spp. is the most frequently isolated organism. Traditionally, discospondylitis was diagnosed based on characteristic radiographic changes together with laboratory findings. A limitation of radiography is the delay of up to a few weeks between the onset of clinical signs and detection of radiographic changes. There is also a discrepancy between clinical and radiographic improvement during recovery.[247]

CT and MRI can be used to confirm a tentative diagnosis of discospondylitis.[248–255] CT features include adjacent endplates erosion, multifocal lytic changes extending into the vertebral bodies, periosteal proliferation adjacent to the affected disc, narrowing or collapse of the disc space.[256] Dorsal and sagittal reformatting is important to identify subtle endplate changes, particularly in juvenile dogs where the only initial change may be a narrowed disc space without significant endplates changes.[257] Compared with CT, MRI can assess the soft tissue components of the vertebral canal including the epidural structures and spinal cord, and thereby provide additional information on degree of involvement of these structures and presence and degree of spinal cord compression. MRI can reveal changes suggestive of discospondylitis in dogs that have normal radiographs, thereby allowing an earlier diagnosis in dogs with supportive clinical signs but equivocal radiographs (Fig. 15.45).[248]

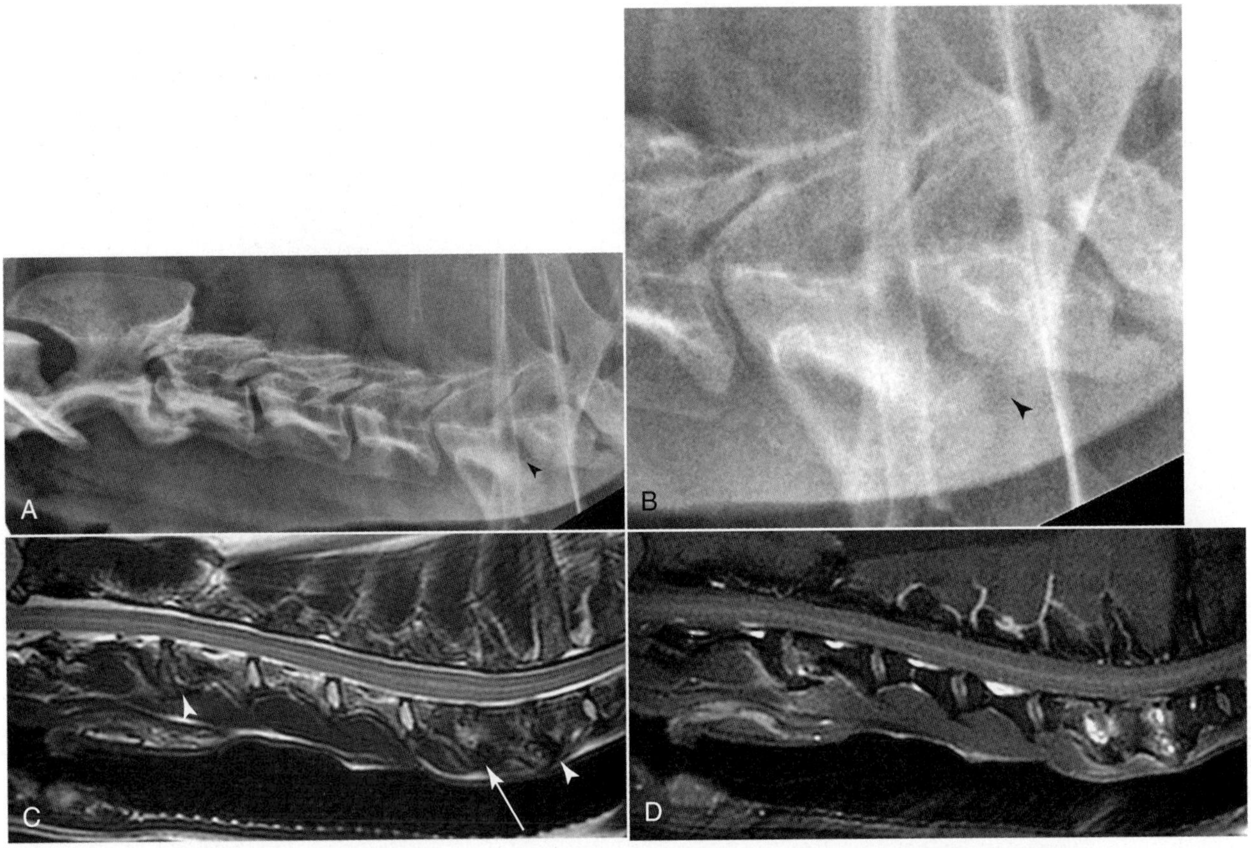

Fig. 15.45 Lateral radiograph of the cervical spine **(A)**, close-up radiograph of C6–C7 **(B)**, sagittal T2-weighted **(C)**, and postcontrast fat saturated T1-weighted **(D)** images in a dog with fever and cervical pain. Characteristic radiographic changes consistent with discospondylitis were present at C6–C7 (*black arrowheads* in **A** and **B**). On the magnetic resonance images, there was irregularity and lysis of the cortical bone around that space (*white arrow* in C), and the bone marrow of C6 and C7 has a mixture of increased and decreased intensity on T2-weighted images **(C)**. However, additional lesions are present at C2–C3 and C7–T1 that are also characterized by loss of integrity of the endplates and abnormal bone marrow signal in the vertebral bodies with loss of the normal structure of the intervertebral disc spaces (*white arrowheads* in **C**). On the postcontrast fat-saturated T1-weighted images **(D)**, there is enhancement of the vertebral bodies around the endplates of these three spaces, as well as of the paravertebral soft tissues ventral to the disc spaces, indicative of inflammation. These changes are consistent with discospondylitis, not only at C6–C7 but also at C2–C3 and C7–T1. Lesions of discospondylitis can be detected earlier with MR images than with radiography.

Typical MRI changes seen with discospondylitis include the following (see Fig. 15.45)[248–252,255,257,258]:

- Abnormal T1 hypointensity and T2 hypointensity of adjacent endplates and bone marrow; these lesions are hyperintense on T2W STIR images
- Hyperintense disc on T2W images
- Contrast enhancement of the intervertebral disc, vertebral endplates, and paravertebral soft tissues
- Endplate erosion is usually present, but in early stages where endplate erosion is absent, the only change may be T2 and STIR hyperintensity of bone marrow adjacent to the end-plates
- Spinal cord compression caused by extension of the infection to the epidural space
- Vertebral subluxation on sagittal images

Discospondylitis caused by *Brucella canis* infection has been reported to cause imaging changes that may be unique to this etiology; affected dogs are often young with multifocal lesions. Smooth, round, central endplate lytic changes, defined as "hole punch" lesions, can be seen on sagittal images and vertebral physitis or spondylitis without discitis may be seen; these can be identified as hyperintense vertebral lesions affecting the vertebral bodies on T2W or STIR images, with enhancement on postcontrast T1W images (best appreciated with fat saturation). Paravertebral inflammation with similar signal characteristics is also frequently seen.[259]

Spinal Epidural Empyema

Spinal epidural empyema is presence of a suppurative lesion in the epidural space.[255,260–263] The clinical signs include fever, pain, and progressive neurologic dysfunction. Spinal empyema is relatively rare in dogs. Causes include extension of adjacent osteomyelitis or discospondylitis or hematogenous spread.

On noncontrast CT, an epidural mass is suspected based on lack of visualization of hypoattenuating epidural fat around the spinal cord, but the epidural mass is best identified with CT myelography.[261,262] Intrathecal contrast medium injection can facilitate spread of the infection in the subarachnoid space because of iatrogenic contamination.

MRI is better for diagnosing spinal empyema, because it does not require subarachnoid injection of contrast medium.[255,260,263] Spinal empyema appears as a well-defined epidural mass in the dorsal or ventral aspect of the vertebral canal. The lesion forms a high or mixed signal mass on T2W images but is usually T1-hypointense. A peripheral, rim-like pattern of contrast enhancement or a diffuse pattern of

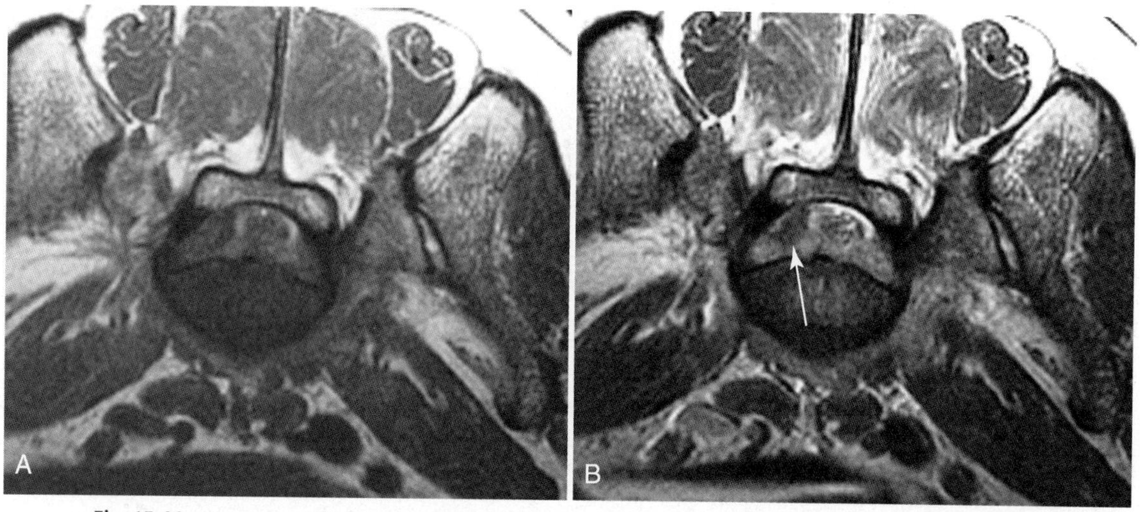

Fig. 15.46 Precontrast **(A)** and postcontrast **(B)** transverse T1-weighted images in the lumbosacral area in a dog with lumbosacral discospondylitis and spinal epidural empyema. The vertebral canal is filled with heterogeneous material that enhances irregularly, with a hypointense nonenhancing area on the right consistent with fluid collection (*white arrow*). Epidural empyema caused by extension of the infectious process from the disc space into the caudal lumbar vertebral canal was confirmed at surgery.

enhancement can be noted (Fig. 15.46). If T2*W gradient recalled echo images are acquired, focal hypointense areas consistent with hemorrhage may be present. Hyperintense lesions in the gray matter of the spinal cord adjacent to the epidural mass can be seen, which may be caused by compression of the spinal cord by the mass or by vascular compromise.[260]

Meningomyelitis

Meningitis and myelitis can have an infectious or noninfectious origin.[264–272] Infectious agents in dogs include viruses (e.g., canine distemper), bacteria (e.g., *Staphylococcus*, *Pasteurella*, *Actinomyces*, and *Nocardia* spp.), fungi (e.g., *Cryptococcus*, *Blastomyces*, *Histoplasma*, and *Coccidioides* spp.), Rickettsiae (e.g., *Ehrlichia* spp., *Rickettsia rickettsii*), protozoa (e.g., *Toxoplasma gondii*, *Neospora caninum*), parasites (e.g., *Dirofilaria immitis*, *Angiostrongylus* spp.), and rarely algae (e.g., *Prototheca wickerhamii*, *Prototheca zopfii*).[267] In cats, feline infectious peritonitis and toxoplasmosis have been reported.[207]

Noninfectious causes of canine meningomyelitis include granulomatous meningoencephalomyelitis, pyogranulomatous meningoencephalomyelitis, and steroid-responsive meningitis arteritis.[265–267,270–272]

CT changes in dogs with meningomyelitis include spinal cord swelling, spinal cord hypoattenuation, and occasionally intramedullary or meningeal contrast enhancement.[266]

General MRI findings in dogs and cats with meningomyelitis include irregular areas of intramedullary T2 hyperintensity (Fig. 15.47), which are isointense or hypointense on precontrast T1W images and have various degrees of contrast enhancement.[264,265,267] Meningeal enhancement may or may not be present. The use of fat suppression on postcontrast spinal images is important in animals with a clinical suspicion of inflammatory pathology, as it may facilitate the recognition of subtle meningeal enhancement.[176,273]

Cervical MRI abnormalities are quite common in dogs with steroid-responsive meningitis arteritis, and include T1W postcontrast enhancement of the meninges, synovium of the articular process joints, and paravertebral muscles with less commonly spinal cord parenchymal enhancement.[273]

Intradural hemorrhage causing cord compression has also been reported (see "Spinal Hemorrhage" section).[242]

In general, MRI changes of meningomyelitis are nonspecific, and other conditions (such as myelomalacia, ischemic myelopathy, or some neoplastic conditions such as histiocytic sarcoma[202] or lymphosarcoma[207,264]) can produce similar changes. Therefore, correlation with clinical signs and laboratory test results is necessary.

VERTEBRAL ANOMALIES

Congenital anomalies of the spine that can be assessed with CT or MRI include atlantoaxial malformation, hemivertebrae, block vertebrae, butterfly vertebrae, transitional vertebrae, and spina bifida (see Fig. 15.30). Most of these anomalies can be diagnosed radiographically (see Chapter 14); however, CT and MRI can provide important additional information. CT provides a better understanding of the bony abnormality and spatial relationship between the abnormal and adjacent vertebrae and effect of the anomaly on the vertebral canal and intervertebral foramina (Fig. 15.48). MRI is indicated when assessment of the spinal cord and associated nerve roots is desired, especially when the consequences of the vertebral anomalies need to be assessed. For example, spina bifida can be associated with focal anomalies of the spinal cord and meninges in the form of a meningocele or myelomeningocele (see Fig. 15.30).[274]

Dysplasia or aplasia of the caudal articular processes in the thoracic spine is common in some breeds such as French and English bulldogs and even more so in pugs.[275] In pugs, several studies have suggested that the condition can be associated with spinal cord pathology in the caudal thoracic spine,[139,276–279] although some studies have questioned that association.[275,280] The spectrum of evidence in that breed, however, suggests that spinal instability associated with the malformation can lead to constrictive myelopathy (dorsal or circumferential) secondary to meningeal fibrosis, and development of compressive arachnoid diverticulum cranial to the constriction.[139,276–279] Concurrent spinal cord compression by disc herniation has also been described.[278] The absence or hypoplasia of the caudal articular processes is best

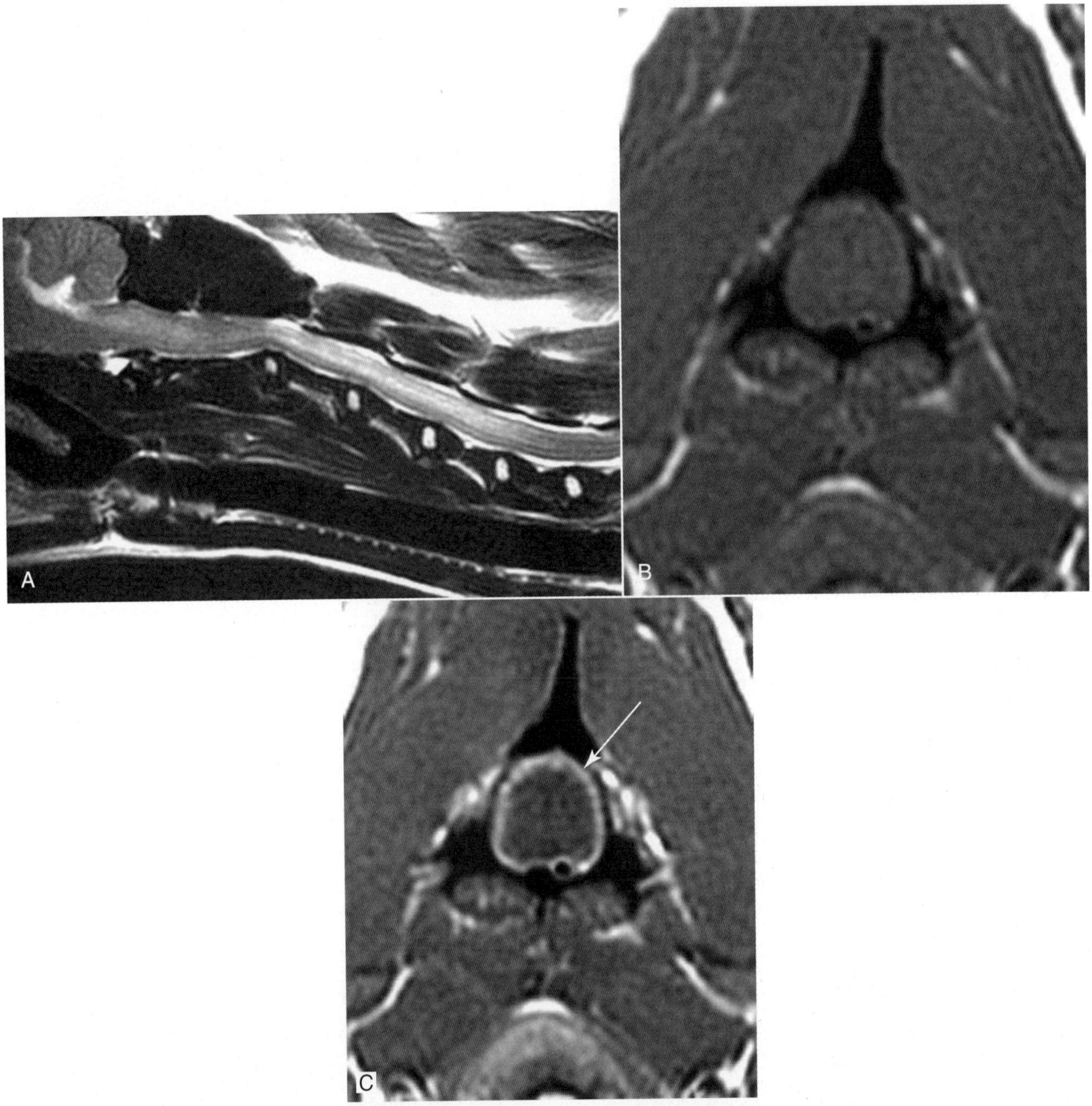

Fig. 15.47 Sagittal T2-weighted **(A)**, transverse precontrast T1-weighted **(B)**, and transverse postcontrast T1-weighted **(C)** images at the level of C2 in a dog with meningomyelitis caused by *Cryptococcus* infection. On the T2-weighted image, extensive ill-defined areas of T2 hyperintensity are present **(A)**. On the postcontrast T1-weighted image, there is strong contrast enhancement (**C,** *white arrow*) of the meninges compared with the precontrast image at the same level **(B)**.

demonstrated with CT given its exquisite bony detail (Fig. 15.49). However, the secondary spinal cord pathology is best demonstrated by MRI. Arachnoid diverticula are easily identified with MRI (see earlier). Meningeal fibrosis causes irregular margination of the subarachnoid space best seen on T2W images, and enhancing meningeal thickening on T1W postcontrast images, located either dorsally or circumferentially.[139,276–279] Focal T2W spinal cord parenchyma hyperintensity is commonly seen. Some studies also reported ventral extradural compression that is V-shaped on transverse images, corresponding histopathologically to areas of fibrosis and chondroid metaplasia.[277]

SYRINGOMYELIA

Syringomyelia is the development of fluid-filled cavities in the spinal cord. It can be caused by various primary problems, including abnormalities of the caudal fossa (Chiari-like malformations), but also other conditions, such as a quadrigeminal cistern cyst, tethered spinal cord, trauma, arachnoiditis, and neoplasia. Any condition that results in altered CSF flow in the caudal fossa of the skull or in the vertebral column can result in the development of a syrinx.[130,281–309]

Chiari-like malformation is common in the Cavalier King Charles spaniel but is reported in other breeds as well.[310] The

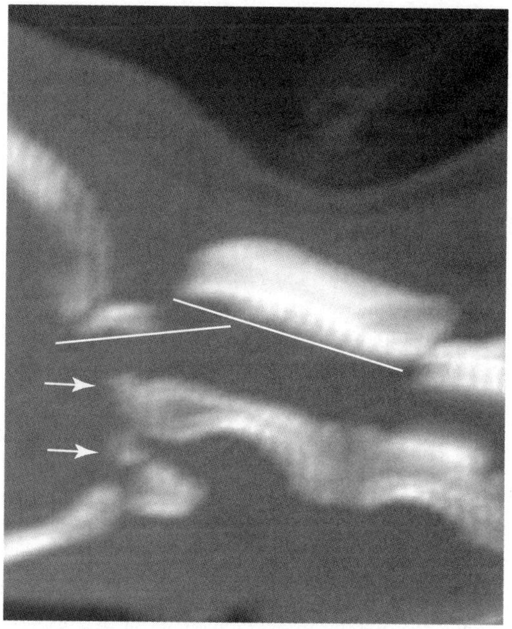

Fig. 15.48 Reformatted sagittal computed tomography (CT) image of the cranial aspect of the cervical spine, in a dog with atlantoaxial instability. The dorsal lamina of C1 is not aligned with the dorsal aspect of the vertebral canal of C2 (*lines*) indicating subluxation. Small bone fragments are associated with the dens (*white arrows*).

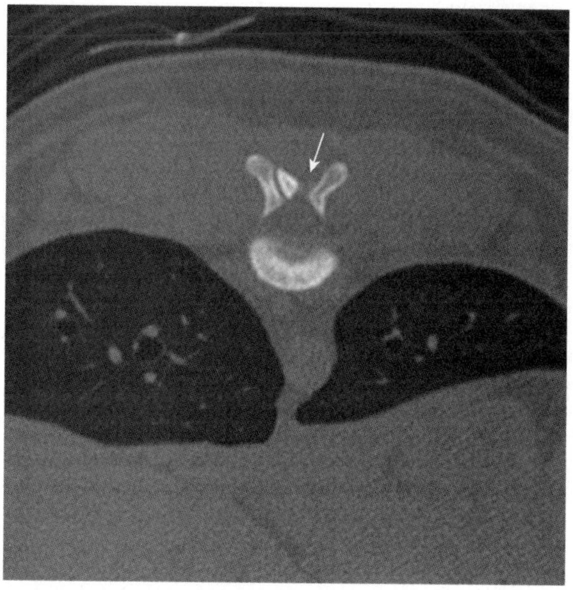

Fig. 15.49 Transverse CT image in a bone window at the level of T11–T12 in a 7-year-old pug. There is complete aplasia of the left caudal articular process of T11 (*arrow*).

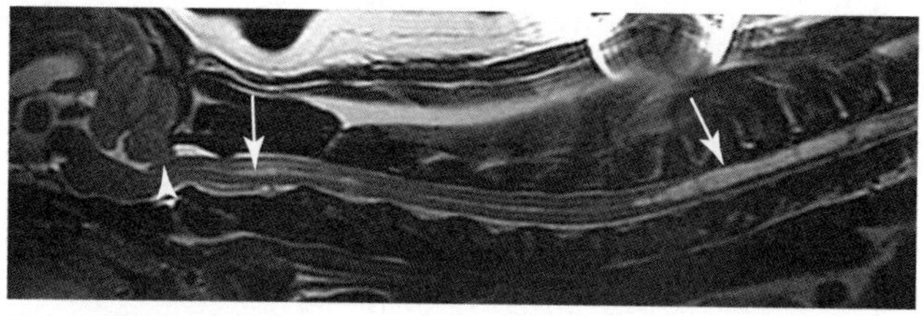

Fig. 15.50 Sagittal T2-weighted image of the caudal brain and cervical spine in a Cavalier King Charles spaniel with Chiari-like malformation and syringomyelia. The caudal fossa is small, causing overcrowding and caudal herniation of the cerebellum into the foramen magnum (*white arrowhead*). There are multiple areas of elongated irregular dilation of the central canal (*white arrows*) in the cervical and cranial thoracic aspects of the spinal cord that form a long syrinx, more pronounced in the thoracic spine.

basioccipital bone is presumed to be short, resulting in a reduced caudal fossa volume. This causes the caudal aspect of the cerebellar vermis and medulla to extend into or through the foramen magnum causing obstruction of CSF flow. CSF displaced by each systolic cycle through the compressed subarachnoid space results in a high-velocity jet, and this causes an abnormal pressure differential between the spinal cord and subarachnoid space in the cervical area.[289,290,293,303] There is a relative increase in intramedullary pressure and decrease in subarachnoid pressure, the consequence of which is repeated mechanical distention of the spinal cord. This in turn results in fluid accumulation in the spinal cord, with cavitation and accumulation of extracellular fluid that coalesces eventually into elongated cavities and syrinx formation; these cavities are commonly separate from the central canal.[289,303]

MRI is a good modality to assess the presence and extent of the syrinx.[284] The syrinx may take the form of a cavity or be complex with septations. A portion of the central canal is usually involved at some level. The longitudinal extent of the syrinx can be evaluated on sagittal images, appearing T2-hyperintense and T1-hypointense (Fig. 15.50). In Chiari-like malformation, the cerebellar vermis and medulla extend into or through the foramen magnum, which is occluded with little or no CSF around neural structures. The magnitude of cerebellar herniation is not correlated with severity. There is typically ventricular dilatation. The cranial cervical and cranial thoracic segments of the spinal cord are typically the most severely affected by the syrinx. Maximum syrinx width is the strongest predictor of pain, scratching behavior, and scoliosis; 95% of Cavalier King Charles spaniels with a maximum syrinx width of 0.64 cm or more will have associated clinical signs,[302] although myelopathic signs develop as soon as the syrinx reaches 4 mm width.[311] Larger syringes with involvement of the dorsal horns of the gray matter of the spinal cord and asymmetrical appearance on transverse images may be associated with persistent neuropathic pain, although the relative contribution of the asymmetry and syrinx size is controversial.[302,312]

REFERENCES

1. Gavin PR. Growth of clinical veterinary magnetic resonance imaging. *Vet Radiol Ultrasound*. 2011;52:S2–S4.
2. Robertson I, Thrall DE. Imaging dogs with suspected disc herniation: pros and cons of myelography, computed tomography, and magnetic resonance. *Vet Radiol Ultrasound*. 2011;52:S81–S84.
3. Evans H. *Miller's Anatomy of the Dog*. 3rd ed. Philadelphia: WB Saunders; 1993.
4. Kent M, Glass EN, Song RB, et al. Anatomic description and clinical relevance of the meningovertebral ligament in dogs. *J Am Vet Med Assoc*. 2019;255:687–694.
5. Pardo A, Morgan J. Myelography in the cat: a comparison of cisternal versus lumbar puncture, using metrizamide. *Vet Radiol*. 1988;29:89.
6. Morgan JP, Atilola M, Bailey CS. Vertebral canal and spinal cord mensuration: a comparative study of its effect on lumbosacral myelography in the dachshund and German shepherd dog. *J Am Vet Med Assoc*. 1987;191:951–957.
7. Scrivani PV, Barthez PY, Leveille R, et al. Subdural injection of contrast medium during cervical myelography. *Vet Radiol Ultrasound*. 1997;38:267–271.
8. Jones JC, Cartee RE, Bartels JE. Computed tomographic anatomy of the canine lumbosacral spine. *Vet Radiol Ultrasound*. 1995;36:91–99.

9. Sharp NJH, Med BV, Cofone M, et al. Computed tomography in the evaluation of caudal cervical spondylomyelopathy of the Doberman Pinscher. *Vet Radiol Ultrasound.* 1995;36:100–108.
10. Adams WH, Daniel GB, Pardo AD, et al. Magnetic resonance imaging of the caudal lumbar and lumbosacral spine in 13 dogs (1990–1993). *Vet Radiol Ultrasound.* 1995;36:3–13.
11. Seiler G, Hani H, Scheidegger J, et al. Staging of lumbar intervertebral disc degeneration in nonchondrodystrophic dogs using low-field magnetic resonance imaging. *Vet Radiol Ultrasound.* 2003;44:179–184.
12. Pease A, Sullivan S, Olby N, et al. Value of a single-shot turbo spin-echo pulse sequence for assessing the architecture of the subarachnoid space and the constitutive nature of cerebrospinal fluid. *Vet Radiol Ultrasound.* 2006;47:254–259.
13. Seiler GS, Robertson ID, Mai W, et al. Usefulness of a half-Fourier acquisition single-shot turbo spin-echo pulse sequence in identifying arachnoid diverticula in dogs. *Vet Radiol Ultrasound.* 2012;53:157–161.
14. Adams WH. The spine. *Clin Tech Sm Anim Pract.* 1999;14:148–159.
15. Chang Y, Dennis R, Platt SR, et al. Magnetic resonance imaging of traumatic intervertebral disc extension in dogs. *Vet Rec.* 2007;160:795–799.
16. Hansen H. A pathologic-anatomical study on disc degeneration in the dog. *Acta Orthop Scand.* 1952;Suppl.
17. Besalti O, Pekcan Z, Sirin YS, et al. Magnetic resonance imaging findings in dogs with thoracolumbar intervertebral disk disease: 69 cases (1997–2005). *J Am Vet Med Assoc.* 2006;228:902–908.
18. De Decker S, Gomes SA, Packer RM, et al. Evaluation of magnetic resonance imaging guidelines for differentiation between thoracolumbar intervertebral disk extrusions and intervertebral disk protrusions in dogs. *Vet Radiol Ultrasound.* 2016;57:526–533.
19. Gomes SA, Volk HA, Packer RM, et al. Clinical and magnetic resonance imaging characteristics of thoracolumbar intervertebral disk extrusions and protrusions in large breed dogs. *Vet Radiol Ultrasound.* 2016;57:417–426.
20. Fenn J, Olby NJ. Consortium. CSCI: classification of intervertebral disc disease. *Front Vet Sci.* 2020;7:579025.
21. Tartarelli CL, Baroni M, Borghi M. Thoracolumbar disc extrusion associated with extensive epidural haemorrhage: a retrospective study of 23 dogs. *J Small Anim Pract.* 2005;46:485–490.
22. Woelfel CW, Robertson JB, Mariani CL, et al. Outcomes and prognostic indicators in 59 paraplegic medium to large breed dogs with extensive epidural hemorrhage secondary to thoracolumbar disc extrusion. *Vet Surg.* 2021;50:527–536.
23. Hay CW, Muir P. Tearing of the dura mater in three dogs. *Vet Rec.* 2000;146:279–282.
24. Kent M, Holmes S, Cohen ELI, et al. CT myelography in a dog with intramedullary intervertebral disc herniation. *Vet Radiol Ultrasound.* 2011;52:185–187.
25. Kitagawa M, Okada M, Kanayama K, et al. Identification of ventrolateral intramedullary intervertebral disc herniation in a dog. *J S Afr Vet Assoc.* 2012;83:103.
26. McConnell JF, Garosi LS. Intramedullary intervertebral disk extrusion in a cat. *Vet Radiol Ultrasound.* 2004;45:327–330.
27. De Risio L, Adams V, Dennis R, et al. Association of clinical and magnetic resonance imaging findings with outcome in dogs with presumptive acute noncompressive nucleus pulposus extrusion: 42 cases (2000–2007). *J Am Vet Med Assoc.* 2009;234:495–504.
28. McKee WM, Downes CJ, Pink JJ, et al. Presumptive exercise-associated peracute thoracolumbar disc extrusion in 48 dogs. *Vet Rec.* 2010;166:523–528.
29. Beltran E, Dennis R, Doyle V, et al. Clinical and magnetic resonance imaging features of canine compressive cervical myelopathy with suspected hydrated nucleus pulposus extrusion. *J Small Anim Pract.* 2012;53:101–107.
30. Hamilton T, Glass E, Drobatz K, et al. Severity of spinal cord dysfunction and pain associated with hydrated nucleus pulposus extrusion in dogs. *Vet Comp Orthop Traumatol.* 2014;27:313–318.
31. Manunta ML, Evangelisti MA, Bergknut N, et al. Hydrated nucleus pulposus herniation in seven dogs. *Vet J.* 2015;203:342–344.
32. Falzone C. Canine acute cervical myelopathy: hydrated nucleus pulposus extrusion or intraspinal discal cysts? *Vet Surg.* 2017;46:376–380.
33. Kang BJ, Jung Y, Park S, et al. Discal cysts of the cervical spine in two dogs. *J Vet Sci.* 2015;16:543–545.
34. Konar M, Lang J, Fluhmann G, et al. Ventral intraspinal cysts associated with the intervertebral disc: magnetic resonance imaging observations in seven dogs. *Vet Surg.* 2008;37:94–101.
35. Drees R, Dennison SE, Keuler NS, et al. Computed tomographic imaging protocol for the canine cervical and lumbar spine. *Vet Radiol Ultrasound.* 2009;50:74–79.
36. Olby NJ, Munana KR, Sharp NJ, et al. The computed tomographic appearance of acute thoracolumbar intervertebral disc herniations in dogs. *Vet Radiol Ultrasound.* 2000;41:396–402.
37. Olby NJ, Dyce J, Houlton JEF. Correlation of plain radiographic and lumbar myelographic findings with surgical findings in thoracolumbar disc disease. *J Small Anim Pract.* 1994;35:345–350.
38. Dennison SE, Drees R, Rylander H, et al. Evaluation of different computed tomography techniques and myelography for the diagnosis of acute canine myelopathy. *Vet Radiol Ultrasound.* 2010;51:254–258.
39. Parry AT, Harris A, Upjohn MM, et al. Does choice of imaging modality affect outcome in dogs with thoracolumbar spinal conditions? *J Small Anim Pract.* 2010;51:312–317.
40. Cooper JJ, Young BD, Griffin JF, Fosgate GT. Comparison between noncontrast computed tomography and magnetic resonance imaging for detection and characterization of thoracolumbar myelopathy caused by intervertebral disk herniation in dogs. *Vet Radiol Ultrasound.* 2014;55:182–189.
41. Noyes JA, Thomovsky SA, Chen AV, et al. Magnetic resonance imaging versus computed tomography to plan hemilaminectomies in chondrodystrophic dogs with intervertebral disc extrusion. *Vet Surg.* 2017;46:1025–1031.
42. Levitski RE, Lipsitz D, Chauvet AE. Magnetic resonance imaging of the cervical spine in 27 dogs. *Vet Radiol Ultrasound.* 1999;40:332–341.
43. Naude SH, Lambrechts NE, Wagner WM, et al. Association of preoperative magnetic resonance imaging findings with surgical features in Dachshunds with thoracolumbar intervertebral disk extrusion. *J Am Vet Med Assoc.* 2008;232:702–708.
44. Mateo I, Lorenzo V, Foradada L, et al. Clinical, pathologic, and magnetic resonance imaging characteristics of canine disc extrusion accompanied by epidural hemorrhage or inflammation. *Vet Radiol Ultrasound.* 2011;52:17–24.
45. Bridges J, Windsor R, Stewart SD, et al. Prevalence and clinical features of thoracolumbar intervertebral disc-associated epidural hemorrhage in dogs. *J Vet Intern Med.* 2022;36:1365–1372.

46. Tidwell AS, Specht A, Blaeser L, et al. Magnetic resonance imaging features of extradural hematomas associated with intervertebral disc herniation in a dog. *Vet Radiol Ultrasound*. 2002;43:319–324.
47. Suran JN, Durham A, Mai W, et al. Contrast enhancement of extradural compressive material on magnetic resonance imaging. *Vet Radiol Ultrasound*. 2011;52:10–16.
48. Furtado ARR, Cherubini GB, Taeymans O. Low-field magnetic resonance changes in the paravertebral musculature of dogs with acute intervertebral disc extrusion. *J Small Anim Pract*. 2019;60:367–373.
49. Morrison EJ, Baron-Chapman ML, Chalkley M. MRI T2/STIR epaxial muscle hyperintensity in some dogs with intervertebral disc extrusion corresponds to histologic patterns of muscle degeneration and inflammation. *Vet Radiol Ultrasound*. 2021;62:150–160.
50. Trampus P, Goepfert C, Welle M, et al. Magnetic resonance imaging signal alterations in paraspinal muscles in dogs with acute thoracolumbar intervertebral disk extrusion. *Front Vet Sci*. 2018;5:16.
51. Beale CC, Secrest SA. MRI assessment of epaxial myosteatosis in dogs with intervertebral disc extrusions and associations with patient factors and outcome. *Vet Radiol Ultrasound*. 2021;62:687–696.
52. Lerer A, Nykamp SG, Harriss AB, et al. MRI-based relationships between spine pathology, intervertebral disc degeneration, and muscle fatty infiltration in chondrodystrophic and non-chondrodystrophic dogs. *Spine J*. 2015;15:2433–2439.
53. Ryan TM, Platt SR, Llabres-Diaz FJ, et al. Detection of spinal cord compression in dogs with cervical intervertebral disc disease by magnetic resonance imaging. *Vet Rec*. 2008;163:11–15.
54. Cherrone KL, Dewey CW, Coates JR, et al. A retrospective comparison of cervical intervertebral disk disease in nonchondrodystrophic large dogs versus small dogs. *J Am Anim Hosp Assoc*. 2004;40:316–320.
55. Hillman RB, Kengeri SS, Waters DJ. Reevaluation of predictive factors for complete recovery in dogs with nonambulatory tetraparesis secondary to cervical disk herniation. *J Am Anim Hosp Assoc*. 2009;45:155–163.
56. Silva S, Genain MA, Khan S, et al. The spinal cord-to-vertebral canal area ratio measured with computed tomography is lower in the thoracolumbar than the cervical region in French bulldogs. *J Am Vet Med Assoc*. 2022:1–4.
57. Penning V, Platt SR, Dennis R, et al. Association of spinal cord compression seen on magnetic resonance imaging with clinical outcome in 67 dogs with thoracolumbar intervertebral disc extrusion. *J Small Anim Pract*. 2006;47:644–650.
58. Gaitero L, Anor S. Cranial thoracic disc protrusions in three German Shepherd dogs. *Vet J*. 2009;182:349–351.
59. Gaitero L, Nykamp S, Daniel R, et al. Comparison between cranial thoracic intervertebral disc herniations in German shepherd dogs and other large breed dogs. *Vet Radiol Ultrasound*. 2013;54:133–138.
60. Jaderlund KJ, Hansson K, Lindberg R, et al. T3-T4 disc herniation in a German shepherd dog. *Vet Rec*. 2002;151:769–770.
61. Israel SK, Levine JM, Kerwin SC, et al. The relative sensitivity of computed tomography and myelography for identification of thoracolumbar intervertebral disk herniations in dogs. *Vet Radiol Ultrasound*. 2009;50:247–252.
62. Levine JM, Fosgate GT, Chen AV, et al. Magnetic resonance imaging in dogs with neurologic impairment due to acute thoracic and lumbar intervertebral disk herniation. *J Vet Intern Med*. 2009;23:1220–1226.
63. Ito D, Matsunaga S, Jeffery ND, et al. Prognostic value of magnetic resonance imaging in dogs with paraplegia caused by thoracolumbar intervertebral disk extrusion: 77 cases (2000–2003). *J Am Vet Med Assoc*. 2005;227:1454–1460.
64. Ruddle TL, Allen DA, Schertel ER, et al. Outcome and prognostic factors in non-ambulatory Hansen Type I intervertebral disc extrusions: 308 cases. *Vet Comp Orthop Traumatol*. 2006;19:29–34.
65. Wang-Leandro A, Siedenburg JS, Hobert MK, et al. Comparison of preoperative quantitative magnetic resonance imaging and clinical assessment of deep pain perception as prognostic tools for early recovery of motor function in paraplegic dogs with intervertebral disk herniations. *J Vet Intern Med*. 2017;31:842–848.
66. Freeman P. Sacrococcygeal intervertebral disc extrusion in a dachshund. *Vet Rec*. 2010;167:618–619.
67. Lawson CM, Reichle JK, McKlveen T, et al. Imaging findings in dogs with caudal intervertebral disc herniation. *Vet Radiol Ultrasound*. 2011;52:487–491.
68. Jones JC, Banfield CM, Ward DL. Association between postoperative outcome and results of magnetic resonance imaging and computed tomography in working dogs with degenerative lumbosacral stenosis. *J Am Vet Med Assoc*. 2000;216:1769–1774.
69. Bresciani L, Trevail R, Clarke S, et al. Lumbosacral intervertebral disk extrusions in 13 dogs. *Vet Surg*. 2021;50:823–832.
70. Jones EC, Sorjonen DC, Simpson ST, et al. Comparison between computed tomographic and surgical findings in nine large-breed dogs with lumbosacral stenosis. *Vet Radiol Ultrasound*. 1996;37:247–256.
71. Jones JC, Inzana KD. Subclinical CT abnormalities in the lumbosacral spine of older large-breed dogs. *Vet Radiol Ultrasound*. 2000;41:19–26.
72. Jones JC, Wilson ME, Bartels JE. A review of high resolution computed tomography and a proposed technique for regional examination of the canine lumbosacral spine. *Vet Radiol Ultrasound*. 1994;35:339–346.
73. Jones JC, Wright JC, Bartels JE. Computed tomographic morphometry of the lumbosacral spine of dogs. *Am J Vet Res*. 1995;56:1125–1132.
74. Ramirez 3rd O, Thrall DE. A review of imaging techniques for canine cauda equina syndrome. *Vet Radiol Ultrasound*. 1998;39:283–296.
75. Suwankong N, Voorhout G, Hazewinkel HA, et al. Agreement between computed tomography, magnetic resonance imaging, and surgical findings in dogs with degenerative lumbosacral stenosis. *J Am Vet Med Assoc*. 2006;229:1924–1929.
76. Rapp M, Ley CJ, Hansson K, et al. Postoperative computed tomography and low-field magnetic resonance imaging findings in dogs with degenerative lumbosacral stenosis treated by dorsal laminectomy. *Vet Comp Orthop Traumatol*. 2017;30:143–152.
77. Bersan E, McConnell F, Trevail R, et al. Cervical intervertebral foraminal disc extrusion in dogs: clinical presentation, MRI characteristics and outcome after medical management. *Vet Rec*. 2015;176:597.
78. Chambers JN, Selcer BA, Sullivan SA, et al. Diagnosis of lateralized lumbosacral disk herniation with magnetic resonance imaging. *J Am Anim Hosp Assoc*. 1997;33:296–299.
79. Fadda A, Lang J, Forterre F. Far lateral lumbar disc extrusion: MRI findings and surgical treatment. *Vet Comp Orthop Traumatol*. 2013;26:318–322.

80. Silva S, Guevar J, Jose-Lopez R, et al. Clinical signs, MRI findings and long-term outcomes of foraminal and far lateral thoracolumbar intervertebral disc herniations in dogs. *Vet Rec*. 2022;190:e1529.
81. Mouradian-Darby AE, Young BD, Griffin JF, et al. Lymphocytic ganglioneuritis secondary to intervertebral disc extrusion in a dog. *J Small Anim Pract*. 2014;55:471–474.
82. Liptak JM, Allan GS, Krockenberger MB, et al. Radiographic diagnosis: intramedullary extrusion of an intervertebral disc. *Vet Radiol Ultrasound*. 2002;43:272–274.
83. Lu D, Lamb CR, Wesselingh K, et al. Acute intervertebral disc extrusion in a cat: clinical and MRI findings. *J Feline Med Surg*. 2002;4:65–68.
84. McKee WM, Downes CJ. Rupture of the dura mater in two dogs caused by the peracute extrusion of a cervical disc. *Vet Rec*. 2008;162:479–481.
85. Sanders SG, Bagley RS, Gavin PR. Intramedullary spinal cord damage associated with intervertebral disk material in a dog. *J Am Vet Med Assoc*. 2002;221:1594–1596, 1574-1595.
86. De Risio L. A Review of fibrocartilaginous embolic myelopathy and different types of peracute non-compressive intervertebral disk extrusions in dogs and cats. *Front Vet Sci*. 2015;2:24.
87. Fenn J, Drees R, Volk HA, et al. Inter- and intraobserver agreement for diagnosing presumptive ischemic myelopathy and acute noncompressive nucleus pulposus extrusion in dogs using magnetic resonance imaging. *Vet Radiol Ultrasound*. 2015;57:33–40.
88. Chow K, Beatty JA, Voss K, et al. Probable lumbar acute non-compressive nucleus pulposus extrusion in a cat with acute onset paraparesis. *J Feline Med Surg*. 2012;14: 764–767.
89. Packer RA, Frank PM, Chambers JN. Traumatic subarachnoid-pleural fistula in a dog. *Vet Radiol Ultrasound*. 2004;45:523–527.
90. Kamishina H, Ogawa H, Katayama M, et al. Spontaneous regression of a cervical intraspinal cyst in a dog. *J Vet Med Sci*. 2010;72:349–352.
91. Casado D, Fernandes R, Lourinho F, et al. Magnetic resonance imaging features of canine intradural/extramedullary intervertebral disc extrusion in seven cases. *Front Vet Sci*. 2022;9:1003042.
92. Kim J, Kim H, Hwang J, et al. Preliminary study of presumptive intradural-intramedullary intervertebral disc extrusion in 20 dogs. *J Vet Sci*. 2020;21:e52.
93. Tamura S, Doi S, Tamura Y, et al. Thoracolumbar intradural disc herniation in eight dogs: clinical, low-field magnetic resonance imaging, and computed tomographic myelography findings. *Vet Radiol Ultrasound*. 2015;56:160–167.
94. Lipsitz D, Levitski RE, Chauvet AE, et al. Magnetic resonance imaging features of cervical stenotic myelopathy in 21 dogs. *Vet Radiol Ultrasound*. 2001;42:20–27.
95. da Costa RC, Parent J, Dobson H, et al. Comparison of magnetic resonance imaging and myelography in 18 Doberman pinscher dogs with cervical spondylomyelopathy. *Vet Radiol Ultrasound*. 2006;47:523–531.
96. da Costa RC, Parent JM. One-year clinical and magnetic resonance imaging follow-up of Doberman Pinschers with cervical spondylomyelopathy treated medically or surgically. *J Am Vet Med Assoc*. 2007;231:243–250.
97. da Costa RC, Parent JM, Partlow G, et al. Morphologic and morphometric magnetic resonance imaging features of Doberman Pinschers with and without clinical signs of cervical spondylomyelopathy. *Am J Vet Res*. 2006;67: 1601–1612.
98. da Costa RC, Samii VF. Advanced imaging of the spine in small animals. *Vet Clin North Am Small Anim Pract*. 2010;40:765–790.
99. Martin-Vaquero P, da Costa RC. Magnetic resonance imaging features of Great Danes with and without clinical signs of cervical spondylomyelopathy. *J Am Vet Med Assoc*. 2014;245:393–400.
100. Martin-Vaquero P, da Costa RC, Drost WT. Comparison of noncontrast computed tomography and high-field magnetic resonance imaging in the evaluation of Great Danes with cervical spondylomyelopathy. *Vet Radiol Ultrasound*. 2014;55:496–505.
101. Martin-Vaquero P, da Costa RC, Lima CG. Cervical spondylomyelopathy in Great Danes: a magnetic resonance imaging morphometric study. *Vet J*. 2014;201:64–71.
102. Bonelli MA, da Costa L, da Costa RC. Magnetic resonance imaging and neurological findings in dogs with disc-associated cervical spondylomyelopathy: a case series. *BMC Vet Res*. 2021;17:145.
103. Bonelli MA, da Costa RC. Neurologic and magnetic resonance imaging features of German shepherd dogs with cervical spondylomyelopathy: 10 cases (2006–2018). *J Am Vet Med Assoc*. 2019;255:1263–1269.
104. Eagleson JS, Diaz J, Platt SR, et al. Cervical vertebral malformation-malarticulation syndrome in the Bernese mountain dog: clinical and magnetic resonance imaging features. *J Small Anim Pract*. 2009;50:186–193.
105. Bonelli MA, da Costa L, da Costa RC. Association of neurologic signs with high-field MRI findings in 100 dogs with osseous-associated cervical spondylomyelopathy. *Vet Radiol Ultrasound*. 2021;62:678–686.
106. Nye C, Hostnik E, Parker E, et al. Long-term clinical and magnetic resonance imaging follow-up of dogs with osseous-associated cervical spondylomyelopathy. *J Vet Intern Med*. 2020;34:2012–2020.
107. Vansteenkiste D, Martin-Vaquero P, Bonelli M, et al. Long-term computed tomography follow-up in Great Danes with or without signs of osseous-associated cervical Spondylomyelopathy. *BMC Vet Res*. 2019;15:90.
108. de Albuquerque Bonelli M, da Costa RC. Clinical and magnetic resonance imaging characterization of cervical spondylomyelopathy in juvenile dogs. *J Vet Intern Med*. 2019;33:2160–2166.
109. De Decker S, Gielen IM, Duchateau L, et al. Intraobserver, interobserver, and intermethod agreement for results of myelography, computed tomography-myelography, and low-field magnetic resonance imaging in dogs with disk-associated wobbler syndrome. *J Am Vet Med Assoc*. 2011;238:1601–1608.
110. De Decker S, Gielen IM, Duchateau L, et al. Low-field magnetic resonance imaging findings of the caudal portion of the cervical region in clinically normal Doberman Pinschers and Foxhounds. *Am J Vet Res*. 2010;71:428–434.
111. De Decker S, Gielen IMVL, Duchateau L, et al. Intraobserver and interobserver agreement for results of low-field magnetic resonance imaging in dogs with and without clinical signs of disk-associated wobbler syndrome. *J Am Vet Med Assoc*. 2011;238:74–80.
112. Penderis J, Dennis R. Use of traction during magnetic resonance imaging of caudal cervical spondylomyelopathy ("wobbler syndrome") in the dog. *Vet Radiol Ultrasound*. 2004;45:216–219.
113. Provencher M, Habing A, Moore SA, et al. Kinematic magnetic resonance imaging for evaluation of disc-associated cervical spondylomyelopathy in Doberman pinschers. *J Vet Intern Med*. 2016;30:1121–1128.

114. Burke JF, Thawani JP, Berger I, et al. Microsurgical treatment of sacral perineural (Tarlov) cysts: case series and review of the literature. *J Neurosurg Spine*. 2016:1–8.
115. Lowrie ML, Platt SR, Garosi LS. Extramedullary spinal cysts in dogs. *Vet Surg*. 2014;43:650–662.
116. Fiorentino E, Gasparinetti N, Falzone C. Clinical, magnetic resonance imaging and histologic findings of canine thoracolumbar discal pseudocyst: 8 cases (2014–2019). *J Small Anim Pract*. 2021;62:28–32.
117. Penning VA, Benigni L, Steeves E, et al. Imaging diagnosis—degenerative intraspinal cyst associated with an intervertebral disc. *Vet Radiol Ultrasound*. 2007;48:424–427.
118. Dyce J, Herrtage ME, Houlton JEF, et al. Canine spinal 'arachnoid cysts. *J Small Anim Pract*. 1991;32:433–437.
119. Foss KD, Berry WL. What is your neurologic diagnosis? Spinal arachnoid cysts. *J Am Vet Med Assoc*. 2009;234:1009–1011.
120. Frykman OF. Spinal arachnoid cyst in four dogs: diagnosis, surgical, treatment and follow-up results. *J Small Anim Pract*. 1999;40.
121. Galloway AM, Curtis NC, Sommerlad SF, et al. Correlative imaging findings in seven dogs and one cat with spinal arachnoid cysts. *Vet Radiol Ultrasound*. 1999;40:445–452.
122. Gnirs K, Ruel Y, Blot S, et al. Spinal subarachnoid cysts in 13 dogs. *Vet Radiol Ultrasound*. 2003;44:402–408.
123. Goncalves R, Hammond G, Penderis J. Imaging diagnosis: erroneous localization of spinal arachnoid cyst. *Vet Radiol Ultrasound*. 2008;49:460–463.
124. Hashizume CT. Cervical spinal arachnoid cyst in a dog. *Can Vet J*. 2000;41:225–227.
125. Itamoto K. A case involving a dog with a cervical arachnoid cyst treated with marsupilization surgery. *J Jpn Vet Med Assoc*. 2010;63:375–378.
126. Jurina K, Grevel V. Spinal arachnoid pseudocysts in 10 Rottweilers. *J Small Anim Pract*. 2004;45:9–15.
127. Mauler DA, De Decker S, De Risio L, et al. Signalment, clinical presentation, and diagnostic findings in 122 dogs with spinal arachnoid diverticula. *J Vet Intern Med*. 2014;28:175–181.
128. McKee WM, Renwick PW. Marsupialisation of an arachnoid cyst in a dog. *J Small Anim Pract*. 1994;35:108–111.
129. Ness MG. Spinal arachnoid cysts in two Shih Tzu littermates. *Vet Rec*. 1998;142:515–516.
130. Oxley W, Pink J. Amelioration of caudal thoracic syringohydromyelia following surgical management of an adjacent arachnoid cyst. *J Small Anim Pract*. 2012;53:67–72.
131. Parker AJ, Adams WM, Zachary JF. Spinal arachnoid cysts in the dog. *J Am Anim Hosp Assoc*. 1983;19:1001–1008.
132. Rohdin C, Nyman HT, Wohlsein P, et al. Cervical spinal intradural arachnoid cysts in related, young pugs. *J Small Anim Pract*. 2014;55:229–234.
133. Rylander H, Lipsitz D, Berry WL, et al. Retrospective analysis of spinal arachnoid cysts in 14 dogs. *J Vet Intern Med*. 2002;16:690–696.
134. Sessums KB, Ducote JM, American College of Veterinary R. What is your diagnosis? Spinal arachnoid cysts. *J Am Vet Med Assoc*. 2006;228:1019–1020.
135. Shamir MH, Shahar R, Aizenberg I. Subarachnoid cyst in a cat. *J Am Anim Hosp Assoc*. 1997;33:123–125.
136. Skeen TM, Olby NJ, Munana KR, et al. Spinal arachnoid cysts in 17 dogs. *J Am Anim Hosp Assoc*. 2003;39:271–282.
137. Vignoli M, Rossi F, Sarli G. Spinal subarachnoid cyst in a cat. *Vet Radiol Ultrasound*. 1999;40:116–119.
138. Webb AA. Intradural spinal arachnoid cyst in a dog. *Can Vet J*. 1999;40:588–589.
139. Driver CJ, Rose J, Tauro A, et al. Magnetic resonance image findings in pug dogs with thoracolumbar myelopathy and concurrent caudal articular process dysplasia. *BMC Vet Res*. 2019;15:182.
140. Berle M, Wester KG, Ulvik RJ, et al. Arachnoid cysts do not contain cerebrospinal fluid: a comparative chemical analysis of arachnoid cyst fluid and cerebrospinal fluid in adults. *Cerebrospinal Fluid Res*. 2010;7:8.
141. Targett MP, McInnes E, Dennis R. Magnetic resonance imaging of a medullary dermoid cyst with secondary hydrocephalus in a dog. *Vet Radiol Ultrasound*. 1999;40:23–26.
142. Davies ESS, Fransson BA, Gavin PR. A confusing magnetic resonance imaging observation complicating surgery for a dermoid cyst in a Rhodesian ridgeback. *Vet Radiol Ultrasound*. 2004;45:307–309.
143. Shamir MH, Lichovsky D, Aizenberg I, et al. Partial surgical removal of an intramedullary epidermoid cyst from the spinal cord of a dog. *J Small Anim Pract*. 1999;40:439–442.
144. Kiviranta AM, Lappalainen AK, Hagner K, et al. Dermoid sinus and spina bifida in three dogs and a cat. *J Small Anim Pract*. 2011;52:319–324.
145. Fatone G, Brunetti A, Lamagna F, et al. Dermoid sinus and spinal malformations in a Yorkshire terrier: diagnosis and follow-up. *J Small Anim Pract*. 1995;36:178–180.
146. Jones S, Adin C, Thompson E, et al. Computed tomography for the diagnosis and characterization of dermoid sinuses in two dogs. *J Am Anim Hosp Assoc*. 2019;55:e55403.
147. Fleming JM, Platt SR, Kent M, et al. Cervical dermoid sinus in a cat: case presentation and review of the literature. *J Feline Med Surg*. 2011;13:992–996.
148. Rahal S, Mortari AC, Yamashita S, et al. Magnetic resonance imaging in the diagnosis of type 1 dermoid sinus in two Rhodesian ridgeback dogs. *Can Vet J*. 2008;49:871–876.
149. Tong T, Simpson DJ. Case report: spinal dermoid sinus in a Burmese cat with paraparesis. *Aust Vet J*. 2009;87:450–454.
150. Bowens AL, Ducote JM, Early PJ. What is your neurologic diagnosis? Type IV dermoid sinus (pilonidal sinus) in the region of the fourth thoracic vertebra. *J Am Vet Med Assoc*. 2005;227:713–715.
151. Motta L, Skerritt G, Denk D, et al. Dermoid sinus type IV associated with spina bifida in a young Victorian bulldog. *Vet Rec*. 2012;170:127.
152. da Costa RC, Cook LB. Cystic Abnormalities of the spinal cord and vertebral column. *Vet Clin North Am Small Anim Pract*. 2015.
153. Dickinson PJ, Sturges BK, Berry WL, et al. Extradural spinal synovial cysts in nine dogs. *J Small Anim Pract*. 2001;42:502–509.
154. Sale CS, Smith KC. Extradural spinal juxtafacet (synovial) cysts in three dogs. *J Small Anim Pract*. 2007;48:116–119.
155. Webb AA, Pharr JW, Lew LJ, et al. MR imaging findings in a dog with lumbar ganglion cysts. *Vet Radiol Ultrasound*. 2001;42:9–13.
156. Bagley RS. Spinal neoplasms in small animals. *Vet Clin North Am Small Anim Pract*. 2010;40:915–927.
157. Morgan JP, Ackerman N, Bailey CS, et al. Vertebral tumors in the dog: a clinical, radiologic, and pathologic study of 61 primary and secondary lesions. *Vet Radiol*. 1980;21:197–212.
158. Marioni-Henry K, Van Winkle TJ, Smith SH, et al. Tumors affecting the spinal cord of cats: 85 cases (1980–2005). *J Am Vet Med Assoc*. 2008;232:237–243.

159. Marioni-Henry K, Vite CH, Newton AL, et al. Prevalence of diseases of the spinal cord of cats. *J Vet Intern Med.* 2004;18:851–858.
160. Schultz RM, Puchalski SM, Kent M, et al. Skeletal lesions of histiocytic sarcoma in nineteen dogs. *Vet Radiol Ultrasound.* 2007;48:539–543.
161. Agut A, Anson A, Navarro A, et al. Imaging diagnosis-infiltrative lipoma causing spinal cord and lumbar nerve root compression in a dog. *Vet Radiol Ultrasound.* 2013;54:381–383.
162. Hobert MK, Brauer C, Dziallas P, et al. Infiltrative lipoma compressing the spinal cord in 2 large-breed dogs. *Can Vet J.* 2013;54:74–78.
163. Kim HJ, Chang HS, Choi CB, et al. Infiltrative lipoma in cervical bones in a dog. *J Vet Med Sci.* 2005;67:1043–1046.
164. McEntee MC, Thrall DE. Computed tomographic imaging of infiltrative lipoma in 22 dogs. *Vet Radiol Ultrasound.* 2001;42:221–225.
165. Morgan LW, Toal R, Siemering G, et al. Imaging diagnosis—infiltrative lipoma causing spinal cord compression in a dog. *Vet Radiol Ultrasound.* 2007;48:35–37.
166. Auger M, Hecht S, Springer CM. Magnetic resonance imaging features of extradural spinal neoplasia in 60 dogs and seven cats. *Front Vet Sci.* 2020;7:610490.
167. Durand A, Keenihan E, Schweizer D, et al. Clinical and magnetic resonance imaging features of lymphoma involving the nervous system in cats. *J Vet Intern Med.* 2022;36:679–693.
168. Lorenzo V, Ribeiro J, Bernardini M, et al. Clinical and magnetic resonance imaging features, and pathological findings of spinal lymphoma in 27 cats. *Front Vet Sci.* 2022;9:980414.
169. Mallol C, Gutierrez-Quintana R, Hammond G, et al. MRI features of canine hemangiosarcoma affecting the central nervous system. *Vet Radiol Ultrasound.* 2022;63:185–196.
170. Moore TW, Bentley RT, Moore SA, et al. Spinal mast cell tumors in dogs: imaging features and clinical outcome of four cases. *Vet Radiol Ultrasound.* 2017;58:44–52.
171. Paek M, Glass E, Kent M, et al. Primary lumbar extradural hemangiosarcoma in a dog. *J Am Anim Hosp Assoc.* 2015;51:191–196.
172. Drost WT, Love NE, Berry CR. Comparison of radiography, myelography, and computed tomography for the evaluation of canine vertebral and spinal cord tumors in sixteen dogs. *Vet Radiol Ultrasound.* 1996;37:28–33.
173. Kippenes H, Gavin PR, Bagley RS, et al. Magnetic resonance imaging features of tumors of the spine and spinal cord in dogs. *Vet Radiol Ultrasound.* 1999;40:627–633.
174. Tam C, Hecht S, Mai W, et al. Cranial and vertebral osteosarcoma commonly has T2 signal heterogeneity, contrast enhancement, and osteolysis on MRI: a case series of 35 dogs. *Vet Radiol Ultrasound.* 2022;63:552–562.
175. Wyatt S, De Risio L, Driver C, et al. Neurological signs and MRI findings in 12 dogs with multiple myeloma. *Vet Radiol Ultrasound.* 2019;60:409–415.
176. D'Anjou MA. Carmel EN, Tidwell AS: value of fat suppression in gadolinium-enhanced magnetic resonance neuroimaging. *Vet Radiol Ultrasound.* 2011;52:S85–90.
177. Dennis R. Optimal magnetic resonance imaging of the spine. *Vet Radiol Ultrasound.* 2011;52:S72–S80.
178. Wheeler SJ, Sharp NJH. Neurological deficits in multiple limbs: spinal disorders. In: Wheeler SJ, ed. *Manual of Small Animal Neurology*. 2nd ed. Cheltenham. British Small Animal Veterinary Association; 1995:143–158.
179. Brewer DM, Cerda-Gonzalez S, Dewey CW, et al. Spinal cord nephroblastoma in dogs: 11 cases (1985–2007). *J Am Vet Med Assoc.* 2011;238:618–624.
180. Gasser AM, Bush WW, Smith S, et al. Extradural spinal, bone marrow, and renal nephroblastoma. *J Am Anim Hosp Assoc.* 2003;39:80–85.
181. Liebel FX, Rossmeisl Jr JH, Lanz OI, et al. Canine spinal nephroblastoma: long-term outcomes associated with treatment of 10 cases (1996–2009). *Vet Surg.* 2011;40:244–252.
182. Macri NP, Van Alstine W, Coolman RA. Canine spinal nephroblastoma. *J Am Anim Hosp Assoc.* 1997;33:302–306.
183. McConnell JF, Garosi LS, Dennis R, et al. Imaging of a spinal nephroblastoma in a dog. *Vet Radiol Ultrasound.* 2003;44:537–541.
184. Nakade T, Inoue A, Shimazaki H, et al. Spinal nephroblastoma in a miniature Dachshund. *J Vet Med Sci.* 2006;68:1383–1385.
185. Sale CS, Skerritt GC, Smith KC. Spinal nephroblastoma in a crossbreed dog. *J Small Anim Pract.* 2004;45:267–271.
186. Terrell SP, Platt SR, Chrisman CL, et al. Possible intraspinal metastasis of a canine spinal cord nephroblastoma. *Vet Pathol.* 2000;37:94–97.
187. Kraft S, Ehrhart EJ, Gall D, et al. Magnetic resonance imaging characteristics of peripheral nerve sheath tumors of the canine brachial plexus in 18 dogs. *Vet Radiol Ultrasound.* 2007;48:1–7.
188. Linzmann H, Brunnberg L, Gruber AD, et al. A neurotropic lymphoma in the brachial plexus of a cat. *J Feline Med Surg.* 2009;11:522–524.
189. Mellanby RJ, Jeffery ND, Baines EA, et al. Magnetic resonance imaging in the diagnosis of lymphoma involving the brachial plexus in a cat. *Vet Radiol Ultrasound.* 2003;44:522–525.
190. Rudich SR, Feeney DA, Anderson KL, et al. Computed tomography of masses of the brachial plexus and contributing nerve roots in dogs. *Vet Radiol Ultrasound.* 2004;45:46–50.
191. Jose-Lopez R, de la Fuente C, Pumarola M, et al. Spinal meningiomas in dogs: description of 8 cases including a novel radiological and histopathological presentation. *Can Vet J.* 2013;54:948–954.
192. McDonnell JJ, Tidwell AS, Faissler D, et al. Magnetic resonance imaging features of cervical spinal cord meningiomas. *Vet Radiol Ultrasound.* 2005;46:368–374.
193. Petersen SA, Sturges BK, Dickinson PJ, et al. Canine intraspinal meningiomas: imaging features, histopathologic classification, and long-term outcome in 34 dogs. *J Vet Intern Med.* 2008;22:946–953.
194. Wall M, Platt S, Selcer B, et al. Multifocal spinal papillary meningioma in a dog. *Vet Radiol Ultrasound.* 2005;46:309–312.
195. Yeomans SM. Short paper – extensive spinal meningioma in a young dog. *J Comp Pathol.* 2000;122:303–306.
196. Pancotto TE, Rossmeisl Jr JH, Zimmerman K, et al. Intramedullary spinal cord neoplasia in 53 dogs (1990–2010): distribution, clinicopathologic characteristics, and clinical behavior. *J Vet Intern Med.* 2013;27:1500–1508.
197. Hammond JJ, deLahunta A, Glass EN, et al. Feline spinal cord gliomas: clinicopathologic and diagnostic features of seven cases. *J Vet Diagn Invest.* 2014;26:513–520.
198. Tamura S, Hori Y, Tamura Y, et al. Long-term follow-up of surgical treatment of spinal anaplastic astrocytoma in a cat. *J Feline Med Surg.* 2013;15:921–926.
199. Gibson AM, Rosser MF, de Oliveira CR, et al. Magnetic resonance imaging findings and antemortem cytologic diagnosis of intramedullary spinal cord ependymoma in a dog. *J Am Vet Med Assoc.* 2021;259:1446–1451.

200. Taylor A, Eichelberger B, Hodo C, et al. Imaging diagnosis—spinal cord histiocytic sarcoma in a dog. *Vet Radiol Ultrasound*. 2015;56:E17–E20.
201. Mariani CL, Jennings MK, Olby NJ, et al. Histiocytic sarcoma with central nervous system involvement in dogs: 19 cases (2006–2012). *J Vet Intern Med*. 2015;29:607–613.
202. Tzipory L, Vernau KM, Sturges BK, et al. Antemortem diagnosis of localized central nervous system histiocytic sarcoma in 2 dogs. *J Vet Intern Med*. 2009;23:369–374.
203. Uchida K, Morozumi M, Yamaguchi R, et al. Diffuse leptomeningeal malignant histiocytosis in the brain and spinal cord of a Tibetan terrier. *Vet Pathol*. 2001;38: 219–222.
204. Bradshaw JM, Pearson GR, Gruffydd-Jones TJ. A retrospective study of 286 cases of neurological disorders of the cat. *J Comp Pathol*. 2004;131:112–120.
205. Lane SB, Kornegay JN, Duncan JR, et al. Feline spinal lymphosarcoma: a retrospective evaluation of 23 cats. *J Vet Intern Med*. 1994;8:99–104.
206. Palus V, Volk HA, Lamb CR, et al. MRI features of CNS lymphoma in dogs and cats. *Vet Radiol Ultrasound*. 2012;53:44–49.
207. Goncalves R, Platt SR, Llabres-Diaz FJ, et al. Clinical and magnetic resonance imaging findings in 92 cats with clinical signs of spinal cord disease. *J Feline Med Surg*. 2009;11:53–59.
208. Allett B, Hecht S. Magnetic resonance imaging findings in the spine of six dogs diagnosed with lymphoma. *Vet Radiol Ultrasound*. 2016;57:154–161.
209. Bush WW, Throop JL, McManus PM, et al. Intravascular lymphoma involving the central and peripheral nervous systems in a dog. *J Am Anim Hosp Assoc*. 2003;39:90–96.
210. Kornder J, Platt SR, Eagleson J, et al. Imaging diagnosis – vertebral polyostotic lymphoma in a geriatric dog. *Vet Radiol Ultrasound*. 2015.
211. Lamagna B, Lamagna F, Meomartino L, et al. Polyostotic lymphoma with vertebral involvement and spinal extradural compression in a dog. *J Am Anim Hosp Assoc*. 2006;42:71–76.
212. Long SN, Johnston PE, Anderson TJ. Primary T-cell lymphoma of the central nervous system in a dog. *J Am Vet Med Assoc*. 2001;218:719–722.
213. Ortega M, Castillo-Alcala F. Hind-limb paresis in a dog with paralumbar solitary T-cell lymphoma. *Can Vet J*. 2010;51:480–484.
214. Veraa S, Dijkman R, Meij BP, et al. Comparative imaging of spinal extradural lymphoma in a Bordeaux dog. *Can Vet J*. 2010;51:519–521.
215. Feeney DA, Sharkey LC, Steward SM, et al. Applicability of 3T body MRI in assessment of nonfocal bone marrow involvement of hematopoietic neoplasia in dogs. *J Vet Intern Med*. 2013;27:1165–1171.
216. Hammond LJ, Hecht S. Susceptibility artifacts on T2*-weighted magnetic resonance imaging of the canine and feline spine. *Vet Radiol Ultrasound*. 2015;56:398–406.
217. Mackenzie GB, Bellah JR, Threatte RM. What is your diagnosis? Hemangiosarcoma of the cervical vertebrae. *J Am Vet Med Assoc*. 2003;222:1075–1076.
218. Reed AL, Payne JT, Aronson E. What is your diagnosis? Primary hemangiosarcoma of the sixth lumbar vertebra in a dog. *J Am Vet Med Assoc*. 1994;204:1749–1750.
219. de la Fuente C, Pumarola M, Anor S. Imaging diagnosis—spinal epidural hemangiosarcoma in a dog. *Vet Radiol Ultrasound*. 2014;55:424–427.
220. Perez-Martinez C, Regueiro-Purrinos M, Fernandez-Martinez B, et al. Magnetic resonance imaging and immunohistochemistry of primary vertebral hemangiosarcoma in a dog and implications for diagnosis and therapy. *Can Vet J*. 2016;57:1247–1250.
221. Kutara K, Maeta N, Kanda T, et al. Magnetic resonance imaging findings of an intradural extramedullary hemangiosarcoma in a dog. *J Vet Med Sci*. 2019;81:1527–1532.
222. Okada M, Kitagawa M, Ito D, et al. Magnetic resonance imaging features and clinical signs associated with presumptive and confirmed progressive myelomalacia in dogs: 12 cases (1997–2008). *J Am Vet Med Assoc*. 2010;237:1160–1165.
223. Platt SR, McConnell JF, Bestbier M. Magnetic resonance imaging characteristics of ascending hemorrhagic myelomalacia in a dog. *Vet Radiol Ultrasound*. 2006;47:78–82.
224. Balducci F, Canal S, Contiero B, et al. Prevalence and risk factors for presumptive ascending/descending myelomalacia in dogs after thoracolumbar intervertebral disk herniation. *J Vet Intern Med*. 2017;31:498–504.
225. Gilmour LJ, Jeffery ND, Miles K, et al. Single-shot turbo spin echo pulse sequence findings in dogs with and without progressive myelomalacia. *Vet Radiol Ultrasound*. 2017;58:197–205.
226. Castel A, Olby NJ, Mariani CL, et al. Clinical characteristics of dogs with progressive myelomalacia following acute intervertebral disc extrusion. *J Vet Intern Med*. 2017;31:1782–1789.
227. Cordle KJ, Seiler GS, Barnes D, et al. MRI features can help to confirm a diagnosis of progressive myelomalacia, but may not be accurate in dogs lacking characteristic clinical signs at the time of imaging. *Vet Radiol Ultrasound*. 2023;64:283–293.
228. da Costa RC, De Decker S, Lewis MJ, et al. Diagnostic imaging in intervertebral disc disease. *Front Vet Sci*. 2020;7:588338.
229. Olby NJ, da Costa RC, Levine JM, et al. Prognostic factors in canine acute intervertebral disc disease. *Front Vet Sci*. 2020;7:596059.
230. Abramson CJ, Garosi L, Platt SR, et al. Magnetic resonance imaging appearance of suspected ischemic myelopathy in dogs. *Vet Radiol Ultrasound*. 2005;46:225–229.
231. De Risio L, Adams V, Dennis R, et al. Magnetic resonance imaging findings and clinical associations in 52 dogs with suspected ischemic myelopathy. *J Vet Intern Med*. 2007;21:1290–1298.
232. De Risio L, Adams V, Dennis R, et al. Association of clinical and magnetic resonance imaging findings with outcome in dogs suspected to have ischemic myelopathy: 50 cases (2000–2006). *J Am Vet Med Assoc*. 2008;233:129–135.
233. Rylander H, Eminaga S, Palus V, et al. Feline ischemic myelopathy and encephalopathy secondary to hyaline arteriopathy in five cats. *J Feline Med Surg*. 2014;16: 832–839.
234. Simpson KM, De Risio L, Theobald A, et al. Feline ischaemic myelopathy with a predilection for the cranial cervical spinal cord in older cats. *J Feline Med Surg*. 2014;16:1001–1006.
235. Theobald A, Volk HA, Dennis R, et al. Clinical outcome in 19 cats with clinical and magnetic resonance imaging diagnosis of ischaemic myelopathy (2000–2011). *J Feline Med Surg*. 2013;15:132–141.
236. MacKay AD, Rusbridge C, Sparkes AH, et al. MRI characteristics of suspected acute spinal cord infarction in two cats, and a review of the literature. *J Feline Med Surg*. 2005;7:101–107.
237. Mai W. Reduced field-of-view diffusion-weighted MRI can identify restricted diffusion in the spinal cord of dogs and cats with presumptive clinical and high-field MRI diagnosis of acute ischemic myelopathy. *Vet Radiol Ultrasound*. 2020;61:688–695.
238. Vernon JC, Durand A, Guevar J, et al. Vertebral venous system abnormalities identified with magnetic resonance imaging in sighthounds. *Vet Radiol Ultrasound*. 2017.

239. Gilbert S, Brooks-Brownlie H, Cardy T. MRI characteristics of ventral vertebral venous plexus occlusion due to lymphoma in a large breed dog. *Vet Radiol Ultrasound*. 2022.
240. Rhue KE, Taylor AR, Cole RC, et al. Bilateral vertebral venous sinus thrombosis causing cervical spinal cord compression in a dog. *Front Vet Sci*. 2017;4:8.
241. Barker A, Williams JM, Chen A, et al. Suspected primary hematomyelia in 3 dogs. *Can Vet J*. 2015;56:278–284.
242. Wang-Leandro A, Huenerfauth EI, Heissl K, et al. MRI findings of early-stage hyperacute hemorrhage causing extramedullary compression of the cervical spinal cord in a dog with suspected steroid-responsive meningitis-arteritis. *Front Vet Sci*. 2017;4:161.
243. Hague DW, Joslyn S, Bush WW, et al. Clinical, magnetic resonance imaging, and histopathologic findings in 6 dogs with surgically resected extraparenchymal spinal cord hematomas. *J Vet Intern Med*. 2015;29:225–230.
244. Kinns J, Mai W, Seiler G, et al. Radiographic sensitivity and negative predictive value for acute canine spinal trauma. *Vet Radiol Ultrasound*. 2006;47:563–570.
245. Johnson P, Beltran E, Dennis R, et al. Magnetic resonance imaging characteristics of suspected vertebral instability associated with fracture or subluxation in eleven dogs. *Vet Radiol Ultrasound*. 2012;53:552–559.
246. Gallastegui A, Davies E, Zwingenberger AL, et al. MRI has limited agreement with CT in the evaluation of vertebral fractures of the canine trauma patient. *Vet Radiol Ultrasound*. 2019;60:533–542.
247. Shamir MH, Tavor N, Aizenberg T. Radiographic findings during recovery from discospondylitis. *Vet Radiol Ultrasound*. 2001;42:496–503.
248. Carrera I, Sullivan M, McConnell F, et al. Magnetic resonance imaging features of discospondylitis in dogs. *Vet Radiol Ultrasound*. 2011;52:125–131.
249. Cherubini GB, Cappello R, Lu D, et al. MRI findings in a dog with discospondylitis caused by *Bordetella* species. *J Small Anim Pract*. 2004;45:417–420.
250. Gendron K, Doherr MG, Gavin P, et al. Magnetic resonance imaging characterization of vertebral endplate changes in the dog. *Vet Radiol Ultrasound*. 2012;53:50–56.
251. Gonzalo-Orden JM, Altonaga JR, Orden MA, et al. Magnetic resonance, computed tomographic and radiologic findings in a dog with discospondylitis. *Vet Radiol Ultrasound*. 2000;41:142–144.
252. Harris JM, Chen AV, Tucker RL, et al. Clinical features and magnetic resonance imaging characteristics of diskospondylitis in dogs: 23 cases (1997–2010). *J Am Vet Med Assoc*. 2013;242:359–365.
253. Kraft SL, Mussman JM, Smith T, et al. Magnetic resonance imaging of presumptive lumbosacral discospondylitis in a dog. *Vet Radiol Ultrasound*. 1998;39:9–13.
254. Lipscomb VJ, Muir P. Magnetic resonance imaging of a dog with sciatic nerve root signature. *Vet Rec*. 2000;147:393–394.
255. Plessas IN, Jull P, Volk HA. A case of canine discospondylitis and epidural empyema due to *Salmonella* species. *Can Vet J*. 2013;54:595–598.
256. Gomes SA, Targett M, Lowrie M. Computed tomography features of discospondylitis in dogs. *J Vet Intern Med*. 2022;36:2123–2131.
257. Kirberger RM. Early diagnostic imaging findings in juvenile dogs with presumed diskospondylitis: 10 cases (2008–2014). *J Am Vet Med Assoc*. 2016;249:539–546.
258. Gomes SA, Behr S, Garosi LS, et al. Imaging features of discospondylitis in cats. *J Feline Med Surg*. 2020;22: 631–640.
259. Long C, Burgers E, Copple C, et al. *Brucella canis* discospondylitis in 33 dogs. *Front Vet Sci*. 2022;9:1043610.
260. De Stefani A, Garosi LS, McConnell FJ, et al. Magnetic resonance imaging features of spinal epidural empyema in five dogs. *Vet Radiol Ultrasound*. 2008;49:135–140.
261. Granger N, Hidalgo A, Leperlier D, et al. Successful treatment of cervical spinal epidural empyema secondary to grass awn migration in a cat. *J Feline Med Surg*. 2007;9:340–345.
262. Nykamp SG, Steffey MA, Scrivani PV, et al. Computed tomographic appearance of epidural empyema in a dog. *Can Vet J*. 2003;44:729–731.
263. Whitty CC, Milner HR, Oram B. Use of magnetic resonance imaging in the diagnosis of spinal empyema caused by a migrating grass awn in a dog. *N Z Vet J*. 2013;61:115–118.
264. Alves L, Gorgas D, Vandevelde M, et al. Segmental meningomyelitis in 2 cats caused by *Toxoplasma gondii*. *J Vet Intern Med*. 2011;25:148–152.
265. Cherubini GB, Platt SR, Anderson TJ, et al. Characteristics of magnetic resonance images of granulomatous meningoencephalomyelitis in 11 dogs. *Vet Rec*. 2006;159: 110–115.
266. Griffin JF, Levine JM, Levine GJ, et al. Meningomyelitis in dogs: a retrospective review of 28 cases (1999 to 2007). *J Small Anim Pract*. 2008;49:509–517.
267. Parry AT, Penning VA, Smith KC, et al. Imaging diagnosis—necrotizing meningomyelitis and polyarthritis. *Vet Radiol Ultrasound*. 2009;50:412–415.
268. Radaelli ST, Platt SR. Bacterial meningoencephalomyelitis in dogs: a retrospective study of 23 cases (1990–1999). *J Vet Intern Med*. 2002;16:159–163.
269. Snook ER, Baker DG, Bauer RW. Verminous myelitis in a pit bull puppy. *J Vet Diagn Invest*. 2009;21:400–402.
270. Tipold A. Diagnosis of inflammatory and infectious diseases of the central nervous system in dogs: a retrospective study. *J Vet Intern Med*. 1995;9:304–314.
271. Tipold A, Schatzberg SJ. An update on steroid responsive meningitis-arteritis. *J Small Anim Pract*. 2010;51: 150–154.
272. Tipold A, Stein VM. Inflammatory diseases of the spine in small animals. *Vet Clin North Am Small Anim Pract*. 2010;40:871–879.
273. Remelli C, Martello A, Valentini A, et al. Magnetic resonance imaging highlights the meningeal involvement in steroid responsive meningitis-arteritis and suggests the inflammation of the surrounding tissues (70 cases). *Front Vet Sci*. 2022;9:957278.
274. Fingeroth JM, Johnson GC, Burt JK, et al. Neuroradiographic diagnosis and surgical repair of tethered cord syndrome in an English bulldog with spina bifida and myeloschisis. *J Am Vet Med Assoc*. 1989;194:1300–1302.
275. Bertram S, Ter Haar G, De Decker S. Caudal articular process dysplasia of thoracic vertebrae in neurologically normal French bulldogs, English bulldogs, and pugs: prevalence and characteristics. *Vet Radiol Ultrasound*. 2018;59:396–404.
276. Longo S, Gomes SA, Lowrie M. Previously unreported magnetic resonance findings of subarachnoid fibrosis leading to constrictive myelopathy in a pug. *J Small Anim Pract*. 2019;60:324.
277. Lourinho F, Holdsworth A, McConnell JF, et al. Clinical features and MRI characteristics of presumptive constrictive myelopathy in 27 pugs. *Vet Radiol Ultrasound*. 2020;61:545–554.
278. Nishida H, Nakata K, Maeda S, et al. Prevalence and pattern of thoracolumbar caudal articular process anomalies and intervertebral disk herniations in pugs. *J Vet Med Sci*. 2019;81:906–910.
279. Rohdin C, Ljungvall I, Haggstrom J, et al. Thoracolumbar meningeal fibrosis in pugs. *J Vet Intern Med*. 2020;34:797–807.

280. Rohdin C, Haggstrom J, Ljungvall I, et al. Presence of thoracic and lumbar vertebral malformations in pugs with and without chronic neurological deficits. *Vet J.* 2018;241:24–30.
281. Carruthers H, Rusbridge C, Dube MP, et al. Association between cervical and intracranial dimensions and syringomyelia in the cavalier King Charles spaniel. *J Small Anim Pract.* 2009;50:394–398.
282. Cerda-Gonzalez S, Bibi KF, Gifford AT, et al. Magnetic resonance imaging-based measures of atlas position: relationship to canine atlantooccipital overlapping, syringomyelia and clinical signs. *Vet J.* 2016.
283. Cerda-Gonzalez S, Olby NJ, Griffith EH. Dorsal compressive atlantoaxial bands and the craniocervical junction syndrome: association with clinical signs and syringomyelia in mature cavalier King Charles spaniels. *J Vet Intern Med.* 2015;29:887–892.
284. Couturier J, Rault D, Cauzinille L. Chiari-like malformation and syringomyelia in normal cavalier King Charles spaniels: a multiple diagnostic imaging approach. *J Small Anim Pract.* 2008;49:438–443.
285. da Costa RC, Parent JM, Poma R, et al. Cervical syringohydromyelia secondary to a brainstem tumor in a dog. *J Am Vet Med Assoc.* 2004;225:1061–1064, 1048.
286. Driver CJ, De Risio L, Hamilton S, et al. Changes over time in craniocerebral morphology and syringomyelia in cavalier King Charles spaniels with Chiari-like malformation. *BMC Vet Res.* 2012;8:215.
287. Driver CJ, Rusbridge C, Cross HR, et al. Relationship of brain parenchyma within the caudal cranial fossa and ventricle size to syringomyelia in cavalier King Charles spaniels. *J Small Anim Pract.* 2010;51:382–386.
288. Driver CJ, Rusbridge C, McGonnell IM, et al. Morphometric assessment of cranial volumes in age-matched Cavalier King Charles spaniels with and without syringomyelia. *Vet Rec.* 2010;167:978–979.
289. Driver CJ, Volk HA, Rusbridge C, et al. An update on the pathogenesis of syringomyelia secondary to Chiari-like malformations in dogs. *Vet J.* 2013;198:551–559.
290. Driver CJ, Watts V, Bunck AC, et al. Assessment of cerebellar pulsation in dogs with and without Chiari-like malformation and syringomyelia using cardiac-gated cine magnetic resonance imaging. *Vet J.* 2013;198:88–91.
291. Fenn J, Schmidt MJ, Simpson H, et al. Venous sinus volume in the caudal cranial fossa in Cavalier King Charles spaniels with syringomyelia. *Vet J.* 2013;197:896–897.
292. Freeman AC, Platt SR, Kent M, et al. Chiari-like malformation and syringomyelia in American Brussels Griffon dogs. *J Vet Intern Med.* 2014;28:1551–1559.
293. Greitz D. Unraveling the riddle of syringomyelia. *Neurosurg Rev.* 2006;29:251–263. discussion 264.
294. Hu HZ, Rusbridge C, Constantino-Casas F, et al. Histopathological investigation of syringomyelia in the cavalier king Charles spaniel. *J Comp Pathol.* 2012;146:192–201.
295. Jung DI, Park C, Kang BT, et al. Acquired cervical syringomyelia secondary to a brainstem meningioma in a Maltese dog. *J Vet Med Sci.* 2006;68:1235–1238.
296. Kirberger RM, Jacobson LS, Davies JV, et al. Hydromyelia in the dog. *Vet Radiol Ultrasound.* 1997;38:30–38.
297. Kromhout K, van Bree H, Broeckx BJ, et al. Low-field magnetic resonance imaging and multislice computed tomography for the detection of cervical syringomyelia in dogs. *J Vet Intern Med.* 2015;29:1354–1359.
298. Loderstedt S, Benigni L, Chandler K, et al. Distribution of syringomyelia along the entire spinal cord in clinically affected Cavalier King Charles Spaniels. *Vet J.* 2011;190:359–363.
299. MacKillop E, Schatzberg SJ, De Lahunta A. Intracranial epidermoid cyst and syringohydromyelia in a dog. *Vet Radiol Ultrasound.* 2006;47:339–344.
300. Plessas IN, Rusbridge C, Driver CJ, et al. Long-term outcome of Cavalier King Charles spaniel dogs with clinical signs associated with Chiari-like malformation and syringomyelia. *Vet Rec.* 2012;171:501.
301. Rusbridge C. Chiari-like malformation with syringomyelia in the Cavalier King Charles spaniel: long-term outcome after surgical management. *Vet Surg.* 2007;36:396–405.
302. Rusbridge C, Carruthers H, Dube MP, et al. Syringomyelia in cavalier King Charles spaniels: the relationship between syrinx dimensions and pain. *J Small Anim Pract.* 2007;48:432–436.
303. Rusbridge C, Greitz D, Iskandar BJ. Syringomyelia: current concepts in pathogenesis, diagnosis, and treatment. *J Vet Intern Med.* 2006;20:469–479.
304. Rusbridge C, Knowler SP. Coexistence of occipital dysplasia and occipital hypoplasia/syringomyelia in the cavalier King Charles spaniel. *J Small Anim Pract.* 2006;47:603–606.
305. Schmidt MJ, Kramer M, Ondreka N. Comparison of the relative occipital bone volume between Cavalier King Charles spaniels with and without syringohydromyelia and French bulldogs. *Vet Radiol Ultrasound.* 2012;53:540–544.
306. Schmidt MJ, Ondreka N, Sauerbrey M, et al. Volume reduction of the jugular foramina in cavalier king Charles spaniels with syringomyelia. *BMC Vet Res.* 2012;8:158.
307. Scrivani PV, Thompson MS, Winegardner KR, et al. Association between frontal-sinus size and syringohydromyelia in small-breed dogs. *Am J Vet Res.* 2007;68:610–613.
308. Shaw TA, McGonnell IM, Driver CJ, et al. Increase in cerebellar volume in Cavalier King Charles Spaniels with Chiari-like malformation and its role in the development of syringomyelia. *PLoS One.* 2012;7:e33660.
309. Wolfe KC, Poma R. Syringomyelia in the Cavalier King Charles Spaniel (CKCS) dog. *Can Vet J.* 2010;51:95–102.
310. Rusbridge C, Knowler SP, Pieterse L, et al. Chiari-like malformation in the Griffon Bruxellois. *J Small Anim Pract.* 2009;50:386–393.
311. Rusbridge C, Stringer F, Knowler SP. Clinical application of diagnostic imaging of Chiari-like malformation and syringomyelia. *Front Vet Sci.* 2018;5:280.
312. Schmidt MJ, Roth J, Ondreka N, et al. A potential role for substance P and interleukin-6 in the cerebrospinal fluid of Cavalier King Charles Spaniels with neuropathic pain. *J Vet Intern Med.* 2013;27:530–535.

ELECTRONIC RESOURCES

Additional information related to the content in Chapter 15 can be found online at eBooks.Health.Elsevier.com.

- Chapter Quiz

SECTION III

The Appendicular Skeleton: Canine, Feline, and Equine

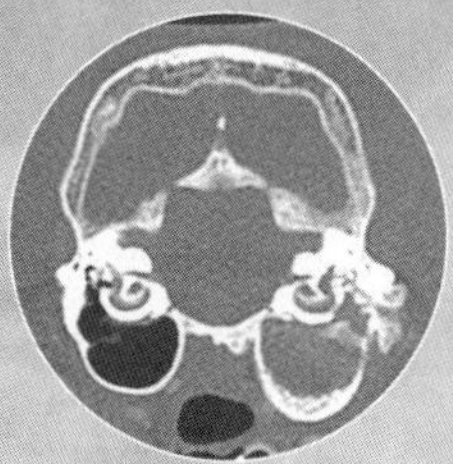
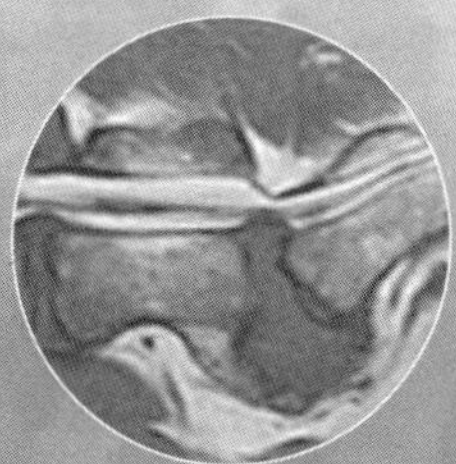
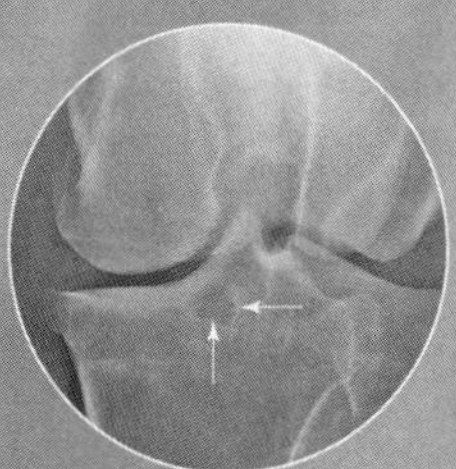
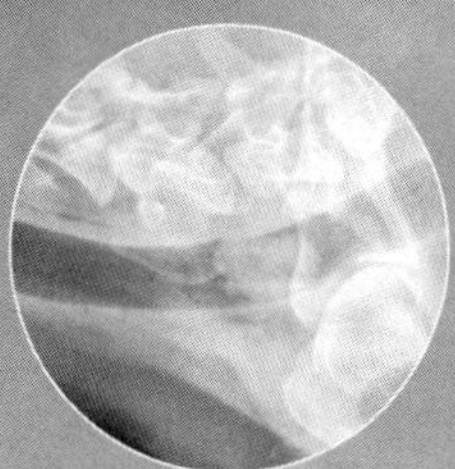
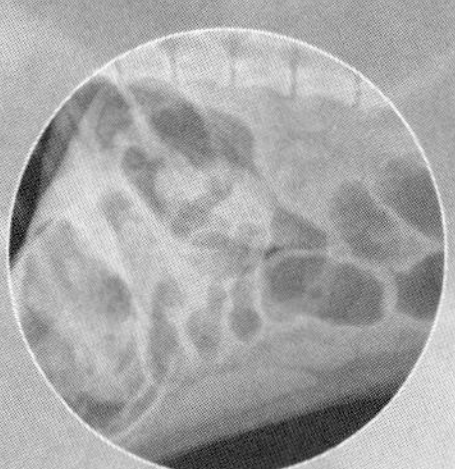

CHAPTER 16

Radiographic Anatomy of the Appendicular Skeleton

Kathy A. Spaulding and Andra K. Voges

To use the roentgen sign method of recognizing abnormal radiographic findings effectively, an understanding of normal radiographic anatomy for the specific area of interest is necessary. The purpose of this chapter is to provide a limited reference for the radiographic anatomy of the appendicular skeleton. Refer to comprehensive textbooks on gross and radiographic anatomy for more detailed information.[1–7]

The radiographic nomenclature used in this chapter was approved by the American College of Veterinary Radiology in 1983.[8] Some equine images in this chapter (Figs. 16.30–16.49 and 16.54–16.57) have been taken from previous publications and are reproduced here with permission of the journals and authors.[9-11]

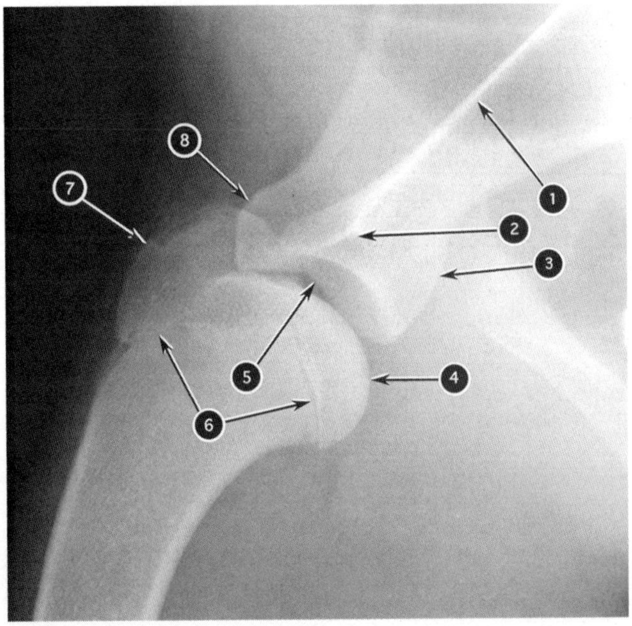

Fig. 16.1 Mediolateral (lateral) radiograph of canine shoulder joint.
1. Spine of scapula
2. Acromion of scapula
3. Infraglenoid tubercle of scapula
4. Head of humerus
5. Glenoid cavity of scapula
6. Proximal physis of humerus
7. Greater tubercle of humerus
8. Supraglenoid tubercle of scapula

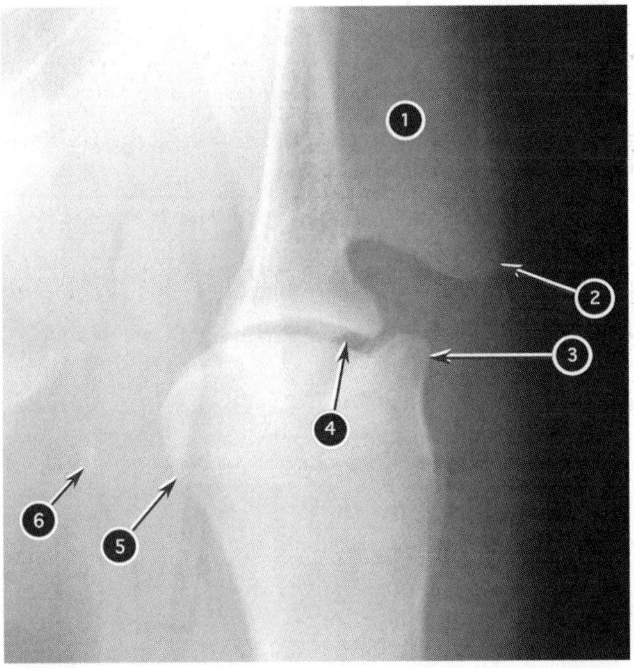

Fig. 16.2 Caudocranial radiograph of canine shoulder joint.
1. Spine of scapula
2. Acromion of scapula
3. Greater tubercle of humerus
4. Humeral (scapulohumeral) joint
5. Lesser tubercle of humerus
6. Clavicle

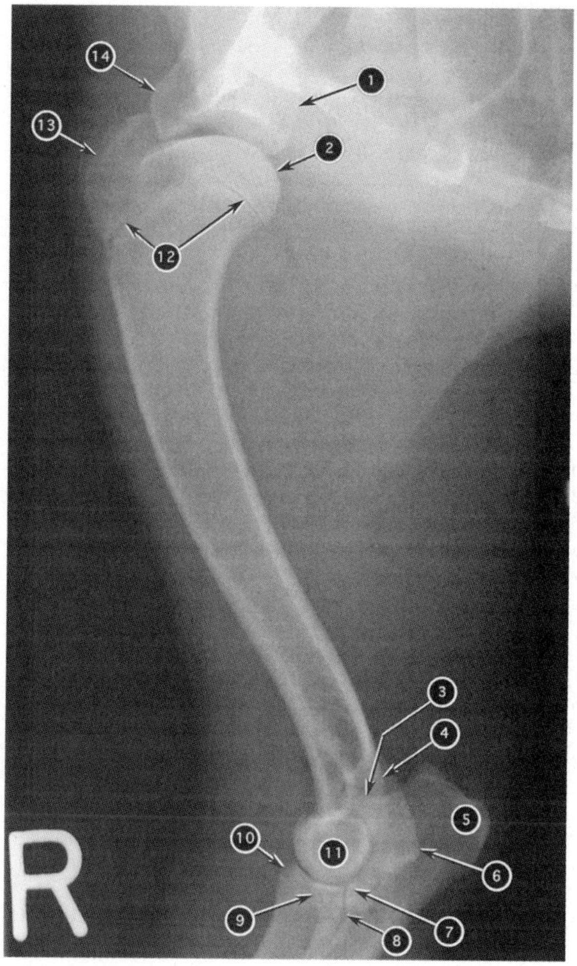

Fig. 16.3 Mediolateral (lateral) radiograph of canine humerus.
1. Infraglenoid tubercle of scapula
2. Head of humerus
3. Anconeal process of ulna
4. Lateral epicondyle of humerus
5. Tuber olecrani
6. Medial epicondyle of humerus
7. Lateral coronoid process of ulna
8. Proximal radioulnar joint
9. Medial coronoid process of ulna
10. Head of radius
11. Condyle of humerus
12. Proximal physis of humerus
13. Greater tubercle of humerus
14. Supraglenoid tubercle of scapula

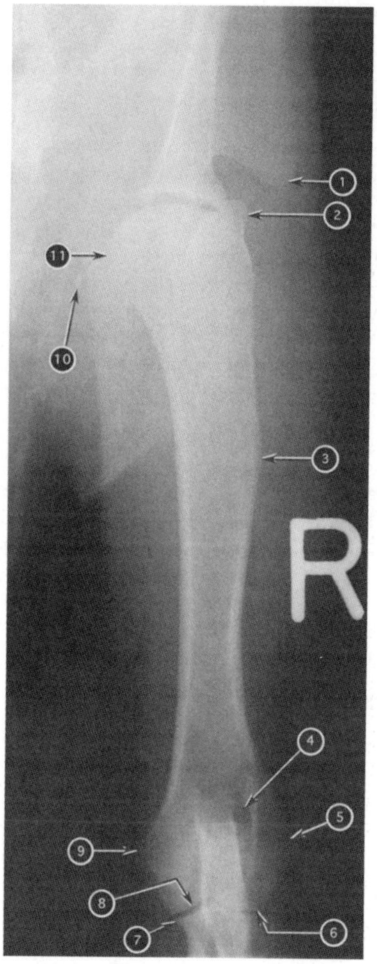

Fig. 16.4 Caudocranial radiograph of canine humerus.
1. Acromion of scapula
2. Greater tubercle of humerus
3. Deltoid tuberosity
4. Supratrochlear foramen of humerus
5. Lateral epicondyle of humerus
6. Capitulum of humeral condyle
7. Medial coronoid process of ulna
8. Trochlea of humeral condyle
9. Medial epicondyle of humerus
10. Clavicle
11. Lesser tubercle of humerus

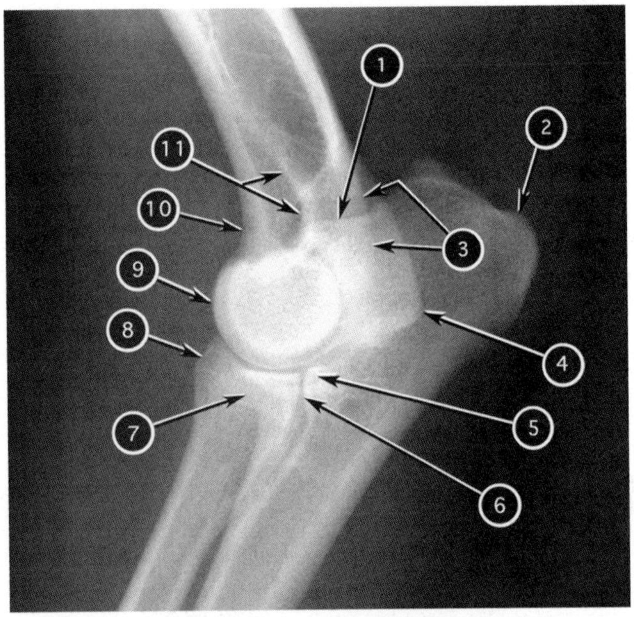

Fig. 16.5 Mediolateral (lateral) radiograph of canine elbow joint.
1. Anconeal process of ulna
2. Tuber olecrani of ulna
3. Caudal border of lateral epicondyle of humerus
4. Caudal border of medial epicondyle of humerus
5. Lateral coronoid process of ulna
6. Proximal radioulnar joint
7. Medial coronoid process of ulna
8. Head of radius
9. Condyle of humerus
10. Cranial border of medial epicondyle of humerus
11. Cranial border of lateral epicondyle of humerus

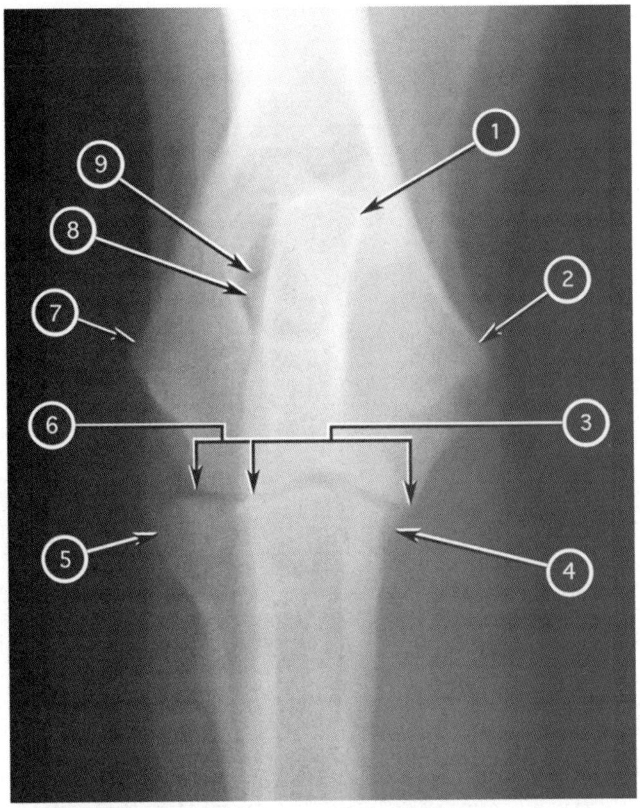

Fig. 16.7 Craniocaudal radiograph of canine elbow joint.
1. Tuber olecrani of ulna
2. Medial epicondyle of humerus
3. Trochlea of humeral condyle
4. Medial coronoid process of ulna
5. Head of radius
6. Capitulum of humeral condyle
7. Lateral epicondyle of humerus
8. Anconeal process of ulna
9. Supratrochlear foramen of humerus

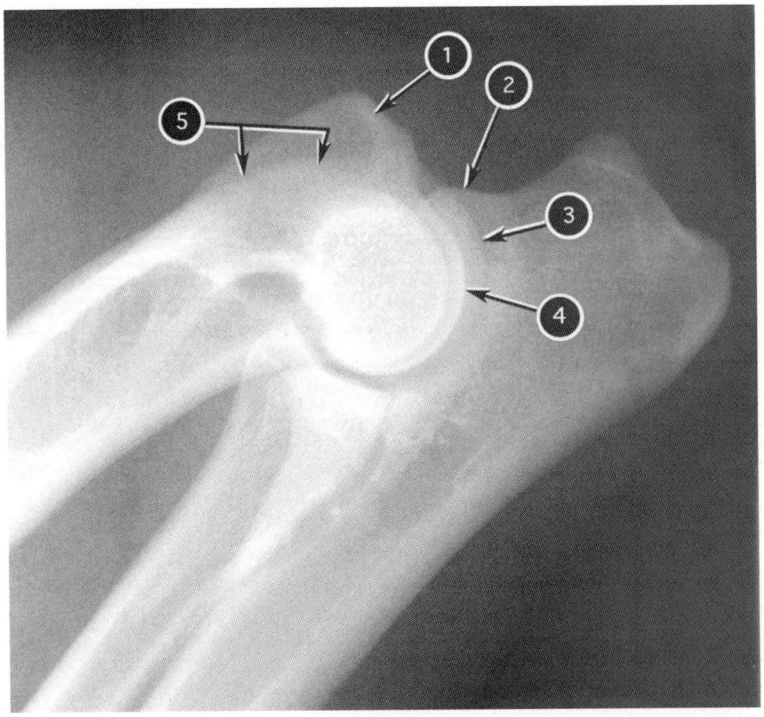

Fig. 16.6 Flexed mediolateral (lateral) radiograph of canine elbow joint.
1. Medial epicondyle of humerus
2. Anconeal process of ulna
3. Medial part of humeral condyle
4. Lateral part of humeral condyle
5. Caudal border of lateral epicondyle of humerus

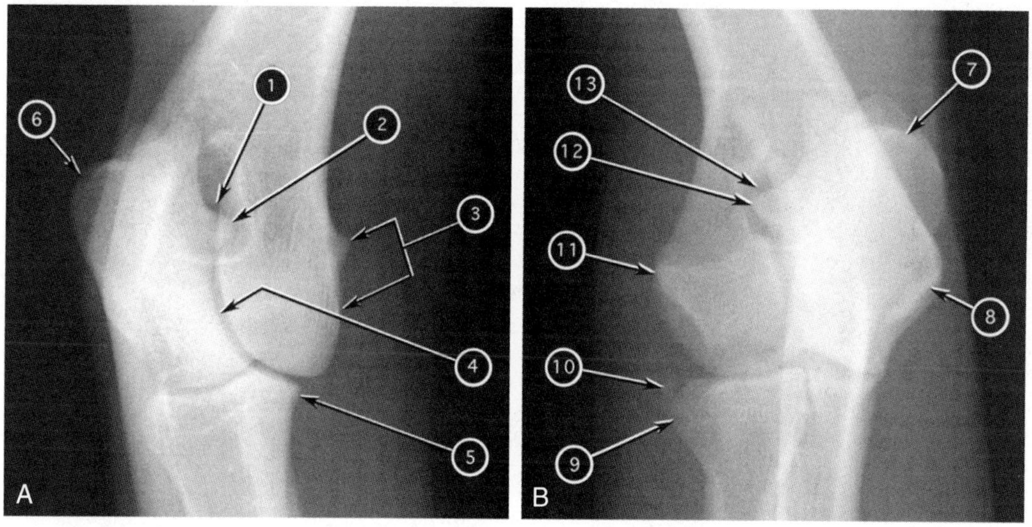

Fig. 16.8 Craniolateral-caudomedial oblique (**A**) and craniomedial-caudolateral oblique (**B**) radiographs of canine elbow joint.

1. Supratrochlear foramen of humerus
2. Anconeal process of ulna
3. Medial epicondyle of humerus
4. Trochlear notch of ulna
5. Medial coronoid process of ulna
6. Tuber olecrani of ulna
7. Tuber olecrani of ulna
8. Medial epicondyle of humerus
9. Head of radius
10. Sesamoid bone of supinator muscle (inconstant)
11. Lateral epicondyle of humerus
12. Anconeal process of ulna
13. Supratrochlear foramen of humerus

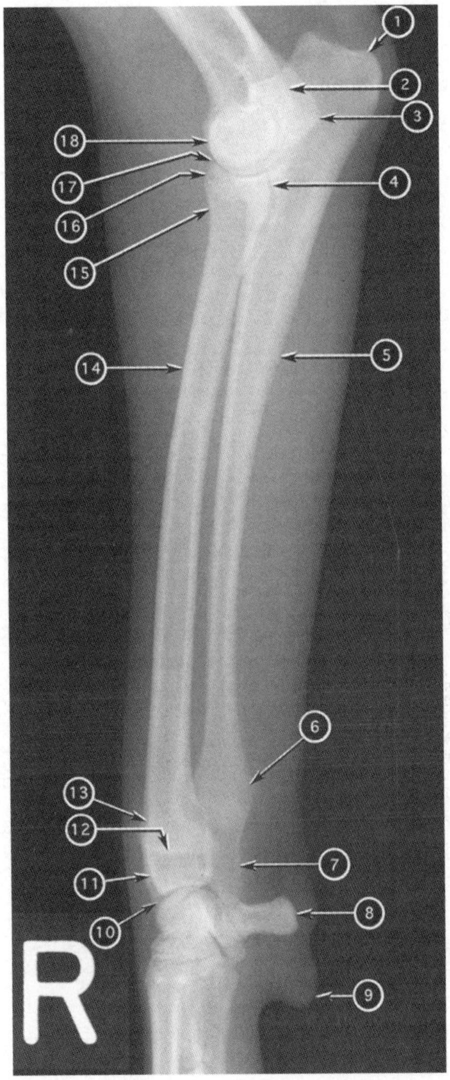

Fig. 16.9 Mediolateral (lateral) radiograph of canine antebrachium.

1. Tuber olecrani of ulna
2. Lateral epicondyle of humerus
3. Medial epicondyle of humerus
4. Proximal radioulnar joint
5. Body of ulna
6. Distal metaphysis of ulna
7. Distal epiphysis of ulna
8. Accessory carpal bone
9. Carpal pad
10. Antebrachiocarpal joint
11. Distal epiphysis of radius
12. Distal physis of radius
13. Distal metaphysis of radius
14. Body of radius
15. Neck of radius
16. Head of radius
17. Elbow (cubital) joint
18. Condyle of humerus

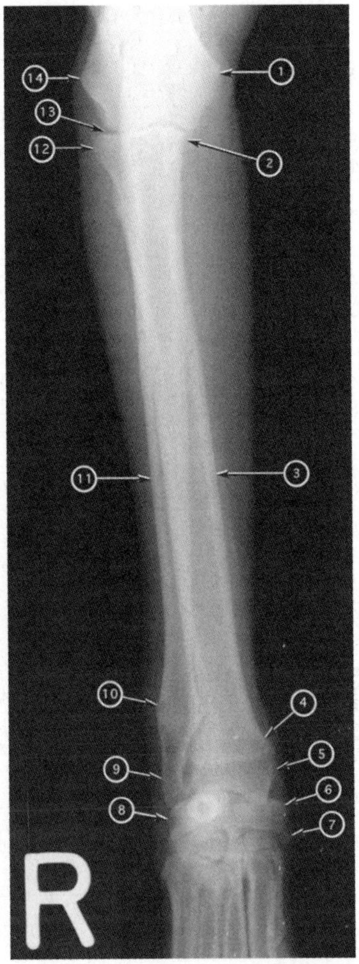

Fig. 16.10 Craniocaudal radiograph of canine antebrachium.

1. Medial epicondyle of humerus
2. Medial coronoid process of ulna
3. Body of radius
4. Distal metaphysis of radius
5. Distal epiphysis of radius
6. Intermedioradial carpal bone
7. Sesamoid bone of abductor pollicis longus
8. Ulnar carpal bone
9. Distal epiphysis (styloid process) of ulna
10. Distal metaphysis of ulna
11. Body of ulna
12. Head of radius
13. Elbow (cubital) joint
14. Lateral epicondyle of humerus

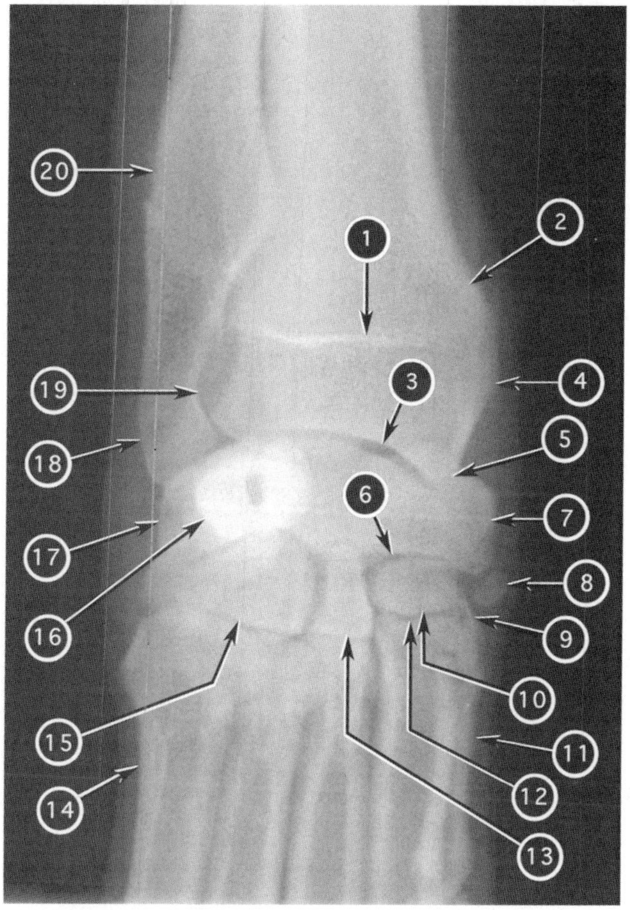

Fig. 16.11 Dorsopalmar radiograph of canine carpus.

1. Distal physis of radius
2. Distal metaphysis of radius
3. Antebrachiocarpal joint
4. Distal epiphysis of radius
5. Styloid process (medial) of radius
6. Middle carpal joint
7. Intermedioradial carpal bone
8. Sesamoid bone of abductor pollicis longus
9. First carpal bone
10. Second carpal bone
11. First metacarpal bone
12. Carpometacarpal joint
13. Third carpal bone
14. Fifth metacarpal bone
15. Fourth carpal bone
16. Accessory carpal bone
17. Ulnar carpal bone
18. Distal epiphysis (styloid process) of ulna
19. Distal radioulnar joint
20. Distal metaphysis of ulna

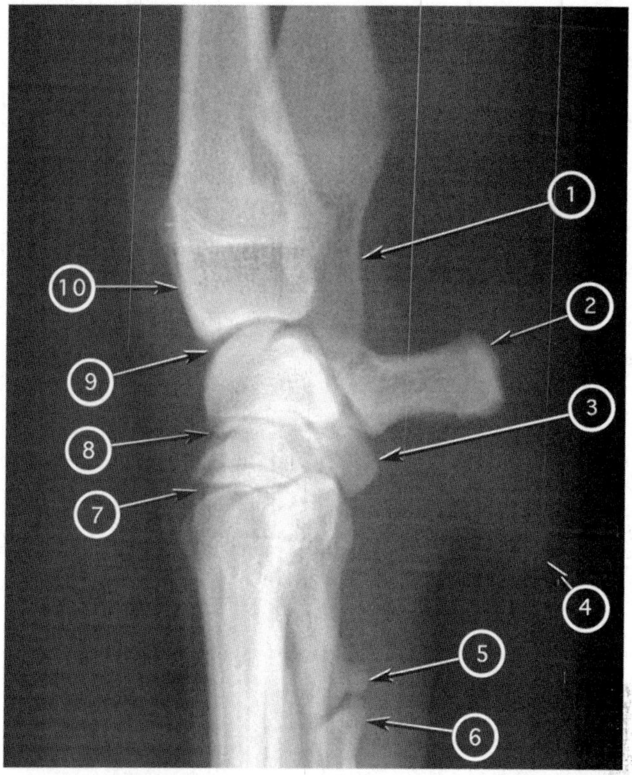

Fig. 16.12 Mediolateral (lateral) radiograph of canine carpus.

1. Distal epiphysis (styloid process) of ulna
2. Accessory carpal bone
3. Ulnar carpal bone
4. Carpal pad
5. Proximal sesamoid bone of first digit
6. Proximal phalanx of first digit
7. Carpometacarpal joint
8. Middle carpal joint
9. Antebrachiocarpal joint
10. Distal epiphysis of radius

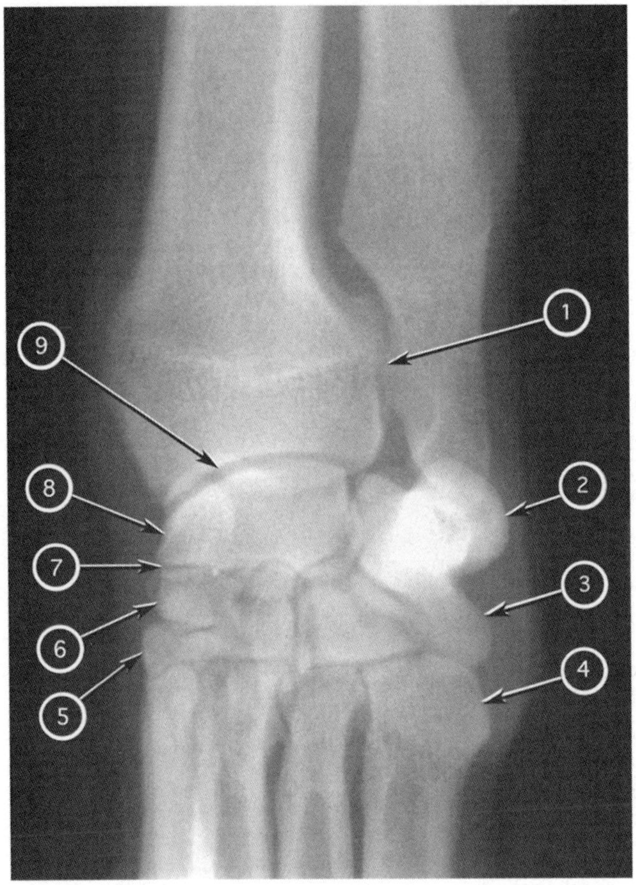

Fig. 16.13 Dorsolateral-palmaromedial oblique radiograph of canine manus.

1. Distal radioulnar joint
2. Accessory carpal bone
3. Ulnar carpal bone
4. Base of metacarpal bone 5
5. First carpal bone
6. Second carpal bone
7. Middle carpal joint
8. Intermedioradial carpal bone
9. Antebrachiocarpal joint

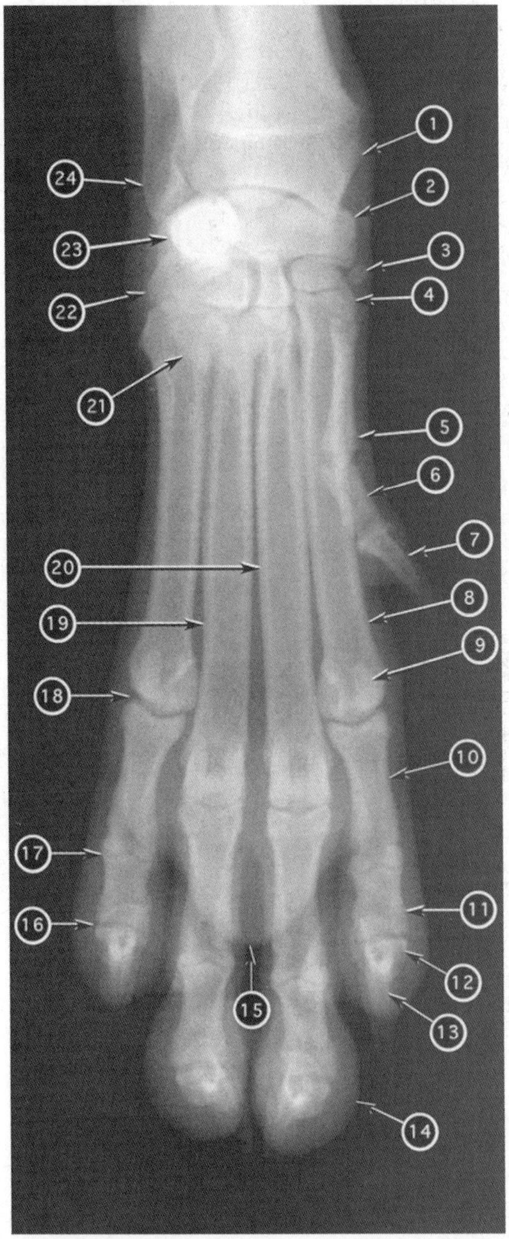

Fig. 16.14 Dorsopalmar radiograph of canine manus.

1. Distal epiphysis of radius
2. Intermedioradial carpal bone
3. Sesamoid bone of abductor pollicis longus
4. First carpal bone
5. Metacarpal bone 1
6. Proximal phalanx of digit 1
7. Distal phalanx of digit 1
8. Second metacarpal bone
9. Abaxial proximal sesamoid bone of digit 2
10. Proximal phalanx of digit 2
11. Middle phalanx of digit 2
12. Unguicular (ungual) crest of distal phalanx of digit 2
13. Unguicular (ungual) process of distal phalanx of digit 2
14. Digital pad of digit 3
15. Metacarpal pad
16. Distal interphalangeal joint of digit 5
17. Proximal interphalangeal joint of digit 5
18. Metacarpophalangeal joint of digit 5
19. Fourth metacarpal bone
20. Third metacarpal bone
21. Carpal pad
22. Ulnar carpal bone
23. Accessory carpal bone
24. Distal epiphysis (styloid process) of ulna

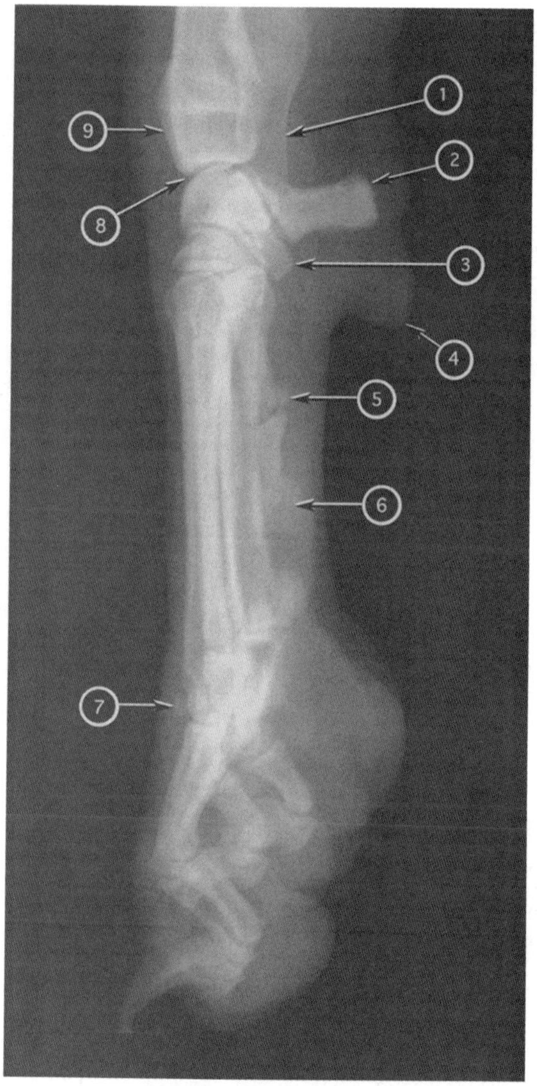

Fig. 16.15 Mediolateral (lateral) radiograph of canine manus.
1. Distal epiphysis (styloid process) of ulna
2. Accessory carpal bone
3. Ulnar carpal bone
4. Carpal pad
5. Proximal sesamoid bone of digit 1
6. Distal phalanx of digit 1
7. Dorsal sesamoid bone
8. Antebrachiocarpal joint
9. Distal epiphysis of radius

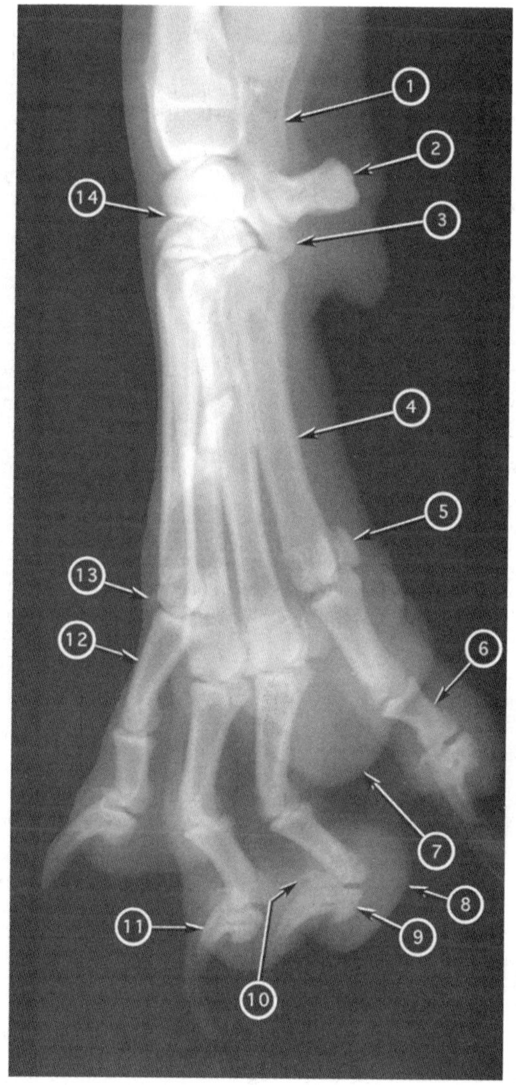

Fig. 16.16 Palmaromedial-dorsolateral oblique radiograph of canine manus.
1. Distal epiphysis (styloid process) of ulna
2. Accessory carpal bone
3. Ulnar carpal bone
4. Body of metacarpal bone 5
5. Abaxial proximal sesamoid bone of digit 5
6. Middle phalanx of digit 5
7. Metacarpal pad
8. Digital pad of digit 4
9. Flexor tubercle of distal phalanx of digit 4
10. Unguicular (ungual) crest of distal phalanx of digit 4
11. Unguicular (ungual) process of distal phalanx digit 3
12. Proximal phalanx of digit 2
13. Dorsal sesamoid bone of digit 2
14. Middle carpal joint

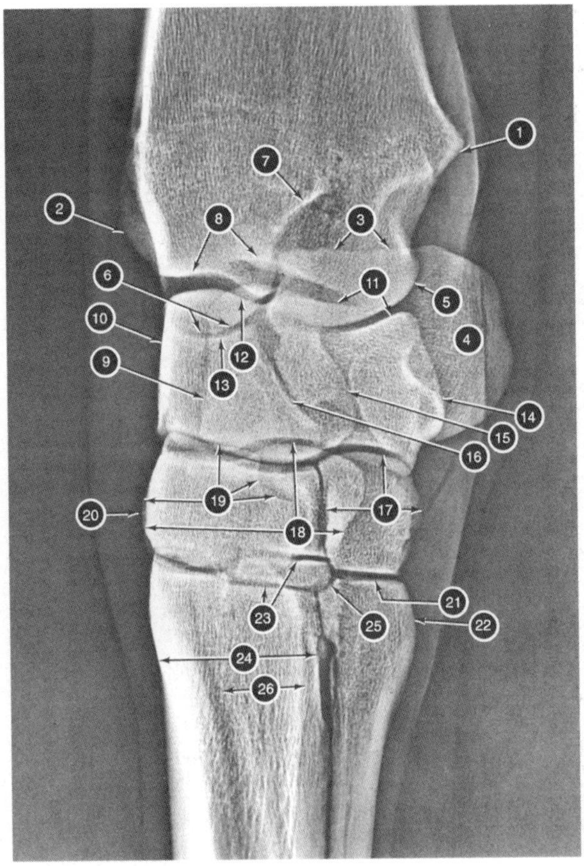

Fig. 16.37 Dorsomedial-palmarolateral oblique xeroradiograph of left equine carpus.

1. Projection of radius for attachment of medial collateral ligament
2. Ridge that forms lateral border of groove for common digital extensor tendon
3. Proximal border of accessory carpal bone
4. Accessory carpal bone
5. Medial styloid process of radius
6. Lateral styloid process
7. Ridge on caudal aspect of radius
8. Ridge at junction of cranial surface of radius with carpal articular surface
9. Dorsolateral border of radial carpal bone
10. Dorsolateral borders of ulnar and intermediate carpal bones
11. Proximal surface of radial carpal bone
12. Proximal surface of intermediate carpal bone
13. Proximal surface of ulnar carpal bone
14. Palmaromedial border of radial carpal bone
15. Palmaromedial border of intermediate carpal bone
16. Palmaromedial border of ulnar carpal bone
17. Second carpal bone
18. Third carpal bone
19. Fourth carpal bone
20. Dorsolateral borders of third and fourth carpal bones
21. Articulation between second carpal bone and metacarpal bone 2
22. Metacarpal bone 2
23. Articulation between third carpal bone and metacarpal bone 3
24. Metacarpal bone 3
25. Inconstant articulation between third carpal bone and metacarpal bone 2
26. Metacarpal bone 4

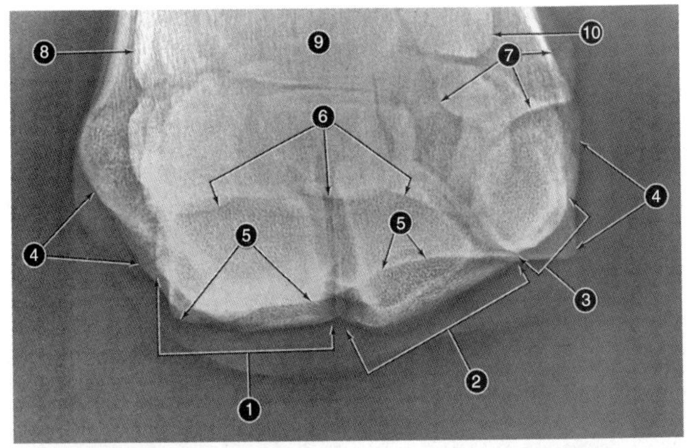

Fig. 16.38 Dorsoproximal-dorsodistal oblique xeroradiograph of proximal row of equine carpal bones.

1. Dorsal surface of radial carpal bone
2. Dorsal surface of intermediate carpal bone
3. Dorsal surface of ulnar carpal bone
4. Radius
5. Carpal articular surface of radial trochlea
6. Dorsal surfaces of distal carpal bones
7. Accessory carpal bone
8. Metacarpal bone 2
9. Metacarpal bone 3
10. Metacarpal bone 4

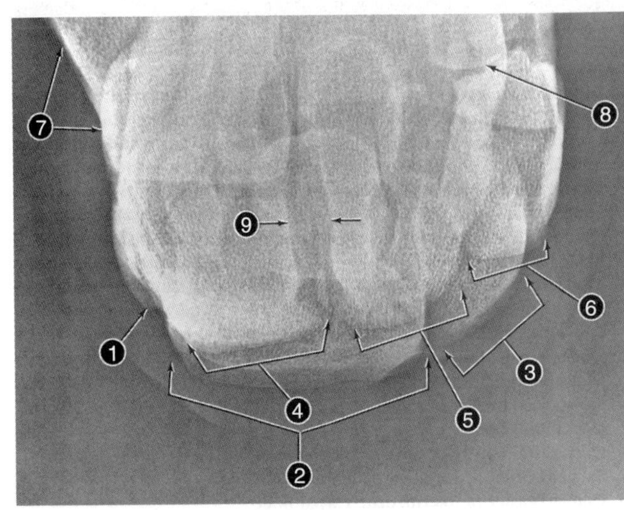

Fig. 16.39 Dorsoproximal-dorsodistal oblique xeroradiograph of distal row of equine carpal bones.

1. Dorsal surface of second carpal bone
2. Dorsal surface of third carpal bone
3. Dorsal surface of fourth carpal bone
4. Dorsal surface of radial carpal bone
5. Dorsal surface of intermediate carpal bone
6. Dorsal surface of ulnar carpal bone
7. Radius
8. Accessory carpal bone
9. Interosseous space between radial and intermediate carpal bones

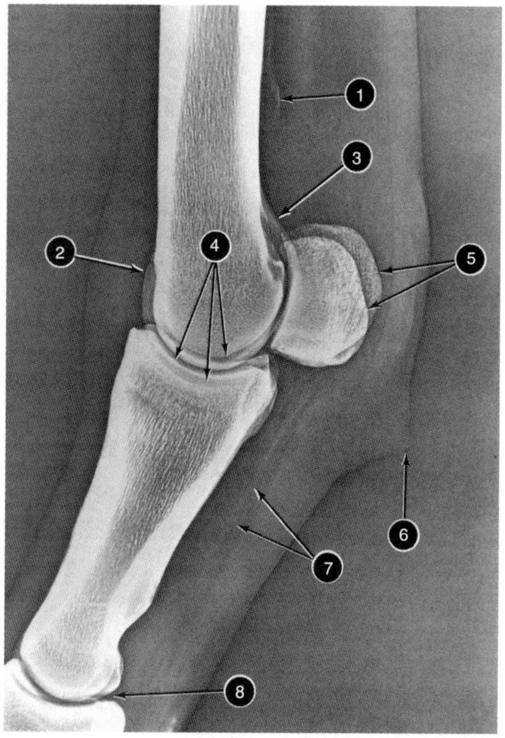

Fig. 16.40 Lateromedial (lateral) xeroradiograph of left equine metacarpophalangeal joint.

1. Distal end (head) of small metacarpal bone
2. Dorsal part of sagittal ridge of metacarpal bone 3
3. Palmar part of sagittal ridge of metacarpal bone 3
4. Metacarpophalangeal joint
5. Proximal sesamoid bones
6. Ergot
7. Straight sesamoid ligament
8. Proximal interphalangeal joint

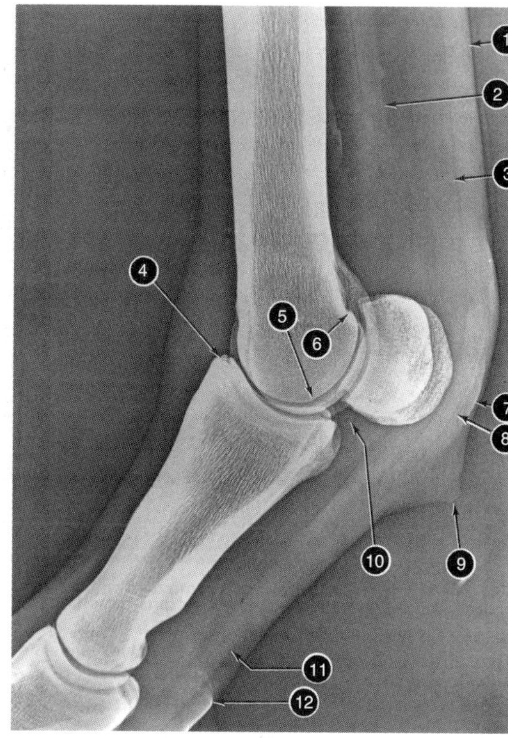

Fig. 16.41 Lateromedial (lateral) xeroradiograph of left equine metacarpophalangeal joint with right limb lifted to increase weight on left limb.

1. Superficial digital flexor tendon
2. Interosseus
3. Deep digital flexor tendon
4. Dorsoproximal aspect of proximal phalanx
5. Subtle transverse ridge on head of metacarpal bone 3
6. Distinct transverse ridge at palmar edge of articular surface
7. Palmar annular ligament of metacarpophalangeal joint
8. Superficial digital flexor tendon
9. Ergot
10. Increased distance between proximal sesamoid bones and proximal phalanx (see Fig. 16.40)
11. Deep distal flexor tendon
12. Distal digital annular ligament

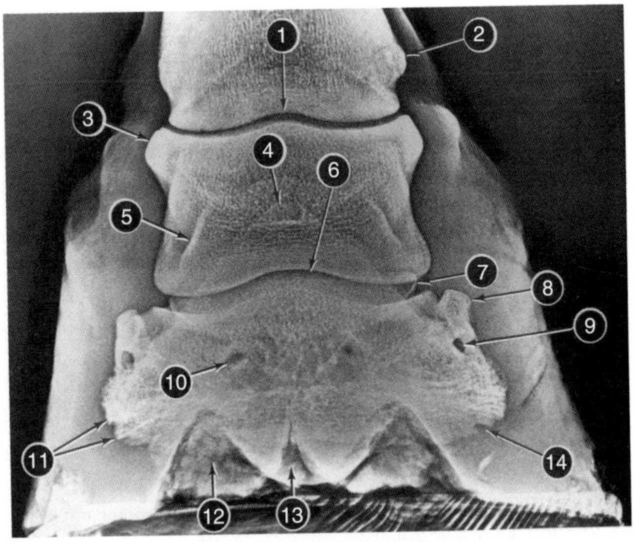

Fig. 16.46 Dorsopalmar xeroradiograph of left equine foredigit.

1. Proximal interphalangeal joint
2. Lateral distal collateral tubercle of proximal phalanx
3. Medial proximal collateral tubercle of middle phalanx
4. Extensor process of distal phalanx
5. Wall of depression in middle phalanx for attachment of medial collateral ligament of distal interphalangeal joint
6. Distal interphalangeal joint
7. Lateral extremity of navicular bone
8. Lateral palmar process of distal phalanx
9. Foramen in lateral palmar process of distal phalanx that accommodates dorsal branches of digital vessels
10. Medial sole foramen of distal phalanx; receives digital vessels as they enter sole canal
11. Sole border of distal phalanx; typically irregular because of notches for vascular channels
12. Medial collateral groove of frog
13. Central groove of frog
14. Notch in sole border associated with vascular channel from sole canal of distal phalanx

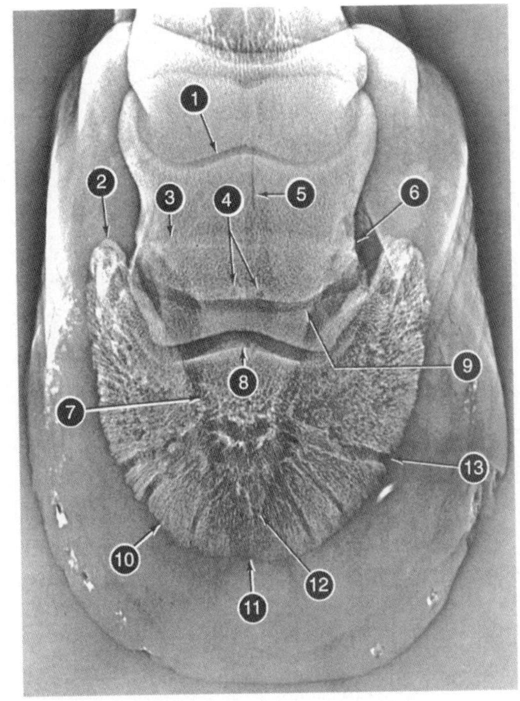

Fig. 16.47 Dorsal 65-degree proximal-palmarodistal oblique xeroradiograph of left equine foredigit.

1. Proximal interphalangeal joint
2. Medial palmar process of distal phalanx
3. Proximal border of navicular bone
4. Vascular foramina and synovial fossae along distal border of navicular bone
5. Air within central groove of frog
6. Lateral extremity of navicular bone
7. Sole canal of distal phalanx
8. Distal interphalangeal joint
9. Articulation of distal phalanx with navicular bone; part of distal interphalangeal joint
10. Sole border of distal phalanx
11. Crena marginis solaris
12. Apex of frog
13. Vascular channel from sole canal to sole border of distal phalanx

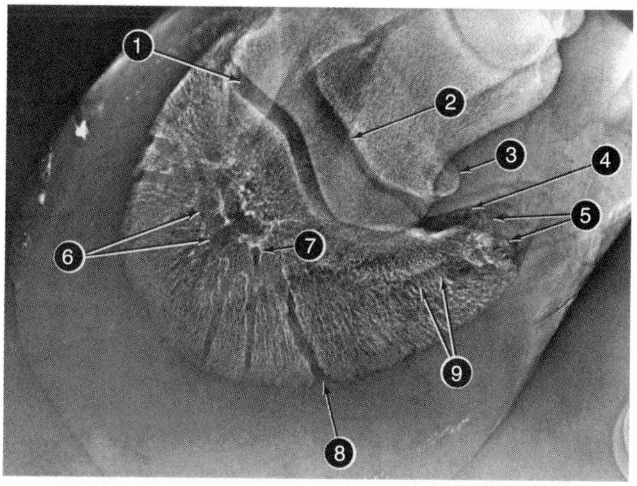

Fig. 16.48 Dorsoproximolateral-palmarodistomedial oblique xeroradiograph of left equine foredigit.

1. Distal interphalangeal joint
2. Articulation of distal phalanx with navicular bone; part of distal interphalangeal joint
3. Lateral extremity of navicular bone
4. Air within lateral collateral groove of frog
5. Lateral palmar process of distal phalanx
6. Sole canal of distal phalanx
7. End-on perspective of vascular channel from sole canal to parietal surface of distal phalanx
8. Vascular channel from sole canal to sole border of distal phalanx
9. Lateral parietal groove of distal phalanx; accommodates dorsal branches of digital vessel

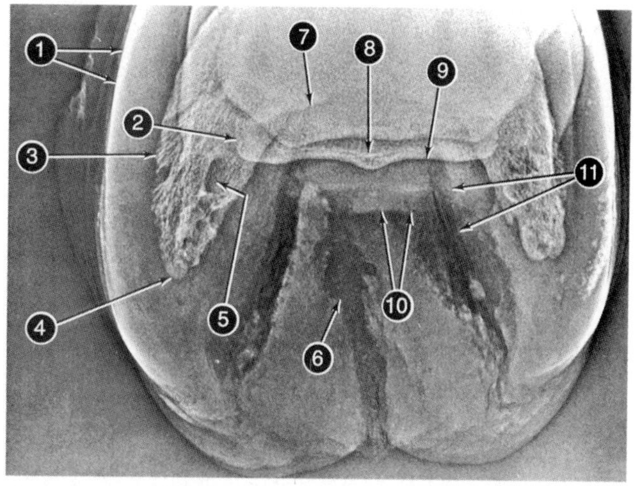

Fig. 16.49 Palmaroproximal-palmarodistal oblique xeroradiograph of left equine foredigit.

1. Proximal border of hoof wall
2. Lateral extremity of navicular bone
3. Sole border of distal phalanx
4. Lateral palmar process of distal phalanx
5. Foramen of lateral palmar process
6. Air within central groove of frog
7. Articulation of middle phalanx with navicular bone; part of distal interphalangeal joint
8. Sagittal ridge of navicular bone
9. Flexor surface of navicular bone
10. Deep digital flexor tendon
11. Air within medial collateral groove of frog

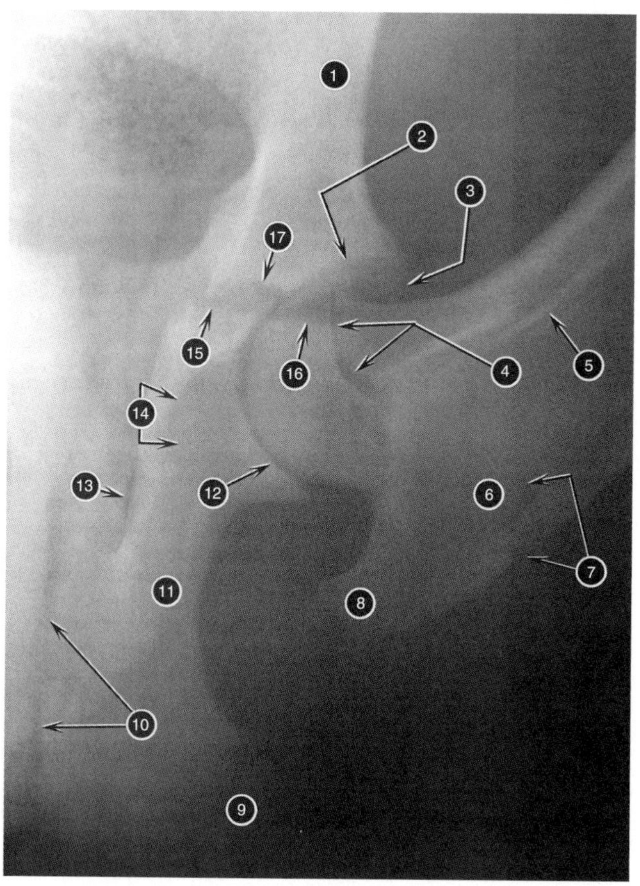

Fig. 16.50 Ventromedial-dorsolateral oblique radiograph of equine hip joint (8 months old).

1. Body of ilium
2. Cranioventral border of acetabulum
3. Craniodorsal border of acetabulum
4. Proximal physis (epiphyseal cartilage) of femur
5. Shadow created by caudal edge of lesser trochanter
6. Radiolucent area created by trochanteric fossa of femur
7. Cartilaginous junction between greater trochanter and femoral body
8. Greater trochanter of femur, caudal part
9. Tuber ischiadicum (ischiatic tuberosity)
10. Cartilaginous pelvic symphysis
11. Body of ischium
12. Caudoventral border of acetabulum
13. Obturator foramen
14. Radiolucent area created by acetabular fossa
15. Radiolucent area created by groove on ventral surface of pubis for accessory ligament of femoral head
16. Radiolucent area created by fovea capitis of femoral head
17. Cranial edge of acetabular notch

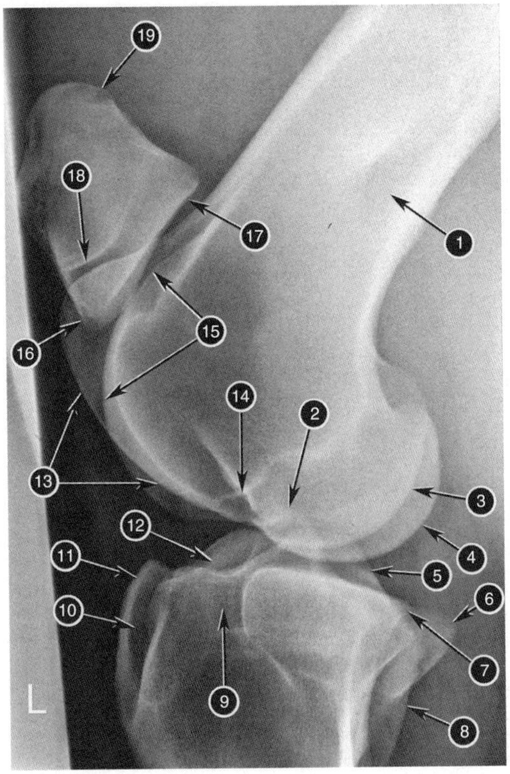

Fig. 16.51 Lateromedial (lateral) radiograph of equine stifle joint.

1. Supracondylar fossa of femur for origin of superficial digital flexor and gastrocnemius muscles
2. Medial tubercle of intercondylar eminence
3. Lateral condyle of femur
4. Medial condyle of femur
5. Lateral tubercle of intercondylar eminence
6. Lateral condyle of tibia
7. Medial condyle of tibia
8. Fibula
9. Extensor groove of tibia
10. Groove for intermediate patellar ligament
11. Lateral part of tibial tuberosity
12. Cranial intercondylar area of tibia
13. Medial ridge of femoral trochlea
14. Extensor fossa of femur
15. Lateral ridge of femoral trochlea
16. Apex of patella
17. Articular surface of patella, gliding part
18. Articular surface of patella, resting part
19. Base of patella

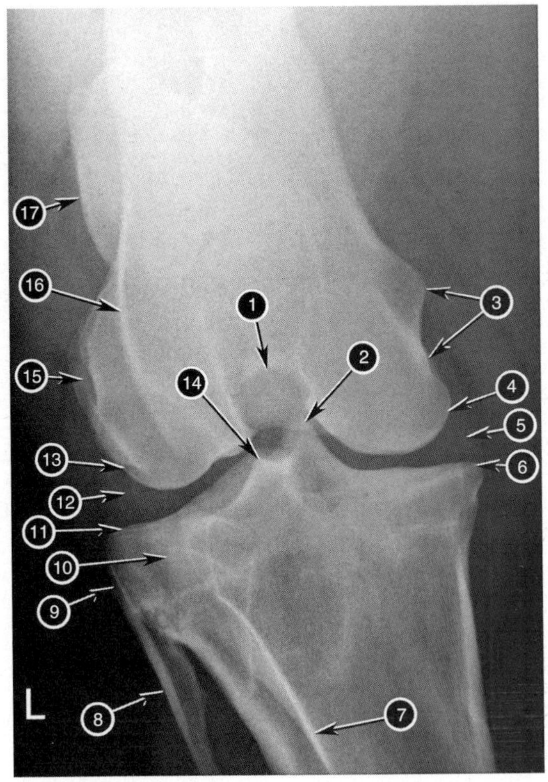

Fig. 16.52 Caudocranial radiograph of equine stifle joint.

1. Intercondylar fossa of femur
2. Medial tubercle of intercondylar eminence
3. Medial epicondyle of femur
4. Medial condyle of femur
5. Medial meniscus and femorotibial joint
6. Medial condyle of tibia
7. Cranial margin of tibia
8. Body of fibula (proximal diaphysis)
9. Head of fibula
10. Lateral part of tibial tuberosity
11. Lateral condyle of tibia
12. Lateral meniscus and femorotibial joint
13. Depression for origin of popliteus muscle
14. Lateral tubercle of intercondylar eminence
15. Lateral epicondyle of femur
16. Lateral ridge of femoral trochlea
17. Patella

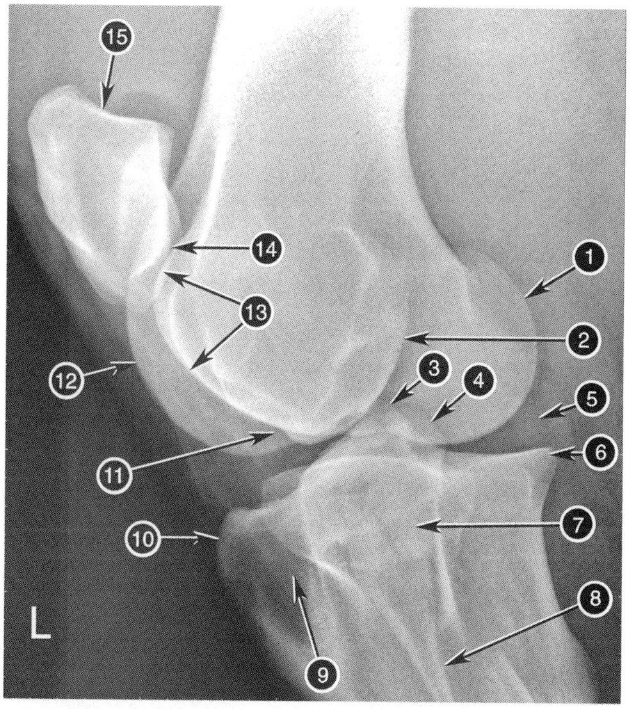

Fig. 16.53 Caudolateral-craniomedial oblique radiograph of equine stifle joint.

1. Medial condyle of femur
2. Lateral condyle of femur
3. Medial tubercle of intercondylar eminence
4. Lateral tubercle of intercondylar eminence
5. Medial meniscus and femorotibial joint
6. Medial condyle of tibia
7. Head of fibula
8. Body of fibula (proximal diaphysis)
9. Extensor groove of tibia
10. Tibial tuberosity
11. Extensor fossa of femur
12. Lateral ridge of femoral trochlea
13. Groove of femoral trochlea
14. Femoropatellar joint
15. Patella

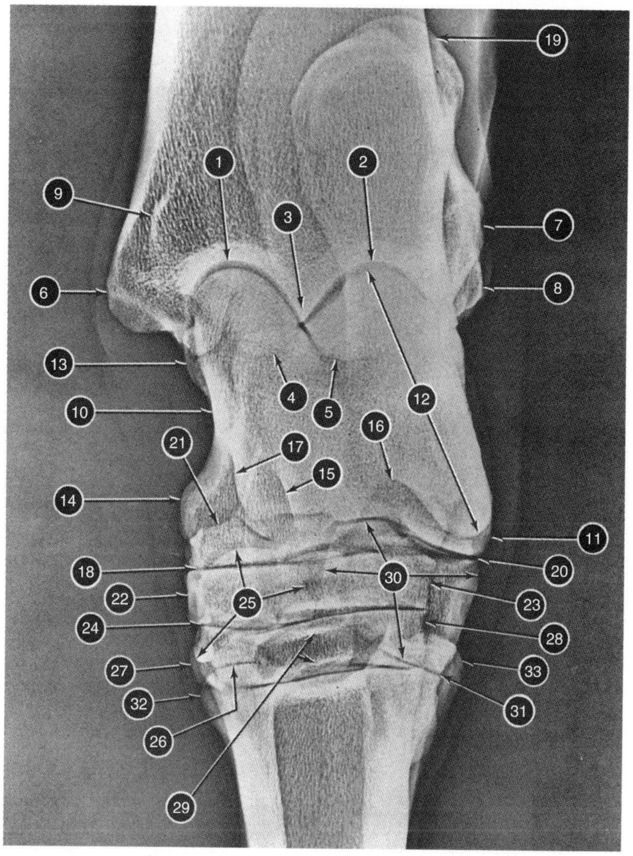

Fig. 16.54 Dorsoplantar xeroradiograph of left equine tarsus.

1. Medial groove of tibial cochlea
2. Lateral groove of tibial cochlea
3. Oblique ridge separating medial and lateral grooves of tibial cochlea
4. Pointed caudal end of oblique ridge
5. Rounded cranial end of oblique ridge
6. Medial malleolus
7. Caudal part of lateral malleolus
8. Cranial part of lateral malleolus
9. Radiopaque shadow
10. Talus
11. Calcaneus
12. Lateral ridge of trochlea tali
13. Proximal tubercle of talus
14. Distal tubercle of talus
15. Medial ridge of trochlea tali
16. Groove between lateral and medial ridges of trochlea tali
17. Medial edge of sustentaculum tali
18. Proximal intertarsal (talocalcaneocentral) joint
19. Tuber calcanei
20. Proximal intertarsal (calcaneoquartal) joint
21. Proximoplantar aspect of central tarsal bone
22. Medial aspect of central tarsal bone
23. Lateral aspect of central tarsal bone
24. Distal intertarsal (centrodistal) joint
25. Fused first and second tarsal bones
26. Articulation between first and second tarsal bones and metatarsal bone 2
27. Medial aspect of third tarsal bone
28. Lateral aspect of third tarsal bone
29. Radiopaque lines produced by walls of nonarticular depressions on third tarsal bone
30. Fourth tarsal bone
31. Tarsometatarsal joints (also articulation between first and second tarsal bones and metatarsal bone 2)
32. Base of metatarsal bone 2
33. Base of metatarsal bone 4

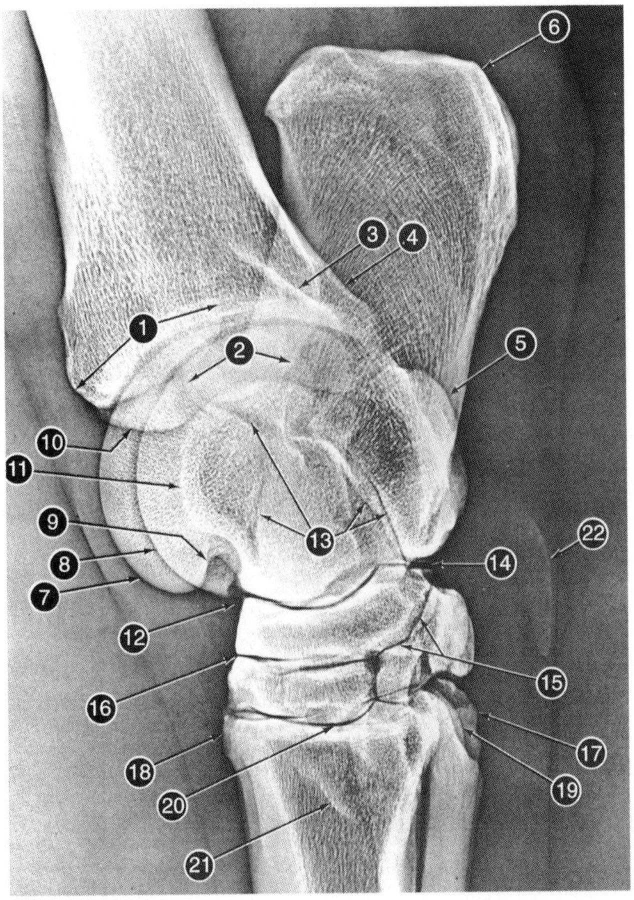

Fig. 16.55 Lateromedial (lateral) xeroradiograph of left equine tarsus.

1. Lateral malleolus
2. Medial malleolus
3. Radiopaque line produced by ridge on caudal surface of tibia
4. Medial part of caudal surface of tibia
5. Sustentaculum tali
6. Tuber calcanei
7. Lateral ridge of trochlea tali
8. Medial ridge of trochlea tali
9. Larger notch associated with lateral ridge of trochlea tali
10. Intermediate part of tibial cochlea
11. Groove of trochlea tali
12. Proximal intertarsal joint
13. Articular facets between talus and calcaneus
14. Plantar aspect of proximal intertarsal joint
15. Articulation between central tarsal bone and fused first and second tarsal bones
16. Distal intertarsal joint
17. Base of metatarsal bone 2
18. Base of metatarsal bone 3
19. Base of metatarsal bone 4
20. Tarsometatarsal joint
21. Groove on metatarsal bone 3 for dorsal metatarsal artery 3
22. Chestnut (torus tarseus)

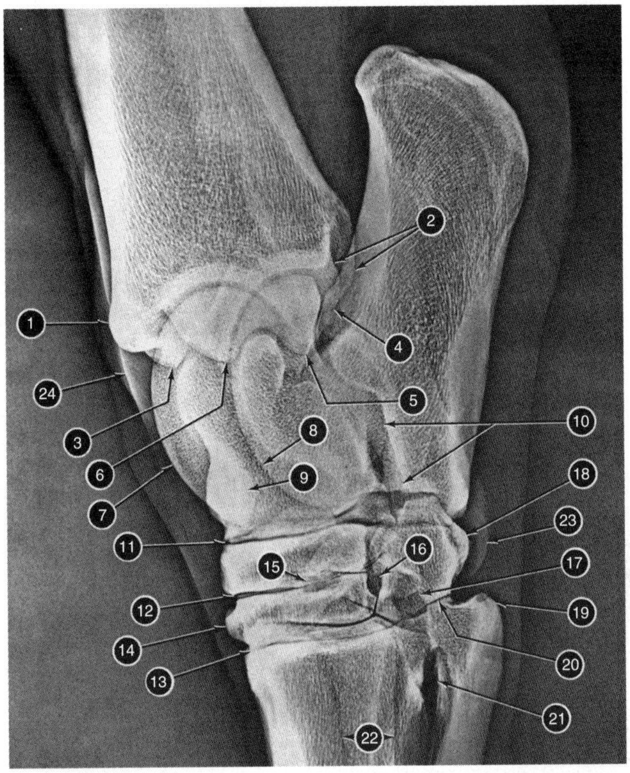

Fig. 16.56 Dorsolateral-plantaromedial oblique xeroradiograph of left equine tarsus.

1. Cranial aspect of medial malleolus
2. Shadows produced by borders of groove in lateral malleolus
3. Distal projection of medial malleolus
4. Distal projection of lateral malleolus
5. Caudal aspect of intermediate ridge of tibial cochlea
6. Cranial aspect of intermediate ridge of tibial cochlea
7. Medial ridge of trochlea tali
8. Lateral ridge of trochlea tali
9. Radiopaque area produced by distal tubercle of talus
10. Sinus tarsi
11. Dorsomedial aspect of proximal intertarsal joint
12. Dorsomedial aspect of distal intertarsal joint
13. Dorsomedial aspect of third tarsometatarsal joint
14. Ridge on dorsomedial aspect of third tarsal bone
15. Nonarticular area between central tarsal bone and third tarsal bone
16. Dorsal opening of tarsal canal
17. Plantar opening of tarsal canal
18. Plantar tuberosity on fourth tarsal bone
19. Base of metatarsal bone 4
20. Articulation between fourth tarsal bone and metatarsal bone 4
21. Interosseous space between metatarsal bones 3 and 4
22. Metatarsal bone 2
23. Chestnut
24. Tendons crossing flexor surface of tarsus

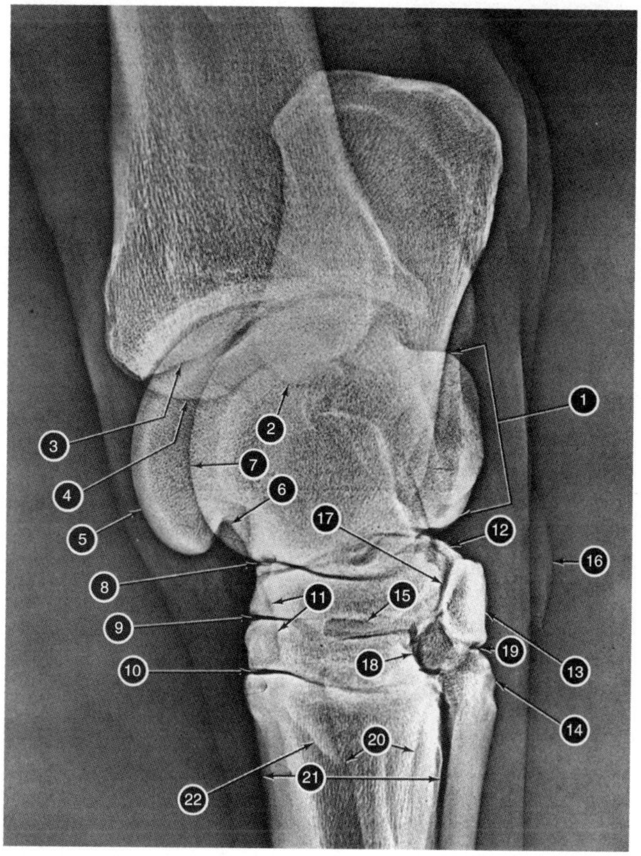

Fig. 16.57 Dorsomedial-plantarolateral oblique xeroradiograph of left equine tarsus.

1. Sustentaculum tali
2. Distal extremity of medial malleolus
3. Distal extremity of lateral malleolus
4. Intermediate ridge of tibial cochlea
5. Lateral ridge of trochlea tali
6. Notch distal to lateral ridge of trochlea tali
7. Medial ridge of trochlea tali
8. Dorsolateral aspect of proximal intertarsal joint
9. Dorsolateral aspect of distal intertarsal joint
10. Dorsolateral aspect of third tarsometatarsal joint
11. Dorsal aspect of fourth tarsal bone
12. Plantaromedial aspect of central tarsal bone
13. Plantaromedial aspect of fused first and second tarsal bones
14. Plantaromedial aspect of metatarsal bone 2
15. Nonarticular depression between central tarsal bone and third tarsal bone
16. Chestnut
17. Articulation between fused first and second tarsal bones and central tarsal bone
18. Articulation between fused first and second tarsal bones and third tarsal bone
19. Articulation between fused first and second tarsal bones and metacarpal bone 2
20. Metacarpal bone
21. Metacarpal bone 3
22. Radiopaque line produced by border of groove for dorsal metatarsal artery 3

REFERENCES

1. Evans HE. *Miller's Anatomy of the Dog*. 3rd ed. Philadelphia: W. B. Saunders Co; 1993.
2. Waibl H, Mayrhofer E, Matis U, et al. *Atlas of Radiographic Anatomy of the Dog*. Stuttgart: Parey Verlag; 2005.
3. Schebitz H, Wilkens H. *Atlas of Radiographic Anatomy of the Horse*. 3rd ed. Philadelphia: Saunders; 1978.
4. Denoix JM. In: *The Equine Distal Limb. An Atlas of Clinical Anatomy and Comparative Imaging*. Boca Raton: CRC Press; 2000.
5. Schebitz H, Wilkens H. *Atlas of Radiographic Anatomy of the Dog and Cat*. 4th ed. Philadelphia: W.B. Saunders Co; 1986.
6. Thrall D, Robertson ID. *Atlas of Normal Radiographic Anatomy and Anatomic Variants in the Dog and Cat*. 2nd ed. St Louis: Elsevier; 2016.
7. Coulson A, Lewis N. *An Atlas of Interpretative Radiographic Anatomy of the Dog and Cat*. 2nd ed. Ames: Blackwell Publishing; 2008.
8. Smallwood JE, Shively MJ, Rendano VT, et al. A standardized nomenclature for radiographic projections used in veterinary medicine. *Vet Radiol*. 1985;26:2.
9. Smallwood JE, Shively MJ. Radiographic and xeroradiographic anatomy of the equine carpus. *Equine Pract*. 1979;1:22.
10. Smallwood JE, Holladay SD. Xeroradiographic anatomy of the equine digit and metacarpophalangeal region. *Vet Radiol*. 1987;28:166.
11. Shively MJ, Smallwood JE. Radiographic and xeroradiographic anatomy of the equine tarsus. *Equine Pract*. 1980;2:19.

CHAPTER 17

Principles of Radiographic Interpretation of the Appendicular Skeleton and Radiographic Features of Bone Tumors

Donald E. Thrall

POSITIONING: DOG AND CAT

Radiographic examination of extremities in dogs and cats should consist of a minimum of two orthogonal projections, a lateral view and a craniocaudal* view. The radiographic field of view should include the joints proximal and distal to the bone of interest. If a joint is being investigated, the primary x-ray beam should be centered on that joint. Occasionally, especially for complex joints like the carpus and tarsus, there are views in addition to the standard orthogonal views that are used for further clarification. These *oblique* views allow evaluation of an edge that is not projected in the standard view. Oblique views are discussed later in the section on equine positioning as they are used more frequently in the horse than in the dog or cat.

There are a few highly specific ancillary projections in dogs that allow evaluation of the edge of surfaces that cannot be assessed in the conventional views. Examples include a cranioproximal/craniodistal view of the bicipital groove for changes associated with bicipital tenosynovitis (Fig. 17.1A) and a flexed dorsoplantar view of the canine tarsus for evaluation of the trochlea of talus without superimposition of calcaneus, for changes associated with osteochondrosis of the talus (see Fig. 17.1B). These specific views are provided only as examples of how changing the orientation of the x-ray beam can lead to projection of clinically important surfaces that cannot be assessed adequately in more standard views. These ancillary views, and others, are discussed throughout the textbook where appropriate.[1]

POSITIONING: HORSE

One aspect of equine radiography that deserves special mention is the common practice of holding the plate by hand. Equine extremity radiographs are almost always acquired with the horse in a standing position, and holding the plate by hand is convenient. However, handholding the plate increases the chance that radiation safety practices will be compromised. Individuals holding a plate by hand should wear protective lead aprons and lead gloves, as well as a thyroid shield and protective lead glasses. And the positioning must be such that no part of the holder is in the primary x-ray beam.

The use of a plate holder for equine extremity radiography is encouraged because it will minimize occupational radiation exposure. A plate holder secures the plate and has an extension handle so that the hands are distant from the primary x-ray beam. A potential disadvantage of a plate holder is the strength needed to position the plate properly.

There are very few instances in the horse where two orthogonal views of a limb will suffice. Two orthogonal views might be adequate for examining the radius or tibia, but even in those sites, *oblique* views are often needed for completeness. Oblique views are intended to project *edges* of a joint or region that cannot be evaluated in standard orthogonal views. More than the edge of a structure can be assessed in any radiograph, but important edge lesions can be overlooked unless they are projected at the periphery of the part. Oblique views maximize the chances of detecting an edge lesion in a complex joint. In oblique views, the point of entrance of the primary x-ray beam is typically moved 30 to 45 degrees medial or 30 to 45 degrees lateral to the point of entrance used for a conventional view. The geometry of oblique projections can be confusing, and this will be explained using the equine carpus as a model (Table 17.1, Figs. 17.2–17.5).[†]

In a dorsopalmar view of the carpus, the x-ray beam strikes the dorsal surface and the medial and lateral edges are projected in an unobstructed fashion (see Fig. 17.2). A palmarodorsal view would be similar.

In a lateromedial view of the carpus, the x-ray beam strikes the lateral surface, and the dorsal and palmar edges are projected in an unobstructed fashion (see Fig. 17.3). A mediolateral view would be similar.

In a dorsolateral-palmaromedial view of the carpus, the x-ray beam strikes the dorsolateral surface (between the true dorsal and lateral surfaces) with the dorsomedial and palmarolateral edges projected in an unobstructed fashion (see Fig. 17.4). A palmaromedial-dorsolateral view would be similar.

In a dorsomedial-palmarolateral view of the carpus, the x-ray beam strikes the dorsomedial surface with the dorsolateral and palmaromedial edges projected in an unobstructed fashion (see Fig. 17.5). A palmarolateral-dorsomedial view would be similar.

AGGRESSIVE VERSUS NONAGGRESSIVE BONE LESIONS

The principle of using roentgen signs to describe radiographic abnormalities was introduced in Chapter 6, and this method is applicable to describing bone lesions located anywhere in the body. However, in addition to describing a bone lesion according to roentgen signs, an important distinction is whether the bone lesion is caused by an aggressive process, such as a tumor or infection, versus a nonaggressive process, such as a bone cyst. Determining whether a bone lesion is aggressive will

*The term *craniocaudal* applies to a view of a limb where the x-ray beam strikes the front of the limb proximal to the antebrachiocarpal or tarsocrural joint. Views distal to these points would be termed *dorsopalmar* and *dorsoplantar*, respectively. A caudocranial (or palmarodorsal or plantarodorsal) view would be comparable.

†In Figs. 17.2 through 17.5, the imaging plate is oriented perpendicular to the primary x-ray beam, but the plate is not shown for the sake of clarity.

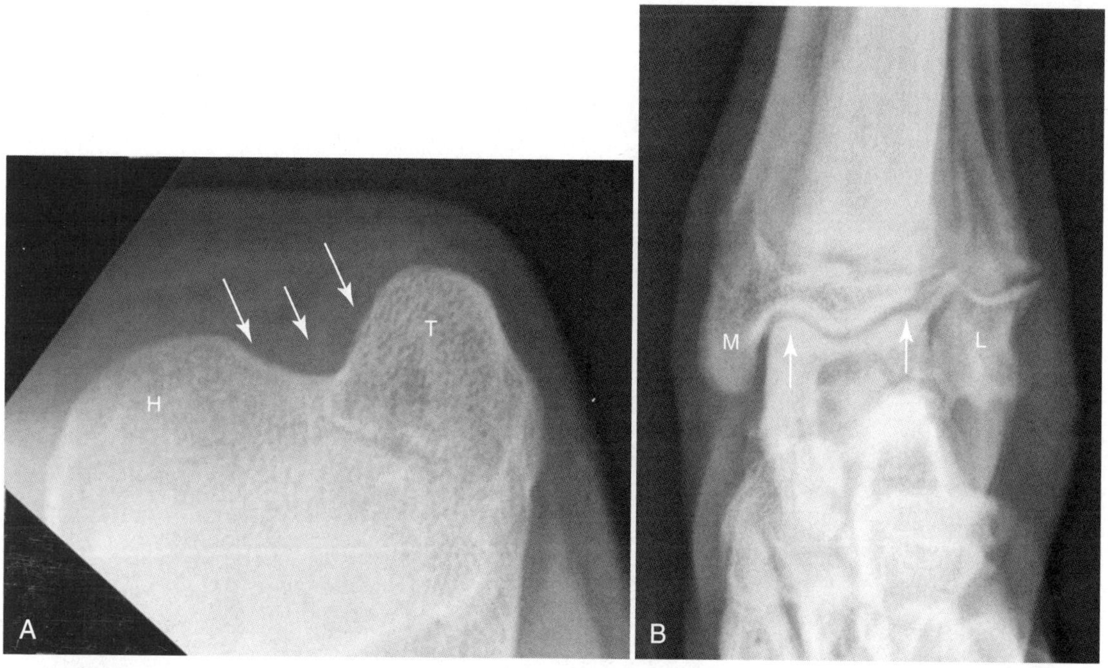

Fig. 17.1 **A,** Cranioproximal/craniodistal view of the proximal humerus to project the bicipital groove (*white arrows*). *H,* Humeral head; *T,* greater tubercle. **B,** Flexed dorsoplantar view of the canine tarsus to project the trochlea of the talus (*white arrows*) without superimposition of the calcaneus. *H,* Humeral head; *L,* lateral malleolus; *M,* medial malleolus; *T,* greater tubercle.

Table • **17.1**

Summary of Edges Projected in Oblique Radiographs.

PROJECTION	STRIKE POINT OF PRIMARY X-RAY BEAM	EDGES PROJECTED
Dorsopalmar	Dorsal	Lateral and medial
Dorsoplantar	Dorsal	Lateral and medial
Craniocaudal	Cranial	Lateral and medial
Palmarodorsal	Palmar	Lateral and medial
Plantarodorsal	Plantar	Lateral and medial
Caudocranial	Caudal	Lateral and medial
Lateromedial	Lateral	Dorsal and palmar, or dorsal and plantar, or cranial and caudal
Mediolateral	Medial	Dorsal and palmar, or dorsal and plantar, or cranial and caudal
Dorsolateral/palmaromedial	Dorsolateral	Dorsomedial and palmarolateral
Palmaromedial/dorsolateral	Palmaromedial	Dorsomedial and palmarolateral
Dorsolateral/plantaromedial	Dorsolateral	Dorsomedial and plantarolateral
Plantaromedial/dorsolateral	Plantaromedial	Dorsomedial and plantarolateral
Craniolateral/caudomedial	Craniolateral	Craniomedial and caudolateral
Caudomedial/craniolateral	Caudomedial	Craniomedial and caudolateral
Dorsomedial/palmarolateral	Dorsomedial	Dorsolateral and palmaromedial
Palmaromedial/dorsomedial	Palmaromedial	Dorsolateral and palmaromedial
Dorsomedial/plantarolateral	Dorsomedial	Dorsolateral and palmaromedial
Plantarolateral/dorsomedial	Plantarolateral	Dorsolateral and palmaromedial

be helpful in directing patient management. For example, a nonaggressive bone lesion could be evaluated sequentially over time for any change. However, sequential evaluation of an aggressive lesion, which is often due to a tumor or an infections process, could jeopardize the patient. Also, if an aggressive bone lesion is present, thoracic radiographs are indicated and an aspirate or biopsy should also be considered. Distinguishing an aggressive from a nonaggressive bone lesion involves the consideration of several specific factors other than basic roentgen signs.

Three criteria are used to determine whether a bone lesion is aggressive: (1) the integrity of the cortex, (2) the character of any periosteal reaction, and (3) the distinctness of the boundary between the bone lesion and the normal bone, called the

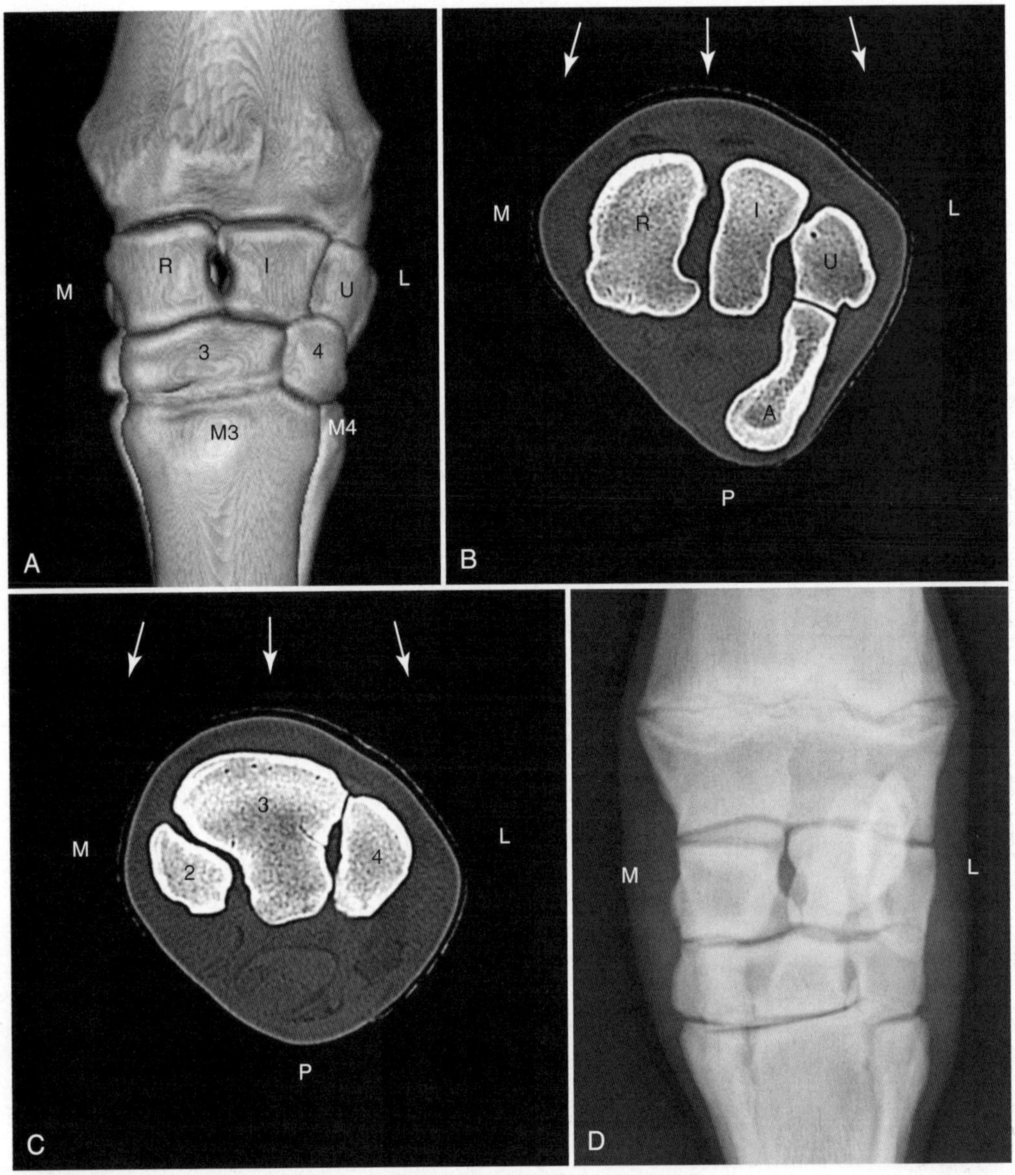

Fig. 17.2 Anatomy of a dorsopalmar radiograph of the equine carpus. **A,** Three-dimensional volume-rendered computed tomography (CT) image of an equine carpus from a dorsal perspective. **B,** Transverse CT image of an equine carpus through the proximal row of carpal bones. **C,** Transverse CT image of an equine carpus through the distal row of carpal bones. **D,** Dorsopalmar equine carpal radiograph. In **B** and **C,** the *white arrows* indicate the direction of the primary x-ray beam. For a dorsopalmar projection, the x-ray beam strikes the dorsal surface of the carpus and the medial and lateral edges of the carpus will be projected. *2,* Second carpal bone; *3,* third carpal bone; *4,* fourth carpal bone; *A,* accessory carpal bone; *I,* intermediate carpal bone; *L,* lateral; *M,* medial; *M3,* third metacarpal bone; *M4,* fourth metacarpal bone; *P,* palmar; *R,* radial carpal bone; *U,* ulnar carpal bone.

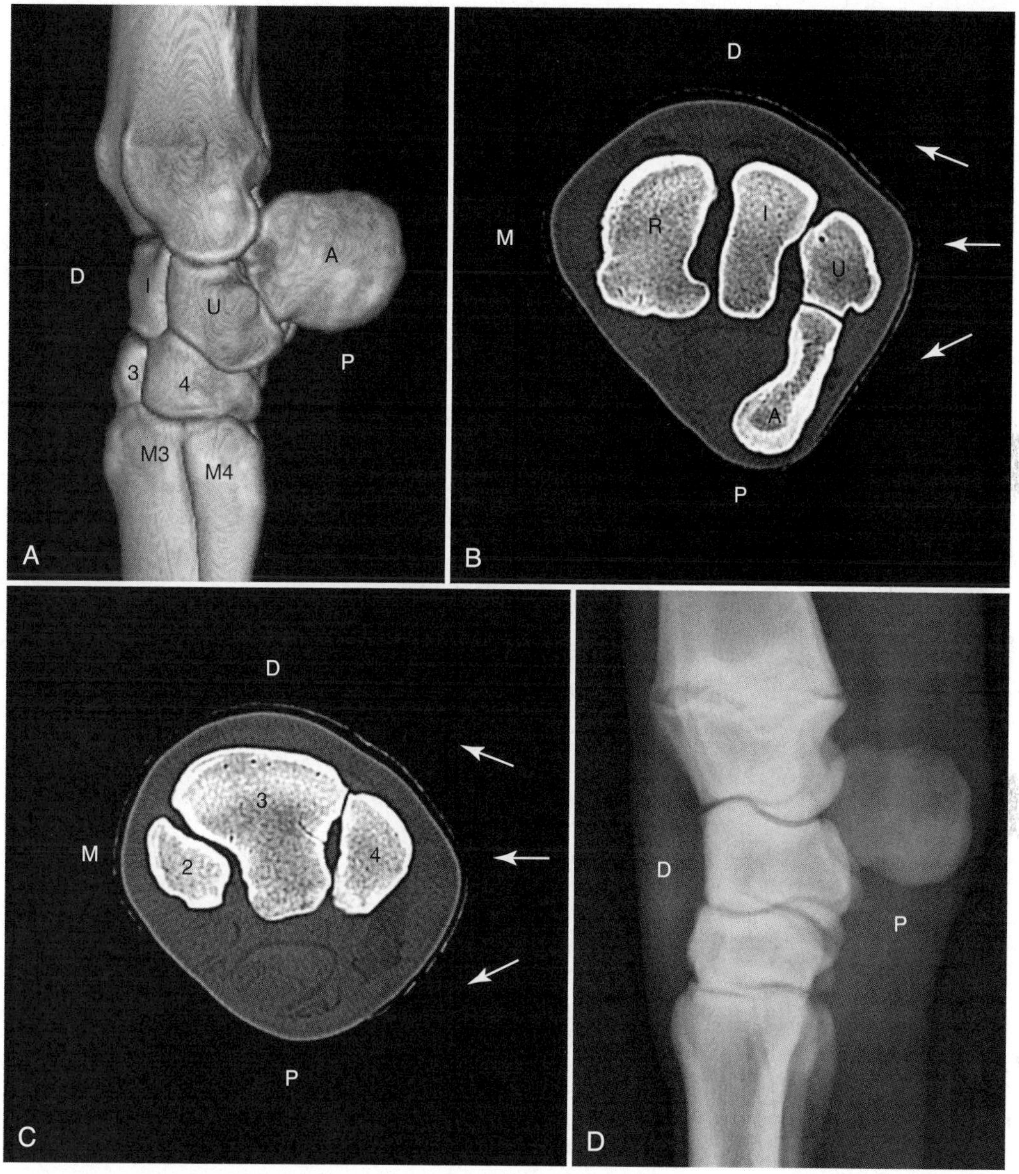

Fig. 17.3 Anatomy of a lateromedial radiograph of the equine carpus. **A,** Three-dimensional volume-rendered computed tomography (CT) image of an equine carpus from a lateral perspective. **B,** Transverse CT image of an equine carpus through the proximal row of carpal bones. **C,** Transverse CT image of an equine carpus through the distal row of carpal bones. **D,** Lateromedial equine carpal radiograph. In **B** and **C,** the *white arrows* indicate the direction of the primary x-ray beam. For a lateromedial projection, the x-ray beam strikes the lateral surface of the carpus and the dorsal and palmar edges of the carpus will be projected. *2,* Second carpal bone; *3,* third carpal bone; *4,* fourth carpal bone; *A,* accessory carpal bone; *D,* dorsal; *I,* intermediate carpal bone; *M,* medial; *M3,* third metacarpal bone; *M4,* fourth metacarpal bone; *P,* palmar; *R,* radial carpal bone; *U,* ulnar carpal bone.

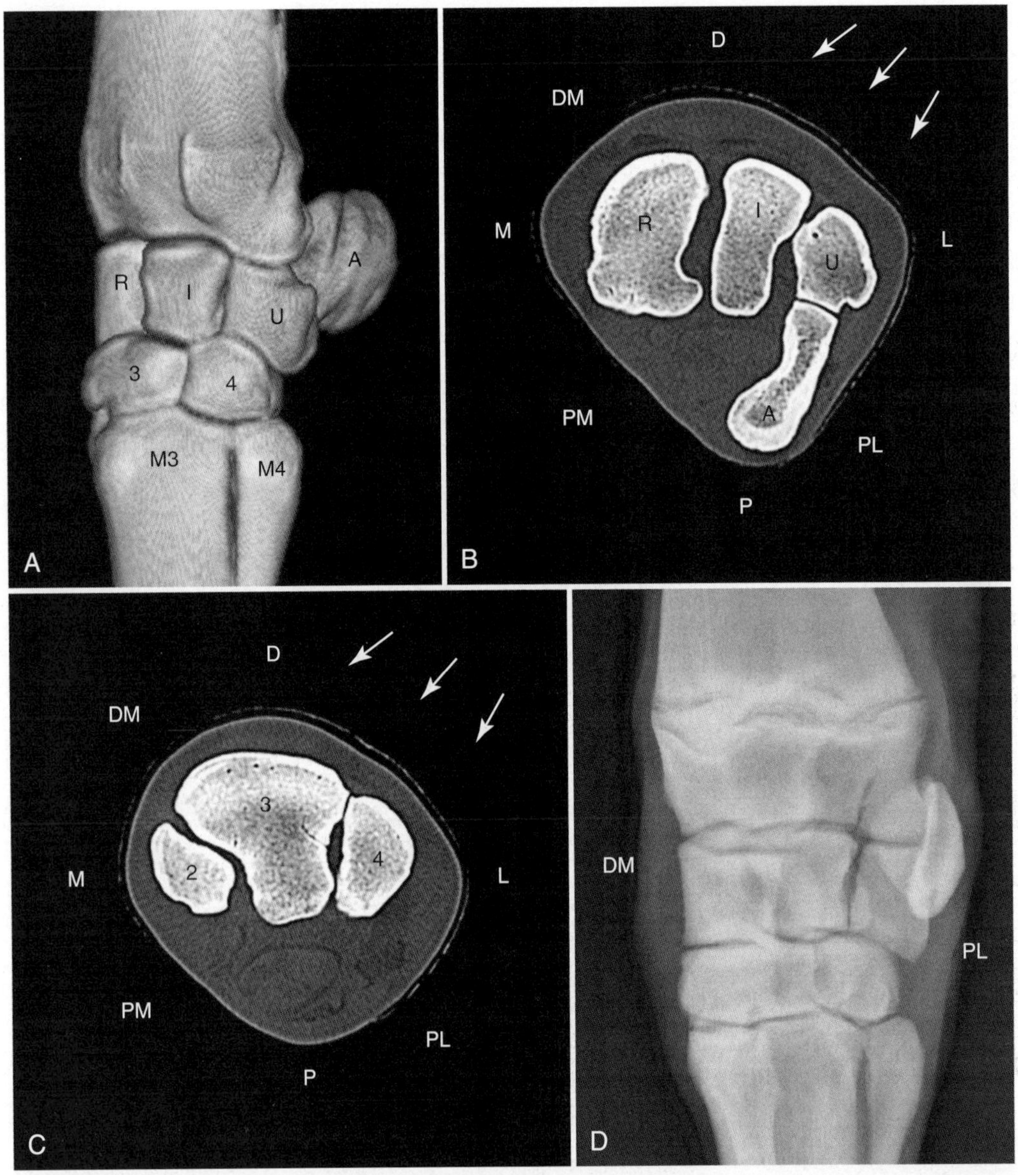

Fig. 17.4 Anatomy of a dorsolateral-palmaromedial radiograph of the equine carpus. **A,** Three-dimensional volume-rendered computed tomography (CT) image of an equine carpus from a dorsolateral perspective. **B,** Transverse CT image of an equine carpus through the proximal row of carpal bones. **C,** Transverse CT image of an equine carpus through the distal row of carpal bones. **D,** Dorsolateral-palmaromedial equine carpal radiograph. In **B** and **C,** the *white arrows* indicate the direction of the primary x-ray beam. For a dorsolateral/palmaromedial radiograph, the x-ray beam strikes the dorsolateral surface of the carpus, and the dorsomedial and palmarolateral edges of the carpus will be projected. *2,* Second carpal bone; *3,* third carpal bone; *4,* fourth carpal bone; *A,* accessory carpal bone; *D,* dorsal; *DM,* dorsomedial; *I,* intermediate carpal bone; *L,* lateral; *M,* medial; *M3,* third metacarpal bone; *M4,* fourth metacarpal bone; *P,* palmar; *PL,* palmarolateral; *PM,* palmaromedial; *R,* radial carpal bone; *U,* ulnar carpal bone.

transition zone (Table 17.2). An aggressive bone lesion will have either an area of cortex destruction **and/or** an active periosteal reaction **and/or** an indistinct transition zone. Therefore, only one criterion of aggressiveness is needed to fulfill the definition of aggressiveness. Importantly, whether a lesion is primarily radiolucent (loss of bone) or radiopaque (production of bone) has no bearing on whether the lesion is aggressive.

Destruction of the Cortex

For cortex destruction, also referred to as *cortex effacement*, to be apparent radiographically, the region of destruction must be hit tangentially by the primary x-ray beam. In other words, the *edge* of the cortex destruction must be visible radiographically, and this depends on the orientation of the cortical destruction with the primary x-ray beam (Figs. 17.6–17.8). If the cortex destruction is not projected tangentially, the affected region of bone will appear more radiolucent, but a discrete area of cortex destruction will not be identified.

Not all bone destruction involves the cortex. Bone loss can be totally within the medullary cavity with preservation of the cortex. Purely medullary bone loss does not mean that the lesion is not aggressive; it means only that one feature of lesion aggressiveness (i.e., cortical destruction) is not present.

A subclassification of bone lysis into geographic, moth-eaten, and permeative patterns has been described.[2] Geographic bone lysis is a large, relatively well-defined region

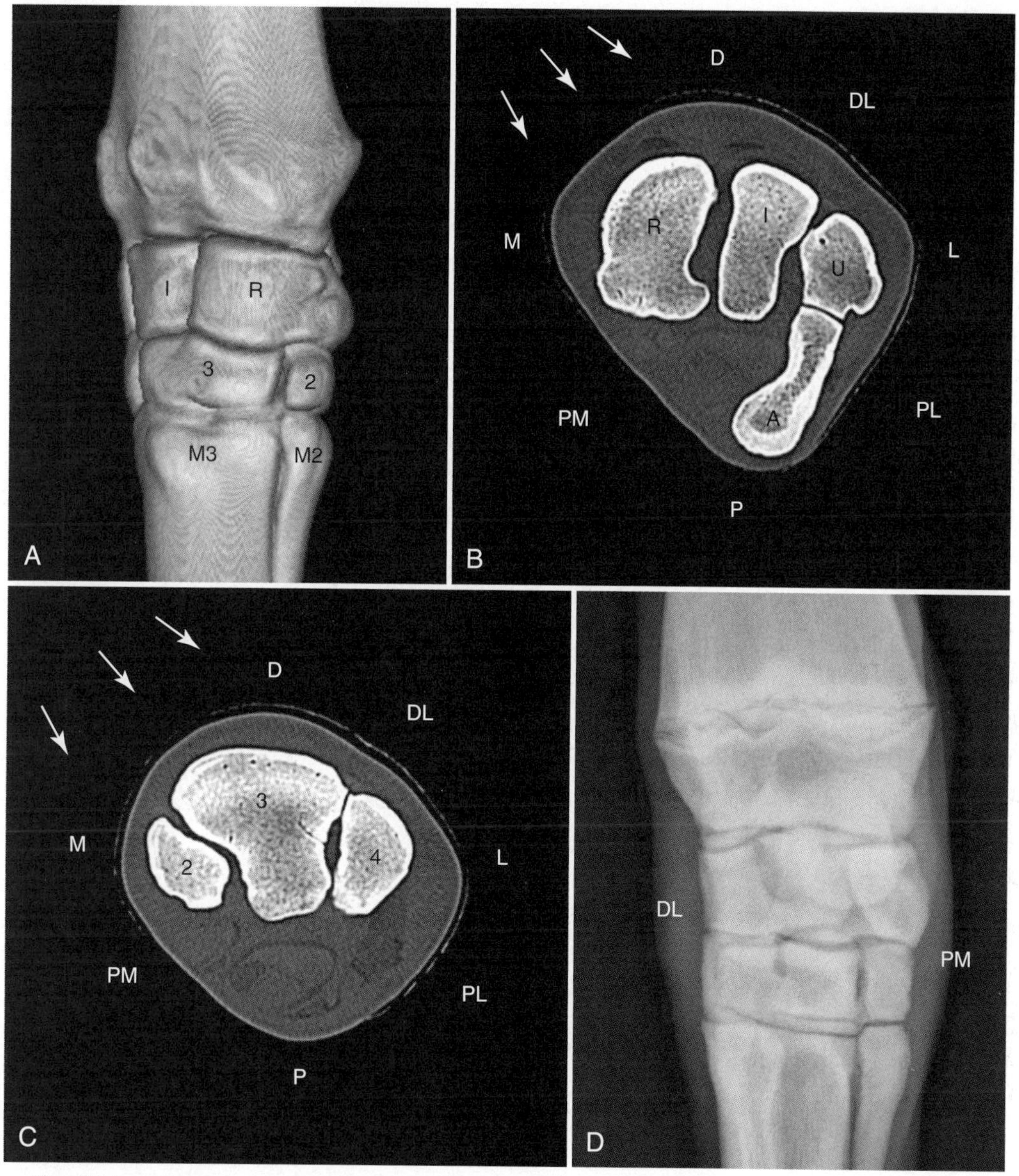

Fig. 17.5 Anatomy of a dorsomedial-palmarolateral radiograph of the equine carpus. **A,** Three-dimensional volume-rendered computed tomography (CT) image of an equine carpus from a dorsomedial perspective. **B,** Transverse CT image of an equine carpus through the proximal row of carpal bones. **C,** Transverse CT image of an equine carpus through the distal row of carpal bones. **D,** Dorsomedial-palmarolateral equine carpal radiograph. In **B** and **C,** the *white arrows* indicate the direction of the primary x-ray beam. For a dorsomedial/palmarolateral projection, the x-ray beam strikes the dorsomedial surface of the carpus, and the dorsolateral and palmaromedial edges of the carpus will be projected. *2,* Second carpal bone; *3,* third carpal bone; *4,* fourth carpal bone; *A,* accessory carpal bone; *D,* dorsal; *DL,* dorsolateral; *I,* intermediate carpal bone; *L,* lateral; *M,* medial; *M2,* second metacarpal bone; *M3,* third metacarpal bone; *P,* palmar; *PL,* palmarolateral; *PM,* palmaromedial; *R,* radial carpal bone; *U,* ulnar carpal bone.

Table • **17.2**

Features of Aggressive and Nonaggressive Bone Lesions.

LESION CLASS	CORTICAL DESTRUCTION	PERIOSTEAL REACTION	TRANSITION ZONE
Aggressive	Yes	Active (irregular)	Not distinct
Nonaggressive	None or expansion of cortex without destruction	None or smooth	Distinct

The presence of any one feature of aggressiveness is sufficient to classify the lesion as such; it is not necessary for all three criteria of aggressiveness to be fulfilled.

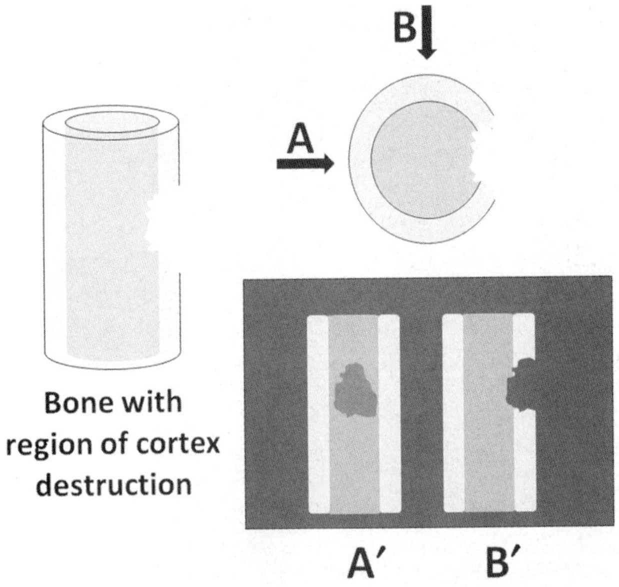

Fig. 17.6 Diagram illustrating the effect of x-ray beam orientation on appearance of cortex destruction. The drawing on the *left* is a bone with a region of cortex destruction. At the *top right* is a cross-section of the bone through the region of cortex destruction. Two orientations of the x-ray beam are shown. In orientation *A*, the x-ray beam strikes the cortex destruction *en face*. In orientation *B*, the x-ray beam strikes the cortex destruction *tangentially*. At the *bottom right* is a diagram of the radiograph resulting from each orientation. In *A′*, the cortex defect will appear as a region of decreased opacity in the center of the bone but the actual defect will not be apparent. In *B′*, the cortex defect is apparent because the defect has been struck tangentially by the x-ray beam. This reemphasizes the importance of having at least two projections of each part being radiographed.

of bone loss (Fig. 17.9). Moth-eaten and permeative patterns of bone lysis are similar and describe the presence of multiple smaller foci, or a less well-defined permeating pattern, of bone lysis (Figs. 17.10 and 17.11). It has been suggested that geographic bone lysis characterizes a less aggressive bone lesion than either moth-eaten or permeative lysis.[2] However, this is not always true and whether a lesion is aggressive should be based only on the criteria noted in Table 17.2. These patterns of lysis should be reserved for descriptive purposes only, as in communication or reports.

In a nonaggressive bone lesion, the cortex may be uninvolved, or it may be expanded without destruction (Fig. 17.12).

Periosteal Reaction

Periosteal bone proliferation is most commonly caused by elevation of the periosteum or regional hyperemia causing activation of bone-forming mesenchymal cells (Fig. 17.13). An active periosteal reaction is a feature of an aggressive bone lesion and is one where the margin of the periosteal reaction is *irregular*, not smooth. There are various degrees of periosteal reactivity and almost innumerable specific appearances of an active periosteal reaction. The presence of an *irregular margin* is the clue that the periosteal reaction is active. Any evidence of periosteal irregularity is consistent with an aggressive bone lesion (Figs. 17.14–17.16). In comparison, a nonaggressive periosteal reaction is characterized by a smooth edge to the periosteal new bone growth (Figs. 17.17 and 17.18) due to remodeling of the periosteal surface after a previous insult or a very slowly proceeding disease process. A smooth periosteal reaction does not mean that the lesion is not aggressive as there may be another finding that characterizes the lesion as aggressive. For example, a lesion with a smooth periosteal reaction but an indistinct transition zone would still be aggressive, as in Fig. 17.17.

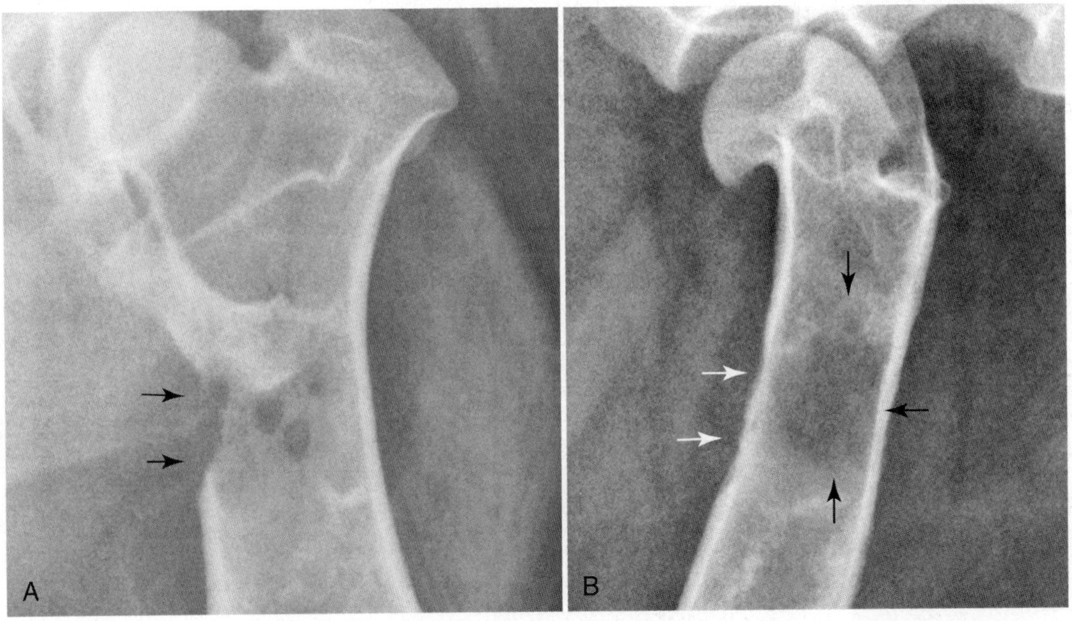

Fig. 17.7 Craniocaudal **(A)** and lateral **(B)** radiographs of the femur of a dog with region of cortex destruction due to metastatic carcinoma. In **A,** the x-ray beam strikes the cortex destruction tangentially (*black arrows*). In **B,** the cortex destruction is superimposed on the bone (*black arrows*) and is not specifically identified. The cranial cortex is irregular (*white arrows*) but is not completely effaced.

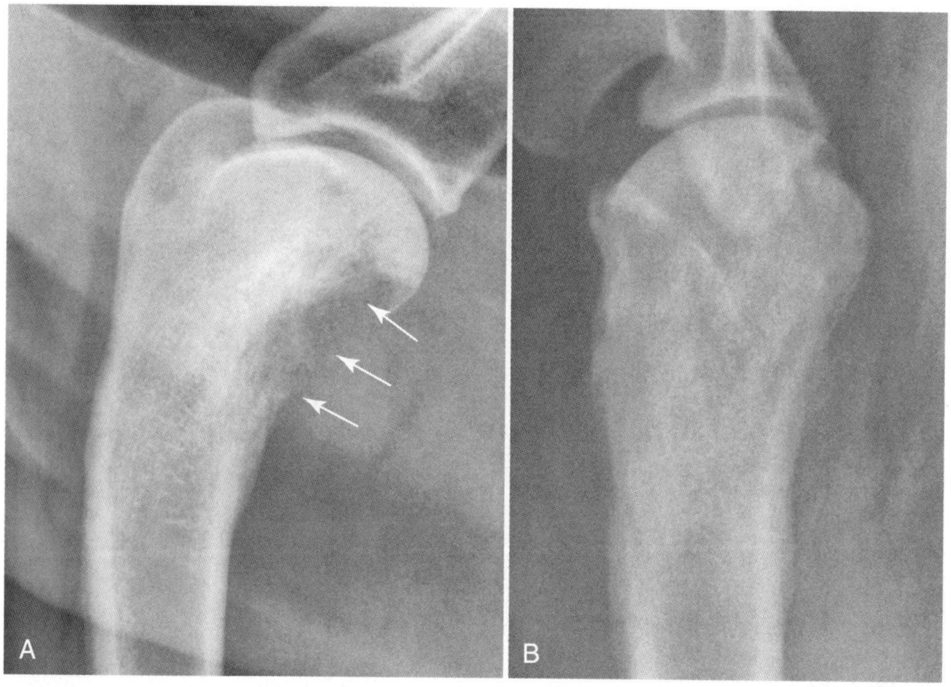

Fig. 17.8 Lateral **(A)** and caudocranial **(B)** views of the proximal aspect of the humerus of a dog with a region of cortex destruction due to osteosarcoma. In **A**, there is obvious destruction of the caudal aspect of the cortex (*white arrows*). In **B**, the cortex destruction is not evident because it is superimposed on the bone.

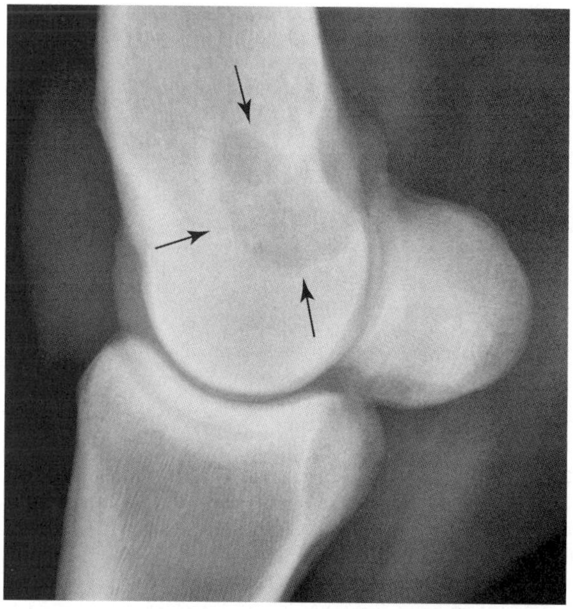

Fig. 17.9 Lateral radiograph of the distal metacarpus of a horse. There is a large region of geographic bone lysis in the third metacarpal bone (*black arrows*). This lesion has a well-defined transition zone (*black arrows*).

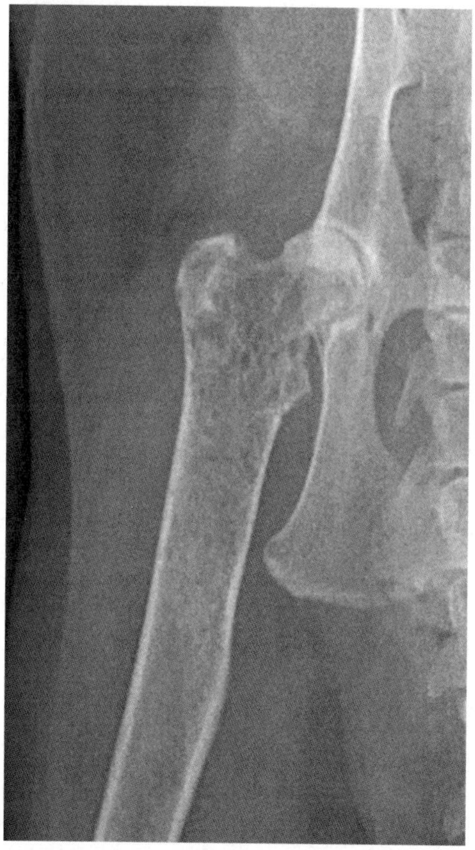

Fig. 17.10 Craniocaudal view of the proximal femur of a cat where multiple small areas of moth-eaten lysis are present. The border of these lesions is not well defined, and this is an aggressive process.

Transition Zone

The character of the junction of the bone lesion with the adjacent normal bone is termed the *transition zone*. The transition zone is typically evaluated in the medullary cavity of the bone. The host bone is usually able to contain a nonaggressive process by forming a sclerotic rim around any area of diseased bone, and the transition zone between the lesion and

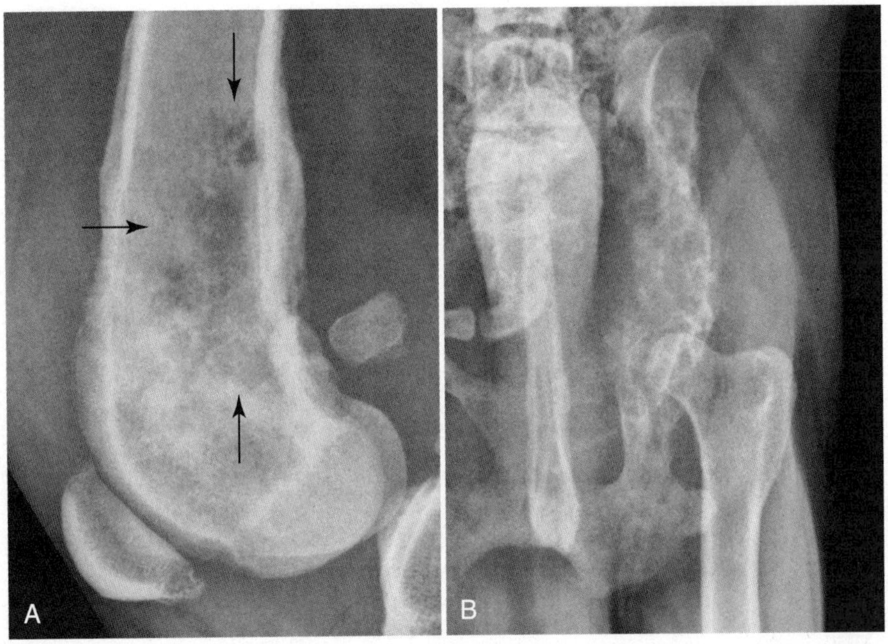

Fig. 17.11 Lateral radiograph of the distal femur in a dog **(A)** and ventrodorsal radiograph of the left hemipelvis of a dog **(B)** with each characterized by permeative lysis. In **A,** the region of lysis is poorly defined (*black arrows*). There is also a sclerotic component and a periosteal reaction. In **B,** the medial cortex of the ilium is also destroyed.

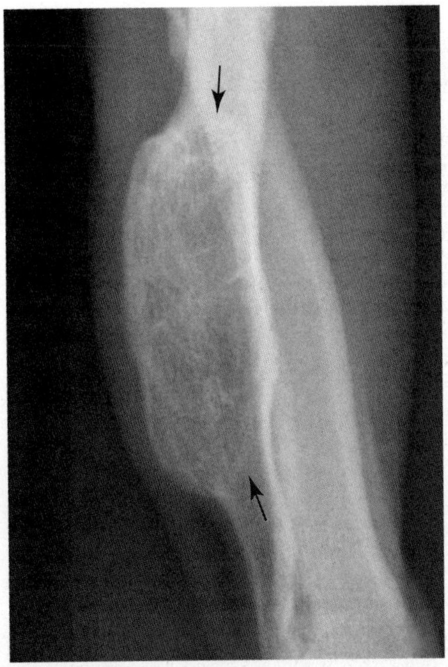

Fig. 17.12 Craniocaudal radiograph of the antebrachium of a dog with a nonaggressive lesion in the ulna. There is expansion of the cortex but not destruction; the edge of the expanded cortex is smooth. There is no active periosteal reaction. Also, the demarcation between abnormal and normal bone, the transition zone, is distinct (*black arrows*).

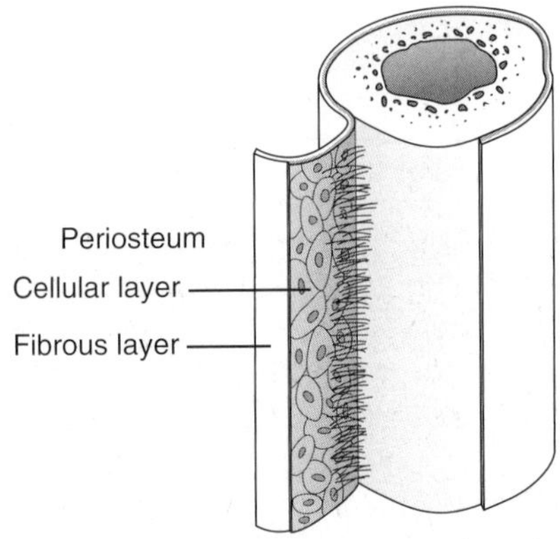

Fig. 17.13 Illustration of the different layers of the periosteum. A cellular layer with mesenchymal cells which have the potential to be activated to produce new bone is covered by a fibrous layer.

the host bone will be easy to define radiographically (Fig. 17.19, see Fig. 17.12). In aggressive bone lesions, the host bone is unable to contain the lesion as the ongoing disease process does not allow for mineral deposition to contain the lesion, and there is no demarcation between the lesion and the host bone (Fig. 17.20, see Fig. 17.17).

As already noted, it is not necessary for a lesion to have all three radiographic features of aggressiveness (cortical destruction, active periosteal reaction, and an indistinct transition zone) to be characterized as aggressive. Any single criterion is sufficient. Moreover, the combined radiographic features of the aggressiveness of a bone lesion are a continuum from a minor alteration in cortex integrity, periosteal response, or transition zone, to major alterations in all three parameters. Importantly, there is not a clinically significant correlation between the number of aggressive features of a lesion, or the extent of their aggressiveness, and the biologic behavior of the lesion. In other words, low radiographic aggressiveness does not mean low biologic aggressiveness. But, importantly, the absence of radiographic evidence of aggressiveness usually means no biologic aggressiveness. Finally, as already mentioned, the categorization of aggressiveness does not take into account whether the lesion is primarily productive or primarily destructive.

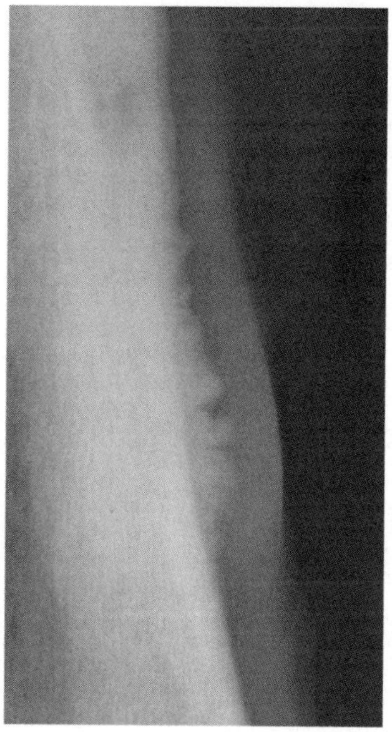

Fig. 17.14 An active periosteal reaction on the radius of a horse with a nondisplaced fracture; the fracture line is not visible in this image. Normal callus is not irregular, and this active periosteal reaction was due to osteomyelitis.

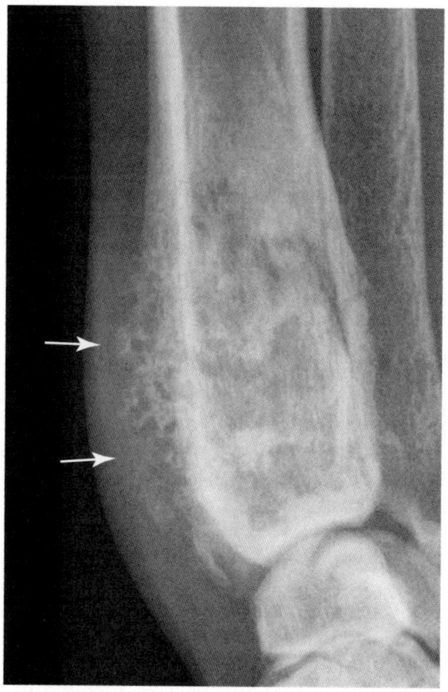

Fig. 17.15 Lateral radiograph of the distal antebrachium of a dog with radial osteosarcoma. There is an active, irregular, periosteal reaction on the radius (*white arrows*). The transition zone between the proximal end of the radial lesion and normal bone in the radius is also poorly defined.

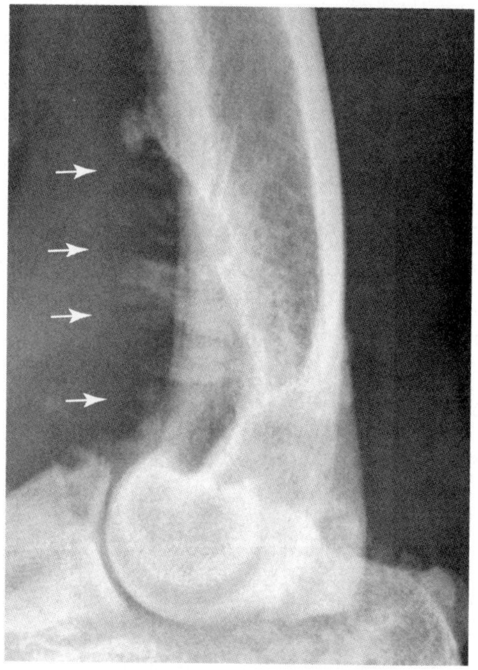

Fig. 17.16 Lateral radiograph of the distal humerus of a dog with an osteosarcoma. There is an active, irregular, periosteal reaction on the humerus (*white arrows*).

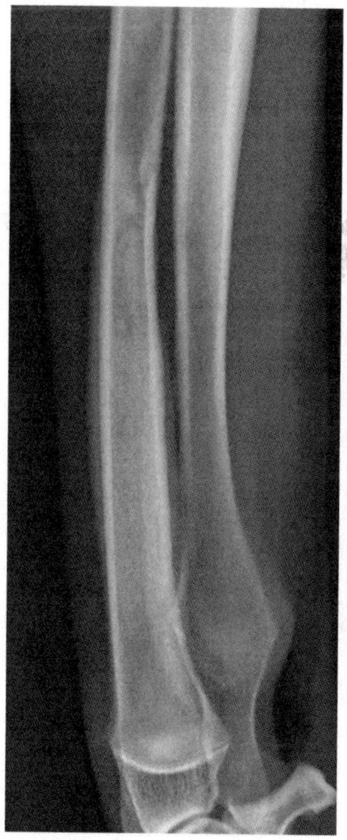

Fig. 17.17 Lateral radiograph of the antebrachium of a 7-month-old German shepherd with canine panosteitis.‡ The panosteitis resulted in poorly defined, increased bone opacity in the medullary cavity of the radius that has an indistinct transition zone, but in this dog, there is also a smooth periosteal reaction on the radius.

‡Canine panosteitis is discussed in Chapter 18.

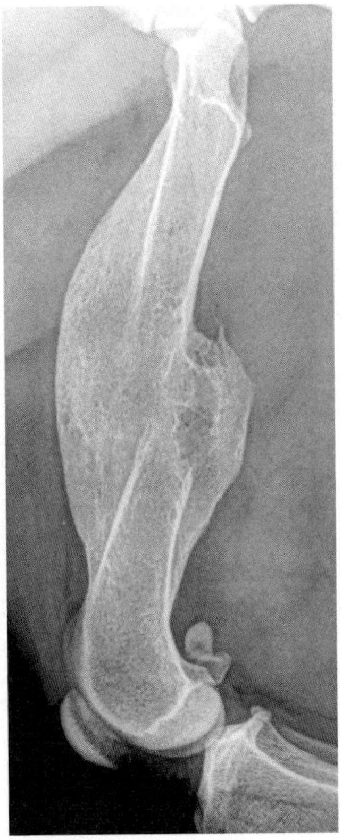

Fig. 17.18 Lateral radiograph of a femur. There is a healed malunion midshaft fracture. There is exuberant smooth periosteal reaction cranial and caudal to the healed fracture representing normal fracture callus.

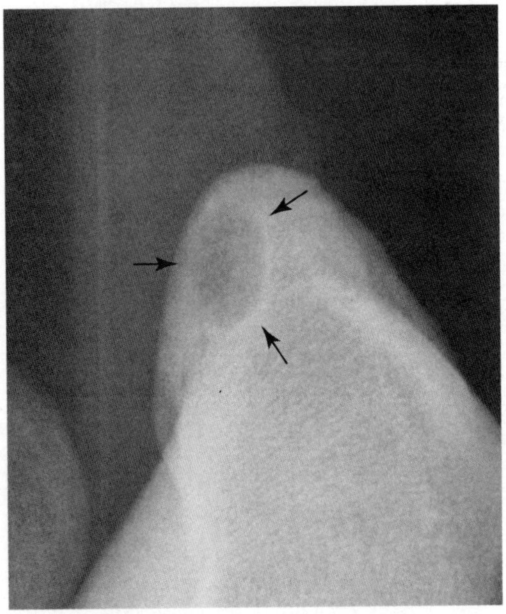

Fig. 17.19 Plantaroproximal-plantarodistal view of an equine calcaneus. There is a well-defined region of bone loss and the edge of the lesion is sharply defined (*black arrows*). This is an example of a well-defined transition zone. There are no other signs of aggressiveness—that is, no cortex destruction and no active periosteal reaction.

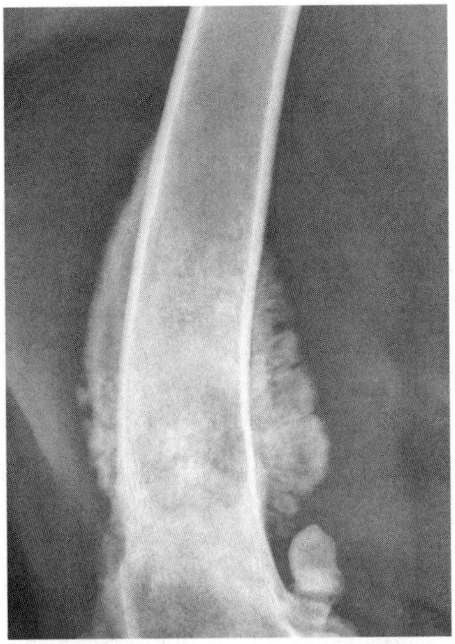

Fig. 17.20 Lateral radiograph of the distal femur of a dog with an osteosarcoma. At the proximal extent of the lesion, it is impossible to identify the point at which the abnormal bone ends and the normal bone begins. This is an indistinct transition zone. An active periosteal reaction is also present.

Causes of an Aggressive Lesion

If an aggressive bone lesion is identified, the DAMNITV (degenerative, anomalous, metabolic, neoplastic, infectious [inflammatory, immune], traumatic, and vascular) approach should be used to formulate the list of possible causes. Of most concern is whether the lesion is neoplastic or infectious. A definitive distinction between neoplastic and infectious bone lesions is impossible by radiographic means. However, the radiographic features of the bone lesion, such as the number of bones involved and the location of the lesions within the bones, along with the signalment, history, and physical and laboratory findings can be used to prioritize the possible causes (Table 17.3). Nevertheless, a biopsy or fine-needle aspirate with histopathologic or cytologic evaluation and possibly microbiologic culture is almost always needed for the definitive diagnosis of any aggressive bone lesion where a diagnosis cannot be assumed from the clinical scenario.

Primary Bone Tumors

There are many types of primary bone tumors in the dog, but osteosarcoma is the most common. Canine osteosarcoma is usually characterized by a single (monostotic) aggressive bone lesion originating in the metaphysis.[3] The age distribution of canine osteosarcoma is bimodal with a small peak in incidence at approximately 2 years of age and then a larger peak in incidence later in adult life.[3] Age distribution in cats is not bimodal and osteosarcoma typically occurs in older cats.[4] Most primary bone tumors enlarge from the metaphysis into the epiphysis or diaphysis, or both. Common osteosarcoma sites in the forelimb are the proximal humerus and the distal radius (away from the elbow), and in the hindlimb the distal femur and proximal tibia (toward the stifle). Tumors in the distal tibia are also relatively common. However, a primary bone tumor can arise at any location in either the axial or appendicular skeleton. Primary

Table • 17.3

Common Features of Neoplastic and Infectious Bone Disease in the Appendicular Skeleton of Small Animals[a].

CRITERION	PRIMARY BONE TUMOR	METASTATIC BONE TUMOR	MYCOTIC OSTEOMYELITIS	BACTERIAL OSTEOMYELITIS: HEMATOGENOUS	BACTERIAL OSTEOMYELITIS: INOCULATION
Patient age	Usually old but occurs in young dogs	Old	Young to middle age	Young	Any
Mono- or polyostotic	Monostotic	Polyostotic[b]	Polyostotic[a,b]	Polyostotic	Monostotic or adjacent bones
Location in bone	Metaphysis[c]	Metaphysis or diaphysis	Metaphysis	Metaphysis	Anywhere
Likelihood of columnar periosteal reaction	+	−	−	−	+++

[a]Tabular features are only guidelines, and findings in individual patients may vary. Features are also based on the experience of the author and have not been substantiated by evidence-based investigations.
[b]The axial skeleton may also be affected.[c]Epiphyseal and diaphyseal tumors also occur.

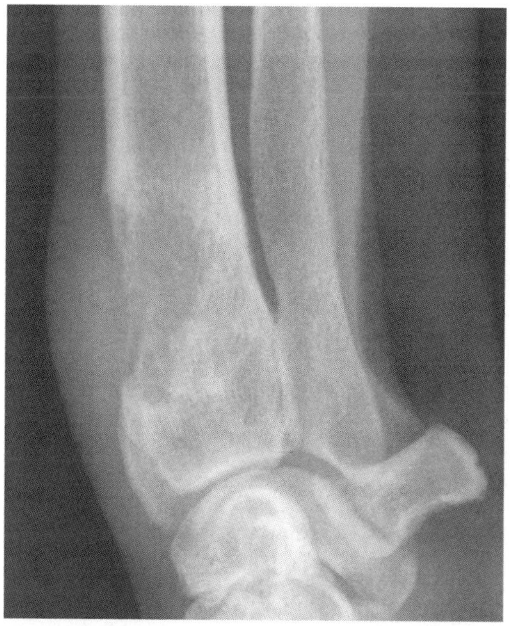

Fig. 17.21 An aggressive lytic lesion (osteosarcoma) in the craniodistal aspect of the radius. There is marked cortex destruction and a poorly defined transition zone between the lytic lesion and normal bone.

bone tumors do not often cross joints or invade adjacent bones but both can occur as the tumor enlarges. Appendicular osteosarcomas may be primarily lytic (Fig. 17.21), primarily productive (also termed *blastic* or *sclerotic*) (Fig. 17.22), or, most commonly, mixed, with both lytic and productive features (Fig. 17.23).

Occasionally, osteosarcoma develops secondary to bone infarction, either idiopathic bone infarction[5] or bone infarction secondary to chronic bone trauma such as surgical intervention with placement of a prosthetic joint or other implants.[6–8] Other, less common primary bone tumors include fibrosarcoma and chondrosarcoma.[3] Chondrosarcoma is most commonly located in flat bones such as the ribs and scapula.

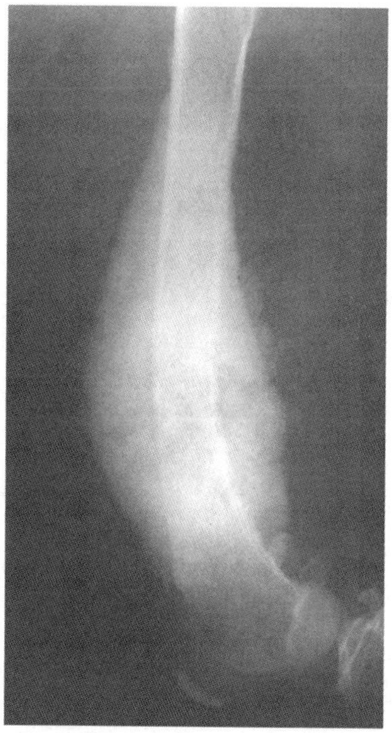

Fig. 17.22 A predominantly productive, or sclerotic, aggressive lesion (osteosarcoma) in the distal diaphysis and metaphysis of the femur. This lesion is composed mainly of smoothly marginated new bone, but there is the lack of a sharp transition zone between normal and abnormal bone.

Metastatic Bone Tumors

Any malignant tumor has the potential to metastasize to the skeleton, but in general bone metastasis from carcinomas is more common than from sarcomas. In dogs, mammary and lung cancers are a common source of bone metastasis. Metastatic tumor sites in the skeleton arise hematogeneously, which usually leads to a polyostotic distribution, either in the axial and/or appendicular skeleton (Fig. 17.24). The lesion distribution is metaphyseal or diaphyseal through the nutrient foramen,

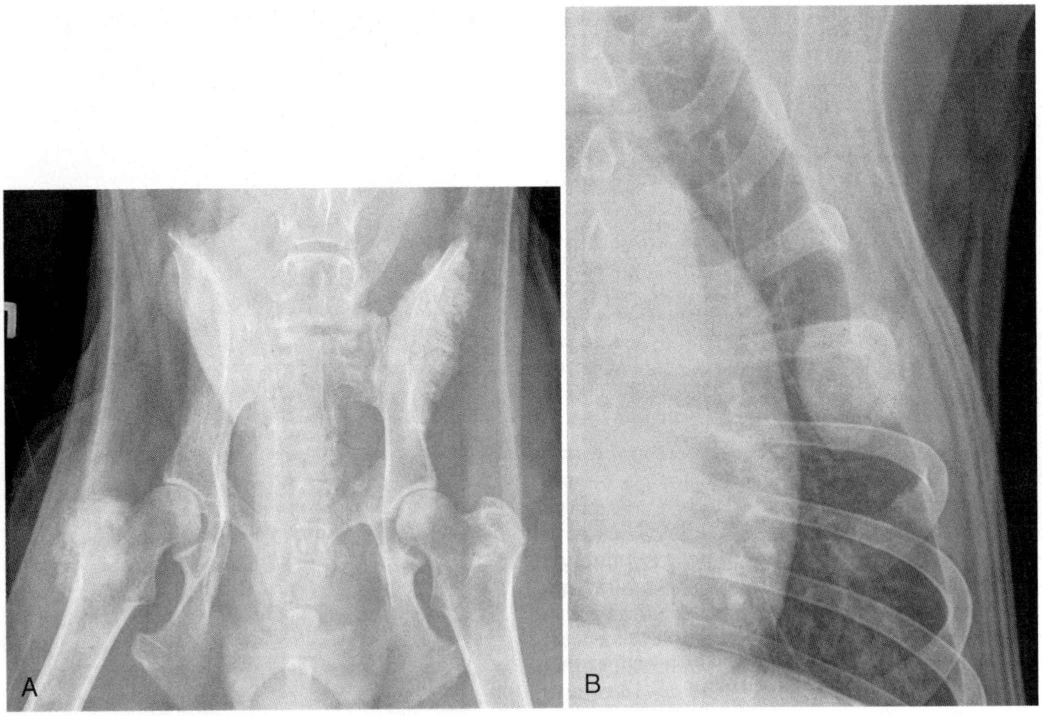

Fig. 17.27 Pelvic **(A)** and thoracic **(B)** radiographs from a 4-year-old pit bull. Aggressive lesions are present in the left ilium, proximal right femur and left fifth rib. Mycotic osteomyelitis is the main consideration for this distribution of aggressive bone lesions. A primary bone tumor would be considered for any of these lesions independently but not in combination. Metastatic neoplasia could have this appearance. Diagnosis: coccidioidomycosis.

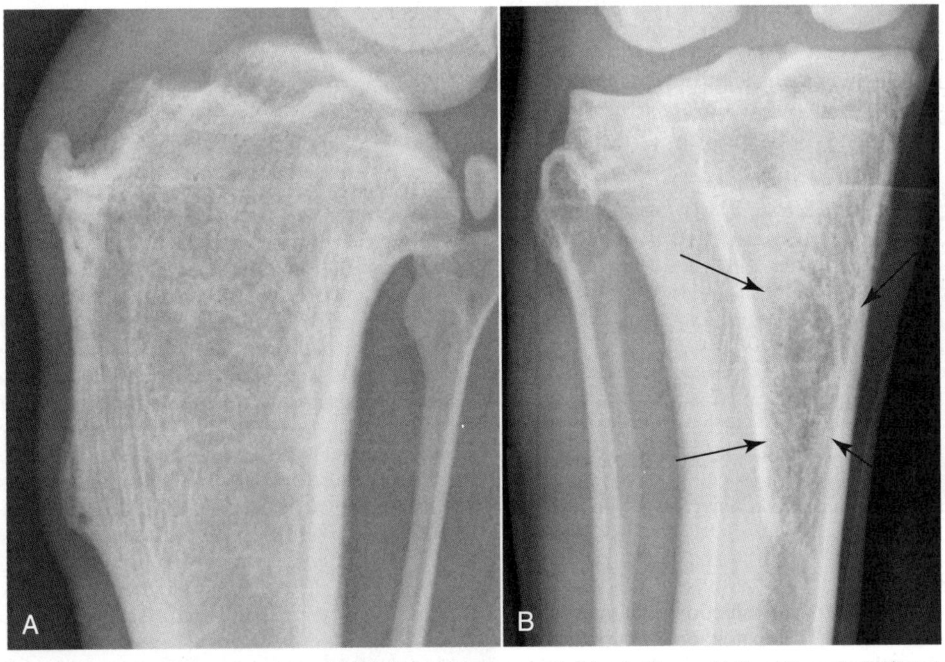

Fig. 17.28 Lateral **(A)** and craniocaudal **(B)** views of the proximal tibia of a 2-year-old Great Dane. In **A,** there is moth-eaten lysis of the proximal tibia. In **B,** there is a region of permeative lysis (*black arrows*) with an indistinct transition zone. This monostotic aggressive lesion is consistent with an osteosarcoma, even in a 2-year-old dog, but was caused by blastomycosis infection.

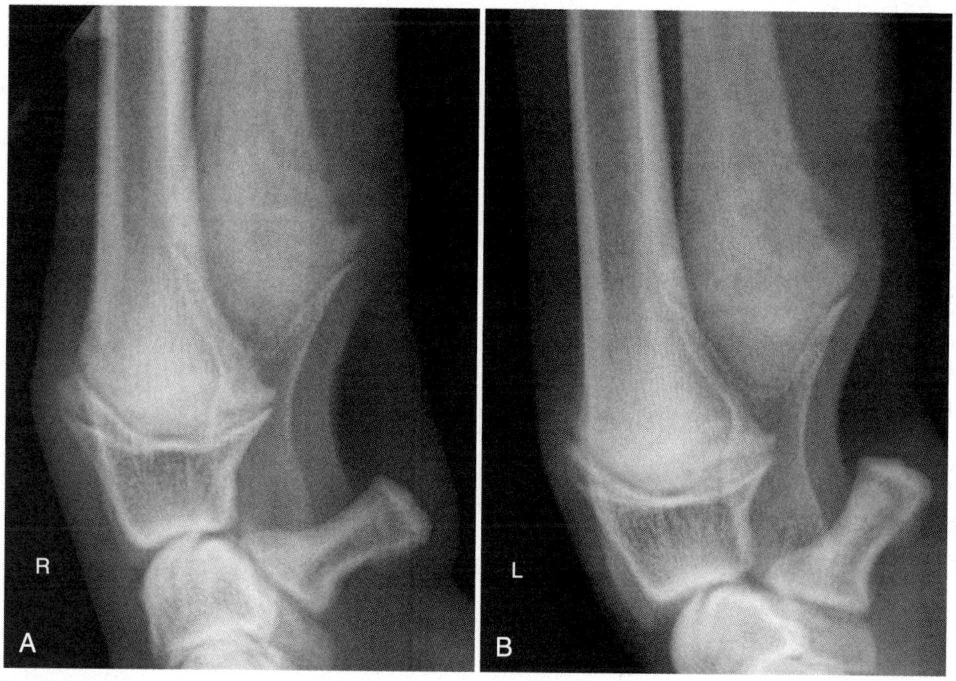

Fig. 17.29 Lateral radiograph **(A)** of the right distal antebrachium of a 5-month-old Irish setter with a right forelimb lameness and pain on carpal palpation. There is an irregular appearance to the distal ulna, especially caudally. It would be easy to misinterpret this as an aggressive lesion, but this is the normal cutback zone resulting from remodeling of the distal ulna as it elongates. If one does not remember that this is a normal finding in young, rapidly growing dogs, radiographing the contralateral left carpal region **(B)** and finding the same appearance lessens the chance that this is a significant lesion.

that may be encountered in the appendicular skeleton of dogs and cats is great and cannot be covered adequately here. Comprehensive references are available.[1] The concept of radiographing the contralateral limb for comparative purposes when a questionable finding is encountered is valuable (Fig. 17.29).

Interpretation Paradigm

Like in all body systems, an organized approach to radiographic interpretation of the appendicular skeleton is needed. This begins with an overview of technique, according the following questions, followed by evaluation for abnormalities.

Are the radiographic views adequate, and are all of the views that are needed present?
Are oblique or other ancillary views needed?
Do the views correspond to the clinical localization of the lesion?
Are the radiographic technique and positioning adequate?
Has a grid been used? Did this affect the quality of the image?
Has sedation or anesthesia been used? If not, how will this affect the utility of the radiographs?
What is the species and breed of the patient?
Was a horizontally directed x-ray beam used with handholding of the cassette or a wall-mounted cassette holder?
Was the cassette held by hand? Is there motion artifact?
Has the joint above and below the location of a suspected bone lesion been included in the imaging study?
Will radiographs of the contralateral limb be helpful?
What congenital anomalies are present that alter the normal appearance of the bone but may not be clinically significant?

After these variables have been considered, the images can be scrutinized for abnormalities. The roentgen sign and DAMNITV methods described in Chapter 6 should be used, along with an assessment of lesion aggressiveness. Unfortunately, bone is very limited in its response to injury. There will be either more or less bone than normal, a periosteal response will be either present or not, and the soft tissues will be either involved or not. Thus, the distribution within the skeleton and the assessment of the patient signalment become extremely important factors in formulating a reasonable differential diagnosis and for formulating a plan (Table 17.4). Regardless, especially for aggressive bone lesions, cytologic and/or microbiologic testing of a tissue sample, from bone or other involved tissue, will be needed for definitive diagnosis.

Experienced radiologists may have a random search pattern, but it is recommended that inexperienced interpreters use an organized approach.[7] Having a mental checklist to guide the order of interpretation will reduce the number of errors (Box 17.1).

In addition to a general examination of the images, it is also helpful to scrutinize appendicular radiographs with a preconception of what disease might be found in a particular region in a particular patient. This is particularly true in young canine and feline patients, where developmental and juvenile bone diseases are often characterized by very specific findings. This is defined as *targeted viewing* and was introduced earlier (see Chapter 6). Examples of targeted viewing are close examination of the (1) proximal margin of the anconeal process in dogs at risk of having elbow dysplasia, (2) proximal margin of the medial ridge of the talus in dogs at risk for tarsal osteochondrosis, and (3) distal radial and ulnar metaphysis in young dogs at risk for hypertrophic osteodystrophy. It is critical that targeted viewing be used as an *ancillary* method. It is a way of double checking that all possibilities have been addressed. Assessing radiographs with only a preconceived idea of what will be present will invariably lead to overlooked lesions and missed diagnoses.

Table • 17.4

Summary of Selected Orthopedic Diseases in Small Animals by Skeletal Distribution and Patient Demographics.

DISEASE	MONOSTOTIC OR POLYOSTOTIC	LOCATION IN BONE	DEMOGRAPHICS
Primary bone cancer	Monostotic	Metaphyseal	Older patients
Metastatic bone cancer	Polyostotic	Metaphyseal or diaphyseal	Older patients
Mycotic osteomyelitis	Polyostotic	Metaphyseal	Middle-aged patients
Bacterial osteomyelitis—hematogenous	Polyostotic	Metaphyseal or diaphyseal	Young patients
Bacterial osteomyelitis—traumatic	Monostotic	Anywhere	Variable
Metabolic bone disease	Polyostotic	Metaphyseal or epiphyseal	Young patients
Panosteitis	Polyostotic	Diaphyseal	Young patients
Hypertrophic osteodystrophy (HOD)	Polyostotic	Metaphyseal	Young patients
Osteochondrosis	Polyostotic	Epiphyseal	Young patients
Hypertrophic osteopathy (HO)	Polyostotic	Epiphyseal and metaphyseal then diaphyseal	Older patients

These data are generalizations and will not apply to all patients.

Box • 17.1

Checklist for Interpretation of Appendicular Skeletal Radiographs

Number of bones involved
Region of bone involved; epiphysis vs. metaphysis vs. diaphysis vs. multiple
Joint involvement
Overall bone opacity
Integrity of the cortex
Presence or absence of a smooth or irregular periosteal reaction
Shape of bones
Character of any transition zone
Character of adjacent soft tissues

REFERENCES

1. Thrall D, Robertson I. *Atlas of Normal Radiographic Anatomy and Anatomic Variants in the Dog and Cat*. 3rd ed. St Louis: Saunders/Elsevier; 2023.
2. O'Donnell P. Evaluation of focal bone lesions: basic principles and clinical scenarios. *Imaging*. 2003;15(4):298–323.
3. Chun R. Common malignant musculoskeletal neoplasms of dogs and cats. *Vet Clin North Am Small Anim Pract*. 2005;35(5):1155–1167.
4. Heldmann E, Anderson M, Wagner-Mann C. Feline osteosarcoma: 145 cases (1990–1995). *J Am Anim Hosp Assoc*. 2000;36(6):518–521.
5. Jimenez IA, Pool Jr RR, Gabrielson KL. Canine idiopathic arteriopathy, appendicular bone infarcts, and neoplastic transformation of bone infarcts in 108 dogs (*Canis lupus familiaris*). *Comp Med*. 2022;72(5):306–319.
6. Marcellin-Little DJ, DeYoung DJ, Thrall DE, Merrill CL. Osteosarcoma at the site of bone infarction associated with total hip arthroplasty in a dog. *Vet Surg*. 1999;28(1):54–60.
7. Sebestyen P, Marcellin-Little DJ, DeYoung BA. Femoral medullary infarction secondary to canine total hip arthroplasty. *Vet Surg*. 2000;29(3):227–236.
8. Arthur EG, Arthur GL, Keeler MR, Bryan JN. Risk of osteosarcoma in dogs after open fracture fixation. *Vet Surg*. 2016;45(1):30–35.
9. Trost ME, Inkelmann MA, Galiza GJN, Silva TM, Kommers GD. Occurrence of tumours metastatic to bones and multicentric tumours with skeletal involvement in dogs. *J Comp Pathol*. 2014;150(1):8–17.
10. Henry CJ, Whitley EM, Tyler JW, Ogilvie GK, Norris A, et al. Canine digital tumors: a veterinary cooperative oncology group retrospective study of 64 dogs. *J Vet Intern Med*. 2005;19(5):720–724.
11. Goldfinch N, Argyle DJ. Feline lung-digit syndrome: unusual metastatic patterns of primary lung tumours in cats. *J Feline Med Surg*. 2012;14(3):202–208.
12. Kerl ME. Update on canine and feline fungal diseases. *Vet Clin North Am Small Anim Pract*. 2003;33(4):721–747.
13. Gieling F, Peters S, Erichsen C, Richards RG, Zeiter S, Moriarty TF. Bacterial osteomyelitis in veterinary orthopaedics: pathophysiology, clinical presentation and advances in treatment across multiple species. *Vet J*. 2019;250:44–54.
14. Ewing SA, Panciera RJ. American canine hepatozoonosis. *Clin Microbiol Rev*. 2003;16(4):688–697.
15. Drost WT, Cummings CA, Mathew JS, Panciera RJ, Ko JCH. Determination of time of onset and location of early skeletal lesions in young dogs experimentally infected with *Hepatozoon americanum* using bone scintigraphy. *Vet Radiol Ultrasound*. 2003;44(1):86–91.

ELECTRONIC RESOURCES

Additional information related to the content in Chapter 17 can be found online at eBooks.Health.Elsevier.com.

- Chapter Quiz

CHAPTER 18

Orthopedic Diseases of Young and Growing Dogs and Cats

Kathryn L. Phillips

Developmental orthopedic disease is a grouping of variable diseases tied together by the population that they affect. This chapter reviews the basic pathophysiology and radiographic appearance of the more common developmental orthopedic diseases in dogs and cats. There are a few trends across this diverse grouping. The lesions are often generalized or at least bilaterally symmetric, for example, affecting all the epiphyses as with congenital hypothyroidism, or all the physes as with rickets, or mirroring lesions on both thoracic or both pelvic limbs as with hypertrophic osteodystrophy (HOD) and osteochondrosis (OC). Because these diseases have known predilection sites, the anatomic distribution of the lesions can be used to make the diagnosis or at least limit the differential list. In this chapter the diseases are grouped based on their anatomic distribution (Table 18.1).

Degenerative joint disease is a common sequela to developmental disorders of the immature skeleton, particularly when the primary lesion involves joints or produces limb deformity. Adult patients will frequently present with lameness attributable to the secondary degenerative joint disease. Advanced degenerative changes can mask the original developmental lesion on radiographs.

DISORDERS PRIMARILY AFFECTING JOINTS

Osteochondrosis and Osteochondrosis Dissecans

Osteochondrosis (OC) is a common cause of lameness in young, rapidly growing, large-breed dogs. Clinical signs usually develop between 6 and 9 months of age. OC occurs from epiphyseal cartilage necrosis, resulting in a failure of normal endochondral ossification. If the vascular bed of the adjacent subchondral bone can envelop and bypass the region of cartilage necrosis, endochondral ossification may resume without development of a clinical lesion. Otherwise, focal failure of endochondral ossification leads to divots within the subchondral bone and progressive chondromalacia may lead to development of clefts or fissures extending from the surface of the cartilage to the subchondral bone. The terms *osteochondrosis* and *osteochondritis* have both been historically used in the literature. Osteochondritis implies inflammation, and inflammation is not a component of the primary developmental disease and the term is therefore not used in this chapter.[1] Osteochondrosis (OC) is further characterized into osteochondrosis dissecans (OCD) when there is a complete fissure through the cartilage creating a flap. As chondral flaps and fragments are of soft tissue opacity, they cannot be radiographically identified. However, when they become ossified and an osteochondral fragment is radiographically apparent, the term *osteochondrosis dissecans* is more specific.

OC occurs at specific anatomic locations and is frequently bilaterally symmetric; thus, if an OC lesion is identified, radiographs of the contralateral limb should be performed. It is rare for a lesion to occur outside of the predilection sites. In dogs the predilection sites are caudal aspect of the humeral head, distomedial humeral trochlea, lateral and medial femoral condyles, and the medial and lateral trochlear ridges of the talus.

Radiographic Signs

Radiographic findings of OC include flattening or concavity of the affected subchondral bone surface with or without subchondral bone sclerosis. This may result in nonuniformity and apparent widening of the joint space. When mineralized, a cartilage flap is sometimes seen within the subchondral defect, and separate osteochondral fragments (joint mice) may migrate within the joint space. Fragments that have migrated often adhere to the synovial lining and may become vascularized and continue to mineralize and enlarge over time. Joint effusion or joint capsule thickening may present as a localized region of soft tissue thickening centered on the affected joint. A subchondral bone defect is occasionally seen involving the articular surface opposite the primary lesion. These defects are called *kissing lesions*. Degenerative joint disease is a common sequel to OC.

Detection of lesions on the caudal humeral head can be difficult as this surface is spherical in shape and the beam must be tangential to the subchondral bone divot to be detected. If a lesion is not identified but clinically suspected, obtaining additional lateral views in varying degrees of supination can aid in detection of focal subchondral bone flattening. OC of the lateral trochlea of the talus can be obscured by superimposition of the calcaneus in the dorsoplantar view. In this instance, a dorsolateral-plantaromedial oblique[2] or a flexed dorsoplantar view can be acquired to provide an unobstructed view of the lesion. In the stifle, the fossa for the origin of the long digital extensor muscle is sometimes mistaken for a lateral femoral condyle OC lesion because it is superimposed on the dorsolateral aspect of the condyle on both the lateromedial and the caudocranial views (Figs. 18.1–18.3, eFig. 18.1).

When a nonmineralized cartilage fragment is present, intra-articular contrast medium (arthrography) can be used to outline the flap if contrast medium dissects between the fragment and the underlying subchondral bone. Arthrography can be performed in conjunction with radiographs or computed tomography (CT) but is infrequently performed as it adds little to the clinical diagnosis, is not as sensitive as arthroscopy, and the presence of a cartilage flap does not change the surgical plan.[3]

Elbow Dysplasia

Dysplasia is the abnormal growth or development of an organ or structure. There are many ways for the elbow joint to be dysplastic; however, there is a triad of common developmental diseases that are encountered so frequently that the term *elbow dysplasia* is used clinically to refer to them. They include ununited anconeal process, medial coronoid process disease of the ulna, and OC of the distomedial aspect of the humeral

Table • 18.1

Juvenile Orthopedic Diseases of Dogs and Cats Based on Anatomic Location.

ANATOMIC LOCATION	DISEASE	ROUGH ESTIMATE OF FREQUENCY OF OCCURRENCE	SPECIES
Diseases primarily affecting joints	Osteochondrosis	Frequent	Large-breed dogs
	Osteochondrosis dissecans		
	Ununited anconeal process	Moderate	Large-breed dogs
	Medial coronoid disease	Extremely frequent	Dogs
	Congenital radial head luxation	Occasional	Bulldogs and chondrodystrophic dogs
	Hip dysplasia	Extremely frequent	Dogs and cats
	Aseptic necrosis of the femoral head	Occasional	Toy breed dogs
	Congenital hypothyroidism	Occasional	Cats and dogs
	Mucopolysaccharidosis	Rare	Cats and dogs
Epiphyseal dysplasia	Multiple epiphyseal dysplasia	Extremely rare	Reported in dogs
	Spontaneous capital physeal fractures of cats	Occasional	Male cats ~2 years of age
	Incomplete ossification of the humeral condyle	Occasional	Dogs
Diseases of the physis	Rickets	Rare	Dogs and cats
	Osteochondrodysplasia of Scottish fold cats	Breed specific	Scottish fold cats
	Breed specific chondrodysplasias	Rare	Dogs
	Hypertrophic osteodystrophy	Moderate	Large-breed dogs
	Multiple cartilaginous exostosis	Rare	Dogs
Disease of the metaphysis	Retained cartilaginous core	Moderate—often not clinical	Dogs
	Panosteitis	Moderate	Large-breed dogs
	Nutritional secondary hyperparathyroidism	Occasional	Dogs, cats, and exotics
Disease of the diaphysis	Osteogenesis imperfecta	Rare	Dogs
Generalized bone disorders	Osteopetrosis	Rare	Cats and dogs
	Knees and teeth syndrome	Rare	Cats

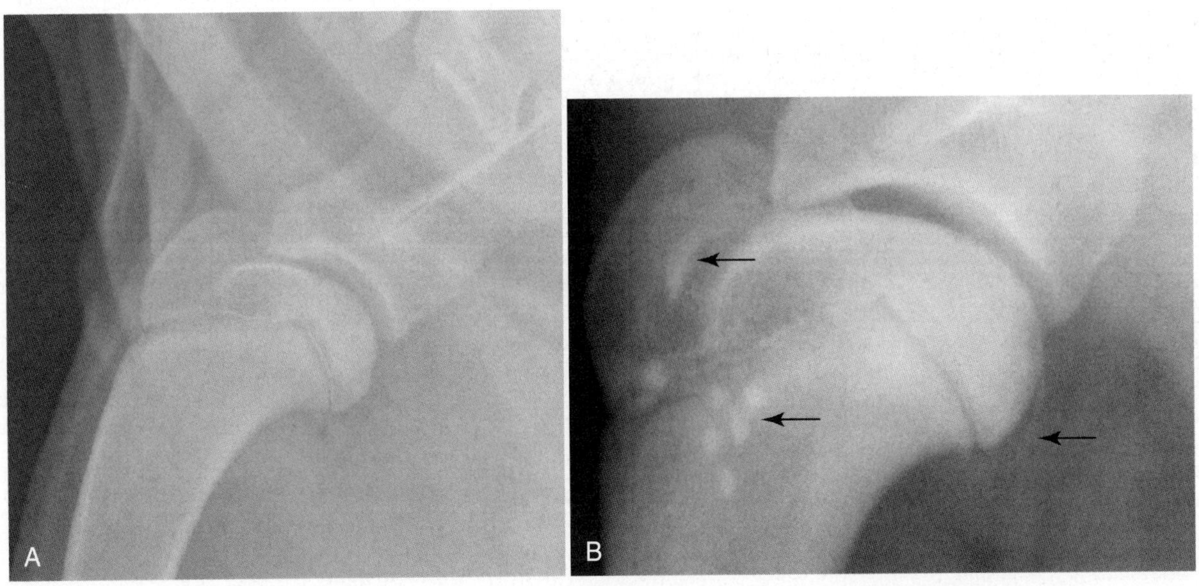

Fig. 18.1 Shoulder osteochondrosis **(A)** and osteochondrosis dissecans **(B)**. The lesions are characterized by concave lucencies of the humeral head and variable surrounding sclerosis. These lesions can sometimes be missed on a straight lateral view due to the rounded surface of the humeral head and several slightly oblique lateral views can be obtained with the limb in varying degrees of internal rotation (pronation). In image **B**, there is a thin flap of mineralized cartilage along the caudal humeral head (*black arrow*) as well as several osteochondral fragments within the bicipital bursa (*black arrows*). In dogs the bicipital bursa and shoulder joint freely communicate. Osteochondral fragments from the humeral head can migrate into the bicipital bursa.

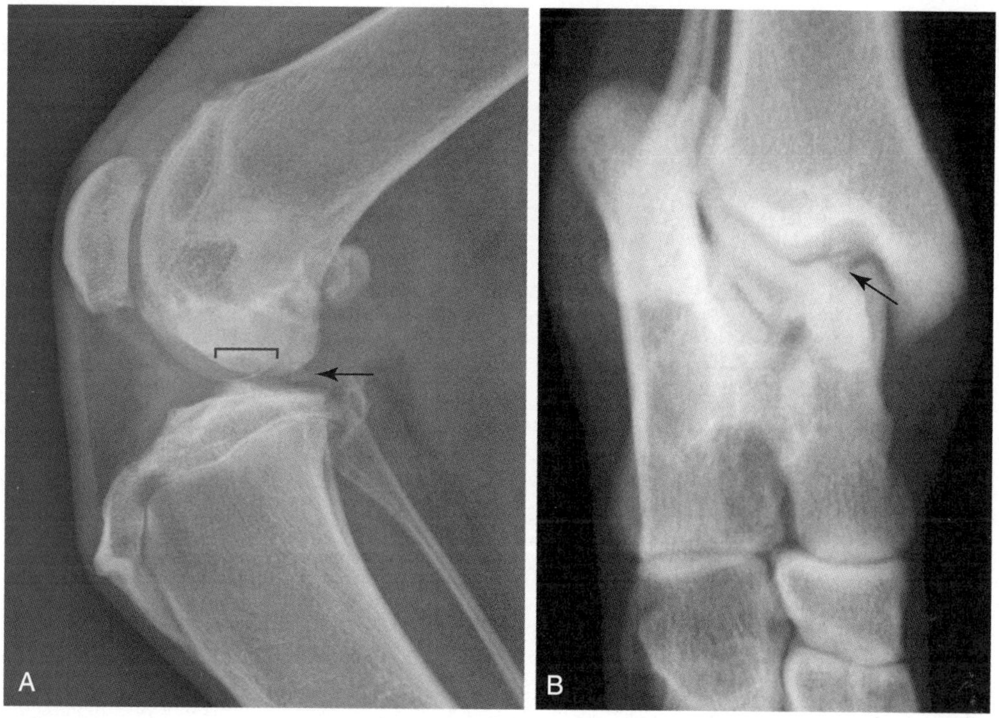

Fig. 18.2 Osteochondrosis dissecans. **A,** Lateral radiograph of the stifle. There is joint effusion. There is an irregularly margined divot so that one of the distal femoral condyles no longer has a round shape (indicated with *brackets*). There is an adjacent osteochondral fragment (*arrow*) in the caudal aspect of the joint. On the dorsoplantar view of the tarsus **(B)**, there is a divot in the medial trochlear ridge of the talus with a rounded osteochondral fragment (*arrow*).

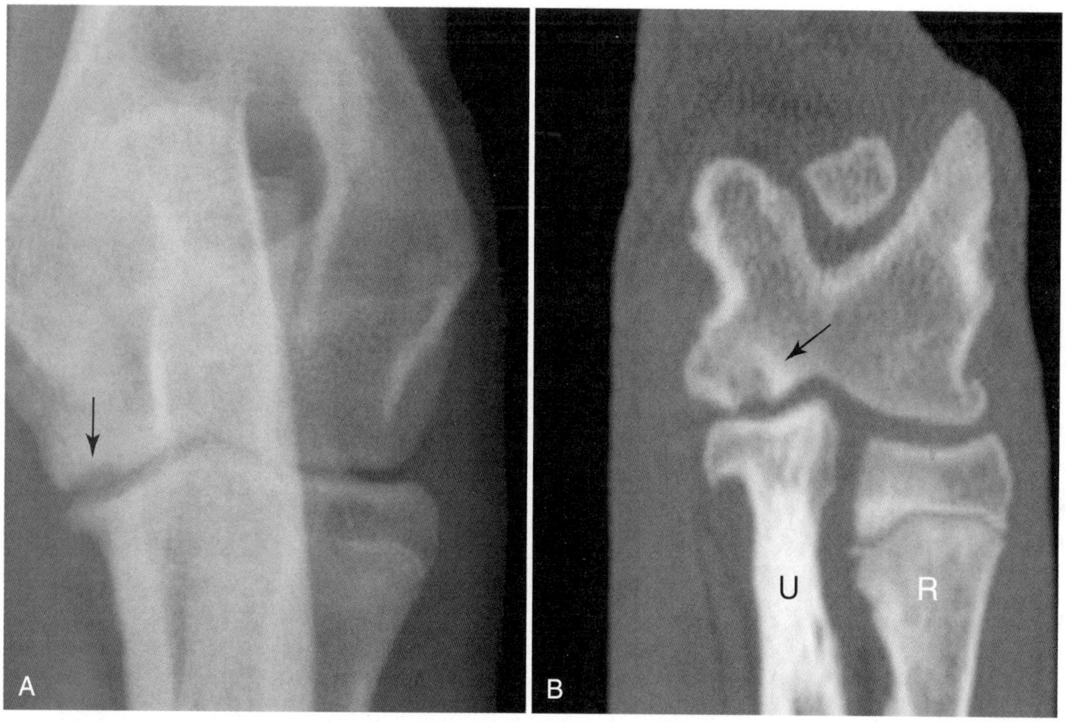

Fig. 18.3 Osteochondrosis of the medial humeral trochlea on radiographs **(A)** and dorsal plane computed tomography (CT) image **(B)**. This is characterized by a well-defined concavity (*arrows*) that can be difficult to identify with radiographs alone due to superimposition.

trochlea (see Osteochondrosis and Osteochondrosis Dissecans section earlier). Elbow joint incongruity is frequently included in the term *elbow dysplasia* as a fourth category. However, joint incongruity is also implicated as the overarching cause for all of the lesions included in elbow dysplasia. When there is disparity between any of the three bones, such as asynchronous growth of the radius and ulna or an elliptically shaped ulnar notch, the result is nonuniform contact of articulating surfaces,

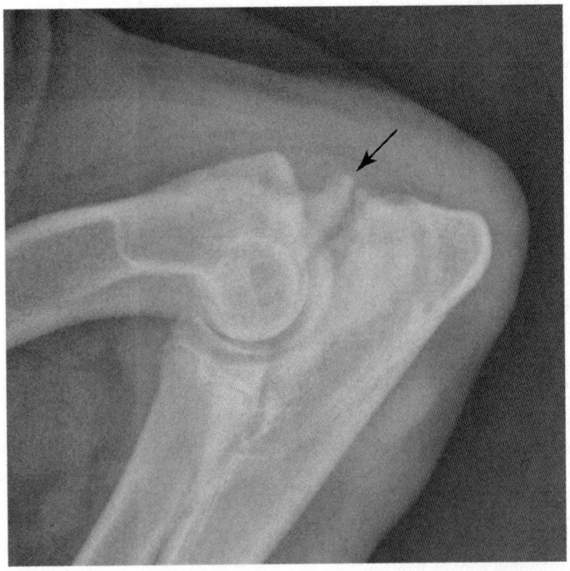

Fig. 18.4 A flexed lateral radiograph of the elbow with an ununited anconeal process. The *arrow* indicates the gap between the anconeal process and the olecranon.

which then leads to cartilage damage, medial coronoid process disease, or ununited anconeal processes. This is typically a bilateral disease, and a patient can have one, two, or all three of the primary lesions simultaneously. A radiographic study of the elbow includes a neutral lateral, a flexed lateral, and a craniocaudal radiograph of both elbow joints. The flexed lateral radiograph facilitates visibility of new bone formation on the proximal margin of the anconeal process and detection of ununited anconeal process since the medial humeral epicondyle is not superimposed. However, flexing the elbow induces a mild degree of rotation that can partially obscure the medial coronoid margin. A slight craniolateral to caudomedial (pronating the limb 15–25 degrees) view can be used to highlight the craniomedial margin and thus the medial coronoid and medial humeral trochlea. CT is now used routinely to evaluate the elbow joint and is more sensitive than survey radiography for detecting medial coronoid disease.

Ununited Anconeal Process

Ununited anconeal processes are a disease of large-breed dogs. A number of large-breed dogs have a normal separate center of ossification at the anconeal process during development.[4,5] Small, separate centers of ossification can be seen radiographically in puppies starting at 13 weeks of age. The anconeal process should be fused normally to the olecranon of the ulna by 150 days (5 months) of age.

Radiographic Signs

The primary radiographic finding is best seen on the flexed lateral view and consists of a radiolucent line separating the anconeal process from the olecranon in dogs older than 150 days (Fig. 18.4, eFig. 18.2). This lucent line is at the base of the anconeal process and can be sharply defined or it may appear irregular and of variable width. Degenerative joint disease of the elbow is a common sequel, and periarticular new bone production from osteoarthrosis may partially obscure the lucency between the ulna and the anconeal process.

Medial Coronoid Process Disease

Medial coronoid process disease is the most common developmental disorder involving the elbow joint and one of the most common causes for thoracic limb lameness in dogs. Medial coronoid process disease includes fragmentation as well as sclerosis and remodeling of the medial coronoid process. It affects medium- and large-breed dogs primarily and has a significantly higher incidence in males. Clinical signs may be apparent as early as 4 to 6 months of age. Radiographic visibility of the medial coronoid is hampered by superimposition of the radius (Fig. 18.5, eFig. 18.3). In most instances, the radiographic diagnosis of fragmented medial coronoid process is made indirectly through recognition of degenerative changes that accompany the primary lesion.

Radiographic Signs

Primary radiographic signs include an abnormal contour or poor definition of the cranial margin of the medial coronoid process on the lateral view. Often the margin, which is radiographically distinct in normal dogs, cannot be followed proximally to the articular surface in affected animals. On the craniocaudal view, the medial margin of the medial coronoid process may appear blunted, rounded, or tipped distally. A separate osseous body, representing the fragmented coronoid process, is seen rarely. Joint incongruity or subluxation may also be present and appears as a stair-step lesion between the ulna and the radial head on the lateral view. However, caution should be used to prevent overinterpretation of this finding. On the lateral view, the normal overlapping lucent lines representing the complex elbow joint margins can be confused with joint incongruity if there is any proximal to distal or vice versa obliquity present.[6,7] Secondary degenerative joint disease is frequent even in young patients. Osteophyte formation on the proximal margin of the anconeal process is one of the earliest signs of degenerative joint disease. Subchondral bone sclerosis also develops along the distal border of the trochlear notch in the region of the lateral coronoid process.[7–10] These secondary findings are best appreciated on the lateral view. A large osteophyte may arise from the medial coronoid margin on the craniocaudal view in addition to the more generalized osteophyte production.

Congenital Radial Head Luxation

Congenital caudolateral radial head luxation has been reported in a variety of dog breeds including bull-dogs, Bouvier de Flandres, Shih Tzu, and Afghan hounds.[11] Affected puppies present with mild forelimb lameness first noticed at 3 to 4 months of age with physical examination findings of pain and reduced range of motion in the affected elbow.

Radiographic Signs

Caudal and lateral luxation of the radius relative to the distal humerus is the primary radiographic finding (Fig. 18.6). The radial epiphysis may appear convex because articulation with the humeral condyle has not resulted in normal development. The articulation of the humerus with the ulna is typically normal and there is no evidence of trauma.

Hip Dysplasia

Hip dysplasia is an extremely common disease caused by abnormal development of the coxofemoral joints. It is a disease that ranges from mild alterations in gait and mobility to debilitating lameness. The majority of the clinical signs are caused by secondary osteoarthritis. Hip dysplasia mainly occurs in large-breed dogs, but it can also affect small dogs and cats.

Canine hip dysplasia is a polygenic inherited disease that is influenced by environmental factors. It is a disease that is not detectable at birth but during growth laxity of the joint develops. As the animal moves, the joints subluxate resulting in altered biomechanical forces on the articular surfaces. Without normal forces applied, the acetabulum does not develop a normal cup-like shape and the femoral head is flattened. This incongruity leads to arthritis later in life.[12] Heritability is a

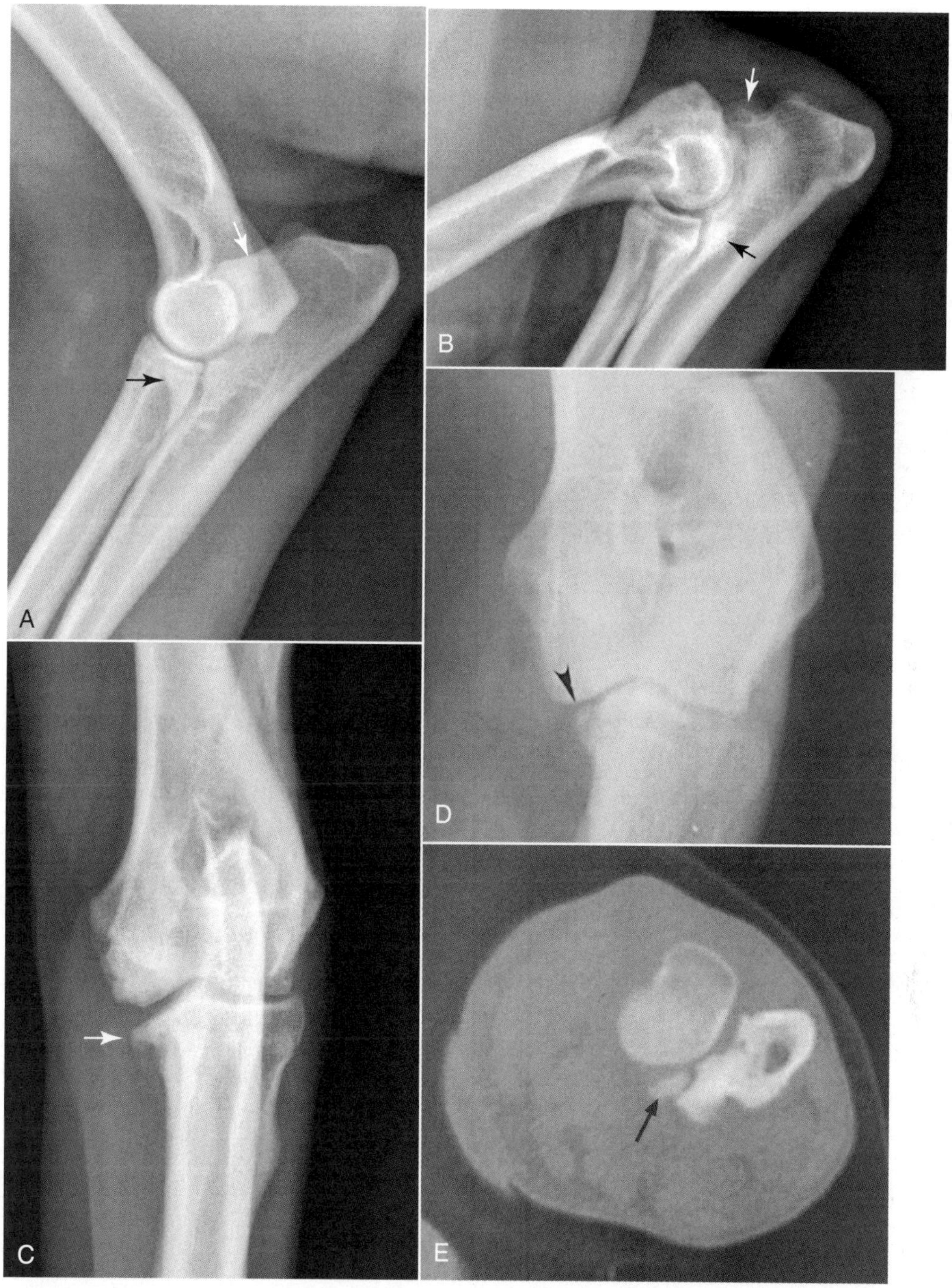

Fig. 18.5 Fragmented medial coronoid process. **A,** Lateral view of a normal elbow. The cranial edge of the medial coronoid process (*black arrow*) has a distinct margin that is superimposed on the head of the radius. The proximal margin of the anconeal process (*white arrow*) is also distinct despite being superimposed on the medial and lateral epicondyles of the humerus. **B,** Fragmented medial coronoid process with degenerative joint disease. The margins of the medial coronoid are indistinct compared with those in **A**. There are osteophytes along the proximal margin of the anconeal process (*white arrow*). Subchondral bone sclerosis is also present adjacent to the ulnar notch (*black arrow*). **C,** An osteophyte arises from the medial margin of the ulna on a craniocaudal view (*white arrow*). This osteophyte should not be misinterpreted as the coronoid fragment. **D,** Fragmentation of the medial coronoid process can occasionally be seen on a craniolateral-caudomedial view (*arrow*). **E,** Computed tomography image of the elbow from a dog with a fragmented medial coronoid process and degenerative joint disease. The fragmented coronoid process (*black arrow*) is easily seen. In addition, the basilar part of the coronoid process is sclerotic and remodeled.

numeric estimate of how much a particular trait is controlled by the genotype; a heritability of 1 indicates that the trait is completely genetically controlled and 0 indicates the trait is not genetically influenced. Heritability numbers have been calculated for different breeds of dogs based on hip scores from ventrodorsal radiographs. This results in a range of heritability numbers for different breeds of dogs, from 0.11 in Boxers to 0.43 in German shepherd dogs.[13] However, hip laxity as measured by the distraction index (DI) has a higher genetic correlation. Heritability estimates for hip laxity are 0.46 in

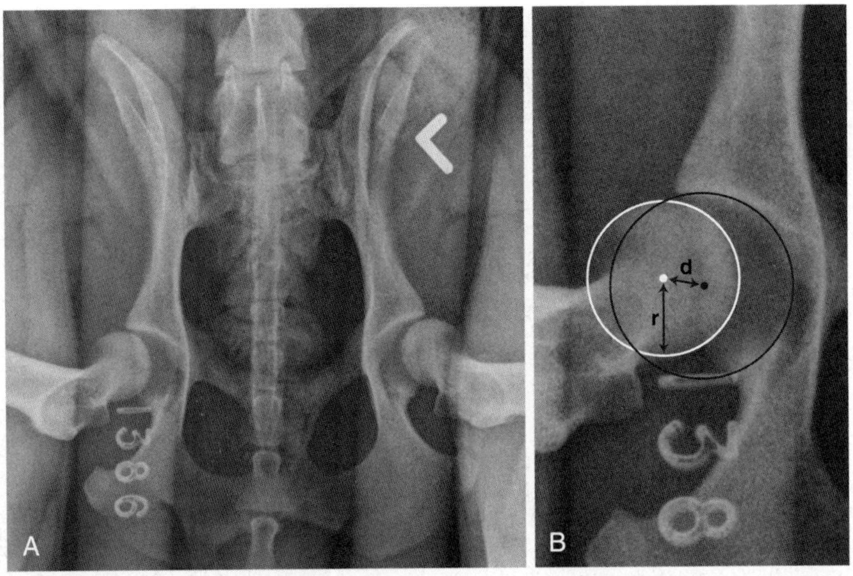

Fig. 18.9 Figure **A** demonstrates a PennHIP distraction view of the coxofemoral joints to assess joint laxity. Figure **B** demonstrates how the distraction index = d/r is determined.

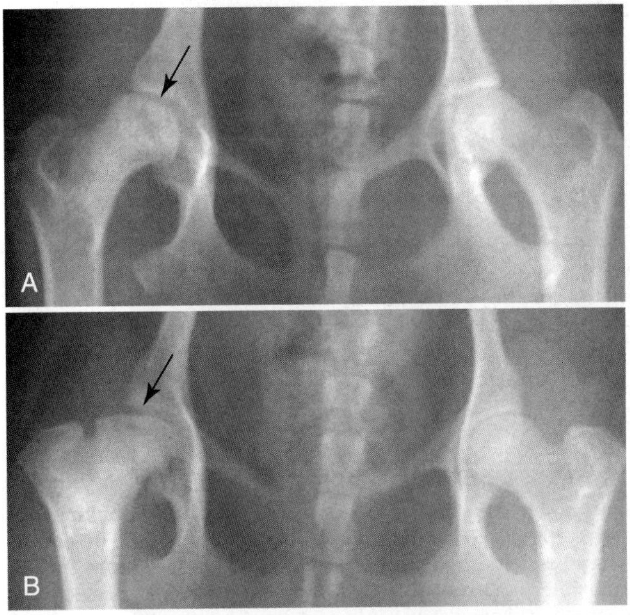

Fig. 18.10 Serial radiographs of a patient with aseptic necrosis of the right femoral head (*arrows*). Image **A** is earlier in the disease process, overtime the femoral head becomes flattened and progressively deformed **(B)**. The left femoral head is normal and remains round in shape.

Aseptic Necrosis of the Femoral Head (Legg-Calvé-Perthes Disease)

Aseptic necrosis of the femoral head occurs in adolescent toy and small-breed dogs (Fig. 18.10, eFig. 18.5). Compromised blood supply to the femoral capital epiphysis causes necrosis of subchondral bone while overlying articular cartilage continues to grow. Revascularization occurs in an attempt to repair the defect, and removal of necrotic bone causes decreased opacity in the affected femoral head. Incomplete removal of necrotic bone and invasion of granulation tissue interferes with healing, resulting in a misshapen femoral head of nonuniform opacity.[18]

Radiographic Signs

As with many of the other developmental skeletal disorders, the radiographic findings of aseptic necrosis of the femoral head vary with the duration of the lesion. Radiographs of the hip joints may appear normal early in the course of the disease. As the disease progresses, lucencies can be detected within the subchondral bone within the femoral head. Areas of decreased opacity may also appear in both the femoral epiphysis and the metaphysis. Flattening and irregularity of the femoral head and neck become apparent as the affected bone remodels and collapses on itself. Remodeling of the femoral head may cause coxofemoral joint space widening and subluxation. Fragmentation of the femoral head may eventually occur from pathologic fracture. Muscle atrophy and radiographic findings associated with degenerative joint disease usually develop. Radiographic evaluation of both hips is indicated because this disease may be bilateral.

EPIPHYSEAL DYSPLASIA

Congenital Hypothyroidism

Congenital hypothyroidism is an uncommon developmental disorder that has been reported in cats, Boxers, Scottish deerhounds, Giant Schnauzers, Affenpinschers, and Great Danes and is caused by thyroid aplasia or hypoplasia (Fig. 18.11, eFigs. 18.6 and 18.7).[19–21] Clinically, the animals are disproportionate, short-limbed dwarves with bowed limbs and long necks and trunks. After identifying an epiphyseal dysplasia radiographically, the diagnosis can be confirmed by measuring thyroid and thyroid stimulating hormone concentrations.

Radiographic Signs

Radiographic findings consist of epiphyseal dysplasia that appears as reduced or delayed ossification of the epiphyseal cartilage model. This is seen most easily in the proximal tibia and the humeral and femoral condyles. Cuboid bone ossification in the carpus and tarsus is also delayed. Vertebral bodies are shorter than normal as a result of endplate dysplasia. The skull may appear shorter and broader than normal. Degenerative joint disease may be seen as a sequel.

Mucopolysaccharidosis

Mucopolysaccharidosis represents a loosely related group of uncommon autosomal recessive inherited disorders that result in a reduction or absence of glycosaminoglycan catabolism. Lysosomal degradation of these mucopolysaccharides is necessary for normal growth in developing animals and the abnormal metabolism leads to chronic, progressive, multisystemic disease. More than 10 forms are recognized in people, each produced by a different enzyme defect. Many of these have also been identified in dogs and cats.[22–24] The best-studied animal form is the feline form of mucopolysaccharidosis VI (MPS-VI). It causes polyarthropathies because of faulty cartilage formation. The morphologic appearance of affected cats ranges from normal to short-legged dwarfs with facial dysmorphism. Feline MPS-VI has two genotypes. The least affected phenotype ranges from being physically and clinically normal to having degenerative joint disease of the shoulder and stifle joints. The classic form produces phenotypic features of dwarfism and facial dysmorphia. These cats tend to have lameness and develop hind limb paresis. The diagnosis is confirmed by an MPS urine spot test that looks for the presence of undegraded glycosaminoglycans in the urine.

Radiographic Signs

Radiographic changes of mucopolysaccharidosis involve both the axial and the appendicular skeleton. Generalized epiphyseal dysplasia is present, involving long bones and vertebral endplates. Severely affected animals are osteopenic. Findings include delayed and incomplete mineralization of the epiphyseal cartilage model. Ossified regions of the epiphyses are smaller than normal and have a nonuniform opacity with a granular appearance. Vertebral bodies appear cuboid and shorter than normal (Fig. 18.12, eFig. 18.8). The maxilla is short and flattened; the frontal sinuses may be small or absent. Progressive degenerative joint disease occurs as a result of the epiphyseal malformations. Coxofemoral subluxation or luxation may result from femoral head epiphysis remodeling. Ventral bridging spondylosis is seen in older animals.

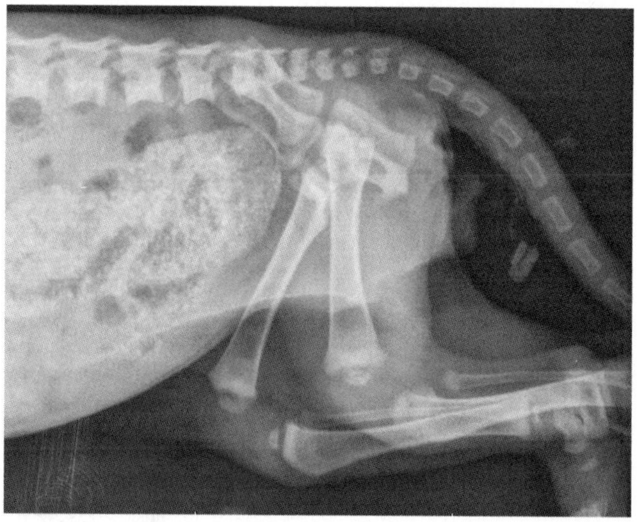

Fig. 18.11 A lateral radiograph of an 11-week-old kitten. The image was obtained for the patient's obstipation but demonstrates epiphyseal dysplasia affecting all epiphyses and endplates, and delayed ossification of the cuboidal and sesamoid bones from congenital hypothyroidism.

Multiple Epiphyseal Dysplasia

Multiple epiphyseal dysplasia is described in people where at least five different familial mutations have been identified and result in variation of inappropriately mineralized epiphyses. Multiple epiphyseal dysplasia is very rare, with only sporadic reports in veterinary medicine including a cohort of Beagles reported in the 1970s and a retrospective evaluation that yielded 19 cases from 10 different litters of Hygenhund, Dunker, Golden Retriever, and English pointers. The breeding of two affected Beagle dogs yielded an autosomal recessive pattern of inheritance.[25–27] The dogs are normal at birth and by 5 to 8 months of age the puppies are chronically lame. Some have angular limb deformities. The disease is characterized by failure of ossification of the epiphyses, apophyses, cuboidal bones, and sesamoids. Affected individuals have delayed growth and never reach normal size. This is a diagnosis of exclusion as specific genetic mutations are not known in dogs. Epiphyseal dysplasia is diagnosed radiographically and the more common causes including congenital hypothyroidism and mucopolysaccharidosis are excluded by measuring serum thyroid concentrations and evaluating for glycosaminoglycans (GAGs) in the urine.

Radiographic Signs

These include stippling of the epiphyses and irregular epiphyseal margins. Affected epiphyses eventually mineralize but are moderately deformed. Aberrant separate centers of ossification that eventually fuse with the normal ossification centers have also been described. Accelerated degenerative joint disease occurs.

DISEASES PRIMARILY AFFECTING THE PHYSIS

Spontaneous Capital Physeal Fracture of Cats

Spontaneous capital physeal fractures are defined as fractures that occur without associated trauma. In cats, spontaneous capital physeal fractures are most commonly seen in male cats

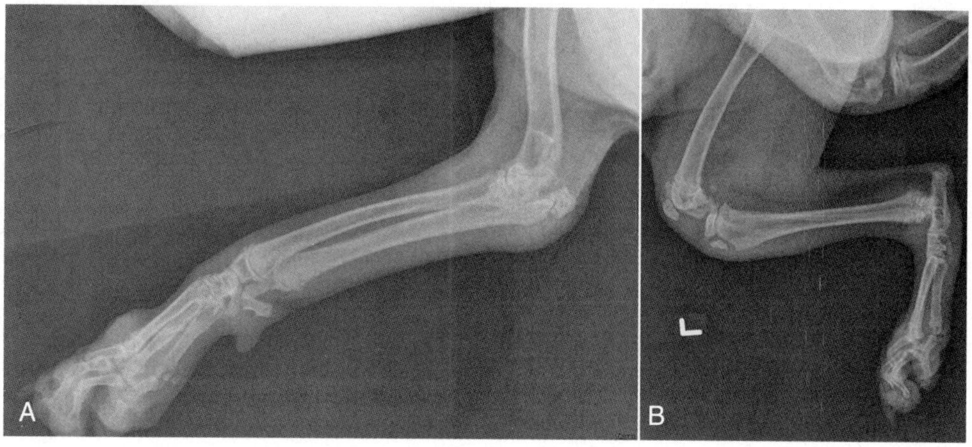

Fig. 18.12 Mucopolysaccharidosis. Lateral radiograph of the elbow (A) and of the stifle (B) of a 5-month-old Alaskan Malamute puppy with small and irregularly shaped epiphyses.

and are associated with early neutering, obesity, and delayed capital physeal closure.[28] A relationship between early neutering and delayed physeal closure is proposed and most cats are approximately 2 years of age at time of presentation. Fractures are frequently bilateral although may occur consecutively rather than simultaneously.

Radiographic Signs

The primary radiographic abnormalities include varying degrees of fragment malalignment, femoral head and neck osteolysis, and regional sclerosis (Fig. 18.13, eFig. 18.9). The physeal fracture precedes metaphyseal resorption and the degree of osteolysis and sclerosis of the femoral head and neck progress with chronicity. The ventrodorsal radiograph provides the best evaluation of the capital physis although multiple projections including flexed "frog-legged" and extended leg radiographs may be necessary for diagnosis. Evaluation of the contralateral femoral head and neck is suggested as delayed physeal closure may be evident and bilateral fractures are frequent.

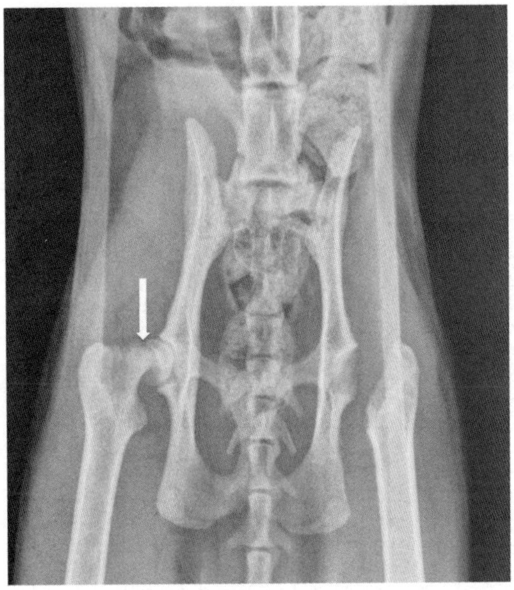

Fig. 18.13 Spontaneous capital physeal fracture in a 23-month-old neutered male cat. The right femoral head is no longer aligned with the femoral neck (*white arrow*). A left-sided femoral head and neck ostectomy was performed previously for capital physeal fracture.

Incomplete Ossification of the Humeral Condyle

Incomplete ossification of the humeral condyle is an inheritable condition of spaniels and French bulldogs resulting in a higher-than-normal incidence of humeral condylar fractures associated with normal physical activity.[29] The incidence of the disorder appears to be higher in males. Sporadic reports have been made of other medium- and large-breed dogs affected by this disorder.[30,31] Two separate centers of ossification in the humeral condyle appear typically by approximately 22 days after birth. The medial and lateral centers of the condyle should fuse by approximately 84 days after birth. Incomplete ossification leads to the presence of a thin fissure separating the medial and lateral halves of the humeral condyle in skeletally mature dogs. The fissure line can be subtle and difficult to detect radiographically, whereas CT is more sensitive. When pathologic fractures occur, approximately half are Y- or T-type fractures affecting the entire epicondylar region; the remainder are limited to fractures of the lateral (35%) or medial (15%) condyle.[29] The incidence of incomplete humeral condylar ossification is high enough that bilateral elbow radiographs or CT should be obtained in any spaniel or French bulldog with a unilateral condylar fracture. An increased incidence of fragmented coronoid processes appears to be associated with this disorder.

Radiographic Signs

The primary radiographic finding in dogs with incomplete humeral condylar ossification is a vertically oriented radiolucent line in the central region of the condyle that may extend from the subchondral bone margin of the trochlea to the distal margin of the supratrochlear foramen (Fig. 18.14). This radiolucency is evident only on the craniocaudal view and may be better seen when the view is obliqued approximately 15 degrees craniomedial to caudolateral, which positions the fissure parallel to the x-ray beam angle. Secondary radiographic signs

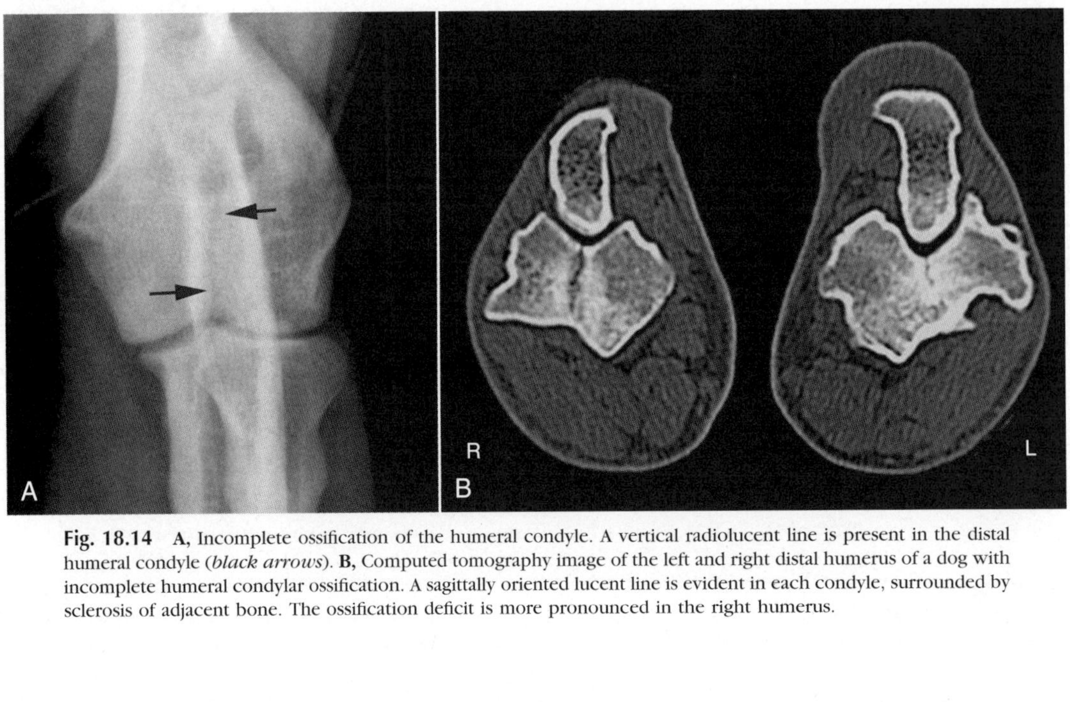

Fig. 18.14 **A,** Incomplete ossification of the humeral condyle. A vertical radiolucent line is present in the distal humeral condyle (*black arrows*). **B,** Computed tomography image of the left and right distal humerus of a dog with incomplete humeral condylar ossification. A sagittally oriented lucent line is evident in each condyle, surrounded by sclerosis of adjacent bone. The ossification deficit is more pronounced in the right humerus.

include smooth periosteal new bone formation along the lateral and caudal aspect of the humeral epicondylar region. This finding may be a response to chronic instability or incomplete, nondisplaced fracture through the nonossified region. Overt, displaced, pathologic condylar fractures may be present in one or both limbs.

Rickets

Rickets is a rare disease of dogs and cats and is defined as osteomalacia of the physes in juvenile patients due to inadequate vitamin D or heritable disorders affecting vitamin D metabolism or utilization. The decreased vitamin D results in insufficient absorption of calcium and phosphorus from the gastrointestinal (GI) tract. Affected juvenile patients present with hypocalcemia, alopecia, thickening at level of metaphyses, bowing or angular deformities, and lameness. Rickets can be concomitant with secondary hyperparathyroidism as the lack of vitamin D will inhibit GI absorption of calcium. Vitamin D can be manufactured in the skin with ultraviolet light in reptiles, amphibians, birds, and herbivores whereas carnivore dogs and cats obtain vitamin D from dietary sources.[32] Fortunately, rickets from dietary deficiencies is rarely seen in dogs and cats. Hereditary disorders of vitamin D metabolism are sporadically reported in both dogs and cats and are categorized as vitamin D–dependent rickets type I, where there is a deficiency in the enzyme that converts vitamin D to its active form. Type II is also known as hereditary vitamin D–resistant rickets where there is an anomaly of the vitamin D receptor on the target organs.[33]

Radiographic Findings

Radiographic findings of rickets include marked widening of the physes creating large, nonmineralized gaps with flaring and cupping of the adjacent epiphyses and metaphyses (Fig. 18.15, eFig. 18.10). Flared osteochondral junctions along the ribs are called "rachitic rosary" and are usually easily palpated. Diffuse osteopenia with thin cortices may be appreciated and can progress to folding fractures.

Chondrodysplasia and Osteochondral Dysplasia

Chondrodysplasia and osteochondral dysplasia result in short limb disproportionate dwarfism. There are multiple dog breeds (and other species) where short, curved limbs are the breed standard. In fact, the 19 different American Kennel Club chondrodysplastic dog breeds all share a common retrogene that encodes fibroblast growth factor 4 (fgf4).[34] Distinguishing between chondrodystrophic breeds that have been bred for many generations to establish a defect as a breed characteristic and chondrodysplastic dwarves that arise sporadically from normal parents is important. Chondrodysplasia and osteochondrodysplasias as undesirable genetic mutations have been reported in a number of breeds (Table 18.2).[35–41] This category of diseases includes a conglomerate of different genetic mutations. These different causes for chondrodysplasia can appear clinically and radiographically similar with widened physes, flared metaphyses, and angular limb deformities. Further characterization is hampered because specific genetic mutations are not described for many of these examples, and the sporadic nature of both the occurrence and the literature reporting them.

Osteochondrodysplasia of Scottish Fold Cats

A single gene variant in the *TRPV₄* that is autosomal dominant results in the folded ear appearance of the breed and osteochondrodysplasia. The degree of limb deformity and degenerative change is variable and appears worst in individuals that are homozygous dominant for this trait. Heterozygous individuals still have folded ears. When blinded radiologists are asked to evaluate radiographs of heterozygous individuals and of those without the mutation, they are largely able to detect the affected cats, although the heterozygous individuals are much less affected than the extreme examples in Fig. 18.16. Affected animals are shorter than normal, with thick inflexible

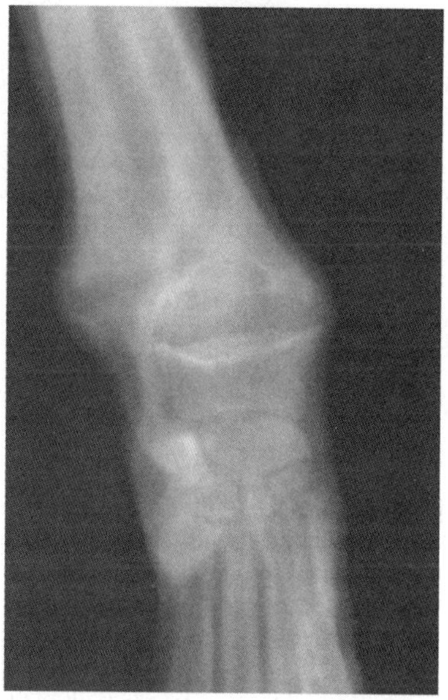

Fig. 18.15 Rickets in a 6-month-old female Pomeranian puppy. There is diffuse osteopenia with marked widening of the physis and flaring of the adjacent epiphysis and metaphysis. The puppy did not respond to high doses of oral calcium supplementation and later genome sequencing was performed and an anomaly of the vitamin D receptor ligand-binding domain was identified, compatible with type II/vitamin D-resistant rickets.

Table • 18.2

Incomplete List of Breed-Specific Chondrodysplasias.

	HERITABILITY	KEY FEATURES	RADIOGRAPHICALLY
Chondrodysplasia of Alaskan Malamutes	Autosomal recessive gene	The skull and spine are not affected	Wide physes, small carpal bones, flared metaphysis
Chondrodysplasia of Norwegian Elkhounds	Autosomal recessive	Front limbs affected more than hind limbs	Similar to the Malamutes, but spine can be affected
Ocular chondrodysplasia of Labrador retrievers	Autosomal recessive	Retinal dysplasia, cataracts	Shortened long bones, asynchronous growth of radius and ulna, large carpal bones, wide ribs

Acknowledgment

With special thanks to prior authors of this chapter for their contributions.

REFERENCES

1. Ytrehus B, Carlson C, Ekman S. Etiology and pathogenesis of osteochondrosis. *Vet Pathol*. 2007;44:429–448.
2. Wisner ER, Berry CR, Morgan JP, et al. Osteochondrosis of the lateral trochlear ridge of the talus in seven rottweiler dogs. *Vet Surg*. 1990;19:435.
3. van Bree HJ, Van Ryssen B. Diagnostic and surgical arthroscopy in osteochondrosis lesions. *Vet Clin North Am Small Anim Pract*. 1998;28:161.
4. Frazho JK, Graham J, Peck JN, et al. Radiographic evaluation of thc anconeal process in skeletally immature dogs. *Vet Surg*. 2010;39:829.
5. Nemanic S, Nixon B, Baltzer W. Analysis of risk factors for elbow dysplasia in giant breed dogs. *Vet Comp Orthop Traumatol*. 2016;29(05).
6. Blond L, Dupuis J, Beauregard G, et al. Sensitivity and specificity of radiographic detection of canine elbow incongruence in an in vitro model. *Vet Radiol Ultrasound*. 2005;46:210.
7. Holsworth IG, Wisner ER, Scherrer WE, et al. Accuracy of computerized tomographic evaluation of canine radio-ulnar incongruence in vitro. *Vet Surg*. 2005;34:108.
8. Hornof WJ, Wind AP, Wallack ST, et al. Canine elbow dysplasia. The early radiographic detection of fragmentation of the coronoid process. *Vet Clin North Am Small Anim Pract*. 2000;30:257.
9. Berry C. Evaluation of the canine elbow for fragmented medial coronoid process. *Vet Radiol Ultrasound*. 1992; 33:273.
10. Heidenreich DC, Fourie Y, Barreau P. Presumptive congenital radial head sub-luxation in a Shih Tzu: successful management by radial head osctectomy. *JSAP*. Oct;56(10):626-629.
11. Riser WH. The dysplastic hip joint: radiologic and histologic development. *Vet Pathology*. 1975;12(4):279–305. https://doi.org/10.1177/030098587501200405.
12. King M. Etiopathogenesis of canine hip dysplasia, prevalence, and genetics. *Vet Clin N Am Small Anim Pract*. 2017;47:753–767.
13. Ginja M, Silvestre A, Gonzalo-Orden J, Ferreira A. Diagnosis, genetic control and preventive management of canine hip dysplasia: a review. *Vet J*. 2010;184(3).
14. Smith G, Meyhew P, Kapatkin A, McKelvie P, Shofer F, Grego T. Evaluation of risk factors for degenerative joint disease associated with hip dysplasia in German shepherd dogs, golden retrievers, labrador retrievers and rottweilers. *JAVMA*. 2001;219(12).
15. Powers M, Biery D, Lawler D, et al. Use of the caudolateral curvilinear osteophyte as an early marker for future development of osteoarthritis associated with hip dysplasia in dogs. *JAVMA*. 2004;225(2).
16. Keller G, Reed A, Lattimer J, Corely E. Hip dysplasia: a feline population study. *Vet Radiol Ultrasound*. 1999;40(4).
17. Lee R. Legg-Perthes disease in the dog: the histological and associated radiological changes. *J Am Vet Radiol Assoc*. 1974;15:24.
18. Lieb AS, Grooters AM, Tyler JW, et al. Tetraparesis due to vertebral physeal fracture in an adult dog with congenital hypothyroidism. *J Small Anim Pract*. 1997;38:364.
19. Crowe A. Congenital hypothyroidism in a cat. *Can Vet J*. 2004;45:168.
20. Konde L, Thrall M, Gasper P, et al. Radiographic changes associated with mucopolysaccharidosis in the cat. *Vet Radiol*. 1987;28:223.
21. Rasmussen PG. Multiple epiphyseal dysplasia in a litter of beagle puppies. *J Small Anim Pract*. 1971;12:91.
22. Rasmussen PG. Multiple epiphyseal dysplasia in beagle puppies. *Acta Radiol Suppl*. 1972;319:251.
23. Rorvik A, Teige J, Ottesen N, Lingaas F. Clinical, radiographic and pathologic abnormalities in dogs with multiple epiphyseal dysplasia: 19 cases (1991–2005). *JAVMA*. 2008;233:4.
24. McNicholas WT, Wilkens BE, Blevins WE, et al. Spontaneous femoral capital physeal fractures in adult cats: 26 cases (1996–2001). JAVMA Dec 15:221(12): 1731-1736.
25. Marcellin-Little DJ, DeYoung DJ, Ferris KK, et al. Incomplete ossification of the humeral condyle in spaniels. *Vet Surg*. 1994;23:475.
26. Rovesti GL, Fluckiger M, Margini A, et al. Fragmented coronoid process and incomplete ossification of the humeral condyle in a Rottweiler. *Vet Surg*. 1998;27:354.
27. Gabriel P, Pfeil A, Ludewig E, et al. Magnetic resonance imaging diagnosis: incomplete ossification of the humeral condyle in a German shepherd dog. *J Small Anim Pract*. 2009;50:92.
28. LeVine D, Zhou Y, Ghiloni R, et al. Hereditary 1,25-dihydroxyvitamin D-resistant rickets in Pomeranian dog caused by a novel mutation in the vitamin D receptor gene. *JVIM*. 2009;23:1278–1283.
29. Parker H, VonHoldt B, Pascale Q, et al. An expressed Fdf4 retrogene is associated with breed-defining chondrodysplasia in domestic dogs. *Science*. 2009;325(5943).
30. Bingel SA, Sande RD. Chondrodysplasia in the Norwegian elkhound. *Am J Pathol*. 1982;107:219.
31. Bingel SA, Sande RD, Wight TN. Chondrodysplasia in the Alaskan malamute. Characterization of proteoglycans dissociatively extracted from dwarf growth plates. *Lab Invest*. 1985;53:479.
32. Malik R, Allan GS, Howlett CR, et al. Osteochondrodysplasia in Scottish fold cats. *Aust Vet J*. 1999;77:85.
33. Allan GS. Radiographic features of feline joint diseases. *Vet Clin North Am Small Anim Pract*. 2000;30:281.
34. Rorden C, Griswold M, Moses N, et al. Radiographical survey of osteochondrodysplasia in Scottish fold cats caused by the $TRPV_4$ gene variant. *Hum Genet*. 2021;140.
35. Gandolfi B, Alamri S, Darby W, et al. A dominant $TRPV_4$ variant underlies osteochondrodysplasia in Scottish fold cats. *Oseoarthritis and Cartilage*. 2016;24:8.
36. Muir P, Dubielzig R, Johnson K, et al. Hypertrophic osteodystrophy and calvarial hyperostosis. *Compendium*. 1996;18:143.
37. Baumgartner W, Boyce RW, Weisbrode SE, et al. Histologic and immunocytochemical characterization of canine distemper-associated metaphyseal bone lesions in young dogs following experimental infection. *Vet Pathol*. 1995; 32:702.
38. Franklin MA, Rochat MC, Broaddus KD. Hypertrophic osteodystrophy of the proximal humerus in two dogs. *J Am Anim Hosp Assoc*. 2008;44:342.
39. Gambardella PC, Osborne CA, Stevens JB. Multiple cartilaginous exostoses in the dog. *J Am Vet Med Assoc*. 1975;166:761.
40. Doige C, Pharr J, Withrow S. Chondrosarcoma arising in multiple cartilaginous exostoses in a dog. *J Am Anim Hosp Assoc*. 1978;14:605.
41. Jacobson LS, Kirberger RM. Canine multiple cartilaginous exostoses: unusual manifestations and a review of the literature. *J Am Anim Hosp Assoc*. 1996;32:45.
42. Paek M, Engilges J, Mai W. Prevalence, association with stifle conditions and histopathologic characteristics of tibial tuberosity radiolucencies in dogs. *Vet rad us*. 2013;54(5).
43. Bohning RHJ, Suter PF, Hohn RB, et al. Clinical and radiologic survey of canine panosteitis. *J Am Vet Med Assoc*. 1970;156:870.

44. Voorhout G. Radiographic features of nutritional secondary hyperparathyroidism in the growing dog and cat [in German]. *Tijdschr Diergeneeskd*. 1981;106:317.
45. Campbell BG, Wootton JA, Krook L, et al. Clinical signs and diagnosis of osteogenesis imperfecta in three dogs. *J Am Vet Med Assoc*. 1997;211:183.
46. Seeliger F, Leeb T, Peters M, Bru M, Gmann FM, Trautwen Hewicker-. Osteogenesis imperfecta in two litters of dashhunds. *Vet Pathol*. 2003;40.
47. Hanel RM, Graham JP, Levy JK, et al. Generalized osteosclerosis in a cat. *Vet Radiol Ultrasound*. 2004; 45:318.
48. Reyes N, Longley M, Bailey S, Langley-Hobbs S. Incidence and types of preceding and subsequent fractures in cat with patellar fracture and dental anomaly syndrome. *J Feline Med Surg*. 2019;21(8).
49. Huchkowsky S. Craniomandibular osteopathy in a bullmastiff. *Can Vet J*. 2002;43:11.
50. Hudson J, Montgomery R, Hathcock J, Jarobe J. Computed tomography of craniomandibular osteopathy in a dog. *Vet rad and ultrasound*. 1994;35(2).
51. Johnson KA. Retardation of endochondral ossification at the distal ulnar growth plate in dogs. *Aust Vet J*. 1981;57(10):474–478.
52. Pastor K, Boulay J, Schelling S, Carpenter J. Idiopathic hyperostisis of the calvaria in five young bullmastiffs. *J Am Anim Hosp Assoc*. 2000;36.

ELECTRONIC RESOURCES

Additional information related to the content in Chapter 18 can be found online at eBooks.Health.Elsevier.com.

- Chapter Quiz

CHAPTER 19

Fracture Healing and Complications

Gabriela S. Seiler

PHYSIOLOGY OF BONE DEVELOPMENT AND HEALING

Bones contain three principal cell types: osteoblasts, osteocytes, and osteoclasts. Osteoblasts synthesize the osteoid bone matrix and become osteocytes following mineralization of the osteoid. Osteoclasts are larger cells that reside on the surface of the mineralized matrix and remove both mineral and matrix by secretion of acids and enzymes. In normal bone, the activities of osteoblasts and osteoclasts are coordinated in response to stress (Wolff's law), allowing adaptation of the bone pattern and shape to withstand varying load placed on the bone. Although bone can react to external stimuli or forces, it is slow to react and has limited methods of reaction: bone production, bone resorption, or a combination of production and resorption.[1–3]

The regulation of mineral ions in the serum is controlled mainly by parathyroid hormone, calcitonin, and vitamin D. Parathyroid hormone increases serum calcium by stimulating osteoclastic bone resorption. Calcitonin inhibits the activity of osteoclasts and inhibits intestinal and renal calcium absorption. Vitamin D acts on the intestine to increase absorption of calcium and phosphorus and directly on bone by both mobilization of calcium and phosphorus from previously formed bone and promotion of maturation and mineralization of bone matrix.[1–3]

There are various bone shapes including long, short (cuboid), flat, irregular (such as vertebrae), and sesamoid bones. The structure of the bone can be described as lamellar, which exists as cortical (also called compact) and trabecular (also called cancellous) bone or as woven bone which is a more haphazard organization of the collagen fibers. Specialized connective tissue called *periosteum* surrounds the outer surface of bones and provides protection and nutrition. Long bones are divided into epiphyseal, physeal, metaphyseal, and diaphyseal regions.[1–4]

Normal bone development is similar to post-traumatic remodeling and fracture healing. Therefore, understanding normal bone development is helpful for assessment and optimization of fracture healing. Bone growth occurs through two mechanisms, intramembranous and endochondral ossification. *Intramembranous ossification* is characterized by synthesis of bone directly from osteogenic mesenchymal cells without a cartilage precursor. Most flat bones such as the skull and mandibles are developed this way and intramembranous ossification plays a role in increasing the width of long bones. In *endochondral ossification*, a cartilage model derived from the mesenchyme is formed and subsequently mineralized to form bone. In contrast to intramembranous ossification, mesenchymal cells are stimulated to differentiate into chondrocytes rather than osteoblasts. Endochondral ossification is the primary mechanism to form the appendicular and portions of the axial skeleton such as the vertebrae, ribs, sternebral, and flat bones of the pelvis. Bone remodeling is a continuous process and consists of bone resorption in concert with new bone formation to repair and replace old bone.[1–3] In people, approximately 2% to 3% of the total skeletal mass is thought to be renewed every year through normal remodeling processes.[5–7]

FRACTURE IDENTIFICATION AND DESCRIPTION

Physical examination is an essential first step in the evaluation of fractures and possible complicating factors. Dealing with immediate life-threatening injuries takes precedence over imaging to look for fractures. Identification of open fractures, spinal fractures, and skull fractures requires careful evaluation and methods for temporary stabilization should be available.

Radiography is the most commonly used imaging tool for fracture evaluation in veterinary medicine. At least two orthogonal views of the area in question are essential for adequate evaluation of a potential fracture; otherwise, important information about presence and nature of an injury can be missed (Fig. 19.1). Pain management and sedation are important to minimize patient motion and discomfort during radiography, except in spinal trauma cases where sedation may lead to destabilization and higher risk of spinal cord injury. For long bones, the proximal and distal joints should be included in the view. Horizontal beam radiographs are helpful in patients with spinal injury or instable fractures where moving the patient could be detrimental. Horizontal beam radiography can also be good for optimal imaging of humeral and femoral fractures where imaging with a vertical beam is difficult. In some patients, oblique views are necessary to define or identify a subtle or complex fracture.[8] With minimal displacement, at least part of the fracture plane must be parallel to the x-ray beam for the radiolucent fracture line to be seen (Fig. 19.2). Small stress fractures or incomplete fractures may not have sufficient displacement immediately following the injury to allow detection. Follow-up radiographs in 7 to 10 days may be needed to detect these fractures as the fracture line becomes more conspicuous due to resorption at the fracture fragments.

Computed tomography (CT) imaging is a valuable imaging tool to assess fractures of complex anatomical structures such as the skull and spine, and for surgical planning (Fig. 19.3).[9–13] Fractures are recognized as a radiolucent line or plane traversing the bone with variable amounts of bone fragmentation, displacement of fracture fragments, and soft tissue injury. Knowledge of normal anatomy and normal variations or aberrant anatomic change is critical for accurate interpretation of

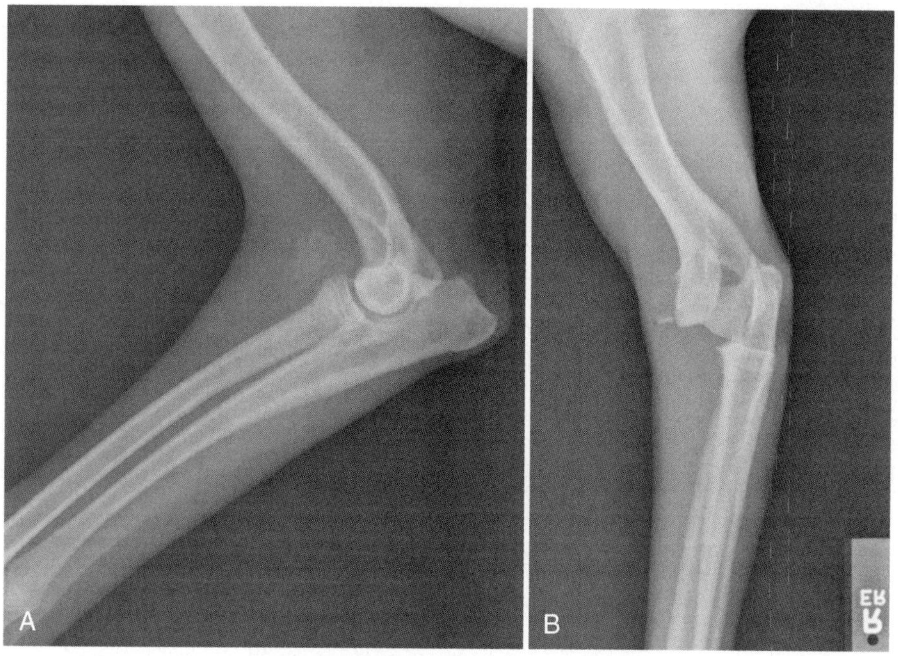

Fig. 19.1 Lateral **(A)** and craniocaudal **(B)** radiographs of the elbow joint of a young hound dog after trauma. Mild joint incongruence and a small osseous body superimposed over the cranial aspect of the radiohumeral joint are visible in the lateral view, whereas joint luxation is and a small fracture fragment are identified when adding the craniocaudal view.

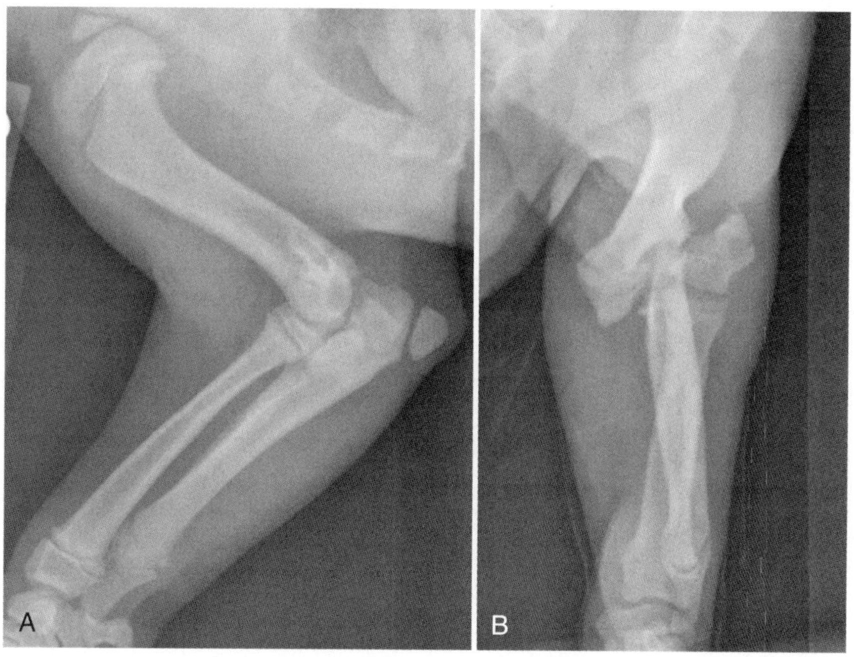

Fig. 19.2 Lateral **(A)** and craniocaudal **(B)** radiographs of the right elbow joint of a 4-month-old French bulldog with a Salter-Harris type IV intercondylar fracture of the distal humerus. The fracture extends through the lateral condyle, physis, and epiphysis into the joint. The fracture is difficult to identify in the lateral view alone.

images. Normal and accessory ossification centers and normal or aberrant nutrient foramina, overlying skin folds, fascial planes, or subcutaneous gas can all mimic fractures.[14,15]

When a fracture is identified, there are several observations that should be considered to optimize fracture assessment and treatment planning.[3]

Location is the first descriptor used in describing a fracture and includes the bone involved and the location in the bone. The location within the bone can be described as diaphyseal, metaphyseal, or epiphyseal. It is important to note the extent of any articular involvement and if there are intra-articular fracture fragments. Concurrent joint luxation or subluxation should be noted

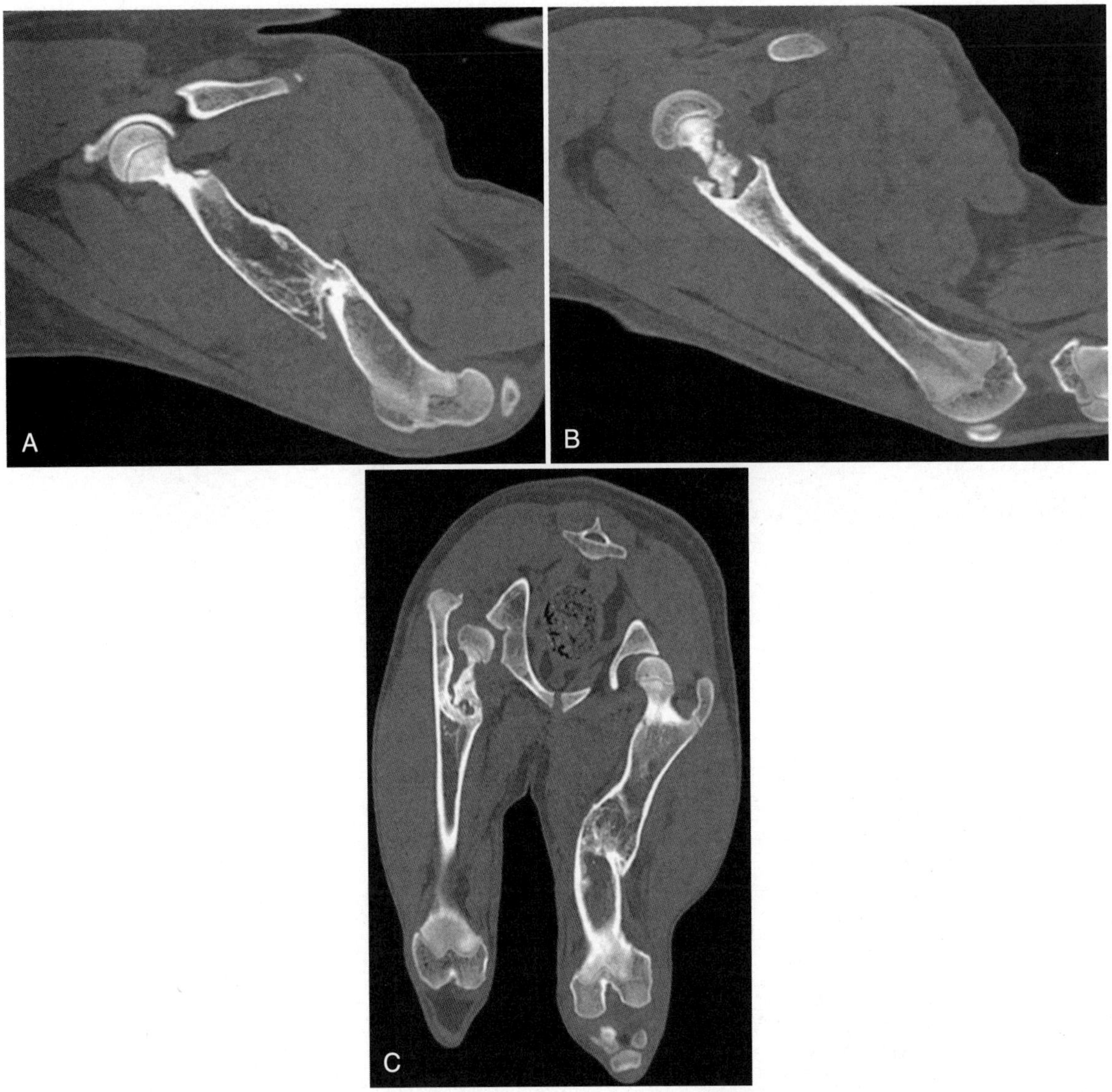

Fig. 19.3 Sagittal (**A**, *left*; **B**, *right*) and dorsal (**C**) plane reconstructed computed tomography (CT) images of the pelvic limbs of a young shepherd mix after unknown trauma. There is a malunion fracture of the left femoral diaphysis and a nonunion fracture of the right femoral neck. Showing the three-dimensional orientation of the fractures is helpful for surgical planning.

as well. If there is growth plate involvement, the Salter-Harris classification system is used, see Box 19.1 (Figs. 19.4–19.6).[16]

Direction of the fracture plane is described as transverse, oblique, longitudinal, or spiral (Figs. 19.7 and 19.8, eFig. 19.1). A fracture can be simple with a single fracture plane, multiple with several fracture planes that are not connecting, or comminuted where there are multiple fragments at a single fracture site (Fig. 19.9, eFig. 19.2). The presence and location of larger fragments should be noted as their presence and degree of displacement may influence treatment choices.

Displacement of fracture fragment components should be mentioned. This is done by noting the location of the distal or caudal fragment relative to the proximal or cranial fragment. Overriding or compression of fracture fragments can result in shortening and increased opacity of the bone at the fracture site; this is particularly important in vertebral fractures. Lengthening of the bone resulting in widening of the fracture gap is uncommon except with avulsion fractures where a piece of bone attached to a tendon or ligament gets pulled away from the bone (Fig. 19.10, eFig. 19.3).

Complete fractures are more common and extend across the entire bone, whereas incomplete fractures involve only a single cortex and are usually very localized. A *greenstick* fracture usually occurs in young animals and is an incomplete fracture of

Box • **19.1**

Salter-Harris Classification

- *Salter-Harris type I*—fracture extends through the physis.
- *Salter-Harris type II*—fractures extends through the physis and a portion of the metaphysis.
- *Salter-Harris type III*—fractures extend through the physis and epiphysis and are usually articular.
- *Salter-Harris type IV*—fractures extend through the epiphysis and cross the physis through the metaphysis. These are usually articular fractures as well.
- *Salter-Harris type V*—crushing or compression fractures that involve the physis. Type V fractures may not be apparent immediately after trauma or could present as increased opacity of the physis without displacement. Comparison with the normal opposite limb may aid in identifying subtle changes. Salter-Harris type V fractures frequently cause premature closure of all or a portion of the physis, leading to angular limb deformities.

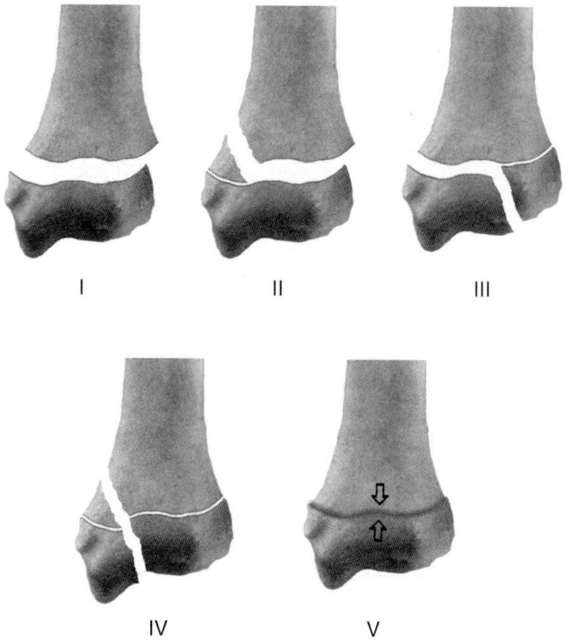

Fig. 19.4 Salter-Harris physeal fracture classification.

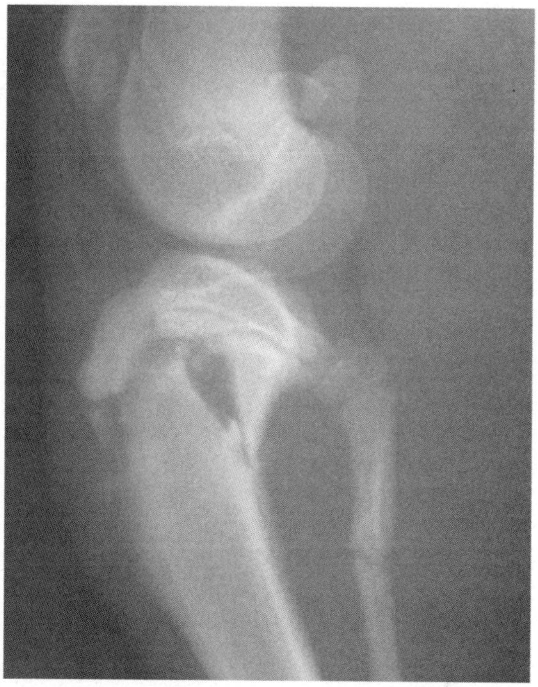

Fig. 19.6 Salter-Harris type II fracture of the proximal tibia.

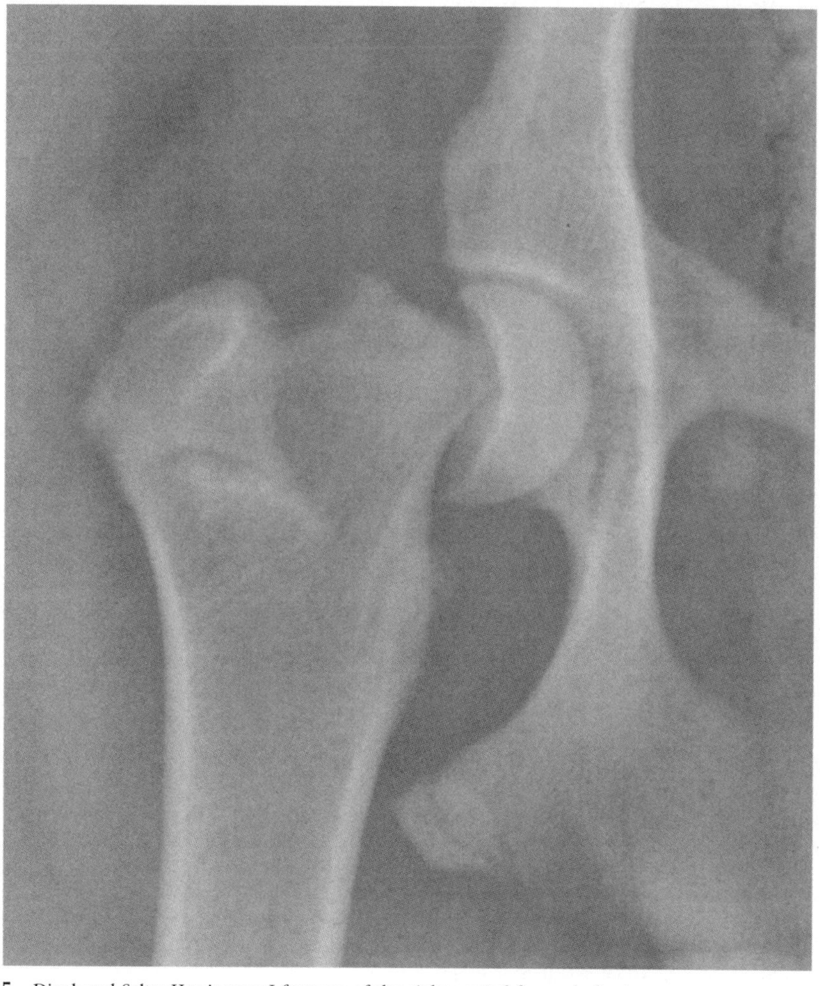

Fig. 19.5 Displaced Salter-Harris type I fracture of the right capital femoral physis.

one side of the bone with bending of the opposite cortex (plastic deformation) (Fig. 19.11). *Fatigue* or *stress* fractures are another type of incomplete fracture. They are typically microfractures caused by repeated trauma over time that exceeds the load capacity of the bone slightly. Stress fractures may not be seen radiographically or may appear as faint, linear, incomplete fractures involving one portion of a bone. Scintigraphy can be used to identify stress fractures when radiographs are normal or inconclusive.[17,18] The term *fissure* is used for thin radiolucent incomplete fracture lines often originating from a complete fracture (see Fig. 19.8, eFig. 19.4). Fissures may develop into complete fractures during repair or during the recovery phase of the injury and are thus important to be recognized.

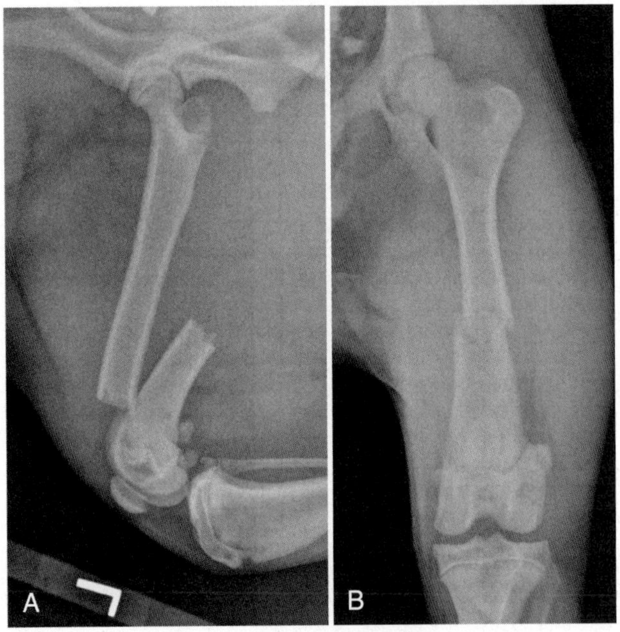

Fig. 19.7 Lateral **(A)** and craniocaudal **(B)** radiographs of an 8-month-old Golden retriever with a transverse fracture of the distal left humeral diaphysis. There is caudal and mild medial displacement of the distal fracture fragment and overriding of the fracture fragments due to contraction of the thigh musculature.

A fracture is described as open (as opposed to closed) when there is evidence of soft tissue trauma with disruption of the skin surface that could expose the fracture to the outside environment with increased risk of infection. A fracture should always be described as open in presence of subcutaneous emphysema indicating compromise of the skin surface (see Fig. 19.9, eFigs. 19.5 and 19.6).

Chronicity of the fracture is usually known from the history but if uncertain can be estimated radiographically. Acute fractures are characterized by sharp, acute fracture margins without evidence of remodeling and by the presence of soft tissue swelling. A few days after trauma, the fracture margins will be less clearly defined due to resorption and periosteal new bone formation may be noticed.

Pathologic fractures occur if the bone is weakened by preexisting disease such as bone neoplasia or metabolic demineralization, such as hyperparathyroidism. A history of minimal trauma associated with a fracture can be a first indicator that a pathologic fracture may be present. Hints that a fracture is pathologic are reduced bone opacity at the fracture site, cortical thinning, presence of a periosteal reaction with an acute fracture, disturbance in the trabecular pattern, and disproportionate swelling (Figs. 19.12 and 19.13, eFig. 19.7).

FRACTURE HEALING

Fracture healing involves the same processes as bone growth and remodeling and occurs by two basic methods: direct or primary and indirect or secondary healing. In contrast to the

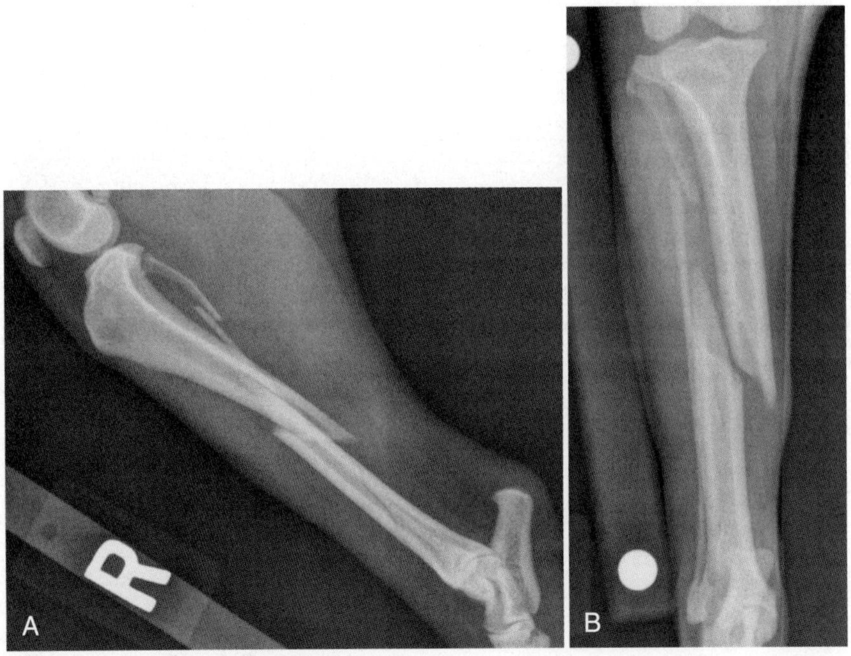

Fig. 19.8 Lateral **(A)** and craniocaudal **(B)** radiographs of a dog with a mid-diaphyseal spiral fracture of the right tibia, and short oblique transverse fracture of the proximal fibular diaphysis. Notice a fissure line that extends distally in a caudoproximal to craniodistal direction.

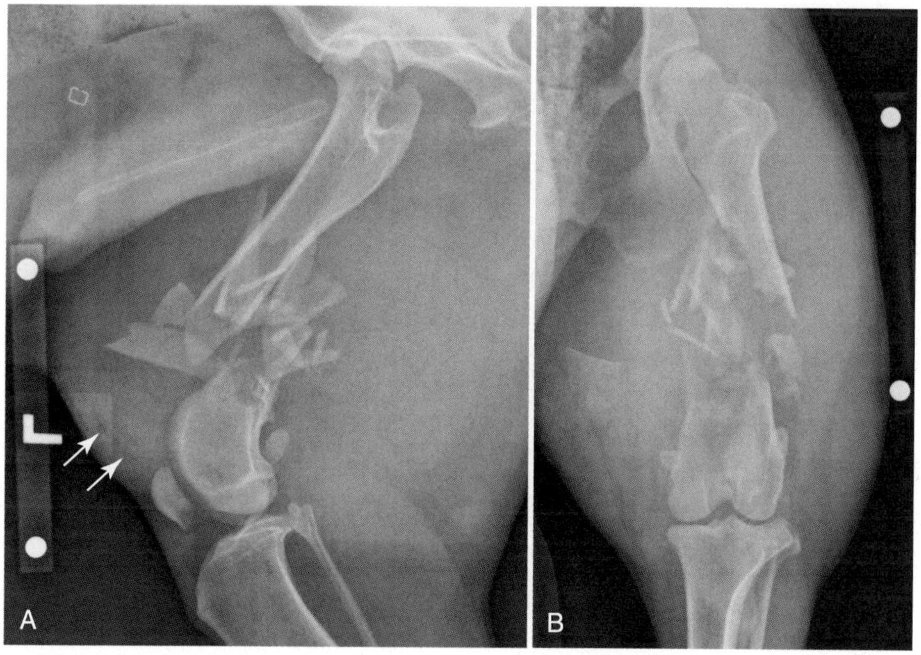

Fig. 19.9 Lateral **(A)** and craniocaudal **(B)** radiographs of a dog with a comminuted fracture of the distal femoral diaphysis and severe soft tissue swelling. Several gas foci along a fascial plane at the cranial aspect of the distal femur (*arrows*) indicate that this is an open fracture.

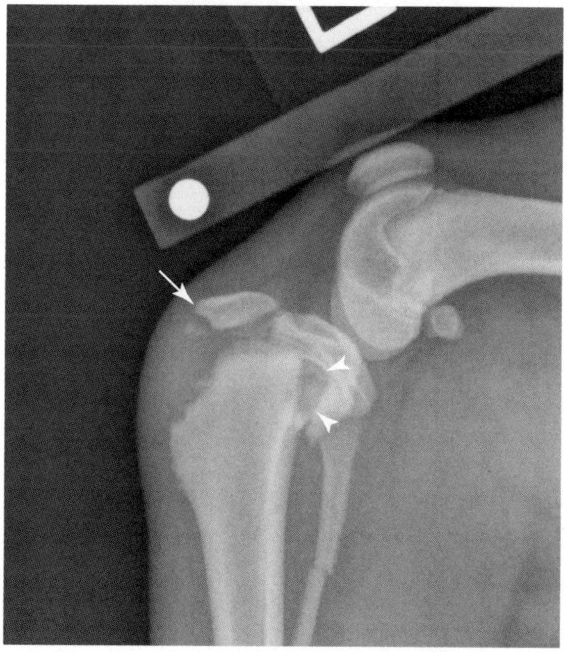

Fig. 19.10 Avulsion fracture of the tibial tuberosity with proximal displacement of the fragment (*arrow*). A Salter-Harris type II fracture of the proximal tibial physis (*arrowheads*) and a transverse fracture of the proximal fibula are also present.

healing process in many other organs where the reparative tissue is of lesser quality than the original tissue, healing bone is at least as strong, and sometimes stronger, than the original bone.

Direct (primary) bone healing occurs when the gap between fracture fragments is less than 0.01 mm and there is less than 2% strain or motion between the fragments. In direct healing, lamellar bone is formed directly between the two fragments where osteoclasts remove dead bone and osteoblasts follow immediately behind and form new bone. Radiographically, direct bone healing is characterized by slow disappearance of a fracture gap without callus formation. This type of healing is most commonly seen after a corrective osteotomy with reapposition that results in a minimal gap (Fig. 19.14). It is rarely observed in the healing of traumatic fractures.

Indirect (secondary) fracture healing is typical in traumatic fractures. The healing process undergoes several stages that have a different radiographic appearance (Box 19.2). Immediately after the fracture, the inflammatory phase is initiated. Ruptured blood vessels cause hemorrhage and hematoma formation, with associated release of tissue growth factures which stimulate inflammatory cells, osteoprogenitor cells, and osteoclasts which lead a concerted effort in cleaning up, revascularizing, and stabilizing the fracture. The hematoma provides some initial stability to the fracture. Additionally, there is muscle contraction caused by pain which adds stability but, depending on muscle mass, may also further aggravate fracture displacement. Muscle contraction plays an important role in stabilizing spinal fractures and minimizing spinal cord damage. Radiographic changes in the inflammatory phase of fracture healing include soft tissue thickening around an acute fracture which is characterized by sharp fracture margins.

The reparative phase is characterized by reduced swelling and formation of a soft, fibrous callus. The fracture gap is bridged by tissues that are more stress tolerant, with replacement of each tissue type by a more rigid type of tissue until a rigid bridge is formed between the fragments. Granulation tissue can withstand 100% stretching before failure, whereas fibrous tissue can withstand only 10% and bone only 2% deformation before failure.[2] The initial hematoma at a fracture site is replaced by granulation tissue followed by fibrous connective tissue that is replaced by fibrocartilage and then endochondral ossification to produce a bony union.[2,19] Radiographically, in this phase the fracture gap may become more obvious. The fracture margins are not sharp and smooth any longer, and may have a rounded appearance. Clinically, a fibrous callus can form a rigid brace for the bone with a stable fracture before there is a mineralized callus (Fig. 19.15A).

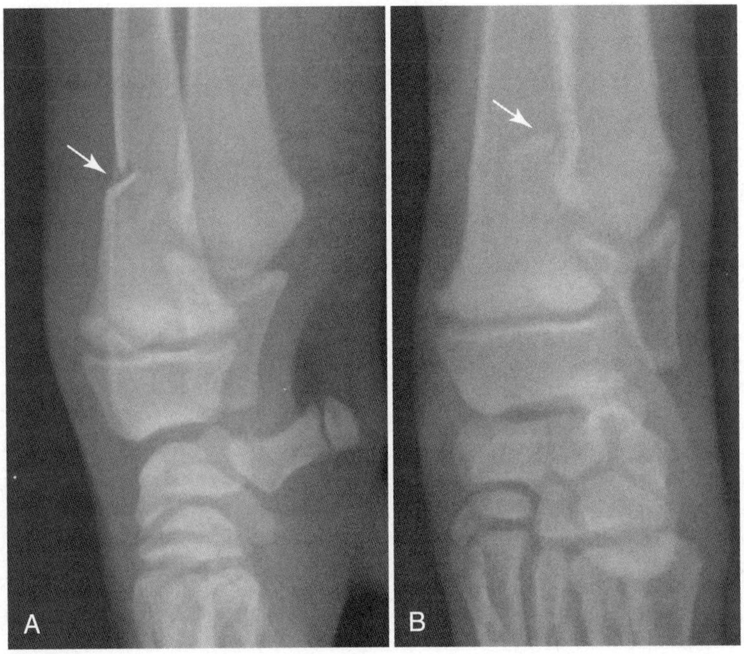

Fig. 19.11 Lateral **(A)** and dorsopalmar **(B)** radiographs of the carpus of a young puppy. There is an incomplete (greenstick) fracture (*arrow*) of the cranial cortex of the distal radial diaphysis.

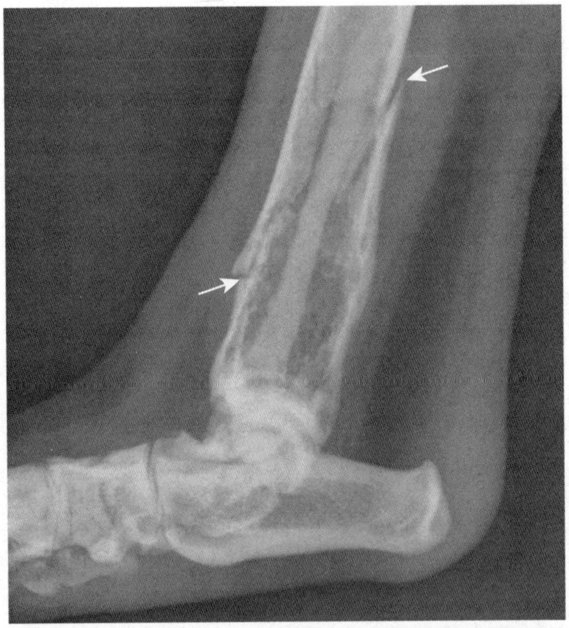

Fig. 19.12 Aggressive lesion of the distal tibia, characterized by cortical thinning, moth eaten lysis and poor margination. A pathologic fracture extends through the cranial and caudal tibial cortex (*arrows*).

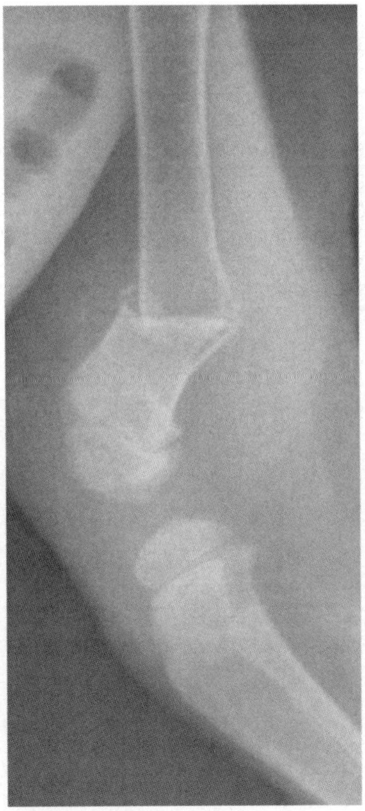

Fig. 19.13 Lateral view of the distal femur of a cat with nutritional secondary hyperparathyroidism. There is a healing malunion fracture of the distal femur. Note the thin cortices and poor contrast between the demineralized bones and adjacent soft tissue.

Wolff's law dictates that bone remodeling adapts to the loads on the bone in *the remodeling phase*.[20] A small degree of motion at the fracture site stimulates formation of an osseous callus which eventually bridges the fracture gap. Osteoblastic bone formation and osteoclastic resorption work together to transform the woven bone of the callus into compact cortical bone, restore the shape of the cortical bone, and reestablish a medullary cavity.

Radiographically, mineralized callus is first visible as a faint mineral opacity between fracture margins, followed by more and more opaque bone deposits and finally a smoothly margined, completely mineralized osseous callus which creates a clinically stable fracture (see Fig. 19.15). The amount of callus is related to the type of fracture, degree of reduction, and fixation. Excessive callus may form in areas of elevation (for example due to subperiosteal hemorrhage) and/or stripping of the

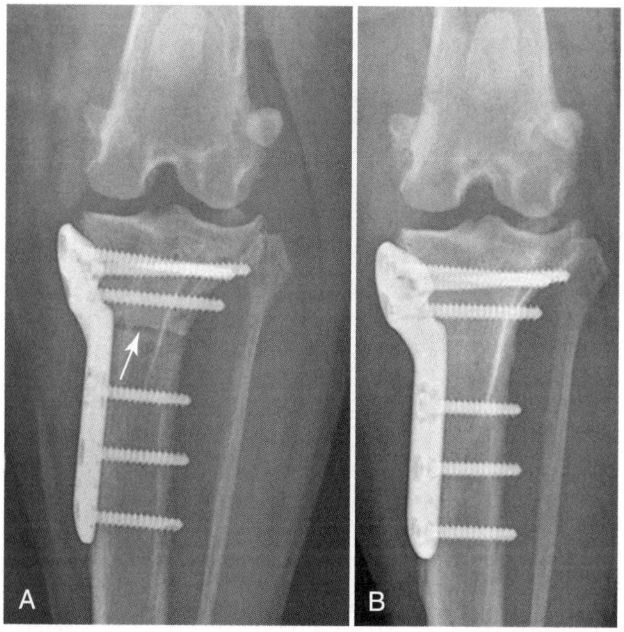

Fig. 19.14 Proximal tibial osteotomy for a tibial plateau leveling osteotomy (TPLO) procedure. Radiographs were obtained after surgery **(A)** and 2 months later **(B)**. The osteotomy site *(arrow)* has healed without callus formation consistent with primary healing.

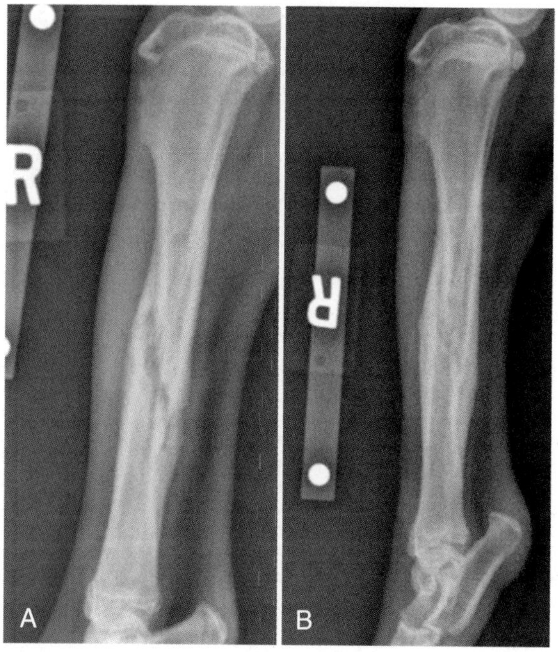

Fig. 19.15 Spiral fracture of the tibial diaphysis of an 8-month old mixed-breed dog 3 weeks **(A)** and 6 weeks **(B)** after trauma. The fracture was treated with a splint. At 3 weeks, a wide fracture gap is visible, and early callus formation is present starting to bridge the cranial fracture gap. At 6 weeks, there is smooth bridging callus present and the fracture gap is starting to disappear, consistent with normal secondary fracture healing.

Box • 19.2

Radiographic Appearance of Secondary Fracture Healing

Acute Fracture
Fracture margins are sharp, soft tissue swelling

5 to 10 Days After Reduction
Fracture fragments lose sharp margins due to resorption
Demineralization of fracture fragment ends may result in slight fracture gap widening

10 to 20 Days After Reduction
Formation of endosteal and periosteal callus
Decreasing size of fracture gap
Variable loss in opacity of free fracture fragments

30 Days or More After Reduction
Fracture lines gradually disappear
External callus increases in opacity and remodels

3 Months or More After Reduction
Continued remodeling of external calluses
Trabecular pattern may develop within the callus
Cortical shadow becomes visible through the callus
Medullary cavity continuity gradually reestablished
Cortical remodeling along the lines of stress

periosteum. Findings to support ongoing remodeling include continuity of the cortex across the fracture gap, disappearance of the fracture gap, flattening of the osseous callus, and finally establishment of a near normal bone outline and structure, which can take several months or years to accomplish.

Radiography should not be used as the sole criterion of fracture healing, but the appearance of the fracture should be considered in concert with clinical findings to assess progression and potential complications. The following factors may influence fracture healing and should be considered in the assessment.

Blood Supply

One of the most important prerequisites for normal fracture healing is a normal blood supply. Deficient vascularity may cause complications such as delayed fracture healing or nonunion fracture. Particularly at risk are fractures which are poorly covered by soft tissues and therefore have reduced potential for recruitment of periosteal blood supply, severely comminuted or displaced fractures with disruption of existing blood supply, or fractures with severe tissue damage such as gunshot wounds.[21,22] The incidence of nonunion fractures for example is high in the distal antebrachium of toy breed dogs treated with external coaptation where decreased intraosseous vascular density and minimal soft tissue coverage contribute to the lack of healing.[23] While the blood supply itself cannot be determined radiographically, potential damage can be estimated based on location and appearance of the fracture.

Stability and Anatomic Reduction

Bone healing depends on a certain degree of stability. While a small amount of instability can actually have a stimulating effect on formation of a fibrous and subsequently an osseous callus, too much instability (>5%) is detrimental to fracture healing and may lead to delayed union, malunion, nonunion, or pseudarthrosis formation. Anatomic reduction with a narrow fracture gap improves the chance of direct or rapid indirect fracture healing.[24–27]

Age

Young age is advantageous for fracture healing, and fracture healing progresses at an astonishing pace, occasionally to the detriment of the patient if a fracture is not treated immediately and fibrous tissues have to be broken down to realign fracture fragments with the risk of disrupting fragile blood supply.

Fracture healing progresses slowly in geriatric patients and this has to be taken into account when making treatment and management decisions, and when assessing fractures for normal healing.[28]

Metabolism

The overall metabolism of a patient plays a role and diseases affecting normal bone turnover, such as hyperadrenocorticism, may lead to delays in bone healing.[29,30]

Infection

Infection of the bone or surrounding tissues can disrupt fracture healing directly, or indirectly by causing loosening of the fixation device or necessitating removal of implants before the fracture has healed.

RADIOGRAPHIC EVALUATION OF FRACTURE HEALING AND ASSOCIATED COMPLICATIONS

After treatment, both normal healing and possible complications should be evaluated. At least two orthogonal radiographs are needed to assess reduction and alignment of the fracture after treatment (Fig. 19.16). Radiographs should be repeated every 4 to 6 weeks during the healing process, sooner if clinical signs indicate presence of complications. The "four A" system can be helpful for systematic evaluation of surgical fracture repair, in addition to systematic evaluation of the entire radiograph, including the soft tissues.

- Apposition or reduction of fracture fragments has the goal of restoring the length and shape of the bone.
- Alignment of the affected bone and adjacent joint should be evaluated and changes in alignment over time are signs of instability or implant failure.
- The Apparatus has to be evaluated for size relative to the bone. Cortical engagement of pins and screws and position relative to joint space should be noted; an implant entering a joint space requires surgical revision.
- Activity of new bone formation over time is assessed for presence of callus formation but also for presence bone lysis with implant instability or active bone proliferation indicative of osteomyelitis.

There are many potential complications of fracture healing that should be considered in every follow-up examination.

Stress Protection and Bone Atrophy

A degree of reduced bone density in a fracture site can be caused by insufficient stimulation of bone turnover due to the implant taking up most of the load. Oversized implants are more prone to provide stress protection. Diffuse osteopenia of the affected limb may be noticeable if the limb is not or only lightly used after a fracture, usually associated with disuse muscle atrophy. These changes will resolve once the patient returns to normal activity but is severe can be a predisposition for a stress fracture.

Delayed Union

Delayed union is a subjective classification for a fracture that is not healing within the expected timeframe, this is one of the most common complications of fracture healing. Determination of delayed vs. normal fracture healing is subjective as many factors influence the progression of normal fracture healing as outlined earlier.[31] Radiographically, delayed union is characterized by some signs of fracture healing over time such as resorption of fracture margins, mineralization of the soft tissues bridging the fracture gap while preserving an open medullary cavity at the fracture gap, or nonbridging callus formation (Fig. 19.17).

Nonunion

A nonunion state is reached when a fracture does not have the potential to heal anymore.[32] The diagnosis of nonunion fracture should be made with caution and only when there is strong evidence for it, as it will necessitate a different and often more aggressive treatment approach than a very slowly healing fracture. Radiographically, the most important indicators for a nonunion fracture are lack of progression of fracture healing over time and this typically requires evaluation of the fracture at multiple time points. Smooth, rounded fracture margins with sclerosis of the medullary cavity at the fracture site are suggestive of a nonunion fracture. There are two types of nonunion fractures: viable and nonviable.[2]

Viable (or reactive, vascular) nonunion fractures are characterized by viable active attempts to heal the fracture with

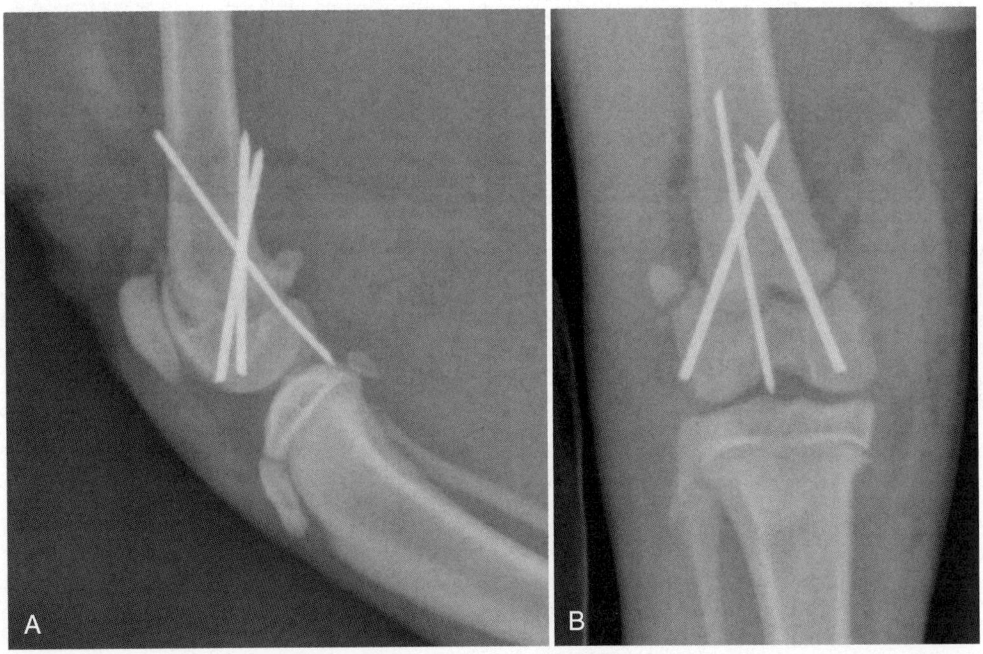

Fig. 19.16 Lateral (A) and craniocaudal (B) postoperative radiographs of a Salter-Harris type II fracture of the distal femur in a cat. One of the pins extends into the caudal aspect of the stifle joint and had to be replaced.

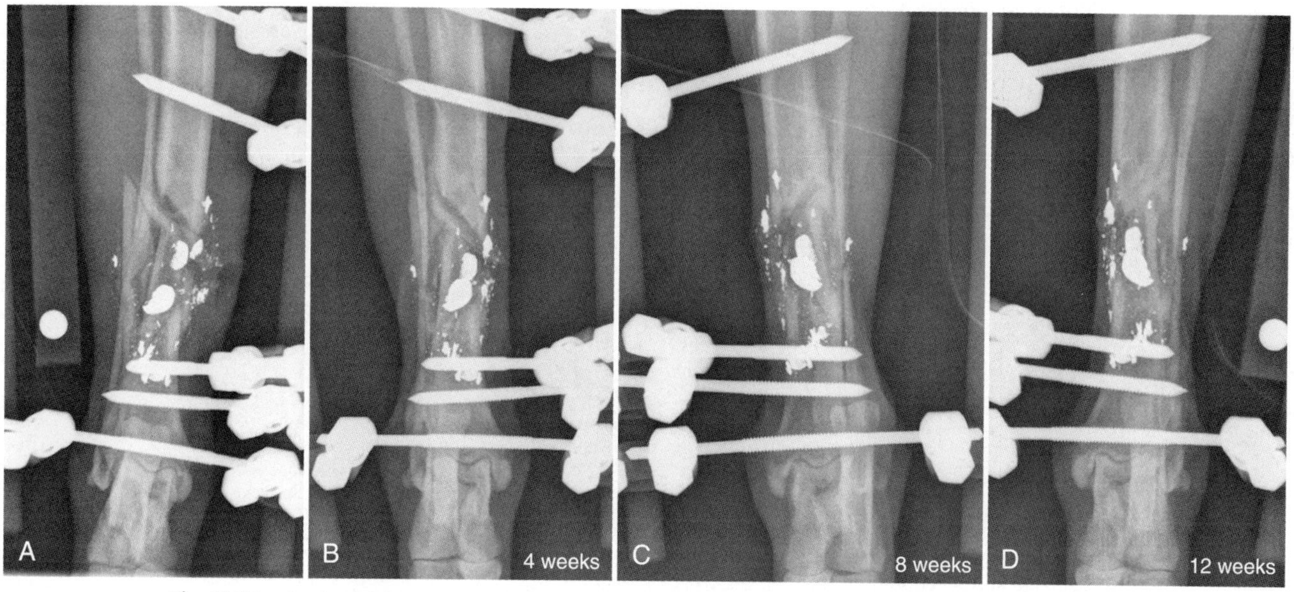

Fig. 19.17 Craniocaudal radiographs of a comminuted fracture of the distal tibia of a 5-year-old dog caused by a gunshot wound, immediately **(A)**, 4 weeks **(B)**, 8 weeks **(C)**, and 12 weeks **(D)** after surgery. The fracture gap is continuously more mineralized, and some callus is slowly added over time. Fracture healing is progressing but at a slow pace consistent with a delayed union, most likely caused by disruption of blood supply due to gunshot trauma.

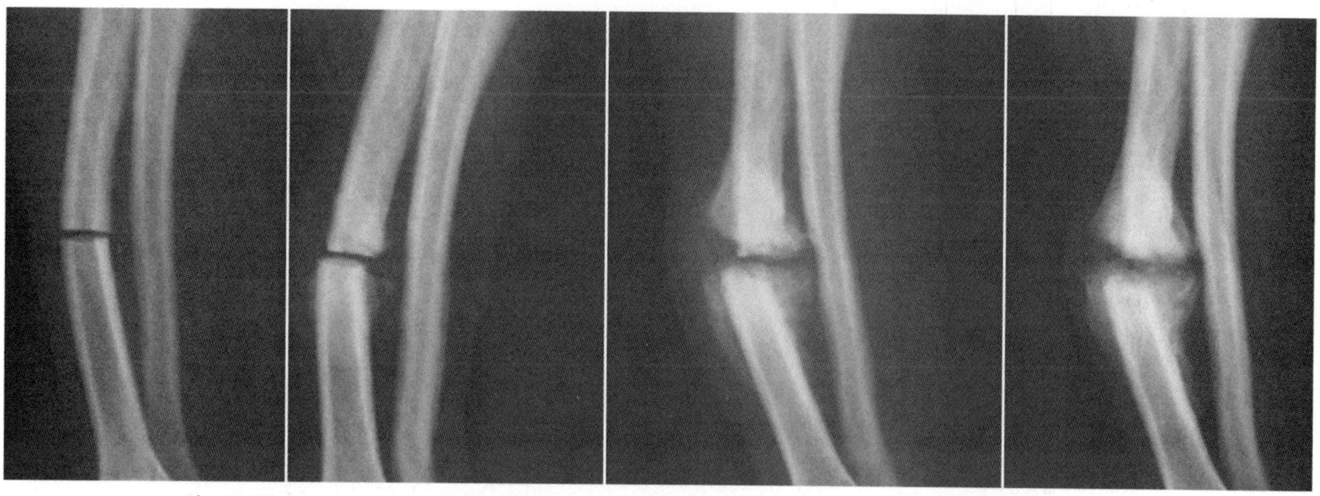

Fig. 19.18 Osteotomy of the radius with lack of fixation develops into a hypertrophic nonunion. Note the exuberant callus around the osteotomy ends with no bridging callus. This appearance is often termed an *elephant foot.*

reactive bone and callus formation. They can be hypertrophic, characterized by abundant callus formation but lack of bridging callus due to excessive motion at the fracture site (Fig. 19.18). Rarely, a pseudoarthrosis may develop because of chronic motion at the fracture site where a fibrous capsule fills with serous fluid (eFig. 19.8). Oligotrophic nonunion fractures have little or no callus with bridging of the fracture fragments by fibrous tissue (Fig. 19.19). These may be difficult to differentiate from a nonviable nonunion fracture because of the lack of callus and reaction at the fracture site. Scintigraphy may be used to detect blood supply to the fracture gap, indicating viable tissue.[33] Generally, some bone reaction at the fragment ends suggests a viable nonunion.

Nonviable nonunion fractures are uncommon and typically occur due to insufficient blood supply at the fracture fragments or an excessive fracture gap between fragments. Nonunion fractures can be dystrophic in nature where there is no bridging callus, a fracture gap, and rounded, sclerotic fracture margins. Necrotic nonunion fractures are associated with sequestrum formation due to complete loss of blood supply; see more details on sequestrum formation later. A large fracture gap that is too wide for bridging callus to form is termed *defect nonunion fracture*. Atrophic nonunion is characterized by thinned, tapering fracture ends without evidence of callus formation and decreased bone opacity, usually a sequela of the other forms of nonviable nonunion fractures. This is most commonly seen in distal antebrachial fractures of toy breeds where there is insufficient blood supply to the fracture (Fig. 19.20).[34,35]

Malunion

Malunion fractures are defined by healing with permanent angular and/or rotational deformity of the affected bone. Malunion can occur due to poor initial reduction and alignment, shifting of fragments during the healing process, implant failure, or premature removal (eFig. 19.9). The clinical relevance of malunion fractures depend on the degree of malunion but also on its influence on associated soft tissue structures such as muscles, tendons, and ligaments which may undergo altered

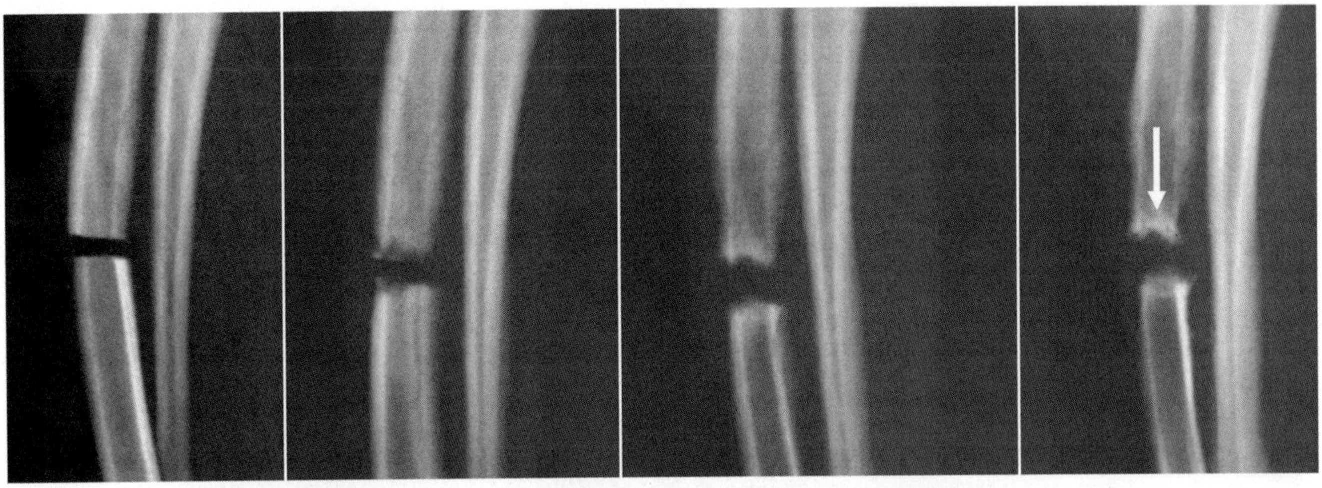

Fig. 19.19 Osteotomy with no fixation develops into an oligotrophic nonunion. Little callus is present at the osteotomy site, with filling in one of the ends of the segments seen as a sclerotic band (*white arrow*).

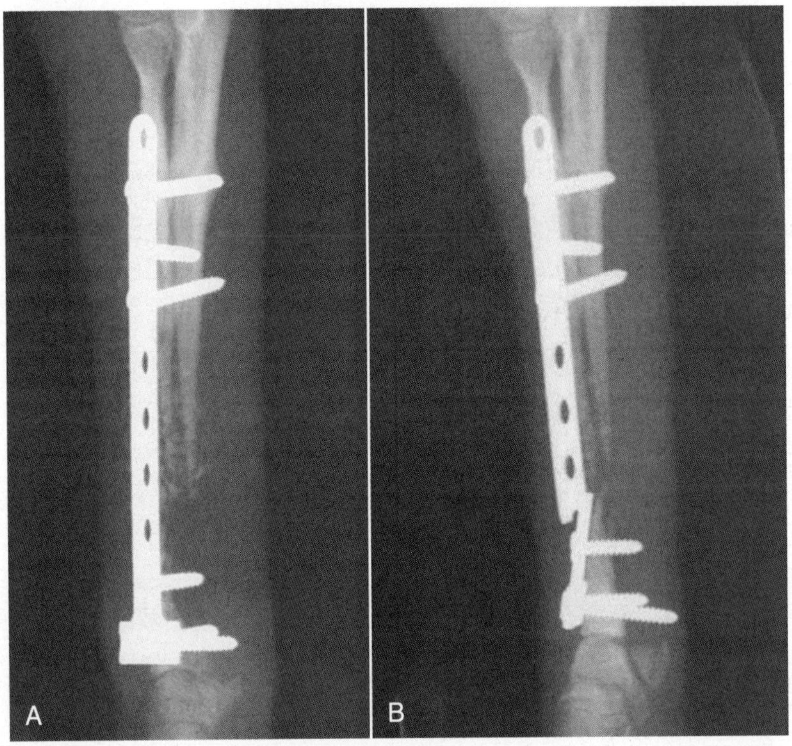

Fig. 19.20 **A,** This toy poodle has atrophic nonunion radial and ulnar fractures at 3 months after the original injury. Note the lack of callus and atrophy of the adjacent ends of the fracture fragments. The small mineral foci overlying the fragments are small islands of cancellous bone grafts placed during fixation. Poor soft tissue environment, including poor blood supply, at the fracture site prevented the formation of callus. **B,** At 4.5 months after the initial injury, bone plate failure from metal fatigue is evident.

stresses and potential injury, as well as adjacent joints (eFig. 19.10). Loadbearing of the bone itself may also be affected in the sense that the main load on the bone may now be shifted from the center to the periphery of the bone. Radiographically, malunion fractures are characterized by abnormal angulation or rotation of the affected bone. Long bone malunion fractures can be classified as *valgus, varus, antecurvatum, recurvatum, torsional,* or *translational* (Fig. 19.21). Cortical thickness may be asymmetrical as one part of the bone may take up more of the load along the axis of force resulting in remodeling and increased cortical thickness (Fig. 19.22).

Implant Instability and Failure

Loosening of fracture of implants can lead to implant failure. Common causes of implant loosening include instability, micromotion of the implants, or infection. Implant motion leads to focal bone resorption around the implant, characterized by a radiolucent area surrounding the implant (Fig. 19.23, eFig. 19.11). This has to be differentiated from an Uberschwinger digital imaging artifact, which is a continuous, thin radiolucent rim around the edges of implants caused by edge enhancement.[36] Resorption due to motion, on the other hand, manifests as asymmetric radiolucency that widens towards the periphery of the bone. Accompanying signs are often soft tissue

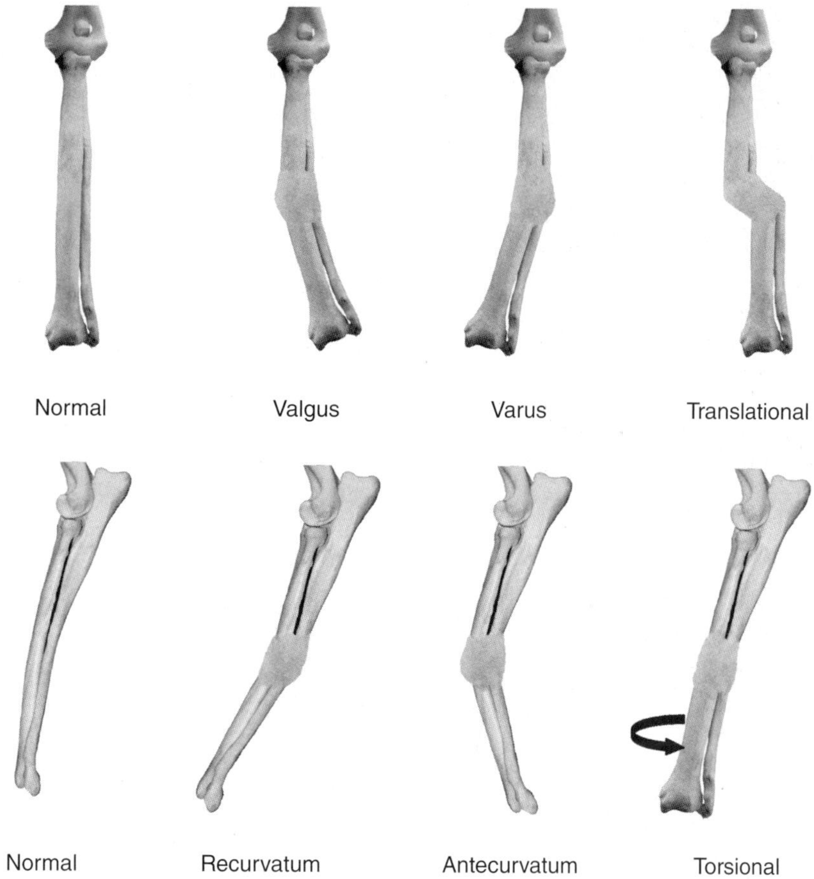

Fig. 19.21 Classification of malunion fractures.

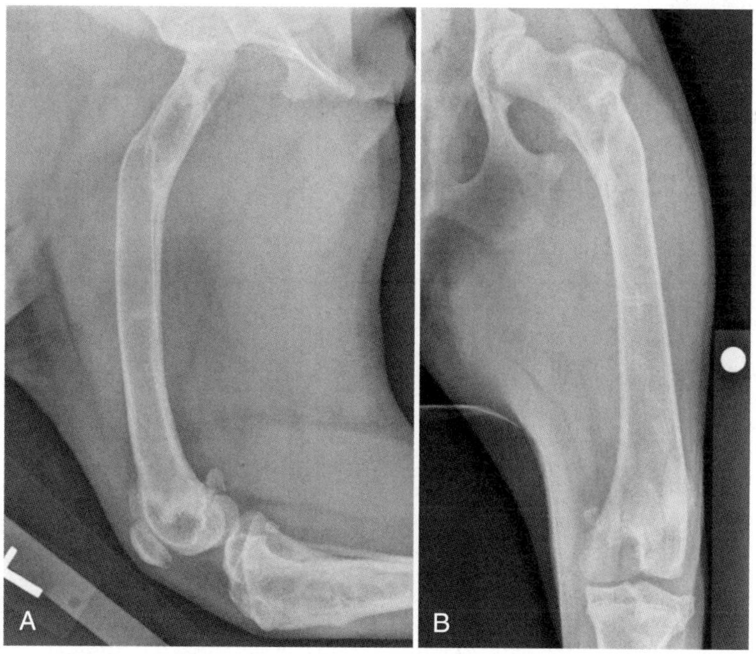

Fig. 19.22 Lateral **(A)** and craniocaudal **(B)** radiographs of a malunion femoral fracture. The fracture has healed but there is abnormal angulation of the proximal femur. Notice that the caudal cortex is thicker due to increased load bearing.

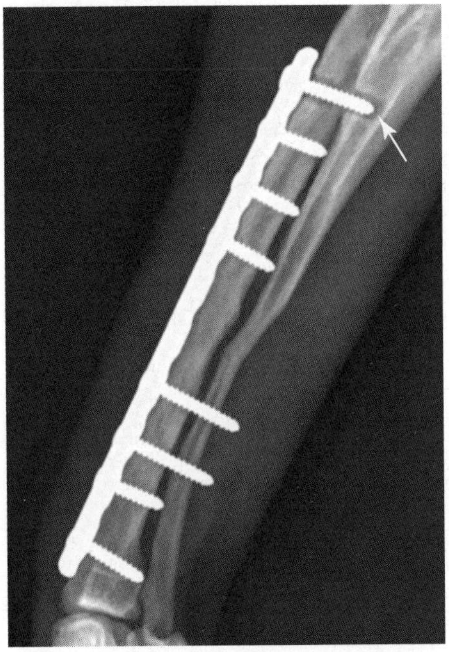

Fig. 19.23 There is uniform peri-implant radiolucency surrounding the most proximal screw (*arrow*) indicating micromotion and loosening of the screw. This is not an Uberschwinger artifact as it is not present at any of the other screws.

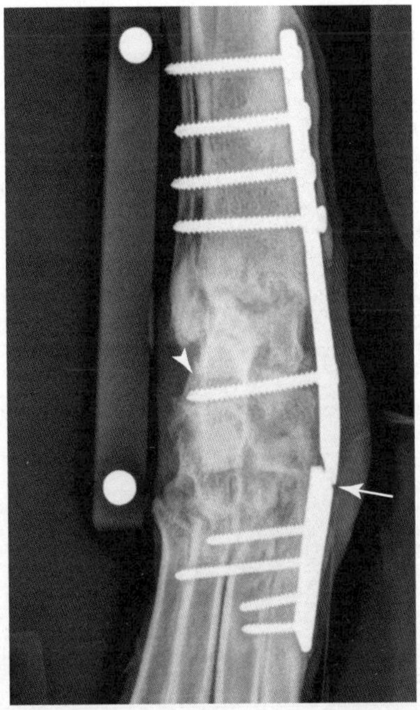

Fig. 19.24 Tarsal arthrodesis with implant failure. The medially applied bone plate is fractured at the level of the distal intertarsal joint (*arrow*). There is a wedge-shaped radiolucent area surrounding the tip of the screw placed into the talus (*arrowhead*) caused by motion and implant loosening.

swelling around the implant in question, and movement of the implant relative to the bone it resides in. Comparison of post-operative radiographs with recheck radiographs is therefore helpful to compare the location and position of the implant relative to the bone, of course taking into account potential bone growth in juvenile animals. Care should be taken when obtaining repeat radiographs, to ensure consistent limb positioning and beam centering so that minimal implant motion can be detected with certainty. Fractures of implants are usually relatively easy to recognize radiographically and need to be evaluated based on their potential impact on stability and overall healing capacity of the fracture (Figs. 19.24 and 19.25, eFigs. 19.12 and 19.13).

Angular Limb Deformity

Abnormal, asynchronous bone growth or premature closure of growth plates in immature animals after trauma may lead to angular limb deformity. The most common site for this complication in the dog is premature closure of the distal ulnar physis (eFig. 19.14). The distal ulnar physis appears more susceptible to injury, potentially due to its conical shape that may concentrate forces into the apex of the physis. The initial compressive growth plate injury is often not visible radiographically and the damage is only noted when angular limb deformity develops. Premature closure of the distal ulna leads to cranial bowing of the radius due to continued growth of this bone, and/or distal subluxation of the ulna at the elbow joint. Subluxation of the ulnar carpal joint and valgus deformity of the manus are also common (Fig. 19.26). Premature closure of the distal radial physis is less common and may involve only one side of the physis (eFig. 19.15). Commonly observed sequela of distal radial closure are humeroradial and humeroulnar subluxation, antebrachiocarpal subluxation, and uncommonly, angulation of the manus (Fig. 19.27).

Infection

All fractures have the potential to get infected, given the presence of damaged tissues which can provide a suitable environment for bacterial growth. Poor blood supply and a compromised immune system adds to the risk of infection. Open fractures should always be considered to be contaminated and therefore at a higher risk of infection than a closed fracture, necessitating different treatment decisions.[37–39] Clinical signs of osteomyelitis such as redness, pain, and acute worsening of lameness may be recognized before radiographic signs are present. As infection continues, signs of an aggressive bone lesion including bone lysis, active, irregular, often palisading periosteal reaction and soft tissue swelling will develop (Figs. 19.28 and 19.29, eFig. 19.16). The definitive diagnosis of osteomyelitis is not possible radiographically, and tissue sampling for culture and cytology as needed. A special case of infection includes sequestrum formation, as described in the next paragraph.

Sequestrum

Devitalization of fracture fragments can occur during trauma. It is a normal occurrence that small fracture fragments lose their blood supply and are subsequently resorbed. When larger fracture fragments are devitalized, the devitalized bone or sequestrum creates a reaction with surrounding inflammation and necrosis. A classic sequestrum is recognized as a sharply marginated sclerotic bone fragment (sequestrum) surrounded by or separated from the parent bone by a radiolucent zone that is surrounded by sclerotic bone (involucrum) (see Figs. 19.30 and 19.31). In some instances, a draining tract (cloaca) arises from the radiolucent necrotic area surrounding the sequestrum and extends to the skin surface. Generally, less reaction occurs surrounding a sterile sequestrum; however, determining radiographically whether the sequestrum is infected is not always possible.[40]

Fracture Associated Tumors

Fracture associated sarcomas are defined as sarcomas occurring at a previous fracture site more than 5 years after the original fracture. The pathophysiology of fracture-associated sarcoma is poorly understood. Chronic inflammation and infection at the fracture site with delayed healing as well as implant degradation have been considered as possible causes (Fig. 19.32, eFig. 19.17).[38,41,42]

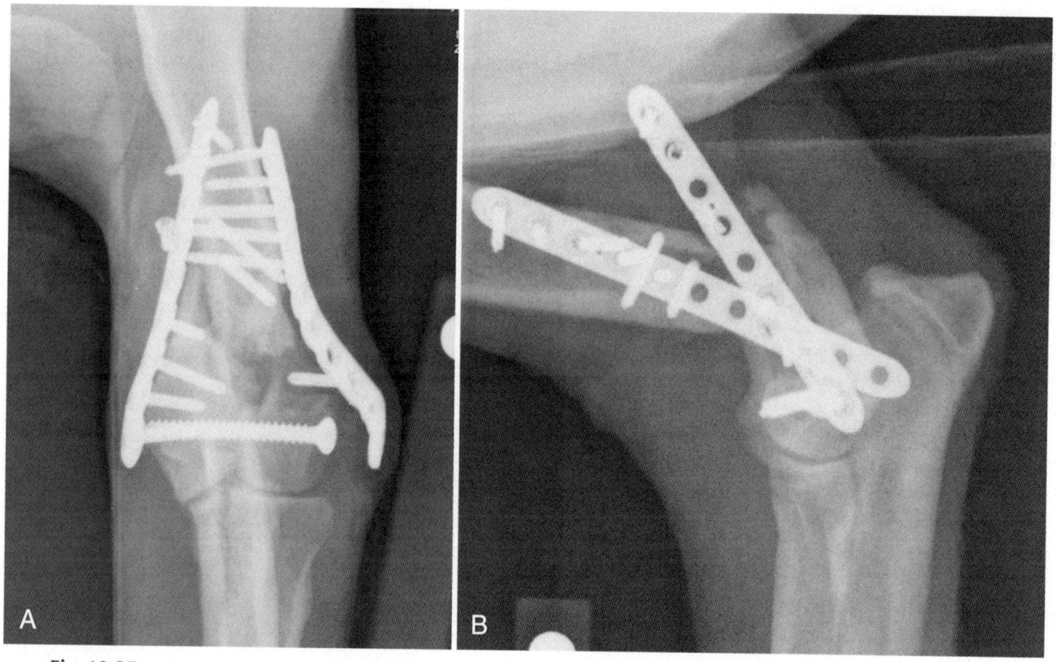

Fig. 19.25 Craniocaudal **(A)** and lateral **(B)** radiographs of a humeral condylar fracture repair with implant failure. The distal portion of the laterally applied bone plate has migrated laterally and there is a large area of radiolucency around the distal most screw that is only partially engaged in the bone. The proximal screws of the medially applied bone plate have fractured, and the plate is removed from the proximal fracture fragment. The fracture is instable with caudal and medial displacement of the distal fracture fragment.

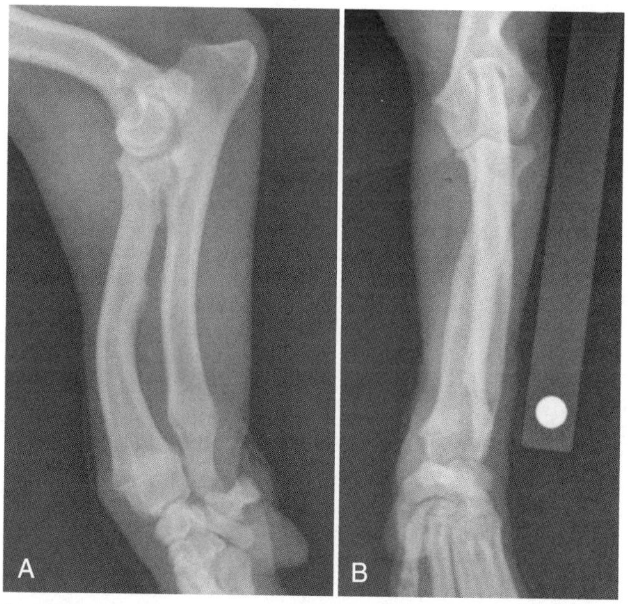

Fig. 19.26 Lateral **(A)** and craniocaudal **(B)** radiographs of the antebrachium of a dog with premature distal ulnar physeal closure which causes shortening of the ulna. Continued growth of the radius results in cranial bowing of the radius and mild carpal valgus.

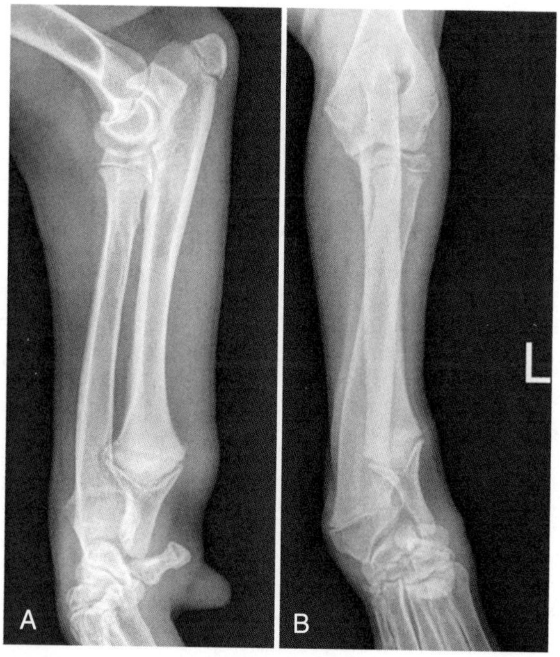

Fig. 19.27 Lateral **(A)** and craniocaudal **(B)** radiographs of the antebrachium of a dog wtih premature partial distal radial physeal closure. The lateral aspect of the distal radial physis is closed whereas there is still growth medially resulting in valgus deformation at the carpus. The radius is shortened relative to the ulna resulting in elbow joint incongruity.

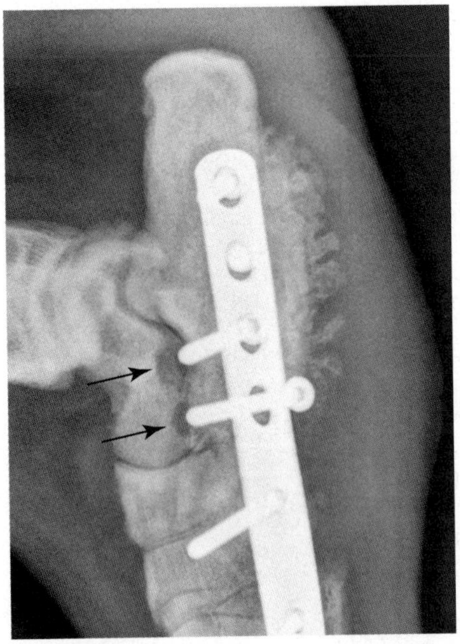

Fig. 19.28 Lateral view of the tarsus of a dog with osteomyelitis. A bone plate is present to provide stabilization of an unstable tarsal joint. There is lysis around the tip of two screws (*black arrows*). The fourth screw from the top is backing out. There is also an irregular active columnar periosteal reaction on the plantar aspect of the calcaneus; this irregular periosteal reaction, which is highly suggestive of osteomyelitis, should never be seen with normal callus. The lysis around the tips of the screws could be caused by motion but considering the columnar periosteal reaction on the calcaneus, screw tract infection is likely.

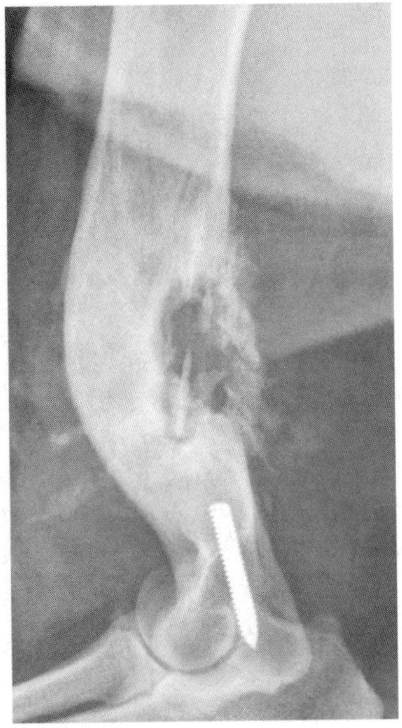

Fig. 19.30 Lateral radiograph of the distal humerus of a dog. There is a healed malunion fracture of the distal humerus with the distal fragment angled caudally (antecurvatum malunion fracture). A piece of a threaded pin is embedded in the distal humerus. There is a sharply margined opaque bone fragment surrounded by a zone of lysis and an active periosteal reaction. The adjacent medullary cavity of the humerus is sclerotic. These are classic findings of a sequestrum with secondary osteomyelitis.

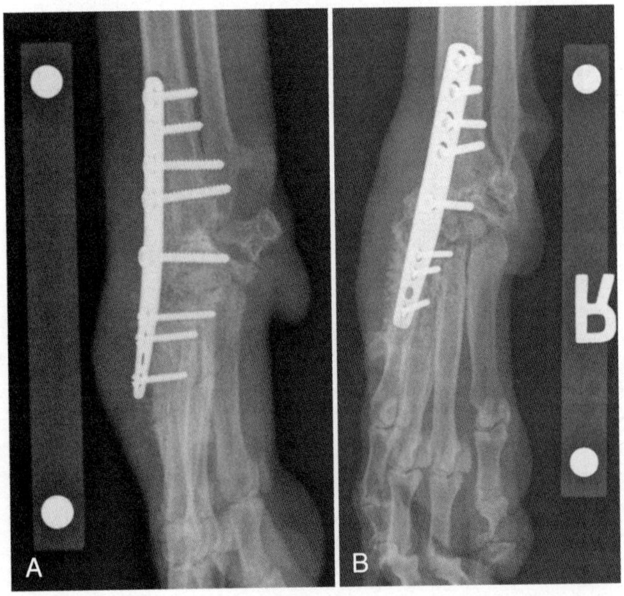

Fig. 19.29 Lateral **(A)** and oblique **(B)** radiograph of the carpus after pancarpal arthrodesis and implant-associated osteomyelitis. The distal most screwhead is disengaged from the plate and the distal aspect of the plate is dorsally displaced. There is spiculated and palisading periosteal reaction along the dorsomedial aspect of the carpus associated with severe soft tissue thickening. There is irregular, palisading periosteal reaction along the cortices of the radius and ulna. There is increased radiolucency surrounding the full pin. The fracture has not healed.

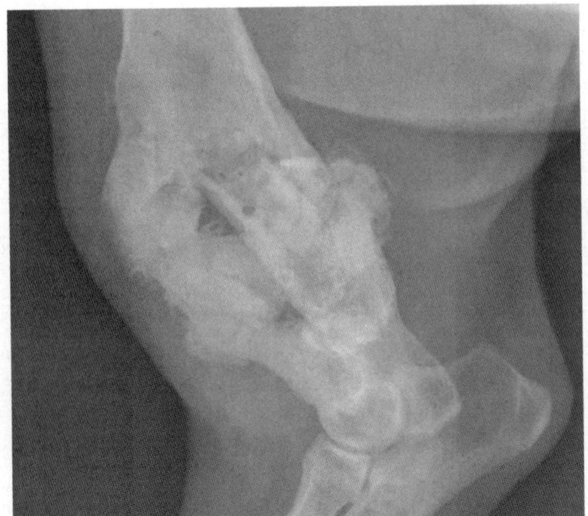

Fig. 19.31 Close-up lateral radiograph of the distal humerus of a dog with an open fracture that was repaired with an external fixator 3 months ago, but an open draining tract remained. The external fixator has been removed. There is a large amount of bridging callus formation. Several angular cortical fragments with no evidence of modeling or periosteal new bone formation are present in the center of the fracture, surrounded by a rim of radiolucency. Bone sequestra were removed surgically.

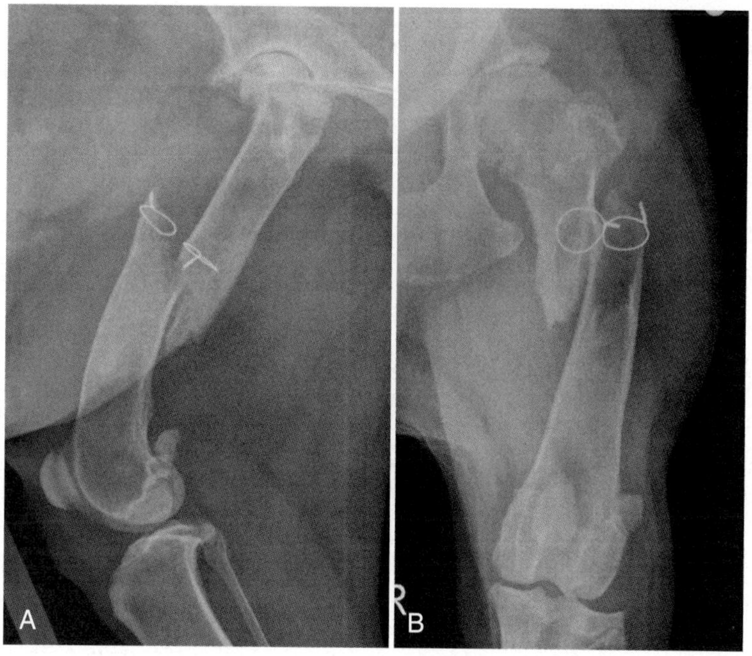

Fig. 19.32 Lateral **(A)** and craniocaudal **(B)** radiographs of the femur of a 12-year-old dog with a pathologic mid-diaphyseal fracture due to osteosarcoma. The dog had a femoral fracture repaired at 2 months of age (see small diameter of cerclage wire). Given the presence of implants and an aggressive lesion in an atypical location for osteosarcoma, implant associated neoplasia was suspected.

Acknowledgment

With special thanks to prior authors of this chapter for their contributions.

REFERENCES

1. Resnick D, Kransdorf MJ. *Bone and Joint Imaging*. 3rd ed. Philadelphia: Elsevier/Saunders; 2005.
2. Slatter D. *Textbook of Small Animal Surgery*. 3rd ed. Vol. 2. Philadelphia: Elsevier/Saunders; 2003.
3. Fossum TW. *Small Animal Surgery*. 5th ed. St Louis: Elsevier/Mosby; 2019.
4. Hedberg EL, Mikos AG. Bone augmentation and repair. In: Buschow KHJ, Cahn RW, Flemings MC, et al., eds. *Encyclopedia of Materials: Science and Technology [Internet]*. Oxford: Elsevier; 2001:782–787.
5. Clarke B. Normal bone anatomy and physiology. *Clin J Am Soc Nephrol*. 2008;3(suppl 3):S131–S139.
6. Palmer RH. External fixators and minimally invasive osteosynthesis in small animal veterinary medicine. *Vet Clin North Am Small Anim Pract*. 2012;42(5):913–934.
7. Elliott DS, Newman KJH, Forward DP, et al. A unified theory of bone healing and nonunion. *Bone Joint Lett J*. 2016;98-B(7):884–891.
8. Sande R. Radiography of orthopedic trauma and fracture repair. *Vet Clin North Am Small Anim Pract*. 1999;29(5):1247–1260.
9. Stieger-Vanegas SM, Senthirajah SKJ, Nemanic S, Baltzer W, Warnock J, Bobe G. Evaluation of the diagnostic accuracy of four-view radiography and conventional computed tomography analysing sacral and pelvic fractures in dogs. *Vet Comp Orthop Traumatol*. 2015;28(3):155–163.
10. Martin TW, LaRue SM, Griffin L. CT characteristics and proposed scoring scheme are predictive of pathologic fracture in dogs with appendicular osteosarcoma treated with stereotactic body radiation therapy. *Vet Radiol Ultrasound*. 2022;63(1):82–90.
11. Kubicek L, Vanderhart D, Wirth K, et al. Association between computed tomographic characteristics and fractures following stereotactic radiosurgery in dogs with appendicular osteosarcoma. *Vet Radiol Ultrasound*. 2016;57(3): 321–330.
12. Draffan D, Clements D, Farrell M, Heller J, Bennett D, Carmichael S. The role of computed tomography in the classification and management of pelvic fractures. *Vet Comp Orthop Traumatol*. 2009;22(3):190–197.
13. Strohmeier UW, Harris KP. Humeral intracondylar fissures in French bulldogs. *Vet Rec*. 2021;189(11):e504.
14. Orsini PG, Rendano VT, Sack WO. Ectopic nutrient foramina in the third metatarsal bone of the horse. *Equine Vet J*. 1981;13(2):132–134.
15. Becht JL, Park RD, Kraft SL. Radiographic interpretation of normal skeletal variations and pseudolesions in the equine foot. *Vet Clin North Am Equine Pract*. 2001;17(1):1–18.
16. Salter R, Harris W. Injuries involving the epiphyseal plate. *J Bone Joint Surg*. 1963;45:587.
17. Valdés-Martínez A, Seiler G, Mai W, et al. Quantitative analysis of scintigraphic findings in tibial stress fractures in Thoroughbred racehorses. *Am J Vet Res*. 2008;69(7): 886–890.
18. Koblik PD, Hornof WJ, Seeherman HJ. Scintigraphic appearance of stress-induced trauma of the dorsal cortex of the third metacarpal bone in racing Thoroughbred horses: 121 cases (1978–1986). *J Am Vet Med Assoc*. 1988;192(3): 390–395.
19. Rockwood CA, Green DP, Heckman JD, et al. *Rockwood and Green's Fractures in Adults*. 7th ed. Philadelphia: Lippincott, Williams & Wilkins; 2009.
20. Frost HM. A 2003 update of bone physiology and Wolff's Law for clinicians. *Angle Orthod*. 2004;74(1):3–15.
21. Karladani AH, Granhed H, Karrholm J, et al. The influence of fracture etiology and type on fracture healing: a review of 104 consecutive tibial shaft fractures. *Arch Orthop Trauma Surg*. 2001;121(6):325–328.

22. Hudson CC, Pozzi A, Lewis DD. Minimally invasive plate osteosynthesis: applications and techniques in dogs and cats. *Vet Comp Orthop Traumatol*. 2009;22(3):175–182.
23. Harasen G. External coaptation of distal radius and ulna fractures. *Can Vet J*. 2003;44(12):101–1011.
24. Epari DR, Schell H, Bail HJ, et al. Instability prolongs the chondral phase during bone healing in sheep. *Bone*. 2006;38(6):864–870.
25. Morgan EF, Gleason RE, Hayward LNM, et al. Mechanotransduction and fracture repair. *J Bone Joint Surg Am*. 2008;90(suppl 1):25–30.
26. Wehner T, Claes L, Niemeyer F. Influence of the fixation stability on the healing time—a numerical study of a patient-specific fracture healing process. *Clin Biomech (Bristol, Avon)*. 2010;25(6):606–612.
27. Lienau J, Schell H, Duda GN, et al. Initial vascularization and tissue differentiation are influenced by fixation stability. *J Orthop Res*. 2005;23(3):639–645.
28. Beale BS. Orthopedic problems in geriatric dogs and cats. *Vet Clin North Am Small Anim Pract*. 2005;35(3): 655–674.
29. Follak N, Kloting I, Merk H. Influence of diabetic metabolic state on fracture healing in spontaneously diabetic rats. *Diabetes Metab Res Rev*. 2005;21(3):288–296.
30. Tack LJW, Tatsi C, Stratakis CA, Lodish MB. Effects of glucocorticoids on bone: what we can learn from pediatric endogenous Cushing's syndrome. *Horm Metab Res Horm Stoffwechselforschung Horm Metab*. 2016;48(11):764–770.
31. Piermattei DL, Flo GL, Brinker WO. *Brinker, Piermattei, and Flo's Handbook of Small Animal Orthopedics and Fracture Repair*. 4th ed. Philadelphia: Elsevier/Saunders; 2006.
32. McCartney WT, MacDonald BJ. Incidence of non-union in long bone fractures in 233 cats. *Intern J Appl Res Vet Med*. 2006;4:209.
33. Goggin JM, Hoskinson JJ, Carpenter JW, Roush JK, McLaughlin RM, Anderson DE. Scintigraphic assessment of distal extremity perfusion in 17 patients. *Vet Radiol Ultrasound*. 1997;38(3):211–220.
34. Saikku-Backstrom A, Raiha JE, Valimaa T, et al. Repair of radial fractures in toy breed dogs with self-reinforced biodegradable bone plates, metal screws, and light-weight external coaptation. *Vet Surg*. 2005;34(1):11–17.
35. Welch JA, Boudrieau RJ, DeJardin LM, et al. The intraosseous blood supply of the canine radius: implications for healing of distal fractures in small dogs. *Vet Surg*. 1997;26(1):57–61.
36. Drost WT, Reese DJ, Hornof WJ. Digital radiography artifacts. *Vet Radiol Ultrasound*. 2008;49(1 suppl 1):S48–S56.
37. Gieling F, Peters S, Erichsen C, Richards RG, Zeiter S, Moriarty TF. Bacterial osteomyelitis in veterinary orthopaedics: pathophysiology, clinical presentation and advances in treatment across multiple species. *Vet J*. 2019;250:44–54.
38. Jackson LC, Pacchiana PD. Common complications of fracture repair. *Clin Tech Small Anim Pract*. 2004;19(3): 168–179.
39. Metsemakers WJ, Kuehl R, Moriarty TF, et al. Infection after fracture fixation: current surgical and microbiological concepts. *Injury*. 2018;49(3):511–522.
40. Maley JR, Mertens WD, Bahr A. Osteomyelitis-related sequestrum formation in association with the combination tibial plateau leveling osteotomy and cranial closing wedge osteotomy procedure. *Vet Comp Orthop Traumatol*. 2010;23(2):141–147.
41. Stevenson S, Hohn RB, Pohler OE. Fracture-associated sarcoma in the dog. *J Am Vet Med Assoc*. 1982;180(10): 1189–1196.
42. Baum JI, Skinner OT, Boston SE. Fracture-associated osteosarcoma of the femur in a cat. *Can Vet J Rev*. 2018;59(10): 1096–1098.

ELECTRONIC RESOURCES

Additional information related to the content in Chapter 19 can be found online at eBooks.Health.Elsevier.com.

- Chapter Quiz

CHAPTER 20

Radiographic Signs of Joint Disease in Dogs and Cats

Graeme Allan • Sarah Davies

Most radiographic signs of joint disease are degenerative in nature and nonspecific for the underlying etiology (Box 20.1, Fig. 20.1). Radiographic signs change as joint disease progresses through different phases. Sound knowledge of joint pathophysiology is as important in the diagnosis of joint disease as the ability to make and interpret radiographs of joints.

RADIOGRAPHIC SIGNS OF JOINT DISEASE

Increased Synovial Volume

A moderate increase in joint capsular or intracapsular soft tissue volume may be detected on good-quality radiographs. The joint cartilage, synovial fluid, synovial membrane, and joint capsule cannot be differentiated, because they are all of soft tissue opacity and silhouette with one another. In most joints, an increase in synovial mass appears as periarticular soft tissue swelling, as it can be difficult to differentiate intracapsular from extracapsular soft tissue thickening.

In the stifle, the infrapatellar fat pad may be used to evaluate synovial volume. The normal infrapatellar fat pad is identified readily on lateral stifle radiographs as a relatively radiolucent triangular region immediately caudal to the patellar ligament (Fig. 20.2). When stifle synovial mass increases, either from increased synovial fluid or soft tissue, a combination of inflammatory response and effusion causes the fat pad to be reduced in size and less defined.

Box 20.1

Radiographic Signs of Joint Disease

- Increased synovial volume
- Compressed infrapatellar fat pad
- Altered thickness of the joint space
- Decreased subchondral bone opacity
- Increased subchondral bone opacity
- Subchondral bone cyst formation
- Altered perichondral bone opacity
- Perichondral bony proliferation
- Mineralization of joint soft tissues
- Intra-articular calcified bodies
- Joint displacement or incongruency
- Joint malformation
- Intra-articular gas

Altered Width of the Joint Space

The joint space is the region of soft tissue opacity between subchondral bone surfaces of opposing weight-bearing surfaces of a joint. This space consists of two layers of articular cartilage separated by a microfilm of synovial fluid. In early joint disease, synovial effusion may cause widening of the joint space. As joint disease progresses, attrition of articular cartilage results in decreased width of the joint space (Fig. 20.3). These changes in joint space width are rarely diagnosed radiographically as small animal patients are not radiographed while bearing weight and also because of inconsistency between the orientation of the primary x-ray beam and joint space.

Decreased Subchondral Bone Opacity and Bone Cyst

Subchondral bone is separated from the synovial fluid by an intact layer of articular cartilage. Any disease that changes the character of synovial fluid, causing the articular cartilage to

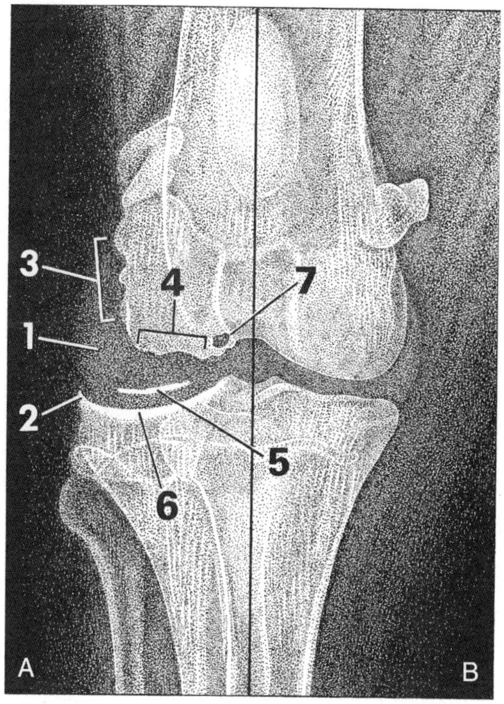

Fig. 20.1 Radiographic signs of joint disease **(A)** compared with a normal joint **(B)**. Increased synovial mass (*1*), perichondral osteophyte (*2*), and enthesophyte formation (*3*) are common radiographic changes. Erosion of the subchondral bone surface (*4*) and joint mice (*5*) are less common, whereas increased subchondral bone opacity (*6*) and subchondral bone cyst formation (*7*) are signs of chronic joint disease.

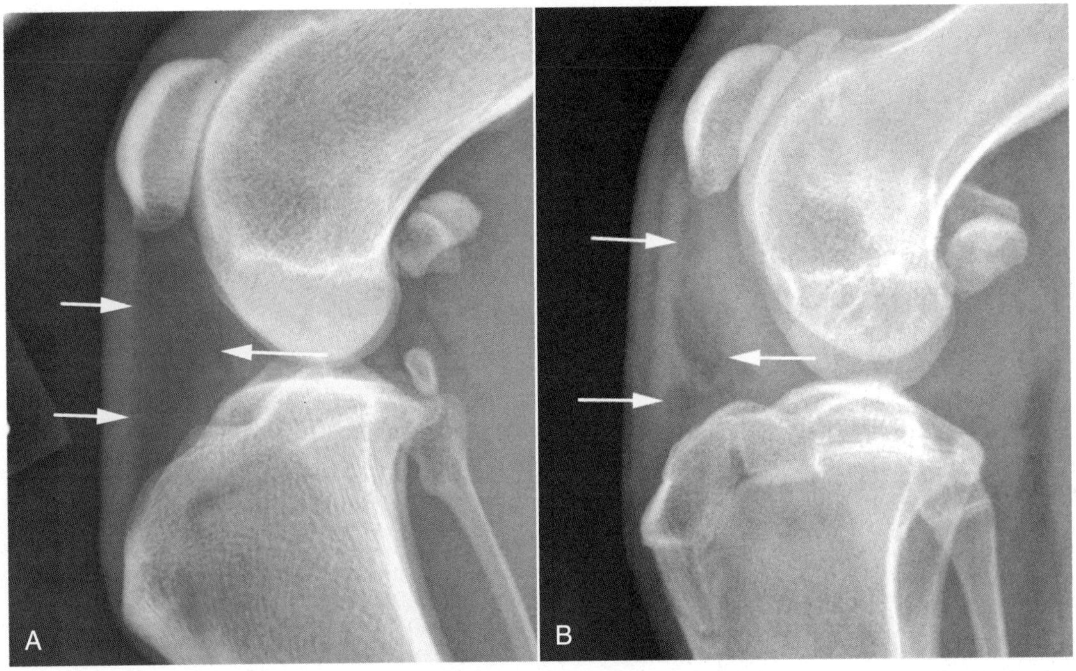

Fig. 20.2 Changes in the shape of the infrapatellar fat pad, located between the *arrows*, is a sensitive indicator of absence **(A)** or presence **(B)** of increased synovial volume in the stifle.

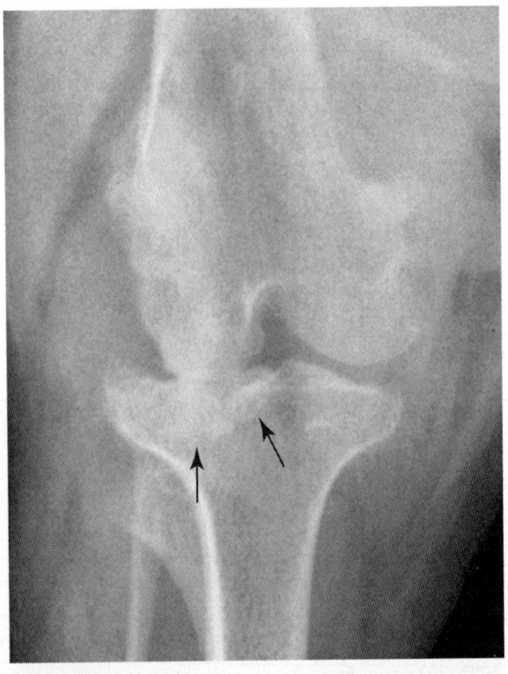

Fig. 20.3 Chronic malalignment of the stifle joint has resulted in narrowing of the lateral aspect of the femorotibial joint, likely because of degeneration of the lateral meniscus. The secondary altered loading of the lateral tibial condyle has resulted in secondary sclerosis (*black arrows*).

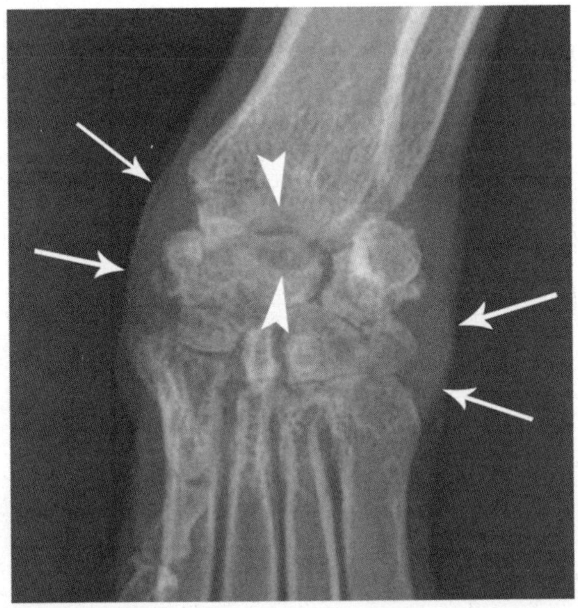

Fig. 20.4 Periarticular soft tissue swelling (*white arrows*) and subchondral bone erosion (*white arrowheads*) in the carpus of a dog with an erosive polyarthropathy. (Courtesy Perth Veterinary Specialists, Perth, Australia.)

erode, potentially threatens the integrity of subchondral bone. In inflammatory joint disease, inflammatory exudates may cause pronounced subchondral bone loss. Infectious arthritis may extend into subchondral bone. Subchondral bone loss appears initially as an irregular margin of subchondral bone, but it may extend to cause marked destruction of bone (Fig. 20.4). When bone loss affects smaller carpal and tarsal bones, these small cuboidal bones may be dramatically reduced in mass.

Increased Subchondral Bone Opacity

In benign joint disease such as degenerative joint disease, subchondral bone may be more opaque than normal because of stress remodeling (see Fig. 20.3). Increased subchondral bone opacity usually appears as a subchondral zone sclerosis 1 to 2 mm wide.

Altered Perichondral Bone Opacity

Articular cartilage merges with the synovial membrane at the chondrosynovial junction. This highly vascular membrane is

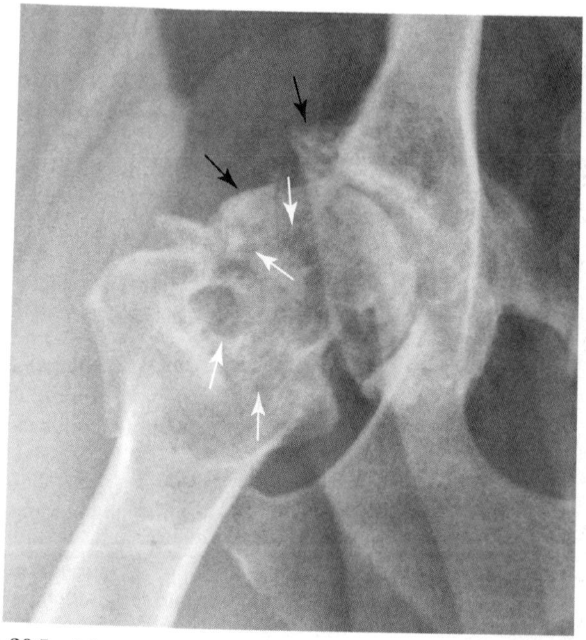

Fig. 20.5 Advanced coxofemoral degenerative joint disease. The femoral neck is thickened, the femoral head is misshapen, and there are numerous osteophytes (*black arrows*). There are multiple small and large radiolucencies (*white arrows*) in the femoral neck because of invasion of bone by hyperplastic synovium.

sensitive to inflammation. Synovial inflammation, or hypertrophy, may result in erosion of bone adjacent to the synovium. Early inflammation causes adjacent bone to appear ragged and spiculated. Longstanding or severe synovial inflammation or hypertrophy may cause pronounced bone erosion (Fig. 20.5).

Articular Soft Tissue Mineralization

Mineralization may occur within the joint capsule, synovial membrane, or synovial fluid as a consequence of chronic joint disease. Occasionally, large accumulations of articular or periarticular calcific material may be observed. Large osteochondromas have been reported within the joints of dogs and cats, and intrameniscal calcification and ossification have been observed in the stifle joints of cats.[1] Pseudogout, or calcium pyrophosphate deposition disease, also causes mineralization of articular and periarticular soft tissues and has been reported in dogs.

Intra-articular Calcified Bodies

Small, well-defined articular and periarticular calcific opacities are occasionally observed in dogs and cats. Such mineralized fragments are sometimes called *joint mice*. Not all such fragments are free within the joint, although they may appear free radiographically; fragments may become adhered to the joint capsule. Articular calcified bodies usually fall into three fairly distinct categories: (1) avulsed fragments of articular or periarticular bone, (2) osteochondral components of a disintegrating joint surface, or (3) small synovial osteochondromas (Table 20.1).[2] They must be differentiated from sesamoid bones.

Joint Displacement or Incongruency

When the normal spatial relation between components of a joint is disturbed, some type of displacement has occurred. A good example is a luxated coxofemoral joint. Other less obvious incongruities, such as the cranial drawer sign in a stifle with a ruptured cranial cruciate ligament and minor elbow incongruity in dogs with elbow dysplasia, can be difficult to see radiographically.[3]

Table • 20.1

Some Common Causes of Calcified Intra-Articular Bodies.

JOINT	ETIOLOGY
Shoulder	Osteochondritis dissecans (OCD) of the head of the humerus
	Mineralization of the bicipital tendon/sheath
	Synovial osteochondroma
	Separate centers of ossification on the glenoid rim
Elbow	Ununited anconeal process
	Fragmented coronoid process
	OCD of the humeral medial condyle
Hip	Avulsion epiphyseal fractures after femoral luxation
	Avascular necrosis of the femoral head
Stifle	OCD of the femoral condyles
	Avulsion fractures of the:
	Origin of the long digital extensor tendon
	Origin or insertion of the cruciate ligaments
	Origin of the popliteus
	Meniscal calcification
	Synovial osteochondroma
	Fragmented or fractured sesamoid bones
Tarsus	OCD of the talus

In all joints, soft tissue periarticular mineralization may occur as a result of degenerative joint disease.

Osteophytes

Osteophytes are bone proliferations covered with fibrocartilage along a joint margin. The proposed pathogenesis of osteophyte formation is that abnormal joint cartilage loading leads to cartilage wear, fibrillation, and loss of cartilage. The products of cartilage degradation mediate synovial hyperplasia and subsequent development of osteophytes.[4,5] Initially, osteophytes consist of cartilage and later become radiographically visible when they become ossified. A fully formed osteophyte is integrated with the subchondral bone and seen as bony outgrowth at the periphery of articular cartilage. Osteophytes occur as a component of degenerative joint disease (see Fig. 20.5).

Entheses and Enthesophytes

An enthesis is the point of insertion of a tendon, ligament, joint capsule, or fascia to bone. During embryogenesis, ligaments and tendons are attached to cartilage, but subsequent metaplasia of fibroblasts at their attachment site results in formation of fibrocartilage. This extends into the tendon or ligament, and endochondral ossification proceeds within the remaining cartilage. Enthesitis is inflammation of the site of tendon or ligament attachment to bone. An enthesophyte is a bony proliferation that develops at an enthesis (Fig. 20.6).[6]

Because enthesophytes and osteophytes appear radiographically similar, confusion in terminology often occurs when referring to these structures on a radiograph. To separate osteophytes around or within joints from enthesophytes, knowing the location of the common entheses is useful information (Figs. 20.6–20.8). In complex joints such as the carpus and tarsus, a large number of intra-articular ligaments are present. Every diarthrodial joint has a joint capsule, and intra-articular and periarticular ligaments and joint capsules insert onto bone at their respective entheses. New bone formations

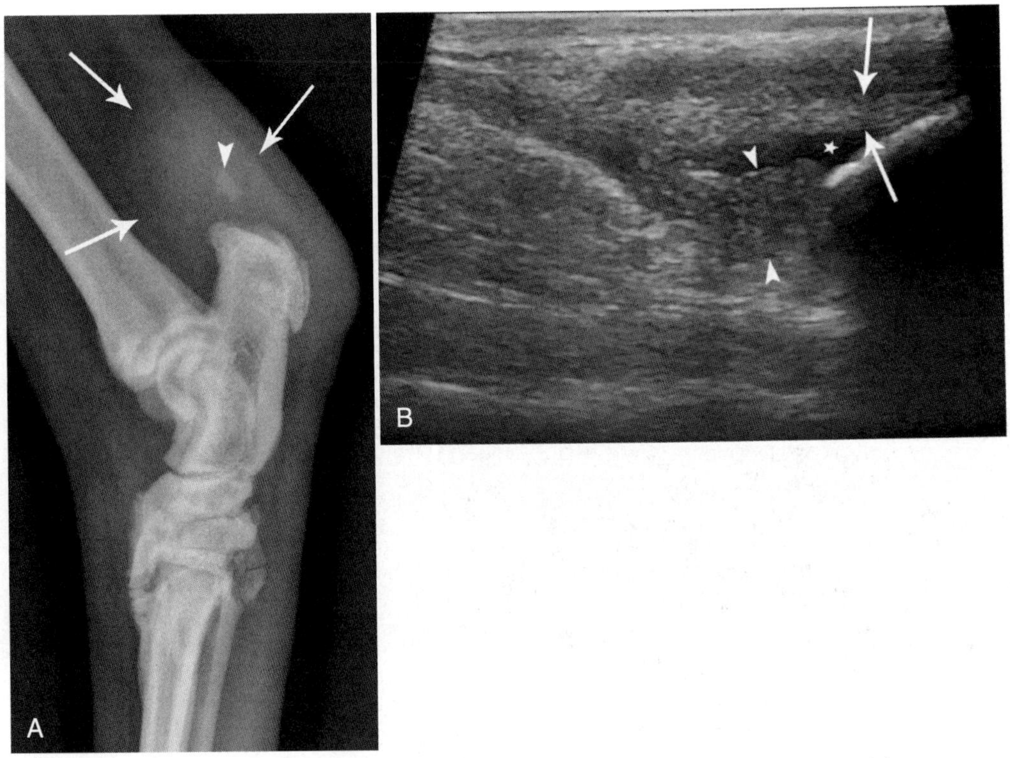

Fig. 20.35 Soft tissue swelling (*arrows*) and dystrophic calcification (*arrowhead*) in the region of the common calcaneal tendon in a dog **(A)**. In the same patient **(B)**, there is sonographic evidence of peritendinous fluid (*star*) and likely fibrinous material (*arrowheads*) in the caudal aspect of the tibiotarsal joint. The gastrocnemius tendon (*arrows*) inserts undisrupted onto the calcaneal tuberosity. (Courtesy North Shore Veterinary Specialist Centre, Sydney, Australia.)

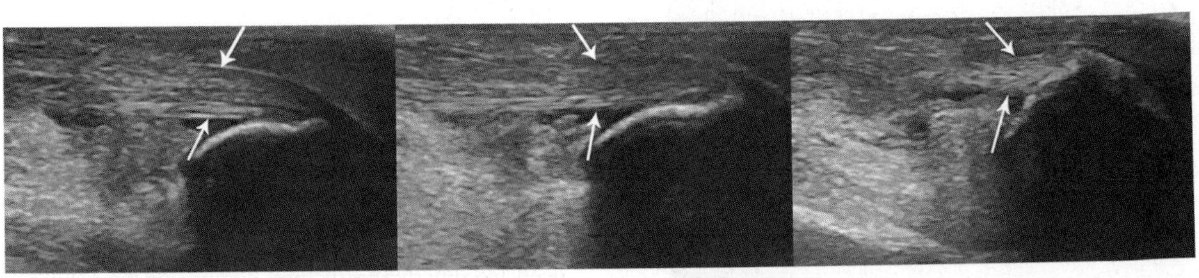

Fig. 20.36 Sonographic study in a dog presented with tarsal swelling after being hit by a car. Sequential images from left to right show progressive extension of the tibiotarsal joint. Attachment of the gastrocnemius tendon (*arrows*) to the calcaneal tuberosity is intact. (Courtesy North Shore Veterinary Specialist Centre, Sydney, Australia.)

THE SYNOVIUM

Villonodular Synovitis

Villonodular synovitis is an intracapsular joint disorder characterized by nodular synovial hyperplasia, which is thought to represent a response to trauma. Experimentally, villonodular synovitis has been reproduced in dogs by repeated intra-articular injections of whole blood. Villonodular synovitis is an established, although uncommon, disorder of people and has also been reported in horses and dogs.[37,38] In dogs, the condition has been identified in the carpus, coxofemoral joint, and stifle. Radiographic signs of villonodular synovitis may be nonspecific but include articular soft tissue swelling alone or with erosion of cortical bone at the chondrosynovial junction (Fig. 20.37). These cortical erosions may appear cyst like, with slightly opaque borders. In severe proximal femoral villonodular synovitis in people, the femoral neck has been described as looking like an apple core. The articular cartilage and subchondral bone are not involved. Differential diagnoses for perichondral erosive lesions, characteristic of villonodular synovitis, include synovial osteochondromatosis, rheumatoid arthritis, and joint neoplasia.

Synovial Osteochondromas

Synovial osteochondromas are islands of cartilage produced by the synovial membrane. Foci of cartilage become pedunculated and may become separated to form loose bodies within the joint. Reports of synovial osteochondromatosis in cats suggest that Burmese cats are overrepresented. The radiographic appearance of mineralized synovial osteochondromas varies. These lesions are usually well-defined, rounded, often multiple intra-articular nodules of calcific opacity (Fig. 20.38). Synovial osteochondromas may also arise from extra-articular foci of synovial tissue (Fig. 20.39).

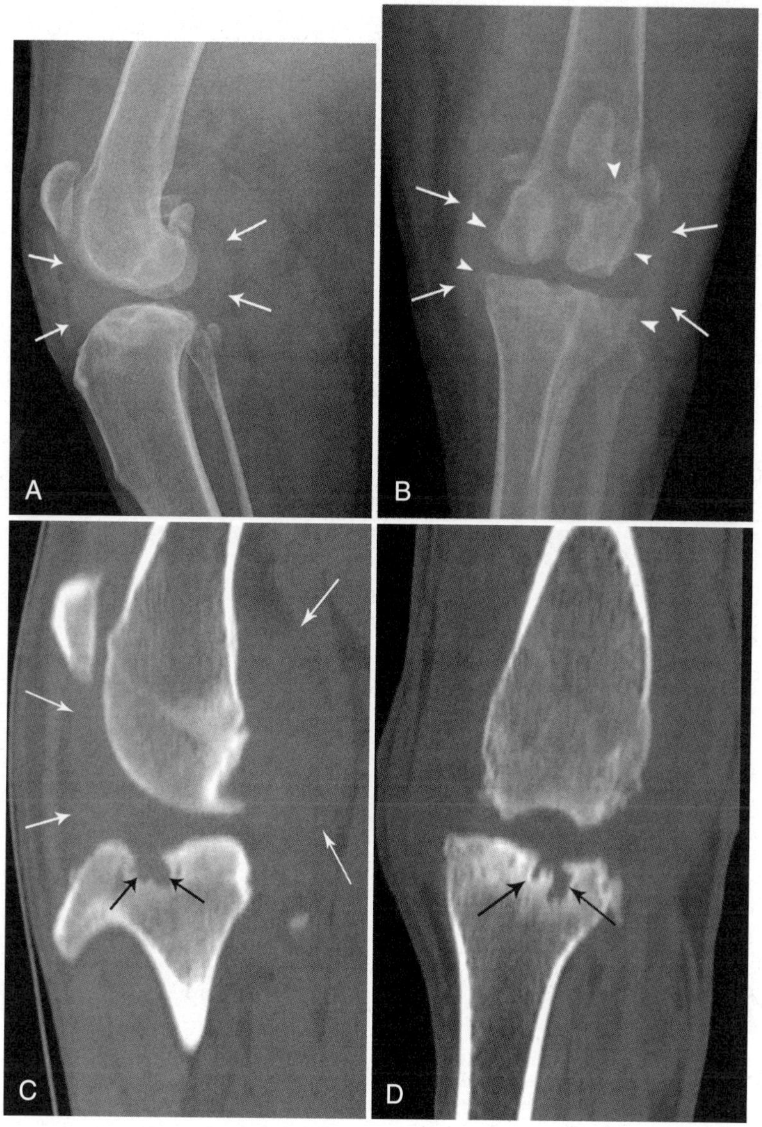

Fig. 20.37 Lateral **(A)** and craniocaudal **(B)** radiographs of the stifle of a dog with a histopathologic diagnosis of villonodular synovitis. There is marked intracapsular soft tissue swelling (*white arrows*) and osteophytes are present on periarticular surfaces (*arrowheads*). Loss of bone (*black arrows*) is detected with computed tomography (CT) in the cranial intercondylar region **(C and D)**. (Courtesy Animal Orthopaedic Specialists, Sydney, Australia.)

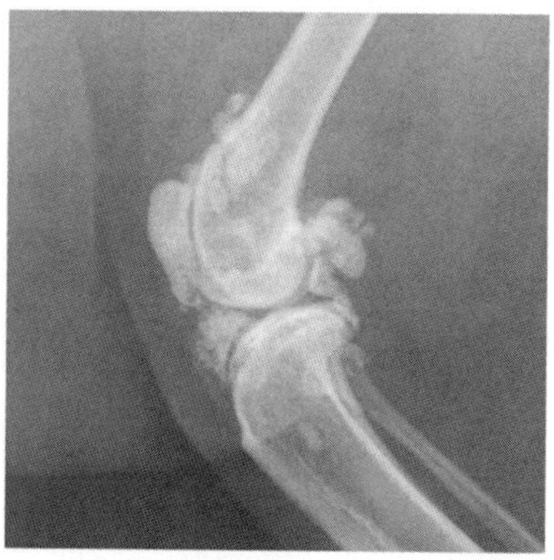

Fig. 20.38 A 5-year-old Burmese cat had bilateral stifle enlargement. Extensive lobular mineralization within the stifle joint was evident radiographically. Histologic diagnosis was synovial osteochondroma. (Courtesy Perth Veterinary Specialists, Perth, Australia.)

Synovial osteochondromas have been reported in the dog and the cat.[39,40] Their cause is unknown, but the theory of synovial metaplasia is generally accepted. These lesions have been reported to cause severe lameness in some dogs. Surgical removal of synovial osteochondromas relieves clinical signs of joint pain and lameness.[39] Other conditions in cats in which intra-articular and periarticular mineralization may be confused with synovial osteochondromatosis are mild forms of mucopolysaccharidosis type VI (MPS VI) and hypervitaminosis A.[41]

IMMUNE-MEDIATED POLYARTHROPATHIES

Rheumatoid Arthritis

Rheumatoid arthritis is a severe, progressive, erosive polyarthritis that has been reported in dogs,[42] and a similar condition has been reported in cats.[43] Radiographic changes usually occur in joints of the distal extremities. The stifle and elbow are affected occasionally. Synovial effusion occurs initially. Radiographs made early are characterized by nonspecific periarticular soft tissue swelling. The joint capsule may be distended. The first radiographic signs of bone involvement may be detected several weeks after the onset of clinical signs. Initial changes are mild, but the radiographic abnormalities become more obvious as the disease advances.

The progression of radiographic changes includes:

1. Subchondral bone destruction and cyst formation (Fig. 20.40)
2. Joint space narrowing
3. Progressive decreased opacity of epiphyses adjacent to affected joints;
4. Destruction of subchondral and perichondral bone
5. Mushrooming of the ends of the metacarpi and metatarsi, which occurs in advanced arthritis and represents collapse of subchondral bone
6. Varying degrees of joint subluxation and luxation (Fig. 20.41, eFig. 20.3)

Other changes more characteristic of degenerative joint disease (osteophytes/enthesophytes, subchondral sclerosis, and calcified periarticular tissues) may also be present.[42]

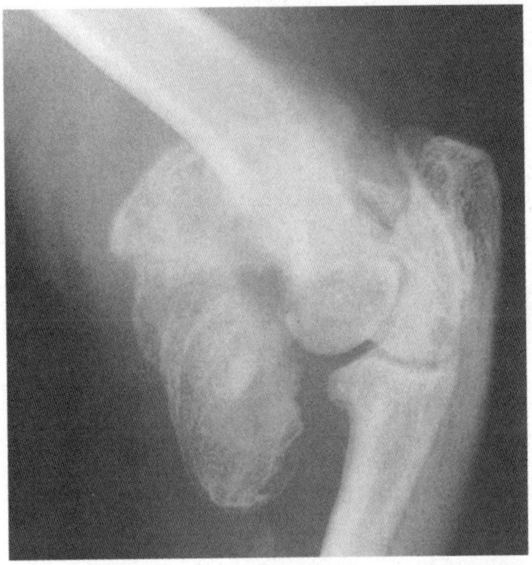

Fig. 20.39 A 6-year-old male (neutered) Burmese cat had progressive lameness of the right forelimb for 6 weeks. Radiographically, a large, well-defined, ossified mass was visible on the craniomedial aspect of the right elbow. Histologic diagnosis was extra-articular synovial osteochondroma.

Systemic Lupus Erythematosus

Systemic lupus erythematosus (SLE) is a multisystemic disease that affects dogs of all breeds, as well as cats. It has a variety of clinical manifestations, including polyarthritis, anemia, nephropathy, skin disease, pericarditis, myocarditis, and lymphadenopathy.[44] Diagnosis of SLE is complicated and is made on the basis of the concurrence of clinical manifestations and serologic evidence. In one study, 121 dogs with a diagnosis of

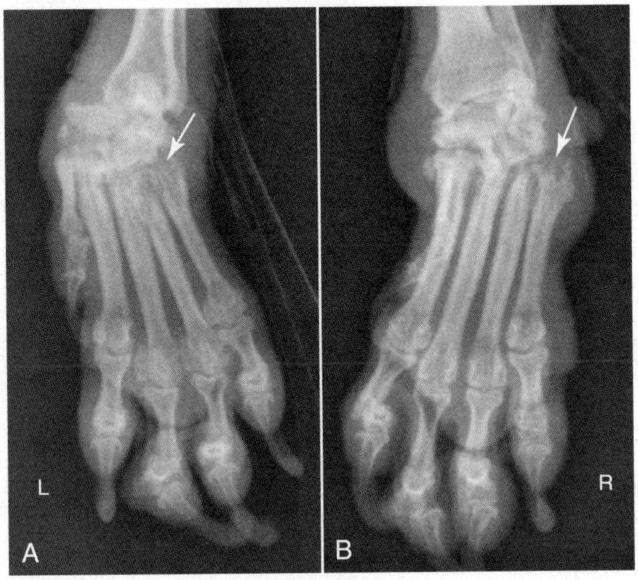

Fig. 20.41 Dorsopalmar radiographs of the left **(A)** and right **(B)** manus of a dog with immune-mediated arthropathy. There is subluxation of the left antebrachiocarpal joint and the right carpometacarpal joint. There is also subluxation of distal interphalangeal joint in each manus. Numerous subchondral lytic erosive lesions are present (*white arrows*).

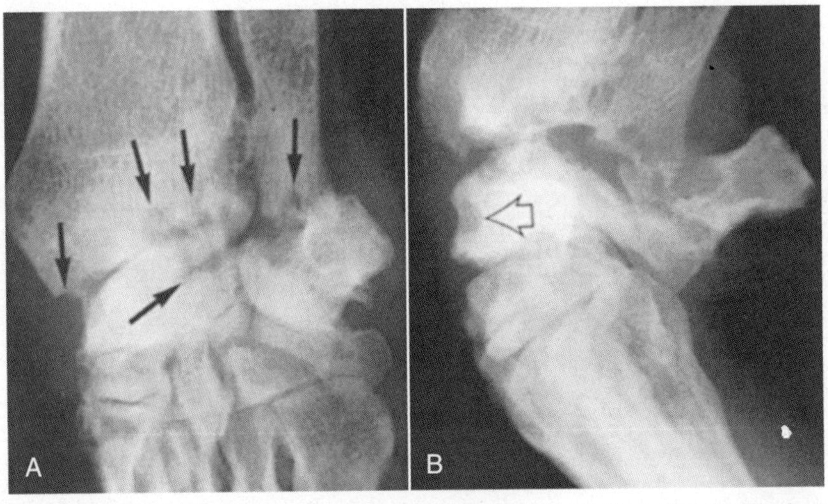

Fig. 20.40 An 8-year-old neutered male corgi crossbreed with rheumatoid arthritis. **A,** Dorsolateral-palmaromedial projection. There is extensive subchondral erosion of the styloid process of the ulna and the articular surfaces of the distal radius and radial carpal bone (*black arrows*). **B,** Lateral projection during flexion. In addition to the changes seen in **A,** note the erosion of the non–weight-bearing dorsal surface of the intermedioradial carpal bone (*open black arrow*). (Courtesy University Veterinary Centre, Sydney, Australia.)

SLE were reviewed, and joint disease was reported to be the most frequent clinical sign (69%), followed by hematologic (53%), renal (50%), cutaneous (33%), and intrathoracic (17%) manifestations. The arthropathy that occurs in canine SLE is usually effusive but nonerosive. Polyarthritis is typical, but monoarticular arthritis has been reported. Affected joints may be swollen, painful, and warm. The joints most commonly affected are the carpus, tarsus, metatarsus, stifle, and elbow. Radiographic signs are usually absent or are minimal. In chronic SLE, the joint space of affected joints may be narrowed, and the joint capsule is distended. A mild periosteal response has been reported at the junction of joint capsule and bone.

Feline Noninfectious Polyarthritis

Feline noninfectious polyarthritis is a disease of male cats aged 1 to 5 years.[43,45] The polyarthritis can be erosive or nonerosive.[46] There are two types of erosive polyarthritis: (1) the periosteal proliferative form and (2) the erosive form. The erosive form is commonly referred to as *feline rheumatoid arthritis*. A group of nonerosive, effusive polyarthropathies thought to be immune mediated also occur in cats and are associated with a variety of conditions.

Periosteal Proliferative Form

Affected cats have fever, malaise, and stiffness, followed by periarticular soft tissue swelling and regional lymphadenopathy. Radiographic changes may be identified in affected joints after a few weeks. Commonly affected joints are the carpi and tarsi. The stifle, elbow, shoulder, and hip joints are affected to a lesser extent. During the first month, periarticular soft tissue swelling is the predominant sign. Swelling may be either intracapsular or extracapsular. One to 3 months after the onset of clinical signs, periosteal new bone production may be identified at site of joint capsule attachment. During this phase, bone adjacent to affected joints may have decreased opacity and a coarse trabecular pattern. Perichondral new bone formation is pronounced 2 to 3 months after onset of the disease. Extensive enthesopathy may bridge smaller joint spaces. More severe radiographic manifestations include perichondral bone erosion and formation of subchondral cysts. Narrowing of affected joint spaces may occur late.[43] Radiographic signs of the periosteal proliferative form of feline chronic progressive polyarthritis include periarticular soft tissue swelling, periosteal new bone formation, perichondral enthesophyte production, perichondral and subchondral erosion, subchondral cysts, osteopenia of bone adjacent to affected joints, and narrowed joint spaces (Fig. 20.42).

Feline Erosive Polyarthritis

A second, more erosive, form of feline noninfectious polyarthritis has been described; it resembles human rheumatoid arthritis and occurs in older cats.[43] This form is characterized radiographically by severe subchondral bone erosion, perichondral bone erosion, and subchondral cyst formation. Perichondral enthesophyte formation, bone destruction at points of ligamentous insertion to bone, and subluxation of small joints of the extremities also occur. A diagnosis of feline rheumatoid arthritis requires a positive rheumatoid factor test, characteristic histologic changes seen on a synovial biopsy, or both. Both test results are negative in cats with feline proliferative polyarthritis.[46]

Feline Nonerosive Polyarthritis

Two categories of nonerosive polyarthritis have been described in cats.[46] They are feline SLE and idiopathic polyarthritis. Idiopathic polyarthritis has four subtypes: (1) uncomplicated polyarthritis; (2) reactive polyarthritis, associated with a disease process elsewhere in the body; (3) enteropathic polyarthritis, associated with gastrointestinal disease; and (4) malignant-related idiopathic polyarthritis, associated with myeloproliferative disease. Radiography is used to distinguish between erosive and nonerosive forms of feline polyarthritis. The latter group is identified as having periarticular soft tissue swelling, joint capsule distention, and synovial fluid accumulation.

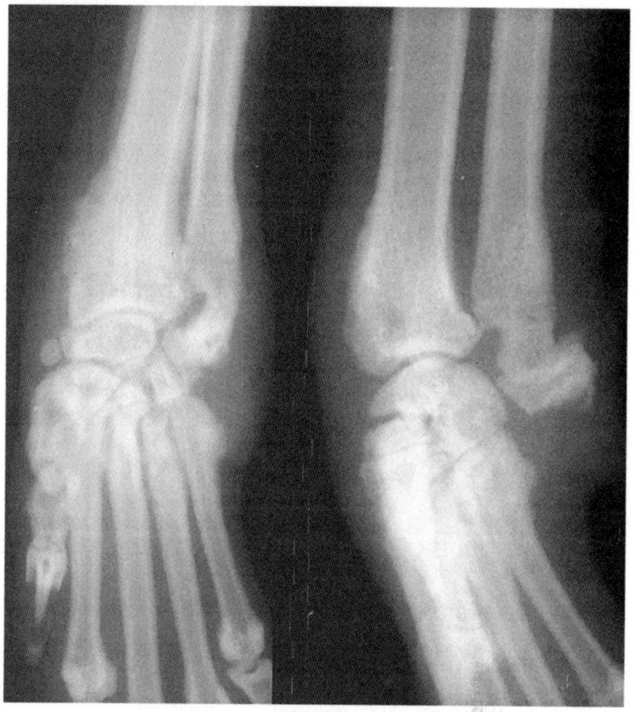

Fig. 20.42 The carpus of a young cat with feline chronic progressive polyarthritis. (Courtesy University Veterinary Centre, Sydney, Australia. Reproduced with permission from Allan GS. Radiographic features of feline joint diseases. *Vet Clin North Am Small Anim Pract*. 2000;30:281.)

Hypertrophic Osteopathy

Hypertrophic osteopathy is a generalized osteoproductive disorder of the periosteum that affects the long and short tubular bones of the extremities. It is usually caused by a thoracic mass or cardiopulmonary disease. Abdominal masses, particularly those of urinary origin, have also been known to cause hypertrophic osteodystrophy. Nonneoplastic causes of hypertrophic osteopathy include inflammatory lung disease (e.g., blastomycosis), intrathoracic foreign bodies, *Dirofilaria immitis* infestation, and spirocercosis. The pathogenesis of hypertrophic osteopathy is understood incompletely. New bone formation typically commences on the distal end of both short and long tubular bones and progresses proximally. Periosteal new bone formation results in cortical thickening. The periosteal surface appears nodular or spiculated when visualized radiographically (Figs. 20.43 and 20.44).

SEPTIC ARTHRITIS

Septic arthritis is diagnosed infrequently in small animals, with the incidence being lower than that of immune-mediated joint disease. Septic arthritis is difficult to diagnose radiographically. Initial radiographic changes are usually limited to joint effusion

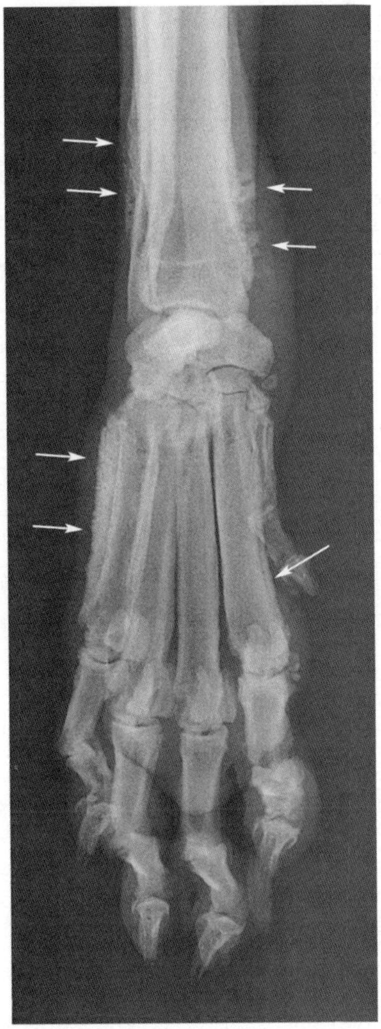

Fig. 20.43 Radiograph of the manus of a dog with hypertrophic osteopathy. There is irregular periosteal reaction (*arrows*) that is most pronounced on the lateral aspect of the fifth metacarpal bone and on the medial aspect of the distal radius. There is less pronounced periosteal reaction on the medial aspect of the manus.

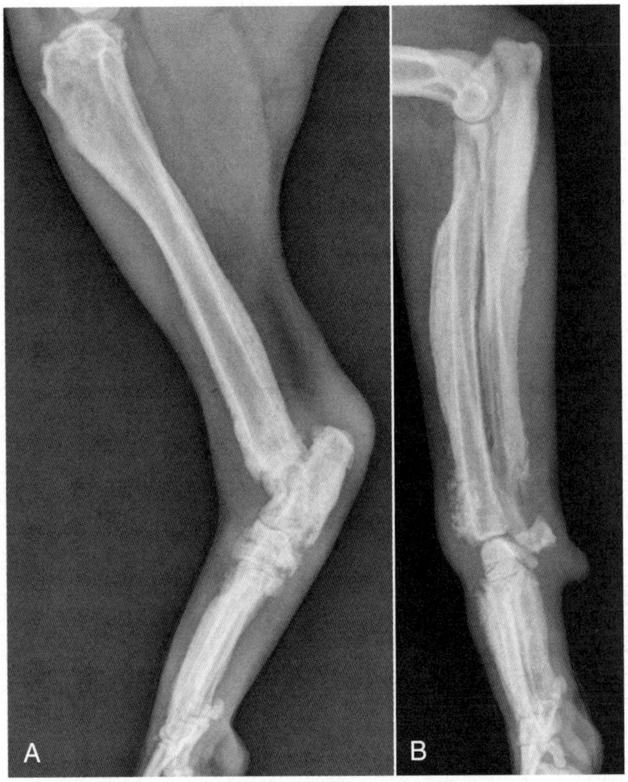

Fig. 20.44 Lateral radiographs of the crus (A) and antebrachium (B) of a dog with hypertrophic osteopathy that is more advanced than in Fig. 20.46. The abnormal periosteum has progressed to involve the more proximal aspect of the long and short tubular bones.

and periarticular swelling. Ideally, the arthritis should be diagnosed and treated successfully before radiographic changes become apparent.[47] Polyarticular septic arthritis may occur as a result of bacteremia associated with an isolated focus of infection (endocarditis, discospondylitis, or omphalophlebitis) or in conjunction with a systemic disease (as in *Mycoplasma* arthritis, canine leishmaniasis, or feline caliciviral lameness).[48] Polyarticular septic arthritis must be differentiated from immune-mediated joint disease. The former is more likely to affect the larger, more proximal joints of the appendicular skeleton, whereas the latter more commonly affects the joints nearer the distal extremities (Box 20.5). Monoarticular septic arthritis most likely results from extension of focal osteomyelitis into an adjacent joint, direct joint trauma, or foreign body penetration (grass seed awns), or it may occur after joint surgery or intra-articular therapy. Hematogenous dissemination of infection to joints is more common in young animals. Septic arthritis as a complication of surgery, particularly addressing cranial cruciate insufficiency, is more common in older animals.

As already noted, the earliest radiographic changes of septic arthritis are synovial effusion and increased synovial mass, which represent an inflammatory response of the synovium. Soft tissue swelling is usually demarcated by the distended joint capsule. Joint capsule distention is identified more easily in carpal, tarsal, and stifle joints. A useful landmark in the stifle is the infrapatellar fat pad. When the fat pad is compressed cranially, it becomes smaller and unclear, indicating synovial effusion is present. In untreated septic arthritis, joint cartilage destruction follows synovial effusion and is followed by subchondral and perichondral bone destruction (Figs. 20.45 and 20.46, eFig. 20.4, Box 20.6).

Septic arthritis is being identified increasingly in joints that have chronic degenerative joint disease. Initial radiographs are characterized by degenerative joint disease, often leading to inappropriate therapy for the infection. Radiographs made 2 to 4 weeks later reveal more aggressive signs of periosteal new bone formation and intra-articular bone destruction. Septic arthritis should be suspected when acute lameness and joint pain are identified in individual animals whose degenerative joint disease has been controlled previously.

Diagnosis of septic arthritis is based on cytologic assessment of synovial fluid and microbiologic examination of synovial fluid and/or synovium and joint capsule. Radiographic assessment alone has low specificity for septic arthritis, but survey radiographs are useful to rule out other conditions, as well as to follow the progress of a joint infection once a diagnosis of septic arthritis is confirmed.

Box • 20.5

Polyarthropathies Affecting the Appendicular Skeleton of Dogs and Cats

- Immune-mediated joint diseases
  - Rheumatoid arthritis
  - Systemic lupus erythematosus (SLE)
  - Feline periosteal proliferative polyarthritis
  - Feline nonerosive immune-mediated polyarthropathy
- Septic arthritis
  - Hematogenous septic arthritis
  - Bacterial or fungal septic arthritis
- Inflammatory arthritides
  - Leishmaniasis
  - Rocky Mountain spotted fever
  - Rickettsia rickettsii
  - Lyme disease
  - *Borrelia burgdorferi*
  - Mycoplasma arthritis
  - Chinese Shar-Pei fever syndrome
  - Feline calicivirus, coronavirus
  - Greyhound polyarthritis
- Hemarthrosis
  - Chronic, recurrent, caused by blood dyscrasias
- Hypervitaminosis A
- Primary degenerative joint disease/osteoarthrosis
- Disseminated idiopathic skeletal hyperostosis syndrome
- Familial or genetic skeletal dysplasias
  - Scottish fold osteochondrodysplasia
  - Feline mucopolysaccharidosis (MPS)
  - Canine hip dysplasia
  - Canine elbow dysplasia
  - Osteochondrosis
- Drug-induced and vaccine-mediated polyarthritis
- Feline osteochondromatosis

Septic Arthritis in Cats

In cats, hematogenously disseminated septic arthritis may be caused by a variety of microorganisms, which include *Mycoplasma gateae*, *Mycoplasma felis*, bacterial L-form infection (*Pasteurella* spp.), calicivirus (transient arthritis in kittens), coronavirus (feline infectious peritonitis), and fungi (cryptococcosis, histoplasmosis). Hematogenously disseminated septic arthritis initially causes a nonerosive polyarthropathy characterized by lameness, synovial effusion, and synovial thickening. Affected cats may be systemically ill. Viremic polyarthropathies tend to be transient, whereas bacterial arthritis can have a protracted course. Direct injection of bacteria from bite wounds can result in mixed infections of microorganisms, which may include anaerobic bacteria.

Septic arthritis from penetrating bite wounds causes lameness that is usually restricted to one joint. Synovial effusion and periarticular soft tissue thickening precede secondary changes (such as, subchondral bone erosion) by weeks or months. CT can facilitate early detection of bone erosions and demonstrate synovitis. Joint infections that extend through the synovium and joint capsule into extracapsular tissue stimulate periosteal new bone formation on bone surfaces adjacent to the joint. Septic arthritis can lead to osteomyelitis in bones on either side of an affected joint.

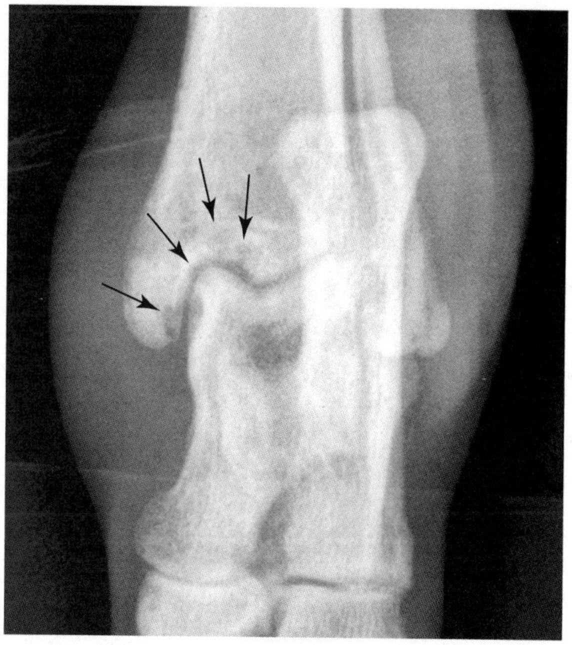

Fig. 20.45 A 1.5-year-old canine mix with lameness and tarsal swelling for 2 weeks. There are focal subchondral lucencies in the distomedial aspect of the tibia (*black arrows*). The swelling is also obvious. Cryptococcus was isolated from synovial fluid.

MISCELLANEOUS POLYARTHROPATHIES

Hypervitaminosis A

Excessive dietary vitamin A produces an ankylosing arthropathy and spondylopathy. Although both dogs and cats can be affected, the disorder is more likely to affect cats. The food mostly associated with hypervitaminosis A is bovine liver, and when fed as an exclusive diet, the clinical syndrome of vitamin A excess can be recognized after a few months. Affected cats become obtunded, apprehensive, reluctant to jump, hypersensitive to neck palpation, and lame. The underlying connective tissue disorder causes vertebral ankylosis and an ankylosing degenerative joint disease of the forelimbs. Recognizable radiographic manifestations of hypervitaminosis A may be seen in as little as 10 weeks after introduction of a diet rich in vitamin A. Changes include ankylosing spondylopathy of the cervical and cranial thoracic vertebral column and periarticular enthesopathy and degenerative joint disease of shoulder and elbow joints (Figs. 20.47 and 20.48). In advanced disease, the additional bone becomes incorporated seamlessly with existing bone so that architecture of the original bones is remodeled completely. Other regions of the vertebral column and other joints of the appendicular skeleton may become involved, but the aforementioned bones and joints appear to be the primary site of bony changes in cats. The ankylosing changes are permanent. They do not resolve once a balanced diet is substituted, but some of the clinical signs of hypervitaminosis A resolve once the dietary imbalance is corrected.

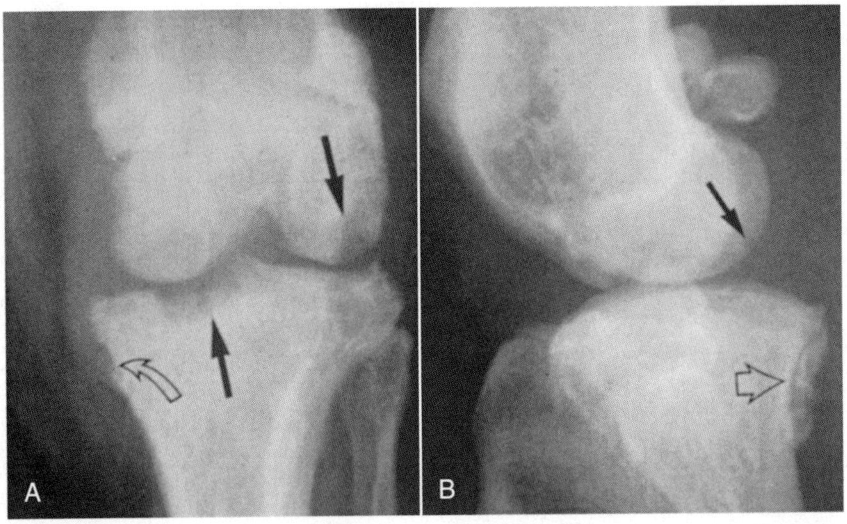

Fig. 20.46 An 8-year-old male Australian cattle dog had stifle swelling and pain that persisted after repair of a ruptured cranial cruciate ligament. **A and B,** Subchondral bone erosion involves the medial condyle of the tibia and the femoral condyles (*solid black arrows*). Periarticular new bone formation is also evident (*open black arrow*). Note the concurrent medial patellar luxation. *Staphylococcus aureus* was isolated from the synovial fluid.

Box • 20.6

Progression of Radiographic Signs of Infectious Arthritis

- Increased synovial mass indicating synovial effusion and widened radiolucent joint space
- Diminished radiolucent joint space indicating destruction of articular cartilage
- Loss of the smooth surface of the subchondral bone plate; an early sign of infectious penetration of subchondral bone
- Radiolucent signs of destruction of subchondral and perichondral bone usually highlighted by a peripheral border of increased osseous opacity
- In advanced infectious arthritis, weight-bearing surfaces may collapse, causing distortion of joint architecture

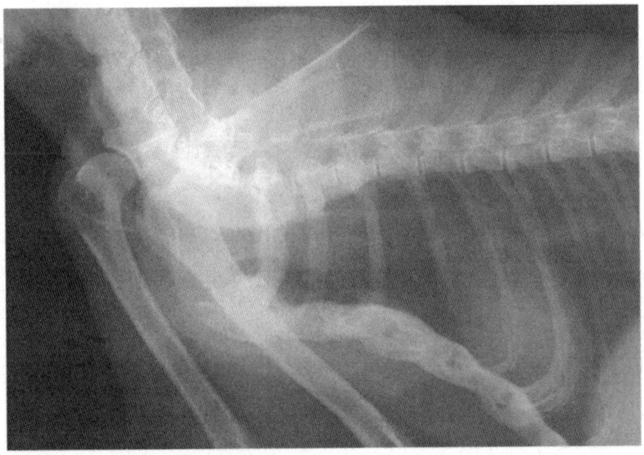

Fig. 20.47 Ankylosing spondylopathy of the cervical and cranial thoracic vertebrae and the sternum of a cat with hypervitaminosis A. (Reproduced with permission from Allan GS. Radiographic features of feline joint diseases. *Vet Clin North Am Small Anim Pract.* 2000;30:281. Courtesy University of Queensland, Brisbane, Australia.)

JOINT NEOPLASIA

Joint tumors are uncommon in dogs and rare in cats.[49,50] The most commonly affected joints are the stifle and elbow in middle-aged, medium-sized to large dogs.[51] The most common tumor types in dogs include histiocytic sarcoma, synovial cell sarcoma, and synovial myxoma. Other types of sarcoma, such as fibrosarcoma or chondrosarcoma, are uncommon.[49] Synovial cell sarcoma arises from primitive mesenchymal precursor cells of the synovial membrane of joints and bursae.[51] Synovial cell sarcomas grow slowly and are first noticeable as a homogeneous soft tissue mass that involves or is near a joint. Portions of the tumor may be calcified, with mineral deposits appearing as hazy and punctate or as linear streaks.

Initial bone involvement usually appears as a spiculated periosteal response followed by ragged erosion of cortical bone adjacent to the tumor. Occasionally, the neoplasm initially appears relatively nonaggressive, mimicking a simple cyst, only to change later into a more extensive and destructive disease (Fig. 20.49, eFig. 20.5). Destruction of cancellous bone may be extensive and most commonly occurs on both sides of the joint. The tumor is locally invasive with a capacity to metastasize.[52] Distant metastasis, particularly to the lungs, occurs in as many as half of reported patients.[51] Histiocytic sarcoma is an aggressive periarticular tumor that can be difficult to differentiate from other joint tumors (Fig. 20.50). It is associated with a high rate of distant metastasis.[53] Bernese mountain dogs and Rottweilers are predisposed and prior joint disease presents an increased risk for development of periarticular histiocytic sarcoma[53] (Fig. 20.51).

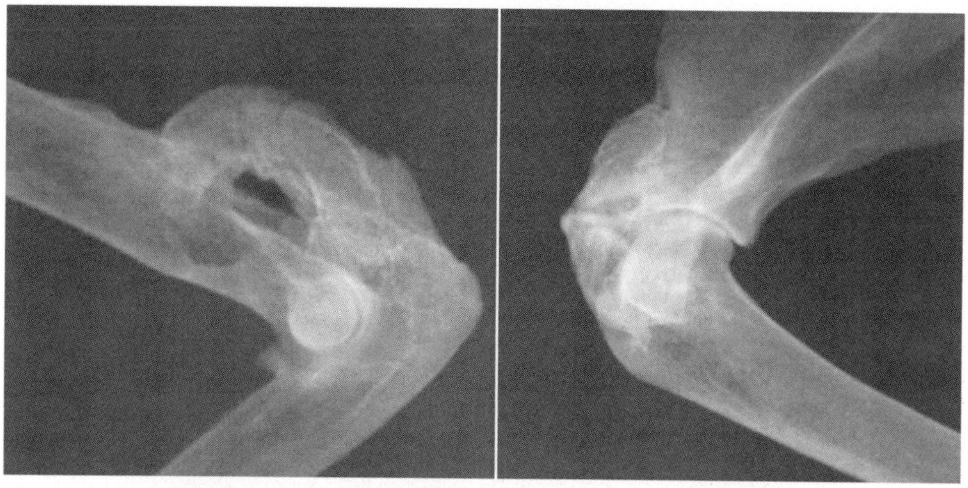

Fig. 20.48 Radiographs of the elbows and a shoulder from the skeleton of a cat that was euthanized because of ankylosing arthropathy caused by hypervitaminosis A.

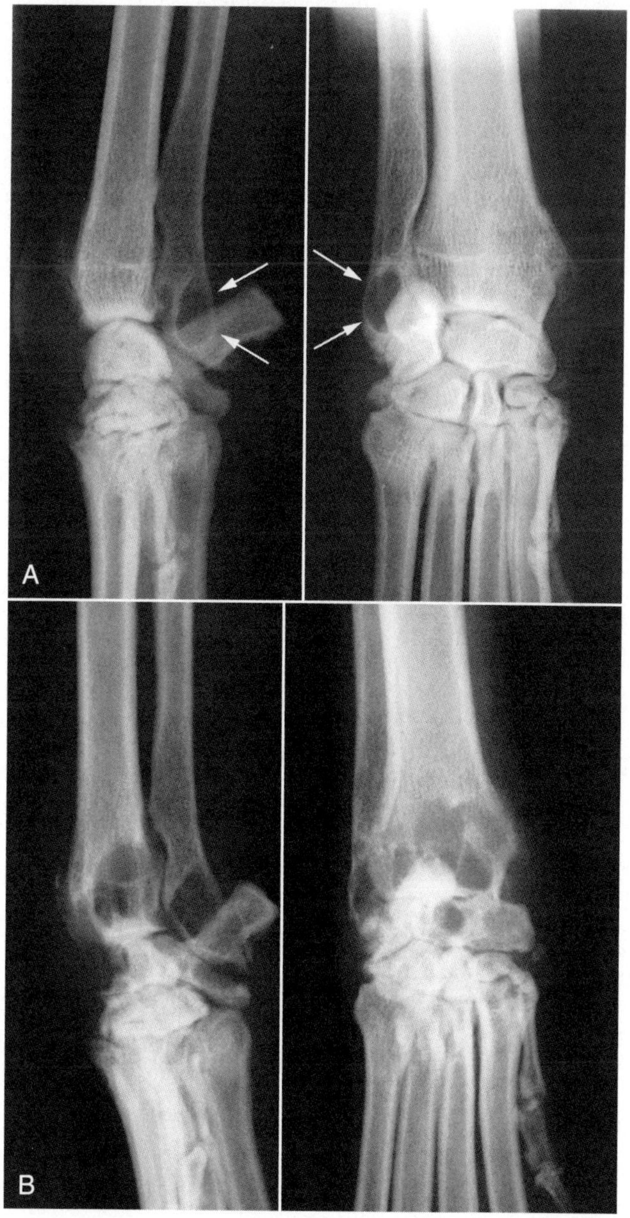

Fig. 20.49 **A,** A cystic lesion was identified in the distal end of the left ulna (*white arrows*) 6 weeks after the onset of soft tissue swelling around the antebrachiocarpal joint. **B,** The lesion progressed over the succeeding 12 months, by which time a multiloculated cyst-like change was present in the distal radius, ulna, and the proximal row of carpal bones. Histologic diagnosis was synovial cell carcinoma. (Courtesy Dr. P. Young, All Pets Veterinary Hospital, Albury, Australia.)

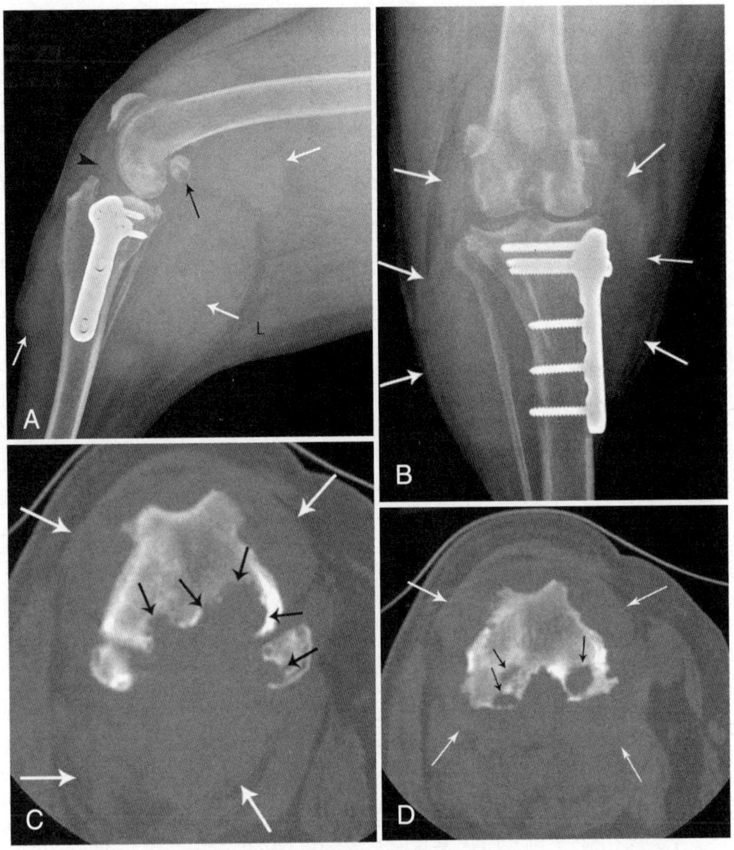

Fig. 20.50 Lateral **(A)** and craniocaudal **(B)** radiographs of the stifle with extensive intracapsular and extracapsular soft tissue swelling. A tibial plateau leveling osteotomy (TPLO) plate is present on the medial aspect of the tibia. *White arrows* indicate the extent of soft tissue swelling. *Black arrowhead* indicates effacement of the infrapatellar fat pad as a sign of increased synovial mass. The distal femur and supracondylar areas have a mottled appearance and lucent foci are present in the fabellae (*black arrow*). The popliteal lymph node is within normal limits for size (*L*). Axial computed tomography (CT) images **(C and D)** show the extent of osteolysis involving the femoral condyles and fabella medial (*black arrows*). Final diagnosis was histiocytic sarcoma. There is no presumed association with the prior TPLO. (Courtesy Animal Orthopaedic Specialists, Sydney, Australia.)

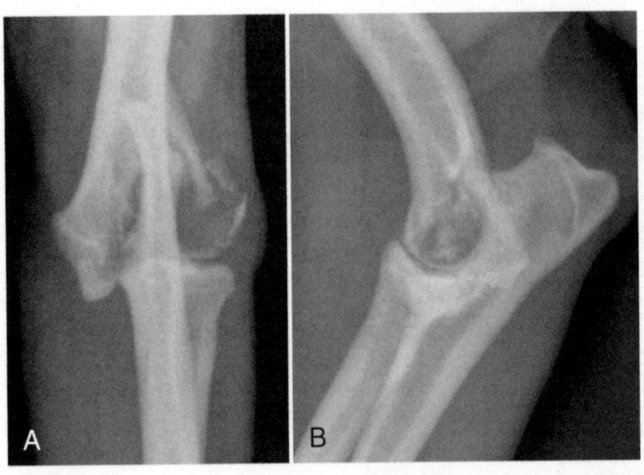

Fig. 20.51 Craniocaudal **(A)** and lateral **(B)** radiographs of a dog with extensive lysis of the lateral aspect of the humeral condyle. There is resulting pathologic fracture in the lateral epicondylar region, extending to involve the joint. Final diagnosis was diffuse mixed cell lymphoma of bone. (Courtesy North Shore Veterinary Specialist Centre, Sydney, Australia.)

REFERENCES

1. Whiting PG, Pool RR. Intrameniscal calcification and ossification in the stifle joints of three domestic cats. *J Am Anim Hosp Assoc*. 1985;21:579.
2. Mahoney PN, Lamb CR. Articular, periarticular and juxtaarticular calcified bodies in the dog and cat: a radiologic review. *Vet Radiol Ultrasound*. 1996;37:3.
3. Mason DR, Schultz KS, Samii VF, et al. Sensitivity of radiographic evaluation of radio-ulnar incongruence in the dog in vivo. *Vet Surg*. 2002;31:125.
4. Widmer WR, Buckwalter KA, Braunstein EM, et al. Radiographic and magnetic resonance-imaging of the stifle joint in experimental osteoarthritis in dogs. *Vet Radiol Ultrasound*. 1994;35:371.
5. Wong SHJ, Chiu KY, Yan CH. Review article: osteophytes. *J Orthopedic Surgery*. 2016;24(3):403–410.
6. McGonagle D, Benjamin M, Marzo-Ortega H, et al. Advances in the understanding of entheseal inflammation. *Curr Rheumatol Rep*. 2002;4:500.
7. Morgan JP. *Radiology of Skeletal Diseases—Principles of Diagnosis in Dogs*. Davis, CA: Veterinary Radiology Associates; 1981:22.

8. van Bree H. Vacuum phenomenon associated with osteochondrosis of the scapulohumeral joint in dogs: 100 cases. *J Am Vet Med Assoc*. 1992;1985–1991(1916):201.
9. *PennHIP Training Manual*. San Diego, CA: Synbiotics Corporation; 1998:22.
10. Hathcock JT. Vacuum phenomenon of the canine spine: CT findings in 3 patients. *Vet Radiol Ultrasound*. 1994;35:285.
11. Weber WJ, Berry CR, Kramer RW. Vacuum phenomenon in 12 dogs. *Vet Radiol Ultrasound*. 1995;36:493.
12. Rendano VT, Dueland R. Variation in location of gastrocnemius sesamoid bones (fabellae) in a dog. *J Am Vet Med Assoc*. 1978;173:200.
13. Cake MA, Read RA. Canine and human sesamoid disease. *Vet Comp Orthop Traumatol*. 1995;8:70.
14. Read RA, Black AP, Armstrong SJ, et al. Incidence and clinical significance of sesamoid disease in Rottweilers. *Vet Rec*. 1992;130:533.
15. Davis PE, Bellenger CR, Turner DM. Fractures of the sesamoid bones in the greyhound. *Aust Vet J*. 1969;45:15.
16. Ljunggren G, Olsson SE. Osteoarthrosis of the shoulder and elbow joints in dogs: a pathologic and radiographic study of necropsy material. *J Am Vet Radiol Soc*. 1975;16:33.
17. Innes JF, Costello M, Barr FJ, et al. Radiographic progression of osteoarthritis of the canine stifle joint: a prospective study. *Vet Radiol Ultrasound*. 2004;45:143.
18. Enomoto M, Baines EA, Roe SC, Marcellin-Little DJ, Lascelles BDX. Defining the rate of, and factors influencing, radiographic progression of osteoarthritis of the canine hip joint. *Vet Record*. 2021;189(10):20–27.
19. Smith GK, Popovitch CA, Gregor TP, et al. Evaluation of risk factors for degenerative joint disease associated with hip dysplasia in dogs. *J Am Vet Med Assoc*. 1995;206:642.
20. Smith GK, Gregor TP, Rhodes WH, et al. Coxofemoral joint laxity from distraction radiography and its contemporaneous and prospective correlation with laxity, subjective score, and evidence of degenerative joint disease from conventional hip-extended radiography in dogs. *Am J Vet Res*. 1993;54:1020.
21. Marshall JL, Olsson SE. Instability of the knee: a long-term experimental study in dogs. *J Bone Joint Surg Am*. 1971;53:1561.
22. Lascelles BDX, Henry JB, Brown J, et al. Cross-sectional study of the prevalence of radiographic degenerative joint disease in domesticated cats. *Vet Surg*. 2010;39:535.
23. Gandolfi B, Alamri S, Darby WG, et al. A dominant TRPV4 variant underlies osteochondrodysplasia in Scottish fold cats. *Osteoarthr Cartil*. 2016;24:1441.
24. Freire M, Brown J, Robertson ID, et al. Meniscal mineralization in domestic cats. *Vet Surg*. 2010;39:545.
25. Walker M, Phalan D, Jensen J, et al. Meniscal ossicles in large non-domestic cats. *Vet Radiol Ultrasound*. 2002;43:249.
26. Salter RB, Harris WR. Injuries involving the epiphyseal plate. *J Bone Joint Surg*. 1963;45:587.
27. Farrow CS. Stress radiography: applications in small animal practice. *J Am Vet Med Assoc*. 1982;181:777.
28. Davidson EB, Griffey SM, Vasseur PB, et al. Histopathological, radiographic, and arthrographic comparison of the biceps tendon in normal dogs and dogs with biceps tenosynovitis. *J Am Anim Hosp Assoc*. 2000;36:522.
29. Kramer M, Gerweng M, Sheppard C, Schimke E. Ultrasonography for the diagnosis of diseases of the tendon and tendon sheath of the biceps brachii muscle. *Vet Surge*. 2001;30(1):64–71.
30. DeBakker E, Saunders JH, vanBree H, Gielen I, Van Ryssen B. Radiographic features of primary and concomitant flexor enthesopathy in the canine elbow. *Vet Radiol Ultrasound*. 2013;54(2):107–113.
31. Streubel R, Geyer H, Montavon PM. Medial humeral epicondylitis in cats. *Vet Surg*. 2012;41(7):795–802.
32. Streubel R, Bilzer T, Grest P, Damur D, Montavon PM. Medial humeral epicondylitis in clinically affected cats. *Vet Surg*. 2015;44(7):905–913.
33. Grundmann S, Montavon PM. Stenosing tenosynovitis of the abductor pollicis longus muscle in dogs. *Vet Comp Orthop Traumatol*. 2001;14:95.
34. Kramer M, Stengel H, Gerwing M, et al. Sonography of the canine stifle. *Vet Radiol Ultrasound*. 1999;40:282.
35. Lamb CR, Duvernois A. Ultrasonographic anatomy of the normal canine calcaneal tendon. *Vet Radiol Ultrasound*. 2005;46(4):326–330.
36. Bellah JR, Weigel JP. Hemarthrosis secondary to suspected warfarin toxicosis in a dog. *J Am Vet Med Assoc*. 1983;182:1126.
37. Mapuvire T, Kandiwa E, Mbiri P, et al. Chronic lymphoplasmacytic villonodular proliferative synovitis in a 10-year-old Jack Russell terrier dog. *Int J Vet Sci Med*. 2020;8(1):100–105.
38. Dempsey LM, Maddox TW, Meiring T, Wustefeld-Janssens B, Comerford EJ. Computed tomography findings of pigmented villonodular synovitis in a dog. *Vet Comp Orthop Traumatol*. 2018;31(4):304–310.
39. Flo GL, Stickle RL, Dunstan RW. Synovial chondrometaplasia in five dogs. *J Am Vet Med Assoc*. 1987;191:1417.
40. Hubler M, Johnson KA, Burling RT, et al. Lesions resembling osteochondromatosis in two cats. *J Small Anim Pract*. 1986;27:181.
41. Crawley AC, Yogalingam G, Muller VJ, et al. Two mutations within a feline mucopolysaccharidosis type VI colony cause three different phenotypes. *J Clin Invest*. 1998;101:109.
42. Bennett D. Immune-based erosive inflammatory joint disease of the dog: canine rheumatoid arthritis: I. Clinical, radiological and laboratory investigations. *J Small Anim Pract*. 1987;28:779.
43. Pedersen NC, Pool RR, O'Brien T. Feline chronic progressive polyarthritis. *Am J Vet Res*. 1980;41:522.
44. Bennett D. Immune-based non-erosive inflammatory joint disease of the dog: I. Canine SLE. *J Small Anim Pract*. 1987;28:871.
45. Moise NS, Crissman JW. Chronic progressive polyarthritis in a cat. *J Am Anim Hosp Assoc*. 1982;18:965.
46. Bennett D, Nash AS. Feline immune-based polyarthritis: a study of thirty-one cases. *J Small Anim Pract*. 1988;29:501.
47. Bennett D, Taylor DJ. Bacterial infective arthritis in the dog. *J Small Anim Pract*. 1988;29:207.
48. Moise NS, Crissman JW, Fairbrother JF, et al. *Mycoplasma gateae* arthritis and tenosynovitis in cats: case report and experimental reproduction of the disease. *Am J Vet Res*. 1983;44:10.
49. Craig LE, Julian ME, Ferracone JD. The diagnosis and prognosis of synovial tumors in dogs: 35 cases. *Vet Pathology*. 2002;39(1):66–73.
50. Silva-Krott IU. Synovial sarcoma in a cat. *J Am Vet Med Assoc*. 1993;203:1430.
51. Vail DM, Powers BE, Getzy DM, et al. Evaluation of prognostic factors for dogs with synovial sarcoma: 36 cases (1986–1991). *J Am Vet Med Assoc*. 1994;205:1300.
52. McGlennon NJ, Houlton JEF, Gorman NT. Synovial sarcoma in the dog—a review. *J Small Anim Pract*. 1988;29:139.
53. Manor EK, Craig LE, Sun X, Cannon CM. Prior joint disease is associated with increased risk of periarticular histiocytic sarcoma in dogs. *Vet Comp Oncol*. 2017;16(1):E83–E88.

ELECTRONIC RESOURCES

Additional information related to the content in Chapter 20 can be found online at eBooks.Health.Elsevier.com.

- Chapter Quiz

CHAPTER 21

The Equine Stifle

Valeria Busoni • Fabrice Audigié

THE STIFLE

Radiographic Examination

Stifle radiographs are acquired frequently in lame patients, presale examinations, and screening radiographic protocols in young horses.[1–3] Most equine radiographic examinations are performed today using digital radiographic (DR) equipment. The greater sensitivity and better dynamic range of DR compared to computed radiographic (CR) systems have led to a significant improvement in quality of stifle radiographs obtained with portable radiographic generators.

Given the large amount of soft tissue in the stifle region, scatter radiation doses to the hands of the detector holder and of the person holding the portable generator may not differ. Lead gloves should therefore be worn by both operators to increase radioprotection.[4] Reducing the number of repeat radiographs is also crucial to increase radioprotection. Because positioning errors are the most common reason for repeat and nondiagnostic radiographs,[5] good knowledge of radiographic technique and anatomy is critical to assess the stifle region.[6]

The lateromedial view is the basic radiographic view of the stifle. The beam is centered 5 to 7 cm proximal to the tibial plateau, between the cranial and middle third of the stifle region. The detector should be vertical to the ground to avoid geometric distortion, and exposure must be sufficient to penetrate the femoral condyles. A lateromedial view of the flexed stifle can be used to examine the cranial and central intercondylar areas of the tibia in more detail.

Depending on the purpose of the radiographic examination or the disease suspected, a caudolateral-craniomedial view and/or a caudocranial view are indicated. The caudolateral-craniomedial view allows good visibility of the two most common sites of disease in the young horse: the lateral femoral trochlear ridge (osteochondrosis site) and the medial femoral condyle (subchondral cyst-like lesion site). Because the femoral condyles are superimposed on the lateromedial view, the caudolateral-craniomedial view is a valuable complement to evaluate the medial femorotibial joint with low exposure factors. The caudolateral-craniomedial view is also helpful for documenting injuries of the articular surface of the patella. The caudocranial view is mainly aimed at the assessment of the femorotibial joints for osteoarthrosis, and it is essential for documenting axial injuries such as enthesopathies or avulsion fractures at the enthesis of the cranial cruciate ligament. The caudocranial view may require the use of a grid for optimal contrast in larger horses, but good diagnostic quality caudocranial radiographs of the stifle can be achieved without a grid with a portable radiographic unit and a DR system if scattering is limited by accurate collimation. This projection should be performed with a 10-degree descending beam to obtain the most accurate assessment of the width of the radiolucent femorotibial joint space, in particular the medial joint space.[7] The caudomedial-craniolateral view requires similar exposure factors to the caudocranial view and is performed less routinely. This projection is also useful to diagnose lateral femorotibial injuries, such as subchondral cyst-like lesions of the lateral femoral condyle and bone remodeling at the proximal or distal insertion of the cranial cruciate ligament.[6] The cranioproximal-craniodistal view of the patella is useful when patellar disease is being investigated. This view can be easily obtained with a portable x-ray unit and the required exposure is relatively low.

With the advent of DR systems and their inherently excellent contrast resolution, radiographic evaluation of the soft tissues of the stifle is possible to a certain extent. Lateromedial radiographs of the stifle allow good visualization of the patellar ligaments and the cranial fat pad (Fig. 21.1). Femoropatellar and femorotibial effusions can be suspected on radiographs (see Figs. 21.1 and 21.2). Localization of soft tissue swelling as being extra-articular or intra-articular is possible by evaluating border effacement of patellar ligaments and fat pad displacement (see Fig. 21.1).

Ultrasonography for Supplemental Stifle Imaging

Subchondral cyst-like lesions and tibial or femoral osteophyte formation as a result of osteoarthrosis are the most common radiographic signs of femorotibial disease. Bone fragments, new bone formation, or radiolucent areas at ligament insertions, suggesting avulsion fractures or enthesopathy, may also be seen.[8–10] However, because of the high incidence of soft tissue lesions involving menisci and ligaments, femorotibial pain may be present with no or minor radiographic signs.[8–10] The severity of the lameness, the midterm prognosis for a return to work, or the long-term prognosis for development of osteoarthrosis depends mainly on the severity of articular cartilage and soft tissue damage, in particular meniscal injury.[11,12] A combination of ultrasonographic and radiographic examination is therefore necessary for a routine more complete assessment of the stifle.[9]

Ultrasonography of the weight-bearing stifle allows easy assessment of the femoropatellar and femorotibial synovial recesses, the femoral trochlea, the patellar ligaments, the menisci, the collateral ligaments, and the medial femorotibial joint margins (Fig. 21.3).[13–16] In the flexed stifle, ultrasonography allows evaluation of the cranial horns of the menisci, the cranial meniscotibial ligaments, and a portion of the articular surface of the medial and lateral femoral condyles (see Fig. 21.3).[17,18] Ultrasonography is the first-line modality to diagnose meniscal and cranial meniscotibial ligament damage (see Fig. 21.19), which frequently affects sport and pleasure horses.[19,20] Although specificity is relatively low using arthroscopy as the gold standard,[19] a good correlation between histologic changes and ultrasonographic images has been suggested for meniscal injuries.[21]

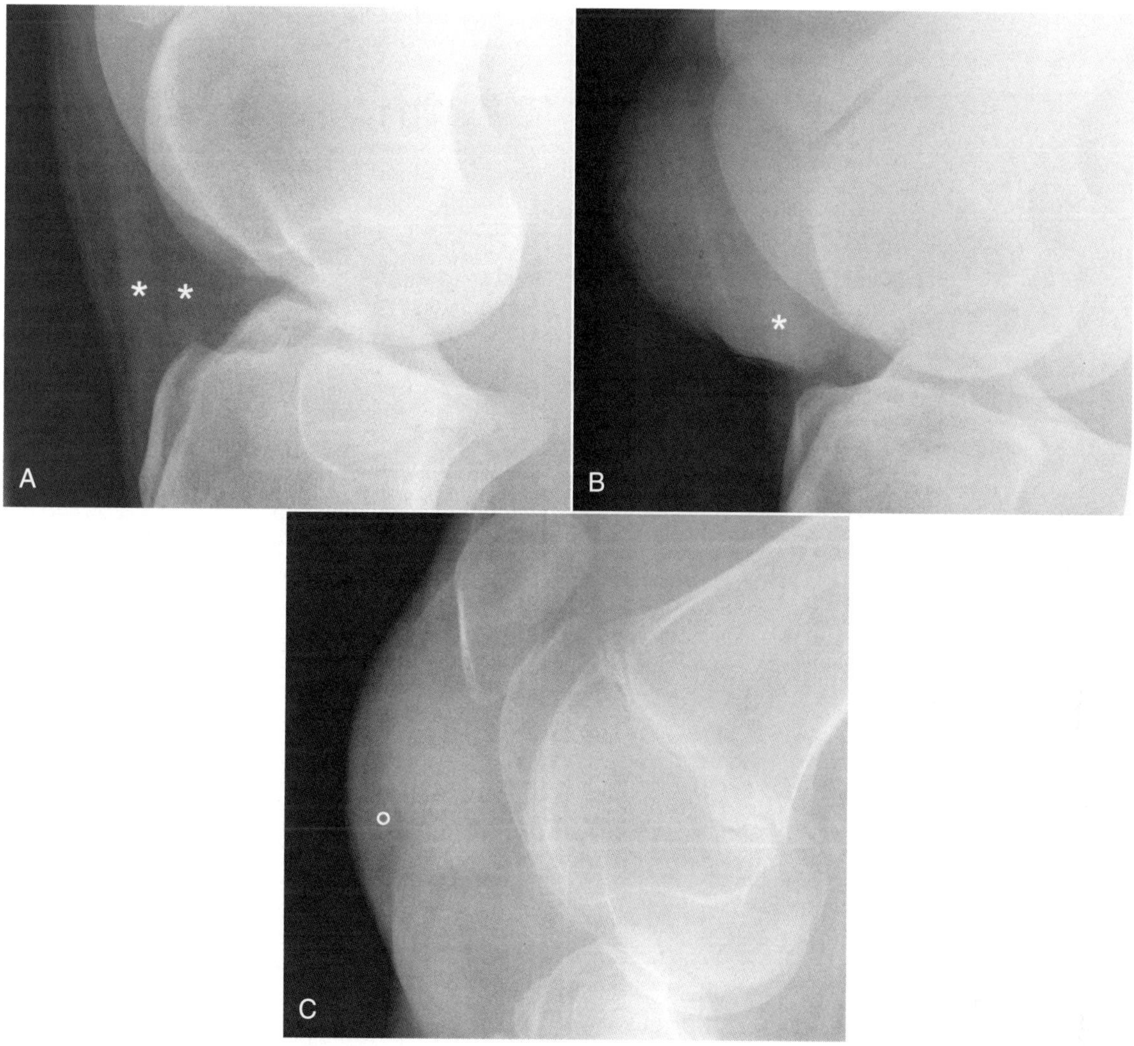

Fig. 21.1 Lateromedial radiographs of three equine stifles. **A,** Normal stifle. The patellar ligaments (*asterisks*) are delineated by the different opacity of the fat pad at the cranial aspect of the joint. **B,** A localized extra-articular soft tissue swelling is present. The middle patellar ligament is still visible (*asterisk*). The horse had an extra-articular abscess. Note that the positioning is not correct for a lateromedial view because it is slightly oblique. **C,** Large soft tissue swelling at the cranial aspect of the stifle. The swelling is intra-articular (femoropatellar and femorotibial), and the patellar ligaments are no longer visible because of border effacement. The fat pad (*open circle*) is displaced cranially.

Advanced Imaging of the Stifle

Because each modality has its limitations depending on lesion location and nature, further comprehensive joint assessment can be carried out using advanced imaging techniques such as computed tomography (CT), CT arthrography and magnetic resonance imaging (MRI).[22–25] The increasing number of large-bore CT machines in equine practice has made the examination of the stifle accessible for all types of horses (Fig. 21.4). The advantage of this modality is the speed of acquisition and the inclusion of both stifle joints allowing the opposite limb to be used as reference in case of unilateral conditions. The short acquisition time also allows the screening of other body parts during the same general anesthesia (for example, other joints of the lame hindlimb in adult horses or both hindlimbs and pelvis in young foals presenting with hematogenous sepsis), and allows the CT examination to be followed by surgical procedures such as arthroscopy. CT examination provides high-resolution three-dimensional (3D) bone imaging while CT-arthrography with intra-articular injection of contrast medium is necessary for an accurate evaluation of articular soft tissues and cartilage.[26,27] Contrary to CT, MRI of the stifle of an adult horse is feasible only in a limited number of magnetic resonance (MR) units. Today, most MR examinations of the stifle are acquired using an open low-field MR unit with a tiltable magnet (see Fig. 21.4).[28] The positioning of the horse in the MR machine remains challenging even in open units and induces compression of the thigh and gluteal muscles of the opposite hindlimb. Therefore, only one stifle can be examined in one session to limit the anesthetic risk and prevent potential anesthetic complications.[28] Knowledge of the 3D anatomy of the stifle is crucial with these modalities and several studies provide reference images.[22,29,30] As documented for other joints, compared to CT, MRI of stifle conditions has the major advantage of documenting soft tissue lesions (including lesions of the articular cartilage) without the use of contrast medium and allows the diagnosis of lesions of the cancellous bone.[26,27] MRI, however, is less sensitive than CT to detect periarticular remodeling and soft tissue mineralization.

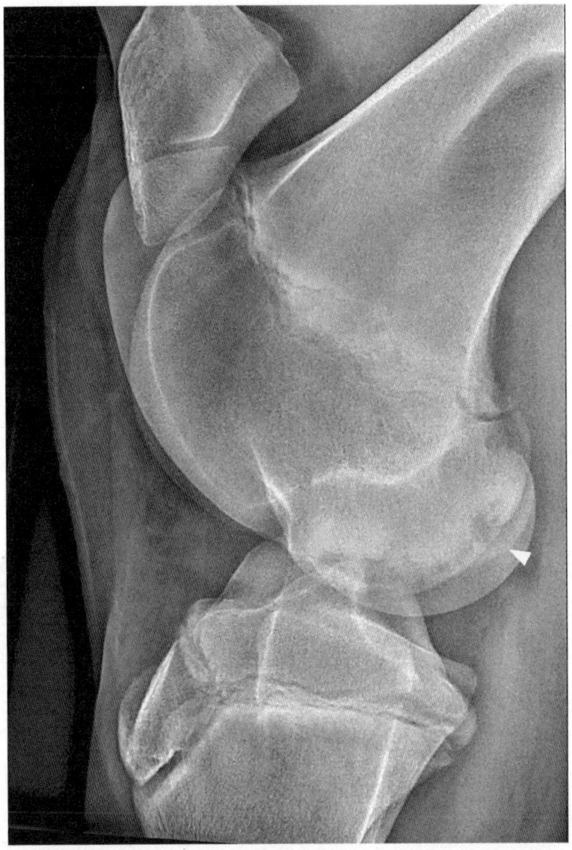

Fig. 21.14 Lateromedial radiograph of the stifle of a 5-month-old Thoroughbred colt with a grade 4/5 lameness showing marked changes in the opacity of the subchondral and adjacent cancellous bone of the lateral femoral condyle extending from its cranial to its caudoproximal aspect. Note the duplication of the caudal articular surface of the lateral femoral condyle compatible with a large osteochondral fragment (*arrowhead*). These changes most likely represent an extensive juvenile osteochondral disease.

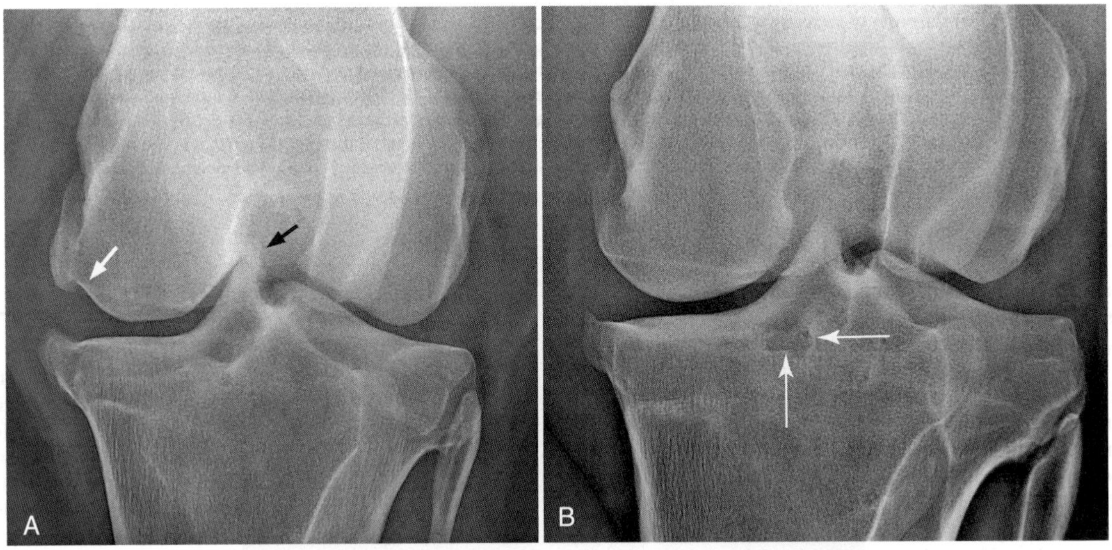

Fig. 21.15 Caudocranial radiographs of the stifle of two horses with meniscal injuries and degenerative joint disease. **A,** Femoral and tibial osteophytes are present on the medial articular margins. Note the change in curvature between the condyle surface and the femoral osteophyte (*white arrow*). Osteophytes are also present on the top of the medial tibial intercondylar eminence and corresponding axial margin of the medial femoral condyle (*black arrow*). **B,** A radiolucent area delineated by a faint sclerotic margin is present in the medial aspect of the cranial intercondylar area at the site of insertion of the cranial meniscotibial ligament (*white arrows*). This radiographic sign indicates a cranial enthesopathy of the medial meniscus. Femoral and tibial osteophytes are also visible. Note the thin horizontal line superimposed over the medial femoral condyle. This line is created by remodeling of the craniomedial margin of the medial femoral condyle and is observed frequently when there is marked-to-severe degenerative joint disease of the medial femorotibial joint (see Fig. 21.16).

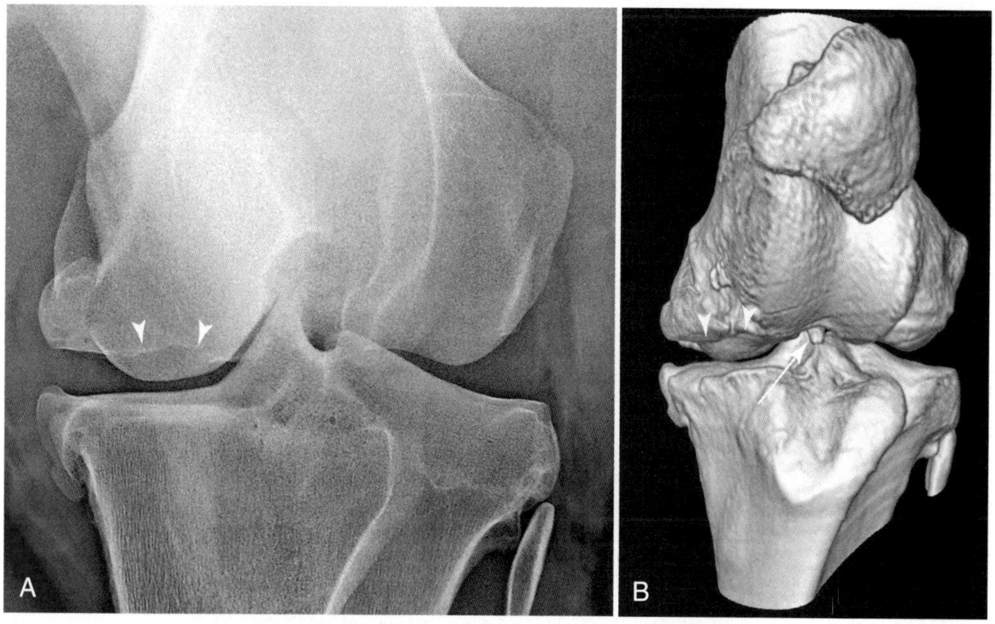

Fig. 21.16 Caudocranial radiograph **(A)** and three-dimensional (3D) volume rendering computed tomography (CT) image **(B)** of the stifle of a horse with advanced medial femorotibial degenerative joint disease. Large broad-based osteophytes are present on the medial femoral and tibial margins. The margin of the femoral osteophyte production extending on the cranial border of the femoral condyle **(B)** creates a thin radiopaque osteophytic line superimposed to the femoral condyle on the caudocranial radiograph **(A, B,** *arrowheads***)**. Note the large remodeling of the cranial aspect of the medial intercondylar tubercule **(B,** *arrow***)**.

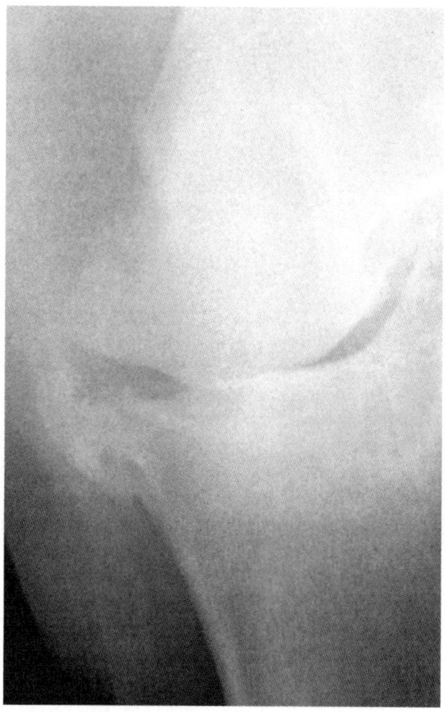

Fig. 21.17 Caudocranial radiograph (close-up view) of the stifle of a horse with severe medial meniscal damage, calcification, and prolapse. The medial femorotibial joint space is narrowed, and the proximal tibial condyle is sclerotic because of a prolapse of the medial meniscus. Calcified meniscal material is present outside the articular space at the medial aspect of the joint. The medial femoral and tibial joint margins have large osteophytes.

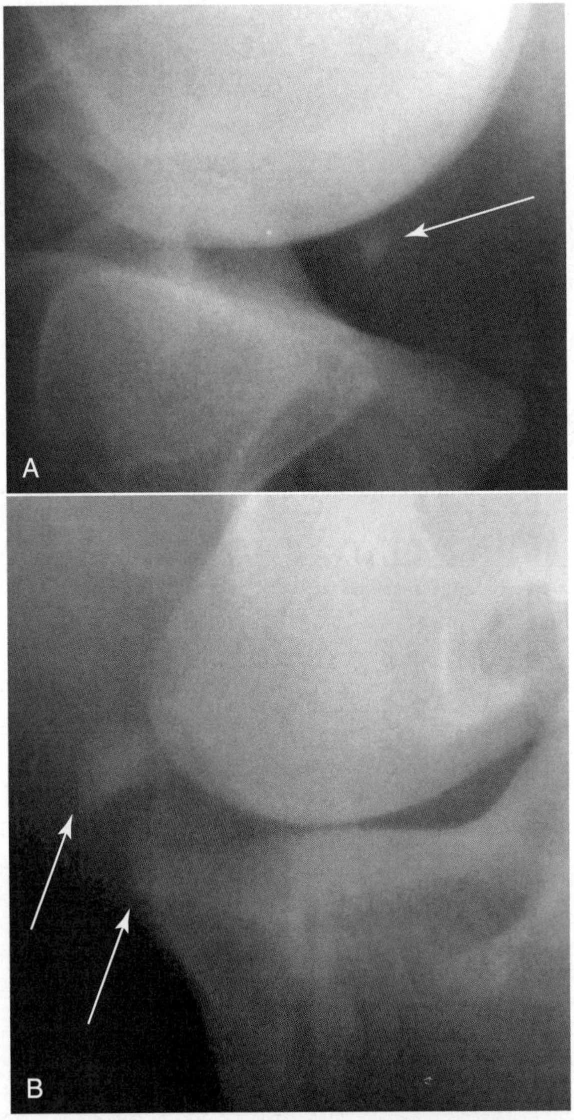

Fig. 21.18 Lateromedial **(A)** and caudocranial **(B)** radiographs (close-up views) of the stifle of two horses with meniscal calcification. **A,** A small radiopaque focus (*white arrow*) is present between the femoral condyle and the caudal aspect of the tibial plateau compatible with calcification in the caudal horn of the medial meniscus. **B,** Two large radiopaque bodies (*white arrows*) at the medial aspect of the medial femorotibial joint correspond to calcified portions of a prolapsed medial meniscus. Note the associated narrowing of the femorotibial joint space.

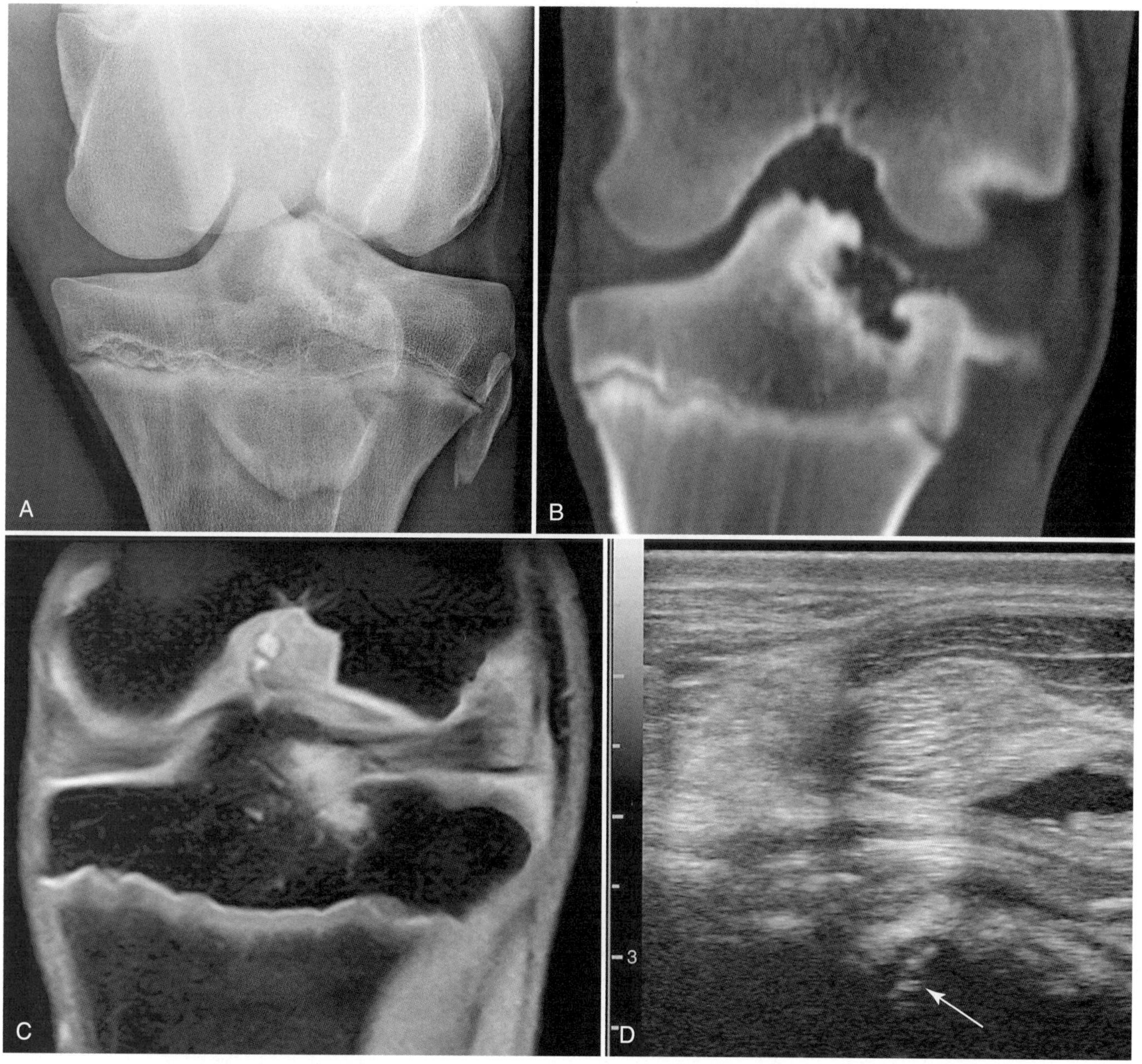

Fig. 21.19 Caudocranial radiograph **(A)**, computed tomography (CT) **(B)**, fat suppressed magnetic resonance (MR) **(C)**, and ultrasonographic **(D)** images of the stifle of a 11-month-old filly with severe cranial meniscotibial ligament enthesopathy of the lateral meniscus. A large semicircular defect with irregular margins surrounded by severe sclerosis is present in the cranial intercondylar area of the tibia at the site of insertion of the lateral cranial meniscotibial ligament. Note the increased signal around the bone defect in the MR image representing bone edema **(C)** and the presence of small mineralization or bony fragments within the meniscotibial ligament **(B–D)**. The ultrasonographic transverse image obtained at the cranial aspect of the medial femorotibial joint in the flexed stifle shows a hypoechoic area in the deep portion of the ligament and the irregular interrupted hyperechoic bone surface at the site of attachment (*arrow*, compare to normal image in Fig. 21.3D).

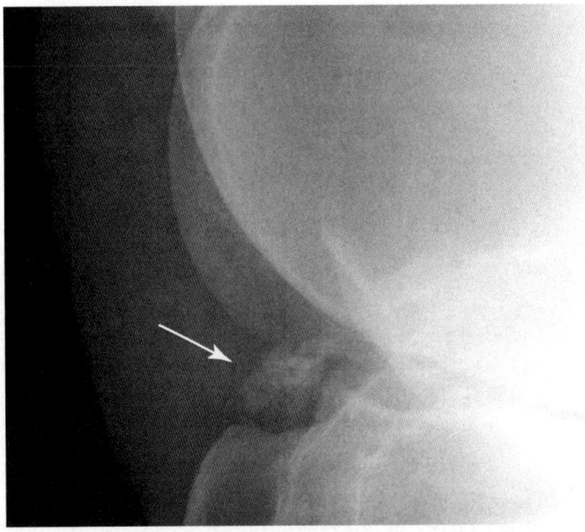

Fig. 21.20 Caudolateral-craniomedial radiograph (close-up view) of the stifle in a horse with severe medial meniscal damage and prolapse. A large bone fragment is visible at the cranial aspect of the femorotibial joint space (*white arrow*), which represents an old avulsion fragment at the cranial meniscotibial ligament attachment.

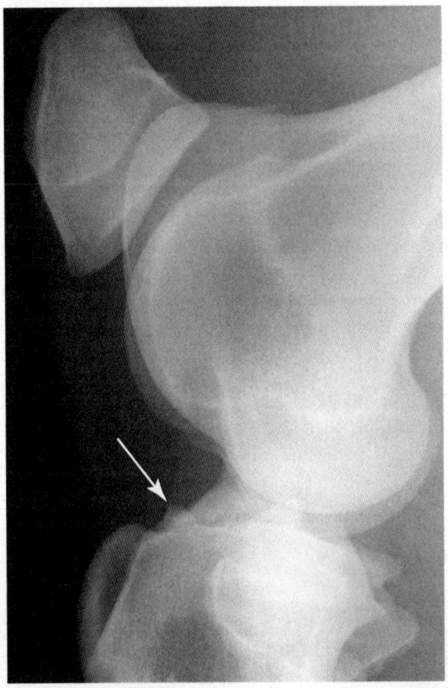

Fig. 21.21 Flexed lateromedial radiograph of an equine stifle. An osseous proliferation is present cranial to the tibial intercondylar eminence (*white arrow*). Ultrasonographically, there was a horizontal fissure and a partial prolapse of the medial meniscus and damage to the medial cranial meniscotibial ligament.

the trochlear ridges of the femur.[36] Ultrasonographic examination adds valuable information in patellar fractures by documenting associated soft tissue injuries and defining the anatomic origin of avulsed fragments, that is, parapatellar fibrocartilages, patellar ligaments, and distal enthesis of the quadriceps femoris muscle.

Tibial and Femoral Fractures

Fractures of the tibial tuberosity are the most commonly reported fractures involving the proximal tibia in adult horses.[36] Trauma with wounds of the tibial tuberosity may lead to sequestrum formation and be associated to lateral patellar ligament damage (Fig. 21.25).[62] In these instances, synovial involvement is uncommon. Fractures involving the intercondylar eminence or the caudal aspect of the proximal tibia are seen in association with cruciate ligament damage and often involve the ligament insertion sites.[57,58,63] The proximal aspect of the tibial diaphysis is the most common site for incomplete fracture of the tibia, which usually begins at the lateral aspect of the bone and spirals distally (eFig. 21.4).[36,64] Radiographic diagnosis of an incomplete fracture may be challenging even if several oblique views are made. Complete rest and repeat radiographs approximately 7 to 10 days after the onset of the acute lameness are indicated. At this stage, the fracture line becomes more visible because of resorption of the fracture margins. In racehorses, tibial fatigue fractures can also be encountered, most commonly in the caudal and proximal metaphyseal region. The most common radiographic signs at

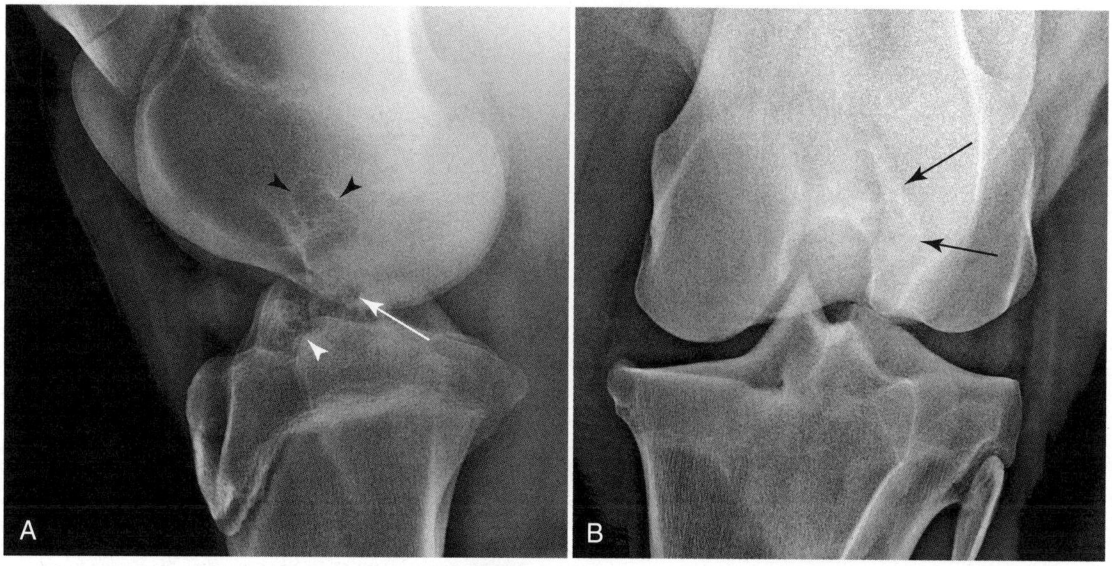

Fig. 21.22 Lateromedial **(A)** and caudocranial **(B)** radiographs of two horses with cruciate ligament injury. **A,** One-year-old colt with a history of trauma 5 months ago. The soft tissue swelling located cranial to the femorotibial joint space without border effacement of the patellar ligaments suggests severe femorotibial joint effusion. Severe opacity changes are visible at the cranial and central tibial intercondylar areas (*white arrowhead*). The caudal aspect of the medial intercondylar eminence is difficult to identify because of increased and heterogeneous opacity seen in the intercondylar area (*white arrow*). In other radiographic views and based on ultrasonographic examination, there were enthesopathies of the cranial meniscotibial ligaments and a fracture of the medial intercondylar eminence suggesting cranial cruciate ligament damage. The large radiolucent area surrounded by a thin sclerotic rim visible in the cranioproximal aspect of the femoral intercondylar fossa (*black arrowheads*) suggests an associated chronic femoral enthesopathy of the caudal cruciate ligament. **B,** Several round coalescing radiolucencies surrounded by sclerosis (*arrows*) are visible at the axial aspect of the lateral femoral condyle in the intercondylar area at the site of femoral attachment of the cranial cruciate ligament and represent the radiographic signs of a severe chronic enthesopathy.

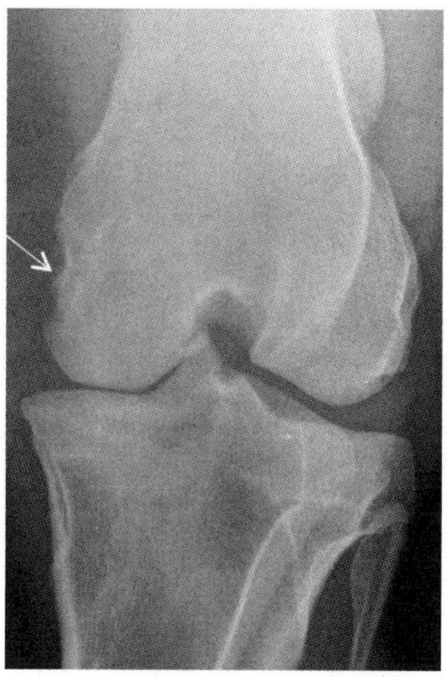

Fig. 21.23 Caudocranial radiograph of the stifle of a horse with a history of previous trauma to the stifle. The medial epicondyle has an irregular surface indicating chronic enthesopathy of the medial collateral ligament (*arrow*). Ultrasound confirmed medial collateral ligament damage by demonstrating a severely enlarged and hypoechoic ligament with loss of its regular fiber architecture.

the site of the stress fracture are periosteal bone proliferation, thickening of the cortical bone, and sclerosis of the adjacent cancellous bone (Fig. 21.26).

Fractures of the femur involving the distal epiphysis are uncommon in adult horses. Trochlear ridge fractures are seen as free sharp fragments and a bone defect in the trochlea or as radiolucent lines in the trochlear ridge in incomplete nondisplaced fractures. These fractures result from direct external trauma and may be associated with patellar fractures.[36] Femoral avulsion fractures of the origin of the common tendon of the peroneus tertius and the extensor digitorum longus are reported in foals (Fig. 21.27).[65,66]

Fibular Fractures

Fibular fractures have been rarely reported as a cause of lameness.[36,67] Care should be taken not to confuse the normal radiolucent line traversing the proximal fibula because of incomplete ossification with a fracture line. Callus formation is a useful radiographic sign of the presence of a fracture.[36,67]

MISCELLANEOUS CONDITIONS INVOLVING THE STIFLE

Calcinosis Circumscripta

Calcinosis circumscripta is localized deposition of calcium in small nodules in subcutaneous tissues or attached to tendons or joint capsules.[68] The lesions of calcinosis circumscripta appear grossly as hard, spherical, nonpainful, subcutaneous, or periarticular swellings. The etiology of calcinosis circumscripta is unknown but thought to be of traumatic origin.[69] In the horse, the predilection site is the lateral aspect of the stifle close to the extensor groove of the tibia.[69] The lesion is visible radiographically as a well-circumscribed, roughly oval accumulation of granular mineral opacities at the lateral aspect of the proximal tibia (Fig. 21.28). Calcinosis circumscripta may be an incidental finding because the lesion rarely causes lameness.[69]

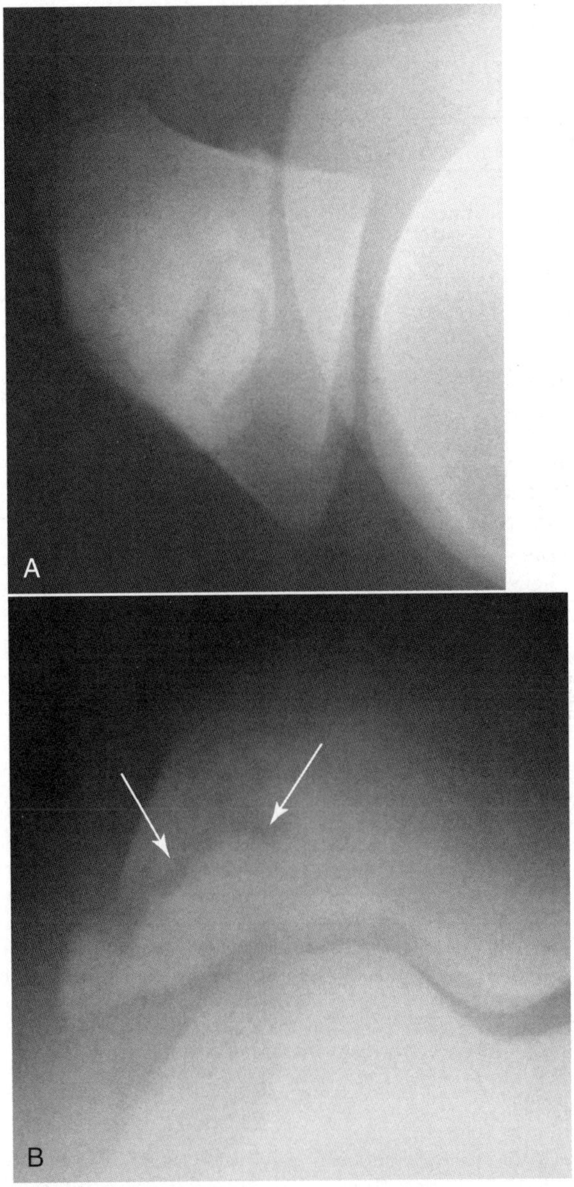

Fig. 21.24 Flexed lateromedial **(A)** and cranioproximal-craniodistal **(B)** radiographs (close-up views) of the stifle of a horse with a chronic nondisplaced fracture of the medial aspect of the patella. **A,** The patella has increased opacity and a radiolucent line at the level of the medial angle. The medial articular surface is irregular and interrupted by the radiolucent line. **B,** The fracture of the medial angle of the patella is seen as an ill-defined radiolucent line (*white arrows*) separating two bone fragments. The fracture involves the medial articular surface of the patella.

Most commonly, there is a firm, nonpainful swelling that has been increasing slowly in size. The lesions are frequently bilateral, and radiographic examination of the contralateral limb is important if surgical removal is considered.

Septic Arthritis and Osteomyelitis

Septic arthritis is inflammation of a joint caused by bacterial invasion and proliferation.[70] Septic arthritis may occur in foals or adult horses. Hematogenous spread is the most common cause of septic arthritis in foals, whereas septic arthritis in adult horses is usually a consequence of penetrating wounds, injection, or surgery.[70]

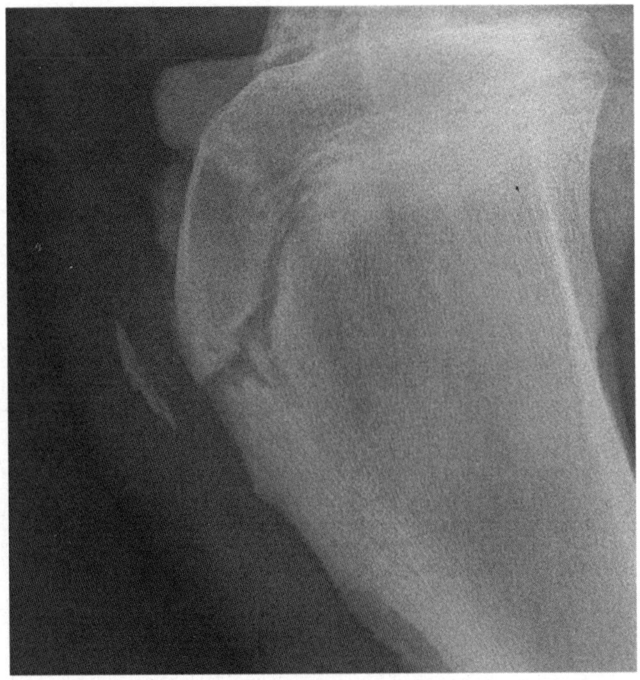

Fig. 21.25 Lateromedial radiograph of the proximal tibia of a young horse who had a trauma of the stifle with several wounds 3 weeks before. A linear radiopaque fragment is visible at a short distance from the tibia cranially and represents a bone sequestrum detached from the tibial tuberosity. Note the soft tissue swelling at the same level and the bone debris between the sequestrum and the tibia. The cranial surface of the tibial tuberosity is slightly irregular. At ultrasonography the horse had a hypoechoic fistulous tract and a traumatic lesion of the lateral patellar ligament.

Infection of the stifle joint in adult horses is rare. Periarticular infection and abscess after trauma and penetrating wounds is more common than bacterial joint invasion.[70] In foals, the femoropatellar joint and the femorotibial joints are common sites of septic arthritis, and the femur is one of the bones most affected by hematogenous osteomyelitis.[71] Bone changes appear late in the condition in adult horses, whereas they occur earlier in foals. Concurrent septic arthritis and osteomyelitis is common in foals, and foals with osteomyelitis without septic arthritis are usually older.[71] In the same way, foals with a single bone lesion tend to be older than those with multiple bone lesions.[71] Bone changes attributable to osteomyelitis may have a physeal or epiphyseal location in foals and are located differently depending on the joints infected concomitantly. When the femoropatellar joint is affected, osteolysis is mainly seen on the femoral trochlea and/or the patellar articular surface (Fig. 21.29). Subchondral bone abnormalities on the femoral trochlea may be more difficult to assess, because the trochlear ridges normally have an irregular bone surface in young foals during ossification. Femorotibial involvement is often uniaxial (medial or lateral) (Fig. 21.30). Bone involvement is seen as ill-defined radiolucent areas in the subchondral bone of the tibial plateau and/or the femoral condyles, with the medial femoral condyle being affected more commonly.[51,71] Another characteristic of these subchondral radiolucent areas is their potential location in the non–weight-bearing part of the femoral condyles. Physeal osteomyelitis in foals appears as widening of the radiolucent physis and ill-defined physeal margins associated with local swelling. Well-defined radiolucent areas in the subchondral bone may remain evident as long-term sequelae of osteomyelitis when infection is eliminated.

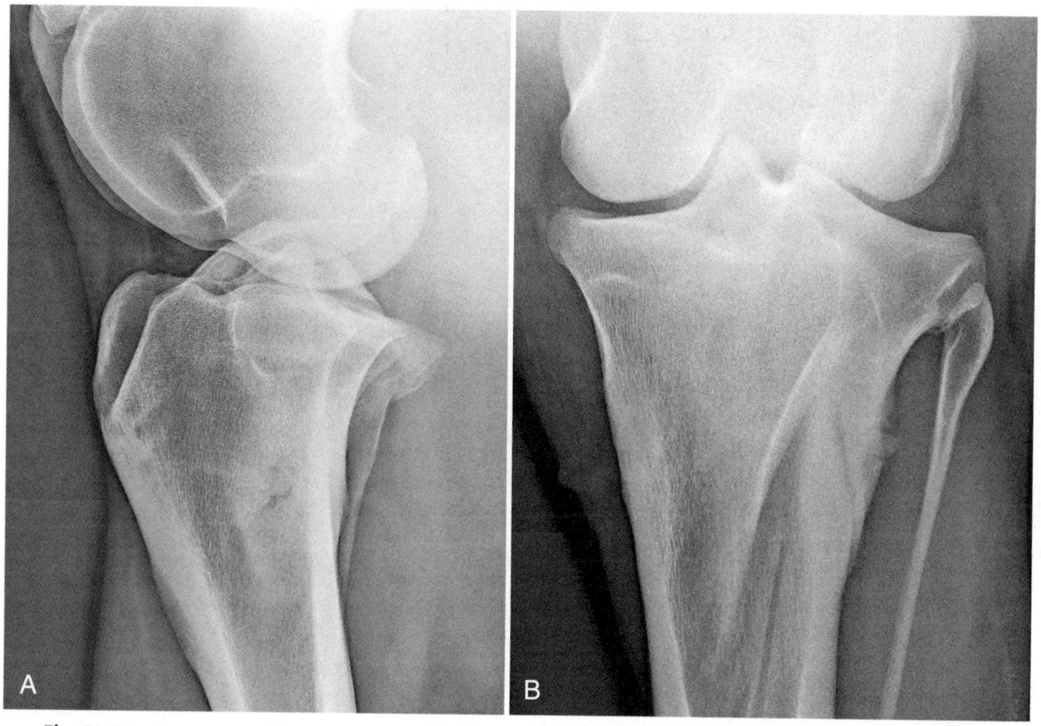

Fig. 21.26 Lateromedial **(A)** and caudocranial **(B)** radiographs of a Thoroughbred horse with a stress fracture of the proximal tibia. The stress fracture is seen as a linear radiolucent line with massive sclerosis of the cancellous bone, thickening of the cortical bone, and focal periosteal bony proliferation in the lateral caudal aspect of the proximal tibial metaphysis.

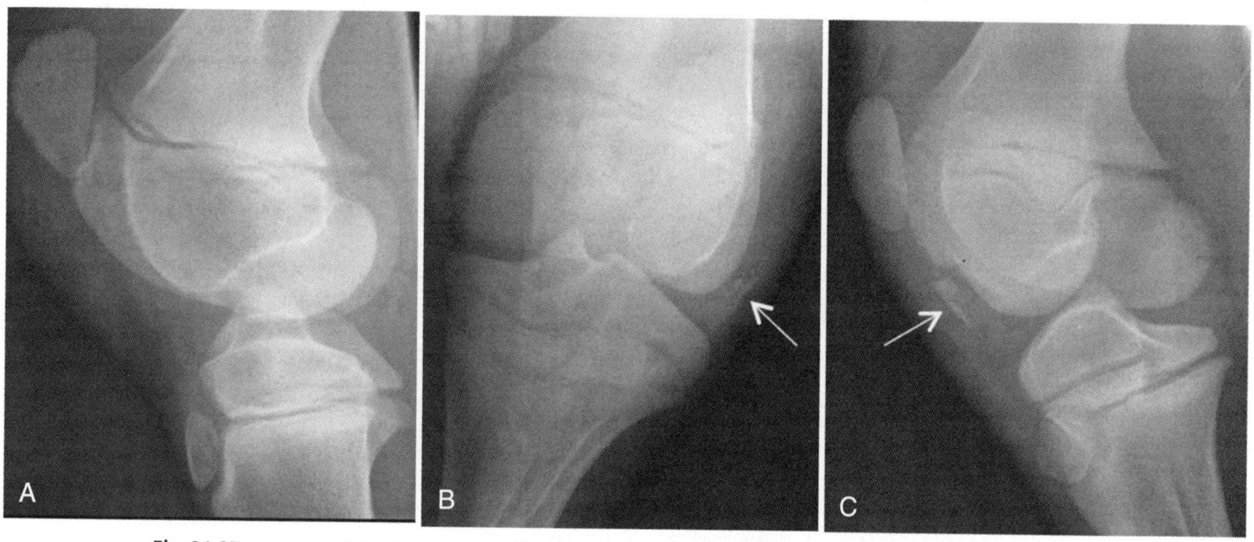

Fig. 21.27 Lateromedial **(A)**, caudocranial **(B)**, and caudolateral-craniomedial oblique **(C)** radiographs of the stifle of a foal with a femoral avulsion fracture at the site of origin of the common tendon of the peroneus tertius and the extensor digitorum longus. Because of its lateral position, the bone fragment is better seen on the caudocranial and on the caudolateral-craniomedial oblique views (*arrows*) but is only visible as a heterogeneous opacity in the area of the extensor fossa superimposed over the femur on the lateromedial radiograph.

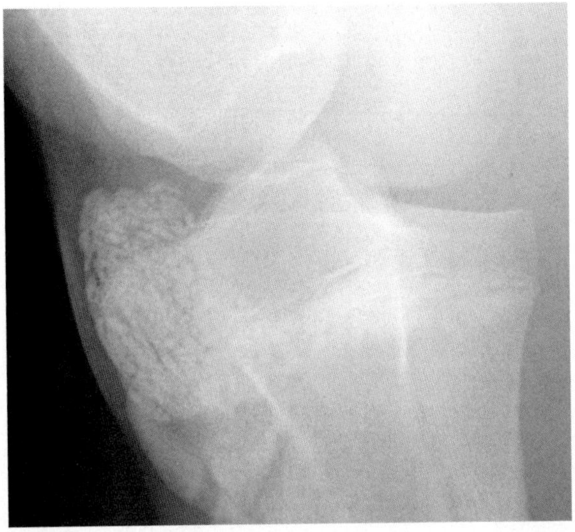

Fig. 21.28 Caudolateral-craniomedial stifle radiograph of a young horse with calcinosis circumscripta. A large cluster of calcified granular material is located at the lateral aspect of the proximal tibia.

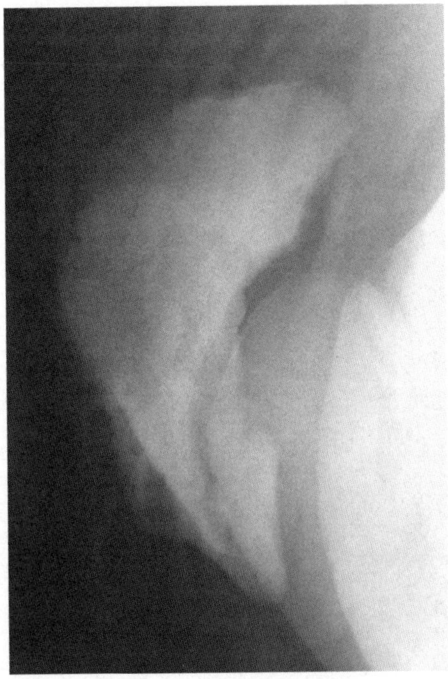

Fig. 21.29 Lateromedial radiograph of the patella of a foal with septic arthritis of the femoropatellar joint. The articular surface of the patella is irregular, and there is severe lysis of the subchondral bone.

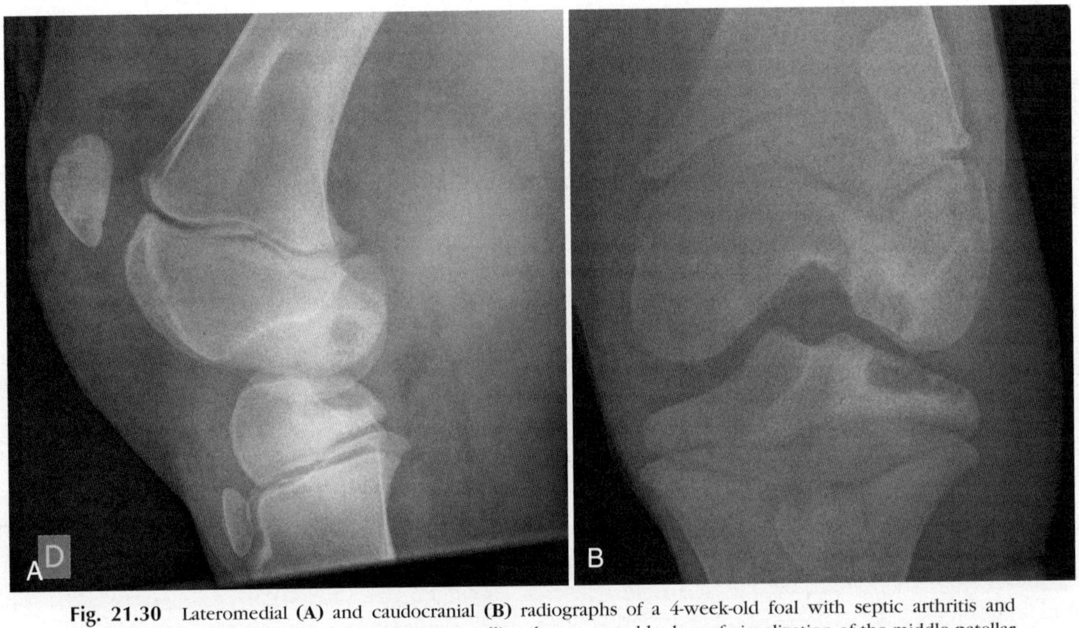

Fig. 21.30 Lateromedial **(A)** and caudocranial **(B)** radiographs of a 4-week-old foal with septic arthritis and osteomyelitis of the stifle. There is severe joint swelling demonstrated by loss of visualization of the middle patellar ligament, lack of visualization of the fat pad, and displacement of the fascial and cutaneous planes. In the caudal aspect of the stifle, two large, slightly heterogeneous, radiolucent areas of infected bone are seen in the axial aspect of the lateral femoral condyle and in the proximal tibia. Surrounding cancellous bone has an increased opacity due to sclerosis.

REFERENCES

1. Preston SA, Zimmel DN, Chmielewski TL, et al. Prevalence of various presale radiographic findings and association of findings with sales price in Thoroughbred yearlings sold in Kentucky. *J Am Vet Med Assoc*. 2010;236(4):440–445.
2. Van Grevenhof EM, Ducro BJ, Van Weeren PR, et al. Prevalence of various radiographic manifestations of osteochondrosis and their correlations between and within joints in Dutch Warmblood horses. *Equine Vet J*. 2009;41(1):11–16.
3. Verwilghen D, Serteyn D, Pille F, et al. Prevalence of radiographic findings in candidate sires (2001–2008). *Vlaams Diergeneeskundig Tijdschrift*. 2009;78:419.
4. Belotta AF, Mayer MN, Waldner CL, et al. X-ray tube operators can be exposed to equal or higher scattered radiation doses to the hand as cassette holders during diagnostic radiographic procedures of the equine vertebral column and limbs. *Am J Vet Res Mar*. 2022 3;83(5):412–418.
5. Jackson MA, Vizard AL, Anderson GA, et al. Identification and prevalence of errors affecting the quality of radiographs submitted to Australian Thoroughbred yearling sale repositories. *Vet Radiol Ultrasound*. 2011;52(3):262–269.
6. Aldrich ED, Goodrich LR, Monahan MK, et al. Radiographic localisation of the entheses of the equine stifle. *Equine Vet J*. 2017;49(4):493–500.
7. Trencart P, Alexander K, De Lasalle J, et al. Radiographic evaluation of the width of the femorotibial joint space in horses. *Am J Vet Res*. 2016;77(2):127–136.
8. Walmsley JP. Diagnosis and treatment of ligamentous and meniscal injuries in the equine stifle. *Vet Clin North Am Equine Pract*. 2005;21(3):651–672.
9. Denoix JM, Audigié F. Imaging of the musculoskeletal system in horses. In: Hinchcliff K, Kaneps AJ, Geor RJ, et al., eds. *Equine Sports Medicine and Surgery—Basic and Clinical Sciences of the Equine Athlete*. Philadelphia: Saunders; 2004:161.
10. De Busscher V, Verwilghen D, Bolen G, et al. Meniscal damage diagnosed by ultrasonography in horses: a retrospective study of 74 femorotibial joint ultrasonographic examinations (2000–2005). *J Equine Vet Sci*. 2006;26:453.
11. Flynn KA, Whitcomb MB. Equine meniscal injuries: a retrospective study of 14 horses. *Proc Am Assoc Equine Pract*. 2002;48:249.
12. Hendrix SM, Baxter GM, McIlwraith CW, et al. Concurrent or sequential development of medial meniscal and subchondral cystic lesions within the medial femorotibial joint in horses (1996–2006). *Equine Vet J*. 2010;42(1):5–9.
13. Coudry V, Denoix JM. Ultrasonography of the femorotibial collateral ligaments of the horse. *Equine Vet Educ*. 2010;17(5):275–279.
14. Denoix JM, Busoni V. Ultrasonography of joints and synovia. In: White NA, Moore JN, eds. *Current Techniques in Equine Surgery and Lameness*. 2nd ed. Philadelphia: Saunders; 1998:643.
15. Hoaglund EL, Barrett MF, Daglish J, et al. Intermediate patellar ligament desmopathy often occurs in conjunction with other stifle abnormalities. *Vet Radiol Ultrasound*. 2019;60(4):416–422.
16. Gottlieb R, Whitcomb MB, Vaughan B, et al. Ultrasonographic appearance of normal and injured lateral patellar ligaments in the equine stifle. *Equine Vet J*. 2016;48(3):299–306.
17. Moiroud CH, Denoix JM. Ultrasound diagnosis of injuries of the cranial meniscotibial ligament of the medial meniscus. *Equine Vet Educ*. 2017;29(11):617–620.
18. Jacquet S, Audigié F, Denoix JM. Ultrasonographic diagnosis of subchondral bone cysts in the medial femoral condyle in horses. *Equine Vet Educ*. 2007;19:47.
19. Cohen JM, Richardson DW, McKnight AL, et al. Long-term outcome in 44 horses with stifle lameness after arthroscopic exploration and debridement. *Vet Surg*. 2009;38(4):543–551.
20. Davis JG, García-López JM. Arthroscopic findings and long-term outcomes in 76 sport horses with meniscal injuries (2008–2018). *Vet Surg*. 2022;51(3):409–417.
21. De Busscher V, Schreder A, Busoni V, et al. Histological study of the horse stifle menisci in relation with ultrasonographic aspect: preliminary study. *Italian J Anat Embryol*. 2006;111:132.
22. Santos MP, Gutierrez-Nibeyro SD, McKnight AL, et al. Gross and histopathologic correlation of low-field magnetic resonance imaging findings in the stifle of asymptomatic horses. *Vet Radiol Ultrasound*. 2015;56(4):407–416.
23. Adrian AM, Barrett MF, Werpy NM, et al. A comparison of arthroscopy to ultrasonography for identification of pathology of the equine stifle. *Equine Vet J*. 2017;49(3):314–321.
24. De Lasalle J, Alexander K, Olive J, et al. Comparisons among radiography, ultrasonography and computed tomography for ex vivo characterization of stifle osteoarthritis in the horse. *Vet Radiol Ultrasound*. 2016;57(5):489–501.
25. Valdés-Martínez A. Computed tomographic arthrography of the equine stifle joint. *Vet Clin North Am Equine Pract*. 2012;28(3):583–598.
26. Aßmann AD, Ohlerth S, Suárez Sánchez-Andráde J, et al. Ex vivo comparison of 3 Tesla magnetic resonance imaging and multidetector computed tomography arthrography to identify artificial soft tissue lesions in equine stifles. *Vet Surg*. 2022;51(4):648–657.
27. Nelson BB, Kawcak CE, Goodrich LR, et al. Comparison between computed tomographic arthrography, radiography, ultrasonography, and arthroscopy for the diagnosis of femorotibial joint disease in western performance horses. *Vet Radiol Ultrasound*. 2016;57(4):387–402.
28. Waselau M, McKnight A, Kasparek A. Magnetic resonance imaging of equine stifles: technique and observations in 76 clinical cases. *Equine Vet Educ*. 2020;32(10):85–91.
29. Daglish J, Frisbie DD, Selberg KT, et al. High field magnetic resonance imaging is comparable with gross anatomy for description of the normal appearance of soft tissues in the equine stifle. *Vet Radiol Ultrasound*. 2018;59(6):721–736.
30. Vekens EV, Bergman EH, Vanderperren K, et al. Computed tomographic anatomy of the equine stifle joint. *Am J Vet Res*. 2011;72(4):512–521.
31. Denoix JM, Jeffcott LB, McIlwraith CW, et al. A review of terminology for equine juvenile osteochondral conditions (JOCC) based on anatomical and functional considerations. *Vet J*. 2013;197(1):29–35.
32. Dik KJ, Enzerink E, Van Weeren PR. Radiographic development of osteochondral abnormalities in the hock and stifle of Dutch Warmblood foals, from age 1 to 11 months. *Equine Vet J*. 1999;31:9–15.
33. Bourzac C, Alexander K, Rossier Y, et al. Comparison of radiography and ultrasonography for the diagnosis of osteochondritis dissecans in the equine femoropatellar joint. *Equine Vet J*. 2009;41(7):685–692.
34. Robert C, Valette JP, Denoix JM. Correlation between routine radiographic findings and early racing career in French trotters. *Equine Vet J Suppl*. 2006;36:473–478.
35. Kane AJ, Park RD, McIlwraith CW, et al. Radiographic changes in Thoroughbred yearlings. Part 1: prevalence at the time of the yearling sales. *Equine Vet J*. 2003;35(4):354–365.

36. Butler JA, Colles CM, Dyson SJ, et al. *Clinical Radiology of the Horse*. 3rd ed. London: Blackwell; 2008.
37. Trostle SS, Casinella LL, Sussman KH, et al. What is your diagnosis? Osseous cystlike lesion of the patella. *J Am Vet Med Assoc*. 2007;230(5):663–664.
38. Jacquet S, Robert C, Valette JP, et al. Evolution of radiological findings detected in the limbs of 321 young horses between the ages of 6 and 18 months. *Vet J*. 2013;197(1):58–64.
39. Santschi EM, Prichard MA, Whitman JL, et al. Stifle radiography in Thoroughbreds from 6 to 18 months of age. *Equine Vet Educ*. 2019;32(10):78–84.
40. Hoey S, O'Sullivan J, Byrne J, et al. Ultrasound screening protocol for osteochondrosis at selected predilection sites in thoroughbred yearlings, Ir. *Vet J*. 2022;75(1):8.
41. Martel G, Crowley D, Olive J, et al. Ultrasonographic screening for subclinical osteochondrosis of the femoral trochlea in foals (28–166 days old): a prospective farm study. *Equine Vet J*. 2018;50(3):312–320.
42. Baccarin RY, Martins EA, Hagen SC, et al. Patellar instability following experimental medial patellar desmotomy in horses. *Vet Comp Orthop Traumatol*. 2009;22(1):27–31.
43. Labens R, Busoni V, Peters F, et al. Ultrasonographic and radiographic diagnosis of patellar fragmentation secondary to bilateral medial patellar ligament desmotomy in a Warmblood gelding. *Equine Vet Educ*. 2005;17:201.
44. McIlwraith CW. Osteochondral fragmentation of the distal aspect of the patella in horses. *Equine Vet J*. 1990;22(3):157–163.
45. Engelbert TA, Tate LP, Richardson DC, et al. Lateral patellar luxation in miniature horses. *Vet Surg*. 1993;22(4):293–297.
46. Pagliara E, Cantatore F, Pallante M, et al. Lateral patellar instability in Standardbred horses at the weanling age: clinical and morphological features in four cases (2017–2019). *Equine Vet Educ*. 2022;34(1):47–53.
47. Hall MS, Jalim SL, Russell TM. Distal luxation of the patella in a horse. *Aust Vet J*. 2010;88(10):396–398.
48. Pérez-Nogués M, Derham A, Marmion J, et al. Progression of shallow medial femoral condyle radiographic lucencies in Thoroughbred repository radiographs and their influence on future racing careers. *Equine Vet J*. 2021;53(2):287–293.
49. Scott GS, Crawford WH, Colahan PT, et al. Arthroscopic findings in the horses with subtle radiographic evidence of osteochondral lesions of the medial femoral condyle: 15 cases (1995–2002). *J Am Vet Med Assoc*. 2004;224(11): 1823–1826.
50. Howard RD, McIlwraith CW, Trotter GW. Arthroscopic surgery for subchondral cystic lesions of the medial femoral condyle in horses: 41 cases (1988–1991). *J Am Vet Med Assoc*. 1995;206(6):842–850.
51. Hance SR, Schneider RK, Embertson RM, et al. Lesions of the caudal aspect of the femoral condyles in foals: 20 cases (1980–1990). *J Am Vet Med Assoc*. 1993;202(4):637–646.
52. Haggett EF, Foote AK, Head MJ, et al. Necrosis of the femoral condyles in a four-week-old foal: clinical, imaging and histopathological features. *Equine Vet J*. 2012;41:91–95.
53. Bonilla AG, Bertone AL, Brokken MT, et al. Concurrent or sequential tibial subchondral cystic lesions in 4 horses with medial femoral condyle subchondral cystic lesions. *J Am Vet Med Assoc*. 2016;249(11):1313–1318.
54. Textor JA, Nixon AJ, Lumsden J, et al. Subchondral cystic lesions of the proximal extremity of the tibia in horses: 12 cases (1983–2000). *J Am Vet Med Assoc*. 2001;218(3):408–413.
55. Audigié F. *Unpublished Data*. 2011.
56. Dillenbeck MB, Whitcomb J, Dechant, et al. Ultrasonographic diagnosis of lateral meniscal rupture in two horses with severe lameness. *Equine Vet Educ*. 2022;34(1): 21–26.
57. Edwards RB, Nixon AJ. Avulsion of the cranial cruciate ligament insertion in a horse. *Equine Vet J*. 1996;28(4): 334–336.
58. Rose PL, Graham JP, Moore I, et al. Imaging diagnosis—caudal cruciate ligament avulsion in a horse. *Vet Radiol Ultrasound*. 2001;42(5):414–416.
59. Dyson S, Wright I, Kold S, et al. Clinical and radiographic features, treatment and outcome in 15 horses with fracture of the medial aspect of the patella. *Equine Vet J*. 1992;24(4):264–268.
60. Dyson SJ. Stifle trauma in the event horse. *Equine Vet Educ*. 1994;6:234.
61. McLellan J, Plevin S, Taylor E. Concurrent patellar fracture and lateral collateral ligament avulsion as a result of trauma in three horses. *J Am Vet Med Assoc*. 2012;240(10): 1218–1222.
62. Gottlieb R, Whitcomb MB, Vaughan B, et al. Ultrasonographic appearance of normal and injured lateral patellar ligaments in the equine stifle. *Equine Vet J*. 2016;48(3): 299–306.
63. Rubio-Martínez LM, Redding WR, Bladon B, et al. Fracture of the medial intercondylar eminence of the tibia in horses treated by arthroscopic fragment removal (21 horses). *Equine Vet J*. 2018;50(1):60–64.
64. Ross MW. The crus. In: Ross MW, Dyson SJ, eds. *Diagnosis and Management of Lameness in the Horse*. 2nd ed. St Louis: Elsevier/Saunders; 2011:526.
65. Blikslager AT, Bristol DG. Avulsion of the origin of the peroneus tertius tendon in a foal. *J Am Vet Med Assoc*. 1994;204(9):1483–1485.
66. Holcombe SJ, Bertone AL. Avulsion fracture of the origin of the extensor digitorum longus muscle in a foal. *J Am Vet Med Assoc*. 1994;204(10):1652–1654.
67. Engiles JB, Orsini JA, Ross MW. What is your diagnosis? Fracture of the fibula. *J Am Vet Med Assoc*. 2004;224(9):1429–1430.
68. Studdert VP, Gay CC. *Blood DC: Saunders Comprehensive Veterinary Dictionary*. 4th ed. St Louis: Elsevier/Saunders; 2012.
69. Milner PI. Calcinosis Circumscripta in the horse. *Equine Vet Educ*. 2009;21:589.
70. Bertone A. Infectious arthritis. In: Ross MW, Dyson SJ, eds. *Diagnosis and Management of Lameness in the Horse*. 2nd ed. St Louis: Elsevier/Saunders; 2011:677.
71. Neil KM, Axon JE, Begg AP, et al. Retrospective study of 108 foals with septic osteomyelitis. *Aust Vet J*. 2010; 88(1–2):4–12.

ELECTRONIC RESOURCES

Additional information related to the content in Chapter 21 can be found online at eBooks.Health.Elsevier.com.

- Chapter Quiz

CHAPTER 22

Equine Tarsus

Jody E. Lawver

TARSAL ANATOMY

The equine tarsus is a complex joint composed of a large centrally located talus that articulates with the tibial cochleae proximally, the calcaneus plantarly and medially, and central and fourth tarsal bones distally. The calcaneus has a large medial rectangular projection, the sustentaculum tali, that forms the osseous boundaries of the tarsal canal for passage of the lateral digital flexor tendon. The elongated calcaneal tuber provides a broad surface for the common calcaneal tendon insertion. The fourth tarsal bone is the largest of the cuboidal bones, located laterally, and spans the height of both the central tarsal and third tarsal bone which are large flat bones stacked upon one another. The smaller first and second tarsal bones are usually fused and located plantaromedially. There are five main joints of the tarsus, including the high motion tibiotarsal (also called tarsocrural) joint and low motion talocalcaneal, talocalcaneal-centroquartal (proximal intertarsal), centrodistal (also called distal intertarsal), and tarsometatarsal joints.[1] The tibiotarsal, talocalcaneal, and proximal intertarsal joints communicate in all horses.[2] The centrodistal and tarsometatarsal joints communicate in approximately a third of horses.

A myriad of tendons and ligaments support and traverse the tarsus. Separation into four quadrants, dorsal, plantar, medial, and lateral, simplifies anatomic understanding (Box 22.1). A recent review of radiographic tarsal soft tissue attachments is available.[3]

Neonatal and Juvenile Tarsus

Normal tarsal cuboidal bones are all present and nearly fully ossified in a skeletally mature foal at birth with only slightly rounded bone margins and mildly widened joint spaces. The talar trochleae should be convex at birth but may have slightly roughed or granular margins. The tibial medial malleolus is incompletely ossified, often with mildly roughened margin but is not a separate apophysis. The tibial lateral malleolus and calcaneal tuber are separate apophyses usually present at birth or shortly after and fuse by 3 months (see Fig. 22.18) and between 16 and 28 months, respectively.[4,5] The third metatarsal bone proximal physis and usually the first and second tarsal bones should be completely fused at birth.[5] The distal tibial physis fuses between 17 and 24 months.[4] Endochondral, apophyseal, and physeal ossification is generally a bilaterally symmetric process and radiographs of both tarsi should be acquired for comparison of questionable abnormalities.

Normal Tarsal Variants and Incidental Findings

- Lateral or medial trochlear ridge of the talus slight flattening or mild focal concavity unassociated with sclerosis and/or fragmentation[6] (Fig. 22.1).
- Medial trochlear talar ridge distal margin varied shape and contour with occasional small rounded osseous fragments, referred to as "dew drop" lesions[1,6] (see Fig. 22.1).
- Fused versus unfused first and second tarsal bones.[4]

TARSAL RADIOGRAPHY

Complete tarsal evaluation requires four projections, including dorsoplantar (DPl), lateromedial (LM, 5°lateroproximal-mediodistal oblique, or 5°LPrMDiO), dorsolateral-plantaromedial (D45°MPlLO, DMPLO, or medial oblique), and dorsomedial-plantarolateral (D60°LPlMO, DLPMO, or lateral oblique) (Box 22.2). Given inherently narrowed distal tarsal joints, the horse should be square and radiographed on a level surface with x-ray beam crosshairs centered on the distal tarsus. When standard views fail to identify the cause of lameness localized to the tarsus,

Box 22.1

Soft Tissues of the Tarsus Separated Into Compartments

Dorsal Quadrant

- Cranialis tibialis musculotendinous portion with medial (cunean) tendon branch and cunean bursa
- Fibularis (peroneus) tertius ligament with lateral branch
- Talometatarsal ligament (dorsal tarsometatarsal ligament)
- Long digital extensor tendon

Medial Quadrant

- Long and three short (superficial, middle, deep) tibiotarsal collateral ligaments
- Medial digital flexor tendon

Lateral Quadrant

- Long and three short (superficial, middle, deep) tibiotarsal collateral ligaments
- Lateral digital extensor tendon

Plantar Quadrant

- Lateral digital flexor within the tarsal sheath
- Long plantar ligament
- Common calcaneal tendon:
  - Superficial digital flexor, gastrocnemius, accessory ligament (composed of the biceps femoris, semitendinosus, and vestigial soleus)
- Calcaneal bursae (subcutaneous, intertendinous, gastrocnemius calcaneal bursae):
  - Intertendinous and gastrocnemius calcaneal bursae are contiguous in all horses
  - Subcutaneous and intertendinous calcaneal bursae communicate in approximately 40% of horses

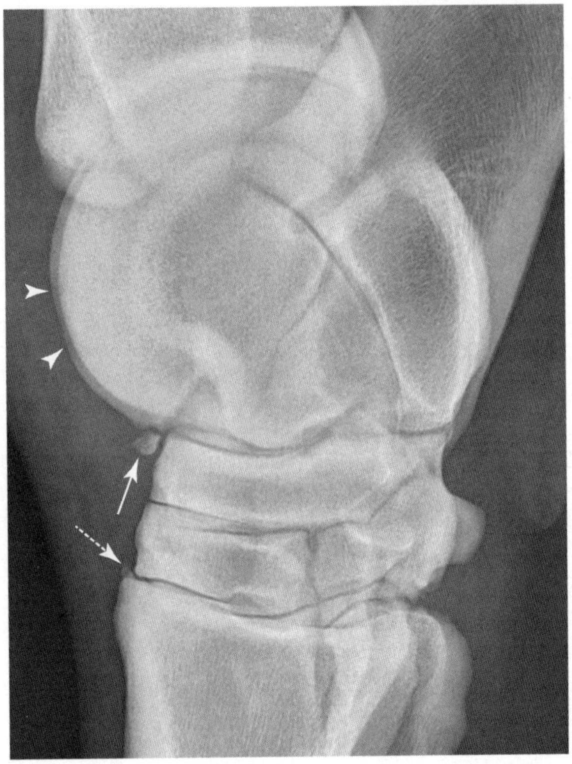

Fig. 22.1 Lateromedial (LM) projection depicting normal variants of slight medial trochlear ridge flattening (*white arrowheads*) and a separate osseous body at the distal medial trochlear ridge (*white arrow*) which should not be mistaken for osteochondrosis. Small, smoothly margined bone proliferation of the dorsal third metatarsal bone (*white dashed arrow*) with smooth margination of the third tarsal bone is generally incidental enthesopathy.

additional oblique and stressed radiographic views often aid lesion characterization (see Box 22.2).

DEVELOPMENTAL OSSEOUS CONDITIONS

Osteochondrosis and Osteochondritis Dissecans

Osteochondrosis (OC) is a common juvenile bone disorder. OC is caused by focal endochondral vascular failures often of unknown etiology,[7] and current investigations of heritable/genetic causes or acquired causes such as sepsis, physiologic or traumatic vascular insult, or metabolic/nutritional imbalances are ongoing.[7,8] Osteochondritis dissecans (OCD) is a condition in which OC leads to the separation of bone and cartilage fragments into the joint resulting in joint inflammation. Separated osteochondral fragments may remain attached or become loose within the joint and may never ossify requiring ultrasound or arthroscopy for identification. OC can occur in any breed, although is most common in Standardbreds (10.5%–35%), Warmbloods (20%), and Thoroughbreds (20%) and uncommon in ponies.[9] Affected yearlings or juvenile horses early in training generally present with variable tibiotarsal joint effusion (bog spavin) and/or variable degrees of lameness. Severity of joint effusion does not always correlate with the degree of lameness. Clinical signs are occasionally absent. Because OC is found in multiple joints in 50% of cases[7] and commonly bilateral, screening radiographs or systematic ultrasound[10] of the contralateral joint and other joints with OC predilection is often performed in racing and performance stock.

The four major tarsal OC predilection sites are within the tibiotarsal joint and include the intermediate cochlear ridge of the tibia (ICRT, also known as DIRT for distal intermediate ridge of the tibia), lateral talar trochlear ridge, medial talar trochlear ridge, and tibial medial malleolus articular margin[11–13] (Figs. 22.2 and 22.3, eFigs. 22.1 and 22.2). DMPLO and D20PLMO are the most helpful projections; thus, acquiring a D20PLMO for evaluation of the medial malleolus articular margin is crucial when evaluating horses for tarsal OC lesions. Other less common OC locations include the proximal weight-bearing portion of the medial trochlear ridge of the talus[14] and medial margin of the intermediate cochlear ridge of the talus[15] (see Fig. 22.2). These unique OC locations often require additional oblique and/or flexed projections for detection. OC of the lateral tibial malleolus and medial proximal tubercle of the talus has been reported although soft tissue avulsion fragments, particularly of the deep collateral ligaments, may mimic OC at these locations.[16]

Tarsal osteochondral lesions identified in young foals with no clinical signs may be monitored for progressive ossification with maturation however bone abnormalities are likely permanent after 5 months of age.[9,17] OC associated with joint effusion or lameness of any aged animal should prompt surgical consultation.

Radiographic features of OC include:

1. Intracapsular swelling of the tibiotarsal joint.
2. Subchondral bone margin flattening, irregularity or concave defect of parent bone generally accompanied by peripheral sclerosis.
3. Faint to well-mineralized rounded osseous fragments, although fragmentation may remain as unossified cartilage requiring ultrasound or arthroscopy for identification.
4. Eventual osteoarthritis (OA).

Fragmentation of the Proximal Talar Tubercle

Osseous fragments originating from the proximomedial tubercle of the talus (Fig. 22.4) are more common in Warmbloods and are occasionally bilateral. They may represent an additional site of OC, although trauma to the medial short deep collateral ligament, medial talocalcaneal or tarsal plantar ligament has also been proposed. Medial fragmentation of this tubercle may be more clinically significant compared to plantar fragmentation, as the medial aspect serves as the insertion site of the medial short deep collateral ligament. A calcaneal dorsoplantar skyline projection can improve localization. However, tubercle fragmentation is often incidental in sound horses without tibiotarsal effusion, so its clinical significance should be carefully weighed against other plausible causes.

Subchondral Osseous Cyst-Like Lesions

Tarsal subchondral osseous cyst-like lesions (SOCLs) are rare and sparsely reported. They occur in both older and younger horses and may be either developmental or acquired. Possible causes include joint sepsis, trauma to the articular cartilage or underlying bone, or OC. The central and third tarsal bones, talus, and distal tibia are most affected, and horses may be lame or sound, with or without joint effusion. Classically, SOCLs are centrally radiolucent or hyperintense on magnetic resonance imaging (MRI) with intense surrounding regional sclerosis (Fig. 22.5). A flexed lateral projection to remove calcaneal summation may assist in identifying talar[18] (Fig. 22.6, eFig. 22.3) or distal tibial SOCLs since standard radiographs occasionally appear normal. As many SOCLs cause intense sclerosis additional evaluation with computed tomography (CT) or MRI is helpful in differentiating a cyst-like lesion from other causes of sclerosis.[19,20]

Incomplete Cuboidal Bone Ossification (Also Termed *Aseptic Necrosis*)

If cuboidal bone ossification is incomplete, typical of premature or dysmature foals, and the foal is allowed to exercise normally, the underdeveloped bones are prone to collapse and crush injury (Fig. 22.7, eFig. 22.4). Wedge shaping that commonly

Box • 22.2

Orthogonal, Oblique, and Stressed Radiograph Projections of the Tarsus and Their Uses

Standard Projections

Dorsoplantar (DPl)

- Elevating the generator 5 to 10 degrees proximally will orient the x-ray beam through the lateral joint spaces.
- Generator at 0 degrees horizontal with the long axis of the tarsus better orients the x-ray beam through the medial joint space. Preferred view as most distal tarsal pathology occurs medially.

Lateromedial (5°lateroproximal-mediodistal oblique or 5°LPrMDiO)

- 5 degrees lateral obliquity of the x-ray generator plantar from midsagittal plane is preferred over true 0 degrees LM projections as it will completely superimpose the talar trochlea, improving talocalcaneal joint space evaluation (Fig. 22.2A).

Dorsolateral-plantaromedial (D45°MPlLO, DMPLO, or medial oblique) (Fig. 22.2C).

Dorsomedial-plantarolateral (D60°LPlMO, DLPMO, or lateral oblique) (Fig. 22.2D).

Additional Projections

Dorso20°lateral to plantaromedial oblique (D20°LPlMO)

- Evaluation of the medial malleolar subchondral bone for osteochondrosis (Fig. 22.2B).
- Detection of incomplete sagittal fractures of the talus in racing breeds (Fig. 22.17B).

Flexed plantar 75 degrees proximal- plantarodistal oblique (Flexed Pl75°PrPDiO or calcaneal skyline)

- Improved visualization of the proximal talar tubercle for fragmentation or avulsion (Fig. 22.4E).
- Plantaroproximal view of the sustentaculum tali, tarsal groove and calcaneal tuber for abnormal osseous remodeling or lysis, or mineralization of the lateral digital flexor tendon.
- Highlights a small portion of the plantar medial trochlear ridge and medial aspect of the talocalcaneal joint.

Flexed lateromedial (Flexed LM)

- Offsets tibial cochleae from the weight-bearing portion of the proximal talar trochleae for proximoplantar osteochondral fragments, fractures, or bone remodeling. Adding mild proximal or distal obliquity to the flexion can additionally reduce medial/lateral talar trochlea superimposition augmenting individual evaluation (Fig. 22.6C).
- Assists in identification of distal tarsal luxations (Fig. 22.11).

Flexed dorsoplantar (Flexed DPl)

- Removes superimposition of the talar trochlea from the calcaneus providing orthogonal plane evaluation of individual trochlea and cochlea subchondral bone margins.
- Challenging to perform.

Dorso 30 degrees medial to plantarolateral oblique (D30°MPlLO)

- Offsets proximal talar tubercle from the talus in cases of tubercle fragmentation (Fig. 22.4D).
- In clinically suspected central tarsal bone sagittal fractures, multiple obliques D30-550°MPlLO at 5 to 10 degree intervals may be necessary to align the x-ray beam tangential to the fracture plane (Fig. 22.15C).

Dorsoplantar (DPl) with medial or lateral limb stress

- Confirms pathologic joint space widening of collateral ligament ruptures and/or osseous malalignment indicative of subluxation/luxation (Fig. 22.14C).

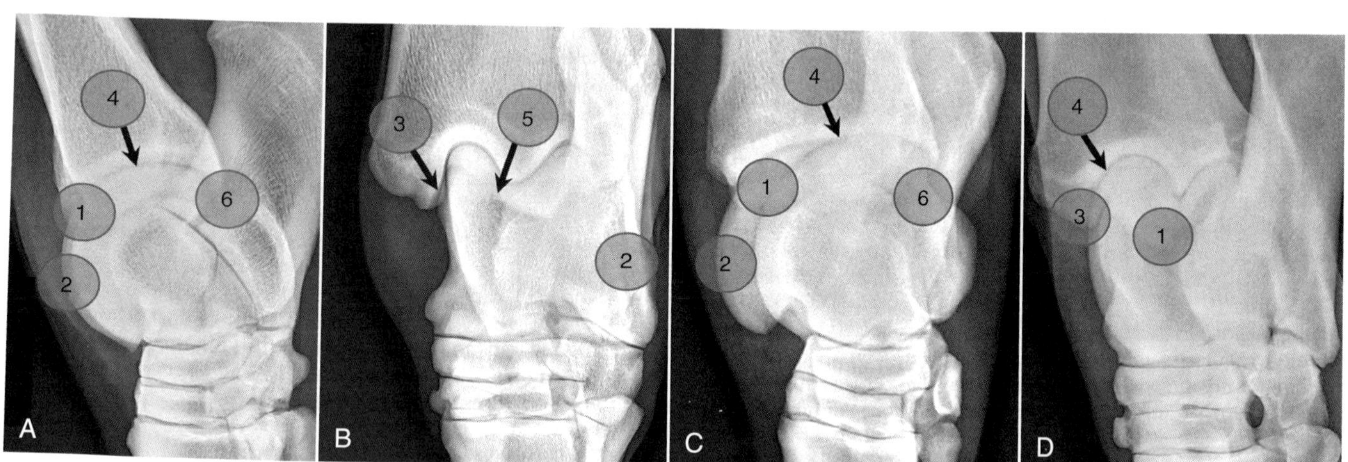

Fig. 22.2 Lateral **(A)**, D20PLMO **(B)**, DMPLO **(C)**, and DPLMO **(D)** normal tarsal radiographs illustrating the predilection sites of osteochondritis dissecans. *1,* Intermediate cochlear ridge of the tibia (ICRT); *2,* lateral talar trochlear ridge; *3,* tibial medial malleolus; *4,* medial talar trochlear ridge (uncommon); *5,* medial margin intermediate cochlear ridge of the tibia (uncommon); *6,* proximal tubercle of the talus (not conclusively osteochondrosis etiology).

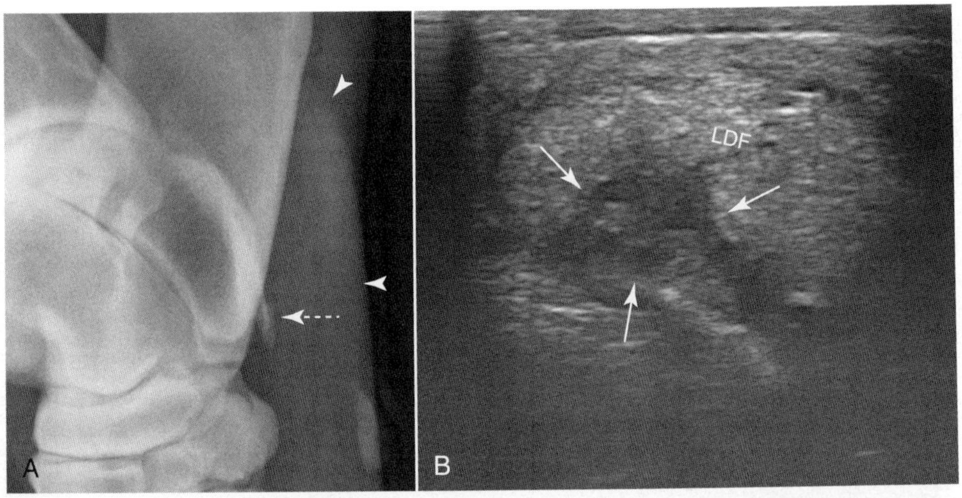

Fig. 22.26 **A,** Lateromedial (LM) radiograph of a 6-year-old Friesian mare with right pelvic limb lameness and progressive plantar tarsal curb-like swelling showing plantar soft tissue convexity (*white arrowheads*) and smoothly margined mineral proliferation distal to the sustentacula tali (*white dashed arrow*). Differentials for the mineral include exostosis or dystrophic mineralization of the tarsal sheath or lateral digital flexor tendon and are often associated with extensive tarsal sheath pathology warranting ultrasound interrogation. **B,** Plantar ultrasound revealed proliferative tarsal sheath effusion along with severe generalized enlargement and central large hypoechoic core lesion (*white arrows*) of the lateral digital extensor just proximal to the chestnut. *LDF,* Lateral digital flexor. (Ultrasound image courtesy Caitlyn Horne, DVM, DACVSMR.)

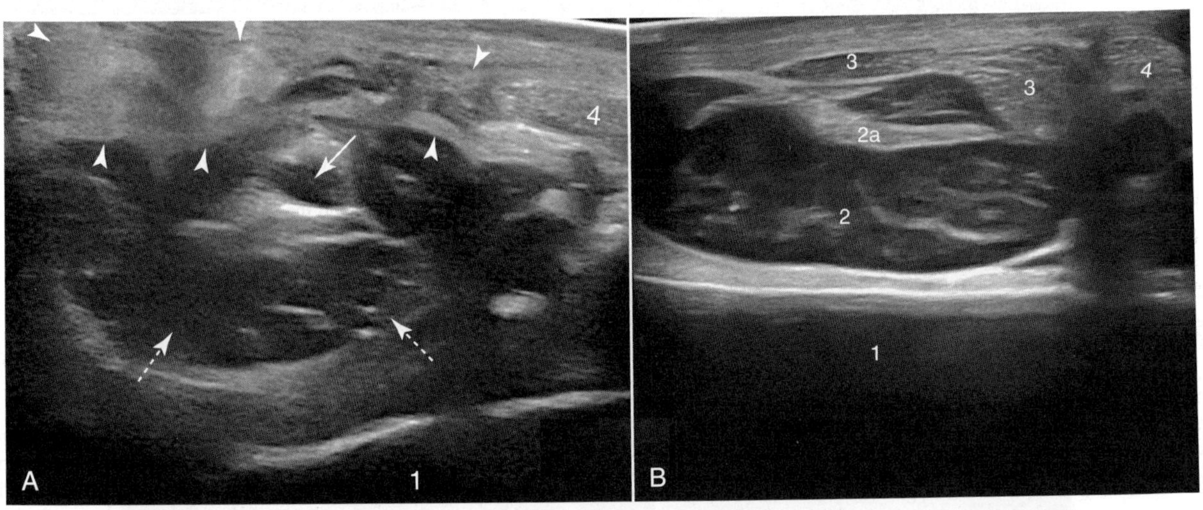

Fig. 22.27 Ultrasound images of a 4-year-old Thoroughbred gelding with recent lameness and dorsal tarsal soft tissue swelling and pain. The tarsus was not able to be extended when the stifle was flexed. In **A and B,** the ultrasound transducer is positioned perpendicular to the long axis of limb just proximal to the tibiotarsal joint, resulting in a short axis (transverse) image of the combined fibularis tertius ligament and cranialis tibialis musculotendinous portion. In **A,** the fibularis tertius ligament (*white arrowheads*) is enlarged and misshapen with complete loss of architecture replaced by heterogeneous tissue and no identifiable normal ligament fibers. The surrounding cranialis tibialis muscle (*white dashed arrows*) is enlarged and rounded with a hypoechoic tear in the central forming tendon (*white arrow*). This clinical picture is compatible with hyperextension injury and severe fibularis tertius desmitis and cranialis tibialis musculotendinitis with small central tear. Compare with the normal contralateral limb in **B**. *1,* Distal tibia; *2,* cranialis tibialis muscular portion; *2a,* cranialis tibialis tendinous portion; *3,* fibularis tertius ligament; *4,* long digital extensor tendon. In both images, medial is to the *left* and cranial is to the *top* of the images.

tendon.[66–68] Ultrasound of the common tendon components, surrounding bursae, and tarsal sheath is important for diagnosis and identification of comorbidities. Ultrasound characteristics of GT tendinitis generally reveal diffuse tendon enlargement and less commonly fiber disruption within the body.[69] The tendon is also prone to complications associated with plantar lacerations and wounds.[70] Injuries of the common calcaneal tendon components particularly if associated with plantar wounds should be evaluated with radiographs, including a flexed calcaneal skyline projection. This is necessary to assess for concurrent calcaneal osteitis, which often indicates a septic process and should be taken seriously given poorer outcomes.[45]

Dorsal Soft Tissue Injuries

Fibularis (Peroneus) Tertius

The fibularis tertius (FT) is entirely tendinous in the horse and represents the cranial arm of the reciprocal apparatus. At the level of the tibiotarsal joint, the FT traverses the dorsal tarsus forming a tunnel for passage of the cranialis tibialis musculotendinous junction. The FT then bifurcates into smaller dorsal and lateral branches which insert on the dorsal metatarsus and dorsal and lateral distal tarsal bones.[71,72] FT complete or partial rupture—or tendinitis are caused by hyperextension injury or trauma and will present with varying degrees of dorsal tarsal or crus swelling and lameness depending on the severity and location of the injury. While radiographs are indicated to rule out concurrent osseous trauma, ultrasound is paramount and may show tendon enlargement, margin irregularity, and variable degrees of fiber disruption (see Fig. 22.27).[73] Complete rupture results in inappropriate extension of the tarsus when the stifle is flexed.[72] Generally, rupture occurs within the mid- or distal portion, although can occur at the origin resulting in femoropatellar effusion and possibly osseous avulsion.[71,74] Dystrophic mineralization or insertional enthesopathy of the FT is occasionally identified radiographically and generally well tolerated when not associated with other changes.

Long Digital Extensor Tenosynovitis

A synovial sheath envelops the long digital extensor tendon (LoDET) as it traverses the dorsal tarsus and is a palpable structure just lateral to the medial trochlear ridge. The proximal, middle, and distal dorsal tarsal retinaculae are situated between the LoDET and skin and generally prevent visualization of LoDET sheath effusion. Distal to the tarsus, the lateral digital extensor tendon, which also has its own sheath, fuses with the LoDET and travels dorsally along the metatarsus to insert on the distal phalanx. Severing of these tendons once conjoined below the metatarsus has a poorer prognosis than more proximal at the tarsus/metatarsus, where they are separated and the retinacular attachments afford collateral stabilization.[75]

Focal Peritarsal Cellulitis

This is a rare, acute, and painful cellulitis localized to the dorsal tarsus and results in severe, sudden-onset lameness. It is characterized by expansion and increased echogenicity of the subcutaneous and peritendinous structures, with diffuse hypoechoic fluid locules,[76] and may be associated with septic tenosynovitis of the LoDET.[77] Early and aggressive diagnosis and treatment without complications of osteomyelitis or laminitis are associated with favorable outcomes.

Acknowledgment

With special thanks to prior authors of this chapter for their contributions.

REFERENCES

1. Espinosa-Mur P, Cote N, Desjardins MR. Arthroscopic removal of osteochondral fragments in the dorsal pouch of the proximal intertarsal joint in 29 horses. *Vet Surg*. 2018;47(4):555–565.
2. Bell BT, Baker GJ, Foreman JH, Abbott LC. In vivo investigation of communication between the distal intertarsal and tarsometatarsal joints in horses and ponies. *Vet Surg*. 1993;22(4):289–292.
3. Casillas JM, Jacobs CC, Manfredi JM. Radiographic localization of the attachments of soft tissue structures in the tarsal region of horses. *Am J Vet Res*. 2020;81(5):406–415.
4. Butler JR, Colles CM, Dyson SJ, Kold SE. *The tarsus. Clinical Radiology of the Horse*. 4th ed. John Wiley & Sons; 2017:349–398.
5. Rogers CW, Gee EK, Dittmer K. Growth and bone development in the horse: when is a horse skeletally mature? *Animals (Basel)*. 2021;11(3):632.
6. Hinkle FE, Johnson SA, Selberg KT, Barrett MF. A review of normal radiographic variants commonly mistaken for pathological findings in horses. *Equine Vet Educ*. 2020;32(12):664–672.
7. Olstad K, Ekman S, Carlson CS. An update on the pathogenesis of osteochondrosis. *Vet Pathol*. 2015;52(5): 785–802.
8. Hendrickson EH, Lykkjen S, Dolvik NI, Olstad K. Prevalence of osteochondral lesions in the fetlock and hock joints of Standardbred horses that survived bacterial infection before 6 months of age. *BMC Vet Res*. 2018;14(1):143.
9. Ortved K. Surgical management of osteochondrosis in foals. *Vet Clin North Am Equine Pract*. 2017;33(2):379–396.
10. Hoey S, O'Sullivan J, Byrne J, Devine S, Toomey W, McAllister H, et al. Ultrasound screening protocol for osteochondrosis at selected predilection sites in Thoroughbred yearlings. *Ir Vet J*. 2022;75(1):3.
11. Grevenhof EM, Ducro BJ, Van Weeren PR, Van Tartwijk JMFM, Van den Belt AJ, Bijma P. Prevalence of various radiographic manifestations of osteochondrosis and their correlations between and within joints in Dutch Warmblood horses. *Equine Vet J*. 2009;41(1):11–16.
12. James O, Payne R, Bathe A, Greet T, Wylie C. Arthroscopy of the dorsal and plantar pouches of the tarsocrural joint for the treatment of osteochondritis dissecans in the horse: clinical features and follow-up. *Vet Surg*. 2016;45(8):1049–1055.
13. Oliver LJ, Baird DK, Baird AN, Moore GE. Prevalence and distribution of radiographically evident lesions on repository films in the hock and stifle joints of yearling Thoroughbred horses in New Zealand. *N Z Vet J*. 2011;59(4):202–209.
14. Simpson CM, Lumsden JM. Unusual osteochondral lesions of the talus in a horse. *Aust Vet J*. 2001;79(11):752–755.
15. Kadic LIM, Rodgerson DH, Newsom LE, Spirito M. Description of a rare osteochondrosis lesion of the medial aspect of the distal intermediate ridge of the tibia in seven Thoroughbred horses (2008-2018). *Vet Radiol Ultrasound*. 2019;60(3):285–290.
16. Espinosa-Mur P, Lacourt M, Alexander K, David F, Laverty S. Fragmentation of the proximal tubercle of the talus in horses: 9 cases (2004–2010). *J Am Vet Med Assoc*. 2013;243(7):984–991.
17. Vanderperren K, Raes E, Van Bree H, Saunders JH. Diagnostic imaging of the equine tarsal region using radiography and ultrasonography. Part 2: bone disorders. *Vet J*. 2009;179(2):188–196.
18. Montgomery LJ, Juzwiak JS. Subchondral cyst-like lesions in the talus of four horses. *Equine Vet Educ*. 2009;21(12): 629–636.
19. Dyson S. Lameness associated with mineralization of the central tarsal bone and a small osseous cyst-like lesion in two sport horses. *J Equine Vet Sci*. 2013;33(1):51–56.
20. Garcia-Lopez JM, Kirker-Head CA. Occult subchondral osseous cyst-like lesions of the equine tarsocrural joint. *Vet Surg*. 2004;33(6):557–564.
21. Baird DH, Pilsworth RC. Wedge-shaped conformation of the dorsolateral aspect of the third tarsal bone in the thoroughbred racehorse is associated with development of slab fractures at this site. *Equine Vet J*. 2001;33(7):617–620.
22. Wong DM, Scarratt WK, Maxwell V, Moon VM. Incomplete ossification of the carpal, tarsal, and navicular bones in a dysmature foal. *Equine Vet Educ*. 2003;15(2):72–81.

23. Suarez-Fuentes DG, Tatarniuk D. Clinical and radiographic findings of septic physitis in foals. *Equine Vet Educ.* 2020;32(3):e134–e139.
24. Sprackman L, Dakin SG, May SAWR. Relationship between the shape of the central and third tarsal bones and the presence of tarsal osteoarthritis. *Vet J.* 2015;203(1): 94–98.
25. Byam-Cook KL, Singer ER. Is there a relationship between clinical presentation, diagnostic and radiographic findings and outcome in horses with osteoarthritis of the small tarsal joints. *Equine Vet J.* 2009;41(2):118–123.
26. Fairburn A, Dyson S, Murray R. Clinical significance of osseous spurs on the dorsoproximal aspect of the third metatarsal bone. *Equine Vet J.* 2010;42(7):591–599.
27. Smith RK, Dyson SJ, Schramme MC, Head MJ, Payne RJ, Platt D, et al. Osteoarthritis of the talocalcaneal joint in 18 horses. *Equine Vet J.* 2005;37(2):166–171.
28. Raes EV, Vanderperren K, Pille F, Saunders JH. Ultrasonographic findings in 100 horses with tarsal region disorders. *Vet J.* 2010;184(2):201–209.
29. Barrett MF, Selburg KT, Johnson SA, Hersman J, Frisbie DD. High field magnetic resonance imaging contributes to diagnosis of equine distal tarsus and proximal metatarsal lesions: 103 cases. *Vet Radiol Ultrasound.* 2018;59(5):587–596.
30. Barker WHJ, Smith MRW, Minshall GJ, Wright IM. Soft tissue injuries of the tarsocrural joint: a retrospective analysis of 30 cases evaluated arthroscopically. *Equine Vet J.* 2013;45(4):435–441.
31. Keller SA, Furst AE, Kircher P, Ringer S, Kuemmerle JM. Locking compression plate fixation of equine tarsal subluxations. *Vet Surg.* 2015;44(8):949–956.
32. Dowling BA, Dart AJ, Hodgson DR. Surgical treatment of tarsometatarsal joint luxation in a miniature horse foal. *Aust Vet J.* 2000;78(10):683–684.
33. Abuja GA, Bubeck KA, Quinteros DD, Garcia-Lopez JM. Surgical treatment of distal tarsal joint luxations in three horses. *Vet Comp Orthop Traumatol.* 2013.
34. Smith MRW. Fractures of the tibial malleoli. *Equine Vet Educ.* 2012;24(10):503–506.
35. Nixon AJ. *Equine Fracture Repair.* Hoboken: John Wiley & Sons; 2020.
36. Katzman SA, Spriet MP, Beck BR, Barrett MF, Hendrickson DA. Incomplete fracture of the talus secondary to maladaptive stress remodeling in a horse. *J Am Vet Med Assoc.* 2019;254(1):102–108.
37. Gunst S, Chicca FD, Furst AE, Kuemmerle JM. Central tarsal bone fractures in horses not used for racing: computed tomographic configuration and long-term outcome of lag screw fixation. *Equine Vet J.* 2016;48(5):585–589.
38. Steel CM, Collins VL, Hance SR, Adkins AR, Hitchens PL. Prevalence, radiographic resolution and outcomes of slab fractures of the third and central tarsal bones in juvenile Thoroughbred horses. *Aust Vet J.* 2019;97(4):108–115.
39. Davidson EJ, Ross MW, Parente EJ. Incomplete sagittal fractures of the talus in 11 racehorses: outcome. *Equine Vet J.* 2005;37(6):457–461.
40. Wright L, Ekstrom CT, Kristoffersen M, Lindegaard C. Haematogenous septic arthritis in foals: short- and long-term outcome and analysis of factors affecting prognosis. *Equine Vet J.* 2017;29(6):328–336.
41. Bryant HA, Dixon JJ, Weller R, Bolt DM. Use of positive contrast radiography to identify synovial involvement in horses with traumatic limb wounds. *Equine Vet J.* 2019;51(1):20–23.
42. Barba M, Lepage OM. Diagnostic utility of computed tomography imaging in foals: 10 cases (2008–2010). *Equine Vet Educ.* 2013;25(1):29–38.
43. Munsterman AS, Alexander K, Samii VF, Latimer FG. Computed tomography in the diagnosis of septic physitis in two foals. *Equine Vet Educ.* 2007;19(4):200–206.
44. Gaschen L, LeRoux A, Trichel J, Riggs L, Bragulla HH, Rademacher N, et al. Magnetic resonance imaging in foals with infectious arthritis. *Vet Radiol Ultrasound.* 2011;52(6):627–633.
45. Post EM, Singer ER, Clegg PD, Smith RK, Cripps PJ. Retrospective study of 24 cases of septic calcaneal bursitis in the horse. *Equine Vet J.* 2003;35(8):662–668.
46. Isgren CM, Salem SE, Singer ER, Wylie CE, Lipreri G, Graham RJTY, et al. A multi-centre cohort study investigating the outcome of synovial contamination or sepsis of the calcaneal bursae in horses treated by endoscopic lavage and debridement. *Equine Vet J.* 2020;52(3):404–410.
47. Hand DR, Watkins JP, Honnas CM, Kemper D. Osteomyelitis of the sustentaculum tali in horses: 10 cases (1992-1998). *J Am Vet Med Assoc.* 2001;219(3):341–345.
48. Tommasa SD, Scharner D, Brehm W, Troillet A. Disorders of the sustentaculum tali and the medial trochlear ridge of the talus in horses: novel findings and surgical management of five cases. *Vet Rec.* 2021;188(5):e144.
49. Sherlock CE, Eggleston RB, Peroni JF, Parks AH. Desmitis of the medial tarsal collateral ligament in 7 horses. *Equine Vet Educ.* 2012;24(2):72–80.
50. Kummerle JM, Kummer MR. Arthroscopically accessible anatomy of the tarsal collateral ligaments in the horse. *Vet Surg.* 2013;42(3):267–274.
51. Whitcomb M. Ultrasonography of the equine tarsus. *AAEP Proceedings.* 2006;52:13–30.
52. Lamb L, Zubrod C, Hague B, Brakenhoff J, Major M. Clinical outcome of collateral ligament injuries of the tarsus. *Can Vet J.* 2012;53(5):518–524.
53. Raes E, Bergman HJ, Van Ryssen B, Vanderperren K, Stock E, Saunders JH. Computed tomographic features of lesions detected in horses with tarsal lameness. *Equine Vet J.* 2014;46:189–193.
54. Biggi M, Dyson SJ. Use of high-field and low-field magnetic resonance imaging to describe the anatomy of the proximal portion of the tarsal region of nonlame horses. *Am J Vet Res.* 2018;79(3):299–310.
55. Ross MW, Genovese RL. Curb. In: Ross MW, Dyson SJ, eds. *Diagnosis and Management of Lameness in the Horse.* 2nd ed. St. Louis: W.B. Saunders; 2011:792–798.
56. Paris A, Beccati F, Pepe M. Plantar fasciitis in 19 endurance horses: diagnosis, treatment and follow-up. *Equine Vet Educ.* 2020;32(1):1–10.
57. Ross MW, Genovese RL, Reef VB. Curb: a collection of plantar tarsal soft tissue injuries. *AAEP Proceedings.* 2002;48:337–342.
58. Emond AL, Seignour VC, Denoix JM. Ultrasonographic examination of the tuber calcanei area: technique and normal ultrasonographic images. *Equine Vet Educ.* 2022;34(4):192–199.
59. Wright IM, Minshall GJ. Injuries of the calcaneal insertions of the superficial digital flexor tendon in 19 horses. *Equine Vet J.* 2012;44(2):136–142.
60. Federici M, Furst AE, Hoey S, Bichofberger AS. Outcome of conservative and surgical treatment for luxations of the equine superficial digital flexor tendon from the calcaneal tuber. *Equine Vet Educ.* 2019;31(2):49–56.
61. Dyson S, Blunden A, Murray R. Magnetic resonance imaging, gross postmortem, and histological findings for soft tissues of the plantar aspect of the tarsus in normal horses. *Vet Radiol Ultrasound.* 2016;57(2):216–227.
62. Davis W, Caniglia CJ, Lustgarten M, Blackwelder T, Robertson I, Redding RW. Clinical and diagnostic imaging characteristics of lateral digital flexor tendinitis within the

tarsal sheath in four horses. *Vet Radiol Ultrasound*. 2013;54(2):166–173.
63. Dyson SJ. Bursae and other soft tissue swellings. In: Ross MW, Dyson SJ, eds. *Diagnosis and Management of Lameness in the Horse*. Philadelphia: Saunders; 2003:705–708.
64. Vanderperren K, Raes E, Hoegaerts M, Saunders JH. Diagnostic imaging of the equine tarsal region using radiography and ultrasonography. Part 1: the soft tissues. *Vet J*. 2009;182(2):179–187.
65. Minshall GJ, Wright IM. Synoviocoeles associated with the tarsal sheath: description of the lesions and treatment in 15 horses. *Equine Vet J*. 2011;43(1):71–75.
66. Jesty SA, Palmer JE, Parente EJ, Schaer TP, Wilkins PA. Rupture of the gastrocnemius muscle in six foals. *J Am Vet Med Assoc*. 2005;227(12):1965–1968.
67. Swor TM, Schneider RK, Ross MW, Hammer EJ, Tucker RL. Injury to the origin of the gastrocnemius muscle as a possible cause of lameness in four horses. *J Am Vet Med Assoc*. 2001;219(3):215–219.
68. Raes EV, Bergman EHJ, van der Veen H, Vanderperren K, Van der Vekens E, Saunders JH. Comparison of cross-sectional anatomy and computed tomography of the tarsus in horses. *Am J Vet Res*. 2011;72(9):1209–1221.
69. Redding RW. The tarsus. In: Baxter GM, ed. *Adam's and Stashak's Lameness in Horses*. 7th ed. John Wiley & Sons; 2020:657–701.
70. Bertuglia A, Puglisi G. Repair of the Achilles mechanism in a miniature horse. *Equine Vet Educ*. 2005;17(1):3–8.
71. Koenig J, Cruz A, Genovese R, Trostle S. Rupture of the peroneus tertius tendon in 27 horses. *Can Vet J*. 2005;46(6):503–506.
72. Deniox J. Peronius tertius anatomy and lesions. *Equine Vet Educ*. 2007;19(8):416–418.
73. Reimer JA, Ruggles AR, Hopper SA. Sonographic abnormalities of the dorsal tarsal region. In: 55. American Association of Equine Practitioners Proceedings; 2009:458–466.
74. Holcombe SJ, Bertone AL. Avulsion fracture of the origin of the extensor digitorum longus muscle in a foal. *J Am Vet Med Assoc*. 1994;204(11):1652–1653.
75. Elliott CRB, Vasey JR, Russell TM. Transection of the lateral and long digital extensor tendons in racehorses. *Aust Vet J*. 2012;90(1–2):20–23.
76. Pilswoth RC, Head MJ. A study of ten cases of focal peritarsal infection as a cause of severe lameness in the Thoroughbred racehorse: clinical signs, differential diagnosis, treatment and outcome. *Equine Vet J*. 2001;33(4):366–370.
77. Kalka T, Harding PG, Cullimore AM. Focal peritarsal cellulitis with long digital extensor tenosynovitis. *Equine Vet Educ*. 2022;34(5):e228–e233.

ELECTRONIC RESOURCES

Additional information related to the content in Chapter 22 can be found online at eBooks.Health.Elsevier.com

- Chapter Quiz

CHAPTER 23

Equine Carpus

Lindsey J. Gilmour

The equine carpus is a complex anatomical region comprised of seven cuboidal bones that are arranged in two rows to create three main joints: antebrachiocarpal (radiocarpal), middle carpal (intercarpal), and carpometacarpal. The proximal row of cuboidal bones contains the radial, intermediate, and ulnar carpal bones. The accessory carpal bone is situated palmar to and articulates with the radius and ulnar carpal bone. The distal row of cuboidal bones contains the second, third, and fourth carpal bones with inconsistent appearance of first and fifth carpal bones. The bulk of the horse's weight-bearing load falls upon the radial, intermediate, and third carpal bones.[1] Small intercarpal joints between articulating cuboidal bones are stabilized by numerous extracapsular and intracapsular ligaments. Range of motion within the carpus is largely limited to flexion and extension of the antebrachiocarpal and middle carpal joints while the carpometacarpal joint is relatively immobile.[2]

Indications for carpal imaging are similar to those in other areas of the equine limb and include a history of regional trauma, external wounds, soft tissue swelling or palpable thickening, pain or lameness that is relieved with regional or intra-articular diagnostic analgesia, and prepurchase examinations plus screening for incomplete ossification of cuboidal bones in foals with suspected prematurity or dysmaturity.[3] Radiographic findings should always be correlated with a complete patient history, physical and lameness exam findings, and the results of diagnostic analgesia, if performed. The focus of this chapter will be radiography of the equine carpus, which is a practical first step for diagnostic imaging of this region.

RADIOGRAPHIC STUDY ACQUISITION

Soft tissues surrounding the carpal region in a full-sized, adult horse are thin enough that the area can be successfully imaged using a standard portable x-ray machine and image receptor. At minimum, a standard radiographic study of the carpus will include four projections made with the x-ray beam centered on the middle carpal joint in a standing and evenly weight-bearing patient. Projections include dorsopalmar, lateromedial, and paired dorsolateral-palmaromedial (DLPMO) and dorsomedial-palmarolateral oblique (DMPLO) views.[3]

In many patients, the addition of one or more special views to the standard carpal study will further aid in radiographic interpretation. A flexed lateromedial projection is obtained to aid in differentiation of the cuboidal bones as the intermediate and fourth carpal bones will move proximally relative to the radial and third carpal bones, respectively. This view allows supplementary evaluation of articular surfaces and joint spaces. Its high clinical utility leads some clinicians to consider this view part of a standard carpal study.[1] Three additional flexed dorsoproximal-dorsodistal oblique projections, also called tangential or "skyline" views, can be made at increasing angles from the horizontal plane (Fig. 23.1). One or more skyline views can be added to a study for the purpose of enhanced evaluation of the dorsal aspects of the distal row of carpal bones, proximal row of carpal bones, and the distal radius.

Radiographic projections made while stress is manually applied to the carpal joints can be used to diagnose and/or characterize joint subluxation that is otherwise suspected based on clinical examination of a patient. The typical flexed lateral radiographic projection can be considered a stress projection, while others include a lateral view with the carpus held in extension and dorsopalmar views made while lateral or medial bending pressure is applied to the carpus. Stress projections are employed in an attempt to demonstrate abnormal dorsopalmar or mediolateral movements within the carpus that result in joint space widening and asymmetry secondary to partial or complete rupture of the supporting soft tissue structures. Manipulation of unstable joints in this manner is expected to be very painful for the patient. Adequate sedation and analgesia are critical to perform stress radiographs humanely in these cases. Radiation safety should not be compromised, and the diagnostician must ensure that patient and equipment handlers are wearing protective equipment with their hands always positioned outside of the primary x-ray beam.[4]

Carpal lesions are bilateral in many instances. Radiographic examination of both carpi can be especially valuable when investigating an equine patient for stress-related pathology, fractures and osteochondral fragments, and developmental disorders. It is also important to note that normal radiographs do not necessarily indicate lack of osseous or soft tissue pathology. There are many reports where radiographic findings (or lack thereof) conflict with findings of other imaging modalities such as ultrasound, computed tomography, magnetic resonance imaging, and arthroscopy.[1]

NORMAL ANATOMICAL VARIANTS AND INCIDENTAL FINDINGS

Medial and Lateral Protrusions on the Caudal Aspect of Distal Radial Physis

The caudomedial and caudolateral aspects of the distal radius have normal osseous projections at the level of the physis that are highlighted on lateral, DLPMO, and DMPLO projections (Fig. 23.2A). A smooth indentation in the caudal aspect of the distal radial epiphysis known as the radial fossa is also apparent on dorsopalmar projections of the carpus (Fig. 23.2B). These normal features should be recognized to avoid a misdiagnosis.

Vestigial Ulna

In some horses, a vestigial ulna is visible as a thin, mineral opacity separated from the caudolateral aspect of the radius. This structure should not be misinterpreted as periosteal proliferation or other disease[5] (Fig. 23.2C).

Incomplete Fusion of the Lateral Styloid Process

Developmentally, the distal aspect of the ulna becomes the lateral styloid process via a separate center of ossification that fuses with the radial epiphysis by 9 months of age.[1] The lateral styloid process is usually completely fused with the radius in skeletally mature horses. Occasionally, horses may have incomplete fusion that is incidental but results in radiographically visible retention of a small radiolucent zone in the distal radial epiphysis without surrounding sclerosis or bone irregularity. This should not be mistaken for an osseous cyst-like lesion or fracture[6] (Fig. 23.2C).

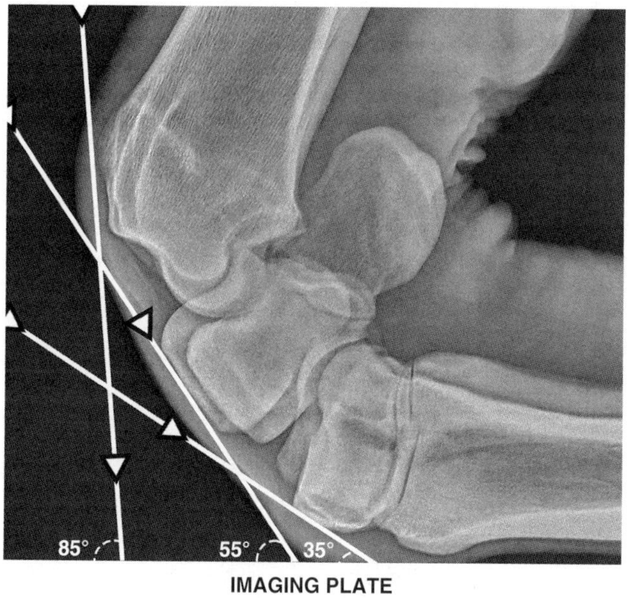

Fig. 23.1 Skyline projections of the equine carpus. To obtain the three skyline projections of the equine carpus, the carpus is flexed and the image receptor is held parallel to the metacarpus. The x-ray tube is positioned dorsal to the carpus and angled distally at approximately 85 degrees to highlight the dorsodistal aspect of the radius, 55 degrees to highlight the dorsal aspect of the proximal row of carpal bones, and 35 degrees to highlight the dorsal aspect of the distal row of carpal bones. *White lines* represent the x-ray beam angle for each projection.

Variable Appearance of Ulnar Carpal Bone

Lucent regions, irregularities, and variable shapes of the axial, non–weight-bearing surface of the ulnar carpal bone and, sometimes, the adjacent fourth metacarpal bone can be seen on the DLPMO images[5] (Fig. 23.3). These lesions are very rarely associated with lameness or joint effusion and are commonly considered as having low clinical significance despite the likelihood of an early traumatic avulsion of the lateral palmar intercarpal ligament. Radiolucencies on the subchondral, weight-bearing surface of the ulnar carpal bone are sometimes associated with lameness but may also heal before 12 months of age and/or respond to conservative management.[7]

First and Fifth Carpal Bones

Vestigial first and fifth carpal bones are inconsistently present in adult horses and should not be mistaken for osteochondral fragments. In a study of radiologic anatomic variation of the carpus, first carpal bones were found in 29% of horses and fifth carpal bones in 1.4% of horses.[5] The fifth carpal bone is usually smaller than the first carpal bone, although their size is highly variable and either bone may be present in one or both limbs. Occasionally, the first carpal bone is incompletely separated from the second carpal bone. Vestigial first and fifth carpal bones can also be associated with incidental, focal concavities or lucent defects in the adjacent cuboidal and metatarsal bones as a result of variable articulation[5] (Fig. 23.4).

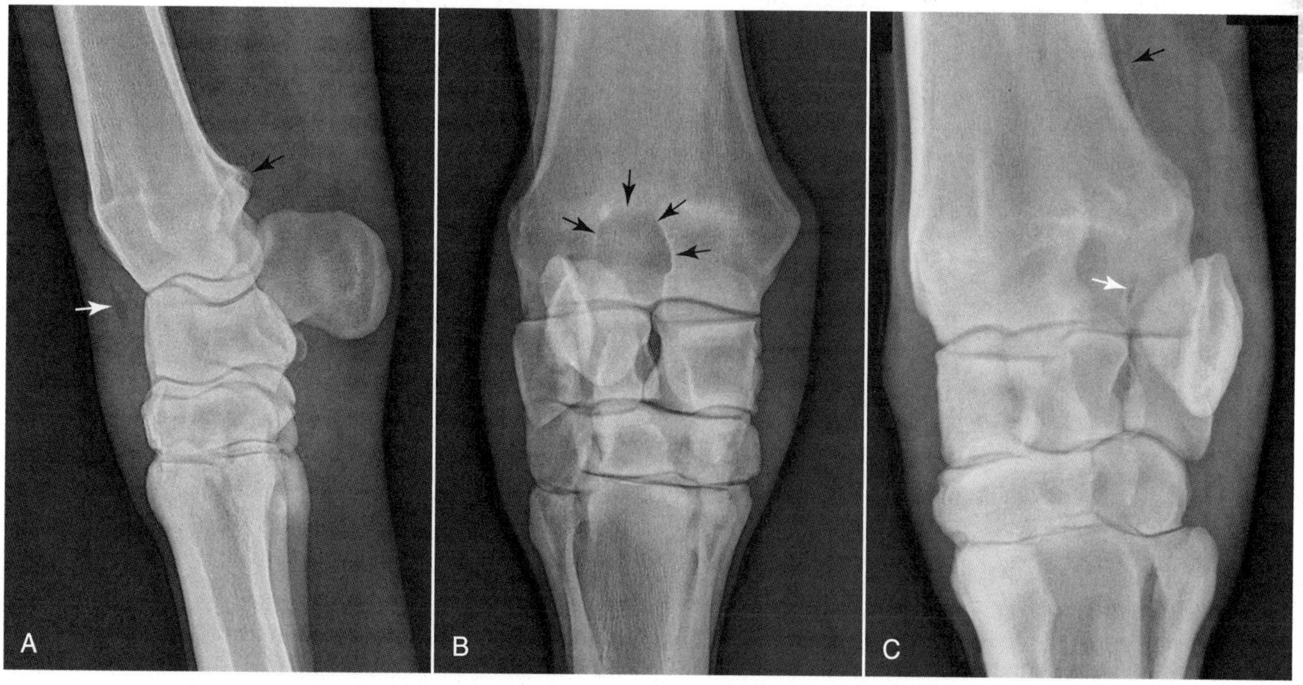

Fig. 23.2 Normal anatomical variants and incidental findings of the distal radius. **A,** Lateral view depicting normal protrusions on the caudodistal radius (*black arrow*) and small dorsal fat pad of the antebrachiocarpal joint (*white arrow*). **B,** Slightly obliqued dorsopalmar projection highlighting the well-defined radial fossa (*black arrows*). **C,** Dorsolateral-palmaromedial oblique (DLPMO) projection of a patient with a vestigial ulna (*black arrow*) represented by a thin, mineral opacity running roughly parallel with the lateral surface of the radius before fusing with it distally. The lateral styloid process of the ulna is also incompletely fused to the radial epiphysis (*white arrow*).

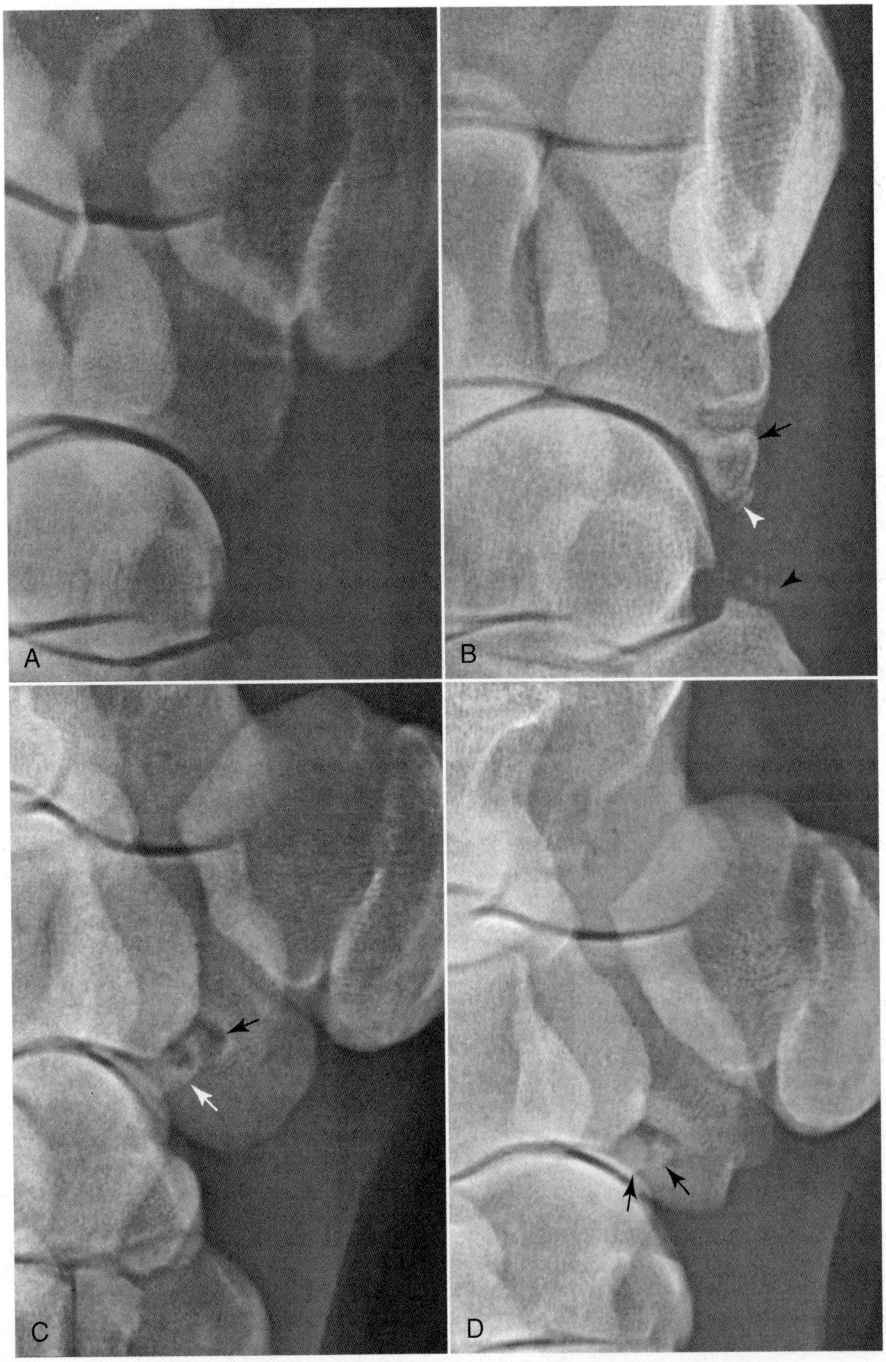

Fig. 23.3 Normal/incidental variants of the ulnar carpal bone on magnified dorsolateral-palmaromedial oblique projections. **A,** Normal/typical ulnar carpal bone. **B,** Atypical configuration of the distal palmar aspect of the ulnar carpal bone (*black arrow*) with a separate center of ossification immediately distal to this (*white arrowhead*). Note also the poorly demarcated mineralization proximal to the base of the fourth metacarpal bone (*black arrowhead*). **C,** There is an osseous cyst-like lesion in the ulnar carpal bone (*black arrow*) with an osseous fragment distal to this (*white arrow*). **D,** There are two well-defined osseous fragments overlying the ulnar carpal bone (*black arrows*) surrounded by a less well-demarcated radiolucent area in the ulnar carpal bone.

RADIOGRAPHIC ABNORMALITIES

Juvenile Orthopedic Conditions

Radiographic examination is useful for both diagnosis of and screening for developmental type orthopedic diseases in young equine patients. Some conditions have the capacity to evolve in patients between 6 and 18 months of age, becoming newly apparent, improved, worsened, or even spontaneously resolved on serial radiographs obtained throughout this timeframe.[8] Therefore, it is important to recognize that use of radiographs for screening purposes at a single time point does have limitations in this population of horses.

Incomplete Ossification

Carpal (and tarsal) cuboidal bones become mineralized via endochondral ossification that occurs in the final 2 to 3 months

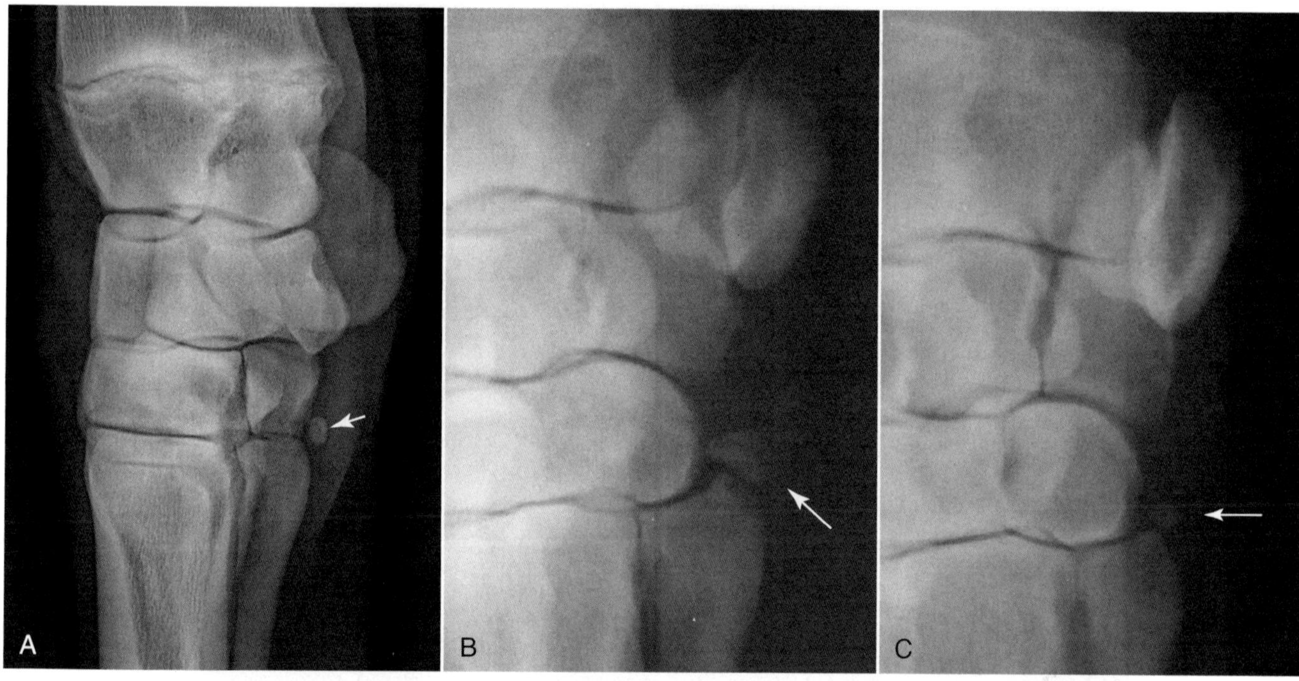

Fig. 23.4 Normal first and fifth carpal bones. **A,** Dorsomedial-palmarolateral view depicting a small, round first carpal bone (*white arrow*) adjacent to a very subtle concavity in the second carpal bone. **B–C,** Magnified dorsolateral-palmaromedial views showing normal variations of a fifth carpal bone (*white arrows*) in two different horses. In **B,** note the associated concavity in the proximal aspect of the fourth metacarpal bone (incidental).

of gestation. Mature carpal bones generally have straight edges with squared corners, congruent joint spaces with uniform width, and a trabecular bone pattern within the medullary cavity. Due to reduced mineralization of the cartilage model, radiographically immature carpal bones have:

- curved corners and rounded contour
- very little medullary trabecular detail
- wide joint spaces without flat apposing bone surfaces (Fig. 23.5A, eFig. 23.1)

Although often associated with neonatal prematurity or dysmaturity in hospitalized foals, variably incomplete ossification of the cuboidal bones has also been reported in a large percentage of full-term, clinically normal foals within 1 week of birth which suggests that cuboidal bone mineralization does not always predictably correlate with gestational length.[7] If a neonatal foal with incomplete ossification of the cuboidal bones is allowed to exercise freely, the relatively soft cartilage model of immature carpal bones can become compressed or crushed, ultimately leading to misshapen bones, angular limb deformity, and/or osteoarthritis later in life (Fig. 23.5B). All of these sequelae can result in reduced athletic performance. Early diagnosis can guide management decisions to favorably reduce the impact of incomplete cuboidal bone ossification.

Physitis/Epiphysitis

Physitis can manifest in the distal radius of young horses up to 2 years old. Physitis may be septic or aseptic in nature, and radiographic features of these two different pathogeneses can overlap. Knowledge of the normal, evolving physeal appearance in growing horses is crucial for radiographic interpretation (Fig. 23.6A). Acquisition of complementary radiographic views of the contralateral limb can be valuable for comparison and diagnosis of physitis. Radiographs have been shown to underestimate the presence and severity of physitis compared to computed tomography.[9]

Sometimes referred to as physeal dysplasia, aseptic physitis is an inflammatory but noninfectious process identified in young horses. It is correlated with nutritional factors and rapid bone growth. Radiographs may be normal in the early stages of physitis, and in more chronic stages may show:

- metaphyseal flaring
- irregularity and widening of the physis
- asymmetry and sclerosis of the metaphysis
- wedge-shaped epiphysis[10] (Fig. 23.6B)

Septic physitis is caused by hematogenous bacterial spread that is most common in younger foals between 1 week and 4 months of age.[10] This process rarely occurs in isolation and is usually associated with septicemia and respiratory, gastrointestinal, or umbilical disease. Foals with failure of passive transfer are at greatest risk for development of septic arthritis and septic physitis. The distinguishing radiographic feature of septic physitis in foals is aggressive osteolysis presenting as a focal irregularity of the physis with irregular radiolucency extending into the adjacent epiphysis and/or metaphysis (Fig. 23.6C). Detection of radiolucency and physeal irregularity is more challenging if the osteolysis extends along the entire length of the physis. The bone adjacent to the physis may be sclerotic and it may have an altered trabecular pattern, flared abaxial contour, and/or periosteal proliferation. Concurrent soft tissue swelling surrounding the affected physis and septic arthritis of the antebrachiocarpal joint or any other synovial joint are other radiographic findings that may be present in foals with septic physitis.[11] Differentiation of aseptic versus septic physitis will be further guided by patient clinical data such as the presence or absence of a fever and other systemic comorbidities.

Angular Limb Deformities

Developmental limb deformities of the carpus are common in young horses and can be congenital or acquired. They are classified into three categories: (1) angular limb deformity in which a portion of the limb is angled medially or laterally from the center line, (2) flexural deformity in which the alignment of the limb is deviated in a cranial or caudal direction, and (3)

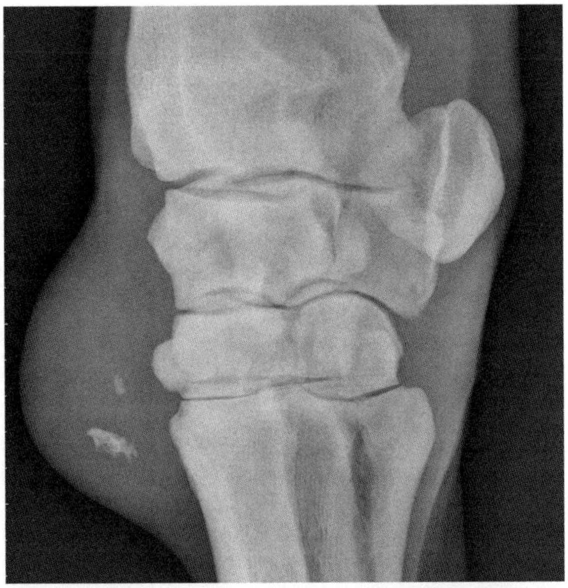

Fig. 23.27 Dorsolateral-palmaromedial projection depicting a chronic carpal hygroma in a 17-year-old mule. The focal soft tissue swelling centered dorsomedial to the carpometacarpal joint contains two foci of dystrophic mineralization. No communication with the regional synovial structures could be identified and the swelling remained static over the course of several years.

may be smooth or palisading, and concurrent enthesopathy on the dorsal aspect of the radial, intermediate, and third carpal bone is also possible.[37]

Carpal Hygroma, Synovial Hernia, and Synovial Fistula

A carpal hygroma is a nonpainful soft tissue swelling on the dorsal aspect of the carpus that is acquired following trauma or repetitive injury (Fig. 23.27).[38] Hygromata are not connected to synovial structures, although they are sometimes called "false bursae" because it is common to identify subcutaneous fluid accumulation deep to the soft tissue swelling.

Synovial hernias result from a defect in the joint capsule through which a portion of the synovial membrane (and synovial fluid) protrudes. This term is sometimes used synonymously with "synovial cyst" or "synovial ganglia," although the three terms are distinct entities as cysts do not necessarily have a patent communication with the joint cavity and ganglia do not have a synovial lining.[39] Synovial hernias are also typically nonpainful and identified as an incidental finding with contrast radiographs, ultrasound, or magnetic resonance imaging (MRI).

Synovial fistulae are communications between two synovial structures (e.g., joints and tendon sheaths) that are often presumed to be secondary to previous, concurrent trauma to the communicating structures. Fistulous communication between a carpal hygroma, the antebrachiocarpal joint, and the extensor carpi radialis tendon sheath has also been reported.[40]

Soft Tissue Trauma, Draining Tracts, Foreign Bodies

Following acute carpal trauma, radiographs are indicated to identify osseous lesions such as fractures, luxations, and avulsions as well as to assess the region for radiopaque foreign bodies. Hematomas and hemarthrosis can result in extra- and intracapsular soft tissue swelling, respectively. In the chronic stages of healing, soft tissue wounds sometimes develop suppurative draining/fistulous tracts secondary to bone sequestra or foreign material that remains embedded within the soft tissues.

Table • 23.2

Soft Tissue Swellings of the Dorsal Carpus and Their Possible Radiographic Findings Following Intralesional Contrast Medium Injection.

ETIOLOGY OF SOFT TISSUE SWELLING	EXPECTED CONTRAST RADIOGRAPHIC FINDINGS
Carpal hygroma	Contrast medium remains extracapsular and within the soft tissue swelling itself
Synovial hernia	Contrast medium can be detected in an underlying synovial cavity (joint space or tendon sheath); occasionally, contrast movement is restricted by a one-way valve effect and communication between the synovial hernia and underlying synovial cavity cannot be confirmed
Synovial fistula	Contrast medium detected in two communicating synovial structures
Draining tracts	Contrast medium may highlight the tract itself, subcutaneous pockets, foreign bodies, and/or communication between the tract and adjacent synovial cavities

Following survey radiographs, contrast medium can be aseptically injected into hygromas, synovial cavities, and draining tracts to better characterize and aid in differentiation of these various soft tissue lesions of the carpus[41] (Table 23.2).

Calcinosis Circumscripta

Calcinosis circumscripta is a collection of calcium salt deposits in the subcutaneous tissue that manifests radiographically as a granular, mineral opaque mass. This is a variation of dystrophic mineralization that is uncommonly identified at sites of previous soft tissue trauma or chronic irritation, over bony prominences and pressure points, or near joint spaces. Calcinosis circumscripta may be intra- or extracapsular.[42]

Hypertrophic Osteopathy

Hypertrophic osteopathy is characterized most commonly by painful lower limb swelling, stiffness and/or lameness, joint effusion, and/or restricted flexibility of affected joints. Radiographically, the metacarpal and metatarsal bones are affected most commonly with symmetrical, palisading periosteal proliferation along the diaphyses and metaphyses without involvement of the subchondral bone or articular surfaces. This bone proliferation can be seen in other bones including the radius and carpal bones. Similar to what is seen in small animal patients, equine hypertrophic osteopathy occurs in tandem with a variety of intrathoracic and, rarely, intra-abdominal pathology including granulomatous disease, pulmonary abscess, pneumonia, pleural space disease, and neoplasia. The osseous lesions of hypertrophic osteopathy may regress or resolve following treatment of the primary disease process.[43]

Acknowledgment

With special thanks to prior authors of this chapter for their contributions.

REFERENCES

1. Wright IM, Butler JA. Radiography and radiology of the mature carpus. *Equine Vet Educ*. 1996;8:37–42.
2. Wright IM, McIlwraith CW. Fractures of the carpus. In: Wright IM, ed. *Fractures in the Horse*. Hoboken: Wiley-Blackwell; 2022.
3. Butler J. Radiography and radiology of the carpus and proximal aspect of the metacarpus of the horse. *Practice*. 2013;35:85–90.
4. Pilsworth RC. Stress radiographs: when, how and why to use them. *Equine Vet Educ*. 2002;14, 16-16.
5. Simon V, Dyson SJ. Radiologic anatomic variation of the carpus in horses with carpal lameness and control horses. *Vet Radiol Ultrasound*. 2010;51:601–606.
6. Hinkle FE, Johnson SA, Selberg KT, Barrett MF. A review of normal radiographical variants commonly mistaken for pathological findings in horses. *Equine Vet Educ*. 2020;32:664–672.
7. Santschi EM, Prichard MA, Whitman JL, et al. Survey radiography of the carpus and tarsus in neonatal thoroughbred foals and appearance at 6 months of age. *J Equine Vet Sci*. 2018;63:55–60.
8. Jacquet S, Robert C, Valette JP, Denoix JM. Evolution of radiological findings detected in the limbs of 321 young horses between the ages of 6 and 18 months. *Vet J*. 2013;197(1):58–64.
9. Glass K, Watts AE. Septic arthritis, physitis, and osteomyelitis in foals. *Vet Clin North Am Equine Pract*. 2017;33(2): 299–314.
10. Tatarniuk DM, Trumble TN, Baxter GM, Ernst NS, McIlwraith CW, Hunt RJ. Lameness in the young horse. In: Baxter GM, ed. *Adams & Stashak's Lameness in Horses*. 7th ed. Hoboken: John Wiley & Sons; 2020.
11. Suarez-Fuentes DG, Tatarniuk DM. Clinical and radiographic findings of septic physitis in foals. *Vet Comp Orthop Traumatol*. 2020;03(02):e134–e139.
12. Stashak TS. Lameness of the proximal limb: the carpus. In: Baxter GM, ed. *Adams & Stashak's Lameness in Horses*. 7th ed. Hoboken: John Wiley & Sons; 2020.
13. Gaughan EM. Flexural limb deformities of the carpus and fetlock in foals. *Vet Clin North Am Equine Pract*. 2017;33(2):331–342.
14. Denoix JM, Jacquet S, Lepeule J, Crevier-Denoix N, Valette JP, Robert C. Radiographic findings of juvenile osteochondral conditions detected in 392 foals using a field radiographic protocol. *Vet J*. 2013;197(1):45–51.
15. Pilsworth R, Head M. Presales radiographic surveys in yearlings 2. Significance of lesions in the carpus, tarsus and stifle. *Practice*. 2010;32:247–253.
16. Graham RJTY, Rosanowski SM, McIlwraith CW. A 10-year study of arthroscopic surgery in racing Thoroughbreds and Quarter Horses with osteochondral fragmentation of the carpus. *Equine Vet J*. 2020;52:225–231.
17. Ramos S, Pinto A, Crespo J, et al. Osteochondrosis (osteochondritis dissecans) in Lusitano horses. *Prevalence and characteristics, J Equine Vet Sci*. 2022;117.
18. Garvican E, Clegg P. Clinical aspects of the equine carpal joints. *Companion Anim*. 2007;12:5–12.
19. Panizzi L, Barber SM, Lang HM, Carmalt JL. Carpometacarpal osteoarthritis in thirty-three horses. *Vet Surg*. 2009;38:998–1005.
20. Malone ED, Les CM, Turner TA. Severe carpometacarpal osteoarthritis in older Arabian horses. *Vet Surg*. 2003;32:191–195.
21. Schneider RK, Bramlage LR, Moore RM, Mecklenburg LM, Kohn CW, Gabel AA. A retrospective study of 192 horses affected with septic arthritis/tenosynovitis. *Equine Vet J*. 1992;24(6):436–442.
22. Steel CM, Hunt AR, Adams PL, et al. Factors associated with prognosis for survival and athletic use in foals with septic arthritis: 93 cases (1987–1994). *J Am Vet Med Assoc*. 1999;215(7):973–977.
23. Hardy J. Etiology, diagnosis, and treatment of septic arthritis, osteitis, and osteomyelitis in foals. *Clin Tech Equine Pract*. 2006;5(4):309–317.
24. Lindegaard C, van Galen G, Aarsvold S, Berg LC, Verwilghen D. Haematogenous septic arthritis, physitis and osteomyelitis in foals. A tutorial review on pathogenesis, diagnosis, treatment and prognosis. Part 1. *Equine Vet Educ*. 2021;33:659–672.
25. Ramzan PHL. A novel radiographic projection for the detection of sagittal plane slab fracture of the equine third carpal bone. *Equine Vet J*. 2019;51(2):258–260.
26. Doering AK, Reesink HL, Luedke LK, et al. Return to racing after surgical management of third carpal bone slab fractures in thoroughbred and Standardbred racehorses. *Vet Surg*. 2019;48:513–523.
27. Minshall GJ, Wright IM. Frontal plane fractures of the accessory carpal bone and implications for the carpal sheath of the digital flexor tendons. *Equine Vet J*. 2014;45(5):579–584.
28. Dyson SJ. Fractures of the accessory carpal bone. *Equine Vet Educ*. 1990;2:188–190.
29. Smith MRW. Management of joint instability. *Equine Vet Educ*. 1990;22(3):112–114.
30. Bailey JV, Barber SM, Fretz PB, Jacobs KA. Subluxation of the carpus in thirteen horses. *Can Vet J*. 1984;25(8):311–314.
31. Russell JW, Hall MS, Kelly GM. Osteochondroma on the cranial aspect of the distal radial metaphysis causing tenosynovitis of the extensor carpi radialis tendon sheath in a horse. *Aust Vet J*. 2017;95(1–2):46–48.
32. Nixon AJ, Schachter BL, Pool RR. Exostoses of the caudal perimeter of the radial physis as a cause of carpal synovial sheath tenosynovitis and lameness in horses: 10 cases (1999–2003). *J Am Vet Med Assoc*. 2004;224(2): 264–270.
33. Wright IM, Minshall GJ. Clinical, radiological and ultrasonographic features, treatment and outcome in 22 horses with caudal distal radial osteochondromata. *Equine Vet J*. 2012;44:319–324.
34. Quiney L, Murray R, Dyson S. Management of primary injuries of the medial collateral ligament of the carpus in two horses. *J Equine Vet Sci*. 2020;86.
35. Vanslambrouck LMA, Whitcomb MB, Vaughan B. Ultrasonographic diagnosis of carpal collateral ligament injuries in 20 horses (2000–2015). *Proceedings of the 62nd Annual Convention of the Am Assoc Equine Pract*. 2016;399.
36. Beinlich CP, Nixon AJ. Radiographic and pathologic characterization of lateral palmar intercarpal ligament avulsion fractures in the horse. *Vet Radiol Ultrasound*. 2004;45(6):532–537.
37. Platt D, Wright IM. Chronic tenosynovitis of the carpal extensor tendon sheaths in 15 horses. *Equine Vet J*. 1997;29:11–16.
38. Schramme M, Schumacher J. Management of Bursitis. In: Auer JA, Kümmerle JM, Prange T, Stick JA, eds. *Equine Surgery*. 5th ed. St. Louis: Elsevier; 2019.
39. Lacourt M, MacDonald M, Rossier Y, Laverty S. Equine articular synovial cysts: 16 cases. *Vet Surg*. 2013;42: 99–106.
40. Rybar M, Fraser BSL. Surgical repair of synovial fistulae between a carpal hygroma, the tendon sheath of the extensor carpi radialis and the antebrachiocarpal joint in a horse. *Equine Vet Educ*. 2020;32:e100–e105.
41. Lamb CR. Contrast radiography of equine joints, tendon sheaths, and draining tracts. *Vet Clin North Am Equine Pract*. 1991;7(2):241–257.

42. Tóth F, Schumacher J, Newman S. Calcinosis circumscripta in the antebrachiocarpal joint of a horse. *Equine Vet Educ.* 1991;21:584–588.
43. Mair TS, Dyson SJ, Fraser JA, Edwards GB, Hillyer MH, Love S. Hypertrophic osteopathy (Marie's disease) in Equidae: a review of twenty-four cases. *Equine Vet J.* 1996;28:256–262.

ELECTRONIC RESOURCES

Additional information related to the content in Chapter 23 can be found online at eBooks.Health.Elsevier.com.

- Chapter Quiz

CHAPTER 24

Equine Metacarpus and Metatarsus

Erin G. Porter

Throughout this chapter, we will refer to the metacarpus and metatarsus collectively as the metacarpus; however, discussion also applies to the metatarsus unless otherwise specified. Relevant anatomical and pathological differences between the metacarpus and metatarsus will be discussed. In order to obtain high quality radiographs of the metacarpus, appropriate patient positioning and restraint is imperative. The patient should stand with all four limbs squarely positioned and equally weight bearing, and light sedation may be necessary. Comprehensive radiographic evaluation of the metacarpus includes the carpometacarpal joint in collimation proximally, and the metacarpophalangeal joint, distally. Depending on the size of the x-ray detector available, this may require a proximally and distally collimated view of each projection. A standard radiographic series includes dorsopalmar (DP), lateromedial, dorsomedial-palmarolateral oblique (DMPLO), and dorsolateral-palmaromedial oblique (DLPMO) projections. In the pelvic limb, the term *palmar* should be replaced by *plantar*. Additional projections may be indicated based on the history, clinical exam, and available imaging findings and these projections will be further discussed where indicated.

RADIOGRAPHIC ANATOMY AND COMMON VARIANTS

The Third Metacarpal Bone (The Cannon Bone)

The third metacarpal bone lies between the second and fourth metacarpal bones and is the largest of the three bones. When there is partial superimposition of two bones, as is seen in radiography of the metacarpus, a linear lucent line can be seen paralleling the region of superimposition. This phenomenon, known at Mach bands or Mach lines, is due to an optical illusion of edge enhancement created by the observer's retina, and should not be mistaken for a fracture line (Fig. 24.1).[1] While all three metacarpal bones articulate with the distal row of carpal bones to form the carpometacarpal joint, it is only the third metacarpal bone that contributes to the articulation of the metacarpophalangeal joint. The third metatarsal bone is slightly longer than the third metacarpal bone and has a more convex dorsal margin and more palmar angulation of the condyle. The principal nutrient foramen is present in the proximal to middle third of the third metacarpal bone. On the dorsopalmar projection, it is easily identified as a well-defined, oval lucency, but on lateral and oblique projections, it is obliquely oriented in the palmar cortex of the third metacarpal bone, and should not be mistaken for a fracture (Fig. 24.2). On the dorsopalmar projection, a variable number of pinpoint nutrient foramina may be seen in the proximal subchondral bone of the third metacarpal bone, just distal to the carpometacarpal joint (see Fig. 24.2). The palmaroproximal cortex of the third metacarpal bone normally has a coarser trabecular pattern than the remainder of the cortex (see Fig. 24.2). The dorsal cortex of the third metacarpal bone is normally thicker than the palmar cortex, as seen on the lateral projection, which should not be mistaken for pathology. A well-defined exostosis or "bone spur," which may be bilateral, may be present at the dorsoproximal aspect of the third metatarsal bone in up to 25% of horses, and although it is not correlated with lameness, it is more frequently seen concurrent with radiologic abnormalities of the distal tarsal joints (Fig. 24.3).[2] The condyle of the third metacarpal bone consists of medial and lateral parts separated by a sagittal ridge, which is the most distal extension of the condyle and articulates with the sagittal groove of the proximal phalanx. The medial portion of the condyle is mildly larger than the lateral portion, which can be helpful for determining laterality on the dorsopalmar projection if necessary. At birth, the proximal physis of the third metacarpal bone should be completely closed and the distal physis closes at 3 to 6 months of age.

The Second and Fourth Metacarpal and Metatarsal Bones (The Splint Bones)

The second and fourth metacarpal bones are attached to the medial and lateral aspect of the third metacarpal bone by small interosseous ligaments. It is common for these ligaments to

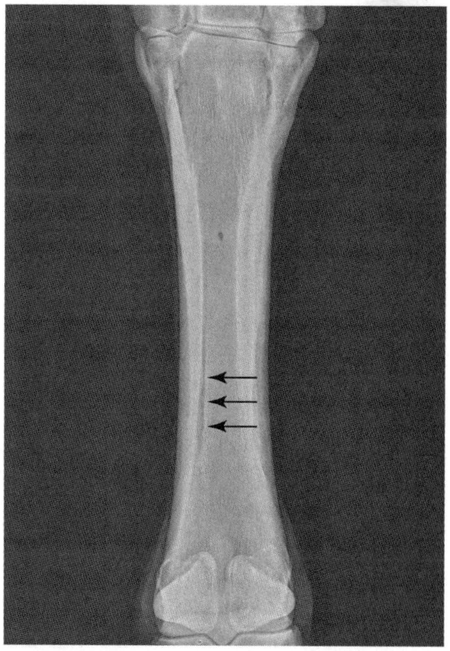

Fig. 24.1 Dorsopalmar radiograph of a metacarpus. Lateral is to the *left.* There is a radiolucent line (*arrows*) on the axial aspect of the fourth metacarpal bone. This is a Mach line artifact created at the margin of the third and fourth metacarpal bones.

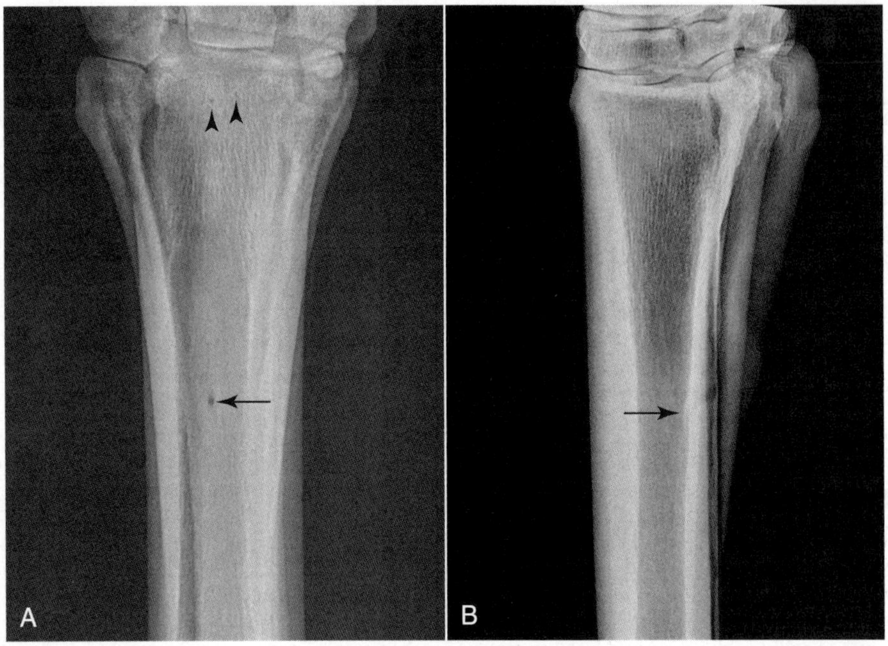

Fig. 24.2 **A,** Dorsopalmar radiograph of the metacarpus. Lateral is to the *left.* The principal nutrient foramen is seen as a well-defined, oval lucency (*arrow*) and pinpoint nutrient foramina are present in the proximal subchondral bone of the third metacarpal bone (*arrowheads*). Note the coarser trabecular pattern of the proximal aspect of the third metacarpal bone. **B,** Lateromedial projection of the metacarpus. Dorsal is to the *left.* The principal nutrient foramen is obliquely oriented in the palmar cortex of the third metacarpal bone and should not be mistaken for a fracture (*arrow*).

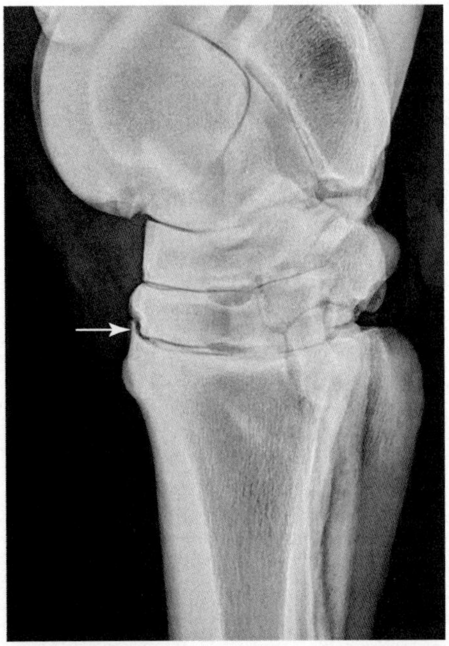

Fig. 24.3 Lateromedial projection of the proximal metatarsus. Dorsal is to the *left.* A well-defined exostosis or "bone spur" is present at the dorsoproximal aspect of the third metatarsal bone (*arrow*). This finding is often incidental and not associated with lameness.

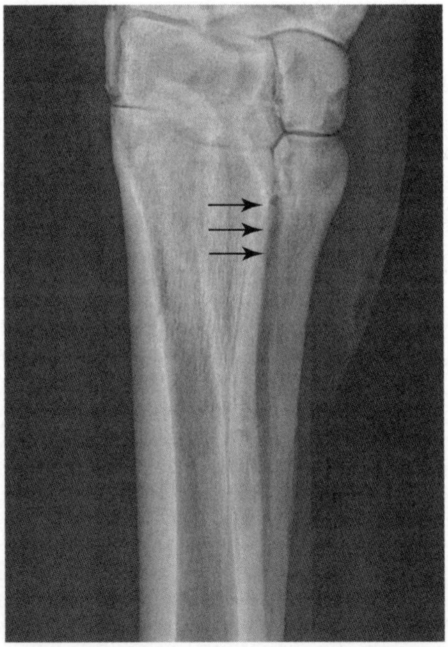

Fig. 24.4 Dorsomedial-palmarolateral oblique projection of the right metacarpus. Dorsal is to the *left.* There is smooth mineralization of the interosseous space between the second and third metacarpal bones (*arrows*). This is a common, incidental finding.

ossify over time, often bilaterally, with the medial interosseous space being more affected (Fig. 24.4).[3] Proximally, the metacarpal bones have a larger base and taper in size along their shaft towards their distal ends or "buttons," which may be bulbous, and can be palpated approximately three-quarters of the way down the metacarpus. In the forelimb, the second metacarpal bone articulates with the second carpal bone as well as a variable portion of the third carpal bone, and the fourth metacarpal bone articulates with the fourth carpal bone (Fig. 24.5). In the hindlimb, the second metatarsal bone articulates with the fused first and second tarsal bones, and the fourth metatarsal bone articulates with the fourth tarsal bone (see Fig. 24.5). In well-positioned, oblique projections of the metacarpus and metatarsus, the interosseous space between

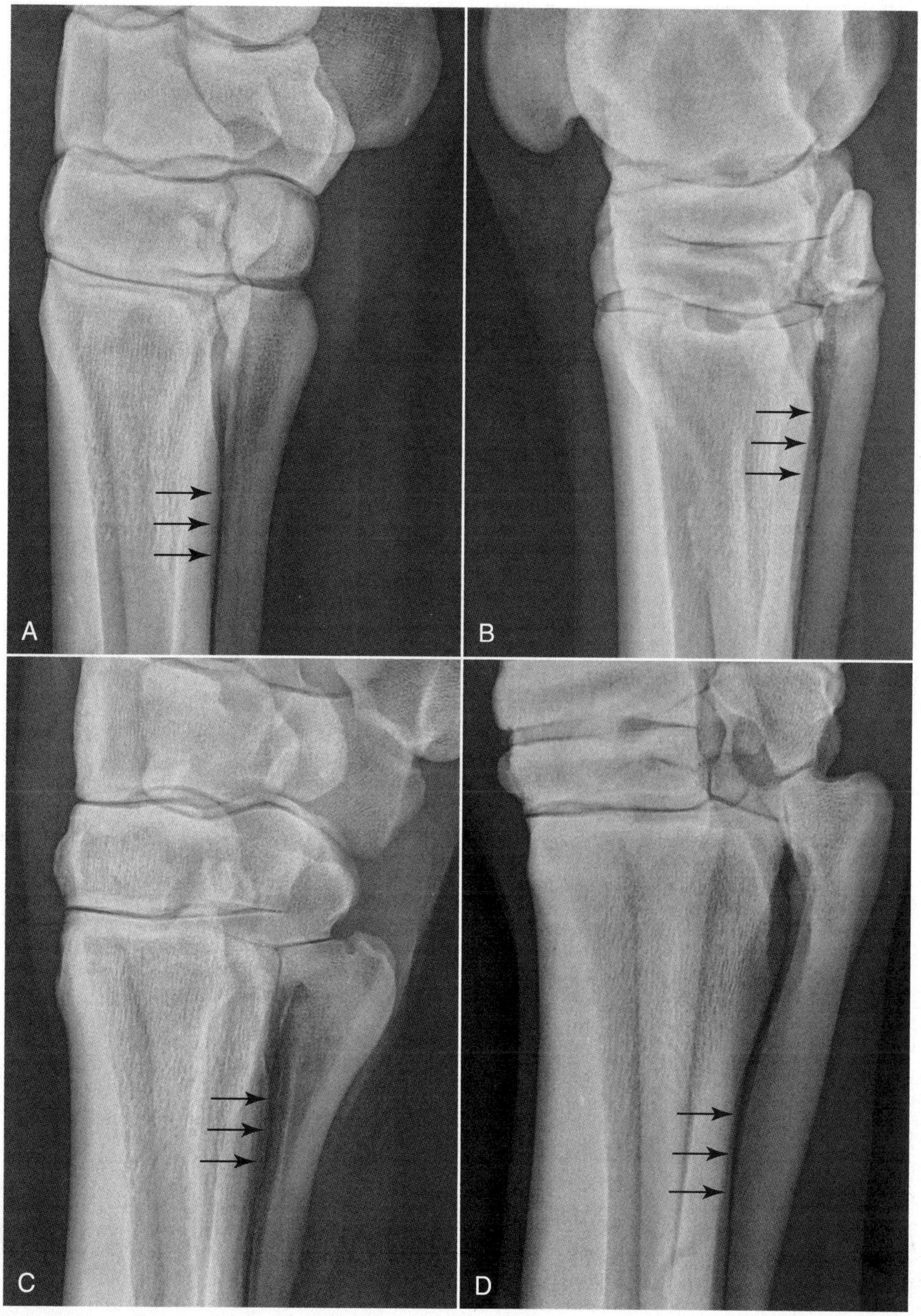

Fig. 24.5 **A,** Dorsomedial-palmarolateral oblique projection of the left proximal metacarpus. Dorsal is to the *left*. The second metacarpal bone articulates with the second and third carpal bone. The interosseous space between the second and third metacarpal bones can be clearly seen. **B,** Dorsomedial-plantarolateral oblique projection of the right proximal metatarsus. Dorsal is to the *left*. The second metatarsal bone can be seen articulating with the fused first and second tarsal bones. The interosseous space between the second and third metatarsal bones can be clearly seen. **C,** Dorsolateral-palmaromedial oblique projection of the left proximal metacarpus. Dorsal is to the *left*. The fourth metacarpal bone articulates with the fourth carpal bone. The interosseous space between the fourth and third metacarpal bones can be clearly seen. **D,** Dorsolateral-plantaromedial oblique projection of the left proximal metatarsus tarsus. Dorsal is to the left. The fourth metatarsal bone can be seen articulating with the fourth tarsal bone. The interosseous space between the fourth and third metatarsal bones can be clearly seen. *Arrows* indicate the interosseous space on all radiographs.

the second and third or fourth and third metacarpal or metatarsal bones is clearly visible (see Fig. 24.5). The fourth metatarsal bone has a prominent base, which can be variably shaped, including having a notched, bilobed or fragmented appearance, often bilaterally, and the base of the fourth metacarpal bone may have a proximal extension or radiolucency (Fig. 24.6).[4] A radiolucent concavity may be seen, in the proximal aspect of the second metacarpal bone, especially when a first carpal bone is present (Fig. 24.7).[4] At birth, the proximal physes of the splint bones should be closed, while the distal epiphyses are cartilaginous and may appear separated from the body of the splint bone as they ossify, which can be mistaken for a fracture.

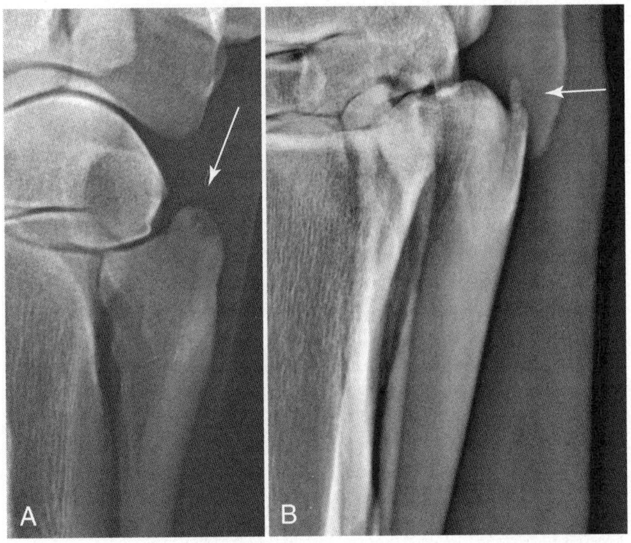

Fig. 24.6 **A,** Dorsolateral-palmaromedial oblique radiograph of a proximal metacarpal region. The base of the fourth metacarpal bone is extended proximally, and there is an ill-defined radiolucent area (*arrow*) in the most proximal aspect. **B,** Dorsolateral-plantaromedial oblique radiograph of the proximal metatarsal region. There is osseous proliferation extending proximally from the plantaroproximal aspect of the fourth metatarsal bone (*arrow*).

Metacarpal Soft Tissues

Multiple tendons, ligaments, and soft tissue structures provide support for the metacarpus and allow for extension and flexion of the digit. The extensor tendons, which lie along the dorsal and lateral aspect of the third metacarpal bone contribute little to the radiographic appearance of the metacarpus and are rarely of clinical relevance. The flexor tendons of the metacarpus include the superficial and deep digital flexor tendons, which run palmar to the third metacarpal bone. At the midmetacarpus, the deep digital flexor tendon is joined dorsally by an accessory (check) ligament which originates from the palmar carpal ligament and palmar aspect of the third and fourth carpal bones in the forelimb.[5] In the pelvic limb, the accessory ligament of the deep digital flexor tendon originates from the plantar aspect of the ligament between the calcaneus and central and third tarsal bones. It is usually smaller, reportedly absent in 6% of hindlimbs, and has more variable morphology than in the thoracic limb.[6] In the distal third of the metacarpus, between the splint bones and the proximal sesamoid bones, is the manica flexoria, a sleeve that wraps dorsally from the superficial digital flexor tendon and encircles the deep digital flexor tendon to maintain both tendons in a central position within the digital sheath.

The third interosseous muscle (suspensory ligament) originates primarily from the palmar or plantar aspect of the third metacarpal or metatarsal bone. It has smaller attachments on the third carpal and metacarpal bone or fourth tarsal bone, calcaneus, and fourth metatarsal bones, and it is bordered by the splint bones.[5,7–9] The proximal portion of the suspensory ligament is bilobed in the forelimb and somewhat triangular in the hindlimb, and it fuses distally to form a flat, oval body before dividing into branches. In the hindlimb, the proximal

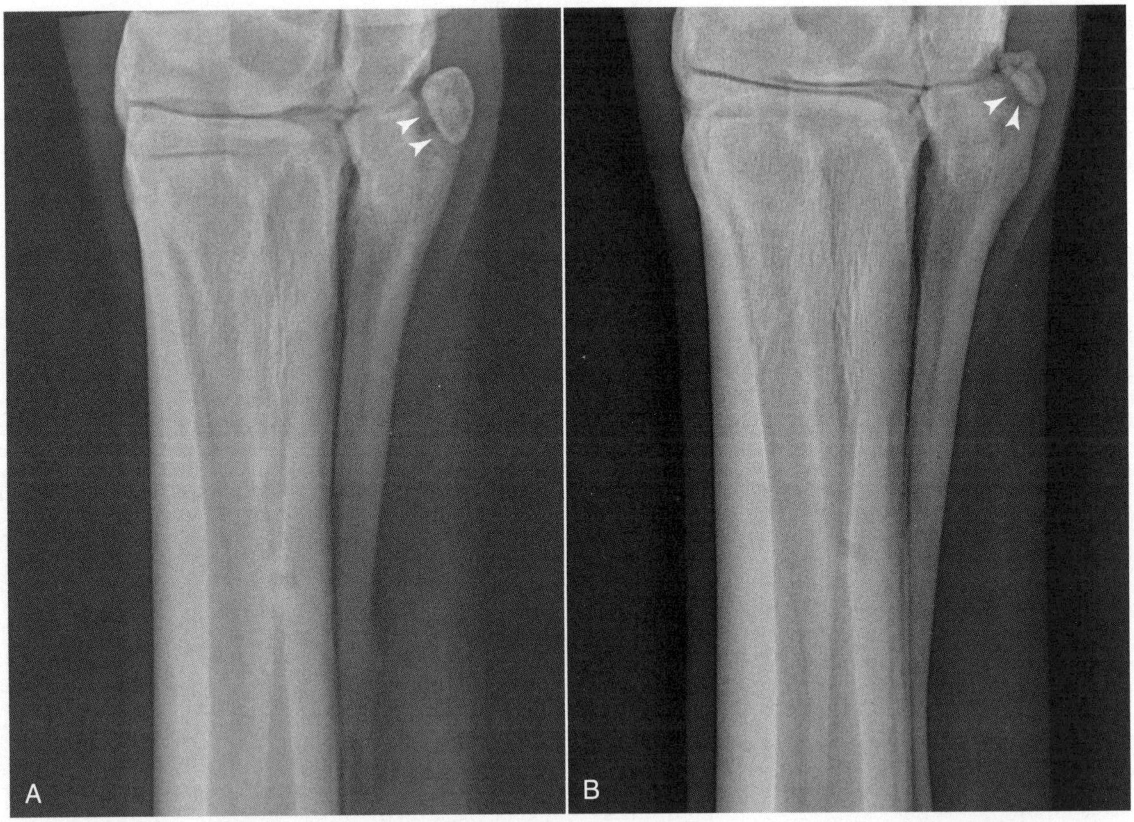

Fig. 24.7 Dorsomedial-palmarolateral oblique projections of the *right* **(A)** and *left* **(B)** proximal metacarpus of the same horse. The palmaroproximal aspect of the second metacarpal bone has a focal, concave margin and radiolucency (*arrowheads*) and a first carpal bone is present bilaterally. The *left* first carpal bone has an incidental, bipartite appearance **(B)**.

aspect of the suspensory ligament is closer to the fourth metatarsal bone with more connective tissue separating it from the second metatarsal bone.[10] A dense band of fascia borders the plantar aspect of the proximal suspensory ligament, connecting to the second and fourth metatarsal bones. In the distal third of the metacarpus, the suspensory ligament body splits into medial and lateral branches which insert on the proximal sesamoid bones. Small, medial and lateral extensor branches wrap dorsally to insert on the extensor tendon. Up to 29.5% of the length of the suspensory ligament branches is subsynovial to the metacarpophalangeal and metatarsophalangeal joints.[11] The suspensory ligament contains variable amounts of fat and muscle, which are typically located in two medial and lateral bundles proximally and become more randomly positioned in a zig-zag pattern within the body of the ligament.[10]

Synovial structures of the metacarpus and metatarsus include the carpal and tarsal sheath, respectively, and the digital flexor tendon sheath. The carpal sheath encircles the superficial and deep digital flexor tendon and accessory ligament of the deep digital flexor tendon and extends to the proximal third of the metacarpus. The tarsal sheath encircles the lateral digital flexor tendon and accessory ligament of the deep digital flexor tendon and extends to the proximal third of the metatarsus. The digital flexor tendon sheath extends from the distal third of the metacarpus to the mid to distal pastern and surrounds the superficial and deep digital flexor tendons.

COMMON RADIOGRAPHIC ABNORMALITIES OF THE METACARPUS

Soft Tissue Structures

When evaluating the metacarpus for soft tissue pathology, it is important to have a thorough understanding of relevant soft tissue anatomy. Due to the limited amount of fat in the metacarpus, soft tissue swelling due to enlargement of the superficial soft tissue structures such as the suspensory ligament branches or superficial digital flexor tendon may be radiographically apparent. Moderate to marked effusion and/or synovitis of the digital flexor tendon sheath may result in the appearance of soft tissue enlargement of the medial and lateral aspect of the distal third of the metacarpus on the DP projection or increased soft tissue opacity between the suspensory ligament branches and digital flexor tendons on the lateral projection (Fig. 24.8). Dystrophic mineralization of soft tissues structures such as the flexor tendons or suspensory ligament branches may be radiographically apparent (see Fig. 24.8).

Soft tissue thickening of the metacarpus may be focal or diffuse. Differentials for focal soft tissue thickening depend on the anatomic location, how extensive the lesion is, and if there is concurrent osseous pathology. Differential diagnoses may include focal edema, hematoma, granuloma formation as secondary to trauma or infectious etiologies such as habronemiasis, fibrosis from prior/chronic soft tissue injury or soft tissue neoplasia (Fig. 24.9). Subcutaneous emphysema may also be seen due to a wound, abscess, or iatrogenic introduction. Thorough evaluation of the osseous structures in the region of the soft tissue pathology is pertinent, and acquiring multiple oblique radiographic projections may be helpful to rule out associated pathology such as sequestrum formation, periosteal proliferation, or osteomyelitis. Differential diagnoses for diffuse soft tissue thickening surrounding the metacarpus may include subcutaneous edema, cellulitis, lymphangitis, and vasculitis and should be prioritized in light of the clinical exam and other imaging findings (see Fig. 24.9).

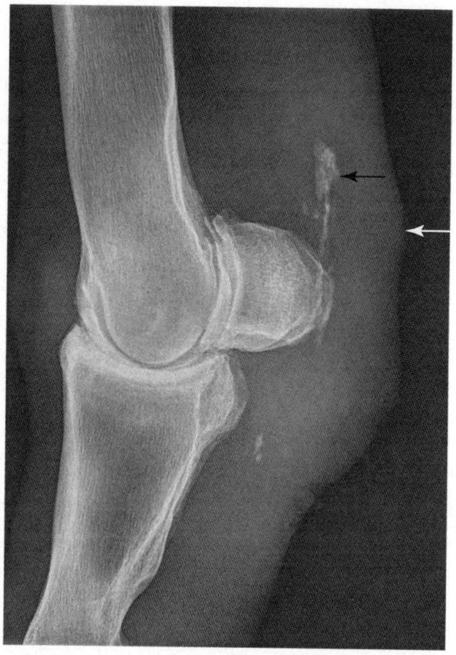

Fig. 24.8 Lateromedial projection of the right distal metatarsus and metatarsophalangeal joint. Dorsal is to the *left*. Increased soft tissue opacity is present in the region of the digital flexor tendon sheath, plantar to the suspensory ligament branches, and there is focal plantar convexity (*white arrow*) due to marked tenosynovitis. A large amount of soft tissue dystrophic mineralization is seen in the region of the digital sheath (*black arrow*).

Periostitis

Periostitis is inflammation of the periosteum which may result in osseous proliferation and can occur due to trauma, infection, or less commonly, neoplasia. The equine metacarpus is a common location for focal periosteal proliferation due to trauma, as there is a limited amount of fat and soft tissue overlying the bone to provide protection. Radiographic evaluation should be performed when firm, osseous thickening is noted in order to rule out fractures and attempt to differentiate between benign and malignant processes. Although these periosteal reactions are not frequently associated with lameness, they will often have persistently increased radiopharmaceutical uptake when evaluated with nuclear scintigraphy.[12]

Focal regions of osseous proliferation may also be seen at the interosseous space between the metacarpal bones, commonly referred to as "splints."[13] These occur due to trauma to the interosseous ligament or syndesmosis between the metacarpal bones, and are very common, especially in young horses as they are started into work. Splints most commonly develop between the second and third metacarpal bones in the forelimb, and between the third and fourth metatarsal bones in the hindlimb. Splints can be difficult to differentiate from periostitis radiographically and may have a similar clinical presentation. In the initial, active phases, these lesions are often warm and painful upon palpation and may have associated soft tissue swelling. After the inflammation resolves, nonpainful osseous proliferation will persist for an extended period of time. The anatomic location of the periosteal proliferation should be considered even after the inflammatory period resolves as the proliferation may impinge on adjacent soft tissue structures such as the suspensory ligament, causing regional desmopathy and adhesion formation.[14] In these cases,

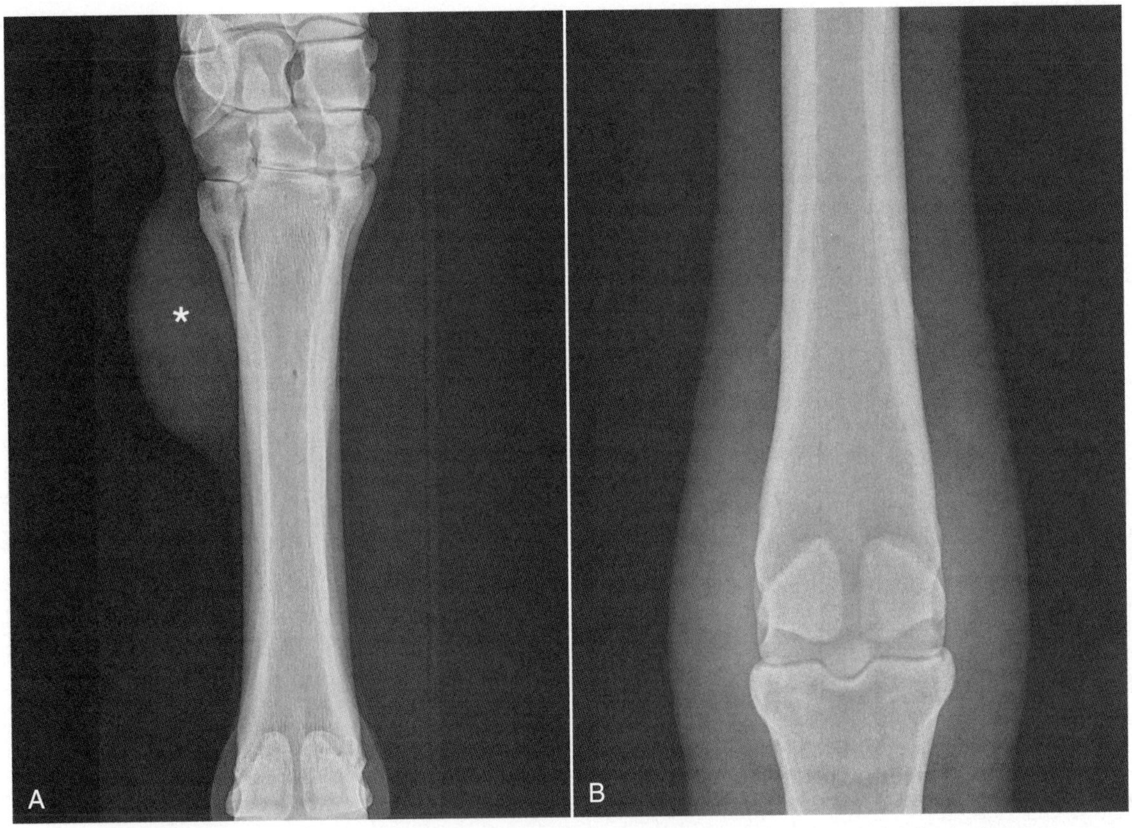

Fig. 24.9 **A,** Dorsopalmar projection of the left metacarpus. Lateral is to the *left*. A large, well-defined soft tissue opaque mass is present along the proximal lateral aspect of the metacarpus (*asterisk*). This lesion was diagnosed as fibrosarcoma. **B,** Dorsoplantar projection of the left distal metatarsus. Lateral is to the *left*. Marked, diffuse soft tissue swelling surrounds the metatarsus, secondary to cellulitis in this case.

ultrasound provides a useful compliment to radiographs for evaluation of concurrent soft tissue pathology. The proliferation may have irregular margins with multiple linear lucent regions, which, when superimposed on the underlying bone, can be difficult to differentiate from fracture formation (Fig. 24.10). Radiographic evaluation should include oblique projections at various angles of obliquity of the metacarpal region as needed to evaluate the interosseous spaces between the metacarpal bones.

Dorsal metacarpal disease, also known as "bucked shins," is a common cause of periostitis, most often seen in 2-year-old Thoroughbred racehorses. It is caused by cyclic fatigue due to excessive compression of the dorsal and dorsomedial aspects of the third metacarpal bone, often bilaterally, and can lead to incomplete (saucer) fractures of the dorsal cortex of the third metacarpal bone. With this disease, the bone undergoes repetitive stress without the necessary amount of time needed to adequately remodel. New, weaker bone is produced at the points of stress on the bone, and the rapid bone formation causes the periosteum to be elevated from the underlying cortex and become inflamed. Diagnosis is often made by the physical exam and history of pain on palpation over the dorsal aspect of the third metacarpal bone and/or soreness after strenuous athletic activity. Radiographic findings may include smooth periosteal proliferation over the dorsal and dorsal medial aspect of the third metacarpal bone and incomplete, dorsal cortical fractures. This region should be carefully evaluated for incomplete fractures (Fig. 24.11).

Hypertrophic osteopathy is a rare condition in horses resulting in symmetrical periosteal proliferation along the diaphysis and metaphysis of long bones, most often affecting the metacarpal and metatarsal bones. This disease process typically occurs in association with other pathology, most commonly intrathoracic disease.[15]

Osteomyelitis and Sequestra

Due to limited fat and soft tissue surrounding the metacarpal bones, this region is especially predisposed to bone trauma, which in some cases, may result in infectious osteitis or osteomyelitis. Radiographically, aggressive processes in bone, such as infection and neoplasia are more likely to result in irregularly margined, ill-defined proliferation and/or lysis with indistinct margins or a long zone of transition between normal and abnormal bone. Sequestrum formation is a common sequela to trauma and infection in the metacarpal region, often affecting the thick dorsal cortex of the third metacarpal bone.[16] Sequestra consist of a central piece of devitalized, sclerotic bone (the sequestrum) which has become separated from the adjacent, healthy bone and surrounded by a radiolucent region consisting of purulent material and granulation tissue encircled by a zone of dense bone (the involucrum). A draining tract (cloaca) may also be present, extending from the sequestrum through the surrounding tissues. The radiographic appearance of sequestra depends on the angle at which it is struck by the x-ray beam (Fig. 24.12, eFig. 24.1). As the sequestrum serves as a nidus for infection, surgical debridement is often necessary to facilitate healing.

Proximal Suspensory Ligament Enthesopathy and Avulsion

Radiographic findings of suspensory ligament enthesopathy may include periosteal proliferation, trabecular or endosteal sclerosis, or osteolysis at the proximal attachment site of the suspensory ligament.[10,17,18] As seen on the dorsopalmar projections, the trabecular pattern of the proximal third metacarpal

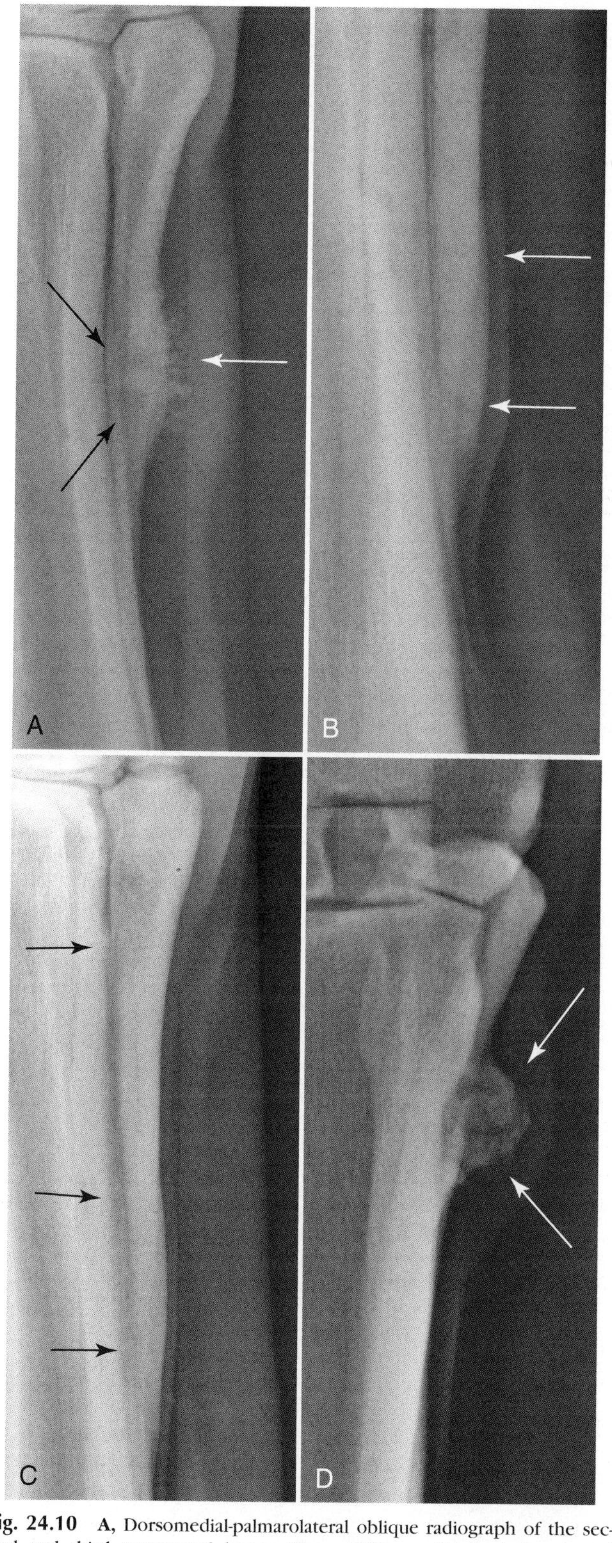

Fig. 24.10 **A,** Dorsomedial-palmarolateral oblique radiograph of the second and third metacarpal bones. The middle one-third of the second metacarpal bone is smoothly enlarged, with irregularly outlined new bone on the palmar aspect of heterogeneous mineral opacity (*white arrow*). Within the second metacarpal bone there are ill-defined radiolucent areas (*black arrows*). Although irregular in appearance, such lesions may not be clinically significant. **B,** Dorsomedial-palmarolateral oblique radiograph of the second and third metacarpal bones. There is a smoothly marginated exostosis (*white arrows*) on the second metacarpal bone of unlikely clinical significance. **C,** Dorsomedial/palmarolateral oblique radiograph of the second and third metacarpal bones. There is mineralization between the two bones in the interosseous space (*black arrows*). This is of unlikely clinical significance. **D,** Dorsoplantar radiograph of a proximal metatarsal region. Lateral is to the *right*. There is a large exostosis of heterogeneous mineral opacity on the lateral aspect of the third metatarsal bone (*white arrows*).

bone normally has a more coarse appearance relative to the remainder of the bone, but the pattern should be uniformly distributed. It is common to see a proximodistally oriented, thin, linear mineral opacity on midline, which may be an incidental finding (Fig. 24.13). Sclerosis of the proximal third metacarpal bone at the attachment of the suspensory ligament may be multifocal or localized to the lateral or medial aspect and can range from mild to severely increased mineral opacity resulting in loss of the normal trabecular bone pattern (Fig. 24.14, eFig. 24.2). Osteolysis may be seen as focal or multifocal regions of decreased mineral opacity at the palmaroproximal cortex of the third metacarpal bone. These radiographic findings may be subtle and more thorough evaluation of the proximal suspensory ligament attachment site may be achieved with collimated projections centered on the proximal one-third of the metacarpus. Abnormal mineral opacity or changes in the trabecular bone pattern will be best seen on the dorsopalmar projection, while endosteal sclerosis and osseous proliferation will be better evaluated on the lateromedial projection. Osseous proliferation or sclerosis at the proximal suspensory ligament attachment site is likely chronic in nature and does not always indicate a source of lameness. When evaluated in Quarter horses, radiographically identified osseous changes on the third metatarsal bone were not predictive of either the presence or severity of proximal suspensory desmopathy, but there was a positive correlation between the severity of radiographic and magnetic resonance imaging (MRI) findings for osseous proliferation and resorption at the ligament attachment site.[19] Avulsion fractures at the attachment site of the suspensory ligament can also occur.[20,21] In these cases, additional projections including collimated dorsopalmar and lateral projections of the proximal aspect of the third metacarpal region can be helpful to better elucidate the fracture line (Fig. 24.15).

Splint Bone Fractures

The second and fourth metacarpal and metatarsal bones will be referred to as the splint bones in this section unless otherwise specified. Similar to the third metacarpal bone, the splint bones are particularly prone to external trauma due to their superficial location and limited soft tissue coverage to offer protection. Trauma such as kicks can result in open fractures of the proximal and mid portions of the splint bones, which can lead to osteomyelitis and sequestration. The distal aspect of the splint bones may be abaxially displaced and even fractured in association with desmopathy of the suspensory ligament branches (Fig. 24.16, eFig. 24.3).[22] Nonunion fractures or unfused separate centers of ossifications may be seen in the distal aspects of the splint bones, without clinical relevance. Management of splint fractures depends on the location of the fracture and the weight-bearing status of the bone.[21,23] When a splint bone fracture is clinically suspected, it may be helpful to obtain radiographs at multiple angles of obliquity between lateromedial and dorsopalmar in order to obtain an image with the primary x-ray beam tangential to the fracture margin. Repeated radiographs over time should be evaluated for fracture healing as well as callus development. The position of any excessive callus formation should be taken into consideration as axial protrusion of the callus can impinge upon the suspensory ligament and result in desmopathy and adhesion formation (Fig. 24.17).[14]

Third Metacarpal/Metatarsal Fractures

The third metacarpal bone is a common location for stress fractures in racehorses and sport horses. Stress fractures occur at specific predilection sites along the bone when damage due to repetitive loading accumulates more quickly than can be repaired by the remodeling process. Common stress fractures in the third metacarpal bone include parasagittal groove condylar fractures,[24] sagittally oriented fractures of the palmar, proximal cortex,[25] transversely oriented stress fractures of the palmar, distal cortex,[26] and frontal[27] and sagittal oblique[28]

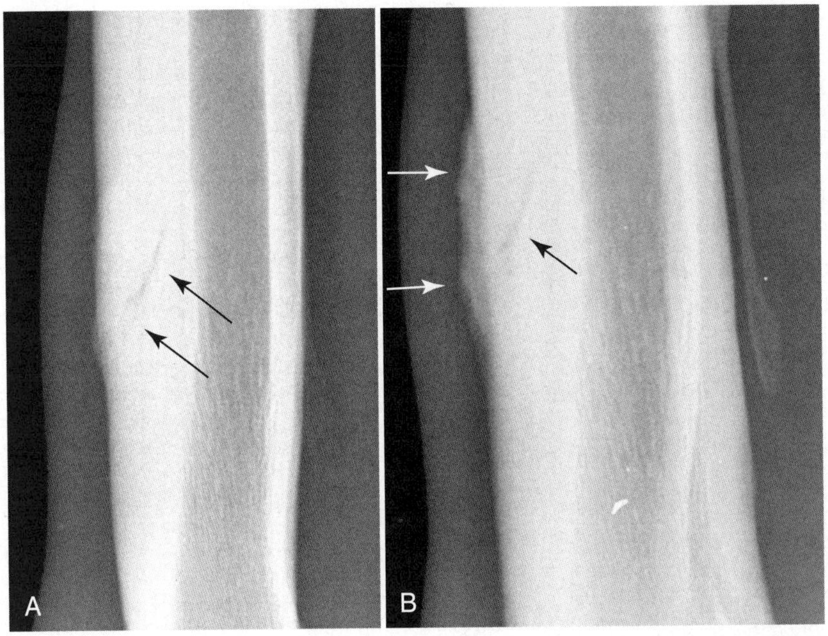

Fig. 24.11 **A,** Lateromedial projection of the mid metacarpus of a 3-year-old Thoroughbred flat racehorse. Dorsal is to the *left.* There is a curved radiolucent line in the dorsal cortex of the third metacarpal bone (*black arrows*), typical of an incomplete dorsal cortical stress or fatigue fracture with mild overlying soft tissue swelling. **B,** Dorsolateral-palmaromedial oblique radiograph of the mid metacarpal region of the same limb as illustrated in **A**. There is an incomplete dorsal cortical stress fracture (*black arrow*), with extensive periosteal callus (*white arrows*) and overlying soft tissue swelling. There is also a mild endosteal reaction.

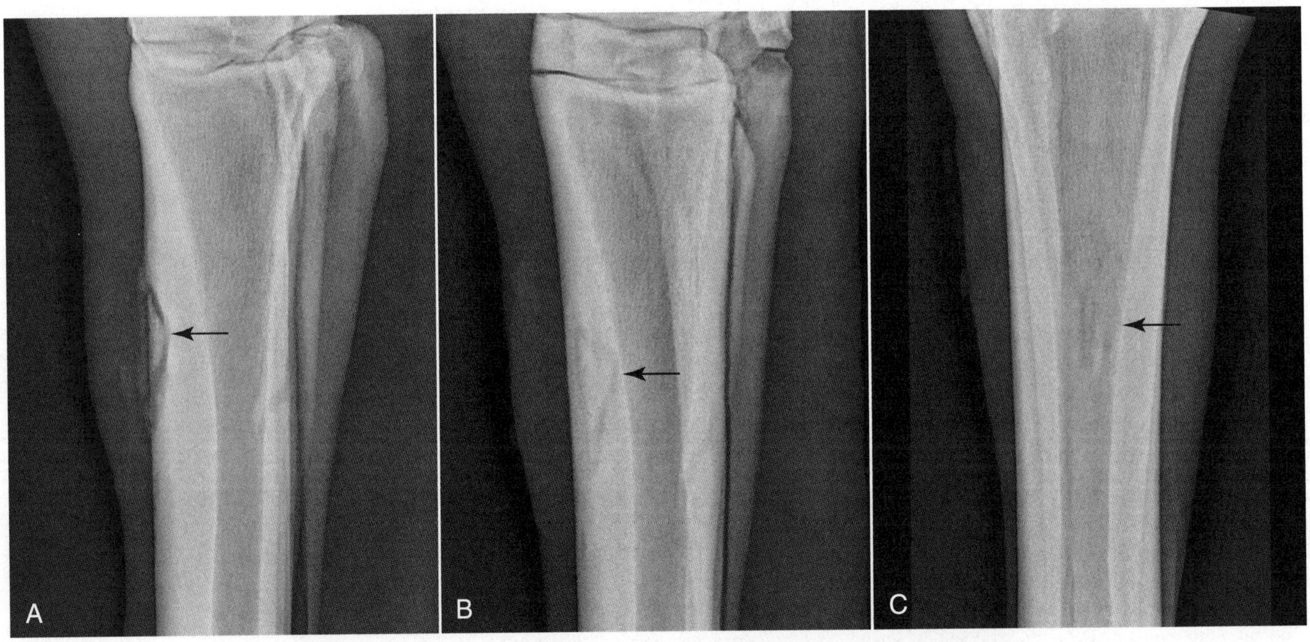

Fig. 24.12 Lateromedial **(A)**, dorsomedial-plantarolateral oblique **(B)**, and dorsoplantar **(C)** projections of the metatarsus. A sequestrum is present on the dorsoproximal aspect of the third metatarsal bone (*arrows*), characterized by a well-defined, thin, oval, sclerotic mineral opacity (sequestrum) surrounded by a radiolucency bordered by sclerotic bone (involucrum), with focal soft tissue thickening and adjacent cutaneous margin irregularity. Note the difference in appearance of the sequestrum depending on the orientation of the x-ray beam relative to the lesion.

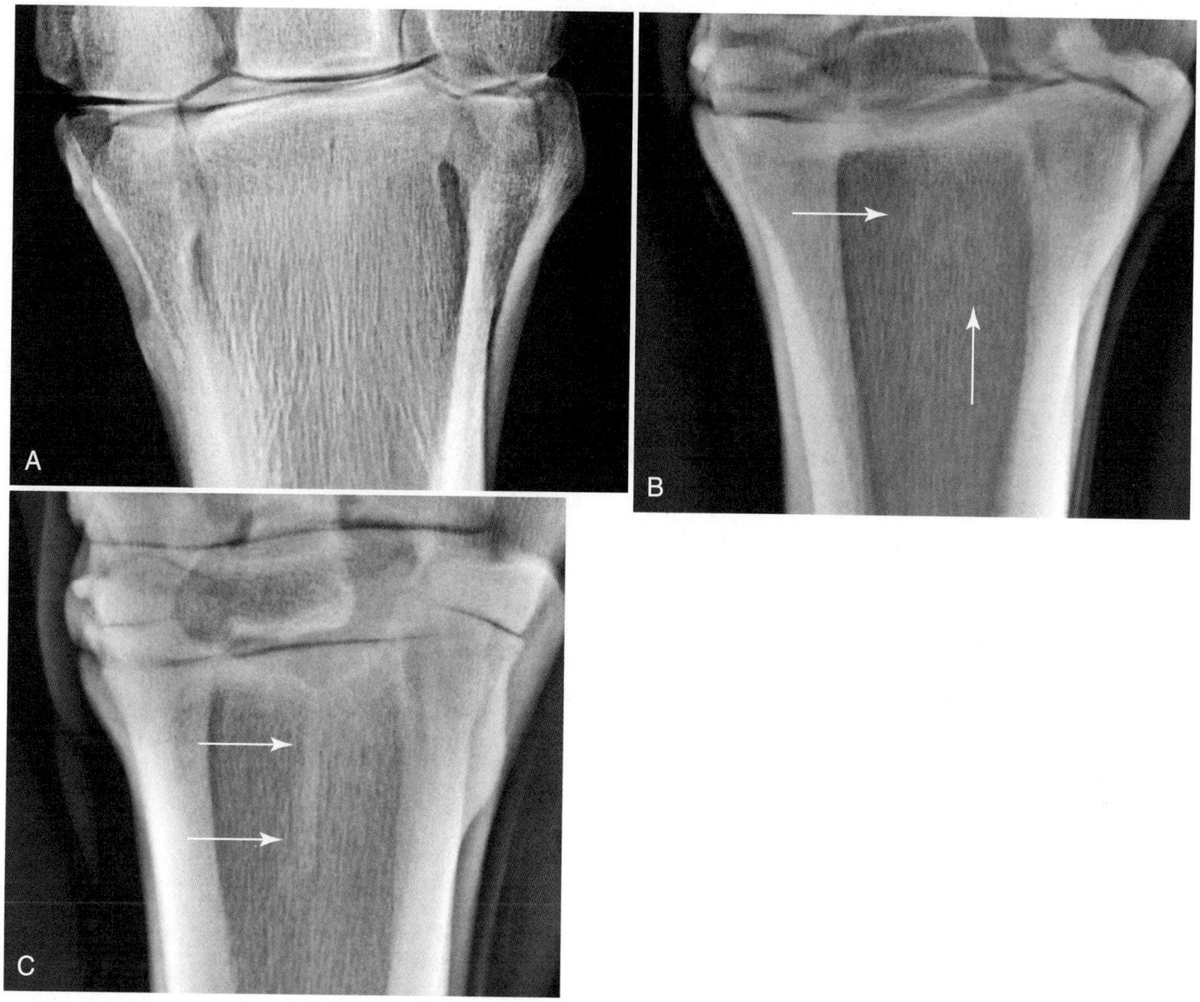

Fig. 24.13 **A,** Dorsopalmar radiograph of a normal proximal metacarpal region. Note the uniform but mildly course trabeculae in the third metacarpal bone. **B,** Dorsoplantar radiograph of a proximal metatarsal region. Lateral is to the *right.* There is mild diffuse increased mineral opacity in the proximolateral aspect of the third metatarsal bone (*white arrows*). This can be an incidental finding. **C,** Dorsoplantar radiograph of a proximal metatarsal region. Lateral is to the *right.* There is a linear axial region of increased opacity in the proximal aspect of the third metatarsal bone (*white arrows*). This can be an incidental finding.

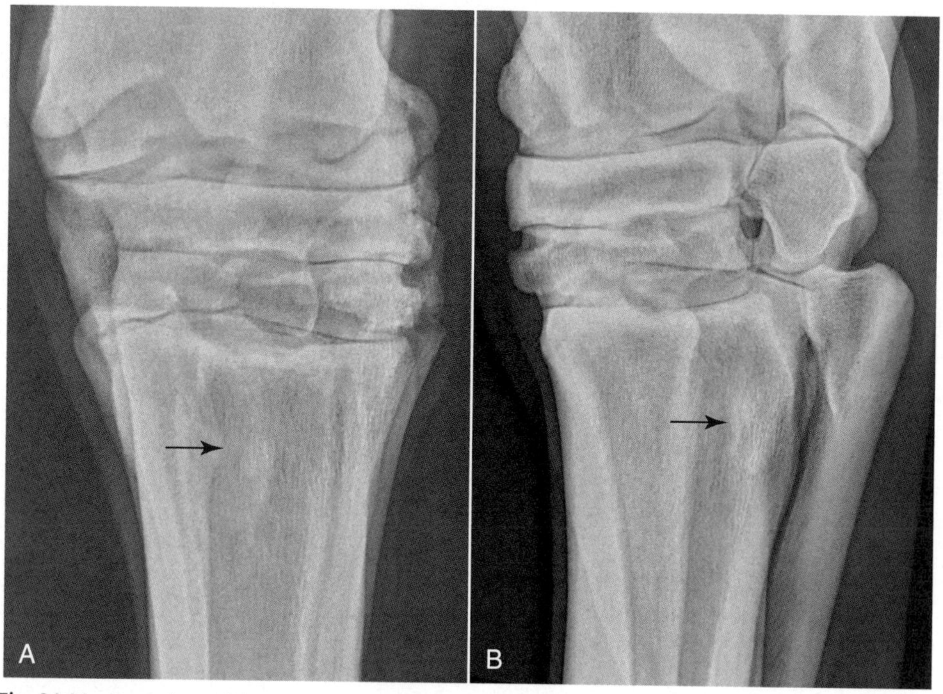

Fig. 24.14 Dorsoplantar **(A)** and dorsolateral-plantaromedial **(B)** projections of the right proximal metatarsus. Lateral is to the *left* on the dorsoplantar projection. There is moderate, ill-defined and irregular sclerosis of the proximal plantarolateral aspect of the third metatarsal bone, representing chronic enthesopathy at the attachment of the proximal suspensory ligament (*arrow*). Mild to moderate proximal suspensory desmopathy and a small avulsion fracture were identified on concurrent ultrasound examination.

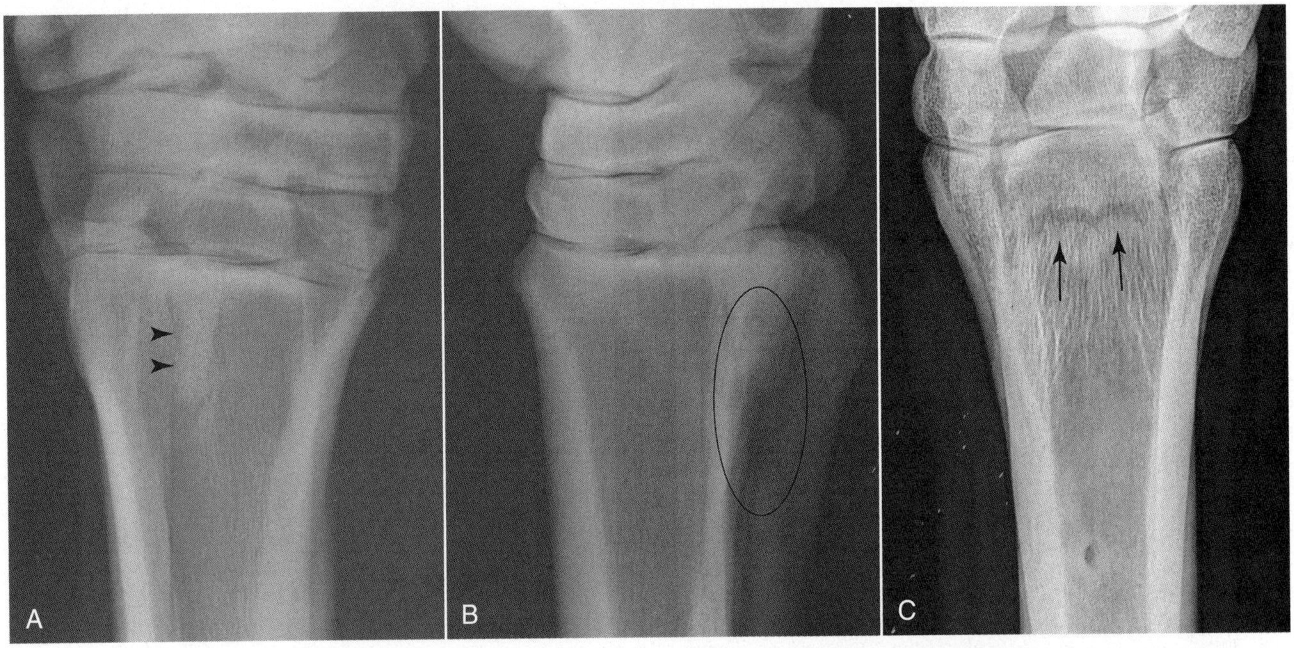

Fig. 24.15 Dorsoplantar (lateral is to the *left*) (**A**) and lateromedial (**B**) projections collimated on the proximal metatarsus. **A,** A sclerotic, ovoid mineral opacity is superimposed on the lateral aspect of the proximal third metatarsal bone (*arrowheads*), with decreased mineral opacity along the distal border. **B,** The lateromedial projection helps to elucidate the fracture margins, and confirms there is an avulsion fracture fragment separated from the plantar cortex of the third metatarsal bone (*circled*). **C,** Dorsopalmar radiograph of a proximal metacarpal region of an elite horse. Lateral is to the *right.* There are broad curved radiolucent lines (*black arrows*) in the proximal aspect of the third metacarpal bone representing avulsion fracture of the origin of the suspensory ligament from the palmar aspect of the third metacarpal bone.

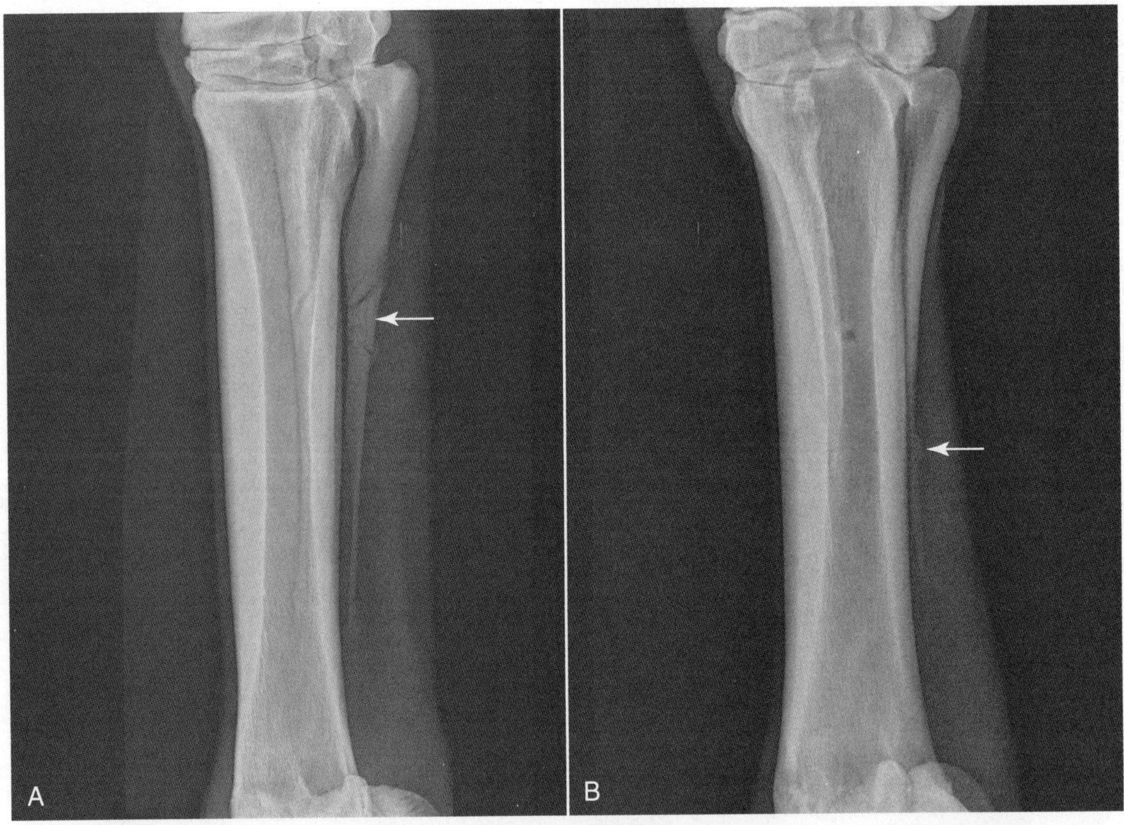

Fig. 24.16 **A,** Dorsolateral-plantaromedial oblique projection of the metatarsus, dorsal is to the *left.* There is a sharply margined, comminuted fracture of the fourth metatarsal bone mid body due to trauma (*arrow*). **B,** Dorsolateral-palmaromedial oblique projection of the right metacarpus of a Standardbred racehorse with a chronic fracture of the distal body of the fourth metacarpal bone (*arrow*) in association with severe, suspensory body and biaxial branch desmopathy. The most distal aspect of the second and fourth metacarpal bones had been previously excised.

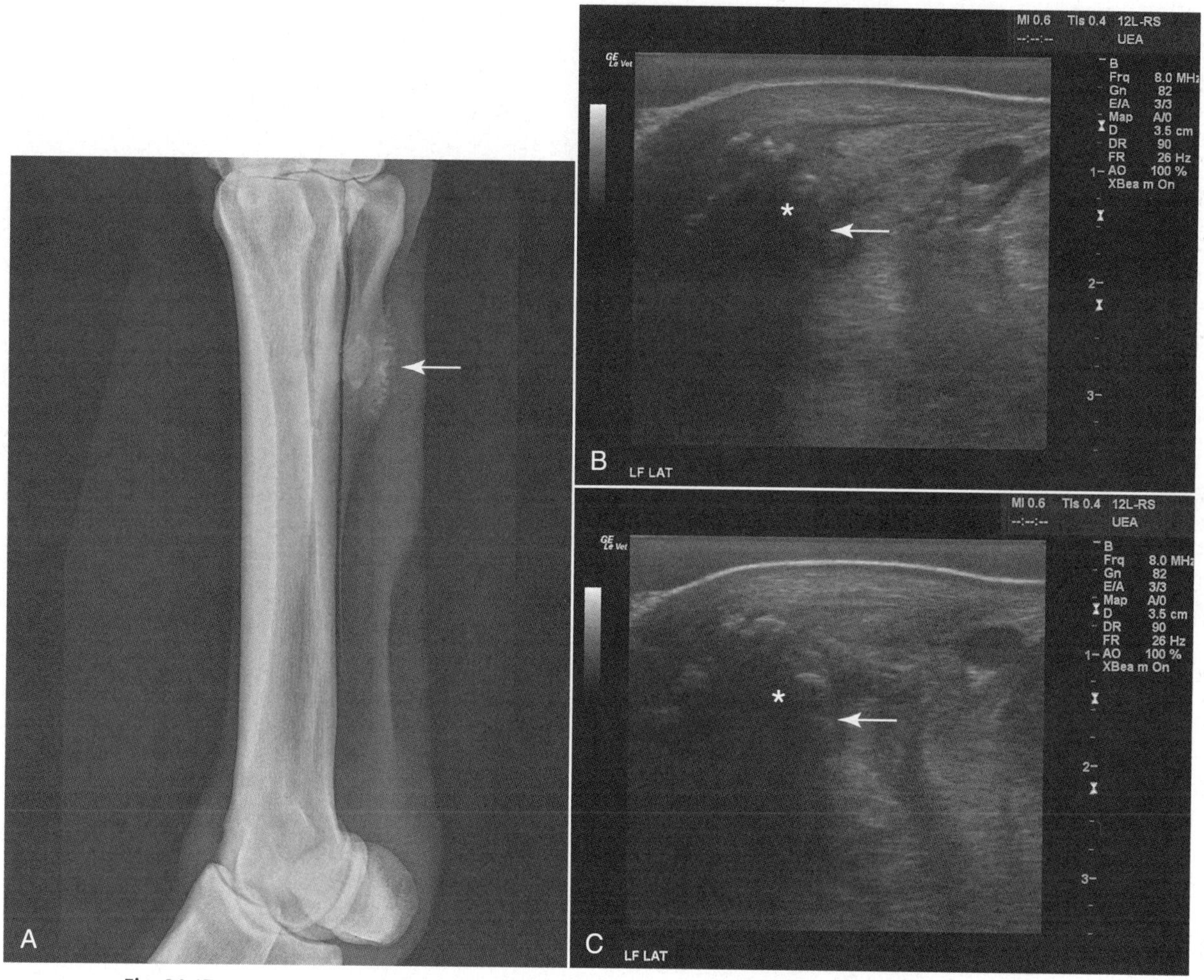

Fig. 24.17 **A,** Dorsolateral-palmaromedial oblique projection of the metacarpus. At the proximal to mid fourth metacarpal bone, there is spiculated, osseous proliferation (*arrow*) and associated, moderate soft tissue thickening. **B,** Transverse plane ultrasound image of the lateral aspect of the suspensory ligament body at the level of the exostosis (*asterisk*), made with a linear transducer. Dorsal is to the *left*. There is focal enlargement of the lateral aspect of the suspensory ligament body, with hypoechogenicity and fiber pattern disruption (*arrow*). **C,** Transverse plane ultrasound image at the same level as **B** using an oblique angle of insonation. Dorsal is to the *left*. The ligament fibers are hypoechoic due to anisotropism and fiber pattern disruption can be seen (*arrow*). The exostosis was surgically removed and marked focal desmopathy of the suspensory ligament was noted intraoperatively.

fractures of the dorsal cortex (Fig. 24.18). Evidence of osseous remodeling may precede fracture formation and includes endosteal or trabecular bone sclerosis, osseous proliferation and/or lysis, and concurrent soft tissue thickening or joint effusion. Recognizing incomplete fractures as early as possible is imperative because they may progress to complete catastrophic fractures. Radiographic projections in which the primary x-ray beam is tangential to the fracture line will be most diagnostic; thus, special radiographic projections may be helpful in addition to the standard series. When evaluating for incomplete condylar fractures, more thorough evaluation includes a dorsopalmar projection of the joint in flexion or a dorsodistal-palmaroproximal oblique projection.[29,30] Even with ideal positioning, however, fractures may not be radiographically apparent for 10 to 14 days and, even then, may be subtle. For thorough evaluation of cases in which stress fractures are clinically suspected, but not identified radiographically, alternative imaging such as nuclear scintigraphy or positron emission tomography (PET) should be considered.

OTHER IMAGING TECHNIQUES

Alternative imaging modalities such as ultrasonography, computed tomography (CT), MRI, nuclear scintigraphy, and PET serve as a complement to radiography in the metacarpus, when clinically indicated and available.

Ultrasonography

Ultrasound is commonly performed of the palmar metacarpus and provides a widely accessible, portable, and practical approach for more thorough evaluation of soft tissues. The superficial nature of the palmar soft tissues of the metacarpus makes ultrasound ideal for evaluation of this region when performed by experienced ultrasonographers.

When preparing for transcutaneous ultrasonography, adequate preparation of the site is imperative and should include clipping the hair, thoroughly cleaning the skin, and applying acoustic coupling agents such as alcohol and/or ultrasound gel. Two techniques are commonly utilized for

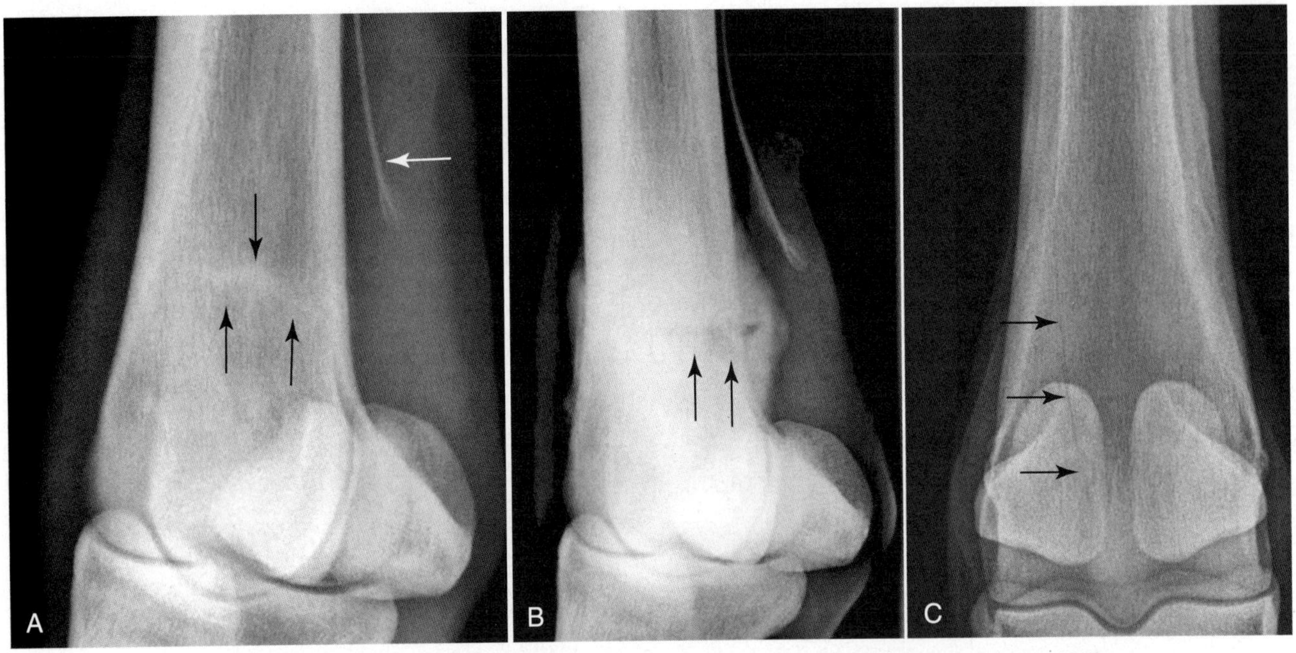

Fig. 24.18 **A,** Dorsolateral/palmaromedial oblique radiograph of a distal metacarpal region of a 3-year-old Thoroughbred flat racehorse, 3 days after the onset of acute severe lameness associated with soft tissue swelling and focal pain in the distal palmarolateral aspect of the metacarpal region. The distal aspect of the fourth metacarpal bone is distorted in shape (*white arrow*) because of the soft tissue swelling. There is an ill-defined transverse radiopaque line (*black arrows*) in the palmar aspect of the third metacarpal bone. This is a distal metaphyseal stress fracture. **B,** Dorsolateral/palmaromedial oblique radiograph of the distal metacarpal region of the same horse as in **A**, 30 days after the onset of acute severe lameness. There is increased bowing of the distal aspect of the fourth metacarpal bone because of extensive periosteal callus on the palmar aspect of the third metacarpal bone. There is also periosteal callus dorsomedially. There is diffuse increased radiopacity of the cancellous bone in the metaphyseal region of the third metacarpal bone and an ill-defined transverse radiolucent line (*black arrows*) toward the palmarolateral aspect of the third metacarpal bone. **C,** Dorsoplantar projection of the right distal metatarsus. Lateral is to the *left*. An ill-defined, incomplete lateral condylar stress fracture is present (*black arrows*). (Image courtesy Dr. Margret Thompson, Cornell University.)

evaluating different regions of the metacarpus and metatarsus, including measuring the distance from the point of the hock or accessory carpal bone to the area of interest or using defined anatomical regions or zones.[10,31] A systematic approach should be followed for each exam. Structures should be evaluated in both transverse (short axis) and longitudinal (long axis) planes, with consistent transducer orientation and comparison to the contralateral limb. For evaluation of the palmar metacarpus, a linear transducer with a frequency range of 8 to 15 megahertz is an ideal starting point; however, it is recommended to use the highest frequency possible while still achieving the depth penetration needed to image the entire area of interest. Use of an acoustic standoff pad is necessary to eliminate the effect of near-field artifact when evaluating more superficial structures. Frequency, focal zones, gain, and depth should be routinely adjusted as needed to maximize image quality. Recognizing ultrasound artifacts including, but not limited to, edge shadowing, distal acoustic enhancement, and distal acoustic shadowing is essential for accurate image interpretation. Anisotropism is a particularly important principle to understand with regard to musculoskeletal imaging. It explains the effect that the incident angle of the ultrasound beam has on the appearance of fibrillar structures such as tendons or ligaments.[31] When the ultrasound beam is perpendicular to such structures, the majority of sound is reflected and echogenicity is maximized, and when the angle of insonation is decreased, the echogenicity of that structure is decreased, and the tendon or ligament will appear hypoechoic (Fig. 24.19).[32] This artifact can be helpful in differentiating tissue types such as fat or fascia surrounding a tendon or ligament. Without a thorough understanding of this phenomenon, areas of hypoechogenicity due to decreased angles of insonation can be falsely interpreted as pathology.

Sonographic anatomy and technique for evaluation of the palmar metacarpus and metatarsus have been described.[8,10,33–36] In the palmar metacarpus, the superficial and deep digital flexor tendons, accessory ligament of the deep digital flexor tendon, and the suspensory ligament are easily identified, and synovial structures such as the digital sheath can be evaluated (Fig. 24.20). In order to optimize imaging parameters, it is ideal to evaluate the more superficial structures (superficial and deep digital flexor tendons) independently of the deeper structures (accessory ligament of the deep digital flexor tendon and suspensory ligament body), and the suspensory ligament branches should be evaluated from the bifurcation of the suspensory ligament to their insertion on the proximal sesamoid bones using a medial and lateral approach.[33] For the more superficial structures, such as the superficial digital flexor tendon and suspensory ligament branches, a standoff pad should be used.[31,33] The metacarpus should be carefully evaluated from a medial and lateral approach in addition to a palmar approach in order to include the peripheral margins of the soft tissue structures, and to evaluate for peritendinous or periligamentous tissue proliferation.

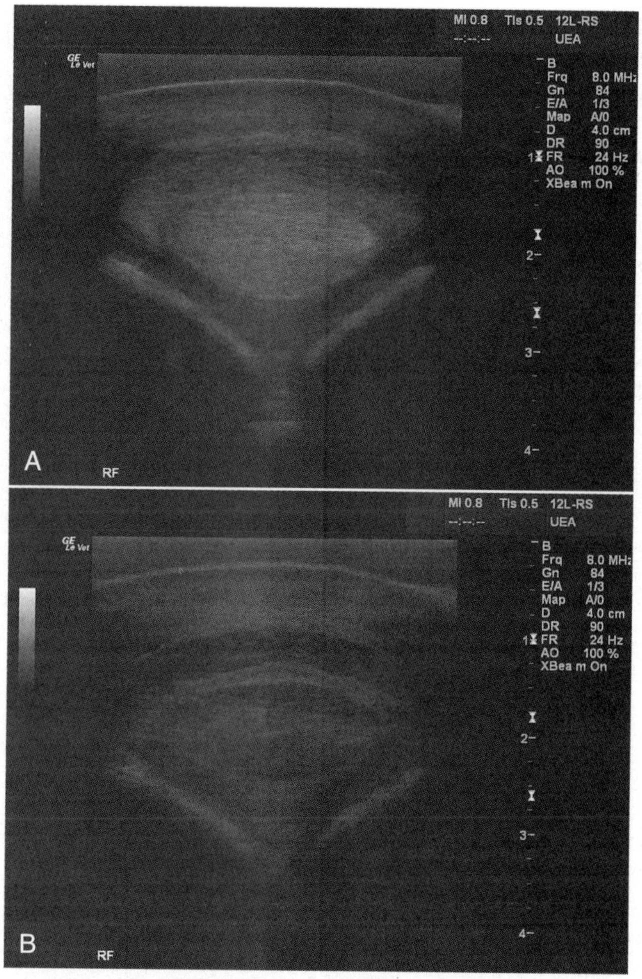

Fig. 24.19 Transverse plane ultrasound images of the distal metacarpus using a linear transducer at the level of the proximal sesamoid bones. Lateral is to the *right*. Images demonstrate the principal of anistropism. **A,** The ultrasound beam is oriented perpendicular to the superficial and deep digital flexor tendon fibers and echogenicity of the flexor tendons is maximized. **B,** The ultrasound beam is oriented obliquely to the long axis of the tendons and the echogenicity of the flexor tendons is decreased relative to **A**.

Abnormal sonographic findings in the equine metacarpus may include focal or diffuse ligament or tendon enlargement, margin irregularity/tearing, or changes in echogenicity. Cross-sectional area measurements can be obtained to objectively measure size and to compare these measurements over time, and normal measurements have been reported in the metacarpus/metatarsus.[37–39] Tendon or ligament hypoechogenicity, termed *core lesions* when they occur centrally, may result from areas of fiber pattern irregularity, edema, or hematoma formation and can be focal or diffuse. Focal regions of increased tendon or ligament echogenicity may result from scar tissue/fibrin formation or mineralization. The use of color and power Doppler interrogation has been described as a complement to B-mode ultrasound evaluation of tendons and ligaments in the metacarpus and may be helpful for assessment of healing[40–42] (Fig. 24.21).

Superficial digital flexor tendinopathy is the most common tendon injury in athletic horses and frequently involves tendon enlargement and palpable heat, pain, and swelling in the mid metacarpus. Sonographic findings often include focal areas of hypoechogenicity centrally or peripherally within the tendon; however, diffuse hypoechogenicity throughout a region of the tendon may also occur (Fig. 24.22). Although the mid metacarpal region is most commonly affected, superficial digital flexor tendinopathy can occur at the most proximal aspect of the tendon,[43] as well as in the carpal canal of middle-aged to older horses, where it is often characterized by focal, palmar hypoechogenicity.[44] Less commonly, lesions of the superficial digital flexor tendon may be seen at the level of the digital sheath.[45]

Deep digital flexor tendinopathy is often located at the level of the digital sheath, and may have concurrent digital sheath effusion and/or tenosynovitis.[46] Most commonly, lesions consist of marginal tears. Hypoechoic lesions, which may extend to the tendon periphery, tendon enlargement, and perilesional tissue proliferation, may be seen (Fig. 24.23).[47] The pathology of the manica flexoria may also be seen in the digital sheath and includes asymmetry, heterogeneous echogenicity, lack of margin definition, partial or complete tears, abnormal sliding of the deep and superficial digital flexor tendons, and displacement of the superficial digital flexor tendon on dynamic exam.[45,48] Complete evaluation of the tendons in the digital sheath is challenging. Evaluation from a medial and lateral approach in addition to a palmar approach is important for margin

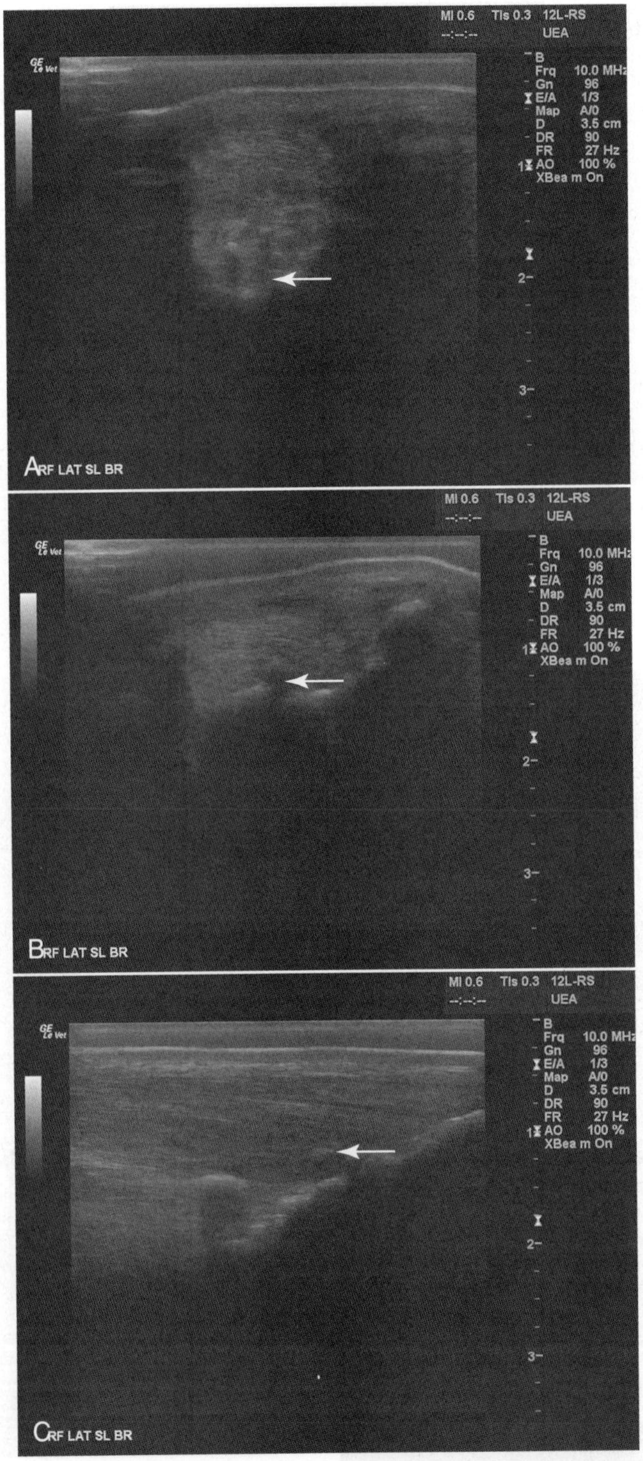

Fig. 24.27 **A and B,** Transverse plane ultrasound images of the lateral suspensory ligament branch made with a linear transducer. Dorsal is to the *left.* **A,** The mid aspect of the lateral suspensory ligament branch has multifocal, mild to moderate fiber abnormalities, hyperechoic foci with distal acoustic shadowing (*arrow*), moderate enlargement and mild to moderate periligamentous tissue proliferation. **B,** The distal aspect of the suspensory ligament branch near the insertion on the proximal sesamoid bone. Mild to moderate fiber abnormalities are present (*arrow*). **C,** Long axis image of the right fore lateral suspensory ligament branch insertion on the lateral, proximal sesamoid bone. Proximal is to the *left.* There is moderate to marked enthesopathy characterized by proliferation, avulsion fragments, and/or dystrophic mineralization (*arrow*) at the attachment to the sesamoid bone.

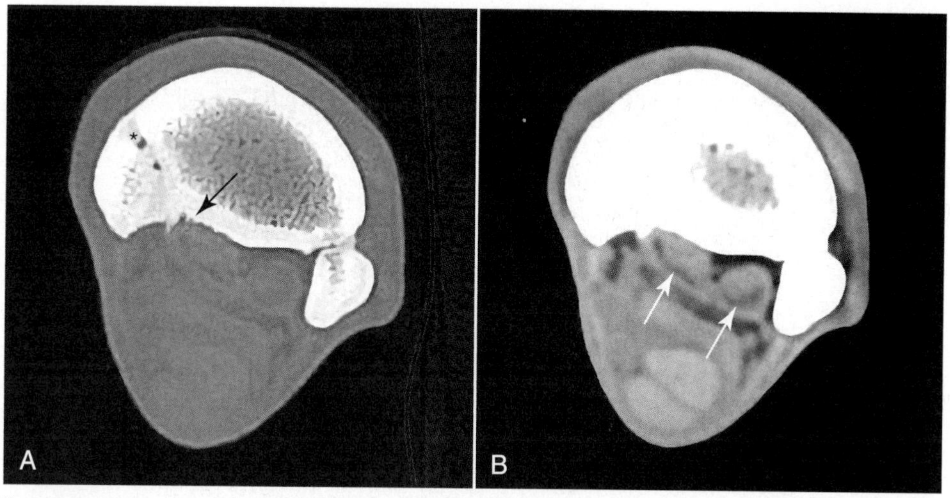

Fig. 24.28 Transverse plane computed tomography (CT) images of the proximal metacarpal region in bone (**A**) and soft tissue (**B**) algorithms. Lateral is to the *right*. **A,** Subtle osseous proliferation and resorption are present along the palmar medial aspect of the third metacarpal bone at the attachment of the medial lobe of the proximal suspensory ligament (*arrow*). Mineralization of the interosseous ligament between the second and third metacarpal bones is also noted (*asterisk*). **B,** Using a soft tissue algorithm, it is possible to differentiate between the ligamentous tissue and the hypoattenuating, fat/muscular portions of the proximal suspensory ligament (*arrows*).

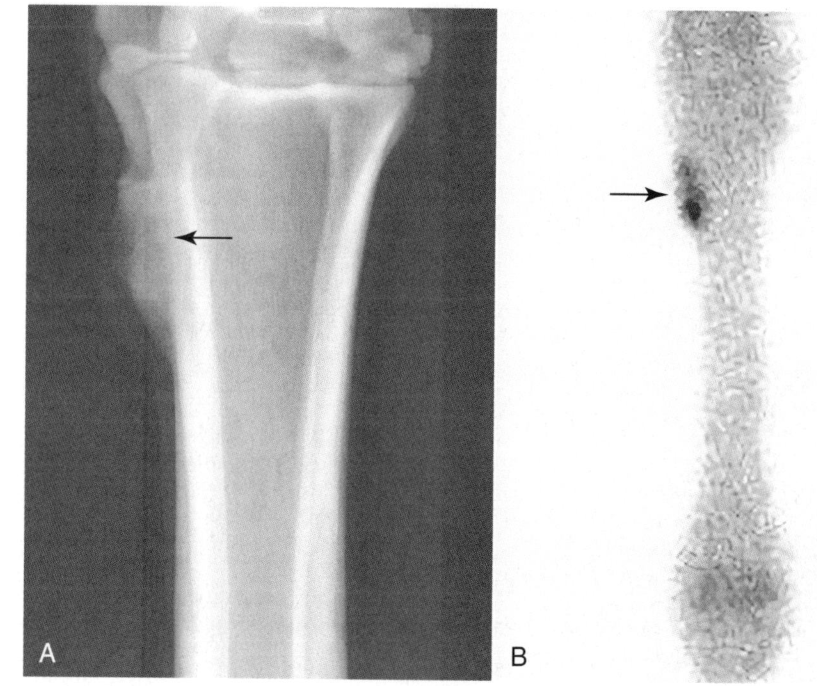

Fig. 24.29 **A**, Dorsoplantar radiograph of the left proximal metatarsus. Lateral is to the *left*. A smooth, well-defined exostosis is present along the proximal lateral aspect of the fourth metatarsal bone. **B,** Plantar nuclear scintigraphic image of the left metatarsus of the same horse. Lateral is to the left. Focal, moderate increased radiopharmaceutical uptake is identified in the region of the exostosis (*arrow*). This lesion was nonpainful on palpation, without associated lameness.

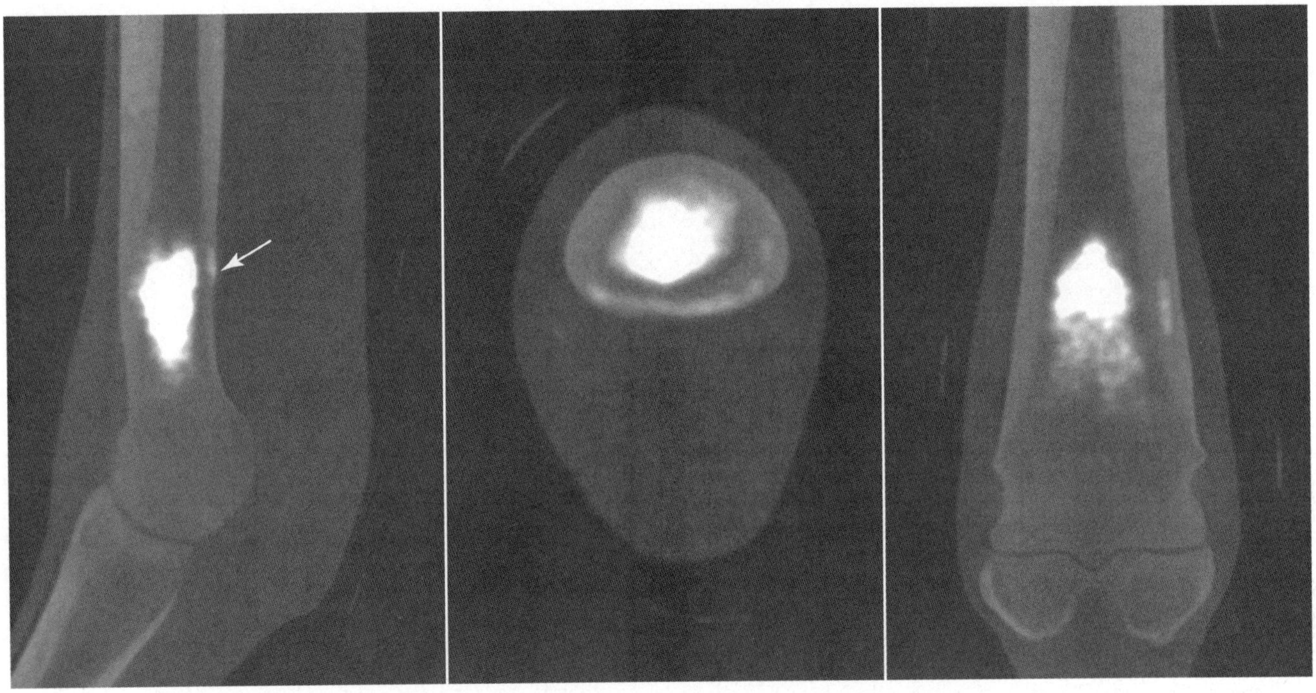

Fig. 24.30 Sagittal (*left*), transverse (*middle*), and dorsal (*right*) plane coregistered standing cone beam computed tomography (CT) and positron emission tomography (PET) images of the distal metacarpal region in a 3-year-old Thoroughbred. On CT images, an ill-defined stress fracture was identified in the palmar cortex of the distal diaphysis of the third metacarpal bone. This corresponds to focal, severe increase in radiopharmaceutical (F^{18}-NaF) uptake in this region on the PET scan (*arrow*). Additionally, there is an increase in radiopharmaceutical uptake within the medullary cavity of the third metacarpal bone at this site, confirming the stress fracture and associated trauma to the trabecular bone in the medullary cavity. (Image courtesy of Dr. Kate Bills, University of Pennsylvania, New Bolton Center.)

Acknowledgment

With special thanks to prior authors of this chapter for their contributions.

REFERENCES

1. Lane EJ, Proto AV, Phillips TW. Mach bands and density perception. *Radiology*. 1976. Published online October 1.
2. Fairburn A, Dyson S, Murray R. Clinical significance of osseous spurs on the dorsoproximal aspect of the third metatarsal bone. *Equine Vet J*. 2010;42(7):591–599.
3. Les CM, Stover SM, Willits NH. Necropsy survey of metacarpal fusion in the horse. *Am J Vet Res*. 1995;56(11):1421–1432.
4. Simon V, Dyson SJ. Radiologic anatomic variation of the carpus in horses with carpal lameness and control horses. *Vet Radiol Ultrasound Off J Am Coll Vet Radiol Int Vet Radiol Assoc*. 2010;51(6):601–606.
5. Nagy A, Dyson S. Anatomical, magnetic resonance imaging and histological findings in the accessory ligament of the deep digital flexor tendon of forelimbs in nonlame horses. *Equine Vet J*. 2011;43(3):309–316.
6. Muylle S, Vanderperren K, Saunders J, Simoens P. Morphometric data on the accessory ligament of the deep digital flexor tendon in the equine hindlimb. *Vet J*. 2010;184:298–302.
7. Nagy A, Dyson S. Magnetic resonance imaging and histological findings in the proximal aspect of the suspensory ligament of forelimbs in nonlame horses. *Equine Vet J*. 2012;44(1):43–50.
8. Bischofberger AS, Konar M, Ohlerth S, et al. Magnetic resonance imaging, ultrasonography and histology of the suspensory ligament origin: a comparative study of normal anatomy of Warmblood horses. *Equine Vet J*. 2006;38(6): 508–516.
9. Nagy A, Dyson S. Magnetic resonance anatomy of the proximal metacarpal region of the horse described from images acquired from low- and high-field magnets. *Vet Radiol Ultrasound*. 2009;50(6):595–605.
10. Werpy NM, Denoix JM. Imaging of the equine proximal suspensory ligament. *Vet Clin North Am Equine Pract*. 2012;28(3):507–525.
11. Minshall GJ, Wright IM. Arthroscopic diagnosis and treatment of intra-articular insertional injuries of the suspensory ligament branches in 18 horses. *Equine Vet J*. 2006;38(1): 10–14.
12. Dyson S. Musculoskeletal scintigraphy of the equine athlete. *Semin Nucl Med*. 2014;44(1):4–14.
13. Rooney J, Prickett M. Foreleg splints in horses. *Cornell Vet*. 1966;56(2):259–269.
14. Zubrod CJ, Schneider RK, Tucker RL. Use of magnetic resonance imaging identify suspensory desmitis and adhesions between exostoses of the second metacarpal bone and the suspensory ligament in four horses. *J Am Vet Med Assoc*. 2004;224(11):1815–1820, 1789.
15. Mair TS, Dyson SJ, Fraser JA, Edwards GB, Hillyer MH, Love S. Hypertrophic osteopathy (Marie's disease) in Equidae: a review of twenty-four cases. *Equine Vet J*. 1996;28(4):256–262.
16. Moens Y, Verschooten F, Moor D, Wouters L. Bone sequestration as a consequence of limb wounds in the horse. *Vet Radiol*. 1980;21(1):40–44.
17. Dyson SJ, Arthur RM, Palmer SE, Richardson D. Suspensory ligament desmitis. *Vet Clin North Am Equine Pract*. 1995;11(2):177–215.
18. Dyson S. Proximal suspensory desmitis in the hindlimb: 42 cases. *Br Vet J*. 1994;150(3):279–291.
19. Hinkle FE, Selberg KT, Frisbie DD, Barrett MF. Radiographic changes of the proximal third metatarsal bone do

not predict presence or severity of proximal suspensory desmopathy in a predominately Quarter Horse population. *Equine Vet J*. 2022;(n/a):1–9.
20. Bramlage LR, Gabel AA, Hackett RP. Avulsion fractures of the origin of the suspensory ligament of the horse. *J Am Vet Med Assoc*. 1980;176(10 pt 1):1004–1010.
21. Kidd J. Management of splint bone fractures in horses. *In Pract*. 2003;25(7):388–395.
22. Verschooten F, Gasthuys F, De MOOR A. Distal splint bone fractures in the horse: an experimental and clinical study. *Equine Vet J*. 1984;16(6):532–536.
23. Seabaugh KA, Hubert JD, Kawcak CE, et al. Effect of sequential removal of parts of the second metacarpal bone on the biomechanical stability of the equine carpus. *Vet Surg*. 2012;41(7):862–868.
24. Riggs CM, Whitehouse GH, Boyde A. Pathology of the distal condyles of the third metacarpal and third metatarsal bones of the horse. *Equine Vet J*. 1999;31(2):140–148.
25. Ross MW, Ford TS, Orsini PG. Incomplete longitudinal fracture of the proximal palmar cortex of the third metacarpal bone in horses. *Vet Surg*. 1988;17(2):82–86.
26. Shan R, Johnston AS, Rosanowski SM, O'Shea J, Riggs CM. Stress fracture of the palmar, distal cortex of the third metacarpal bone: a diagnostic challenge with a good prognosis. *Equine Vet J*. 2022;54(1):74–81.
27. Ross MW, Martin BB. Dorsomedial articular fracture of the proximal aspect of the third metacarpal bone in Standardbred racehorses: seven cases (1978–1990). *J Am Vet Med Assoc*. 1992;201(2):332–335.
28. Watt BC, Foerner JJ, Haines GR. Incomplete oblique sagittal fractures of the dorsal cortex of the third metacarpal bone in six horses. *Vet Surg*. 1998;27(4):337–341.
29. Kawcak CE, Bramlage LR, Embertson RM. Diagnosis and management of incomplete fracture of the distal palmar aspect of the third metacarpal bone in five horses. *J Am Vet Med Assoc*. 1995;206(3):335–337.
30. Pilsworth RC, Hopes R, Greet TR. A flexed dorso-palmar projection of the equine fetlock in demonstrating lesions of the distal third metacarpus. *Vet Rec*. 1988;122(14):332–333.
31. Werpy NM, Denoix JM, McIlwraith CW, Frisbie DD. Comparison between standard ultrasonography, angle contrast ultrasonography, and magnetic resonance imaging characteristics of the normal equine proximal suspensory ligament. *Vet Radiol Ultrasound*. 2013;54(5):536–547.
32. Fornage BD. The hypoechoic normal tendon. A pitfall. *J Ultrasound Med*. 1987;6(1):19–22.
33. Whitcomb MB. Ultrasonographic evaluation of the metacarpus, metatarsus, and pastern. *Clin Tech Equine Pract*. 2004;3(3):238–255.
34. Wood AK, Sehgal CM, Polansky M. Sonographic brightness of the flexor tendons and ligaments in the metacarpal region of horses. *Am J Vet Res*. 1993;54(12):1969–1974.
35. Denoix JM, Busoni V. Ultrasonographic anatomy of the accessory ligament of the superficial digital flexor tendon in horses. *Equine Vet J*. 1999;31(3):186–191.
36. Denoix JM, Farres D. Ultrasonographic Imaging of the proximal third interosseous muscle in the pelvic limb using a plantaromedial approach. *J Equine Vet Sci*. 1995;15(5):346–350.
37. Smith RKW, Jones R, Webbon PM. The cross-sectional areas of normal equine digital flexor tendons determined ultrasonographically. *Equine Vet J*. 1994;26(6):460–465.
38. Gillis C, Meagher DM, Cloninger A, Locatelli L, Willits N. Ultrasonographic cross-sectional area and mean echogenicity of the superficial and deep digital flexor tendons in 50 trained thoroughbred racehorses. *Am J Vet Res*. 1995;56(10):1265–1269.
39. Gillis C, Sharkey N, Stover SM, Pool RR, Meagher DM, Willits N. Ultrasonography as a method to determine tendon cross-sectional area. *Am J Vet Res*. 1995;56(10):1270–1274.
40. Rabba S, Grulke S, Verwilghen D, Evrard L, Busoni V. B-mode and power Doppler ultrasonography of the equine suspensory ligament branches: a descriptive study on 13 horses. *Vet Radiol Ultrasound*. 2018;59(4):453–460.
41. Lacitignola L, Rossella S, Pasquale DL, Crovace A. Power Doppler to investigate superficial digital flexor tendinopathy in the horse. *Open Vet J*. 2020;9(4):317.
42. Murata D, Misumi K, Fujiki M. A preliminary study of diagnostic color Doppler ultrasonography in equine superficial digital flexor tendonitis. *J Vet Med Sci*. 2012;74(12):1639–1642.
43. Chesen AB, Dabareiner RM, Chaffin MK, Carter GK. Tendinitis of the proximal aspect of the superficial digital flexor tendon in horses: 12 cases (2000–2006). *J Am Vet Med Assoc*. 2009;234(11):1432–1436.
44. Gates S, Hinnigan G, Rich A, Ricci E, Owen K. A case series of five horses with superficial digital flexor tendon lesions in the carpal canal. *J Equine Vet Sci*. 2021;103:103656.
45. Garcia da Fonseca RM, Evrard L, Rabba S, Salciccia A, Busoni V. Dynamic flexion/extension and non-weight bearing ultrasonography is helpful for identifying manica flexoria tears in horses. *Vet Radiol Ultrasound*. 2019;60(1):65–74.
46. Barr ARS, Dyson SJ, Barr FJ, O'Brien JK. Tendonitis of the deep digital flexor tendon in the distal metacarpal/metatarsal region associated with tenosynovitis of the digital sheath in the horse. *Equine Vet J*. 1995;27(5):348–355.
47. Smith MRW, Wright IM. Noninfected tenosynovitis of the digital flexor tendon sheath: a retrospective analysis of 76 cases. *Equine Vet J*. 2006;38(2):134–141.
48. Kent AV, Chesworth MJ, Wells G, et al. Improved diagnostic criteria for digital flexor tendon sheath pathology using contrast tenography. *Equine Vet J*. 2020;52(2):205–212.
49. McDiarmid AM. Eighteen cases of desmitis of the accessory ligament of the deep digital flexor tendon. *Equine Vet Educ*. 1994;6(1):49–56.
50. van den Belt AJ, Becker CK, Dik KJ. Desmitis of the accessory ligament of the deep digital flexor tendon in the horse: clinical and ultrasonographic features. A report of 24 cases. *Zentralbl Veterinarmed A*. 1993;40(7):492–500.
51. Dyson SJ. Desmitis of the accessory ligament of the deep digital flexor tendon: 27 cases (1986–1990). *Equine Vet J*. 1991;23(6):438–444.
52. Dyson S. Proximal injuries of the accessory ligament of the deep digital flexor tendon in forelimbs and hindlimbs: 12 horses (2006–2010). *Equine Vet Educ*. 2012;24(3):134–142.
53. Dyson S, Murray R, Pinilla MJ. Proximal suspensory desmopathy in hindlimbs: a correlative clinical, ultrasonographic, gross post mortem and histological study. *Equine Vet J*. 2017;49(1):65–72.
54. Brokken MT, Schneider RK, Sampson SN, Tucker RL, Gavin PR, Ho CP. Magnetic resonance imaging features of proximal metacarpal and metatarsal injuries in the horse. *Vet Radiol Ultrasound*. 2007;48(6):507–517.
55. Powell SE, Ramzan PHL, Head MJ, Shepherd MC, Baldwin GI, Steven WN. Standing magnetic resonance imaging detection of bone marrow oedema-type signal pattern associated with subcarpal pain in 8 racehorses: a prospective study. *Equine Vet J*. 2010;42(1):10–17.
56. Ehrlich PJ, Dohoo IR, O'Callaghan MW. Results of bone scintigraphy in racing Standardbred horses: 64 cases (1992–1994). *J Am Vet Med Assoc*. 1999;215(7):982–991.

57. Markel MD, Snyder JR, Hornof WJ, Meagher DM. Nuclear scintigraphic evaluation of third metacarpal and metatarsal bone fractures in three horses. *J Am Vet Med Assoc.* 1987;191(1):75–77.
58. Koblik PD, Hornof WJ, Seeherman HJ. Scintigraphic appearance of stress-induced trauma of the dorsal cortex of the third metacarpal bone in racing Thoroughbred horses: 121 cases (1978–1986). *J Am Vet Med Assoc.* 1988;192(3):390–395.
59. Weekes JS, Murray RC, Dyson SJ. Scintigraphic evaluation of the proximal metacarpal and metatarsal regions in clinically sound horses. *Vet Radiol Ultrasound.* 2006;47(4):409–416.
60. Dyson SJ, Weekes JS, Murray RC. Scintigraphic evaluation of the proximal metacarpal and metatarsal regions of horses with proximal suspensory desmitis. *Vet Radiol Ultrasound.* 2007;48(1):78–85.
61. Spriet M, Edwards L, Arndt S, et al. Validation of a dedicated positron emission tomography scanner for imaging of the distal limb of standing horses. *Vet Radiol Ultrasound Off J Am Coll Vet Radiol Int Vet Radiol Assoc.* 2022;63(4): 469–477.
62. Spriet M. Positron emission tomography: a horse in the musculoskeletal imaging race. *Am J Vet Res.* 2022;83(7). ajvr.22.03.0051.
63. Spriet M, Espinosa P, Kyme AZ, et al. Positron emission tomography of the equine distal limb: exploratory study. *Vet Radiol Ultrasound.* 2016;57(6):630–638.
64. Spriet M, Espinosa-Mur P, Cissell DD, et al. 18 F-sodium fluoride positron emission tomography of the racing Thoroughbred fetlock: validation and comparison with other imaging modalities in nine horses. *Equine Vet J.* 2019;51(3):375–383.
65. Wilson S, Spriet M, Mur PE, et al. 18Fluorine-fluorodeoxyglucose positron emission tomography for assessment of deep digital flexor tendinopathy: an exploratory study in eight horses with comparison to CT and MRI. *Vet Radiol Ultrasound.* 2021;62(5):610–620.

ELECTRONIC RESOURCES

Additional information related to the content in Chapter 24 can be found online at eBooks.Health.Elsevier.com.

- Chapter Quiz

CHAPTER 25

Equine Fetlock Joint

Kathryn W. Bills

ANATOMY

The equine fetlock, or metacarpophalangeal (MCP) and metatarsophalangeal (MTP) articulations are high motion hinge joints, formed by the distal end of the metacarpal (or metatarsal) bone and the proximal end of the proximal phalanx. It is not possible to reliably differentiate the right from the left or the forelimb from the hindlimb on unlabeled radiographs. The articular surface of the proximal phalanx is concave and has a sagittal groove opposing the sagittal ridge at the distal end of the third metacarpal (MC III) or the third metatarsal (MT III) bone. This ridge and groove divide the weight-bearing surface into two unequal parts, the third metacarpal/metacarpal condyles and the proximal phalanx medial and lateral fovea. The largest surface is on the medial (or axial) side, where loading is greatest. The sagittal ridge of MC III or MT III is received into a depression at the palmar* surface that is created by the proximal sesamoid bones and the intersesamoidean ligament. The joint has two radii of articulation. The dorsal radius serves the weight-bearing portion, and the palmar radius conforms to the articulation with the proximal sesamoid bones.[1] The junction of these radii of articulation often appears flat in lateral radiographs and may be confused with a lesion of the articular surface and subchondral bone, which is complicated by the fact that pathology occurs in the same location.

The joint capsule attachments at the proximal end of the proximal phalanx are immediately periarticular, with a palmarodistal recess between the proximal phalanx and the distal sesamoidean ligaments. The capsule attaches to the distal end of MC III or MT III at the periarticular margins. Dorsally, a large recess extends proximally and forms a pouch. The palmar joint capsule extends proximal to the sesamoid bones between the suspensory ligament and MC III or MT III.[1] Ligaments associated with the MCP and MTP articulations are described elsewhere.[2]

RADIOGRAPHIC EXAMINATION

The examination of the fetlock joint should include the proximal interphalangeal joint and the distal third of the metacarpal or metatarsal bones. Identification markers are essential in radiographic examination of the MCP or MTP articulation; right versus left and front versus hind should be designated clearly. If oblique views are obtained, the direction of the x-ray beam designates the name of the projection from point-of-entrance to point-of-exit. Markers should be placed at the lateral aspect of the anatomic part of interest on all views, except for the lateromedial view for which markers should be placed dorsally.[3]

*"Palmar(o)" is used throughout this chapter with the understanding that "plantar(o)" should be substituted if reference is being made to the hindlimb.

Survey radiographic examination of the joint should include a lateromedial, a dorsopalmar, and two oblique projections (dorsal 15-degree proximal 45-degree lateral-palmarodistomedial and dorsal 15-degree proximal 45-degree medial-palmarodistolateral), with the limb bearing weight if possible. In the author's opinion, using a horizontal oblique projection has less utility than the incorporation of 15-degree proximal to distal angle as palmar fragments are easily missed on the horizontal oblique projections. The survey examination should precede any special radiographic projections or contrast studies of the joint. The lateromedial projection should be made with the primary beam centered at the articulation and directed parallel to an imaginary line connecting the condylar fossae at the distal end of MC III or MT III. A true lateromedial projection is essential to properly assess the sagittal ridge of distal MC III or MT III.[4] For the dorsopalmar projection, because the plane of the joint is at an angle to the solar surface of the hoof, the primary beam is directed from dorsoproximal to palmarodistal at least 10 to 15 degrees (forelimb 10, hindlimb 15). This should result in the projection of the proximal sesamoid bones over the distal aspect of MC III or MT III and the joint space projected with maximal width.[5] The dorsal 15-degree proximal 45-degree lateral/palmarodistomedial and dorsal 15-degree proximal 45-degree medial/palmarodistolateral projections should be a routine part of the survey examination. These oblique views are necessary to view the abaxial aspects of the articular surfaces, the periarticular margins, and the proximal sesamoid bones. Oblique views made in a dorsal 60-degree lateral/palmaromedial or dorsal 60-degree medial/palmarolateral direction allow the best visibility of the dorsal eminence of the proximal phalanx, which is located near midline, and the axial aspect of the proximal sesamoid bones as well as the joint space between the dorsal margin of the proximal sesamoid bone and the palmar condyle. Some prefer using the 60-degree oblique view as the routine oblique view rather than the oblique views made at 45 degrees because of improved delineation of the axial margin of the proximal sesamoid bones (Fig. 25.1).[6]

Additional projections of the joint may be indicated according to the information gained from the routine survey radiographs or based on discipline-specific indications, such as the flexed dorsopalmar projection for the Thoroughbred racehorse.[4,7] The lateromedial projection during flexion is performed while the foot is held off the ground as if the sole of the hoof were being inspected visually. Alternate positions include variations in the degree of flexion and flexed oblique views. These projections may provide better visibility of subarticular surfaces at the dorsal aspect of distal MC III or MT III, the proximal part of the proximal phalanx, and the articular margins of the proximal sesamoid bones.[5]

A dorsal 30-degree proximal 70-degree lateral-palmarodistomedial oblique projection, or "elevated angle oblique," can be used to assist in the evaluation of the palmar condyle of the third metacarpal bone, the base of the proximal sesamoid bones, and the palmar processes of the proximal phalanx, particularly in cases of comminuted fracture of the latter.[4]

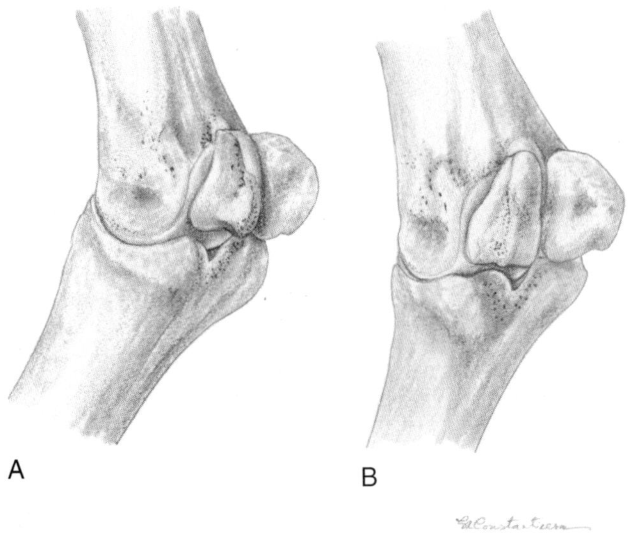

Fig. 25.1 The effect of angle of obliquity on the different aspects of the proximal sesamoid bones that will be projected. **A,** The dorsal 30-degree proximal, 45-degree medial (or lateral)/palmarodistolateral (or medial) view of the metacarpophalangeal (MCP) joint best demonstrates the abaxial aspect of the sesamoid bones where the branches of the suspensory ligament attach. **B,** Dorsal 30-degree proximal, 60-degree medial (or lateral)/palmarodistolateral (or medial) view of the joint maximizes the evaluation of the dorsal eminence of P1. (Drawing courtesy Gheorghe M. Constantinescu, DVM, University of Missouri, Columbia.)

The dorsodistal-palmaroproximal projection is made while the limb is extended and weight bearing. In this projection, a tangential view of the articular margin of the distal aspect of MC III or MT III is created. The foot is elevated on a block, and the limb is extended. The primary beam direction is approximately 125 degrees to the axis of the metacarpal or metatarsal bone.[8] The angle of the primary beam determines the tangent of the joint surface that is visible. In an ideally positioned radiograph, the distal third of the proximal sesamoid bones will be superimposed with the articular margin. This projection is particularly helpful for identifying incomplete condylar fractures and characterizing palmar comminution.

The palmaroproximal-palmarodistal projection is used to see the palmar articular surface of MC III or MT III and the proximal sesamoid bones. Positioning of the patient requires that the x-ray tube be placed close to the horse's body. The limb should be positioned as far caudal as possible, and the foot is placed on a supporting tunnel containing a cassette.[5] Inherent magnification results from the use of this projection because of the distance between the proximal sesamoid bones and the detector.

The abaxial surfaces of the proximal sesamoids may be examined further by placing the detector medial or lateral to the joint on the affected side. The x-ray beam is then directed in a dorsal 50-degree proximal, 45-degree lateral/distopalmaromedial or dorsal 50-degree proximal, 45-degree medial/distopalmarolateral direction, respectively, to create a tangential view of the proximal sesamoid bones.[9] This positioning results in the x-ray beam being directed downward at the sesamoid bones at an angle of 50 degrees from horizontal. This tangential projection is beneficial in assessing whether articular involvement is present with sesamoid lesions and to better characterize occult suspensory ligament avulsions or basilar sesamoid fractures. The results can affect the surgical approach (Fig. 25.2A,C).

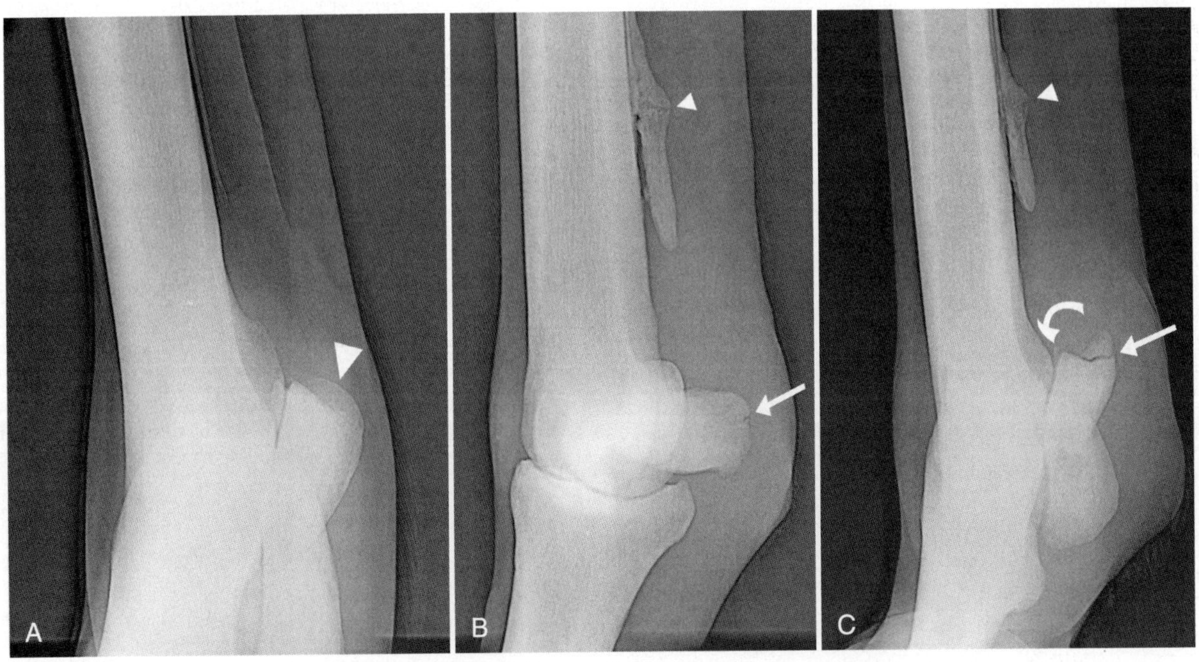

Fig. 25.2 **A,** A dorsal 50-degree proximal, 45-degree medial/distopalmarolateral view; note the normal appearance of the proximal abaxial aspect of the sesamoid bone on this tangential view (*white arrowhead*). **B and C,** Oblique views of an apical sesamoid fracture. **B,** A dorsal 30-degree proximal, 60-degree lateral/palmarodistomedial oblique view. A fracture of the lateral sesamoid bone is visible (*white arrow*) and the fracture appears incomplete. A chronic fracture of the distal MC IV is also present (*white arrowhead*). **C,** A dorsal 50-degree proximal, 45-degree medial/distopalmarolateral view of the same horse. From this projection it is apparent that the sesamoid fracture is both complete and articular (*straight white arrow*) with a small articular fragment (*curved white arrow*). The chronic distal MC IV fracture is also visible (*white arrowhead*). (Courtesy Scott E. Palmer, VMD, Dipl. ABVP-Equine, New Jersey Equine Clinic, Clarksburg, New Jersey.)

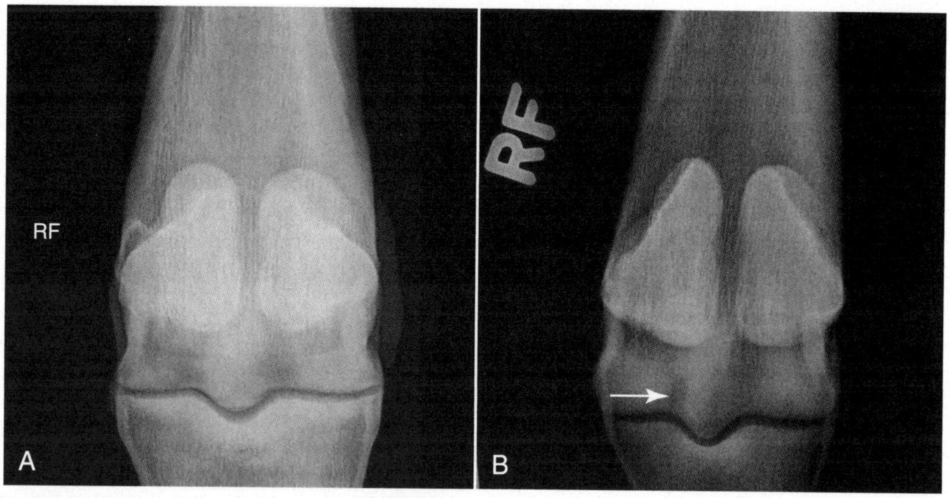

Fig. 25.3 Dorsopalmar **(A)** and flexed dorsopalmar **(B)** radiographs of the right metacarpophalangeal joint from the same horse. A lucent line (*white arrow*) is present in the lateral parasagittal groove and is only noted on the flexed projection. Also note the increased conspicuity of the marked surrounding lateral parasagittal groove sclerosis.

A flexed dorsopalmar projection is acquired by positioning the foot in a block (e.g., Hickman navicular block) to provide a more predictable degree of fetlock flexion. The primary beam is angled between 0 and 35 degrees depending on the tangential surface of the condyle attempting to be imaged.[10] The projection is particularly useful for identifying unicortical condylar fractures, palmar comminution of said condylar fractures, and axial sesamoid lesions (Fig. 25.3).[11]

The dorsoproximal-dorsodistal projection is used to improve visualization of the dorsal margin of the metacarpal/metatarsal condyles. With the metacarpus aligned perpendicular to the ground, the fetlock is held in a flexed position with the detector held horizontal to the ground under the joint. The beam is variably angled, between 45 and 70 degrees, to create a tangential image of the dorsodistal metacarpal condyle and helps to characterize the dorsal articular margin (Fig. 25.4). The ideal projection angle will depend upon where a particular lesion is located along the curvature of the condyle, most commonly in the dorsal to mid-thirds of the medial aspect.[12]

Contrast arthrography of the MCP or MTP joint and intrathecal injection of the digital flexor tendon sheath is sometimes useful but has largely been replaced by ultrasonographic assessment. For contrast arthrography, 5 to 10 mL of water-soluble contrast medium containing 300 mg/mL of iodine is injected using aseptic technique. Injection of contrast medium should follow arthrocentesis and withdrawal of an equal volume of synovial fluid. Injection is made into the lateral pouch of the joint, proximal to the lateral sesamoid bones and dorsal to the suspensory ligament or into the dorsal synovial recess. The joint should be flexed, extended, and massaged vigorously before radiography to distribute the contrast medium throughout the joint.

ALTERNATIVE IMAGING MODALITIES

Ultrasound offers detailed evaluation of soft tissues surrounding the MCP or MTP joint and is used frequently to complement the radiographic examination. Portable ultrasound machines can be used to image the extensor and flexor tendons, manica flexoria, the suspensory and distal sesamoidean ligaments, the intersesamoidean ligament, the synovial lining and joint recesses, collateral ligaments, cortical margins, and portions of the articular cartilage of standing horses at rest.[13] More recently, non–weight-bearing and dynamic ultrasound of the suspensory branches and digital flexor tendon sheath has been performed.[14,15] The normal sonographic features of the MCP and MTP joints have been described.[16]

Nuclear scintigraphy for evaluation of bone utilizing ^{99m}Tc-methylene diphosphonate (MDP) or ^{99m}Tc-hydroxymethylene disphosphonate (HDP) has been performed for decades. It is highly sensitive for detecting osseous fetlock pathology in many disciplines.[17,18] Pathologic changes and nonpathologic manifestations of adaptive remodeling of bone can be identified, so knowledge of discipline-specific patterns of uptake is imperative for correct interpretation.[19]

In addition to conventional radiography, computed tomography (CT) may be useful in selected patients to image the MCP or MTP joint.[20] CT excels in the evaluation of bone and is useful in imaging condylar and complex fractures, developmental orthopedic disease, and manifestations of early joint disease, such as small osteophytes, subchondral and trabecular sclerosis, osseous cyst-like lesions (OCLLs), subchondral bone injury secondary to repetitive trauma, and ill-defined lysis as found in joint sepsis and septic osteomyelitis[21,22] (Fig. 25.5). There is wider availability of standing fan- and cone-beam CT systems with similar performance in identification of osseous fetlock pathology in various disciplines.[23–25] The speed of image acquisition is also a benefit compared to other standing cross-sectional imaging modalities, such as low-field magnetic resonance imaging (MRI). Finally, similar to certain MRI sequences, CT volume data acquisition allows for multiplanar reconstruction and reformatting of images such that an infinite number of planes can be evaluated with a single scan of the region of interest.

MRI is commonly used to evaluate the equine distal limb, including the MCP or MTP joints.[21,26–31] A distinct advantage of MRI is the exceptional soft tissue contrast resolution and ability to evaluate articular cartilage (Figs. 25.6–25.8). Magnetic resonance (MR) examinations usually include several types of acquisition sequences to allow evaluation of different anatomic and pathologic features, based on the composition of each tissue. MR systems employing high-field magnets require that horses be under general anesthesia for imaging. Low-field MR

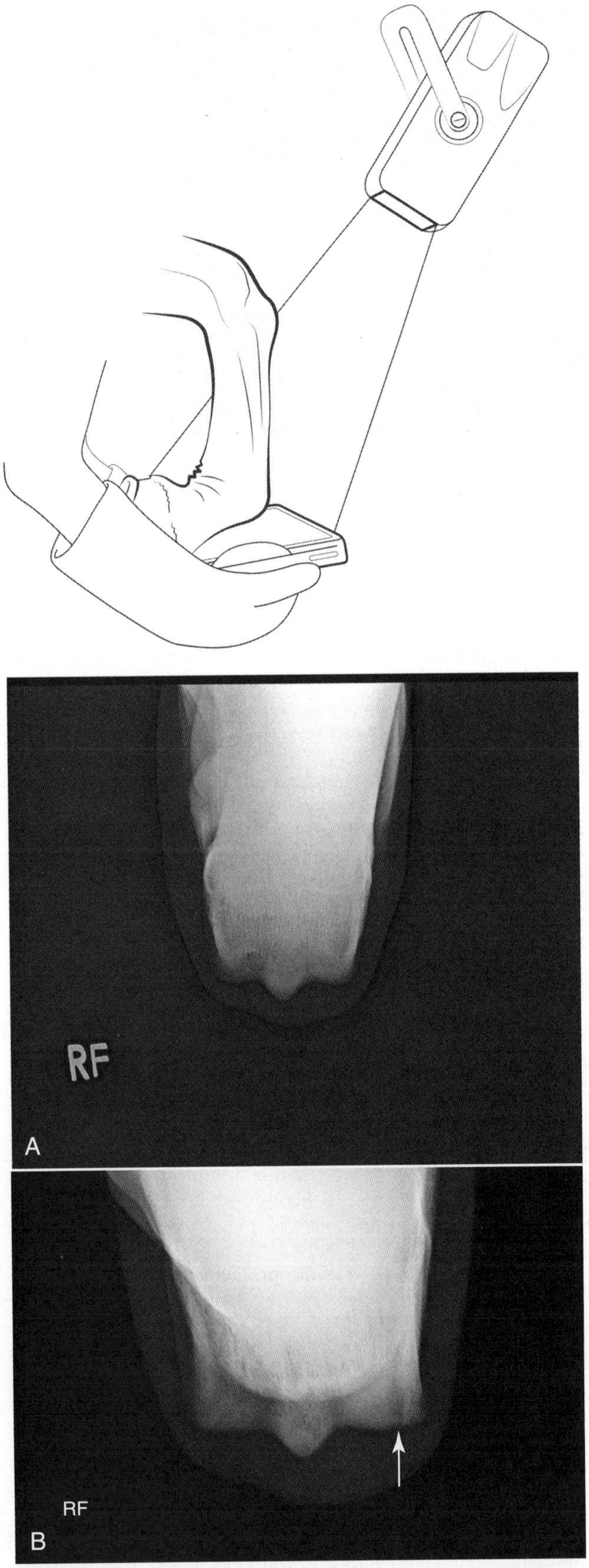

Fig. 25.4 **A,** Schematic drawing for positioning the limb and detector to acquire the flexed dorsoproximal-dorsodistal oblique projection (*top image*) of the fetlock and resultant well-positioned radiograph (*bottom image*). The tangential projection allows isolation of the dorsal margin of the metacarpal condyle to increase the detection of subchondral bone disease **(B)**, which manifests radiographically as regions of sclerosis with central demineralization/lucent regions (*white arrow*). (Images courtesy of Dr. Laura Faulkner, Watermark Equine, Ridgefield, CT, USA. Line drawing in (A) is contributed by Beth Mellor.)

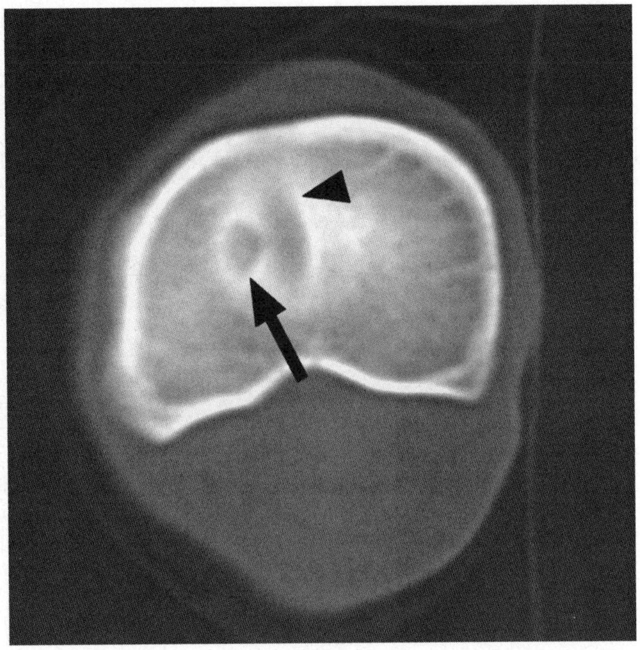

Fig. 25.5 A transverse 1.5-mm-thick computed tomography (CT) image of the proximal aspect of the proximal phalanx. A small, oval, hypoattenuating subchondral demineralization lesion (*black arrow*) is surrounded by hyperattenuating sclerotic bone just lateral parasagittal to the sagittal groove (*black arrowhead*).

systems are available for imaging the limbs of standing horses. However, volume averaging and motion artifact remain limitations of these, especially proximal to the distal phalanx, although motion correction techniques improve resolution.[32]

Finally, the most recently developed imaging modality for evaluating the equine fetlock is positron emission tomography (PET), utilizing both ^{18}F-NaF and ^{18}F-FDG tracers for bone and soft tissue imaging, respectively. As a cross-sectional imaging modality, PET combines the benefits of tomographic imaging with the high sensitivity and physiologic information from scintigraphy and has the highest lesion detection and agreement amongst specialty and general practitioners compared to other modalities.[33] PET has already demonstrated an ability to detect injuries at sites unable to be diagnosed by radiographs, such as the dorsal aspect of the proximal sesamoid bone (Fig. 25.9).

RADIOGRAPHIC INTERPRETATION OF DISEASES OF THE METACARPOPHALANGEAL/ METATARSOPHALANGEAL ARTICULATION

Joint disease in many horses is often associated with training-associated repetitive trauma and the pathologic changes may be characteristic of the joint or function of the horse. A study of racetrack injuries has provided an overview of pathologic findings and pathogenesis of MCP or MTP joint disease.[34] Lameness and distension of a joint are the initial clinical signs that typically precede the request for radiographic examination following localization with diagnostic analgesia. The earliest signs of joint disease may remain obscure on radiographs, because wear lines in the articular cartilage or synovial hypertrophy are usually unrecognized. Radiographs of the contralateral joint are helpful for comparison. Although pathologic change is often bilateral, it is usually in different stages of development between limbs.

Joint Effusion

Joint effusion is usually a result of trauma and subsequent joint debris and not necessarily due to permanent degenerative

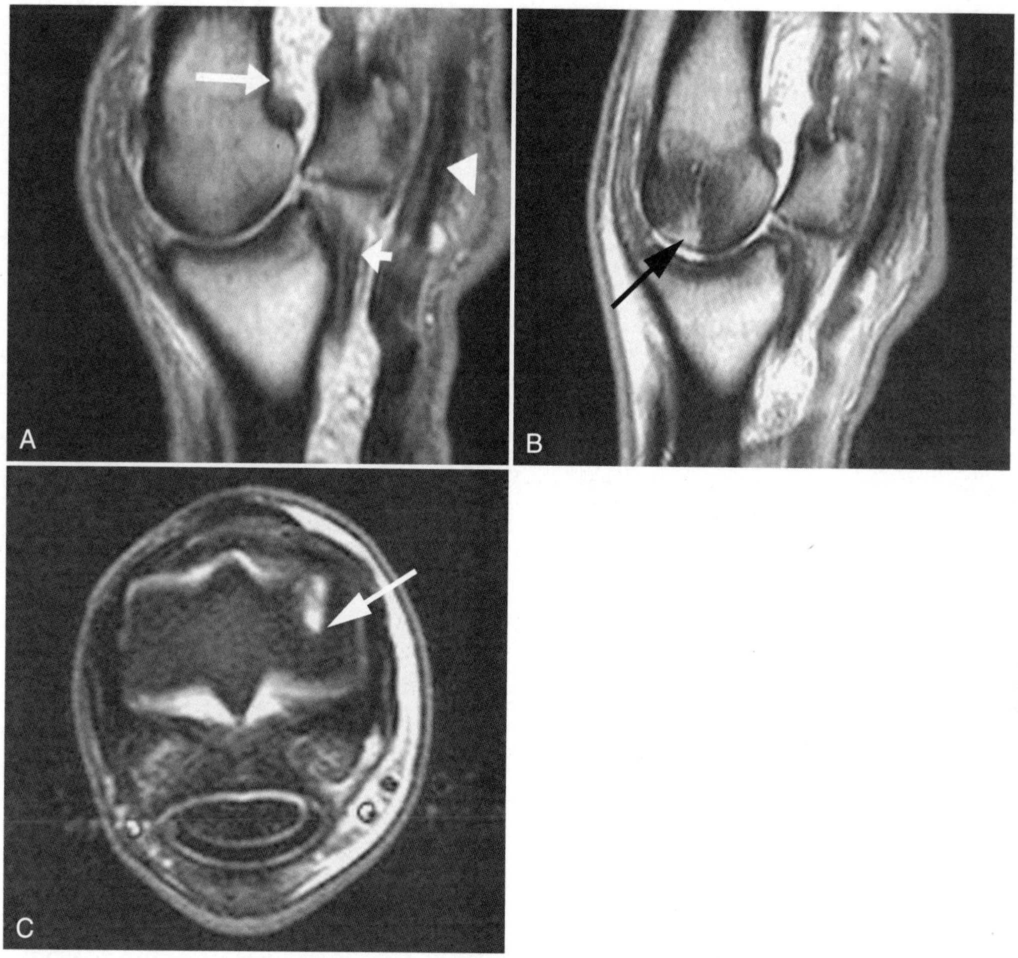

Fig. 25.6 Magnetic resonance (MR) images of right and left distal MC III. **A,** Sagittal proton density-weighted MR image of the metacarpophalangeal (MCP) joint. The deep digital flexor tendon courses along the palmar aspect (*white arrowhead*) and the distal sesamoidean ligaments originate on the distal margin of the proximal sesamoid bone (*short white arrow*). The synovial fluid in the palmar pouch can be visualized clearly (*long white arrow*). **B,** Sagittal proton density-weighted MR image of the contralateral MCP joint. Distal MC III medial condyle high fluid signal (*black arrow*) is consistent with subchondral injury, with an associated articular cartilage defect. **C,** Transverse spectral presaturation with inversion recovery weighted image of the affected area in **B** that removes signal derived from fat. This increases the visibility of the MC III medial condyle lesion (*white arrow*).

changes of the articular surfaces.[35] Radiographic signs include soft tissue swelling and joint distention. With chronic insults, dystrophic calcification of the periarticular soft tissues may also be present.[36]

Villonodular Synovitis

Villonodular synovitis leads to a firm, nonfluctuating swelling located primarily at the dorsoproximal aspect of the joint. Villonodular masses arise from enlargement of the synovial pad of the joint capsule and are associated with repetitive trauma. The condition is usually diagnosed by clinical signs, history, palpation, and ultrasound. With time, the radiographic signs will include mild to severe smooth erosion of distal MC III or MT III at the region just distal to the dorsal joint capsule attachment (Fig. 25.10). Periarticular bone proliferation may be present. With arthrography, radiolucent, space-occupying masses resulting from synovial villus hypertrophy can usually be identified in the dorsal recess of the joint (Fig. 25.11). Erosion occurring along the palmar/plantar surface of the distal MC III or MT III is termed *supracondylar lysis.*

Supracondylar Lysis

In MC III or MT III, the radiographic features of supracondylar lysis are similar to those in villonodular synovitis affecting the dorsoproximal aspect of the joint, except that supracondylar lysis occurs at the palmar (or plantar) surface of the bone. Changes are caused by chronic proliferative synovitis. Radiographic signs are joint distention and smooth osteolysis at the distal palmar cortex of MC III or MT III, distal to the joint capsule attachment (see Fig. 25.10B). Arthrography may be difficult to perform because of the presence of hypertrophied synovium and diminished synovial joint space. The erosive concavity formed in the bone is usually readily apparent (see Fig. 25.11).

Degenerative Joint Disease

Degenerative joint disease, also termed *osteoarthritis* or *osteoarthrosis*, is a nonspecific term describing the deterioration of articular and periarticular structures. It is a chronic disorder characterized by progressive deterioration of articular cartilage that results in a radiographic loss in joint space and proliferative changes in the joint margin and capsule.[34]

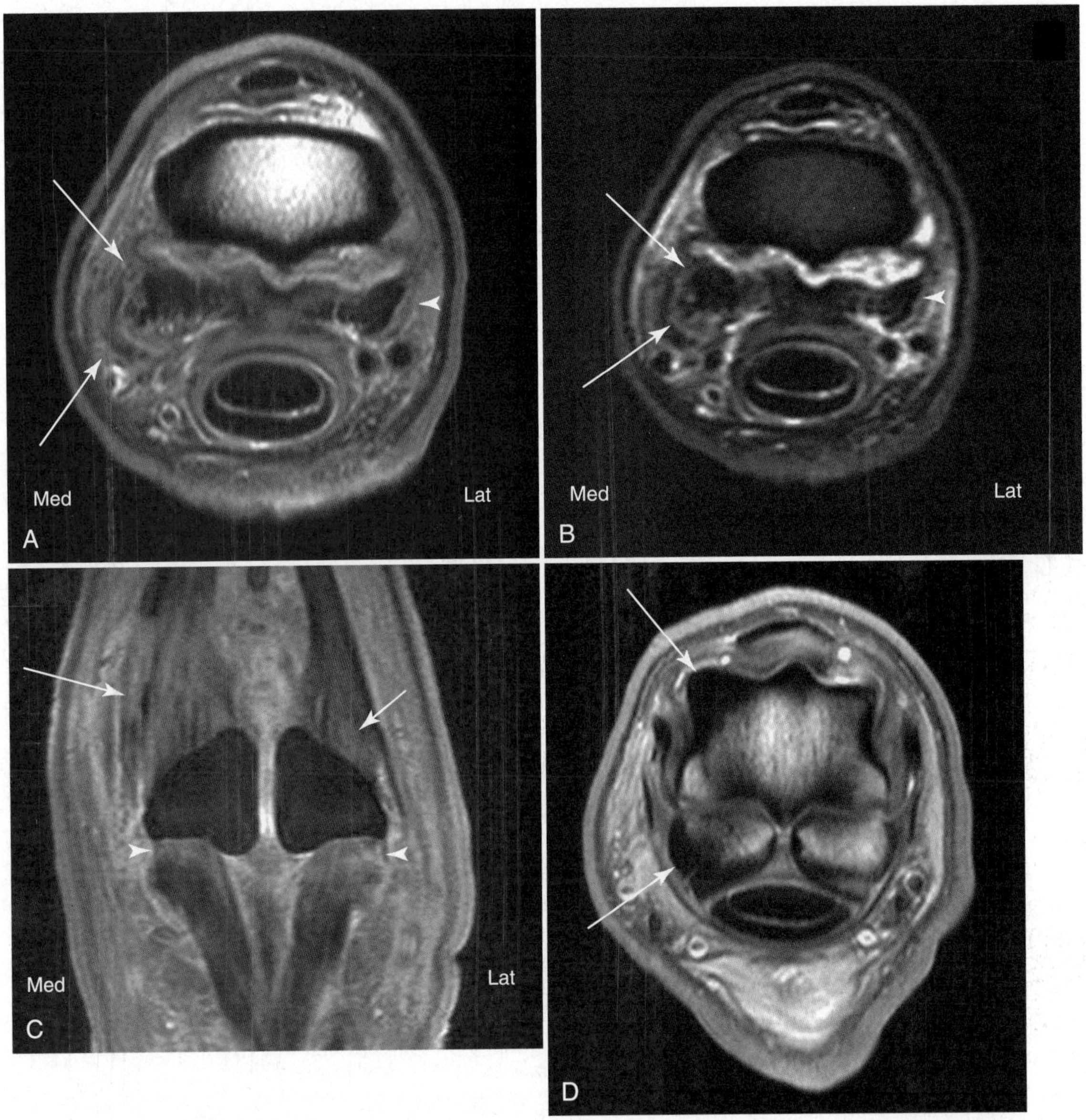

Fig. 25.7 Magnetic resonance (MR) images of a 12-year-old male Friesian with right metatarsophalangeal (MTP) joint swelling and lameness. Radiographically, there was marked periarticular soft tissue swelling, especially along the medial and plantar aspects, but no bone changes were present. Transverse proton density image **(A)** and transverse short time inversion recovery image **(B)** of the joint immediately proximal to the proximal sesamoid bones. There is marked enlargement and abnormal signal of the medial branch of the suspensory ligament (*white arrows*) with surrounding periligamentous fibrosis and soft tissue swelling. The abaxial margin of the lateral branch of the suspensory ligament has an abnormal hyperintensity (*white arrowhead*). **C,** Dorsal gradient recalled echo image of the proximal sesamoid bones. There is diffuse disruption and enlargement of the medial branch of the suspensory ligament (*large white arrow*) and focal disruption of the lateral branch of the suspensory ligament at the insertion to the sesamoid bone (*small white arrow*). In addition, there is abnormal signal and morphology of the proximal aspect of the oblique distal sesamoidean ligaments (*white arrowheads*). **D,** Transverse proton density image at the level of the mid-body of the proximal sesamoid bones. There is sclerosis in the dorsal medial condyle of the third metatarsal bone and along the abaxial margins of the medial proximal sesamoid bone (*white arrows*). *Lat,* Lateral; *Med,* medial.

The first stages include cartilage degeneration and formation of wear lines characteristic of hinge joints. The most common joint in the horse to develop spontaneous osteoarthritis is the metacarpo(tarso) phalangeal joint due to the relatively thin articular cartilage compared to other joints. The articular surfaces develop linear erosions that form grooves oriented parallel to the direction of joint motion.[37] Cartilaginous fibrillation and erosions form on the surface, and subsequent wear results in narrowing of the joint space. If reduction in the width of a joint space is confirmed on two radiographic views, cartilage thinning is likely. Progressive loss of joint width is a subjective finding and must be assessed in conjunction with clinical signs to determine its significance (Fig. 25.12).

Radiographic signs of degenerative joint disease are soft tissue swelling, narrowed joint space, and bone remodeling, including lysis and proliferation (e.g., osteophytes and

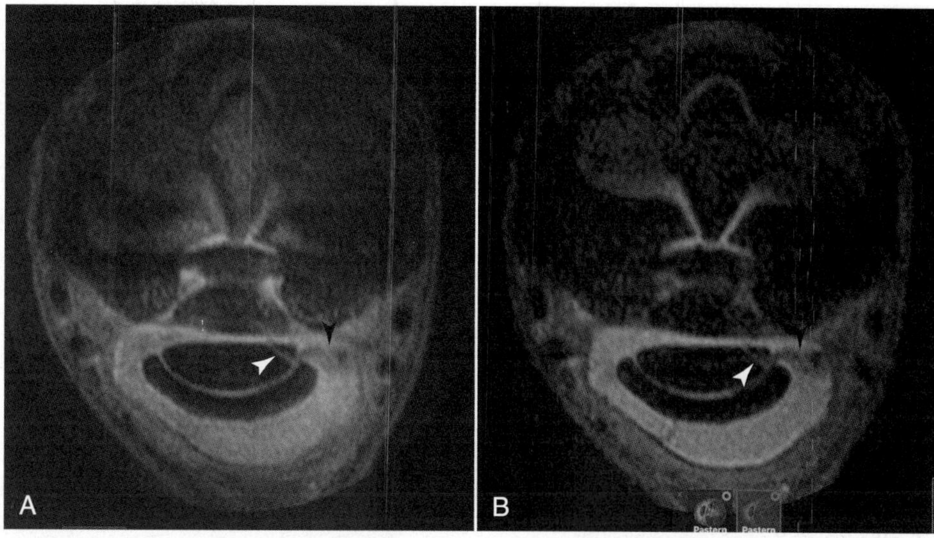

Fig. 25.8 A 9-year-old Arabian with acute digital flexor tendon sheath tenosynovitis: transverse proton density **(A)** and T2-weighted fast-spin echo (T2W FSE) **(B)** images. There is moderate to marked digital flexor tendon sheath effusion secondary to an oblique dorsolateral peripheral tear of the deep digital flexor tendon (DDFT) just distal to the metacarpophalangeal joint (*white arrowhead*). Also note the amorphous heterogeneous intermediate intensity tissue lateral to the tear, consistent with torn DDFT fibers (*black arrowhead*). This type of lesion is best visualized on the T2W images due to partial mitigation of magic angle artifact.

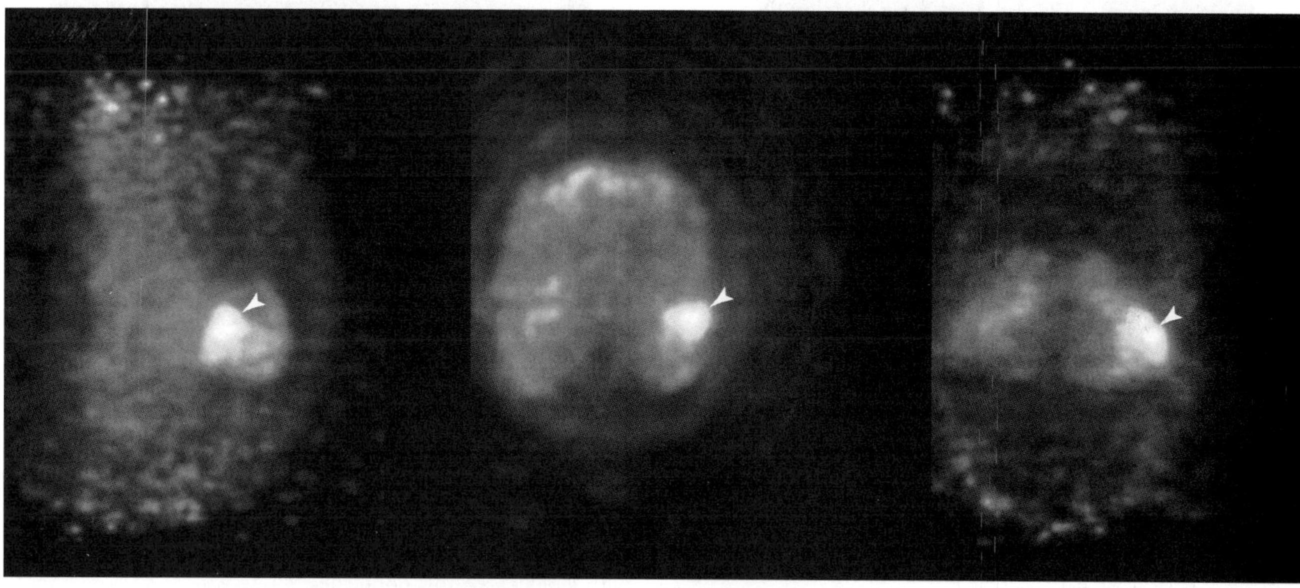

Fig. 25.9 Sagittal (*left*), transverse (*middle*), and dorsal (*right*) ^{18}F-NaF positron emission tomography of a Thoroughbred racehorse fetlock. Dorsal is to the left in the sagittal image. Medial is to the right in the transverse and dorsal plane images. Marked, focal radioavidity (*white arrowheads*) is present in the dorsal, abaxial midaspect of the medial proximal sesamoid bone, a known site of demineralization that acts as a stress riser to proximal sesamoid fracture in Thoroughbred racehorses. (Courtesy of Mathieu Spriet, DVM, MS, DACVR, DECVDI, DACVR-EDI, University of California at Davis, Davis, California, USA.)

enthesophytes) (see Fig. 25.12). These findings may occur in any combination. Joint capsule thickening may be suspected but is rarely visualized, even on high-detail radiographs. Soft tissue swelling results from synovial effusion, as well as hypertrophy and proliferation of other periarticular soft tissues.

Chronic osteoarthritis is characterized by sclerosis or eburnation of subchondral bone, with loss of trabecular architecture because of erosion of the overlying articular cartilage. Repetitive stress or trauma at the joint capsule attachments results in enthesophyte formation (see Fig. 25.10). Similar, but not identical, are periarticular osteophytes that form at the margin of narrowed joints in response to damage to the articular surface as the disease progresses (Fig. 25.13, eFig. 25.1). Of note, many joint disorders can progress to a common end point having the stereotypic features of chronic degenerative joint disease.[34] The initiating factors of degenerative joint disease may be difficult or impossible to determine in the late stages of the disease.

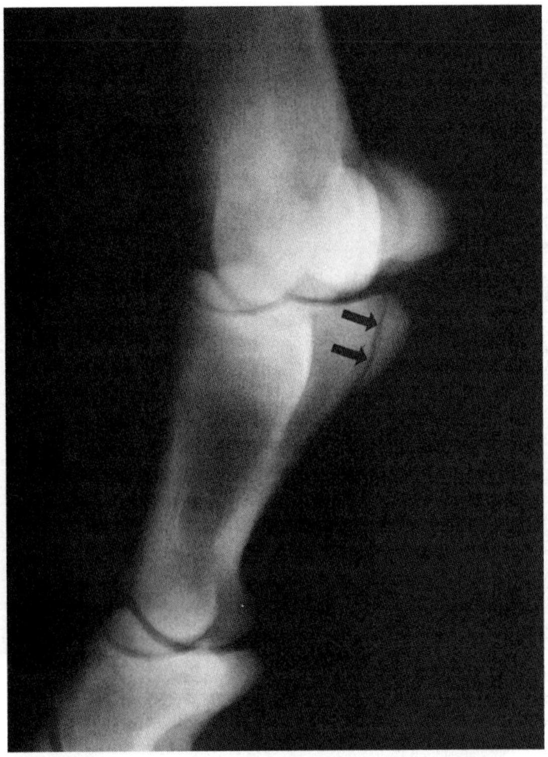

Fig. 25.15 Dorsal 45-degree medial/palmarolateral radiograph of the metacarpophalangeal (MCP) joint with a large type II fragment (*black arrows*) originating from the medial palmar eminence of the proximal phalanx.

Osteochondrosis of the sagittal ridge of MC III or MT III is usually diagnosed in young horses and occurs with variable radiographic expression (Fig. 25.18, eFig. 25.2). Radiographic signs may vary from small areas of flattening to large excavations of subchondral bone of the sagittal ridge and free osseous fragmentation. Lesions are best seen on flexed lateral projections of the MCP or MTP joint and can also be seen on dorsopalmar projections. Detached osteochondral fragments may be found in close association to the bone defect or may be nestled in distant recesses of the joint.[50]

Osseous Cyst-Like Lesions

Ovoid lucent regions with thin rims of surrounding sclerosis can be found in the distal metacarpal condyle and proximal aspect of the proximal phalanx and variably can be a cause of lameness (Fig. 25.19, eFig. 25.3). The etiology is uncertain with both developmental and juvenile trauma etiologies proposed. Subchondral OCLLs can also occur at the proximal end of the proximal phalanx and are often difficult to see radiographically.

Septic Arthritis

Septic arthritis may be associated with hematogenous spread of microorganisms, such as occurs with omphalophlebitis, or by direct contamination because of trauma or nonsterile invasive techniques. Radiographic signs of early septic arthritis are periarticular soft tissue swelling and distention of the joint. Progression of the disease results in malalignment, subluxation, or collapse of the joint (Fig. 25.20) and subchondral bone lysis and periosteal proliferation at the joint margins (Fig. 25.21). The cartilage space may appear increased at areas of subchondral bone lysis. Diminished joint space is evidence of the loss of articular cartilage that typically precedes subchondral bone change.

The radiographic signs of increased apparent joint space must be analyzed critically. Incomplete ossification of the cartilage model is normally present in young, developing animals. The large soft tissue space at articular margins diminishes progressively with skeletal maturity. Furthermore, radiographs made in non—weight-bearing horses will cause joint spaces to be widened compared with weight-bearing projections. Whenever possible, the horse should bear normal weight on the joint at the time of radiography. Increased thickness of the articular cartilage has not been documented in animals. Excessive fluid or soft tissue in the joint space, as occurs with immune-mediated arthritis, results in a wider joint space. However, such diseases have not been documented in the horse.

Nonseptic inflammatory joint diseases have varied causes and may be difficult to classify. Radiographic signs are distension of the joint and displacement of periarticular soft tissues. If the condition is chronic, periarticular osteoproliferation may develop.

Subchondral Bone Disease

Historically erroneously referred to as *traumatic osteochondrosis*, a consensus term of "subchondral bone disease" has been recommended by experts to describe an osseous injury that occurs due to repetitive cyclic stress leading to marked trabecular sclerosis and variably shaped central demineralization.[51] The most common site of subchondral bone injury is found in the distal aspect of MC III or MT III of Thoroughbred racehorses.[34,39] The radiographic findings are an ill-defined or well-demarcated radiolucent region with variable thickness rim of surrounding sclerosis that may extend several centimeters deep to the articular margin. A lateromedial radiograph of the joint may best demonstrate the depth of the lesion in the condyle, although the lesions are typically best visible on the flexed dorsopalmar projection. The shape of the defect may be a linear defect, shallow concavity, a deep concavity, crescentic, oval, or circular. The ovoid/circular changes are typically at the junction of the radii of articulation between the MCP or the MTP joint and the metacarposesamoidean or metatarsosesamoidean articular surface while the linear lesions are most commonly identified in the parasagittal grooves (see Fig. 25.3). Cavitation of the joint surface may exist, although advanced degenerative subchondral bone changes can also be found with the overlying cartilage intact at the articular surface.

There is increasing recognition that nonracing sport horses are afflicted by subchondral bone disease in discipline-specific patterns, but the imaging manifestation of regions of sclerosis with central demineralization is conserved across breeds and disciplines. The sagittal groove, medial fovea of the proximal phalanx, and the dorsomedial MC III/MT III condyles are overrepresented in nonracing sport horses[17,52] (Fig. 25.22). Variable angle dorsopalmar projections can improve the conspicuity of sagittal groove lesions, while the dorsoproximal to dorsodistal oblique projection is best to characterize medial condylar injury (see Fig. 25.4). These lesions can sometimes be miscategorized as OCLLs, but from an etiologic standpoint, differ from OCLLs as described previously.[53]

Condylar Fractures

Fractures in the distal condyle of MC III or MT III occur most commonly in Thoroughbred racehorses due to acute exacerbation of underlying subchondral bone disease. The forelimbs are more affected than the hind. The palmar aspect of the lateral parasagittal groove is the most commonly affected site and lesions can be difficult to identify radiographically until more advanced disease is present. The flexed dorsopalmar projection and 125 dorsodistal-palmaroproximal projections are

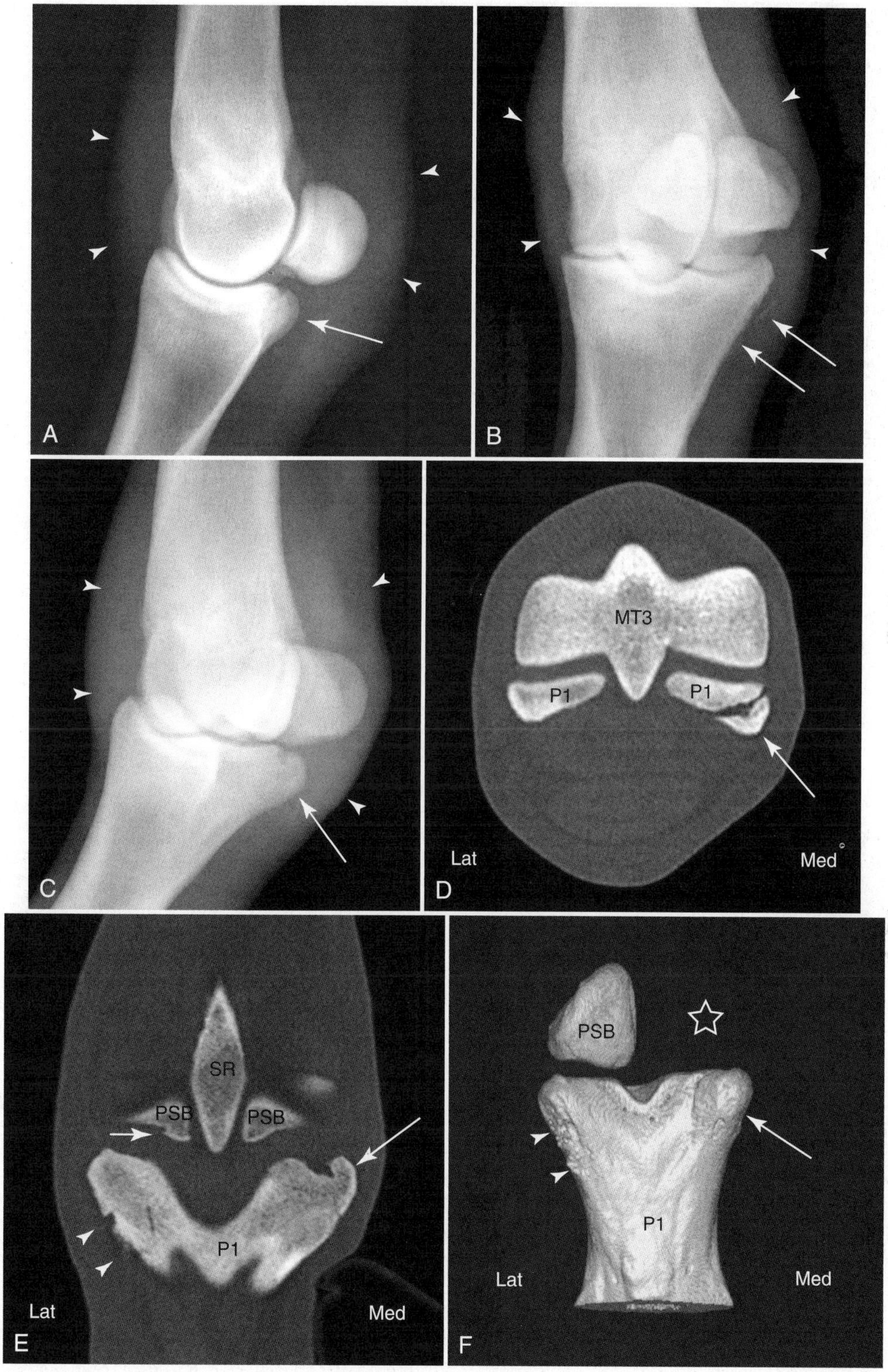

Fig. 25.16 Radiography and computed tomography (CT) images of a 1-year-old male Quarter horse. **A,** Lateral radiograph of the right metatarsophalangeal (MTP) joint. There is diffuse soft tissue swelling (*white arrowheads*) with osseous remodeling and fragments associated with the plantar process of the proximal phalanx (*large white arrow*). **B,** Dorsolateral/plantaromedial radiograph. Note the soft tissue swelling (*white arrowheads*) and periosteal proliferation and fragmentation associated with the proximal lateral first phalanx (*white arrows*). **C,** Dorsomedial/plantarolateral radiograph. Note the soft tissue swelling (*white arrowheads*) and slight defect of the medial plantar process of the first phalanx (*large white arrow*). **D,** Transverse CT image at the level of MTP joint. Note the slightly displaced fragment of the medial plantar process of the proximal phalanx (*white arrow*). **E,** Reconstructed dorsal CT image of the plantar aspect of the metacarpophalangeal (MCP) joint. Note the large osteophyte associated with the medial plantar process (*large white arrow*), the osseous proliferation immediately distal to the lateral plantar process (*white arrowheads*), and a small enthesophyte off the axial aspect of the distal margin of the lateral proximal sesamoid bone (*small white arrow*). **F,** Three-dimensional surface rendering of the plantar aspect of the MTP joint following digital elimination of the medial proximal sesamoid bone (*star*). Note the attached osseous fragment of the medial plantar process (*long white arrow*) and periosteal proliferation along the proximal lateral cortex of the proximal phalanx (*white arrowheads*). *MT3,* Third metatarsal bone; *P1,* first phalanx; *PSB,* proximal sesamoid bones; *SR,* sagittal ridge of third metatarsal bone.

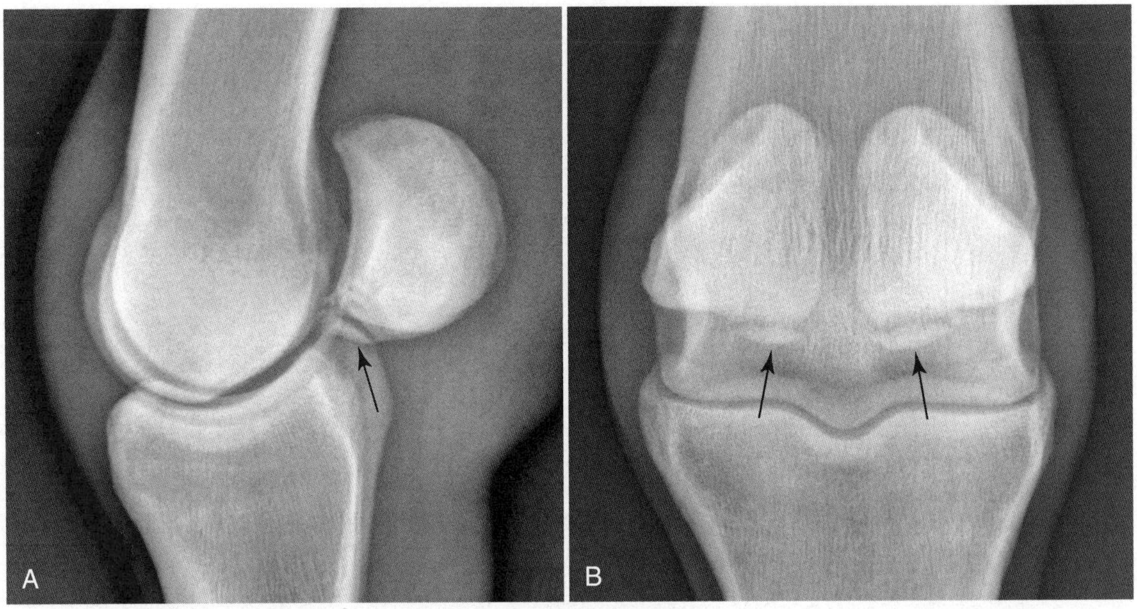

Fig. 25.17 Flexed lateromedial and dorsopalmar radiographs of a metacarpophalangeal (MCP) joint with bilateral type III fractures originating from the basilar margin of the proximal sesamoid bones. A crescent-shaped fragment **(A)** is present along the distal aspect of the proximal sesamoid bones; and on **B,** it is apparent that both proximal sesamoid bones are affected (*black arrows*).

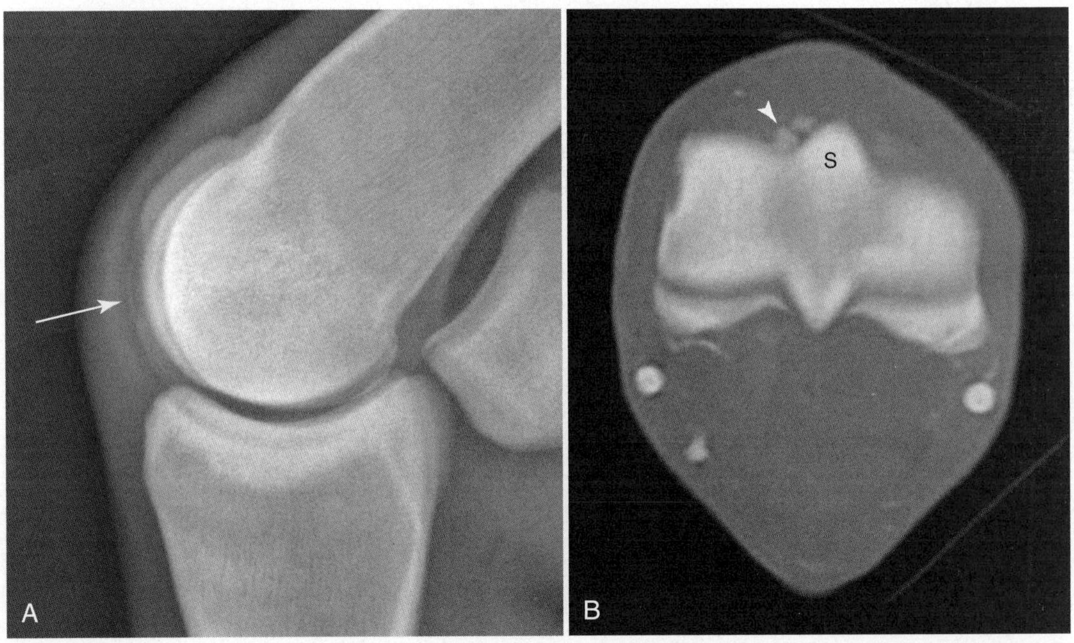

Fig. 25.18 **A,** Flexed metacarpophalangeal (MCP) joint with osteochondrosis of the sagittal ridge of MC III. There is excavation of subchondral bone (*white arrow*). **B,** Transverse computed tomography (CT) image at the distal edge of the sagittal ridge of the third metacarpal bone with two adjacent osteochondral fragments (*white arrowhead*). These fragments came from the proximal aspect of the proximal phalanx, and therefore, the sagittal ridge is smooth. *S,* Sagittal ridge of third metatarsal bone. (**A,** Courtesy John C. Janicek, DVM, MS, DACVS, Weems and Stephens Equine Hospital, Aubrey, Texas, USA.)

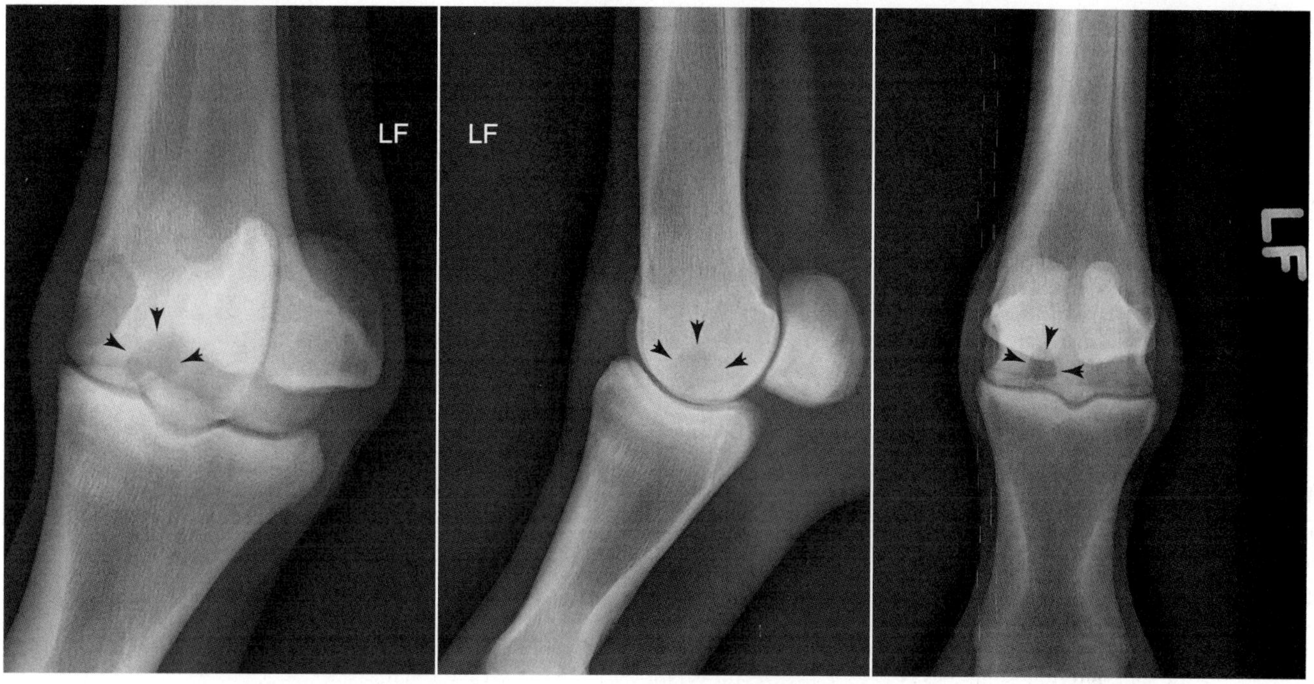

Fig. 25.19 Dorsolateral-palmaromedial oblique (*left*), lateromedial (*middle*), and dorsopalmar (*right*) radiographs of a horse with a distal third metacarpal osseous cyst-like lesion. An ovoid lucent structure with surrounding radiopaque sclerosis (*black arrowheads*) is visible on all three images, demonstrating that the lesion involves the medial condyle of the distal metacarpus. Periarticular remodeling is also seen on all three views.

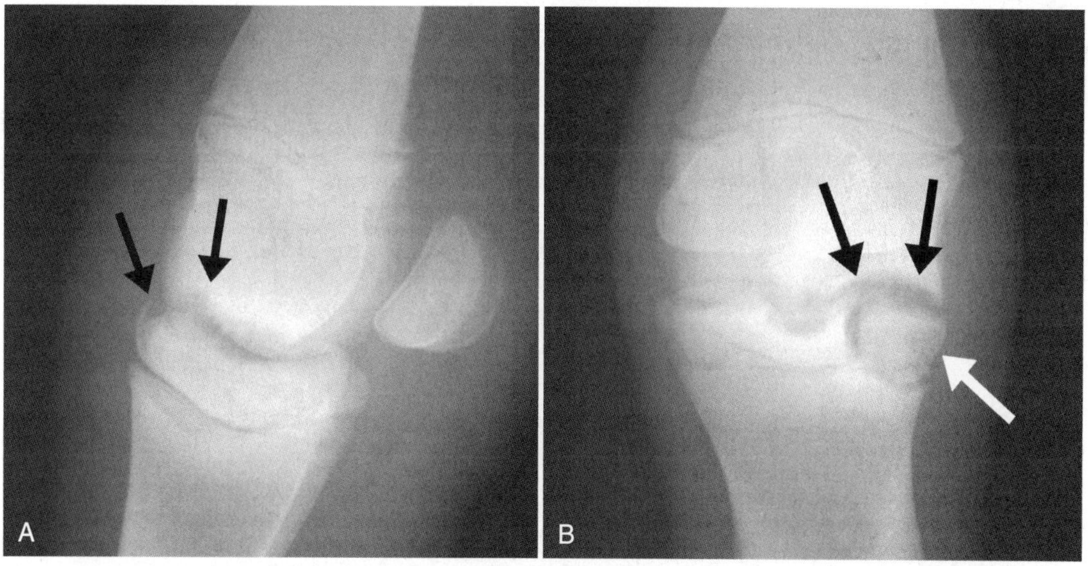

Fig. 25.20 Lateromedial and dorsopalmar views of a 1-month-old filly with soft tissue swelling, septic arthritis, and osteomyelitis. **A,** There is severe osteolysis of the subchondral bone of the distal aspect of the third metatarsal bone and the proximal epiphysis of the proximal phalanx (*black arrows*). **B,** There is severe erosion of the subchondral bone of the distal aspect of the third metatarsal bone (*black arrows*) and a large osteolytic fragment involving the medial side of the proximal epiphysis of the proximal phalanx (*white arrow*). These changes are consistent with advanced septic arthritis and septic epiphysitis with a pathologic Salter-Harris type III fracture of the epiphysis.

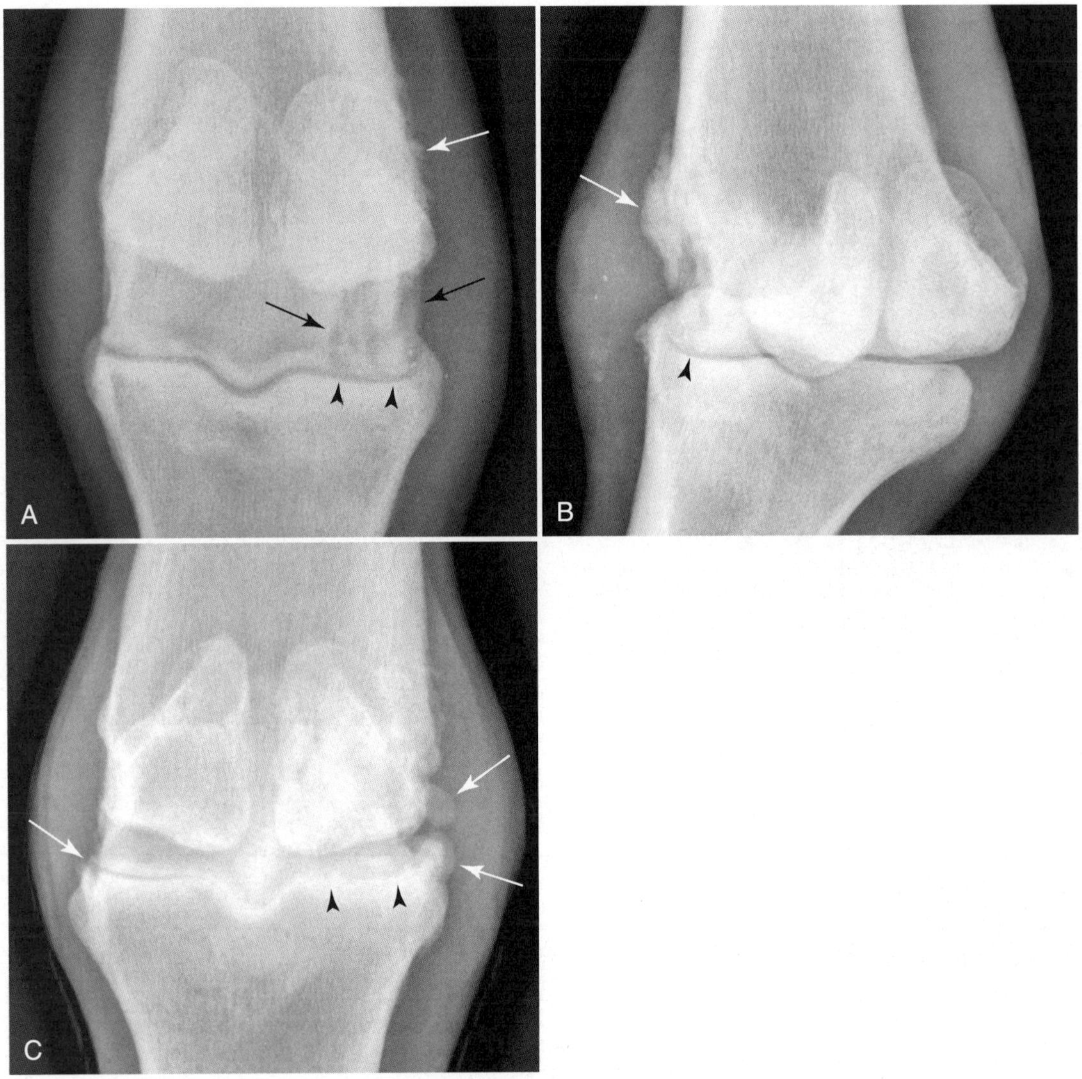

Fig. 25.21 Dorsopalmar **(A)** and dorsolateral/palmaromedial **(B)** radiographs of a horse with active septic arthritis. There is lysis of cortical and subchondral bone of the medial condyle of the third metacarpal bone (*black arrows*), irregular periosteal proliferation (*white arrows*), and mild joint space narrowing (*black arrowheads*). **C,** Dorsopalmar radiograph of a horse with chronic septic arthritis that is no longer active. There is severe erosion of subchondral bone of the opposing joint surfaces with resulting sclerosis and joint space collapse (*black arrowheads*). Smooth bone proliferation is evident on all periarticular surfaces (*white arrows*). Generalized soft tissue swelling is present surrounding the joint on all three radiographs.

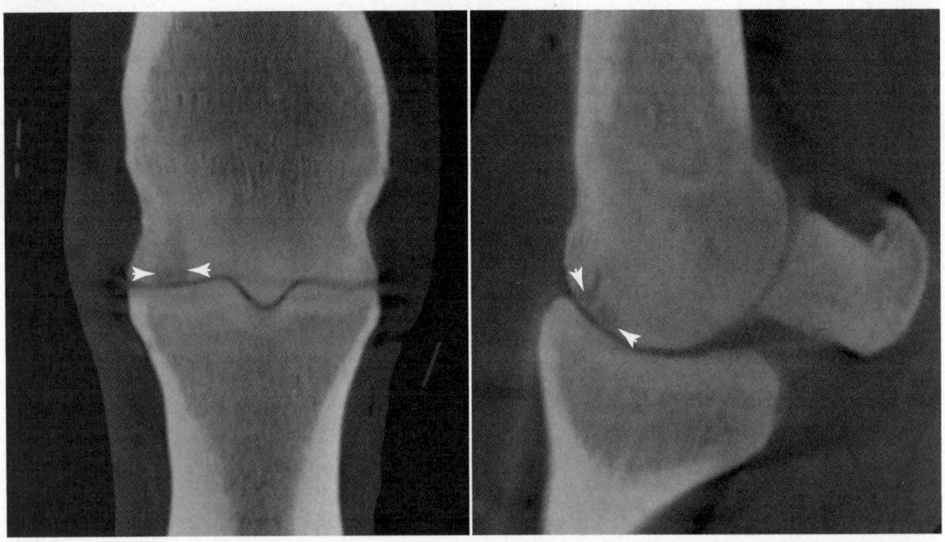

Fig. 25.22 Dorsal plane (*left*) and sagittal plane (*right*) reformatted standing cone-beam computed tomography (CT) images of dorsomedial third metacarpal condylar subchondral bone disease (demineralization [*white arrowheads*]) in an aged Warmblood. For the dorsal image, medial is to the *left*. Note the somewhat ill-defined ovoid region of hypoattenuation with marked adjacent trabecular sclerosis that extends palmar and proximal to the lesion.

the most sensitive for incomplete fracture identification and characterization of palmar comminution that is not apparent on standard radiographic series[7,8,11] (see Fig. 25.3). Lateral condylar fractures most commonly propagate proximally and laterally toward the lateral cortex while medial fractures are more likely to spiral proximally; thus, radiographic evaluation of the latter requires radiograph acquisition of the entire metacarpus/metatarsus. With the exception of Standardbred racehorses, distal MC III or MT III condyle fractures in other breeds are typically the result of a single traumatic event. Radiographic signs include uneven joint surface, interruption of the metaphyseal cortex, and the presence of a radiolucent fracture line extending from the joint surface to the cortex. The fractures in Thoroughbred racehorses (Fig. 25.23) may be displaced, complete but nondisplaced, or incomplete and in a lower percentage of horses, associated with axial fracture of the ipsilateral sesamoid bone.[54,55] Prognosis after surgical treatment varies but is best for fractures without concurrent sesamoid fracture, palmar comminution, or intra-articular fragmentation.[55–57] A dorsal 20-degree medial-palmarolateral projection can improve the sensitivity of detection for this lesion.[58]

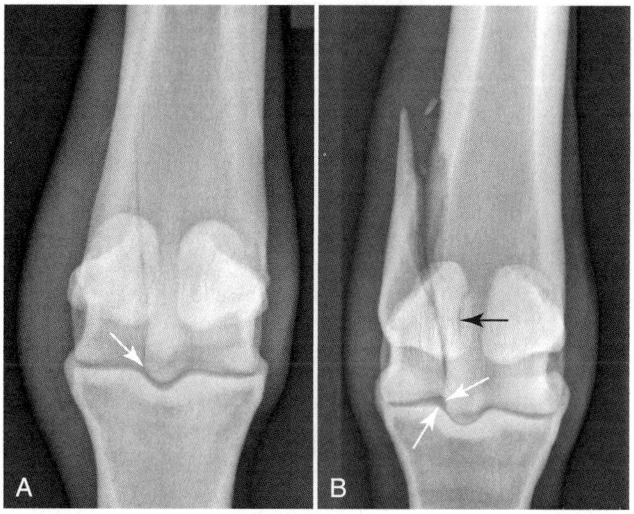

Fig. 25.23 Dorsopalmar radiographs of two horses with third metacarpal lateral condylar fractures. **A,** Incomplete, nondisplaced articular fracture (*white arrow*). **B,** Complete, displaced fracture resulting articular incongruity (*white arrows*). Concurrent axial fracture of the lateral proximal sesamoid is present (*black arrow*).

Sagittal or parasagittal fractures of the proximal phalanx in racehorses often result from prodromal accumulated microtrauma.[59] If there is distal extension of the fracture, this may extend to the proximal interphalangeal joint or obliquely through the lateral cortex of the proximal phalanx.[60] Highly comminuted proximal phalanx fractures resulting from rotational or torsional forces are not uncommon in nonracing sport and pleasure horses. Fracture location and severity must be considered relative to surgical repair and prognosis.[61]

Traumatic Osteochondral Fragmentation, Chip Fractures

Traumatic osteochondral fragmentation is most common in racehorses, with the forelimbs and the medial periarticular eminence of the proximal phalanx highly overrepresented. This is the result of repetitive impact of the proximal phalanx with the dorsodistal metacarpus/tarsus in extension.[62–64] Acute chip fractures may have sharp borders and angular configurations. Chronic chip fractures undergo remodeling and have smooth, rounded borders. The latter are usually attached to the joint capsule or to the joint margin as an exostosis (Fig. 25.24, eFig. 25.4). Free joint bodies may displace or move about within the joint.

Osteochondral fragments arising from the palmarolateral/plantarolateral or palmaromedial/plantaromedial eminences of the proximal phalanx (Fig. 25.25, eFig. 25.5) have been reported as chronic or juvenile avulsion fractures[34,40,45,65] but are considered by some to be manifestations of osteochondrosis as described earlier.[41–49,66,67]

Fractures of the Proximal Sesamoids

Proximal sesamoid fractures are consistently of three types: apical, midbody, or basilar. Some may be found as osteochondral fragments separated from the sesamoid apex (apical

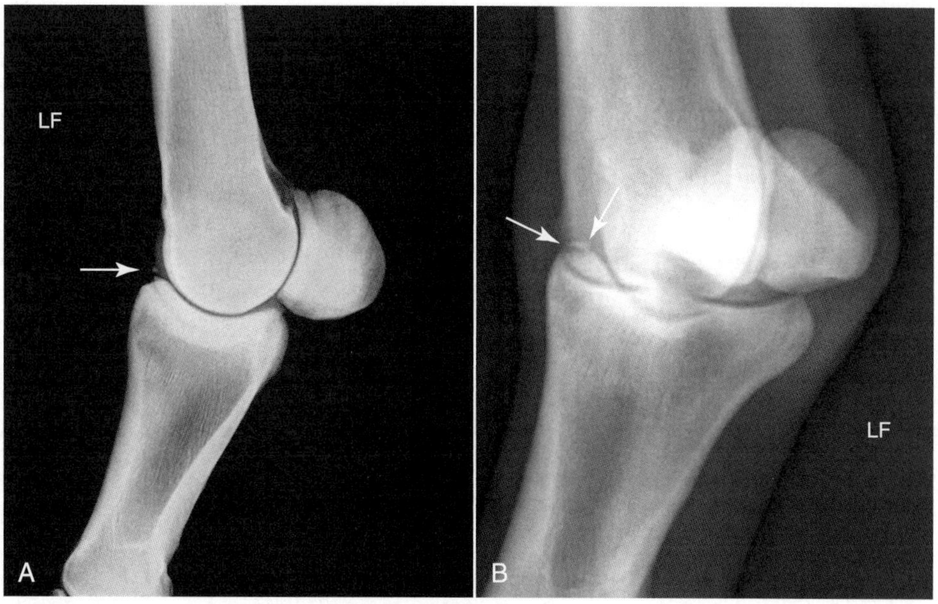

Fig. 25.24 Lateromedial **(A)** and dorsolateral-palmaromedial oblique **(B)** radiographs of a 3-year-old Thoroughbred racehorse. An osteochondral (chip) fracture (*white arrows*) is present at the dorsoproximomedial periarticular rim of the proximal phalanx with adjacent concave fragment bed within the parent bone.

fractures; see Fig. 25.2) or base (basilar fractures; see Fig. 25.17). Fractures through the body of a sesamoid may have a narrow cleavage line, indicating that the suspensory apparatus remains intact (Fig. 25.26A). Wide separation of sesamoid fragments usually indicates bilateral sesamoid fractures and disruption of the fibers of the suspensory ligament (see Fig. 25.26B). Hyperextension of the MCP or MTP joint is apparent if stress is applied to the joint or if the limb is bearing weight with disruption of the suspensory ligament.

Abaxial fractures are detected by using special radiographic projections. These fractures result from avulsion of bone by a portion of the attachment of the branches of the suspensory ligament on the medial or lateral abaxial aspects of the respective proximal sesamoid (Fig. 25.27, eFig. 25.6, see Fig. 25.2A,C).

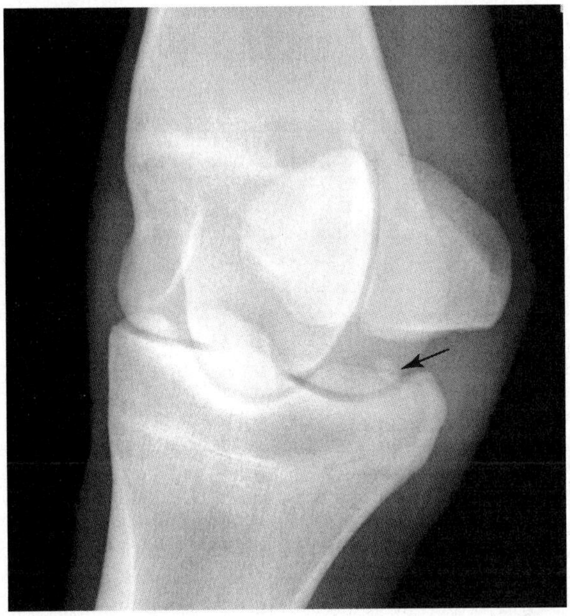

Fig. 25.25 Dorsolateral/plantaromedial radiograph of the metatarsophalangeal (MTP) joint of a horse with an osteochondral fragment arising from the plantarolateral eminence of the proximal phalanx (*black arrow*). These fragments have features of chip fractures but are still often lumped with the osteochondrosis complex of lesions.

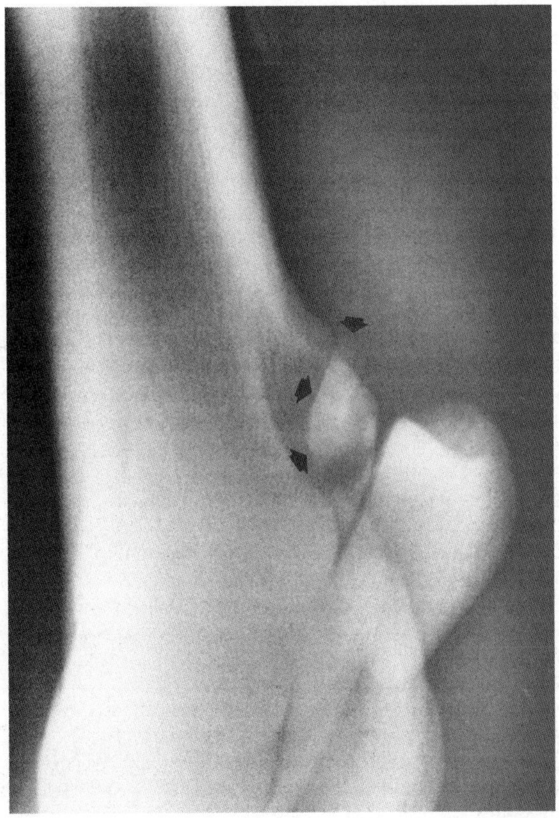

Fig. 25.27 Dorsal 50-degree proximal, 45-degree medial/palmarodistolateral radiograph of a horse with an apical, articular fracture of the medial proximal sesamoid bone (*black arrowheads*). The fracture originates at an articular surface and emerges at the abaxial surface of the sesamoid bone.

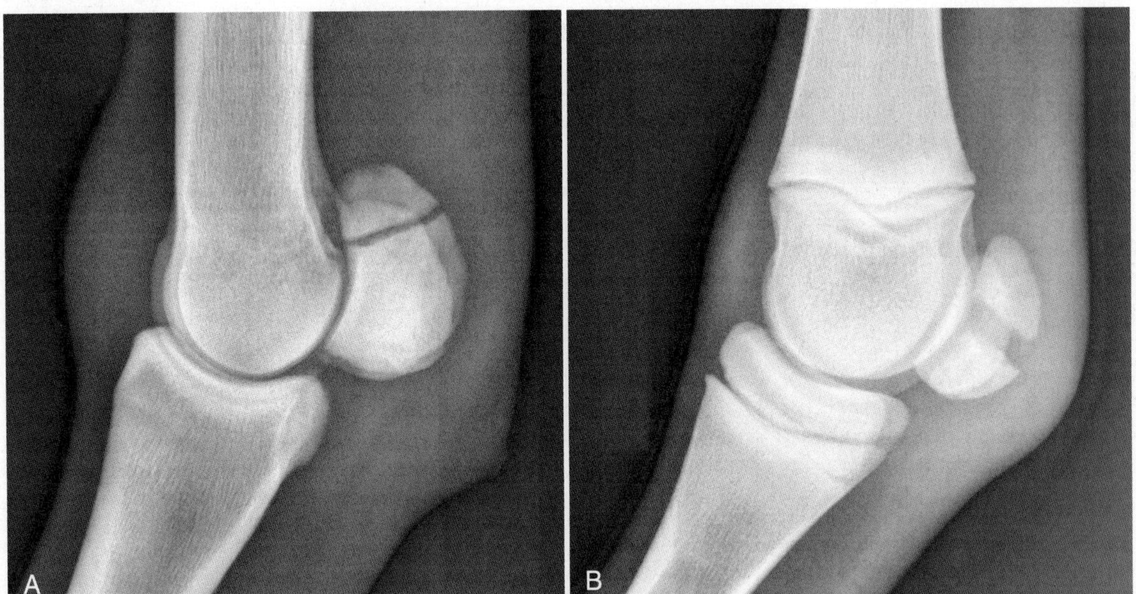

Fig. 25.26 **A,** Large apical fracture of one of the proximal sesamoid bones with mild displacement. **B,** Midbody fracture of a proximal sesamoid bone with displacement. (**A,** Courtesy John C. Janicek, DVM, MS, DACVS, Weems and Stephens Equine Hospital, Aubrey, Texas, USA.)

Recently, dorsal subchondral bone injury of the proximal sesamoid bones has been implicated as the underlying cause of midbody sesamoid fractures in racehorses.[68] However, these lesions are essentially impossible to detect radiographically and require cross-sectional imaging for diagnosis (i.e., CT, MRI, PET).

The prognosis of sesamoid fractures is correlated to the type of fracture and damage to the associated structures. Reviews of the clinical aspects of apical[69] and basilar[70] sesamoid fractures are available.

Sesamoiditis, Suspensory Enthesopathy

Sesamoiditis is characterized radiographically by bone proliferation on nonarticular surfaces of the proximal sesamoid bones.[71] Sesamoiditis is usually associated with degenerative change in the suspensory ligament and degenerative remodeling or fracture at the distal ends of MC II or MT IV. Linear or ovoid lysis may appear to penetrate the sesamoid from the abaxial surface. The linear lesions typically represent widened vascular channels while ovoid or cyst-like lesions represent suspensory branch enthesis resorption (Fig. 25.28, eFig. 25.7). Axial sesamoiditis is somewhat rare with numerous speculative etiologies, including infarction, infection, and trauma.[72] Axial and intersesamoidean sesamoid pathology is notoriously painful typically with a poor prognosis for athletic soundness regardless of the underlying etiology.

Disuse Atrophy of Bone

The earliest manifestation of disuse atrophy is typically in the proximal sesamoid bones but may also be recognized in the long bones as a reduction in medullary opacity and cortical thinning. Trabeculae within the bone become large and coarse. This change occurs because of altered stress or axial weight bearing and may not signify primary pathologic change in the joint (Fig. 25.29).

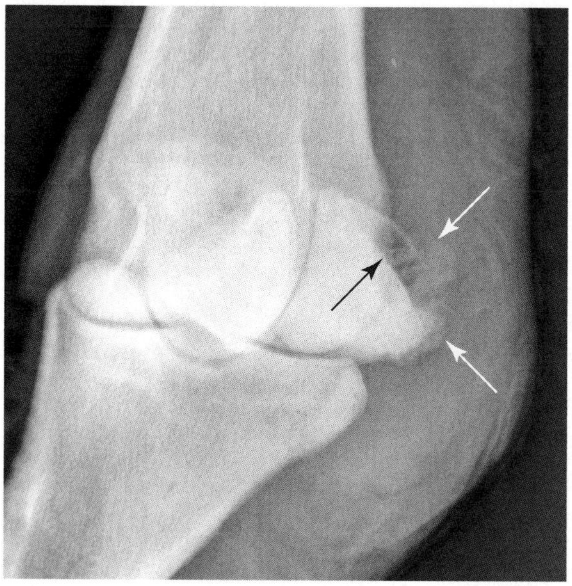

Fig. 25.28 Dorsal 45-degree medial/palmarolateral radiograph of a horse with sesamoiditis of the medial proximal sesamoid bone. Degenerative remodeling is present with increased size of vascular channels within the sesamoid bone and enthesis resorption (*black arrow*) and palmar enthesophytosis (*white arrows*). Soft tissue swelling surrounds the metacarpophalangeal (MCP) joint.

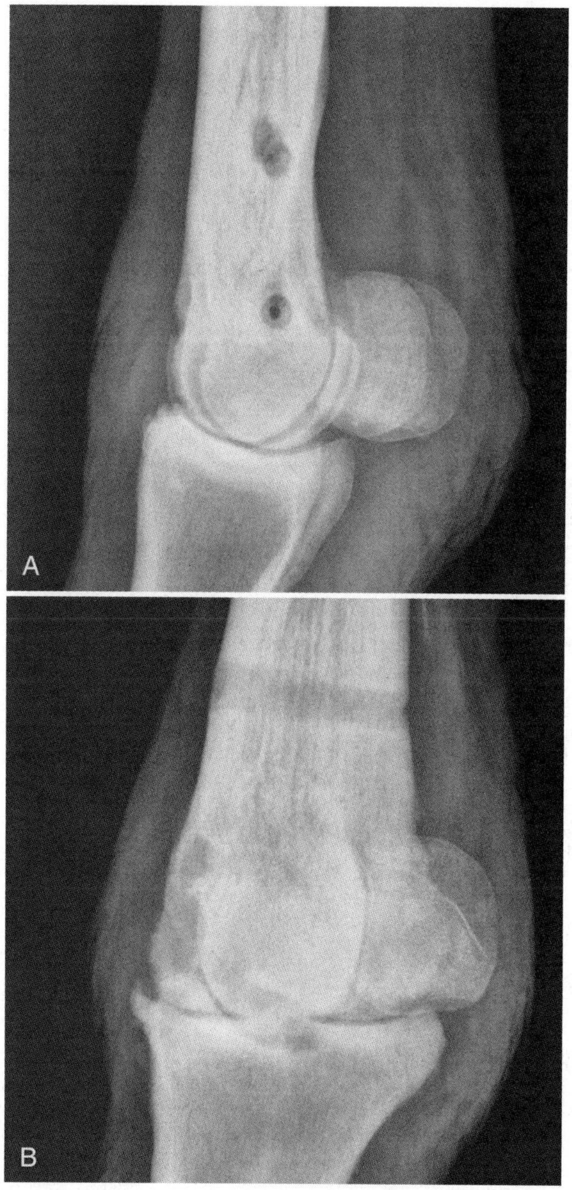

Fig. 25.29 Lateromedial **(A)** and dorsal 45-degree medial/palmarolateral **(B)** radiographs of the distal third metacarpal bone and the proximal phalanx of a horse recently having external support removed from the leg. Sclerosis surrounds the transverse pin tracts, but the remaining bone has advanced osteopenia. Generalized remodeling of bone has occurred, and the cortices are thin. Osseous trabeculae are coarse and irregular, with no organized pattern and linear radiolucent lines running the length of included portion of the third metacarpal bone. The sesamoid bones have a sponge-like appearance. There is generalized soft tissue swelling and periarticular remodeling along the dorsal aspect of the metacarpophalangeal (MCP) joint.

Acknowledgment

With special thanks to prior authors of this chapter for their contributions.

REFERENCES

1. Getty RS. *Grossman's the Anatomy of the Domestic Animals*. 5th ed. Philadelphia: Saunders; 1975:357–360.
2. Weaver JC, Stover SM, O'Brien TR. Radiographic anatomy of soft tissue attachments in the equine metacarpophalangeal and proximal phalangeal region. *Equine Vet J*. 1992;24(4):310–315.
3. Rendano VT. Equine radiology. The fetlock. *Mod Vet Pract*. 1977;58(10):871–875.
4. Butler JA, Colles CM, Dyson SJ, et al. *Clinical Radiology of the Horse*. London: Blackwell; 2017:175–215.
5. Morgan JP. *Techniques of Veterinary Radiography*. 5th ed. Ames: Iowa State University; 1993.
6. O'Brien T. *Radiography for the Ambulatory Equine Practitioner*. Jackson, WY: Teton; 2005.
7. Davis A, Fan X, Shen L, Robinson P, Riggs C. Improved radiological diagnosis of palmar osteochondral disease in the Thoroughbred racehorse. *Equine Vet J*. 2017;49(4): 454–460.
8. Hornof WJ, O'Brien TR. Radiographic evaluation of the palmar aspect of the equine metacarpal condyles: a new projection. *Vet Radiol*. 1980;21:161.
9. Palmer SE. Radiography of the abaxial surface of the proximal sesamoid bones of the horse. *J Am Vet Med Assoc*. 1982;181(3):264–265.
10. Pilsworth RC, Hopes R, Greet TR. A flexed dorso-palmar projection of the equine fetlock in demonstrating lesions of the distal third metacarpus. *Vet Rec*. 1988;122(14): 332–333.
11. Ramzan P, Palmer L, Powell S. Unicortical condylar fracture of the Thoroughbred fetlock; 45 cases (2006–2013). *Equine Vet J*. 2015;47(6):680–683.
12. De Guio C, Segard-Weisse E, Thomas-Cancian A, Schramme M. Bone marrow lesions of the distal condyles of the third metacarpal bone are common and not always related to lameness in sports and pleasure horses. *Vet Radiol Ultrasound*. 2018;60(2):167–175.
13. Seignour M, Coudry V, Norris R, et al. Ultrasound examination of the palmar/plantar aspect of the fetlock in the horse. Technique and normal images. *Equine Vet J*. 2012;24:18–29.
14. DiGiovanni DL, Radmacher N, Riggs LM, et al. Dynamic sonography of the equine metacarpo (tarso) phalangeal digital flexor tendon sheath. *Vet Radiol Ultrasound*. 2016;57(6):621–629.
15. Werpy N, Chapman K, Griffith L. Non-weight bearing ultrasonographic examination allows the diagnosis of longitudinal fiber disruption (split) in the equine suspensory ligament branches not visible on weight bearing examination. *Vet Radiol Ultrasound*. 2020;62(1):84–97.
16. Denoix JM, Jacot S, Bousseau B, et al. Ultrasonographic anatomy of the dorsal and abaxial aspects of the equine fetlock. *Equine Vet J*. 1996;28(1):54–62.
17. Trope GD, Anderson GA, Whitton RC. Patterns of scintigraphic uptake in the fetlock joint of Thoroughbred racehorses and the effect of increased radiopharmaceutical uptake in the distal metacarpal/tarsal condyle on performance. *Equine Vet J*. 2011;43(5):509–515.
18. Dyson S, Murray R. Osseous trauma in the fetlock region in mature sport horses. *AAEP Proceedings*. 2006;52:443–456.
19. Twardock AR. Equine bone scintigraphic uptake patterns related to age, breed, and occupation. *Vet Clin N Am-Equine*. 2001;17(1), 75-04.
20. Vanderperren K, Ghaye B, Snaps FR, et al. Evaluation of computed tomographic anatomy of the equine metacarpophalangeal joint. *Am J Vet Res*. 2008;69(5):631–638.
21. Olive J, D'Anjou MA, Alexander K, et al. Comparison of magnetic resonance imaging, computed tomography, and radiography for assessment of noncartilaginous changes in equine metacarpophalangeal osteoarthritis. *Vet Radiol Ultrasound*. 2010;51(3):267–279.
22. Morgan J, Santschi E, Zekas L, et al. Comparison of radiography and computed tomography to evaluate metacarpo/metatarsophalangeal joint pathology of paired limbs of thoroughbred racehorses with severe condylar fracture. *Vet Surg*. 2006;35(7):611–617.
23. Curtiss A, Ortved K, Dallap-Schaer B, et al. Validation of standing cone beam computed tomography for diagnosing subchondral fetlock pathology in the Thoroughbred racehorse. *Equine Vet J*. 2020;53(3):510–523.
24. Johnston GCA, Ahern BJ, Palmieri C, Young A. Imaging and gross pathologic appearance of changes in the parasagittal groove of Thoroughbred racehorses. *Animals*. 2021; 11(12):3366.
25. Brounts SH, Lund J, Whitton RC, Ergun D, Muir P. Use of a novel helical fan beam imaging system for computed tomography of the distal limb in sedated standing horses. 167 cases (2019–2020). *J Am Vet Med A*. 2022;260(11): 1351–1360.
26. Tucker RL, Sande RD. Magnetic resonance imaging and computed tomography: evaluation of equine musculoskeletal conditions. *Vet Clin North Am Equine Pract*. 2001;17:145.
27. Smith M, Dyson S. In: Murray R, Equine MRI, eds. *Normal Anatomy: The Fetlock Region*. West Sussex, UK: Wiley-Blackwell; 2011:173–189.
28. Powell S. In: Murray R, Equine MRI, eds. *The Fetlock Region*. West Sussex, UK: Wiley-Blackwell; 2011:315–360.
29. Dyson S, Murray R. Magnetic resonance imaging of the equine fetlock. In: Orsini J, ed. *Clinical Techniques in Equine Practice*. Philadelphia: Elsevier/Saunders; 2007: 62–78.
30. Brama PA, Tekoppele JM, Bank RA, et al. Topographical mapping of biochemical properties of articular cartilage in the equine fetlock joint. *Equine Vet J*. 2000;32(1):19–26.
31. Smith S, Dyson SJ, Murray RC. Magnetic resonance imaging of distal sesamoidean ligament injury. *Vet Radiol Ultrasound*. 2008;49(6):516–528.
32. McKnight AL, Manduca A, Felmlee JP, et al. Motion correction techniques for standing equine MRI. *Vet Radiol Ultrasound*. 2004;45(6):513–519.
33. Spriet M, Arndt S, Pige C, et al. Comparison of skeletal scintigraphy and standing 18F-NaF positron emission tomography for imaging the fetlock in 33 Thoroughbred racehorses. *Vet Radiol Ultrasound*. 2022;1–8 (published online).
34. Pool RR, Meagher DM. Pathologic findings and pathogenesis of racetrack injuries. *Vet Clin North Am Equine Pract*. 1990;6(1):1–30.
35. Bramlage L. Part 1. Operative orthopedics of the fetlock joint of the horse: traumatic and developmental diseases of the equine fetlock joint. *Milne Lecture AAEP Annual Convention*. 2009;55.
36. Gillette EL, Thrall DE, Lebel JL. *Carlson's Veterinary Radiology*. 3rd ed. Philadelphia: Lea & Febiger; 1977:435.
37. McIlwraith CW, Frisbie DD, Kawcak CE. The horse as a model of naturally occurring osteoarthritis. *Bone Joint Res*. 2012;1(11):297–309.
38. Declercq K, Martens A, Maes D, Boussauw B, Forsyth R, Boening KJ. Dorsoproximal proximal phalanx osteochondral fragmentation in 117 Warmblood horses. *Vet Comp Orthop Traumatol*. 2009;22(1):1–6.

39. O'Brien TR, Hornof WJ, Meagher DM. Radiographic detection and characterization of palmar lesions in the equine fetlock joint. *J Am Vet Med Assoc*. 1981;178(3):231–237.
40. Petterson H, Ryden G. Avulsion fractures of the caudoproximal extremity of the first phalanx. *Equine Vet J*. 1982;14(4):333–335.
41. Carlsten J, Sandgren B, Dalin G. Development of osteochondrosis in the tarsocrural joint and osteochondral fragments in the fetlock joints of Standardbred trotters. I. A radiological survey. *Equine Vet J*. 1993;16:42. suppl.
42. Grøndahl AM, Engeland A. Influence of radiographically detectable orthopedic changes on racing performance in Standardbred trotters. *J Am Vet Med Assoc*. 1995;206(7):1013–1017.
43. Gaschen L, Burba DJ. Musculoskeletal injury in thoroughbred racehorses: correlation of findings using multiple imaging modalities. *Vet Clin North Am Equine Pract*. 2012;28(3):542–551.
44. Kawack CE, McIlwraith CW. Proximodorsal first phalanx osteochondral chip fragmentation in 336 horses. *Equine Vet J*. 1994;26(5):392–396.
45. Dalin G, Sandgren B, Carlsten J. Plantar osteochondral fragments in the fetlock joints of Standardbreds: result of osteochondrosis or trauma? *Equine Vet J*. 1993;suppl 16:62.
46. Philipsson J, Andréasson E, Sandgren B, et al. Osteochondrosis in the tarsocrural joint and osteochondral fragments in the fetlock joints in Standardbred trotters. II. Heritability. *Equine Vet J*. 1993;suppl 16:38.
47. Sandgren B, Dalin G, Carlsten J, et al. Development of osteochondrosis in the tarsocrural joint and osteochondral fragments in the fetlock joints of Standardbred trotters. II. Body measurements and clinical findings. *Equine Vet J*. 1993;suppl 16:48.
48. Sandgren B, Dalin G, Carlsten J. Osteochondrosis in the tarsocrural joint and osteochondral fragments in the fetlock joints in Standardbred trotters. I. Epidemiology. *Equine Vet J*. 1993;suppl 16:31.
49. Fortier LA, Foerner JJ, Nixon AJ. Arthroscopic removal of axial osteochondral fragments of the plantar/palmar proximal aspect of the proximal phalanx in horses: 119 cases (1988–1992). *J Am Vet Med Assoc*. 1995;206(1):71–74.
50. Yovich JV, McIlwraith CW, Stashak TS. Osteochondritis dissecans of the sagittal ridge of the third metacarpal and metatarsal bones in horses. *J Am Vet Med Assoc*. 1985;186(11):1186–1191.
51. Smith MWR, Kawcak CE, McIlwraith CW. Science in brief: report on the Havermeyer Foundation workshop on subchondral bone problems in the equine athlete. *Equine Vet J*. 2016;48:6–8.
52. Gold S, Werpy N, Gutierrez-Nibeyro S. Injuries of the sagittal groove of the proximal phalanx in Warmblood horses detected with low-field magnetic resonance imaging: 19 cases (2007–2016). *Vet Radiol Ultrasound*. 2017;58(3):344–353.
53. Ammann L, Ohlerth S, Furst AE, Jackson MA. Differences of morphological attributes between 62 proximal and distal subchondral cystic lesions of the proximal phalanx as determined by radiography and computed tomography. *J Am Vet Med A*. 2022;83(12).
54. Zekas LJ, Bramlage LR, Embertson RM, et al. Characterization of the type and location of fractures of the third metacarpal/metatarsal condyles in 135 horses in central Kentucky (1986–1994). *Equine Vet J*. 1999;31(4):304–308.
55. Rick MC, O'Brien TR, Pool RR, et al. Condylar fractures of the third metacarpal bone and third metatarsal bone in 75 horses. Radiographic features, treatments, and outcome. *J Am Vet Med Assoc*. 1983;183(3):287–296.
56. Zekas LJ, Bramlage LR, Embertson RM, et al. Results of treatment of 145 fractures of the third metacarpal/metatarsal condyles in 135 horses (1986–1994). *Equine Vet J*. 1999;31(4):309–313.
57. Cianci JM, Wulster KB, Richardson DW, Stefanovski D, Ortved KF. Computed tomographic assessment of fracture characteristics and subchondral bone injury in Thoroughbred racehorses with lateral condylar fractures and their relationship to outcome. *Vet Surg*. 2022;51(3):426–437.
58. Labbe K, Pigott JH. Radiographic technique to improve diagnosis of sagittal axial sesamoid fracture in racing Thoroughbreds with lateral condylar fracture. *Equine Vet Edu*. 2022;34(4):200–206.
59. Ramzan PHL, Powell SE. Clinical and imaging features of suspected prodromal fractures of the proximal phalanx in three Thoroughbred racehorses. *Equine Vet J*. 2010;42(2):164–169.
60. Smith MRW, Corletto FC, Wright IM. Parasagittal fractures of the proximal phalanx in Thoroughbred racehorses in the UK: outcome of repaired fractures in 113 cases (2007–2011). *Equine Vet J*. 2017;49(6):784–788.
61. Holcombe SJ, Schneider RK, Bramlage LR, et al. Lag screw fixation of noncomminuted sagittal fractures of the proximal phalanx in racehorses: 59 cases (1973–1991). *J Am Vet Med Assoc*. 1995;206(8):1195–1199.
62. Yovich JV, McIlwraith CW. Arthroscopic surgery for osteochondral fractures of the proximal phalanx of the metacarpophalangeal and metatarsophalangeal (fetlock) joints in horses. *J Am Vet Med Assoc*. 1986;188(3):273–279.
63. Ramzan PHL, Wylie CE. Nonsurgical and surgical management of metacarpo/metatarsophalangeal joint dorsal chip fracture in the Thoroughbred racehorse. *Equine Vet J*. 2020;52:399–403.
64. Walsh R, Smith MRW, Wright IM. Frequency distribution of osteochondral fragmentation of the dorsoproximal articular surface of the proximal phalanx in racing Thoroughbreds in the UK. *Equine Vet J*. 2018;50(5):624–628.
65. Nixon AJ, Pool RR. Histologic appearance of axial osteochondral fragments from the proximoplantar/proximopalmar aspect of the proximal phalanx in horses. *J Am Vet Med Assoc*. 1995;207(8):1076–1080.
66. Barclay WP, Foerner JJ, Phillips TN. Lameness attributable to osteochondral fragmentation of the plantar aspect of the proximal phalanx in horses. 19 cases (1981–1985). *J Am Vet Med Assoc*. 1987;191(7):855–857.
67. Grøndhal AM. Incidence and development of ununited proximoplantar tuberosity of the proximal phalanx in Standardbred trotters. *Vet Radiol Ultrasound*. 1992;33:18.
68. Schaffer SK, To C, Garcia T, Fyhrie DP, Uzal FA, Stover SM. Subchondral focal osteopenia associated with proximal sesamoid bone fracture in Thoroughbred racehorses. *Equine Vet J*. 2021;53:294–305.
69. Spurlock GH, Gabel AA. Apical fractures of the proximal sesamoid bones in 109 Standardbred horses. *J Am Vet Med Assoc*. 1983;183(1):76–79.
70. Parente EJ, Richardson DW, Spencer P. Basal sesamoidean fractures in horses: 57 cases (1980–1991). *J Am Vet Med Assoc*. 1993;202(8):1293–1297.
71. Blevins WE, Widmer WR. Radiology in racetrack practice. *Vet Clin North Am Equine Pract*. 1990;6(1):31–61.
72. Le Roux C, Carstens A. Axial sesamoiditis in the horse: a review. *J S Afr Vet Assoc*. 2018;89:1544.

ELECTRONIC RESOURCES

Additional information related to the content in Chapter 25 can be found online at eBooks.Health.Elsevier.com.

- Chapter Quiz

CHAPTER 26

Equine Pastern

Elizabeth Biscoe • Dana A. Neelis

OVERVIEW

The proximal phalanx (P1) and middle phalanx (P2) are the osseous structures of the equine pastern region. In the horse, the proximal phalanx is the longest of the phalanges, with the middle phalanx being approximately half of the length of the proximal phalanx. The proximal interphalangeal (pastern) joint is a diarthrodial joint formed where the proximal and middle phalanges meet. The pastern region is supported by multiple soft tissue structures, including the medial and lateral collateral ligaments, straight and oblique distal sesamoidean ligaments, superficial and deep digital flexor tendons, collateral sesamoidean ligament (suspensory ligament of the navicular bone), abaxial and axial palmar (plantar) ligaments, proximal and distal digital annular ligaments, and the extensor tendons. The digital flexor tendon sheath is also located along the palmar/plantar aspect of the pastern region. No muscle is present in the pastern region and there is very little fat delineating these soft tissue structures on radiographs. Detailed radiographic anatomy of this region is illustrated in Chapter 16 and can be found in multiple published sources, including comparative images of the anatomy on multiple imaging modalities (i.e., ultrasound, magnetic resonance imaging [MRI]) for reference.[1–4]

INDICATIONS FOR RADIOGRAPHY

Radiographs of the pastern are often included on survey images of the foot and/or fetlock; however, radiographs centered on the proximal interphalangeal joint are necessary to minimize distortion and obtain a more detailed assessment of this joint and the middle phalanx if disease is localized to this region. Imaging of the pastern may be pursued when clinically indicated from the history, findings from physical or lameness examinations, or results of diagnostic analgesia (i.e., palmar digital, abaxial, or basi-sesamoid nerve blocks).

ALTERNATE IMAGING OF THE PASTERN

Alternate imaging modalities (i.e., standing low-field vs. high-field MRI, computed tomography [CT], ultrasound) are very often used to assess the pastern region, especially when there is concern for abnormalities of the soft tissue structures. These modalities will not be discussed in detail in this chapter but will be referenced when applicable.

TECHNICAL FACTORS

Patient Preparation

Preparation of the pastern region for radiographic examination is similar to preparation of the foot. Removal of any dirt, debris, or iodine-containing substances from the skin or haircoat of the pastern region is needed to avoid artifacts. Elevation of the foot with the use of positioning devices (i.e., wooden blocks) is helpful to center the radiographic beam on the proximal interphalangeal joint.

Recommended Views

Lateromedial, dorsopalmar,* dorsomedial-palmarolateral oblique, and dorsolateral-palmaromedial oblique views are routinely obtained for assessment of the pastern. Flexed lateromedial and/or oblique views may be used for assessment of the periarticular margins of the proximal interphalangeal joint.[3] Obtaining the dorsopalmar view with a 5- to 10-degree angle from proximal to distal, with corresponding mild angulation of the imaging plate, may also be helpful for assessing this joint.

NORMAL RADIOGRAPHIC ANATOMY AND ANATOMICAL VARIATIONS

A few normal anatomic and incidental variants are present in the pastern region and should be noted to avoid misinterpreting these areas as pathologic during radiographic assessment.[3,5,6] On the dorsopalmar view of the distal limb, the proximal interphalangeal joint space is normally mildly wider than the fetlock joint, but narrower when compared to the distal interphalangeal joint (Fig. 26.1). If the patient is properly positioned with even weight bearing on the foot, the proximal interphalangeal joint space should be symmetric in width from medial to lateral; however, if the patient is placing more weight on one side of the limb or the other, this may create the appearance of asymmetric joint space narrowing.[7]

An area devoid of trabeculae is present centrally within the proximal phalanx, and occasionally a similar, but smaller, region is present centrally within the middle phalanx. On radiographs, this area appears more radiolucent than the remainder of the medullary cavity and is most apparent on the dorsopalmar view (Fig. 26.2). This radiolucent area may appear circular or ovoid and is variable in size. On the dorsopalmar view of the proximal phalanx, thin radiopaque lines, extending from proximal to distal, are visible along the medial and lateral aspects of this radiolucent region in the medullary cavity. These are the sites of attachment of the oblique distal sesamoidean ligaments and should not be misinterpreted as a lesion. On the lateromedial view, the distal aspect of the insertion of the oblique distal sesamoidean ligaments is also commonly visible as a small area of irregular bone along the palmar cortex of the distal third of the proximal phalanx. This area may be more prominent in older and/or larger horses.[3]

*Palmar/dorsopalmar is used throughout this chapter with the understanding that plantar/dorsoplantar should be substituted if referencing the hindlimb.

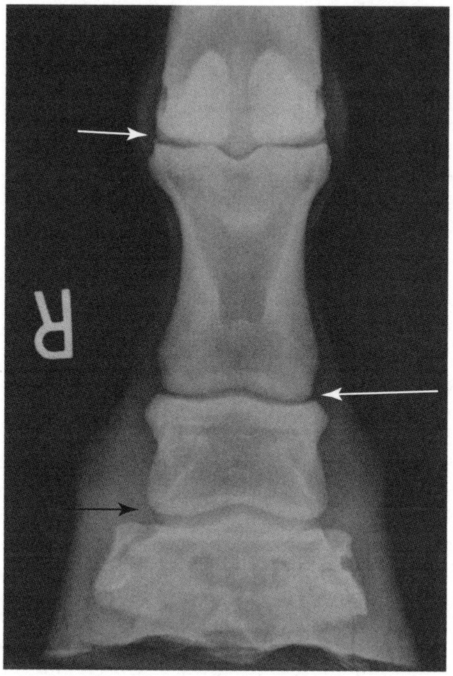

Fig. 26.1 Dorsopalmar view of the distal limb. On this view, the width of the joint spaces of the fetlock joint (*short white arrow*), proximal interphalangeal joint (*long white arrow*), and distal interphalangeal joint (*short black arrow*) can be compared. The distal interphalangeal joint space is typically the widest, followed by the proximal interphalangeal joint, with the fetlock joint being the narrowest.

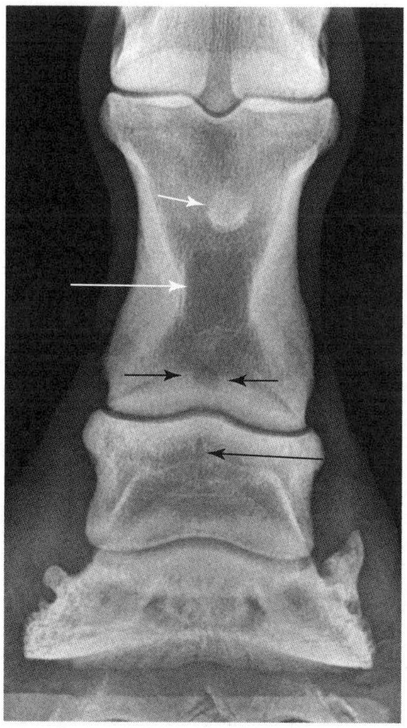

Fig. 26.2 Dorsopalmar view of the distal limb. A small, round, mineral opacity that corresponds to the ergot is present summating with the proximal phalanx (*short white arrow*). A round radiolucency is present in the mid medullary cavity of the proximal phalanx (*long white arrow*), often where the cortices of the bone are thickest. A thin radiopaque rim may be seen around this central region of radiolucency. A small, round radiolucency is present along the distal aspect of the proximal phalanx, which is associated with the small concavity in the distal palmar aspect of the bone and should not be confused for a cyst (*between the short black arrows*). The nutrient foramen appears as a small linear lucency along the proximal aspect of the middle phalanx, near midline (*long black arrow*).

The ergot can be visible as a round soft tissue to mineral opacity superimposed with the proximal phalanx on the dorsopalmar view (see Fig. 26.2). On the corresponding lateromedial view, the ergot will be located along the palmar aspect of the skin.

A small palmar concavity is present between the medial and lateral condyles of the distal aspect of the proximal phalanx. This concavity may create another round radiolucent region near midline on dorsopalmar radiographs and should not be mistaken for a cyst in the distal aspect of the bone (see Fig. 26.2).

A nutrient foramen may be identified radiographically in the proximal phalanx but can be variable in position. The position of the nutrient foramen of the proximal phalanx on forelimb radiographs has been characterized in two studies.[8,9] A nutrient foramen was identified radiographically in the majority of forelimbs reviewed (77% of Thoroughbreds and 69.5% of Standardbreds) and was present either within the dorsal or palmar cortex. The appearance of the nutrient foramen can be bilaterally symmetrical in some horses but asymmetrical in others. A nutrient foramen was not found in both the dorsal and palmar cortex of the same limb; however, both were occasionally present in the proximal phalanx of foals (Fig. 26.3). In another review of dorsal foramina in the proximal phalanx, the nutrient foramen was found in the dorsal cortex of 27.5% of the forelimbs and hindlimbs evaluated.[10] In this study, three breeds of horses (Standardbreds, Warmbloods, and Friesians) were included, and in most of the horses the dorsal foramen was identified unilaterally.

The nutrient foramen in the dorsal aspect of the proximal phalanx is best seen on the lateromedial view and most commonly courses obliquely from proximal to distal at the level of the mid diaphysis (see Fig. 26.3, also see Fig. 26.6B). On the dorsopalmar view, the foramen in the dorsal cortex appears as a thin lucent line in the medullary region near midline (see Fig. 26.6A). When in the palmar cortex, the foramen is typically

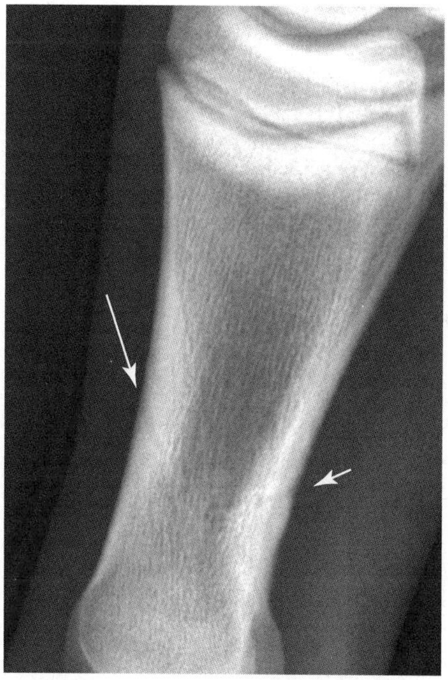

Fig. 26.3 Lateromedial view of the proximal phalanx in a 2-month-old foal. Linear radiolucencies are present along the dorsal (*long white arrow*) and palmar (*short white arrow*) cortices of the diaphysis. These are normal nutrient foramina and were bilaterally symmetric in the forelimbs of this patient.

in the distal third of the bone and courses in a shorter oblique to transverse direction.

RADIOGRAPHIC ABNORMALITIES

Osseous Lesions

Osteochondrosis/Osteochondral Fragments

Developmental disease, such as osteochondrosis, does not occur as commonly in the proximal interphalangeal joint as in other joints of the horse. Osteochondral fragments, secondary to osteochondrosis, are occasionally found in the proximal interphalangeal joint. In one study assessing presale radiographs of Warmbloods, an osteochondral fragment was present in the proximal interphalangeal joint in 0.9% of horses.[11] Osteochondral fragments have been described along the dorsal/dorsomedial and palmar/plantar aspects of the proximal interphalangeal joint, originating from the distal aspect of the proximal phalanx (most common) or proximal aspect of the middle phalanx.[12–17] Dorsal fragments have been suggested to be developmental in origin, whereas palmar fragments have been proposed to be due to partial avulsion fractures of the soft tissue attachments along the proximal interphalangeal joint during hyperextension of the joint.[3,12,13,17] Osteochondral fragments in the proximal interphalangeal joint may be incidental findings but have also been associated with lameness. In these horses, removal of the fragments is often recommended and return to previous levels of athletic performance has been reported.[12,17,18]

Osseous Cyst-Like Lesions

Osteochondrosis can also manifest as subchondral cystic lesions along the proximal interphalangeal joint, especially in a juvenile patient with no history of trauma.[19,20] Osseous cyst-like lesions (also known as subchondral cystic lesions or cysts, osseous cysts, or subchondral cyst-like osteochondrosis) can occur in the pastern region and are typically found in the subchondral bone near, and often communicating with, the proximal interphalangeal joint[21] (Fig. 26.4, eFig. 26.1). These cysts are most commonly identified unilaterally in the distal condyle of the proximal phalanx, although bilateral lesions are possible. These lesions are more common in the hindlimb.[15,19,22,23] Radiographically, these lesions may initially appear as a small depression, flattening or concavity in the articular margin but can later progress to a round, ovoid, conical-shaped or multichambered radiolucency in the subchondral bone.[3,21] Single cysts or multiple cysts may be present, with varying degrees of surrounding sclerosis. In addition to osteochondrosis, these cystic lesions can develop secondary to osteoarthritis, infection, or trauma; however, the etiology of these cysts is still debated.[19–23]

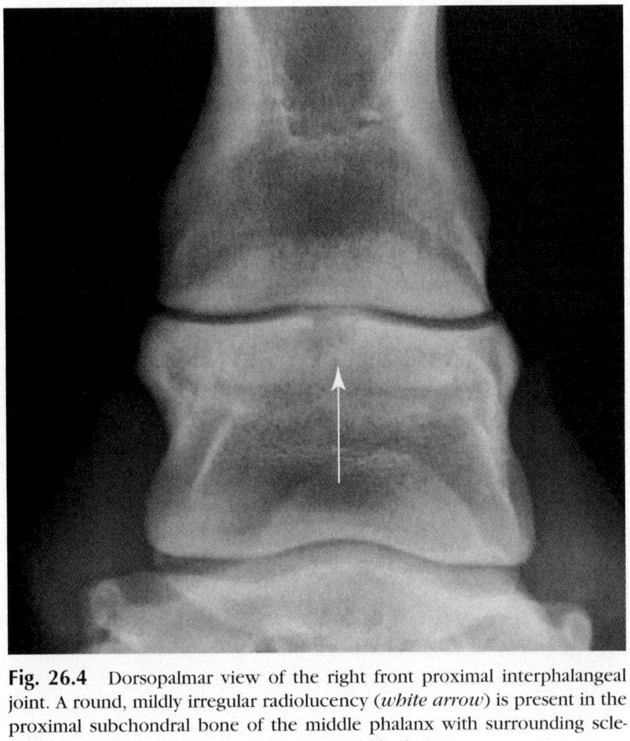

Fig. 26.4 Dorsopalmar view of the right front proximal interphalangeal joint. A round, mildly irregular radiolucency (*white arrow*) is present in the proximal subchondral bone of the middle phalanx with surrounding sclerosis, most consistent with an osseous cyst-like lesion.

Variable degrees of lameness have been reported in patients with osseous cyst-like lesions, likely associated with the extent of joint involvement. These lesions are typically more clinically significant when the cyst communicates with the joint; therefore, careful assessment of the radiographs for any involvement of the articular surface, such as a thin cloaca or a wider, broader area of radiolucency between the cyst and articular margin, is advised. Advanced imaging (i.e., MRI) may be needed in some horses to confirm the diagnosis of a cyst and/or to determine if the cyst is communicating with the joint. In young horses, small subchondral cysts can be identified incidentally on survey radiographs and may resolve or cause minimal clinical signs; however, others will progress with secondary osteoarthritis and be associated with clinically significant lameness.[22,24,25]

Fractures

Fractures of the proximal and middle phalanges are relatively common, and radiography is often the initial imaging modality used for diagnosis. These fractures can be identified in all breeds/types of horses; however, fractures of the proximal phalanx occur most commonly in racehorses (i.e., Thoroughbreds, Standardbreds), while middle phalanx fractures are more common in Western performance horses (Quarter horses).[15,17,26] These fractures can be simple (noncomminuted) or comminuted, incomplete or complete, monoarticular or biarticular, and course primarily in a sagittal or dorsal plane relative to the long axis of the bone. Fig. 26.5 illustrates the various configurations of fractures in the proximal and middle phalanges. Lameness associated with an incomplete fracture may vary from minimal to severe, but horses with complete or comminuted fractures typically have an acute onset of severe lameness. Fractures may initially be nondisplaced and difficult to diagnose radiographically; therefore, if a fracture is suspected, several oblique views should be performed to identify the fracture and determine its complexity. Repeat radiographs 10 to 14 days after an injury will often allow better visualization of a nondisplaced fracture as the fracture line may be slightly wider due to resorption of the fracture margins. Periosteal new bone formation, suggestive of callus formation, can be present along the cortices of the phalanges, especially if the fracture is more chronic. Advanced imaging (i.e., CT or MRI) may be needed to identify the fracture (usually if the fracture is nondisplaced), determine the exact fracture configuration, and for surgical planning.[27,28] In one study comparing radiography and CT, CT was able to diagnose 4 of 20 fractures that were not identified radiographically.[29]

Proximal Phalanx. Fractures of the proximal phalanx at the level of the fetlock joint, such as osteochondral fragments, chip fractures, or palmar/plantar proximal tuberosity fractures, are common, especially in racehorses.[26] These fractures are described in detail in Chapter 25.

Sagittal (midsagittal or parasagittal) fractures of the proximal phalanx are frequently diagnosed and can have multiple configurations, most often originating from the midsagittal groove of the proximal articular surface.[26,30–32] These fractures can be (1) short or long incomplete fractures, (2) complete monoarticular or biarticular fractures, or (3) comminuted fractures. These fractures are typically best visible on the dorsopalmar

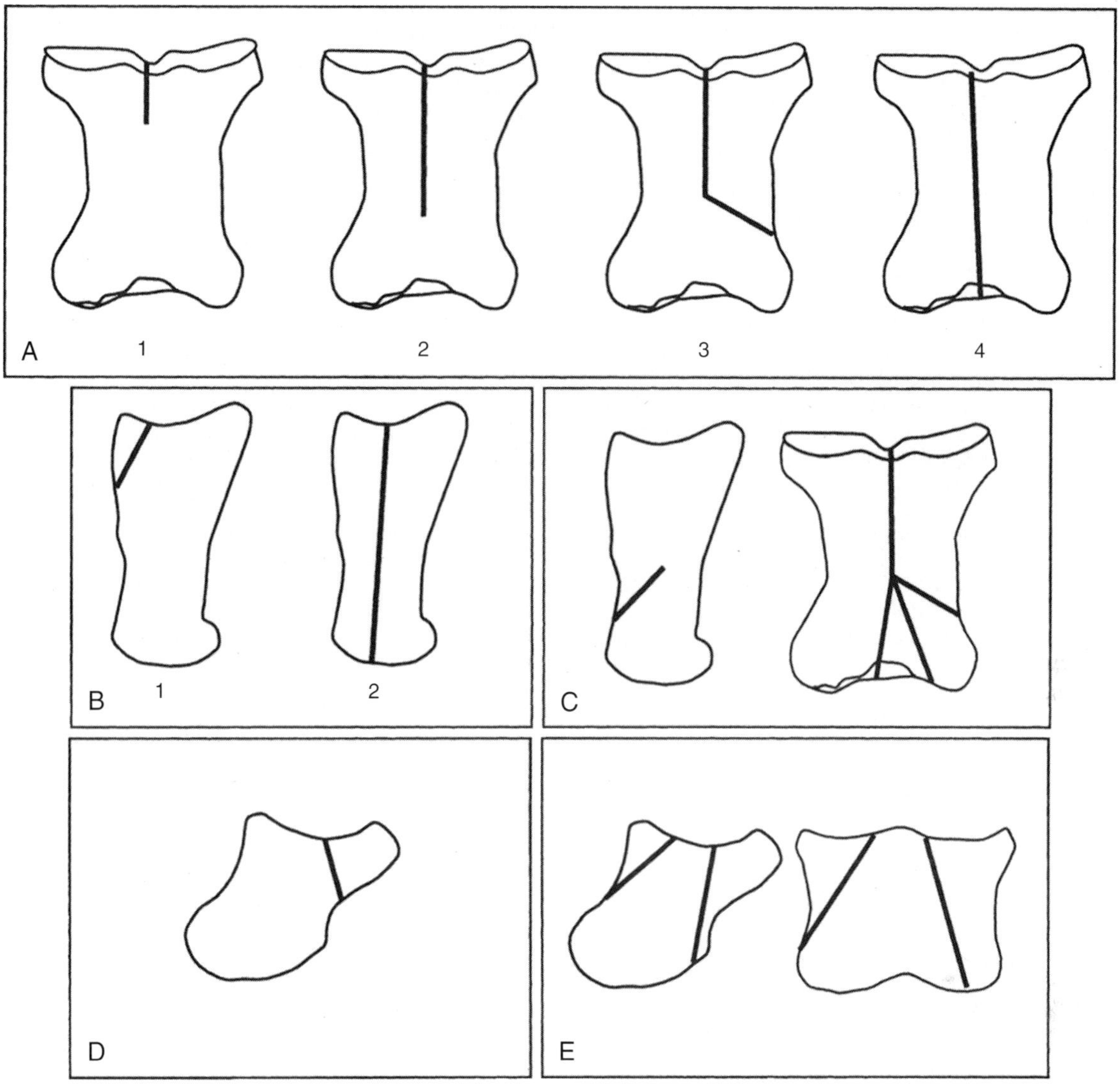

Fig. 26.5 **A–E,** Common fracture configurations of the proximal and middle phalanges. *Proximal phalanx:* **A,** Sagittal plane fractures, noncomminuted. *1,* Incomplete, monoarticular (short, <30 mm variation); *2,* incomplete, monoarticular (long, >30 mm variation); *3,* complete, monoarticular; *4,* complete, biarticular. **B,** Dorsal plane fractures, noncomminuted. *1,* Complete, monoarticular; *2,* complete, biarticular. **C,** Comminuted, complete, biarticular, dorsal, and/or sagittal plane. *Middle phalanx:* **D,** Palmar/plantar eminence (monoarticular, complete). **E,** Comminuted, complete, biarticular.

views; however, oblique views (i.e., 5–15 degrees medial or lateral to the midsagittal plane) may be needed for identification.

The incomplete, monoarticular sagittal fracture is the most common configuration[30,33] (Figs. 26.6 and 26.7). This fracture type is most often identified in young (2- to 3-year-old) racehorses, actively racing and/or training, although can also be seen in endurance or sporthorses.[15] These fractures are more common in the forelimbs of Thoroughbreds and hindlimbs of Standardbreds. The fracture typically originates at the level of the fetlock joint, near midline, within the sagittal groove of the proximal articular margin and then propagates distally.[26,30,31,34,35] Two variations of incomplete sagittal fractures have been reported, including a (1) short fracture (<30 mm extension into the diaphysis) and (2) long fracture (>30 mm extension in the diaphysis). These sagittal fractures may course in a slightly spiral or oblique manner and are often seen as parallel or offset radiolucent fracture lines on the dorsopalmar view due to the dorsal and palmar/plantar aspects of the fracture being in slightly different planes (see Fig. 26.7). Subchondral cystic lesions have been reported to occur with incomplete fractures, particularly the short variation.[34,35] Horses with incomplete fractures of the proximal phalanx may present with more subtle lameness but many have a severe, acute lameness. Most of these horses often have fetlock effusion as the fractures frequently involve the fetlock joint.

With increasing evidence to indicate that these fractures can be the result of repetitive stress and adaptive failure, careful radiographic assessment of the proximal articular margins of the proximal phalanx is recommended, especially in performance horses.[36] These subtle early changes, such as small subchondral fissures or changes in subchondral bone thickness, may represent increased risk for a development of a fracture in the future.[33,36–38]

Complete sagittal fractures, either biarticular or monoarticular, are less common than incomplete fractures. This type of fracture is most commonly reported in the Western

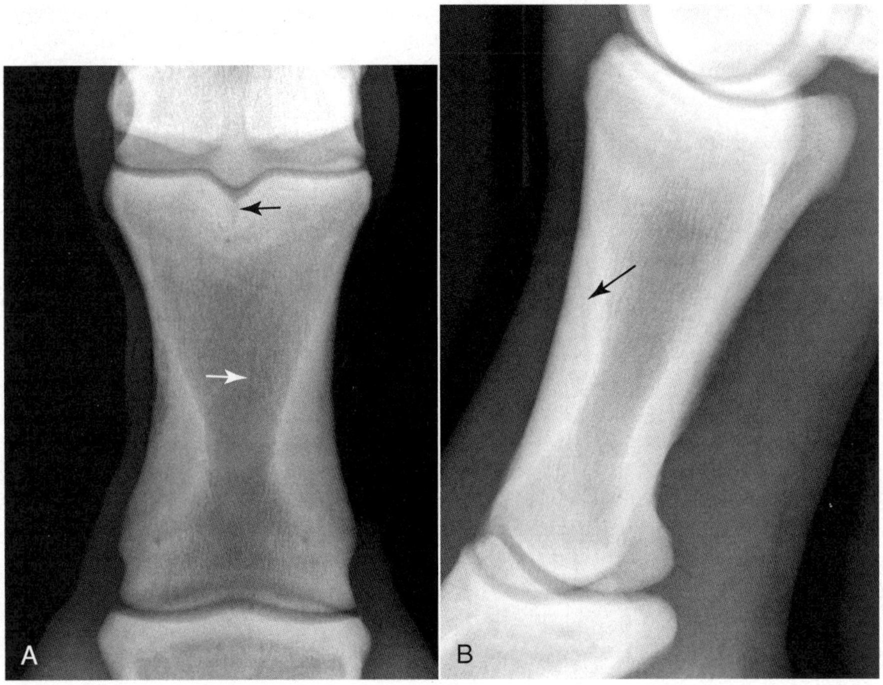

Fig. 26.6 Dorsopalmar **(A)** and lateromedial **(B)** views of the proximal phalanx in an adult horse. **A,** Incomplete short sagittal fracture (*short black arrow*) in the proximal phalanx, originating in the midsagittal groove, with surrounding sclerosis. The normal nutrient foramen is visible on this view and should not be misinterpreted as a fracture (*short white arrow*). **B,** The normal nutrient foramen is seen as a thin linear radiolucency coursing obliquely in a proximal to distal orientation (*black arrow*).

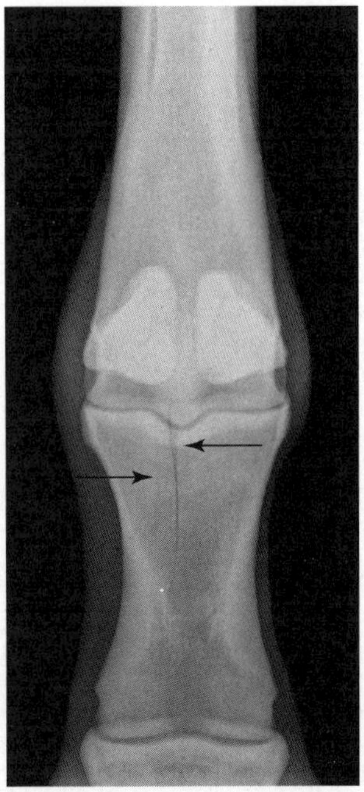

Fig. 26.7 Dorsopalmar view of the fetlock in the forelimb of a 2-year-old racehorse. Noncomminuted, incomplete, monoarticular long sagittal fracture of the proximal phalanx, originating from the midsagittal groove of the proximal articular margin. Two linear radiolucent fracture lines (*black arrows*) are identified on this view, corresponding to the slightly different location of the fracture in the dorsal and palmar cortices. (Image courtesy Dr. Samantha Morello, University of Wisconsin-Madison, WI.)

performance horse. Two variations of this fracture occur: (1) biarticular fracture involving the fetlock and proximal interphalangeal joints and (2) monoarticular fracture, often exiting through the lateral distal palmar/plantar cortex.

Comminuted fractures of the proximal phalanx are also relatively common. These fractures typically involve the fetlock and proximal interphalangeal joints (biarticular) and more frequently exit the lateral cortex. These fractures may involve the entire length of the proximal phalanx or only be found in the proximal or distal portion. Not surprisingly, these fractures have the most guarded prognosis for survival and poor prognosis for return to performance.[30,35,39]

Dorsal plane fractures of the proximal phalanx are less common and are best seen on lateromedial views. There are three different configurations for dorsal plane fractures: (1) incomplete proximal dorsal articular fractures, (2) complete proximal dorsal articular fractures, and (3) fractures that extend from the midportion of the proximal articulation into the proximal phalanx, toward the proximal interphalangeal joint.[15,40] Proximal dorsal fractures occur most commonly in the hindlimb of Standardbred and Thoroughbred racehorses.[15,26,41]

Other infrequently reported fractures of the proximal phalanx include physeal fractures (typically Salter-Harris type II) in foals and weanlings and incomplete distal articular fractures.[15] Avulsion fractures of the proximal annular ligament in the hindlimb have also been described.[42] These fractures are identified along the proximal plantar aspect of the proximal phalanx, at the proximal site of attachment of the proximal digital annular ligament, and are associated with variable degrees of lameness.

Middle Phalanx. Fractures of the middle phalanx are most common in Western performance or working horses, polo ponies, and jumpers during activity; however, fractures have also developed during light/leisure activity or paddock turnout.[17,27,43–45] Most middle phalanx fractures are thought to occur due to the extreme simultaneous compression and torsion forces placed on the middle phalanx while the foot is fixed to the ground, such as during tight turns and sudden stops.[44,45] These horses are typically lame with variable swelling of the

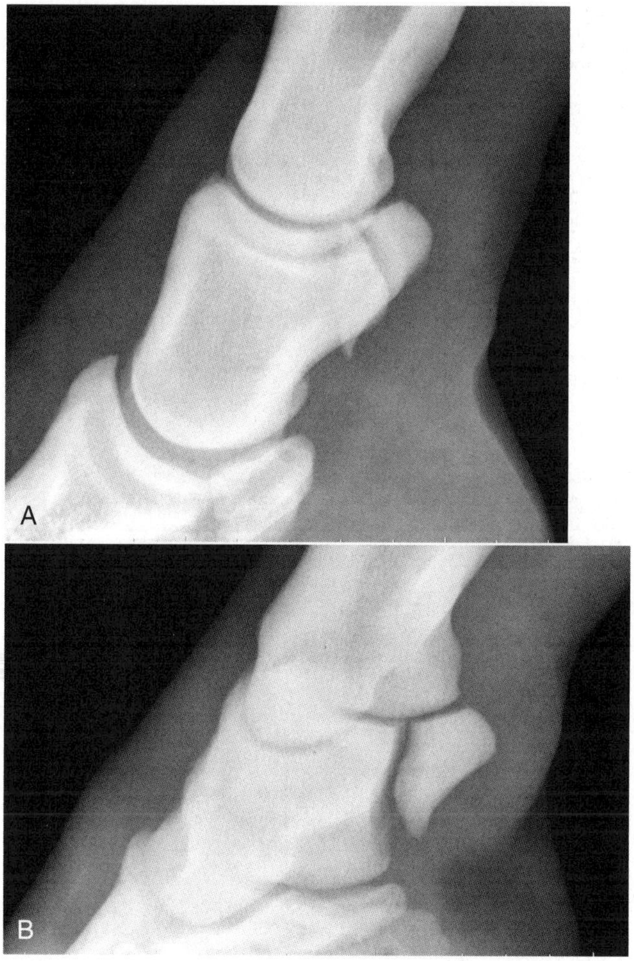

Fig. 26.8 A–B, Lateromedial and oblique views of the distal limb. Noncomminuted, complete, monoarticular fracture of the medial palmar eminence of the middle phalanx. The oblique view (B) aids in displaying the fracture plane and involvement of the proximal interphalangeal joint.

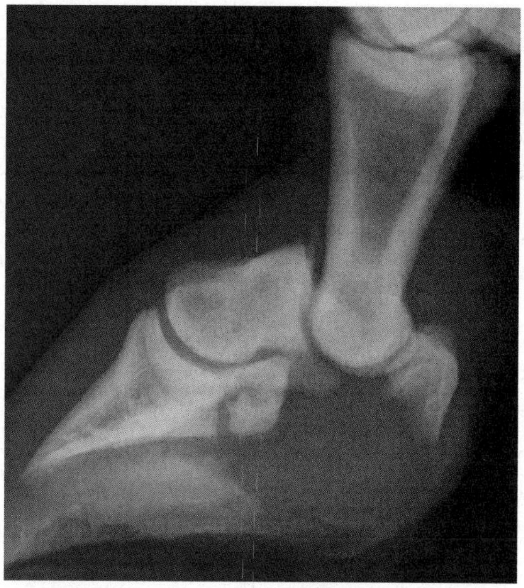

Fig. 26.9 Lateromedial view of the distal limb. Complete, monoarticular biaxial fracture of the middle phalanx in the hindlimb. The medial and lateral plantar eminences are both fractured with plantar displacement of the fracture fragments, resulting in instability and luxation of the proximal interphalangeal joint.

pastern region. Fractures of the middle phalanx more commonly affect the hindlimbs; however, forelimb fractures are more frequently comminuted.[15,17,43,45] Fractures of the middle phalanx can be: (1) comminuted (most common), (2) involving the palmar/plantar eminences (uni- or biaxial), and, less frequently, (3) osteochondral (chip) fractures. Physeal fractures have been reported in young horses but are rare.

Fractures of the palmar (plantar) eminences more commonly involve both eminences (biaxial).[17] When the distal palmar (plantar) eminences are fractured, without comminution, the fragments are displaced in a palmar or plantar direction (Fig. 26.8). This is most often identified in the hindlimb. Biaxial eminence fractures typically result in instability of the joint and, in severe cases, the proximal interphalangeal joint is luxated with proximal displacement and overriding of the middle phalanx relative to the proximal phalanx (Fig. 26.9, eFig. 26.2).

The comminuted fractures are typically biarticular, involving both the proximal and distal interphalangeal joints (Fig. 26.10, eFig. 26.3). Additionally, comminution of the fracture may only be present in the proximal aspect of the bone with one or more fracture lines extending distally to the distal interphalangeal joint.[17,43] Involvement of the distal interphalangeal joint significantly affects the prognosis, and treatment of this type of fracture and multiple radiographic views or advanced imaging may be needed to identify involvement of this joint. Additional imaging (i.e., CT) may be needed to better determine the degree of comminution and joint involvement or to assist with surgical planning.[46]

Osteomyelitis

Infection of the pastern region is most common secondary to trauma, a complication of surgery, or less commonly, due to hematogenous dissemination. Penetrating trauma and lacerations can result in a secondary infection of the soft tissue and/or bone. Additionally, sequestrum formation can occur in the pastern region, often associated with a history of a draining wound. There is one report of osteomyelitis developing after proximal interphalangeal arthrodesis due to a fracture where osteolysis and osteoproliferation of the proximal and middle phalanges occurred with sequestrum formation.[47] Increased rates of infection have also been reported after surgical repair of highly comminuted fractures of the proximal phalanx.[35] Hematogenous osteomyelitis and septic physitis are much more common in foals (Fig. 26.11, eFig. 26.4). In a study of foals, hematogenous osteomyelitis was frequently identified in the distal limb but more commonly in the distal phalanx than the more proximal phalanges.[48] One case of fungal osteomyelitis caused by *Cryptococcus gattii* has been reported in the proximal phalanx of an adult horse.[49]

New Bone Formation

Enthesophyte formation can occur at the sites of ligament attachments along the pastern region. Bone proliferation is often identified along the palmar aspect of the mid to distal aspect of the proximal phalanx associated with the distal sesamoidean ligaments. These changes may be associated with desmopathy and should prompt further assessment of the soft tissue structures in this region.

Focal periosteal new bone formation/periostitis and regional soft tissue swelling in the diaphyseal region of the proximal or middle phalanges not corresponding to ligament or capsular attachments are most likely secondary to trauma. The bone generally remodels with time, although periosteal new bone may persist after resolution of the soft tissue component and

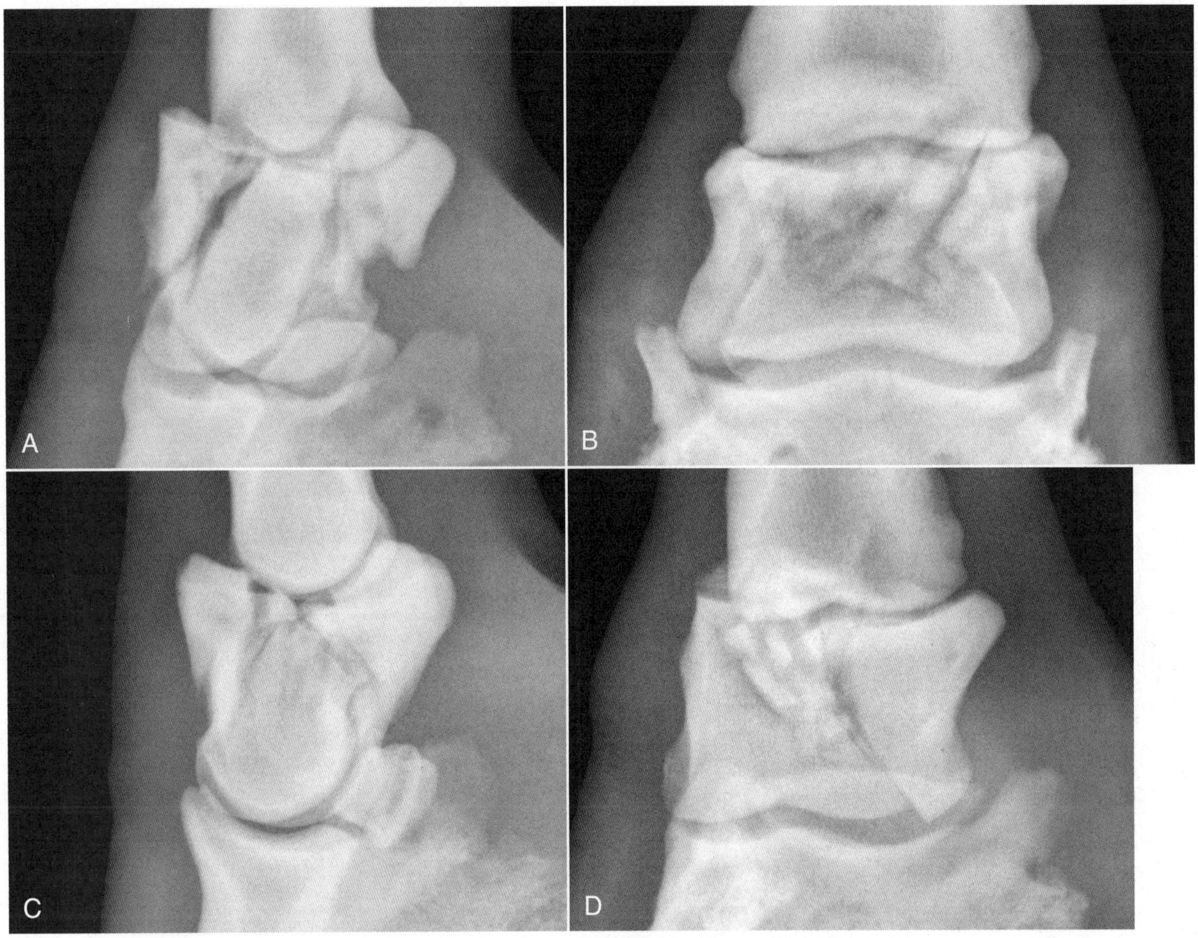

Fig. 26.10 **A–D,** Lateromedial, dorsopalmar, and oblique views of the distal limb. Comminuted, multiplane, biarticular middle phalanx fracture. The oblique views are helpful to confirm the involvement of both the proximal and distal interphalangeal joints. The horse was not bearing weight for the images. With weight bearing, the proximal interphalangeal joint would be luxated.

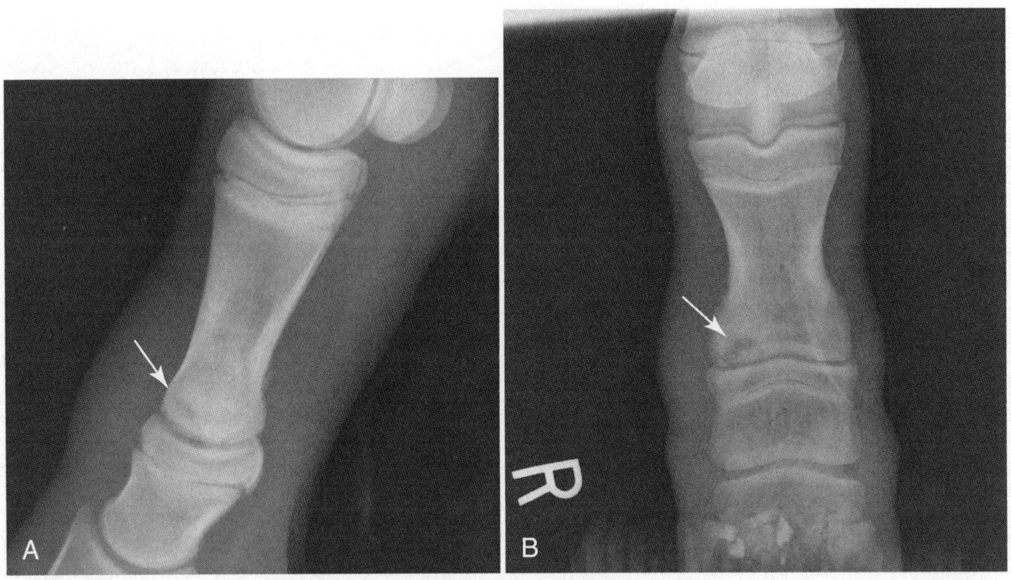

Fig. 26.11 Lateromedial **(A)** and dorsopalmar **(B)** views of the distal limb in a foal. A large radiolucency is present in the subchondral bone of the distodorsal lateral condyle of the proximal phalanx (*white arrows*) with adjacent soft tissue swelling. The diagnosis was osteomyelitis. (Images courtesy Dr. Tom Wilkinson Jr., Washington State University, WA.)

can enlarge with chronic repetitive trauma, such as continued focal impingement along the medial aspect of the pastern by the contralateral limb.

Bone Marrow Lesions

Horses with an acute onset of severe lameness localized to the pastern region may not have radiographic evidence of disease. In these horses, advanced imaging (i.e., MRI) is often pursued for further assessment. MRI is helpful to better exclude the possibility of a fracture and to look for evidence of a bone marrow lesion, which is a lesion characterized by increased fluid signal (high signal on fat- suppressed or inversion recovery sequences) and reduced T1 signal within the bone (Fig. 26.12).

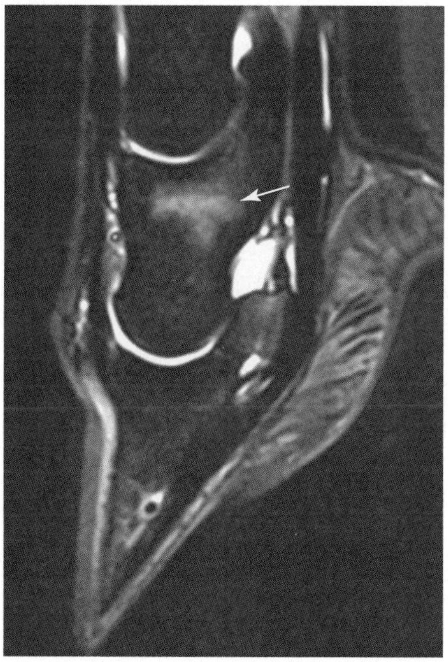

Fig. 26.12 Magnetic resonance imagery (MRI) of the distal forelimb, sagittal short tau inversion recovery (STIR) sequence. On this sequence, the normal fat in the bone marrow is nulled or black. Note the large area of increased signal in the proximal aspect of the middle phalanx (*white arrow*). This is consistent with a bone marrow lesion.

Bone marrow lesions, also known as bone edema or edema-like change, can be secondary to an osseous contusion (bone bruise), bone edema, fibrosis, or osteonecrosis, and often, these lesions are clinically significant. Many of these lesions will resolve with rest and time; however, some will be persistently lame due to development of osteonecrosis, subchondral and trabecular bone loss, and progressive joint pathology.[50–52]

Joint Pathology

Osteoarthritis

Osteoarthritis a chronic degenerative disorder of synovial joints that occurs when articular cartilage deteriorates, over time resulting in radiographically detectable changes including periarticular new bone formation, subchondral sclerosis and/or lucency, and changes in the width of the joint space. Regional soft tissue swelling may also be seen, associated with the adjacent ligaments/tendons, joint effusion, capsular and synovial thickening, or periarticular fibrosis. Periarticular new bone can present as osteophytes (new bone arising along the articular margins) and enthesophytes (new bone at the attachments of periarticular soft tissues, including ligaments, tendons, and the joint capsule). Causes of osteoarthritis include chronic age-related degeneration, acute or chronic repetitive trauma, infection/septic arthritis, abnormal limb conformation, or developmental joint disease. The inciting underlying cause of proximal interphalangeal osteoarthritis may not be evident radiographically, with limb deformity a notable exception.

The proximal interphalangeal joint is commonly affected by osteoarthritis. It is a low-motion joint which bears a high load, particularly in Western performance horses.[24] Since the proximal interphalangeal joint does not have a high range of motion during athletic activity, a smaller region of the joint surface has higher weight-bearing load for a longer time period. This results in articular cartilage and subchondral bone damage, and initiates the cascade of inflammation leading to osteoarthritis.[15,24] Small periarticular osteophytes along the dorsoproximal aspect of the middle phalanx are often the initial radiographic indicator of proximal interphalangeal degenerative joint disease (Fig. 26.13A). As disease progresses, subchondral bone modeling, sclerosis, and demineralization may become evident (see Fig. 26.13B). Late-stage changes include joint space narrowing, progressive lysis of the subchondral bone, advancing sclerosis, and more extensive periarticular osteophytosis (see Fig. 26.13C). Over time, ankylosis or partial ankylosis of the joint can develop (see Fig. 26.13D, eFig. 26.5).

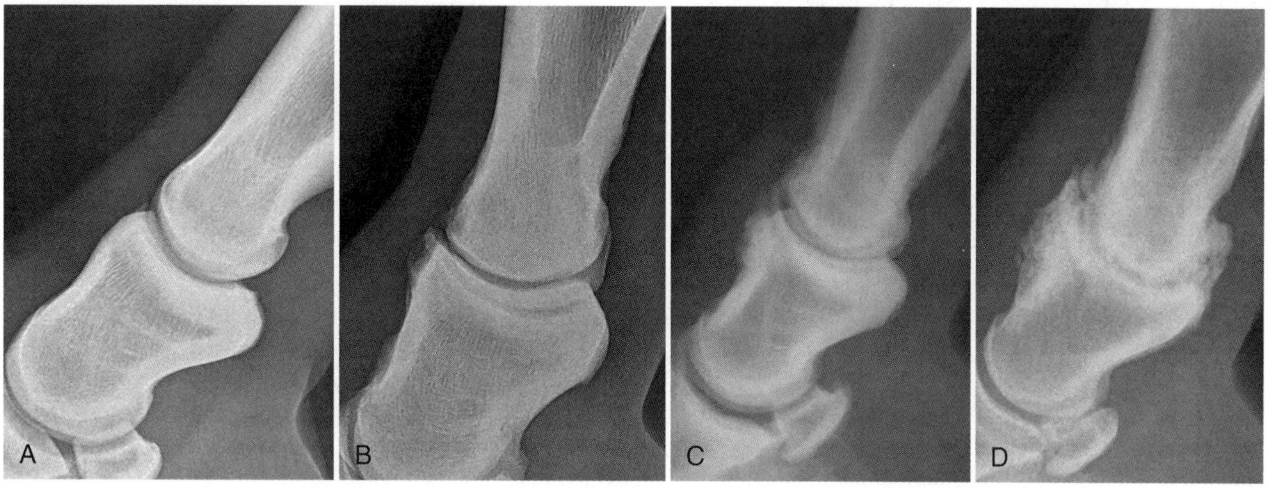

Fig. 26.13 Lateromedial projections of the proximal interphalangeal joint, with progressive osteoarthritis: mild **(A)**, moderate **(B)**, moderate-severe **(C)**, and severe with near ankylosis **(D)**. Note progressive periarticular osteophyte and enthesophyte formation, sclerosis, subchondral lysis, and joint space narrowing **(D)**.

The early radiographic changes indicative of proximal interphalangeal osteoarthritis (small periarticular osteophytes and enthesophytes at ligamentous or capsular attachments) can be incidental in some cases, however these lesions could predict future or developing problems and should be considered in light of the clinical exam and response to regional anesthesia, as well as the onset of lameness (acute versus chronic).

Subchondral Bone Trauma

Severe acute-onset lameness can be seen with trauma and secondary articular cartilage and subchondral bone injury in the proximal interphalangeal joint. The radiographic manifestations can be subtle, and MRI is more sensitive in identifying and characterizing these injuries, particularly in the acute phase (Fig. 26.14A). These lesions also demonstrate marked focal radiopharmaceutical uptake on bone scintigraphy (see Fig. 26.14B). If visible radiographically, lesions can be seen as elongated horizontal or focal circular regions of subchondral lucency in the proximal aspect of the middle phalanx (see Fig. 26.14C, eFig. 26.6), which may become more evident over time and can extend into the trabecular bone.[3] Periosteal proliferation and periarticular osteophyte formation can be seen secondary to this articular cartilage and subchondral bone damage, representing developing degenerative joint disease. The prognosis is guarded in these cases.

Subchondral bone trauma also occurs focally in the distal dorsal aspect of the middle phalanx, either medially or laterally, and is only diagnosed with MRI as increased fluid signal (hyperintensity on fat-suppressed images and hypointensity on T1-weighted images). No radiographic abnormalities are identified in association with this syndrome.

Septic Arthritis

Joint infection arises from penetrating wounds, iatrogenic injections, or hematogenous spread (most commonly in foals). The proximal interphalangeal joint is uncommonly involved in septic polyarthritis in foals.[53–55] Sepsis of the proximal interphalangeal joint should be considered with any lacerations near the joint in conjunction with persistent substantial lameness. Initially, no radiographic changes may be evident with septic arthritis. Synovial proliferation and effusion may cause intracapsular soft tissue swelling although this is difficult to detect radiographically as the proximal interphalangeal joint pouch is relatively small. Positive contrast arthrography and/or contrast fistulography can be helpful to confirm communication between the joint and a wound/wound tract. Early osseous changes include proliferative bone at the joint capsular attachments and/or along the chondro-osseous junctions at the joint periphery. With progressive cartilage deterioration, joint space narrowing can be seen, although care should be taken to ensure even weight bearing when assessing joint space width radiographically.[7] Subchondral irregularity, lysis, and sclerosis can be identified as intra-articular infection progresses (Fig. 26.15A,B). Periosteal new bone also develops along the articular margins. The prognosis is always guarded.

Subluxation/Luxation

Dorsal displacement of the distal aspect of the proximal phalanx with increased flexion of the proximal interphalangeal joint is generally referred to as subluxation. This is most commonly seen in younger horses although it can occur in older horses, is more common in the hindlimbs, and may be unilateral or bilateral.[3] Potential causes include flexor deformities caused by contracture of the deep digital flexor tendon and straight distal sesamoidean ligament, injuries to the suspensory ligament and extensor branches, or injuries to the palmar/plantar ligaments of the proximal interphalangeal joint. Dorsal subluxation may be appreciated on physical examination as abnormal dorsal movement of the distal end of the proximal phalanx at a walk and can occasionally be appreciated at rest. An audible click is sometimes heard when the subluxation is reduced upon full weight bearing. In lateral radiographic projections there is mild dorsal displacement of the distal aspect of the proximal phalanx and increased flexion of the proximal interphalangeal joint. No additional radiographic changes are generally apparent. Palmar/plantar subluxation is typically associated with acute trauma and rupture of the distal sesamoidean ligaments or injury to the superficial digital flexor tendon branches or middle scutum, and there may be associated avulsion fragments or enthesophytes at ligament insertions.[15] Ultrasound examination of the soft tissues of the pastern is indicated in such horses for further evaluation. Degenerative joint disease may also develop with chronic subluxation.

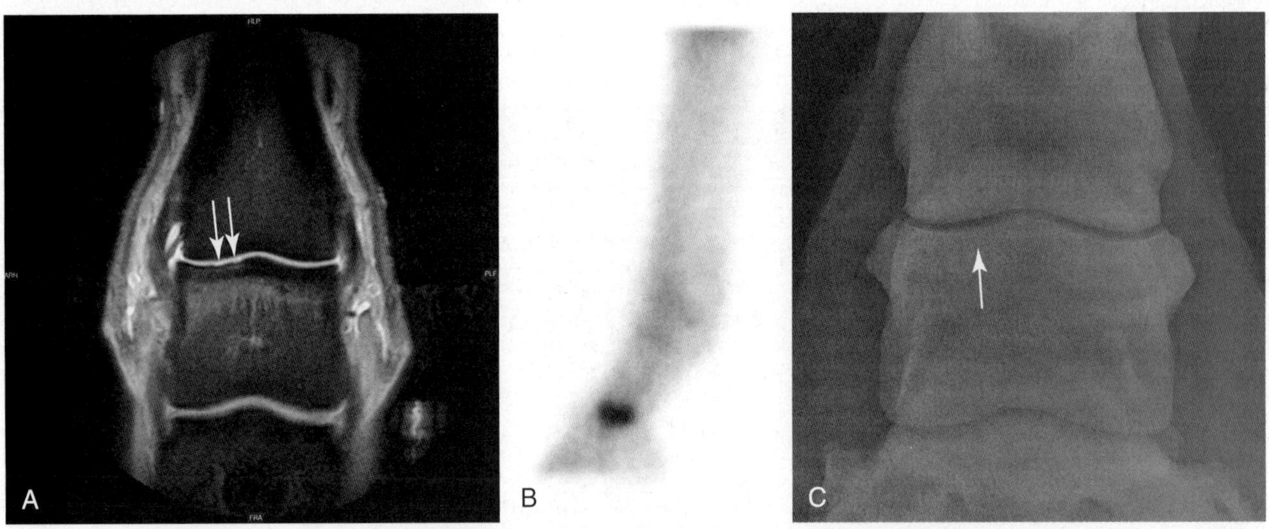

Fig. 26.14 **A–C,** Acute subchondral bone injury of the middle phalanx. **A,** Dorsal plane fat-suppressed magnetic resonance image (MRI) with extensive increased fluid signal in the proximal to mid portion of the middle phalanx and subchondral bone and cartilage defects (*white arrows*). **B,** Lateral nuclear scintigraphic image of the same patient with marked focal increased radiopharmaceutical uptake in the proximal aspect of the middle phalanx, corresponding to the region of subchondral bone injury. **C,** Dorsopalmar radiographic image of the same horse, with subtle subchondral lucency along the proximal aspect of the middle phalanx (*white arrow*).

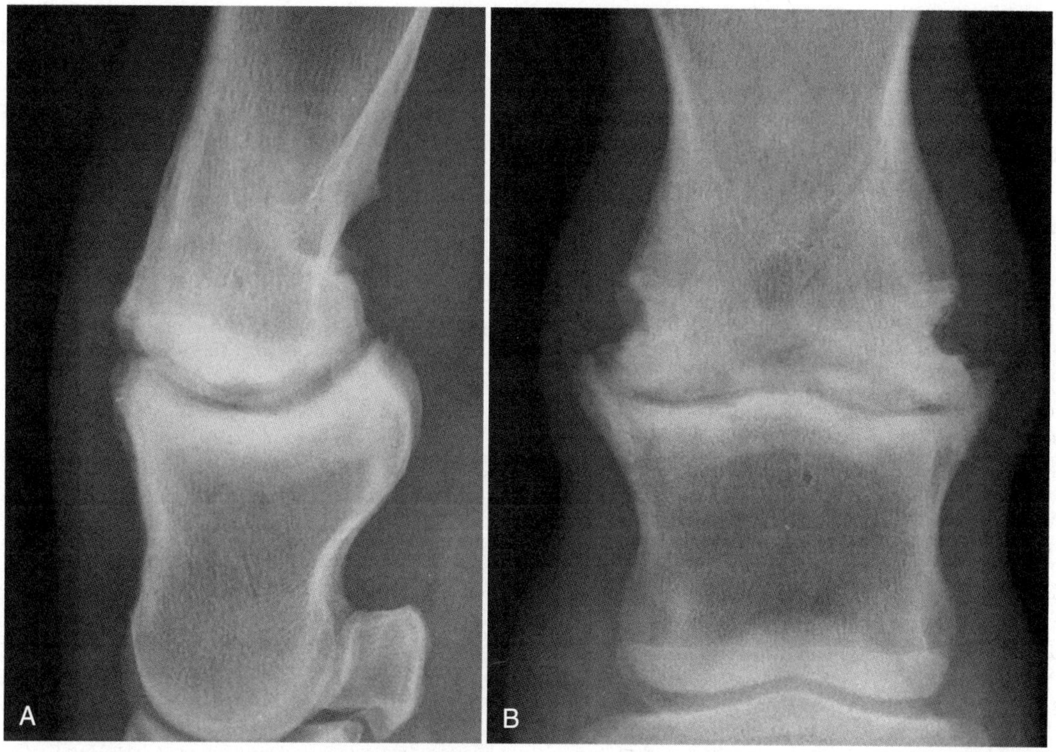

Fig. 26.15 Lateromedial **(A)** and dorsopalmar **(B)** images of the proximal interphalangeal joint of an adult horse with chronic proximal interphalangeal sepsis. There is extensive periarticular remodeling, subchondral sclerosis, subchondral lysis, and joint space narrowing. Mild soft tissue swelling is seen dorsally, primarily intracapsular. This horse also has mild dorsal subluxation of the proximal interphalangeal joint.

Luxation of the proximal interphalangeal joint is typically evident clinically and can be seen with significant trauma to the limb, such as large fractures of the proximal and middle phalanges and/or with avulsion fractures at supporting ligament attachments (see Fig. 26.9).

Hyperextension of The Proximal Interphalangeal Joint

Hyperextension of the proximal interphalangeal joint is uncommon although can be seen with rupture of both the straight distal sesamoidean ligament and the superficial digital flexor tendon. Hyperextension of the proximal interphalangeal joint can also be seen with concomitant hyperextension of the metacarpophalangeal and distal interphalangeal joints, either in foals as a congenital deformity or secondary to weak flexor tendons (resulting from poor nutrition, systemic disease, or after prolonged splinting or casting of the limb) or as an acquired deformity secondary to rupture or avulsion of the deep digital flexor tendon.

Soft Tissue Lesions

Soft tissue changes detectable radiographically can include thickening, altered shape/contour, or abnormal opacity. Increased soft tissue can be seen surrounding joints, either confined to the region of the joint capsule (intracapsular fluid and/or synovial thickening) or external to the joint capsule (extracapsular inflammation, fluid, fibrosis, or cellular infiltrates). Increased extracapsular soft tissue can obscure intracapsular soft tissue changes. Soft tissue thickening or abnormal contour away from the joint may indicate trauma, infection, tendon/ligament injury, acute or chronic wound, granulation tissue, or a soft tissue mass/neoplasm.

Injuries to the tendons and ligaments of the pastern region are common but cannot be accurately diagnosed radiographically. Ultrasound, MRI, and to some degree CT (particularly contrast-enhanced) are superior to radiographs for detecting soft tissue injuries. Regions of osseous proliferation can be seen in association with ligament injury, typically present at the attachment sites as enthesophytes. A thorough knowledge of the soft tissue attachments in the region is necessary for accurate radiographic interpretation; several detailed references for soft tissue attachments are available.[3,4,56] The most common sites for enthetic new bone in the pastern region include the attachments of the oblique distal sesamoidean ligaments (Fig. 26.16), the collateral ligaments of the proximal and distal interphalangeal joints, the proximal and distal digital annular ligaments, the ligaments between the proximal phalanx and the ungular cartilages, and the palmar/plantar ligaments of the proximal interphalangeal joint (Fig. 26.17). Enthesophytes may be of variable to no clinical significance, although indicate an area of potential active or historical injury. Enthetic bone production does not typically resolve following resolution of associated soft tissue injury. Occasionally, avulsion fragmentation can occur at tendinous/ligamentous insertions.

Dystrophic mineralization can develop within tendons or ligaments secondary to chronic injury or may be seen in pericapsular soft tissues associated with previous corticosteroid injections or focal necrosis associated with prior neurectomy. Intraligamentous mineralization is most commonly seen in the distal sesamoidean ligaments (see Fig. 26.16). This is of variable/equivocal significance and should be correlated with ultrasound and clinical examination.

Gas opacity in the regional soft tissues is also sometimes identified, most commonly secondary to regional anesthesia or open skin wounds (Fig. 26.18). Infection with gas-producing organisms is rare.

Miscellaneous Diseases of the Pastern

Hypertrophic osteopathy (Marie's disease) is uncommon but does occur.[57–60] This condition is characterized by soft tissue swelling of the limbs and periosteal bone proliferation along the diaphyses and epiphyses of affected long bones.[58] Concurrent intrathoracic disease is typically the cause of hypertrophic osteopathy; however, occasionally the syndrome is idiopathic or associated with extrathoracic disease. If the underlying disease can be successfully treated, the signs associated with hypertrophic osteopathy can improve and even completely regress. However, in general, many horses with this condition have a poor prognosis as the underlying disease is often serious or fatal.

Cutaneous neoplasms occur in the pastern region, including mast cell tumors,[61–64] carcinomas,[65] and sarcoids (Fig. 26.19).[66] Mast cell tumors, also known as mastocytosis or mastocytomas, are uncommon neoplasm. In one series of mast cell tumors, Arabians were overrepresented.[61] These tumors are most commonly identified as a solid mass arising from the skin, similar to cutaneous mast cell tumors in other animals, and are typically benign, well-demarcated and slow growing. The mast cell tumors on the distal limbs tend to be nonpainful, firm and immobile, and in close proximity to a joint.[63] Additionally, these masses are often calcified.[62]

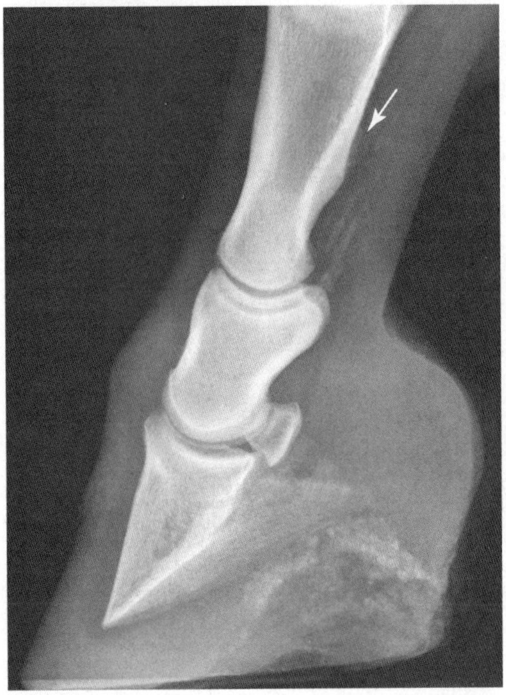

Fig. 26.16 Lateromedial view of the pastern region. Soft tissue mineralization is evident in the superficial digital flexor tendon and straight distal sesamoidean ligament. There is mild smooth enthesopathy at the insertion of the oblique distal sesamoidean ligament on the mid-aspect of the proximal phalanx (*arrow*). This horse also has a mild distal interphalangeal flexural deformity.

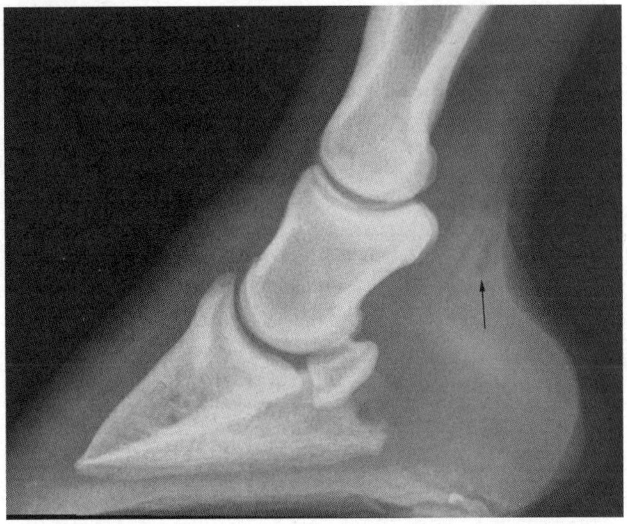

Fig. 26.18 Lateromedial view of the pastern region. Gas is present in the palmar soft tissues (*arrow*) secondary to diagnostic nerve block.

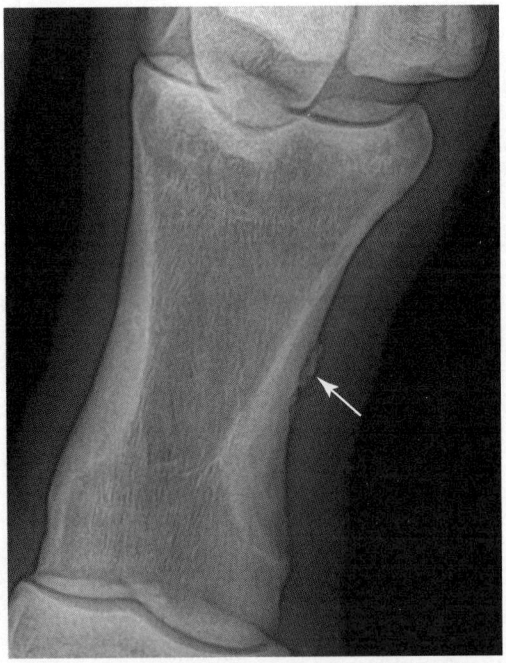

Fig. 26.17 Dorsomedial palmarolateral oblique projection with mild osseous proliferation (*arrow*) at the attachment of the medial abaxial palmar ligament of the proximal interphalangeal joint.

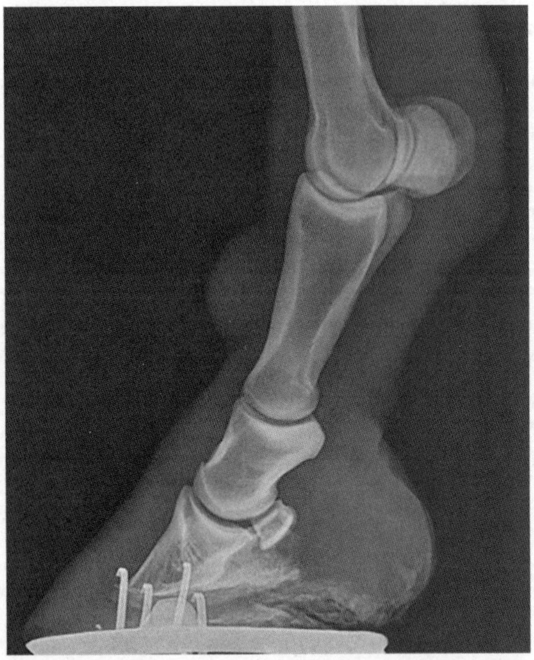

Fig. 26.19 Lateromedial view of the pastern region of a 26-year-old Arabian. A broad-based convex soft tissue opaque mass is present along the dorsal aspect of the mid diaphysis of the proximal phalanx. The adjacent bone is normal. A sarcoid was diagnosed histopathologically.

Osseous neoplasia is uncommon in the distal limb of horses but can include benign (i.e., osteoma, ossifying fibroma) and malignant (i.e., osteosarcoma) etiologies. An osteosarcoma has been reported in the middle phalanx of a horse.[67] In this horse, an aggressive bone lesion was identified radiographically throughout the middle phalanx, with a pathologic fracture. An ossifying fibroma has been described in the proximal phalanx of a horse.[68] Radiographically, multifocal areas of osteolysis with surrounding sclerosis were identified in the distomedial aspect of the proximal phalanx, involving the distal articular margin and subchondral bone. A traumatic osseous cyst-like lesion was the primary differential as many of these areas were well defined; however, an ossifying fibroma was diagnosed histopathologically.

Benign mineralization, such as dystrophic mineralization or osseous metaplasia, have also been described in the distal limb and typically occur secondary to previous trauma or soft tissue injury. One report of focal osseous metaplasia described a focal, well-circumscribed extraskeletal mineralized mass in the plantar pastern of the right hindlimb causing a chronic lameness.[69] This mass was suspected to be causing lameness due to compression on the adjacent plantar digital nerve.

REFERENCES

1. Schebitz H, Wilkens H. *Atlas of Radiographic Anatomy of the Horse*. Philadelphia: Saunders; 1978.
2. Smallwood JE, Holliday SD. Xeroradiographic anatomy of the equine digit and metacarpophalangeal region. *Vet Radiol*. 1987;28:166.
3. Butler JA, Colles CM, Dyson SJ, et al. *Clinical Radiology of the Horse*. 3rd ed. Oxford, UK: Blackwell; 2008.
4. Denoix JM. *The Equine Distal Limb Atlas of Clinical Anatomy and Comparative Imaging*. Ames: Iowa State University; 2002.
5. Becht JL, Park RD, Kraft SL, et al. Radiographic interpretation of normal skeletal variations and pseudolesions in the equine foot. *Vet Clin North Am Equine Pract*. 2001;17(1):1–18.
6. Hinkle FE, Johnson SA, Selberg KT, Barrett MF. A review of normal radiographical variants commonly mistaken for pathological findings in horses. *Equine Vet Educ*. 2020;12:664–672.
7. Contino EK, Barrett MF, Werpy NM. Effect of limb positioning on the radiographic appearance of the distal and proximal interphalageal joint spaces of the forelimbs of horses during evaluation of dorsopalmar radiographs. *J Am Vet Med Assoc*. 2014;244(10):1186–1190.
8. Losonsky JM, Kneller SK. Variable location of nutrient foramina of the proximal phalanx in the forelimbs of Standardbreds. *J Am Vet Med Assoc*. 1988;193(6): 671–673.
9. Kneller SK, Losonsky JM. Variable locations of nutrient foramina of the proximal phalanx in the forelimbs of Thoroughbreds. *J Am Vet Med Assoc*. 1990;197(6):736–738.
10. Frietman S, van Proosdij R, ter Braake F, de Heer N. A detailed radiographic description of the nutrient foramen of the dorsal cortex of the proximal phalanx in horses. *Equine Vet Educ*. 2020;32(suppl 10):72–77.
11. Stock K, Hamann H, Distl O. Prevalence of osseous fragments in distal and proximal interphalangeal, metacarpo- and metatarsophalangeal and tarsocrural joints of Hanoverian Warmblood horses. *J Vet Med*. 2005;52: 388–394.
12. Schneider RK, Ragle CA, Carter BG, et al. Arthroscopic removal of osteochondral fragments from the proximal interphalangeal joint of the pelvic limb in three horses. J Am Vet Med *Assoc*. 1994;205:79–82.
13. Fjordbakk CT, Strand E, Milde AK, et al. Osteochondral fragments involving the dorsomedial aspect of the proximal interphalangeal joint in young horses: 6 cases (1997–2006). *J Am Vet Med Assoc*. 2007;230:1498–1501.
14. Modransky PD, Grant BD, Rantanen NW, et al. Surgical treatment of a palmar midsagittal fracture of the proximal second phalanx in a horse. *Vet Surg*. 1982;4:129–131.
15. Ross MW, Dyson SJ. *Diagnosis and Management of Lameness in the Horse*. ed 2. St Louis: Saunders/Elsevier; 2011.
16. Welch RD, Watkins JP. Osteochondral fracture of the proximal palmar middle phalanx in a Thoroughbred. *Equine Vet J*. 1991;23:67–69.
17. Watkins JP. Fractures of the middle phalanx. In: Nixon AJ, ed. *Equine Fracture Repair*. Philadelphia: WB Saunders Co; 1996.
18. Radcliffe RM, Cheetham J, Bezuidenhout AJ, et al. Arthroscopic removal of palmar/plantar osteochondral fragments from the proximal interphalangeal joint in four horses. *Vet Surg*. 2008;37(3):733–740.
19. Trotter GW, McIlwraith CW, Norrdin RW, et al. Degenerative joint disease with osteochondrosis of the proximal interphalangeal joint in young horses. *J Am Vet Med Assoc*. 1982;180:1312–1318.
20. Nixon AJ. In: Auer JA, Stick JA, Surgery E, eds. *Phalanges and the Metacarpophalangeal and Metatarsophalangeal Joints*. 3rd ed. St Louis: Saunders Elsevier; 2006.
21. Sherlock C, Mair T. Osseous cyst-like lesions/subchondral bone cysts of the phalanges. *Equine Vet Educ*. 2011;23(4):191–204.
22. McIlwraith CW. Subchondral bone cysts in the horse: aetiology, diagnosis and treatment options. *Equine Vet Educ*. 1998;10(6):3131–3317.
23. Ammann L, Ohlerth S, Fürst AE, Jackson MA. Differences of morphological attributes between 62 proximal and distal subchondral cystic lesions of the proximal phalanx as determined by radiography and computed tomography. *Am J Vet Res*. 2023;83(12).
24. McIlwraith CW, Frisbie DD, Kawcak C, Van Weeren R, eds. *Joint Disease in the Horse*. St. Louis: Elsevier; 2016.
25. Kol'vek F, Krešáková L, Vdoviaková K, et al. Modified proximal interphalangeal joint arthrodesis in a yearling filly with an osseous cyst-like lesion in the proximal phalanx. *Animals (Basel)*. 2021;11(4):948.
26. Richardson DW. Fractures of the proximal phalanx. In: Nixon AJ, ed. *Equine Fracture Repair*. Philadelphia: WB Saunders Co; 1996.
27. Rose PL, Seeherman H, O'Callaghan MO. Computed tomographic evaluation of comminuted middle phalangeal fractures in the horse. *Vet Radiol Ultrasound*. 1997;38:424.
28. Brunishoz HP, Hagen R, Furst AE, et al. Radiographic and computed tomographic configuration of incomplete proximal fractures of the proximal phalanx in horses used for racing. *Vet Surg*. 2015;44(7):809–815.
29. Crijns CT, Martens A, Bergman HJ, et al. Intramodality and intermodality agreement in radiography and computed tomography of equine distal limb fractures. *Equine Vet J*. 2014;46(1):92–96.
30. Ellis DR, Simpson DJ, Greenwood RE, Crowhurst JS. Observations and management of fractures of the proximal phalanx in young Thoroughbreds. *Equine Vet J*. 1987;19(1):43–49.
31. Holcombe SJ, Schneider RK, Bramlage LR, et al. Lag screw fixation of noncomminuted sagittal fractures of the proximal phalanx in racehorses: 59 cases (1973–1991). *J Am Vet Med Assoc*. 1995;206:1195–1199.
32. Tetens J, Ross MW, Lloyd JW. Comparison of racing performance before and after treatment of incomplete, mid sagittal

fractures of the proximal phalanx in Standardbreds: 49 cases (1986–1992). *J Am Vet Med Assoc*. 1997;210:82–86.
33. Smith MRW, Wright IM. Radiographic configuration and healing of 121 fractures of the proximal phalanx in 120 Thoroughbred racehorses (2007–2011). *Equine Vet J*. 2014;46(1):81–87.
34. Kümmerle JM, Auer JA, Rademacher N, et al. Short incomplete sagittal fractures of the proximal phalanx in ten horses not used for racing. *Vet Surg*. 2008;37(2):193–200.
35. Markel MD, Richardson DW, Nunamaker DM. Comminuted first phalanx fractures in 30 horses: surgical vs nonsurgical treatments. *Vet Surg*. 1985;14(2):135–140.
36. Ramzan PHL, Powell SE. Clinical and imaging features of suspected prodromal fracture of the proximal phalanx in three Thoroughbred racehorses. *Equine Vet J*. 2010; 42:164.
37. Dyson S, Nagy A, Murray R. Clinical and diagnostic imaging findings in horses with subchondral bone trauma of the sagittal groove of the proximal phalanx. *Vet Radiol Ultrasound*. 2011;52(6):596–604.
38. Powell SE. Low-field standing magnetic resonance imaging findings of the metacarpo/metatarsophalangeal joint of racing Thoroughbreds with lameness localized to the region: a retrospective study of 131 horses. *Equine Vet J*. 2012;44(169):2–12.
39. Markel MD, Martin BB, Richardson DW. Dorsal frontal fractures of the first phalanx in the horse. *Vet Surg*. 1985;14:36–40.
40. Kraus BM, Richardson DW, Nunamaker DM, Ross MW. Management of comminuted fractures of the proximal phalanx in horses: 64 cases (1983–2001). *J Am Vet Med Assoc*. 2004;224:254–263.
41. Wright IM, Minshall GJ. Short frontal plane fractures involving the dorsoproximal articular surface of the proximal phalanx: description of the injury and a technique for repair. *Equine Vet J*. 2018;50:54–59.
42. O'Brien EJO, McAlpine JM, Schramme MC, et al. Avulsion of the proximal digital annular ligament in five hindlimbs. *Equine Vet Educ*. 2018;30(8):427–432.
43. Colahan PT, Wheat JD, Meagher DM. Treatment of middle phalangeal fractures in the horse. *J Am Vet Med Assoc*. 1981;178:1182–1185.
44. Rick MC. Fractures of the middle phalanx. In: White NA, Moore JN, eds. *Current Practice of Equine Surgery*. Philadelphia: Lippincott; 1990.
45. Stashak TS. *Adams' Lameness in Horses*. 5th ed. Philadelphia: Lippincott Williams & Wilkens; 2002.
46. Perrin RAR, Launois MT, Brogniez L, et al. The use of computed tomography to assist orthopaedic surgery in 86 horses (2002–2010). *Equine Vet Educ*. 2011;23:306.
47. Brasche SU, Rick MC, Herthel DJ. Treatment of a horse with osteomyelitis following repair of a middle phalangeal fracture via pastern arthrodesis. *Equine Vet Educ*. 2004;16(5): 262–266.
48. Neil KM, Axon JE, Begg AP, et al. Retrospective study of 108 foals with septic osteomyelitis. *Aust Vet J*. 2010;88(1–2):4–12.
49. Lenard ZM, Lester NV, O'Hara AJ, et al. Disseminated cryptococcosis including osteomyelitis in a horse. *Aust Vet J*. 2007;85(1–2):51–55.
50. Dyson SJ, Murray R, Schramme MC. Lameness associated with foot pain: results of magnetic resonance imaging in 199 horses (January 2001–December 200) and response to treatment. *Equine Vet J*. 2005;37:113–121.
51. Olive J, Mair TS, Charles B. Use of standing low-field magnetic resonance imaging to diagnose middle phalanx bone marrow lesions in horses. *Eq Vet Educ*. 2009;21:116–123.
52. Werpy N. Diagnosis of middle phalanx bone marrow lesions in horses using magnetic resonance imaging and identification of phase effect cancellation for proper image interpretation. *Equine Vet Educ*. 2009;21(3):125–130, 2009.
53. Steel CM, Hunt AR, Adams PL, et al. Factors associated with prognosis for survival and athletic use in foals with septic arthritis: 93 cases (1987–1994). *J Am Vet Med Assoc*. 1999;215(7):973–977.
54. Vos NJ, Ducharme NG. Analysis of factors influencing prognosis in foals with septic arthritis. *Ir Vet J*. 2008;61(2):102–106.
55. Wright L, Ekstrom CT, Kristoffersen M, et al. Haematogenous septic arthritis in foals: short- and long-term outcome and analysis of factors affecting prognosis. *Equine Vet Educ*. 2017;29(6):328–336.
56. Weaver JCB, Stover SM, O'Brien TR. Radiographic anatomy of soft tissue attachments in the equine metacarpophalangeal and proximal phalangeal region. *Equine Vet J*. 1992;24(4):310–315.
57. Levoie J, Carlson GP, George L. Hypertrophic osteopathy in three horses and a pony. *J Am Vet Med Assoc*. 1992;201: 1900–1904.
58. Mair TS, Dyson SJ, Frasser JA, et al. Hypertrophic osteopathy (Marie's disease) in Equidae: a review of twenty-four cases. *Equine Vet J*. 1996;28(4):256–262.
59. Schleining JA, Voss ED. Hypertorphic osteopathy secondary to gastric squamous cell carcinoma in a horse. *Equine Vet Educ*. 2004;16:304–307.
60. Tomlinson JE, Divers TJ, McDonough SP, et al. Hypertrophic osteopathy secondary to nodular pulmonary fibrosis in a horse. *J Vet Intern Med*. 2011;25(1):153–157.
61. McEntee MF. Equine cutaneous mastocytoma: morphology, biological behavior and evolution of the lesion. *J Comp Pathol*. 1991;104:171–178.
62. Samii VF, O'Brien TR, Stannard AA. Radiographic features of mastocytosis in the equine limb. *Equine Vet J*. 1997;29(1):63–66.
63. Scott DW, Miller WH. Mast cell tumor. In: Scott D, Miller W, eds. *Equine Dermatology*. 2nd ed. St. Louis Missouri: Elsevier; 2003.
64. Mair TS, Krudewig C. Mast cell tumours (mastocytosis) in the horse: a review of the literature and report of 11 cases. *Equine Vet Educ*. 2008;20(4):177–182.
65. Dörner CA, Castellón CH, Yañez D. Clinical presentation and treatment of multifocal epitrichial sweat gland carcinoma in a horse. *Austral J Vet Sci*. 52(3):109-112.
66. Sloet van Oldruitenborgh-Oosterbaan MM, Grinwis GCM. Equine sarcoidosis: clinical signs, diagnosis, treatment and outcome of 22 cases. *Vet Dermatol*. 2013;24(1): 218–224.e48.
67. Cillan-Garcia E, Kearns LJ, Hetzel U, et al. Osteosarcoma of the middle phalanx in a horse. *Equine Vet Educ*. 2010;22:535.
68. Balducci J, Selberg K, Pool R, Radue RP. Primary ossifying fibroma of the proximal phalanx in a horse. *Equine Vet Educ*. 2020;32(6):O41–O44.
69. Grabski M, Fews D, Busschers E. Hindlimb lameness associated with a focal osseous metaplasia in an 18-year-old Welsh Section D mare. *Eq Vet Educ*. 2017;29(3):121–124.

ELECTRONIC RESOURCES

Additional information related to the content in Chapter 26 can be found online at eBooks.Health.Elsevier.com.

- Chapter Quiz

CHAPTER 27

Equine Foot

Myra F. Barrett • Elizabeth Acutt • Federica Morandi

OVERVIEW

The equine digit is comprised of the three phalanges and associated proximal and distal interphalangeal joints; the podotrochlear (navicular) apparatus, including the navicular bone and navicular bursa; the distal termination of the flexor and extensor tendons; other supporting soft tissues; and the hoof capsule.[1–3] This chapter focuses specifically on the structures of the foot.

INDICATIONS FOR RADIOGRAPHY

Radiography is the primary imaging modality for evaluation of the foot. Indications for radiographs of the digit include prepurchase examinations; lameness localized to the foot with regional analgesia (palmar digital and/or abaxial or basisesamoid nerve block) or intra-articular analgesia of the distal interphalangeal joint; assessment of osseous and/or synovial involvement in foot wounds or abscesses; suspected trauma; and monitoring the progression or resolution of known abnormalities.

TECHNICAL FACTORS

Patient Preparation

Pertinent information obtained from the patient's history and physical examination is crucial to determine the significance of many radiographic abnormalities of the equine foot. The results of diagnostic nerve blocks should also be considered, whilst noting the growing body of literature suggesting that these blocks may diffuse beyond previously described boundaries.[4,5] Dirt, skin lesions, specialized shoes, pads, and foot packing material can all produce artifactual opacities that complicate radiographic interpretation. All external material should be removed from the haircoat and hoof wall. Whenever possible, shoes and pads should be removed. The sole and sulci of the frog should be cleaned thoroughly. The sulci may then be filled uniformly with a material of soft tissue opacity (e.g., Play-Doh, Hasbro, Pawtucket, RI) to the level of the solar surface (Fig. 27.1). Packing the central and collateral sulci can help eliminate radiolucent linear regions created when the air-filled sulci are superimposed on the distal phalanx in the dorsal 65-degree proximal-palmarodistal (D65Pr-PaDiO)* or other views, which may imitate the appearance of fracture lines (see

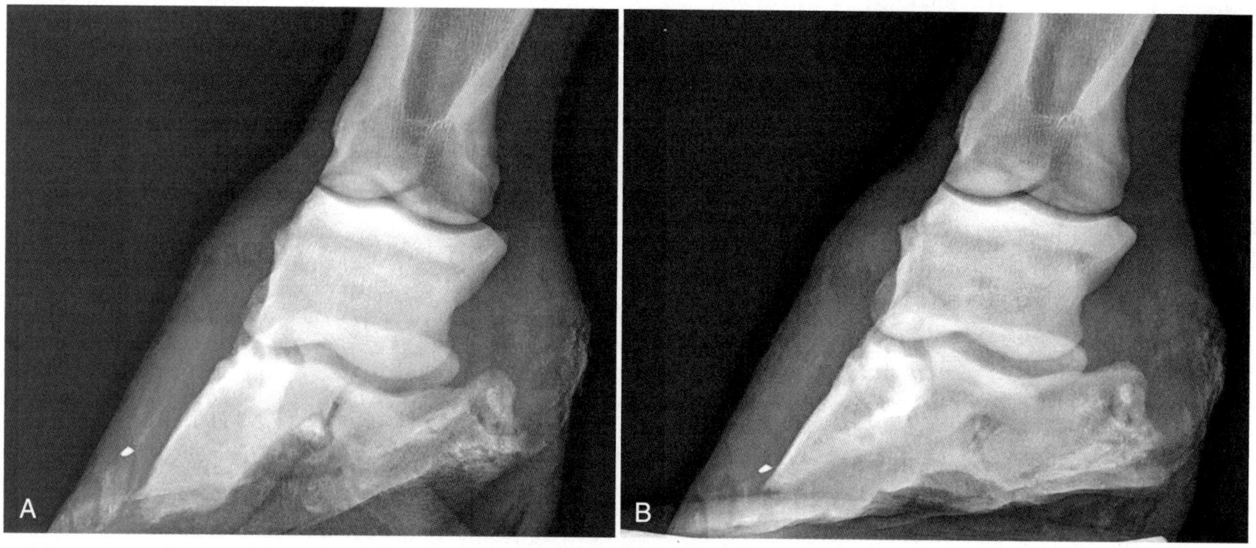

Fig. 27.1 A, Dorsolateral-palmaromedial oblique view of a normal foot without the sulci packed. Note the linear gas lucency in one of the sulci that can appear as a fracture line within the distal phalanx. **B**, The same foot as **A** with the sulci packed, resulting in resolution of the appearance of distal phalanx fracture.

*Palmar(o) is used throughout this chapter with the understanding that plantar(o) should be substituted if reference is being made to the hind digit.

Fig. 27.1). However, occasionally, packing can also increase the number of artifacts, especially if insufficient packing material is applied; therefore, in some cases, leaving the foot unpacked is preferred. The horse should be positioned with both feet on even wooden blocks so as to elevate the feet and facilitate the inclusion of the entire hoof capsule within the field of view. Additional positioning aids, such as a cassette tunnel or upright pedal block, should be used to assist in radiographic evaluation of the navicular bone (Fig. 27.2). When possible, an upright pedal block is preferred to a cassette tunnel for the D65Pr-PaDiO and dorsal 65-degree proximal 45-degree lateral(medial)-palmarodistomedial(lateral) oblique (D65Pr45L[M]-PaDiM[L]O) views since it allows for a tangential orientation of the x-ray beam to the plate, thereby limiting distortion and magnification artifacts. Not all patients are cooperative with placing their feet in the upright blocks, and in those cases a tunnel can suffice.

Recommended Views

The standard views included in a series for assessment of the foot and pastern are included in Table 27.1. Excellent descriptions of positioning are available for additional information.[6,7]

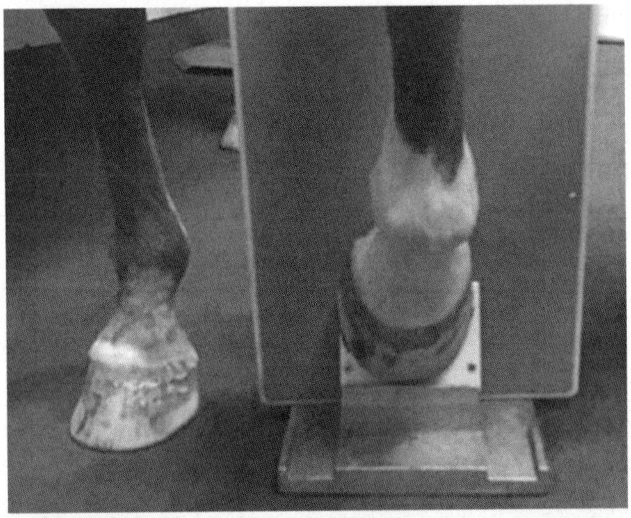

Fig. 27.2 Positioning of the foot for acquisition of dorsal 60–65-degree proximal to palmarodistal oblique radiograph using a Redden navicular block, NANRIC, Lawrenceburg KY.

Alternate Imaging of the Foot

Ultrasound, nuclear scintigraphy, magnetic resonance imaging (MRI), and computed tomography (CT) are used to enhance the assessment of foot lameness. Standing open and conventional open and closed magnets are being used with increasing frequency to assess the soft tissues and bone of the foot. Although these modalities are not discussed in detail in this chapter, specific notation will be made regarding important alternate imaging findings where applicable.

NORMAL RADIOGRAPHIC ANATOMY (INCLUDING VARIATIONS)

Osseous Structures

The appearance of the dorsal margin of the distal interphalangeal joint can vary in several ways, and this is a common area of radiographic misinterpretation. The shape of the extensor process of the distal phalanx (P3) and the dorsodistal margin of the middle phalanx (P2) may vary among individual animals from rounded to pointed (Fig. 27.3).[8] Pointed margins may be mistaken for periarticular osteophytes. Closely examining the joint for other signs of degenerative changes and comparing with the contralateral limb to assess for symmetry can help to distinguish between osteoarthritis changes and normal variation. The dorsal cortex of P2 should be smooth on a straight lateral view. If the lateromedial view is slightly oblique, the eminences for attachment of the collateral ligaments of the distal interphalangeal joint become more conspicuous and can be misinterpreted as abnormal (Fig. 27.4).

The radiographic appearance of the normal P3 in the D65Pr-PaDiO view varies in several respects.[7,9] The most obvious is the number and distribution of vascular channels (Fig. 27.5). The number of vascular channels is typically greater in rear P3 than in front P3.[8] All vascular channels radiate from the solar canal to the solar border.

A smoothly rounded concavity in the toe of the distal phalanx may be present in the normal horse (see Fig. 27.5). This notch is referred to as the *crena marginalis solaris* or, more commonly, the *crena*. In a radiographic study of the foredigit of the developing Quarter horse, a crena was identified in foals between 4 and 22 weeks of age in 83% of the distal phalanges evaluated.[10] The depth of this notch usually does not exceed 1.5 cm.[2] The crena is more conspicuous in front than in hind feet.[9] Ninety percent of sound racing Thoroughbreds have bilateral symmetry in the presence of the crena in the front feet,

Table • 27.1

Views for Equine Foot Evaluation.

STRUCTURES EVALUATED	VIEWS
Distal phalanx	Dorsopalmar view with horizontal beam (0-degree) and foot on block to include soft tissues of the sole on the radiograph
	Lateromedial view with horizontal beam (0-degree) and foot on block to include soft tissues of the sole on the radiograph
	Dorsal 65-degree proximal-palmarodistal oblique
Distal interphalangeal joint	Dorsal 65-degree proximal-palmarodistal oblique
	Dorsopalmar view with horizontal beam (0-degree)
	Lateromedial view with horizontal beam (0-degree)
	Two oblique views: dorsal 65-degree proximal, 45-degree lateral-palmarodistomedial and dorsal 65-degree proximal, 45-degree medial-palmarodistolateral oblique
Navicular bone	Dorsal 65-degree proximal-palmarodistal oblique
	Palmar 45-degree proximal-palmarodistal oblique

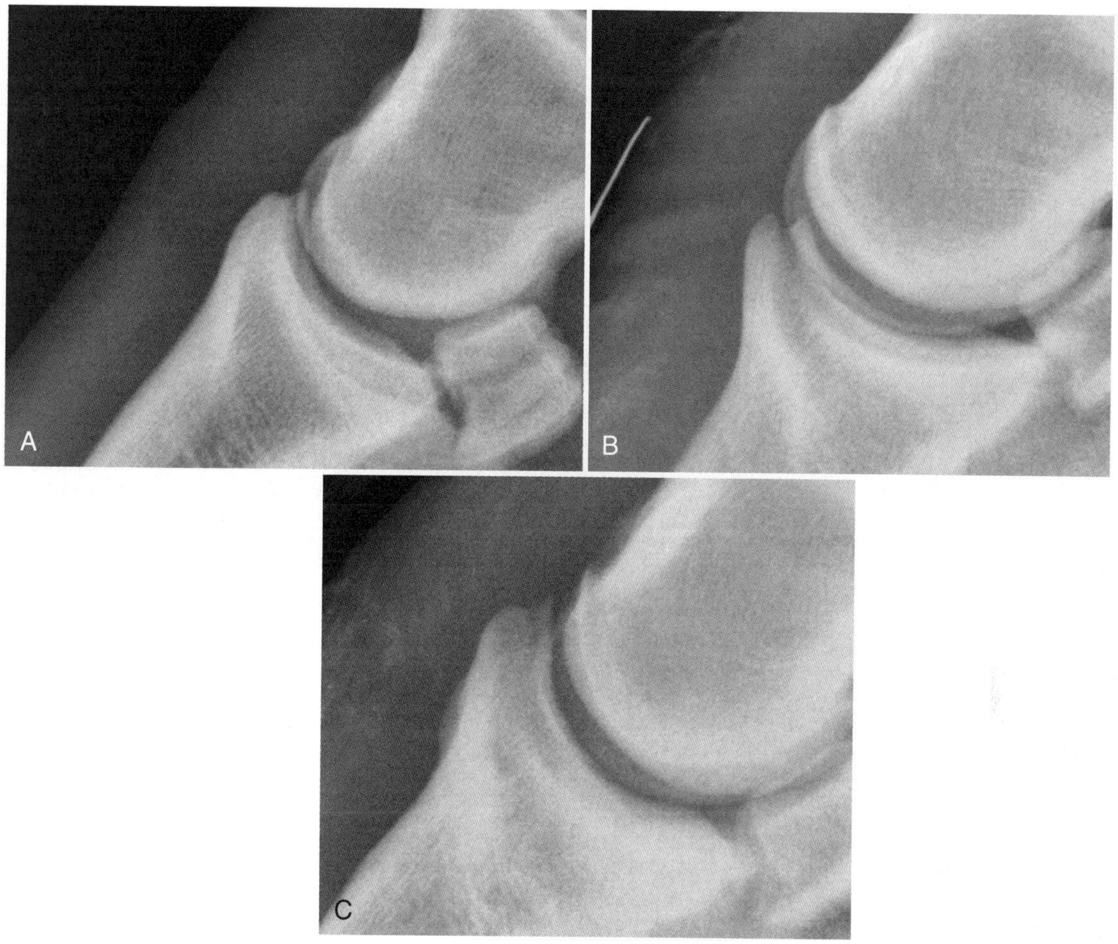

Fig. 27.3 **A–C,** Normal variations in the shape of the extensor process of the distal phalanx, as might be seen on the lateromedial view.

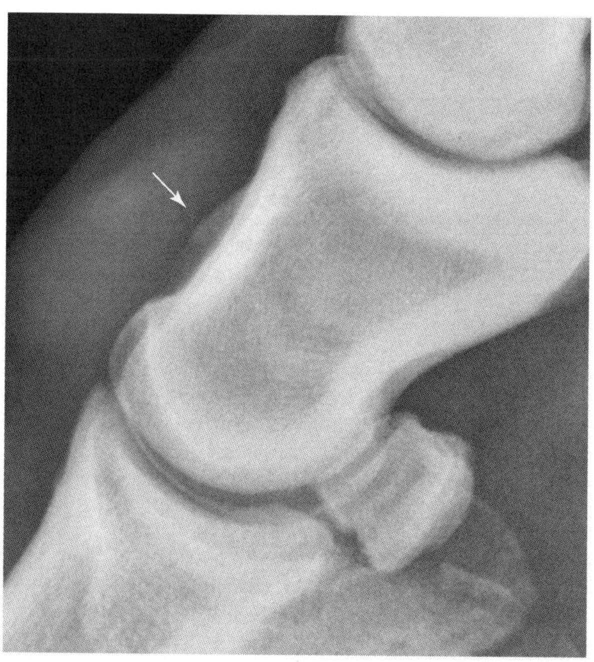

Fig. 27.4 Smooth eminences associated with the origins of the distal interphalangeal joint collateral ligaments on dorsal P2 (*arrow*) are highlighted by the slight dorsopalmar obliquity of this lateromedial radiograph. This is a normal finding that should not be confused with abnormal osseous proliferation.

5% asymmetry in the front feet, and 5% in neither front foot.[9] Heavier breed horses such as drafts and Friesians tend to have more prominent crena than light breed horses. Space occupying lesions within the hoof capsule, such as keratomas, discussed later in this chapter, may also give rise to regions of smooth concavity at the distal phalanx solar margin. However, these will be asymmetric between feet, may be present anywhere along the solar margin, and may be of variable depth. Comparing with the contralateral limb and correlating with clinical signs help to differentiate a normal crena from resorption due to a space occupying mass.

The palmar processes of the P3 become ossified more extensively with age (Fig. 27.6) and it is not uncommon to identify a separate osseous body of one or both palmar processes as an incidental radiographic variant (Fig. 27.7).

The flexor cortex of the navicular bone should be smooth with sharp definition between the cortex and spongiosa. The opacity of the flexor cortex should be uniform, aside from a small, well-defined crescent-shaped radiolucency that can be found in the central eminence (a.k.a. sagittal ridge). This lucent region is due to a normal area of decreased mineral density and/or a synovial fossa. This fossa is occasionally seen as a dimple on the flexor surface on the lateral view. A lucent crescent can also exist without a prominent synovial fossa due to a trabecular bone island interposed between two parallel cortical bone plates of the central eminence (Fig. 27.8).[11] This should not be confused with flexor cortical lysis, discussed later.

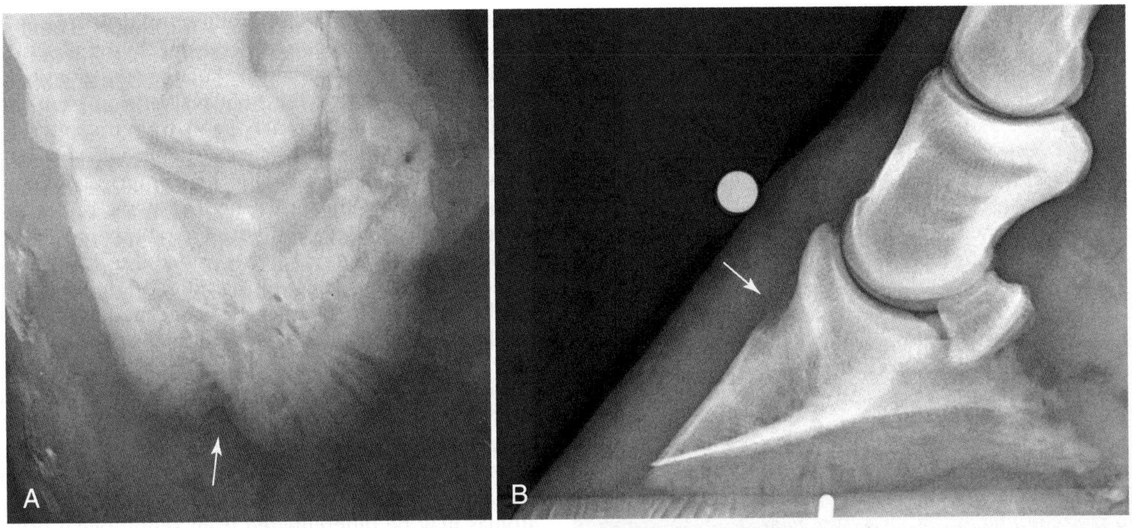

Fig. 27.11 **A,** Classic keratoma resulting in smooth concave osseous resorption at the solar margin of P3 (*arrow*). **B,** Atypical keratoma resulting in smooth concave osseous resorption at the dorsal cortex of P3 (*arrow*).

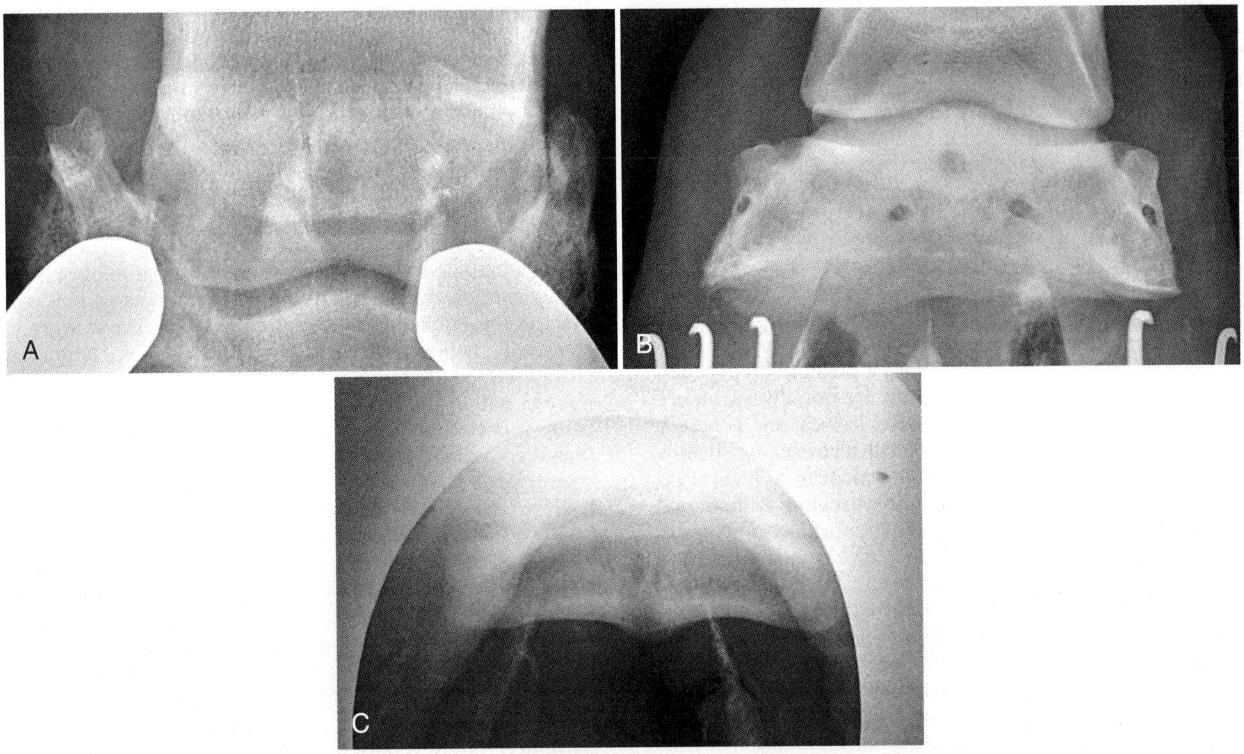

Fig. 27.12 Rounded lucent region within the mid aspect of the navicular bone on the D65Pr-PaDiO **(A)** and horizontal dorsopalmar (DP) **(B)** views, confirmed as flexor cortical erosion on the skyline view **(C)**.

Fractures

Phalangeal fractures occur in a wide variety of horse breeds and after varied activities. Radiography is the most often used mode of screening for identification. Knowing the common distribution of phalangeal fractures associated with breed and discipline can guide a thorough assessment of those areas in the lame horse.[37,38] It is now recognized that some diagnostic imaging changes are prodromal features of potential impending fractures, particularly in racing and sport horses. In a study comparing agreement in fracture evaluation between radiography and CT, CT identified 4 of 20 fractures that were not identified by radiography.[39] CT evaluation of fracture complexity is superior to that of radiography, particularly when planning surgical treatment. Intraoperative CT is being used in some facilities.[40,41]

Navicular Bone

True navicular fractures are uncommon.[42] The most frequently reported type is complete, minimally displaced parasagittal fractures, although other configurations, including comminuted fractures, can occur. Traumatic etiologies are considered most likely. It can be challenging to distinguish fractures from the developmentally abnormal bipartite (or even tripartite) navicular bones. Bi- or tripartite navicular bones are often found bilaterally (Fig. 27.13). These horses are frequently sound and

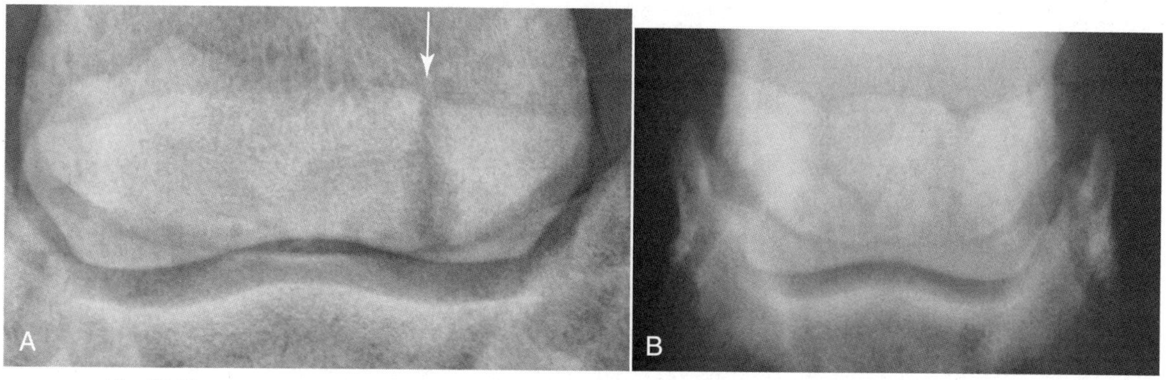

Fig. 27.13 **A,** Complete navicular bone fracture (*white arrow*). **B,** Tripartite navicular bone; notice the smooth margins of the navicular fragments. This was a mature horse with tripartite navicular bones in both front feet and minimal lameness. (Courtesy Dr. Robert J. Bahr, Oklahoma State University, Stillwater, OK.)

in athletic work, although the developmental abnormality can also lead to degenerative bone remodeling. Navicular bone fractures generally form a fibrous union resulting in radiographically persistent fracture lines, even in chronic cases.[43] Complete fractures are more commonly seen in the forelimb.[42] In the authors' experience, the athletic outcome from navicular bone fractures is variable and likely depends on other comorbidities sustained at the time of trauma or as a sequela to the fracture. An incidence of 1.5% was reported for "clinically silent" navicular fractures during radiographic screening of 200 Warmblood yearlings.[42]

Fragments of the distal border of the navicular bone are seen with relative frequency but are more likely to represent a developmental anomaly or feature of navicular syndrome (discussed later) than traumatic fractures (Fig. 27.14). They are commonly seen alongside other degenerative navicular changes and have been identified more commonly in lame than sound horses in some population studies.[42] However, their frequent presence in nonlame horses makes their clinical significance questionable in the absence of additional navicular changes.[44] These have been postulated to represent dystrophic mineralization or osseous metaplasia within the distal sesamoidean impar ligament, or separate centers of ossification. The accompanying concave defect in the distal border of the navicular bone suggests they may be avulsed fragments. Larger fragments are relatively well identified on radiographs, although the sensitivity of this modality for their identification is lower than cross-sectional modalities.

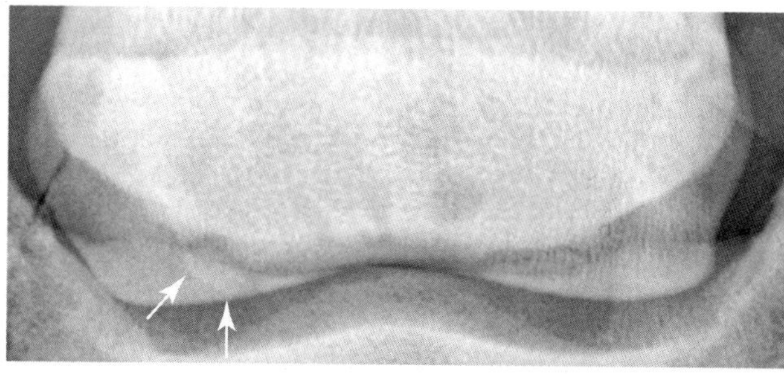

Fig. 27.14 Chip fracture at the distal navicular border. The small fragment (*white arrows*) and the underlying fracture bed can be seen. A medullary cyst-like lesion is also present.

Distal Phalanx

A fracture classification system (types I through VII; illustrated in Fig. 27.15F) describes the fractures of the distal phalanx.[45] Fractures are classified based on region of the bone affected, articular or nonarticular involvement, and anatomic plane of the fracture, as follows:

I. Nonarticular fracture of palmar or plantar process
II. Articular fracture, extending from distal interphalangeal joint to solar margin (Fig. 27.16)
III. Articular fracture, midsagittal, divides distal phalanx into equal parts (Fig. 27.17)
IV. Articular fracture, extensor process (Fig. 27.18)
V. Articular fracture, comminuted body fracture (not of type II, III, or IV)
VI. Solar margin fracture (see Fig. 27.40B,C)
VII. Palmar process fracture in foals (Fig. 27.19)

Trauma is the most common cause of distal phalanx fractures; however, they also occur as pathologic fractures secondary to infective pedal osteitis and laminitis. Because the hoof wall restricts displacement of bone fragments, diagnosis of the distal phalanx fracture depends on visualization of the fracture line. If the plane of the primary x-ray beam is not parallel to the fracture plane, the superimposed parts of the bone obscure the fracture line. Therefore, a comprehensive series of foot radiographs, as outlined in Table 27.1, is recommended. A recent study found that radiographic identification of palmar/plantar process fractures (types I and II) was improved via the inclusion of oblique projections (palmaro 50-degree proximal 45-degree medial(lateral)-dorsodistolateral(medial) oblique (Pa50Pr45M[L]-DdiL[M]O views; Fig. 27.20) and therefore it may be helpful to include these views in cases with a suspicion of distal phalanx fracture.[46] Occasionally, the horizontal beam oblique views (dorsal 45-degree lateral[medial]-palmaromedial[lateral] (D45L[M]-PM[L]O)) typically used to assess the proximal interphalangeal joint may more effectively demonstrate the articular component of a fracture. Identification of type VI fractures requires careful assessment of the solar margin. Overexposure of the image makes this fracture difficult to see.

Two large retrospective studies have reported the prevalence of distal phalanx fracture types. In a predominantly Warmblood population, type I fractures were most often seen, followed by type II. In contrast, in a population in which Quarter horses were the most common breed, type VI fractures predominated. In Thoroughbred racehorses, type II fractures appear to be the most frequently reported configuration.[41,45,47] Type II fractures are often distributed in accordance with the direction of racing; the forelimb that bears the most weight in turns is at greatest risk. In addition, since racehorses in North America race in a counterclockwise direction, fractures tend to involve the lateral aspect of the left front limb or the medial aspect of the right front limb.[6] Fractures of the extensor process (type IV) can result in small or quite large (>25% of the joint surface) fragments.[12,48,49] A question exists as to whether the smaller lesions are true fractures or a result of developmental defect. Larger fragments are more likely of traumatic

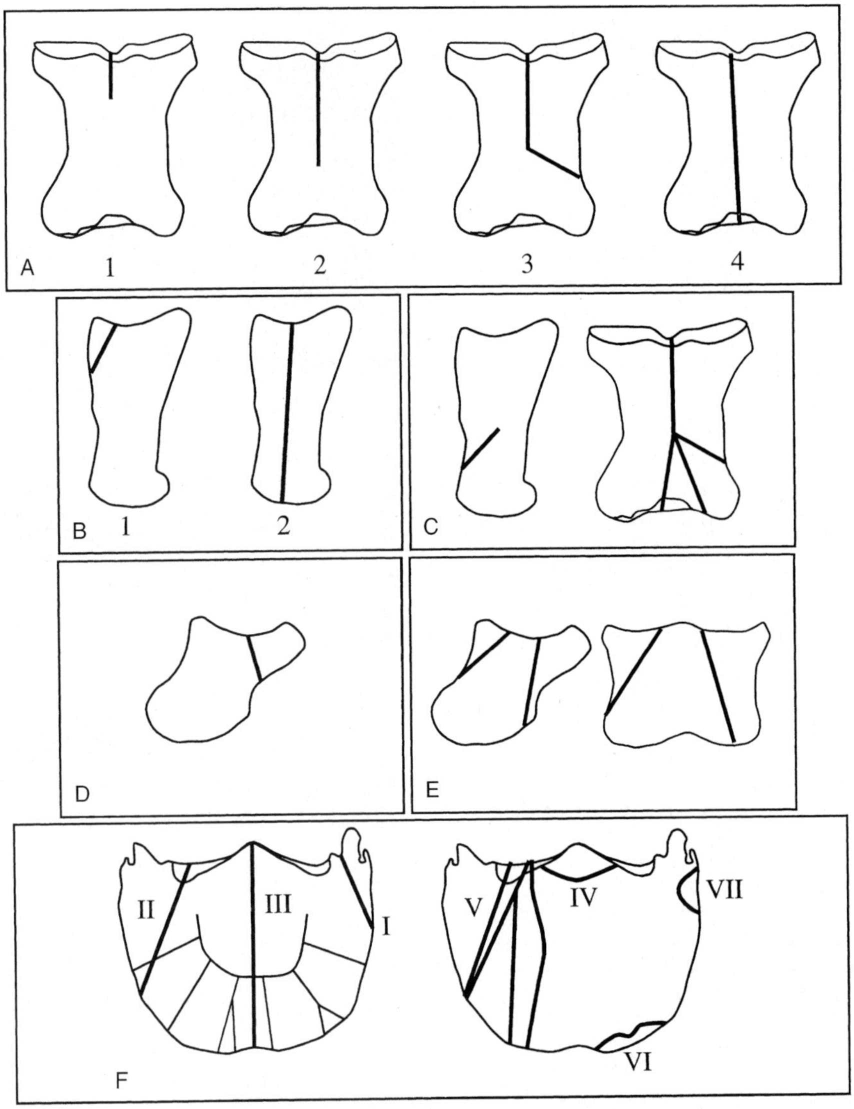

Fig. 27.15 Common fractures of the phalanges. *Proximal phalanx:* **A,** Sagittal plane fractures, noncomminuted. *1,* Incomplete, monoarticular (short, less than 30 mm variation); *2,* incomplete, monoarticular (long, more than 30 mm variation); *3,* complete, monoarticular; *4,* complete, biarticular. **B,** Dorsal plane fractures, noncomminuted. *1,* Complete, monoarticular; *2,* complete, biarticular. **C,** Comminuted, complete, biarticular, dorsal, and/or sagittal plane. *Middle phalanx:* **D,** Palmar/plantar eminence (monoarticular, complete). **E,** Comminuted, complete, biarticular. *Distal phalanx:* **F,** *I,* Nonarticular, palmar/plantar process; *II,* articular, extending from distal interphalangeal joint to solar margin; *III,* articular, midsagittal, divides into equal parts; *IV,* articular, extensor process; *V,* articular, comminuted body fracture

origin. Front limbs are more often affected than hindlimbs. Type V fractures require cross-sectional imaging to identify the various fracture planes. The type VI fracture is often found in association with radiographic signs of laminitis (32% of type VI fractures in one study) (see Fig. 27.40B,C).[45]

The progression of healing of a distal phalanx fracture is difficult to determine radiographically because of the minimal amount of external (periosteal) osseous callus produced by this bone. The periosteum of the distal phalanx is poorly developed and does not respond with abundant proliferation to the stimulation of direct trauma. From a multicenter study of 285 horses with distal phalanx fractures, those that had radiographic follow-up assessment showed evidence of healing of types I to III on average by 16 weeks with a range of 2 to 87 weeks from the start of their treatment.[50] Mean time of bone union was significantly shorter for horses 3 years old or younger. Bone union began at the solar margin and progressed to the articular surface in these horses; this is speculated to be due to improved blood supply in the periphery of the bone.[51] Because of the fibrous component of healing, radiographic bone union and clinical soundness do not correlate accurately.[50] Nonarticular type I fractures had the best prognosis for return to original or expected level of work or performance than type III followed by type II fractures. Surgical fixation has been advocated in articular fractures to maximize congruity of the joint surface and mitigate against the development of secondary osteoarthritic changes.[41]

Fractures of the extensor process generally produce more proliferative bone than other types of distal phalangeal fractures (see Fig. 27.18B). However, large extensor process fragments may not heal by bone union but by fibrous union, making them predisposed to loosening with additional trauma. In horses with

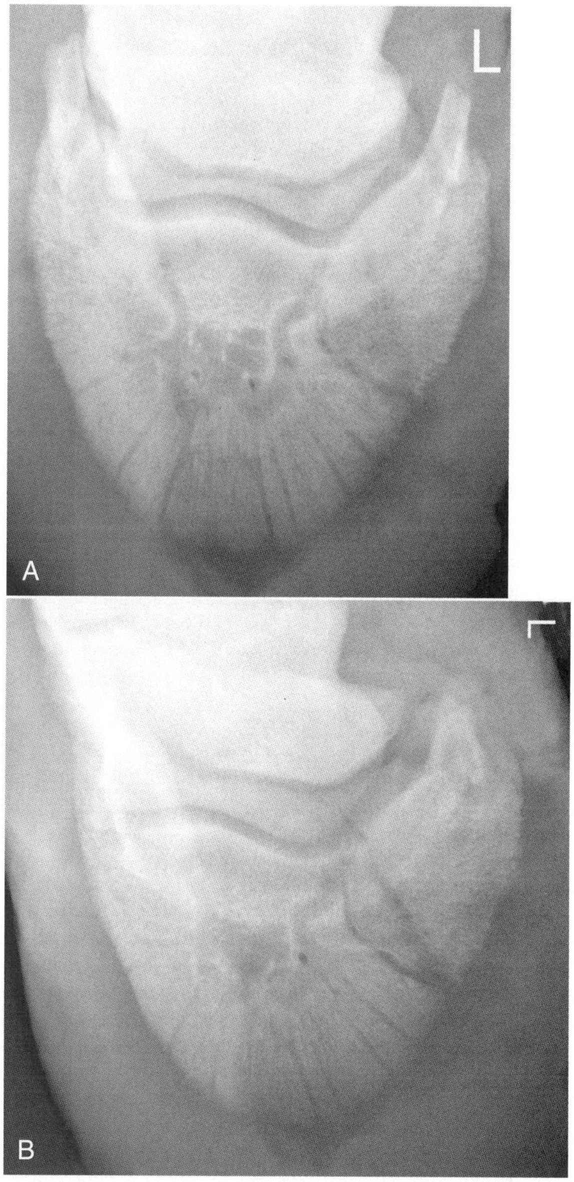

Fig. 27.16 Oblique fracture of the lateral wing of the distal phalanx. **A,** The fracture is subtle in the standard dorsal 65-degree proximal/palmarodistal view. Because there is minimal distraction, the x-ray beam must pass parallel through the fracture gap for optimal depiction. The curvature of the foot necessitates oblique projections to identify these fractures, particularly at the acute stage. **B,** This is a dorsal 65-degree proximal 45-degree lateral/palmarodistal view. The fracture is evident and approaches but does not disrupt the subchondral bone. However, the location along the joint contour makes this a type II fracture.

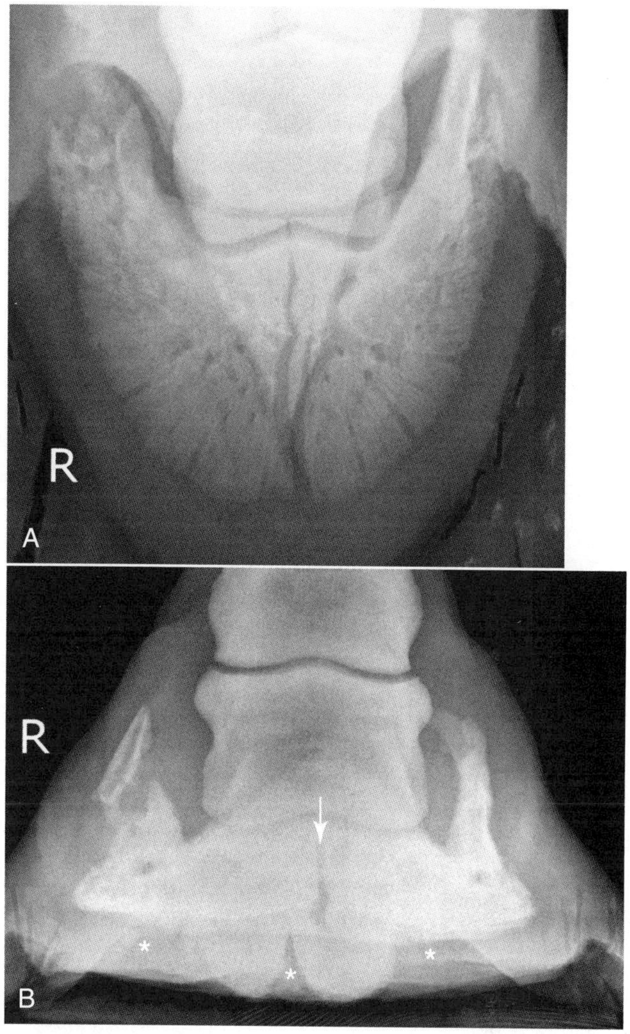

Fig. 27.17 **A,** Midsagittal, articular fracture (type III) of the distal phalanx. The fracture is seen easily in the dorsal 65-degree proximal/palmarodistal view, and a small offset is evident at the articular border. **B,** In the horizontal (0-degree) dorsopalmar view, the fracture may have been mistaken for air in the heel crevice or as an extension of the air in the central sulcus of the frog. The fracture line has been marked with a *white arrow* and *asterisks* placed in the sulci of the frog. This horse also has grade 5 ossification of the collateral cartilages. The lateral ossification is separated at the base.

chronic, recurrent lameness, surgical removal of the extensor process fragment has been recommended. In a study of 18 Friesian horses treated by surgical removal, the long-term outcome was good in 82% and was best in those horses used for pleasure riding and low-level dressage or driving competition.[12] In the radiographic follow-up evaluations, some horses had filling of the fragment defect with subchondral bone.

The type VII palmar process fracture of foals has been described in Arabian, Quarter horse, Thoroughbred, and Warmblood horses (see Figs. 27.15F and 27.19).[52,53] Fractures may be uni- or biaxial and may be seen in one or both forelimbs. Whilst the microradiographic and histologic appearance in most foals studied is consistent with fracture healing, rather than a separate center of ossification, affected foals are rarely lame and this finding is often incidental. Foals through 12 weeks old have a lucent line between the proximal and distal angles of the palmar process. This line is normal and should not be mistaken for a fracture (Fig. 27.21). In the horses studied from 1 week to 12 months, fracture identification is more evident after 3 months and most are healed without intervention at 12 months. The etiology is undetermined, with most recent theories related to effect of genetics, normal process of foot development, hoof conformation, and foot balance.[53] The long-term effects of these fractures have not been assessed.

Pedal Osteitis

The term *equine pedal osteitis* is typically used to refer to chronic remodeling and demineralization of the solar margin of the distal phalanx, generally seen in response to repetitive concussive trauma.[54] Radiographically, this may appear as

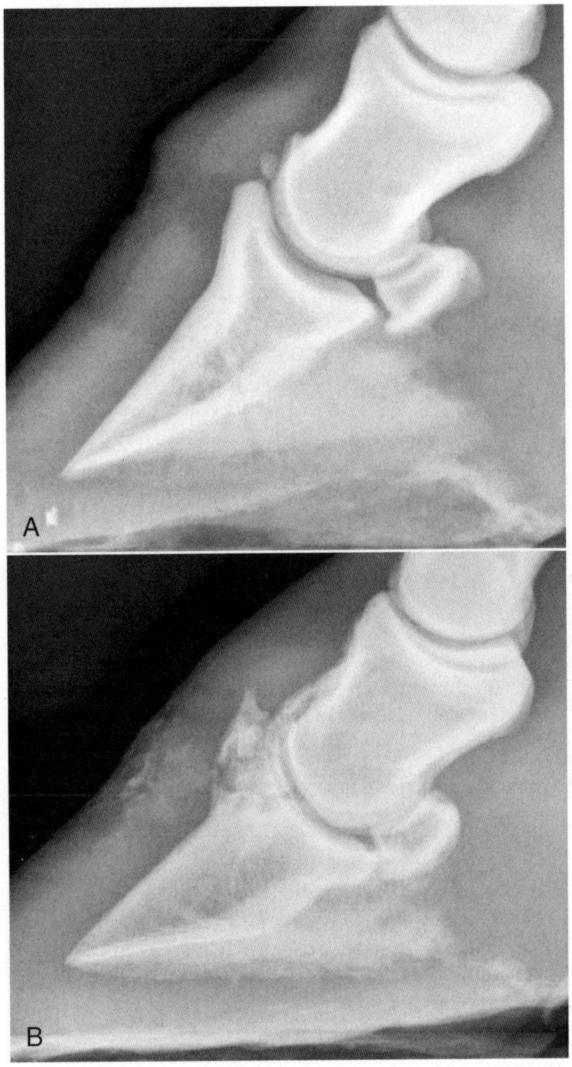

Fig. 27.18 Fractures of the extensor process in two horses. **A,** 2-year-old male Standardbred with a small rounded fragment separated from the extensor process of a front distal phalanx. There is enlargement of the soft tissue at the coronary band. There is no evident deficit in the contour of the extensor process, suggesting that this may have been of developmental origin. This horse developed fragmentation in the opposite front extensor process approximately 1 year later during race training. **B,** 20-year-old Quarter horse gelding with a large extensor process fracture. Circular lucencies in the distal phalanx at the distal palmar aspect of the fracture line, rounding of the fragment edges at the articular border, and the new bone on the dorsal surface of the middle phalanx are indicative of a chronic nonunion or fibrous union.

diffuse roughening of the solar border creating a ragged, lacy appearance when viewed on the lateromedial or D65Pr-PaDiO projection (Fig. 27.22). Once the primary insult and pedal osteitis become inactive, little change in the appearance of the roughened contour of the solar margin is seen. The normal appearance of the solar surface of the distal phalanx varies considerably, and a mild degree of incidental irregularity may be misinterpreted as disease. A positive response to hoof testers, positive response to softer footing or sole padding, an increased number and diameter of vascular channels seen concomitantly with demineralization of the bone, and thinning of the sole of the foot increase the probability of pedal osteitis being the cause of lameness. Thus, clinical signs must be considered in the determination of whether a radiographically irregular margin of the distal phalanx is an indicator of active remodeling. Whilst typically a diffuse change, pedal osteitis can be a localized change due to chronic medial-lateral imbalance or secondary to another lesion within the hoof capsule, such as a subsolar abscess. It is difficult to determine radiographically if such focal pedal osteitis is associated with localized infection. In these cases, MRI can provide additional information for differentiating disease processes and thereby help determine the appropriate management plan.

Infection

Osteomyelitis and Septic Osteitis

Septic pedal osteitis refers to infection of the distal phalanx. The most common cause is penetrating foreign objects through the sole. Common radiographic changes are discrete areas of lysis, irregular margin, and decreased opacity of the distal phalanx, typical of chronic inflammation (Fig. 27.23, eFig. 27.2). Gas may be present in the soft tissue adjacent to the surface of the distal phalanx. Separation of a piece of the distal phalanx may represent a pathologic fracture or sequestrum (see Fig. 27.23). Clinically, a draining tract at the sole or coronary band may be found. Contrast fistulography or images made with a radiopaque stylet in the tract can be helpful to assess if the tract includes involvement of bone, tendons, ligaments, or regional synovial structures (distal interphalangeal joint and/or navicular bursa), which necessitates aggressive treatment. If a metallic foreign body is evident at physical examination, radiographs should be made before removal to determine the depth of its penetration and its relation to the regional bone (Fig. 27.24). In one study of penetrating injuries to the frog, septic osteitis of the distal phalanx was cited as a reason for euthanasia.[55] These injuries are discussed in more detail at the end of this chapter.

Another possible cause of septic pedal osteitis is hematogenous spread. Of 108 Thoroughbred foals with 141 sites of hematogenous osteomyelitis, there were a significant number with phalangeal involvement.[56] This included 25 distal phalanx lesions in 21 foals. None of the foals with a solar margin lesion had visible evidence of sole bruising or a penetrating wound. Radiographic lysis was present in four foals with a sequestrum. The hindlimb was affected more commonly (62% of lesions). Three of four foals with extensor process lesions had concurrent septic arthritis. Although the proximal physis and epiphysis of the proximal and middle phalanges are common potential locations for hematogenous osteomyelitis, the distal phalanx has not typically been evaluated. Eighty-six percent of the foals with distal phalanx lesions were discharged from the hospital, and 50% of those that trained for racing had official race starts. Septic osteomyelitis of the navicular bone can also occur, with the majority of cases occurring secondary to penetrating injury to the foot.[55]

Bone Marrow Lesions

Bone marrow edema, edema-like signal, bone bruises, contusions, and bone marrow lesions (BMLs) are all terms used to refer to trabecular changes resulting in the increased presence of fluid within bone. These lesions cannot be identified radiographically, and diagnosis is almost always via MRI. Lesions may be visible on nuclear scintigraphy but cannot be differentiated from other lesions causing focal intraosseous increased radiopharmaceutical uptake. The appearance on MRI is that of a region of low signal on T1- and T2*-weighted sequences that has high signal on fat-suppressed sequences, such as the short tau inversion recovery (STIR). Multiples patterns of BML have been identified, including BML associated with joint pathology,

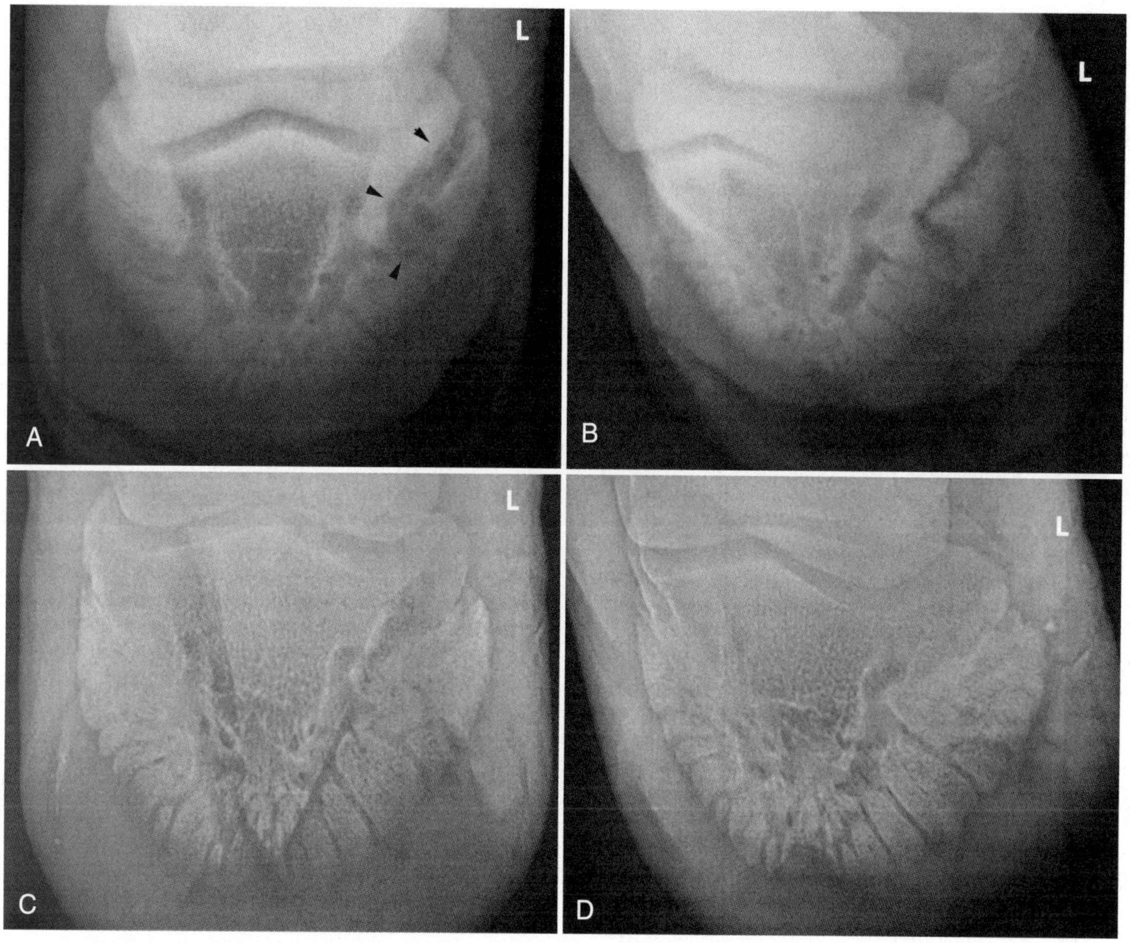

Fig. 27.19 A palmar process fracture in the distal phalanx of a foal (type VII in Fig. 27.15F). **A and B** were obtained at 3 months; **C and D** are at age 5 months. *Black arrowheads* in **A** indicate one edge of the fracture extending from the incisure of the palmar process to the solar margin. **B** is the dorsal 65-degree proximal, 45-degree medial/palmarodistolateral oblique projection that better demonstrates the fracture gap and separated triangular fragment. In **C and D,** (the oblique projection) the fracture is minimally visible and was considered clinically healed. *L* marks the lateral side of the foot.

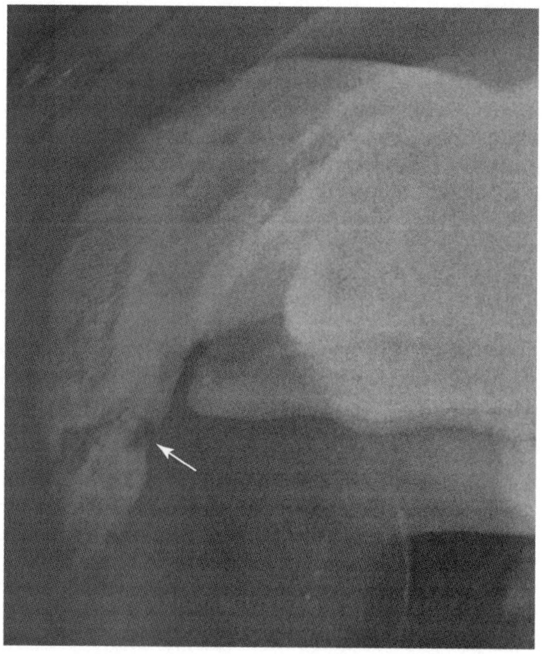

Fig. 27.20 PaPrM(L)-DDiL(M)O view of P3 palmar process fracture (*white arrow*).

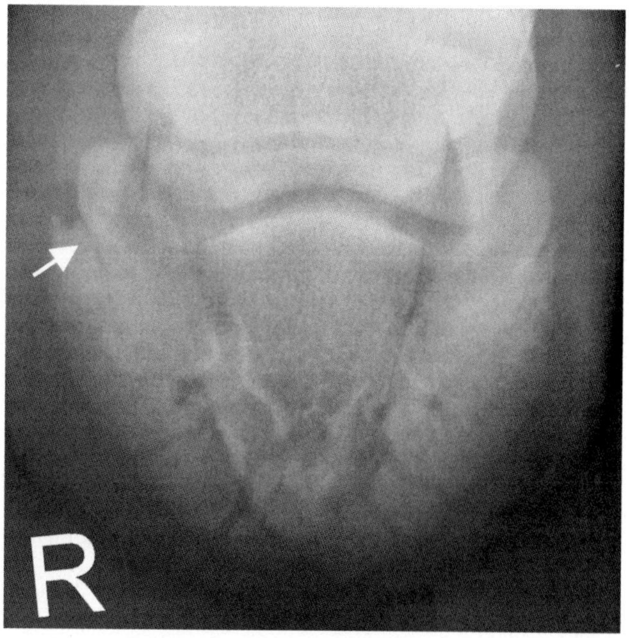

Fig. 27.21 Dorsal 65-degree proximal/palmarodistal view of the distal phalanx of a normal foal. Note the normal radiolucent line in the palmar process (*white arrow*), which should not be confused with a fracture.

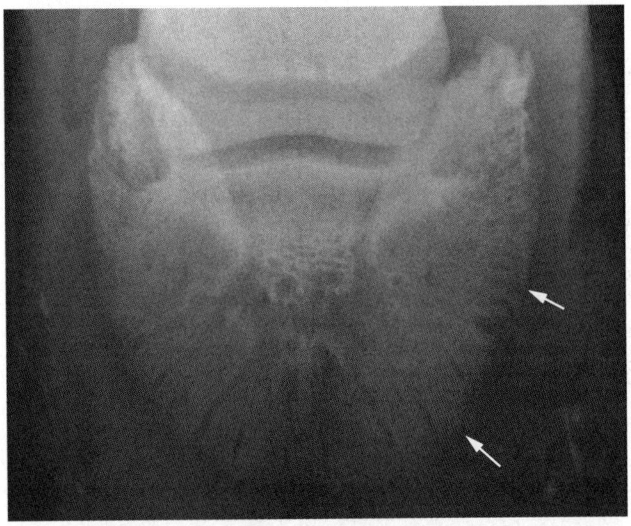

Fig. 27.22 Dorsal 65-degree proximal/palmarodistal view of the distal phalanx of a horse with pedal osteitis. The solar border between the *arrows* is irregular compared with the opposite margin. The horse was sensitive to hoof testers in this region, and no lesions were found in the sole. Gas lucencies in the peripheral soft tissues are the result of the recently pulled shoe and nails.

BML associated with soft tissue injury, BML associated with acute trauma, and BML that is unassociated with other injury in the absence of current lameness.[57] Whilst the clinical significance of this latter group of lesions in some horses has been debated, it is the authors' experience that the majority of BMLs have clinical relevance and, where extensive and/or associated with particularly pronounced signal abnormalities, can be a source of profound pain. In addition, if such a lesion is identified in a nonlame leg, such horses may subsequently develop lameness and progressive arthrosis in the proceeding months.[58] Although some BMLs can resolve quickly (within 3–4 months), with an accompanying rapid improvement in lameness, severe injury can result in the development of osteonecrosis of the trabecular and subchondral bone and progressive articular pathology. These horses remain lame during the rehabilitation period and have a poorer prognosis for return to athletic activity.[58] BM edema-type pattern seen at the entheses of the distal interphalangeal joint (DIPJ) collateral ligament without associated ligament desmopathy has a reportedly good to excellent prognosis for return to activity.[59]

It is worth noting that diffuse increased signal throughout the distal phalanx on fluid-sensitive sequences, particularly within the flexor surface, can also be seen with demineralization associated with disuse osteopenia. This is frequently found in horses with chronic lameness or those that have undergone extensive layup.

Palmar endosteal fluid signal is a common finding within the navicular bone on MRI. This fluid signal may indicate edema, inflammatory infiltrate, trabecular remodeling, fibrosis, hemorrhage, or necrosis. These various etiologies cannot technically be differentiated based upon the MRI appearance; however, these differential diagnoses can be ranked based upon severity and extent of fluid signal and when interpreted in light of clinical history (including lameness severity and chronicity), other changes of the navicular bone, and additional regional pathology (e.g., navicular bursitis, deep digital flexor tendinopathy etc.)

Navicular Syndrome

Navicular syndrome, also known as navicular disease, is a chronic, often progressive condition characterized by a spectrum of changes within the navicular bone and surrounding podotrochlear apparatus. Osseous navicular changes are described here, while the pathology of the soft tissues of the podotrochlear apparatus is discussed in more detail later in the chapter. Navicular syndrome primarily occurs in forelimbs and changes are frequently bilateral, even in cases presenting for unilateral lameness.[60] Breed predispositions are observed, although it is unknown whether a true genetic component of disease exists, or rather if it is a feature of the differences in foot conformation between breeds. The syndrome is seen most commonly in Quarter horses, which often have small, upright feet.[61]

Early or mild navicular bone changes that may be detected radiographically include characteristic dilation of the synovial invaginations present along the distal border (eFig. 27.3). These invaginations can vary in size, shape, and number. In a normal horse, these structures appear as a low number (in the region of 3–7) of small (less than a couple of millimeters), concave indentations of uniform or tapering width with a broad base. In navicular syndrome, several larger invaginations with a narrow base and bulbous proximal portion, a so-called "lollipop" shape, may be seen. It is important to note that there is a variation in size and number across different breeds. A greater number of larger synovial invaginations may be seen in Warmbloods without other evidence of navicular degeneration or lameness.[62] Enlarged synovial invaginations have been shown to be associated not only with primary remodeling of the navicular bone but can also result due to pathology of the distal interphalangeal joint.[63]

Medial and lateral triangular bone production of the proximal border of the navicular bone indicates enthesopathy of the collateral sesamoidean ligament (see eFig. 27.3). This change alone is often incidental but may be considered to fall within the spectrum of navicular syndrome. A more reliable indicator of navicular bone degenerative remodeling at the proximal cortex is dilation of the proximal vascular channels. This can be difficult to identify radiographically unless more advanced, but is easily appreciated with MRI.

Sclerosis of the navicular bone spongiosa rarely occurs as a form of adaptive remodeling and is an indication of degenerative change. A hallmark finding for this change is loss of distinction between the flexor cortex and sclerotic medullary bone. The loss of distinction can be focal or diffuse. A focal area of loss of distinction is often found in conjunction with an adjacent focal area flexor cortical erosion. Care should be taken when interpreting skyline views since superimposition of the most proximal and distal aspects of the curved flexor cortex of the navicular bone can give the false appearance of linear sclerosis of the palmar medullary cavity.

Flexor cortical lysis is found with more advanced cases of navicular syndrome and is often associated with greater lameness and a more guarded prognosis.[7,64,65] Flexor cortical lysis may be seen as ill-defined, often rounded to ovoid lucent regions within the bone on the D65Pr-PaDiO view. To confirm their location, erosions may also be seen as decreased mineral density within the flexor cortex on a skyline view (Fig. 27.25). These should be differentiated from the aforementioned normal, crescent-shaped lucency within the sagittal ridge. Skyline views obtained at multiple degrees of proximodistal obliquity may be required in order for the x-ray beam to be tangential to the region of lysis. Flexor cortical erosions most

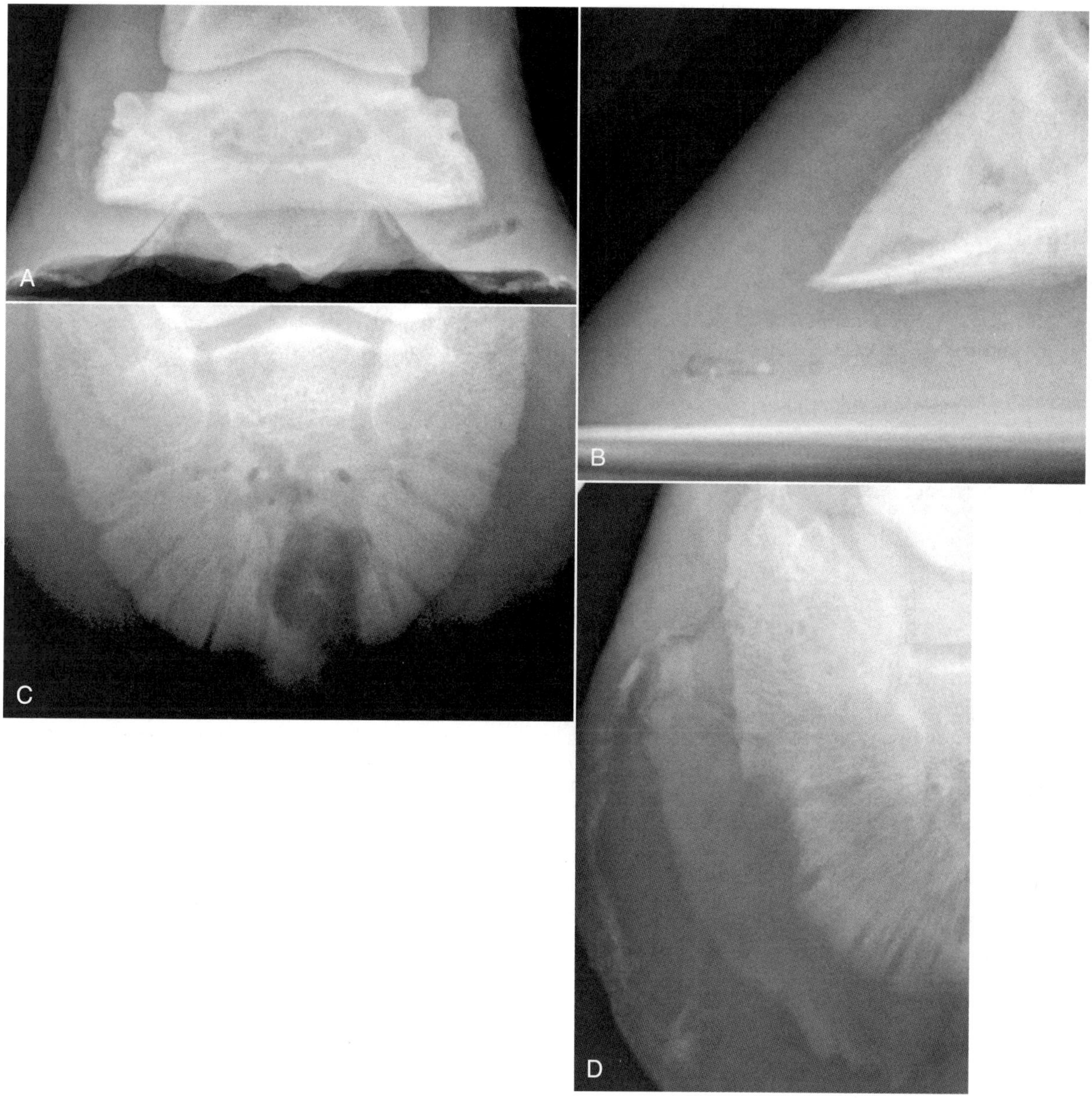

Fig. 27.23 Variations seen with infective pedal osteitis associated with foot abscesses in three horses. Horse 1 **(A)** has only gas in the subsolar soft tissues with no bone lesion. Images **B and C** are the second horse. In **B,** there is subsolar gas at the toe. The dorsal border of the distal phalanx from the toe to midbody is abnormally thin and has an irregular surface. In **C,** a large circular osteolytic area is present on the midline toe. A small mineralized opacity consistent with a sequestrum is present in the lytic area. In horse 3 **(D)**, there is a smoothly marginated concave defect in the solar border of the quarter region. This was associated with a resolving abscess.

commonly occur within the distal portion of this bone and therefore more shallow projections can help to highlight this region.[66] Flexor cortical erosions may also be seen as regions of decreased cortical bone density and associated loss of corticomedullary distinction on a well-positioned lateromedial foot radiograph.

The presence of fluid within the navicular bone is a common finding on MRI, both in horses with other evidence of navicular syndrome and as an isolated finding. When trabecular fluid signal is seen within an otherwise normal navicular bone, this likely represents mild trabecular bone remodeling, transient inflammation, edema, or, less likely, hemorrhage and is of variable clinical significance. This type of bone fluid signal often resolves with rest. Fluid signal of the navicular bone in conjunction with other degenerative changes is more likely to be associated with trabecular bone remodeling, osteofibrosis and potentially osteonecrosis. The only way to definitively differentiate between these varied causes of navicular bone fluid is to monitor its progression or resolution on sequential MRI scans (Fig. 27.26).

ARTICULAR PATHOLOGY

Disease of the proximal interphalangeal joint of the digit is discussed in Chapter 26; therefore, this section will focus on

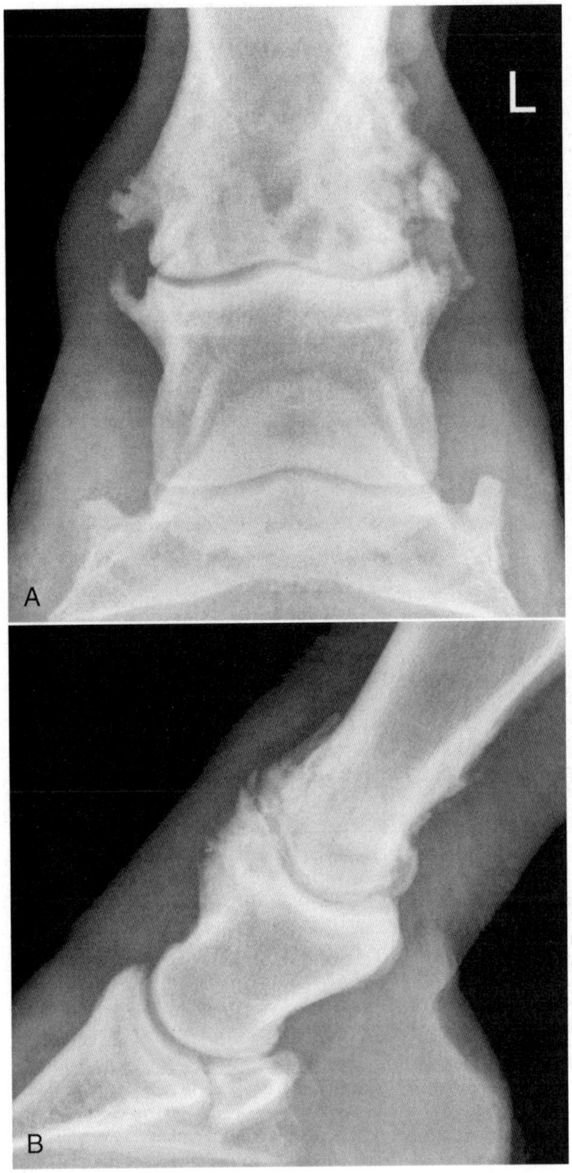

Fig. 27.27 **A and B,** These images depict the typical radiographic features of chronic proximal interphalangeal osteoarthritis. Osteophytes, enthesophytes, joint space narrowing (asymmetric in this example), subchondral sclerosis, and subchondral cysts are evident.

without associated trabecular bone changes.[72] In 11 lame horses evaluated with MRI, subchondral trabecular bone damage was found that was not evident radiographically.[73] These changes consisted of subchondral fluid signal with and without cyst formation. Subchondral remodeling is less commonly found in the distal interphalangeal joint than the proximal interphalangeal and fetlock joints. There can be extensive articular cartilage damage in the distal interphalangeal joint without identifiable subchondral bone changes.

Septic Arthritis

Infective agents are most commonly introduced into the distal interphalangeal joint by penetrating wounds or iatrogenic injections. Any laceration near a joint that is associated with significant and persistent lameness warrants concern for extension to the joint and infection. The joint pouches of the distal interphalangeal joint are large, extending proximal to the midplane of the middle phalanx.[3] One large retrospective study of heel bulb lacerations found that the distal interphalangeal joint was involved in 13% of these injuries.[74] During the initial stage of infection, no radiographic changes may be present. Inflammation of the synovium and effusion may create a focal enlargement at or just proximal to the coronary band (Fig. 27.29).

Options for assessing the likelihood of joint involvement secondary to an acute penetrating wound or laceration on radiographs include firstly assessing for soft tissue swelling and radiolucent gas foci within the region of the joint recesses. If none is identified or if the gas cannot be definitively localized to the joint, placement of a sterile metallic probe within the wound/tract and repeating radiographs may be valuable to assess the trajectory and depth of injury. Additionally, use of positive contrast techniques may assist in demonstrating or ruling out joint communication. A fistulogram may be performed in which contrast medium is instilled directly into the wound prior to radiographic assessment. Documenting the subsequent dispersal of contrast medium may demonstrate extension into the region of the joint. However, it can be difficult to generate sufficient pressure to distend the tract with contrast medium, particularly if the wound is not fresh. An alternative is positive-contrast arthrography. This was successful at identifying communication of the contrast medium from the joint to the external wound in one study of horses suspected to have joint infection but no bone changes.[64] This is the authors' preferred contrast technique in cases such as these.

In the nonacute stage, one of the earliest radiographic signs of septic arthritis is irregularity at the joint capsule insertion or chondro-osseous junction on the perimeter of the joint surfaces. As cartilage begins to deteriorate, thinning of the joint space is seen. As the infection invades the deeper regions of the cartilage and reaches the subchondral bone, the subchondral bone margin becomes irregular because of lysis (see Fig. 27.28). Lysis of the subchondral bone causes the joint to be widened unevenly. At this stage, periosteal new bone should be evident at the joint margins (Fig. 27.30). Septic arthritis always has a guarded prognosis. Ultrasound evaluation of the dorsal joint pouch can be used to identify severe septic distal interphalangeal synovitis and may also be used for ultrasound guided collection of fluid, which can be difficult in proliferative joints. Typically, septic effusion will be slightly more echogenic than the fluid seen with nonseptic inflammation and is often associated with a greater degree of synovial proliferation. MRI provides the ability to detect septic osteoarthritis at an early stage via the identification of features such as diffuse hyperintensity within the adjacent tissues, severe, contrast-enhancing synovial proliferation[75] and is also valuable for more rapid identification of secondary osteomyelitis via the detection of intraosseous fluid.

Deformity of the Distal Interphalangeal Joint

The clinical appearance of DIPJ flexural deformity varies with the degree of hyperflexion from mild to an almost vertical orientation of the hoof wall to the ground (Fig. 27.31). Flexural deformity may be either congenital or acquired in the foal. Older horses may develop a flexural deformity secondary to lesions of the accessory ligament of the DDFT or chronic damage resulting in contracture of the DDFT.[76] Radiography is used to assess changes in the distal phalanx and screen for possible concurrent bone or joint lesions. Changes in the distal phalanx range from none to widened vascular channels and bone resorption at the solar margin. If the deformity is corrected early, the bone changes can resolve.

Hyperextension of the distal interphalangeal joint may occur in newborn foals as a congenital abnormality affecting all three joints of the foot. Weakened flexor tendons may also be a result of poor nutrition, slow or incomplete recovery from a systemic disease, or after prolonged periods of external support (splinting or casting) of the leg. Acquired hyperextension to the point

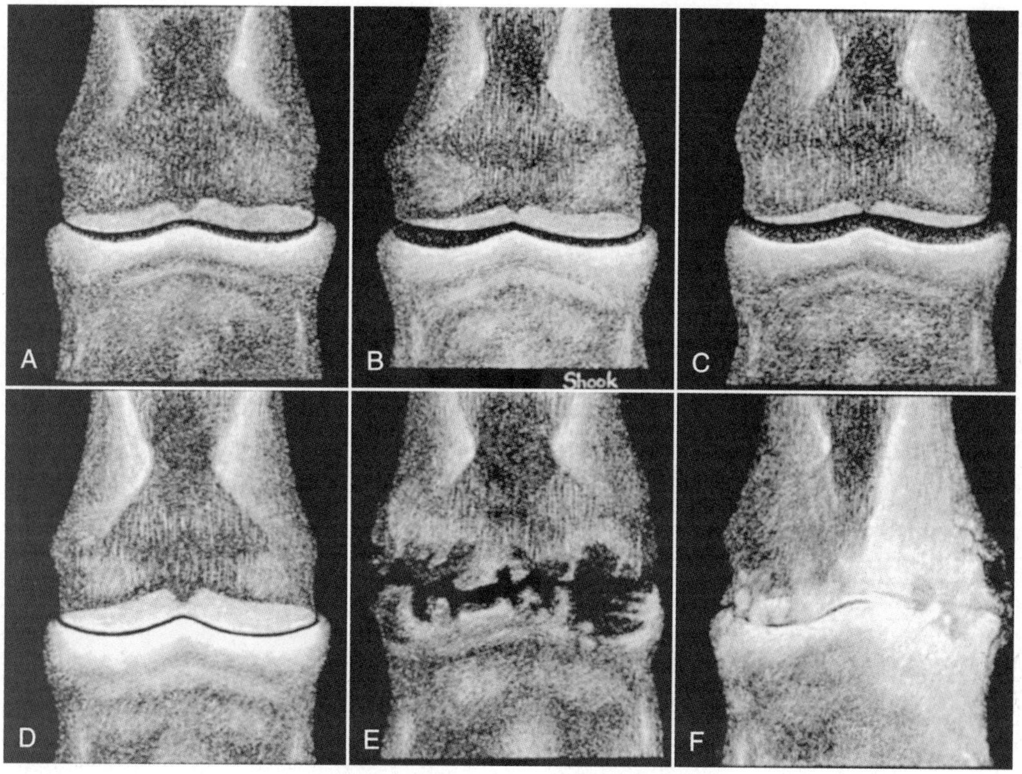

Fig. 27.28 Changes in joint space width, subchondral bone opacity, or both, as seen in the dorsopalmar view of the proximal interphalangeal joint, and likely causes. **A,** Normal joint space and subchondral bone. **B,** Widened joint space on the lateral or medial side, no subchondral bone changes. Artifact is caused by asymmetric weight distribution on the foot or unbalanced hoof trimming. **C,** Widened joint space, no subchondral bone changes; not weight bearing at time of radiography or increased intra-articular fluid volume. **D,** Uniformly narrowed joint space, no subchondral bone changes. Artifact caused by x-ray beam angulation, asymmetric foot placement, or uniform degenerative wearing and loss of articular cartilage. **E,** Widened joint space, lysis of the subchondral bone; active septic arthritis. **F,** Narrowed joint space, irregular opacity, and contour of subchondral bone; chronic low-grade septic arthritis or chronic osteoarthritis caused by trauma-related instability or poor conformation. (Illustration courtesy Richard A. Shook, DVM.)

of joint (sub)luxation is also caused by rupture of the DDFT or avulsion of its insertion (Fig. 27.32). Subluxation has also been reported following severe lacerations of the common digital extensor tendon and rupture of the distal interphalangeal joint collateral ligaments.[77–79] Stress views may be needed to detect subluxation. Secondary changes expected with subluxation are enthesophyte formation at the ligament insertion sites and osteoarthritis. The range of change will depend on the severity of the initial injury and the frequency of recurring subluxation, but severe osteoarthrosis and/or ankylosis is a sequela with an associated poor prognosis.

SOFT TISSUE PATHOLOGY

Soft Tissue Structures

Although the soft tissues of the equine foot are generally poorly visualized radiographically, indirect evidence of soft tissue injury can be gained by associated osseous changes. Therefore, knowledge of the attachment sites of the joint capsules, tendons, and ligaments is imperative. The DDFT can often be seen in the lateromedial view as a slightly more opaque soft tissue band as it passes between the level of the proximal aspect of the middle phalanx and the proximal margin of the navicular bone. The most common radiographic finding to provide direct evidence of damage to the DDFT in the foot is the presence of mineral within the tendon.

To adequately assess the soft tissues of the distal limb, imaging modalities other than radiography must be employed. Ultrasound and MRI are well recognized for their value in assessing soft tissue injuries, although the use of ultrasound for assessing injuries of the foot is limited by the hoof capsule. CT, particularly with the use of contrast medium, is also valuable for assessing soft tissue damage in the foot. Comparing the results of advanced imaging to radiographs improves the interpretation of radiographs. The radiographic signs of abnormal soft tissue include alteration of thickness, contour, or opacity. A diffuse increase in soft tissue thickness in the region of the foot and pastern may indicate edema and/or cellulitis, whilst more focal, localized swelling may indicate trauma or, depending on proximity to a synovial structures, intracapsular effusion or synovial proliferation. An irregular surface contour suggests acute laceration or chronic granulation tissue. Increased opacity within soft tissue is usually caused by dystrophic mineralization (Fig. 27.33). Decreased opacity within the soft tissues is caused by gas, which may be secondary to recent diagnostic nerve block, open skin wounds or abscessation due to a gas-producing organism (Fig. 27.34).

Soft Tissue Enthesopathy

Stress at the point of attachment of a tendon, ligament, joint capsule, or other soft tissue structure onto an osseous structure is termed *enthesopathy* and is often radiographically apparent. Changes may manifest as osseous proliferation, resorption, or a

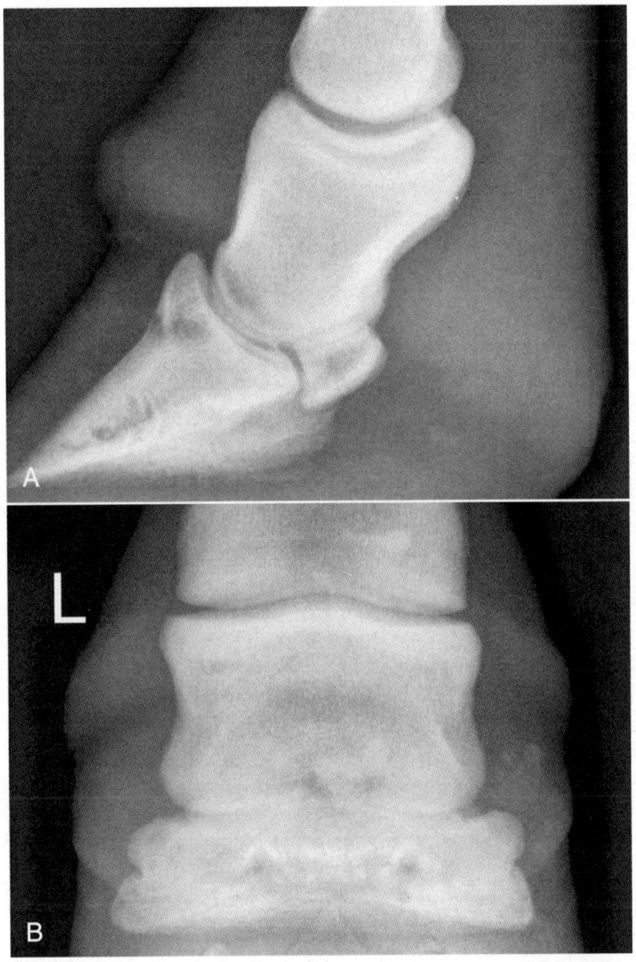

Fig. 27.29 **A and B,** This yearling sustained unknown trauma to the foot causing a significant lameness. The following day a draining tract developed at the dorsal coronary band. One and a half weeks later, the lameness persisted, and radiographs were acquired. There is evident swelling at the coronary band, as well as thinning of the distal interphalangeal joint space (narrower than the proximal interphalangeal joint space), subchondral lucency of distal dorsal half of the middle phalanx, and a separation of a large extensor process fragment from the distal phalanx. No new bone formation is evident. These changes are indicative of septic arthritis with osteomyelitis of the middle and distal phalanges with fracture and probable sequestrum formation of the extensor process.

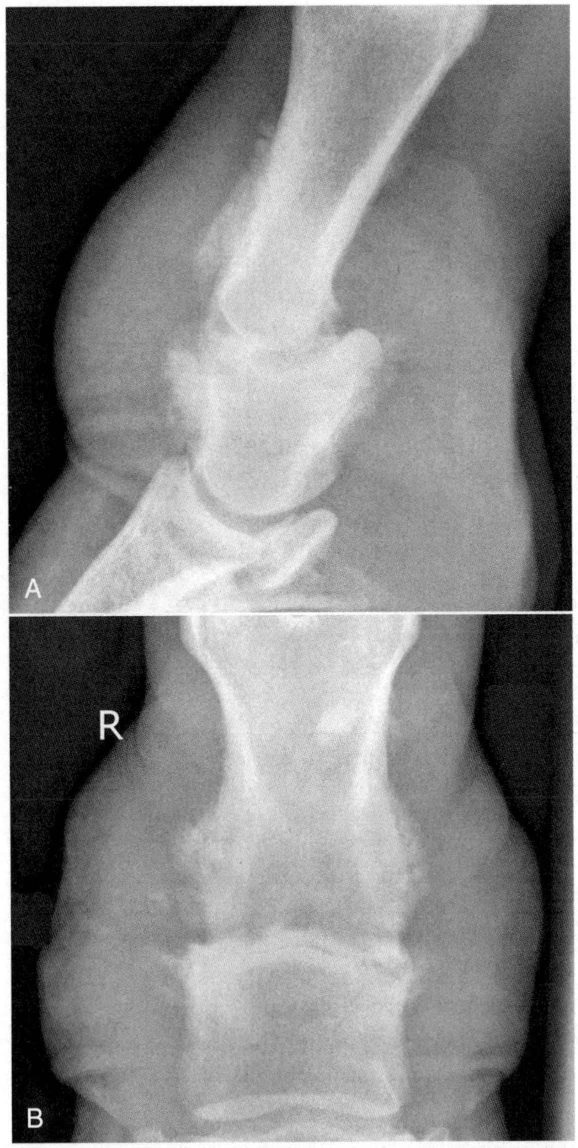

Fig. 27.30 **A and B,** The proximal interphalangeal joint is narrowed dramatically with mild palmar subluxation. Focal areas of subchondral lysis are evident in the proximal aspect of the middle phalanx. The periosteal new bone formation has a palisading appearance, and there is soft tissue swelling. These features are typical of chronic active infection and joint instability.

combination of the two. Avulsion fracture at soft tissue attachment sites occurs uncommonly and will be evident as a bone fragment displaced in the direction of traction of the tendon/ligament. Regions of new bone formation (enthesophytes) are commonly seen on the cortical surfaces of the phalanges. Early or mild enthesopathy manifests as often focal or smooth undulating bone production. With further progression, the enthesophyte may form a smooth, hook-like, or spur-like shape, projecting in the direction of tension or traction. The significance of enthesophytes varies depending upon location. Enthesophytosis of the distal interphalangeal joint capsule on the dorsal cortex of the middle phalanx is frequently an indicator of other significant joint pathology. Enthesopathy can also present as bone loss, which is often seen in the collateral fossae of the distal phalanx, although substantial bone loss can occur before it is identified radiographically. When visible, it presents as regions of rounded bone loss, seen best on D65Pr-PaDiO and D65Pr45L(M)-PaDiM(L)O views (Fig. 27.35, eFig. 27.4). Lesions at the site of insertion of the distal sesamoidean impar ligament on the flexor surface of the distal phalanx have been characterized histopathologically as a resorptive bone cavity containing cellular debris and chondroid metaplasia.[80] This lucency is best identified in the dorsal 60-degree proximal/palmarodistal oblique view, occurring most frequently in the central region of the distal phalanx just distal to the distal border of the navicular bone in this view (Fig. 27.36). If large, enough, these lesions can also be identified on lateromedial projections (see Fig. 27.36). However, similar to the resorptive lesions of the collateral fossae, bone loss at the distal sesamoidean impar ligament attachment is often not well seen radiographically when compared to CT and MRI.

Collateral Ligaments

Desmopathy of the collateral ligaments of the distal interphalangeal joint is a significant cause of foot lameness, which may present in the absence of the radiographic changes. Ultrasound in the region of the coronary band may detect changes in the proximal third of the ligament; however, damage is more

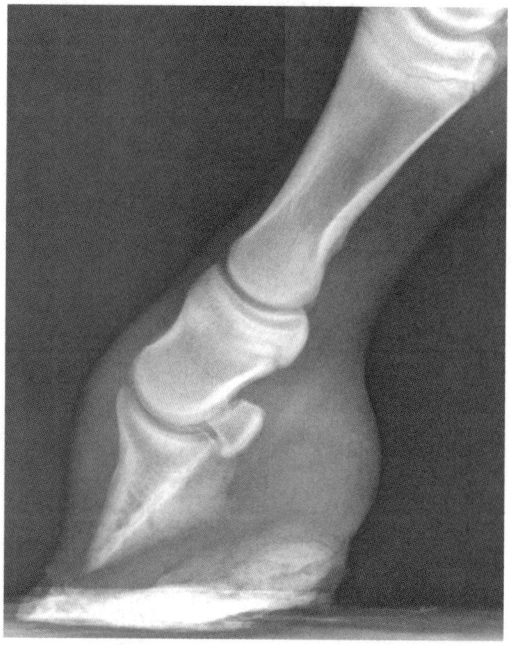

Fig. 27.31 Flexural deformity of the distal interphalangeal joint in a 4-month-old foal. The dorsal surface of the distal phalanx remains parallel to the dorsal hoof wall; however, both structures assume an abnormally vertical position. There is mild modeling of the toe of the distal phalanx. The straight course of the deep digital flexor tendon (DDFT) is visible.

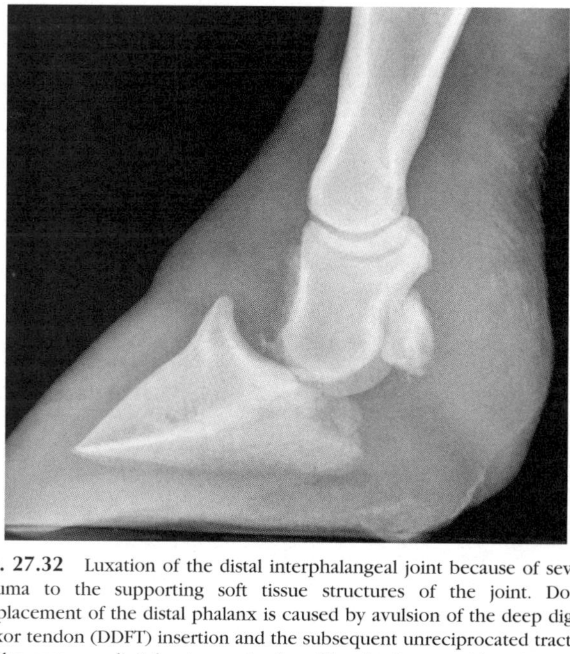

Fig. 27.32 Luxation of the distal interphalangeal joint because of severe trauma to the supporting soft tissue structures of the joint. Dorsal displacement of the distal phalanx is caused by avulsion of the deep digital flexor tendon (DDFT) insertion and the subsequent unreciprocated traction of the common digital extensor tendon. The distal sesamoidean impar ligament is also ruptured, allowing proximal displacement of the navicular bone.

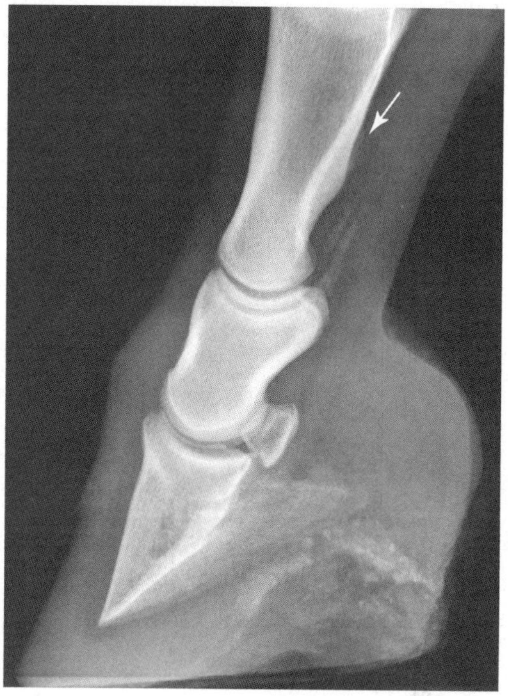

Fig. 27.33 Soft tissue mineralization is evident in the superficial digital flexor tendon and straight sesamoidean ligament. There is mild smooth enthesopathy at the insertion of the oblique sesamoidean ligament on the midaspect of the proximal phalanx (*arrow*). This horse also has a mild distal interphalangeal flexural deformity.

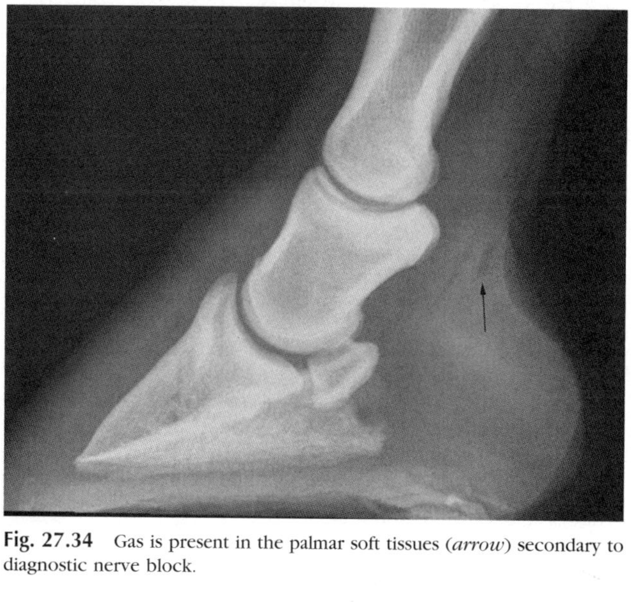

Fig. 27.34 Gas is present in the palmar soft tissues (*arrow*) secondary to diagnostic nerve block.

frequently found in the distal portion. MRI is the most useful imaging modality to define the changes in these ligaments (eFig. 27.5).[77,81] Knowledge of the appearance of magic angle artifact in these ligaments, particularly on low-field MRI, will prevent overdiagnosis of collateral ligament injury.[82–84] Imaging may also be used to direct targeted treatment of collateral ligaments injuries, such as radiograph-guided injection of the collateral ligament fossae or MRI- or ultrasound-guided intralesional or periligamentous injection.[85–88]

Tendinopathy and Desmopathy

Strain injury results from damage to ligaments or tendons induced by overuse or overstress. Radiographically, localized soft tissue swelling may be the only finding. Dystrophic mineralization can develop in a chronically inflamed tendon and may be visible on radiographs (see Fig. 27.33), although dystrophic mineral within several soft tissue structures has also been reported as an incidental finding and depends in part on the location of the mineralization.[89] Tendon and ligament injury can be best imaged by ultrasound, MRI, contrast-enhanced CT, and, less commonly, vascular and soft tissue pool phase scintigraphy.[64,90–92] Ultrasound is the most commonly available modality for soft tissue assessment of the pastern but is limited in the foot region by poor access through the hoof and sole. The increasing availability of low-field standing magnetic resonance (MR) scanners has resulted in increased use of MRI in horses and thereby the identification of numerous tendon and ligament abnormalities. MRI has become the modality of choice when lameness is persistent and the other modalities have negative or equivocal findings. Injuries to specific soft tissues of the foot are discussed in more detail below.

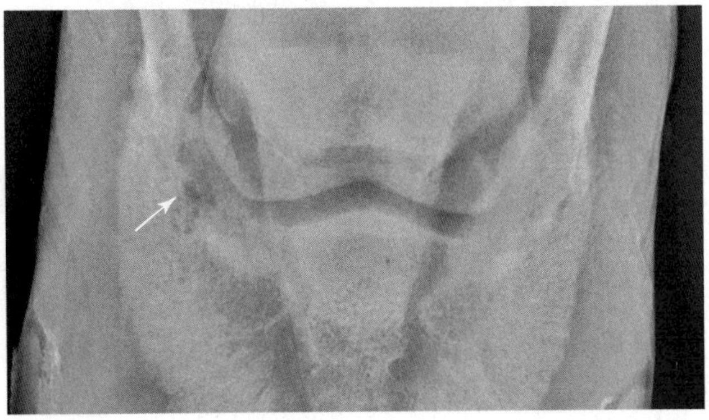

Fig. 27.35 Region of irregular osseous resorption of the distal interphalangeal joint lateral collateral ligament fossa of P3 (*white arrow*), representing insertional resorptive enthesopathy of this ligament.

Injuries to the DDFT are common within the foot and are categorized in four forms: (1) dorsal border tears; (2) core lesions; (3) sagittal or parasagittal splits; or (4) tendinosis.[64,92] The distribution of these lesions varies by location (Fig. 27.37). Dorsal border fibrillations are most common at the level of the proximal recess of the navicular bursa (also referred to as *suprasesamoidean location*) and navicular bone. Core lesions are common in the pastern and suprasesamoidean regions, and distal to the navicular bone. Sagittal/parasagittal splits are common at the navicular bone level (region 2 in Fig. 27.37). Insertional tendinopathies occurring immediately proximal to the insertion of the tendon on P3 can have a variety of configurations.[93,94] DDF tendinopathy in the pastern is readily identified on ultrasound; more distal tendinopathy is limited by the hoof capsule. Transcuneal ultrasonography has been reported but is technically challenging and provides limited visualization.[95–97] Lesions of the DDFT have been identified by (contrast-enhanced) CT, but MRI is generally considered the superior modality for full characterization of tendinopathy and any additional changes within the foot.[91] It is worth noting that three-quarters of horses with DDFT injuries in the pastern were shown to have additional injuries to this tendon within the foot; therefore, if a lesion is detected on pastern ultrasound, MRI of the foot for assessment of further tearing is particularly warranted.[98]

Podotrochlear Apparatus

The term *podotrochlear apparatus* has been used to refer to the regional structures of the palmar/plantar foot, in particular

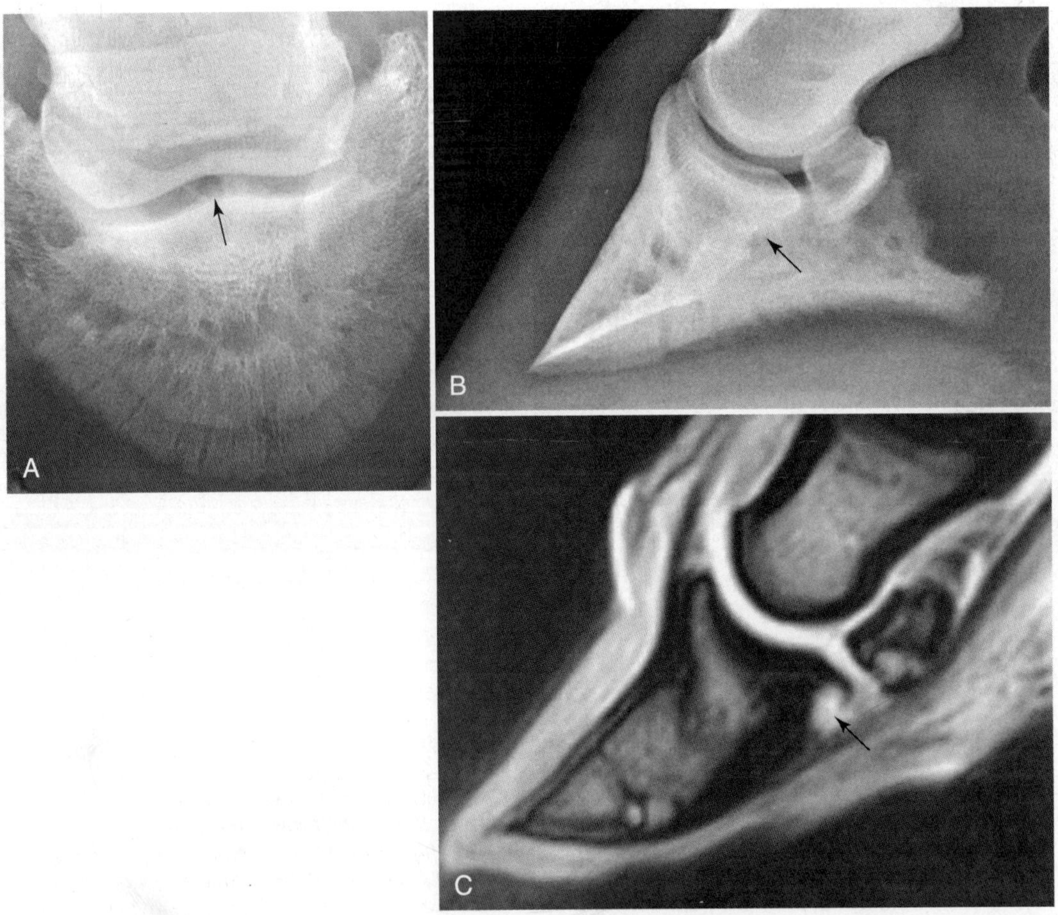

Fig. 27.36 Resorptive enthesopathy of the impar ligament (*black arrows*) on D65Pr-PaDiO **(A)** and lateromedial **(B)** radiographic views, and on a sagittal T2*-weighted magnetic resonance (MR) image **(C)**.

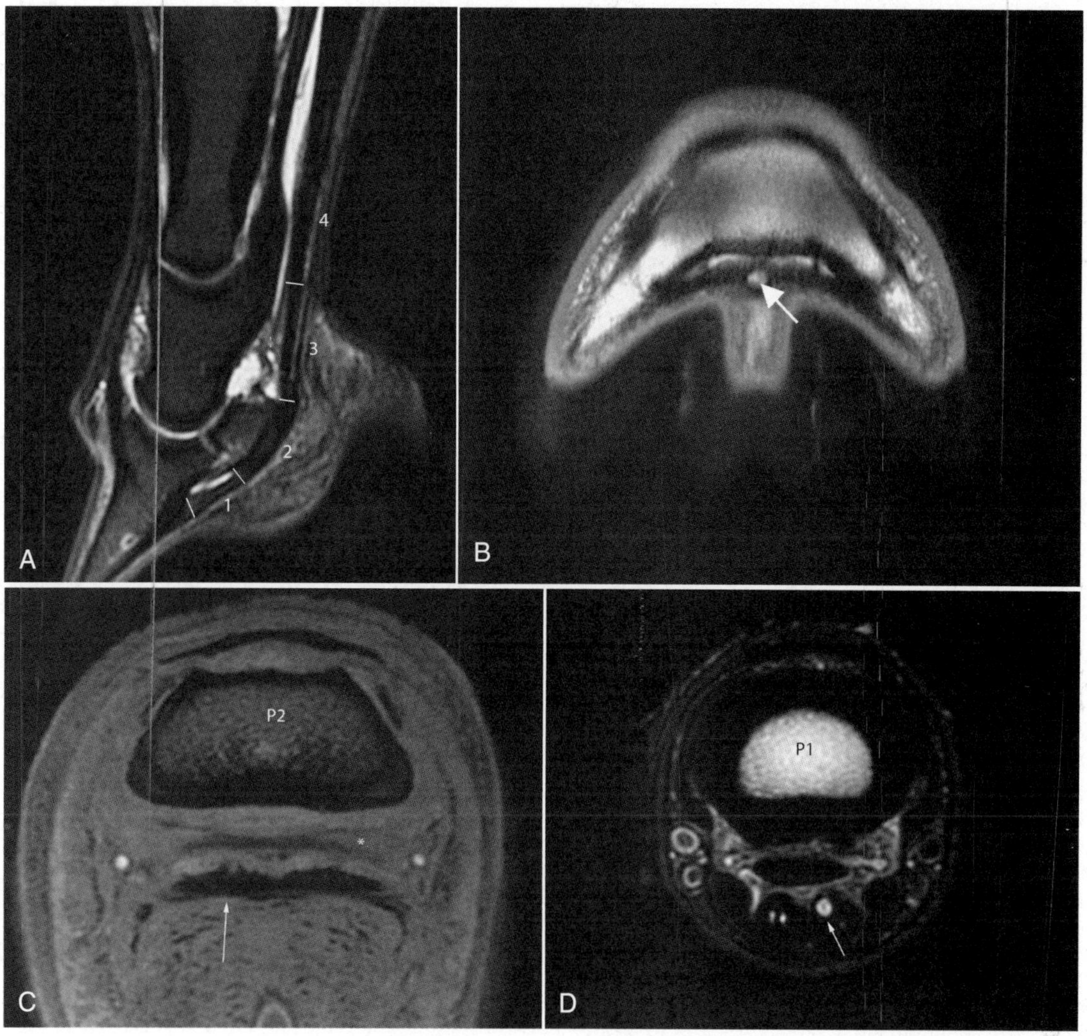

Fig. 27.37 This grouping shows common lesions of the deep digital flexor tendon (DDFT) in the foot region, as seen on magnetic resonance imagery (MRI). The sagittal **(A)** plane indicates the regions of the tendon as relates to where different types of tendon lesions are identified. **B through D** images are transverse planes with lateral on the left of the image. **B** is a proton density sequence that shows a core lesion (*white arrow*) in the insertional region 1. **C** is a T2-weighted gradient echo sequence that shows dorsal border fibrillations of the lateral lobe in the suprasesamoidean region 3 (*arrow* points to the palmar border of the tendon). In **C**, the *asterisk* is within the medial portion of the collateral distal sesamoidean ligament. **D** is a T2-weighted fast spin–echo sequence that shows bilobed core lesions (larger in the medial lobe [*arrow*]) within the pastern region 4.

those in close association with the navicular bone. These include the collateral sesamoidean ligament, distal sesamoidean (impar) ligament, distal digital annular ligament, navicular bursa, and the DDFT within the hoof capsule. Fiber disruption of the dorsal border of the DDFT at the level of the proximal recess of the navicular bursa is a relatively common finding on horses undergoing MRI of the foot. Mild fibrillation in this region may be considered to be of limited clinical significance since it has been seen in the sound limb of unilaterally lame horses. However, cleft-shaped tears are a clinically relevant finding and may often occur in combination with other changes to the podotrochlear apparatus, most notably, erosions of the navicular bone flexor cortex and/or inflammation of the navicular bursa. This association between flexor cortical lysis and DDFT dorsal border abrasions is a part of the reason as to why this is a particularly concerning radiographic finding.

Navicular bursitis can be generally categorized into two main types: proliferative bursitis, in which synovial proliferation predominates, and effusive bursitis, characterized primarily by an abundance of synovial fluid. Proliferative synovium can develop into intrabursal adhesions, most frequently in association with tearing of the dorsal border of the DDFT.

The ligaments of the podotrochlear apparatus are susceptible to the desmopathy changes previously described. One unique feature of the impar ligament is its fenestrated appearance in the absence of pathology. In horses with navicular syndrome, this ligament may lose these fenestrations and become thickened, and may contact the dorsal border of the DDFT at its insertion. This feature, along with the other described changes of the podotrochlear apparatus, is best identified on MRI.[80,99–101] Ultrasound performed between the heel bulbs with a microconvex probe can be used to visualize the suprasesamoidean DDFT, proximal recess of the navicular bursa, collateral sesamoidean ligament, and distal digital annular ligament.[98] However, because the ultrasound beam is not tangential to the structures of interest, assessment of echogenicity is limited. Transcuneal ultrasound, in which the structures of the foot are visualized via a window through the frog, may also be performed.[102,103]

THE HOOF

The hoof wall consists of the epidermis and the dermis (or corium), the latter bound to the parietal surface of the distal phalanx. The epidermal layers are the stratum externum (tectorium), the stratum medium, and the stratum internum (lamellatum and white line at the ground surface). The lamellae of the stratum internum interdigitate with the dermal lamellae. Between the dermal lamellae and the parietal surface of P3 is a dense network of fibers that includes vessels and nerves (stratum reticulare). Because of the composition of these layers, there is a distinct radiographic opacity difference visible at the junction of the stratum medium and stratum internum and the superficial more radiopaque layer and less radiopaque deep layer are readily differentiated (Fig. 27.38) and correlate with MRI depiction of the layers.[104] The complex anatomic connection between the stratum internum, the corium, and the ridges of the parietal surface of the distal phalanx forms a functional suspensory apparatus of the distal phalanx.[105] The junction of the coronary band and the most proximal extent of the hoof wall is not always clearly distinct in lateromedial and dorsopalmar views.

Hoof Balance

Unbalanced trimming and improper shoeing of the foot can result in lameness. Lateromedial and dorsopalmar radiographic views of the foot can be used to assess foot balance.[106,107] When radiographic views are used in this manner, particular attention must be paid to positioning of the foot, the center of the x-ray beam, and degree of weight bearing on the limb being assessed. The measurements used to assess foot balance radiographically are shown in Fig. 27.39. In the lateromedial view, the dorsal hoof wall should be parallel to the wall at the heel. The pastern axis, as seen in the lateromedial view, is a line that divides the middle phalanx into equal dorsal and palmar halves. Ideally, this line similarly bisects the proximal phalanx and is parallel to the dorsal cortex of the distal phalanx. When this line is carried through to intercept with a line on the bearing surface of the hoof wall, it should create an angle of 45 to 55 degrees (front foot) or 50 to 55 degrees (hind foot) with the bony solar margin.[106] Significant differences were induced in the angles of the interphalangeal joints when the hoof angle was altered.[106] The greatest difference in angle occurred in the distal interphalangeal joint. Clinically, such a change in the angle of the distal interphalangeal joint may influence the strain on the DDFT.[106] The angle of intercept of a line parallel to the solar margin of the distal phalanx and the line of the weight-bearing surface of the hoof wall should be 5 to 10 degrees.[7] The length of the toe region compared with the heel region of the bearing surface of the hoof wall is judged by comparison with the distal interphalangeal joint. A line from the center of the best-fit circle of curvature of the joint space, when drawn perpendicular to the weight-bearing surface, should be at the middle of the weight-bearing surface.[7,106] The lateral and medial portions of the hoof wall should be of equal length. An

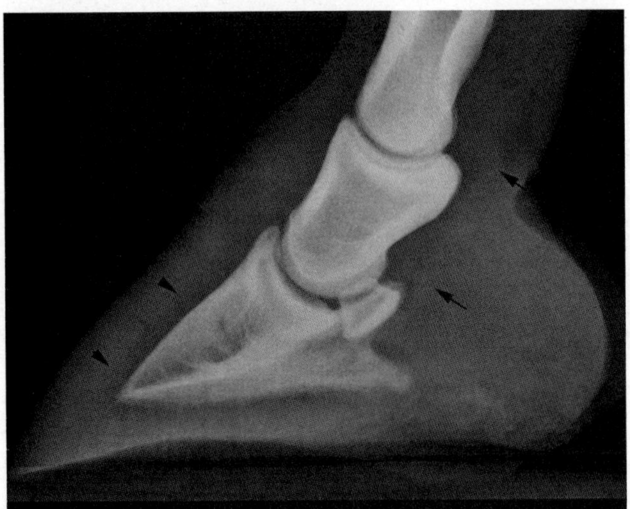

Fig. 27.38 Lateral view of the foot showing the delineation of the deep digital flexor tendon (DDFT; *arrows*). The distinct opacity difference in the dorsal hoof wall allowing identification of two layers is evident. The *arrowheads* mark the interface between the superficial stratum medium and deeper stratum internum.

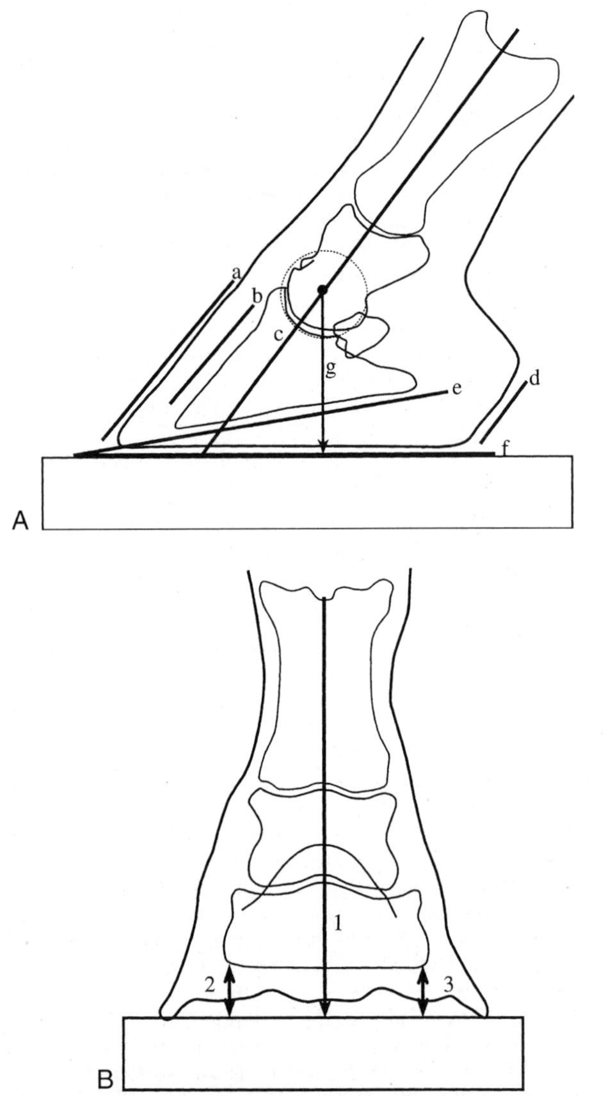

Fig. 27.39 Radiographic measurements for foot balance. **A,** Assessment from the lateromedial view of normal foot. *a,* Line parallel to dorsal hoof wall; *b,* line parallel to dorsal cortex of the distal phalanx; *c,* line that bisects the middle phalanx into equal dorsal and palmar halves; *d,* line drawn parallel to the bulbs of the heel; *e,* line drawn parallel to the solar surface of the distal phalanx; *f,* line drawn parallel to the bearing surface of the hoof wall; *g,* line from center of best-fit circle for the distal interphalangeal joint drawn perpendicular to the bearing surface of the hoof wall. Line *a* should be parallel to lines *b, c,* and *d.* Line *g* should intersect at the midpoint of the bearing surface of the hoof wall. Angle *af,* 45 to 55 degrees in a front foot; 50 to 55 degrees in a hind foot; angle *ef,* 5 to 10 degrees. **B,** Assessment from dorsopalmar view of the normal foot. *1,* Line bisecting the phalanges; *2 and 3,* lines from respective lateral and medial solar margins of the distal phalanx to bearing surface of the hoof wall. These lines should be parallel to line *1.* Distance *2* = *3.*

elaborate set of measurements has been made on the dorsopalmar view to assess the effects of uneven mediolateral hoof wall trimming.[106,107] This method was used to assess the effects of using the corrective full rolling shoe in horses that were lame because of interphalangeal degenerative joint disease.[108]

The distal border of the distal phalanx should be at an angle of 3 to 10 degrees relative to the sole of the hoof. A neutral or negative so-called "palmar angle" puts strain on the soft tissues supporting the palmar/plantar soft tissues on the limb and has been associated with scintigraphic evidence of subchondral bone injury in the palmar/plantar third metacarpal/tarsal condyles, in addition to hindlimb lameness originating from both the tarsi and stifles.[109,110]

Laminitis

The normal orientation of the distal phalanx to the hoof is maintained by the complex structure of the interplay between the epidermal, dermal, and parietal surface of P3 forming the suspensory apparatus of the distal phalanx as noted in the description of the normal soft tissues of the foot.[105] Insult to this unique anatomic structure can result in the loss of mechanical support of the distal phalanx within the hoof capsule. *Laminitis* is the general clinical term used to refer to the complex of signs expressed by the horse and its effects on the structural relations of the hoof wall, the distal phalanx, and sole from a variety of insults. Most horses that develop clinical laminitis do so because of a systemic illness, typically equine metabolic syndrome.[111] Horses with protracted, severe, unilateral limb lameness are at risk for developing supporting limb laminitis in the contralateral limb, particularly those in full limb or transfixation casts for a long duration.[112,113] The development of supporting limb laminitis often occurs as rapid, severe failure of the suspensory apparatus of the distal phalanx manifesting as full sinking of the distal phalanx within the hoof capsule and has associated high mortality.[114]

Although differences of opinion exist regarding the terminology and categorization of this complex condition, several clinical phases or stages of laminitis are recognized: developmental, acute, and chronic.[115] *Developmental laminitis* is defined as the period between the initial insult to the first expression of lameness. It may be as short as 24 hours or as long as 60 hours.[115] This is likely an imperceptible stage to the owner unless access to excessive grain or grass is known to have occurred or a systemic disease or other condition is present that warrants concern for initiation of laminitis. This period is a prevention phase for mechanical failure of the foot complex.[115] *Acute laminitis* represents the phase from the first expression of lameness through 72 hours without evidence of mechanical collapse or at any time that signs of mechanical collapse occur.[115] Radiographs in either the developmental or the acute phase will rarely show signs of laminar inflammation and instead serve as a baseline for future comparison. Horses may recover fully from either developmental or acute laminitis with no loss of mechanical support. If, however, radiographic or clinical signs of distal phalanx displacement are seen, the phase of chronic laminitis has begun.[115]

Radiographic Evaluation of Laminitis

Radiographic evaluation of any horse with a clinical impression of pain and lameness caused by laminitis is justified. The goals of radiography are to detect changes indicative of mechanical failure and observe changes that contribute to formulation of prognosis and therapy. Front feet are affected most commonly. Placement of radiopaque markers on the foot has been advocated, but variation in normal measurements across patient types, in addition to variability in marker positioning may decrease their utility.[116,117]

The earliest radiographically detectable signs of laminitis involve the dorsal laminae. Thickening of the more radiolucent, sensitive laminae such that this layer represents more than one-third to one-half of the width of the whole dorsal wall and loss of distinction between this layer and the overlying radiopaque, keratinized hoof wall are both early radiographic signs of laminar inflammation. Crucially, these changes are often irreversible, thus their presence on radiographs is merely evidence of a laminitic episode, which may be the cause of the current lameness, or a residual change from a prior insult.

In the normal foot, the dorsal cortex of the distal phalanx should be parallel to the dorsal margin of the hoof wall in the lateromedial view. Divergence of these surfaces, with the toe region of the distal phalanx deviating or rotating in a palmar direction, is an indication of mechanical separation of the dermal and epidermal laminae (Figs. 27.40 and 27.41). This is the easiest of the distal phalanx displacements to detect radiographically. The angle at the point of convergence can be measured and is referred to as the *degree of rotation* (see Fig. 27.41C). Phalangeal malalignment (broken forward hoof pastern axis) due to rotation of the distal phalanx may be exacerbated by contraction of the DDFT, or if the more rapid growth of the hoof wall at the heel is managed improperly. Vertical displacement or "sinking" of the distal phalanx can be difficult to detect, especially earlier in the progression of disease. In the normal foot, the proximal edge of the extensor process of the distal phalanx is positioned roughly at the same plane or just proximal to the junction of the hoof wall and coronary band. Subjective distal displacement of the extensor process in combination with a concave defect and/or radiolucent "halo" in the soft tissues at the level of the coronary band can be radiographic indicators of sinking. Uniaxial distal displacement of the distal phalanx can occur and is most frequently seen medially.[118] Serial radiographs are often used to monitor laminitic changes and comparison between time points can help to better identify vertical displacement.

Other radiographic changes that can be seen with chronic and progressive laminitis include a very thin sole. The change in the position of the toe of the distal phalanx may cause a convex bulge in the sole contour, or the toe may penetrate through the sole. Lateral foot radiographs that are centered at the sole rather than at the coronary band are better for assessing these changes. Separation of the dorsal laminae can be seen as a single lucent line between the layers of the hoof wall on the lateral view (see Fig. 27.40D) and as a series of vertically oriented, thin, parallel lucent lines in the D65Pr-PaDiO view. This may progress to laminar necrosis, with eventual dissection of gas between the laminae once necrosis erodes through to the coronary band or white zone of the sole. Larger regions of radiolucency are more likely to be associated with secondary soft tissue infection.

In addition to the laminar changes, the distal phalanx undergoes characteristic changes associated with laminitis. These changes include bone production along the dorsal cortex of the distal phalanx dome-shaped contour, lipping or ski-slope-shaped bone formation at the toe, enlargement of the vascular channels, solar margin lysis, resorption of the palmar cortex, and/or angular orientation of a solar margin fracture (type VI) (see Fig. 27.40).

Because of the severe morbidity and protracted treatment required for chronic laminitis, indicators of prognosis for success or failure of treatment are desired. Various radiographic measurements have been assessed retrospectively to define reliable predictors of outcome for horses with chronic laminitis. Fig. 27.41 and eFig. 27.6 illustrate several of these measurements. Sole thickness (sole depth), not included in these illustrations, is measured from the toe of the distal phalanx to the ground surface, or top of the shoe, or to the distal soft tissue border of the sole if the horse has a prominent cup-shaped bottom of the foot (see Fig. 27.40A). The normal sole thickness should be greater than 15 mm in normal horses and greater

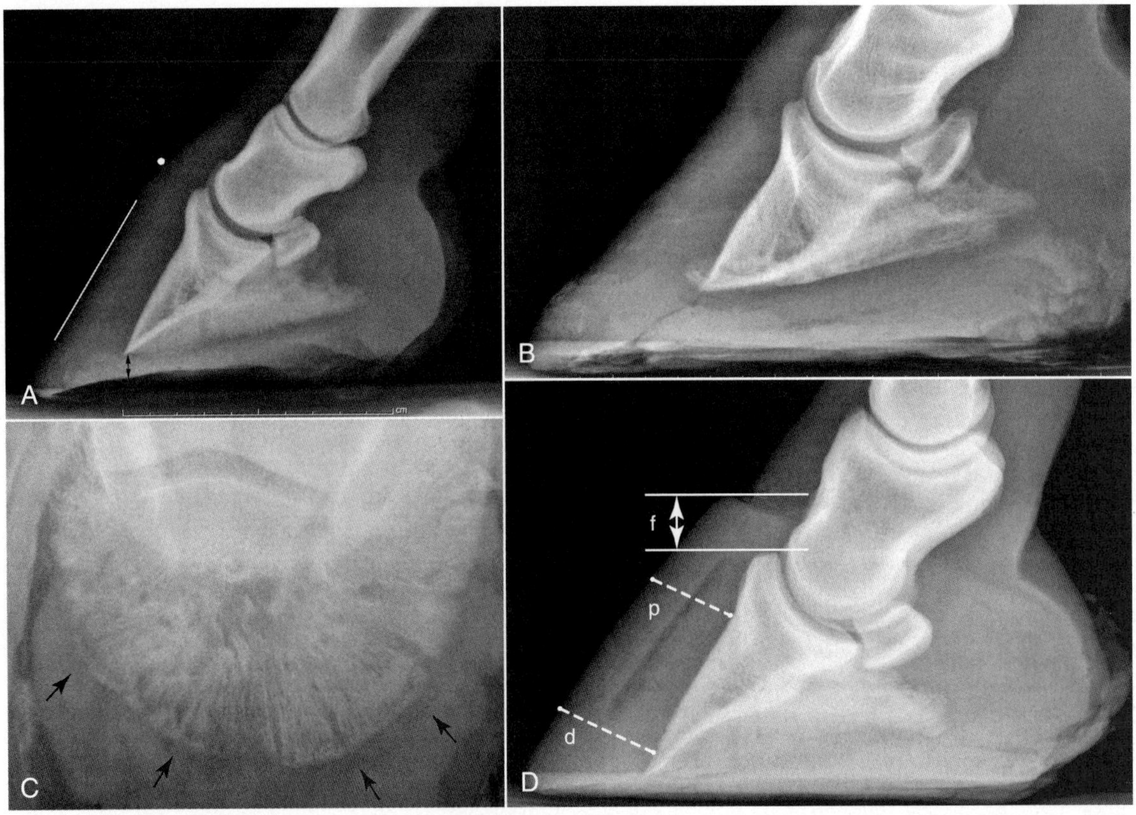

Fig. 27.40 Three variations of chronic laminitis. **A** is a horse with supporting limb laminitis with mild palmar rotation of the distal phalanx. The *white line* simulates the position for placement of a radiopaque marker on the dorsal hoof wall surface. The *white dot* simulates the location for placement of a marker at the coronary band. Palpation of the hoof wall and coronary band junction is important to achieve proper placement of this marker. The *double-headed arrow* shows the location for measuring sole depth or sole thickness. **B and C** are images of a horse with more chronic laminitis. In addition to rotation of the distal phalanx, there is a linear gas shadow extending from the sole to the toe. A bone fragment is present at the toe because of pathologic distal phalanx fractures along the medial and lateral solar margins (type VI) as seen in **C** (*arrows*). Punctate radiolucencies in the trabecular region are end-on vessels increased in number and diameter. **D** is a horse that developed plantar rotation and vertical displacement of the distal phalanx within 3 weeks of a severe injury to the contralateral limb. There is a marked indentation at the coronary band. The sole is extremely thin at the toe. Gas is also evident at the laminar junction. Measurements made on the images indicated a founder distance *(f)* of 18 mm, proximal dorsal hoof wall distance *(p)* of 28 mm, and distal dorsal hoof wall distance *(d)* of 33 mm.

than 10 mm in normal ponies and more thin-soled Thoroughbred racehorses.[119,120] Even though none has been completely reliable when used as the only indicator, trends have been identified. In general, the more deviant from normal, the more guarded the prognosis. The vertical distance between the proximal limit of the dorsal hoof wall and the proximal limit of the extensor process of the distal phalanx has been measured to generate a *founder distance* (Fig. 27.41B).[116] When corrected for magnification, this distance in 25 normal horses was an average of 4 mm (range, −2 to 11 mm) in the front feet and an average of 4.6 mm (range, −2 to 9 mm) in the hind feet.[116] The wide variation in these measurements reflects the spectrum of equine foot conformation and a single measurement alone is of limited value. Serial measurements in repeated radiographic studies may give more meaningful information about progression of laminitis in that individual patient. Evaluating a large number of horses for prognostic indicators of poor outcome, distal displacement of the distal phalanx was the only radiographic variable associated with an increased probability of death.[120] However, the severity of the lameness was the single best predictor of outcome. Others concur that radiographic assessment is important in establishing and monitoring bone stability within the hoof but should not be used as an isolated indicator of outcome.[121]

Digital venography can be used to evaluate several foot problems, most notably laminitis. This procedure is described in detail within the literature and involves the administration of positive contrast medium via a palmar digital vein followed by rapid acquisition of lateromedial and dorsopalmar radiographs of the foot.[7,122] In a normal horse, the contrast medium is maintained within the vasculature and the tip of the distal phalanx is located proximal to the circumflex vein. In horses with laminitis, there may be compression of vasculature, failure of adequate filling, rapid extravascular diffusion of contrast medium, and/or an altered (more distal) position of the tip of the distal phalanx relative to the circumflex vein.[7,123] This technique has been used to guide treatment recommendations and inform prognostication; however, imaging findings should be considered in the context of the clinical appearance when making decisions.[124]

MRI can be used to detect laminitis, even in the acute stages. A study of active phase laminitis was performed using a 4.7 T magnet, and it was possible to detect changes in laminar and corium structure and signal intensity that correlated strongly with the histologic diagnosis of acute laminitis.[124] In this study the sensitivity of MRI for detecting these changes was 95% to 100%, compared with just 48% to 58% for radiography. Changes such as laminar fibrillation and signal alterations within the

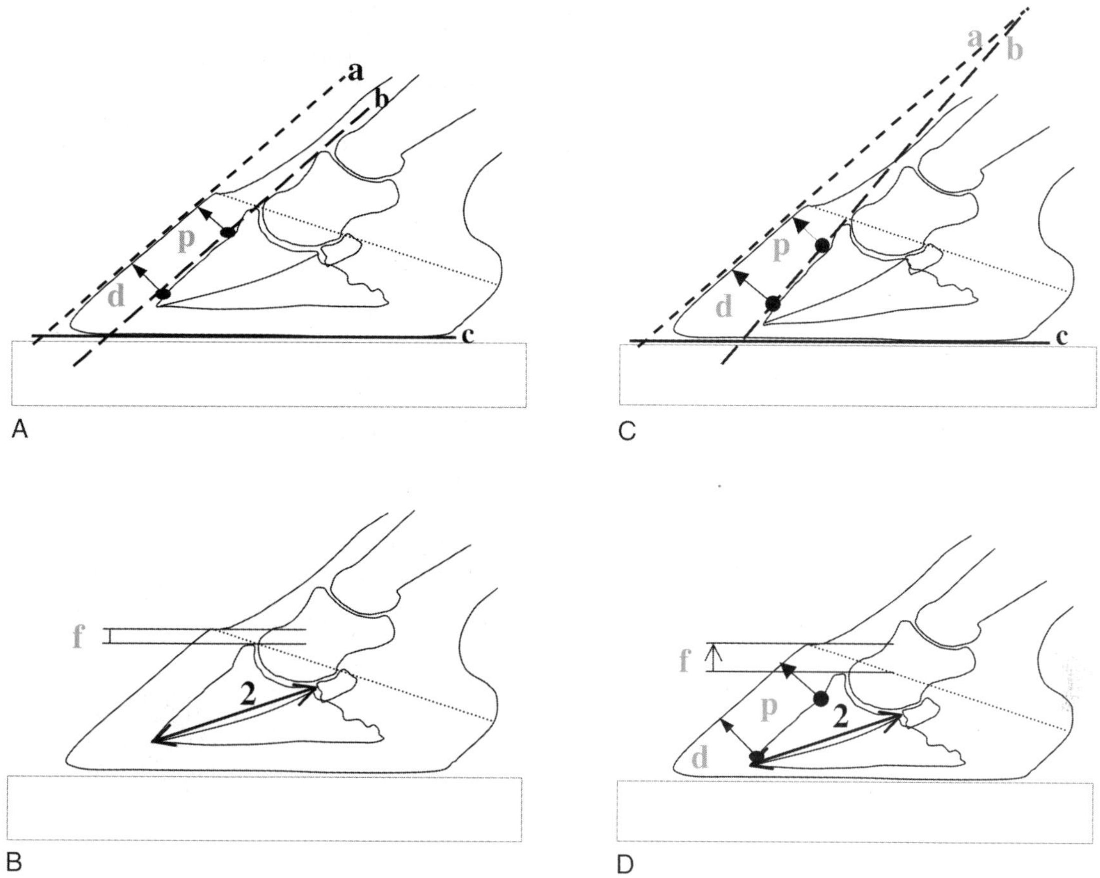

Fig. 27.41 **A and B,** Radiographic measurements of the normal foot. **A,** Line *a* is parallel to the hoof wall. Line *b* is parallel to the dorsal cortex of the distal phalanx. Line *c* is parallel to the weight-bearing surface of the hoof wall. Angle *ac* is the hoof axis. Angle *bc* is the foot axis. Distance *p* is the thickness of the dorsal soft tissues measured 5 mm distal to the junction of the extensor process with the dorsal cortex. Distance *d* is the thickness of the dorsal soft tissues measured 6 mm proximal to the most distal point of the dorsal cortex. **B,** Line *2* is the length of the palmar cortex measured from the solar margin at the distal toe to the palmar articular edge between the distal phalanx and the distal sesamoid bone. Distance *f* is the vertical distance or "founder" distance measured between coronary band and proximal edge of the extensor process. **C and D,** Radiographic measurements of the foot with chronic laminitis. **C,** Foot with chronic laminitis exhibiting displacement of the distal phalanx as rotation only. Lines *a* and *b* are no longer parallel and converge proximally, forming angle *ab* or the rotation angle. Distance *d* is greater than distance *p*. **D,** Foot with chronic laminitis exhibiting distal phalanx displacement as vertical displacement (sinking) only. Founder distance *f* is increased. Distance *p* equals *d*, but both are greater than normal. The percentage that *d* is of line *2* will be greater than normal. (See text for normal and abnormal values.) (Reproduced with permission from Lindford RL, O'Brien TR, Trout DR. Qualitative and morphometric radiographic findings in the distal phalanx and digital soft tissues of sound Thoroughbred racehorses. *Am J Vet Res.* 1993;54:38; and Cripps PJ, Eustace RA. Radiological measurements from the feet of normal horses with relevance to laminitis. *Equine Vet J.* 1999;31:427.)

corium are also detectable with other high-field systems in more common clinical use (1−3 T).

Ungual (Collateral) Cartilages

The ungual cartilages extend in a proximopalmar direction from the palmar processes of the distal phalanx. There are multiple ligaments associated with these cartilages which anchor them to adjacent osseous structures. These include the chondropedal (attach to the proximal phalanx), chondrocoronal (attach to the middle phalanx), chondrotendinous (attach to the extensor process of the distal phalanx), chondroungular (attach to the palmar processes of the distal phalanx), and chondrosesamoidean ligaments (attach to the navicular bone). In addition, fibers of the distal interphalangeal collateral ligaments connect to the dorsal aspect of these cartilages.[3,125]

Tears of the Ungual Cartilages

Tears of the unossified ungual cartilages can occur and are frequently associated with severe injury of the adjacent soft tissues, particularly the collateral ligaments of the distal interphalangeal joint. This diagnosis can only be made definitively on MRI or high-quality contrast-enhanced CT.

Ossification/Calcification (Sidebones)

This is a common finding in radiographs of the distal part of the digit, especially in draft-breed horses. Ascribing clinical significance of ossified cartilages can be difficult. Many consider this finding to be incidental or, if asymmetric within a foot, indicative of increased stress on the ossified portion.[126] A grading scheme has been used to grade the ossification as depicted in the weight-bearing horizontal dorsopalmar view (see Fig. 27.42).[56] Generally, ossification begins at the base of the

89. O'Brien EJ, Smith RWK. Mineralization can be an incidental ultrasonographic finding in equine tendons and ligaments. 2018;59(5):613–623.
90. Mair TS, Kinns J. Deep digital flexor tendonitis in the equine foot diagnosed by low-flied magnetic resonance imaging in the standing patient: 18 cases. *Vet Radiol Ultrasound*. 2005;46(6):458–466.
91. Vallance SA, Bell RJW, Spriet M, et al. Comparison of computed tomography, contrast-enhanced computed tomography and standing low-field magnetic resonance imaging in horses with lameness localized to the foot. Part 2: lesion identification. *Equine Vet J*. 2012;44(2):149–156.
92. Bolt DM, Dixon JJ. Deep digital flexor tendon lesions in the foot—a career-ending injury for the equine athlete? *Livestock*. 2016;21:196.
93. Dyson s, Murray R. Magnetic resonance imaging evaluation of 264 horses with foot pain: the podotrochlear apparatus, deep digital flexor tendon and collateral ligaments of the distal interphalangeal joint. *Equine Vet J*. 2007;39(4):340–343.
94. Sampson SN, Schneider RK, Gavin PR, et al. Magnetic resonance imaging findings in horses with recent onset navicular syndrome but without radiographic abnormalities. *Vet Radiol Ultrasound*. 2009;50(4):339–346.
95. Busoni V, Lahaye B, Denoix JM. Transcuneal ultrasonographic findings in the podotrochlear apparatus: comparison with postmortem in 14 equine digits. *J Equine Vet Sci*. 2006;26(3):113–119.
96. Jacquet S, Denoix JM. Ultrasonographic examination of the distal podotrochlear apparatus of the horse: a transcuneal approach. *Equine Vet Educ*. 2011;24(2):90–96.
97. Evrard L, Joostens Z, Vandersmissen M, et al. Comparison between ultrasonographic and standing magnetic resonance imaging findings in the podotrochlear apparatus of horses with foot pain. *Front Vet Sci*. 2021;8(675180):1–13.
98. Acutt EV, Contino EK, Frisbie DD, et al. Deep digital flexor tendon lesions in the pastern are associated with the presence of distal tendinopathy. *Equine Vet J*. 2021;54(3):502–512.
99. Biggi M, Dyson S. Comparison between radiological and magnetic resonance imaging lesions in the distal border of the navicular bone with particular reference to distal border fragments and osseous cyst-like lesions. *Equine Vet J*. 2010;42(8):707–712.
100. Dyson S, Pool R, Blunden T, et al. The distal sesamoidean impar ligament: comparison between its appearance on magnetic resonance imaging and histology of the axial third of the ligament. 2010;42(4), 332-229.
101. Barrett MF, Frisbie DD, King MR, et al. A review of how magnetic resonance imaging can aid in case management of common pathological conditions of the equine foot. 2017;29(12):683–693.
102. Whitcomb MB. Ultrasonographic appearance and distribution of deep digital flexor injuries in the pastern region. *AAEP Proc*. 2008;54:453–454.
103. Kidd JA, Lu KG, Frazer ML, eds. *Atlas of Equine Ultrasonography*. 2nd ed. Chichester, West Sussex, UK: John Wiley & Sons Inc; 2022.
104. Grundmann IN, Drost WT, Zeas LJ, et al. Quantitative assessment of the equine hoof using digital radiographs and magnetic resonance imaging. *Equine Vet J*. 2015;47(5):542–547.
105. Pollitt CC. Collins SN: the suspensory apparatus of the distal phalanx in normal horses. *Equine Vet J*. 2016;48(4):496–501.
106. Caudron I, Grulke S, Farnir F, et al. Radiographic assessment of equine interphalangeal joints asymmetry: articular impact of phalangeal rotations (part I). *J Vet Med*. 1998;45(6–7):319–325.
107. Caudron I, Grulke S, Farnir F, et al. Radiographic assessment of equine interphalangeal joints asymmetry: articular impact of asymmetric bearings (part II). *J Vet Med*. 1998;45(6–7):327–335.
108. Caudron I, Miesen M, Grulke S, et al. Radiological assessment of the effects of a full rolling motion shoe during asymmetrical bearing. *Equine Vet J Suppl*. 1997;23: 20–22.
109. Pezzanite L, Bass L, Kawcak C, et al. The relationship between sagittal hoof conformation and hindlimb lameness in the horse. *Equine Vet J*. 2018;51(4):464–469.
110. Walmsley EA, Jackson M, Wells-Smith L, et al. Solar angle of the distal phalanx is associated with scintigraphic evidence of subchondral bone injury in the palmar/plantar aspect of the third metacarpal/tarsal condyles in Thoroughbred racehorses. *Equine Vet J*. 2019;51(6):720–726.
111. Pollitt CC. Laminitis pathophysiology. In: Floyd AE, Mansmann RA, eds. *Equine Podiatry*. St Louis: Saunders/Elsevier; 2007:313.
112. Virgin JE, Goodrich LR, Baxter GM, et al. Incidence of support limb laminitis in horses treated with half limb, full limb or transfixation pin casts: a retrospective study of 113 horses (2000-2009). *Equine Vet J*. 2011;40:7–11.
113. van Eps A, Collins SN, Pollitt CC. Supporting limb laminitis. *Vet Clin North Am Equine Pract*. 2010;26(2): 287–302.
114. Hood DM. Laminitis in the horse. *Vet Clin North Am Equine Pract*. 1999;15(2):287–294.
115. Floyd AE, Mansmann RA, eds. *Equine Podiatry*. St Louis: Saunders/Elsevier; 2007.
116. Cripps PJ, Eustace RA. Radiological measurements from the feet of normal horses with relevance to laminitis. *Equine Vet J*. 1999;31(5):427–432.
117. Thieme K, Ehrle A, Lixcher C. Radiographic measurements of the hooves of normal ponies. *Vet J*. 2015;206(3):332–337.
118. Sherlock C, Parks A. Radiographic and radiological assessment of laminitis. *Equine Vet Educ*. 2013;25(10):524–535.
119. Kummer M, Geyer H, Imboden I, et al. The effect of hoof trimming on radiographic measurements of the front feet of normal Warmblood horses. *Vet J*. 2006;172(1):58–66.
120. Orsini JA, Parsons CS, Capewell L, et al. Prognostic indicators of poor outcome in horses with laminitis at a tertiary care hospital. *Can Vet J*. 2010;51(6):623–628.
121. Hunt RJ, Wharton RE. Clinical presentation, diagnosis, and prognosis of chronic laminitis in North America. *Vet Clin North Am Equine Pract*. 2010;26(1):141–153.
122. Rucker A. Equine venography and its clinical application in North America. *Vet Clin North Am Equine Pract*. 2010;26(1):167–177.
123. Kramer J, Rucker A, Leise B. Venographic evaluation of the circumflex vessels and lamellar circumflex junction in laminitic horses. *Equine Vet Educ*. 2018;32(7):386–392.
124. Arble JB, Mattoon JS, Drost WT, et al. Magnetic resonance imaging of the initial active stage of equine laminitis at 4.7 T. *Vet Radiol Ultrasound*. 2009;50(1):3–12.
125. Ruohoniemi M, Makela O, Eskonen T. Clinical significance of ossification of the cartilages of the front feet based on nuclear bone scintigraphy, radiography and lameness examinations in 21 Finnhorses. *Equine Vet J*. 2004; 36:143–148.
126. Ross MW, Dyson SJ. *Diagnosis and Management of Lameness in the Horse*. 2nd ed. St Louis: Saunders/Elsevier; 2011.
127. Dakin SG, Robson KE, Dyson SJ. Fractures of ossified cartilages of the foot: 10 cases. *Equine Vet Educ*. 2006;18:130.
128. Selberg K, Werpy N. Fractures of the distal phalanx and associated soft tissue and osseous abnormalities in 22 horses with ossified sclerotic ungual cartilages diagnosed

with magnetic resonance imaging. *Vet Radiol Ultrasound*. 2011;52(4):394–401.
129. Smith MRW. Infection of the cartilages of the foot. *Equine Vet Educ*. 2014;26(11):580–583.
130. Meehan LJ, Taylor SE, Labens R, et al. Magnetic resonance imaging assisted management in five cases of suspected quittor. *Vet Comp Orthop Traumatol*. 2016;29(1):75–82.
131. del Junco CI, Mair TS, Powell SE, et al. Magnetic resonance imaging findings of equine solar penetration wounds. *Vet Radiol Ultrasound*. 2012;53(1):71–75.
132. Ogden NKE, Milner PI, Stack JD, et al. CT more accurately detects foreign bodies within the equine foot than MRI or digital radiography. *Vet Radiol Ultrasound*. 2020;62(2): 225–235.
133. Urraca del Junco CI, Mair TS, Powell SE, et al. Magnetic resonance imaging findings of equine solar penetration wounds. *Vet Radiol Ultrasound*. 2012;53(1):71–75.
134. Findley JA, Pinchbeck GL, Milner PI, et al. Outcome of horses with synovial structure involvement following solar foot penetrations in four UK veterinary hospitals: 95 cases. *Equine Vet J*. 2014;46(3):352–357.
135. Schiavo S, Cillán-García E, Elce Y, et al. Horses with solar foot penetration, deep digital flexor tendon injury, and absence of concurrent synovial sepsis can have a positive outcome. *Vet Radiol Ultrasound*. 2018;59(6): 697–704.

ELECTRONIC RESOURCES

Additional information related to the content in Chapter 27 can be found online at eBooks.Health.Elsevier.com.

- Chapter Quiz

SECTION IV

The Thoracic Cavity Canine, Feline and Equine

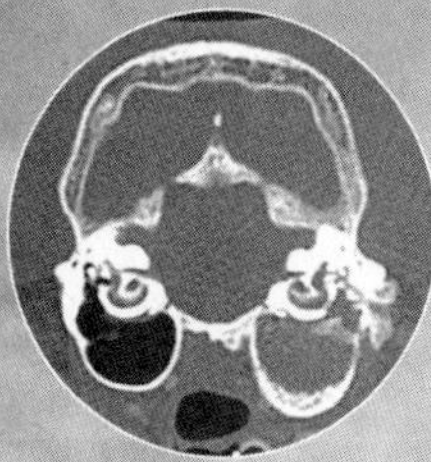
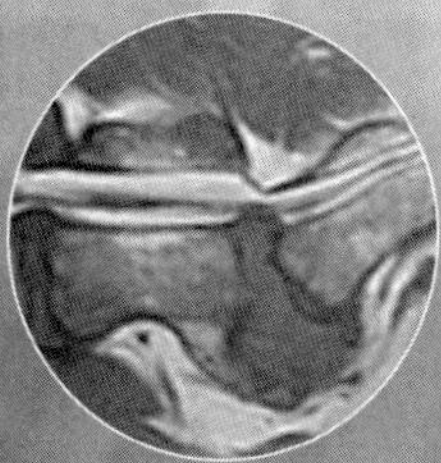
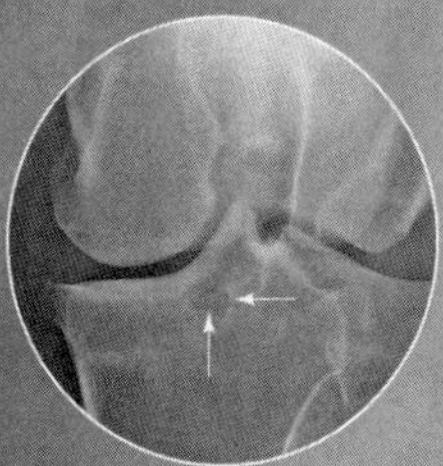
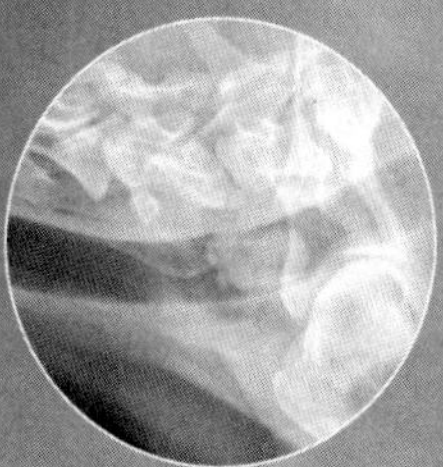
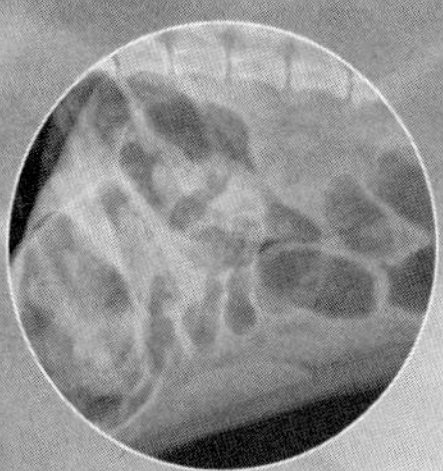

CHAPTER 28

Principles of Radiographic Interpretation of the Thorax

Donald E. Thrall

Acquisition of thoracic radiographs is a common radiographic examination in small animal practice. Radiographs of at least part of the thorax can also be obtained in foals and in most adult horses.

NOMENCLATURE

In daily practice, the naming of conventional lateral thoracic radiographs made with the patient lying on their side and a vertically directed x-ray beam violates the point-of-entrance to point-of-exit nomenclature system described in Chapter 6. If the patient was on the left side, for example, the correct name for this view would be a *right-left* lateral because the x-ray beam enters on the right side and exits on the left. But in daily practice, the naming of such a view is abbreviated to designate the side the patient is lying on; in this case a *left lateral*. Similarly, a thoracic radiograph made with the patient lying on the right side would be a *right lateral* view.

In the adult horse, lateral thoracic radiographs are made with the patient standing and a horizontally directed x-ray beam. Therefore, the point-to-entrance to point-of-exit system should still be used, and lateral radiographs should be designated as either left-right or right-left laterals.

In all species, ventrodorsal (VD) and dorsoventral (DV) radiographs of the thorax are named according to the point-of-entrance to point-of-exit of the x-ray beam.

RADIOGRAPHIC TECHNIQUE: DOG AND CAT

A relatively low contrast image of the thorax is preferred. The air in the lung will provide the necessary level of contrast and there is not a need to enhance contrast using technical factors. With analog technology, a low-contrast image is obtained by using a high kilovoltage peak (kVp)—low milliampere-seconds (mAs), combination, and this approach can also be used with digital systems. However, in digital imaging the contrast of the image is controlled primarily by the processing algorithm that is applied to the raw image data. Therefore, it is important that the correct processing parameters are assigned to thorax studies when the digital image system is compiled. For patients thicker than 10 cm, a grid should be used to remove scattered x-rays from the beam.

Exposure time is critical when radiographing the thorax. Motion is the biggest enemy of image detail in veterinary radiology. Respiratory motion can induce blurring and lead to reduced detail. This reduces the ability to interpret the radiograph accurately. To minimize the effects of motion, the shortest exposure time and highest milliamperes (mA) setting possible should be used to produce the needed mAs.

Ideally, the respiratory pattern of the patient should be observed for a few seconds before the radiographic exposure is made so that the exposure can be coordinated with peak inspiration. The increased lung aeration at peak inspiration will optimize pulmonary contrast and reduce the false impression of pulmonary disease caused by poor aeration (Fig. 28.1).

RADIOGRAPHIC TECHNIQUE: HORSE

The same technical principles relating to radiography of the canine and feline thorax also apply to the horse. Radiographing the equine thorax does not require the massive exposure factors that might be expected based on the sheer size of the thorax because of the large volume of air present in the equine lungs. However, obtaining radiographs of all regions of the equine thorax when using a grid will require more output than typically available from a portable x-ray unit, such as those used commonly to radiograph equine extremities. It may be possible to obtain diagnostic-quality radiographs of the dorsocaudal portion of the equine thorax with a portable x-ray machine and without a grid, but obtaining suitable radiographs in other regions of the thorax with this type of equipment will not be possible because of the thickness of the horse, and the amount of scatter produced from intervening soft tissue.

POSITIONING: DOG AND CAT

The routine thoracic radiographic examination in the dog and cat should consist of left lateral, right lateral, and either VD or DV projections. The entire thoracic cavity should be included in the image. This seems obvious, but omitting the cranial or caudal part of the thorax from the field of view is a common error, which increases the chance of missing a lesion. The field of view should extend from just cranial to the thoracic inlet, to a few centimeters caudal to the last rib. The dorsocaudal tips of the caudal lobes extend further caudally than anticipated. Even in the largest dogs, including the entire thoracic cavity in one 14-inch by 17-inch image is usually possible. For the occasional huge dog where this is not possible, then each projection (left lateral, right lateral, VD or DV) should be divided into cranial and caudal portions.

For lateral and VD/DV views of the thorax, the forelimbs should be pulled cranially to remove the brachial muscles from being superimposed on the cranial aspect of the thorax. Failure to do this will cause an artificial increase in radiographic opacity and lead to errors in interpretation of the cranial mediastinum and cranial lung lobes. This is a common mistake. Poor attention to positioning and technique will result in incorrect assessments and potentially unnecessary emotional and financial stress for the animal owner (Fig. 28.2).

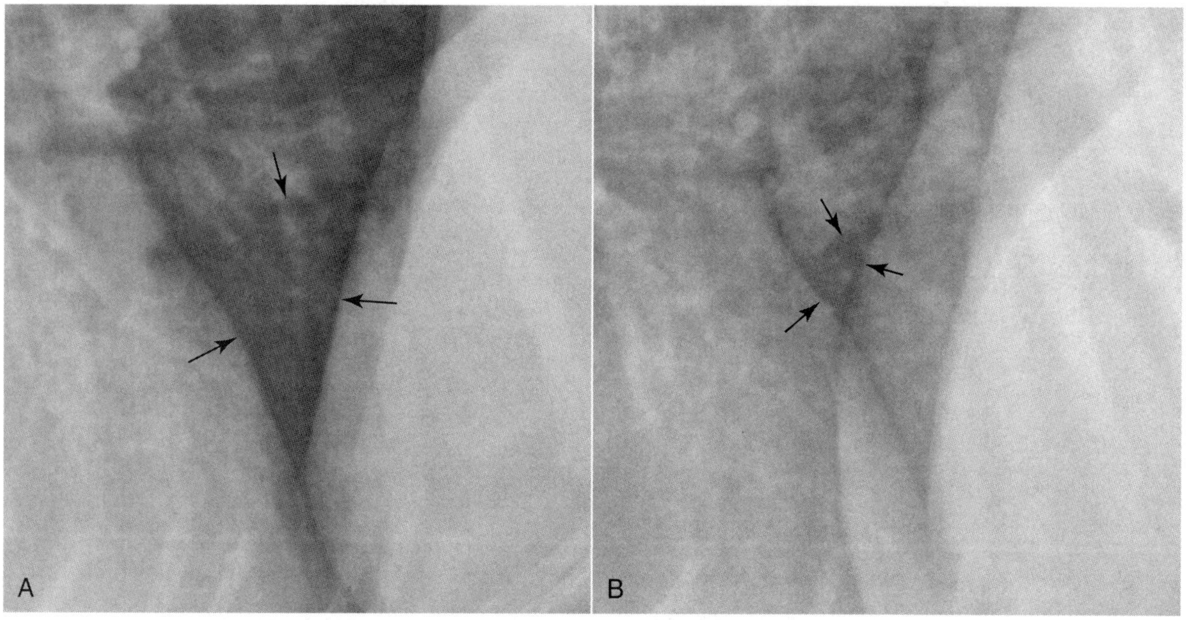

Fig. 28.1 Close-up view of the caudoventral aspect of the thorax in a dog at inspiration **(A)** and expiration **(B)**. The size of the triangular region of lung between the caudal vena cava, heart, and diaphragm (*arrows*) can be used as an indicator of the degree of lung inflation that was present when the radiograph was acquired. Note the reduction in size of this region of lung and the overall increased lung opacity, in **B** versus **A**. Poor ventilation is a common cause of overdiagnosis of pulmonary disease.

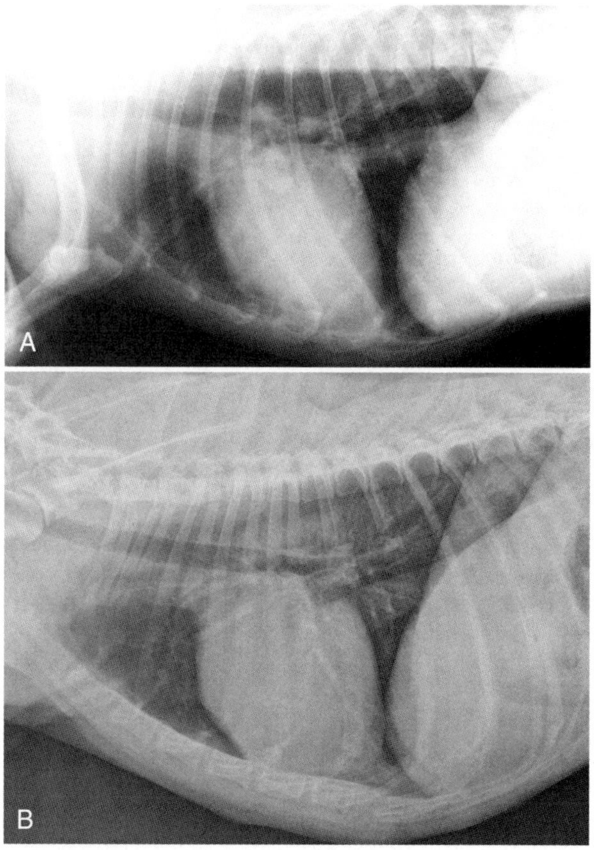

Fig. 28.2 **A,** Initial thoracic radiograph of a dog. A diagnosis of multiple pulmonary nodules was made. There are numerous technical problems with this radiograph. The patient is rotated, the image contrast is too high, and the thoracic limbs are superimposed on the cranial aspect of the thorax. The patient was referred to an oncologist. **B,** Repeat thoracic radiograph where the positioning and technique are excellent. The radiograph is normal. The poor technique used in the initial radiograph resulted in unnecessary financial burden and emotional stress for the owner.

POSITIONING: HORSE

In small foals or miniature horses, it may be possible to acquire lateral thoracic radiographs by restraining the subject on a small-animal x-ray table and using a vertically directed x-ray beam. However, obtaining conventional VD or DV thoracic radiographs in a horse can only be accomplished in the smallest and most compliant patients. If a VD view is able to be acquired, the cardiac silhouette will appear very large due to magnification (Fig. 28.3), and this is often misinterpreted as cardiac enlargement.

Most thoracic radiographs of horses are acquired with the horse standing. Lateral views are therefore acquired with a horizontally directed x-ray beam, and DV or VD views are not obtained. The plate should not be held by hand when radiographing the equine thorax. The light field that corresponds to the primary x-ray beam is visible only on the side of the horse closest to the x-ray tube, meaning that no part of the light field can be seen on the plate. Therefore, aligning the x-ray beam with the plate is impossible when the plate is held by hand. This invariably results in the primary x-ray beam striking the person holding the plate. A wall-mounted plate holder, as described in Chapter 9, or a floor-mounted mobile plate holder should be used for equine thoracic radiography. When using these devices, the x-ray beam can be aligned with the plate before the horse is brought into position next to the plate.

Given the large size, it is not possible to obtain a radiograph of the entire equine thoracic cavity in one image, except in young foals or miniature horses. For lateral radiographs of an adult horse, four images are usually acquired: (1) craniodorsal, (2) caudodorsal, (3) cranioventral, and (4) caudoventral. The approximate location for each of these views is illustrated in Fig. 28.4.

Radiographic magnification is an important consideration when interpreting equine thoracic radiographs. This has already been discussed relative to the appearance of the heart of a foal in a VD radiograph. But, also as a result of the large diameter of the

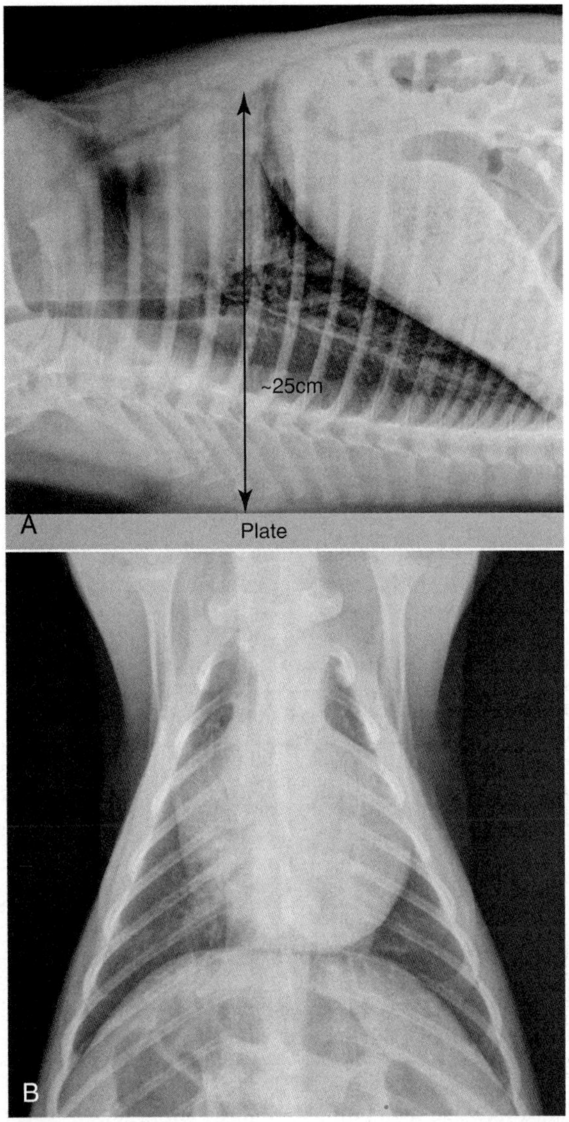

Fig. 28.3 **A,** Illustration of the geometry for obtaining a ventrodorsal (VD) view of the thorax in a foal. Due to the shape of the foal thorax, the cardiac apex may be approximately 25 cm from the plate, resulting in marked magnification of the heart. **B,** VD radiograph of a normal 4-week-old mule; the heart appears large for the reasons described in **A** of this illustration.

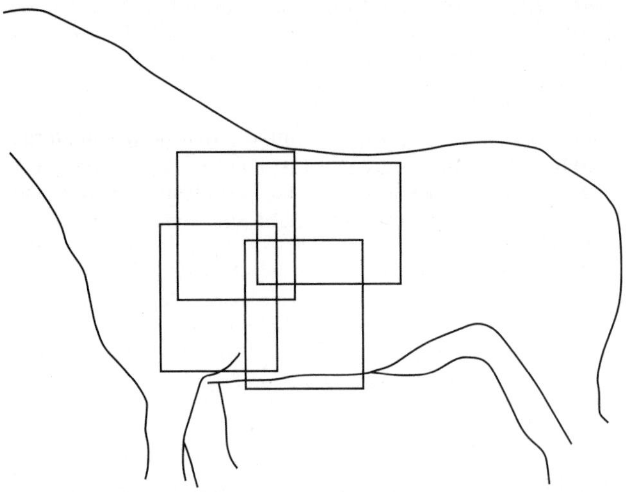

Fig. 28.4 Outline of a horse showing the approximate locations of the plate for a four-view radiographic examination that would include the entire thoracic cavity.

thorax of an adult horse, a lesion in the lung on the side closest to the x-ray tube could be approximately 35 cm from the plate. This would lead to the lesion being magnified by approximately 1.5 times. At this level of magnification, the resultant blurring could result in the lesion being inconspicuous, especially if the lesion is small. To rule out the presence of a small lesion, left-right *and* right-left thoracic radiographs should be obtained.* This means that eight exposures would be necessary for complete radiographic examination of the thorax. Alternatively, the x-ray tube can be moved further from the cassette to reduce geometric magnification, but this will require an increase in the mAs that is proportional to the square of the distance.[1] Whether this approach is feasible depends on the capacity of the x-ray equipment.

WHY ARE BOTH LEFT AND RIGHT LATERAL THORACIC VIEWS NEEDED ROUTINELY IN SMALL ANIMALS?

When an animal is in lateral recumbency, the dependent lung partially collapses due to the heart compressing the lung, and cranial excursion of the dependent side of the diaphragm. This pulmonary collapse, which causes the lung to have increased opacity, occurs rapidly in awake, sedated, and anesthetized dogs and cats after being placed in lateral recumbency. The extent of this lung collapse can be illustrated in a thoracic radiograph made with the dog in lateral recumbency and using a horizontally directed x-ray beam. This view is correctly termed a *right* (or *left*) *recumbent horizontal-beam VD* (Fig. 28.5). The amount of collapse of the down lung is pronounced but is not seen specifically in a conventional lateral radiograph because the aerated nondependent lung is superimposed on the collapsed dependent lung. Recumbency-associated atelectasis also occurs in the dorsocaudal aspect of the caudal lung lobes when the patient is placed in dorsal recumbency for the VD view (Fig. 28.6), but to a lesser extent than in lateral recumbency (compare with Fig. 28.5B).

The reduced aeration of the down, dependent, lung is problematic for two reasons. First, in lateral radiographs, the increased opacity of the partially collapsed dependent lung results in the overall opacity of the lung field being increased over that present in VD or DV radiographs where there is less or no atelectasis, respectively. Overinterpreting this increased opacity in lateral radiographs as lung disease is a common mistake (Fig. 28.7). If an increase in overall lung opacity is suspected from one or both lateral views, it is critical that this be confirmed in the VD view to rule out that the suspected lung disease is artifactual, caused by atelectasis. The use of sedation or anesthesia for the radiographic examination will exacerbate the amount of recumbency-associated atelectasis that is present. If thoracic radiographs are made of an anesthetized patient, positive pressure ventilation helps to reduce the amount of atelectasis that occurs.

Second, the increased opacity of the collapsed dependent lung will silhouette with any soft tissue lesion in that lung. This renders the lesion inconspicuous in the radiograph (Figs. 28.8–28.10).[2,3] If only one lateral view is acquired and there is a lesion that is not visible in the VD view, it could be missed depending on which lateral view is acquired. Clearly, three-view thoracic radiographic examinations are needed to prevent significant lesions from being missed.[3]

*For an example of how a lesion in a large patient can be missed due to magnification please see Fig. 38.5. This example is in the abdomen but the same principle applies to the thorax.

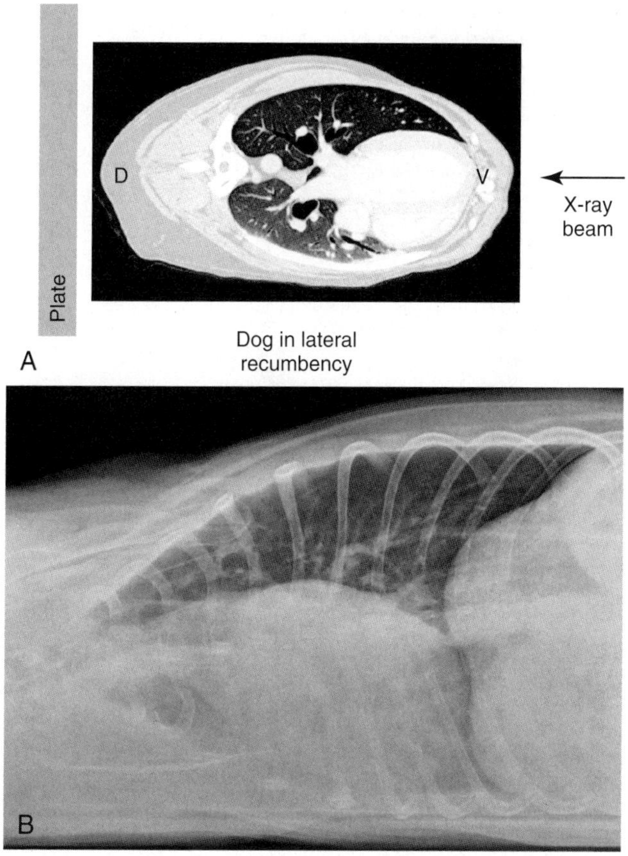

Fig. 28.5 **A,** Method of acquiring a horizontal-beam ventrodorsal (VD) radiograph of the thorax. The transverse computed tomography (CT) image of the thorax represents the dog being radiographed. This dog is in right recumbency. The x-ray beam is directed onto the ventral surface and the plate positioned dorsally. **B,** Radiograph resulting from the positioning illustrated in part **A**. This radiograph would be termed a right recumbent horizontal-beam VD view. Note the marked collapse of the dependent right lung. The heart is shifted into the dependent right hemithorax and is compressing the lung. The diaphragm is also displaced cranially, also compressing the lung. *D,* Dorsal; *V,* ventral.

SPECIFIC FEATURES OF CANINE AND FELINE THORACIC RADIOGRAPHS

Pulmonary Vessels

The pulmonary artery and vein in the right cranial lobe are used commonly as a basis for assessing the pulmonary circulation.[4] This is done by comparing the respective size of these vessels, which requires that other structures are not superimposed. These specific pulmonary vessels are isolated, and more conspicuous, in a left lateral than in a right lateral radiograph (Fig. 28.11). In right recumbency the right cranial lobe vessels are displaced dorsally and become superimposed on the left-sided vessels, whereas in left recumbency the left- and right-sided vessels are not superimposed.

The left cranial lobe pulmonary vessels cannot usually be assessed or compared accurately in either the left or right lateral view, because they are located more dorsally in the thorax and usually superimposed on other vessels or the thicker dorsal portion of the mediastinum.

Pulmonary arteries and veins can also be compared in the caudal lung lobes. This is best accomplished in a DV view. The caudal lobe pulmonary vessels are more conspicuous in DV compared to VD radiographs for two main reasons: (1) a perpendicular orientation with the primary x-ray beam and (2) less adjacent pulmonary atelectasis (Figs. 28.12 and 28.13).

Diaphragm

The diaphragm consists of a left crus and a right crus (collectively the crura) dorsally and a dome ventrally. The diaphragmatic hiatus for the caudal vena cava is located slightly to the right of midline and passes through the right diaphragmatic crus. In the left lateral view, the two dorsal crura of the diaphragm diverge from each other, whereas in the right lateral view they are more parallel (Fig. 28.14). In the right lateral view, the dependent right crus will be cranial to the left crus because of pressure from abdominal contents, and therefore the caudal vena cava will silhouette, or merge, with the more cranial right crus. In the left lateral view, the left crus will be cranial to the right crus, and the caudal vena cava will be superimposed on the left crus before silhouetting, or merging, with the more caudally located right crus that contains the caval hiatus (see Fig. 28.14). Therefore, the appearance of the junction of the caudal vena cava with the diaphragm can be used as a way to distinguish a left lateral from a right lateral radiograph if an external marking system has not been used. However, this principle is not 100% accurate, because occasionally, the left crus will be cranial to the right crus in the right lateral view, and vice versa.

Cardiac Silhouette

There is only a minor difference in the appearance of the cardiac silhouette in left vs. right lateral views. In general, the cardiac silhouette will appear slightly rounder and the apex may be slightly elevated from the sternum in the left lateral view compared with the right lateral view (Fig. 28.15). Comparatively, there is a major difference in the appearance of the cardiac silhouette in VD versus DV radiographs. In sternal recumbency for the DV radiograph, the ventral aspect of the diaphragm is displaced cranially where it contacts the heart and displaces it, typically to the left. The heart is also more upright in the thoracic cavity when the patient is in sternal recumbency, making it appear rounder (Fig. 28.16). The rounder appearance and displacement to the left that occur normally in DV radiographs are commonly misinterpreted as cardiomegaly. The extent of leftward cardiac displacement in DV radiographs is more pronounced in large dogs and will not be as obvious in small dogs or cats.[5–7]

Accessory Lung Lobe

The cranial excursion of the diaphragm that occurs in sternal recumbency also impinges on the territory of the accessory lung lobe. This diminishes the ability to evaluate the accessory lobe and caudal mediastinum, and significant disease in this area can be missed in DV radiographs because of this impingement (see Fig. 28.16). As with cardiac displacement, the amount of impingement on the accessory lobe and caudal mediastinal regions in DV radiographs caused by cranial excursion of the diaphragm is more noticeable in large dogs and is not as significant in small dogs or cats.

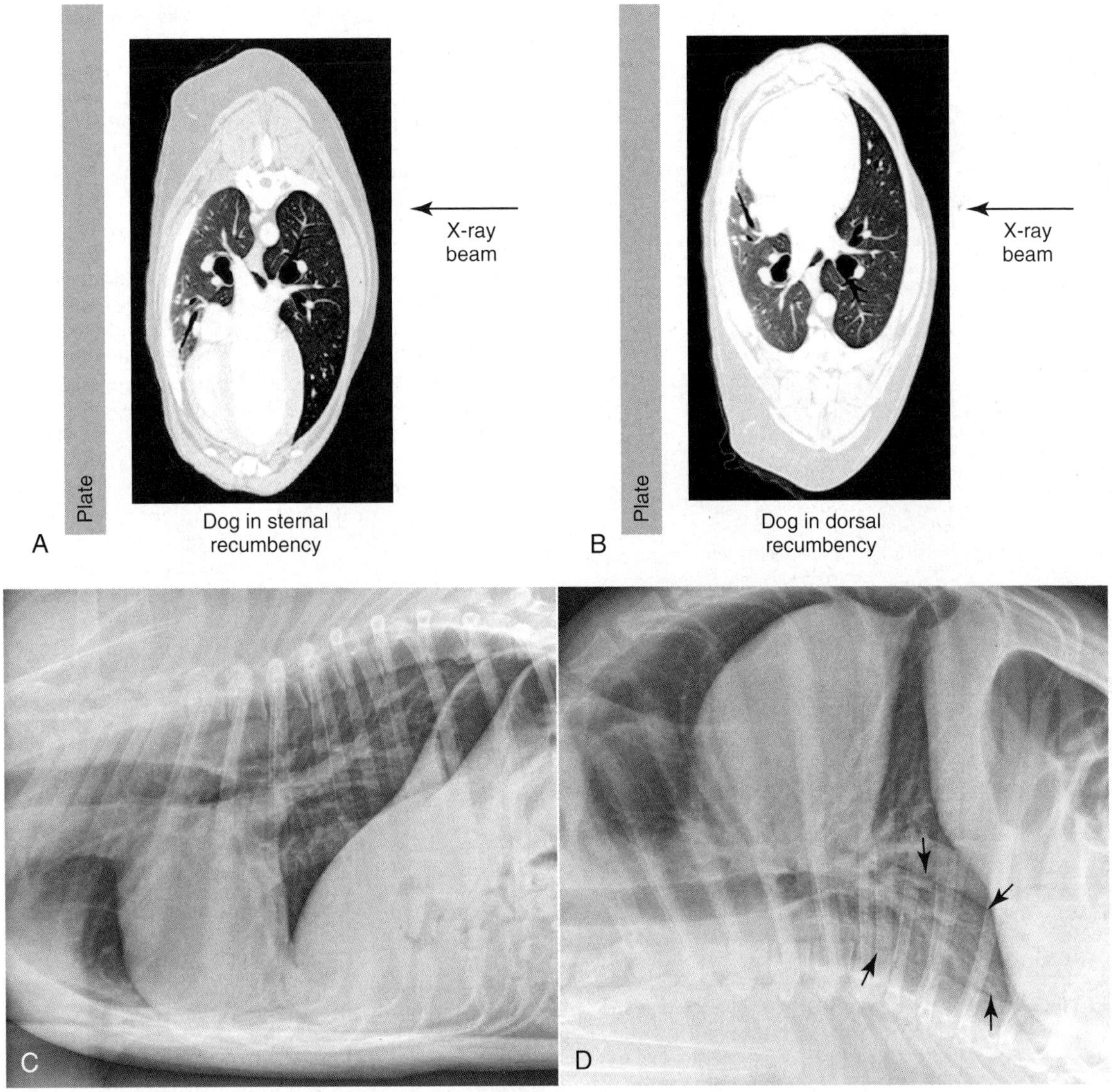

Fig. 28.6 Horizontal-beam lateral thoracic radiographs. **A,** Geometry for acquiring a horizontal-beam lateral thoracic radiograph with a dog in sternal recumbency. This is the body position used for a conventional dorsoventral (DV) radiograph, but the plate would be beneath the dog, with the x-ray beam striking the dorsal surface of the dog. **B,** Geometry for acquiring a horizontal-beam lateral thoracic radiograph with a dog in dorsal recumbency. This is the body position used for a conventional ventrodorsal (VD) radiograph, but the plate would be beneath the dog with the x-ray beam striking the ventral surface of the dog. **C,** Radiograph made with geometry illustrated in **A** with the dog in sternal recumbency. Note the absence of recumbency-associated atelectasis in the dependent ventral aspect of the lung. **D,** Radiograph made with geometry illustrated in **B** with the dog in dorsal recumbency. There is a small amount of atelectasis of the dependent caudal-dorsal aspect of the lung (*black arrows*) but not to the extent seen in the dependent lung in a dog in lateral recumbency (compare with Fig. 28.5B). In **D,** note that the caudal lobe pulmonary vessels are surrounded by atelectasis. This will cause silhouetting and render them more difficult to identify in the VD view compared with the DV view.

Ancillary Factors

The body habitus and presence of cutaneous lesions are ancillary factors that have a significant effect on the appearance of canine and feline thoracic radiographs.

Body Habitus

The volume of extrathoracic soft tissue will influence the overall radiographic opacity of the lung (Fig. 28.17), and can result in overdiagnosis of lung disease. The opacity created by excessive tissue in the body wall will be especially problematic with film-screen technology, because the contrast resolution of the film-screen system is not capable of compensating for the opacity created by this tissue (Fig. 28.18).

Intrathoracic fat accumulation can also be problematic. One common example is an accumulation of mediastinal fat being

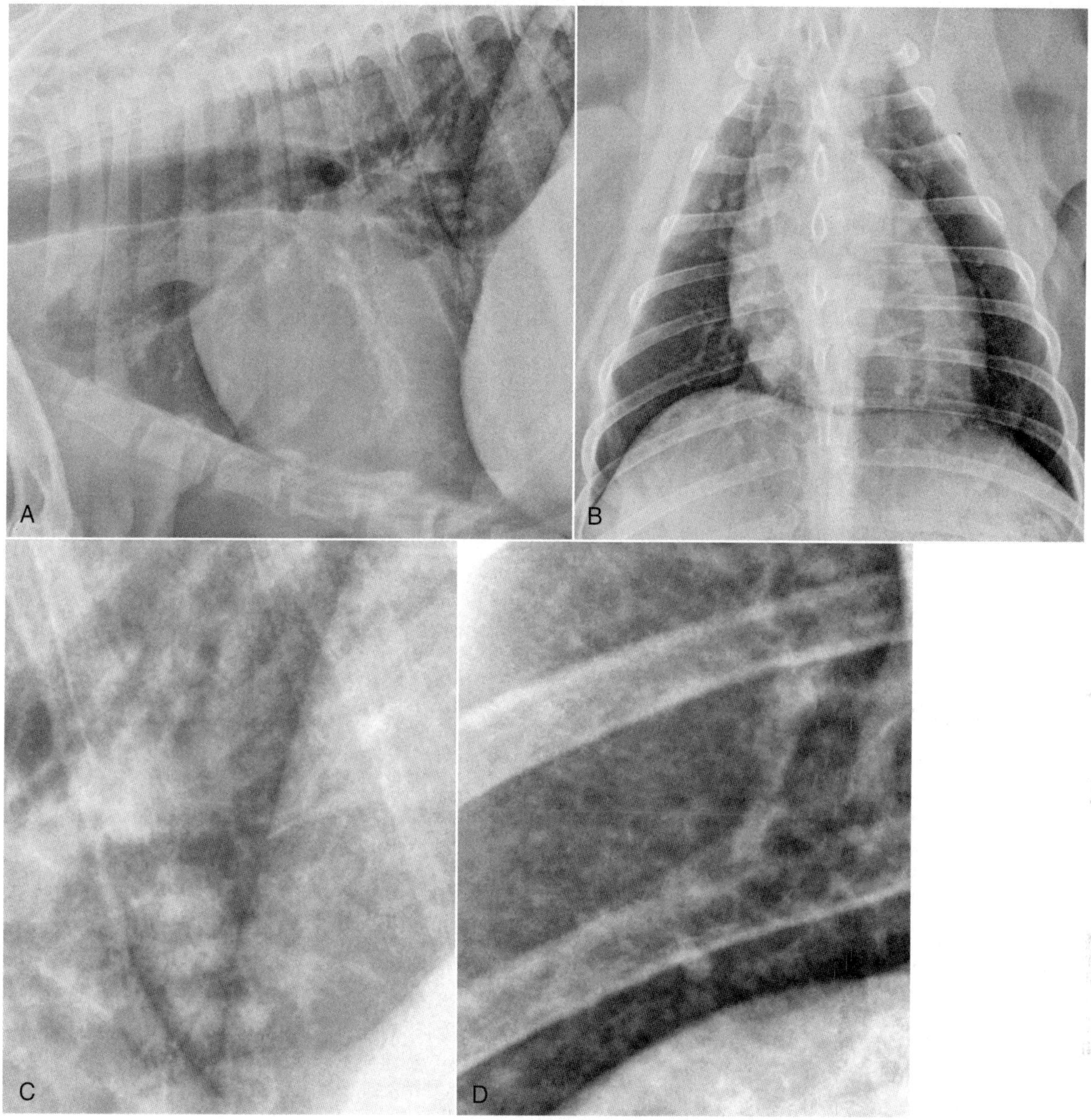

Fig. 28.7 Left lateral **(A)** and dorsoventral (DV) **(B)** thoracic radiographs of a dog, and close-up views of the dorsocaudal lung field from the lateral radiograph **(C)** and the right-caudal lung field from the DV radiograph **(D)**. The increased atelectasis that occurs in lateral views results in an overall increased opacity to the lungs **(A and C).** In the DV projection, where lungs are better aerated, they are more radiolucent **(B and D)**, confirming that the increased pulmonary opacity seen in the lateral view was an artifact of poor ventilation. The increased lung opacity commonly encountered in lateral views is often misinterpreted as lung disease.

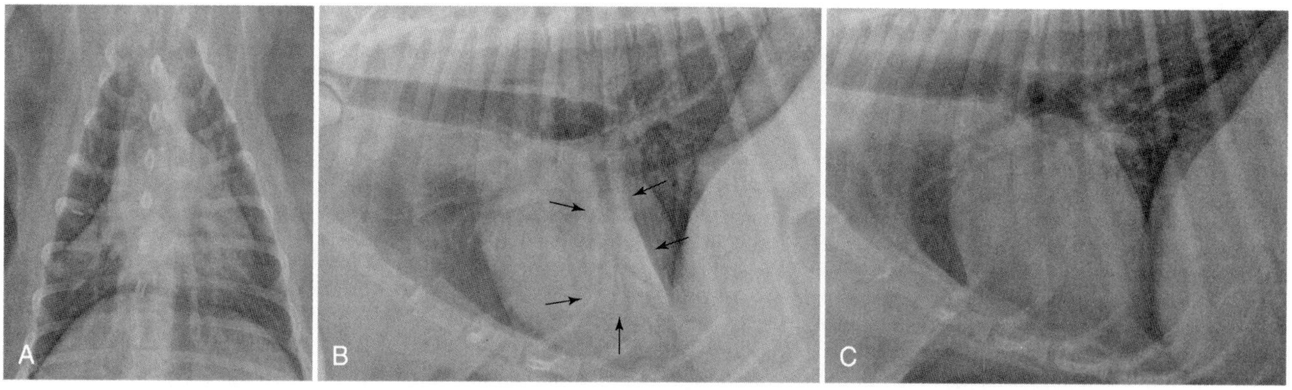

Fig. 28.8 **A,** Dorsoventral (DV) radiograph of a dog with pneumonia in the right middle lung lobe. **B,** Left lateral radiograph. Superimposed on the cardiac silhouette are multiple air bronchograms created by the alveolar nature of the disease in the right middle lung lobe (*black arrows*). The lung lesion is highly conspicuous in this view because the pneumonia is in the upper, nondependent, lung surrounded by aerated lung to provide contrast. **C,** Right lateral radiograph. The pneumonia is in the down, dependent, lung, which is atelectatic. The increased opacity of the atelectatic lung silhouettes with the pneumonia, and it is not visible.

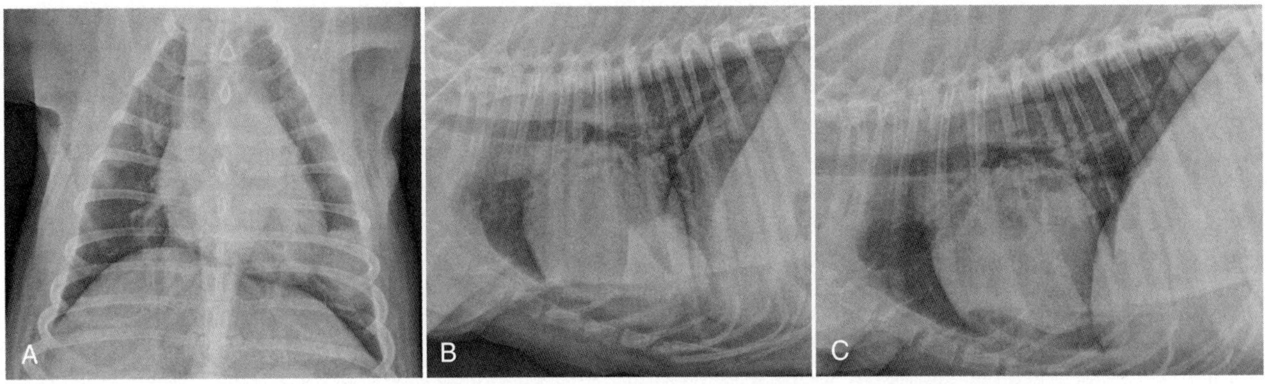

Fig. 28.9 **A,** Dorsoventral (DV) radiograph of a dog with a large mass in the left caudal lung lobe. **B,** Right lateral radiograph of the same dog. The mass is in the up, nondependent, lung and surrounded by aerated lung, making is highly visible. **C,** Left lateral radiograph of the same dog. The mass is now in the collapsed down, dependent, lung and is not visible because of silhouetting by the surrounding atelectatic lung.

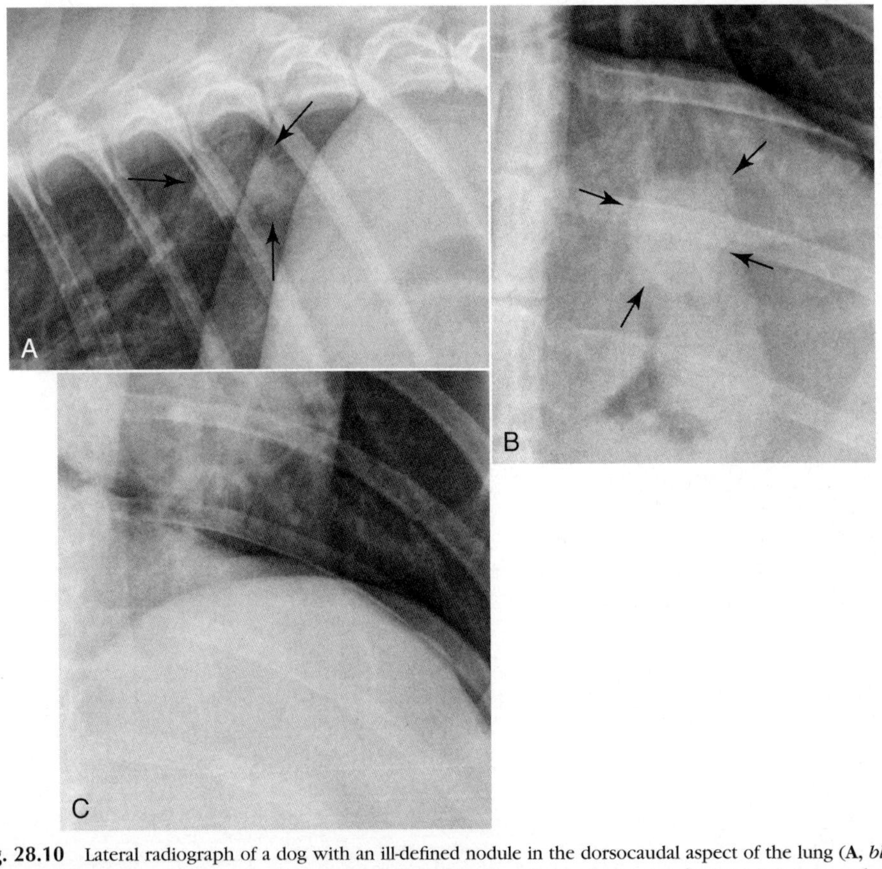

Fig. 28.10 Lateral radiograph of a dog with an ill-defined nodule in the dorsocaudal aspect of the lung (**A,** *black arrows*). This nodule is clearly seen in a dorsoventral (DV) view (**B,** *black arrows*), because it is surrounded by aerated lung. The nodule is not visible in the ventrodorsal (VD) view **(C)**, because it is surrounded by atelectatic lung in the dependent (dorsal) aspect of the thorax.

misinterpreted as a mediastinal mass in VD or DV radiographs (Fig. 28.19). This is particularly common in brachycephalic dogs. In contrast to a large mediastinal mass, mediastinal fat does not lead to tracheal deviation or lateral rounding of the mediastinal contour. Mediastinal fat can also give the false impression of cardiac enlargement, particularly right-sided cardiomegaly. Often, in this instance, the fat is not visible per se, and the distinction between cardiomegaly and adjacent fat may have to be made using echocardiography or with computed tomography (CT) (Fig. 28.20).

Cutaneous Lesions

Normal thoracic wall structures, or lesions superimposed on the thorax, can appear as a pulmonary lesion. Common

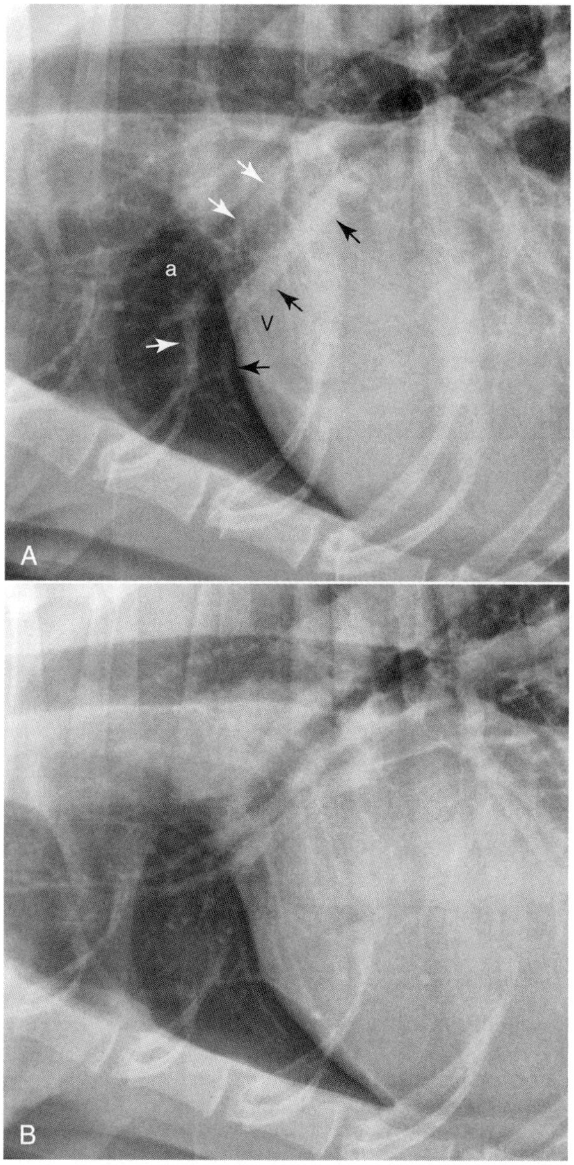

Fig. 28.11 Left (**A**) and right lateral (**B**) radiographs of the cranioventral aspect of the thorax of a dog. The right cranial lobe pulmonary artery (*a, white arrows*) and vein (*V, black arrows*) can be distinguished clearly in the left lateral view. In the right lateral view, these two vessels are superimposed with each other and with the vessels from the left cranial lobe and cannot be identified individually. In **A**, the pulmonary artery and vein in the left cranial lobe are dorsal to the right cranial lobe vessels.

examples include summation opacities created by nipples (Fig. 28.21), cutaneous lesions such as a pedunculated tumor or engorged tick (Fig. 28.22), and costochondral junctions (Fig. 28.23). All of these can be misinterpreted as a pulmonary nodule. The basis of cutaneous lesions creating such a conspicuous opacity was discussed in Chapter 6.

INTERPRETATION PARADIGM

Like in all body systems, an organized approach to radiographic interpretation of the thorax is needed. This begins with an overview of technique, according the following questions, followed by evaluation for abnormalities.

- Are the radiographic views adequate, and are all of the views that are needed present?
- Is the positioning adequate?
- Are the images overexposed or underexposed?
- Were the images acquired using an antiscatter grid? Should an antiscatter grid have been used?
- Was the patient sedated or anesthetized for the radiographic examination, and did this affect the appearance of the images?
- Were the images obtained at peak inspiration or during expiration, and did this affect pulmonary opacity?
- What is the breed and body habitus of the patient, and how is this going to affect the appearance of the images?
- Were the images acquired with a vertically directed x-ray beam with the cassette in an x-ray table, or was a horizontally directed x-ray beam used with the cassette in a mobile or a wall-mounted cassette holder?
- Are there morphologic aspects of the patient that are going to influence the appearance of the radiographs? These include things like a missing limb or cutaneous nodules or masses that will be superimposed on the thorax.

After these variables have been considered, the images can be scrutinized for abnormalities. The roentgen sign and DAMNITV (degenerative, anomalous, metabolic, neoplastic, infectious [inflammatory, immune], traumatic, vascular) methods described in Chapter 6 should be used. Inexperienced interpreters often begin by looking at the lungs, because a suspicion of pulmonary disease is a common reason that thoracic radiographs are acquired. This is a mistake and will lead to other lesions being overlooked. The search pattern is also important. A random search pattern may be appropriate for experienced radiologists, but beginning interpreters should develop an organized approach to searching radiographs.[8] Having a mental checklist to guide the order of interpretation will reduce the number of errors (Box 28.1).

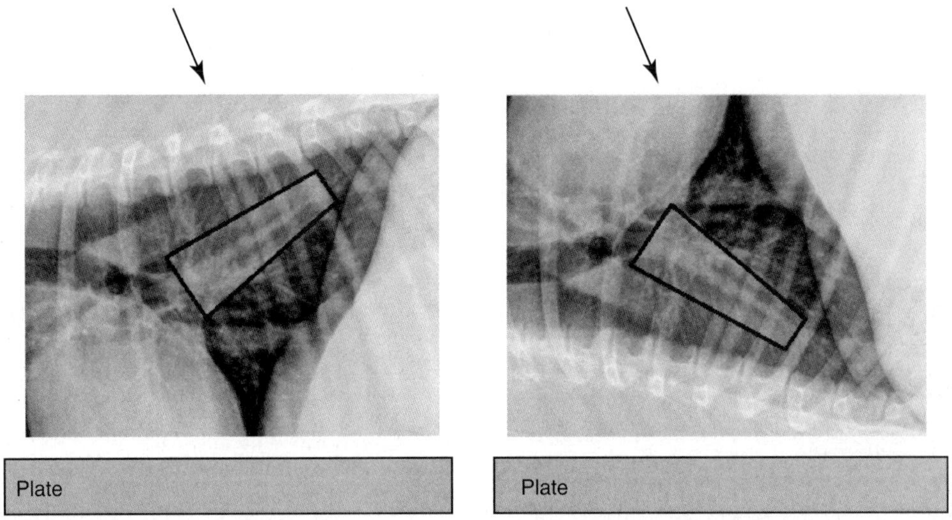

Fig. 28.12 Effect of dorsal versus sternal recumbency on the orientation of the caudal lobe pulmonary vessels with respect to the primary x-ray beam. As the center of the primary x-ray beam is approximately at the level of the cardiac silhouette, the beam (*arrows*) will be diverging at the level of the caudal lobe pulmonary vessels. In the *left panel*, the dog is positioned for a dorsoventral (DV) radiograph. In this view the caudal lobe vessels, shown *outlined,* are nearly perpendicular to the x-ray beam and will not be distorted. In the *right panel*, the dog is in position for a ventrodorsal (VD) radiograph. In this view, the caudal lobe vessels, shown *outlined*, are at an angle with respect to the primary x-ray beam and will be distorted. There is also more surrounding atelectasis in the VD view, which further reduces visibility of the caudal lobe vessels.

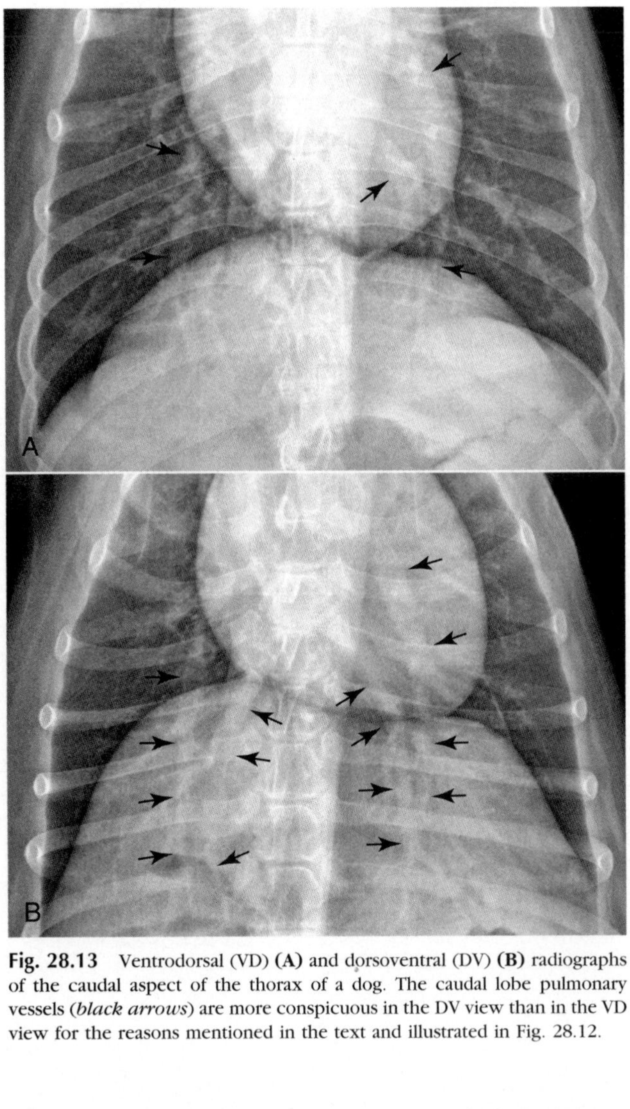

Fig. 28.13 Ventrodorsal (VD) **(A)** and dorsoventral (DV) **(B)** radiographs of the caudal aspect of the thorax of a dog. The caudal lobe pulmonary vessels (*black arrows*) are more conspicuous in the DV view than in the VD view for the reasons mentioned in the text and illustrated in Fig. 28.12.

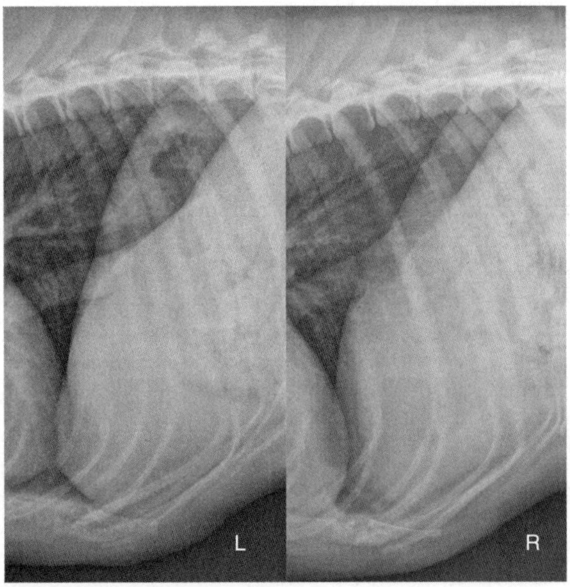

Fig. 28.14 Left (L) and right (R) lateral radiographs of the caudal thorax of a dog. In the left lateral view, the dorsally located diaphragmatic crura diverge more than in the right lateral view. Also, in the left lateral view, the left crus is more cranial, and the caudal vena cava is superimposed on it before joining the right crus that contains the caval hiatus. In the right lateral view, the right crus of the diaphragm that contains the caval hiatus is more cranial, and the caudal vena cava joins this more cranial crus.

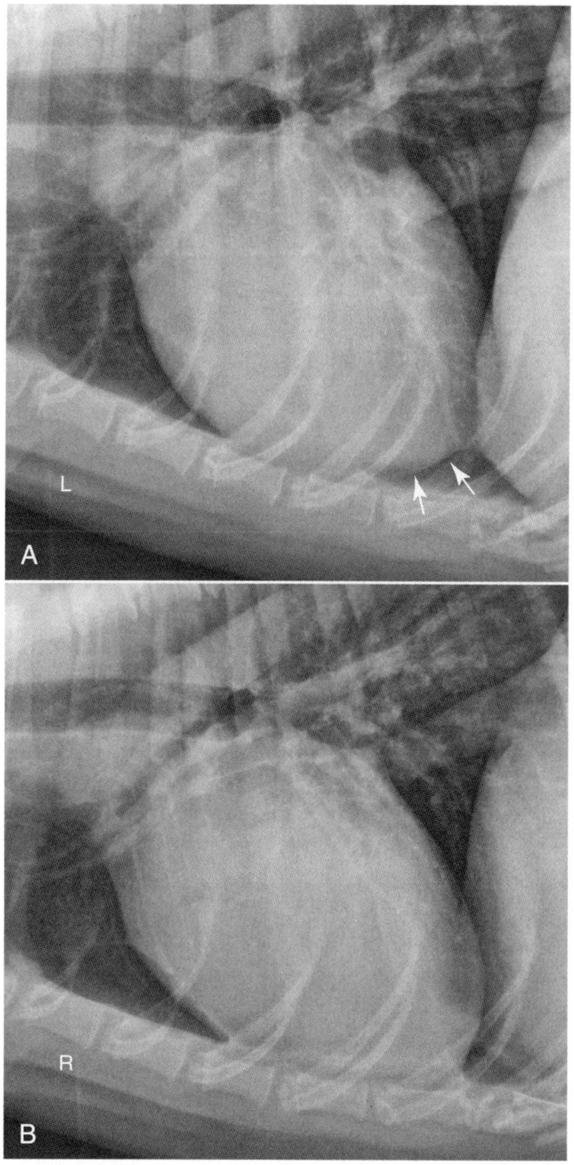

Fig. 28.15 Left lateral **(A)** and right lateral **(B)** thoracic radiographs of the cardiac silhouette in a dog. In the left lateral view, the cardiac silhouette will usually appear slightly rounder, and there will be some slight separation of the cardiac apex from the sternum (*white arrows* in **A**).

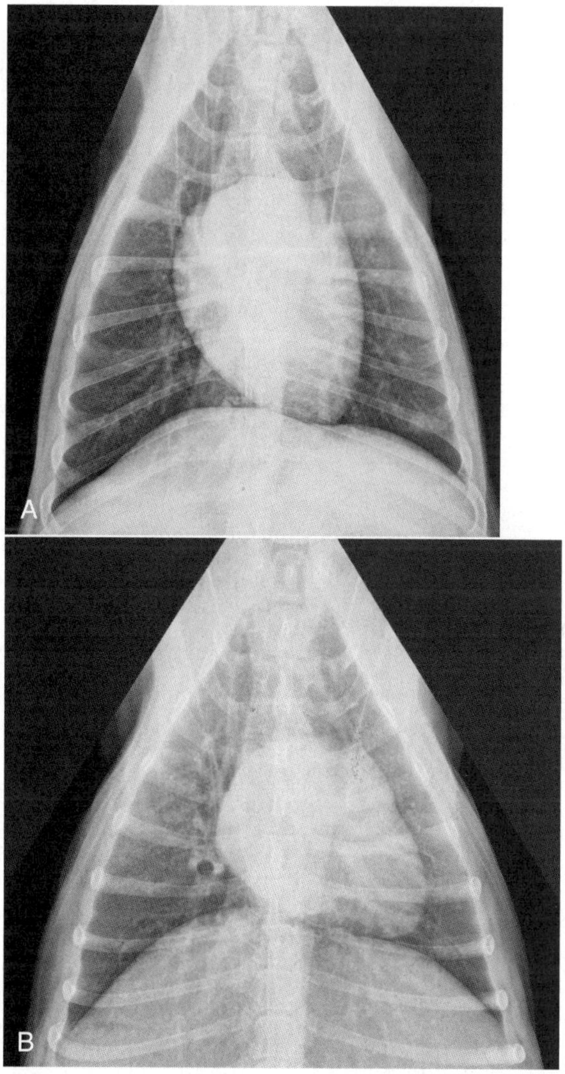

Fig. 28.16 Ventrodorsal (VD) **(A)** and dorsoventral (DV) **(B)** thoracic radiographs. In the DV radiograph, the diaphragm is displaced cranially where it contacts the heart and pushes it into the left hemithorax. The cardiac silhouette is also smaller and rounder, because it is more upright in the thoracic cavity. In a DV view, the cranial excursion of the diaphragm also impinges on the territory of the accessory lung lobe and interferes with the evaluation of that region.

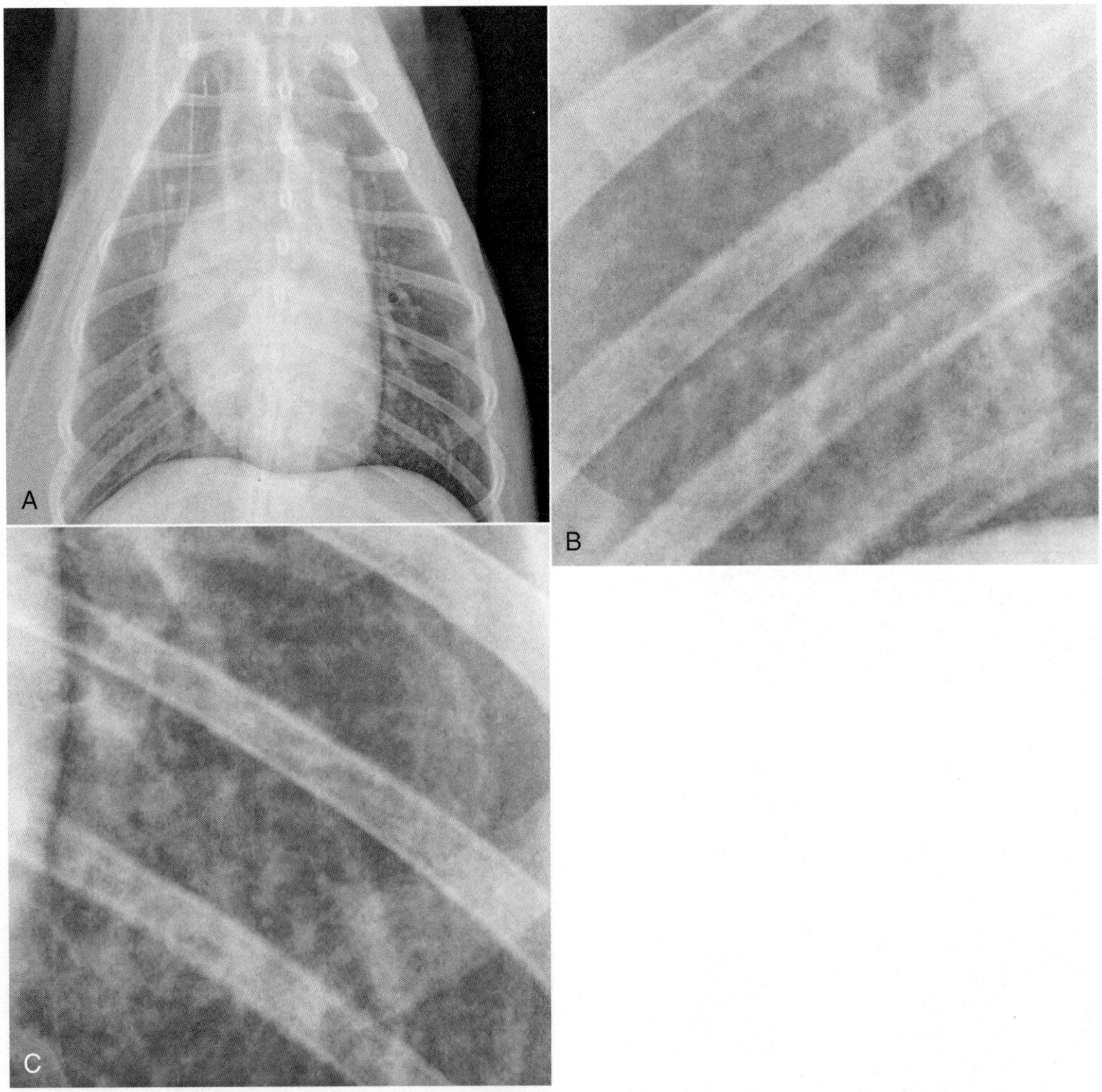

Fig. 28.17 **A,** Ventrodorsal (VD) thoracic radiograph of a dog having undergone a left forelimb amputation. The soft tissues of the left thoracic wall are thinner due to the missing limb and secondary disuse atrophy. This leads to a difference in opacity of the left vs. right hemithorax that can be misinterpreted as a difference in lung opacity. In close-up views from the right **(B)** and left **(C)** caudal lobes, the lung opacity appears increased on the right side. This illustrates how the amount of thoracic wall soft tissue can influence the radiographic opacity of the lung. The right lung could easily be misdiagnosed as having an increase in interstitial opacity.

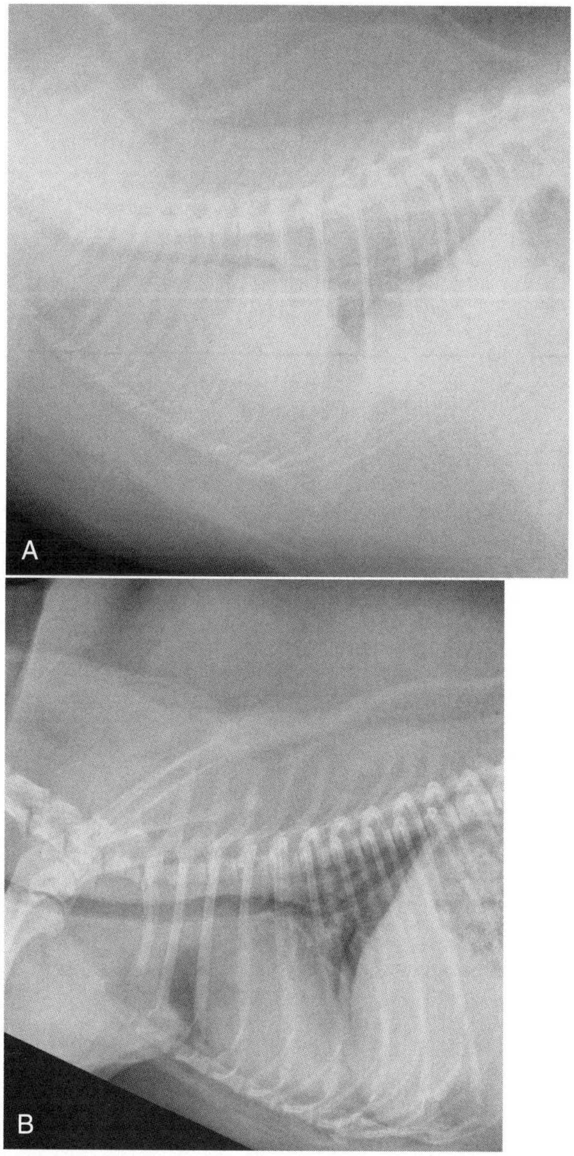

Fig. 28.18 Lateral thoracic radiographs of a morbidly obese cat made using a film-screen system **(A)** and of a morbidly obese dog made using a direct digital system **(B)**. The contrast resolution of the film-screen system cannot accommodate for the huge volume of fat, and the lungs cannot be assessed. With the digital system the lungs remain relatively radiolucent, but there will still be some background opacity created by the fat that could be misinterpreted as lung disease.

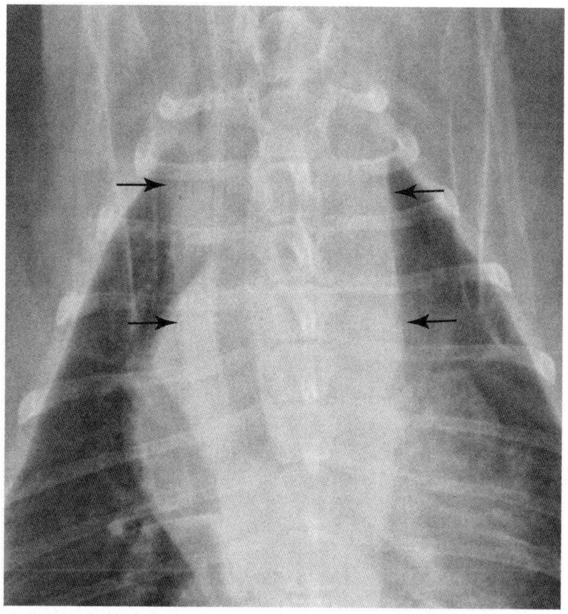

Fig. 28.19 Ventrodorsal (VD) radiograph of an obese dog. Fat deposition causes widening of the cranial mediastinum (*black arrows*), which could be misinterpreted as a mass. Notice, however, that the outlines of the cranial mediastinum are not rounded. There was no evidence of a cranial mediastinal mass in the lateral projections.

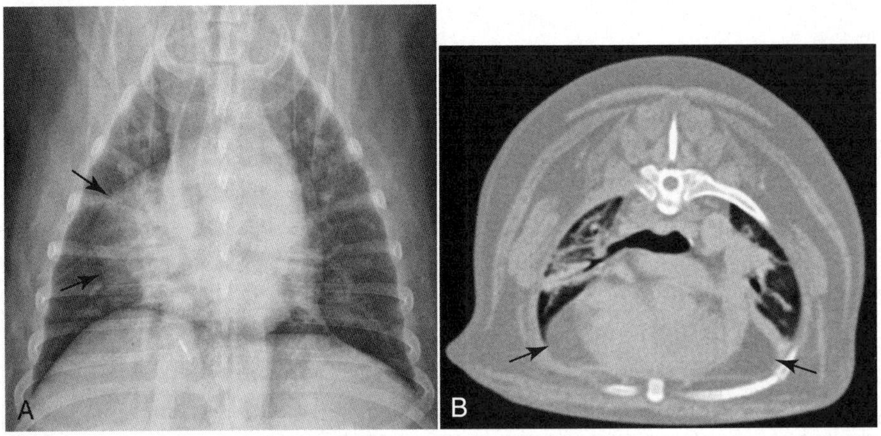

Fig. 28.20 **A,** Ventrodorsal (VD) thoracic radiograph. The cardiac silhouette is enlarged, especially on the right side (*black arrows*). **B,** Computed tomography (CT) image of the same patient. There is a large volume of mediastinal fat (*black arrows*) that is the cause of the enlargement of the cardiac silhouette in the radiograph.

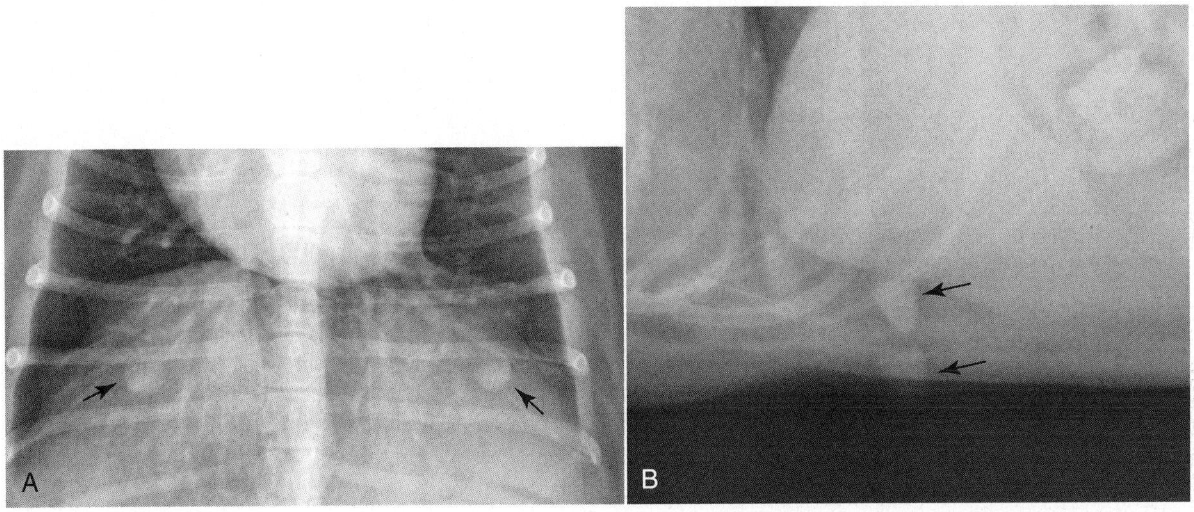

Fig. 28.21 **A,** Ventrodorsal (VD) radiograph of the caudal aspect of the thorax of a dog with two opacities that appear as pulmonary nodules (*black arrows*). These are caused by enlarged nipples on the cranial abdominal mammary glands. The bilaterally symmetric nature of these opacities would be unusual for pulmonary nodules, and enlarged nipples can be seen in the lateral view (*black arrows* in **B**). If the enlarged nipple is unilateral and cannot be seen in the lateral view, the body wall should be examined clinically. If necessary, a radiopaque marker can be applied to the nipples on the patient and the radiograph repeated to determine if the questionable lung opacity is caused by a nipple or by a pulmonary nodule.

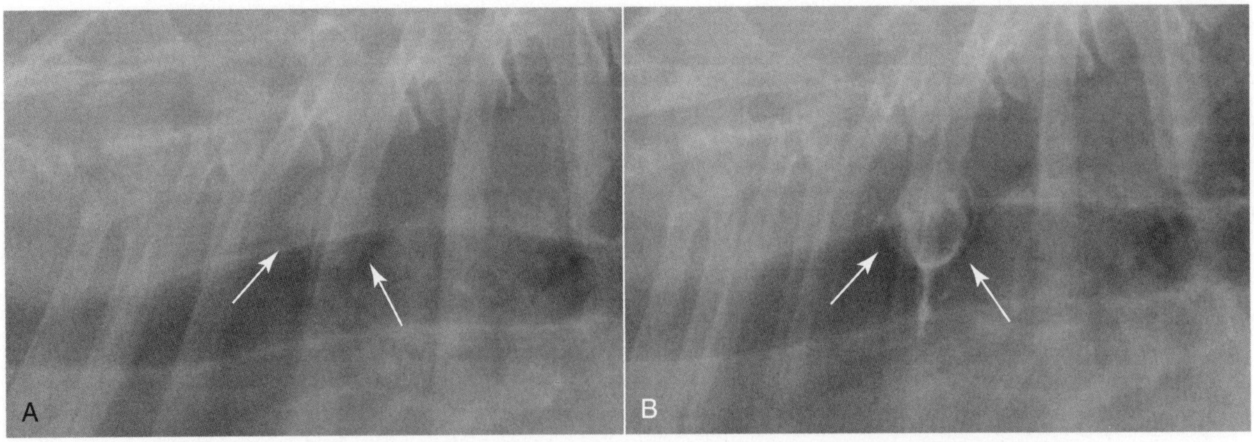

Fig. 28.22 **A,** Close-up from a right lateral thoracic radiograph of a dog where there is a nodular opacity that has the appearance of a pulmonary nodule (*white arrows*). A cutaneous nodule was discovered in a corresponding area on the thoracic wall and it was marked with a small amount of barium and the radiograph repeated. **B,** The barium is confined to the nodular opacity (*white arrows*), confirming that it is not a pulmonary nodule but a superimposition opacity from the cutaneous nodule.

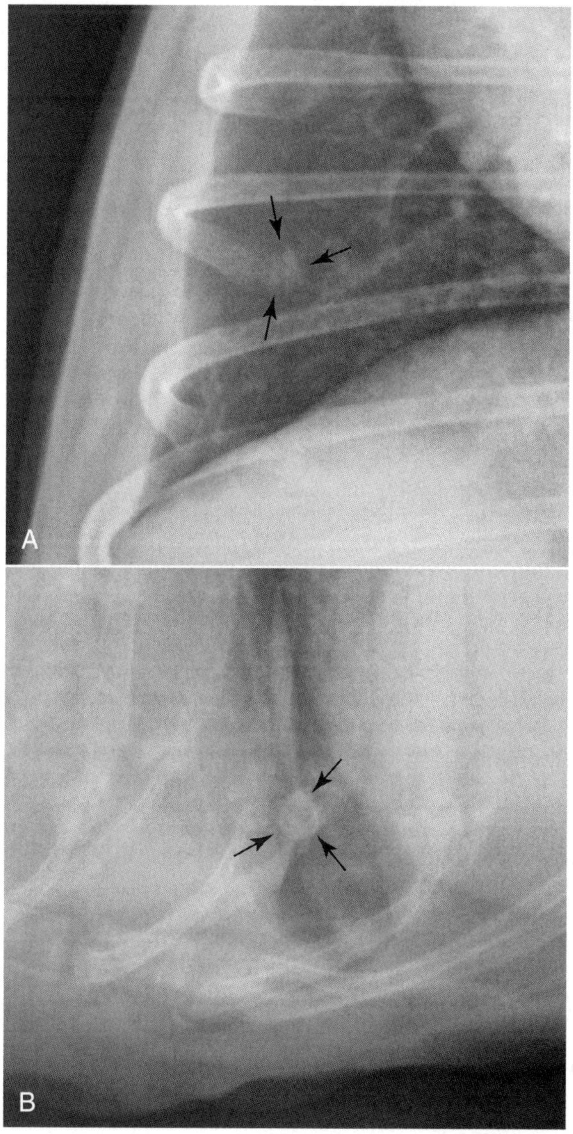

Fig. 28.23 Lateral **(A)** and ventrodorsal (VD) **(B)** radiographs of a dog with a nodular opacity (*black arrows*) that could be misinterpreted as a pulmonary nodule. In each radiograph, the suspicious opacity is located at the end of a rib and is caused by remodeling of the costochondral junction. This is a common change, especially in older dogs.

REFERENCES

1. Feeney D, Gordon B, Johnston G, et al. A 200 centimeter focal spot-film distance (FFD) technique for equine thoracic radiography. *Vet Radiol Ultrasound*. 1982;23(13).
2. Spencer C, Ackerman N, Burt J. The canine lateral thoracic radiograph. *Vet Radiol Ultrasound*. 1981;22:262.
3. Ober CP, Barber D. Comparison of two- vs. three-view thoracic radiographic studies on conspicuity of structured interstitial patterns in dogs. *Vet Radiol Ultrasound*. 2006;47(6):542–545.
4. Thrall D, Losonsky J. A method for evaluating canine pulmonary circulatory dynamics from survey radiographs. *J Am Anim Hosp Assoc*. 1976;12:457.
5. Brinkman EL, Biller D, Armbrust L. The clinical usefulness of the ventrodorsal versus dorsoventral thoracic radiograph in dogs. *J Am Anim Hosp Assoc*. 2006;42(6):440–449.
6. Carlisle C, Thrall D. A comparison of normal feline thoracic radiographs made in dorsal versus ventral recumbency. *Vet Radiol Ultrasound*. 1982;23(3).
7. Ruehl W, Thrall D. The effect of dorsal versus ventral recumbency on the radiographic appearance of the canine thorax. *Vet Radiol Ultrasound*. 1981;22(10).
8. Halvorsen JG, Swanson D. Interpreting office radiographs. A guide to systematic evaluation. *J Fam Pract*. 1990;31(6):602–610.

Box • 28.1

Checklist for Interpretation of Thoracic Radiographs

- Heart
- Major vessels
- Pulmonary vasculature
- Lung parenchyma
- Pleural space
- Mediastinum
- Esophagus
- Diaphragm
- Trachea
- Thoracic wall and bones
- Visible portion of neck
- Cranial abdomen

ELECTRONIC RESOURCES

Additional information related to the content in Chapter 28 can be found online at eBooks.Health.Elsevier.com

- Chapter Quiz

CHAPTER 29

Canine and Feline Larynx and Trachea

Randi Drees

ANATOMIC CONSIDERATIONS: NORMAL ANATOMY

The upper respiratory system comprises the air-filled pharynx, the larynx, and trachea. Typically, the pharynx has the widest lumen, followed by the larynx and the trachea, which is slightly smaller in diameter.

Pharynx: The soft palate divides the pharynx into the dorsally located nasopharynx and ventrally located oropharynx. The caudally adjacent larger laryngopharynx is divided from the nasopharynx by the palatopharyngeal arches, which form the soft tissue line extending caudodorsally from the soft palate, and from the oropharynx by the epiglottis (Fig. 29.1).[1] The piriform recesses are caudodorsally oriented extensions of the laryngopharynx.

Larynx: The epiglottis is usually surrounded by gas and extends to just overlap the tip of the soft palate dorsally or ventrally.[2] In larger dogs, the cuneiform process, which is the rostral portion of the arytenoid cartilage, is occasionally visible. The other laryngeal cartilages are represented by an indistinct soft tissue opacity superimposed on the laryngeal lumen. Gas-filled ventricular saccules are seen occasionally.

In older dogs, and even younger large-breed dogs, laryngeal cartilages may become mineralized, the cricoid cartilage often being the most evident (Fig. 29.2).[3] In brachycephalic dog breeds, the larynx can be positioned slightly more caudally compared to mesaticephalic dogs.[4]

Anatomic structures of interest surrounding the pharyngolarynx with potential secondary effects on the upper respiratory tract are:

- Rostrally: base of the tongue and mandibular lymph nodes
- Laterally: hyoid bones, mandibular and parotid salivary glands
- Caudodorsally: medial retropharyngeal lymph nodes and esophagus
- Caudoventrally: thyroid glands

The hyoid apparatus is paired, except for the basihyoid bone, which facilitates identification of unilateral abnormalities. The normal cricopharyngeus muscle representing the cranial esophageal sphincter sometimes appears as a distinct soft tissue structure dorsal to the larynx and can be misinterpreted as a soft tissue mass.

Trachea: The tracheal lumen is normally gas filled and the luminal diameter is similar between the cervical and thoracic regions. In large-breed dogs, it sometimes widens in the caudal cervical region. The diameter of the normal trachea can also vary mildly between inspiration and expiration. The ratio between tracheal diameter and thoracic inlet height is proportionally larger in dogs with greater body weight and smaller in brachycephalic breeds.[5] The cranial thoracic trachea is approximately parallel to the vertebral column and slightly closer to the vertebral column at the level of the thoracic inlet. In the mid-thorax, the trachea deviates ventrally relative to the vertebral column in most patients (Fig. 29.3). Tracheal rings may mineralize with age and become visible.

RADIOGRAPHIC TECHNIQUE

Pharyngolarynx

The lateral view with the head in neutral position and padding under the nose to avoid angulation is most useful.[6] Any degree

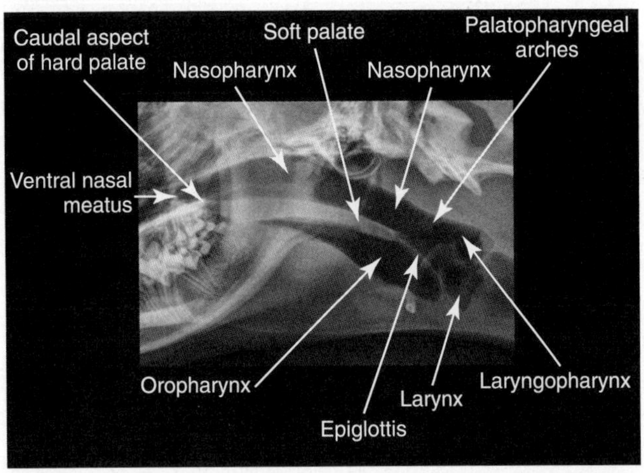

Fig. 29.1 Normal lateral canine pharyngeal/laryngeal region.

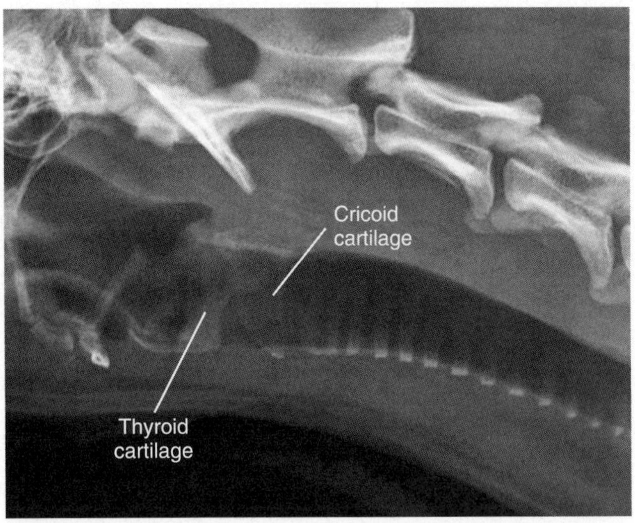

Fig. 29.2 Lateral radiograph of a 9-year-old dog. The laryngeal and tracheal cartilages are mineralized, which aids in their differentiation. This is a normal variant and not pathologic.

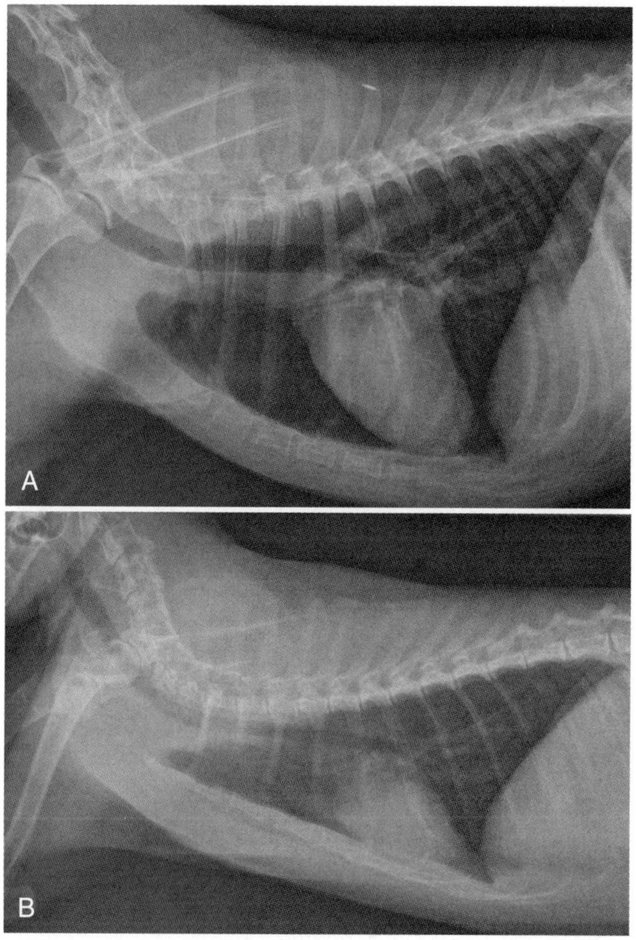

Fig. 29.3 Lateral radiographic view of the normal trachea of a dog **(A)** and a cat **(B)**. Note the similar tracheal luminal size in the cervical and thoracic region and ventral deviation of the trachea from the vertebral column in the thoracic region, in comparison to a relatively parallel position further cranially.

of obliquity results in underestimation of luminal diameter and overestimation of the surrounding soft tissue structures, such as the soft palate and laryngeal cartilages, which can mimic a mass. Superimposition of the ear cartilages with the pharyngolarynx should be avoided.

Ventrodorsal (VD) and oblique views are complementary to establish lesion laterality yet are limited by superimposition of the skull and cervical spine.

Technique parameters offering high-contrast images (relatively low kilovoltage peak [kVp] and high milliampere second [mAs] if using an analog system) selected according to the thickness of the ventral cervical soft tissues are recommended. If possible, the endotracheal tube should be withdrawn during radiography. Differentiation of the various structures is more difficult in obese patients because of narrowing of the air-filled compartments.

Trachea

The lateral view with the head mildly extended is most useful for evaluation of the trachea (see Fig. 29.3). The position of the thoracic portion of the trachea can vary with patient positioning: when the patient's head is ventroflexed, focal dorsal displacement of the trachea can mimic a cranial mediastinal mass (Fig. 29.4). Conversely, extreme extension of the neck can cause tracheal narrowing.

On a dorsoventral radiograph, the thoracic portion of the trachea is located on or curves mildly to the right of midline.[7] In brachycephalic breeds and obese dogs with mediastinal widening, the trachea curves more markedly to the right due to the larger amount of mediastinal fat, and this should not be confused with displacement from a mass, such as from a heart base tumor (Fig. 29.5).

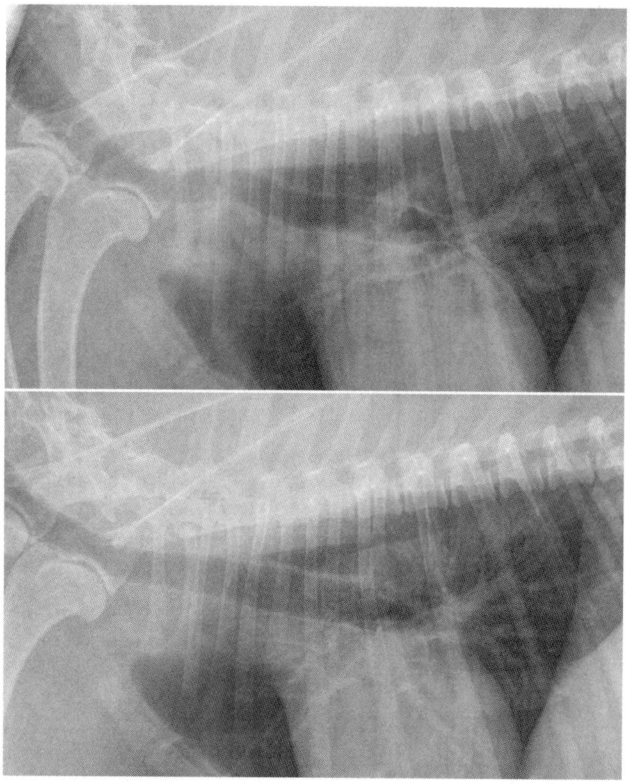

Fig. 29.4 Right lateral (*top*) thoracic radiograph with ventroflexion of the head: Patient positioning has affected the appearance of the trachea. There is focal dorsal elevation of the cranial aspect of the thoracic trachea that can be misinterpreted as being caused by a mediastinal mass. The trachea has a normal course in the left lateral (*bottom*) radiograph where the head is extended.

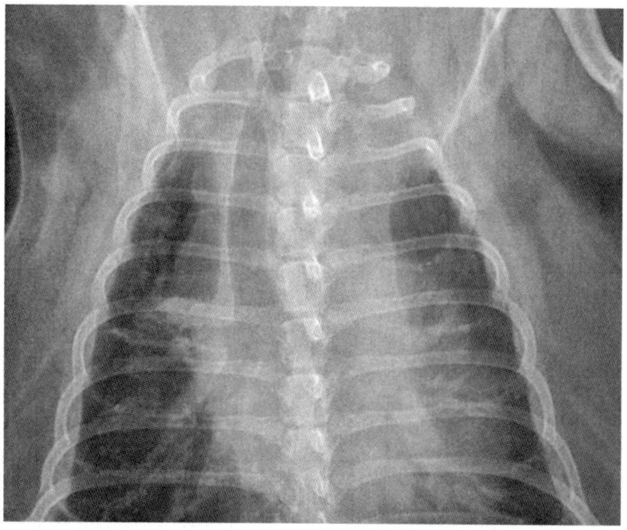

Fig. 29.5 Dorsoventral thoracic radiograph of an obese dog. There is rightward deviation of the thoracic trachea caused by the large amount of mediastinal fat. This is a normal variation and not significant.

RADIOGRAPHIC SIGNS OF DISEASE

Pharyngolarynx

Indications for radiography of the pharyngolarynx include respiratory difficulty and stertor caused by a suspected upper respiratory obstruction, ptyalism, gagging, dysphagia, dysphonia, a palpable mass or swelling, or a visible draining tract. Although ultrasound is useful for evaluating the soft tissues surrounding the upper respiratory tract, radiography is better suited for assessing their impact on the upper respiratory tract lumen. In addition, radiography can help screening for nonpalpable masses.[8] Ultimately, cross-sectional imaging such as computed tomography (CT) is often needed to assess the pharyngolarynx.

Masses

Pharyngolaryngeal masses may be extramural, mural, or intraluminal.

Extramural masses can originate from any of the structures surrounding the pharyngolarynx (Box 29.1) and may be neoplastic (Fig. 29.6, eFig. 29.1), infectious/inflammatory (Fig. 29.7, eFig. 29.2) traumatic, or hemorrhagic in nature. Radiographically, extramural masses usually present as soft tissue thickening which is poorly delineated from the surrounding soft tissues and may cause displacement and/or narrowing of the respiratory tract lumen. Their interface with the air-filled lumen is smoothly marginated and broad based. Their origin is determined based on their location relative to the pharyngolarynx.

Box • 29.1

Differential Diagnoses for Pharyngolaryngeal Masses

Extramural

- Lymph nodes: adenitis, neoplasia
- Salivary glands: sialocele, sialoadenitis, neoplasia
- Esophagus: neoplasia, granuloma
- Thyroid neoplasia (carcinoma) (including ectopic, base of the tongue)
- Malignant nerve sheath tumor
- Carotid body tumor
- Soft tissue trauma, penetrating wound and/or foreign body (hematoma, seroma, cellulitis, abscess)
- Coagulation disorder (hematoma)

Mural

- Neoplasia: adenocarcinoma, squamous cell carcinoma, lymphoma, plasmacytoma, rhabdomyoma, rhabdomyosarcoma, chondrosarcoma, granular cell tumor, mast cell tumor
- Tonsillitis, tonsillar neoplasia
- Granuloma/abscess: fungal (blastomycosis, cryptococcosis, pythiosis), granulomatous laryngitis (cats), lymphoplasmacytic inflammation (cats), chronic foreign body, *Cuterebra* migration
- Polyps: nasopharyngeal (cats), laryngeal
- Chondritis, laryngitis, viral papillomatosis
- Laryngeal cyst
- Brachycephalic syndrome: elongated, edematous soft palate

Intraluminal

- Foreign body (especially if soft tissue opacity)

Mural masses tend to be smaller when clinical signs appear, given that their impact on the respiratory lumen is more direct. Thus, they can be very difficult to identify radiographically, and endoscopy or direct pharyngolaryngoscopic examination as well as CT may be more useful.

- In cats, the two most common forms of pharyngolaryngeal mural neoplasia are lymphoma and squamous cell carcinoma, and in the larynx the arytenoid cartilage is most often involved.[9,10]
- In dogs, in the pharynx, squamous cell carcinoma (in particular tonsillar) is most common, with sarcoma, melanoma, and lymphoma also reported.[11–13] In the larynx, epithelial tumors and rhabdomyoma/rhabdomyosarcoma are most frequent, although mast cell tumor, various sarcomas, oncocytoma, plasma cell tumor, and melanoma are also seen.[10,14,15]

Superimposition of the normal laryngeal cartilage can make laryngeal masses difficult to detect. Laryngeal masses are

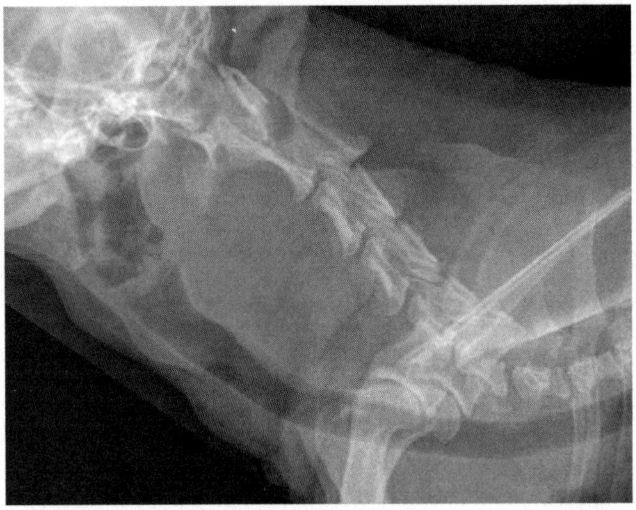

Fig. 29.6 Radiograph of a dog evaluated for a cervical mass. A mass located dorsal to the pharynx, larynx, and cervical portion of the trachea displaces these structures ventrally. There is effacement of the fascial planes in the cervical region. Carcinoma of salivary or sebaceous origin was diagnosed.

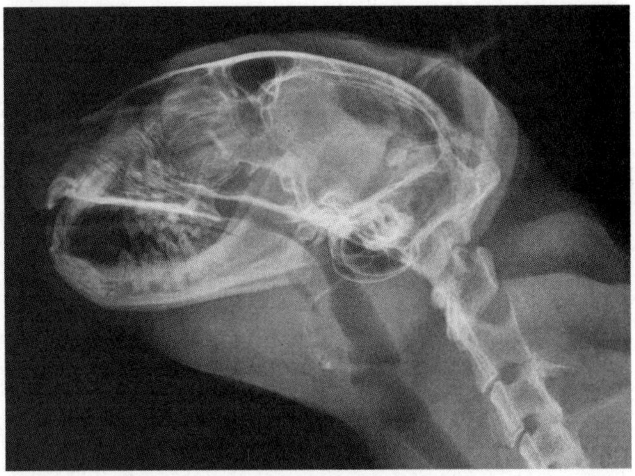

Fig. 29.7 Radiograph of an anesthetized cat with acute dyspnea and a submandibular mass. Ill-defined soft tissue thickening is present ventral and caudal to the mandibular and pharyngeal region, compatible with cellulitis. Complete reduction of the air-filled volume of the oropharynx and incomplete reduction in volume of the nasopharynx are present.

characterized primarily by an increase in soft tissue opacity with diffuse thickening, decreased margination of (pharyngo) laryngeal structures, and/or airway stenosis (Fig. 29.8).[9] They can also appear well defined (Fig. 29.9, eFig. 29.3) and/or lobulated if surrounded by air.[10] Horizontal epiglottic displacement can occur.[16]

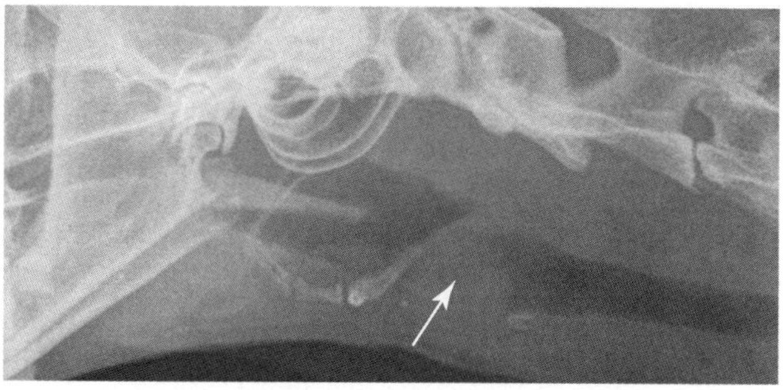

Fig. 29.8 Radiograph of a cat with inspiratory difficulty and change in meow. There is a round increased soft tissue opacity in the midventral aspect of the laryngeal lumen (*white arrow*). A laryngeal squamous cell carcinoma was diagnosed.

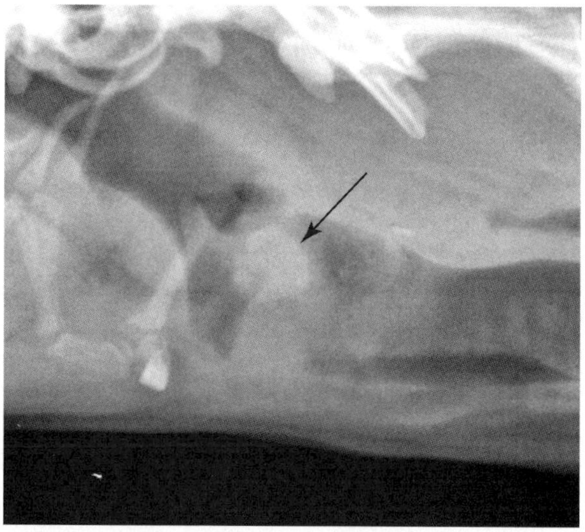

Fig. 29.9 Lateral radiograph of a dog with progressive inspiratory noise. There is a well-defined soft tissue mass (*black arrow*) at the dorsal aspect of the larynx. The diagnosis was benign hyperplastic fibroepithelial polyp.

Ectopic thyroid tissue can be found anywhere along the thyroglossal tract, from the base of the tongue to the base of the heart, and may undergo malignant transformation. Ectopic thyroid carcinoma resulting in effacement of the basihyoid bone and creating a ventral cervical mass has been recognized as a specific syndrome.[17] These tumors are strongly vascularized, heterogeneous masses with foci of mineralization and areas of colloid material accumulation. These tumors result in severe lysis of the basihyoid bone and infiltration of the laryngeal wall (Fig. 29.10, eFig. 29.4).

Trauma and Foreign Body

Pharyngolaryngeal trauma occurs most often because of a penetrating wound originating either internally from the upper respiratory tract or esophagus, due to a stick injury, or externally, such as a bite or gunshot wound, less commonly from blunt trauma. Soft tissue thickening representing swelling and/or a mass may be found with hematoma, cellulitis, granuloma, myositis, and/or abscess. Gas opacities in the subcutaneous tissues and between muscle and tissue planes represent emphysema if linear. Focal rounded gas accumulation may represent an abscess (Fig. 29.11). The sublingual area is reported as the most common entry site for stick injuries in dogs.[18] Emphysema has been reported in 83% of dogs with acute oropharyngeal stick injury and can extend to pneumomediastinum, pneumothorax, mediastinitis, and pleural effusion.[19] Pharyngeal diverticulum,[20] stenosis, cervical swelling, and draining sinus tracts[18] can be complications of trauma.

In addition to other surrounding bone structures, hyoid bone fracture and laryngeal cartilage fracture can occur, particularly when the region has been crushed.[21] These structures should be examined for symmetry and normal contour. Oblique projections may help evaluation of the hyoid apparatus. Hyoid bone fractures may be open to the upper respiratory tract and therefore contaminated.

Foreign bodies are visible when they are mineral or metallic, such as gunshot particles, needles, fishhooks, and bones. Plant material is usually only visible radiographically when large, containing (dry wood) or surrounded by gas (Fig. 29.12). CT[22] or magnetic resonance imaging (MRI)[23] can aid the localization of smaller plant material foreign bodies. In patients with a draining tract, fistulography with iodinated contrast medium can aid in foreign body detection.

Brachycephalic Syndrome

Brachycephalic syndrome comprises a complex of static and dynamic upper respiratory disorders in brachycephalic breeds

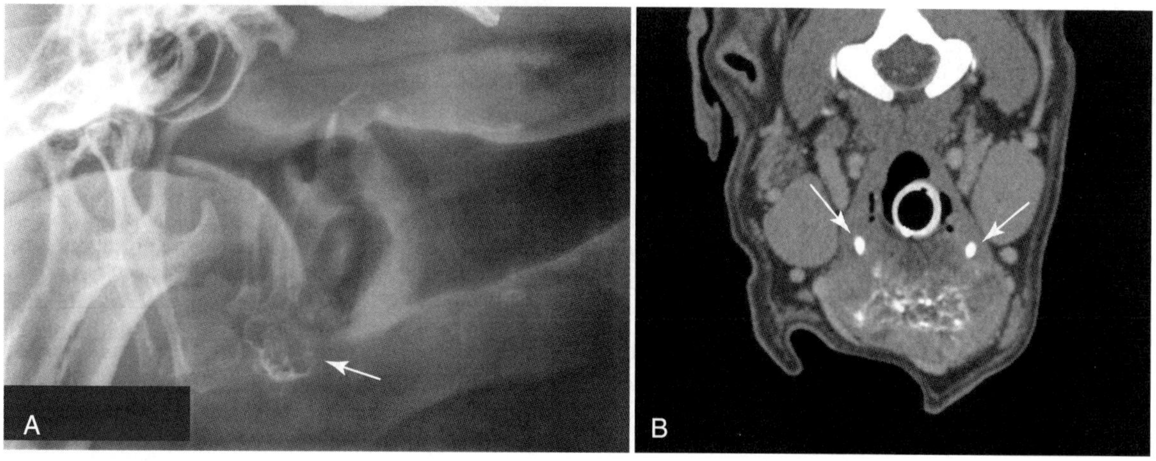

Fig. 29.10 **A,** Lateral cervical radiograph of a dog with an early ectopic basihyoid thyroid carcinoma. There is irregularity and expansion of the basihyoid bone. **B,** Transverse, precontrast, computed tomography (CT) image of the hyoid region of a dog with more advanced ectopic basihyoid thyroid carcinoma. There is a large mass with extensive mineralization that has caused effacement of the basihyoid bone. The normal paired thyrohyoid bones, just caudal to the location of the normal basihyoid bone, are visible and not involved (*white arrows*).

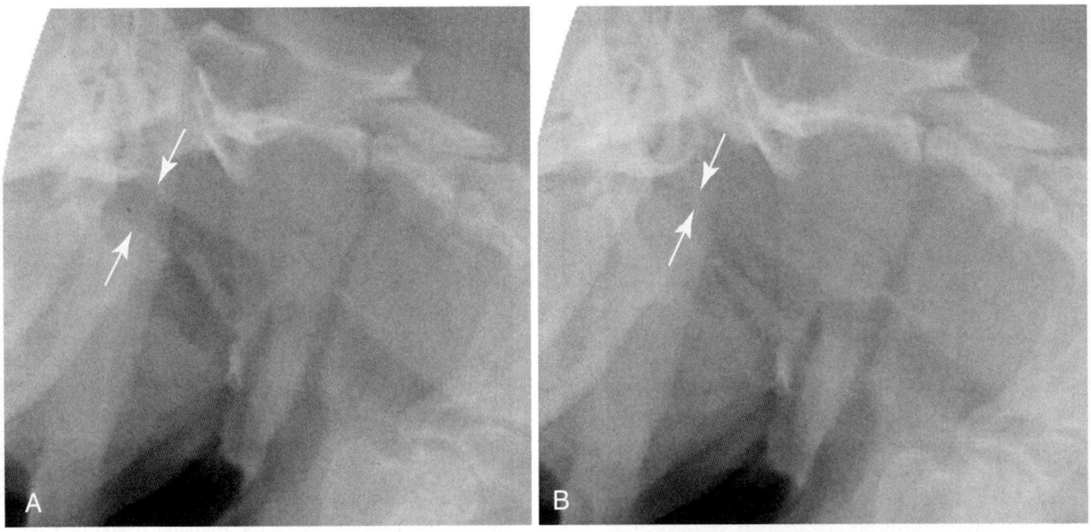

Fig. 29.17 Lateral dynamic digital radiographs of a pug with brachycephalic syndrome and dynamic pharyngeal collapse. In **A,** the nasopharynx is normally open, and the lumen is clearly visible (*white arrows*). In **B,** the lumen of the nasopharynx (*arrows*) is completely collapsed. Collapse was initiated at the beginning of inspiration and opening on the beginning of expiration.

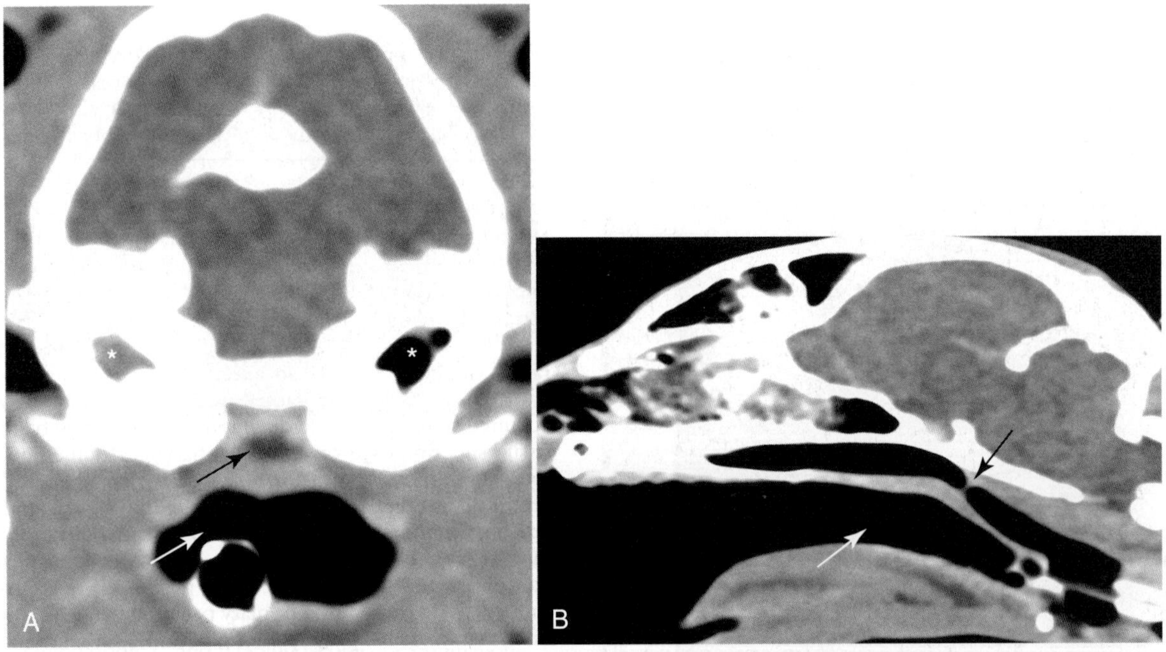

Fig. 29.18 Transverse plane **(A)** and sagittal reformatted **(B)** computed tomography (CT) image of a 9-month-old cat with intermittent and progressive episodes of reverse sneezing and increased respiratory effort. There is marked focal narrowing of the mid nasopharyngeal lumen (*black arrow*), consistent with nasopharyngeal stenosis. The oropharyngeal lumen is normal (*white arrow*). Endoscopy confirmed a most likely congenital soft tissue stricture in the region and additional inflammatory changes. The patient also had bilateral otitis media (*white asterisks*).

narrowing include thyroid carcinoma, cervical or thoracic lymphadenopathy, other mediastinal masses such as thymoma, heart base tumors, or, particularly in cats, mediastinal cysts. Heart base tumors tend to cause deviation of the trachea to the right.[45] Dorsal displacement of the caudal thoracic trachea and carina is seen with left-sided cardiomegaly and ventral displacement with tracheobronchial lymphadenomegaly (Table 29.1). Peritracheal or intramural hemorrhage from rodenticide toxicity[46] (Fig. 29.19) and a peripheral nerve sheath tumor[47] have been reported to cause tracheal luminal narrowing in the dog. Additionally, with persistent right fourth aortic arch, a mild-to-marked focal leftward displacement of the trachea is often seen on a dorsoventral radiograph.[7]

Mural tracheal masses are uncommon but when present are most often neoplastic. Benign tracheal tumors in dogs include osteochondroma, most commonly found in young dogs, followed by chondroma and leiomyoma.[10] Malignant tumors include lymphoma (cats particularly), sarcoma (fibrosarcoma, chondrosarcoma, histiocytic sarcoma), adenocarcinoma, squamous cell carcinoma, and plasmacytoma.[10,48] Other considerations are hematoma secondary to trauma or coagulation disorders including rodenticide toxicity, amyloidosis,[49]

Table • 29.1

Considerations for Radiographically Detectable Deviation of the Trachea in the Lateral Projection.

LOCATION OF DEVIATION	DIRECTION OF DEVIATION	CONSIDERATIONS
Cervical	Ventral	Thyroid mass Retropharyngeal lymphadenomegaly Vertebral/paravertebral mass
Cranial mediastinum	Dorsal	Cranial mediastinal mass (including cranial mediastinal lymphadenomegaly, thymoma, mediastinal cyst, etc.) For a complete list of mediastinal masses, please refer to Chapter 33. Neck position during radiography
Cranial mediastinum	Ventral	Neurogenic tumor Esophageal enlargement/mass
Heart base	Dorsal	Heart base mass Pulmonary artery enlargement Right atrial enlargement
Carina	Dorsal	Left atrial enlargement Tracheobronchial lymphadenomegaly (usually ventral but can be dorsal) Generalized cardiomegaly
Carina	Ventral	Tracheobronchial lymphadenomegaly

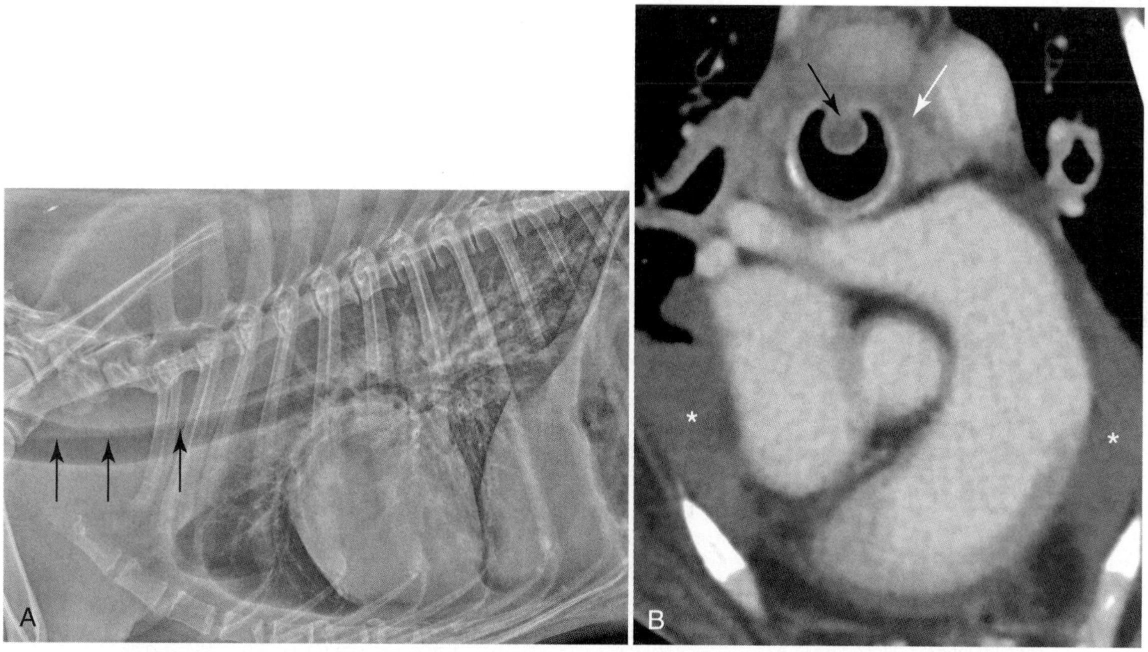

Fig. 29.19 Lateral radiograph **(A)** and transverse plane post contrast CT examination **(B)** of a dog presenting with productive frothy and hemorrhagic cough after rodenticide ingestion. There is a thin, soft tissue band superimposed over the dorsal aspect of the trachea (*black arrows*), which corresponded to submucosal hemorrhage in the dorsal tracheal membrane as seen on the CT examination as marked redundancy and thickening of the dorsal tracheal membrane. There is evidence of additional peritracheal hemorrhage (*white arrow*), mild pleural effusion (*asterisks*), and hemorrhagic pulmonary infiltrates.

inflammatory polyp,[50] and granuloma secondary to foreign body migration, mycobacterial infection, zygomycosis,[51] and parasitic disease. In particular, *Oslerus (Filaroides) osleri* granulomas can be seen near the carina in the dog, and aberrant tracheal *Cuterebra* migration has been reported in a cat.[52] Tracheal masses are usually solitary and distinct, protruding into the lumen, and are well seen because of the contrast provided by the surrounding air (Fig. 29.20).

Masses may be mineralized when they are of cartilage origin, such as osteochondromas.[10]

Foreign Bodies

Tracheal foreign bodies usually result from orotracheal aspiration, such as a tooth, kibble, stone (Fig. 29.21), bone, plant material, or a severed endotracheal tube. Rarely, foreign bodies can migrate from the surrounding soft tissues.[53–55] Young cats and hunting dogs are affected most commonly, possibly because of the small diameter of their trachea and the nature of their activity, respectively.[53,54] The negative contrast afforded by intraluminal tracheal air helps in the detection of both mineral and soft tissue opacity foreign bodies. Since inhaled foreign bodies are most often lodged at the carina, particular attention should be paid to this area (eFig. 29.7). As an alternative to bronchoscopy, fluoroscopic guidance of forceps can be used for tracheal foreign body retrieval.[54,55]

Rupture/Avulsion and Stenosis

Tracheal rupture is a tear in the tracheal wall or the tissues lining the tracheal wall, and may be caused by endotracheal intubation, a penetrating wound (dog bites particularly), blunt trauma, or a foreign body.[56–58] Iatrogenic rupture can be caused by a tube stylet, inappropriately sized endotracheal tube, rotation of the anesthetized patient without disconnecting the tube, and/or excessive dilatation of the tube cuff.[59] Subcutaneous emphysema and pneumomediastinum can be severe and are more readily identified than the actual tracheal tear, which may not be visible radiographically (Fig. 29.22).[57,59] Intratracheal fluid, mural hematoma, and stenosis are seen occasionally.[57]

Tracheal avulsion is a complete severance of the trachea, most commonly in intrathoracic location in cats, following blunt trauma with severe hyperextension of the head and neck. Paradoxically, patients are often presented 1 to 3 weeks following the traumatic event, when signs of pneumomediastinum and soft tissue emphysema have resolved.[60] Most commonly, there is complete circumferential tracheal wall discontinuity 1 to 4 cm cranial to the carina, resulting in focal, well-defined, spherical dilation of the tracheal lumen outlined by a thin, soft tissue opacity margin representing either intact tracheal adventitia or surrounding mediastinal tissue and termed *pseudoairway* (Fig. 29.23).[60,61] This finding is usually associated with stenosis of the tracheal lumen at the margins of the avulsed trachea.[60] Mainstem bronchial avulsion has also been reported.[62]

Stenosis and tracheal diverticulum are complications of the same causes that predispose to tracheal rupture/avulsion, in addition to tracheal surgery.[63,64] A focal, static area of tracheal narrowing or widening is seen. Stenosis can also be seen with neoplasia causing annular tracheal narrowing.[10]

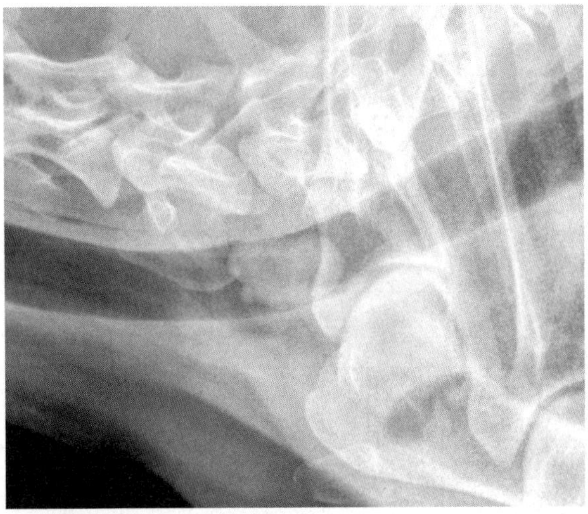

Fig. 29.20 Lateral radiograph of a dog with a small oval intratracheal mass at the thoracic inlet. Tracheal masses extending into the lumen will be sharply outlined by the contrast from surrounding air. This lesion was first thought to be a foreign body but was determined endoscopically to be a pedunculated mass. The diagnosis was B-cell tumor. As this radiograph is slightly oblique, one of the transverse processes of C6 is superimposed on the trachea, just cranial to the mass.

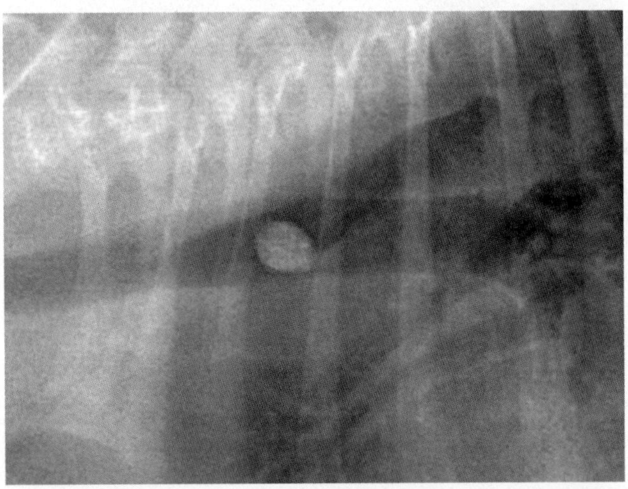

Fig. 29.21 Radiograph of a dog that developed a cough after being observed eating rocks. A well-defined granular mineral opacity structure is present in the caudal aspect of the trachea. A rock was removed endoscopically.

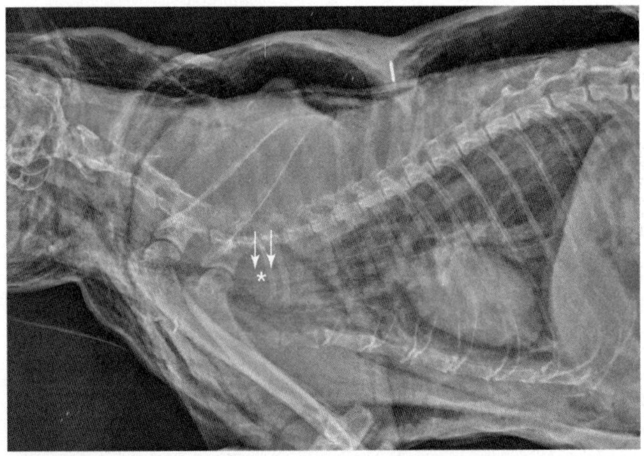

Fig. 29.22 Lateral radiograph of a cat presenting with extensive subcutaneous edema 3 days following a routine dental prophylaxis treatment. There is focal loss of the dorsal outline of the trachea (*white arrows*) and a fusiform soft tissue opacity (*white asterisk*) superimposed over the dorsal tracheal lumen, representing a markedly redundant (considered torn) tracheal membrane, indicating a tracheal tear. There is also extensive subcutaneous emphysema in the cervical and thoracic region, pneumomediastinum and partial atelectasis of the lungs.

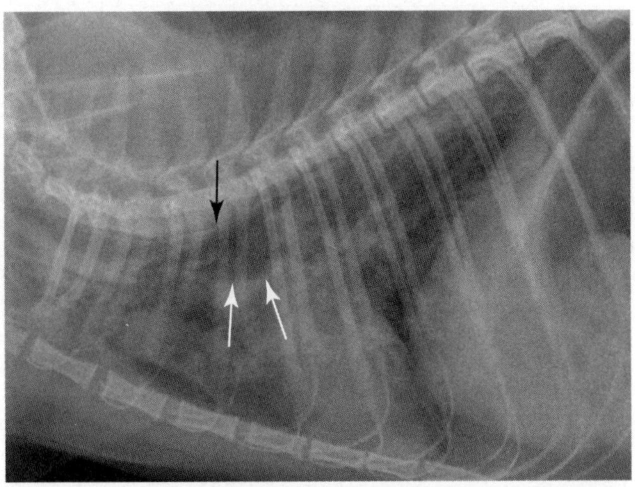

Fig. 29.23 Lateral radiograph of a cat 48 hours after being hit by car. There is a gas-filled saccular structure representing a pseudoairway (*white arrows* indicate ventral margin of sac). The caudal margins of the avulsed trachea can be seen (*black arrow*). There is also evidence of pneumomediastinum, pulmonary contusions, esophageal gas dilation, and aerophagia.

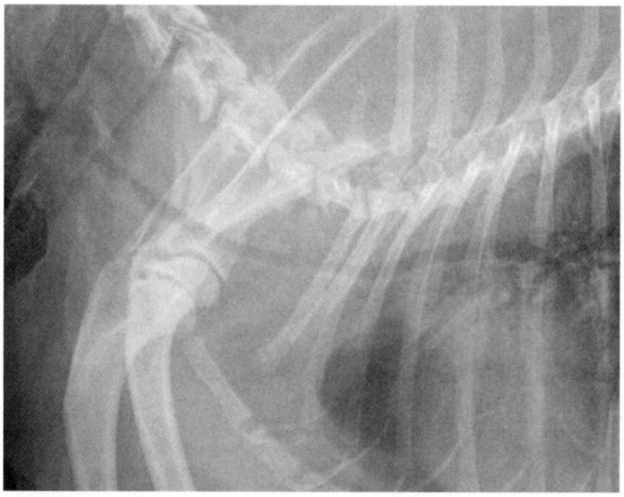

Fig. 29.24 Radiograph of a pug that presented for seizures and a cough. Generalized tracheal narrowing is present, measuring 8% of the height of the thoracic inlet, compatible with tracheal hypoplasia.

Hypoplasia

Tracheal hypoplasia is characterized by generalized reduction in tracheal diameter (Fig. 29.24) due to apposed or overlapping tracheal cartilages and a shortened or absent dorsal tracheal membrane. Approximately 39% of brachycephalic dogs with signs of brachycephalic airway obstruction syndrome have tracheal hypoplasia,[65] and in 10% of dogs, the diagnosis of tracheal hypoplasia is incidental.[66] The diagnosis is made more difficult by the fact that non-bulldog brachycephalic breeds, both with and without respiratory signs, have a smaller average tracheal-diameter-to-thoracic-inlet-height ratio (16% ± 3%) than nonbrachycephalic dogs (20% ± 3%). English bulldogs have an even smaller ratio (13% ± 4%).[5] The smallest ratio in asymptomatic bulldogs was 9%. More recently, tracheal-diameter to thoracic-inlet—height ratio was measured in 32 asymptomatic/grade 1 English bulldogs and found to be 17% ± 3% on radiographs and 26% ± 3% on CT, which is greater than previous measurements.[67] The ratio between tracheal diameter and cricoid cartilage height is also smaller for brachycephalic breeds.[5]

Normal tracheal diameter:thoracic inlet height in cats is 18% in domestic short-haired cats and 20% in Persians.[68] Tracheal hypoplasia has been reported in a kitten with mucopolysaccharidosis VII.[69]

Tracheitis

Generalized tracheal narrowing may be caused by severe tracheitis that leads to thickening of the tracheal mucosa. Tracheitis can be difficult to differentiate from tracheal hypoplasia, and the conditions can occur concurrently. Common causes of tracheitis are inhalation of toxic or chemical irritants, trauma, and upper respiratory infection (Fig. 29.25).

Redundant Tracheal Membrane

The presence of a dorsal tracheal luminal soft tissue opacity in dogs between the midcervical and midthoracic portions of the trachea can be caused by the dorsal tracheal membrane, representing the trachealis muscle and connective tissue bridging the gap between the aspect of the tracheal cartilages.[70] The dorsal tracheal membrane can usually be differentiated from the slightly opaquer dorsal tracheal wall. Visibility of the tracheal membrane dorsally does not necessarily indicate abnormal redundancy, but it can be caused by contraction, or invagination, of the membrane.[70] The opacity caused by a visible dorsal tracheal membrane can be dynamic, depending on phase of respiration (Fig. 29.26, Video 29.1). Its prominence can also be influenced by patient obliquity, displacement of the esophagus

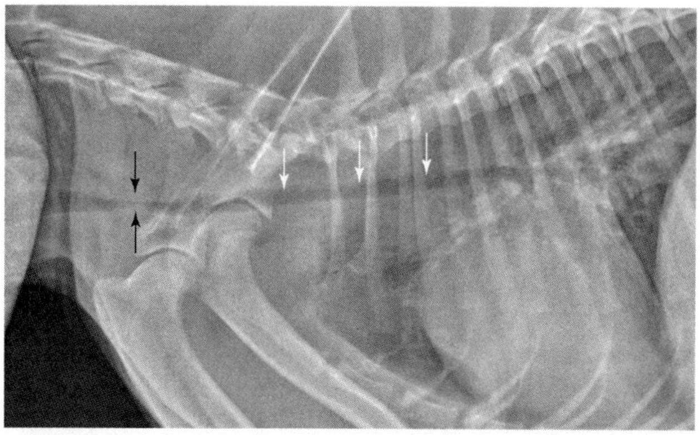

Fig. 29.25 Lateral radiograph of a dog with acute onset of cough following anesthesia for routine spay procedure. There is focal narrowing of the cranial cervical tracheal lumen due to luminal soft tissue thickening (*black arrows*) and an undulating soft tissue opacity superimposed on the dorsal tracheal lumen (*white arrows*) in the caudal cervical and thoracic trachea. Endoscopy confirmed marked inflammation and hemorrhage in the cranial cervical tracheal region, presumed due to trauma related to prior intubation, and associated moderate tracheal inflammation in the further caudal trachea.

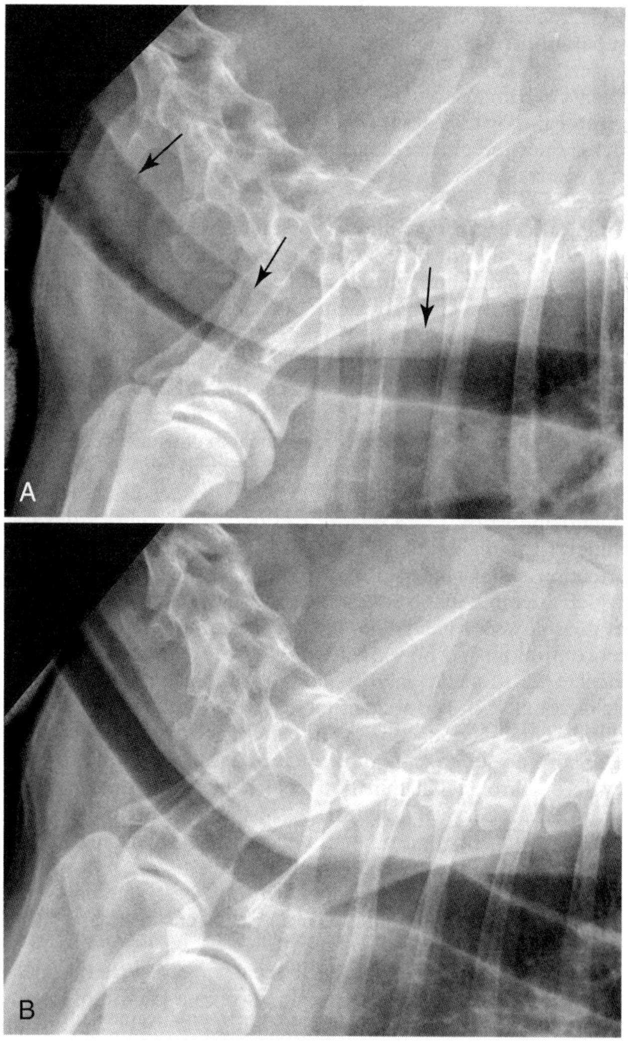

Fig. 29.26 **A,** Lateral view of the cervicothoracic region showing the tracheal lumen dorsally opacified by a visible dorsal tracheal membrane. The dorsal wall is the trachea is also visible (*black arrows*). In **B,** the gas column is wider as the membrane has moved dorsally. There is also a small amount of gas in the cranial cervical and caudal thoracic esophagus.

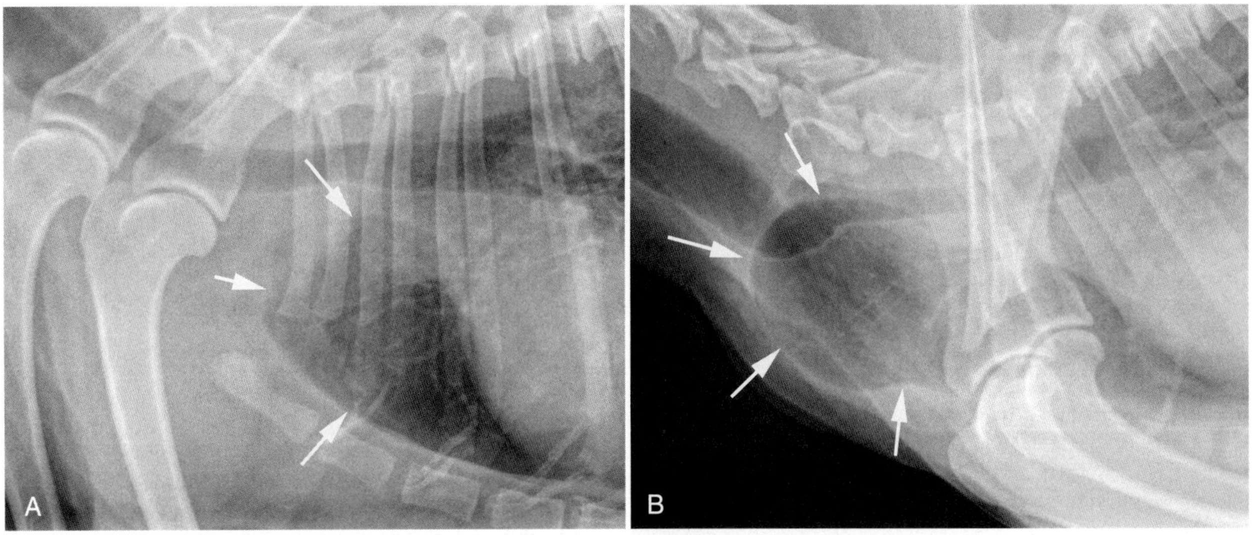

Fig. 29.31 Inspiratory **(A)** and expiratory **(B)** radiographs of a dog with marked collapse of the principal bronchi, which occurs on expiration. In **A,** the cranial lung lobes (*white arrows*) are within the thoracic cavity, extending only a very small distance cranial to the first rib. In **B,** the cranial lung lobes (*white arrows*) have herniated through the thoracic inlet and the cranial margin extends cranially to the level of the C5 to C6 disc space. The lung lobes herniate because the airway collapse that occurs on expiration prevents air from leaving the lungs and as the thoracic cavity becomes smaller the lungs do not reduce in volume as they normally would and are forced through the thoracic inlet. There is also kinking of the trachea superimposed on the herniated lung lobes.

identified.[94,95] Ultrasound may be beneficial for identification of extramural mass lesions and determination of their origin if not obscured by air in the pharyngolarynx, and allows for tissue sampling.[94]

COMPUTED TOMOGRAPHY AND MAGNETIC RESONANCE IMAGING

CT and MRI are both excellent for evaluating the soft tissues surrounding the upper respiratory tract. With faster multidetector units, many CT examinations can be done under sedation, thereby avoiding the need for anesthesia and interference with lesion detection through endotracheal intubation.[96] Examination with the mouth opened to approximately 30 to 45 degrees improves visualization of the pharyngeal structures and is particularly important when evaluating patients for nasopharyngeal stenosis.[97] Three-dimensional virtual endoscopic reformatting can be useful and is essential for CT evaluation of laryngeal collapse/paralysis.[29] Images should be acquired sufficiently caudally to include the medial retropharyngeal lymph nodes. Intraluminal air as well as typically the need for general intubation with placement of an endotracheal tube can limit the usefulness of MRI.[98]

Pharyngolaryngeal Masses

CT examination is well suited to evaluate extramural, mural, and intraluminal abnormalities. Lymph node involvement and osteolysis associated with aggressive pharyngolaryngeal neoplastic or infectious processes, such as squamous cell carcinoma and tonsillar neoplasia, can also be identified using CT.[12,13,99] The tonsillar fossa of the oropharynx is the most common location of pharyngeal neoplasia, specifically squamous cell carcinoma, which can also be bilateral. Tumor mineralization is reported in squamous cell carcinoma and pharyngeal osteosarcoma and can occur in both the mass and regional lymph nodes. Hyoid bone lysis can be a feature of tonsillar squamous cell carcinoma[12] and also as a result of ectopic basihyoid thyroid carcinoma, as described earlier.[17] Marked medial retropharyngeal lymph node enlargement, rounded shape, and heterogeneous enhancement have been reported in most cases of pharyngeal neoplasia, and isolated medial retropharyngeal lymphadenomegaly can be seen in tonsillar neoplasia without tonsillar enlargement.[12,13]

Trauma and Foreign Body

The layered linear appearance of oropharyngeal stick foreign bodies and their contrast-enhancing surrounding inflammatory reaction are well seen on CT.[100] Similarly, MRI readily identifies the inflammatory reaction and regional lymph node enlargement in addition to well-defined linear areas of low-signal intensity representing wooden foreign bodies.[101,102] Spatial understanding of the location of the foreign body is more intuitive using cross-sectional imaging in comparison to ultrasound, thereby helping subsequent surgical planning.[100,102] CT sinography can also be helpful.[103]

CT is also described for hyoid bone fractures and malformation, laryngeal cartilage fracture,[21] and tracheal rupture.[104] In tracheal and left mainstem bronchial avulsion, airway discontinuity and pseudoairway formation can be seen, and CT is useful for measuring the extent of the lesion for planning endotracheal intubation and surgical repair.[84]

Upper Airway Collapse and Tracheal Hypoplasia

CT has been reported in dogs with respiratory distress due to laryngeal paralysis, brachycephalic syndrome, including tracheal hypoplasia, laryngeal collapse and saccule eversion, tracheal/bronchial collapse, and tracheal stenosis. Multiple scans and three-dimensional virtual endoscopic rendering were necessary for detecting laryngeal collapse and laryngeal paralysis.[29]

CT has also been suggested as providing greater accuracy for stent measurement for tracheal collapse with less interobserver variability than fluoroscopy.[105] Tracheal measurements in normal dogs are on average 1 mm larger on CT than on radiographs under equivalent positive pressure manual ventilation.[106] CT can detect pharyngeal soft tissue thickening (mucosal proliferation), a smaller cross-sectional area of the nasopharynx, in addition to osseous abnormalities in feline acromegaly.[107] Everted saccules and diffuse tracheal narrowing can be seen with feline laryngotracheitis.[96,108]

Acknowledgment

With special thanks to prior authors of this chapter for their contributions.

REFERENCES

1. Gaskell CJ. The radiographic anatomy of the pharynx and larynx of the dog. *J Small Anim Pract*. 1974;15(2):89–100.
2. Aron DN, Crowe DT. Upper airway obstruction. General principles and selected conditions in the dog and cat. *Vet Clin North Am Small Anim Pract*. 1985;15(5):891–917.
3. O'Brien J, Harvey C, Tucker J. The larynx of the dog: its normal radiographic anatomy. *Vet Radiol*. 1969;10(38).
4. Plotsky K, Rendall D, Chase K, Riede TL. Cranio-facial remodeling in domestic dogs is associated with changes in larynx position. *J Anat*. 2016;228(6):975–983.
5. Harvey C, Fink E. Tracheal diameter: analysis of radiographic measurements in brachycephalic and nonbrachycephalic dogs. *J Am Animal Hosp Assoc*. 1982; 18:570.
6. Ha Y, Kim J, Chung K, Yoon H, Eom K. Fluoroscopic evaluation of laryngopharyngeal anatomic variations attributable to head posture in dogs. *Am J Vet Res*. 2021;82(1):55–62.
7. Buchanan JW. Tracheal signs and associated vascular anomalies in dogs with persistent right aortic arch. *J Vet Intern Med*. 2004;18(4):510–514.
8. Holt D, Brockman D. Diagnosis and management of laryngeal disease in the dog and cat. *Vet Clin North Am Small Anim Pract*. 1994;24(5):855–871.
9. Jakubiak MJ, Siedlecki CT, Zenger E, et al. Laryngeal, laryngotracheal, and tracheal masses in cats: 27 cases (1998–2003). *J Am Anim Hosp Assoc*. 2005;41(5):310–316.
10. Carlisle C, Bierry D, Thrall D. Tracheal and laryngeal tumors in the dog and cat: literature review and 13 additional patients. *Vet Radiol*. 1991;32:229.
11. Todoroff RJ, Brodey RS. Oral and pharyngeal neoplasia in the dog: a retrospective survey of 361 cases. *J Am Vet Med Assoc*. 1979;175(6):567–571.
12. Carozzi G, Zotti A, Alberti M, et al. Computed tomographic features of pharyngeal neoplasia in 25 dogs. *Vet Radiol Ultrasound*. 2015;56(6):628–637.
13. Thierry F, Longo M, Peccu E, et al. Computed tomographic appearance of canine tonsillar neoplasia: 14 cases. *Vet Radiol Ultrasound*. 2018;59(1):54–63.
14. Venker-van Haagen AJ. Diseases of the larynx. *Vet Clin North Am Small Anim Pract*. 1992;22(5):1155–1172.
15. MacPhail C. Laryngeal disease in dogs and cats. *Vet Clin North Am Small Anim Pract*. 2014;44(1):19–31.
16. Wheeldon EB, Suter PF, Jenkins T. Neoplasia of the larynx in the dog. *J Am Vet Med Assoc*. 1982;180(6):642–647.
17. Rossi F, Caleri E, Bacci B, et al. Computed tomographic features of basihyoid ectopic thyroid carcinoma in dogs. *Vet Radiol Ultrasound*. 2013;54(6):575–581.
18. Griffith LG, Tiruneh R, Sullivan M, Reid SW. Oropharyngeal penetrating injuries in 50 dogs: a retrospective study. *Vet Surg*. 2000;29(5):383–388.
19. Doran IP, Wright CA, Moore AH. Acute oropharyngeal and esophageal stick injury in forty-one dogs. *Vet Surg*. 2008;37(8):781–785.
20. Ober CP, Spotswood TC, Hancock R. Fatal venous air embolism in a cat with a retropharyngeal diverticulum. *Vet Radiol Ultrasound*. 2006;47(2):153–158.
21. Francis KA, Goggin JM, Hoskinson JJ. Imaging diagnosis—laryngeal collapse due to cricoid cartilage fracture. *Vet Radiol Ultrasound*. 2008;49(4):360–361.
22. Lamb CR, Pope EHW, Lee KCL. Results of computed tomography in dogs with suspected wood foreign bodies. *Vet Radiol Ultrasound*. 2017;58(2):144–150.
23. Dobromylskyj MJ, Dennis F, Ladlow FJ, Adams VJ. The use of magnetic resonance imaging in the management of pharyngeal penetration injuries in dogs. *J Small Anim Pract*. 2008;49(2):74–79.
24. Krainer D, Dupré G. Brachycephalic obstructive airway syndrome. *Vet Clin North Am Small Anim Pract*. 2022;52(3):749–780.
25. Jones BA, Stanley BJ, Nelson NC. The impact of tongue dimension on air volume in brachycephalic dogs. *Vet Surg*. 2020;49(3):512–520.
26. Hobson HP. Brachycephalic syndrome. *Semin Vet Med Surg*. 1995;10(2):109–114.
27. Auger M, Alexander K, Beauchamp G, Dunn M. Use of CT to evaluate and compare intranasal features in brachycephalic and normocephalic dogs. *J Small Anim Pract*. 2016;57:529–536.
28. Hara Y, Teshima K, Seki M, Kazushi A, Yamaya Y. Pharyngeal contraction secondary to its collapse in dogs with brachycephalic airway syndrome. *J Vet Med Sci*. 2020;82(1):64–67.
29. Stadler K, Hartman S, Matheson J, et al. Computed tomographic imaging of dogs with primary laryngeal or tracheal airway obstruction. *Vet Radiol Ultrasound*. 2011;52(4): 377–384.
30. Johnson LR, Mayhew PD, Steffey MA, et al. Upper airway obstruction in Norwich terriers: 16 cases. *J Vet Intern Med*. 2013;27(6):1409–1415.
31. Skerrett SC, McClaran JK, Fox PR, et al. Clinical features and outcome of dogs with epiglottic retroversion with or without surgical treatment: 24 cases. *J Vet Intern Med*. 2015;29(6):1611–1618.
32. Flanders JA, Thompson MS. Dyspnea caused by epiglottic retroversion in two dogs. *J Am Vet Med Assoc*. 2009;235(11):1330–1335.
33. Rubin JA, Holt DE, Reetz JA, et al. Signalment, clinical presentation, concurrent diseases, and diagnostic findings in 28 dogs with dynamic pharyngeal collapse (2008–2013). *J Vet Intern Med*. 2015;29(3):815–821.
34. Pollard RE, Johnson LR, Marks SL. The prevalence of dynamic pharyngeal collapse is high in brachycephalic dogs undergoing videoflouroscopy. *Vet Radiol Ultrasound*. 2018;59:529–534.
35. Davis A, Khorzad R, Whelan M. Dynamic upper airway obstruction secondary to severe feline asthma. *J Am Anim Hosp Assoc*. 2013;49(2):142–147.
36. Fujiwara-Igarashi A, Yu Y, Hamamoto Y, Hasegawa D, Fujita M. Dynamic pharyngeal collapse in three cats with different pharyngeal pathology. *J Vet Med Sci*. 2019;81(7): 1012–1016.
37. Zaid MS, Prorat-Mosenco Y, Mosenco AS. Dynamic collapse of the common pharynx in a cat. *J Vet Intern Med*. 2011;25:1458–1460.
38. Coolman BR, Marretta SM, McKiernan BC, et al. Choanal atresia and secondary nasopharyngeal stenosis in a dog. *J Am Anim Hosp Assoc*. 1998;34(6):497–501.
39. Berent AC. Diagnosis and management of nasopharyngeal stenosis. *Vet Clin Small Anim*. 2016;(46):677–689.
40. Burdick S, Berent A, Weisse C, et al. Interventional treatment of benign nasopharyngeal stenosis and imperforate nasopharynx in dogs and cats: 46 cases (2005–2013). *J Am Vet Med Assoc*. 2018;253(10):1300–1308.
41. Boswood A, Lamb CR, Brockman DJ, et al. Balloon dilatation of nasopharyngeal stenosis in a cat. *Vet Radiol Ultrasound*. 2003;44(1):53–55.

42. Kirberger RM, Steenkamp G, Spotswood TC, et al. Stenotic nasopharyngeal dysgenesis in the dachshund: seven cases (2002–2004). *J Am Anim Hosp Assoc.* 2006;42(4):290–297.
43. Peterson K, Beymer J, Rudloff E, et al. Airway obstruction in a dog after *Dieffenbachia* ingestion. *J Vet Emerg Crit Care.* 2009;19(6):635–639.
44. Dixon A, Tivers MS, Packham L, Black V. Infiltrative laryngeal disease in dogs. *J Small Anim Pract.* 2020;61(9):568–575.
45. Zekas LJ, Adams WM. Cranial mediastinal cysts in nine cats. *Vet Radiol Ultrasound.* 2002;43(5):413–418.
46. Berry B, Gallaway A, Thrall D, et al. Thoracic radiographic features of anticoagulant rodenticide toxicity in fourteen dogs. *Vet Radiol Ultrasound.* 1993;34:391.
47. Essman SC, Hoover JP, Bahr RJ, et al. An intrathoracic malignant peripheral nerve sheath tumor in a dog. *Vet Radiol Ultrasound.* 2002;43(3):255–259.
48. Stann SE, Bauer TG. Respiratory tract tumors. *Vet Clin North Am Small Anim Pract.* 1985;15(3):535–556.
49. Besancon MF, Stacy BA, Kyles AE, et al. Nodular immunocyte-derived (AL) amyloidosis in the trachea of a dog. *J Am Vet Med Assoc.* 2004;224(8):1302–1306.
50. Sheaffer KA, Dillon AR. Obstructive tracheal mass due to an inflammatory polyp in a cat. *J Am Anim Hosp Assoc.* 1996;32(5):431–434.
51. Snyder KD, Spaulding K, Edwards J. Imaging diagnosis—tracheobronchial zygomycosis in a cat. *Vet Radiol Ultrasound.* 2010;51(6):617–620.
52. Fitzgerald SD, Johnson CA, Peck EJ. A fatal case of intrathoracic cuterebriasis in a cat. *J Am Anim Hosp Assoc.* 1996;32(4):353–357.
53. Volta A, Piccionello AP, Bonazzi M, et al. What is your diagnosis? Bronchial foreign body. *J Am Vet Med Assoc.* 2007;230(2):191–192.
54. Tivers MS, Moore AH. Tracheal foreign bodies in the cat and the use of fluoroscopy for removal: 12 cases. *J Small Anim Pract.* 2006;47(3):155–159.
55. Nutt LK, Webb JA, Prosser KJ, et al. Management of dogs and cats with endotracheal tube foreign bodies. *Can Vet J.* 2014;55(6):565–568.
56. Hardie EM, Spodnick GJ, Gilson SD, Benson JA, Hawkins EC. Tracheal rupture in cats: 16 cases (1983–1998). *J Am Vet Med Assoc.* 1999;214(4):508–512.
57. Basdani E, Papazoglou LG, Patsikas MN, et al. Upper airway injury in dogs secondary to trauma: 10 dogs (2000–2011). *J Am Anim Hosp Assoc.* 2016;52(5):291–296.
58. Lotti U, Niebauer G. Tracheobronchial foreign bodies of plant origin in 153 hunting dogs. *Compend Cont Educ Pract Vet.* 1992;14:900.
59. Mitchell SL, McCarthy R, Rudloff E, et al. Tracheal rupture associated with intubation in cats: 20 cases (1996–1998). *J Am Vet Med Assoc.* 2000;216(10):1592–1595.
60. White RN, Burton CA. Surgical management of intrathoracic tracheal avulsion in cats: long-term results in 9 consecutive cases. *Vet Surg.* 2000;29(5):430–435.
61. White RN, Milner HR. Intrathoracic tracheal avulsion in three cats. *J Small Anim Pract.* 1995;36(8):343–347.
62. Schmierer PA, Schwarz A, Bass DA, et al. Novel avulsion pattern of the left principal bronchus with involvement of the carina and caudal thoracic trachea in a cat. *J Feline Med Surg.* 2014;16(8):695–698.
63. Mattoon JS, Drost WT. Radiographing the trachea in small animals. *Vet Med.* 2004;72.
64. Griffiths LG, Sullivan M, Lerche P. Intrathoracic tracheal avulsion and pseudodiverticulum following pneumomediastinum in a cat. *Vet Rec.* 1998;142(25):693–696.
65. Fasanella FJ, Shivley JM, Wardlaw JL, et al. Brachycephalic airway obstructive syndrome in dogs: 90 cases (1991–2008). *J Am Vet Med Assoc.* 2010;237(9):1048–1051.
66. Coyne BE, Fingland RB. Hypoplasia of the trachea in dogs: 103 cases (1974–1990). *J Am Vet Med Assoc.* 1992;201(5):768–772.
67. Kaye BM, Boroffka SAEB, Haagsman AN, et al. Computed tomographic, radiographic, and endoscopic tracheal dimensions in English bulldogs with grade 1 clinical signs of brachycephalic airway syndrome. *Vet Radiol Ultrasound.* 2015;56(6):609–616.
68. Hammond G, Geary M, Coleman E, et al. Radiographic measurements of the trachea in domestic shorthair and Persian cats. *J Feline Med Surg.* 2011;13(12):881–884.
69. Schultheiss PC, Gardner SA, Owens JM, et al. Mucopolysaccharidosis VII in a cat. *Vet Pathol.* 2000;37(5):502–505.
70. Lindl-Bylicki BJ, Johnson LR, Pollard RE. Comparison of the radiographic and tracheoscopic appearance of the dorsal tracheal membrane in large and small breed dogs. *Vet Radiol Ultrasound.* 2015;56(6):602–608.
71. Johnson L. Tracheal collapse. Diagnosis and medical and surgical treatment. *Vet Clin North Am Small Anim Pract.* 2000;30(6):1253–1266.
72. Violette NP, Weisse C, Berent AC, Lamb KE. Correlations among tracheal dimensions, tracheal stent dimensions, and major complications after endoluminal stenting of tracheal collapse syndrome in dogs. *J Vet Intern Med.* 2019;33(5):2209–2216.
73. Weisse C, Berent AC, Violette NP, et al. Short-, intermediate-, and long-term results for endoluminal stent placement in dogs with tracheal collapse. *J Am Vet Med Assoc.* 2019;254(3):380–392.
74. Johnson LR, Pollard RE. Tracheal collapse and bronchomalacia in dogs: 58 cases (7/2001–1/2008). *J Vet Intern Med.* 2010;24(2):298–305.
75. Macready DM, Johnson LR, Pollard RE. Fluoroscopic and radiographic evaluation of tracheal collapse in dogs: 62 cases (2001–2006). *J Am Vet Med Assoc.* 2007;230(12):1870–1876.
76. Maggiore AD. An update on tracheal and airway collapse in dogs. *Vet Clin North Am Small Anim Pract.* 2020;50(2):419–430.
77. Heng HG, Lim CK, Gutierrez-Crespo B, Guptill LF. Radiographic and computed tomographic appearance of tracheal collapse with axial rotation in four dogs. *J Small Anim Pract.* 2018;59:53–58.
78. Johnson LR, Singh MK, Pollard RE. Agreement among radiographs, fluoroscopy and bronchoscopy in documentation of airway collapse in dogs. *J Vet Intern Med.* 2015;29(6):1619–1626.
79. Marolf A, Blaik M, Specht A. A retrospective study of the relationship between tracheal collapse and bronchiectasis in dogs. *Vet Radiol Ultrasound.* 2007;48(3):199–203.
80. Leonard CD, Johnson LR, Bonadio CM, et al. Changes in tracheal dimensions during inspiration and expiration in healthy dogs as detected via computed tomography. *Am J Vet Res.* 2009;70(8):986–991.
81. Sura PA, Krahwinkel DJ. Self-expanding nitinol stents for the treatment of tracheal collapse in dogs: 12 cases (2001–2004). *J Am Vet Med Assoc.* 2008;232(2):228–236.
82. Moritz A, Schneider M, Bauer N. Management of advanced tracheal collapse in dogs using intraluminal self-expanding biliary Wallstents. *J Vet Intern Med.* 2004;18(1):31–42.
83. Fujita M, Miura H, Yasuda D, et al. Tracheal narrowing secondary to airway obstruction in two cats. *J Small Anim Pract.* 2004;45(1):29–31.
84. Hendricks JC, O'Brien JA. Tracheal collapse in two cats. *J Am Vet Med Assoc.* 1985;187(4):418–419.
85. Mims HL, Hancock RB, Leib MS, et al. Primary tracheal collapse in a cat. *J Am Anim Hosp Assoc.* 2008;44:149.

86. Nafe LA, Robertson ID, Hawkins EC. Cervical lung lobe herniation in dogs identified by fluoroscopy. *Can Vet J.* 2013;54(10):955–959.
87. Guglielmini C, Simone AD, Valbonetti L, Dina A. Intermittent cranial lung herniation in two dogs. *Vet Radiol Ultrasound.* 2007;48(3):227–229.
88. Lee J, Yun S, Lee I, Choi M, Yoon J. Fluoroscopic characteristics of tracheal collapse and cervical lung herniation in dogs: 222 cases (2012-2015). *J Vet Sci.* 2017;18(4): 499–505.
89. Arndt JW, Marks SL, Kneller SK. What is your diagnosis? Hiatal hernia due to laryngeal squamous cell carcinoma. *J Am Vet Med Assoc.* 2006;228(5):693–694.
90. Schachter S, Norris CR. Laryngeal paralysis in cats: 16 cases (1990–1999). *J Am Vet Med Assoc.* 2000;216(7): 1100–1103.
91. Mattoon JS, Drost WT. Pharyngeal and laryngeal radiography in small animals. *Vet Med.* 2004;50.
92. Kurosawa TA, Ruth JD, Steurer J, et al. Imaging diagnosis—acquired pectus excavatum secondary to laryngeal paralysis in a dog. *Vet Radiol Ultrasound.* 2012;53(3):329–332.
93. Bray JP, Lipscombe VJ, White RA, Rudorf H. Ultrasonographic examination of the pharynx and larynx of the normal dog. *Vet Radiol Ultrasound.* 1998;39(6):566–571.
94. Rudorf H, Barr F. Echolaryngography in cats. *Vet Radiol Ultrasound.* 2002;43(4):353–357.
95. Rudorf H, Barr FJ, Lane JG. The role of ultrasound in the assessment of laryngeal paralysis in the dog. *Vet Radiol Ultrasound.* 2001;42(4):338–343.
96. Stadler K, O'Brien R. Computed tomography of nonanesthetized cats with upper airway obstruction. *Vet Radiol Ultrasound.* 2013;54:231–236.
97. Laurenson MP, Zwingenberger AL, Cissell DD, et al. Computed tomography of the pharynx in a closed vs. open mouth position. *Vet Radiol Ultrasound.* 2011;52(4): 357–361.
98. Vázquez JM, Arencibia A, Gil F, et al. Magnetic resonance imaging of the normal canine larynx. *Anat Histol Embryol.* 1998;27(4):263–270.
99. Gendler A, Lewis JR, Reetz JA, et al. Computed tomographic features of oral squamous cell carcinoma in cats: 18 cases (2002–2008). *J Am Vet Med Assoc.* 2010;236(3): 319–325.
100. Nicholson I, Halfacree Z, Whatmough C, et al. Computed tomography as an aid to management of chronic oropharyngeal stick injury in the dog. *J Small Anim Pract.* 2008;49(9):451–457.
101. Potanas CP, Armbrust LJ, Klocke EE, et al. Ultrasonographic and magnetic resonance imaging diagnosis of an oropharyngeal wood penetrating injury in a dog. *J Am Anim Hosp Assoc.* 2011;47(1):e1–e6.
102. Dobromylskyj MJ, Dennis R, Ladlow JF, et al. The use of magnetic resonance imaging in the management of pharyngeal penetration injuries in dogs. *J Small Anim Pract.* 2008;49(2):74–79.
103. Jones JC, Ober CP. Computed tomographic diagnosis of nongastrointestinal foreign bodies in dogs. *J Am Anim Hosp Assoc.* 2007;43(2):99–111.
104. Bhandal J, Kuzma A. Tracheal rupture in a cat: diagnosis by computed tomography. *Can Vet J.* 2008;49(6):595–597.
105. Williams JM, Krebs IA, Riedesel EA, et al. Comparison of fluoroscopy and computed tomography for tracheal lumen diameter measurement and determination of intraluminal stent size in healthy dogs. *Vet Radiol Ultrasound.* 2016;57(3):269–275.
106. Montgomery JE, Mathews KG, Marcellin-Little DJ, et al. Comparison of radiography and computed tomography for determining tracheal diameter and length in dogs. *Vet Surg.* 2015;44(1):114–118.
107. Fischetti AJ, Gisselman K, Peterson ME. CT and MRI evaluation of skull bones and soft tissues in six cats with presumed acromegaly versus 12 unaffected cats. *Vet Radiol Ultrasound.* 2012;53(5):535–539.
108. Lamb CR, Ciasca TC, Mantis P, et al. Computed tomographic signs of acromegaly in 68 diabetic cats with hypersomatotropism. *J Feline Med Surg.* 2014;16(2): 99–108.

ELECTRONIC RESOURCES

Additional information related to the content in Chapter 29 can be found online at eBooks.Health.Elsevier.com

- Chapter Quiz
- Videos

CHAPTER 30

Pharynx, Upper Esophageal Sphincter, and Esophagus

Rachel E. Pollard

INTRODUCTION

Clinical signs related directly to pharyngeal, cricopharyngeal, and esophageal diseases include gagging, retching, regurgitation, painful swallowing, and dysphagia.[1] Signs developing secondary to esophageal disease include pharyngeal and upper airway inflammation, nasal discharge, weight loss, pneumomediastinum, pneumothorax, pleural effusion, and respiratory disease. Acute respiratory signs may develop secondary to compression of the trachea by an esophageal foreign body or as a result of aspiration of regurgitant material. A strong link between a variety of respiratory diseases and digestive disorders has recently been established.[2–4]

ANATOMIC AND PHYSIOLOGIC FEATURES

Swallowing is an essential and complex process that results in bolus delivery from the oral cavity to the stomach. The actions involving lapping of liquid and prehension and chewing of food are voluntary and require coordinated movements of the tongue and jaws. Once a bolus is propelled into the pharyngeal region, the swallowing reflex occurs involuntarily requiring input from the sensory and motor branches of the trigeminal, the hypoglossal, facial, and glossopharyngeal nerves.[5] The pharynx contracts caudally against the base of the tongue to push the bolus toward the upper esophageal sphincter (UES) (Fig. 30.1). To protect the larynx and airway, the epiglottis flips upward. In coordination with pharyngeal contraction, the paired cricopharyngeus and thyropharyngeus muscles that make up the UES relax to allow passage of the bolus into the proximal esophagus. Subsequently, the UES closes to prevent retrograde movement of the bolus back into the pharynx and the epiglottis returns to its relaxed position so that normal respiration may resume.

The esophagus is a distensible tube responsible for the transport of the bolus from the UES to the stomach. Similar to the rest of the gastrointestinal tract, the esophagus is a layered structure with the innermost surface being lined by mucosa. The submucosa, muscularis, and externally the adventitia are the remaining layers.[6] In the dog, the muscularis layer consists of striated muscle. In the cat, the muscularis layer consists of striated muscle cranially but changes to smooth muscle in the caudal third, resulting in the characteristic "herring bone" appearance on contrast esophagography (Fig. 30.2). A bolus may be transported from the proximal esophagus to the lower esophageal sphincter (LES) by primary or secondary peristaltic waves.[7] A primary peristaltic wave is a continuation of pharyngeal contraction that will propel the bolus directly to the stomach. If primary peristalsis fails, then the bolus is transported

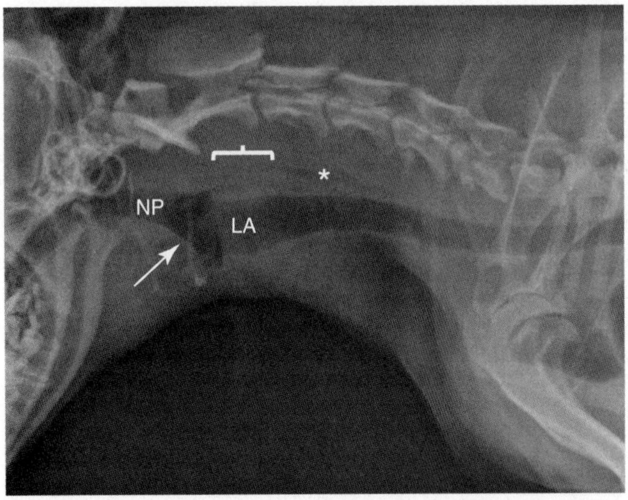

Fig. 30.1 Lateral radiograph of dog showing normal cervical anatomy. *White bracket* = upper esophageal sphincter; *white arrow* = epiglottis. *Asterisk* = air in the proximal esophagus. *LA*, Larynx; *NP*, nasopharynx.

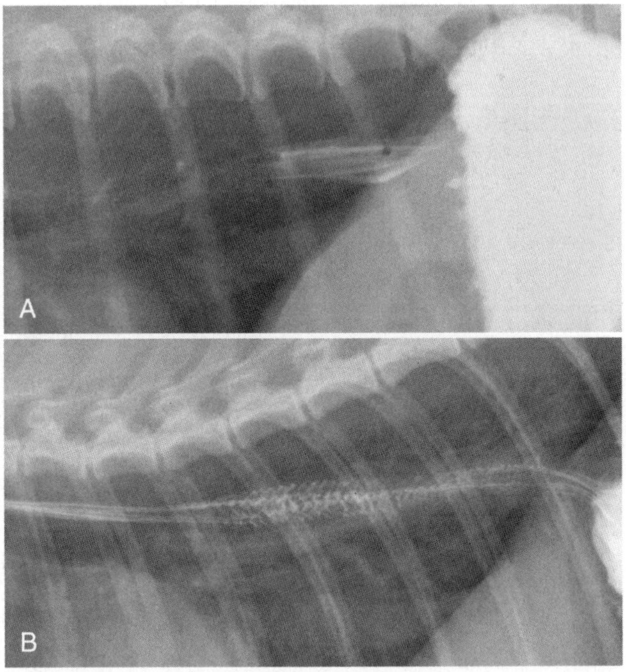

Fig. 30.2 **A,** Barium-contrast esophagram of the caudal esophagus in a normal dog. Note the linear arrangement of the mucosal folds. **B,** Barium-contrast esophagram of the caudal esophagus in a normal cat. Note the herringbone appearance to the mucosa in the caudal aspect of the esophagus that is created by the obliquely oriented smooth muscle in this region.

to the stomach either by secondary peristalsis or with the ensuing primary peristaltic wave generated by the next bolus.

In the cervical region, the esophagus is located slightly to the left of the trachea, gradually becoming completely left sided at the thoracic inlet (Fig. 30.3A).[7] The left common carotid artery, vagosympathetic trunk, internal jugular vein, and tracheal duct course through the angle between the esophagus and the longus capitis muscle. The right common carotid artery, vagosympathetic trunk, internal jugular vein, and tracheal duct are lateral to the trachea on the right side. The thoracic portion of the esophagus is in close proximity to the trachea. The esophagus is to the left of the trachea at the thoracic inlet (see Fig. 30.3B), but gradually courses dorsally over the point of bifurcation of the trachea at the level of the fifth and sixth thoracic vertebrae (see Fig. 30.3C). At its dorsal location, it lies to the right of the aortic arch and ventral to the longus colli muscles. Between the tracheal bifurcation and caudal esophageal sphincter, the esophagus lies in the median plane (see Fig. 30.3D). The vagal nerves run dorsocaudally across the sides of the esophagus and unite at the dorsal aspect of the esophagus a few centimeters cranial to the esophageal hiatus to form the vagal trunk, which passes through the hiatus with the esophagus.

The LES is a focal narrowing of the esophagus at the junction with the stomach that is toned at rest to prevent retrograde movement of gastric contents. The sphincter is made up of a focal thickening of the muscularis layer of the esophagus, a confluence of gastric rugae at the gastroesophageal junction oriented transversely to the sphincter, and a muscular sling created by the diaphragm.[6] A short segment of the esophagus

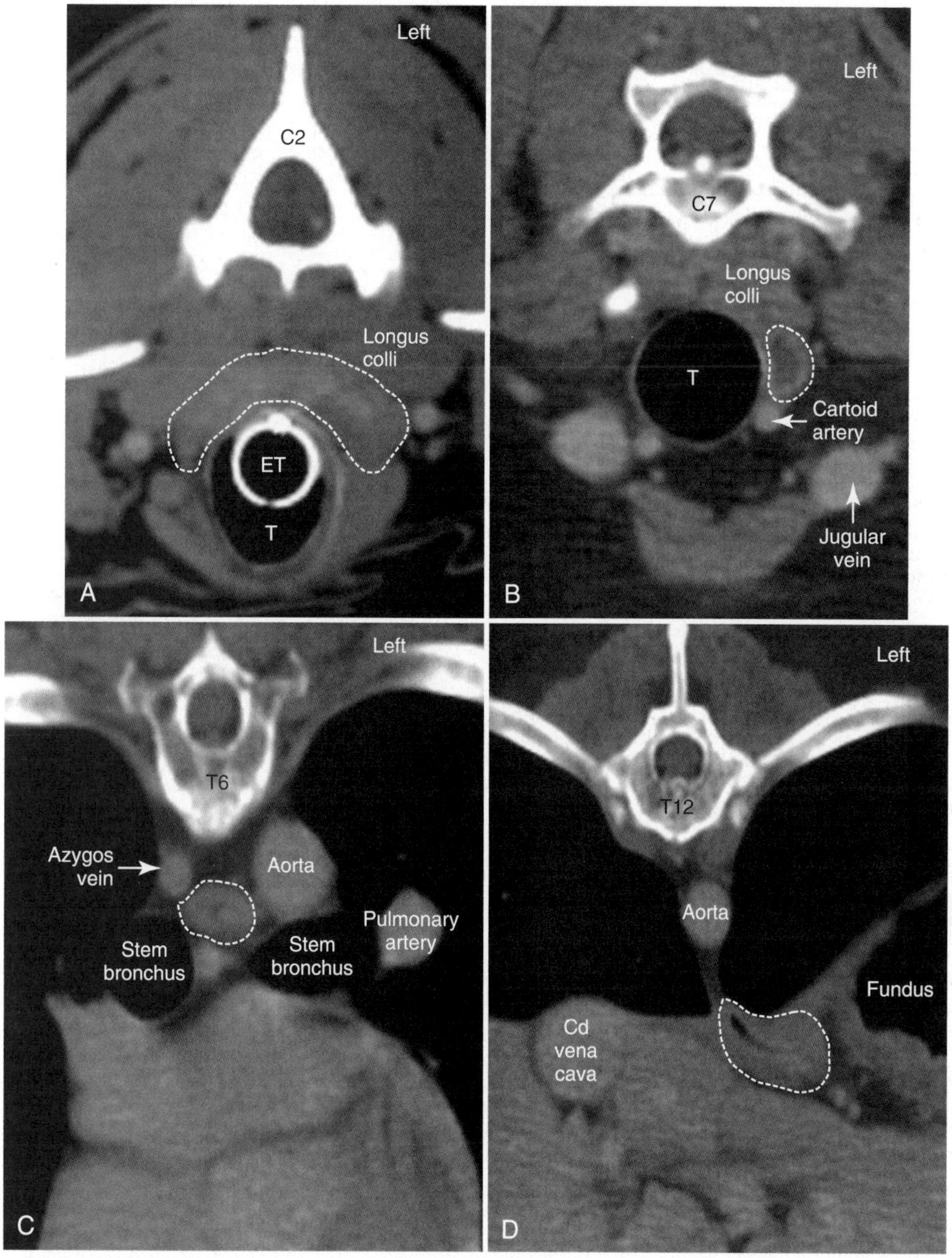

Fig. 30.3 Transverse computed tomography (CT) images of the thorax of a dog at the level of the cricopharyngeal sphincter **(A)**, the thoracic inlet **(B)**, the base of the heart **(C)**, and the level of caudal esophageal sphincter **(D)**, illustrating the relationship of the esophagus (outlined with *dotted line*) to surrounding structures. *C2,* Second cervical vertebra; *C7,* seventh cervical vertebra; *Cd,* caudal; *ET,* endotracheal tube; *T6,* sixth thoracic vertebra; *T12,* twelfth thoracic vertebra, *T,* trachea.

resides on the abdominal side of the diaphragm where the relatively positive intra-abdominal pressure compresses it. When a bolus is transported caudad by the esophagus, the LES relaxes to allow passage into the stomach.

Vascular supply to the esophagus is complicated and begins in the cervical region with branches of the thyroid arteries. The bronchoesophageal artery is the main source to the cranial two-thirds of the thoracic portion. Esophageal branches of the aorta and/or intercostal arteries supply the remainder of the esophagus, and the terminal portion is supplied by the left gastric artery. The azygous vein and left gastric vein drain the thoracic portion. Lymphatic drainage is through the medial retropharyngeal, deep cervical, cranial mediastinal, bronchial, portal, splenic, and gastric lymph nodes.

Innervation of the esophagus is complex and involves 25 paired spinal ganglia from C2 to L5. Neurologic control of swallowing is coordinated by cranial nerves V (trigeminal), VII (facial), IX (glossopharyngeal), X (vagus), and XII (hypoglossal), and their nuclei in the brainstem that, in turn, are controlled by areas of the reticular formation referred to as the swallowing center.[8]

RADIOGRAPHY

Survey radiography of the thorax and neck is often the first imaging step for the evaluation of an animal with suspected pharyngeal, UES, or esophageal disease. This should include three projections of the thorax (dorsoventral or ventrodorsal [VD], right, and left lateral) and at least one lateral projection of the neck. Care should be taken to ensure that the radiograph of the neck is adequately positioned. More specifically, the lateral cervical study must not be rotated and the head should be extended as poor positioning can distort anatomy and seriously compromise interpretation. The pharynx, larynx, and UES should be included.

The normal esophagus is usually empty and rarely visible on thoracic radiographs in cats and dogs because of its location within the mediastinum and silhouetting with adjacent muscles and mediastinal structures. On left lateral thoracic radiographs, the normal caudal thoracic esophagus sometimes contains a small amount of fluid and can be seen as a faint tubular soft tissue opacity between the descending aorta and caudal vena cava (Fig. 30.4A); this appearance is rare in right lateral radiographs. Gas can accumulate focally in the esophagus in animals that are excited, sedated or anesthetized, and dyspneic; this gas accumulation is usually minimal, and the most commonly located just cranial to the tracheal bifurcation (see Fig. 30.4B). The tissue band between the trachea and esophagus (*white arrows*) is termed the *tracheal stripe sign*, also called the *tracheoesophageal stripe sign* and *esophageal stripe sign*. This is created by summation of the ventral aspect of the esophageal wall with the dorsal aspect of the tracheal wall, each outlined by gas in their respective lumen. The tracheal stripe sign is a

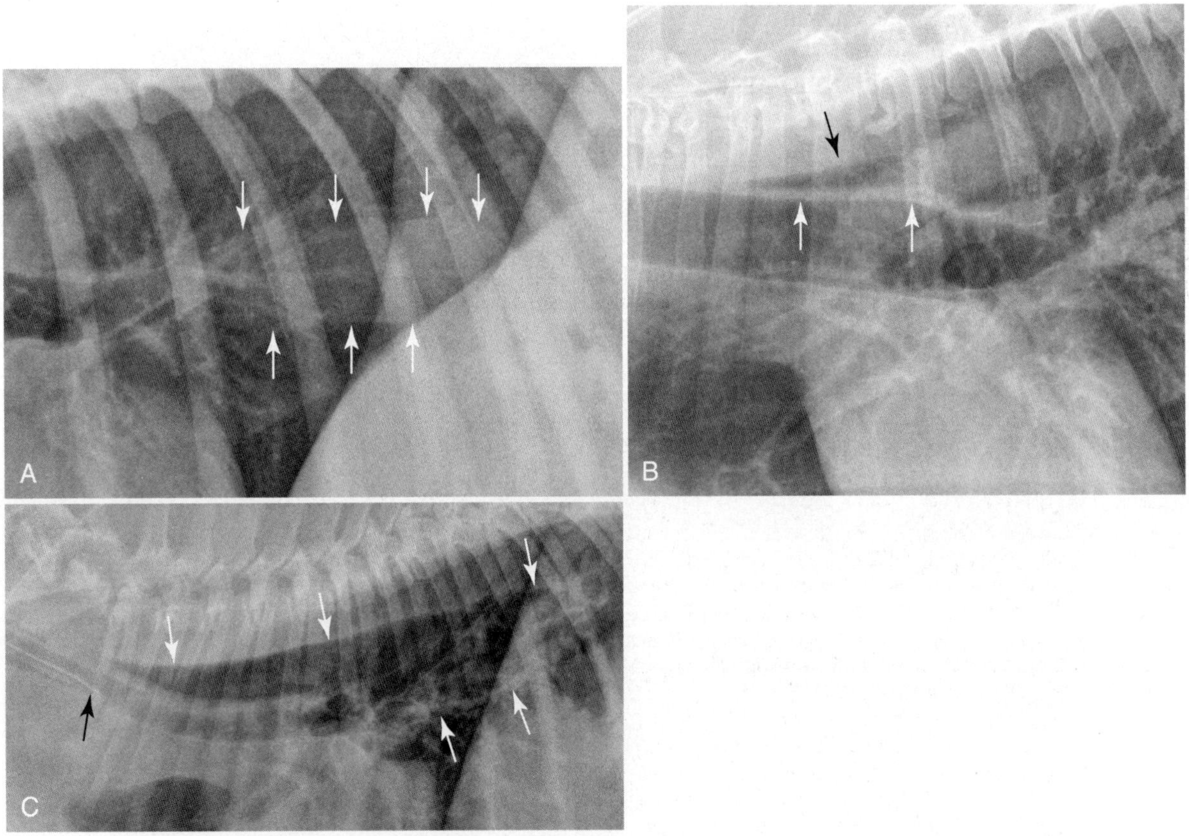

Fig. 30.4 Variations in the appearance of the normal esophagus. **A,** Left lateral radiograph of a normal adult dog. The caudal one-third of the esophagus is visible as a soft tissue band between the aorta and caudal vena cava (*white arrows*). This finding is usually not present on right lateral radiographs of normal dogs. **B,** Left lateral radiograph of a normal adult dog where there is a small amount of gas in the esophagus just cranial to the tracheal bifurcation (*black arrow*). This will not be visible in the ventrodorsal (VD) view. The tissue band between the trachea and esophagus (*white arrows*) is termed the *tracheal stripe sign,* also called the tracheoesophageal stripe sign and esophageal stripe sign. This is created by summation of the ventral aspect of the esophageal wall with the dorsal aspect of the tracheal wall, each outlined by gas in their respective lumen. The tracheal stripe sign is a reliable sign of esophageal gas. **C,** Left lateral radiograph of an anesthetized dog. The endotracheal tube is visible (*black arrow*). There is generalized megaesophagus (*white arrows*) because of the anesthesia. The enlarged esophagus is causing ventral displacement of the intrathoracic trachea. Radiographically, this cannot be distinguished from pathologic megaesophagus.

reliable sign of esophageal gas (see Fig. 30.4B). Focal esophageal gas collections are dynamic and may appear differently or be absent in other radiographs acquired during the same study. General anesthesia or aerophagia may lead to severe dilation of the esophagus, which can appear identical to pathologic megaesophagus (see Fig. 30.4C). Anesthesia-related megaesophagus will resolve spontaneously when the patient is awake again.

Survey radiographs will help define if aspiration pneumonia is present. Aspiration pneumonia is common in animals with swallowing disorders and typically involves the dependent aspect of the right and left cranial and right middle lung lobes. Since the right middle lung lobe is a common site for aspiration, the left lateral thoracic view is essential for complete assessment of the lung.[9] When megaesophagus is identified, the presence of aspiration pneumonia has a negative association with survival time.[10]

The absence of abnormal findings on survey radiographs of the esophagus does not eliminate the possibility of esophageal disease. In animals with appropriate clinical signs of esophageal disease, contrast studies of the esophagus should be considered. However, in cases where severe aspiration pneumonia is present, contrast studies should be delayed until such time as pneumonia is resolved as aspiration of barium during the imaging procedure will further compromise lung function.

CONTRAST RADIOGRAPHY

Survey radiographs of the thorax and cervical region are ideally performed immediately before a contrast esophagram. Box 30.1 contains a list of contrast study techniques used for examination of the esophagus. The type of contrast medium selected to perform contrast radiography depends on several factors.[11] Barium paste or cream is viscous and may adhere best to mucosal irregularities. However, due to the viscosity of these agents, barium paste and cream may not flow well around intraluminal lesions and are contraindicated in animals at increased risk for aspiration, because aspirated paste can cause airway obstruction.[6] Liquid barium (60% weight-volume) is the most common medium used for contrast radiography of the pharynx and esophagus.[12] Dosage is related to size so that cats should receive 5 to 7 mL boluses, small- to medium-sized dogs should receive 15 mL boluses, while larger dogs should receive 20 to 30 mL boluses of liquid barium orally.[12]

When endoscopy is likely to follow or if perforation of the pharynx, cricopharynx, or esophagus is suspected, nonionic iodinated contrast agents are preferable to barium so as to avoid the granulomatous reaction associated with leakage into the cervical soft tissues or mediastinum.[13] Ionic, iodinated contrast agents are specifically contraindicated due to the potential for life-threatening pulmonary edema that can result from aspiration into the lungs. Esophageal perforation should be suspected when survey radiographs identify gas in the cervical soft tissues or mediastinum but no external wounds are present. Soft tissue swelling in the cervical region with regional emphysema is suggestive of perforation. Opacification and widening of the mediastinum may accompany pneumomediastinum when perforation of the thoracic esophagus has resulted in mediastinitis.[14] In these instances, nonionic, iodinated contrast medium should be diluted 50:50 with sterile water and 10 to 15 mL boluses are administered orally.[15] Sedation should generally be avoided unless absolutely necessary since tranquilizers result in significant alterations in swallowing function.[15] However, should sedation be required, acepromazine may be administered but may increase esophageal transit times, particularly at higher doses.[16]

Regardless of the type of contrast medium used, the animal is restrained in right lateral recumbency and liquid contrast medium is administered orally using a catheter-tipped syringe.

Box 30.1

Techniques for Esophageal Contrast Studies

Static Barium Esophagram

Special Considerations

No sedation

Contraindicated for esophageal perforation

Use barium paste instead of barium suspension for evaluating mucosa

Aspiration potential

Procedure

Survey lateral and ventrodorsal (VD) radiographs of the neck and thorax

Orally administer via syringe in lateral recumbency

- Small dog: 15 mL of 60% weight/volume preformulated barium sulfate suspension
- Large dog: 20–30 mL of 60% weight/volume preformulated barium sulfate suspension
- Cat: 5–7 mL of 60% weight/volume preformulated barium sulfate suspension

Lateral radiographs of the neck and thorax immediately after oral administration

VD radiographs of thorax immediately

Right and left oblique VD thoracic radiographs

Repeat entire procedure if amount of contrast medium in esophagus is insufficient

Static Barium Meal Esophagram

Special Considerations

Can identify small or incomplete obstructions that allow liquid to pass

Should be used if the esophagram with liquid barium is negative

Should be used if the patient can swallow liquids but not solid food clinically

Should not be performed if perforation is suspected

Procedure

Dogs: 1 cup dry kibble mixed with 20 mL barium sulfate suspension

Cats: 1/2 cup dry kibble or soft food mixed with 10 mL barium sulfate suspension

Perform following the swallowing study using liquid barium suspension

Provide the food mixture while in lateral recumbency or place in mouth

Perform same sequence of radiographs as for liquid barium

Static Iodinated Esophagram

Special Considerations

Can be used before endoscopy or if perforation is suspected

Do not use ionic contrast medium because it can cause pulmonary edema if aspirated

Procedure

Dog: 10–15 mL of a 50:50 mixture of nonionic iodinated contrast medium and water

Cat: 5–10 mL of a 50:50 mixture of nonionic iodinated contrast medium and water

Administer the liquid via syringe in lateral recumbency

Perform radiographic procedures as for liquid barium

From Wallack ST. Static barium esophagram. In: *The Handbook of Veterinary Contrast Radiography*. Solana Beach, CA: San Diego Veterinary Imaging; 2003:45–53.

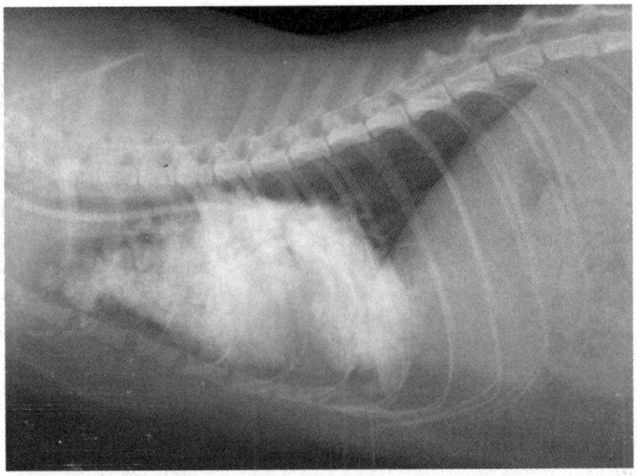

Fig. 30.5 Right lateral radiograph of a cat where barium was injected into the trachea postmortem to demonstrate the appearance of barium accumulation in the airways and lung parenchyma.

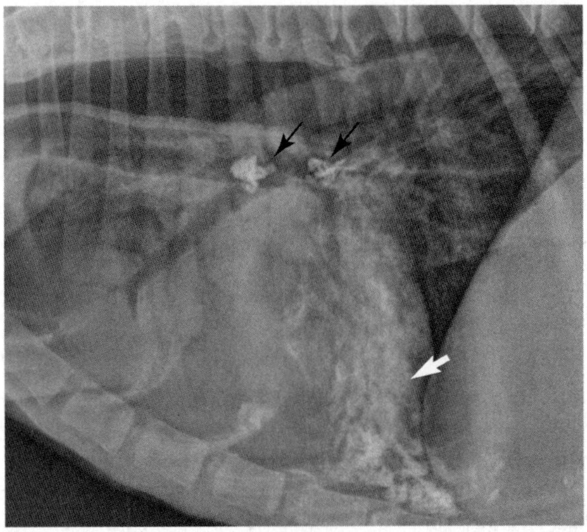

Fig. 30.6 Lateral thoracic radiograph of a 9-year-old standard poodle. Barium aspiration occurred in the right middle lung lobe 1 year prior (*white arrow*). The regional lymph nodes have an amorphous mineral opacity (*black arrows*) because of lymphatic transport of aspirated barium. Active pneumonia, unrelated to barium aspiration, is present in the right cranial lung lobe.

Lateral and dorsoventral radiographs of the neck and thorax should be obtained during swallowing or as soon after swallowing as possible. It is wise to obtain images of multiple swallows and to confirm the presence of a suspected lesion on multiple projections. When perforation is unlikely, kibble is then soaked in barium and administered orally.[12] Additional lateral and VD radiographs of the neck and thorax should be obtained. Barium-soaked kibble is particularly helpful when trying to identify esophageal strictures through which liquid barium may pass unimpeded. Mixing iodinated contrast agents with kibble is not advised since iodinated agents are typically used when perforation is suspected and esophageal leakage of kibble is undesirable.[15]

Barium or iodine aspiration is a potential complication of performing esophageal contrast studies. Aspiration of a small amount of liquid barium is usually insignificant. Pneumonia and lung granuloma formation are rare complications of barium aspiration. Aspirated barium is cleared from the airways by ciliary action, as well as coughing. If barium enters the alveolar space, it may remain there permanently (Fig. 30.5). Lymphatic uptake of aspirated barium will also be evident as amorphous mottled opacities in the region of the mediastinal and tracheobronchial lymph nodes, which may also be a permanent finding (Fig. 30.6).

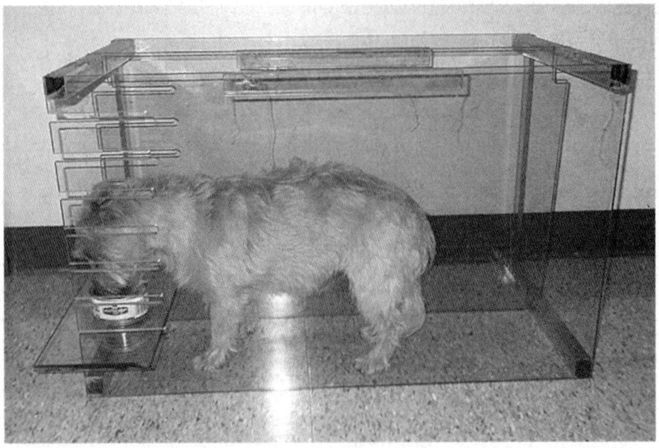

Fig. 30.7 A radiolucent squeeze cage made of polycarbonate can be used to examine the swallowing phases in a dog in a standing position with reduced radiation exposure to personnel and mimic a normal swallowing posture.

CONTRAST VIDEOFLUOROSCOPIC SWALLOWING STUDIES

When a functional or transient disorder of swallowing is suspected and cannot be defined by survey or contrast radiography, contrast videofluoroscopic assessment of swallowing is indicated. When performing dynamic fluoroscopic swallowing studies, it is essential to protect personnel involved in the study from scattered radiation by establishing barriers of lead-impregnated rubber or other shielding between the primary beam and the attending personnel.[8]

In preparation for a videofluoroscopic swallowing study (VFSS), the animal is ideally fasted for 12 hours prior to the procedure. Liquid barium (60% weight-volume) is the most common contrast medium used but, similar to contrast radiography, nonionic iodinated medium diluted 50:50 with sterile water can be used in cases where perforation of the pharynx or esophagus is suspected. The animal is then positioned on the fluoroscopy table. The animal can either be restrained in lateral recumbency on the fluoroscopy table or imaged in sternal or standing position using a cross-table imaging orientation. The differences between sternal and lateral body positioning during VFSS have been reported in the dog and cervical esophageal transit times are significantly delayed in laterally recumbent dogs.[17] However, a specific positioning device is ideal to minimize patient motion during sternally positioned or standing studies (Fig. 30.7) and, in the authors' experience, head motion remains problematic during these examinations, particularly in dogs with dysphagia. As with contrast radiography, sedation should be avoided when performing contrast-enhanced videofluoroscopy due to the inherent alteration in swallowing function that results from tranquilization.

Standardization of videofluoroscopic contrast swallowing studies is essential for accurate interpretation, because bolus size and form (solid vs. liquid) can significantly alter many of the quantitative and qualitative features.[18] Measurements of pharyngeal constriction ratio (PCR), time to maximum pharyngeal contraction, time to cricopharyngeal sphincter opening, time to epiglottis reopening, and the percentage of secondary peristaltic waves do not differ with body position but other esophageal transit times and frequency of peristaltic waves do.[17] Regardless of body position, liquid barium should be administered orally in small (5–10 mL) boluses using a catheter-tipped syringe. At least three complete swallows should be observed and at least one bolus should be followed all the way to the stomach. Barium-soaked soft food followed by barium-soaked kibble should also be given orally and bolus propulsion observed fluoroscopically to rule out abnormalities that allow liquid passage but affects passage of solid foods. Recording the study and performing frame-by-frame analysis can provide quantitative measures of swallowing function.

Many quantitative parameters have been reported as valuable assessments of pharyngeal and cricopharyngeal function.[17–21] These include the interswallow interval ([ISI]; time in seconds between two successive, uninterrupted swallows from the onset frame of swallow 1 to the onset frame of the subsequent swallow), swallow rate (the number of swallows per 3-second interval of uninterrupted prehension), jaw cycles per swallow ratio (the number of licks from maximum jaw excursion to the following maximum jaw excursion), time from swallow onset (Fig. 30.8A) to proximal esophageal sphincter/UES opening (Fig. 30.8B), time to maximum laryngeal excursion (Fig. 30.8C), time to maximum pharyngeal contraction (Fig. 30.8D), time to air column reopening/epiglottis reopening (Fig. 30.8E), and time to proximal esophageal sphincter/UES closure (Fig. 30.8F). When making quantitative measures, videos are viewed frame by frame where each frame represents 1/30th of a second. The frame in which the epiglottis is observed to close over the larynx is considered as the starting point for all time measurements. The swallow is considered completed when the epiglottis is observed to reopen. Once the number of frames to each point in the swallow is calculated, that number can be divided by 30 to obtain the number of seconds from the initiation of the swallow to each particular event within that swallow. The contraction of the pharynx can also be assessed using frame-by-frame analysis to facilitate calculation of the PCR.[19] From the digitized videofluoroscopic studies, a hold frame and a maximum contraction frame are selected. The hold frame is identified as a frame in which the larynx appeared at rest without rostral or caudal motion. The maximum contraction frame is identified as a frame in which the dorsal pharyngeal wall had reached its most

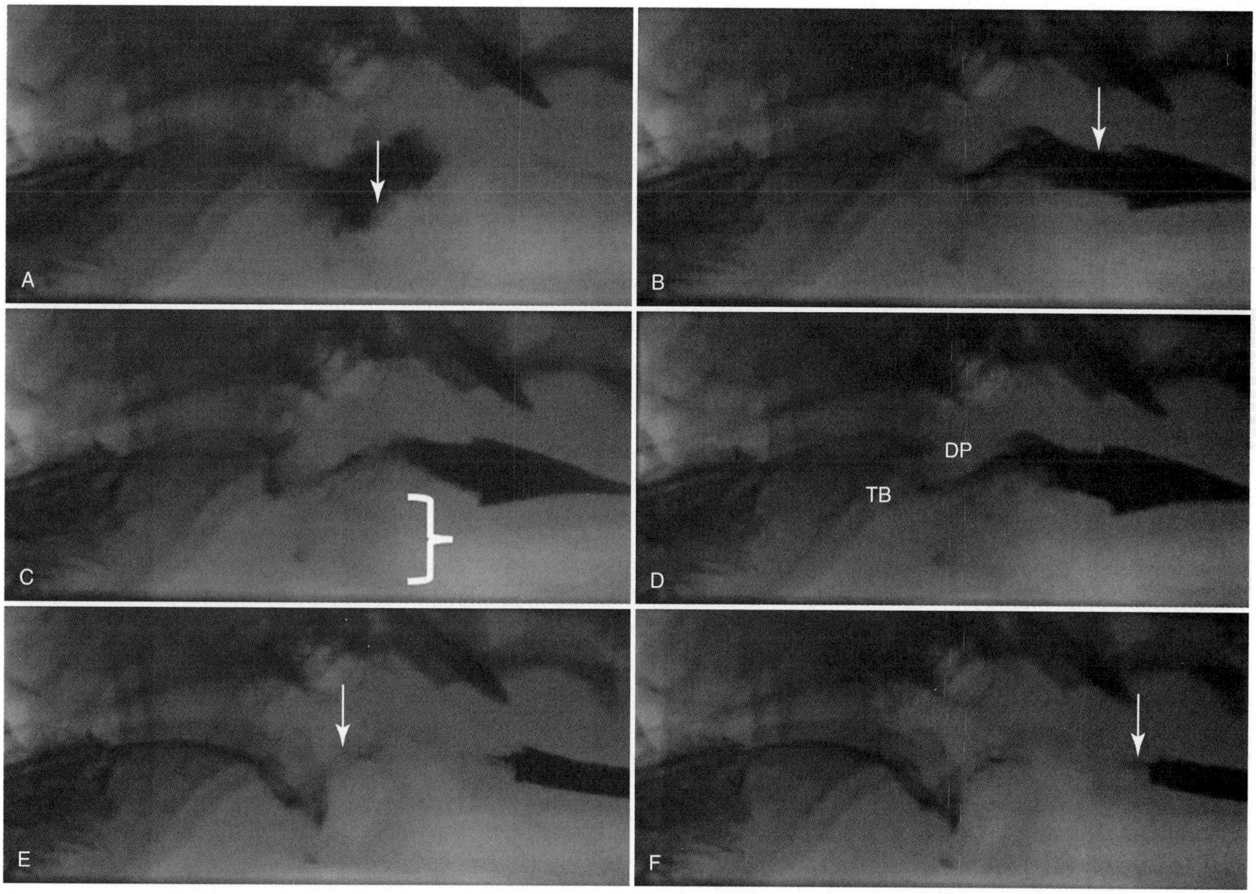

Fig. 30.8 Representative images are shown from a contrast videofluoroscopic evaluation of swallowing obtained from a healthy dog. Typically, the number of frames is counted from onset of swallowing to specified events and converted to seconds based on a 30-frame-per-second image acquisition. **A,** Swallow onset frame indicated by closure of the epiglottis (*white arrow*) *a*nd perpendicular movement of the bolus toward the pharynx. **B,** First frame in which the upper/proximal esophageal sphincter (*white arrow*) is open. **C,** Frame in which the larynx is in its most rostral position (*white bracket*). **D,** Frame obtained at maximal pharyngeal contraction where tongue base (*TB*) and dorsal pharyngeal wall (*DP*) are in contact and have their most ventral and caudal position. **E,** Frame in which the air column in the pharynx has reappeared (*white arrow*) due to opening of the epiglottis and relaxation of the pharynx. **F,** Frame in which the bolus has completely passed into the proximal esophagus and the upper/proximal esophageal sphincter is closed (*white arrow*). (Reproduced with permission from Pollard RE. Videofluoroscopic evaluation of the pharynx and upper esophageal sphincter in the dog: a systematic review of the literature. *Front Vet Sci.* 2019;6:117.)

ventral and caudal position. For the hold frame, a region of interest (ROI) is drawn around the airspace beginning dorsal to the soft palate then rostrally to the hyoid apparatus and tympanic bulla, dorsally to the dorsal aspect of the pharyngeal wall, caudally along the dorsal aspect of the pharyngeal wall to the UES, and ventrally around the corniculate process of the arytenoid cartilage to include the vallecula, finally connecting the epiglottis to the starting point (Fig. 30.9A). The UES is specifically defined as the region in the cranial esophagus that remained the narrowest through the study.[22] For the maximum contraction frame, an ROI is drawn around any residual barium or airspace identified within the pharyngeal area (see Fig. 30.9B). ROIs are expressed in pixel numbers and the PCR is calculated by dividing the number of pixels in the maximum contraction frame by the number of pixels in the hold frame. Normal reference ranges for quantitative measures are outlined in Table 30.1, including measurements made with animals in different body positions, consuming different bolus sizes and of various ages.

Techniques for VFSS in dogs with megaesophagus have been reported with the intent of defining LES function, assess for any evidence of peristalsis, and to determine the optimal dietary consistency for expedition of esophageal clearance.[23,24] Dogs are fasted for 12 hours prior to imaging and positioned in a size appropriate Bailey chair with the photon beam directed horizontally to yield a lateral projection of the cervical and thoracic esophagus to the level of the LES (Fig. 30.10A,B). Bolus consistencies are similar to above and include liquid barium, barium-soaked soft food/slurry and barium-soaked kibble. VFSS is performed along the entire length of the esophagus at baseline, for the first 20 seconds or until complete esophageal clearance, and then every 5 minutes for up to 15 minutes following liquid administration and 30 minutes after each food type. Fluoroscopic evaluation is discontinued if all material clears from the esophagus or after 15 minutes for liquid and 30 minutes for slurry and kibble, whichever comes first.

Regardless of the VFSS study performed, in normal animals, there should be no retention of barium in the oral or pharyngeal cavity during swallowing. Some coating of the mucosa is normal. No contrast medium should be present in the pharynx, larynx, or trachea after swallowing. Small volumes of contrast medium may accumulate in the proximal esophagus if bolus size is inadequate for stimulation of a primary peristaltic wave. However, larger boluses should trigger primary peristalsis, or secondary peristalsis should initiate once boluses accumulate to an adequate size.

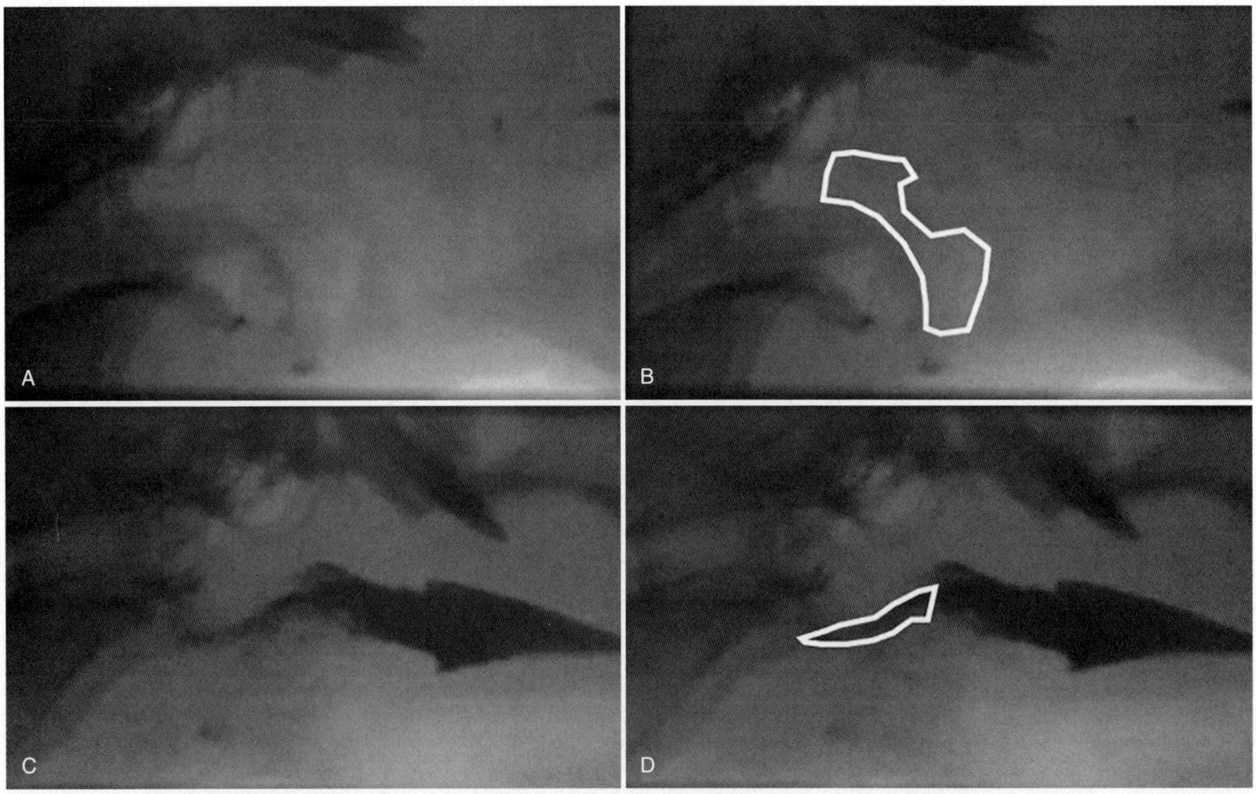

Fig. 30.9 The pharyngeal constriction ratio (PCR) is a metric of pharyngeal function and is calculated by measuring the area in the pharynx at maximal contraction (maximal contraction frame) and dividing that by the area of the pharynx at rest (hold frame). **A,** Hold frame from a contrast videofluoroscopic evaluation of swallowing obtained from a healthy dog. **B,** Same image as in **A** with the area of pharynx outlined including the airspace beginning dorsal to the soft palate then rostrally to the hyoid apparatus and tympanic bulla, dorsally to the dorsal aspect of the pharyngeal wall, caudally along the dorsal aspect of the pharyngeal wall to the cranial esophageal sphincter, ventrally around the corniculate process of the arytenoid cartilage to include the vallecula, and finally connecting the epiglottis to the starting point. **C,** Maximal contraction frame from the same dog as in **A** and **B**. **D,** Maximal contraction frame from the same dog as in **A** and **B** with the area of the pharynx defined. (Reproduced with permission from Pollard RE. Videofluoroscopic evaluation of the pharynx and upper esophageal sphincter in the dog: a systematic review of the literature. *Front Vet Sci.* 2019;6:117.)

Table • 30.1

Summary of Quantitative Parameters Obtained From Videofluoroscopic Swallowing Studies.

	BONADIO ET AL.[17]		CHENEY ET AL.[18]			HARRIS ET AL.[21]		
PARAMETER	LATERAL	STANDING	SMALL BOLUS	MEDIUM BOLUS	LARGE BOLUS	JUVENILE	ADULT	GERIATRIC
UES open	0.10 ± 0.02	0.11 ± 0.02	0.09 ± 0.02	0.08 ± 0.02	0.08 ± 0.02	0.04 ± 0.02	0.05 ± 0.03	0.03 ± 0.02
Max LE	NA	NA	NA	NA	NA	0.07 ± 0.03	0.08 ± 0.04	0.10 ± 0.06
Max PC	0.11 ± 0.04	0.10 ± 0.03	0.15 ± 0.04	0.16 ± 0.04	0.17 ± 0.04	0.11 ± 0.06	0.12 ± 0.04	0.11 ± 0.02
Epi open	0.24 ± 0.04	0.25 ± 0.05	0.22 ± 0.05	0.23 ± 0.04	0.25 ± 0.04	0.28 ± 0.06	0.26 ± 0.06	0.30 ± 0.05
UES close	0.25 ± 0.04	0.27 ± 0.04	0.25 ± 0.06	0.26 ± 0.05	0.29 ± 0.05	0.33 ± 0.03	0.31 ± 0.06	0.35 ± 0.06
PCR	0.11 ± 0.35	0.14 ± 0.04	0.13 ± 0.03	0.13 ± 0.03	0.13 ± 0.04	NA	NA	NA
ISI	NA	NA	NA	NA	NA	1.51 ± 1.97	1.14 ± 0.53	1.19 ± 0.69
Swallow rate (per 3 seconds)	NA	NA	NA	NA	NA	1.65 ± 1.20	2.65 ± 0.70	2.35 ± 0.65
Jaw cycles per swallow ratio	NA	NA	NA	NA	NA	2.70 ± 2.68	2.85 ± 1.15	3.00 ± 1.25

Epi, epiglottis; *ISI,* interswallow interval; *LE,* laryngeal excursion; *Max,* maximum; *NA,* not assessed; *PC,* pharyngeal contraction; *PCR,* pharyngeal constriction ratio; *UES,* upper esophageal sphincter.
Modified from Pollard RE. Videofluoroscopic evaluation of the pharynx and upper esophageal sphincter in the dog: a systematic review of the literature. *Front Vet Sci.* 2019;6:117.

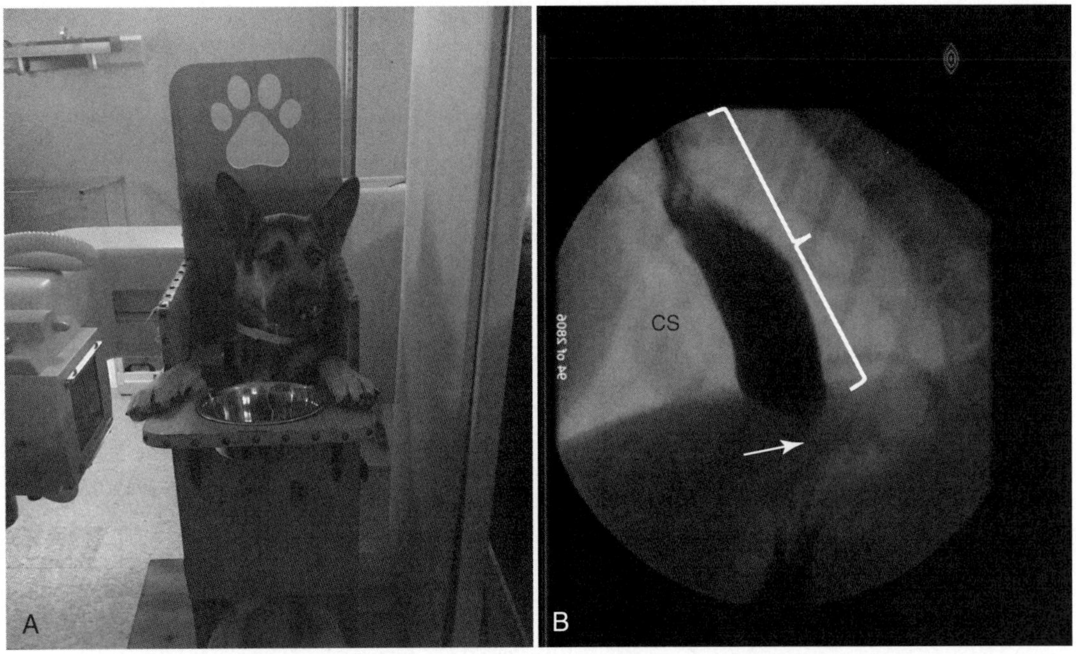

Fig. 30.10 A, Dog with megaesophagus positioned in a Bailey chair with the fluoroscopic unit oriented so as to image horizontally through the thorax. **B,** Lateral fluoroscopic image of the same dog as in **A** showing barium accumulation in the dilated caudal thoracic esophagus (*white bracket*) with the lower esophageal sphincter remaining closed (*white arrow*). *CR,* Cardiac silhouette.

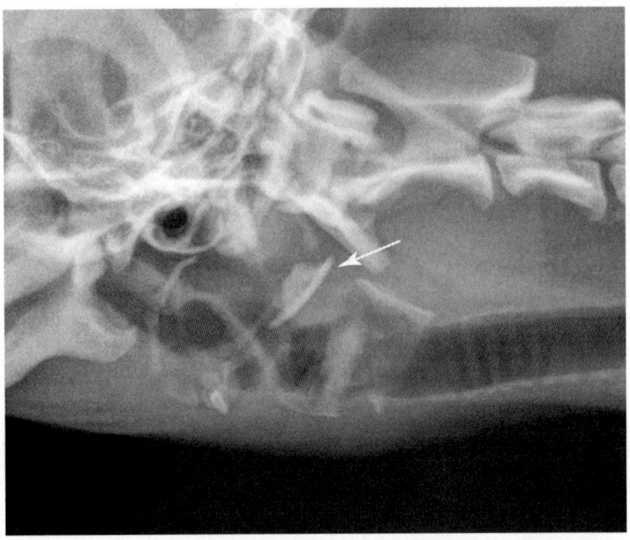

Fig. 30.11 Lateral cervical radiograph of an adult dog. An ingested bone is lodged in the pharynx (*white arrow*).

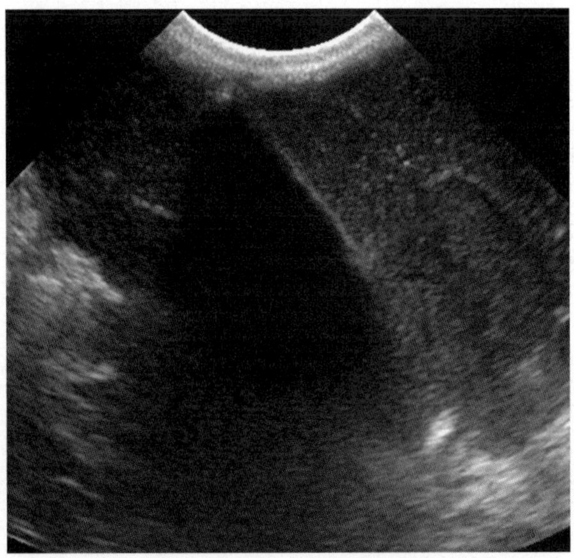

Fig. 30.12 Ultrasound image of the cervical region of a dog with nonspecific swelling of the cranioventral aspect of the neck. There is a large subcutaneous fluid accumulation and multiple, linear, hyperechoic shadowing structures that were determined to be splinters of wood.

PHARYNGEAL AND CRICOPHARYNGEAL DYSPHAGIA

Dysphagia can be morphologic or functional in origin. Morphologic causes include trauma, foreign body, an oral or pharyngeal mass, and regional lymphadenopathy. Lateral and VD survey radiographs of the pharyngeal and cervical region and thorax are indicated to screen for radiopaque foreign bodies, such as bones, needles, and fish hooks (Fig. 30.11). Soft tissue swelling and gas pockets can be seen with perforating pharyngeal trauma, abscesses, or nonradiopaque foreign bodies, such as wooden sticks. Ultrasonography can be useful to determine the source of nonspecific pharyngeal swelling and to identify nonradiopaque foreign bodies (Fig. 30.12).

When a morphologic cause for dysphagia cannot be found, VFSS is indicated to assess function (Table 30.2). Dogs with oral phase dysphagia have difficulty with prehension and bolus formation and with transport to the pharynx. Oral dysphagia is usually characterized by the animal dropping food or liquid from its mouth and drooling.[19] The oral phase of swallowing is the only voluntary portion of the swallowing process. In oral dysphagia, there is failure of aboral transport of liquid or food and lack of bolus formation to induce the swallowing reflex. These disorders are typically diagnosed by watching the animal eat and rarely require imaging. However, if VFSS is performed, liquid contrast medium pools in the dependent vestibule of the

Table • 30.2

Types of Dysphagia, Causes, and Fluoroscopy Findings.

TYPE	CAUSES	FLUOROSCOPIC FEATURES
Oral	Neuromuscular disease Inflammation Oral foreign body Tongue abscess	Bolus not formed or delayed formation Bolus not propelled caudally to pharynx Weak plunger-like movement of tongue Weak pharyngeal contractions Subsequent stages are normal
Pharyngeal	Myositis and myopathy Post-cricopharyngeus myectomy Neuromuscular disease Inflammation Trauma Idiopathic	Normal oral stage Remains synchronous with cricopharyngeal phase Retention of contrast medium in the pharynx No change in time to cricopharyngeal sphincter opening Inadequate pharyngeal contraction Pharyngeal constriction ratio prolonged (0.6) Misdirection of the bolus into larynx or nasopharynx
Cricopharyngeal chalasia	Cricopharyngeus myotomy Radiation therapy Myasthenia gravis	Relaxation or incompetence of the cricopharyngeal sphincter Cricopharyngeal sphincter may appear air-filled Prolonged time to cricopharyngeal sphincter opening (28 seconds) Weak pharyngeal contractions may also be present Aspiration into larynx or trachea possible
Cricopharyngeal achalasia	Idiopathic	Incomplete or lack of opening of cricopharyngeal sphincter Vigorous attempts to pass bolus to cricopharyngeal sphincter Synchrony of timing of the opening of the cricopharyngeal sphincter Delayed time to cricopharyngeal sphincter opening Barium retention in pharynx Aspiration into larynx or trachea possible
Esophageal dysmotility	Delayed maturation Esophagitis	Megaesophagus may be present in young dogs Abnormal primary wave (bolus moves <5 cm aborally) Abnormal secondary wave (bolus retention after two or more subsequent swallows) Retrograde >10 cm Prolonged esophageal transit time >5 seconds

mouth or flows out of the mouth. The backward and forward movement of the tongue will be normal or reduced. The bolus will not be formed and propelled aborally, or its formation will be delayed. The onset of the pharyngeal phase of swallowing may also be delayed. If a swallow is achieved, the pharyngeal and esophageal phases of swallowing are usually normal.

Pharyngeal dysphagia is often characterized by nonspecific signs, such as gagging, retching, and the necessity for multiple swallowing attempts before movement of a bolus into the esophagus.[20] Pharyngeal dysphagia is diagnosed when the contraction of the dorsal pharyngeal wall against the tongue base is weak so that presentation of the bolus to the UES lacks vigorous momentum. The cricopharyngeal phase may or may not be normal. Pharyngeal dysphagia is often the result of neuromuscular disorders that result in weakness or as a result of pharyngeal inflammation. Videofluoroscopic abnormalities include (1) slow contraction of the pharynx, (2) incomplete enclosure of the bolus, (3) incomplete rostral and dorsal movement of the larynx, and (4) absence of forceful contraction of the pharynx to propel the bolus through the cricopharyngeal sphincter. The UES may not open or open to a reduced diameter because of the weakness of the pharyngeal contraction, and this could be misinterpreted as a cricopharyngeal disorder. The PCR was developed to identify dogs with weak pharyngeal contraction that would make them poor candidates for myotomy when cricopharyngeal dysphagia is diagnosed and to better differentiate them from those with cricopharyngeal dysphagia.[19] Dogs with decreased pharyngeal contraction have a significantly higher PCR compared with healthy dogs, but this can also be present in dogs with cricopharyngeal dysphagias. The discerning factor between pharyngeal dysphagia and cricopharyngeal dysphagia is the time to opening of the cricopharyngeal sphincter, which is significantly shorter in pharyngeal dysphagia.[19]

Cricopharyngeal dysphagia is a functional abnormality involving failure of the cricopharyngeal sphincter to open fully (cricopharyngeal achalasia) or at the appropriate time (cricopharyngeal dyssynchrony). The clinical signs of cricopharyngeal dysphagia are similar to those of pharyngeal dysphagia (Fig. 30.13).[19] Although specific breed predilections have not been reported, cricopharyngeal achalasia is often associated with toy breeds.[25] The exact etiology has not been determined, but most affected patients develop clinical signs soon after weaning, suggesting that cricopharyngeal achalasia is a congenital disorder.[26] Critical to the diagnosis is the documentation of delayed or nonopening of the UES and a lack of coordination between pharyngeal contraction and opening of the UES, which requires fluoroscopy (Fig. 30.14). Time from onset of swallowing to opening of the UES is delayed in dogs with cricopharyngeal achalasia compared with normal dogs (0.31 ± 0.14 vs. 09 ± 0.02 seconds for liquids and 0.37 ± 0.06 vs. 0.10 ± 0.03 seconds for kibble).[19] The same is true for UES

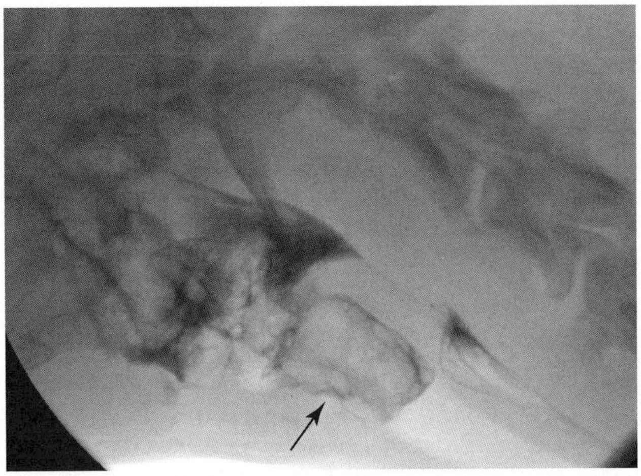

Fig. 30.13 Lateral digital fluoroscopic image of barium swallow in a 2-year-old Border collie with cricopharyngeal dysphagia. The timing of the pharyngeal and cricopharyngeal phases was abnormal, a tight bolus is not present, and barium has been aspirated into the laryngotrachea (*black arrow*). The cricopharyngeal phase was normal but delayed.

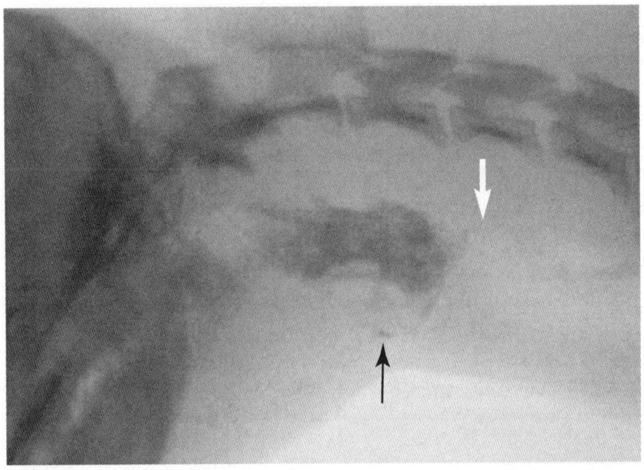

Fig. 30.14 Lateral videofluoroscopic image of a barium swallow in a 1.5-year-old Peekapoo that had severe cricopharyngeal dysphagia. A large bolus (*black arrow*) is present cranial to the closed cricopharyngeal sphincter (*white arrow*). The cricopharyngeal sphincter opened after many swallowing attempts.

closure times. No differences exist in time to maximal pharyngeal contraction and epiglottic reopening between normal dogs and those with cricopharyngeal achalasia with either liquid or kibble meals.

In cricopharyngeal chalasia, the UES does not maintain positive resting pressure between swallows. On survey radiographs, air will often be present in the UES (Fig. 30.15). Cricopharyngeal chalasia can be found in dogs with myasthenia gravis. Barium administration is contraindicated in the presence of a statically open UES because of the increased risk of aspiration.

Dysphagia in cats is less commonly reported than in dogs. Esophageal phase dysphagia is the most common type occurring in cats, with hiatal hernia, dysmotility, and stricture being the most common causes.[27] Quantitative evaluation of the PCR, time to maximal pharyngeal contraction, time to opening of the epiglottis, as well as proximal esophageal sphincter opening and closing times in cats with esophageal dysphagia are similar to that reported in healthy dogs.[27] However, studies in a healthy cat cohort are lacking.

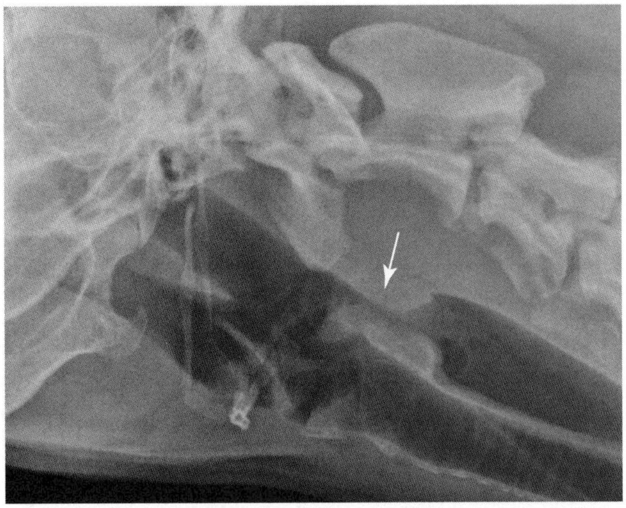

Fig. 30.15 Lateral cervical radiograph of a 5-year-old mastiff with cricopharyngeal chalasia. The cricopharyngeal sphincter is open and contains gas (*white arrow*), as does the cervical esophagus. Cricopharyngeal and cranial esophageal gas is often seen with cricopharyngeal chalasia. The administration of barium is contraindicated in this instance because of increased risk for aspiration.

ESOPHAGEAL DISORDERS

Esophageal motility disorders may result in abnormal peristalsis, transport, and motor function, and clinical signs of regurgitation are common. Survey radiographs can help detect structural abnormalities, such as segmental or generalized dilation of the esophagus, abnormal esophageal content because of lack of normal peristalsis, and the presence of aspiration pneumonia. If survey radiographs are negative in animals with regurgitation, contrast studies are necessary to rule out esophageal disease. Peristaltic abnormalities, hypomotility, strictures, or radiolucent foreign bodies causing obstruction can go undetected on survey radiographs. Mechanical obstruction because of foreign body or stricture can be diagnosed with a static barium esophagram, but accurate assessment of motility requires fluoroscopy. Following passage of a bolus through the UES, a primary peristaltic wave should propel the bolus to the stomach. If this process is interrupted, a secondary peristaltic wave may propel the bolus to the LES in normal animals. It is important to note that, when assessed with VFSS, cervical esophageal transit time is significantly shorter for dogs in sternal recumbency compared to lateral.[17] The percentage of primary waves is significantly greater in liquid and kibble studies when done in sternal recumbency compared with lateral recumbency. Also, the percentage of swallows that have no associated primary peristaltic waves is higher in lateral recumbency. The percentage of secondary waves, however, does not differ between the two positions.[17]

Primary peristalsis can be disrupted by hypomotile segments, and secondary peristalsis may be absent in disease. Dogs with laryngeal paralysis may also have esophageal dysfunction.[28] Esophageal dysmotility in young dogs in the absence of megaesophagus is characterized by abnormal primary waves that move the bolus less than 5 cm aborally, and abnormal secondary waves that allow bolus retention in the esophagus after two subsequent swallows.[29] Retrograde flow of more than 10 cm is another finding associated with hypomotility, as is prolonged esophageal transit time (>5 seconds).[29] Esophageal dysmotility can be caused by delayed maturation, and spontaneous improvement after 1 year of age can occur because of maturation of the neuromuscular system.[30] Esophagitis is another cause of abnormal esophageal motility. Gastroesophageal reflux occurs when gastric and duodenal contents enter aborally into the esophagus, and this can lead to dysmotility secondary to resultant esophagitis.[30]

Esophageal Dilation

Esophageal dilatation can be segmental or generalized depending on the cause and location of disease, and the dilatation can be either functional or mechanical. Generalized dilatation is typically caused by functional disease, whereas segmental dilatation is usually caused by foreign body, infiltrative disease such as neoplasia or inflammation, hiatal diseases, segmental motor disease, stricture, vascular ring anomaly, or redundant esophagus (Fig. 30.16).

Megaesophagus

The term *megaesophagus* describes a dilated and hypomotile esophagus resulting from neuromuscular dysfunction; this type of esophageal dilation is often idiopathic in dogs.[31]

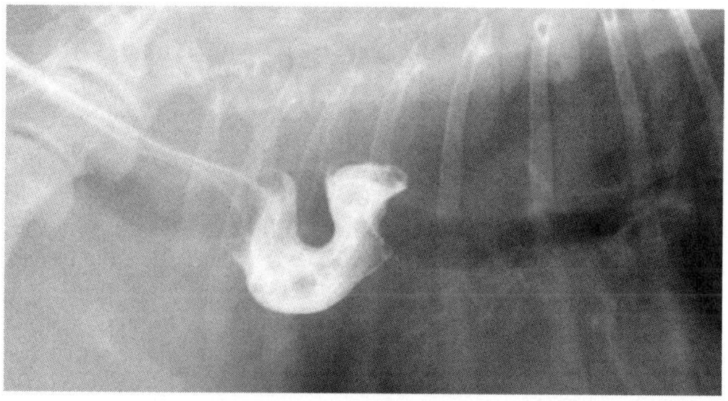

Fig. 30.16 Barium swallow in an 8-year-old Shar-Pei. There is a focal redundancy of the esophagus at the thoracic inlet. This redundancy may be insignificant, but in some dogs, there is diminished contractility with retention of ingesta in this region. A dynamic esophagram is needed to assess the significance of esophageal redundancy.

Megaesophagus in dogs can also result from LES achalasia-like syndrome (LES-AS).[32] Megaesophagus is the most common cause of regurgitation in dogs and the most frequently reported motility disorder affecting the canine esophagus.[33] Megaesophagus is not common in cats but has been described in instances of pylorospasm. Predominant clinical signs in esophageal neuromuscular dysfunction are effortless regurgitation of tubular-formed, undigested food. Megaesophagus can be segmental (cervical or thoracic) or generalized and occurs secondary to diseases of the neuromuscular junction (myasthenia gravis), striated muscle (myositis), peripheral nerves (polyneuropathy), or central nervous system (inflammatory, toxic, and neoplastic).[31]

Radiographic signs of megaesophagus include dilatation of the esophagus with gas, retention of food or fluid, tracheal stripe sign, visibility of the longus colli muscle, ventral displacement of the intrathoracic trachea, ventral displacement of the heart, and aspiration pneumonia (Fig. 30.17; see Figs. 30.4C and 30.5). A cranial mediastinal mass may be present in dogs with thymoma and paraneoplastic myasthenia gravis (eFig. 30.1). When generalized megaesophagus is present, the thoracic segment of the esophagus is usually more severely dilatated than the cervical portion because of surrounding negative intrathoracic pressure. When gas filled, the esophagus can be difficult to discern because of the lucency of the surrounding lung. On lateral thoracic radiographs, two thin soft tissue opaque, parallel bands coursing from cranial to caudal in the dorsal aspect of the thorax represent the wall of the gas-filled esophagus. A focal indentation of the dorsal esophageal wall is caused by the azygous vein crossing over on the right. In the VD radiograph, the wall of the gas-filled esophagus is most often identified as a thin, soft tissue band to the left of the vertebral column. If the dilation is severe enough, a second band can also be seen on the right, converging with the left one at the caudal esophageal sphincter (see Fig. 30.17). When imaged with VFSS in a Bailey chair, dogs with LES-AS can be distinguished from dogs with idiopathic megaesophagus due to the presence of a "bird-beak" appearance to the LES.[32]

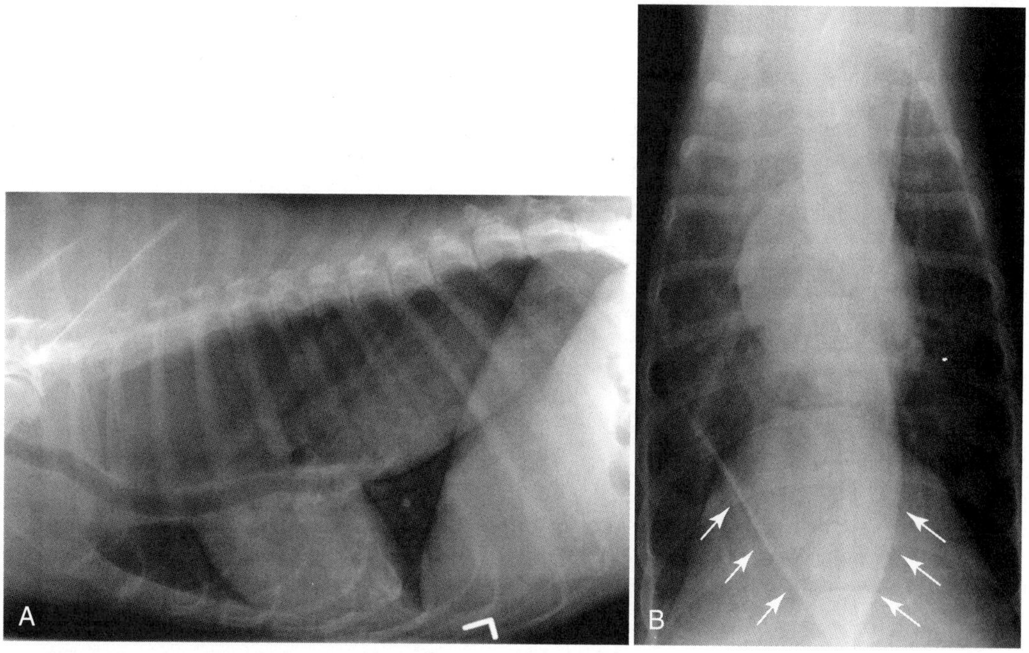

Fig. 30.17 **A,** Lateral radiograph of a 3-year-old German shepherd dog. The esophagus is severely dilated such that the trachea and heart are displaced ventrally. An alveolar pattern because of aspiration pneumonia is present in the periphery of the right middle lung lobe. **B,** Ventrodorsal (VD) radiograph of the same dog. The borders of the enlarged esophagus extend to the left and right side of the thorax and converge in a V shape near the caudal esophageal sphincter (*white arrows*).

Hiatal Diseases

Esophageal hiatal diseases include dynamic esophageal and paraesophageal hernias, gastroesophageal intussusception, and gastroesophageal reflux. Clinical signs may be absent, or dogs may have recurrent gastrointestinal signs, such as regurgitation, retching, and possibly vomiting. Esophageal hernias can be congenital or acquired. The congenital form has been reported in shar-pei dogs.[34] In the acquired form, weakness of the diaphragm, elevated abdominal pressure, and upper airway obstruction are predisposing factors.

In dynamic hiatal hernias, the caudal esophageal sphincter and part of the gastric fundus move in and out of the caudal mediastinum through a weakened esophageal hiatus of the diaphragm. In most dogs and cats, this may happen intermittently and randomly making radiographic identification challenging. Brachycephalic breeds are prone to hiatal hernias in affiliation with brachycephalic upper airway obstruction due to excess negative thoracic pressure needed to respire against the obstructed upper airway.[35,36] In these breeds, hiatal herniation often accompanies inspiration and is more frequent, thereby making radiographic identification more likely.

If captured radiographically, there is a soft tissue, or mixed soft tissue and gas opacity between the aorta and caudal vena cava on lateral radiographs that silhouettes with the cranial diaphragmatic contour (Fig. 30.18, eFig. 30.2 and 30.3). If persistent on the VD view, the opacity has a midline location and is slightly on the left of the vertebral column. Dynamic esophageal hernia may be confirmed with static barium esophagraphy; however, VFSS is often necessary. If the fundus is herniated along with the esophagus, rugal folds outlined by barium may be visible. The caudal esophageal sphincter will also be located cranial to the diaphragm, and barium can be seen to reflux from the stomach into the caudal esophagus with VFSS.

Paraesophageal hernias are caused by the fundus being herniated into the mediastinum alongside of the esophagus with the caudal esophageal sphincter remaining in the abdomen (Fig. 30.19A). On VD radiographs, the herniated fundus is to the left of the esophagus, and hernia contents may move in and out with respiration (see Fig. 30.19B,C).

Gastroesophageal intussusception occurs when part of the stomach and possibly other abdominal organs, such as the spleen, evert into the esophageal lumen. The intussusceptum may be of homogeneous soft tissue opacity or may be a mixed soft tissue and gas opacity if there is gas trapped in the herniated portion of the stomach (Fig. 30.20). A feature that distinguishes gastroesophageal intussusception from a sliding or paraesophageal hernia is the sharply marginated cranial edge of the intussusceptum contrasted against a gas-filled esophageal lumen. Gastroesophageal intussusception is often acquired and secondary to esophageal dilatation or previous surgery at the caudal esophageal sphincter resulting in chalasia.

Gastroesophageal reflux occurs when gastric acid enters the esophagus; this usually results in esophagitis. Survey radiographs are usually normal, or there may be increased soft tissue opacity between the aorta and vena cava on both lateral projections. With increasing severity, the caudal esophagus may become enlarged and contain either air or fluid. Contrast esophagram studies are usually negative unless severe ulceration is present that leads to adherence of the contrast medium to the mucosa. Focal dilatation of the esophagus with contrast medium and/or obliteration of the linear folds normally outlined with barium can occur if the esophagitis is severe. Scarring and stricture can develop.

Redundant Esophagus

Redundant esophagus is often an incidental finding in brachycephalic breeds, such as bulldogs and Shar-Peis (see Fig. 30.16).

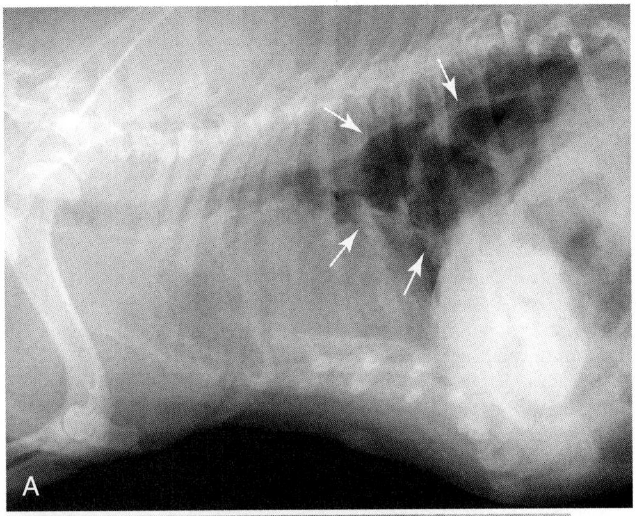

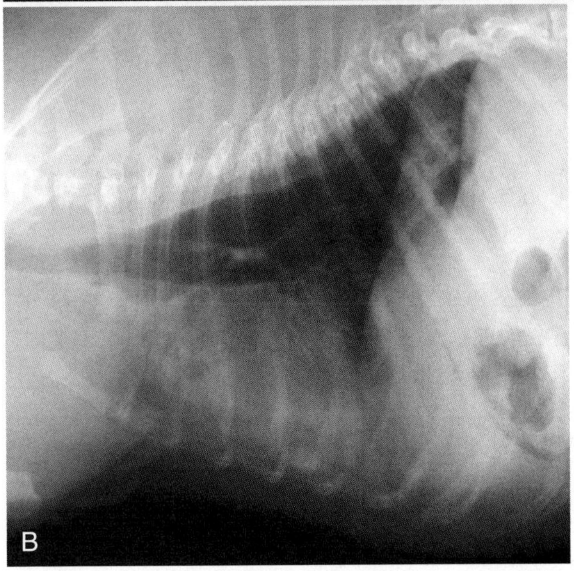

Fig. 30.18 **A,** Lateral thoracic radiograph of a 2-year-old bulldog with upper airway obstruction. There is cranial displacement of the stomach into the thorax (*white arrows*) and dorsal deviation of the sternum and ribs with a small lung volume. **B,** Same dog after endotracheal intubation and under anesthesia. The sternum resumes a normal position, the diaphragm is flatter and in a more caudal position, and the stomach is no longer displaced into the thorax. Residual gas dilatation of the esophagus could be caused by anesthesia or from previous aerophagia. The increase in intrathoracic pressure associated with alleviation of the airway obstruction allowed the stomach to reduce spontaneously into the abdomen.

Survey radiographs may be normal, or focal dilatation of the esophagus with gas can be seen at the thoracic inlet. In static barium esophagrams, the esophagus has a tortuous course at the thoracic inlet that appears as a diverticulum ventral to the trachea. The accumulation of contrast medium in a redundant esophagus is usually only temporary, and the esophagus will appear normal on subsequent radiographs. With VFSS, the redundant segment typically has normal motility. Occasionally, there will be a clinically significant motility disorder associated with the redundant region of the esophagus.

FOREIGN BODIES

Esophageal foreign bodies are more common in dogs than cats, and some terrier breeds appear to be predisposed.[37] Survey radiography should include the region from the base of the

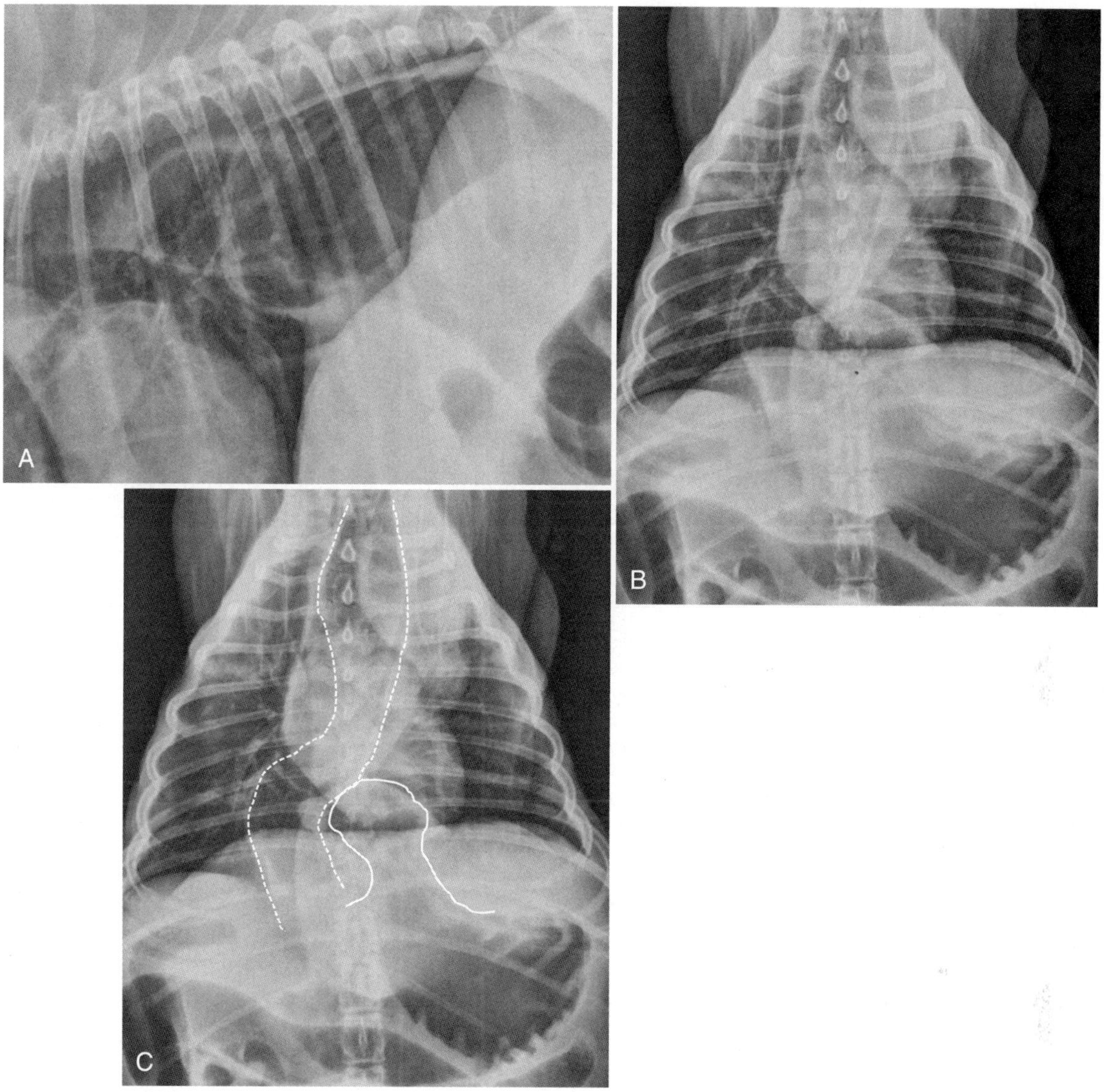

Fig. 30.19 **A,** Lateral thoracic radiograph of a 13-year-old miniature schnauzer. A compartmentalized, gas-filled structure is present in the caudodorsal thorax. This appearance could be caused by either a paraesophageal hernia or a sliding hiatal hernia. Ventrodorsal (VD) radiograph **(B)** and annotated VD radiograph **(C)** of the same dog. The gas-filled structure, which is the fundus (*solid line*), is to the left of midline and adjacent to the gas-filled and dilatated esophagus (*dotted line*), which takes on a tortuous course and is displaced to the right. The soft tissue mass in the left cranial thoracic quadrant is a thymoma.

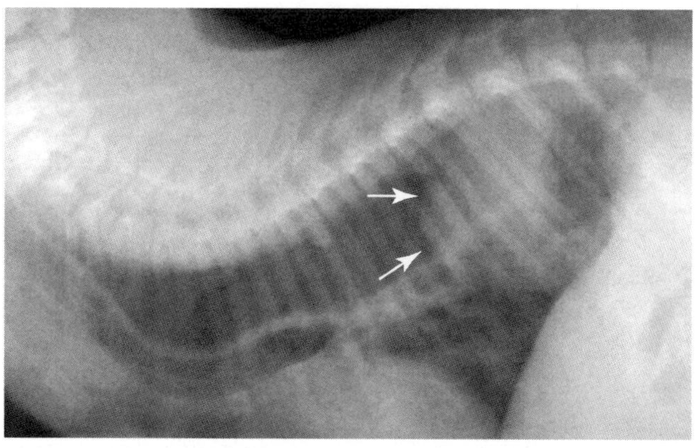

Fig. 30.20 Lateral thoracic radiograph of an 8-week-old Bengal kitten. The thoracic esophagus is gas dilatated with ventral displacement of the trachea and heart. A mixed soft tissue and gas mass with a sharply defined round cranial border (*white arrows*) is present in the dorsocaudal aspect of the thorax. This appearance of a gas-filled esophagus with a caudally located intraluminal mass having a sharply marginated cranial border is characteristic of gastroesophageal intussusception.

tongue to the diaphragm. Foreign bodies are most often located at the thoracic inlet, base of the heart, or just cranial to the diaphragm, sites where the esophagus is limited in its ability to distend. Common radiographic features are visibility of the distinct foreign material, gas in the esophagus contrasting with the foreign body, esophageal dilation orad to the obstruction, and signs of perforation (pleural or mediastinal effusion or pneumomediastinum).[38] Nonobstructive foreign bodies, such as fishhooks and other sharp objects, tend to lodge in the pharyngeal region (Fig. 30.21; see Fig. 30.11). Radiopaque foreign material, such as bones or metal, is recognized easily compared with nonradiopaque material, such as plastic and cartilage, which appears as focal soft tissue opacity in the region of the esophagus (Fig. 30.22, eFig. 30.4). A soft tissue opaque esophageal foreign body may appear similar to an esophageal neoplasm, an esophageal abscess, mediastinal mass, paraesophageal hernia, or lung mass (see Fig. 30.22). A static contrast esophagram can help to differentiate these conditions. Contraindications for a barium swallow include survey radiographic evidence of pneumothorax, pneumomediastinum, and mediastinal or pleural fluid, which are signs of potential esophageal perforation (Fig. 30.23).

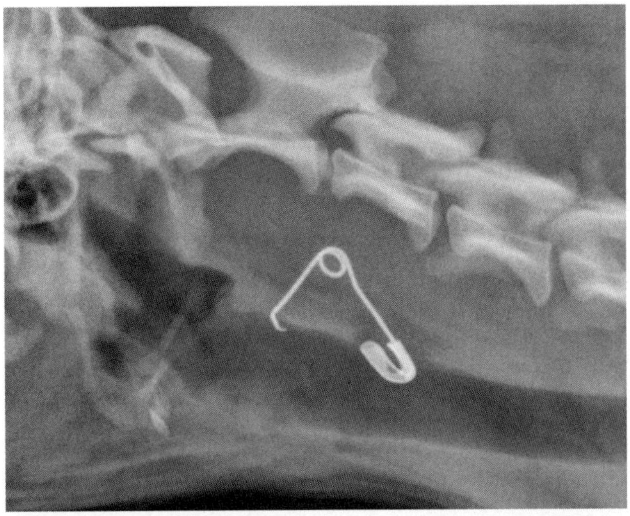

Fig. 30.21 Open safety pin obstructing the cervical esophagus caudal to the cricopharyngeal sphincter.

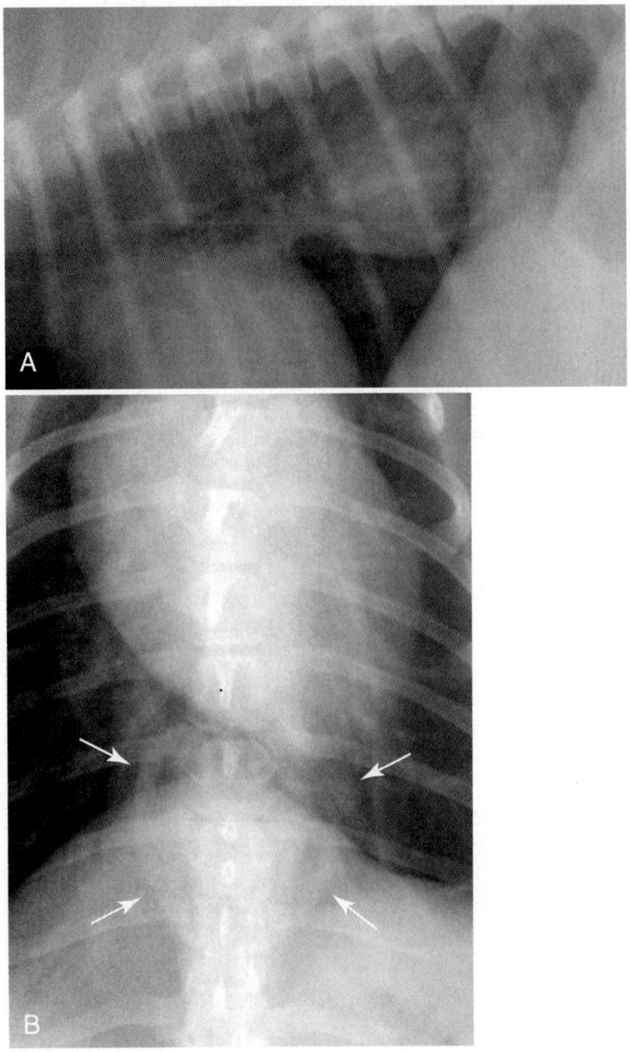

Fig. 30.22 **A,** Lateral thoracic radiograph of a 4-year-old Chihuahua. There is a soft tissue mass in the caudodorsal aspect of the thorax between the aorta and caudal vena cava with its caudal border superimposed with the diaphragm. Based on this appearance, the considerations are esophageal foreign body, esophageal mass, paraesophageal hernia, or pulmonary mass. **B,** Ventrodorsal (VD) radiograph of the same dog. The mass is on the midline (*white arrows*), making a pulmonary mass unlikely. Endoscopy was performed, and a hard, cartilaginous foreign body was removed.

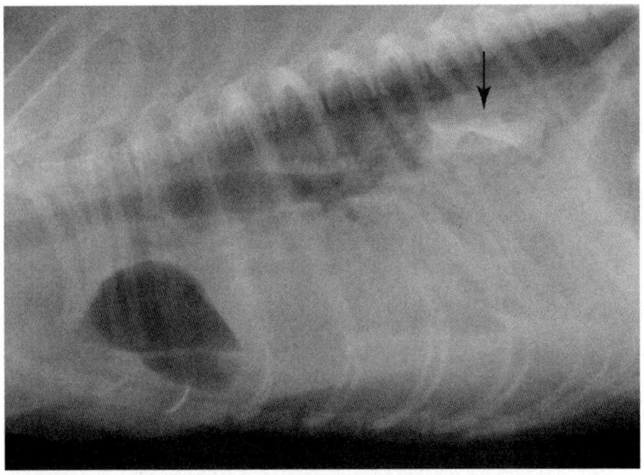

Fig. 30.23 Right lateral radiograph of a dog with a bone lodged in the caudal aspect of the esophagus (*black arrow*). There is also pleural fluid and pneumothorax. A barium esophagram should not be done in this situation because of the high likelihood of esophageal perforation. If an esophagram is necessary, water-soluble contrast medium should be used.

VASCULAR RING ANOMALIES

Regurgitation due to vascular ring anomalies presents at an early age in most instances; however, it can have late-onset occurrence in both cats and dogs.[39–41] Under normal conditions, the aorta is derived from the left fourth aortic arch while the right fourth aortic arch typically regresses. Anomalous development of the aortic arches can lead to secondary extrinsic esophageal compression. Esophageal compression secondary to a vascular malformation is termed *vascular ring anomaly*. Of the seven types of vascular ring anomalies that are described, types I through III have a persistent right aortic arch, type IV has a double aortic arch, and types V through VII have a left aortic arch with combinations of persistent right ligamentum arteriosum and right subclavian arteries, all of which cause entrapment of the esophagus.[42–44]

Development of the aortic arch from the right fourth aortic arch with regression of the left fourth aortic arch, termed *persistent right fourth aortic arch*, is the most common vascular ring anomaly that leads to entrapment of the esophagus. In the normal situation where the aorta is derived from the left fourth arch, the aorta, main pulmonary artery, and interconnecting ligamentum arteriosum are all on the left side of the trachea and esophagus.[42] When the aorta is derived from the right fourth aortic arch rather than the left, the aorta is on the right side of the trachea and esophagus, whereas the main pulmonary artery is on the left side. In this configuration, the ligamentum arteriosum compresses the esophagus against the trachea and base of the heart as it passes from right (aorta) to left (pulmonary artery) (Fig. 30.24). The compression results in esophageal dilation cranial to the base of the heart. Survey radiographs may be normal if the esophagus is not dilated, but this is unusual. The dilated portion of the esophagus cranial to the heart base creates a mass effect that contains air and/or ingesta and usually displaces the trachea ventrally (Figs. 30.25 and 30.26), although occasionally the enlarged esophagus will slide laterally and become positioned ventral to the trachea (Fig. 30.27). In some dogs, it is possible to see the trachea being deviated focally toward the left on VD projections (see Fig. 30.25), and the normal left lateral margin of the aorta may not be evident. In a static barium esophagram, the narrowing of the esophagus at the heart base can be confirmed (see Fig. 30.30). Keep in mind that a single narrowed area in the esophagus may represent a peristaltic wave and strictures or

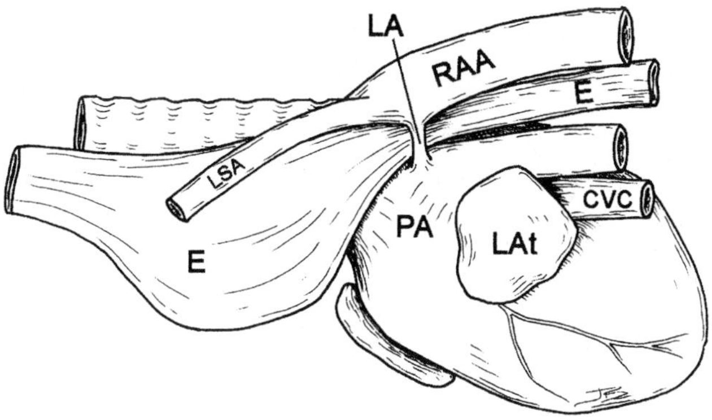

Fig. 30.24 Schematic of persistent right aortic arch. This view from the left shows the ligamentum arteriosus (*LA*) connecting the descending right aortic arch (*RAA*) to the main pulmonary artery (*PA*) causing constriction of the esophagus (*E*) between these structures and the heart base. *CVC,* Caudal vena cava; *LAt,* left atrium; *LSA,* left subclavian artery. (Figure courtesy Dr. Barbara Watrous, DACVR.)

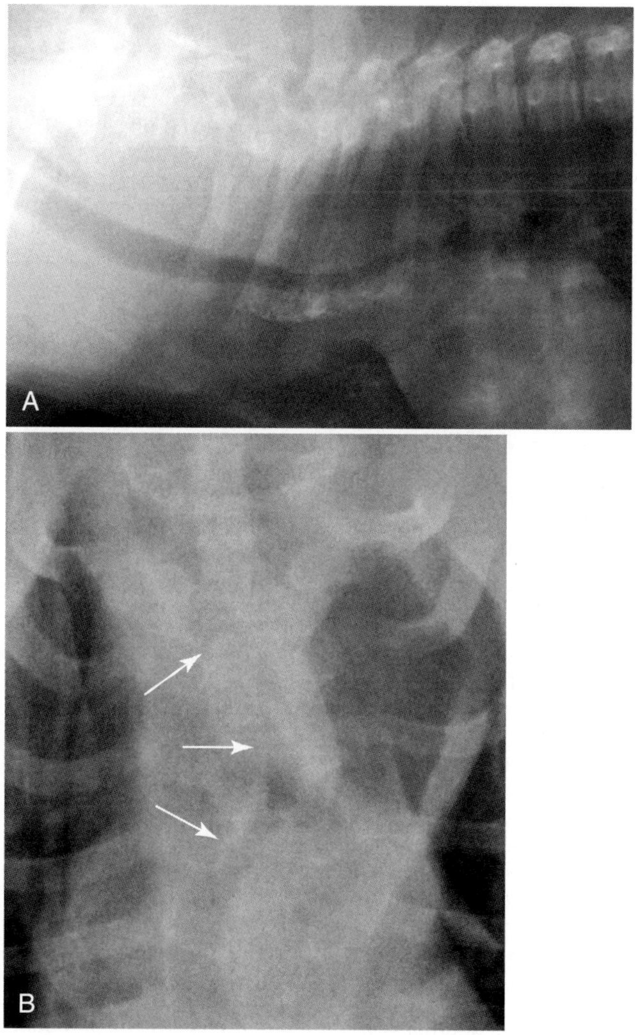

Fig. 30.25 **A,** Lateral thoracic radiograph of a 2-month-old German shepherd with a persistent right fourth aortic arch. The thoracic trachea is displaced ventrally, and there is a superimposed mottled mineral opacity because of foreign material in the enlarged esophageal segment cranial to the heart base. The caudal thoracic esophagus appeared normal. **B,** Ventrodorsal (VD) radiograph of the same dog. The trachea is displaced to the left (*white arrows*).

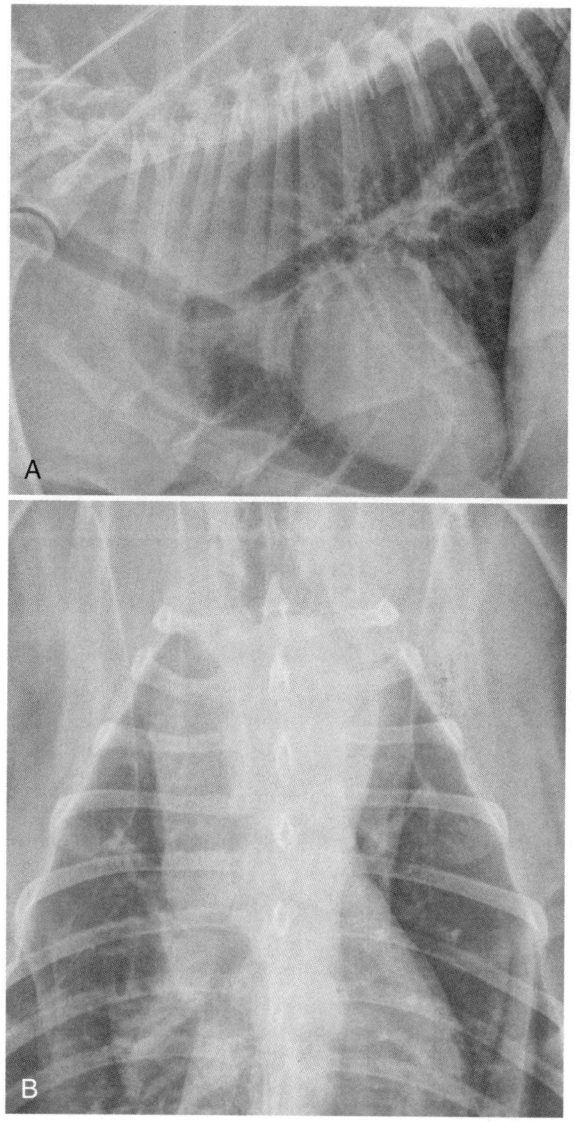

Fig. 30.26 Lateral **(A)** and dorsoventral (DV) **(B)** radiographs of a dog with a persistent right fourth aortic arch. There is dilatation of the cranial aspect of the thoracic esophagus that causes ventral displacement of the trachea. In the DV view, there is a mass effect in the cranial mediastinum. The caudal aspect of the thorax is normal.

vascular ring anomalies should only be diagnosed if persistent narrowing is present on several projections and abnormal dilation of the esophagus is present. VFSS can be useful to assess whether esophageal peristalsis orad to the vascular ring is present as this may influence likelihood of recovery. A persistent left cranial vena cava can accompany persistent right fourth aortic arch and is important that the abnormal left vena cava is recognized at the heart base when a left-thoracotomy is performed to correct the vascular ring constriction.[45]

An aberrant right subclavian artery can also lead to a vascular ring compression of the esophagus. Normally, the right subclavian artery branches from the brachiocephalic trunk but may instead arise directly from the aortic arch, distal to the origin of the left subclavian artery. The right subclavian artery then crosses over the dorsal aspect of the esophagus as it travels from the left side of the median plane, where the normal aortic arch resides, to supply the right forelimb (Figs. 30.28 and 30.29). The site of compression caused by an aberrant subclavian artery is usually slightly more cranial than that caused by a persistent right fourth aortic arch (see Fig. 30.29), and the

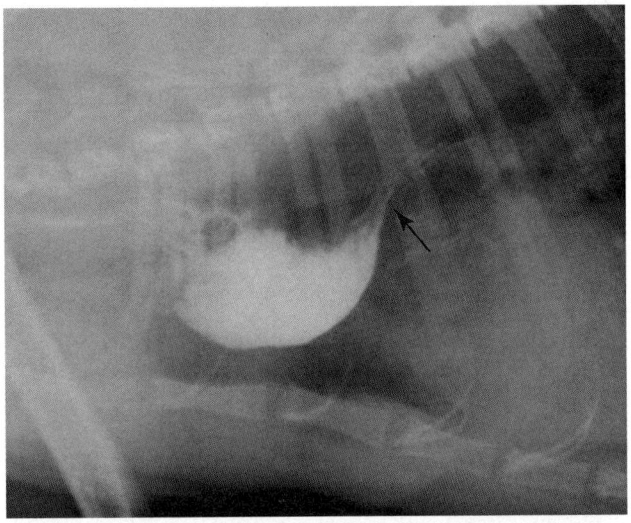

Fig. 30.27 Lateral radiograph of a barium esophagram in an 11-month-old cat with a persistent right fourth aortic arch. Focal dilatation and ventral displacement of the esophagus is present between the thoracic inlet and heart. The contrast column tapers off and narrows at the heart base (*black arrow*) because of the vascular ring constriction.

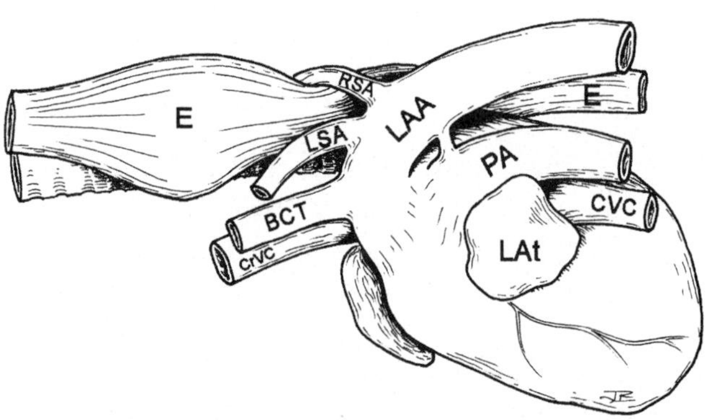

Fig. 30.28 Schematic of aberrant right subclavian artery. This view, from the left side, shows the right subclavian artery (*RSA*) arising from the left-sided aortic arch (*LAA*) and coursing over the top of the esophagus (*E*), causing compression of the esophagus. *BCT,* Brachiocephalic trunk; *CrVC,* cranial vena cava; *CVC,* caudal vena cava; *LAt,* left atrium; *LSA,* left subclavian artery; *PA,* pulmonary artery. (Figure courtesy Dr. Barbara Watrous, DACVR.)

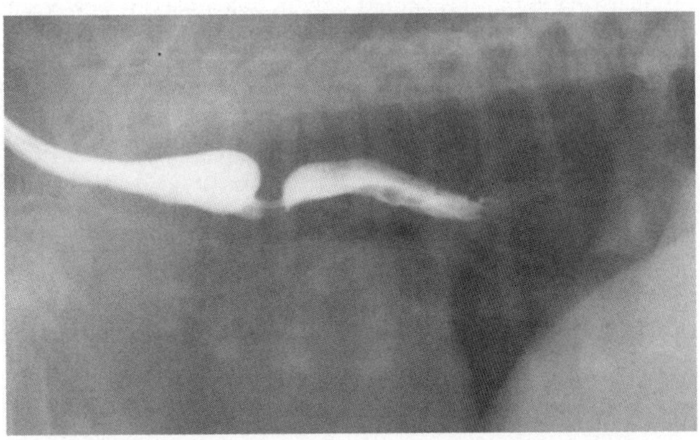

Fig. 30.29 Barium esophagram in a dog with esophageal compression caused by an aberrant right subclavian artery. The indentation in the dorsal aspect of the esophagus results from the compression created by the right subclavian artery passing dorsal to the esophagus as it courses from the left-sided aortic arch to the right forelimb.

compression may not be as severe because the esophagus is not trapped against a solid organ ventrally as it is with persistent right fourth aortic arch.

INFLAMMATORY DISEASES

Esophagitis

Esophagitis can result from infection, ingestion of hot or corrosive substances, vomiting, gastroesophageal reflux, megaesophagus, and foreign body obstructions. Survey radiography is usually unremarkable. Aspiration pneumonia can be identified, but the diagnosis of esophagitis usually requires endoscopy. The esophagus may have reduced motility and therefore be dilated with gas or fluid, but this is a nonspecific finding. Ulcerations, motility disorders, or mechanical obstruction secondary to inflammation requires contrast procedures to be characterized further. If severe esophagitis is present, then segmental narrowing, irregular mucosal contours, indistinct folds of the esophageal wall, and thickening of the wall may be present in static barium contrast studies. Fluoroscopic contrast studies may be characterized by segmental spasticity and minor dilation. Gastroesophageal reflux may be identified with VFSS.

Strictures

Esophageal strictures usually result from foreign body or gastroesophageal reflux. Esophageal strictures thought to be related to gastroesophageal reflux during anesthesia are usually located at the caudal portion of the thoracic esophagus, caudal to the base of the heart.[46] Strictures of the esophagus typically have a smoothly bordered, tapered appearance caudally (Fig. 30.30). Survey radiography may be unremarkable, or there may be segmental or generalized dilatation of the esophagus, depending on the site and extent of the stricture. Contrast esophagraphy is used to determine the location, size, and length of the stricture for treatment planning (see Fig. 30.30). Moreover, the contrast study helps to determine if the stricture is mural, extramural, or luminal. Smoothly bordered mucosal surfaces outlined with contrast medium and having a circumferential narrowing on lateral and VD projections are the typical appearance of a mural stenosis caused by chronic inflammation or scarring. An irregularly bordered mucosal surface can be seen with neoplastic infiltration of the wall or severe ulceration because of inflammation. Extramural compressions have a smoothly bordered contrast column that is convex and tapering toward the narrowing in one projection with the narrowed portion appearing widened in the orthogonal projection. Thyroid masses, enlarged lymph nodes, and cervical abscesses can impinge on or invade the cervical esophagus, causing obstruction. If liquid barium passes through the narrowed region or no abnormality is seen, then barium-soaked kibble can be used to identify a stricture that allows fluid but not solids to pass. Esophageal neoplasms are rare in dogs and cats. Osteosarcoma and fibrosarcoma of the esophagus are reported in areas endemic for *Spirocerca lupi*.[47] Squamous cell carcinoma, adenocarcinoma, branchioma, branchial cleft cysts, papilloma, angioleiomyosarcoma, and leiomyosarcoma have also been reported but are rare.[48–52] If the neoplasm is large enough, it may be recognized on survey radiographs as a soft tissue mass associated with the esophagus (Fig. 30.31, eFig. 30.5). The esophagus may be dilatated cranial to the mass, but this is not always present. Differentiation of esophageal masses from an esophageal foreign body or a nonesophageal mass may require esophagraphy, CT, or endoscopy (see Fig. 30.31). Dystrophic mineralization of esophageal masses is rare, but its presence can be associated with neoplasia, *Spirocerca* infection, or oral administration of radiopaque medication. Esophageal dilation cranial to an esophageal mass may also be present. Obstruction or stenosis at the tumor site, mucosal irregularity caused by

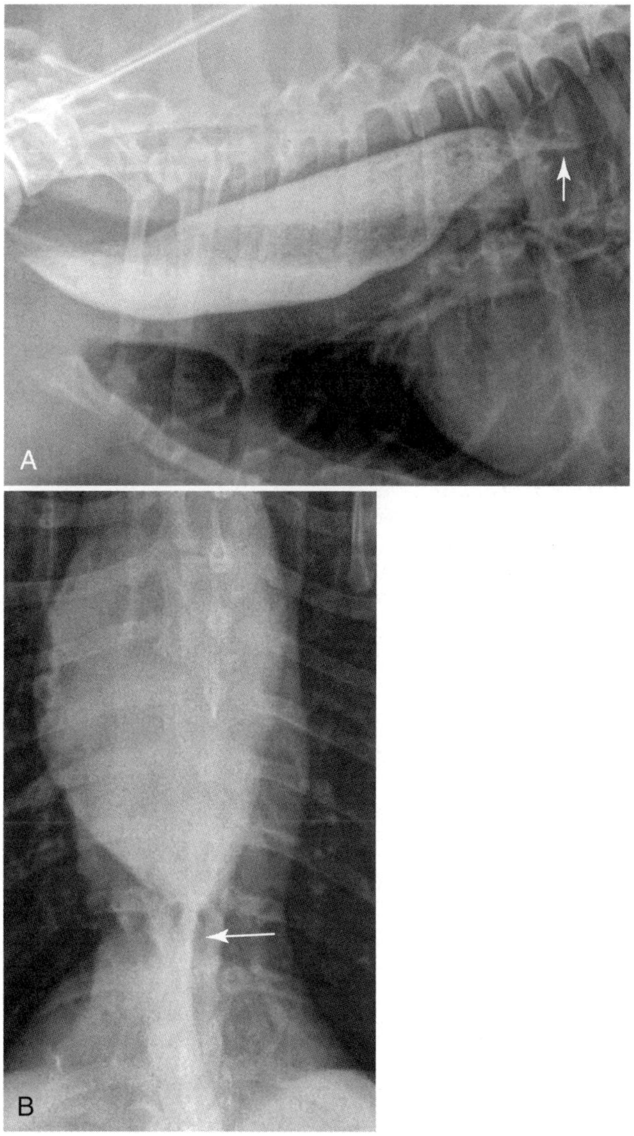

Fig. 30.30 **A,** Lateral radiograph of a barium swallow in a 3.5-year-old Siberian husky with an esophageal stricture. There is dilatation of the esophagus cranial to the carina that tapers smoothly caudally at the site of the stricture (*white arrow*). No contrast medium entered the caudal esophagus. **B,** Ventrodorsal (VD) radiograph of the same dog. The dilated, barium-filled esophagus tapers to a narrow point just caudal to the base of the heart (*white arrow*).

infiltration and ulceration, and/or the location and extent of the infiltration can be evaluated with static esophagraphy. Temporary or persistent retention of barium may occur because of lack of secondary peristalsis where the wall is stiffened because of tumor infiltration. Mural thickening, asymmetry of the lumen, absence of the mucosal folds, ulceration of the mucosa with barium retention, and a locally enlarged or dilated esophagus are suggestive of neoplasia. Infection of dogs and other carnivores with the nematode *S. lupi* occurs in tropical and subtropical regions throughout the world.[53] The parasite infects mainly the esophagus and aorta, leading to gastrointestinal, respiratory, and circulatory signs.[54] In survey radiographs, there may be a mediastinal mass in the region of the caudal thoracic esophagus because of granuloma formation (Fig. 30.32). The inflammatory esophageal mass can become neoplastic, with osteosarcoma and fibrosarcoma being reported. There may be new bone formation on the ventral aspect of thoracic vertebrae dorsal to the mass and also enlargement of the descending aorta.[55–57] *S. lupi* has also caused spinal cord chondrosarcoma.[58] Radiographic abnormalities of the aorta are rare, but dilatation of the proximal descending aorta and aortic mineralization have been reported.[59] In spirocercosis-endemic areas, dorsoventral and right lateral projections are recommended, because they also allow for better visualization of descending aortic aneurysms and prevent interpreting the potentially normally visible esophagus in left lateral images as a mass.[60] However, as noted in Chapter 28, obtaining both left and right lateral views of the thorax should be routine procedure. Contrast studies of the esophagus confirm the granuloma to be originating from the esophagus and are usually characterized by an irregular mucosal border with outpouchings and filling defects. Endoscopy provides similar information, and the parasite may be visualized directly in some dogs.[14] Computed tomography (CT) provides information in confirming nonesophageal or extraesophageal masses to be spirocercosis related because of earlier detection of aortic mineralization and spondylitis.[61] CT angiography perfusion analysis of esophageal nodules can be used to help differentiate nonneoplastic from neoplastic nodules associated with *S. lupi*. *S. lupi*–induced esophageal sarcomas are statistically significantly less perfused than nonneoplastic granulomatous nodules.[62]

DIVERTICULA, PERFORATION, AND FISTULA FORMATION

Esophageal diverticula are pouches of variable size that are either acquired or congenital. The acquired form is caused by a thinning of the esophageal wall that allows it to bulge. Causes include esophagitis, strictures, ulceration from a foreign body, vascular ring anomaly, hiatal hernia, parasites, and periesophageal inflammation. Esophageal diverticula can be classified as either pulsion or traction types. Increased intraluminal pressure from a foreign body or chronic functional obstruction can cause a pulsion diverticulum. Pulsion diverticula are located most commonly between the heart and diaphragm. Traction diverticula are formed because of adhesions on the esophageal wall and are often located in the cranial and midthoracic esophagus.

With an esophageal diverticulum, survey radiographs are characterized by a circumscribed soft tissue mass or outpouching of the esophagus, impacted ingesta, or a mixed gas and soft tissue content (Fig. 30.33). Following survey radiography, further imaging may include endoscopy, CT, or contrast esophagraphy. Contrast medium retention in the outpouching on serial radiographs helps to confirm the diagnosis. Endoscopy is indicated to fully assess the mucosal lining and the size of the opening into the diverticulum for surgical planning.

Perforation of the esophagus occurs either acutely because of a sharp foreign body or chronically because of slow pressure necrosis from a foreign body or neoplasia.[63,64] Perforations can communicate with the mediastinum and/or the pleural space. Bony foreign bodies, a bodyweight of less than 10 kg, and esophageal foreign body present for more than 3 days are considered significant risk factors for complications.[63] Complication rates of esophageal foreign bodies are reported to be

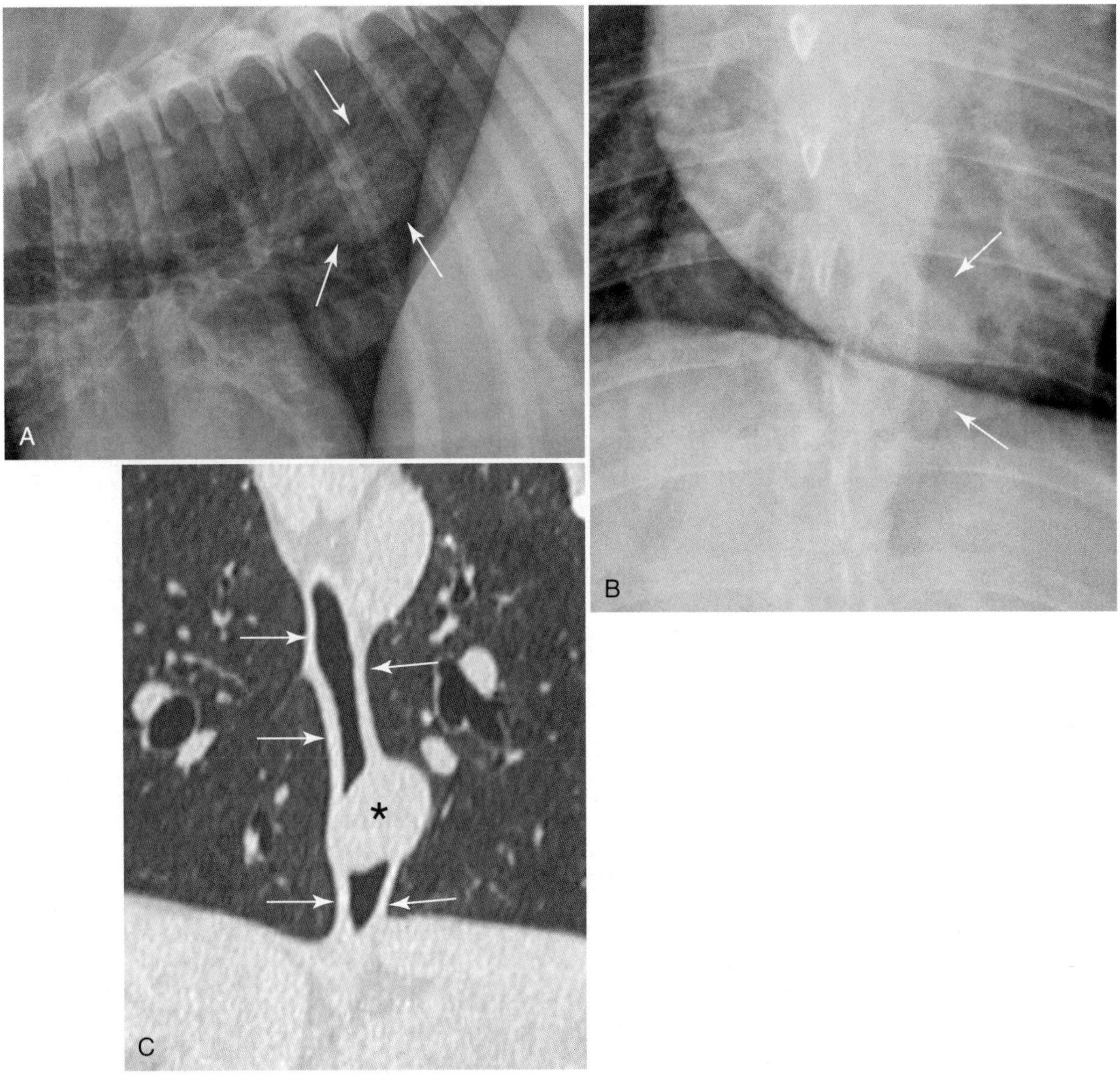

Fig. 30.31 Lateral **(A)** and ventrodorsal (VD) **(B)** radiographs of a dog with a small mass (*white arrows*) in the caudal aspect of the thorax. This mass is in a position consistent with esophagus but could also be a pulmonary or a nonesophageal mediastinal mass. A barium esophagram would be helpful in this patient, but a computed tomography (CT) was done instead. **C,** Dorsal plane reconstructed CT image of the caudal thorax in a plane through the esophagus. The esophagus is mildly dilated with gas (*white arrows*), and there is a mass arising from the left wall (*asterisk*). The mass appears benign because of its smooth margins. The histologic diagnosis of this mass is not known.

12.7% and include perforation, stricture, diverticula, periesophageal abscess, pneumothorax, pleural effusion, and respiratory arrest.[65] Cervical perforations have a better prognosis than thoracic perforations because of the development of septic mediastinitis, pleuritis, and pyothorax when there is perforation of the thoracic esophagus. Radiographically, mediastinal widening caused by inflammation or abscess formation, pneumomediastinum, and extension of gas along the fascial planes of the neck, pneumothorax, and pleural effusion may be present (Fig. 30.34; see Fig. 30.23, eFig. 30.6). A multimodality approach (radiography, contrast esophography, CT, esophagoscopy) to diagnosing esophageal perforations is often warranted.[64] Pleural fluid analysis, thoracic ultrasound, or thoracic CT may be helpful to confirm the presence of a perforation and determine the source of pleural fluid or pneumomediastinum and to best assess the mediastinal structures before performing a contrast esophagram or endoscopy. An esophageal contrast study with nonionic iodinated water-soluble contrast medium can be considered to confirm the perforation. However, water-soluble contrast medium may have poor adherence to devitalized tissue, may not coat the foreign material, and may even bypass an obstruction, giving a false-negative diagnosis.

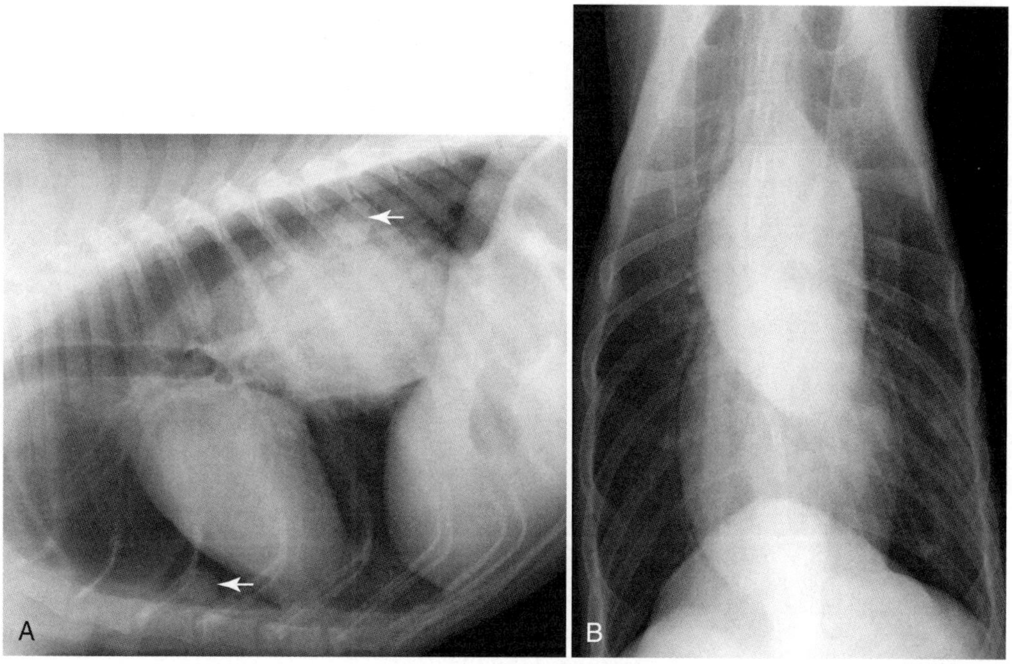

Fig. 30.32 **A,** Right lateral thoracic radiograph of a 2-year-old dog. There is a large mass caused by *Spirocerca lupi* infection in the region of the caudal esophagus. Several lung nodules are present (*white arrows*). The lung nodules suggest malignant transformation of the esophageal mass with secondary pulmonary metastasis. **B,** Ventrodorsal (VD) radiograph of same dog. The mass is midline, and the aorta is not visible. (Image courtesy the Department of Companion Animal Clinical Sciences, Faculty of Veterinary Science, University of Pretoria.)

Esophageal fistulas can be congenital or acquired.[65] Congenital forms are typically bronchoesophageal communications, but tracheoesophageal communications also occur.[66] Acquired forms are typically due to esophageal perforation resulting in communication with the airways of the trachea or lung.[67] Survey radiographs may be characterized by an ill-defined soft tissue or mixed pulmonary opacity. The diagnosis of an esophageal fistula relies upon demonstrating a communication between the esophagus and the airway with contrast medium or bronchoscopy. A swallow with liquid barium will usually show communication from the esophagus into the airway via a fistulous tract.

ESOPHAGEAL VARICES

Esophageal and paraesophageal varices may result from portal hypertension that generates reversal of portal blood flow, which diverts venous blood in a cranial direction through the left gastric vein to the venous plexus of the esophagus.[68,69] Obstructions of the cranial vena cava can also lead to the formation of esophageal and paraesophageal varices. The varices can drain into the azygous vein, the caudal vena cava, or into the portal system, depending on the site of the obstruction. Gallbladder and choledochal varices, omental varices, duodenal varices, phrenicoabdominal varices, colic varices, and abdominal wall varices drain into the caudal vena cava and result from portal hypertension. CT angiography is necessary for determining the origin, course, and termination of these vessels, and their underlying cause (Fig. 30.35). Of note is that bronchoesophageal artery hypertrophy should be included in the differential diagnosis of esophageal and paraesophageal varices in dogs as the two diseases appear similarly on CT angiography.[70] Both portal hypertension causing varices and bronchoesophageal artery hypertrophy secondary to chronic pulmonary or thromboembolic disease can occur concomitantly and can make imaging interpretation challenging. High-quality CT-angiography scans together with knowledge of the anatomy and possible physiopathology changes are essential for the diagnosis of these complex vascular anomalies.

AERODIGESTIVE DISORDERS

Aerodigestive disorders are a group of diseases which arise as a result of the close link between the digestive and respiratory tracts. Typically, animals with aerodigestive disease will present with symptoms of respiratory dysfunction (cough, recurring pneumonia) without typical gastrointestinal signs. However, with further exploration, gastrointestinal dysfunction such as pharyngeal weakness, esophageal dysmotility, or reflux emerges as the underlying pathology ultimately leading to laryngeal penetration-aspiration (P-A) and/or aspiration pneumonia.[4,71] As many as 81% of dogs with respiratory signs and with no evidence of gastrointestinal symptoms have been reported to have abnormalities on VFSS.[4] Therefore, VFSS is indicated in dogs with respiratory disease for which an underlying cause is nebulous. A grading scheme for laryngeal P-A of contrast material as visualized on VFSS has been developed so as to determine the prevalence and clinical significance of this process. Pathologic P-A has been defined as a score ≥ 3 which indicates contrast medium entering or surpassing the supraepiglottic space during VFSS. Some animals will have clinically silent P-A and dogs with pharyngeal disease and esophago-oropharyngeal reflux are prone to pathologic P-A.[72]

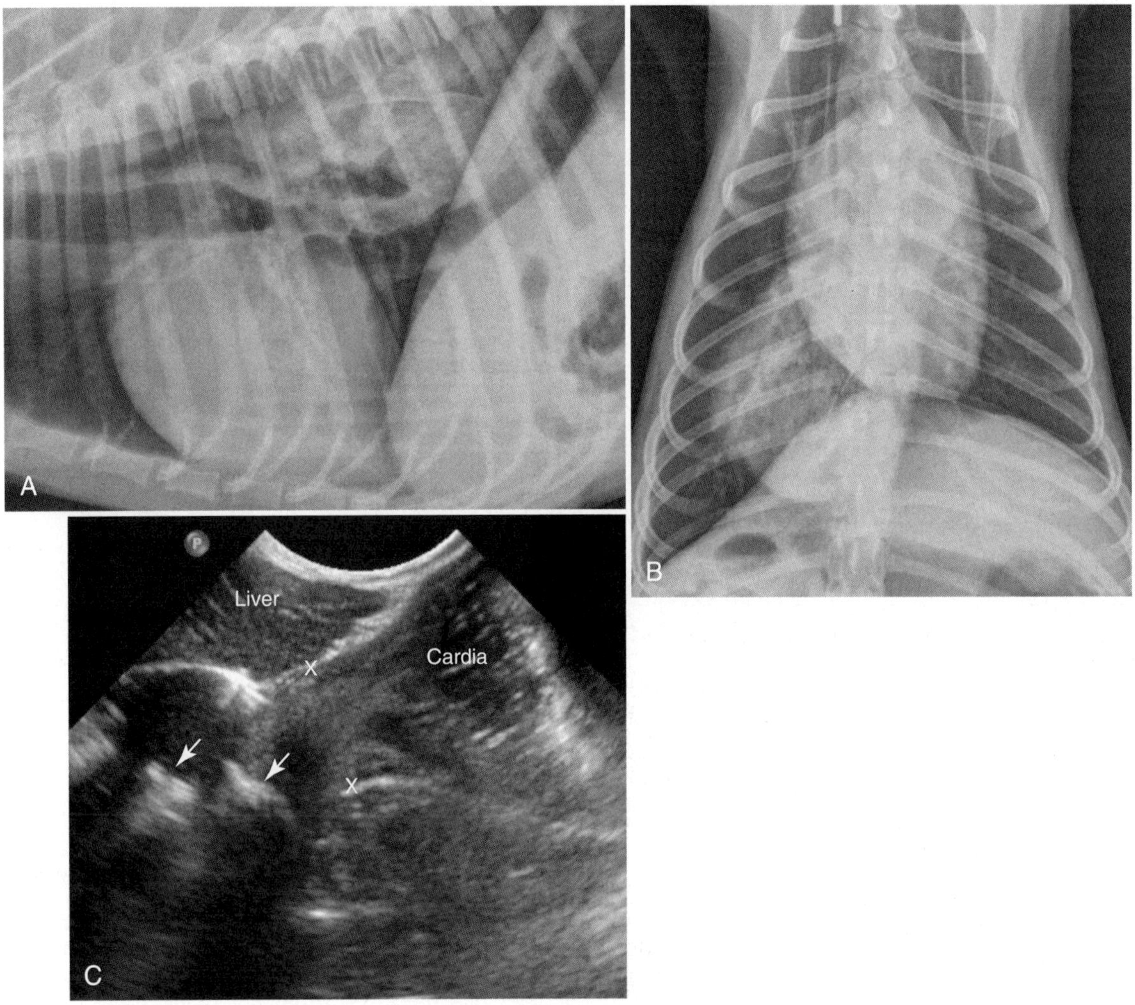

Fig. 30.33 **A,** Lateral radiograph of an 8-year-old Papillon. There is a mixed soft tissue and mineral opacity between the aorta and caudal vena cava in the caudodorsal aspect of the thorax. **B,** Ventrodorsal (VD) radiograph of the same dog. There is a large, right-sided mixed soft tissue and mineral opaque mass with a sharply defined right lateral border at the midline and to the right of the spine. An esophageal diverticulum containing bony foreign material was suspected. **C,** Ultrasound image of the same dog. The probe is positioned at the ventral midline pointing cranially and to the left to visualize the diaphragm and esophageal hiatus (calipers). The esophagus is dilatated at the hiatus and multiple linear, hyperechoic shadowing structures (*white arrows*) and mixed echogenic fluid can be seen filling the caudal esophagus.

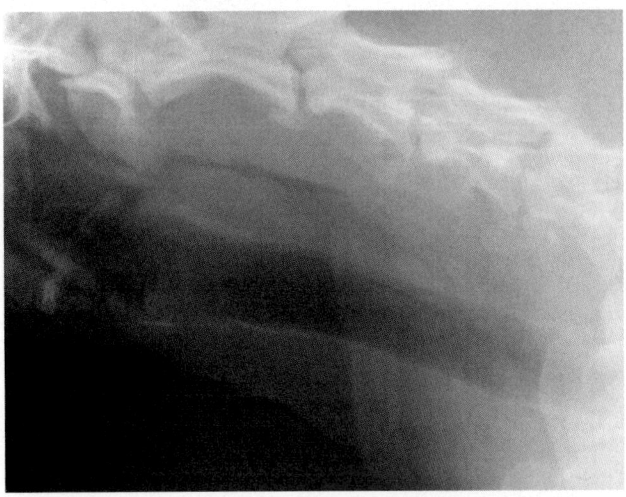

Fig. 30.34 Lateral cervical radiograph in a dog with acute ptyalism and vocalizing. Linear gas opacities are present dorsal to the cricopharyngeal sphincter and trachea. Perforating wood splinters were found on inspection of the mouth.

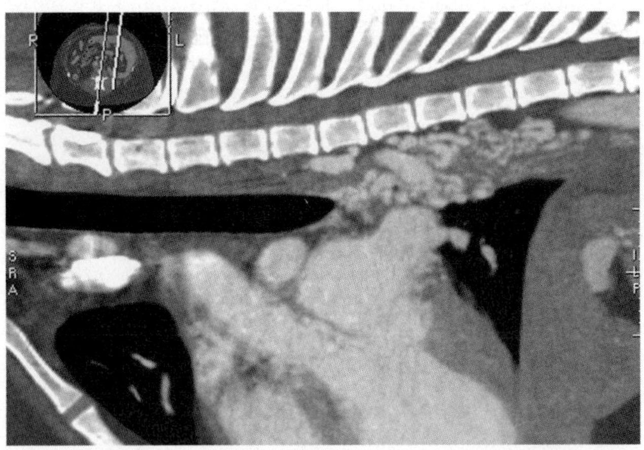

Fig. 30.35 Sagittal plane reconstruction of a computed tomography (CT) image of a dog with esophageal varices caused by portal hypertension. (Image courtesy Dr. Giovanna Bertolini, Clinica Veterinaria San Marco.)

Acknowledgment

With special thanks to prior authors of this chapter for their contributions.

REFERENCES

1. Suter PF. Swallowing problems and esophageal abnormalities. In: Suter PF, Lord PF, eds. *Thoracic Radiography: Thoracic Diseases of the Dog and Cat.* Wettswil, Switzerland; 1984:295–349.
2. Poncet CM, Dupre GP, Freiche VG, et al. Long-term results of upper respiratory syndrome 516 surgery and gastrointestinal tract medical treatment in 51 brachycephalic dogs. *J Small Anim Pract.* 2006;47:137–142.
3. Poncet CM, Dupre GP, Freiche VG, et al. Prevalence of gastrointestinal tract lesions in 73 519 brachycephalic dogs with upper respiratory syndrome. *J Small Anim Pract.* 2005;46:273–279.
4. Grobman ME, Masseau I, Reinero CR. Aerodigestive disorders in dogs evaluated for cough using respiratory fluoroscopy and videofluoroscopic swallow studies. *Vet J.* 2019;251:105344.
5. Gengler W. Gagging. In: Ettinger SJ, Feldman EC, eds. *The Textbook of Veterinary Internal Medicine.* St Louis, Mo, USA: Saunders Elsevier; 2010:189–191.
6. Watrous BJ. The esophagus. In: Thrall DE, ed. *Veterinary Diagnostic Radiology.* 5th ed. St. Louis, Mo, USA: Saunders Elsevier; 2007:495–511.
7. Jergens AE. Diseases of the esophagus. In: Ettinger SJ, Feldman EC, eds. *The Textbook of Veterinary Internal Medicine.* St Louis, Mo, USA: Saunders Elsevier; 2010:1487–1499.
8. Suter PF, Watrous BJ. Oropharyngeal dysphagia in the dog: a cinefluorographic analysis of experimentally induced and spontaneously occurring swallowing disorders; I. Oral stage and pharyngeal stage dysphagias. *Vet Radiol Ultrasound.* 1980;21:24–39.
9. Kogan DA, Johnson LR, Sturges BK, Jandrey KE, Pollard RE. Etiology and clinical outcome in dogs with aspiration pneumonia: 88 cases (2004–2006). *J Am Vet Med Assoc.* 2008;233(11):1748–1755.
10. McBrearty AR, Ramsey IK, Courcier EA, Mellor DJ, Bell R. Clinical factors associated with death before discharge and overall survival time in dogs with generalized megaesophagus. *J Am Vet Med Assoc.* 2011;238(12):1622–1628.
11. O'Brien TR. Esophagus. In: O'Brien TR, ed. *Radiographic Diagnosis of Abdominal Disorders in the Dog and Cat: Radiographic Interpretation, Clinical Signs, Pathophysiology.* Philadelphia, Pa, USA: WB Saunders; 1978:141.
12. Wallack ST. Introduction to barium sulfate. In: Wallack ST, ed. *The Handbook of Veterinary Contrast Radiography.* 2003:1–4. San Diego Veterinary Imaging, Solano Beach, Calif, USA.
13. Seiler G, Rytz U, Gaschen L. Radiographic diagnosis—cavitary mediastinal abscess. *Vet Radiol Ultrasound.* 2001;42(5):431–433.
14. Dvir E, Kirberger RM, Malleczek D. Radiographic and computed tomographic changes and clinical presentation of spirocercosis in the dog. *Vet Radiol Ultrasound.* 2001;42(2):119–129.
15. Wallack ST. Iodinated esophagram-dog. In: Wallack ST, ed. *The Handbook of Veterinary Contrast Radiography.* San Diego Veterinary Imaging. Solano Beach, Calif, USA; 2003:52.
16. Gaynor F, Hoffer RE, Nichols MF, et al. Physiologic features of the canine esophagus: effects of tranquilization on esophageal motility. *Am J Vet Res.* 1980;41(5):727–732.
17. Bonadio CM, Pollard RE, Dayton PA, Leonard CD, Marks SL. Effects of body positioning on swallowing and esophageal transit in healthy dogs. *J Vet Intern Med.* 2009;23(4):801–805.
18. Cheney DM, Marks SL, Pollard RE. Effect of bolus size on deglutition and esophageal transit in healthy dogs. *Vet Radiol Ultrasound.* 2016;57:359–365.
19. Pollard RE, Marks SL, Davidson A, Hornof WJ. Quantitative videofluoroscopic evaluation of pharyngeal function in the dog. *Vet Radiol Ultrasound.* 2000;41(5):409–412.
20. Pollard RE, Marks SL, Leonard R, Belafsky PC. Preliminary evaluation of the pharyngeal constriction ratio (PCR) for fluoroscopic determination of pharyngeal constriction in dysphagic dogs. *Vet Radiol Ultrasound.* 2007;48(3):221–226.
21. Harris RA, Grobman ME, Allen MJ, et al. Standardization of a videofluoroscopic swallow study protocol to investigate dysphagia in dogs. *J Vet Intern Med.* 2017;31:383–393.
22. Leonard R, Kendall K, McKenzie S. UES opening and cricopharyngeal bar in nondysphagic elderly and nonelderly adults. *Dysphagia.* 2004;19(3):182–191.
23. Haines JM, Khoo A, Brinkman E, Thomason JM, Mackin AJ. Technique for evaluation of gravity-assisted esophageal transit characteristics in dogs with megaesophagus. *J Am Anim Hosp Assoc.* 2019 Jul/Aug;55(4):167–177.
24. Lyngby JG, Haines JM, Guess SC. Use of a videofluoroscopic feeding evaluation to guide management of dogs with congenital idiopathic megaesophagus. *Vet Med Sci.* 2022 Jul;8(4):1434–1442.
25. Simpson KW. Disease of the esophagus. In: Ettinger SJ, Feldman EC, eds. *Textbook of Veterinary Internal Medicine: Diseases of the Dog and Cat.* 7th ed. Philadelphia: Saunders; 2023:1487–1500.
26. Watrous BJ. Clinical presentation and diagnosis of dysphagia. *Vet Clin North Am Small Anim Pract.* 1983;13(3):437–459.
27. Levine JS, Pollard RE, Marks SL. Contrast videofluoroscopic assessment of dysphagic cats. *Vet Radiol Ultrasound.* 2014;55(5):465–471.
28. Stanley BJ, Hauptman JG, Fritz MC, et al. Esophageal dysfunction in dogs with idiopathic laryngeal paralysis: a controlled cohort study. *Vet Surg.* 2010;39(2):139–149.
29. Bexfield NH, Watson PJ, Herrtage ME. Esophageal dysmotility in young dogs. *J Vet Intern Med.* 2006;20(6):1314–1318.
30. Diamant N, Szczepanski M, Mui H. Idiopathic megaesophagus in the dog: reasons for spontaneous improvement and a possible method of medical therapy. *Can Vet J.* 1974;15(3):66–71.
31. Kyles AE. Swallowing disorders. In: Bojrab MJ, ed. *Disease Mechanisms in Small Animal Surgery.* 3rd ed. Philadelphia: Lea & Febiger; 2010:205–209.
32. Grobman ME, Schachtel J, Gyawali CP, Lever TE, Reinero CR. Videofluoroscopic swallow study features of lower esophageal sphincter achalasia-like syndrome in dogs. *J Vet Intern Med.* 2019 Sep;33(5):1954–1963.
33. Guilford WG. Diseases of swallowing. In: Guilford G, Center SA, Strombeck DR, et al., eds. *Strombeck's Small Animal Gastroenterology.* 3rd ed. Philadelphia: Saunders; 1996:211–238.
34. Callan MB, Washabau RJ, Saunders HM, et al. Congenital esophageal hiatal hernia in the Chinese shar-pei dog. *J Vet Intern Med.* 1993;7(4):210–215.
35. Reeve EJ, Sutton D, Friend EJ, Warren-Smith CMR. Documenting the prevalence of hiatal hernia and oesophageal abnormalities in brachycephalic dogs using fluoroscopy. *J Small Anim Pract.* 2017;58(12):703–708.
36. Luciani E, Reinero C, Grobman M. Evaluation of aerodigestive disease and diagnosis of sliding hiatal hernia in

brachycephalic and nonbrachycephalic dogs. *J Vet Intern Med*. 2022 Jul;36(4):1229–1236.
37. Houlton JEF, Herrtage ME, Taylor PM, et al. Thoracic esophageal foreign bodies in the dog: a review of ninety cases. *J Small Anim Pract*. 1985;7:521–536.
38. Thompson HC, Cortes Y, Gannon K, et al. Esophageal foreign bodies in dogs: 34 cases (2004–2009). *J Vet Emerg Crit Care*. 2012;22(2):253–261.
39. Buchanan JW. Tracheal signs and associated vascular anomalies in dogs with persistent right aortic arch. *J Vet Intern Med*. 2004;18(4):510–514.
40. Yoon H, Kim J, Kwon GB, et al. Imaging diagnosis—computed tomographic angiography characteristics of multiple vascular anomalies in a senior dog with late-onset regurgitation. *Vet Radiol Ultrasound*. 2018;59(5):E44–E49.
41. Shannon D, Husnik R, Fletcher JM, et al. Persistent right aortic arch with an aberrant left subclavian artery, Kommerell's diverticulum and bicarotid trunk in a 3-year-old cat. *JFMS Open Rep*. 2015;1(2):2055116915614590.
42. Kyles AE. Vascular ring anomalies. In: Bojrab MJ, ed. *Disease Mechanisms in Small Animal Surgery*. 3rd ed. Philadelphia: Lea & Febiger; 2010:350–354.
43. Holt D, Heldmann E, Michel K, et al. Esophageal obstruction caused by a left aortic arch and an anomalous right patent ductus arteriosus in two German Shepherd littermates. *Vet Surg*. 2000;29(3):264–270.
44. Hurley K, Miller MW, Willard MD, et al. Left aortic arch and right ligamentum arteriosum causing esophageal obstruction in a dog. *J Am Vet Med Assoc*. 1993;203(3):410–412.
45. Larcher T, Abadie J, Roux FA, et al. Persistent left cranial vena cava causing oesophageal obstruction and consequent megaoesophagus in a dog. *J Comp Pathol*. 2006;135:150–152.
46. Adamama-Moraitou KK, Rallis TS, Prassinos NN, et al. Benign esophageal stricture in the dog and cat: a retrospective study of 20 cases. *Can J Vet Res*. 2002;66(1):55–59.
47. Dvir E, Clift SJ, Williams MC. Proposed histological progression of the *Spirocerca lupi*-induced oesophageal lesion in dogs. *Vet Parasitol*. 2010;168:71–77.
48. Gibson CJ, Parry NM, Jakowski RM, et al. Adenomatous polyp with intestinal metaplasia of the esophagus (Barrett esophagus) in a dog. *Vet Pathol*. 2010;47(1):116–119.
49. Wray JD, Blunden AS. Progressive dysphagia in a dog caused by a scirrhous, poorly differentiated peri-oesophageal carcinoma. *J Small Anim Pract*. 2006;47(1):27–30.
50. Ranen E, Shamir MH, Shahar R, et al. Partial esophagectomy with single layer closure for treatment of esophageal sarcomas in 6 dogs. *Vet Surg*. 2004;33(4):428–434.
51. Gualtieri M, Monzeglio MG, Di Giancamillo M. Oesophageal squamous cell carcinoma in two cats. *J Small Anim Pract*. 1999;40(2):79–83.
52. Teo LH, Cahalan SD, Benigni L, et al. Oesophageal angioleiomyosarcoma in a cat. *J Feline Med Surg*. 2014;16(10):846–852.
53. Fisher MM, Morgan JP, Krecek RC, et al. Radiography for the diagnosis of spirocercosis in apparently healthy dogs, St. Kitts, West Indies. *Vet Parasitol*. 2009;160:337–339.
54. Harrus S, Harmelin A, Markovics A, et al. *Spirocerca lupi* infection in the dog: aberrant migration. *J Am Anim Hosp Assoc*. 1996;32(2):125–130.
55. Gaschen L, Kircher P, Lang J. Endoscopic ultrasound instrumentation, applications in humans, and potential veterinary applications. *Vet Radiol Ultrasound*. 2003;44(6):665–680.
56. Berry WL. *Spirocerca lupi* esophageal granulomas in 7 dogs: resolution after treatment with doramectin. *J Vet Intern Med*. 2000;14(6):609–612.
57. Kirberger RM, Clift SJ, van Wilpe E, et al. *Spirocerca lupi* associated vertebral changes: a radiologic-pathologic study. *Vet Parasitol*. 2013;195:87–94.
58. Lindsay N, Kirberger R, Williams M. Imaging diagnosis—spinal cord chondrosarcoma associated with spirocercosis in a dog. *Vet Radiol Ultrasound*. 2010;51(6):614–616.
59. Kirberger RM, Stander N, Cassel N, et al. Computed tomographic and radiographic characteristics of aortic lesions in 42 dogs with spirocercosis. *Vet Radiol Ultrasound*. 2013;54(3):212–222.
60. Kirberger RM, Dvir E, van der Merwe LL. The effect of positioning on the radiographic appearance of caudodorsal mediastinal masses in the dog. *Vet Radiol Ultrasound*. 2009;50(6):630–634.
61. Kirberger RM, Cassel N, Stander N, et al. Triple phase dynamic computed tomographic perfusion characteristics of spirocercosis induced esophageal nodules in non-neoplastic versus neoplastic canine cases. *Vet Radiol Ultrasound*. 2015;56(3):257–263.
62. Doran IP, Wright CA, Moore AH. Acute oropharyngeal and esophageal stick injury in forty-one dogs. *Vet Surg*. 2008;37(8):781–785.
63. Paradise H, Mathews KG, Cohen EB. Imaging diagnosis—use of radiography, computed tomography, and endoscopy in the diagnosis of esophageal perforation by an extraluminal tracheal ring prosthesis in a golden retriever. *Vet Radiol Ultrasound*. 2017;58(4):E37–E41.
64. Gianella P, Pfammatter NS, Burgener IA. Oesophageal and gastric endoscopic foreign body removal: complications and follow-up of 102 dogs. *J Small Anim Pract*. 2009;50(12):649–654.
65. Basher AW, Hogan PM, Hanna PE, et al. Surgical treatment of a congenital bronchoesophageal fistula in a dog. *J Am Vet Med Assoc*. 1991;199(4):479–482.
66. Della Ripa MA, Gaschen F, Gaschen L, et al. Canine bronchoesophageal fistulas: case report and literature review. *Compend Contin Educ Vet*. 2010;32(4):E1.
67. Dodman NH, Baker GJ. Tracheo-oesophageal fistula as a complication of an oesophageal foreign body in the dog. *J Small Anim Pract*. 1978;19(5):290–296.
68. Bertolini G. Acquired portal collateral circulation in the dog and cat. *Vet Radiol Ultrasound*. 2010;51(1):25–33.
69. Ledda G, Caldin M, Mezzalira G, et al. Multidetector-row computed tomography patterns of bronchoesphageal artery hypertrophy and systemic-to-pulmonary fistula in dogs. *Vet Radiol Ultrasound*. 2015;56(4):347–358.
70. Wallack ST. Static barium esophagram. In: *The Handbook of Veterinary Contrast Radiography*. Solana Beach, CA: San Diego Veterinary Imaging; 2003:45–53.
71. Grobman M. Aerodigestive disease in dogs. *Vet Clin North Am Small Anim Pract*. 2021;51(1):17–32.
72. Grobman M, Carlue E, Reinero CR. Incidence, clinical signs and videofluoroscopic swallow study abnormalities associated with airway penetration and aspiration in 100 dogs. *J Vet Intern Med*. 2022;36(6):2149–2159.
73. Pollard RE. Videofluoroscopic evaluation of the pharynx and upper esophageal sphincter in the dog: a systematic review of the literature. *Front Vet Sci*. 2019;6:117.

ELECTRONIC RESOURCES

Additional information related to the content in Chapter 30 can be found online at eBooks.Health.Elsevier.com.

- Chapter Quiz

CHAPTER 31

Canine and Feline Thoracic Wall

Gabriela S. Seiler

The thoracic wall is composed of rigid structures such as the spine, sternum ribs, and costal cartilages as well as the interconnecting soft tissue structures including the skin, subcutaneous fat, subcutaneous and intercostal musculature, as well as the parietal pleura, blood vessels, nerves, and lymphatics. The thoracic wall plays an important role in protecting the thoracic soft tissue structures and is an integral part of pulmonary ventilation. Careful inspection of the thoracic wall structures is an important part of the interpretation of thoracic radiographs and other imaging modalities. Radiographs are typically indicated for initial evaluation of a thoracic wall lesion, and additional imaging methods are selected based on findings. Thoracic ultrasound is an excellent method to evaluate the layers of the thoracic wall, and investigate peripheral thoracic masses to determine if they are pulmonary or extrapleural in origin. Ultrasound-guided fine needle aspirates or biopsy of soft tissue or bone lesions may be obtained. Contrast-enhanced computed tomography (CT) is often used to get a more global assessment of the thoracic cavity and thoracic wall, and for surgical or radiation therapy planning.

THE NORMAL THORACIC WALL

Dogs and cats both have 13 thoracic vertebrae and paired ribs, although transitional vertebrae are common anomalies. The appearance and orientation of the ribs are somewhat dependent on breed and thoracic conformation in dogs, whereas it is more consistent in cats. Typically, the first few ribs are positioned vertically and perpendicular to the spine in the lateral and ventrodorsal (VD) projections, respectively. Towards the caudal thoracic spine, the ribs become progressively caudally oriented proximally with a more or less pronounced craniomedial curvature of the costal cartilages. The orientation of the ribs depends on the phase of respiration and the depth of inspiration. At full inspiration the ribs are in a more perpendicular orientation to the spine, whereas they are more caudally oriented during expiration (Fig. 31.1). In dogs, variations in thoracic wall conformation can be breed related. Costochondral conformation in chondrodystrophic breeds can lead to misdiagnosis of pneumothorax or pleural effusion as discussed in Chapter 34 (Fig. 31.2).

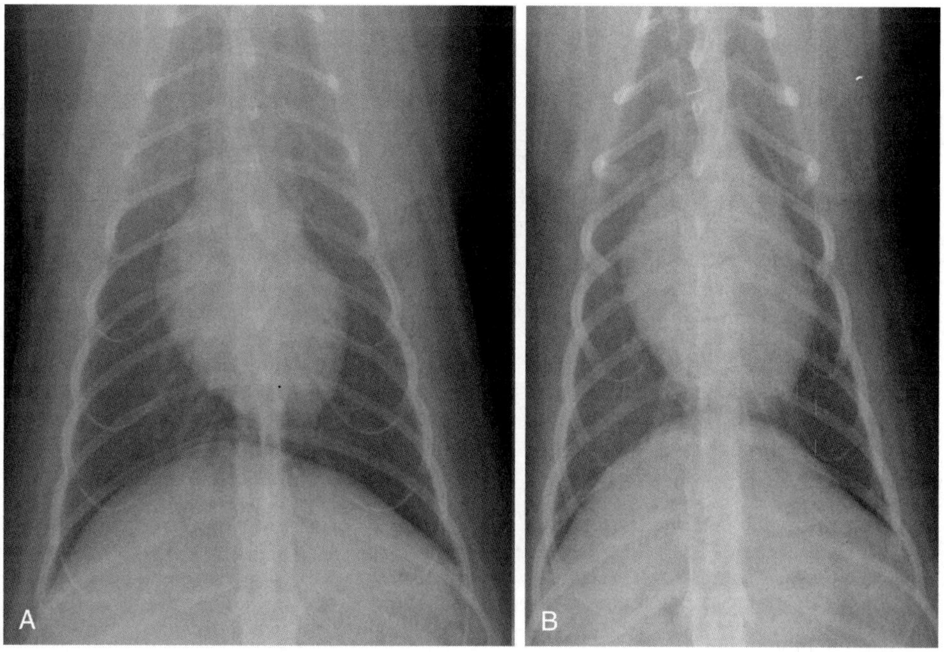

Fig. 31.1 Inspiratory **(A)** and expiratory **(B)** ventrodorsal (VD) thoracic radiographs of an adult cat. Notice the different more cranial orientation of the ribs and flattened shape of the diaphragm during inspiration compared with expiration.

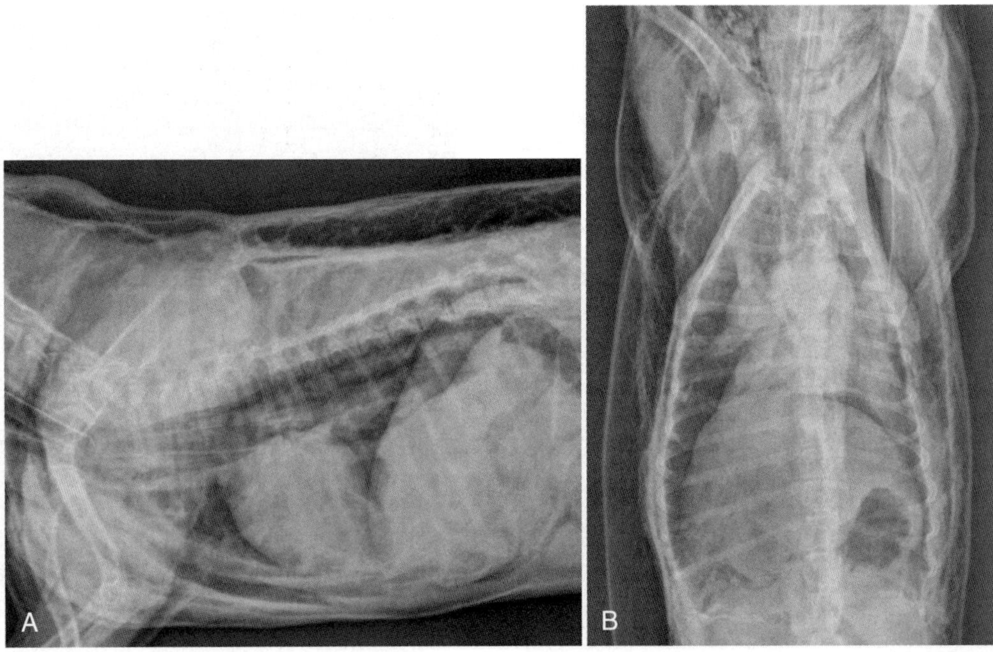

Fig. 31.13 Left lateral **(A)** and dorsoventral (DV) **(B)** thoracic radiographs of a 6-year-old Jack Russell terrier with severe subcutaneous emphysema pneumomediastinum and pneumothorax following anesthesia. Tracheal laceration was confirmed endoscopically.

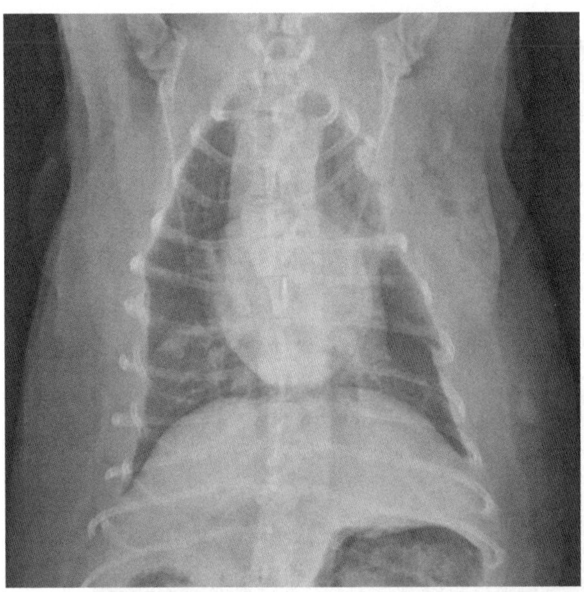

Fig. 31.14 Ventrodorsal (VD) radiograph of a 12-year-old Shih Tzu with tearing of the left cranial thoracic wall intercostal musculature, resulting in increased distance between the third and fourth ribs. Notice also the soft tissue swelling and subcutaneous emphysema of the thoracic wall at this level.

changing the hanging protocol of thoracic radiographs with 90- or 180-degree rotation will improve detection of rib fractures, but this is not recommended, as only a small improvement in accuracy of novice readers was shown with 90-degree rotation.[6] It is more important to include careful evaluation of the ribs in the standard search pattern of thoracic radiographic interpretation. Acute rib fractures are recognized by their sharp margins, whereas rounding and remodeling of the fracture margins and smooth new bone formation are indicative of the healing process (Fig. 31.15, eFigs. 31.2 and 31.3). Traumatic rib fractures have to be differentiated from pathologic fractures due to aggressive lesions. Aggressive rib lesions are discussed in more detail later. Ultrasound can be helpful in evaluating questionable rib fractures since soft tissue masses associated with aggressive lesions as well as irregular lysis can be easier to identify, and tissue sampling can be performed (Fig. 31.16). Spontaneous rib fractures, without external trauma, may occur in cats with chronic respiratory disease. This is presumed to be due to mechanical failure (a form of pathologic fracture), perhaps combined with age-related osteopenia[7] (Fig. 31.17). Typically, the midportion of the caudal ribs is affected. Flail chest is caused by segmental rib fractures of at least two adjacent ribs at two different levels or five or more sequential single rib fractures which results in separation of a thoracic wall segment from the normal respiratory bellows. The resulting destabilized thoracic wall segment moves paradoxically to the normal thoracic wall with inlet displacement during inspiration and outward displacement during expiration[8,9] (Fig. 31.18). Sternal trauma most commonly manifests as luxation rather than fracture and can be painful and associated with soft tissue swelling when acute (Fig. 31.19).

THORACIC WALL MASS LESIONS

The Extrapleural Sign

The extrapleural sign relates to any mass arising outside the parietal pleural, for example in the ribs or soft tissues of the thoracic wall. All extrapleural masses are characterized by growth into rather than expansion within the thoracic cavity. As long as the parietal pleura is intact, the smooth surface of the mass is preserved, and there is often a draping appearance at the junction of the mass with the thoracic wall. Loss of the sharp delineation of an extrapleural lesion can be a sign of

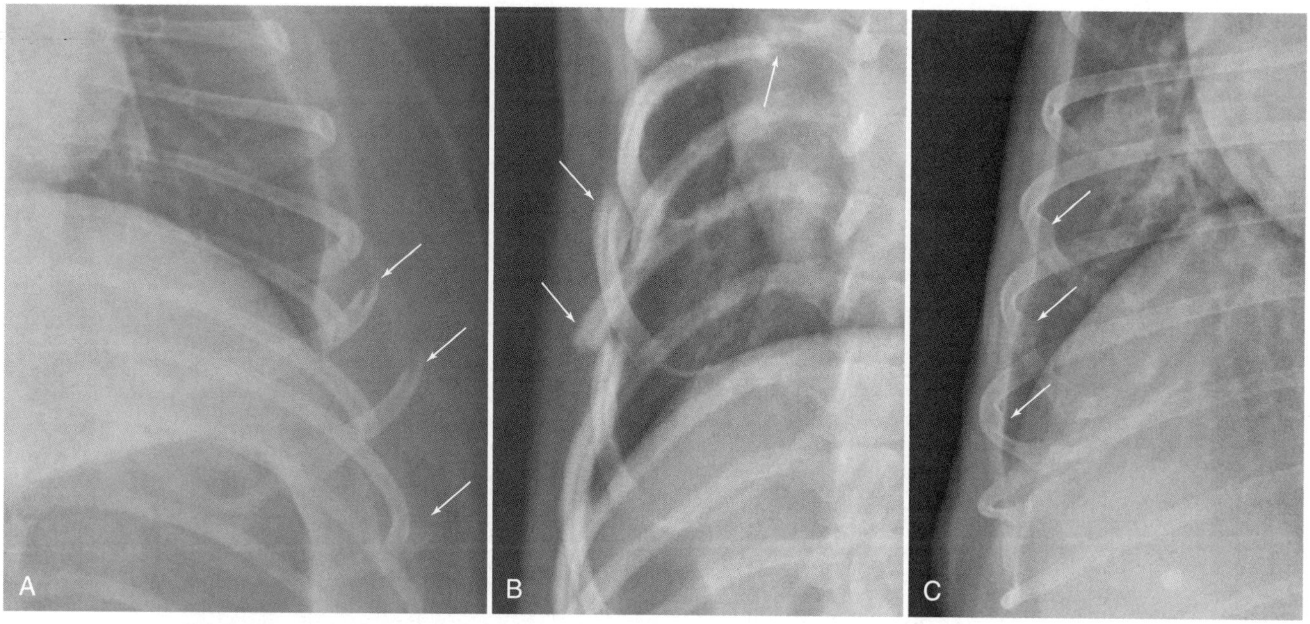

Fig. 31.15 Ventrodorsal (VD) thoracic radiographs of three different dogs with rib fractures in various stages of healing, indicated by *white arrows*. **A,** Acute rib fractures are characterized by sharp margins and regional soft tissue swelling. **B,** Healing rib fractures with remodeling and periosteal reaction along the fracture fragments. **C,** Healed rib fractures with smooth bridging callus causing focal widening of the ribs.

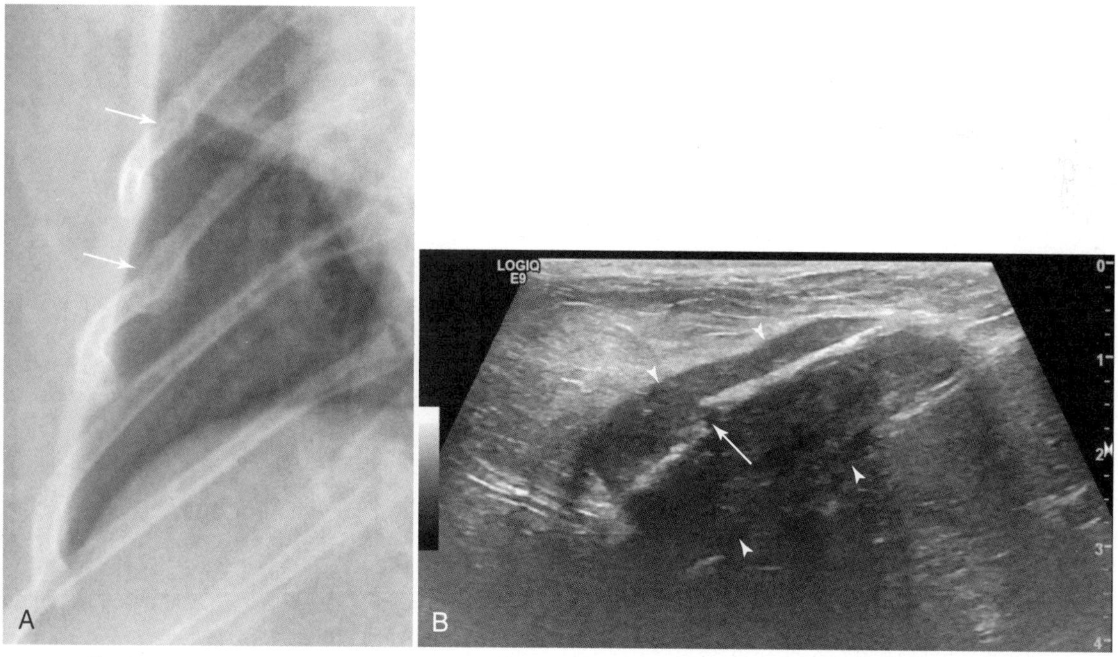

Fig. 31.16 Ventrodorsal (VD) radiograph (**A**) of an 8-year-old cat with a fracture of the right ninth rib with focal surrounding bone proliferation. A second focal osseous proliferation is seen on the eighth rib (*white arrows*). **B,** Ultrasound image of the right ninth rib in the same orientation as on the radiograph; dorsomedial is to the *right* of the image. The ultrasound image shows a hypoechoic mass lesion (*arrowheads*) surrounding the rib fracture (*arrow*). The distal fracture fragment has an irregular periosteal outline consistent with lysis. Fine needle aspirates confirmed metastatic fibrosarcoma.

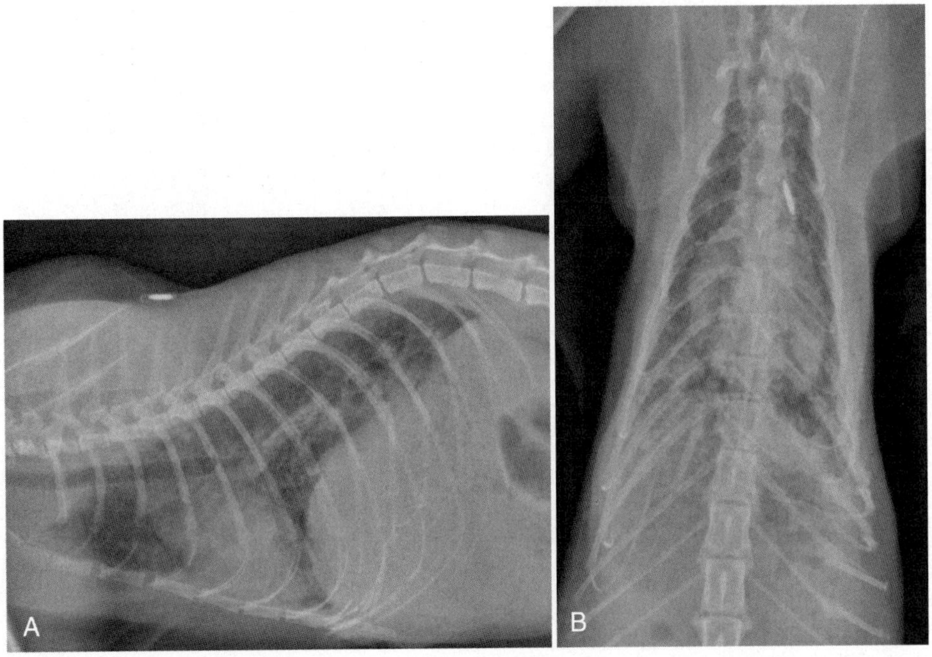

Fig. 31.17 Right lateral **(A)** and ventrodorsal (VD) **(B)** thoracic radiographs of an adult Siamese cat with severe inflammatory airway disease. There are multiple chronic, healing fractures of the left caudal ribs. No trauma was known and the fractures were thought to be caused by chronic increased respiratory effort.

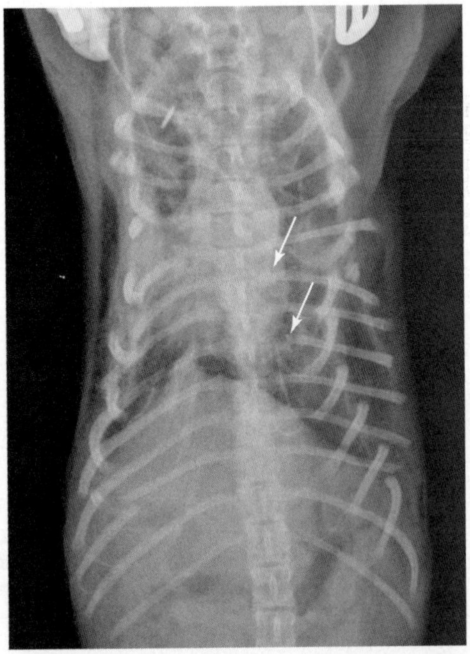

Fig. 31.18 Ventrodorsal (VD) thoracic radiographs of a mixed-breed dog with bilateral multiple rib fractures. Several ribs are fractured at two levels (*white arrows*) and more than five ribs in a row are fractured, resulting in flail chest formation.

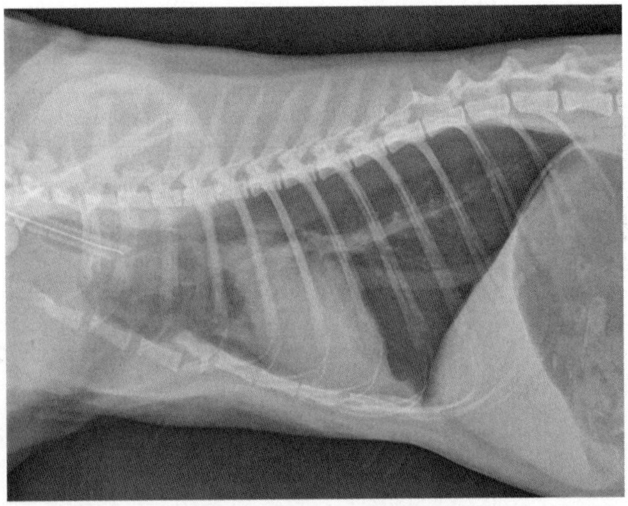

Fig. 31.19 Right lateral thoracic radiograph of an adult cat with sternal luxation after trauma. An endotracheal tube is present.

invasion through the parietal pleura and potentially into the lung (Fig. 31.20). An extrapleural sign is only visible if the x-ray beam encounters the lesion perpendicularly. Radiographic signs of extrapleural lesions are listed in Box 31.1. When using ultrasound to differentiate an extrapleural from a pulmonary mass lesion, it is important to observe respiratory motion. A pulmonary lesion will glide along the thoracic wall in synchrony with respiration, unless there are adhesions present, whereas a thoracic wall mass will remain static against the gliding lung surface.

Soft Tissue Lesions

Soft tissue masses of the thoracic wall are common in older patients. Lipomas are most commonly located subcutaneously and are characterized by fat opacity and smooth margins, although they may be infiltrative[10] (Fig. 31.21). Fibrosarcomas

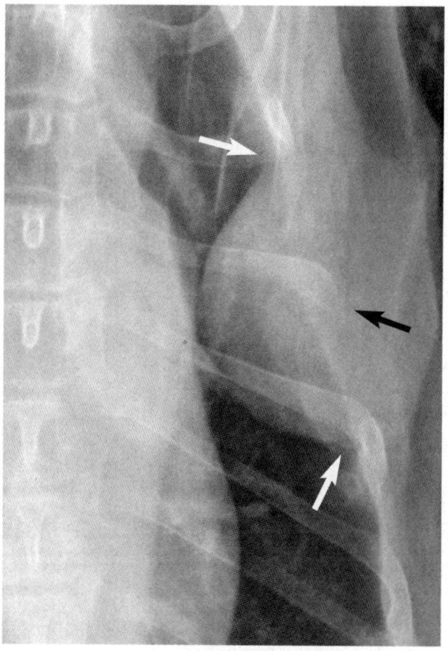

Fig. 31.20 Ventrodorsal (VD) thoracic radiograph of a dog. There is lysis of the distal aspect of the left fourth rib (*black arrow*) with a poorly defined extrathoracic mass and a well-defined intrathoracic mass. The intrathoracic component of the mass is broad based along the intrathoracic wall surface and has a convex margin. The cranial and caudal margins of the mass taper along the thoracic wall (*white arrows*). These radiographic findings are characteristic of an extrapleural sign.

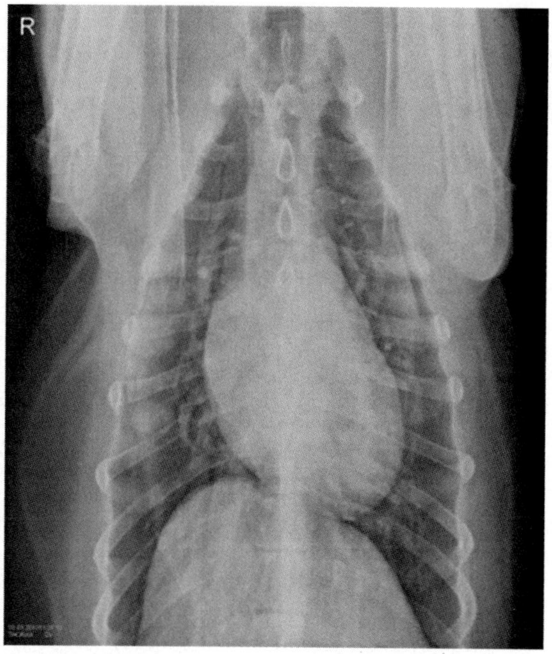

Fig. 31.21 Dorsoventral (DV) thoracic radiograph of a dog with a right-sided thoracic wall lipoma. Notice the fat opacity of the mass lesion that expands the right thoracic wall.

Box • 31.1

Radiographic Signs of Extrapleural Lesions

- Broad base along the thoracic wall
- Well-defined convex surface facing the lung parenchyma
- Tapered cranial and caudal edges of the lesion, merging with the pleural surface
- Widening of the intercostal space and splaying of the adjacent ribs
- Periosteal reaction and/or lysis of ribs or sternebrae
- Soft tissue thickening of the thoracic wall adjacent to and continuous with the extrapleural mass lesion
- Disruption of the fascial planes of the thoracic wall
- Abnormalities of the pleural space such as effusion occur late in the disease process

at sites of known vaccination, especially in the interscapular region, may be identified radiographically as convex soft tissue swelling dorsal to the thoracic spinous processes (Fig. 31.22). Soft tissue masses such as soft tissue sarcomas and adenocarcinomas are soft tissue opaque and often more irregular in outline, and may occur anywhere in the thoracic wall. Secondary bone invasion or destruction is possible. CT imaging is needed to evaluate the full extent of these lesions and determine the presence of bone lysis[11] (Fig. 31.23). Thoracic wall infection and cellulitis of the thoracic wall are most commonly caused by penetrating trauma and migrating foreign bodies such as grass awns. Fistulography, using either radiography or CT imaging, may be helpful to determine the extent of a superficial draining tract and the connection with intrathoracic structures[12] (Fig. 31.24).

Lesions of the Ribs and Sternum

Mass lesions associated with the ribs or sternum can be benign or malignant in nature. The majority of primary rib tumors are osteosarcomas and chondrosarcomas with a smaller portion of other sarcomas (fibrosarcoma, hemangiosarcoma).[13,14] They usually arise near the costochondral junction, are aggressive in nature, and cause lysis and irregular periosteal reaction of the affected ribs. Amorphous mineralization of the associated soft tissue mass is common. The extent of the lesion is often underestimated radiographically and clinically, as most of the tumor mass is intrathoracic. CT gives a much more detailed assessment of the size and origin of a rib mass, effect on adjacent structures, and presence of metastatic lesions (Fig. 31.25, eFig. 31.4). The intrathoracic portion of a rib tumor may be misinterpreted as a pulmonary mass if the adjacent ribs are not examined for the presence of lysis or periosteal reactions (Fig. 31.26) Primary rib tumors typically affect a single rib, although the adjacent ribs can be affected by the mass and have signs of periostitis, compression atrophy, or invasion (eFigs. 31.5 and 31.6). Differential diagnoses for multiple aggressive rib lesions include metastatic neoplasia or marrow-associated tumors such as multiple myeloma (Fig. 31.27, eFig. 31.7). Metastatic neoplasia is often more lytic or expansile than proliferative with variable degree of periosteal reaction (eFig. 31.8).

Cartilaginous exostoses or osteochondromas are benign bone perforations characterized by a cartilage cap and can be singular or multiple (multiple cartilaginous exostoses or osteochondromatosis) (Fig. 31.28). Single osteochondromas most commonly occur in growing dogs and growth of the mass stops with skeletal maturation. They appear as well-defined, thin-walled bony expansile lesions proliferating from the cortical

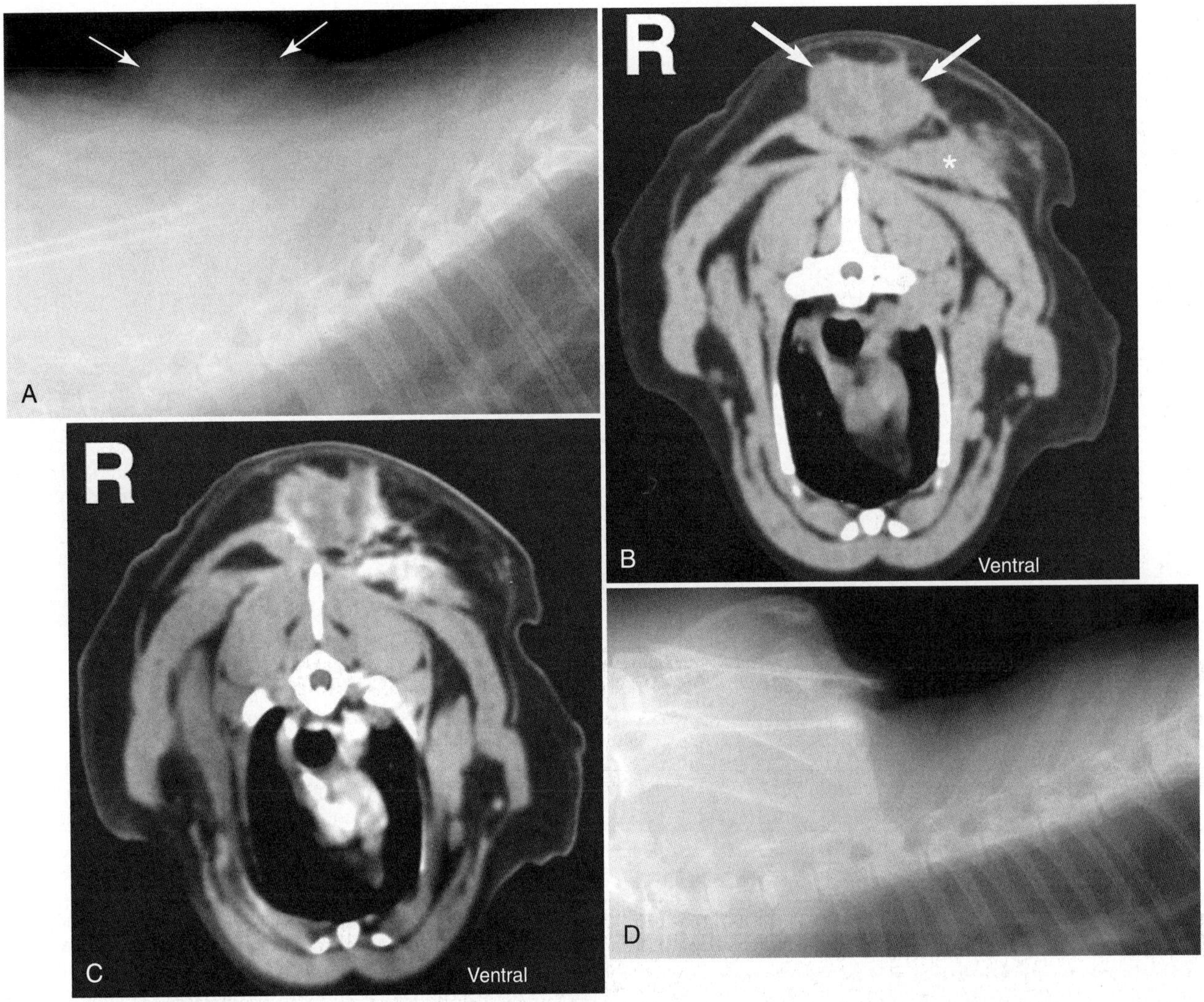

Fig. 31.22 Right lateral radiograph **(A)** and precontrast **(B)** and postcontrast **(C)** computed tomography (CT) images of a cat with a vaccine-associated interscapular fibrosarcoma. A soft tissue mass with a dorsal convex margin is present in the subcutaneous tissues dorsal to the proximal margin of the scapulae (*white arrows*) on the thoracic radiograph **(A)**. On the precontrast CT image **(B)** acquired just caudal to the scapulae, the irregularly margined mass is seen clearly in the fat just dorsal to a thoracic spinous process (*white arrows*). In addition, soft tissue opaque stranding is identified in the fat surrounding the mass and just lateral to the left trapezius muscle (*asterisk*), which is also thickened and irregular in contour. After intravenous administration of iodinated contrast medium, heterogeneous enhancement of the dorsal subcutaneous mass, left trapezius muscle, and soft tissue stranding within the regional fat are present, consistent with neoplastic infiltration and associated inflammation. Contrast-medium opacification of the great vessels cranial to the heart is also seen. Although lysis and remodeling of osseous structures were not identified, soft tissue contrast opacification was observed along the peripheral surfaces of the caudal scapulae and multiple spinous processes. In the interest of obtaining a complete surgical excision, large portions of the scapulae and thoracic spinous processes 2 through 6 were removed **(D)**.

surface of ribs or vertebrae and can cause regional mass effect and compression atrophy of adjacent structures. Multiple cartilaginous exostoses are more common in cats than in dogs. Malignant transformation is possible and then the radiographic appearance will be similar to a primary rib tumor.[15]

Primary or metastatic sternebral tumors are rare and usually of mesenchymal origin. Aggressive sternal neoplasia may be difficult to differentiate from destructive sternebral osteomyelitis and tissue sampling is needed to obtain a diagnosis (Fig. 31.29). Hematogenous infection may affect the sternebral space, and appear similar to discospondylitis in the spine. Sternal osteomyelitis can be a result of trauma or a migrating foreign body, prior trauma, or surgery[16,17] (Fig. 31.30, eFig. 31.9). It is important to closely evaluate the sternum for signs of an aggressive lesion as sternal degenerative changes are common and subtle irregular periosteal reactions or focal lysis may be dismissed. Rib infection is uncommon and most commonly the result of trauma with a penetrating wound. Severe pyothorax may result in rib periostitis which is characterized by periosteal reaction without a soft tissue mass. Hypertrophic osteopathy is a rare differential diagnosis for periosteal reactions along multiple ribs without lysis (Fig. 31.31). However, the differentiation between rib infection and neoplasia is difficult and often impossible.

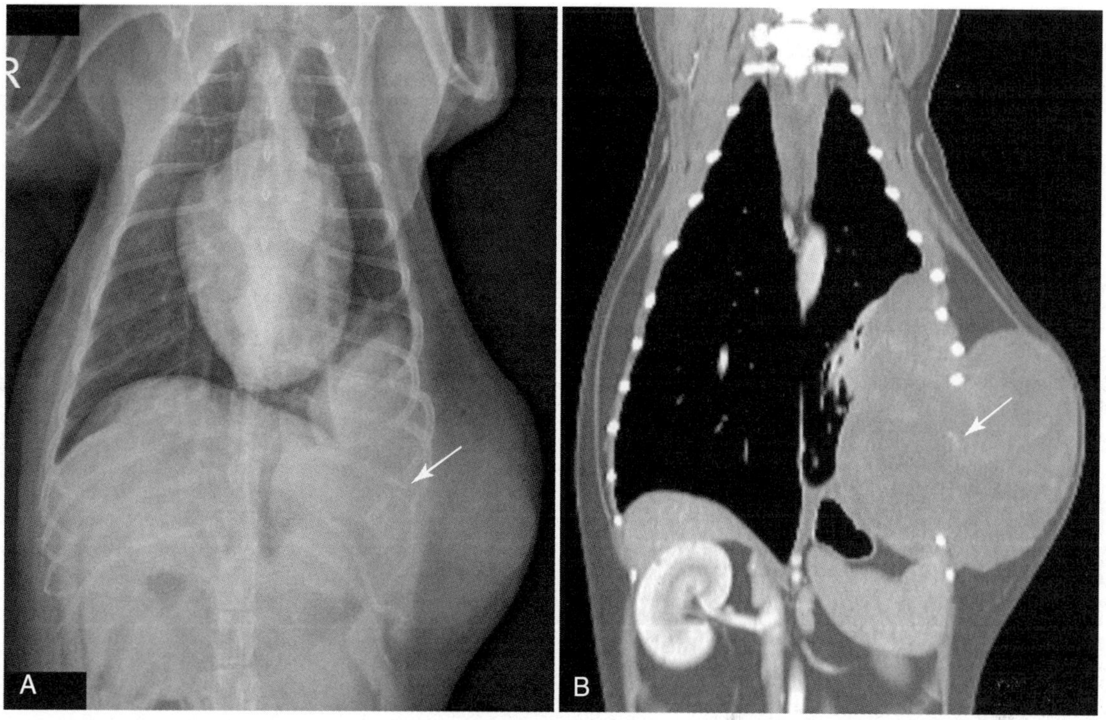

Fig. 31.23 Ventrodorsal (VD) thoracic radiograph **(A)** and corresponding computed tomography (CT) image reformatted in a dorsal plane **(B)** of a Cairn terrier with a thoracic wall mass. There is a large lobulated soft tissue mass in the left caudal thoracic wall that extends into the thorax causing displacement and compression of the adjacent lung. The rib spaces are widened at the level of the mass and there is focal lysis of the left 11th rib (*white arrows*).

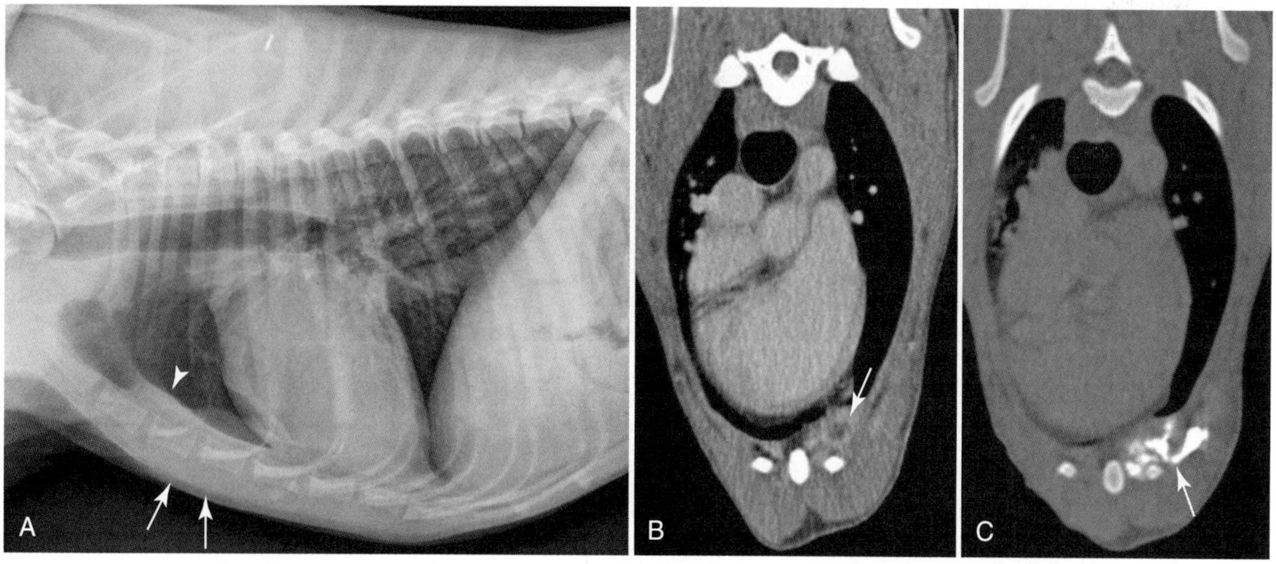

Fig. 31.24 Right lateral thoracic radiograph **(A)** of a 3-year-old Irish setter with a fistulous draining tract at the level of the third sternebral. Focal soft tissue thickening is noted at this level (*white arrows*) and there is focal retrosternal soft tissue thickening in the region of the sternal lymph nodes (*arrowhead*). **B,** Contrast-enhanced computed tomography (CT) image of the thorax. A peripherally contrast-enhancing round structure is seen subpleurally to the left of the sternum (*arrow*). **C,** CT-fistulogram, iodinated contrast medium was injected into the external fistulous tract. Contrast medium extends from the thoracic wall to the subpleural structure (*arrow*), confirming the connection of this structure with the external draining tract. A grass awn was removed surgically.

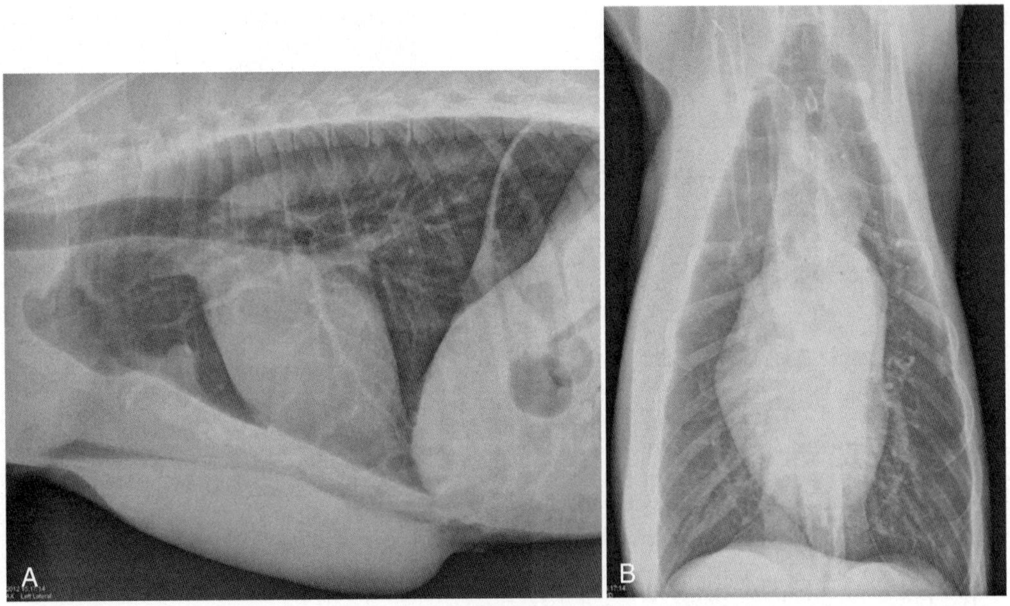

Fig. 31.29 Left lateral **(A)** and ventrodorsal (VD) **(B)** thoracic radiograph of a dog with osteosarcoma of the third sternebra. The sternebra is decreased in radiopacity with an irregular periosteal reaction. A pathologic compression fracture has caused shortening of the sternebra. There is a large amount of soft tissue swelling ventral to the sternum.

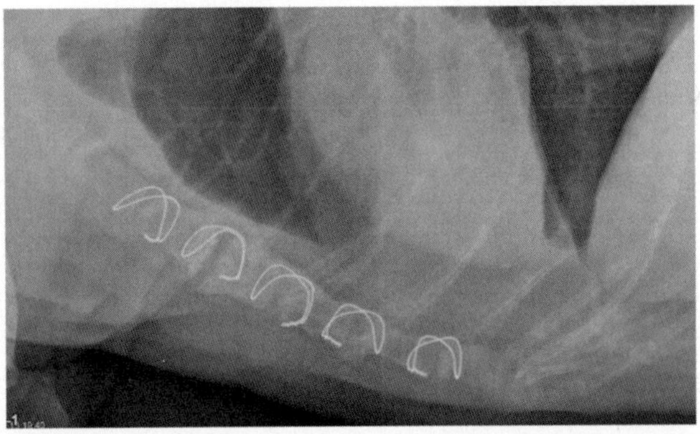

Fig. 31.30 Osteomyelitis of the third and fourth sternebrae after a median sternotomy. The endplates are irregularly margined and sclerotic, and the intersternebral space is narrowed. There is increased radiolucency surrounding the cerclage wires within these sternebrae.

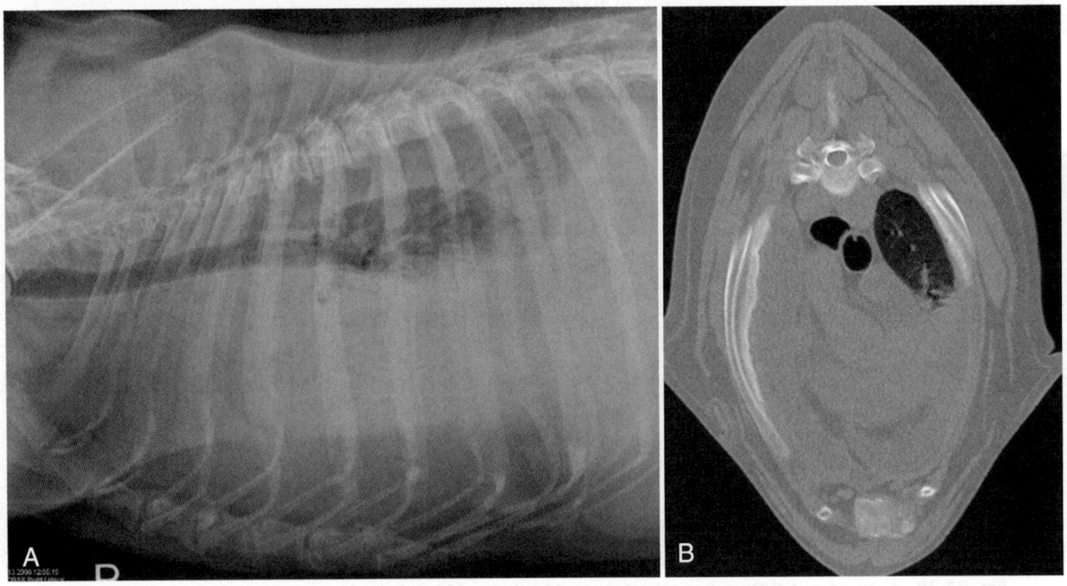

Fig. 31.31 Right lateral thoracic radiograph **(A)** and transverse computed tomography (CT) image **(B)** of a dog with chronic mesothelioma and bilateral pleural effusion. There are extensive, irregular periosteal reactions present along all ribs, predominantly along the medial cortical surface of the ribs. There is no evidence of cortical lysis. Hypertrophic osteopathy secondary to intrathoracic disease was suspected.

Acknowledgment

With special thanks to prior authors of this chapter for their contributions.

REFERENCES

1. Evans SM, Biery DN. Congenital peritoneopericardial diaphragmatic hernia in the dog and cat: a literature review and 17 additional case histories. *Vet Radiol.* 1980;21(3):108–116.
2. Bąkowska J, Proks P, Stehlik L, Irova K, Bugyiova K. Pectus excavatum in seven dogs. *J Comp Pathol.* 2017;156(1):87.
3. Kurosawa TA, Ruth JD, Steurer J, Austin B, Heng HG. Imaging diagnosis—acquired pectus excavatum secondary to laryngeal paralysis in a dog. *Vet Radiol Ultrasound.* 2012;53(3):329–332.
4. Nganvongpanit K, Yano T. Prevalence of swimming puppy syndrome in 2,443 puppies during the years 2006–2012 in Thailand. *Vet Med Int.* 2013;2013:617803.
5. Cabon Q, Deroy C, Ferrand FX, et al. Thoracic bite trauma in dogs and cats: a retrospective study of 65 cases. *Vet Comp Orthop Traumatol VCOT.* 2015;28(6):448–454.
6. Lamb CR, Parry AT, Baines EA, Chang YM. Does changing the orientation of a thoracic radiograph aid diagnosis of rib fractures? *Vet Radiol Ultrasound.* 2011;52(1):75–78.
7. Hardie EM, Ramirez IIIO, Clary EM, et al. Abnormalities of the thoracic bellows: stress fractures of the ribs and hiatal hernia. *J Vet Intern Med.* 1998;12(4):279–287.
8. Cappello M, De Troyer A. Actions of the inspiratory intercostal muscles in flail chest. *Am J Respir Crit Care Med.* 1997;155(3):1085–1089.
9. Olsen D, Renberg W, Perett J, Hauptman JG, et al. Clinical management of flail chest in dogs and cats: a retrospective study of 24 cases (1989–1999). *J Am Anim Hosp Assoc.* 2002;38(4):315–320.
10. McEntee MC, Thrall DE. Computed tomographic imaging of infiltrative lipoma in 22 dogs. *Vet Radiol Ultrasound.* 2001;42(3):221–225.
11. Saba CF. Vaccine-associated feline sarcoma: current perspectives. *Vet Med Res Rep.* 2017;8:13–20.
12. Lamb CR, Pope EHW, Lee KCL. Results of computed tomography in dogs with suspected wooden foreign bodies. *Vet Radiol Ultrasound.* 2017;58(2):144–150.
13. Baines SJ, Lewis S, White RAS. Primary thoracic wall tumours of mesenchymal origin in dogs: a retrospective study of 46 cases. *Vet Rec.* 2002;150(11):335.
14. Chun R. Common malignant musculoskeletal neoplasms of dogs and cats. *Vet Clin North Am Small Anim Pract.* 2005;35(5):1155–1167.
15. Czerwik A, Olszewska A, Starzomska B, et al. Multiple cartilaginous exostoses in a Swiss Mountain dog causing thoracolumbar compressive myelopathy. *Acta Vet Scand.* 2019;61(1):1–6.
16. Wainberg SH, Brisson BA, Hayes GM, Mackenzie S. Use of gentamicin sulfate-impregnated sponges as adjuvant therapy for the treatment of chronic foreign body associated sternal osteomyelitis in a dog. *Can Vet J.* 2015;56(11): 1161–1165.
17. Gilding T, Guilliard MJ. What is your diagnosis? Osteomyelitis of the fourth sternebra. *J Small Anim Pract.* 2003;44(7):297–335.

ELECTRONIC RESOURCES

Additional information related to the content in Chapter 31 can be found online at eBooks.Health.Elsevier.com
- Chapter Quiz

CHAPTER 32

Canine and Feline Diaphragm

Elissa K. Randall

The diaphragm is the musculotendinous partition between the thoracic and abdominal cavities. Embryologically, the diaphragm is formed by the septum transversum ventrally and by the mesentery of the foregut and two pleuroperitoneal folds dorsally.

Movement of the diaphragm provides approximately 75% of the change in intrathoracic volume during quiet respiration, with the intercostal muscles providing the remainder.[1] The diaphragm also acts as a mechanical partition between the thorax and the abdomen. Lymph vessels from the abdomen penetrate the diaphragm and drain into the thoracic lymph nodes and vessels. Thus, inflammatory or neoplastic abdominal disease may spread to the mediastinum and pleural space. Lymph flow from the abdomen is primarily cranially with the final destination being the thoracic trunks, but there are lymphatic vessels in the thorax that drain to the abdomen.[2]

The diaphragm consists of a tendinous center and three thin peripheral muscles: (1) the pars lumbalis, (2) the pars costalis, and (3) the pars sternalis. The pars lumbalis consists of the right and left crura, which attach to the cranial ventral border of L4 and the body of L3. The attachment area on these vertebrae occasionally has a concave indistinct ventral margin that may be mistaken for bone lysis (Fig. 32.1). The pars costalis attaches in an oblique direction to the 13th through 8th ribs, and the pars sternalis attaches to the xiphoid cartilage.[3] The diaphragm is convex and extends into the thorax from its attachments, creating the phrenicocostalis and phrenicolumbalis recesses.

There are three openings through the diaphragm: (1) the dorsally located aortic hiatus encloses the aorta, azygos and hemiazygos veins, and the lumbar cistern of the thoracic duct; (2) the centrally located esophageal hiatus encloses the esophagus and vagus nerve trunks; and (3) the caudal vena cava foramen is located at the junction of the muscular and tendinous portions of the diaphragm.

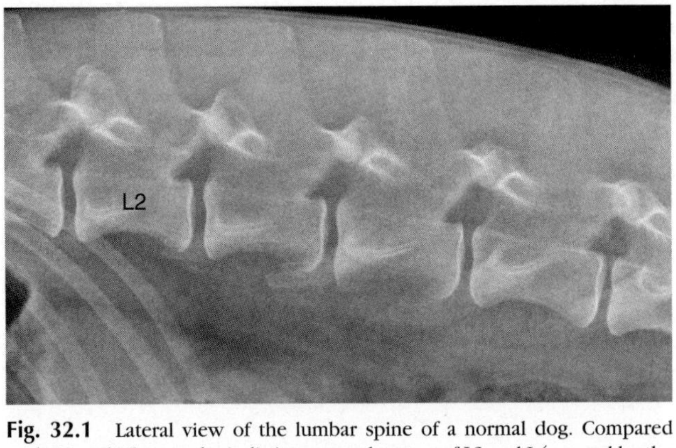

Fig. 32.1 Lateral view of the lumbar spine of a normal dog. Compared with L2 and L5, note the indistinct ventral cortex of L3 and L4 caused by the diaphragm attachment site. This can be misinterpreted as lysis if this normal appearance is not understood. *L2,* Second lumbar vertebra.

NORMAL RADIOGRAPHIC ANATOMY

Radiographically, only a portion of the diaphragm can be seen on any one view. Radiographic visualization of the diaphragm depends on adjacent structures being of different opacity. Most of the thoracic diaphragmatic surface is visible because of the adjacent gas-filled lungs. The phrenicocostalis and phrenicolumbalis recesses are not in contact with the lungs and therefore not outlined. A large portion of the abdominal diaphragmatic surface is not seen because it silhouettes the adjacent liver. The ventral abdominal diaphragmatic surface is visible on the lateral view when fat is present within the falciform ligament. The dorsal aspect of the left diaphragmatic crus and the gastric wall appear as one linear structure when gas is present in the gastric cardia.

Diaphragmatic structures that may be seen distinctly on a radiograph are the right and left crura and the cupula (body) (Figs. 32.2–32.5). Associated structures that may also be seen are the caudal vena cava and the caudal ventral mediastinum. On the lateral view, the caudal vena cava is confluent with the right crus, and the gastric fundus may be seen adjacent to the

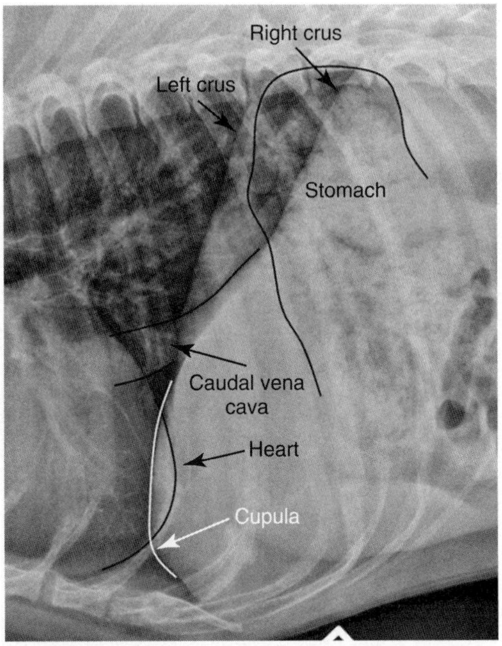

Fig. 32.2 Left lateral radiograph of the diaphragmatic region of a normal dog. In left recumbency, the dependent left crus is usually positioned cranial to the nondependent right crus. The right crus is identified by the confluence of the caudal vena cava, which bypasses the left crus before silhouetting with the right crus. These positional relationships are more consistent in large dogs and less consistent in small dogs and cats.

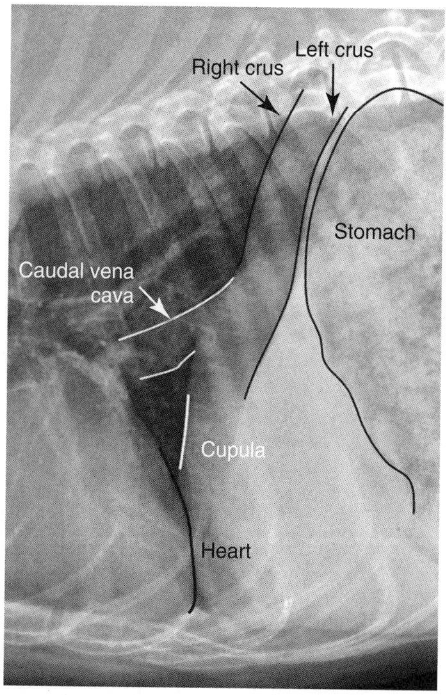

Fig. 32.3 Right lateral radiograph of the diaphragmatic region of a normal dog. In right recumbency, the dependent right crus is usually positioned cranial to the nondependent left crus. The cranially located right crus is identified by the confluence of the caudal vena cava. These positional relationships are more consistent in large dogs and less consistent in small dogs and cats.

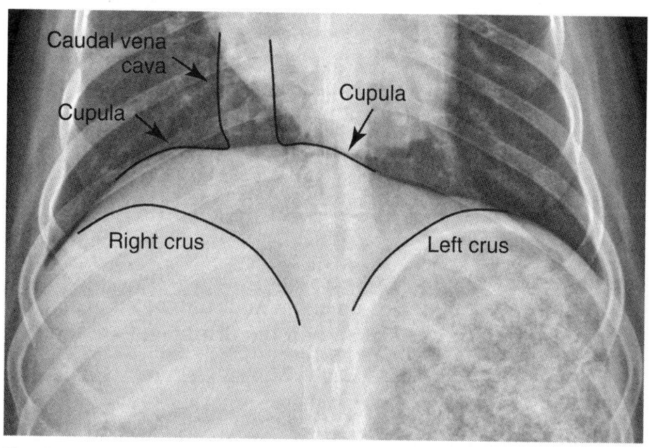

Fig. 32.4 Ventrodorsal (VD) radiograph of the diaphragmatic region of a normal dog with the cupula and both crura projecting into the thorax.

abdominal surface of the left crus (see Figs. 32.2 and 32.3). The cupula is the most cranial convex portion of the diaphragm on both the lateral and the dorsoventral (DV) or ventrodorsal (VD) views. The thoracic surface of the diaphragm may be visible as one, two, or three convex projections into the thoracic cavity (see Figs. 32.4 and 32.5).

Several normal variations of diaphragmatic position and shape may be seen radiographically. Factors that cause this variable appearance are both real and apparent. Real factors consist of breed, age, obesity, phase of respiration, and gravity. Apparent factors are x-ray beam centering and animal positioning during radiographic examination. Many combinations are possible when all permutations of these variables are considered.[4] Most of these variables are not radiographically significant; however, some must be recognized and understood

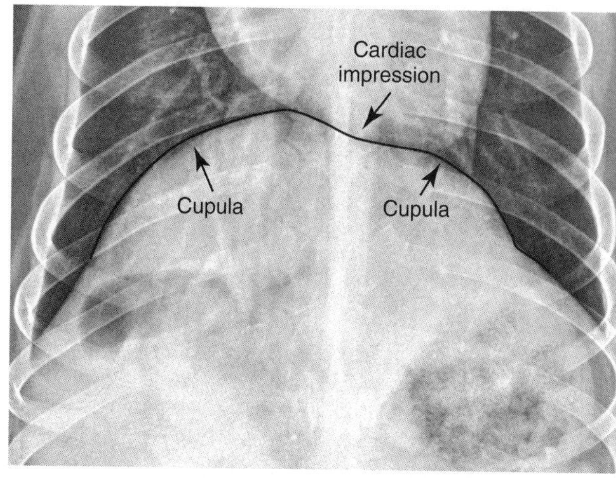

Fig. 32.5 Dorsoventral (DV) radiograph of the diaphragmatic region of a normal dog with only one convex shape projecting into the thorax.

to avoid confusion. Changes most apparent radiographically are the position, shape, and appearance of the cupula and crura. The relative position of the crura depends mostly on the position and size of the animal and primary x-ray beam centering.

The diaphragm usually looks different in left versus right lateral thoracic radiographs. The most dependent crus is usually displaced cranially when an animal is in lateral recumbency since the dependent lung is less inflated and abdominal contents displace the dependent diaphragm cranially. In right lateral recumbency, the crura usually appear to be parallel (see Fig. 32.3); in left lateral recumbency, they sometimes appear to cross. The crura also appear to be more extensively separated, by up to 2.5 vertebral lengths, if the animal is rotated slightly or if the x-ray beam is centered over the mid or cranial thorax.[4] As already mentioned, the confluence of the caudal vena cava with the diaphragm can be used to distinguish the left from right crus.

The radiographic appearance of the diaphragm in VD or DV projections varies with x-ray beam centering. The diaphragm may appear as two or three separate dome-shaped structures (see Fig. 32.4) or as a single dome-shaped structure (see Fig. 32.5). The three structures represent the cupula and two crura. A single domed diaphragm may be seen on a VD view when the x-ray beam is centered on the mid-abdomen or on a DV view when the x-ray beam is centered mid-thorax. Two or three separate domed structures are seen on a VD view with the x-ray beam is centered mid-thorax or on a DV view with the x-ray beam centered mid-abdomen.[4]

Diaphragmatic position and shape vary with phase of respiration, and intra-abdominal pressure. The normal intersection point of the diaphragm and spine is between T11 and T13 but may vary between T9 and L1. The diaphragm changes position with normal respiration from one-half to two vertebral lengths. On a lateral thoracic view made in extreme inspiration, the diaphragm is oriented more vertically; the shape changes from convex to straight (Fig. 32.6). The diaphragm is displaced cranially by increased intra-abdominal pressure, which may be caused by obesity, ascites, gastric or intestinal distention, abdominal pain, or abdominal masses.

Separate diaphragmatic structures are not seen as distinctly in the cat, probably because of the relatively small thoracic size (Fig. 32.7). On extreme inspiration, particularly if the animal is in respiratory distress, of if there is a large volume of free pleural air as with a tension pneumothorax, small symmetric muscle projections are noted from the thoracic diaphragmatic surface in the VD or DV view (Fig. 32.8, eFig. 32.1). This has been referred to as *tenting* of the diaphragm and is discussed in Chapter 36 in reference to pulmonary hyperinflation.

Table • 32.1

Radiographic Signs of Diaphragmatic Disease.

RADIOGRAPHIC SIGNS	CAUSES
General loss of diaphragmatic thoracic surface outline	Bilateral pleural fluid Generalized pulmonary disease in caudal lung lobes
Localized or partial loss of the thoracic surface outline	Thoracic masses adjacent to the diaphragm Diaphragmatic hernias Focal pulmonary disease in caudal lung lobes
Shape changes	Thoracic masses adjacent to the diaphragm Hiatal hernias Small diaphragmatic hernias Pleural reaction on the diaphragmatic surface Neoplasia arising from the diaphragm Hemiparalysis of the diaphragm Unilateral tension pneumothorax
Position Changes	
Cranial displacement	Obesity Peritoneal fluid Abdominal pain Abdominal masses or organ enlargement; liver enlargement and masses frequently cause cranial displacement Generalized diaphragmatic paralysis Cranial displacement of the cupula caused by a diaphragmatic defect with the peritoneum and pleura intact
Caudal displacement	Severe respiratory distress—ventilation or perfusion problems Tension pneumothorax Caudal displacement of the cupula caused by contact with the heart

currently or are more difficult and are therefore used rarely (Fig. 32.11).[12–15]

Ultrasonographic examination of the diaphragm may add diagnostic information, particularly for patients with pleural fluid that obliterates soft tissue. The examination is best done transhepatically.[16] Ultrasonographic signs of a diaphragmatic hernia include identification of abdominal structures within the thorax, particularly the liver, and an interruption in the diaphragmatic outline.[16–18] An interruption in the diaphragmatic outline may not be seen consistently with diaphragmatic hernia.[19]

CT examination of the thorax will add diagnostic information, although CT is usually not necessary for a diagnosis of a diaphragmatic hernia. Contrast-enhanced CT will better define which organs are herniated and the location of the hernia, and it can distinguish hernia from caudal thoracic or diaphragmatic masses (Fig. 32.12). CT may be more useful in more unusual cases, such as herniations through the aortic hiatus, esophageal hiatus, or caval foramen or peritoneopleural hernia.[20,21]

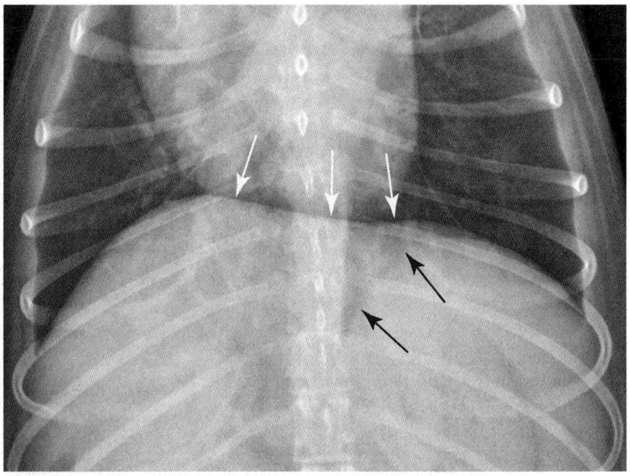

Fig. 32.9 Ventrodorsal (VD) view of the diaphragmatic region of a normal dog. A cardiac impression (*white arrows*) is present on the diaphragmatic body (cupula). The left diaphragmatic crus (*black arrows*) is visible. The right crus is not visible as a separate structure.

Box • 32.1

Radiographic Signs Associated With Traumatic Diaphragmatic Hernia

Abdominal Viscera Within the Thorax
- Gas- or ingesta-filled bowel
- Gas- or ingesta-filled stomach
- Identifiable parenchymal organs, such as the liver and spleen

Displacement of Abdominal Structures—Cranial
- Liver
- Small bowel
- Stomach
- Spleen

Displacement of Thoracic Structures—Generally Displaced Cranially and Laterally Away From an Abnormal Opaque Area in the Thorax
- Heart
- Mediastinum
- Lungs

Partial or Complete Loss of the Thoracic Diaphragmatic Surface Outline
- Pleural fluid or mass
- Lung fluid or mass

Divergence of Diaphragmatic Crura or Cranial Angulation of Diaphragm
- Pleural fluid

Traumatic Diaphragmatic Hernias

In one study, only half of the animals with a trauma-induced diaphragmatic hernia had a history of known trauma.[6] Traumatic diaphragmatic hernias usually involve the muscular portion of the diaphragm.[6,22] It has been suggested that right

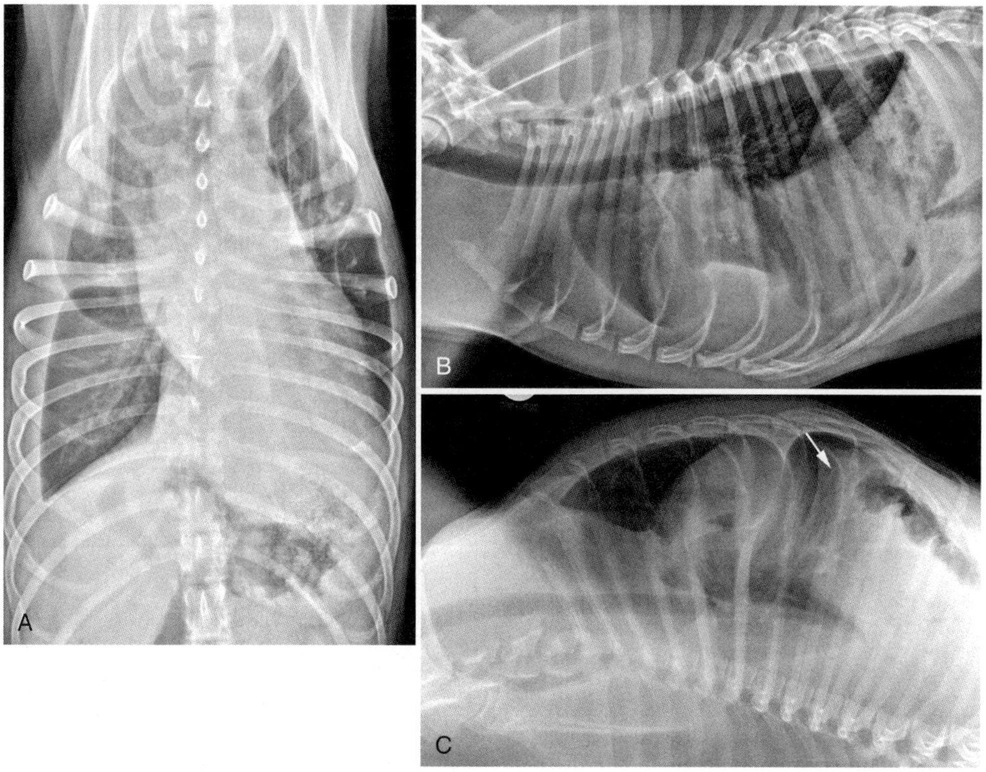

Fig. 32.10 Ventrodorsal (VD) **(A)**, lateral **(B)**, and horizontal beam lateral **(C)** views of a dog with a traumatic diaphragmatic hernia. **A,** An increased opacity in the left caudal thorax is apparent. There is loss of the thoracic diaphragmatic surface outline over the cupula and left crus and partial loss of the cardiac silhouette outline. Bilateral pleural effusion is present. **B,** The outline of the cardiac silhouette and ventral diaphragm are indistinct due to focal increased soft tissue opacity. There is ventral soft tissue opacity and rounded and retracted lung lobes, consistent with pleural effusion. **C,** There is increased soft tissue opacity dorsally, consistent with pleural effusion gravitating to the dependent portion of the thorax. However, an abnormal soft tissue opacity remains in the caudal ventral thorax and the ventral diaphragmatic outline is still not visible in its expected location (*white arrow*), consistent with a diaphragmatic hernia.

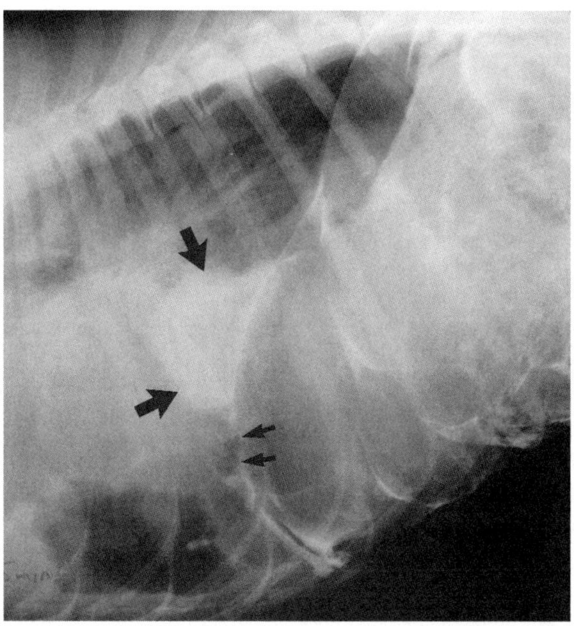

Fig. 32.11 A lateral abdominal radiograph of a positive-contrast peritoneogram. The abdominal surface of the diaphragm has an indistinct outline (*small black arrows*), with contrast medium visible in the pleural cavity (*large black arrows*). These are reliable radiographic signs of a diaphragmatic defect and a diaphragmatic hernia.

and left incidence distribution is equal,[16] but a higher incidence on the right side has been reported in the dog.[6] Most frequently herniated organs are, in order of prevalence, the liver, small bowel, stomach, spleen, and omentum.[6,9,22–24] In patients with a chronic diaphragmatic hernia, the liver and small intestine are the most frequently herniated, followed by omentum, spleen, stomach, colon, and pancreas. Strangulation of organs may be found at surgery.[25]

The most consistent radiographic signs of traumatic diaphragmatic hernia are:

- Abdominal viscera within the thorax
- Displacement of abdominal or thoracic organs, or both
- Partial or complete loss of the thoracic diaphragmatic surface outline
- Asymmetry or altered slope to the diaphragm on the lateral projection[11]
- Presence of pleural fluid (Fig. 32.13, eFigs. 32.2–32.4)

Identification of abdominal structures in the thorax is a conclusive sign of diaphragmatic hernia. Small bowel is easily identified when it is gas filled; when fluid filled, it appears as a tubular structure. The stomach may be filled with gas, fluid, or ingested material. In addition, gastric rugal folds may provide a marker for identifying the stomach within the thorax. A herniated, gas-distended stomach can be mistaken for a unilateral left pneumothorax, and the stomach should be decompressed and repositioned immediately by surgical intervention (Fig. 32.14).[6] Such instances are life-threatening because of potential or actual cardiovascular tamponade.

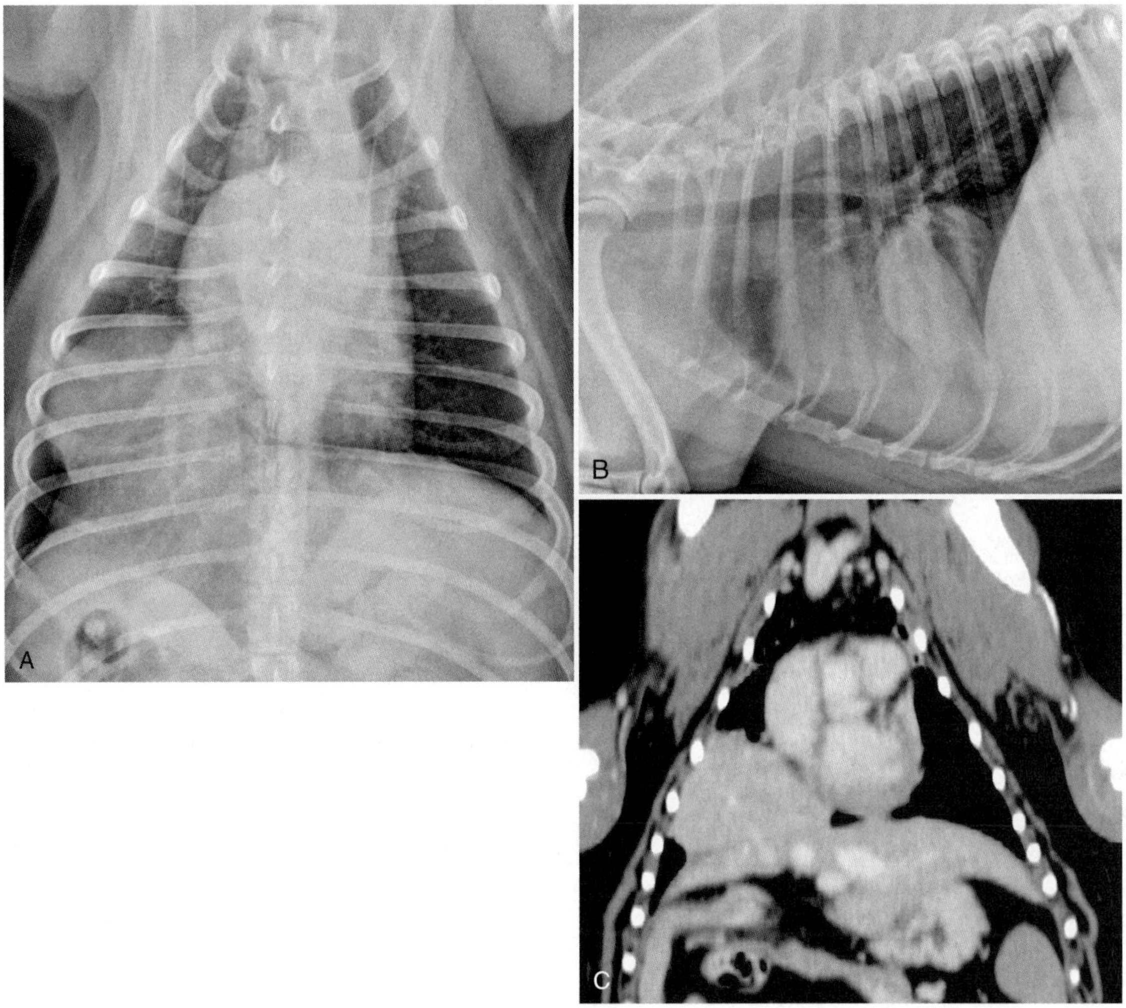

Fig. 32.12 Right lateral **(A)**, ventrodorsal (VD) **(B)** thoracic radiographs and a dorsally reformatted computed tomography (CT) image **(C)** of a dog with a diaphragmatic hernia. **A,** There is a rounded soft tissue mass in the mid-caudal thorax and focal loss of the outline of the ventral aspect of the cardiac silhouette and ventral diaphragm. **B,** The medial and caudal margins of the soft tissue mass in the right caudal thorax are less distinct, and there is loss of the outline of the right crus of the diaphragm. **C,** CT confirmed that the soft tissue opacity in the right caudal thorax was a liver lobe that had herniated through the caval foramen.

Herniated solid abdominal parenchymal organs are difficult to distinguish from localized pleural fluid, pulmonary opacity, or both. Omentum is the most difficult to detect unless it is herniated in association with other abdominal organs. In such instances, it helps outline abdominal visceral organs.

In the absence of finding abdominal organs in the thorax, cranial abdominal organ displacement or absence of abdominal organs from their normal location is an indirect sign of diaphragmatic hernia. The liver, spleen, small bowel, and stomach must be assessed closely for displacement. Barium sulfate may also be administered to identify the stomach and help detect mild to moderate gastric displacement not observed on survey radiographs.

The heart, mediastinum, and lungs may also be displaced, depending on the size and position of abdominal organs within the thorax. The heart and lungs are usually displaced cranially and either medially or laterally by herniated abdominal viscera, and the mediastinum is usually shifted from its midline position. A localized diaphragmatic surface outline loss usually indicates the area through which the hernia has occurred. Abdominal viscera and/or pleural fluid adjacent to the thoracic diaphragmatic surface cause the outline loss. This occurrence must be distinguished from the many other thoracic conditions that produce soft tissue opacity adjacent to the diaphragm. Pleural fluid is present consistently with chronic diaphragmatic hernias, or if a herniated abdominal organ, most usually the liver, is strangulated through a small diaphragmatic opening.[24] Pleural fluid is a nonspecific sign of diaphragmatic hernia and often masks other more important radiographic signs. Thoracocentesis and aspiration of the pleural fluid may be necessary before the hernia can be detected radiographically. The use of a small amount of barium can be highly specific and provide the diagnosis (Fig. 32.15).

Congenitally Predisposed Diaphragmatic Hernias

Approximately 15% of all diaphragmatic hernias are congenitally predisposed.[9] Included in this group are peritoneopericardial diaphragmatic hernias (PPDHs), hiatal hernias, and peritoneopleural hernias. Herniation in association with congenital diaphragmatic defects may occur in an animal of any age after abdominal trauma or transitory increase in intra-abdominal pressure. Defects in diaphragmatic development may be present and never result in a hernia.

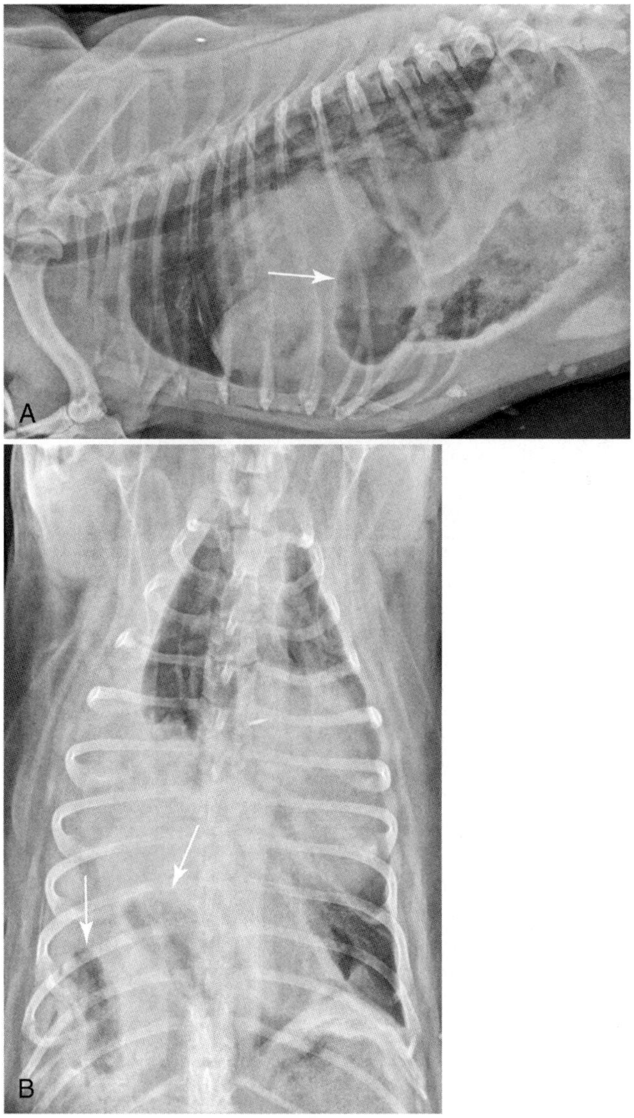

Fig. 32.13 Lateral **(A)** and ventrodorsal (VD) **(B)** radiographs of the thorax of a dog with a traumatic diaphragmatic hernia. Radiographic signs of a diaphragmatic hernia in **A** are gas-filled stomach (*white arrow*) within the thorax, cranial displacement of abdominal structures, and a cranially displaced diaphragmatic segment. Radiographic signs in **B** are the mediastinal shift to the left, away from the herniated viscera; gas-filled stomach and bowel within the thorax (*white arrows*); cranially displaced abdominal structures; and loss of the right diaphragmatic surface outline.

Peritoneopericardial Diaphragmatic Hernias

A PPDH occurs when abdominal viscera herniate into the pericardial sac through a congenital hiatus formed between the tendinous portion of the diaphragm and the pericardial sac. This has been reported to occur in littermates,[26] and a predisposing trait may be carried on a simple autosomal recessive gene in cats, with a 1:500 to 1:1500 rate of incidence.[27] Domestic long-hair cats, Himalayans, and Maine Coon cats appear to be overrepresented, as do Weimaraner dogs.[28,29] The hernia may have been present from birth or is acquired. Mild increases in intra-abdominal pressure may cause abdominal organs to herniate through a congenital hiatus.

Peritoneopericardial hernias may produce clinical signs, but are often an incidental radiographic finding in old or young animals.[5,28–34] The liver is herniated most frequently; the stomach, omentum, and small bowel have a less frequent occurrence of herniation.[35] Hepatic cysts have also been reported to be associated with liver herniation into the pericardial sac.[36]

Radiographic signs associated with peritoneopericardial hernias are listed in Box 32.2. Herniated abdominal organs in the pericardial sac are usually caudal, or caudal and lateral, to the heart. Gas- or ingesta-filled hollow visceral organs are not difficult to identify within the pericardial sac, but the conspicuity of the gas-containing viscus may be a function of body position during radiography (Fig. 32.16, eFig. 32.5). Radiographically, gas within the bowel is in abrupt contrast to the adjacent structures of soft tissue opacity. Solid parenchymal organs, unless surrounded by omentum, are difficult to distinguish as separate structures within the pericardium. When abdominal organs are herniated into the pericardial sac, cranial and ventral organ displacement within the abdomen may be seen, but this displacement is usually not as pronounced as that noted with traumatic diaphragmatic hernias.

A large, round cardiac silhouette and a cardiac silhouette with an abnormal convex projection on the caudal border are signs consistent with PPDHs. These two signs depend on the amount of abdominal viscera within the pericardial sac. Large amounts of viscera produce a large, round cardiac silhouette, whereas smaller amounts, such as a portion of the liver, falciform fat, or stomach, may produce only an abnormal convex caudal cardiac border. A large, round silhouette must be differentiated from pericardial effusion, generalized heart enlargement, or both. An abnormally convex caudal cardiac border must be differentiated from neoplasia, pleural granulomas, or localized pleural fluid.

An indistinguishable outline to the ventral diaphragmatic surface and the caudal ventral cardiac silhouette is produced by the communication between the two structures. This finding must be differentiated from normal contact between the heart and diaphragm, pleural fluid, localized pleuritis, and pleural granulomas. On the lateral view, identification of the dorsal peritoneopericardial mesothelial remnant between the heart and diaphragm is a consistent radiographic sign of peritoneopericardial hernia in cats (Fig. 32.17, eFig. 32.6).[37] Sternal abnormalities may also be present.[34]

Additional radiographic studies that may be performed to confirm a diagnosis include oral administration of barium sulfate, nonselective angiography,[38] and peritoneography. Barium sulfate may be used to demonstrate gastrointestinal structures within the pericardial sac or cranial ventral displacement of abdominal structures (Fig. 32.18).

Ultrasonography has been successfully used to diagnose PPDHs.[16–19] Ultrasonography is a reliable imaging modality to use for documentation of a peritoneopericardial hernia in patients where soft tissue opaque abdominal structures are in the pericardial sac and difficult to differentiate from the heart on radiographs. If available, an ultrasound examination should be considered before contrast examinations are performed to assist in the diagnosis of PPDH.

CT can assist in determining which structures are herniated, and it can confirm a PPDH in cases in which radiographs are not conclusive or when more information is desired prior to surgery.

Hiatal Hernias

Hiatal hernias occur when a portion of stomach enters the thorax through the esophageal hiatus and can be congenital or acquired. Two recognized types of hiatal hernias exist: sliding (or dynamic) and paraesophageal.[39–41] The gastroesophageal sphincter and a portion of the stomach, usually the cardia, are herniated into the thorax with sliding hiatal hernias.[42] Sliding hiatal hernias are usually congenital and found in younger animals.[41] They are often associated with esophagitis from gastroesophageal reflux. As the name implies, the caudal esophagus and the cardia slide intermittently from the abdomen into the thorax, causing temporary cranial displacement of the thoracic esophagus. Because the hernia is dynamic, it may not

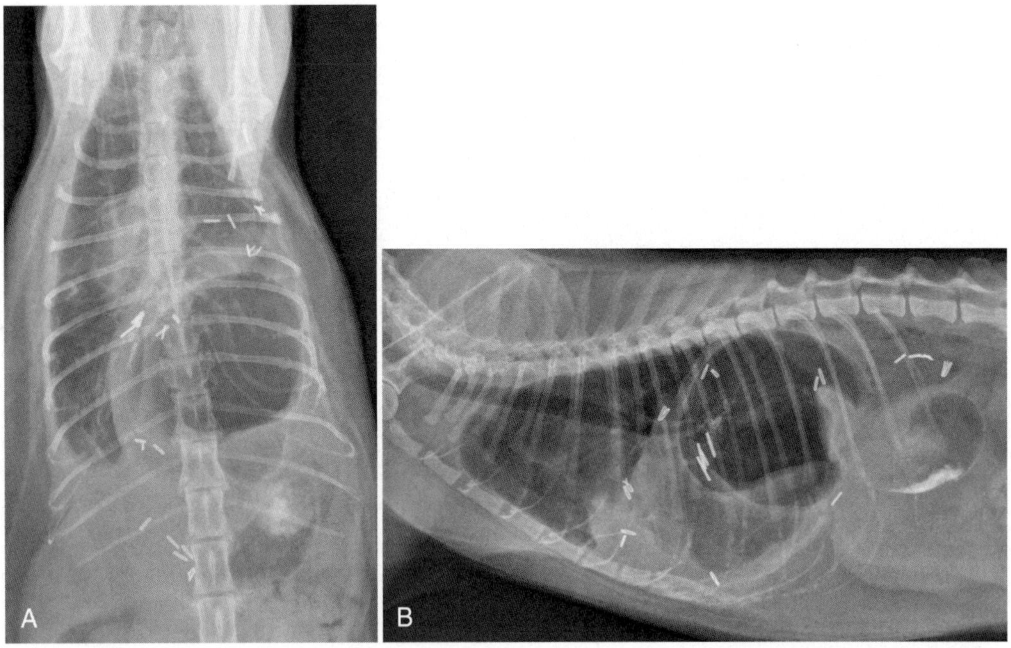

Fig. 32.14 Ventrodorsal (VD) **(A)** and lateral **(B)** views of the thorax of a cat with a traumatic diaphragmatic hernia of the stomach. Hemoclips are present from a previous surgery. **A,** The gas-filled stomach is herniated into the left hemithorax, displacing the heart and lungs to the *right*. The normal gastric and left diaphragmatic outlines are not present. **B,** The severely gas-distended stomach occupies the majority of the caudal thorax and obscures the cardiac silhouette.

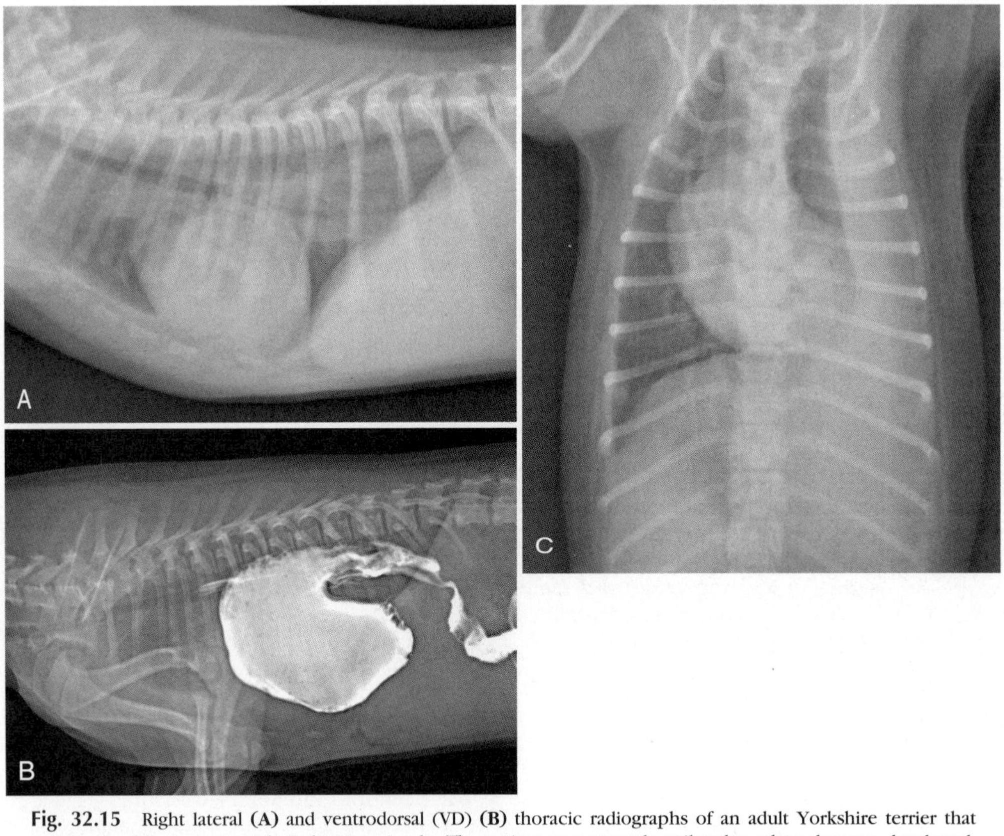

Fig. 32.15 Right lateral **(A)** and ventrodorsal (VD) **(B)** thoracic radiographs of an adult Yorkshire terrier that sustained a fall approximately 7 days previously. The patient was normal until today when dyspnea developed. There is only a mild nonspecific increase in thoracic radiographic opacity in the lateral view. In the VD view, there is a homogeneous increase in opacity along the left thoracic wall and border effacement of the diaphragm. This could be a hernia but a hematoma in the pleural space could also be considered. Following administration of a small amount of barium **(C)**, it is apparent that the stomach is herniated into the thorax, confirming a diaphragmatic hernia.

Box • 32.2

Radiographic Signs Associated With Peritoneopericardial Diaphragmatic Hernias

- Abdominal organs identified in the pericardial sac; gas, ingested material, or structures of soft tissue opacity may be present
- Large, round cardiac silhouette
- Convex projection of the caudal cardiac silhouette
- Indistinguishable border of the ventral thoracic diaphragmatic surface and the caudal ventral cardiac silhouette
- Confluent silhouette between the diaphragm and the heart
- Dorsal peritoneopericardial mesothelial remnant between the heart and diaphragm on the lateral view in cats
- Sternal changes

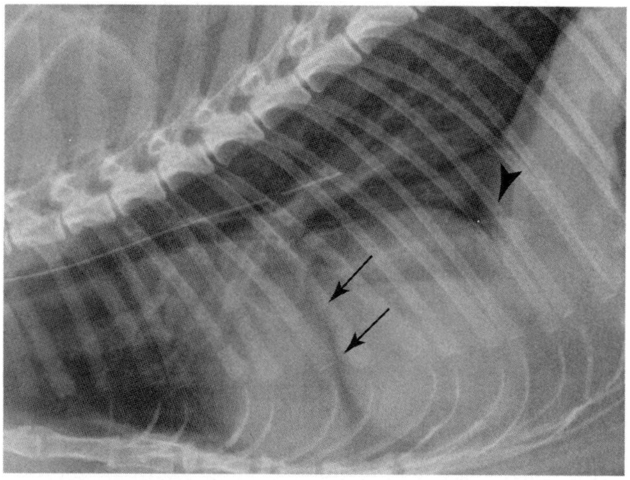

Fig. 32.17 Lateral view of a cat with a peritoneopericardial diaphragmatic hernia. The outline of a dorsal peritoneopericardial mesothelial remnant is visible cranial to the diaphragm (*black arrowhead*). The liver and omentum are herniated into the pericardial sac. The caudal border of the heart is visible (*black arrows*) because of fat in the adjacent omentum.

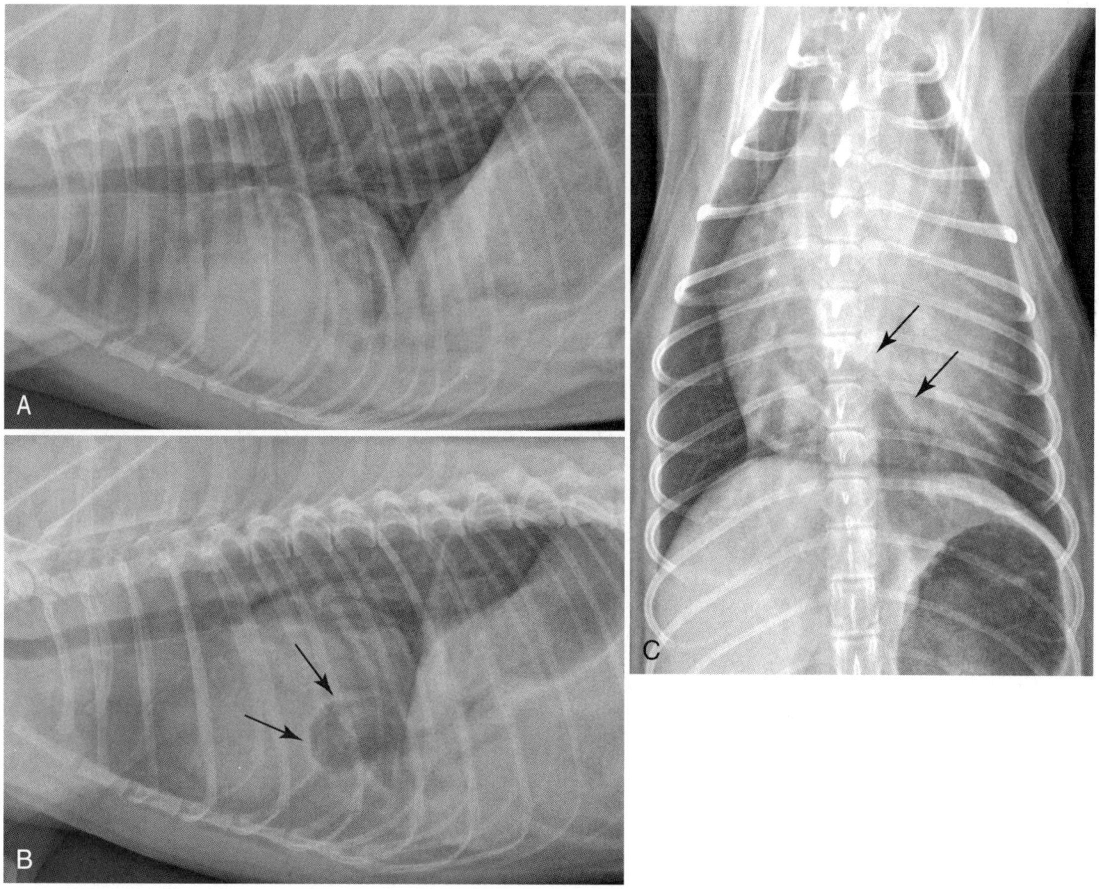

Fig. 32.16 Right lateral **(A)**, left lateral **(B)**, and ventrodorsal (VD) **(C)** radiographs of a dog with a peritoneopericardial diaphragmatic hernia. Various opacities are visualized in the pericardial sac, including gas, soft tissue, and fat. The gas filled herniated portion of the stomach is better visualized on the left lateral and VD views (*black arrows*). The amount of gas within organs in the pericardial sac will change depending on the position of the patient; no gas may be visible in some positions.

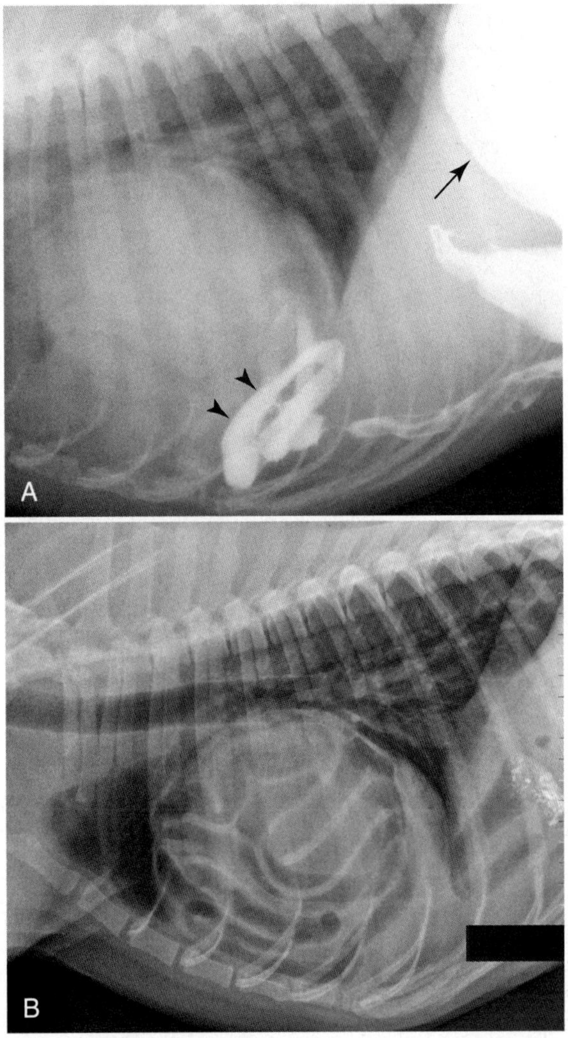

Fig. 32.18 Right lateral **(A)** and left lateral **(B)** views of the thorax of a dog with a peritoneopericardial diaphragmatic hernia. **A,** Barium is present in the normally positioned stomach (*black arrow*), as well as in small intestines (*black arrowheads*) that are herniated into the pericardial sac. **B,** Radiographs of the same patient made at a later time reveal diffuse gas filling of the small intestines, which provides negative contrast that allows easy identification of small intestines within the pericardial sac. (Courtesy Dr. Amy Habing, Ohio State University, Columbus, OH.)

be seen on any one radiograph; fluoroscopic examination is often necessary to make a diagnosis. Patients with nonsliding hiatal hernias have been reported, with the gastroesophageal sphincter and the gastric cardia displaced through the esophageal hiatus and fixed within the thorax.[42]

A paraesophageal hiatal hernia is produced when the cardia or cardia and fundus of the stomach or other soft tissue structures herniate through, or alongside, the esophageal hiatus and become positioned adjacent to the esophagus. They are usually static and do not slide between the thorax and abdomen, and the gastroesophageal sphincter is in a normal position.[40,42] The herniated stomach may cause esophageal obstruction from external pressure on the caudal esophagus.

Hiatal hernias have also been classified as types I through IV. Type I represents a sliding hiatal hernia, type II represents a paraesophageal hernia, and type III represents a combination of type I and type II. Type IV has been described two ways: (1) as a type III hernia combined with herniation of another organ rather than the stomach or (2) as a gastroesophageal intussusception. Other complicated hernias, such as a hernia through

Box • 32.3

Radiographic Signs Associated With Sliding Hiatal Hernias

Survey Radiographs

- Soft tissue mass adjacent to the left diaphragmatic crus close to midline
- Loss of thoracic surface outline on the left diaphragmatic crus
- Cranial displacement of the gastric cardia producing an abnormal gastric shape
- Dilated esophagus
- Pneumonia

Esophagram

- Dilated esophagus
- Hypomotile esophagus
- Gastroesophageal sphincter within the thorax represented by a circumferentially narrowed area of the esophagus
- Gastric cardia within the thorax
- Gastroesophageal reflux

the esophageal hiatus combined with a second, separate gastric herniation through a defect in the diaphragm have been reported.[41]

Hiatal hernias occur in both the dog and the cat.[43] They can be associated with other esophageal conditions in shar-pei dogs.[43] There may be no clinical signs, or vomiting, regurgitation, excessive salivation, dysphagia, and dyspnea may be observed.[43–45] Hiatal hernias can be associated with esophageal dysmotility and are seen more frequently in brachycephalic dogs, especially French bulldogs. Decreased intrathoracic pressure associated with increased respiratory effort may be the cause of these hernias in brachycephalic dogs.[46] Hiatal hernia may be suspected from the clinical signs and survey radiographic findings but must be confirmed by an esophagram.

Radiographic signs of a sliding hiatal hernia are listed in Box 32.3. The most consistent survey radiographic sign is stomach displacement. The cardia appears to be stretched toward the diaphragm or may extend into the thorax. This displacement produces an abnormal shape to the cardia and fundus remaining in the abdomen. The caudal esophagus may or may not be distended, and a soft tissue mass may be seen adjacent to the left diaphragmatic crus (Fig. 32.19, eFig. 32.7, Video 32.1). The size and visibility of this mass depend on the amount of stomach that has herniated into the thorax. The soft tissue mass associated with a hiatal hernia must be differentiated from pulmonary or diaphragmatic masses. Diaphragmatic tumors occur but are rare.[47]

A dilated caudal esophagus is usually best detected and evaluated with an esophagram. An esophagram is also helpful for differentiating the type of hiatal hernia. The caudal esophageal sphincter and a portion of the cardia are cranial to the diaphragm with a sliding hiatal hernia.[48] The caudal esophageal sphincter can be identified as a concentric, smooth, 1- to 2-cm narrowing in the caudal esophagus (Fig. 32.20). Displacement and narrowing of the caudal esophagus by the cardia and fundus can be seen with paraesophageal hiatal hernias. Barium outlining the caudal esophagus can also be seen superimposed over the herniated paraesophageal soft tissue (Fig. 32.21, eFig. 32.8, Video 32.2).

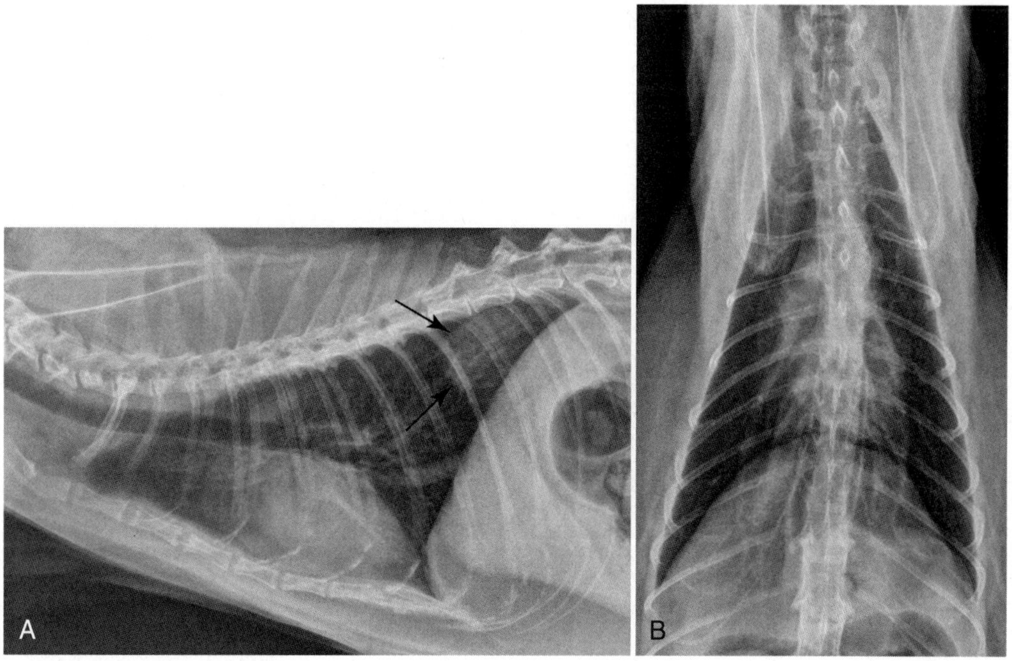

Fig. 32.19 **A,** Lateral thoracic view with a soft tissue opacity in the caudodorsal thorax (*black arrows*). The soft tissue opacity is suspect for a hiatal hernia. **B,** Ventrodorsal (VD) view at the same time is normal, which supports the diagnosis of sliding hiatal hernia.

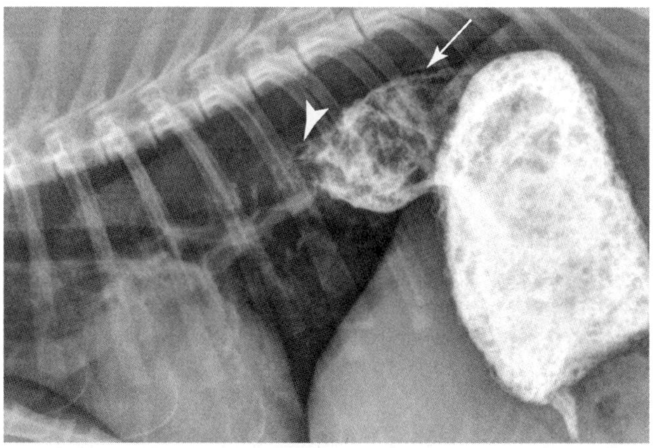

Fig. 32.20 Right lateral view of barium esophagram in a cat with a sliding hiatal hernia. Contrast medium is present in the stomach including the gastric cardia (*white arrow*), which tapers cranially (*white arrowhead*). The gastroesophageal sphincter and gastric cardia are displaced cranial to the diaphragm through the esophageal hiatus.

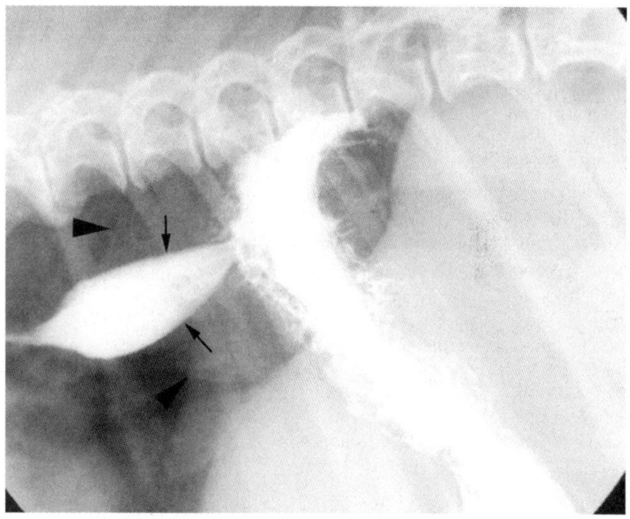

Fig. 32.21 Lateral view of the thorax. Barium is filling and outlining the caudal esophagus (*black arrows*). The barium-filled caudal esophagus is superimposed over a soft tissue organ (*black arrowheads*) cranial to the diaphragm and adjacent to one side of the esophagus. This is consistent with a paraesophageal hiatal hernia.

Gastroesophageal Intussusception

Gastroesophageal intussusception occurs when the stomach, with or without the spleen, duodenum, pancreas, and omentum, invaginates through the esophageal hiatus into the caudal esophagus.[40,42,49,50] They occur most frequently in male and German shepherd dogs and in animals with a pre-existing dilated esophagus.[50] Gastroesophageal intussusception usually produces an esophageal obstruction, which results in rapid deterioration of the animal's condition with a high mortality rate; a timely diagnosis is therefore essential.[50]

On survey radiographs, a large soft tissue mass is seen adjacent to the diaphragm, usually accompanied by a dilated esophagus. There is also usually a sharp air/soft tissue interface between the displaced stomach in the caudal esophagus and the gas in the distended cranial aspect of the esophagus (Fig. 32.22). With an esophagram, gastroesophageal intussusceptions produce a large intraluminal filling defect within the caudal esophagus, rugal folds may be outlined with barium, and barium does not usually enter the stomach (Box 32.4).

Peritoneopleural Hernias

Congenital diaphragmatic defects resulting in peritoneopleural hernias are rare in the dog and cat[51–55] and have been confused with pulmonary masses.[56] The defects are created when the septum transversum or the pleural peritoneal folds do not develop and fuse to form a complete diaphragm. The diaphragmatic defect allows abdominal viscera to enter the

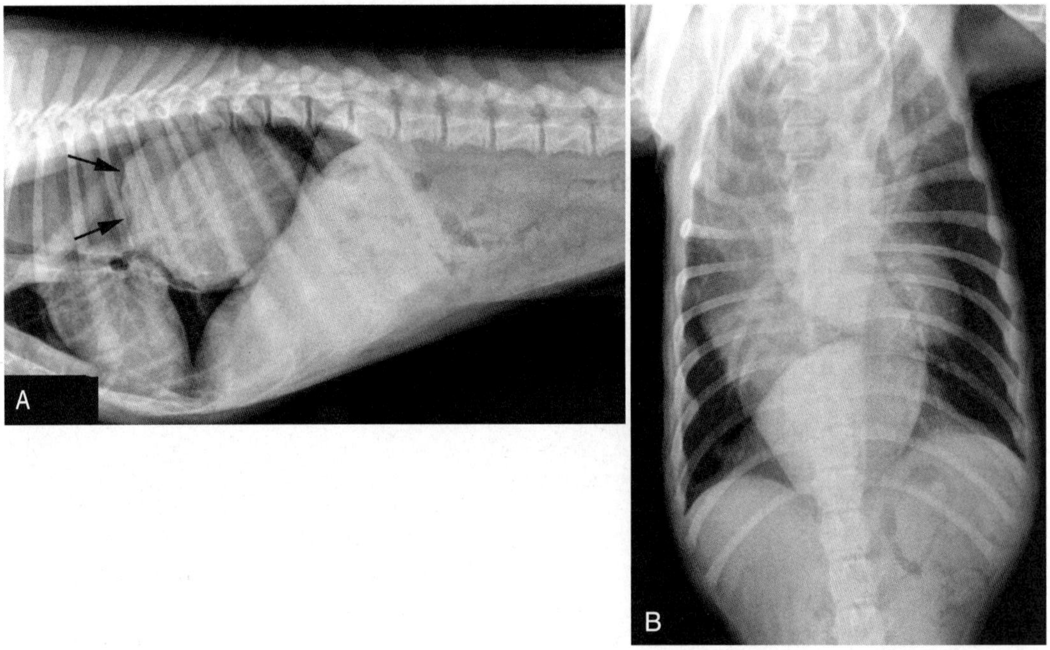

Fig. 32.22 Lateral **(A)** and ventrodorsal (VD) **(B)** views of a juvenile German shepherd with a gastroesophageal intussusception. There is a large soft tissue mass in the caudal thorax, centered on the midline. This represents the stomach herniated into the caudal aspect of the esophagus. The cranial aspect of the esophagus is dilated and there is a sharp air/gas interface in the lateral view (*black arrows*) outlining the cranial margin of the herniated stomach.

Box • 32.4

Radiographic Signs Associated With Gastroesophageal Intussusception

Survey Radiographs

- Soft tissue mass adjacent to the diaphragm
- Cranial displacement of the stomach with or without the spleen or duodenum
- Dilated esophagus
- Convex of tissue/air interface between herniated stomach and gas in cranial esophagus

Esophagram

- Intraluminal filling defect in the caudal esophagus
- Barium outline of rugal folds
- No barium within the stomach

thoracic cavity but they remain contained by serosa or pleura, producing a pleuroperitoneal hernia. These are also called true diaphragmatic hernias.[57]

In human beings, diaphragmatic defects have a familial incidence with a multifactorial mode of inheritance.[58] Congenital defects in dogs have been reported in the muscular diaphragm, dorsolateral in position at the site of the pleuroperitoneal canal,[55] and in the membranous diaphragm associated with umbilical hernias.[5,52] Bochdalek hernias are common peritoneopleural hernias in children, but are rarely reported in veterinary medicine. These are hernias at the dorsolateral margins of the diaphragm through the lumbocostal trigone, due to a failure of closure of the pleuroperitoneal canal in children. There is also a report of extension of a retroperitoneal lipoma through the lumbocostal trigone.[59]

The radiographic signs of peritoneopleural hernias associated with muscular diaphragmatic defects can be the same as for traumatic diaphragmatic hernias (Fig. 32.23, eFig. 32.9), although pleural effusion typically only occurs with traumatic hernias. With membranous defects, however, the liver (in dogs) or the falciform fat (in cats) is displaced cranially, while remaining in the caudal ventral thorax, and is often confined to the mediastinum because the peritoneal membrane and pleura are intact (Fig. 32.24).[60]

Foraminal Hernias

Herniations may occur through the aortic hiatus, esophageal hiatus, or caval foramen. These are rare in humans and veterinary patients. Caval foramen hernias can look like caudal pulmonary masses and may cause compression of the caudal vena cava. CT may be required for correct diagnosis.[20,21]

Motor Disturbances of the Diaphragm

The diaphragm is the principal muscle of respiration and is innervated by the phrenic nerve.

Motor disturbances of the diaphragm consist of unilateral paralysis, bilateral paralysis, and diaphragmatic flutter.[1] Diaphragmatic paralysis may result from pneumonia, trauma, myopathies, and neuropathies, or the cause may be unidentified.[1] Transient post-traumatic hemidiaphragmatic paralysis has been reported in cats.[61] Diaphragmatic paralysis should be suspected when one or both diaphragmatic crura are displaced cranially (Fig. 32.25). Confirmation of paralysis is best achieved with fluoroscopy. Unequal movement between the crura is seen with unilateral paralysis. With bilateral paralysis, minimal or no diaphragmatic movement or a paradoxic cranial displacement of the flaccid diaphragm may occur during inspiration.[62] Bilateral paralysis may be more difficult to confirm with fluoroscopy, because diaphragmatic movement is sometimes produced by compensatory abdominal muscle contraction during respiration. The term *diaphragmatic eventration* is sometimes used for focal weakening of the diaphragm with

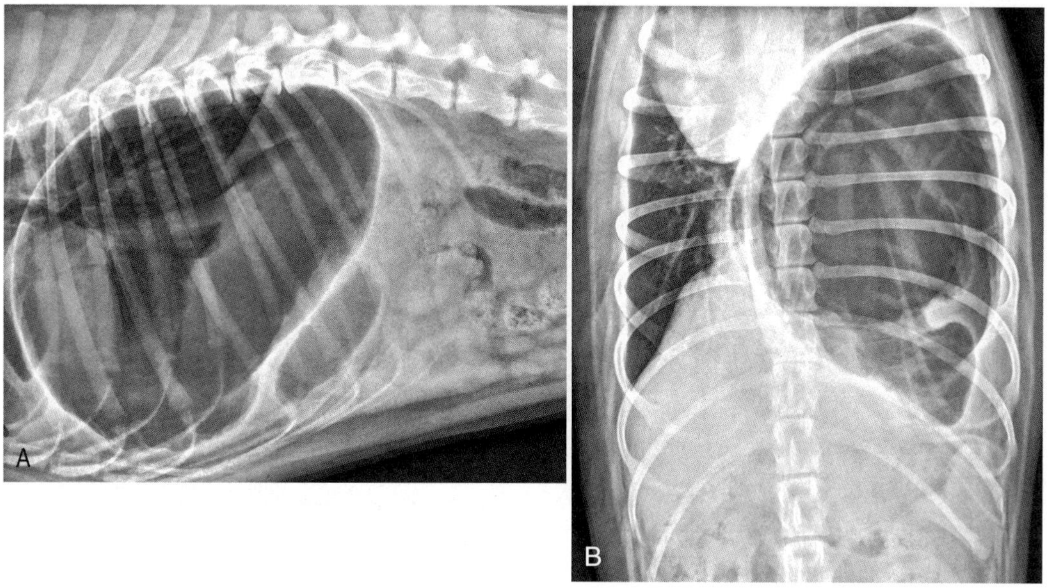

Fig. 32.23 Right lateral **(A)** and ventrodorsal (VD) **(B)** views of a dog. A defect in the left dorsolateral aspect of the muscular portion of the diaphragm resulted in a congenital diaphragmatic hernia. The gas-filled stomach is within the thorax.

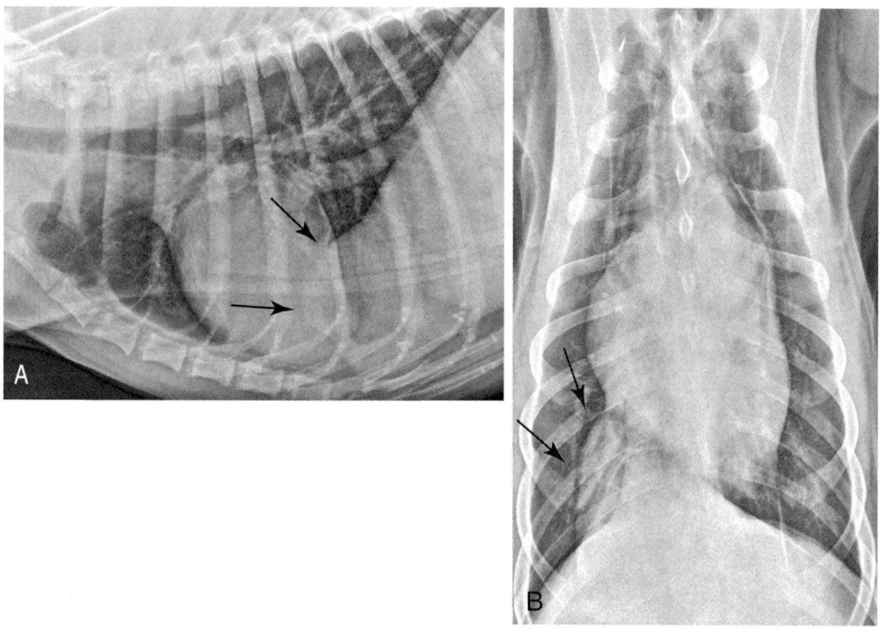

Fig. 32.24 Right lateral **(A)** and ventrodorsal (VD) **(B)** views of a dog thorax. A defect is present in the membranous portion of the diaphragm. A portion of liver is displaced cranially into the right ventral thorax (*arrows*) and surrounded with intact peritoneum and parietal pleura.

cranial displacement of the affected portion of the diaphragm. This condition is difficult to diagnose radiographically.

Diaphragmatic flutter is most often associated with contractions of the diaphragm synchronous with the heartbeat. It is usually transient in nature and can be easily diagnosed with fluoroscopy by observing contractions of the diaphragm in synchrony with the heartbeat.[63]

Muscular Dystrophy

Muscular dystrophy caused by dystrophin deficiency occurs rarely in dogs[64] and cats.[65,66] In dogs with muscular dystrophy, radiographic abnormalities include diaphragmatic asymmetry, diaphragmatic undulation, and gastroesophageal hiatal hernia.[67,68] In cats an irregular, scalloped appearance of the diaphragm, particularly along the ventral margin, was a consistent finding observed on radiographs after 7 months of age.[65] The scalloped margin, noted best on the lateral view, should not be confused with the normal scalloping observed on the VD view in cats on maximal inspiration (see Fig. 32.7). The scalloped appearance is caused by muscular hypertrophy, which can be confirmed by ultrasound.[65] Muscular hypertrophy produced with feline muscular dystrophy has also been reported to cause megaesophagus from extraluminal hiatal obstruction. Definitive laboratory tests, such as immunofluorescence or immunoblot tests, are necessary to establish the diagnosis of muscular dystrophy.

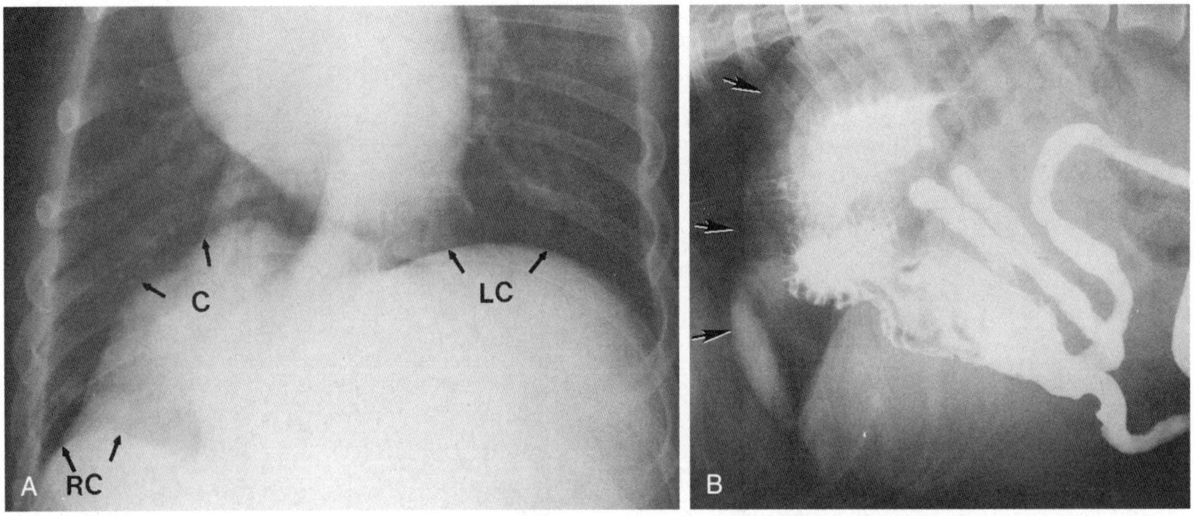

Fig. 32.25 Ventrodorsal (VD) **(A)** and lateral **(B)** radiographs of the cranial abdomen. Hemiparalysis of the left diaphragm is present. **A,** The left diaphragmatic crus (*LC*) is cranial to the right crus (*RC*). The cupula (*C*) and *RC* are in a normal inspiratory position. **B,** The cranial position of the left diaphragmatic crus (*black arrows*) causes the gastric cardia and fundus to be displaced cranially.

REFERENCES

1. Ganong W. *Review of Medical Physiology*. 22nd ed. New York: McGraw-Hill; 2005:652.
2. Baum H. The Lymphatic System of the Dog. Original German text translated by Mayer M, Bettin L, Bellamy K, Stamm I. USask Open Press; 2021. https://openpress.usask.ca/k9lymphaticsystem/.
3. Evans HE. *Miller's Anatomy of the Dog*. 4th ed. Philadelphia: Saunders; 2013:222.
4. Grandage J. The radiology of the dog's diaphragm. *J Small Anim Pract*. 1974;15(1):1–18.
5. Schulman J. Peritoneopericardial diaphragmatic hernia in a dog. *Mod Vet Pract*. 1979;60(4):306–308.
6. Garson HL, Dodman NH, Baker GJ. Diaphragmatic hernia: analysis of fifty-six cases in dogs and cats. *J Small Anim Pract*. 1980;21(9):469–481.
7. Farrow CS. Radiographic diagnosis of diaphragmatic hernia. *Mod Vet Pract*. 1983;64:979.
8. Silverman S, Ackerman N. Radiographic evaluation of abdominal hernias. *Mod Vet Pract*. 1977;58(9):781–785.
9. Wilson 3rd GP, Hayes Jr HM. Diaphragmatic hernia in the dog and cat: a 25-year overview. *Semin Vet Med Surg*. 1986;1(4):318–326.
10. Levine SH. Diaphragmatic hernia. *Vet Clin North Am Small Anim Pract*. 1987;17(2):411–430.
11. Stokhof AA, Wolvekamp WTC, Hellebrekers LJ, et al. Traumatic diaphragmatic hernia in the dog and cat. *Tijdschr Diergeneeskd*. 1986;111(Suppl 1):62S.
12. Rendano VT. Positive contrast peritoneography: an aid in the radiographic diagnosis of diaphragmatic hernia. *J Am Vet Radiol Soc*. 1979;20(67).
13. Stickle RL. Positive-contrast celiography (peritoneography) for the diagnosis of diaphragmatic hernia in dogs and cats. *J Am Vet Med Assoc*. 1984;185:325.
14. Williams J, Leveille R, Myer CW. Imaging modalities used to confirm diaphragmatic hernia in small animals. *Compend Small Anim*. 1998;20:1199.
15. Choi J, Kim H, Kim M, Yoon J. Imaging diagnosis – positive contrast peritoneographic features of true diaphragmatic hernia. *Vet Radiol Ultrasound*. 2009;50:185–187.
16. Lamb CR, Mason GD, Wallace MK. Ultrasonographic diagnosis of peritoneopericardial diaphragmatic hernia in a Persian cat. *Vet Record*. 1989;125(8):186.
17. Hay WH, Woodfield JA, Moon MA. Clinical, echocardiographic, and radiographic findings of peritoneopericardial diaphragmatic hernia in two dogs. *J Am Vet Med Assoc*. 1989;195(9):1245–1248.
18. Hashimoto A, Kudo T, Sawashima I. Diagnostic ultrasonography of noncardiac intrathoracic disorders in small animals. *Res Bull*. 1990;55:235.
19. Hodges RD, Tucker RL, Brace JJ. Radiographic diagnosis (peritoneopericardial diaphragmatic herniation in a dog). *Vet Radiol Ultrasound*. 1993;34:249.
20. Kim J, Kim S, Jo J, Lee S, Eom K. Radiographic and computed tomographic features of caval foramen hernias of the liver in 7 dogs: mimicking lung nodules. *J Vet Med Sci*. 2016;78(11):1693–1697.
21. Park J, Lee H, Jeong S. Caval foramen hernia in a dog: preoperative diagnosis and surgical treatment. *J. Vet Med Sci.* 2020;82(11):1602–1606.
22. Carb A. Symposium on surgical techniques in small animal practice. Diaphragmatic hernia in the dog and cat. *Vet Clin North Am*. 1975;5(3):477–494.
23. Wilson GP, Newton CD, Burt JK. A review of 116 diaphragmatic hernias in dogs and cats. *J Am Vet Med Assoc*. 1971;159(9):1142–1145.
24. Boudrieau RJ, Muir WW. Pathophysiology of traumatic diaphragmatic hernia in dogs. *Compend Contin Educ Pract Vet*. 1987;9:379.
25. Minihan AC, Berg J, Evans KL. Chronic diaphragmatic hernia in 34 dogs and 16 cats. *J Am Anim Hosp Assoc*. 2004;40(1):51–63.
26. Feldman DB, Bree MM, Cohen BJ. Congenital diaphragmatic hernia in neonatal dogs. *J Am Vet Med Assoc*. 1968;153(7):942–944.
27. Saperstein G, Harris S, Leipold HW. Congenital defects in domestic cats. *Feline Pract*. 1976;6(18).
28. Reimer SB, Kyles AE, Filipowisz DE, et al. Long-term outcome of cats treated conservatively or surgically for peritoneopericardial diaphragmatic hernia: 66 cases (1987–2002). *J Am Vet Med Assoc*. 2004;224(5):728–732.
29. Banz A, Gottfried S. Peritoneopericardial diaphragmatic hernia: a retrospective study of 31 cats and eight dogs. *J Am Anim Hosp Assoc*. 2010;46:398–404.
30. Björck GR, Tigerschiöld A. Peritoneo-pericardial diaphragmatic hernia in a dog. *J Small Anim Pract*. 1970;11(9):585–590.

31. Gourley IM, Popp JA, Park RD. Myelolipomas of the liver in a domestic cat. *J Am Vet Med Assoc.* 1971;158(12):2053–2057.
32. Rendano VT, Parker RB. Polycystic kidneys and peritoneopericardial diaphragmatic hernia in the cat: a case report. *J Small Anim Pract.* 1976;17(7):479–485.
33. Weitz J, Tilley LP, Moldoff D. Pericardiodiaphragmatic hernia in a dog. *J Am Vet Med Assoc.* 1978;173(10):1336–1338.
34. Evans SM, Biery DN. Congenital peritoneopericardial diaphragmatic hernia in the dog and cat. *Vet Radiol.* 1980;21:108.
35. Neiger R. Peritoneopericardial diaphragmatic hernia in cats. *Compend Contin Educ Pract Vet.* 1996;18:461.
36. Liptak JM, Bissett SA, Allan GS, et al. Hepatic cysts incarcerated in a peritoneopericardial diaphragmatic hernia. *J Feline Med Surg.* 2002;4(2):123–125.
37. Berry CR, Koblik PD, Ticer JW. Dorsal peritoneopericardial mesothelial remnant as an aid to the diagnosis of feline congenital peritoneopericardial diaphragmatic hernia. *Vet Radiol.* 1990;31:239.
38. Willard MD, Aronson E. Peritoneopericardial diaphragmatic hernia in a cat. *J Am Vet Med Assoc.* 1981;178(5):481–483.
39. Edwards MH. Selective vagotomy of the canine oesophagus: a model for the treatment of hiatal hernia. *Thorax.* 1976;31(2):185–189.
40. Teunissen GHB, Happ RP, Van Toorenburg J, et al. Esophageal hiatal hernia: case report of a dog and a cheetah. *Tijdschr Diergeneeskd.* 1978;103:742.
41. Ellison GW, Lewis DD, Phillips L, et al. Esophageal hiatal hernia in small animals: literature review. *J Am Anim Hosp Assoc.* 1984;20:783.
42. Ellis Jr FH. Controversies regarding the management of hiatus hernia. *Am J Surg.* 1980;139(6):782–788.
43. Stickle R, Sparschu G, Love N, et al. Radiographic evaluation of esophageal function in Chinese Shar Pei pups. *J Am Vet Med Assoc.* 1992;201(1):81–84.
44. Miles KG, Pope ER, Jergens AE. Paraesophageal hiatal hernia and pyloric obstruction in a dog. *J Am Vet Med Assoc.* 1988;193(11):1437–1439.
45. Gordon LC, Friend EJ, Hamilton MH. Hemorrhagic pleural effusion secondary to an unusual type III hiatal hernia in a 4-year-old Great Dane. *J Am Anim Hosp Assoc.* 2010;46(5):336–340.
46. Eivers C, Chicon Rueda R, Luiti T, Salavati Schmitz S. Retrospective analysis of esophageal imaging features in brachycephalic versus non-brachycephalic dogs based on videofluoroscopic swallowing studies. *J Vet Int Med.* 2019;33:1740–1746.
47. Anderson GM, Miller DA, Miller SW. Peripheral nerve sheath tumor of the diaphragm with osseous differentiation in a one-year-old dog. *J Am Anim Hosp Assoc.* 1999;35:319.
48. Steiner GM. Gastro-oesophageal reflux, hiatus hernia, and the radiologist with special reference to children. *Br J Radiol.* 1977;50(591):164–174.
49. Pollock S, Rhodes WH. Gastroesophageal intussusception in an Afghan hound. *J Am Vet Radiol Soc.* 1970;11(5).
50. Leib MS, Blass CE. Gastroesophageal intussusception in the dog: a review of the literature and a case report. *J Am Anim Hosp Assoc.* 1984;20:783.
51. Bath GF. Congenital diaphragmatic hiatus in a dog. *J S Afr Vet Assoc.* 1976;47(1):55–56.
52. Nicholson C. Defective diaphragm associated with umbilical hernia. *Vet Rec.* 1976;98(21):433–434.
53. Sawyer SL. Defective diaphragm associated with umbilical hernia. *Vet Rec.* 1976;98(24):490.
54. Swift BJ. Defective diaphragm associated with umbilical hernia. *Vet Rec.* 1976;98(25):511.
55. Valentine BA, Cooper BJ, Dietze AE, et al. Canine congenital diaphragmatic hernia. *J Vet Intern Med.* 1988;2(3):109–112.
56. White JD, Tisdall PL, Norris JM, et al. Diaphragmatic hernia in a cat mimicking a pulmonary mass. *J Feline Med Surg.* 2003;5(3):197–201.
57. Cariou M, Shihab N, Kenny P, Baines S. Surgical management of an incidentally diagnosed true pleuroperitoneal hernia in a cat. *J Fel Med Surg.* 2009;11:873–877.
58. Wolff G. Familial congenital diaphragmatic defect: review and conclusions. *Hum Genet.* 1980;54(1):1–5.
59. Klosterman E, Heng H, Freeman L, Childress M. Transdiaphragmatic extension of a retroperitoneal lipoma into the intrathoracic extrapleural space via the lumbocostal trigone in a dog. *J Am Vet Med Assoc.* 2012;240:978–982.
60. Voges AK, Bertrand S, Hill RC, et al. True diaphragmatic hernia in a cat. *Vet Radiol Ultrasound.* 1997;38(2):116–119.
61. Vignoli AM, Toniato M, Rossi F, et al. Transient port-traumatic hemidiaphragmatic paralysis in two cats. *J Small Anim Pract.* 2002;43(7):312–316.
62. Greene CE, Basinger RR, Whitfield JB. Surgical management of bilateral diaphragmatic paralysis in a dog. *J Am Vet Med Assoc.* 1988;193(12):1542–1544.
63. Mainwaring CJ. Post-traumatic contraction of the diaphragm synchronous with the heartbeat in a dog. *J Small Anim Pract.* 1988;32:329.
64. Cooper BJ, Winand NJ, Stedman H, et al. The homologue of the Duchenne locus is defective in X-linked muscular dystrophy of dogs. *Nature.* 1988;334(6178):154–156.
65. Berry CR, Gaschen FP, Ackerman H. Radiographic and ultrasonographic features of hypertrophic feline muscular dystrophy in two cats. *Vet Radiol Ultrasound.* 1992;33:357.
66. Gaschen FP, Haugh PG, Swendrowske MA. Hypertrophic feline muscular dystrophy. A unique clinical expression of dystrophin deficiency. *Feline Pract.* 1994;22(23).
67. Brumitt JW, Essman SC, Kornegay JN, et al. Radiographic features of Golden Retriever muscular dystrophy. *Vet Radiol Ultrasound.* 2006;47(6):574–580.
68. Jones BR, Brennan S, Mooney CT, et al. Muscular dystrophy with truncated dystrophin in a family of Japanese Spitz dogs. *J Neurol Sci.* 2004;217(2):143–149.

ELECTRONIC RESOURCES

Additional information related to the content in Chapter 32 can be found online at eBooks.Health.Elsevier.com.

- Chapter Quiz
- Videos

CHAPTER 33

Canine and Feline Mediastinum

Federica Morandi • Donald E. Thrall

NORMAL ANATOMY

There is one pleural sac on each side of the thoracic cavity, and the mediastinum is the space between them (Table 33.1). The pleural layer bounding the mediastinum on each side is termed *mediastinal pleura*. Other components of the pleural sac are the *costal parietal pleura*, which is attached to the thoracic wall; the *diaphragmatic parietal pleura*, which is attached to the diaphragm; and the *visceral pleura*, which covers the lung. All of these pleural layers are contiguous. The connection between the mediastinal and visceral pleural layers occurs at the hilus of the lung, where the mediastinal pleura is reflected onto the surface of the lung as visceral pleura (Figs. 33.1 and 33.2).

The mediastinum extends from the thoracic inlet to the diaphragm and is located mainly in the midsagittal plane, thereby dividing the thoracic cavity into right and left halves (see Figs. 33.1 and 33.2). The mediastinum is arbitrarily subdivided into a cranial portion, cranial to the heart; a middle portion at the level of, and containing the heart; and a caudal portion, caudal to the heart. The mediastinum is also divided into dorsal and ventral portions by a dorsal plane coursing through the tracheal bifurcation. The mediastinum is not a closed space. It communicates cranially with the fascial planes of the neck by way of the mediastinal structures passing through the thoracic inlet, such as the esophagus and trachea and some major vessels. Caudally, the mediastinum communicates with the retroperitoneal space through the aortic hiatus. These communications enable the spread of mediastinal disease to the neck and retroperitoneal space, and vice versa. The mediastinum does not normally communicate with the peritoneal cavity.

In most dogs and cats, the mediastinal pleural layers do not form an anatomic barrier between the left and right pleural spaces, because normal mediastinal pleura contain fenestrations. Thus, unilateral pleural fluid or gas is not usually contained to one side by the mediastinum. For example, 22 of 24 dogs having air injected into one pleural space quickly developed bilateral pneumothorax.[1] Pleural fluid or gas may remain unilateral if the mediastinal pleura is not fenestrated; if the normal fenestrations become closed because of inflammation or plugging, such as with purulent or neoplastic effusion; or if the pleural fluid is too viscous to pass through a normal fenestration.

Of all of the structures in the mediastinum (see Table 33.1), only the heart, trachea, caudal vena cava, aorta, and, in young animals, the thymus are visible normally. Occasionally, a portion of the normal esophagus may be seen (see Chapter 30). The other mediastinal structures are not seen normally, because they are either too small or there is insufficient interposed fat to provide contrast, leading to border effacement.

The cranial mediastinum immediately ventral to the trachea normally is of homogeneous soft tissue opacity in a lateral radiograph. The structures in this portion of the mediastinum (left subclavian artery, brachiocephalic trunk, cranial vena cava mediastinal lymph nodes) are not visible individually because they are in contact with each other and there is insufficient interposed fat to provide contrast (Fig. 33.3). In lateral radiographs, the mediastinum just ventral to the trachea is thicker and thus more radiopaque than the mediastinum just dorsal to the sternum (Fig. 33.4).

In ventrodorsal (VD) or dorsoventral (DV) thoracic radiographs, most of the cranial mediastinum is superimposed on the spine in the midsagittal plane (Fig. 33.5). In obese patients, particularly brachycephalic patients, the cranial mediastinum is increased in width because of fat accumulation, and this can be misdiagnosed as a pathologic mass (Fig. 33.6). Contrary to a mediastinal mass, the borders of the mediastinum tend to remain straight with mediastinal fat only, whereas they tend to be laterally convex in the presence of a mediastinal mass. Other imaging modalities, such as ultrasound or computed tomography (CT), may be necessary to confirm that fat deposition is the cause of increased mediastinal width in obese patients.

The mediastinum normally deviates from the midline in three locations: (1) the cranioventral mediastinal reflection, (2) the caudoventral mediastinal reflection, and (3) the vena caval mediastinal reflection (*plica venae cavae*). The first two are visible in thoracic radiographs of many dogs and cats, although not universally. The plica venae cavae is not seen radiographically in normal dogs or cats.

The cranioventral mediastinal reflection appears in VD or DV radiographs as a curving radiopaque line, just to the left of midline, extending from approximately T1 or T2 to the region of the main pulmonary artery. The concave side of the line is to the right (see Figs. 33.4 and 33.5). The cranioventral mediastinal reflection is caused by extension of the apex of the right cranial lobe across midline, pushing the mediastinum to the left (see Fig. 33.4). The thickness of the cranioventral mediastinal reflection is affected by the amount of fat it contains (see Fig. 33.6). On the lateral view, the cranioventral mediastinal reflection is often identified approximately midway between the thoracic inlet and the heart (see Fig. 33.3). The thymus lies in the cranioventral mediastinal reflection and can sometimes be identified in VD or DV radiographs of young animals as a triangular soft tissue opacity (Fig. 33.7). The normal thymus is in close contact with the cranial contour of the cardiac silhouette and may lead to a false impression of cardiomegaly when visible in a lateral projection. The internal thoracic arteries and veins are also located in the cranioventral mediastinal reflection and are not visible radiographically.

The caudoventral mediastinal reflection is seen only on VD or DV radiographs, but not in lateral views. It is created by extension of the accessory lobe of the right lung across midline to the left, thereby pushing the mediastinum to the left

Table • 33.1

Mediastinal Organs.

ORGAN	CRANIAL MEDIASTINUM	MIDDLE MEDIASTINUM	CAUDAL MEDIASTINUM
Cranial vena cava	X		
Thymus	X		
Sternal lymph nodes	X		
Aortic arch	X		
Brachiocephalic artery	X		
Left subclavian artery	X		
Mediastinal lymph nodes	X		
Trachea	X	X	
Right and left vagosympathetic trunk	X	X	
Dorsal intercostal arteries and veins	X	X	X
Internal thoracic arteries and veins	X	X	X
Esophagus	X	X	X
Thoracic duct	X	X	X
Right and left sympathetic trunks	X	X	X
Right and left phrenic nerves	X	X	X
Descending aorta		X	X
Bronchoesophageal arteries and veins		X	X
Azygos vein		X	X
Heart		X	
Tracheobronchial lymph nodes		X	
Main pulmonary artery		X	
Main pulmonary veins		X	
Principal bronchi		X	
Caudal vena cava			X
Right and left vagus nerves			X

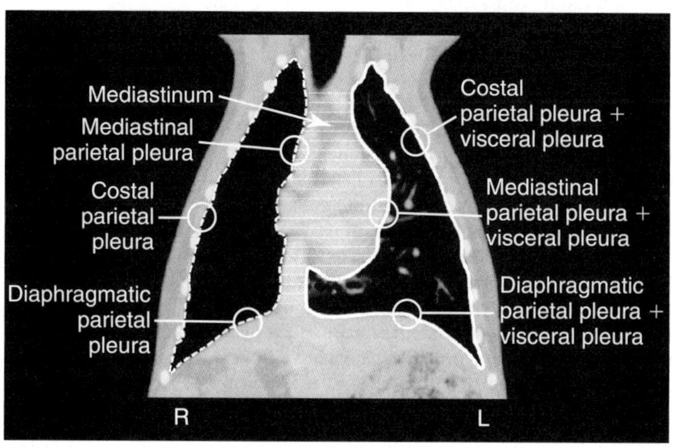

Fig. 33.1 Dorsal plane computed tomography (CT) image of a canine thorax at the level of the base of the heart. The right lung and thus the visceral component of the right pleural sac have been photographically removed from the image. Thus, the *dotted line* in the right hemithorax represents the parietal portion of the right pleural sac. The designation of mediastinal versus costal versus diaphragmatic parietal pleura is based on the location of the pleural layer, and these pleural layers are contiguous. The left lung has not been photographically removed from the image. As the left lung is covered in visceral pleura, the *solid line* designates contact between the visceral and parietal pleural layers of the left pleural sac. The pleural space is the potential space between the parietal and visceral pleural layers. Under normal circumstances the parietal and visceral pleural layers are in contact and the pleural space is only a potential space. The mediastinum, shown here with *horizontal white lines*, is a real space and is located between the two pleural sacs. *L*, Left; *R*, right.

(see Fig. 33.2). The caudoventral mediastinal reflection consists of four pleural layers, which are, from right to left: (1) the visceral pleura of the accessory lobe, (2) the mediastinal parietal pleura of the right pleural sac, (3) the mediastinal parietal pleura of the left pleural sac, and (4) the visceral pleura of the left caudal lobe (see Fig. 33.2). The caudoventral mediastinal reflection appears as a relatively straight radiopaque line in the caudal left hemithorax, extending from the region of the cardiac apex in a caudolateral direction toward the gastric fundus (Fig. 33.8). The caudoventral mediastinal reflection has been incorrectly termed the *phrenicopericardial ligament* (also called the *cardiophrenic* or *sternopericardiac ligament*); however, this ligament, which is a continuation of the apex of the fibrous pericardium and is contained within the caudoventral mediastinum, is not visible radiographically as an individual structure.[2] As for the cranioventral mediastinal reflection, the thickness of the caudoventral mediastinal reflection depends on the amount of fat it contains (Fig. 33.9).

PATHOLOGIC MEDIASTINAL CONDITIONS

Mediastinal abnormalities can be divided into three general classifications: (1) mediastinal shift, (2) mediastinal mass(es), and (3) pneumomediastinum.

Mediastinal Shift

The most common causes of an ipsilateral mediastinal shift are lung atelectasis caused by reduced ventilation or prolonged lateral recumbency. Therefore, mediastinal shift is often seen in

Table • 33.2

Causes of Mediastinal Masses.

CAUSE OF MASS	MEDIASTINAL LOCATION
Vascular ring anomaly (segmental cranial esophagomegaly)	Craniodorsal*
Neurogenic tumor	Craniodorsal or dorsal
Hematoma	Variable, but may have a craniodorsal predilection
Mediastinal lymphadenopathy	Cranioventral
Sternal lymphadenopathy	Cranioventral
Thymoma	Cranioventral
Mediastinal cyst (branchial cyst)	Cranioventral
Ectopic thyroid or parathyroid tumor	Cranioventral, perihilar
Mediastinal abscess—usually caused by esophageal perforation	Cranioventral, caudoventral, caudal, dorsal
Hilar lymphadenopathy	Middle
Heart base mass†	Middle, cranioventral to tracheal bifurcation
Mid-esophageal foreign body	Middle, dorsal to tracheal bifurcation
Paraspinal tumor	Dorsal
Generalized megaesophagus	Dorsal
Spirocerca lupi	Caudodorsal
Caudal esophageal mass or foreign body	Caudodorsal
Mediastinal diaphragmatic hernia	Caudoventral
Hiatal hernia	Caudal to caudodorsal
Diaphragmatic eventration	Caudal, caudoventral, caudodorsal

*Marked segmental esophagomegaly may lead to a cranioventral mediastinal mass as the enlarged esophagus gravitates ventral to the trachea.
†Heart base mass as used here is nonspecific and could apply to a tumor of the base of the heart, a right atrial tumor, or enlargement of the main pulmonary artery.

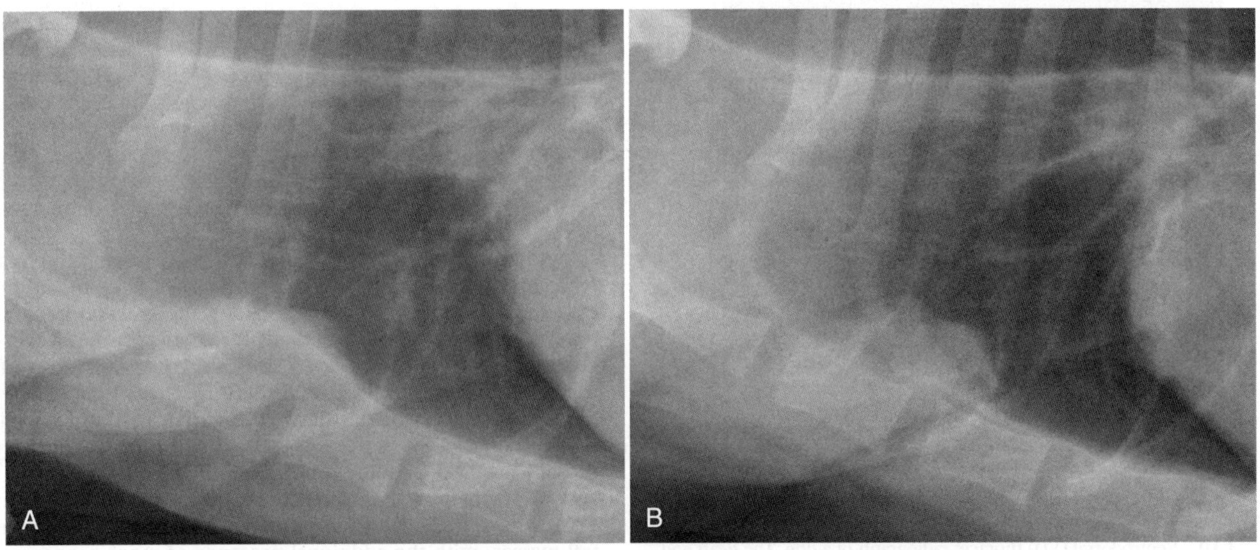

Fig. 33.12 Left **(A)** and right **(B)** lateral radiographs of a dog with mild enlargement of the sternal lymph node. The enlarged lymph node appears as a small mass dorsal to the second and third sternebra. Finding a slightly different size and shape of an enlarged sternal lymph in left versus right lateral views is common. Note the typical broad base of contact of the ventral margin of the sternal lymph node with the thoracic wall.

lymph nodes also receive efferent lymphatics from the intercostal, sternal, middle, and caudal deep cervical, tracheobronchial, and pulmonary lymph nodes.[3] The cranial mediastinal lymph nodes do not enlarge secondary to abdominal disorders.

The thymus is another common source of a cranioventral mediastinal mass. As previously noted, the normal thymus can be seen in young dogs as a triangular or sail-like opacity in the cranioventral mediastinal reflection in VD or DV views (see Fig. 33.7). The thymus undergoes involution as animals age, and should be radiographically inconspicuous in most dogs by approximately 1 year of age. Rebound thymic hyperplasia, in which the thymus atrophies during illness, and undergrows excessive regrowth in the recovery phase, results in thymic enlargement with normal shape, and has been occasionally

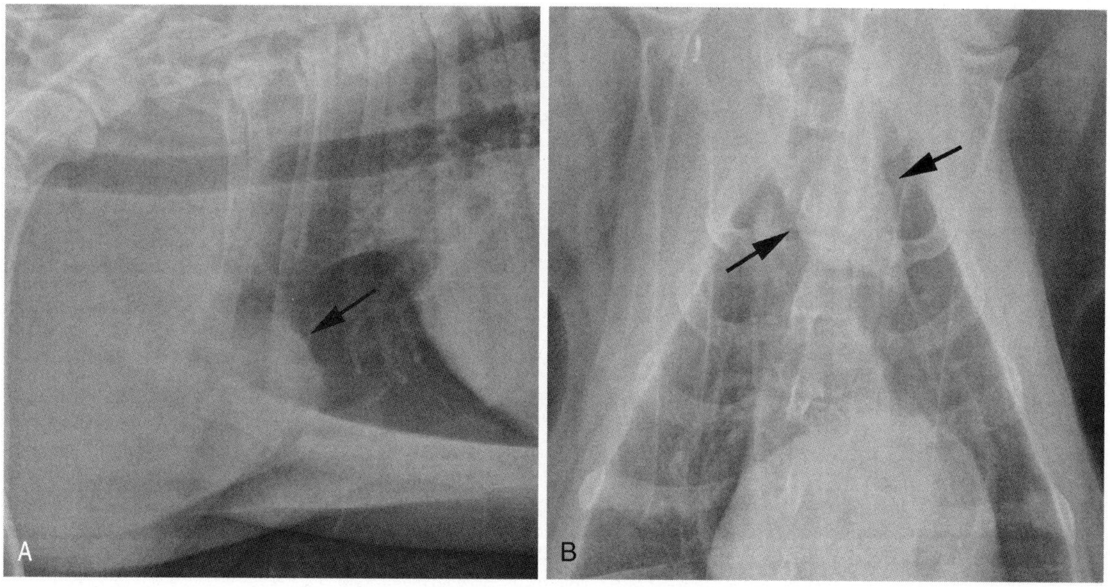

Fig. 33.13 Lateral **(A)** and ventrodorsal (VD; **B**) radiographs of the thorax of a dog with enlargement of the sternal lymph node. There is a soft tissue mass dorsal to the cranial aspect of the sternum in **A** (*black arrow*) and widening of the cranial mediastinum in **B** (*black arrows*). The diagnosis was histiocytic sarcoma. Note the broad ventral base of contact of the enlarged sternal lymph node with the thoracic wall in the lateral view.

described in animals.[8] A thymoma can reach enormous proportions in the cranioventral mediastinum and then extend caudolaterally, adjacent to the heart, as in Fig. 33.17 and eFig. 33.4.

Occasionally, cranioventral pulmonary masses located near midline can be difficult to differentiate from cranial mediastinal masses; in such cases, CT is needed to determine the exact origin of the mass.

Dorsal Mediastinal Masses

Dorsal mediastinal masses, whether in the cranial, middle, or caudal aspect of the mediastinum, cause widening of the mediastinum in the VD or DV view (Figs. 33.18 and 33.19). The caudal mediastinum can be evaluated more thoroughly in a VD view, compared with a DV view, because cranial excursion of the diaphragm in the DV view leads to compression of the caudal mediastinum.[9,10]

The most common cause of a dorsal mediastinal mass is enlargement of the esophagus, which can be generalized or segmental. Enlargement of the cranial aspect of the thoracic esophagus, such as from a vascular ring anomaly, typically causes a craniodorsal mediastinal mass with ventral displacement of the trachea in the lateral view, and widening of the cranial mediastinum in the VD or DV view. The presence of esophageal gas (see Fig. 33.18), or a heterogeneous opacity created by esophageal contents, differentiates esophageal enlargement from other dorsal mediastinal masses. If a dorsal mediastinal mass is homogeneous, it is usually impossible to determine the origin of the mass from survey radiographs alone (Fig. 33.20).

The presence of regurgitation is not necessarily helpful in establishing the origin of a dorsal mediastinal mass as esophagus, because any mass in this location can compress the esophagus and lead to regurgitation. Radiographic signs of esophageal enlargement are discussed more completely in Chapter 30. If the esophagus is suspected as the origin of a dorsal mediastinal mass, an esophagram can be helpful for positive identification.

Craniodorsal Mediastinal Masses

Craniodorsal mediastinal masses are rare (see Table 33.1). A craniodorsal mediastinal mass typically causes ventral and rightward displacement of the trachea (see Fig. 33.19).

Hilar-Region Mediastinal Masses

The main causes of a mediastinal mass in the hilar region are enlargement of the tracheobronchial lymph nodes or a mass arising from the base of the heart (see Table 33.2).

The tracheobronchial lymphocenter is subdivided into the right, left, and middle tracheobronchial lymph nodes. The right and left lymph nodes lie on the lateral side of their respective bronchus and are also in contact with the trachea. The right lymph node is ventral to the azygos vein, and the left lymph node is ventral to the aorta. The middle tracheobronchial lymph node is the largest of the group, and it has the form of a V with the point lying in the angle formed by the tracheal bifurcation. Afferent lymphatics to the tracheobronchial lymph nodes come primarily from the lungs and bronchi, but they also come from the thoracic parts of the aorta, esophagus, trachea, heart, mediastinum, and diaphragm.[3]

Enlargement of the tracheobronchial lymph nodes classically results in a soft tissue mass located dorsocaudal to the tracheal bifurcation on the lateral view, which usually causes cranioventral displacement of a principal bronchus or tracheal bifurcation. If the enlarged lymph nodes reside primarily ventral to the tracheal bifurcation, dorsal displacement of the bifurcation will result instead, which can be confused with left atrial dilation; however, this is very uncommon. Both tracheobronchial lymph node enlargement and left atrial dilation can cause lateral divergence or splaying of the principal bronchi on the VD or DV view (Fig. 33.21); therefore, a lateral view is required to differentiate lymphadenopathy from left atrial enlargement. The extent of the hilar mass effect and degree of splaying of the principal bronchi depend on the magnitude of enlargement of the tracheobronchial lymph nodes, or the extent of left atrial dilation. With mild tracheobronchial lymph node enlargement, displacement of a principal bronchus in a

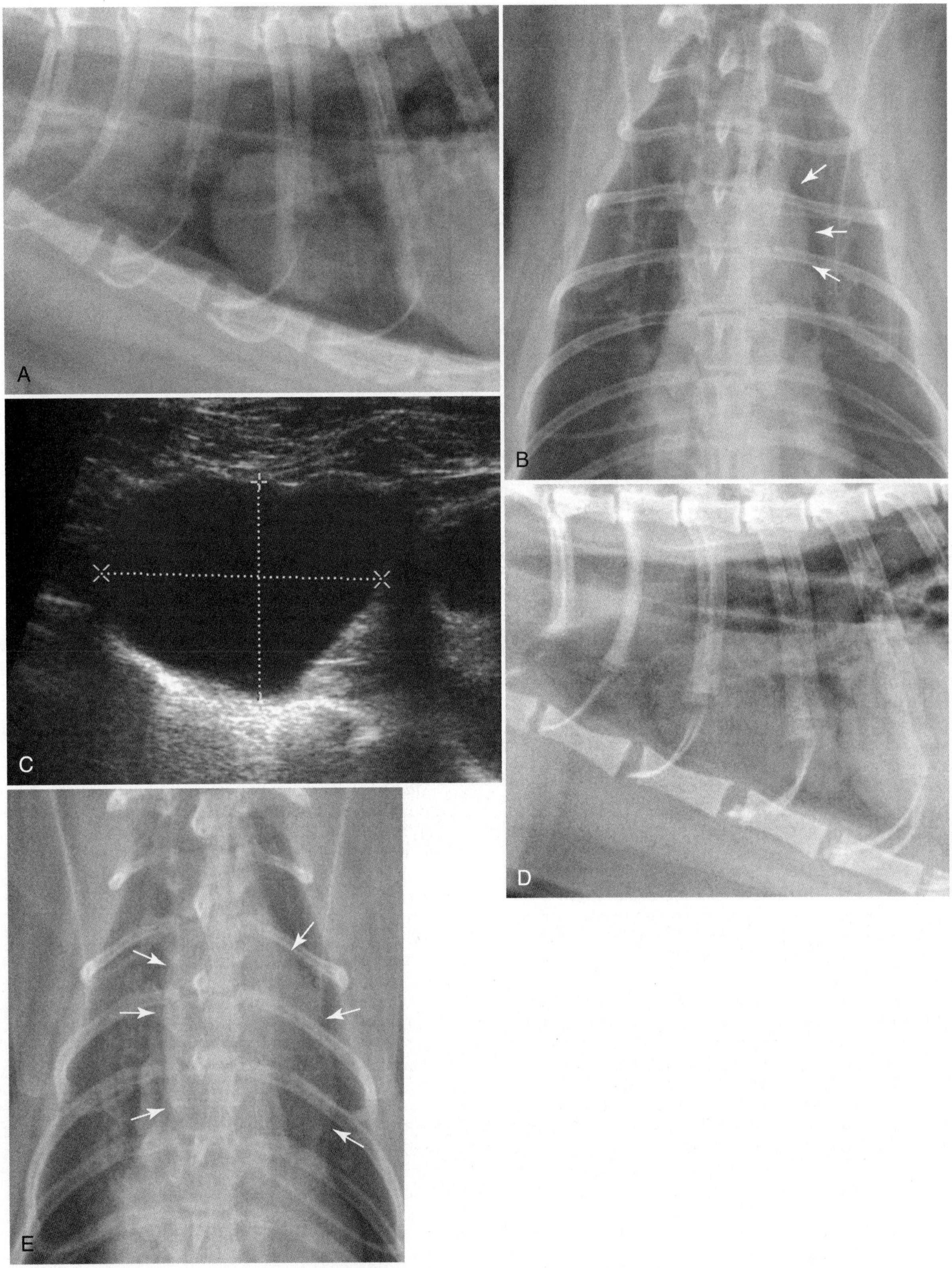

Fig. 33.14 Left lateral **(A)** and ventrodorsal (VD; **B**) thoracic radiographs of a cat. There is a well-defined mass in the cranioventral aspect of the mediastinum. The mass is very conspicuous in the lateral view and causes an ill-defined left mass effect in the VD view (*white arrows*). This cat has mild pneumomediastinum secondary to a tracheal puncture that occurred during blood draw from the jugular vein, and this may have increased the conspicuity of the mass slightly. The mass is more caudal than expected for a cranial mediastinal lymph node or a sternal lymph node and does not have the broad base of ventral contact with the sternum that is typical of sternal lymph node enlargement. Ultrasound imaging **(C)** allows identification of the hypoechoic cystic contents and establishes the diagnosis of mediastinal cyst. The *dotted lines* in **C** are the electronic calipers of the ultrasound machine being used to obtain measurements of the mass, which in this cat were 1.8 cm cranial/caudal and 2.5 cm dorsal/ventral. The cyst in this cat was not drained or removed; and in left lateral **(D)** and VD **(E)** radiographs made 18 months later, the cyst has enlarged (*white arrows*). This cyst is not large enough to require excision but should be monitored subsequently to avoid complications resulting from enlargement and organ compression.

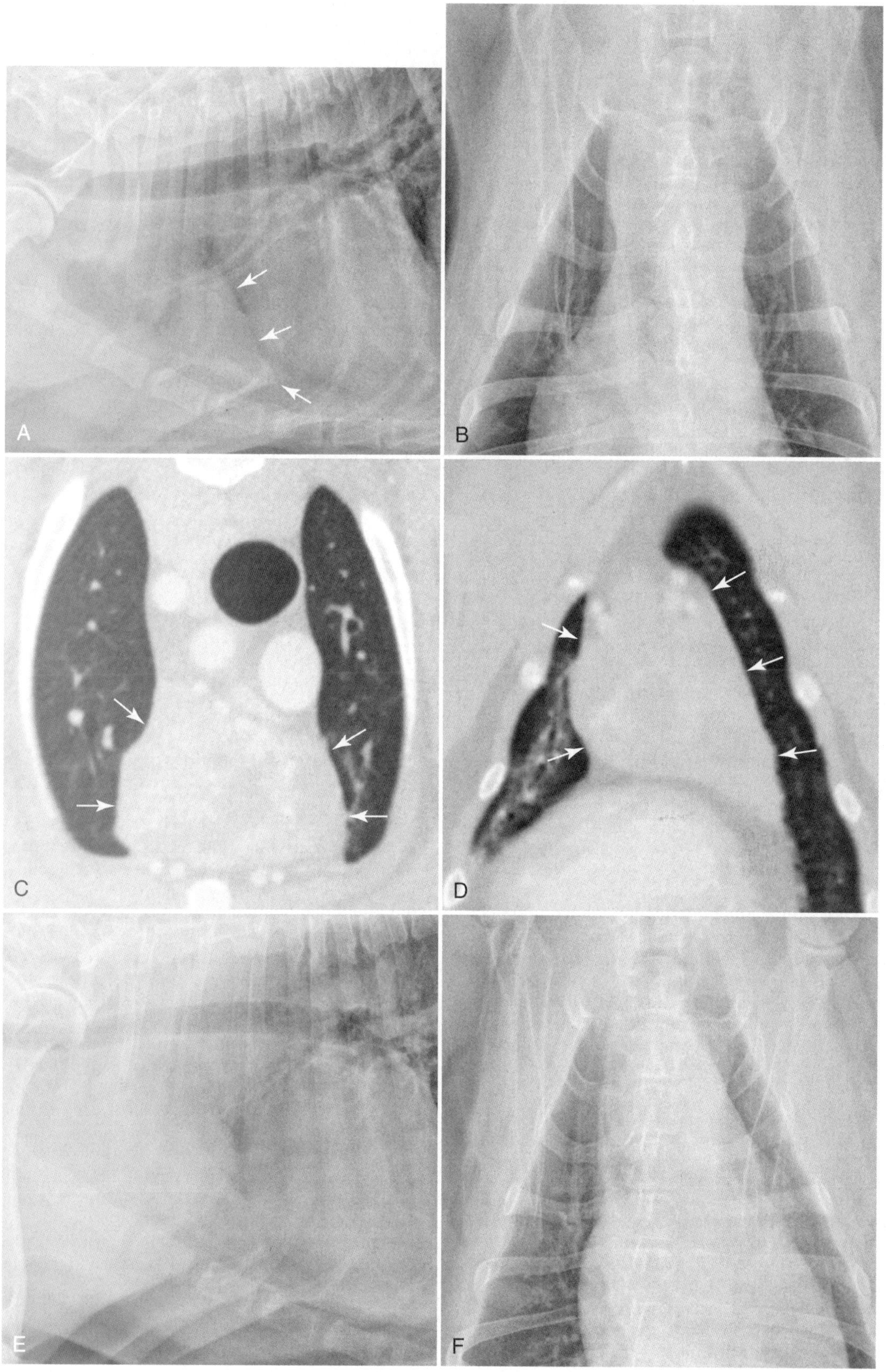

Fig. 33.15 Right lateral **(A)** and ventrodorsal (VD; **B**) radiographs of a dog with a mass in the cranioventral mediastinum. In **A**, the cranioventral mediastinum has overall increased opacity, and the edge of a mass is visible caudoventrally (*white arrows*), contrasted by lung. In **B**, the cranial mediastinum is wide. The trachea is not displaced in either **A** or **B**. This patient was not obese, and mediastinal fat would therefore not be a likely cause for this appearance. Transverse **(C)** and dorsal **(D)** contrast-enhanced computed tomography (CT) images of the thorax were acquired a few days after the images in **A** and **B**. The mass is clearly visible in the ventral aspect of the cranial mediastinum (*white arrows*). Right lateral **(E)** and VD **(F)** radiographs acquired 4 months after those in **A** and **B**. The mass is larger and more obvious, displacing the trachea dorsally and to the right. The mass was removed completely by transsternal thoracotomy, and the histologic diagnosis was thymoma.

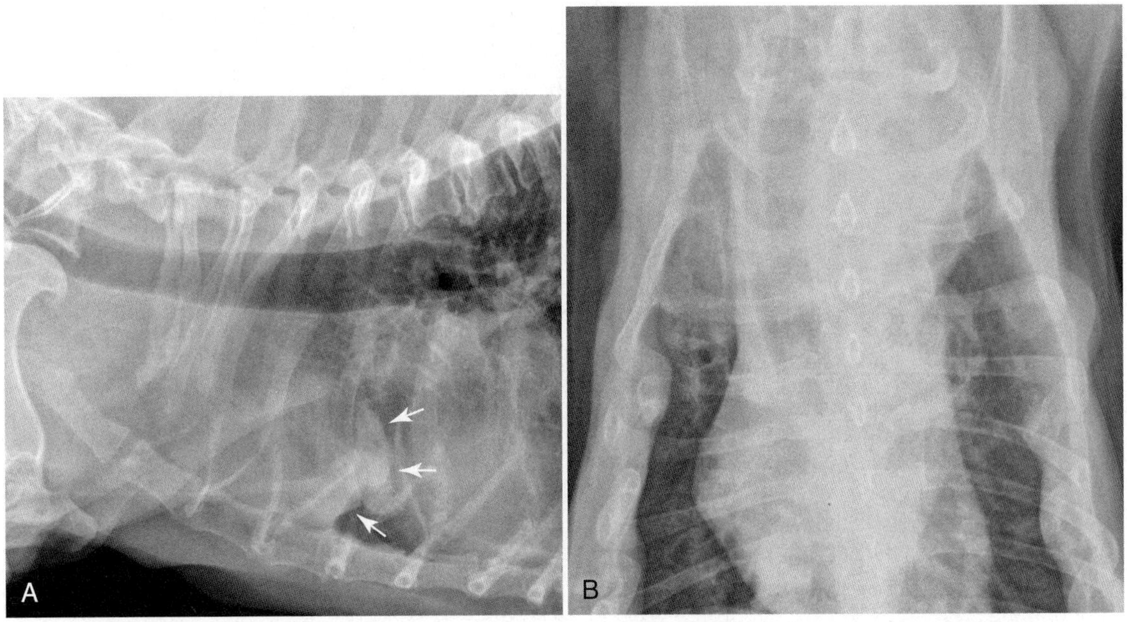

Fig. 33.16 Lateral (**A**) and ventrodorsal (VD; **B**) thoracic radiographs of a Basset hound with a moderately sized mediastinal mass. **A,** The mediastinum ventral to the trachea has increased opacity, and the edge of a mass is visible caudally (*white arrows*), contrasted by lung. The mass has caused mild dorsal displacement of the trachea, which is now parallel to the vertebrae. The mass also causes border effacement of the cranial aspect of the cardiac silhouette. **B,** The cranial mediastinum is wide, and there is border effacement of the cranial margin of the heart. The trachea is displaced slightly to the right. This patient is not obese; thus excessive mediastinal fat is an unlikely cause of this radiographic appearance, and a cranioventral mediastinal mass is the most likely diagnosis. Considerations for this mass are cranial mediastinal lymph node, thymus, and branchial cyst. Sonography or computed tomography (CT) could provide more information about the character of the mass, but an aspirate may be needed for definitive diagnosis.

cranioventral direction in the lateral view may be the most conspicuous abnormality (Fig. 33.22). With progressive enlargement of the tracheobronchial lymph nodes, the mass effect becomes more pronounced and splaying of principal bronchi becomes evident in the VD or DV view (Fig. 33.23, eFig. 33.5).

Masses arising from the base of the heart tend to be relatively inconspicuous since much of the mass is surrounded by other soft tissue structures, resulting in border effacement. These lesions usually create an ill-defined mass effect, rather than a distinct mass, and may become very large before being detectable on survey radiographs. Heart base region masses typically cause rightward displacement of the trachea just cranial to the bifurcation, which may be the most conspicuous finding (Fig. 33.24, eFig. 33.6). As the heart base mass enlarges, the tracheal displacement becomes more pronounced, but the mass itself is still not likely to be seen (Fig. 33.25). A heart base mass may represent a heart base tumor, a right atrial tumor, a tumor arising from ectopic thyroid tissue, or an enlarged main pulmonary artery.

Caudoventral Mediastinal Masses

Caudoventral mediastinal masses are uncommon, and most are associated with the diaphragm, such as a diaphragmatic eventration, or a hernia (see Table 33.1; Fig. 33.26). Caval foramen hernia may also cause a caudoventral mediastinal mass effect. Caudoventral mediastinal masses may cause border effacement of the diaphragm and/or cardiac displacement. In VD or DV views, caudoventral mediastinal masses are often located to the left of midline because of the normal left-sided location of the caudoventral mediastinal reflection (see Fig. 33.26).

As the accessory lung lobe is located on midline, a mass arising from the accessory lobe can appear identical to a caudoventral mediastinal mass[11] (Fig. 33.27). Large accessory lobe masses will cause border effacement of the caudal vena cava, because the accessory lobe surrounds this structure (see Fig. 33.27). However, border effacement of the caudal vena cava can occur with any large caudoventral mediastinal mass; therefore, this sign cannot be used to differentiate accessory lobe masses from caudoventral mediastinal masses. Visibility of the caudal vena cava may be preserved with small caudoventral mediastinal masses, even if of accessory lobe origin (see Fig. 33.26). CT is usually needed to differentiate caudoventral mediastinal masses from accessory lobe masses.

Caudodorsal Mediastinal Masses

The mediastinal serous cavity is a normal, mesothelium-lined anatomic space in the caudodorsal mediastinum. It is located to the right of the esophagus and extends from the diaphragm to the heart base. Purulent material can accumulate in this cavity forming paraesophageal empyema, possibly due to foreign material migration or extension of infectious disease from the adjacent accessory lung lobe (Fig. 33.28).[12] Mediastinal serous cavity mesothelioma has also been reported in dogs.[13] Esophageal foreign bodies can have the appearance of a caudodorsal mediastinal mass but are typically associated with a degree of esophageal gas dilation cranial to the foreign material (see Fig. 33.20).

Some Facts About Mediastinal Lymph Nodes

The drainage patterns of mediastinal lymph nodes were defined in the section dealing with mediastinal masses. Mediastinal lymph node enlargement can be associated with a variety of diseases, but the most common causes are primary lymphoid neoplasia and mycotic infection. Spread of peritoneal disease to the sternal lymph node was discussed earlier.

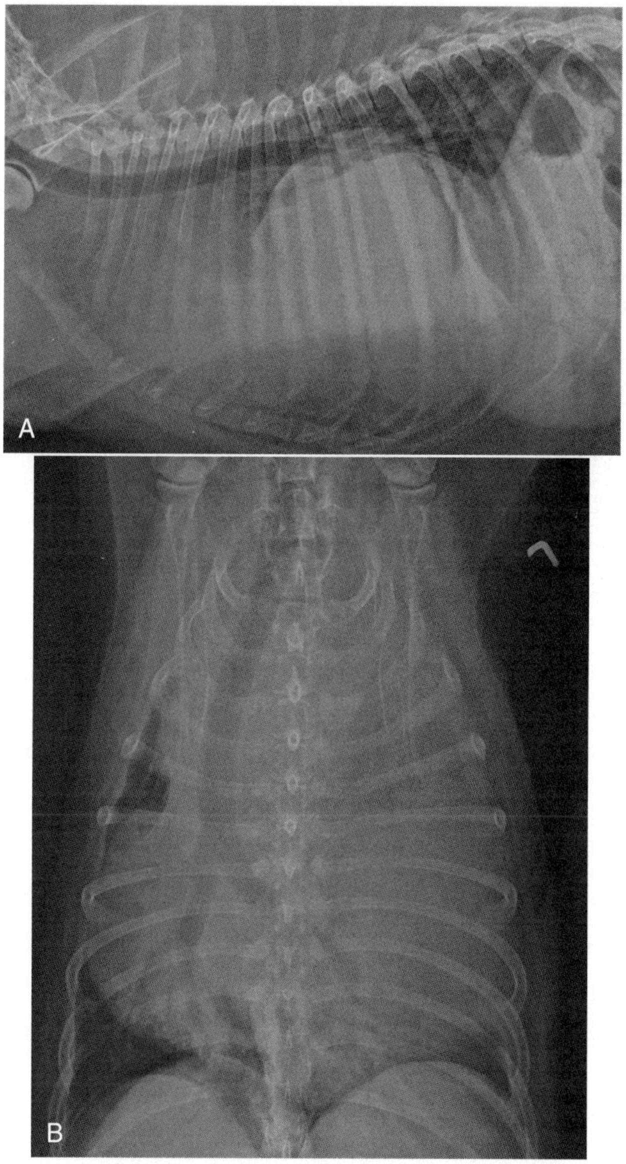

Fig. 33.17 Right lateral (**A**) and ventrodorsal (VD; **B**) radiographs of a dog with a massive, lobular mass arising from the left cranioventral mediastinum. The trachea is severely displaced dorsally and to the right, and the heart is displaced caudodorsally and to the right. There is marked border effacement of the cardiac silhouette in both **A** and **B**. In **B**, the mass extends caudally along the left margin of the heart, and contacts the diaphragm. This dog presented with minor exercise intolerance and muffled left-sided heart sounds; the paucity of clinical signs coupled with the extremely large mass is most consistent with a slow-growing thymoma.

In the cat, lymphoma is a common cause of enlargement of the cranial mediastinal lymph nodes. The thymus may also be affected. In the dog, lymphoma results in enlargement of the sternal lymph nodes in slightly over half of affected patients, but enlargement of cranial mediastinal or tracheobronchial lymph nodes is uncommon.[14] Other reticuloendothelial malignancies, such as pulmonary lymphomatoid granulomatosis[15,16] and disseminated histiocytic sarcoma,[17] are also characterized by a high frequency of lymph node enlargement, particularly the tracheobronchial lymph nodes. In pulmonary lymphomatoid granulomatosis and disseminated histiocytic sarcoma, there is usually accompanying pulmonary parenchymal disease, and isolated mediastinal lymph node enlargement is unusual. Pulmonary mycoses, especially blastomycosis and coccidioidomycosis, are associated with a high prevalence of mediastinal lymph node enlargement. Interestingly, there are a variety of diseases that one might expect to result in mediastinal lymph node enlargement but rarely do, at least to the extent that the enlarged lymph nodes are visible radiographically (Box 33.1).

Distinguishing a Mediastinal Mass From a Lung Mass

Radiographic differentiation of a lung mass from a mediastinal mass is not always possible. Many lung masses can be distinguished from mediastinal masses, because the lung mass is lateral to the mediastinum, surrounded by air-filled lung, and is therefore more sharply marginated (Fig. 33.29). Some mediastinal masses, however, may protrude laterally (Fig. 33.30), or be in a thin portion of the mediastinum (Fig. 33.31) and be surrounded by air making them sharply margined and easily mistaken for a lung mass. In addition, lung masses located in the more medial part of the lung can contact the margin of the mediastinum, particularly in the cranioventral thorax, and not be completely surrounded by gas. For these reasons, definitive localization of many intrathoracic masses is not always possible based on radiographs alone. If thoracotomy is being considered, and the location of the mass is not obvious from radiographs, a presurgical CT scan can assist in determining the origin, location, and extent of the mass and can guide the surgical approach (e.g., intercostal vs. median thoracotomy).

Confounding Effects of Pleural and Mediastinal Fluid

As previously noted, cranial mediastinal masses often cause elevation of the trachea. Elevation of the trachea may also result from a large amount of pleural fluid that results in lung displacement from buoyancy (Fig. 33.32).[18] A small volume of pleural fluid does not result in tracheal elevation unless a mediastinal mass is also present. If pleural fluid is present, definitive radiographic identification of a concurrent mediastinal mass is usually not possible. However, if the mass is large enough to compress the trachea and/or displace the tracheal bifurcation caudally, the presence of a mass can be inferred.

Mediastinal fluid can be difficult to differentiate from pleural effusion that has accumulated in the cranial thorax along the mediastinum. Mediastinal effusion is most commonly caused by hemorrhage, either secondary to trauma with rupture of thymic vessels in young dogs, or secondary to coagulopathies such as rodenticide toxicity.

If pleural fluid obscures the mediastinum, and a mediastinal mass is suspected, various interventions can be used. The easiest and often the most successful is to remove the pleural fluid and repeat the radiographs. Positioning the patient upright and using a horizontally directed x-ray beam to take advantage of gravity, which causes pleural fluid to move away from the area of the suspected mediastinal mass, is often not successful or informative. If available, ultrasound or CT can be used to evaluate for a mass in the mediastinum.[19,20] Pleural fluid provides an excellent acoustic window for sonographic examination, and ultrasound-guided aspiration or biopsy aid in achieving a definitive diagnosis.

Pneumomediastinum

Pneumomediastinum denotes free gas in the mediastinum. The radiographic findings of pneumomediastinum depend on the volume of gas present. Regardless of the amount of gas present, pneumomediastinum is rarely visible in VD or DV views because the overall size of the mediastinum is not increased, and the mediastinal gas is superimposed on the midline and obscured by other structures. Lateral views are typically the most useful for detecting pneumomediastinum. With a large volume of mediastinal gas, organs and structures not normally seen (such as the esophagus, brachiocephalic trunk, and left subclavian artery) become visible because of the contrast

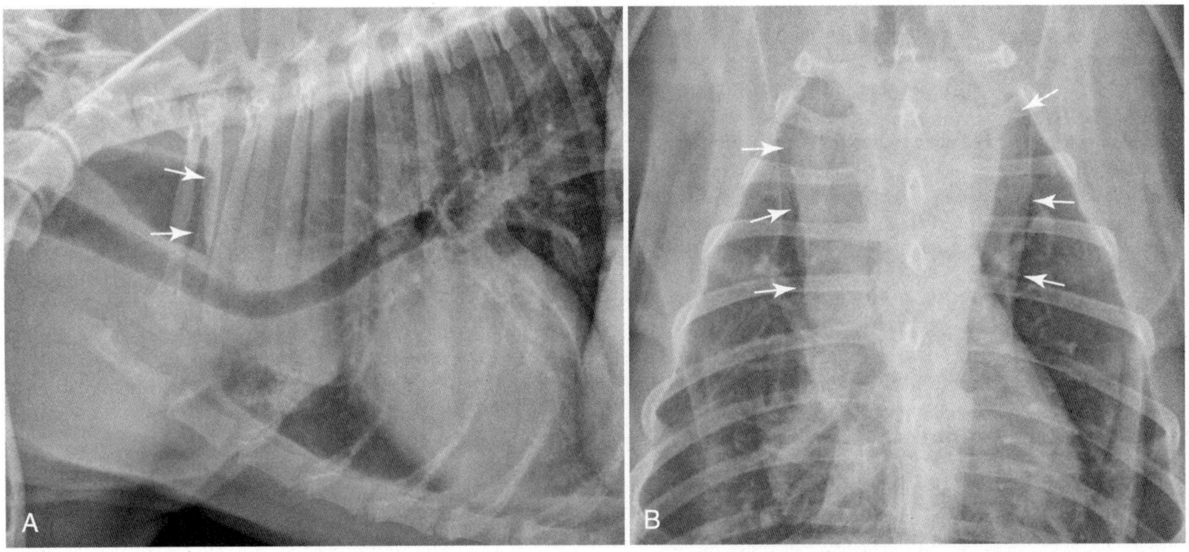

Fig. 33.18 Lateral **(A)** and dorsoventral (DV; **B**) radiographs of a dog with a craniodorsal mediastinal mass caused by a vascular ring anomaly leading to segmental megaesophagus. The enlarged esophagus displaces the trachea ventrally. In **A,** an interface between esophageal contents and gas trapped in the cranial esophagus (*white arrows*) lends support to the mass being of esophageal origin. In **B,** the mass causes widening of the cranial mediastinum (*white arrows*) as expected. From the DV view, the mass cannot be diagnosed as esophagus or localized to the dorsal versus ventral aspects of the mediastinum.

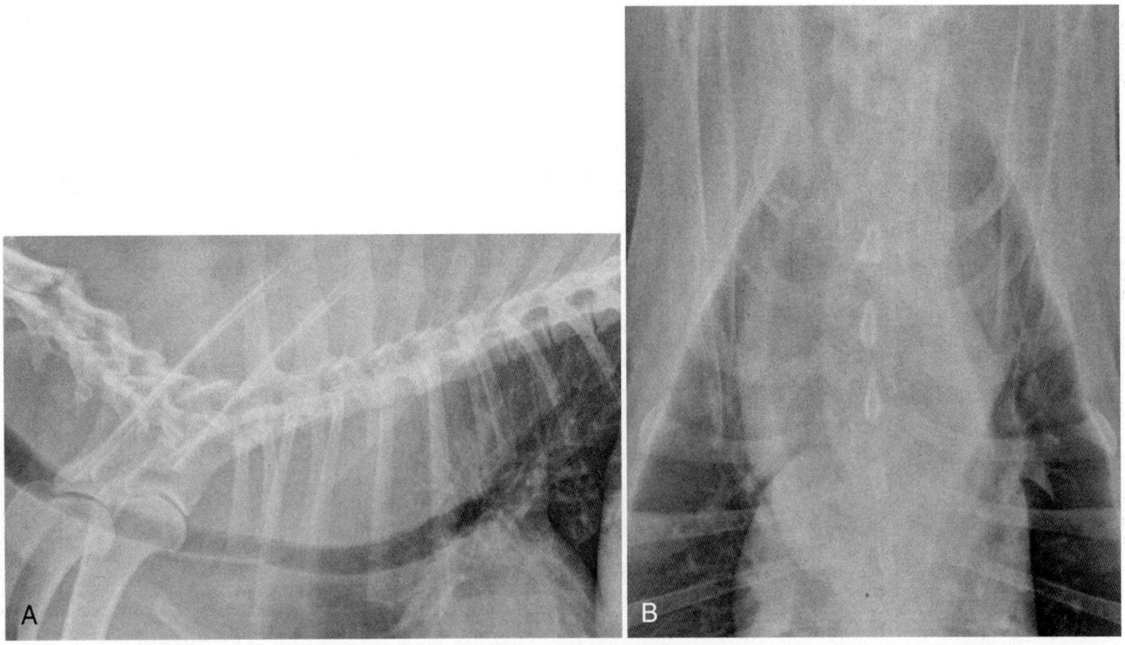

Fig. 33.19 Lateral **(A)** and ventrodorsal (VD; **B**) thoracic radiographs of a dog with a craniodorsal mediastinal abscess. In **A,** there is a homogeneously opaque mass in the craniodorsal aspect of the mediastinum that displaces the trachea ventrally. The mass extends into the cervical region, dorsal to the trachea. In **B,** the cranial mediastinum is wider than normal, and the trachea is displaced to the right. The origin of this mass cannot be determined from these radiographs; esophageal origin cannot be ruled out.

afforded by the adjacent gas (Fig. 33.33, eFig. 33.7). With smaller amounts of mediastinal gas, the changes are less dramatic; for example, the only abnormality may be visualization of the adventitial surface of the trachea (Fig. 33.34A), or a heterogeneous appearance to the cranioventral mediastinum due to gas pocketing (see Fig. 33.34B). If there are large amounts of subcutaneous gas in addition to pneumomediastinum, the superimposed subcutaneous gas creates a very heterogeneous opacity in lateral views, which can lead to overestimation of the volume of gas present in the mediastinum, or even a misdiagnosis of pneumomediastinum (Fig. 33.35).

Pneumomediastinum may progress to pneumothorax if mediastinal gas dissects through the mediastinal pleura into the pleural space. Conversely, pneumothorax does not progress to pneumomediastinum. Dyspnea is usually not seen with pneumomediastinum, unless it results in pneumothorax.

Because of the communication of the mediastinum with the neck and retroperitoneal space, pneumomediastinum may result in subcutaneous emphysema and/or pneumoretroperitoneum (Fig. 33.36, eFig. 33.8). Alternatively, gas in the retroperitoneal space or fascial planes of the neck may diffuse into the mediastinum.

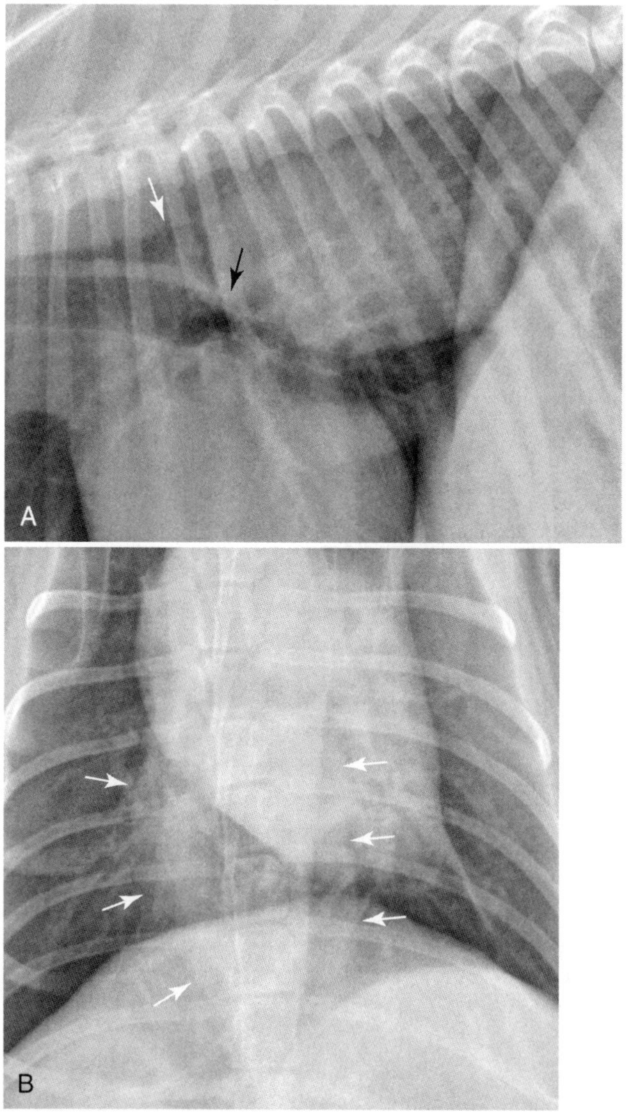

Fig. 33.20 Lateral (**A**) and ventrodorsal (VD; **B**) thoracic radiographs of a dog with a caudal esophageal foreign body. The foreign body is homogeneous and causes a caudodorsal mediastinal mass that in **A** displaces the tracheal bifurcation slightly in a cranioventral direction (*black arrow*). There is also a focal gas collection in the esophagus cranial to the mass (*white arrow* in **A**). In **B**, the mass has caused widening of the caudal mediastinum (*white arrows*). It is not possible to determine from these radiographs whether the mass is esophageal in origin. The small esophageal gas collection could be secondary to extrinsic compression of the esophagus by a soft tissue mass of another origin.

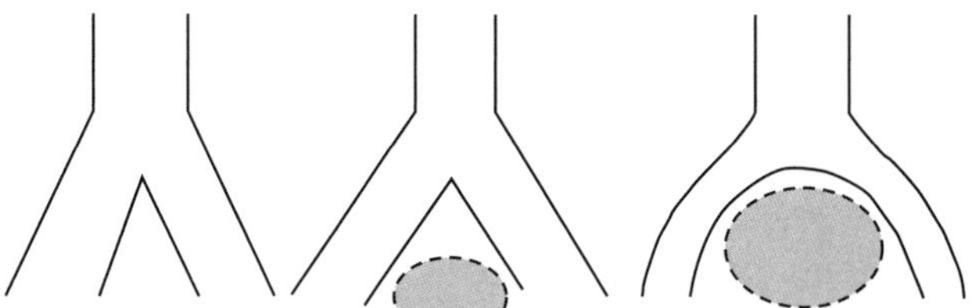

Fig. 33.21 The shape of the principal bronchi in a ventrodorsal (VD) radiograph in the normal state (*left*) and when a mass is present between them (*middle* and *right*). An enlarged left atrium or tracheobronchial lymph node between the principal bronchi may result in the principal bronchi being displaced laterally (*middle*) or, more commonly, assuming a curved appearance (*right*).

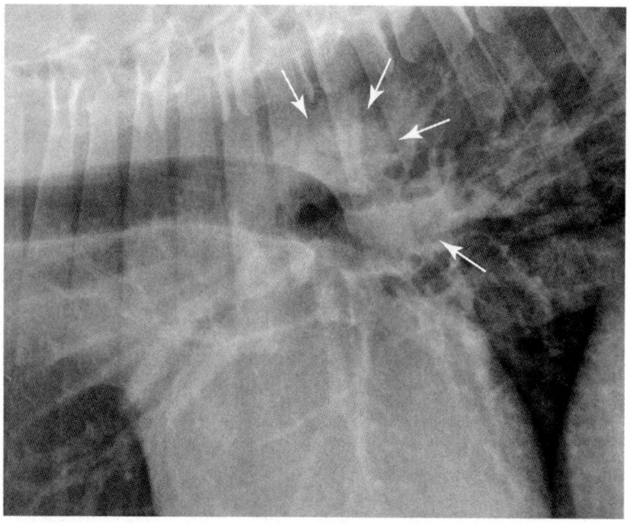

Fig. 33.22 Right lateral radiograph of a dog with mild enlargement of the tracheobronchial lymph nodes. There is a small mass effect caudodorsal to the tracheal bifurcation (*white arrows*) that has caused cranioventral displacement of the bifurcation. Splaying of the principal bronchi was not evident in the ventrodorsal (VD) view.

Pneumomediastinum can result from a variety of causes. It is common for air to escape into the pulmonary interstitium from sites of intrapulmonary alveolar rupture that do not involve the visceral pleural surface of the lung. These intrapulmonary ruptures can be microscopic, with air leaking into the mediastinum and tracking in a retrograde direction in the loose connective tissue adjacent to bronchi and vessels into the mediastinum.[21,22] This phenomenon, called the *Macklin effect*, is a relatively frequent occurrence following blunt thoracic trauma,[23,24] such as a motor vehicle accident, and also after iatrogenic pulmonary hyperinflation during anesthesia or resuscitation.[25] Pneumothorax is not present when pneumomediastinum results from the Macklin effect, unless the visceral pleura becomes torn, or the mediastinal air accumulation extends to the pleural space.

Another common cause of pneumomediastinum is dissection of gas from the fascial planes of the neck into the mediastinum. Gas in the neck commonly results from neck trauma, such as a bite wound. Intrafascial cervical gas can also result from a tracheal perforation. In cats, the trachea can easily be perforated inadvertently during jugular venipuncture, and this can lead to air leaks and pneumomediastinum, as gas tracks down the neck. If a tracheal tear is intrathoracic, air enters the mediastinum directly. Tracheal rupture in anesthetized cats associated with overdistention of the endotracheal tube cuff is a noteworthy cause of pneumomediastinum.[26,27] Cuff overdistention may cause rupture of the trachealis muscle at the point of attachment to the tracheal cartilages. Tracheal rupture may occur at a modest cuff volume and may not be immediately apparent to the anesthetist. Development of subcutaneous emphysema occurs quickly following tracheal rupture from cuff over distention, and the amount of subcutaneous gas is usually pronounced. If subcutaneous emphysema develops during a surgical procedure, the anesthetist must be aware of this potentially fatal complication.

Other less common causes of pneumomediastinum are esophageal perforation as a result of trauma, foreign body, neoplasia, inflammation, or malposition of a feeding tube[28]; extension of retroperitoneal gas into the mediastinum; and presence of gas-producing organism in the mediastinum.

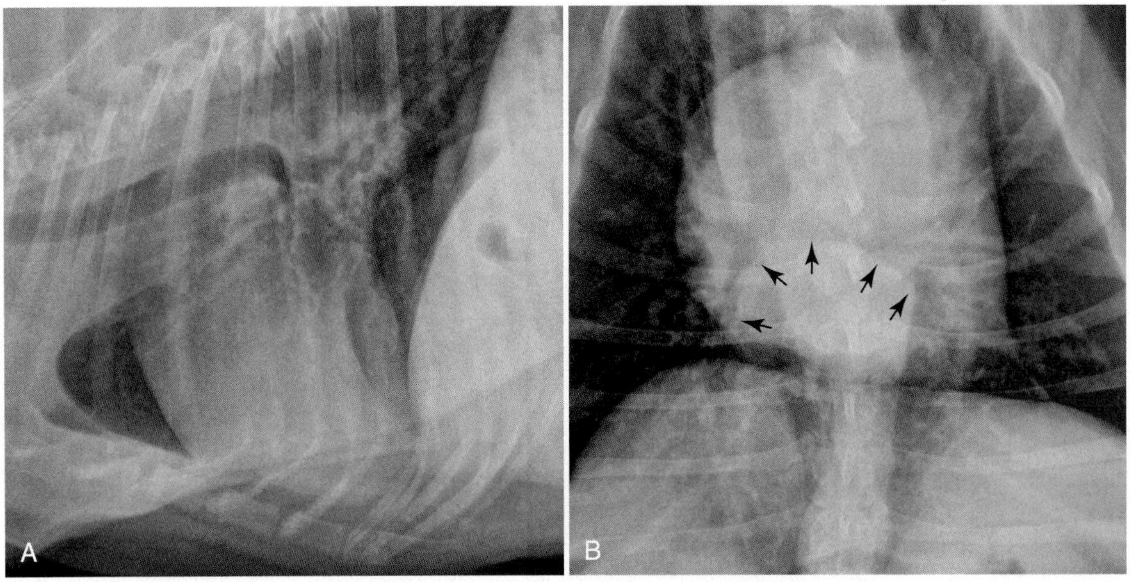

Fig. 33.23 Right lateral (**A**) and ventrodorsal (VD; **B**) radiographs of a dog with pronounced enlargement of the tracheobronchial lymph nodes. In **A**, there is a mass caudodorsal to the tracheal bifurcation that has displaced the bifurcation cranioventrally. In **B**, there is splaying of the principal bronchi (*black arrows*) because of the interposed enlarged tracheobronchial lymph nodes.

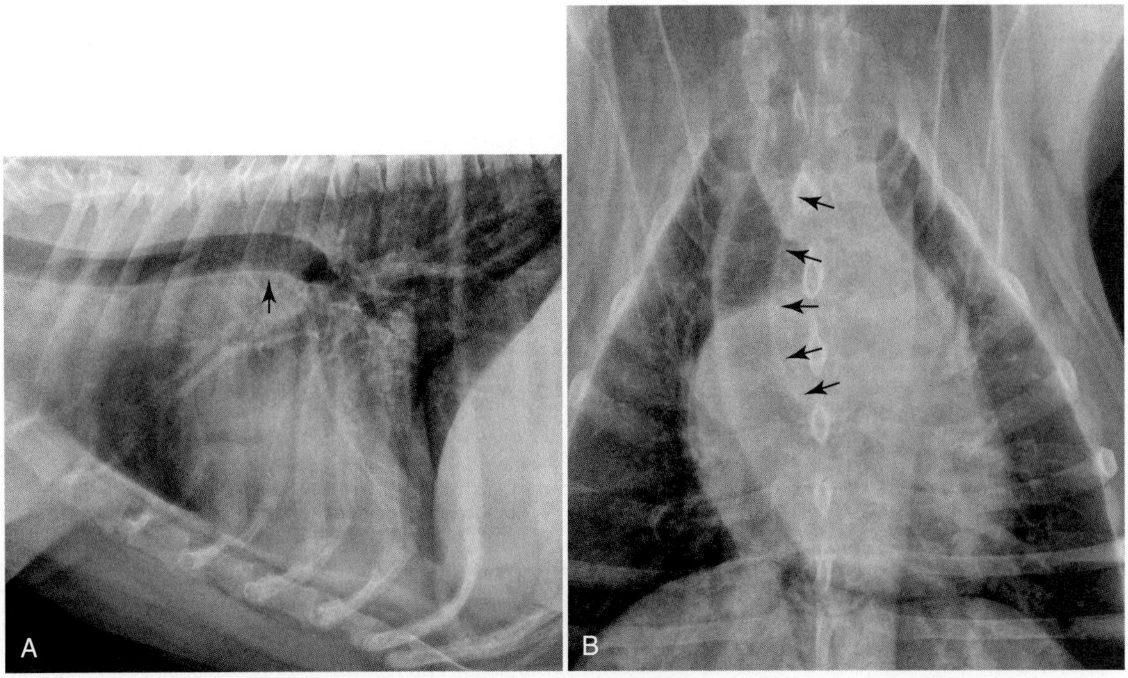

Fig. 33.24 Right lateral (**A**) and ventrodorsal (VD; **B**) radiographs of a dog with a heart base tumor (chemodectoma). In **A**, there is slight focal elevation of the trachea just cranial to the bifurcation (*black arrow*). Enlargement of the left and/or right tracheobronchial lymph nodes could also produce this appearance, but there is no evidence of enlargement of the middle tracheobronchial lymph node, which detracts from the tracheobronchial lymph nodes being the cause of the tracheal elevation seen here. Also, in **B**, there is sharp deviation of the intrathoracic trachea to the right (*black arrows*), which is not usually seen with tracheobronchial lymph node enlargement. The chemodectoma itself is not visible. These tracheal changes are often the only radiographic sign of the presence of a heart base mass.

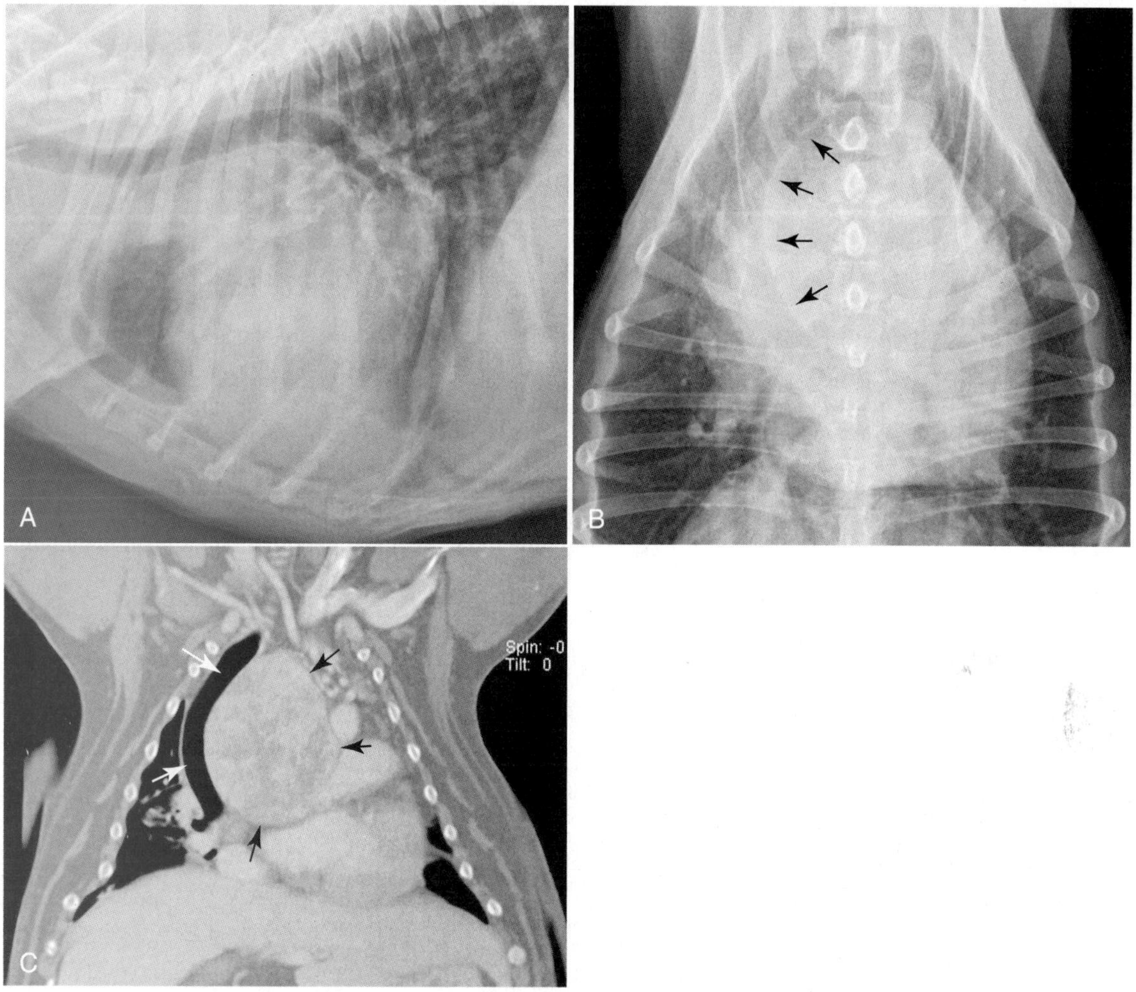

Fig. 33.25 Right lateral **(A)** and ventrodorsal (VD; **B**) radiographs of a dog with a chemodectoma that is larger than the one illustrated in Fig. 33.24. In **A,** there is elevation of the trachea over the base of the heart, and in **B,** there is rightward displacement of the majority of the intrathoracic trachea (*black arrows*). These findings are typical of a large heart base mass. In this dog, the mass itself, even though larger than the one illustrated in Fig. 33.24, is still not overtly conspicuous. **C,** Dorsal plane contrast-enhanced computed tomography (CT) image of another dog with a large chemodectoma (*black arrows*). The image plane is through the level of the heart base. The tumor displaces the trachea (*white arrows*) to the right. The mass is in the mediastinum and contacts the heart. This leads to border effacement, and this is the reason heart base tumors are so inconspicuous radiographically.

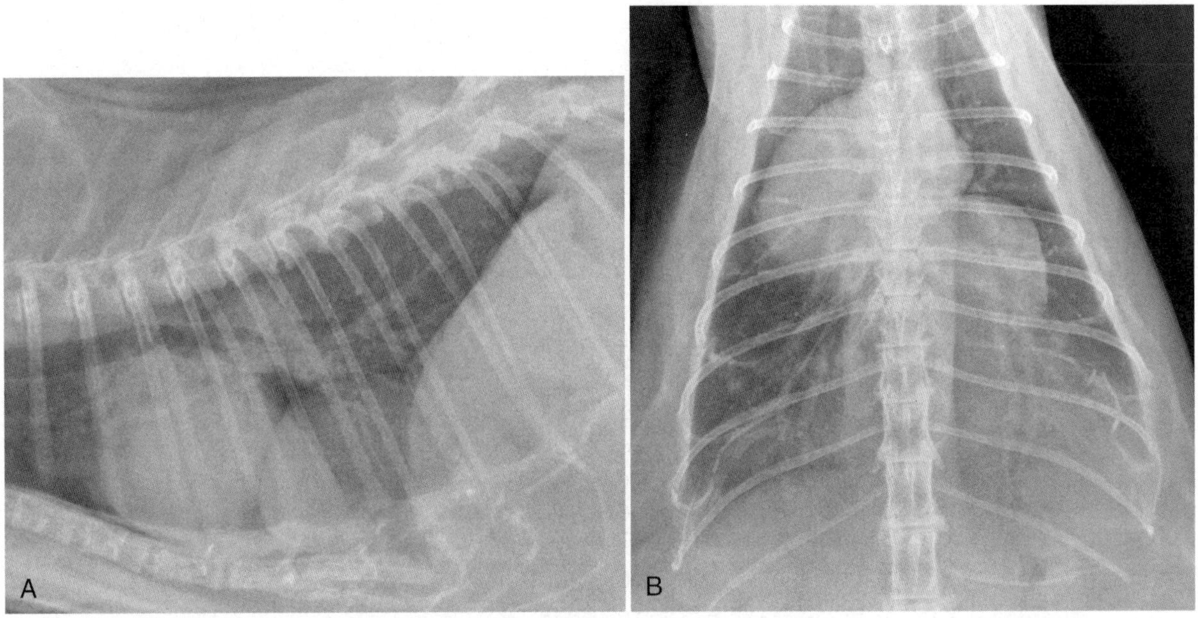

Fig. 33.26 Right lateral **(A)** and dorsoventral (DV; **B**) radiographs of a cat with a lipoma in the caudoventral mediastinum. In **B,** this mass causes border effacement of the diaphragm and is located to the left of midline because of the caudoventral mediastinal reflection being on the left. The heart is displaced to the right. In **A,** the opacity of the mass is slightly less than expected for soft tissue, but making the definitive diagnosis of lipoma from these radiographs is not possible and an aspirate would be required. Visualization of the caudal vena cava has been preserved in **A** due to the ventral location of the mass.

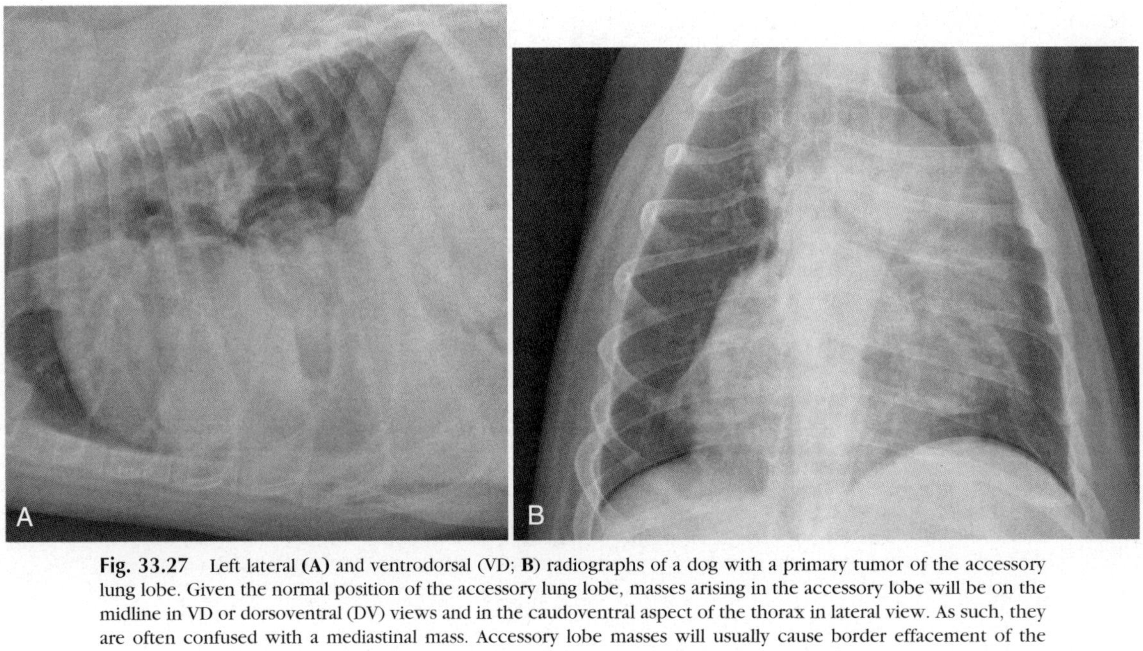

Fig. 33.27 Left lateral **(A)** and ventrodorsal (VD; **B**) radiographs of a dog with a primary tumor of the accessory lung lobe. Given the normal position of the accessory lung lobe, masses arising in the accessory lobe will be on the midline in VD or dorsoventral (DV) views and in the caudoventral aspect of the thorax in lateral view. As such, they are often confused with a mediastinal mass. Accessory lobe masses will usually cause border effacement of the caudal vena cava, as seen here due to the caudal vena cava running through the center of the accessory lung lobe. This mass is also causing border effacement of the diaphragm and displacement of the cardiac apex to the left.

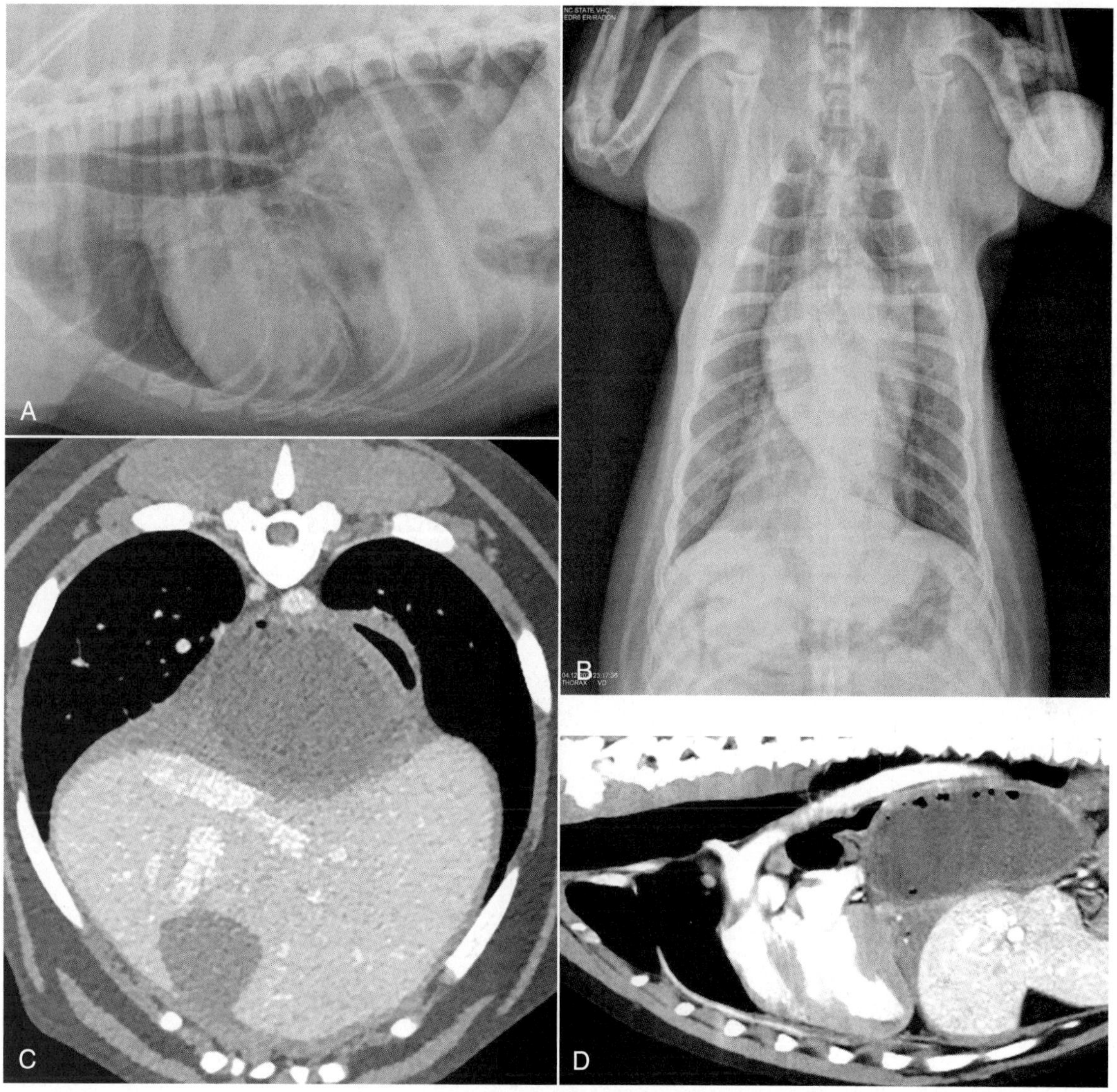

Fig. 33.28 Left lateral **(A)** and ventrodorsal (VD, **B**) radiographs of a dog with empyema of the mediastinal serous cavity. A large ovoid soft tissue opacity is present in the caudodorsal mediastinum at the level of the esophagus. A small amount of gas is present in the cranial thoracic esophagus. In **B**, the soft tissue mass lesion expands the caudal mediastinum to the right of midline. Transverse **(C)** and sagittal reformatted **(D)** contrast-enhanced computed tomography image of the same dog. A large fluid-filled centrally non-contrast-enhancing structure is present in the caudal mediastinum to the right of the mildly gas distended esophagus. Small gas bubbles are present in the dorsal aspect of the cavitary lesion.

Box • 33.1

Diseases Not Typically Associated With Radiographically Detectable Mediastinal Lymph Node Enlargement

- Primary lung tumor
- Metastatic lung tumor
- Bacterial pneumonia
- Pyothorax
- Rib tumors

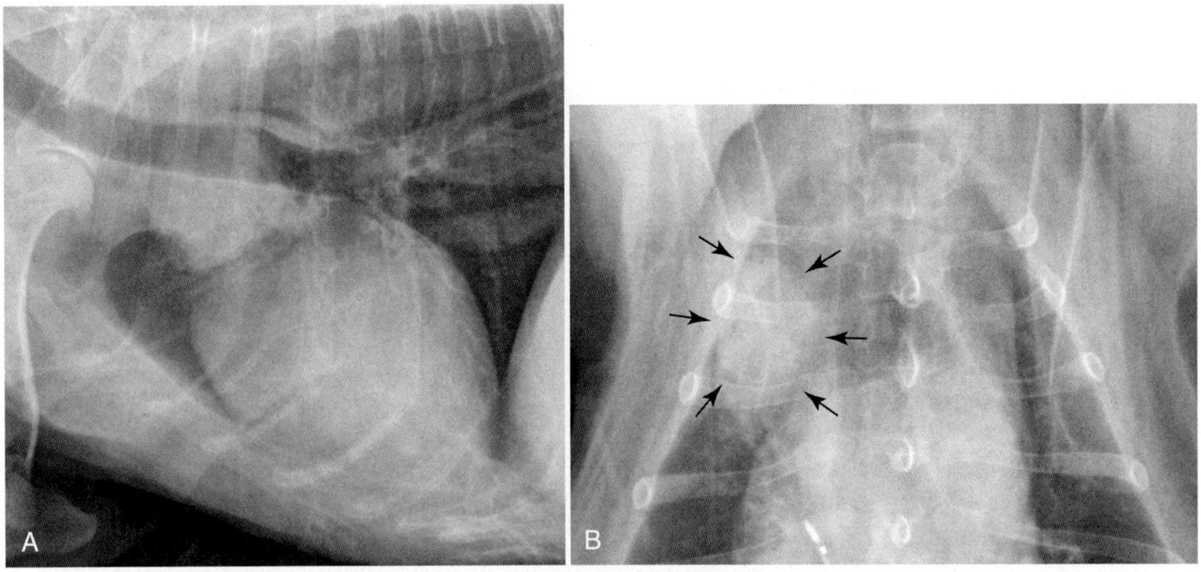

Fig. 33.29 Right lateral (**A**) and ventrodorsal (VD; **B**) radiographs of a dog. In **A**, there is a mass in the cranial aspect of the thorax, ventral to the trachea and just cranial to the tracheal bifurcation. This mass is well marginated ventrally but poorly marginated dorsally. The sharp margination ventrally suggests a pulmonary location for the mass, but a mediastinal mass extending laterally where it would be surrounded by lung cannot be ruled out. In **B**, the mass is located in the right cranial aspect of the thorax (*black arrows*). Because no part of the mediastinum is present normally in this region, the most likely diagnosis is pulmonary mass.

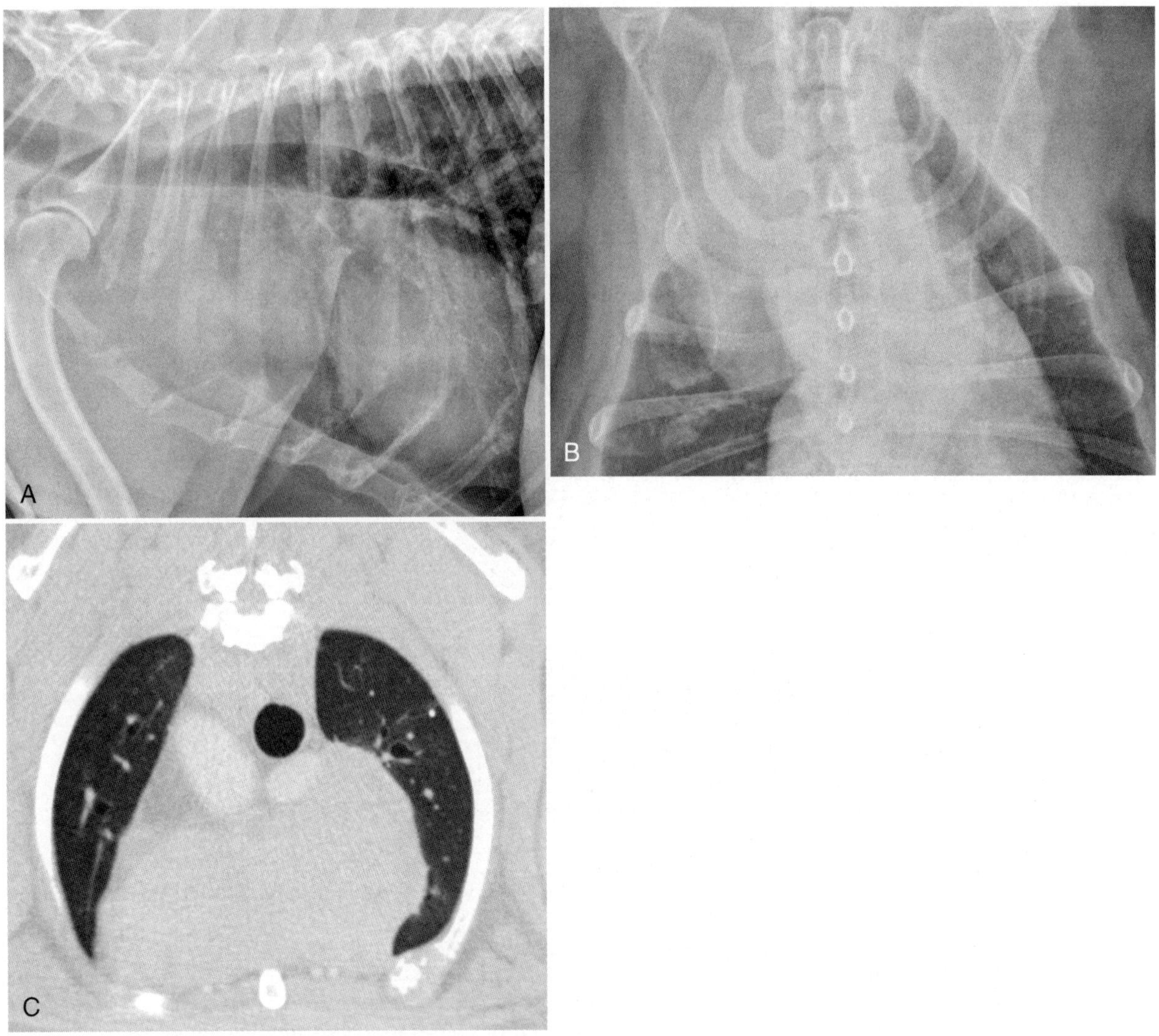

Fig. 33.30 Left lateral (**A**) and dorsoventral (DV; **B**) radiographs of a dog with a large mass in the cranial thorax. In **A**, there is a mass ventral to the trachea, but the trachea is not elevated. In **B**, the mass is to the right of midline, and the caudal border is sharply outlined by air. These findings are consistent with the mass being in the right cranial lung lobe. However, in a computed tomography (CT) image of the thorax (**C**), it was clear that the mass was in the cranial mediastinum. Lobular mediastinal masses can be surrounded by more air than expected, providing for sharp margination leading to misdiagnosis of the mass as pulmonary rather than mediastinal.

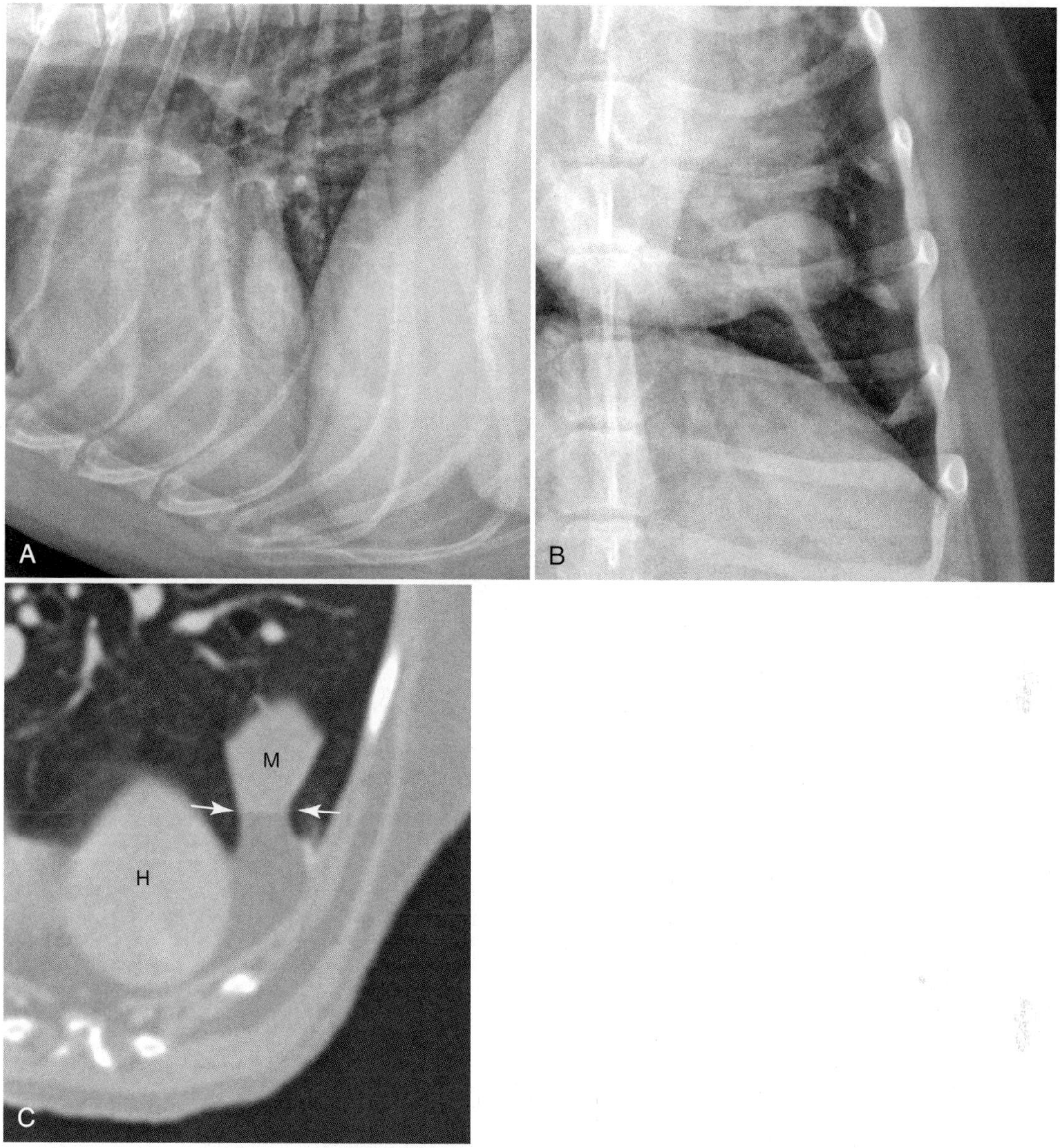

Fig. 33.31 Right lateral **(A)** and ventrodorsal (VD; **B**) radiographs of a dog with a mass in the left caudal thorax. The mass is sharply marginated, making it most consistent with a lung mass. In a computed tomography (CT) image **(C)** of the thorax, the mass (*M*) can be seen to be located in the mediastinum where the caudal mediastinal reflection (*arrows*) envelops the mass. *H*, Heart.

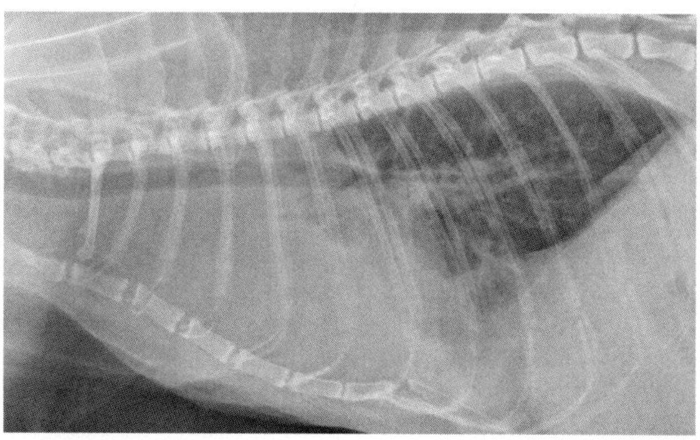

Fig. 33.32 Lateral radiograph of the thorax of a cat with pleural effusion. The trachea is displaced dorsally, but the presence of a mediastinal mass cannot be confirmed radiographically because pleural fluid may be accompanied by tracheal elevation when no mediastinal mass is present because of the lungs floating in the effusion. A thoracic mass cannot be seen, and the trachea is not compressed. Radiography after fluid removal, ultrasonography, or computed tomography (CT) would be more sensitive for determining whether a mediastinal mass was present in this cat.

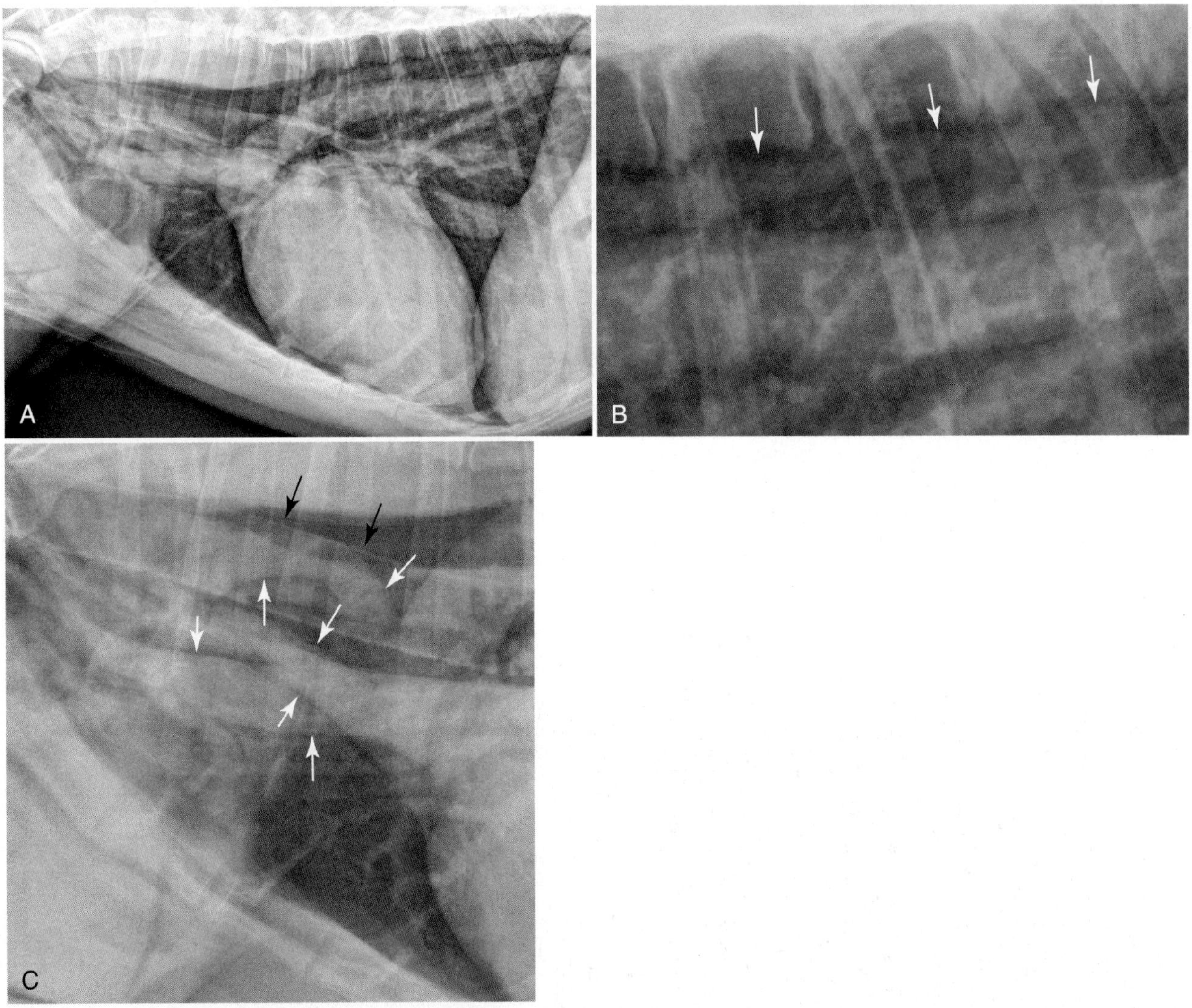

Fig. 33.33 Lateral **(A)** thoracic radiograph of a dog with pronounced pneumomediastinum. The undulating path of the aorta is an aging change and is an incidental finding not related to the pneumomediastinum. The mediastinal gas provides increased contrast that increases the conspicuity of mediastinal structures. **B** is a close-up view of the descending aorta. Mediastinal gas in this region provides contrast for visualization of the azygos vein, dorsal to the aorta (*white arrows*). The azygos vein is not normally seen in thoracic radiographs. **C** is a close-up view of the cranial mediastinum. The mediastinal gas in this region results in very sharp delineation of the adventitial surface of the trachea (*black arrows*). The mucosal and adventitial surfaces of the trachea each have adjacent gas, and therefore both surfaces are highly conspicuous. Also in **C**, the gas in the cranial mediastinum has created a heterogeneous appearance, and large mediastinal vessels can be seen (*white arrows*) as individual structures. Normally, this region has a homogeneous appearance (see Fig. 33.3).

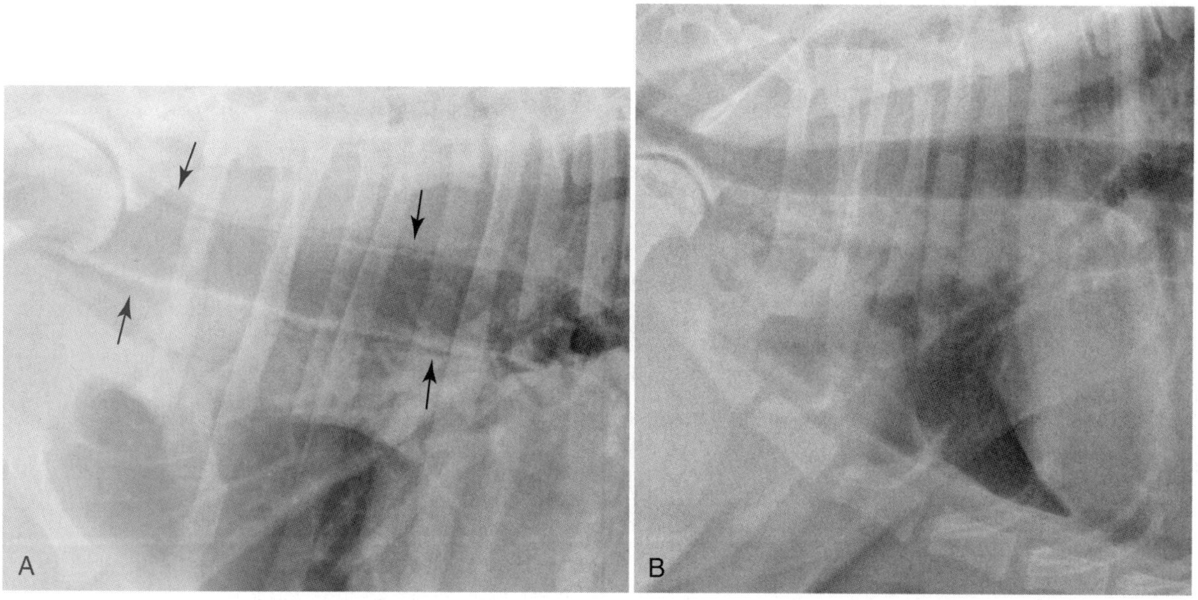

Fig. 33.34 Lateral radiographs of two dogs with a minimal pneumomediastinum. In **A,** the gas is localized around the trachea, leading to increased conspicuity of its adventitial surface (*black arrows*). In **B,** the gas has collected in pockets in the cranioventral aspect of the mediastinum, creating an unstructured mottled radiolucency. With regard to the appearance in **B,** the ventrodorsal (VD) view should be consulted to make sure that the mottling is not caused by superimposition of pockets of subcutaneous emphysema.

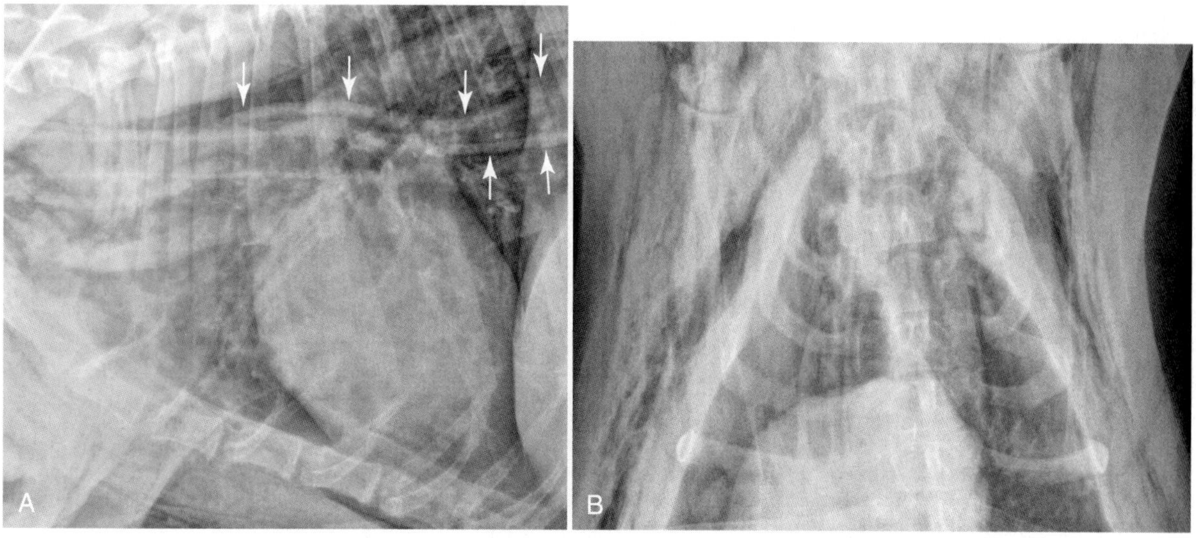

Fig. 33.35 Lateral **(A)** and ventrodorsal (VD; **B**) radiograph of a dog with pneumomediastinum and a large amount of coexisting subcutaneous emphysema. In **A,** the adventitial margin of the trachea and cranial mediastinal vessels are seen because of the contrast afforded by the mediastinal air. The adventitial surface of the esophagus is also visible (*white arrows*). In addition, the cranioventral mediastinum has a mottled appearance. This mottling can be caused by air pocketing in the mediastinum; but in this patient, much of it is caused by superimposition of the subcutaneous emphysema, as can be seen in **B**. In **A,** the mottling extends ventral to the thorax, which is also evidence of coexisting subcutaneous emphysema.

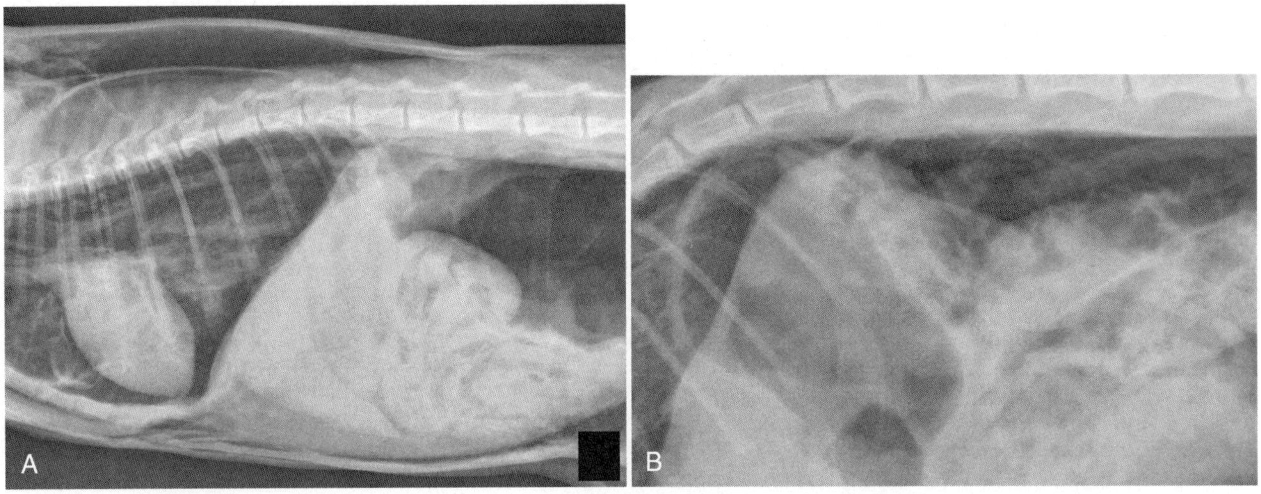

Fig. 33.36 **A,** Lateral radiograph of a cat with pneumomediastinum that has resulted in massive pneumoretroperitoneum. There is also subcutaneous emphysema. **B,** Lateral radiograph of a cat with pneumomediastinum where the extent of pneumoretroperitoneum is less.

REFERENCES

1. Kern D, Carrig C, Martin R. Radiographic evaluation of induced pneumothorax in the dog. *Vet Radiol Ultrasound*. 1994;35:411.
2. Burk R. Radiographic definition of the phrenicopericardiac ligament. *J Am Vet Radiol Soc*. 1976;17:216.
3. Bezuidenhout AJ. The lymphatic system. In: Evans H, ed. *Miller's Anatomy of the Dog*. 3rd ed. Philadelphia: Saunders; 1993:545–550.
4. Tompkins M. Lymphoid system. In: Hudson L, Hamilton W, eds. *Atlas of Feline Anatomy for Veterinarians*. Philadelphia: Saunders; 1993.
5. Kirberger RM, Avner A. The effect of positioning on the appearance of selected cranial thoracic structures in the dog. *Vet Radiol Ultrasound*. 2006;47(1):61–68.
6. Hopper B, Lester N, Irwin P, et al. Imaging diagnosis: pneumothorax and focal peritonitis in a dog due to migration of an inhaled grass awn. *Vet Radiol Ultrasound*. 2004;45(2):136–138.
7. Zekas LJ, Adams WM. Cranial mediastinal cysts in nine cats. *Vet Radiol Ultrasound*. 2002;43(5):413–418.
8. Cordella A, Saunders JS, Stock E. CT characteristics of the thymus in adult dogs with non-thymic neoplasia compared to young dogs. *Vet Sci*. 2023;10(3):192.
9. Ruehl Jr WW, Thrall D. The effect of dorsal versus ventral recumbency on the radiographic appearance of the canine thorax. *Vet Radiol*. 1981;22(10).
10. Brinkman EL, Biller D, Armbrust L. The clinical usefulness of the ventrodorsal versus dorsoventral thoracic radiograph in dogs. *J Am Anim Hosp Assoc*. 2006;42(6): 440–449.
11. Lora-Michiels M, Biller DS, Olsen D, et al. The accessory lung lobe in thoracic disease: a case series and anatomical review. *J Am Anim Hosp Assoc*. 2003;39(5): 452–458.
12. Gendron K, McDonough SP, Flanders JA, Tse M, Scrivani PV. The pathogenesis of paraesophageal empyema in dogs and constancy of radiographic and computed tomography signs are linked to involvement of the mediastinal serous cavity. *Vet Radiol Ultrasound*. 2018;59(2): 169–179.
13. McDonough SP, Scrivani PB, Gendron K, Tse M. Mediastinal serous cavity mesothelioma in two dogs. *J Am Anim Hosp Associ*. 2022;58(4):194–202.
14. Ackerman N, Madewell BR. Thoracic and abdominal radiographic abnormalities in the multicentric form of lymphosarcoma in dogs. *J Am Vet Med Assoc*. 1980;176(1): 36–40.
15. Berry CR, Moore PF, Thomas WP, et al. Pulmonary lymphomatoid granulomatosis in seven dogs (1976–1987). *J Vet Intern Med*. 1990;4(3):157–166.
16. Fitzgerald SD, Wolf DC, Carlton WW. Eight cases of canine lymphomatoid granulomatosis. *Vet Pathol*. 1991;28(3): 241–245.
17. Fulmer AK, Mauldin GE. Canine histiocytic neoplasia: an overview. *Can Vet J*. 2007;48(10):1041–1043.
18. Snyder P, Sato T, Atkins C. The utility of thoracic radiographic measurement for the detection of cardiomegaly in cats with pleural effusion. *Vet Radiol*. 1990;31(89).
19. Reichle JK, Wisner ER. Non-cardiac thoracic ultrasound in 75 feline and canine patients. *Vet Radiol Ultrasound*. 2000;41(2):154–162.
20. Konde L, Spaulding K. Sonographic evaluation of the cranial mediastinum in small animals. *Vet Radiol*. 1991;32:178.
21. Macklin C. Transport of air along sheaths of pulmonic blood vessels from alveoli to mediastinum: clinical implications. *Arch Intern Med*. 1939;64:913.
22. Macklin M, Macklin C. Malignant interstitial emphysema of the lungs and mediastinum as an important occult complication in many respiratory diseases and other conditions: an interpretation of the clinical literature in the light of laboratory experiment. *Medicine (Baltimore)*. 1944;23:281.
23. Baharudin A, Sayuti RM, Shahid H. The Macklin effect—pneumomediastinum and pneumopericardium following blunt chest trauma. *Med J Malaysia*. 2006;61(3):371–373.
24. Wintermark M, Schnyder P. The Macklin effect: a frequent etiology for pneumomediastinum in severe blunt chest trauma. *Chest*. 2001;120(2):543–547.
25. Brown DC, Holt D. Subcutaneous emphysema, pneumothorax, pneumomediastinum and pneumopericardium associated with positive-pressure ventilation in a cat. *J Am Vet Med Assoc*. 1995;206(7):997–999.

26. Mitchell S, McCarthy R, Rudloff E, et al. Tracheal rupture associated with intubation in cats: 20 cases (1996–1998). *J Am Vet Med Assoc*. 2000;216(10):1592–1595.
27. Hardie EM, Spodnick GJ, Gilson SD, et al. Tracheal rupture in cats: 16 cases (1983–1998). *J Am Vet Med Assoc*. 1999;214(4):508–512.
28. Kelly S, Bandt C. Inadvertent placement of an esophagostomy tube into the mediastinum of a cat. *Can Vet J*. 2022;63(11):1124–1128.

ELECTRONIC RESOURCES

Additional information related to the content in Chapter 33 can be found online at eBooks.Health.Elsevier.com.

- Chapter Quiz

CHAPTER 34

Canine and Feline Pleural Space

Gabriela S. Seiler

PLEURAL ANATOMY AND PHYSIOLOGY

The pleural space is the space between two pleural layers, the visceral and parietal pleura. The visceral pleura covers the lung, whereas the parietal pleura covers the mediastinum, diaphragm, and thoracic wall. There are two distinct pleural sacs dividing the left and right thorax; however, mediastinal fenestrations allow fluid and air to travel between the pleural sacs in the majority of dogs and cats (Fig. 34.1) The pleural space normally contains a few milliliters of fluid which facilitates gliding of the lung surface against the thoracic wall during respiration and maintains negative pressure in the pleural space, which is thought to prevent or reduce atelectasis in normal animals. Pleural fluid is produced by the mesothelial cells of the pleural layer and is reabsorbed by the pleura and associated lymphatics.

NORMAL RADIOGRAPHIC APPEARANCE OF PLEURA AND PLEURAL THICKENING

Normal pleura is usually not visible radiographically. Pleura is very thin and also silhouettes with adjacent soft tissue everywhere except in interlobar fissures, where two layers of visceral pleura are in contact only with lung. Thin pleural lines between lobes are sometimes visible radiographically, particularly in the caudoventral thorax. These thin pleural lines may be because of the x-ray beam striking normal interlobar pleura exactly head-on, resulting in absorption of a sufficient number of x-rays for the pleura to be seen, or because of slightly thickened pleura or a trace pleural effusion (Fig. 34.2). Accessory pleural fissures are common in dogs and may result in atypical fissure lines being visible in addition to the interlobar fissure lines.[1] Radiographic determination of whether isolated,

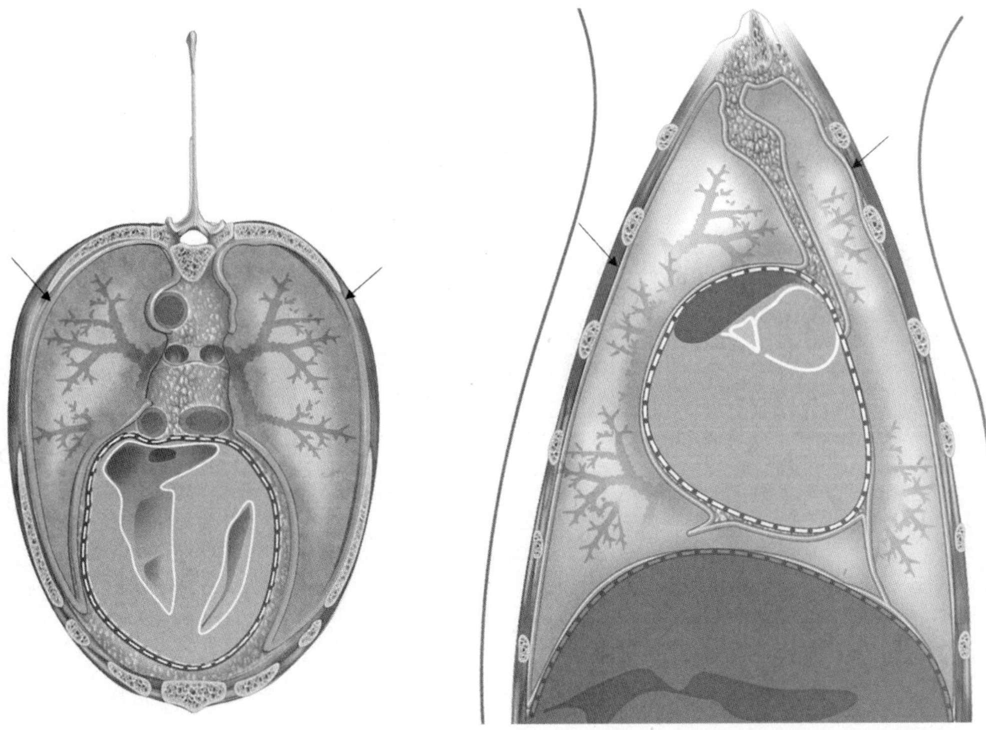

Fig. 34.1 The thorax in transverse **(A)** and dorsal **(B)** planes illustrating the relationship of the pleural layers. There are two distinct pleural sacs (*arrows*). **A,** Note how the mediastinal pleura is reflected onto the lung to become pulmonary pleura. **B,** Note the continuity of the costal, mediastinal, and diaphragmatic parts of each parietal sac. The heart is depicted by the *dotted line*. Also note that the pleural space is not continuous with the mediastinum. (Courtesy Harvey Medical Production.)

thin pleural lines are normal or are caused by mild thickening is impossible. In either instance, this finding is usually of no clinical significance. When pleural thickening is more advanced, wider pleural fissure lines between lung lobes may be seen (Fig. 34.3).

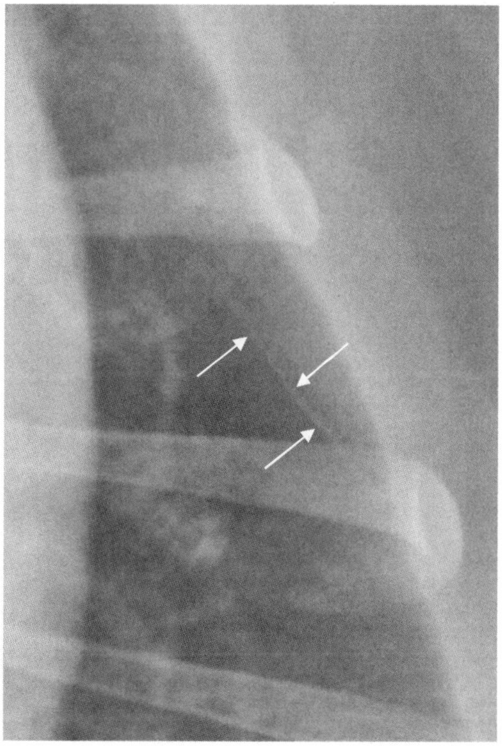

Fig. 34.2 Close-up view of a portion of the left hemithorax of a dog. A thin pleural fissure is visible (*white arrows*). Distinguishing radiographically whether this is caused by x-rays striking a normal fissure or by slight pleural thickening is impossible. This distinction is usually not clinically necessary.

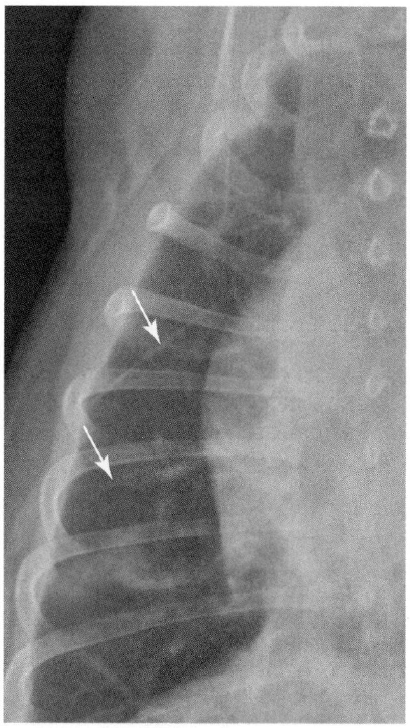

Fig. 34.3 Close-up view of the right hemithorax of a dog with multiple mildly widened pleural fissures (*white arrows*). The cranially located fissure line is thicker than normal (compare with Fig. 34.2) and may be caused by either pleural thickening or a small amount of pleural fluid.

PLEURAL FLUID

Causes of Pleural Fluid

Normal homeostasis of pleural fluid is maintained by the difference of hydrostatic pressures between the systemic and pulmonary circulations and by drainage through the lymphatic vessels. Pleural effusion is therefore the result of either high production and/or increased vascular permeability, decreased reabsorption, decreased lymphatic drainage, or a combination of thereof. Fluid in the pleural space can be an exudate, transudate, or modified transudate, chyle, or hemorrhage and can result from many causes (Table 34.1). The radiographic changes associated with pleural fluid depend on the volume of fluid, the position of the animal in relation to the x-ray beam, the distribution of the fluid, and whether the fluid is free or trapped, so-called *loculated fluid.* There are no radiographic criteria that allow differentiation of an exudate from a transudate, although an exudate may be more asymmetrically distributed. Measurement of Hounsfield units in computed tomography (CT) has a limited ability to predict the characteristics of pleural fluid in dogs.[2] It is often not possible to determine the cause of pleural effusion radiographically, particularly since even large intrathoracic lesions can be obscured, but radiographs should always be evaluated for the presence of additional findings that may help in determining the most likely cause as outlined in Table 34.1. Making additional radiographs after removal of the fluid may provide important information. Any amount of pleural fluid is clinically significant, and attempts should be made to reach a definitive diagnosis. Thoracocentesis with appropriate fluid analysis should be considered if pleural fluid is identified. Ultrasound can be used to determine the presence of pleural effusion if radiographs are equivocal and to guide needle placement for diagnostic or therapeutic thoracocentesis. This is especially helpful in patients with chronic effusion that may be loculated with fibrin strands that tend to adhere to the needle. Ultrasound may also be able to identify mass lesions or cardiac changes which are obscured by the pleural effusion radiographically. The improved contrast resolution of CT imaging and lack of superimposition allow detection of concurrent or causative lesions including mass lesions, lung lobe torsions, and traumatic lesions.

Radiographic Appearance of Pleural Fluid

Regardless of the cause, if the negative pressure in the pleural space is not maintained, elastic recoil leads to retraction of the lung lobe margins and separation of the lobar margins from each other, which is the main radiographic finding associated with pleural space disease.[3] Pleural fluid distributes itself according to gravity and the ability of the lung to expand—that is, lung compliance.[4] It is important to realize that the radiographic appearance of pleural fluid in ventrodorsal (VD) versus dorsoventral (DV) radiographs is different. In DV radiographs, with the dog in sternal recumbency, fluid gravitates ventrally and causes border effacement of the heart. In VD radiographs, with the dog in dorsal recumbency, pleural fluid does not obscure the heart because the fluid gravitates to the dorsal aspect of the thorax, where it does not make contact with the heart and does not cause border effacement (Fig. 34.4). Also, the overall opacity of the thorax will be greater in DV radiographs in patients with pleural fluid because the fluid depth is greater (see Fig. 34.4). Radiographic signs of free pleural fluid are listed in Box 34.1.

Interlobar Fissures

The width and number of interlobar fissures seen with pleural fluid depend on the amount of fluid and the relative position of the patient and the x-ray beam (Fig. 34.5, eFigs. 34.1 and 34.2). Approximately 100 mL of fluid must be present in the pleural space of a medium-sized dog before widened interlobar fissures become visible radiographically.[4] Thus, any radiographic evidence of pleural fluid signifies a relatively large fluid volume,

Table • 34.1

Causes of Pleural Fluid.

CAUSE	FLUID TYPE	POSSIBLE ADDITIONAL RADIOGRAPHIC FINDINGS
Congestive heart failure Dog: right-sided cardiac disease, pericardial effusion Cat: left-sided cardiac disease	T, M, CH	Dogs: right-sided or globoid cardiomegaly, dilated caudal vena cava Cats: left-sided cardiomegaly, sometimes dilated pulmonary veins
Pyothorax • Dog: Nocardia, actinomyces • Cat: Pasteurella, bacteroides, fusobacterium	E	Often unilateral or loculated effusion. Look for thoracic wall trauma, foreign material, esophageal rupture, pulmonary abscess
Feline infectious peritonitis	E	Abdominal effusion commonly present
Mediastinal neoplasia • Lymphoma • Thymoma	M, E, CH	Cranial mediastinal mass
Pulmonary Neoplasia • Pulmonary carcinoma • Metastatic carcinoma • Hemangiosarcoma	M, E, CH, H	Pulmonary mass or nodules
Pleural or thoracic wall neoplasia • Mesothelioma • Rib tumors	M, E	Extrapleural sign, pleural nodules, rib lysis, and/or periosteal reaction
Chylothorax • Idiopathic • Thoracic duct rupture	CH	Rounded lung lobes, effusion may be loculated
Trauma • Diaphragmatic hernia • Thoracic wall trauma • Surgical intervention	M, E, H	Thoracic wall defect, emphysema, or swelling Discontinuous diaphragm, cranial displacement of abdominal organs
Heartworm disease	M, CH	Enlarged pulmonary arteries, right heart enlargement
Pulmonary disease • Pneumonia, pulmonary abscess • Lung lobe torsion	E, H	Pneumonia: ventral alveolar pattern without mediastinal shift Abscess: cavitary lesion with surrounding consolidation Lung lobe torsion: vesicular gas pattern, enlarged lung lobe, discontinuous bronchus
Hypoalbuminemia	T	Concurrent abdominal effusion
Abdominal disease • Pancreatitis • Bile peritonitis	E	Peritoneal effusion, possible cranial abdominal mass effect
Mediastinitis, mediastinal abscess	E	Mediastinal mass effect, mediastinal effusion
Coagulopathies Von Willebrand Rodenticide toxicity	H	May have mediastinal or tracheal wall hemorrhage

CH, Chyle; *E*, exudate; *H*, hemorrhage; *M*, modified transudate; *T*, transudate.

and one that can be sampled by thoracocentesis. Visibility of fluid-containing interlobar fissures results when the x-ray beam strikes the fissure in a parallel fashion, or head-on. Some fluid-containing fissures may not be seen, because their relation to the x-ray beam is not head-on. Pleural fissure lines caused by fluid rather than pleural thickening or fortuitous alignment of the x-ray beam with the pleural space may widen towards the periphery of the thorax with a triangular appearance, caused by rounding of the lung margins. With a *small amount of fluid*, interlobar fissures are more likely to be seen on VD rather than DV radiographs, because when in dorsal recumbency for a VD radiograph, there is a tendency for fluid to enter interlobar fissures (see Fig. 34.3). This is opposed to sternal recumbency for a DV radiograph where the fluid collects dorsal to the sternum (see Fig. 34.4).[2,3] A small amount of pleural fluid usually results in visible interlobar fissures in lateral views as well, commonly superimposed on the cardiac silhouette.

Retraction of Lung Margins

With moderate or pronounced pleural fluid, the number and width of interlobar fissures increase, and fluid also collects between the thoracic wall and the lung, resulting in lung retraction (Figs. 34.6 and 34.7). Retraction of lung from the thoracic wall is characterized by a soft tissue opacity rim between the lung lobe margins and the thoracic wall, and mild rounding of the lung lobe margins. The pleural fluid surrounds the lung, but the fluid will be most apparent radiographically where the x-ray beam strikes the fluid/lung interface in a parallel fashion (see Fig. 34.5). Therefore, more pleural fluid is present than

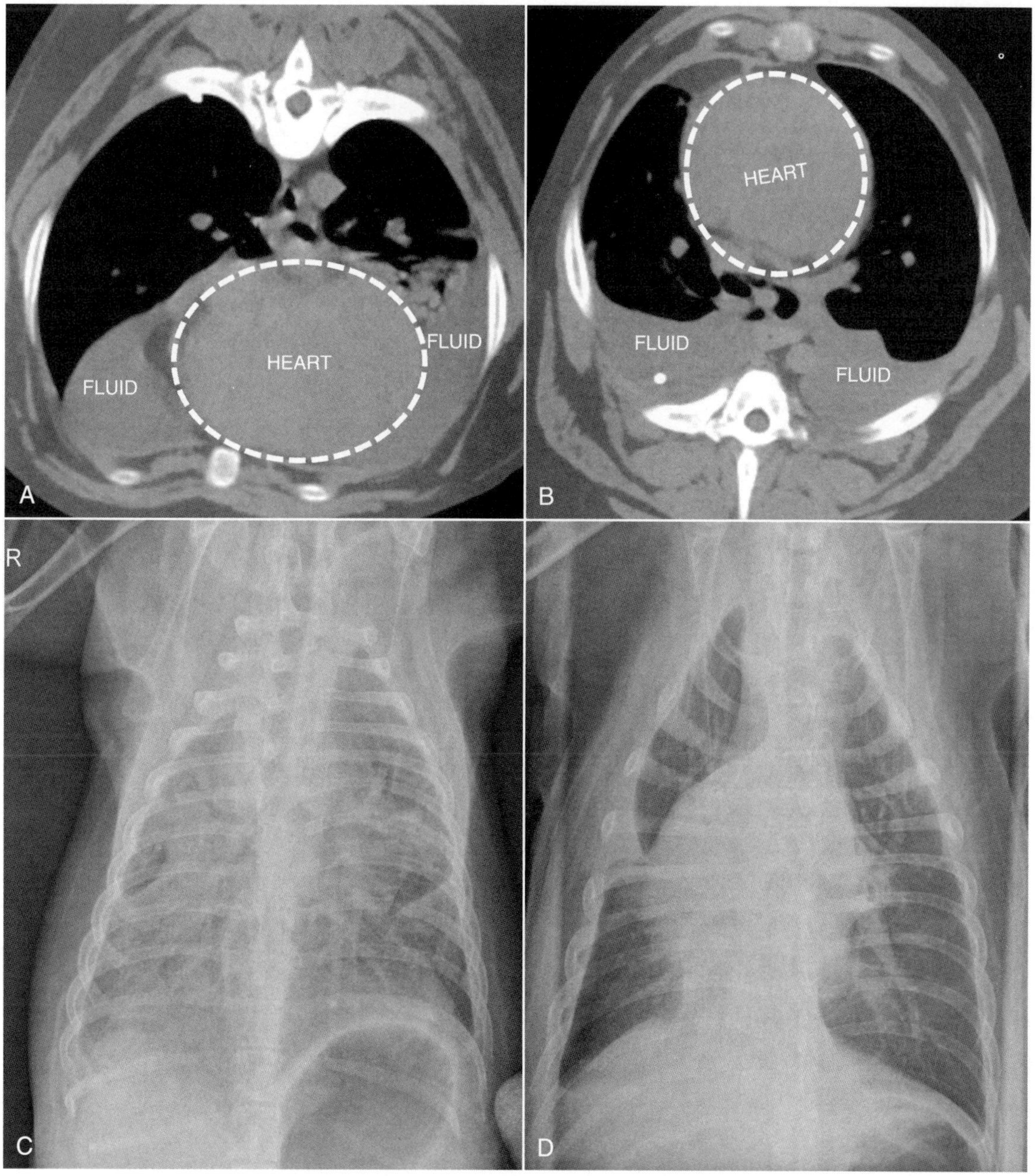

Fig. 34.4 Transverse computed tomography (CT) images of the thorax imaged in ventral **(A)** and dorsal **(B)** recumbency, and dorsoventral (DV) **(C)** and ventrodorsal (VD) **(D)** radiographs of the thorax of a dog with pleural fluid. **A and C,** The patient is in ventral recumbency and fluid gravitates ventrally. The fluid is in contact with the heart, thus obscuring the heart radiographically because of border effacement (i.e., the silhouette sign). When the patient is in dorsal recumbency for the VD radiograph **(B, D)**, the fluid gravitates dorsally and is not in contact with the heart; thus, the cardiac silhouette is visible because it is surrounded by air-filled lung that provides contrast. The overall thoracic opacity is greater because the absolute depth of the fluid is greater when the patient is in ventral recumbency **(A, C)** because the ventral part of the thoracic cavity is narrower, and the fluid rises to a higher level.

predicted based on the amount of lung retraction (Fig. 34.8). Pleural fluid may cause blunting of the costophrenic angle in VD radiographs if fluid is present between the dorsocaudal aspect of the lung and diaphragm. Rounding of the costophrenic angles will seldom be the only radiographic sign of pleural fluid.

Retrosternal Soft Tissue Opacity and Silhouette Sign

In lateral radiographs, pleural fluid can also result in a region of homogeneously increased opacity dorsal to the sternum (Fig. 34.9; also see Figs. 34.6C and 34.7B). This opacity results from fluid having collected in the ventral aspect of the thorax and layered against the mediastinum in the nondependent hemithorax. The margin of this retrosternal opacity often appears *scalloped* because of adjacent, partially collapsed lung that alters the configuration of the fluid. It is important to differentiate retrosternal pleural fluid from mediastinal fat. In presence of pleural fluid, the borders of the cardiac silhouette and diaphragm are effaced, whereas mediastinal fat will create contrast with the diaphragmatic and cardiac margins.

Box 34.1

Roentgen Signs of Free Pleural Fluid

1) Widened interlobar fissures that are of soft tissue opacity
   a) Usually most conspicuous in ventrodorsal (VD) and lateral radiographs
2) Retraction of pleural surface of lung away from pleural surface of thoracic wall, with interposed soft tissue opacity
   a) Seen first in VD radiographs
3) Increased soft tissue opacity with scalloped margins dorsal to sternum
   a) Seen in lateral radiographs
4) Increased opacity of the pulmonary parenchyma
   i) Seen in all views, caused by atelectasis and superimposed fluid
5) Decreased cardiac silhouette visualization
   a) Usually seen in dorsoventral (DV) radiographs
6) Obscured diaphragmatic outline
   a) Seen in all views
7) Blunting of costophrenic sulci
   a) Seen rarely, only in VD radiographs
   b) Expansion of thoracic cavity, diaphragm is flattened
      i) Only with large volume of fluid, seen in all views

Asymmetric Distribution of Pleural Fluid

Pleural fluid is usually relatively equally distributed between the right and left pleural spaces. Some patients, however, have asymmetric fluid distribution. Causes of unilateral or asymmetric pleural fluid include a difference in compliance between lung lobes, the closing of mediastinal fenestrations from inflammation or a mass, and an anatomically complete mediastinum (eFig. 34.3). Pyothorax is a common cause of unilateral or asymmetric pleural fluid because of the viscous nature of the exudate (Fig. 34.10), but other types of fluid can also be asymmetric. Chronic pleural effusions, particularly with exudative, hemorrhagic, or chylous effusions, result in pleural thickening and entrapment of fluid in fibrous capsules. Pleuritis causes the lung lobe margins to be markedly rounded or scalloped (see Fig. 34.10B). Lung reexpansion can be reduced in presence of pleuritis, and this can result in lung rupture and pneumothorax if the pleural fluid is rapidly removed during thoracocentesis (eFig. 34.4). Parenchymal disease or bronchial obstruction of a single lung lobe can also result in focal unilateral accumulation of pleural fluid due to decreased fluid absorption and decreased pleural pressure.

Horizontal-Beam Radiography

Identification of a small amount of pleural fluid may not be possible on survey radiographs if the x-ray beam fails to strike a fluid/lung interface head-on (see Fig. 34.8). If identification of a small amount of pleural fluid is critical, a horizontally directed

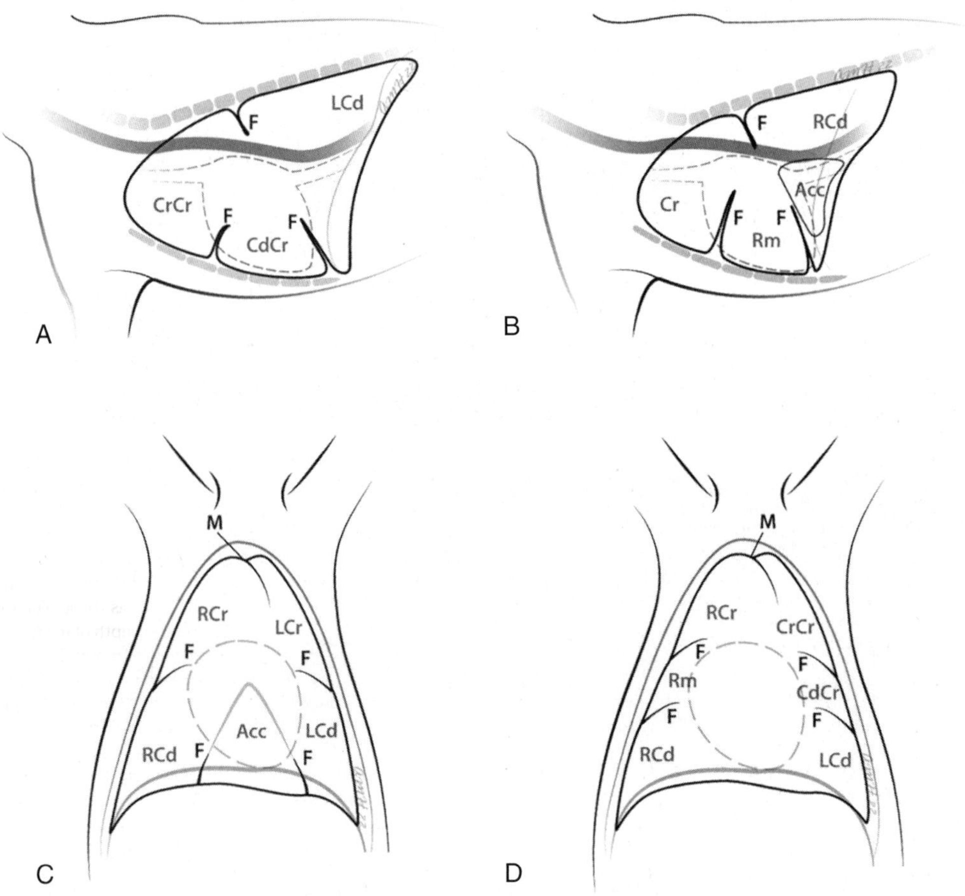

Fig. 34.5 The location of interlobar fissures. The exact fissures visible when pleural fluid is present depends on the position of the patient, the volume of fluid, and whether the x-ray beam strikes the fissure in a parallel orientation. Only fluid-filled fissures that are struck in a parallel fashion will be seen. **A,** Fissures of the lateral aspect of the left lung. These fissures are more likely to be seen when the patient is in left recumbency. **B,** Fissures of the lateral aspect of the right lung, best seen when the patient is in right recumbency. **C,** Fissures on the dorsal aspect of the lungs, best seen when the patient is in dorsal recumbency. The costophrenic sulcus may become rounded when patients with pleural fluid are in dorsal recumbency. **D,** Fissures on the ventral aspect of the lungs, best seen when the patient is in ventral recumbency. *Acc,* Accessory lobe; *Cd,* caudal lobe; *CdCr,* caudal part of left cranial lobe; *Cr,* right cranial lobe; *CrCr,* cranial part of left cranial lobe; *F,* interlobar fissure; *L,* left; *M,* mediastinal reflection; *R,* right; *Rm,* right middle lobe.

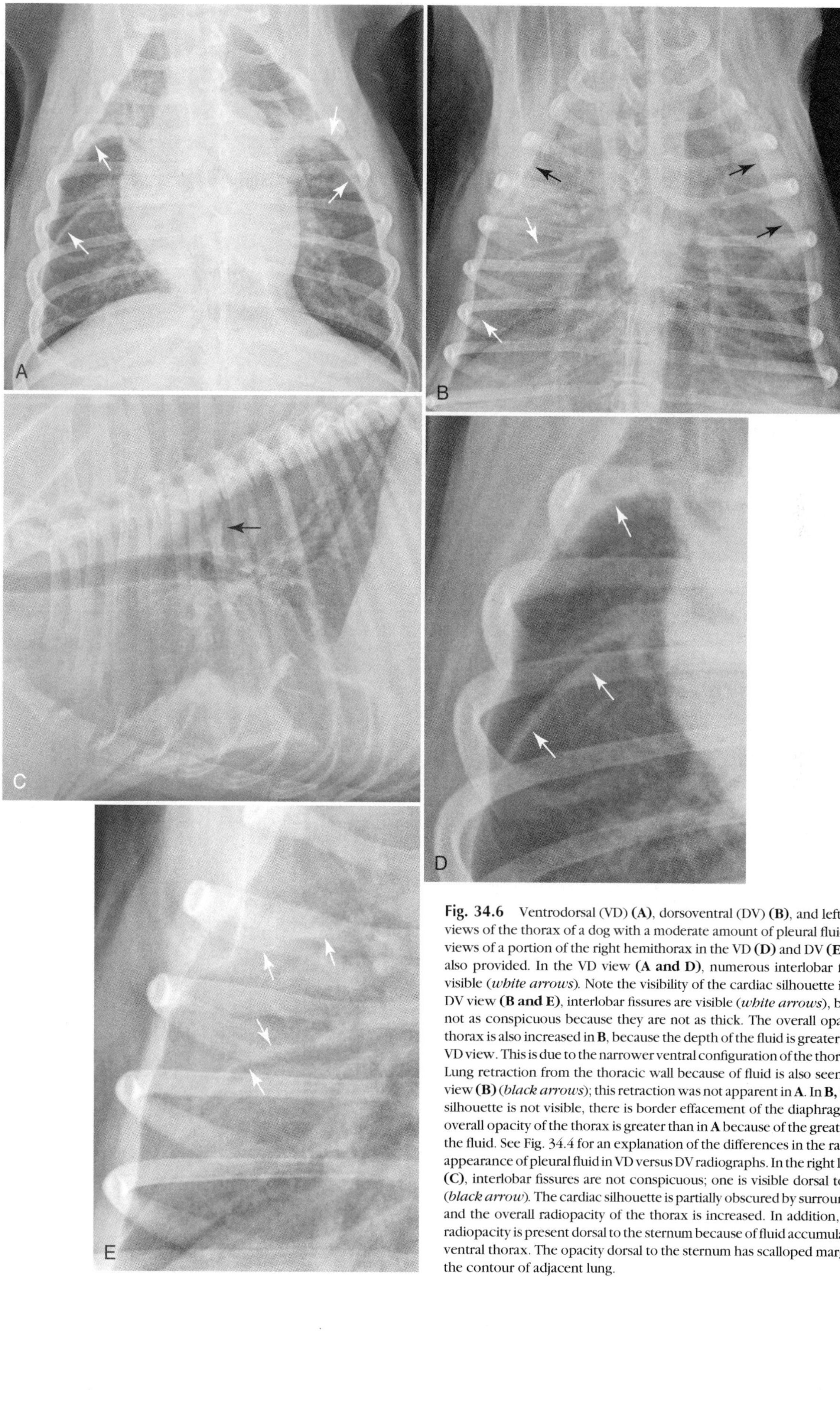

Fig. 34.6 Ventrodorsal (VD) **(A)**, dorsoventral (DV) **(B)**, and left lateral **(C)** views of the thorax of a dog with a moderate amount of pleural fluid. Close-up views of a portion of the right hemithorax in the VD **(D)** and DV **(E)** views are also provided. In the VD view **(A and D)**, numerous interlobar fissures are visible (*white arrows*). Note the visibility of the cardiac silhouette in **A**. In the DV view **(B and E)**, interlobar fissures are visible (*white arrows*), but they are not as conspicuous because they are not as thick. The overall opacity of the thorax is also increased in **B**, because the depth of the fluid is greater than in the VD view. This is due to the narrower ventral configuration of the thoracic cavity. Lung retraction from the thoracic wall because of fluid is also seen in the DV view **(B)** (*black arrows*); this retraction was not apparent in **A**. In **B**, the cardiac silhouette is not visible, there is border effacement of the diaphragm, and the overall opacity of the thorax is greater than in **A** because of the greater depth of the fluid. See Fig. 34.4 for an explanation of the differences in the radiographic appearance of pleural fluid in VD versus DV radiographs. In the right lateral view **(C)**, interlobar fissures are not conspicuous; one is visible dorsal to the heart (*black arrow*). The cardiac silhouette is partially obscured by surrounding fluid, and the overall radiopacity of the thorax is increased. In addition, an area of radiopacity is present dorsal to the sternum because of fluid accumulation in the ventral thorax. The opacity dorsal to the sternum has scalloped margins due to the contour of adjacent lung.

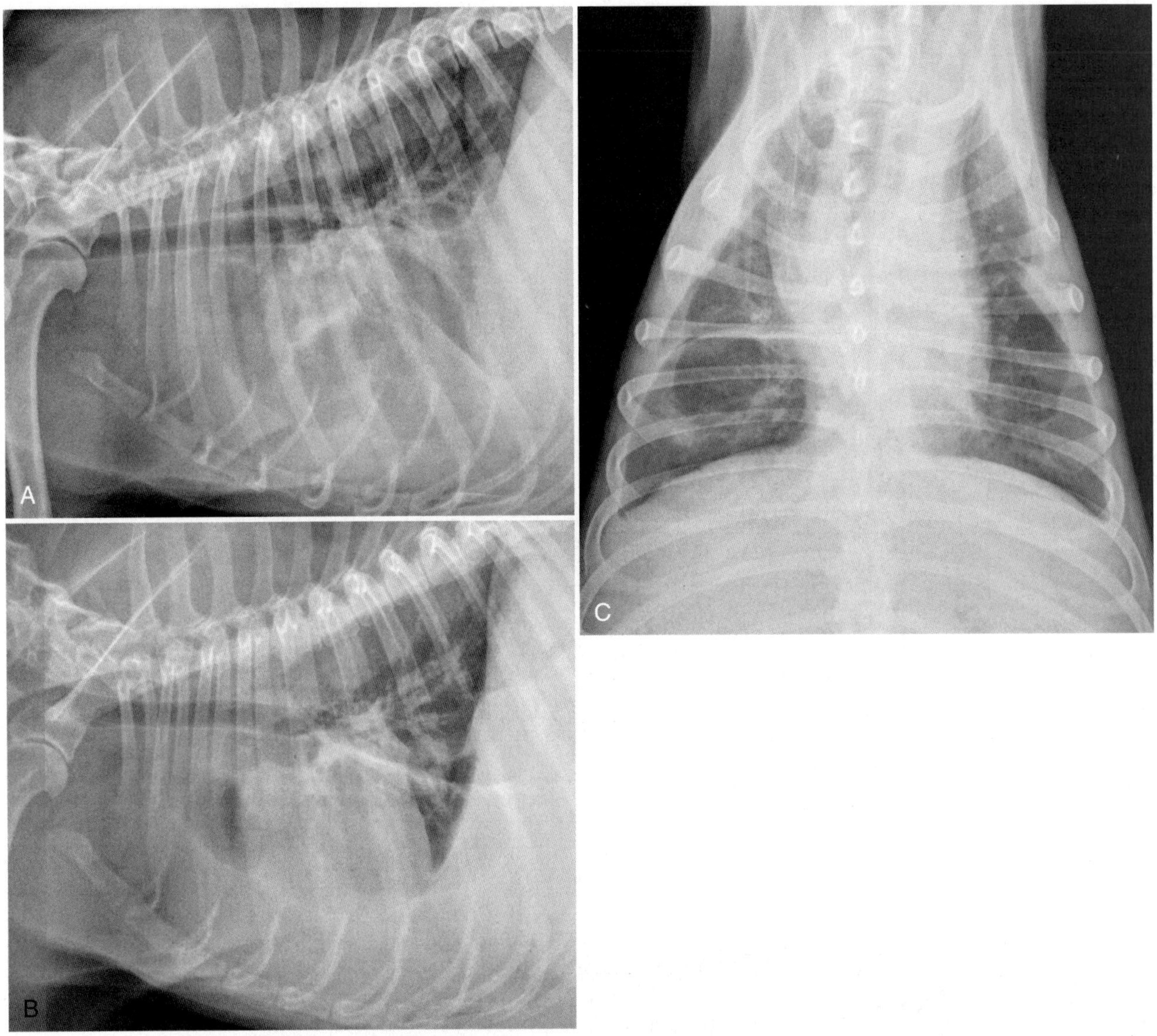

Fig. 34.7 Left lateral **(A)**, right lateral **(B)**, and ventrodorsal (VD) **(C)** radiographs of a dog with a large volume of pleural fluid. In the VD view **(C)**, the lungs are markedly retracted from the thoracic wall by the fluid. The heart is visible, as expected. In the lateral views, the fluid has obscured much of the normal thoracic detail. This volume of fluid could obscure significant lesions in the thoracic cavity. In **C**, note especially the inability to evaluate the cranial mediastinum because of the fluid. The ribs should always be scrutinized carefully in patients with pleural fluid to ensure that the fluid is not the result of a rib tumor. Thoracic ultrasonography or computed tomography (CT) may be helpful in deciding if an underlying mass is present in the thorax.

x-ray beam may be used to ensure a head-on relation between the x-ray beam and the fluid/lung interface. If free pleural fluid is present, it gravitates dependently where the x-ray beam strikes it in a parallel fashion (Fig. 34.11). A sharply demarcated, straight fluid line is only seen when there is a free fluid/free air interface, such as with coexisting pleural fluid and pneumothorax. Horizontal-beam radiographs may also be useful in distinguishing pleural fluid from an intrathoracic mass as the cause of an intrathoracic opacity, as discussed before (see Fig. 34.9).

Pitfalls in Pleural Fluid Diagnosis

Various normal structures can be misinterpreted as pleural fluid. Thickened pleura may have an appearance identical to pleural fluid (see Fig. 34.3). A distinction may be made by using a horizontally directed x-ray beam or with sonography.[4] A mineralized costal cartilage is sometimes confused with an interlobar fissure. The position of these two structures is similar, but their shape is different. Pleural fissure lines are distinctly curving, with the concave surface on the caudal aspect of the fissure line. Costal cartilages are more linear and can usually be seen to attach to the end of a rib (Fig. 34.12). Thoracic wall deformities, as found in chondrodystrophic breeds, such as the Basset hound, may result in increased radiopacity at the margin of the lung field. Without knowledge of this fact, the opacity may be misinterpreted as retraction of the lung from the thoracic wall because of pleural fluid (Fig. 34.13). Accumulation of pleural fluid along the cranial mediastinum can mimic presence of the mediastinal mass. Evaluation of tracheal shape and position of the carina is helpful for differentiating mediastinal masses from pleural effusion. While large volumes of pleural effusion can lead to dorsal

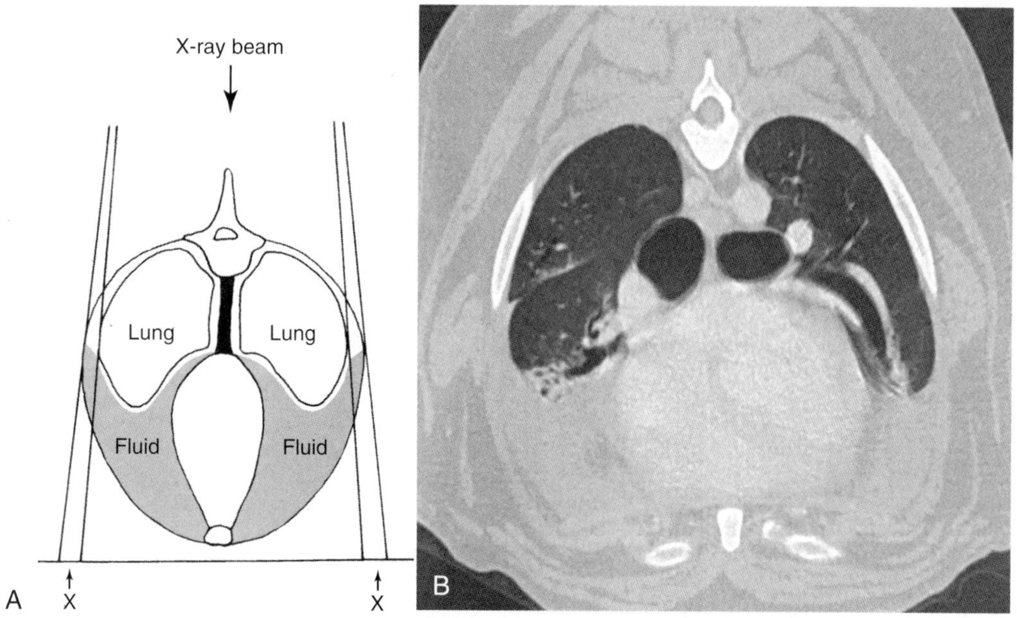

Fig. 34.8 Principle of lung retraction as a result of pleural fluid. **A,** Diagram of a patient with a large amount of pleural fluid being radiographed in ventral recumbency for a dorsoventral (DV) view. Fluid has gravitated ventrally, causing lung retraction. The full extent of the lung retraction is not apparent radiographically because the main fluid/lung interface, ventral to the lung, is not being struck in a parallel fashion by the x-ray beam. The only lung retraction that will be seen is in the regions indicated by (*X*) because here the fluid/lung interface is struck head-on by the x-ray beam. In the central portion of the thorax, the overall radiopacity will increase, and the heart will be obscured, but the lung retraction will not be apparent. **B,** Transverse computed tomography (CT) image of the thorax of a dog in sternal recumbency with pleural fluid. The fluid has pooled ventrally causing lung retraction from the ventral aspect of the thoracic cavity. However, the fluid is not dissecting between the lungs and the thoracic wall; thus, no part of the fluid/lung interface will be struck in a parallel fashion by the oncoming x-ray beam, and there will not be evidence of lung retraction in a DV radiograph of this patient even though there is a large amount of pleural fluid.

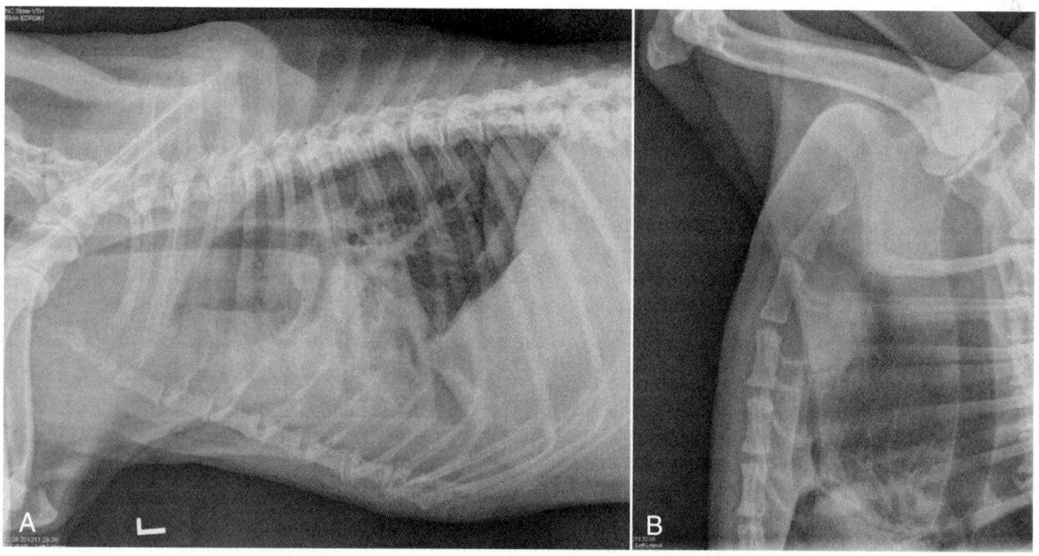

Fig. 34.9 **A,** Conventional lateral radiograph made with a vertically directed x-ray beam. **B,** Lateral radiograph made with a horizontally directed x-ray beam with the patient held in a sitting, upright position. In the conventional right lateral radiograph **(A)**, there is an opacity dorsal to the sternum and it is uncertain whether this opacity represents a mass or pleural fluid. In the radiograph made with a horizontal beam and the patient in upright position **(B)**, there is a rounded retrosternal soft tissue opacity mass visible consistent with an enlarged sternal lymph node. Note that a sharp horizontal fluid line is not present in the horizontal-beam radiograph **(B)** because sharp fluid lines are seen only when there is a free fluid/free air interface.

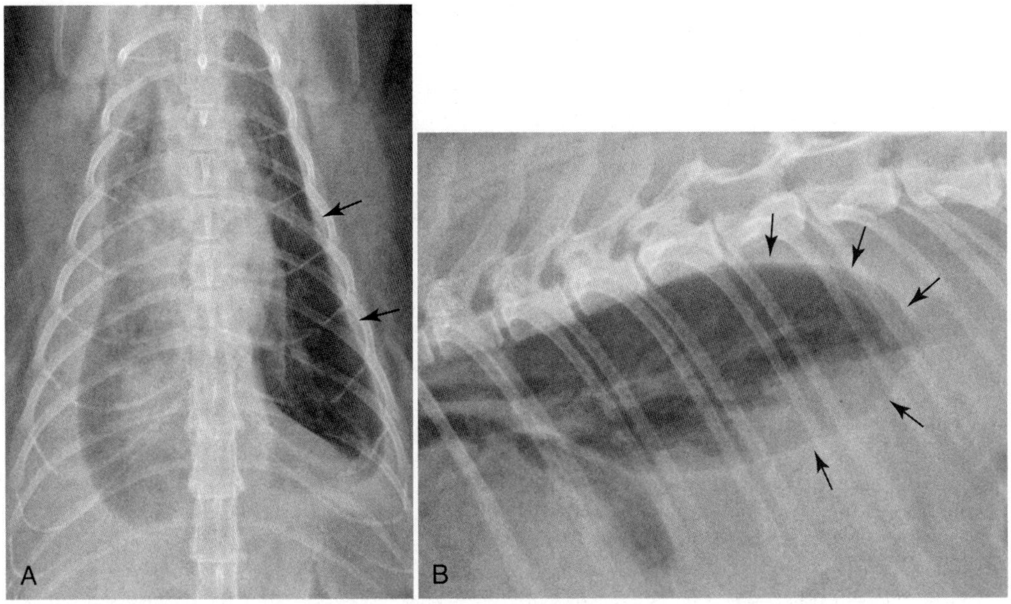

Fig. 34.10 **A,** Ventrodorsal (VD) thoracic radiograph of a cat with asymmetric pleural fluid. There is a small amount of pleural fluid on the left, evidenced by lung retraction (*black arrows*). On the right, there is extensive lung retraction. An asymmetric distribution of pleural fluid such as seen here occurs commonly with an exudate, but any fluid can be asymmetric if the inciting factor is unilateral and mediastinal fenestrations are closed. Ultrasound imaging or computed tomography (CT) would be useful in further characterizing the cause of the unilateral fluid in this patient. Thoracocentesis will also be valuable. **B,** Close-up view of the dorsocaudal aspect of the thorax of the same cat. The retracted lung margin is round rather than having a normal sharp triangular border, indicating pleural fibrosis (*black arrows*). Pleural fibrosis will develop with chronic pleural fluid and will limit the ability of the lung to expand following subsequent fluid removal.

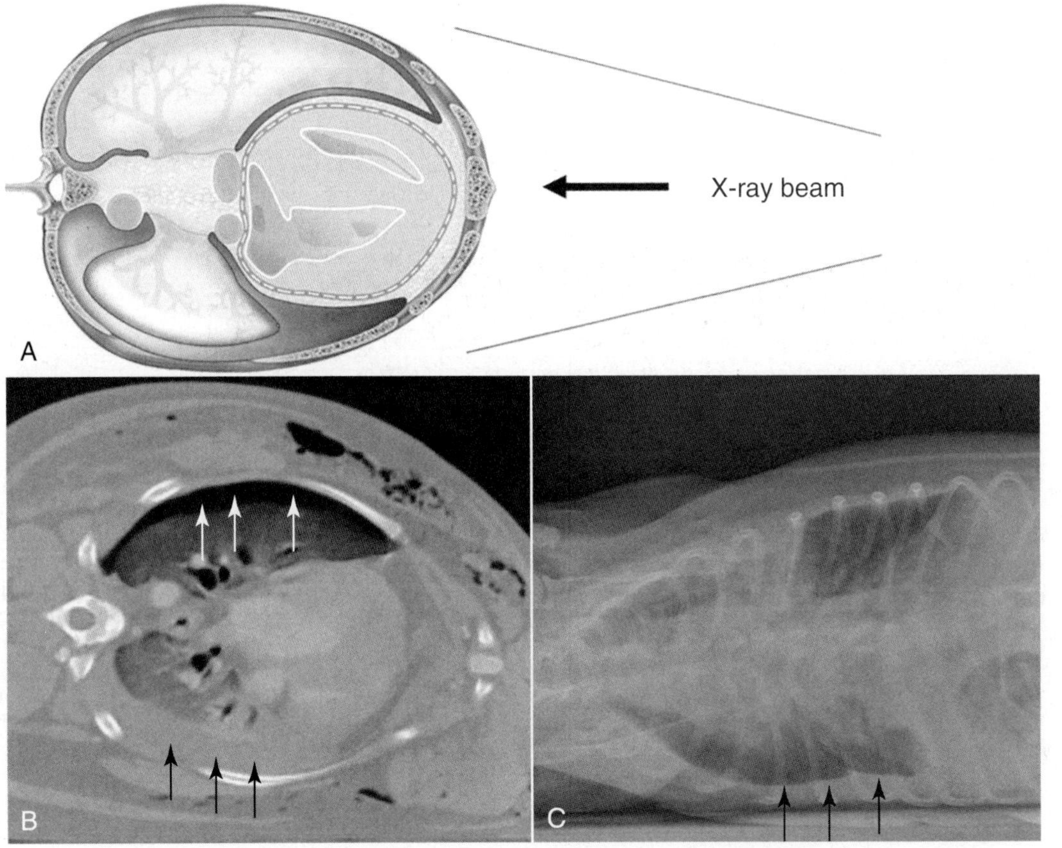

Fig. 34.11 **A,** Drawing illustrating the principle of using a horizontal-beam radiograph to detect pleural fluid. If the mediastinum is complete, fluid in the nondependent hemithorax layers against the mediastinum and is not detectable radiographically. Fluid in the dependent hemithorax, or fluid in the nondependent hemithorax that can move through the mediastinum, gravitates between the lung and the thoracic wall, where the horizontally directed x-ray beam strikes it in a parallel fashion. **B,** Computed tomography (CT) image of a patient with pleural effusion (*black arrows*) and a small amount of pneumothorax (*white arrows*) after trauma. The patient was imaged in lateral recumbency as illustrated in **A**. Pleural fluid accumulates in the dependent thorax whereas free pleural air accumulates in the nondependent thorax. Subcutaneous emphysema is also present. **C,** Horizontal-beam ventrodorsal (VD) thoracic radiograph of a different dog with pleural fluid. The dog was in left lateral recumbency and a horizontally oriented x-ray beam directed onto the sternum. Fluid has pooled against the left thoracic wall causing lung retraction (*black arrows*).

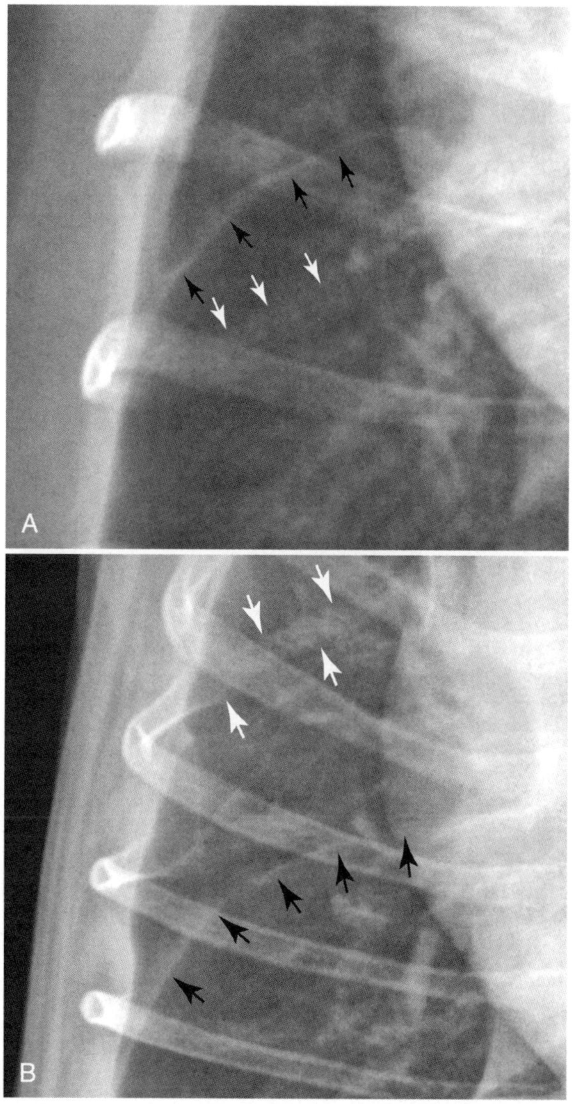

Fig. 34.12 **A and B,** Ventrodorsal (VD) radiographs of two dogs with mild pleural fluid. Interlobar fissures can be seen in each dog; the fissure lines are curving with the caudal aspect of the fissure being concave (*black arrows*). In these dogs, the costal cartilages (*white arrows*) are larger and more linear, and they can be followed laterally to attach to a rib.

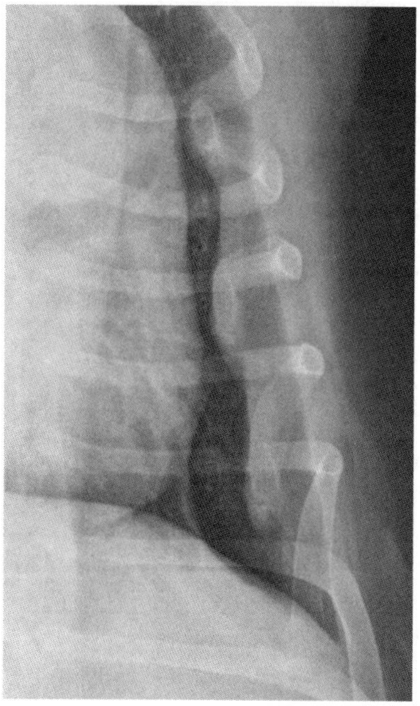

Fig. 34.13 Ventrodorsal (VD) view of the left caudolateral aspect of the thorax of a normal Basset hound. An area of soft tissue opacity is present medial to the left thoracic wall; this is caused by the irregular thoracic wall conformation in this chondrodystrophic dog. The location and appearance of this opacity may result in it being confused with pleural fluid; however, interlobar fissures are not seen and this is a tip-off that this opacity is an artifact.

displacement of the trachea, it remains straight and parallel to the spine whereas mediastinal masses often cause a curved displacement of the trachea. Even large amounts of pleural effusion are not able to caudally displace the cardiac silhouette and carina. Horizontal-beam radiography with the patient in the upright position as well as ultrasonography are useful to differentiate between masses and effusions.

Simultaneous Pleural and Peritoneal Fluid

The detection of simultaneous pleural and peritoneal fluid is an important finding. Of 48 dogs with simultaneous peritoneal and pleural fluid, 32 had either neoplastic or cardiovascular disease. Simultaneous pleural and peritoneal fluid is an indicator of severe disease with poor prognosis.[5]

PNEUMOTHORAX

Causes of Pneumothorax

Air or gas in the pleural space is termed *pneumothorax*. Air can enter the pleural space through a thoracic wall defect or from the lung or mediastinum (Box 34.2). Radiographs should be evaluated for the presence of thoracic wall or mediastinal trauma, and for the presence of cavitary lung lesions. CT imaging is more sensitive for detecting cavitary lesions, and positive pressure ventilation during CT can improve detection of pulmonary bullae.[5,6] In most animals, pneumothorax is bilateral, and this relates either to a bilateral source of pleural air or to movement of air through the mediastinum. When unilateral pneumothorax was induced in 24 dogs, bilateral pneumothorax was observed immediately after air instillation in 22 dogs, indicating rapid movement of air through fenestrations in the mediastinum.[7] Unilateral pneumothorax, however, can occur for the same reasons as for unilateral pleural fluid.

Box • 34.2

Causes of Pneumothorax

- Tear in lung involving visceral pleura
- Thoracic wall rent
- Extension of pneumomediastinum into pleural space
- Rupture of cavitary lung lesion

Radiographic Appearance of Pneumothorax

The character of the radiographic changes resulting from air in the pleural space depends on the volume of air and the relative position of the patient and the x-ray beam. In general, lateral views are more sensitive for detection of pneumothorax than VD or DV views.[8] Roentgen signs of pneumothorax are listed in Box 34.3.

Box • 34.3

Radiographic Signs of Pneumothorax

1. Retraction of pleural surface of lung away from pleural surface of thoracic wall, with interposed radiolucency; lung markings do not extend to thoracic wall
   a. Seen first in lateral radiographs
2. Focal air collection around cardiac apex
3. Appearance of dorsal displacement of the heart
   a. Seen in lateral views

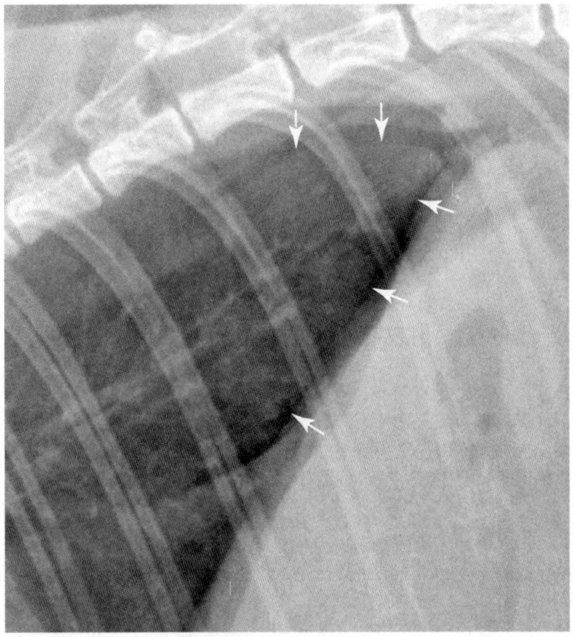

Fig. 34.14 Lateral radiograph of a cat with mild pneumothorax. The air in the nondependent hemithorax collects around the dorsocaudal aspect of the lung, causing the lung to collapse slightly (*white arrows*), creating a thin radiolucency between the lung and thoracic wall.

Lung Retraction From Pneumothorax

With a small volume of pleural air, separation of the lung from the thoracic wall is small and appears as a thin radiolucent line (Fig. 34.14). As in pleural fluid, air surrounds the lung but is most apparent radiographically when the air/lung interface is struck in a parallel fashion by the x-ray beam. The lack of pulmonary vascular markings within the pleural gas allows differentiation from normal air-filled pulmonary parenchyma in many but not all cases. Air-containing interlobar fissures are almost never seen with pneumothorax, because air does not dissect between lung lobes as fluid usually does. A mild pneumothorax may also result in air collection against the cardiac apex. This occurs when the air is trapped against the mediastinum, most often in the dependent hemithorax (Fig. 34.15). With increasing amounts of pleural air, these changes become more pronounced in lateral views, but the changes in the VD or DV view may remain inconspicuous or minimal (Fig. 34.16, eFigs. 34.5 and 34.6). With pronounced pneumothorax, lung collapse is visible in VD or DV radiographs as well, usually best seen in the caudal thorax (Fig. 34.17). The secondary lung collapse leads to the lung becoming more opaque than normal. The degree of increased lung opacity is directly related to the degree of collapse. This increased opacity resulting from atelectasis can interfere with radiographic evaluation of the lung parenchyma. If the pneumothorax is open (i.e., with no valve at the site of air entrance), air may continue to enter the pleural space until pleural pressure equals atmospheric pressure. At this point, the lung is maximally collapsed but still maintains roughly the shape of a normal lung because of its elasticity.

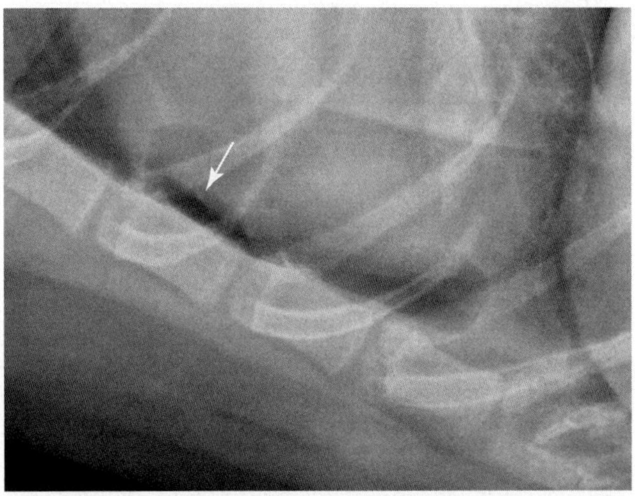

Fig. 34.15 Lateral radiograph of a dog with mild pneumothorax. In this patient, the air is trapped in the dependent hemithorax against the cardiac apex (*white arrow*). There were no regions of lung retraction at the periphery of the thorax in this dog, and this was the only radiographic evidence of pneumothorax.

"Elevation" of the Heart From the Sternum

The appearance of dorsal displacement, or elevation, of the heart from the sternum is seen commonly in lateral radiographs of patients with pneumothorax (see Fig. 34.16). The heart is not actually elevated but displaced into the dependent hemithorax because of a lack of underlying inflated lung to support the heart in its normal midline position. As the heart falls into the dependent hemithorax, it slides dorsally, creating the appearance of elevation on a lateral radiograph (Fig. 34.18). Although pneumothorax is the most common cause of the appearance of elevation of the cardiac silhouette on the lateral view, this can also occur with decreased heart size, in normal dogs with an extremely deep thoracic cavity, in hypovolemic patients, and in patients with hyperinflated lungs (Fig. 34.19).

Tension Pneumothorax

Tension pneumothorax occurs when pleural space pressure exceeds atmospheric pressure during both phases of respiration. Tension pneumothorax results from a check-valve mechanism at the origin of pleural space air. Air enters the thorax with each breath but cannot escape. In tension pneumothorax, increased pleural pressure causes the lung to collapse to a greater degree than even its maximal collapse in an open pneumothorax. Thus, it may no longer maintain the shape of a lung but may assume the appearance of an amorphous opacity compressed against the midline (Fig. 34.20). With unilateral tension pneumothorax, the increased pleural space pressure will cause a contralateral mediastinal shift (Fig. 34.21, eFig. 34.7). Tension pneumothorax may also result in caudal displacement of the diaphragm to the degree that its

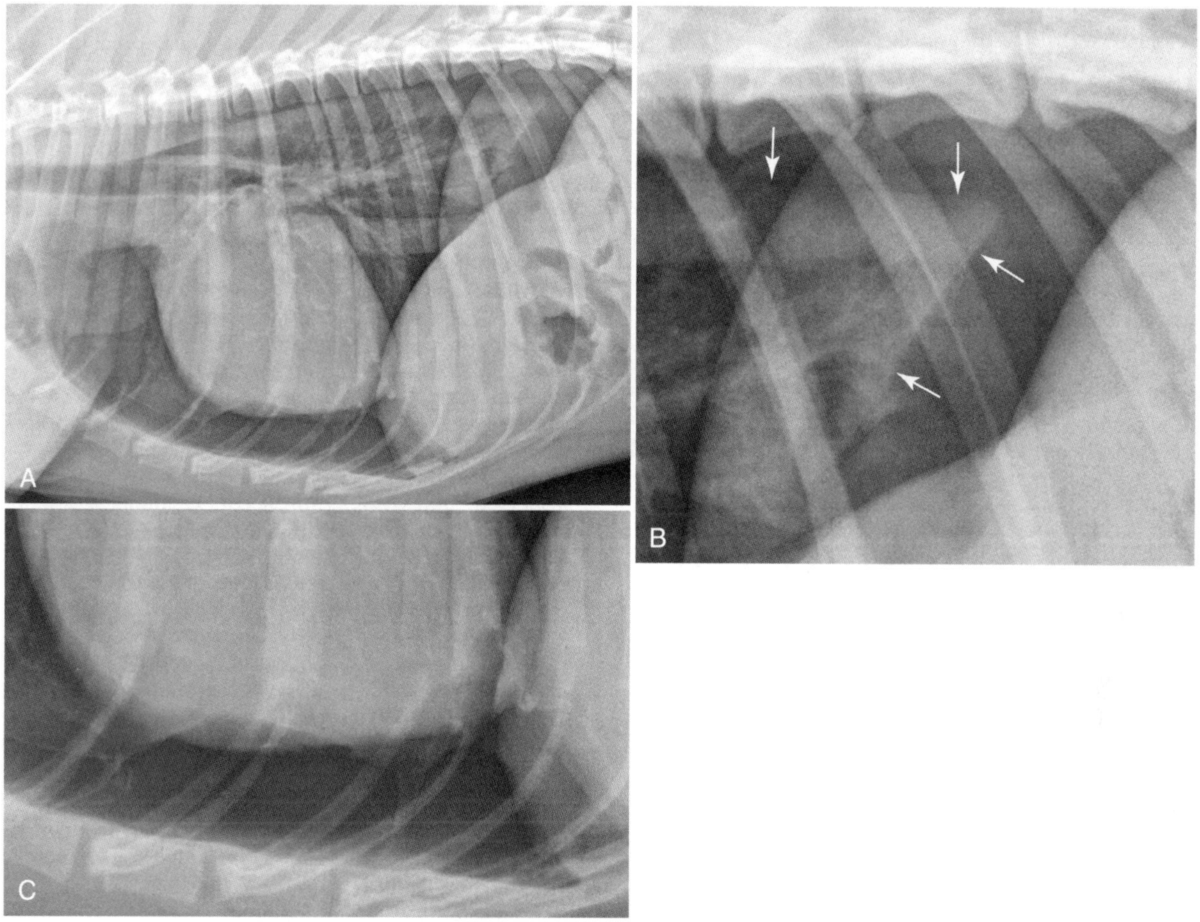

Fig. 34.16 **A,** Left lateral radiograph of a dog with moderate pneumothorax, with close-up views of the dorsocaudal **(B)** and ventral **(C)** aspects of the thorax. There was no evidence of pneumothorax in the ventrodorsal view. **B,** Air in the nondependent hemithorax has risen to the dorsocaudal aspect of the thorax, causing retraction of the caudal lobe from the thoracic wall and diaphragm (*white arrows*). **C,** Secondary atelectasis in the dependent lung allows the heart to slide into the dependent hemithorax, creating a space between the heart and sternum. The air in this region makes this space highly radiolucent.

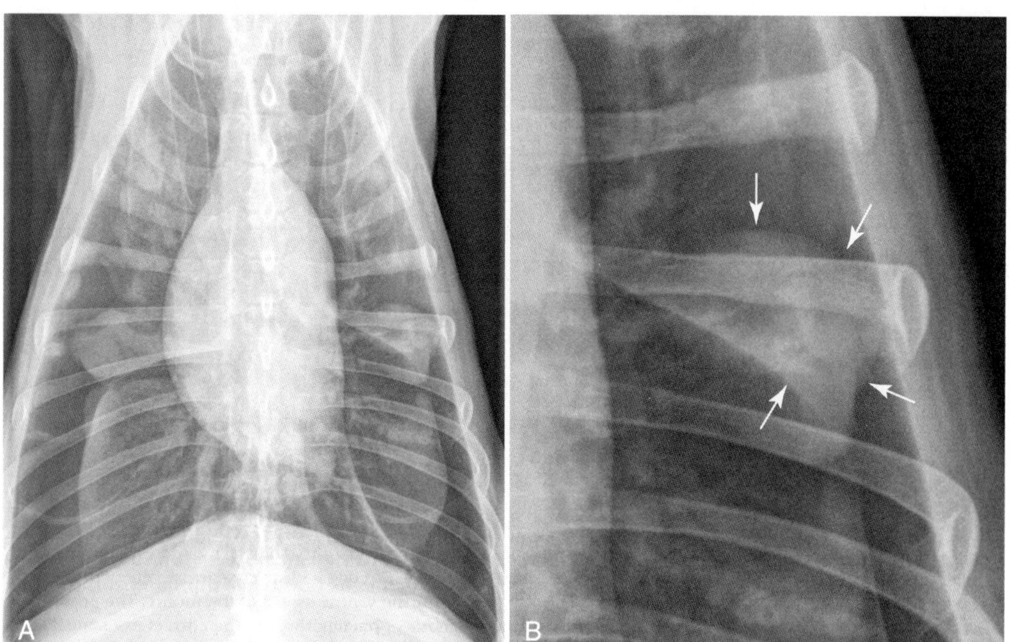

Fig. 34.17 **A,** Ventrodorsal (VD) thoracic radiograph of a dog with a large volume of air in the right and left pleural cavity. The lungs are partially collapsed and therefore of increased radiopacity. **B,** The caudal part of the left cranial lobe is very opaque (*white arrows*); it cannot be determined radiographically whether this is because of atelectasis or pulmonary disease.

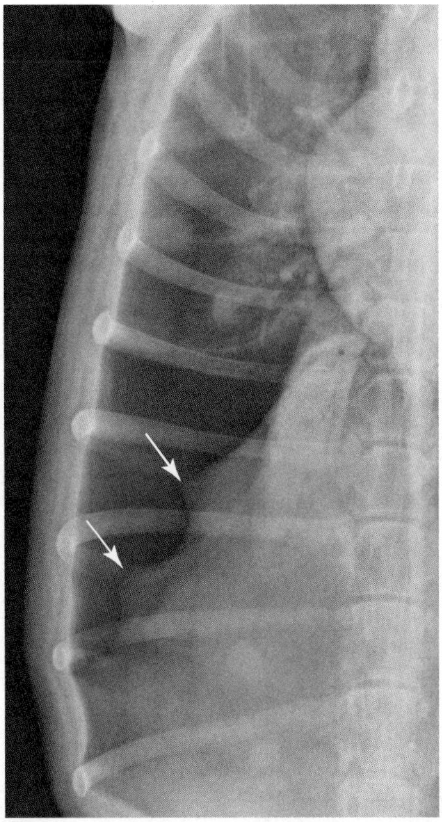

Fig. 34.22 Close-up view of the caudal aspect of the right hemithorax of a dog with tension pneumothorax. The increased pleural space pressure has displaced the right aspect of the diaphragm caudally, causing tension at the costal attachment sites and creating a tented appearance (*white arrows*). Tenting can also occur with pulmonary hyperinflation; but if seen with pneumothorax, it is a reliable sign of tension pneumothorax.

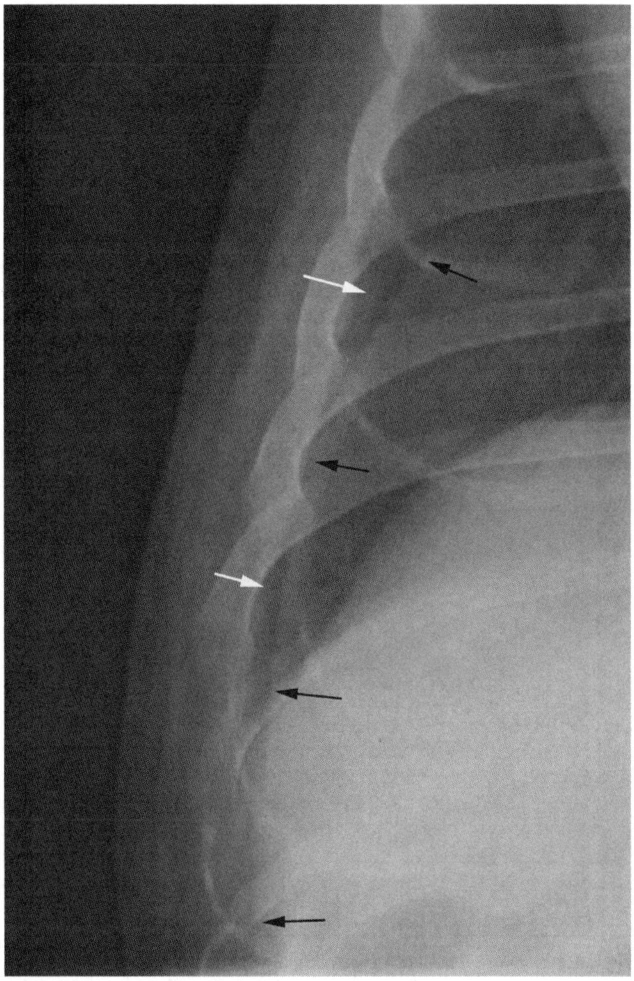

Fig. 34.23 Close-up ventrodorsal (VD) view of the right caudal aspect of the thorax of a dog in which a skin-fold artifact is visible. There is a very radiolucent region just beneath the right thoracic wall with a sharp delineation to a more radiopaque region of the lung that could have the appearance of pneumothorax (*white arrows*). However, faint vascular markings are visible within the more radiolucent region (*white arrows*) and the medial margin of this area is formed by an opaque line that extends caudally beyond the limits of the thoracic cavity (*black arrows*), confirming a skin-fold artifact.

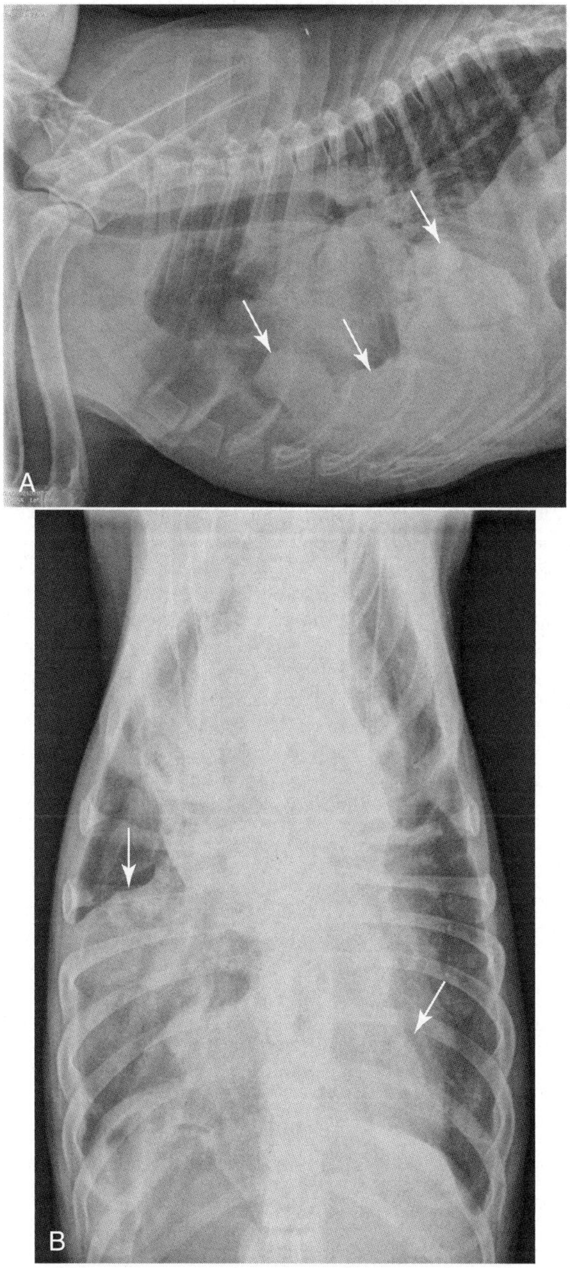

Fig. 34.24 **A,** Left lateral radiograph of a dog with pleural masses suspected to be mesothelioma cytologically. A large lobular soft tissue mass extends to the level of the 5th ribs and silhouettes with the diaphragm caudally (*white arrows*). The mass is outlined by a small amount of free gas in the pleural space. **B,** Dorsoventral radiograph of the same dog. A soft tissue opacity mass fills the right caudal thorax and crosses midline to the left (*white arrows*).

Acknowledgment

With special thanks to prior authors of this chapter for their contributions.

REFERENCES

1. Mendoza P, Giglio RF, Olmo C, Abbott JR, Johnson RD, Berry CR. Anatomic characterization of pulmonary accessory fissures in canine cadavers. *Anat Histol Embryol.* 2019;48(2):157–163. https://doi.org/10.1111/ahe.12424.
2. Woods SJ, Spriet M, Safra N, Cissell DD, Borjesson DL. Hounsfield units are a useful predictor of pleural effusion cytological type in dogs but not in cats. *Vet Radiol Ultrasound Off J Am Coll Vet Radiol Int Vet Radiol Assoc.* 2018;59(4):405–411. https://doi.org/10.1111/vru.12618.
3. Mitrouska I, Klimathianaki M, Siafakas N. Effects of pleural effusion on respiratory function. *Can Respir J.* 2004;11(7):499–503. https://doi.org/10.1155/2004/496901.
4. Groves T, Ticer J. Pleural fluid movement: its effect on appearance of ventrodorsal and dorsoventral radiographic projections. *Vet Radiol Ultrasound.* 1983;24:99.
5. Reetz JA, Caceres AV, Suran JN, Oura TJ, Zwingenberger AL, Mai W. Sensitivity, positive predictive value, and interobserver variability of computed tomography in the diagnosis of bullae associated with spontaneous pneumothorax in dogs: 19 cases (2003–2012). *J Am Vet Med Assoc.* 2013;243(2). https://doi.org/10.2460/javma.243.2.244.
6. Toshima A, Fulkerson CV, Kagawa Y, Murakami M. Positive pressure ventilation computed tomography in dogs with recurrent spontaneous pneumothorax. Abstract ACVR Annual Conference 2022, Reno NV.
7. Kern D, Carrig C, Martin R. Radiographic evaluation of induced pneumothorax in the dog. *Vet Radiol Ultrasound.* 1995;35:411.
8. Aronson E, Reed A. Radiology corner – pneumothorax: ventrodorsal or dorsoventral view. *Vet Radiol Ultrasound.* 36:109.
9. McDonough SP, Scrivani PV, Gendron K, Tse M. Mediastinal serous cavity mesothelioma in two dogs. *J Am Anim Hosp Assoc.* 2022;58(4):194–202. https://doi.org/10.5326/JAAHA-MS-7016.
10. Weston PJ, Baines SJ, Finotello R, Mortier JR. Clinical, CT, and ultrasonographic features of canine and feline pleural and peritoneal carcinomatosis and sarcomatosis. *Vet Radiol Ultrasound Off J Am Coll Vet Radiol Int Vet Radiol Assoc.* 2021;62(3):331–341. https://doi.org/10.1111/vru.12951.
11. Reetz JA, Buza EL, Krick EL. CT features of pleural masses and nodules. *Vet Radiol Ultrasound Off J Am Coll Vet Radiol Int Vet Radiol Assoc.* 2012;53(2):121–127. https://doi.org/10.1111/j.1740-8261.2011.01883.x.
12. Kakkar C, Koteshwara P, Kadavigere R. Round atelectasis. *Lung India.* 2015;32(6):646–647. https://doi.org/10.4103/0970-2113.168105.
13. Woodring JH. Pleural effusion is a cause of round atelectasis of the lung. *J Ky Med Assoc.* 2000;98(12):527–532.
14. Tran DT, Donovan TA, Le Roux A. Computed tomography features of rounded atelectasis in chronic inflammatory pleural effusions in cats and dogs. Abstract ACVR Annual Conference 2022, Reno NV.

ELECTRONIC RESOURCES

Additional information related to the content in Chapter 34 can be found online at eBooks.Health.Elsevier.com.

- Chapter Quiz

CHAPTER 35

Canine and Feline Cardiovascular System

Elodie Huguet • Clifford Berry

INTRODUCTION

High-quality thoracic radiographs are essential for the interpretation of the cardiovascular system. The cardiovascular system in the dog and cat is complex, and basic patterns of recognition are critical for correct radiographic evaluation. Computed tomography (CT) and magnetic resonance imaging (MRI) provide superior spatial and temporal resolution of cardiac structures but are less widely available and require anesthesia or sedation in patients who may be at risk of cardiovascular compromise. Echocardiography is the most practical, safe, and widely used imaging modality for evaluation of cardiovascular morphology and function. While echocardiography is best for assessing the heart, radiographs provide other information, such as vascular status and presence of heart failure. Hence, a comprehensive evaluation of the cardiovascular structures is best routinely achieved with the complementary use of thoracic radiographs and echocardiography.

RADIOGRAPHIC PROJECTIONS AND TECHNICAL CONSIDERATIONS

Three-view thoracic radiographs including right lateral, left lateral, and dorsoventral (DV) and/or ventrodorsal (VD) projections are the standard. For assessment of cardiovascular structures, a DV projection may be preferred to the VD to minimize cardiac magnification and optimize aeration of the caudal lung lobes and caudal lobar pulmonary vasculature. When possible, radiographs should be obtained before echocardiography to avoid atelectasis from prolonged lateral recumbency and wet-hair artefacts due to the presence of gel or alcohol. When positioning the patient for thoracic radiographs, the primary x-ray beam should be centered on the heart to avoid distortion of the cardiovascular structures, and radiographs should be acquired during peak inspiration to avoid atelectasis being misinterpreted as pulmonary disease. The effects of positioning on the appearance of the normal cardiac silhouette and associated vasculature are further discussed in Chapter 28.

INTERPRETATION PARADIGM FOR THE CARDIOVASCULAR STRUCTURES

A systematic evaluation for the thorax is essential. Initially, an interpretation paradigm for the cardiovascular system involves four basic questions related to the various roentgen signs (size, shape, margin, position, number, and opacity) to help formulate a differential diagnosis list, as depicted in Fig. 35.1. These

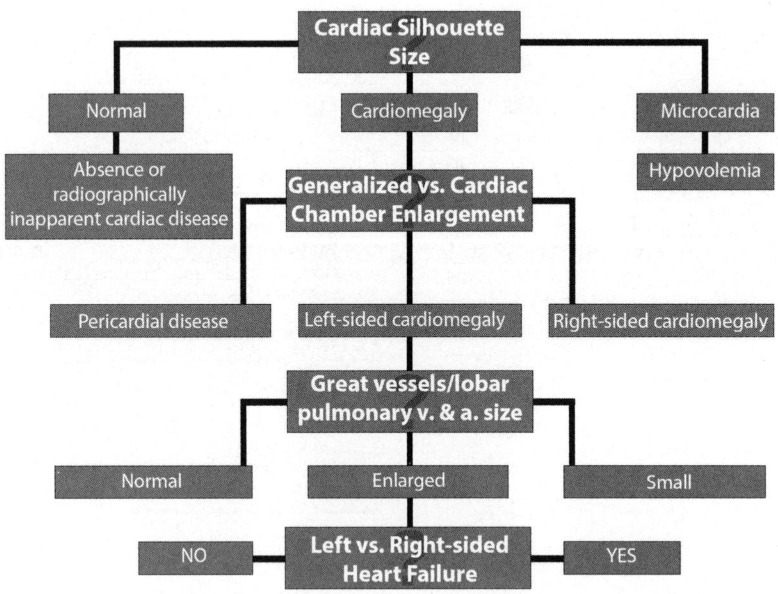

Fig. 35.1 Interpretation paradigm for the cardiovascular system.

questions should be answered in combination with each other to prioritize differential diagnoses. These questions are as follows:

1. Is there a size change of the cardiac silhouette?
2. Is enlargement pericardial disease or localized to the right and/or left cardiac chambers?
3. Are there any changes noted to the great vessels? This is particularly important for the evaluation of the aortic arch and descending thoracic aorta, main pulmonary artery, and the caudal vena cava. Also, are there changes associated with the lobar pulmonary vasculature? If so, is the lobar pulmonary vasculature small or enlarged? If enlarged, are both the pulmonary artery and vein enlarged or is one enlarged relative to the other?
4. Is there radiographic evidence of left- or right-sided congestive heart failure?

EVALUATION OF CARDIAC SILHOUETTE SIZE

Because fluid and soft tissue opacities are radiographically indistinguishable, the heart and pericardial sac are interpreted as a single unit, termed the *cardiac silhouette*. Vascular changes and pericardial disease may also affect cardiac silhouette size and margination. It is also important to keep in mind that absence of cardiomegaly does not exclude the presence of cardiac disease. When evaluating the cardiac silhouette for size, qualitative and quantitative methods are utilized. Comparisons of both methods did not find a significant increase in interpretation accuracy when the quantitative method was used in conjunction with qualitative means of evaluating heart size.[1] A higher confidence level and degree of accuracy may be expected with increased experience and severity of cardiomegaly.[1] In all instances, inherent variations in cardiac silhouette size should be considered between different breeds of dogs. For example, the cardiac silhouette in deep-chested dogs may appear abnormally small, whereas the cardiac silhouette in barrel-chested dogs may look abnormally large (Fig. 35.2A–F). Cats have a more uniform body conformation, which may facilitate the evaluation of feline cardiac silhouette size.[1] The cardiac silhouette in kittens may look enlarged in the absence of disease. Qualitative assessment of cardiac silhouette size is often facilitated by the recognition of specific cardiac chamber enlargement, described in the following section.

Multiple techniques are proposed for the evaluation of cardiac silhouette size. The most common of these is the vertebral heart scale (VHS), which was instituted to take into account the influence of body conformation on the size of the cardiac silhouette.[2] The VHS is obtained by measuring the length of the long and short axes of the heart on a high-quality right lateral radiograph and scaling these measurements against the length of the vertebral bodies starting at T4 to quantify heart size in terms of corresponding vertebral number. Based on 100 clinically normal dogs, the normal mean VHS $\pm$ 2 SD was 9.7 $\pm$ 1 vertebrae. To further reduce variation, VHS measurements specific to particular breeds of dogs have been established and are listed in eTable 35.1. The influence of respiration and the cardiac cycle can affect obtained VHS measurements by up to 1.0 vertebral body length and should be kept in mind when assessing the cardiac silhouette using this method (Video 35.1).[3] Normal VHS measurements (7.5 $\pm$ 0.3 vertebrae) are also available in cats.[4] While the VHS may be a useful adjunct method for the assessment of cardiac silhouette size, it is of particular use for the longitudinal assessment of cardiac disease progression and treatment within an individual patient.

An alternative and more efficient method of assessing the cardiac silhouette size using a heart to single vertebra ratio (HSVR) was recently proposed, taking into account the potential presence of vertebral anomalies, which may affect VHS measurements. Using a similar approach, the length and width

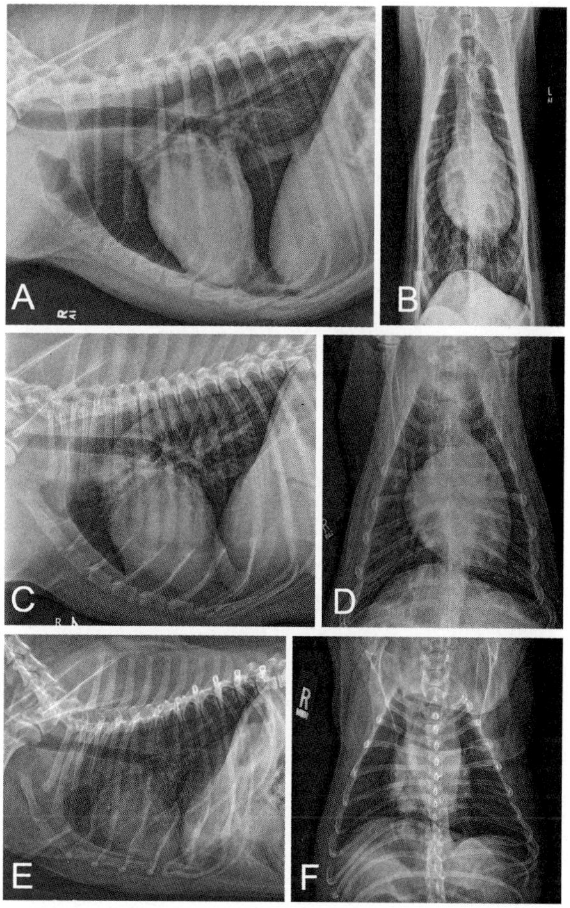

Fig. 35.2 Right lateral and ventrodorsal thoracic radiographs from a normal Borzoi **(A and B)**, a normal Labrador retriever **(C and D)**, and a normal pug **(E and F)**, illustrating the effect of body conformation on the appearance of the cardiac silhouette.

of the cardiac silhouette are measured and added before subtracting from the length of a single morphologically normal vertebra at T4–T8, including the caudal intervertebral disc space.[5] Obtained measurements are comparable to reported normal VHS measurements, although a higher accuracy is reported with HSVR measurements calculated using T7 as a reference vertebra.[5] Other quantitative measurements of cardiac size are proposed and mostly anecdotal (Table 35.1); therefore, these methods should be applied with caution given the lack of research to support their accuracy and unclear effect of patient conformation on obtained measurements.

With advanced age, the long axis of the cardiac silhouette in cats may gradually rotate and be in a plane that is more horizontal to the sternum. Cats with such variation to the orientation of their cardiac silhouette are said to have a "lazy heart." When obtaining measurements of the cardiac silhouette in older cats, the orientation of the cardiac silhouette should be taken into consideration. Additionally, the aortic arch may be enlarged and redundant in older cats, as characterized by the presence of a bulge at the cranial aspect of the cardiac silhouette (e.g., aortic knob). While these findings commonly represent normal age variants, systemic hypertension and hyperthyroidism may also be contributing factors.[6]

Microcardia is sometimes identified on thoracic radiographs in dogs and cats, and is rarely associated with primary cardiac disease. Rather, microcardia is primarily indicative of hypovolemia with reduced circulating cardiovascular volume from dehydration, blood loss, or hypoadrenocorticism (Fig. 35.3A,B).[7] Radiographically, the cardiac silhouette becomes abnormally

Table • **35.1**

Additional Quantitative Methods for the Assessment of Cardiac Silhouette Size.

DOGS			
Lateral projections	Height of cardiac silhouette/dorsoventral height of thoracic cavity	<2/3 at the same level	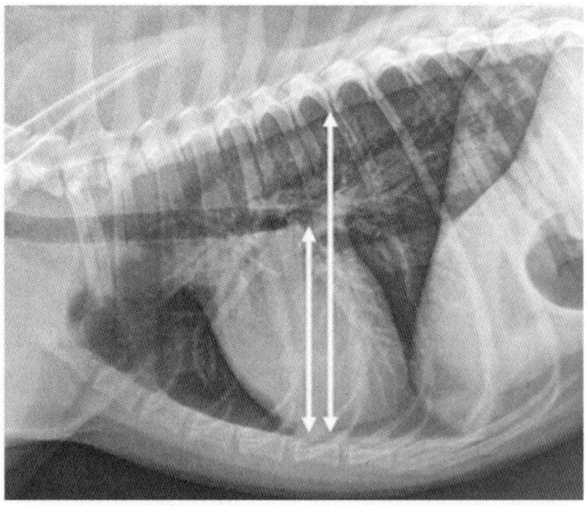
	Cardiac silhouette width to number of equivalent intercostal spaces*	2.5–3.5	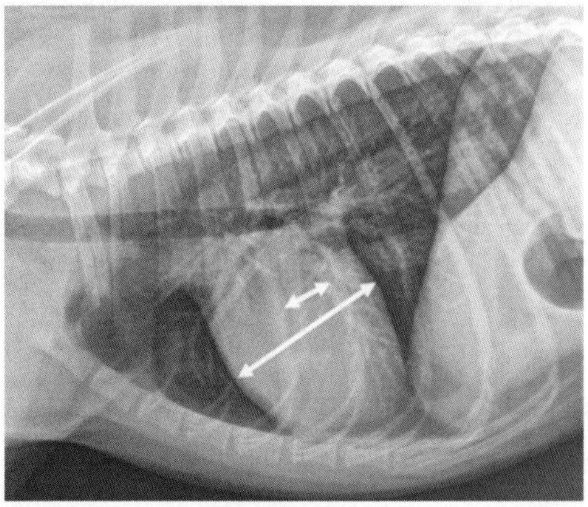
Ventrodorsal/Dorsoventral projections	Maximal width of the cardiac silhouette/width of the thoracic cavity	<1/2 at ninth rib <2/3 at the same level	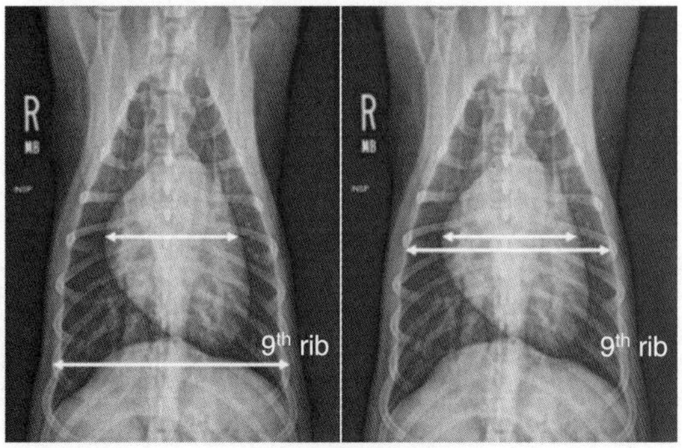
CATS			
Lateral projections	Cardiac silhouette width to number of equivalent intercostal spaces*	2–3	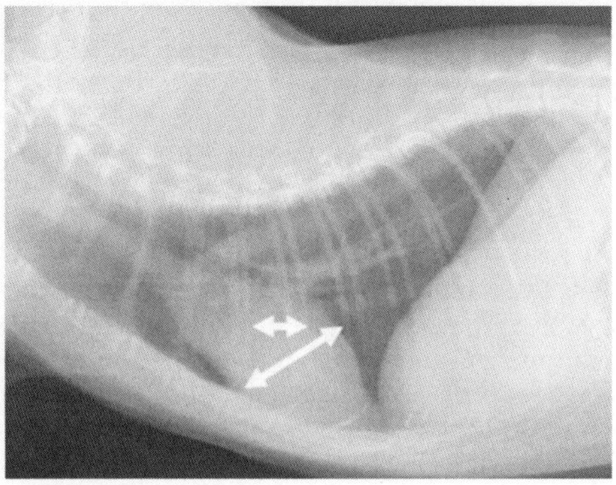

Continued

Table • 35.1

***Additional Quantitative Methods for the Assessment of Cardiac Silhouette Size.*—cont'd**

Ventrodorsal/ Dorsoventral projections	Maximal width of the cardiac silhouette/width of the thoracic cavity	<1/2	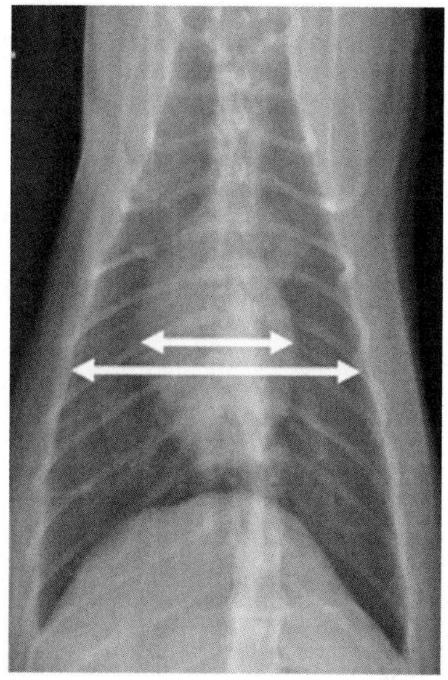

*Width is the measurement obtained at the widest point perpendicular to the long axis of the cardiac silhouette.

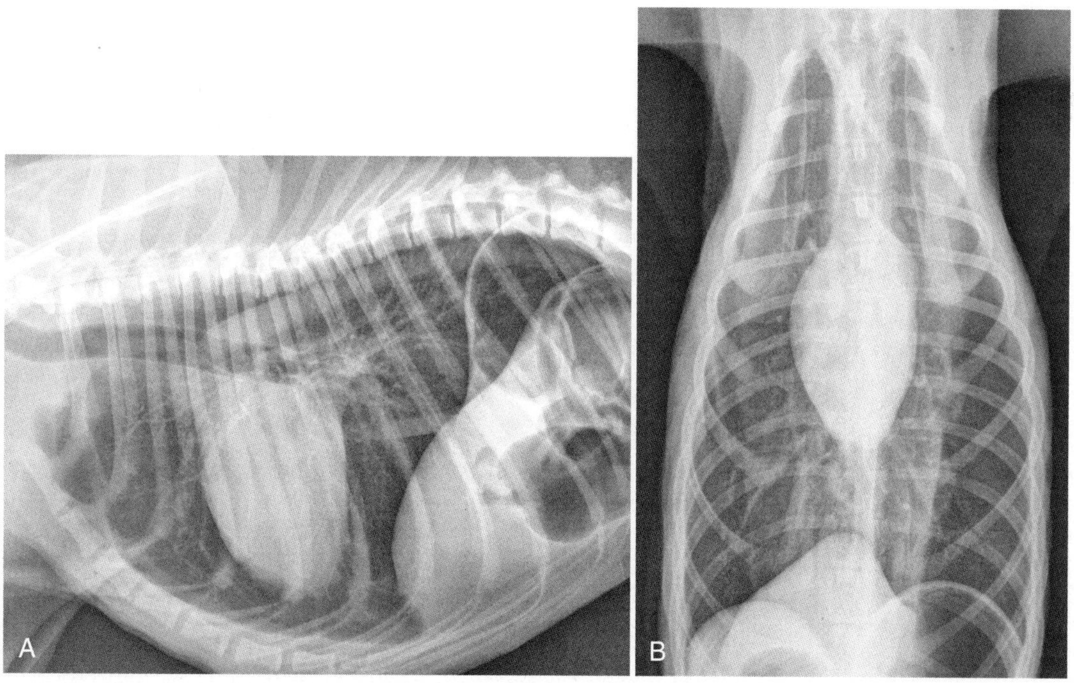

Fig. 35.3 Lateral **(A)** and ventrodorsal **(B)** radiographs of a dog with hypovolemia secondary to hypoadrenocorticism. The cardiac silhouette is small and subsequently elevated from the sternum. The lobar pulmonary vessels and the caudal vena cava are thinned. The lungs are hyperlucent with the false impression of increased lung volume secondary to the microcardia.

small in size with normal margins. The lobar pulmonary vasculature will often be concurrently thinned with subsequent diffuse hyperlucency of the lungs. The caudal vena cava may also be undercirculated with increased severity and will be persistently narrowed.

SPECIFIC PATTERNS OF CARDIAC CHAMBER ENLARGEMENT

Because individual cardiac chambers, sites of great vessel emergence/convergence, and the pericardium are radiographically indistinguishable, evaluation of the cardiac silhouette margins is essential to localize alterations to specific cardiac chambers or the great vessels in the dog based on their relative positioning. For this purpose, a "clock face" analogy is commonly used to correlate alterations to the cardiac silhouette at specific sites to corresponding anatomical cardiovascular structures on both lateral and VD/DV projections (Fig. 35.4A,B). The positioning of the feline heart and subtlety of specific cardiac chamber enlargement on thoracic radiographs limits the use of this approach in cats.

Left Atrium

Enlargement of the left atrium is the most frequently encountered cardiac enlargement in the dog due to the high prevalence of myxomatous mitral valve disease. On lateral projections, enlargement of the left atrium in the dog causes bulging of the dorsocaudal margin of the cardiac silhouette at the 12–2 o'clock position. The caudal border is subsequently flattened to mildly concave, resulting in a loss of the caudal "cardiac waist" (Fig. 35.5). On the VD/DV projection, this bulge corresponds to a rounded focal region of increased soft tissue opacity caudal to the tracheal bifurcation. Superimposition and summation of the enlarged left atrium over the cardiac silhouette can create the appearance of a double wall due to distinction of both the caudal border of the left atrium and cardiac silhouette (Fig. 35.6A,B).

With left atrial enlargement, splaying of the principal bronchi may be observed on the VD/DV projections (Figs. 35.7 and 35.8A,B). Similar splaying of the principal bronchi may occur secondary to tracheobronchial lymphadenopathy but this typically causes ventral displacement of the tracheal bifurcation in lateral views (see Chapter 33). In contrast, left atrial enlargement typically causes dorsal displacement of the tracheal bifurcation. Some dogs with a dorsally displaced

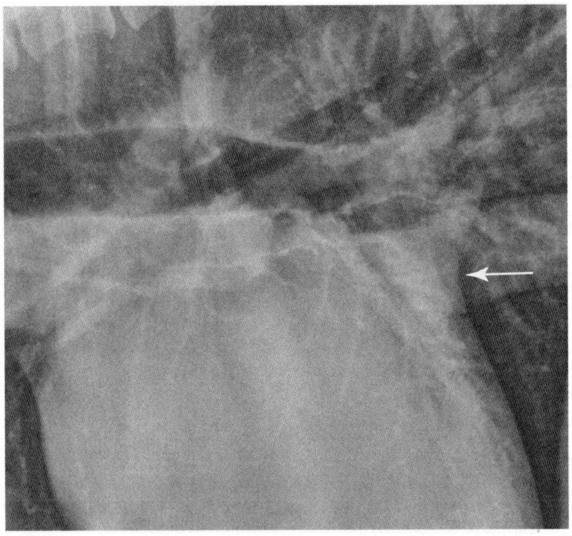

Fig. 35.5 Lateral radiograph of a dog with an enlarged left atrium. Along the caudodorsal aspect of the cardiac silhouette, in the region of the left atrium at the 12–2 o'clock position, a bulge is identified and is associated with concavity of cardiac silhouette margin caudally (*white arrow*).

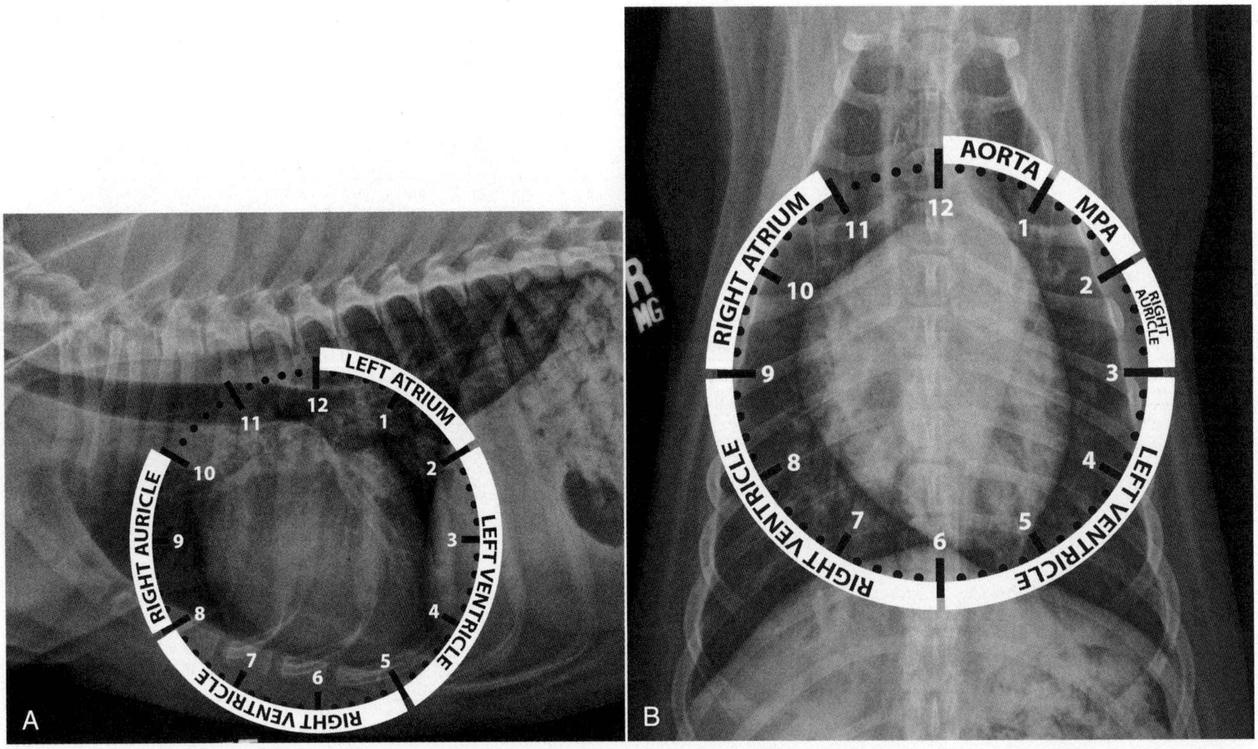

Fig. 35.4 Lateral **(A)** and ventrodorsal **(B)** projections centered on the cardiac silhouette illustrating the clockface analogy for the localization of individual cardiac chambers are sites of emergence or convergence of the great vessels.

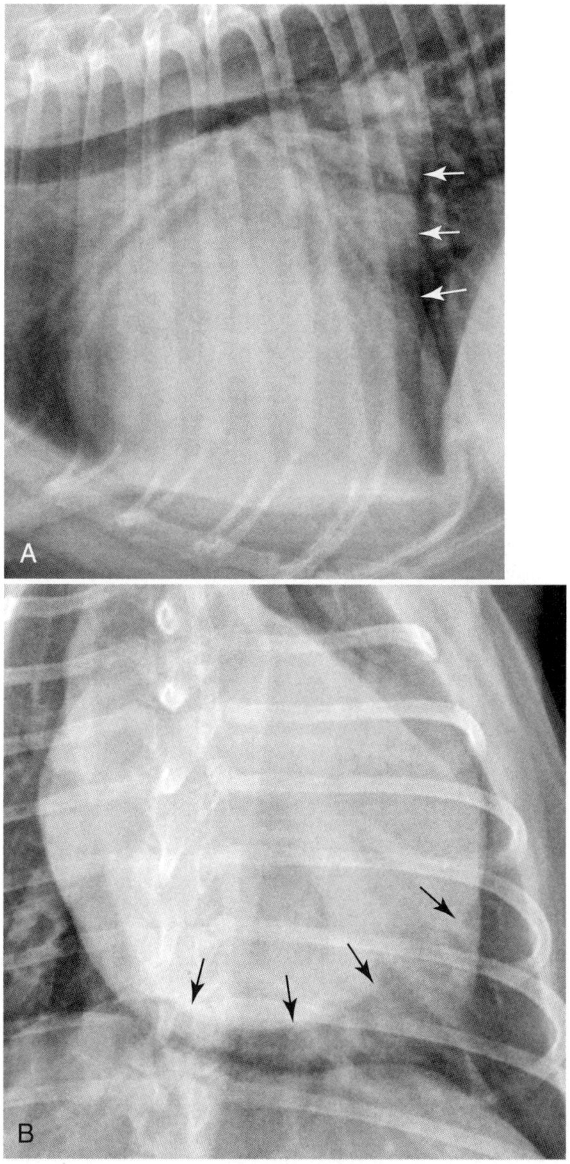

Fig. 35.6 Lateral **(A)** and dorsoventral **(B)** projections of a dog with severe left atrial enlargement. On the lateral projection **(A)**, a large bulge is seen along the caudodorsal aspect of the cardiac silhouette with associated concavity of the caudal cardiac silhouette margin (*white arrows*). On the dorsoventral projection **(B)**, the enlarged left atrium corresponds to a focal region of increased soft tissue opacity (*black arrows*) superimposed on the remainder of the heart with a caudal margin separate from the caudal margin of the cardiac silhouette, resulting in a double wall appearance.

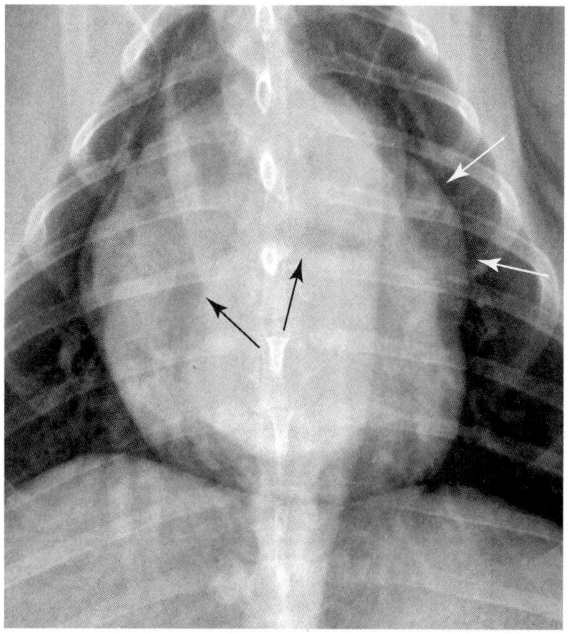

Fig. 35.7 Dorsoventral projection of a dog with pronounced left atrial dilation. The enlarged left atrium has caused abaxial displacement of the principal bronchi (*black arrows*). There is also a bulge on the left aspect of the cardiac silhouette that is consistent with left auricular enlargement (*white arrows*).

tracheal bifurcation will also have narrowing of the left principal bronchus (see Fig. 35.8A,B). A compressive effect on the left and right principal bronchi has been described in the presence of left atrial enlargement due to the spatial relationship between the vertebral column, aorta, left principal bronchus, and left atrium.[8] While the bronchial narrowing may be attributed to direct impingement from the adjacent enlarged left atrium, coexisting bronchomalacia may facilitate this process as a result of altered bronchial wall integrity and/or cause bronchial collapse (Video 35.2).[9] Coughing in dogs with left atrial enlargement is common and can be attributed to tracheal narrowing versus pulmonary edema.[9,10] The absence of cough receptors within the alveoli and interstitium is a likely explanation; however, in dogs, coughing is to be expected in the presence of large amounts of cardiogenic pulmonary edema infiltrating into the larger bronchial structures.[9] Therefore, causes of a cough other than heart failure should always be considered in dogs with a heart murmur. In cats, coughing due to pulmonary edema is very uncommon.

Enlargement of the left auricle is less readily identified than left atrial enlargement and is most prevalent when a higher degree of left atrial enlargement is present. On the VD/DV projection, enlargement of the left auricle may create a focal bulge along the left cardiac border in the 2–3 o'clock position (see Fig. 35.7).

While left atrial enlargement is most commonly evaluated subjectively, the vertebral left atrial size (VLAS) can be used to quantify left atrial enlargement in dogs with good repeatability.[11,12] On either a left or right lateral projection, VLAS indexes are obtained by measuring the distance from the mid ventral aspect of the carina to the most caudal margin of the left atrium at the intersection with the dorsal border of the caudal vena cava. This measurement is transposed to the vertebral column, starting at the cranial margin of T4, to count the equivalent vertebral body number.[13] In 80 healthy dogs, the normal medial VLAS was 1.9 with a reference interval of 1.4 to 2.2.[12] A cutoff value of $\geq$2.3 may support a diagnosis of left atrial enlargement in dogs.[12,13]

Left atrial enlargement in cats is much less conspicuous, and in many cats there are no radiographic changes. In some instances, a bulge may be observed along the caudodorsal margin of the cardiac silhouette and is associated with concavity of the caudal margin (Fig. 35.9). Left atrial enlargement in the cat is also associated with an increase in width of the cardiac silhouette in the region of the cardiac base on the VD/DV projections. In the presence of marked left atrial enlargement, the cardiac silhouette may be "valentine shaped" (Fig. 35.10). While a "valentine-shaped" cardiac silhouette may be associated with the presence of biatrial enlargement, it is most often observed with left atrial enlargement alone.[14]

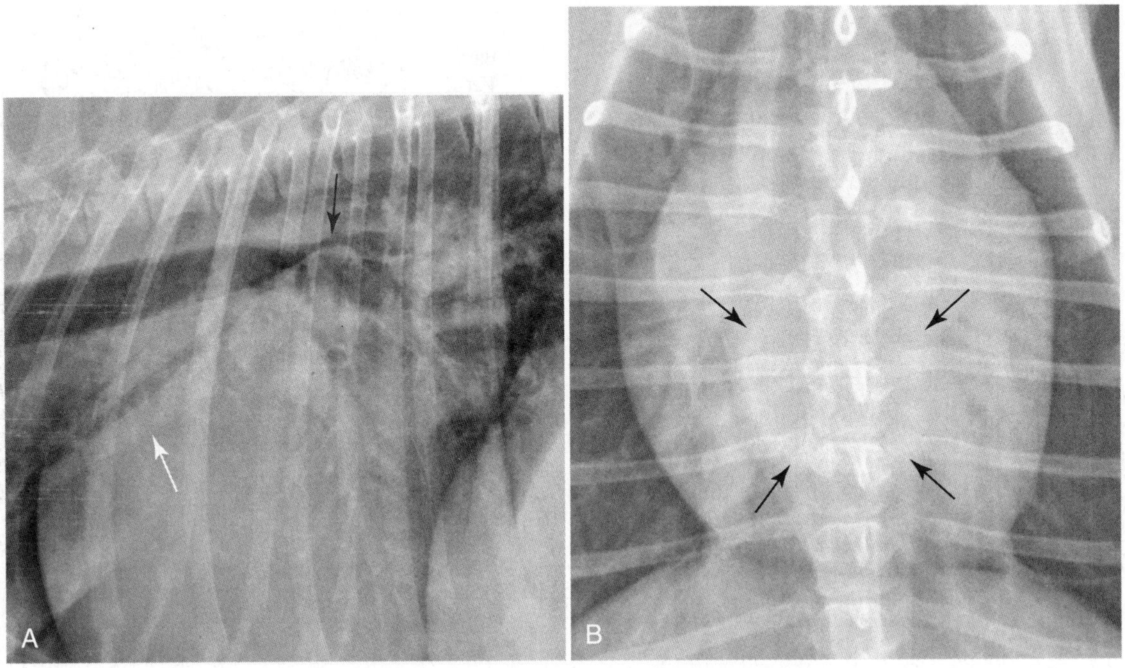

Fig. 35.8 Lateral **(A)** and dorsoventral **(B)** projections of a dog with marked left atrial enlargement. In **A,** there is dorsal displacement of the trachea and narrowing of the left principal bronchus (*black arrow*). The left cranial lobe pulmonary vein is also distended (*white arrow*) compared with the corresponding artery, consistent with pulmonary venous hypertension secondary to mitral insufficiency. In **B,** the dilated left atrium represents a region of increased soft tissue opacity caudal to the tracheal bifurcation (*black arrows*) causing splaying of the principal bronchi.

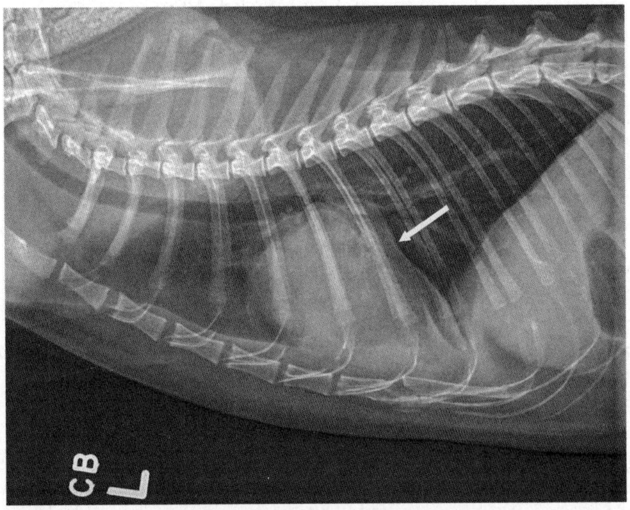

Fig. 35.9 Lateral projection of a cat with left atrial enlargement. A concave depression is present along the caudodorsal margin of the cardiac silhouette (*white arrow*), similar to that seen in many dogs. This is less commonly observed in cats with left atrial dilation than in dogs but is occasionally seen.

Left Ventricle

In both cats and dogs, concentric hypertrophy of the ventricular wall is most commonly seen as a response to pressure overload and mainly occurs at the expense of lumen volume. Therefore, the cardiac margins in the left ventricular region will often maintain a normal contour. In comparison, eccentric hypertrophy is mostly seen in compensation to volume overload and can result in radiographically detectable left

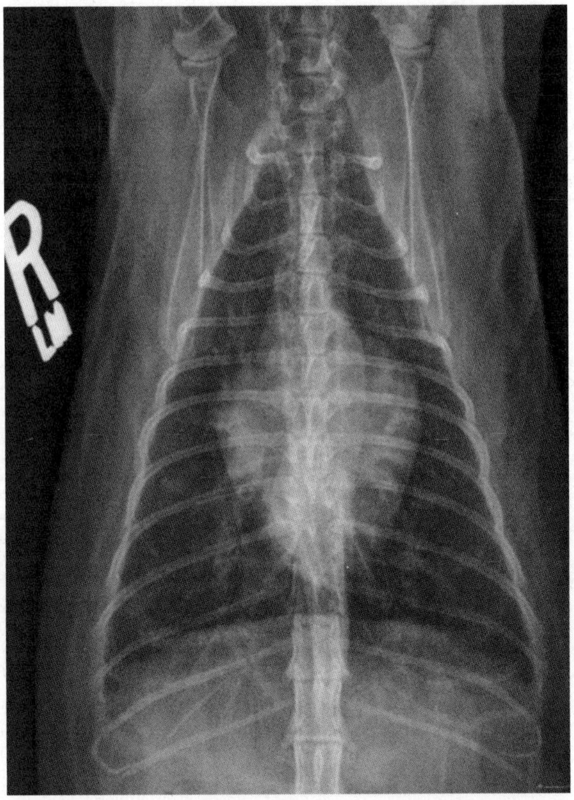

Fig. 35.10 Dorsoventral projection of a cat with marked enlargement of the left atrium. The cardiac silhouette is increased in width in the base region (*black arrows*) and is therefore referred to being "valentine shaped."

ventricular enlargement. In more severe cases of left ventricular enlargement, possibly exacerbated by the concurrent presence of left atrial enlargement, the cardiac silhouette may be increased in apical to basilar length with subsequent dorsal displacement of the trachea at the level of the carina. On VD/DV projections, the cardiac apex may have a rounded contour and may be displaced to the right.

Enlargement of the left ventricle is a likely response to chronically increased preload and may decompensate into left-sided congestive heart failure

Right Atrium

Right atrial enlargement is uncommonly isolated as an independent entity, especially in cats, but may be occasionally seen in dogs with tricuspid dysplasia. Interpretation of right atrial enlargement is supported by the concurrent presence of a bulge at the 9–11 o'clock position along the cardiac silhouette on the VD/DV projection (Fig. 35.11A,B). Enlargement of the right auricle may be associated with a soft tissue bulge along the cranial margin of the cardiac silhouette on the lateral projections. Nonspecific enlargement of the cardiac silhouette may be seen in cats with right atrial enlargement and is usually associated with other cardiac chamber changes.

Right Ventricle

Similar to the left ventricle, the right ventricle may enlarge as a result of both concentric and eccentric hypertrophy. Isolation of right ventricular enlargement in cats is very rare. The right ventricle undergoes concentric hypertrophy in response to pressure overload, as with pulmonic stenosis or pulmonary hypertension, as with heartworm disease. Hypertrophy mainly occurs at the expense of lumen volume and may lead to no or minimal change in the appearance of the cardiac silhouette. On lateral projections, rounding of the cardiac margin in the 5–8 o'clock position may be seen and associated with dorsal displacement or elevation of the cardiac apex from the sternum (Fig. 35.12B,C). On the VD/DV projections, this is further supported by rounding of the cardiac silhouette in the 6–9 o'clock position with an associated leftward apical shift, giving the cardiac silhouette a pronounced "reversed-D" shape (see Fig. 35.12A).

Care should be taken to not over-read the more rounded appearance of the cranial and right lateral margins of the cardiac silhouette as it may be artefactual on expiratory radiographs or may represent a normal variation in some breed of dogs, such as brachycephalic dogs. Additionally, the cranial and right lateral margins of the cardiac silhouette may be rounded in the presence of severe left-sided cardiomegaly due to morphological distortion of cardiac anatomy from the severe left atrial and ventricular enlargement.[15] A more rounded appearance of the right margin of the cardiac silhouette and leftward displacement of the cardiac silhouette may be seen on DV projections when compared to VD projections.

Generalized Cardiomegaly

A generalized enlargement of the cardiac silhouette without apparent cardiac chamber enlargement should raise concerns for pericardial disease in both dogs and cats. With generalized cardiomegaly, the heart occupies a larger portion of the thoracic cavity while maintaining smooth and rounded margins on all projections. The rounded shape of the cardiac silhouette is commonly referred to as being "globoid" in appearance. The cardiac margins may also be better defined due to separation of

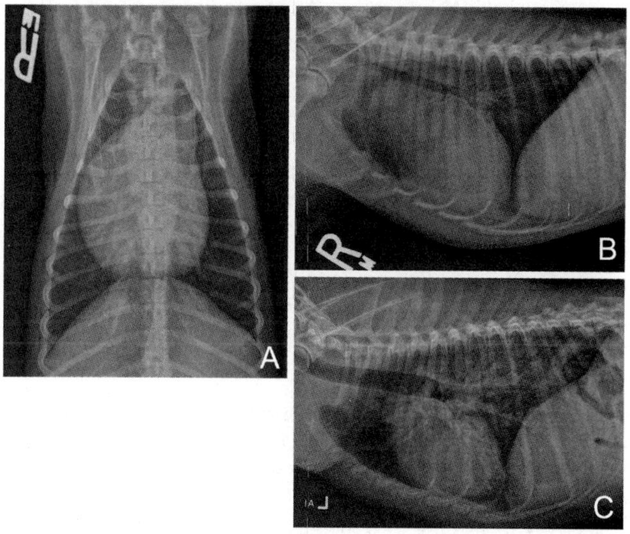

Fig. 35.12 Ventrodorsal (**A**) and right lateral (**B**) projections of a dog with pulmonic stenosis and right ventricular hypertrophy, and left lateral projection of a dog with heartworm disease (**C**). In **A**, the right lateral margin of the cardiac silhouette is moderately rounded with leftward displacement of the cardiac apex and a reversed-D appearance of the cardiac silhouette. Enlargement of the main pulmonary artery is also visible and correlated with a bulge at the 1–2 o'clock position along the cardiac silhouette. In **B**, the right ventricle correlates to rounding of the cranioventral margin of the cardiac silhouette. Similar rounding of the cranioventral margin of the cardiac silhouette is seen in **C** and is associated with increased elevation of the cardiac apex from the sternum.

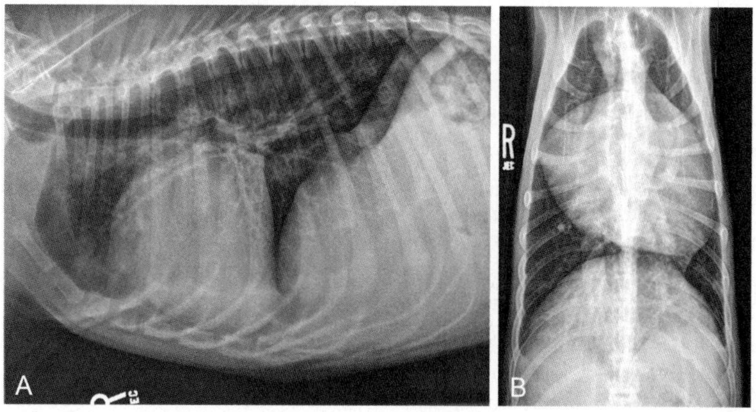

Fig. 35.11 Right lateral (**A**) and dorsoventral (**B**) projections of a Doberman pinscher with tricuspid dysplasia. A bulge is visible in the region of the right atrium consistent with right atrial enlargement.

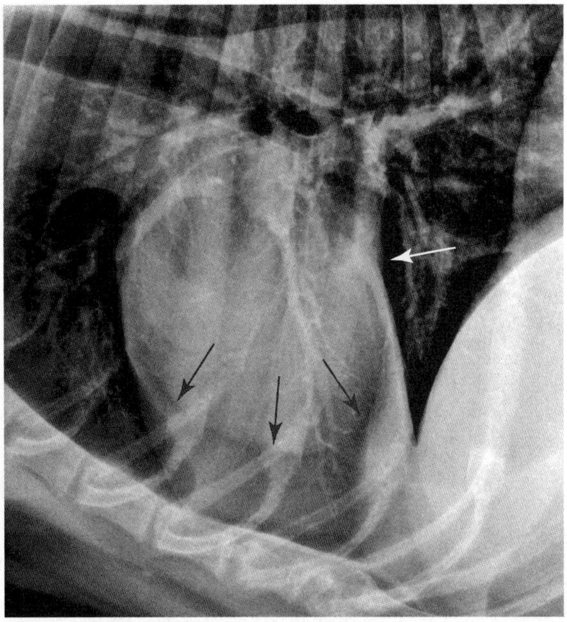

Fig. 35.13 Lateral projection of a Doberman pinscher. The presence of fat in the pericardium results in a generalized enlargement of the cardiac silhouette. The less opaque fat creates contrast for visualization of the actual margin of the heart (*black arrows*). This dog also has left atrial enlargement, as characterized by the presence of a bulge along the caudodorsal aspect of the cardiac silhouette associated with concavity of the cardiac silhouette margin caudodorsally (*white arrow*).

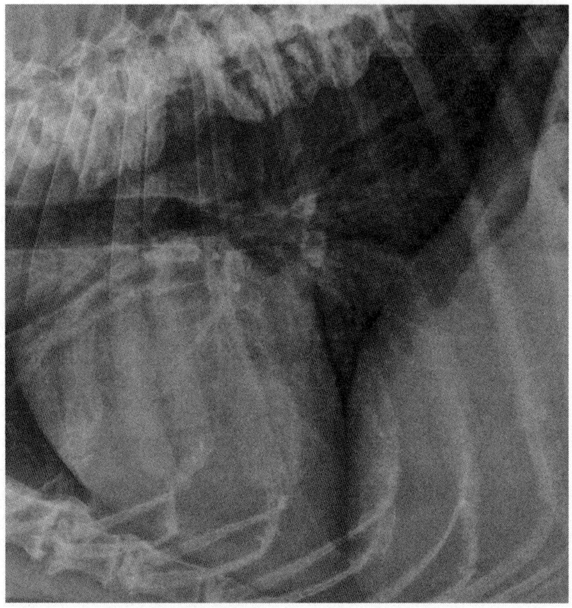

Fig. 35.14 Right lateral projection of a dog with kinking of the caudal vena cava, presumed to be recumbency dependent in the absence of apparent cardiovascular disease and neoplasia.

the pericardium from the cardiac margins and reduced motion artefacts. If the cardiac structures maintain a homogeneous soft tissue opacity, pericardial effusion should be considered, keeping in mind the heart may have an enlarged and rounded appearance due to the presence of increased pericardial fat in dogs and cats (Fig. 35.13). On the other hand, if the opacity of the cardiac silhouette is heterogeneous, especially with continuity of the cardiac silhouette and ventral aspect of the diaphragm, a peritoneopericardial diaphragmatic hernia should be considered.

Obtaining high-quality radiographs on peak inspiration is important for the assessment of cardiomegaly as a decrease in thoracic volume is observed with pulmonary underinflation and the cardiac silhouette may subsequently appear larger relative to the amount of aerated lung surrounding it (see Chapter 28).

SPECIFIC PATTERNS OF GREAT VESSEL ENLARGEMENT

Caudal Vena Cava

The caudal vena cava is variable in size depending on the phase of respiration and cardiac cycle. The caudal vena cava size is commonly assessed subjectively for size; however, the normal caudal vena cava should be less than 1.5 times the diameter of the descending aorta.[16,17] The caudal vena cava can enlarge in response to increased central venous pressure, but the size of the caudal vena cava is not an accurate way to evaluate central venous pressure. Valid inferences on cardiovascular disease cannot typically be made based on the size of the caudal vena cava only.

Kinking of the caudal vena cava is occasionally observed on lateral projections in dogs and may represent a recumbency-dependent change due to a positional shift of the cardiovascular structures, or an association with trauma, cardiovascular disease, or neoplasia (Fig. 35.14).[17,18] While kinking of the caudal vena cava may be a primary cause for postsinusoidal obstruction of venous flow (e.g., Budd-Chiari syndrome), it may also represent a secondary change seen in response to crowding of the caudal intrathoracic structures from cardiomegaly and/or an increase in intra-abdominal pressure, such as secondary to peritoneal effusion or organomegaly/presence of a mass.[17,18]

Narrowing of the caudal vena cava is primarily seen with hypovolemia and is commonly identified in conjunction with microcardia. The caudal vena cava may be intermittently narrowed with the phase of the cardiac cycle; therefore, a diagnosis is best supported by persistent narrowing of the caudal vena cava on both lateral projections (see Fig. 35.3A,B).

Aorta

Widening of the cranial and middle mediastinum in proximity to the heart base can indicate dilation of the aortic arch in both dogs and cats. On the VD/DV projections, a focal bulge in the descending aorta is suggestive of aortic dilation, as seen in patients with aortic stenosis and patent ductus arteriosus, and may correlate with an increase in soft tissue opacity at the cranial aspect of the cardiac silhouette on lateral projections (Fig. 35.15A,B). In older cats, redundancy of the aortic arch and tortuosity of the descending aorta are described to likely represent a normal age variant although systemic hypertension and hyperthyroidism may also contribute (Fig. 35.16A).[6] On the VD/DV projections, the aorta is occasionally projected end-on within the left side of the mediastinum and should not be misinterpreted as a pulmonary nodule (see Fig. 35.16B).[6]

Main Pulmonary Artery

Under normal conditions, the main pulmonary artery cannot be delineated on evaluation of the cardiac silhouette. In the presence of main pulmonary artery enlargement, a bulge at the 1–2 o'clock position in the region of the main pulmonary artery may be isolated on VD/DV projections (Fig. 35.17). With increased severity, the trachea may be displaced to the right at the level of the heart base. An increase in soft tissue opacity may also be

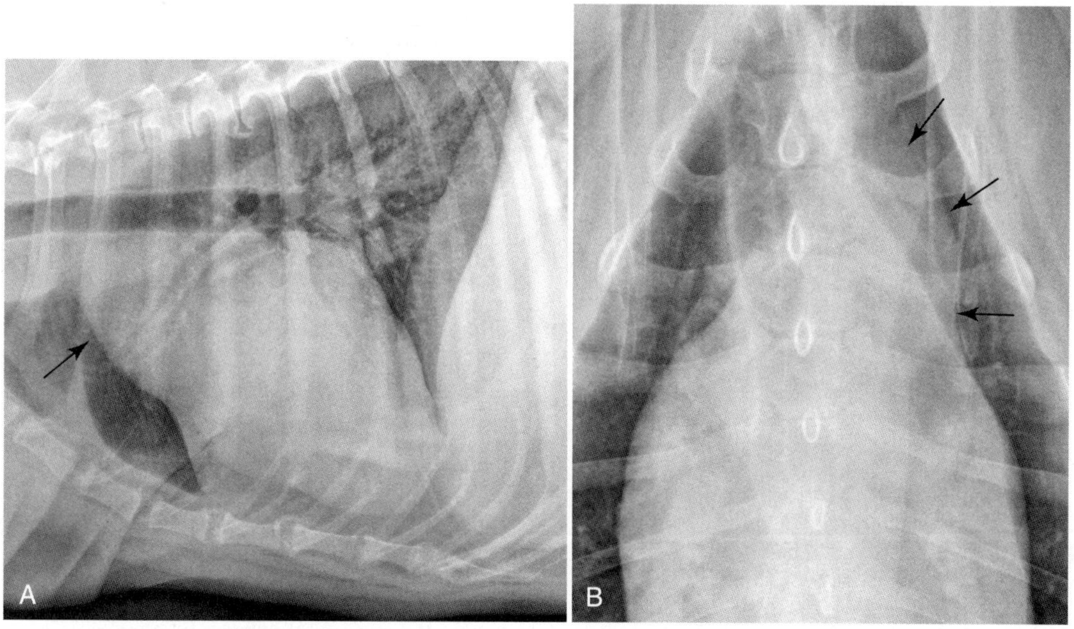

Fig. 35.15 Lateral **(A)** and dorsoventral **(B)** projections of a dog with aortic stenosis. In **A,** the dilated aortic arch represents a bulge on the craniodorsal aspect of the cardiac silhouette (*black arrow*). In **B,** the enlarged aortic arch is seen bulging at the cranial, and slightly left, aspect of the cardiac silhouette (*black arrows*).

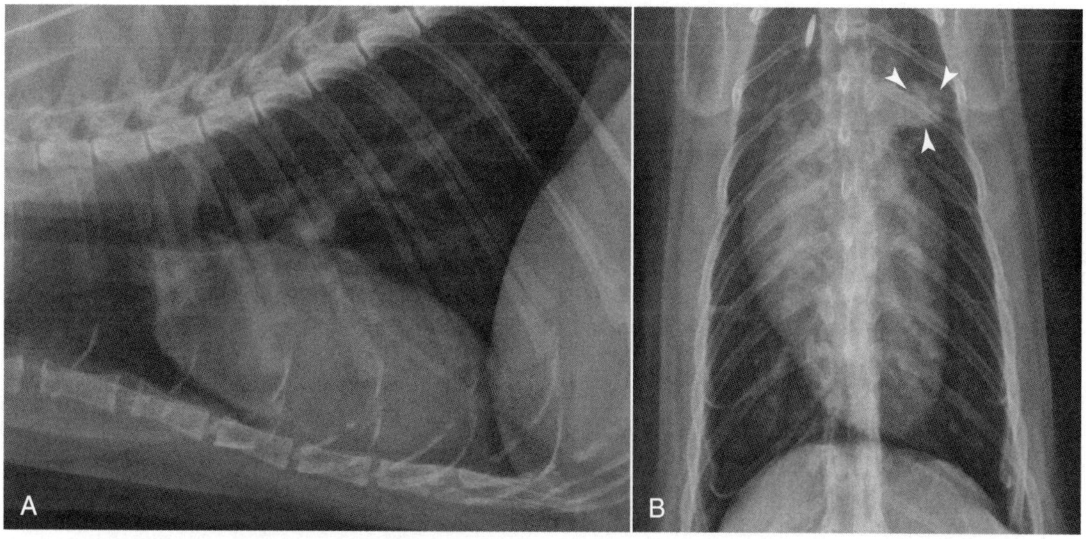

Fig. 35.16 Lateral **(A)** and ventrodorsal **(B)** projections of two different cats with age-associated redundancy and tortuosity of the aorta. In **A,** the aortic arch extends more cranial than normal, and the descending aorta is tortuous. In **B,** the aortic arch is projection end-on, representing a focal soft tissue opacity to the left of midline (*white arrowheads*), which should not be misinterpreted as a pulmonary mass.

seen on the lateral projections at the heart base where the left and right pulmonary arteries converge and are seen end-on. Enlargement of the main pulmonary artery is not recognized routinely on lateral projections. Identification of main pulmonary enlargement in cats may be more difficult due to a less pronounced elevation of the main pulmonary artery margin from the cardiac silhouette in cats and some variations in the orientation of the main pulmonary artery at the heart base in comparison to dogs. Considered causes for main pulmonary artery enlargement in dogs and cats include pulmonary hypertension, as from heartworm infection, and turbulence, as from pulmonic stenosis or patent ductus arteriosus.

SPECIFIC PATTERNS OF LOBAR PULMONARY VESSEL CHANGES

A thorough evaluation of the lobar pulmonary vasculature is integral to the assessment of the cardiovascular structures. The cranial lobar pulmonary arteries and veins are best visible on the lateral projections and most prominent in the nondependent lung lobe. Superimposition of the lobar pulmonary artery and veins on the VD/DV projections limits interpretation. Separation of the left and right cranial lobar pulmonary arteries and veins is greatest on the left lateral projection: therefore, evaluation of the right cranial lobar pulmonary vasculature in the better inflated nondependent right cranial lung lobe is usually easiest (Fig. 35.18A,B). The caudal lobar pulmonary vasculature is best evaluated on VD/DV projections and optimized on the DV projection due to better inflation of the nondependent caudal lung lobes and increased magnification (Fig. 35.19A,B). Additionally, the caudal lobar pulmonary vessels are more perpendicular to the diverging x-ray beam, resulting in less distortion. The lobar pulmonary arteries and veins are located on opposite sides of their corresponding lobar bronchus. On lateral projections, the cranial lobar arteries are dorsal and the veins are ventral to the bronchus, whereas the caudal lobar pulmonary arteries are lateral and veins are medial to their corresponding bronchus on the VD/DV projections.[19] As a simplified means to recall the relative positioning of the lobar pulmonary arteries and veins to each other, the lobar pulmonary arteries may be expressed as being "up and away," while the veins are "ventral and central."

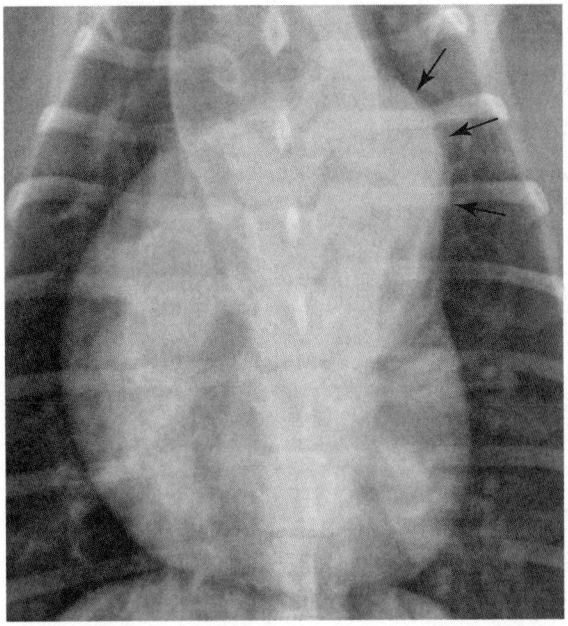

Fig. 35.17 Dorsoventral projection of a dog with dilation of the main pulmonary artery (*black arrows*).

Under normal conditions, the lobar pulmonary arteries and veins should be symmetrical in size.[19] Additionally, normal lobar pulmonary arteries and veins follow a generally straight path as they gradually taper in the periphery of the lung field. The size of the cranial lobar pulmonary vessels may be assessed by comparing vessel diameter to the width of the fourth rib just ventral to the vertebral column on lateral projections and the width of the ninth rib in the VD/DV projections.[19,20] Variable rib conformation and a wide range of normal values limit the clinical usefulness of these comparisons.

Certain diseases cause predictable changes in the size or shape of either pulmonary arteries alone or pulmonary veins alone, or both simultaneously, and are associated with the following conditions:

- *Enlarged lobar pulmonary arteries and veins:* Volume overload is the most common cause for lobar pulmonary vessel enlargement and may be iatrogenic, such as from overzealous intravenous fluid administration. Other causes may include left-to-right shunting congenital cardiovascular anomalies, peripheral arteriovenous fistula, and decreased cardiac output resulting in fluid retention (Fig. 35.20A,B). The concurrent presence of lobar pulmonary vein congestion and pulmonary hypertension can be a cause for simultaneous lobar pulmonary artery and vein enlargement.
- *Small lobar pulmonary arteries and veins*: Diffuse thinning of the lobar pulmonary vasculature results in a generalized hyperlucency of the pulmonary parenchyma due to pulmonary undercirculation. Causes may include dehydration, diuretic administration, or blood loss and are often associated with concurrent caval undercirculation and microcardia (see Fig. 35.3A,B). Pulmonary undercirculation with thinning of the lobar pulmonary arteries and veins is also seen in dogs and cats with right-to-left shunting congenital heart anomalies (Fig. 35.21A,B). Such changes are less conspicuous and uncommonly recognized in cats.

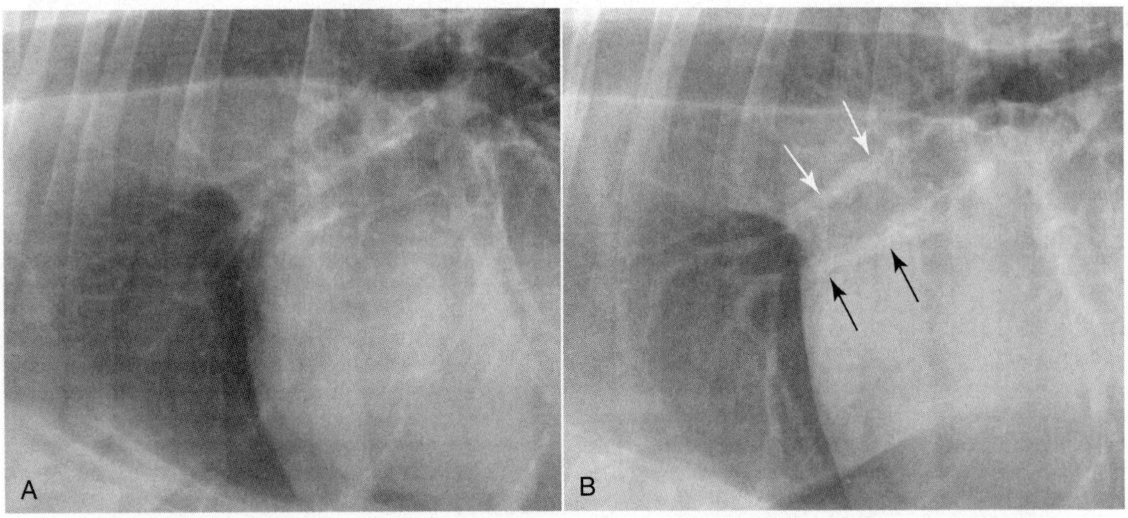

Fig. 35.18 Close-up from right **(A)** and left **(B)** lateral projections of a normal dog. On the right lateral projection **(A)**, the left and right cranial lobar pulmonary arteries and veins are superimposed and cannot be evaluated. On the left lateral projection **(B)**, the right cranial lobar pulmonary artery (*white arrows*) and right cranial lobar pulmonary vein (*black arrows*) are more clearly seen. The ability to distinguish the right cranial artery from the vein is typically easier on a left lateral projection. Note the similar size of the artery and vein in **B**.

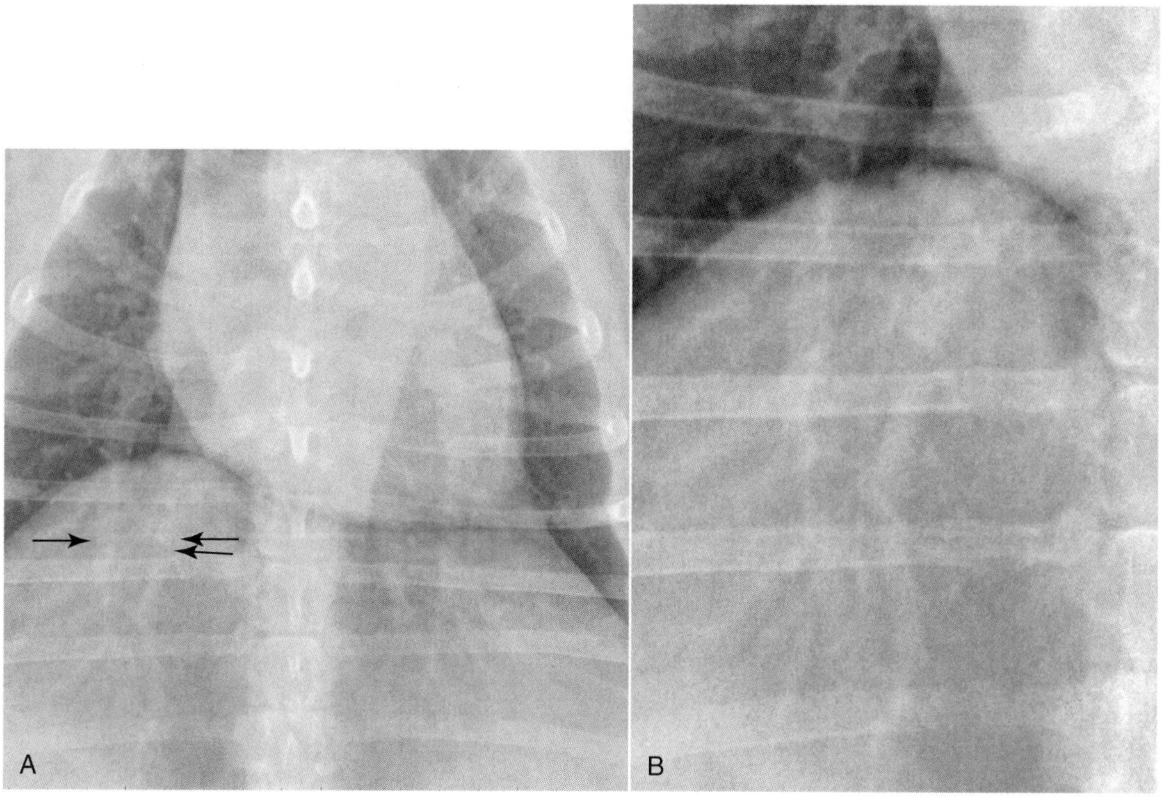

Fig. 35.19 Dorsoventral **(A)** projection of a normal dog with a close-up view **(B)** of the right caudal lobar pulmonary vessels. The right caudal lobe pulmonary artery (*single black arrow*) is lateral to the bronchus, whereas the right caudal lobe pulmonary vein is medial (*double black arrows*). On close inspection, the mineralized wall of the caudal lobe bronchus can be seen between the artery and vein. Note that in this dog, as in most, the bronchus does not occupy the entire space between the artery and vein. When the bronchus is not mineralized, inferring that it occupies the entire distance between its associated artery and vein is inaccurate.

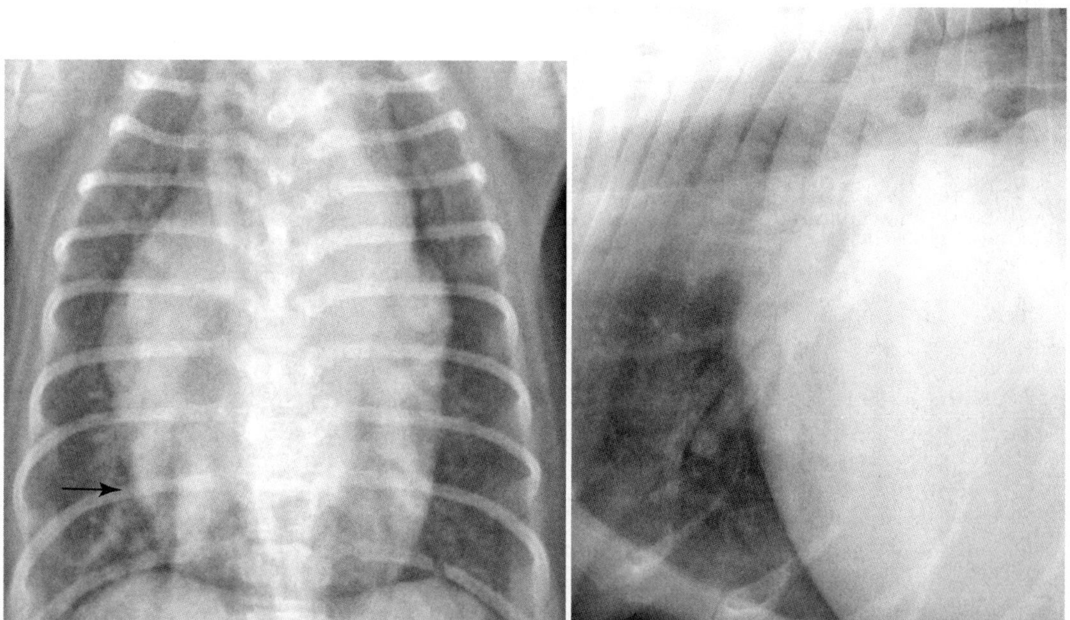

Fig. 35.20 Dorsoventral **(A)** and lateral **(B)** projections of two different dogs with a patent ductus arteriosus. The caudal lobar pulmonary arteries and veins are both enlarged as a result of overcirculation of the pulmonary vascular system. Note the size of the summation shadow where the vessels cross the right ninth rib (*black arrow*) in **A** and compare to Fig. 35.17. The shape of these summation shadows indicates that both the right caudal lobar pulmonary artery and vein are enlarged.

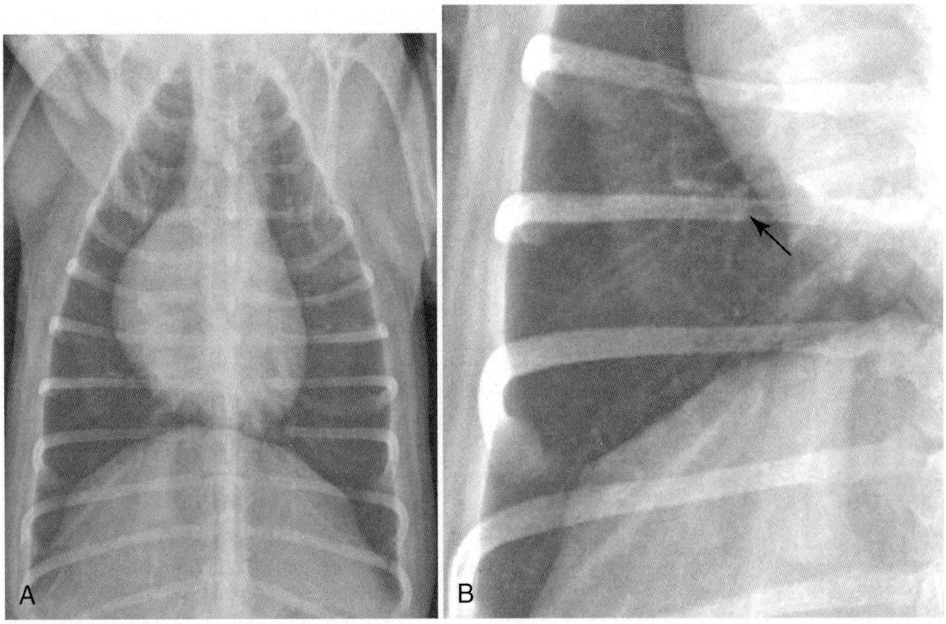

Fig. 35.21 Ventrodorsal **(A)** projection of a dog with pulmonary undercirculation from multiple congenital cardiac anomalies with close-up image of the right caudal lung lobe **(B)**. The pulmonary vessels are small and poorly defined. In **B,** note the small size of the right caudal lobe pulmonary vein where it crosses the right ninth rib (*black arrow*).

- *Enlarged lobar pulmonary arteries with normal veins*: The most common cause in the dog is pulmonary hypertension. Depending on the patient's demographic (e.g., southeastern states), heartworm disease may be the most likely etiology (eFigs. 35.1–35.3). In cats, feline asthma is most prevalent, although heartworm disease is also occasionally identified (see eFig. 35.2).
- *Enlarged lobar pulmonary veins with normal arteries*: Lobar pulmonary vein enlargement is most seen in dogs with mitral valve insufficiency resulting in left-sided volume overload and subsequent pulmonary venous hypertension. A similar finding is inconsistently observed in cats.
- Tortuous pulmonary vessels: Tortuosity of the pulmonary vessels is most commonly seen in dogs and cats with pulmonary hypertension. The most common causes are heartworm disease in dogs and shunting congenital cardiovascular abnormalities in cats (see eFig. 35.3D). Peripherally, the lobar pulmonary arteries may also be blunted (Fig. 35.22).

In some instances, perivascular disease in the adjacent lung parenchyma can partially or completely border efface and reduce the conspicuity of the pulmonary vasculature rendering interpretation difficult. This may be especially encountered in dogs and cats with left-sided congestive heart failure.

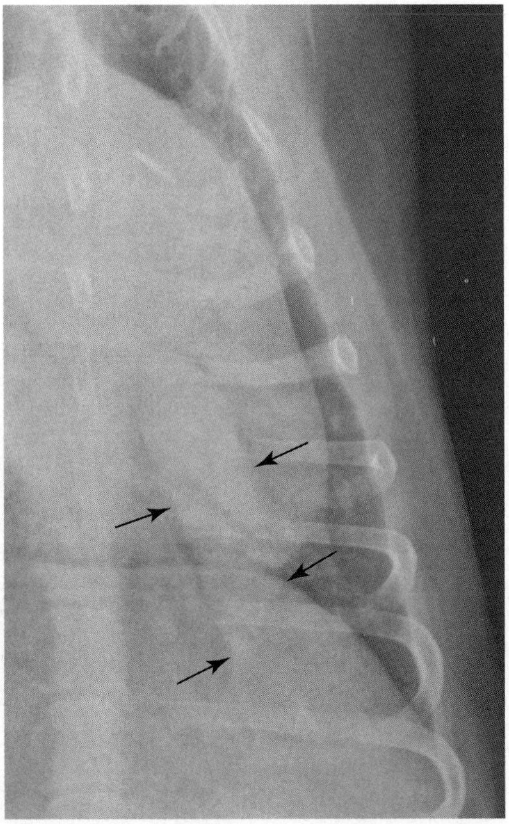

Fig. 35.22 Close-up view of the left caudal thorax of a dog with severe heartworm disease. The left caudal lobe pulmonary artery is severely dilated (*black arrows*). At the most caudal pair of arrows, the vessel ends abruptly, or is truncated. This is due to an intravascular thrombus completely obstructing the lumen at this level with marked reduction in vessel diameter distal to the obstruction.

FEATURES OF CONGESTIVE HEART FAILURE

Left-Sided Congestive Heart Failure

Volume and pressure overload of the left ventricle may result in backward congestion (hypertension) of the lobar pulmonary veins. Pulmonary venous hypertension may ultimately result in the development of cardiogenic pulmonary edema due to transudation of fluid from the pulmonary capillaries into the lung interstitium. In very early left-sided heart failure, poorly defined interstitial pulmonary edema may be observed, but more commonly an alveolar pattern develops. It is important to note that lobar pulmonary vein enlargement is not commonly present when there is cardiogenic pulmonary edema. Pulmonary arterial hypertension is also common in dogs with left-sided heart disease; this may or may not lead to pulmonary arterial enlargement (eFigs. 35.4–35.6).

Cardiogenic pulmonary edema in dogs is most commonly caudodorsally distributed. However, a perihilar, diffuse, or multifocal distribution is also possible but less prevalent. The pattern of pulmonary edema distribution in dogs with mitral valve insufficiency has been associated with the direction of the regurgitant jet. A symmetric distribution was associated predominantly with a central mitral regurgitant jet, whereas an asymmetric distribution was usually associated with an eccentric jet.[21] When asymmetric in distribution, more severe cardiogenic pulmonary edema is identified in the right caudal lung lobe in relation to the left caudal lung lobe. In dogs with cardiogenic pulmonary edema due to dilated cardiomyopathy (DCM), a diffuse unstructured to alveolar pulmonary pattern with a ventral distribution is observed at a higher frequency (Fig. 35.23). Cardiogenic pulmonary edema more often has a multifocal to diffuse distribution in cats. Many cats with left heart failure also have pleural effusion in addition to pulmonary edema.

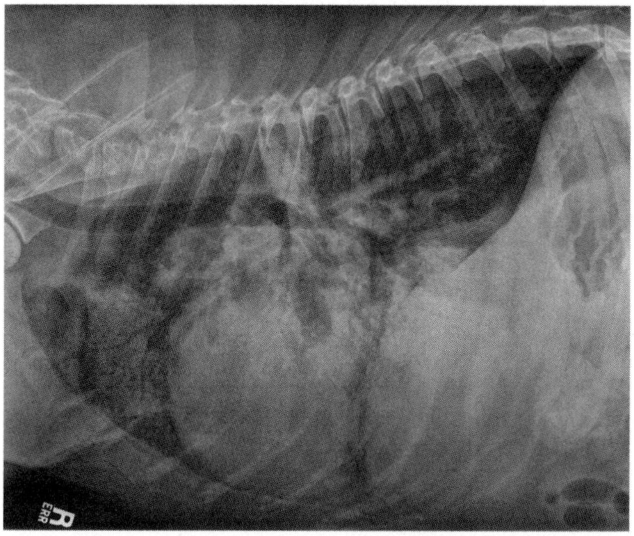

Fig. 35.23 Right lateral projection of a dog with dilated cardiomyopathy and left-sided congestive heart failure. The bulge along the caudodorsal aspect of the cardiac silhouette is indicative of left atrial enlargement and results in straightening of the caudal margin of the cardiac silhouette. The lobar pulmonary veins are enlarged due to left-sided volume overload from myocardial failure. A diffuse unstructured interstitial pulmonary pattern is seen throughout the pulmonary parenchyma and is greater in severity ventrally, where it coalesced into an alveolar pulmonary pattern. This distribution represents a more typical manifestation of cardiogenic pulmonary edema in dogs with dilated cardiomyopathy. (Image courtesy Rachel Lee, DVM.)

Right-Sided Congestive Heart Failure

Right-sided heart disease may result in right ventricular volume and pressure overload with subsequent caudal vena cava and hepatic enlargement. With progression, abdominal effusion, and sometimes pleural effusion, develops (Fig. 35.24A,B).

ABNORMAL OPACITY OF THE CARDIAC SILHOUETTE

In the absence of a peritoneopericardial diaphragmatic hernia, alterations to the normal homogeneous soft tissue opacity of the cardiac silhouette are rare and more commonly associated with the presence of aortic root mineralization and the presence of intraventricular gas. Aortic root mineralization is much more common in dogs than cats.[22] On lateral projections, a poorly to well-defined irregular to curvilinear region of mineralization is present at the level of the aortic root, superimposed over the craniodorsal aspect of the cardiac silhouette (Fig. 35.25). Aortic root mineralization may represent a normal age-associated change and is usually of no clinical significance.[22]

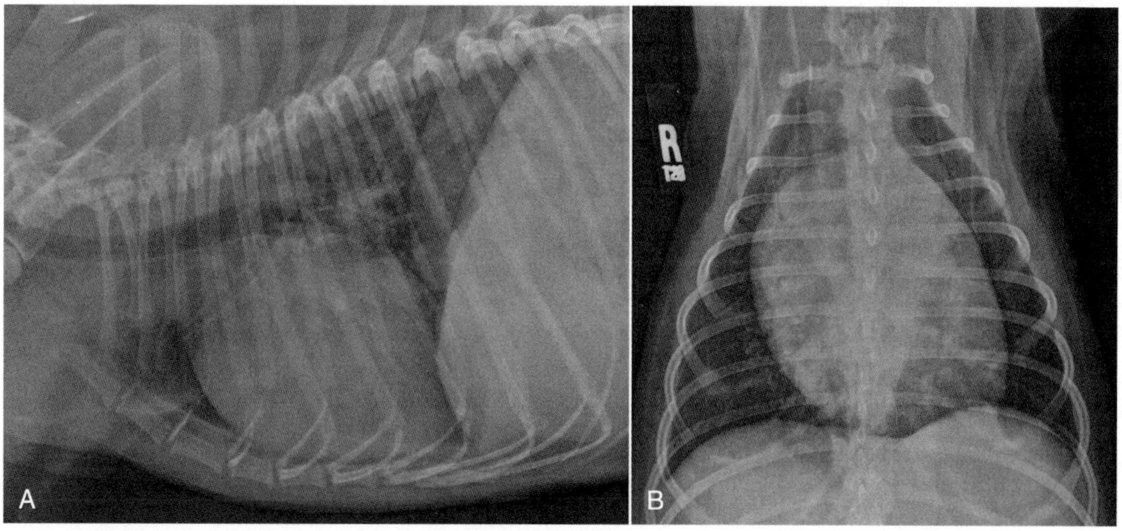

Fig. 35.24 Left lateral **(A)** and ventrodorsal **(B)** projections of a dog with right-sided cardiomegaly and right-sided congestive heart failure. The cranial and right lateral margins of the cardiac silhouette are rounded with leftward displacement of the cardiac apex and a "reversed-D" shape on the ventrodorsal projection. The caudal vena cava is distended and the liver is enlarged due to backward congestion. In combination with the presence of scant pleural effusion, the poor abdominal serosal detail is secondary to the presence of peritoneal effusion and indicative of right-sided congestive heart failure.

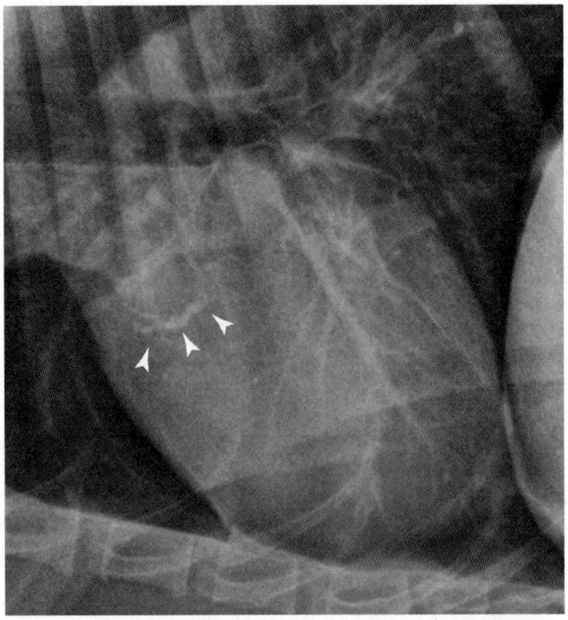

Fig. 35.25 Right lateral radiograph of a dog with aortic root mineralization (*white arrowheads*), representing an incidental age-associated change.

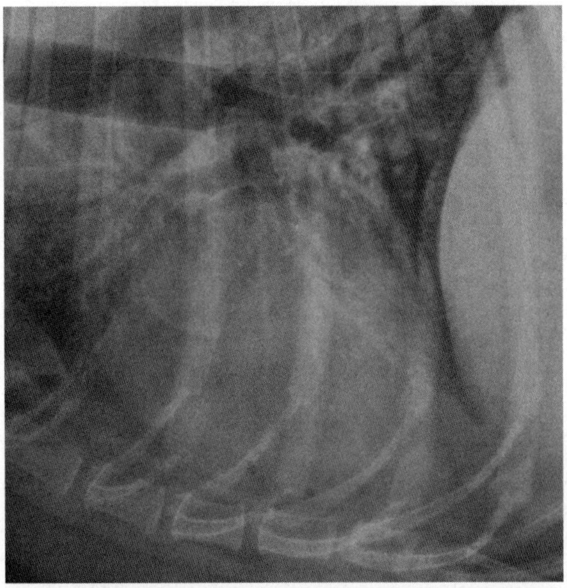

Fig. 35.26 Right lateral projection of a dog with a small amount of intraventricular gas due to recent cephalic vein injection.

A small amount of gas in the plane of the right atrium is occasionally identified on lateral projections (Fig. 35.26). This is usually iatrogenic. While small amounts of gas are unlikely to cause clinical signs, air embolization can be fatal.[23,24] Maintaining the patient in left lateral recumbency may be advantageous to prevent dissemination of gas into the lobar pulmonary arteries.

Acquired Cardiovascular Diseases

Acquired cardiovascular diseases are more prevalent than congenital heart diseases in dogs and cats, reported to represent up to 94.05% of all cardiac abnormalities.[25] Of these, valvular disease is most common in dogs, whereas cats more often have myocardial failure. Factors, such as age, breed, and diet, may increase the risk of acquired heart disease in both dogs and cats. Early diagnosis of acquired disease is important to avoid irreversible cardiac damage.

Myxomatous Mitral Valve Disease

Myxomatous mitral valve disease is the most common acquired heart disease in dogs, representing approximately 75% of all cardiac disease in small animal practice.[26] Myxomatous mitral valve disease is highly prevalent in older small breed dogs, reported in 85% of 13-year-old dogs at necropsy, and may be inherited in certain dog breeds, such as the Cavalier King Charles spaniel.[26,27]

Valve leaf degeneration often leads to left-sided cardiac decompensation and heart failure.[28] Rupture of chordae tendineae and atrial rupture may result in a rapid clinical decline.[28,29] Radiographic signs of myxomatous mitral valve disease include (eFigs. 35.7 and 35.8):

- Left atrial, and sometimes auricular enlargement, as described earlier.
- The sole or combined presence of left atrial and ventricular enlargement will result in an increase in apical to basilar length of the cardiac silhouette.
- Distention of lobar pulmonary veins can result from pulmonary venous hypertension.
- Cardiogenic pulmonary edema from left-sided heart failure. This usually develops in the absence of lobar pulmonary venous enlargement.
- Distention of the pulmonary arteries with an artery to vein ratio >1.1 has been described as supportive of pulmonary hypertension in patients with myxomatous mitral valve disease.[30]

Myxomatous Tricuspid Valve Disease

Approximately 54% of patients with myxomatous mitral valve degeneration have concurrent myxomatous tricuspid valve degeneration.[31] Minor tricuspid valve regurgitation may be negligible; however, severe tricuspid valve degeneration can result in valvular insufficiency and right-sided volume overload. The right atrium and ventricle will become enlarged with associated eccentric hypertrophy. Backward congestion may decompensate into right-sided heart failure with pleural and abdominal effusion developing from the increased hydrostatic pressure.

Radiographic signs of myxomatous tricuspid valve disease include (Fig. 35.27A,B):

- Right atrial and ventricular enlargement is more likely to be radiographically recognized in the presence of at least moderate cardiac chamber enlargement.
- Distention of the caudal vena cava and generalized hepatomegaly are indicative of systemic venous hypertension.
- Peritoneal and/or pleural effusion will develop due to right-sided cardiac decompensation.

Cardiomyopathies

Cardiomyopathies are diseases of the heart muscle and have variable etiologies and presentation in both dogs and cats.

Dilated cardiomyopathy (DCM) is most prevalent in large breed male dogs and is also seen in cats. Canine breeds predisposed to DCM include the Doberman Pinscher, Great Dane, Irish Wolfhound, and Boxer. Although the cause for myocardial failure is not fully understood, genetic mutation, systemic disease, toxins, and nutritional deficiencies (including a more recent correlation between DCM and grain-free diets) are possible etiologies.[32] Failure of the myocardium results in progressive concentric dilation of the left ± right cardiac chambers. The heart becomes volume overloaded, and mitral valve dysfunction may result from a change in shape of the mitral annulus because of cardiac dilation. Enlargement of the pulmonary arteries and veins is commonly seen due to intravascular fluid retention, and may be followed by the development

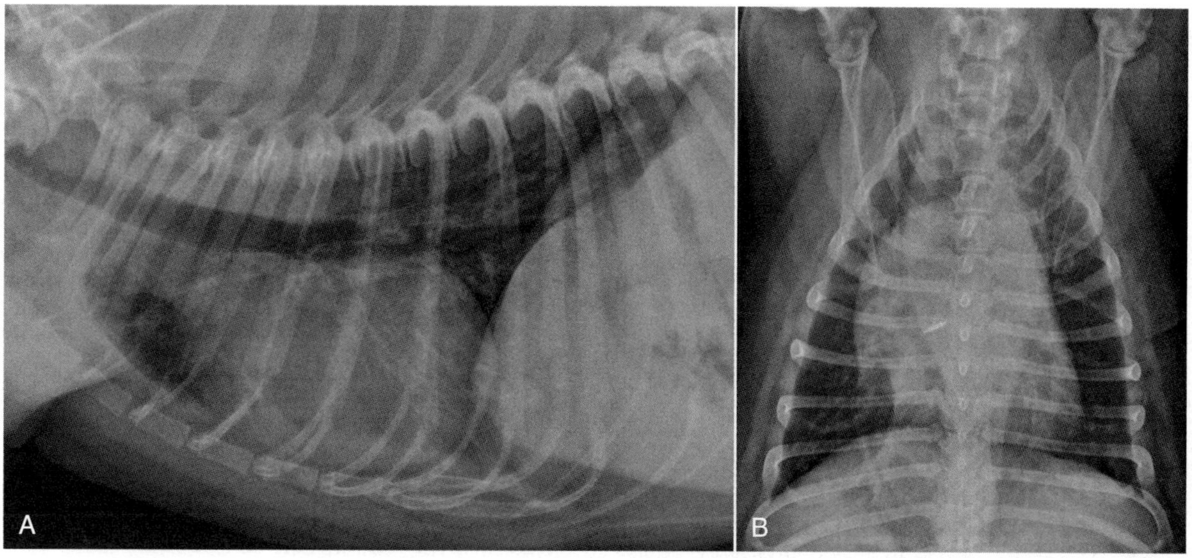

Fig. 35.27 Left lateral (**A**) and ventrodorsal (**B**) projections of a dog diagnosed with myxomatous tricuspid valve disease. The cranial and right lateral margins of the cardiac silhouette are rounded and the cardiac apex is displaced to the left with a "reversed-D" shape of the cardiac silhouette due to right atrial and ventricular enlargements. No evidence of right-sided congestive failure is seen.

of cardiogenic pulmonary edema. Dilation of the pulmonary arteries may also be associated with the development of pulmonary hypertension from activation of the renin-angiotensin system in response to decreased renal perfusion and/or the presence of chronic heart failure.[33]

Radiographic features of DCM include (see Fig. 35.23, Fig. 35.28, eFig. 35.9):

- Left atrial and ventricular enlargement. Cardiomegaly is the most common radiographic abnormality in dogs with DCM and is reported in up to 80% of dogs.[34] However, given the large size and variable thoracic conformation of dogs typically affected with DCM, breed variations need to be taken into account when evaluating the cardiac silhouette for cardiomegaly. The cardiac silhouette may be normal in some dogs. A mean VHS of 11.8 (range 11.0–12.6) may be suggestive of cardiomegaly in dogs with DCM.[33] In cats, the cardiac silhouette may be "valentine shaped."
- Concurrent enlargement of the right heart is observed in more advanced cases and may not be apparent on thoracic radiographs if mild in severity.
- Cardiogenic pulmonary edema due to left-sided heart failure is identified in the majority of dogs (74%) at the time of radiographic evaluation.[34] Most dogs in heart failure from DCM will have a bronchointerstitial pattern, rather than the typical dorsocaudal alveolar pattern seen in dogs with left heart failure from mitral valve disease. A ventral distribution of an interstitial, coalescing into alveolar pattern can be seen in a subset of dogs with DCM, possibly attributed to chronicity.[32,33]
- The presence of pleural effusion, caval distention, hepatomegaly, and/or peritoneal effusion from right-sided heart failure is often seen.

Arrhythmogenic right ventricular cardiomyopathy, also known as ARVC or Boxer cardiomyopathy, is a familial myocardial disease in Boxer dogs but can also affect other breeds of dogs and cats. The myocardium of the right ventricle is affected primarily; however, involvement of the left ventricle and atria is also possible. The myocardium becomes inflamed (e.g., myocarditis) and replaced by fat ± fibrosis, leading to the development of potentially fatal ventricular arrhythmias.[35] With disease progression and not necessarily before the emergence of arrhythmias, the cardiac chambers may undergo eccentric hypertrophy and become volume overloaded. When in excess, the heart will decompensate into right-sided congestive heart failure.[36]

Radiographic features of ARVC include:

- Commonly, there are no thoracic radiographic abnormalities.
- Right-sided cardiomegaly is seen with more advanced systolic dysfunction and congestion.
- Right-sided congestive heart failure is occasionally observed.

Hypertrophic cardiomyopathy (HCM) is the most common acquired heart disease in cats and is familial in some breeds, such as the Maine Coon and Norwegian Forest cat.[37] HCM is seen occasionally in dogs with a much lower prevalence than in cats. Concentric hypertrophy of the left ventricle causes a decrease in ventricular volume capacity and increase in left ventricular filling pressure.[38] The decrease in stroke volume is counteracted by tachycardia, which in turn further limits filling of the left ventricle. Therefore, the left atrium becomes overloaded with further backward hypertension of the lobar pulmonary veins as the disease progresses. In some instances, the papillary muscles may become thickened and result in mitral valve insufficiency, further exacerbating dilation and hypertension of the left atrium. The mitral valve may have altered motion and deviate toward the left ventricular outflow tract, causing dynamic outflow obstruction of the left ventricle during systole.[39] Other diseases, such as systemic arterial hypertension, hyperthyroidism, and aortic stenosis, should be ruled out as a cause for ventricular hypertrophy.

Radiographic features of feline HCM include the following (Fig. 35.29A,B):

- Left atrial dilation is characterized by increased length and width of the cardiac silhouette. The dorsocaudal margin of the cardiac silhouette may be rounded with concavity of the caudal margin. In the presence of moderate to severe left atrial enlargement, the cardiac silhouette may have a "valentine-shaped" heart on VD/DV projections. This is enhanced by the absence of left ventricular enlargement, because the hypertrophy is constrictive (concentric), or

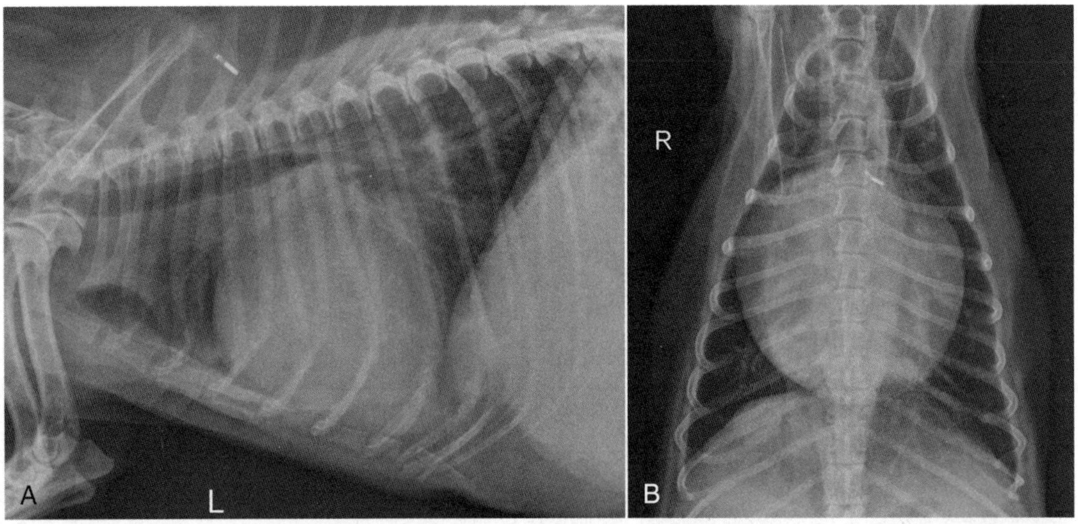

Fig. 35.31 Left lateral **(A)** and dorsoventral **(B)** projections of a dog with cardiomegaly and a globoid cardiac silhouette. This appearance is consistent with pericardial effusion, but based on the radiographs, a peritoneal-pericardial hernia or generalized cardiomegaly cannot be eliminated. This dog had pericardial effusion, along with hepatomegaly, peritoneal and scant pleural effusion due to right-sided heart failure from cardiac tamponade.

and can be life-threatening.[46,47] Pericardial effusion is diagnosed more frequently in dogs than cats and is most often neoplastic in etiology or due to idiopathic pericarditis. Less common causes include cardiac chamber rupture from volume overload or trauma, or infectious processes.[46] Congestive heart failure is reported to be the most cause of pericardial effusion in cats.[48] Regardless of the cause, diastolic function is altered by tamponade. Jugular vein distention is seen in response to the increased pressure, and caudal vena cava and hepatic enlargement may also be observed and followed by the development of peritoneal and pleural effusion due to cardiac decompensation into right-sided heart failure.[46,47]

Radiographic features of pericardial effusion include the following (Fig. 35.31A,B, eFig. 35.10):

- Enlargement and rounding of the cardiac silhouette are seen with larger amounts of pericardial effusion, creating a globoid contour. This finding has been reported in up to 80% of dogs with pericardial effusion.[47] With smaller amounts of pericardial effusion, the cardiac silhouette may maintain a normal contour. Cardiomegaly and rounding of the cardiac silhouette on thoracic radiographs are poorly sensitive and specific for the presence of cardiac tamponade.[49]
- Distention of the caudal vena cava and hepatomegaly are signs of increased central venous pressure if pericardial tamponade is severe enough to prevent diastolic filling of the right atrium and ventricle. The concurrent presence of peritoneal ± pleural effusion is suggestive of right-sided congestive heart failure.

Neoplasia

Cardiac tumors have a low incidence in dogs, representing 0.121% and 4.33% of all tumor types, and an even lower incidence is reported in cats.[50] The most common cardiac tumor reported in dogs is hemangiosarcoma (69% prevalence), followed by aortic body tumors (chemodectoma and paraganglioma) and lymphoma. Lymphoma is the most common neoplastic disease of the feline heart. Both dogs and cats can have metastatic lesions to the heart from tumors of other tissue origin.[50,51] While most cardiac tumors are diagnosed in middle-aged to older patients, lymphoma can affect dogs and cats of any age.[50] Hemangiosarcoma most commonly originates from the right atrium/auricle and is highly metastatic. On the other hand, heart base tumors are less aggressive and are primarily identified at the aortic root.[50,51] Brachycephalic dogs are predisposed to heart base tumors, and it is speculated that chronic hypoxia may be an inciting etiology.[50] Hemangiosarcoma may also be identified at the aortic root, and lymphoma may affect any part of the heart. When larger in size, right atrial/auricular and heart base masses can obstruct the right cardiac chambers and cause vena caval and hepatic hypertension with risks of right-sided cardiac decompensation. Pericardial effusion may develop in some cases and result in cardiac tamponade. Cardiac tumors may be difficult to identify on thoracic radiographs, and echocardiography and advanced imaging (CT or MRI) are superior for the diagnosis and characterization of cardiac neoplasms in dogs and cats.[50,51] However, radiographs remain a good screening tool and should be scrutinized for the presence of a mass even in asymptomatic cases as they may often be found incidentally.

Radiographic features of cardiac neoplasia include the following (Fig. 35.32A,B):

- Heart base and right atrial/auricular tumors cannot be differentiated on thoracic radiographs. When larger in size, a soft tissue opaque mass may be seen at the base of the cardiac silhouette, causing dorsal and rightward displacement of the trachea.
- Cardiomegaly with rounding (globoid appearance) is indicative of pericardial effusion.
- Distention of the caudal vena cava and hepatomegaly are seen secondary to obstruction of venous return to the right heart.
- Peritoneal ± pleural effusion is suggestive of right-sided heart failure.

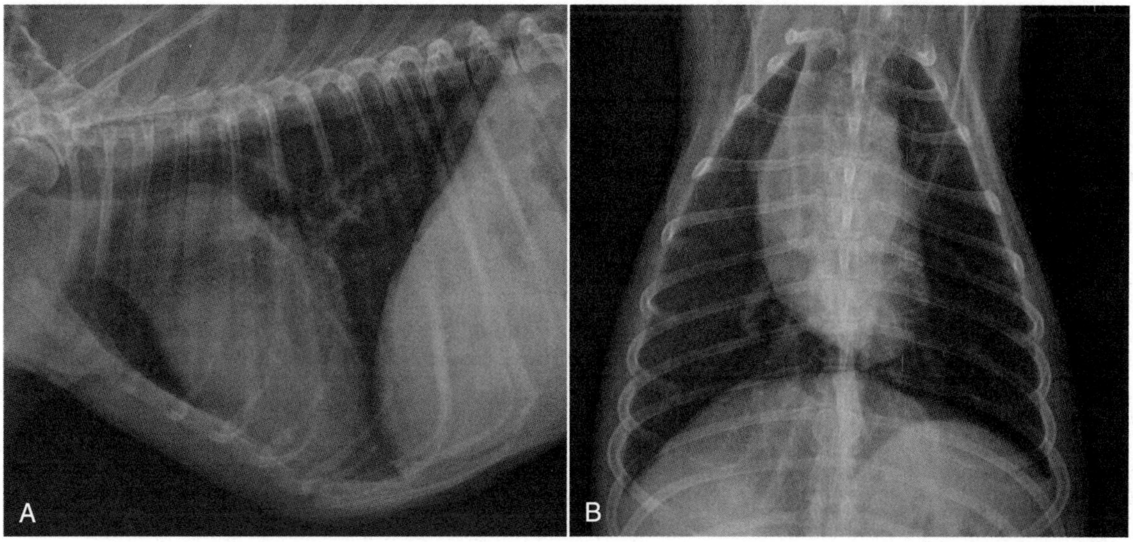

Fig. 35.32 Left lateral **(A)** and dorsoventral **(B)** projections of a dog with a heart base mass. In the region of the heart base, an ill-defined, homogeneously soft tissue opaque mass causes moderate to severe, focal and dorsal displacement of the intrathoracic trachea and moderate widening of the cranial mediastinum. This mass border effaces the cranial margin of the cardiac silhouette, widens the cranial mediastinum, and causes caudal displacement of the proximal descending aorta.

Acknowledgment

With special thanks to prior authors of this chapter for their contributions.

REFERENCES

1. Lamb CR, Tyler M, Boswood A, et al. Assessment of the value of the vertebral heart scale in the radiographic diagnosis of cardiac disease in dogs. *Vet Rec*. 2000;146(24): 687–690.
2. Buchanan JW, Bucheler J. Vertebral scale system to measure canine heart size in radiographs. *J Am Vet Med Assoc*. 1995;206(2):194–199.
3. Olive J, Javard R, Specci S, et al. Effect of cardiac and respiratory cycles on vertebral heart score measured on fluoroscopic images of healthy dogs. *J Am Vet Med Assoc*. 2015;246:1091.
4. Litster AL, Buchanan JW. Vertebral scale system to measure heart size in radiographs of cats. *J Am Vet Med Assoc*. 2000;216(2):210–214.
5. Costanza D, Greco A, Piantedosi D, et al. The heart to single vertebra ratio: a new objective method for radiographic assessment of cardiac silhouette size in dogs. *Vet Radiol Ultrasound*. 2022.
6. Moon ML, Keene BW, Lessard P, et al. Age related changes in the feline cardiac silhouette. *Vet Radiol Ultrasound*. 1993;34:315.
7. Melian C, Stefanacci J, Peterson ME, Kintzer PP. Radiographic findings in dogs with naturally-occurring primary hypoadrenocorticism. *J Am Anim Hosp Assoc*. 1999;35(3):208–212.
8. Côté E, Weisse C, Lamb K, Tozier E. Computed tomographic assessment of principal bronchial anatomy in dogs of various thoracic conformations: 93 cases (2012–2017). *J Am Vet Med Assoc*. 2022;1:1–10.
9. Lebastard M, Le Boedec K, Howes M, et al. Evaluation of bronchial narrowing in coughing dogs with heart murmurs using computed tomography. *J Vet Intern Med*. 2021;35(3):1509–1518.
10. Ferasin L, Crews L, Biller DS, Lamb KE, Borgarelli M. Risk factors for coughing in dogs with naturally acquired myxomatous mitral valve disease. *J Vet Intern Med*. 2013;27(2):286–292.
11. Keene BW, Atkins CE, Bonagura JD, et al. ACVIM consensus guidelines for the diagnosis and treatment of myxomatous mitral valve disease in dogs. *J. Vet. Intern. Med*. 2019;33(3):1127–1140.
12. Vezzosi T, Puccinelli C, Tognetti R, Pelligra T, Citi S. Radiographic vertebral left atrial size: a reference interval study in healthy adult dogs. *Vet Radiol Ultrasound*. 2020;61(5):507–511.

13. Malcolm EL, Visser LC, Phillips KL, Johnson LR. Diagnostic value of vertebral left atrial size as determined from thoracic radiographs for assessment of left atrial size in dogs with myxomatous mitral valve disease. *J Am Vet Med Assoc*. 2018;253(8):1038–1054.
14. Oura TJ, Young AN, Keene BW, et al. A valentine-shaped cardiac silhouette in feline thoracic radiographs is primarily due to left atrial enlargement. *Vet Radiol Ultrasound*. 2015;56(3):245–250.
15. Huguet EE, Vilaplana Grosso F, Lamb WR, et al. Interpretation of cardiac chamber size on canine thoracic radiographs is limited and may result in the false identification of right-sided cardiomegaly in the presence of severe left-sided cardiomegaly. *Vet Radiol Ultrasound*. 2021; 62(6):637–646.
16. Lehmukhl LB, Bonagura JD, Biller DS, Hartman WM. Radiographic evaluation of caudal vena cava size in dogs. *Vet Radiol Ultrasound*. 1997;38(2):94–100.
17. Cornelius L, Mahaffey M. Kinking of the intrathoracic caudal vena cava in five dogs. *J Small Anim Pract*. 1985;26(2):67–80.
18. Pelosi A, Prinsen JK, Eyster GE, Schall W, Olivier NB. Caudal vena cava kinking in dogs with ascites. *Vet Radiol Ultrasound*. 2012;53(3):233–235.
19. Thrall DE, Losonsky JM. A method for evaluating canine pulmonary circulatory dynamics from survey radiographs. *J Am Anim Hosp Assoc*. 1976;12:457.
20. Oui H, Oh J, Keh S, et al. Measurements of the pulmonary vasculature on thoracic radiographs in healthy dogs compared to dogs with mitral regurgitation. *Vet Radiol Ultrasound*. 2015;56(3):251–256.
21. Diana A, Guglielmini C, Pivetta M, et al. Radiographic features of cardiogenic pulmonary edema in dogs with mitral regurgitation: 61 cases (1998–2007). *J Am Vet Med Assoc*. 2009;235(9):1058–1063.
22. Schwarz T, Sullivan M, Störk CK, Willis R, Harley R, Mellor DJ. Aortic and cardiac mineralization in the dog. *Vet Radiol Ultrasound*. 2002;43(5):419–427.
23. Josephson S, Ovenfors CO. Experimental pulmonary air embolism: angiographic study in dogs. *Invest Radiol*. 1970;5(4):220–231.
24. Verstappen FTJ, Bernards JA, Kreuzer F. Effects of pulmonary gas embolism on circulation and respiration in the dog. *Pflügers Archiv*. 1970;368(1):89–96.
25. Baisan RA, Condurachi E, Turcu CA, Vu V. Prevalence of cardiac diseases in small animals: a five-year single-centre retrospective study. *Rev Rom Med Vet*. 2021;31(2):35–40.
26. Atkins C, Bonagura J, Ettinger S, et al. Guidelines for the diagnosis and treatment of canine chronic valvular heart disease. *J Vet Intern Med*. 2009;23(6):1142–1150.
27. Bionda A, Cortellari M, Bagardi M, et al. A genomic study of myxomatous mitral valve disease in Cavalier King Charles Spaniels. *Animals*. 2020;10(10):1895.
28. Fox PP. Pathology of myxomatous mitral valve disease in the dog. *J Vet Cardiol*. 2012;14(1):103–126.
29. Serres F, Chetboul V, Tissier R, et al. Chordae tendineae rupture in dogs with degenerative mitral valve disease: prevalence, survival, and prognostic factors (114 cases, 2001–2006). *J Vet Intern Med*. 2007;21(2):258–264.
30. Lee SK, Choi J. Caudal pulmonary artery to vein ratio on radiography can predict pulmonary hypertension in dogs with mitral regurgitation. *Vet Radiol Ultrasound*. 2022.
31. Borgarelli M, Buchanan JW. Historical review, epidemiology and natural history of degenerative mitral valve disease. *J Vet Cardiol*. 2012;14(1):93–101.
32. Lee RP, Huguet EH, Adin DB, Hernandez JA, Vilaplana Grosso FR. Radiographic features of cardiogenic pulmonary edema in dogs with dilated cardiomyopathy [abstract]. In: *ACVR Annual Meeting*. NV: Reno; 2022.
33. Ames MK, Atkins CE, Pitt B. The renin-angiotensin-aldosterone system and its suppression. *J Vet Intern Med*. 2019;33(2):363–382.
34. Martin MWS, Stafford Johnson MJ, Celona B. Canine dilated cardiomyopathy: a retrospective study of signalment, presentation and clinical findings in 369 cases. *Journal of Small Animal Practice*. 2009;50(1):23–29.
35. Cunningham SM, Dos Santos L. Arrhythmogenic right ventricular cardiomyopathy in dogs. *J Vet Cardiol*. 2022;40:156–169.
36. Schober KE, Wetli E, Drost WT. Radiographic and echocardiographic assessment of left atrial size in 100 cats with acute left-sided congestive heart failure. *Vet Radiol Ultrasound*. 2014;55(4):359–367.
37. Häggström J, Fuentes VL, Wess G. Screening for hypertrophic cardiomyopathy in cats. *J Vet Cardiol*. 2015;17: S134–S149.
38. Rohrbaugh MN, Schober KE, Rhinehart JD, Bonagura JD, Habing A, Yildiz V. Detection of congestive heart failure by Doppler echocardiography in cats with hypertrophic cardiomyopathy. *J Vet Intern Med*. 2020;34(3):1091–1101.
39. Abbott JA. Feline hypertrophic cardiomyopathy: an update. *Vet Clin North Am Small Anim Pract*. 2010;40(4): 685–700.
40. Guglielmini C, Diana A. Thoracic radiography in the cat: identification of cardiomegaly and congestive heart failure. *J Vet Cardiol*. 2015;17:S87–S101.
41. Chetboul V, Passavin P, Trehiou-Sechi E, et al. Clinical, epidemiological and echocardiographic features and prognostic factors in cats with restrictive cardiomyopathy: a retrospective study of 92 cases (2001–2015). *J Vet Intern Med*. 2019;33(3):1222–1231.
42. Ferasin L, Sturgess CP, Cannon MJ, Caney SM, Gruffydd-Jones TJ, Wotton PR. Feline idiopathic cardiomyopathy: a retrospective study of 106 cats (1994–2001). *J Feline Med Surg*. 2003;5(3):151–159.
43. Reinero C, Visser LC, Kellihan HB, et al. ACVIM consensus statement guidelines for the diagnosis, classification, treatment, and monitoring of pulmonary hypertension in dogs. *J Vet Intern Med*. 2020;34(2):549–573.
44. Adams DS, Marolf AJ, Valdés-Martínez A, Randall EK, Bachand AM. Associations between thoracic radiographic changes and severity of pulmonary arterial hypertension diagnosed in 60 dogs via Doppler echocardiography: a retrospective study. *Vet Radiol Ultrasound*. 2017;58(4): 454–462.
45. Rolph KE, Cavanaugh SM. Feline pulmonary hypertension: are we overlooking an important comorbidity? *J Feline Med Surg*. 2022;24(12):e636–e646.
46. Scollan KF, Bottorff B, Stieger-Vanegas S, Nemanic S, Sisson D. Use of multidetector computed tomography in the assessment of dogs with pericardial effusion. *J Vet Intern Med*. 2015;29(1):79–87.
47. Johnson MS, Martin M, Binns S, Day MJ. A retrospective study of clinical findings, treatment and outcome in 143 dogs with pericardial effusion. *J Small Anim Pract*. 2004;45(11):546–552.
48. Hall DJ, Shofer F, Meier CK, Sleeper MM. Pericardial effusion in cats: a retrospective study of clinical findings and outcome in 146 cats. *J Vet Intern Med*. 2007;21(5): 1002–1007.

49. Côté E, Schwarz LA, Sithole F. Thoracic radiographic findings for dogs with cardiac tamponade attributable to pericardial effusion. *J Am Vet Med Assoc*. 2013;243(2): 232–235.
50. Treggiari E, Pedro B, Dukes-McEwan J, Gelzer AR, Blackwood L. A descriptive review of cardiac tumours in dogs and cats. *Vet Comp Oncol*. 2017;15(2):273–288.
51. Aupperle H, März I, Ellenberger C, Buschatz S, Reischauer A, Schoon HA. Primary and secondary heart tumours in dogs and cats. *J Comp Pathol*. 2007;136(1): 18–26.

ELECTRONIC RESOURCES

Additional information related to the content in Chapter 35 can be found online at eBooks.Health.Elsevier.com

- Chapter Quiz
- Videos
- References

CHAPTER 36

Canine and Feline Lung

Isabelle Masseau

LUNG ANATOMY AND RADIOGRAPHIC APPEARANCE

To fulfill its role as the sole oxygen provider, the lungs contain a large amount of air, which provides contrast to the soft tissue opaque heart, major vessels (e.g., aorta, caudal vena cava), and pulmonary vasculature (Fig. 36.1). Additional opacity is provided by the musculoskeletal structures of the thorax, summating with the lungs (eFig. 36.1). The location of lung lobes is fairly constant among dogs and cats and their expected location can be extrapolated on standard three-view thoracic radiography, keeping in mind that lung lobes overlap considerably. The left lung is separated into cranial and caudal lung lobes (Fig. 36.2A). The left cranial lung lobe is further subdivided in cranial and caudal segments, connected to each other dorsally. The right lung is separated into cranial, middle, caudal, and accessory lung lobes (see Fig. 36.2B, inset, and C). The accessory lung lobe occupies a midline position, caudal to the heart, as seen on a ventrodorsal (VD) image of the thorax (see Fig. 36.2C, right bottom panel) and overlaps with the right caudal lung lobe on the left lateral view (see Fig. 36.2B).

Airways

A flowchart indicates the travel of air through the conduit airways up to the pulmonary parenchyma, where gas exchange occurs (Fig. 36.3). In general, the bronchial walls are too thin to be seen on radiography, unless they are mineralized or abnormally thick (Fig. 36.4).[1] Dogs >10 years old are more likely to have bronchial cartilage calcification, which may not be of clinical significance.[1] When the thickness allows their detection, the bronchial walls tend to taper as the bronchus courses away from its origin.

Parenchyma

The acinus constitutes the terminal respiratory unit where gas exchange occurs. This unit includes everything beyond the terminal bronchiole, that is, in the order of the incoming air flow, respiratory bronchioles, alveolar ducts, alveolar sacs, and alveoli (see Fig. 36.3). Alveoli are surrounded by a thin alveolar wall composed of epithelial cells, some of which produce surfactant, preventing collapse of alveoli during exhalation. A thin layer of connective tissue composed of collagen and elastic reticular fibers and occasional fibroblasts constitutes the supporting tissue (i.e., the interstitial space) of the pulmonary parenchyma. The sum of all terminal respiratory units with associated vessels and lymphatics and supporting connective tissue constitutes the pulmonary parenchyma. In many species (e.g., humans, pigs, cattle, and to a lesser extent horses, sheep, and goats), the lungs are further subdivided into pulmonary lobules, surrounded by connective tissue, known as interlobular septa, and disserved by a tertiary bronchus and its paired pulmonary artery.[2] Dogs and cats lack interlobular septa and thus do not share an organization into secondary pulmonary lobules.

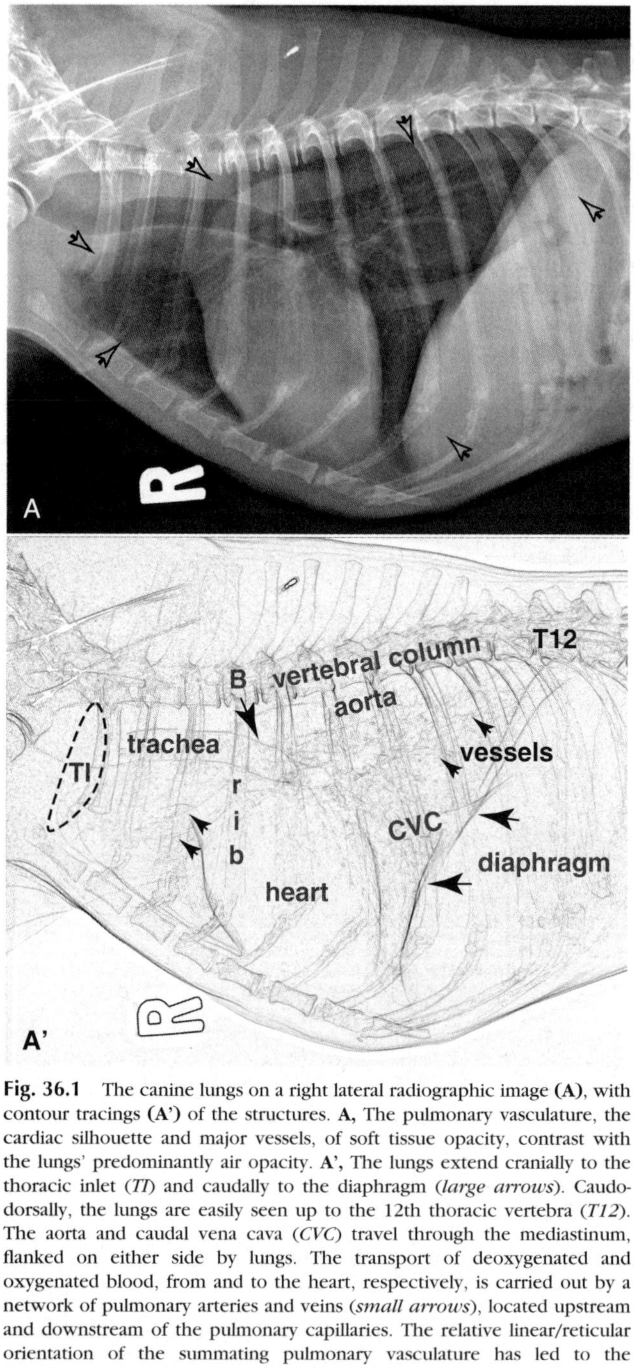

Fig. 36.1 The canine lungs on a right lateral radiographic image **(A)**, with contour tracings **(A')** of the structures. **A**, The pulmonary vasculature, the cardiac silhouette and major vessels, of soft tissue opacity, contrast with the lungs' predominantly air opacity. **A'**, The lungs extend cranially to the thoracic inlet (*TI*) and caudally to the diaphragm (*large arrows*). Caudodorsally, the lungs are easily seen up to the 12th thoracic vertebra (*T12*). The aorta and caudal vena cava (*CVC*) travel through the mediastinum, flanked on either side by lungs. The transport of deoxygenated and oxygenated blood, from and to the heart, respectively, is carried out by a network of pulmonary arteries and veins (*small arrows*), located upstream and downstream of the pulmonary capillaries. The relative linear/reticular orientation of the summating pulmonary vasculature has led to the description of canine and feline lungs appearing on radiography as "a network of radiopacities" or "normal pulmonary markings."

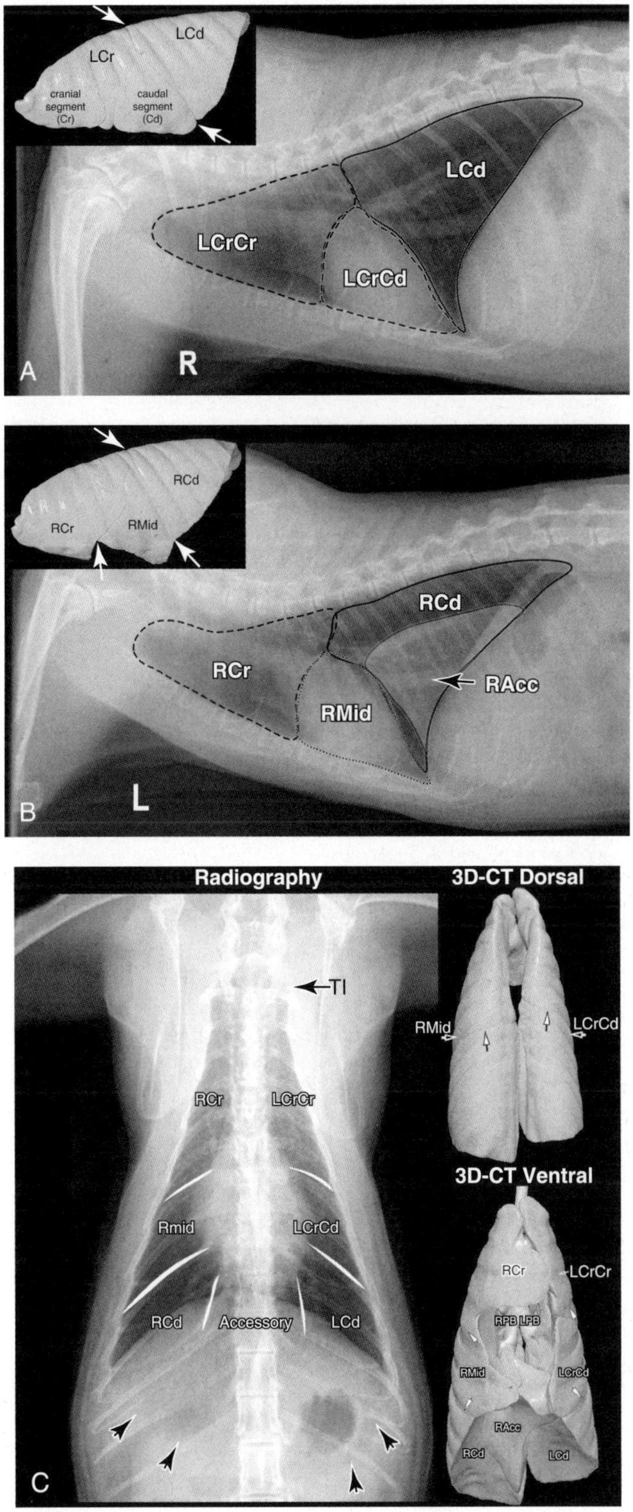

Fig. 36.2 Three-view recumbent thoracic radiography and three-dimensional (3D) computed tomography (CT) images of the lungs. Approximate location of the lung lobes or segments is indicated on the radiographic images. **A,** The left lung is divided into cranial *(LCr)* and caudal *(LCd)* lobes by deep fissures *(arrows)*. The cranial lung lobe is further subdivided into left cranial lobe cranial (*LCrCr*) and left cranial lobe caudal (*LCrCd*) subsegments, united dorsally. On a right lateral recumbent view, the caudal segment of the *LCrCd* summates with the cardiac silhouette. **B,** The right lung is separated by fissures (*inset, white arrows*) into four lobes: the right cranial (*RCr*), the right middle (*RMid*), the right caudal (*RCd*), and the accessory (*RAcc*) lung lobes. On a left lateral view, superimposed over the cardiac silhouette, is the right middle lung lobe. **C,** Dorsoventral view showing the lung lobation. The caudal lungs extend caudodorsally (*arrows*) to the attachment of the left and right diaphragmatic crura. *Right panels,* Dorsal (*top*) and ventral (*bottom*) 3D CT images of the lungs showing the fissures between the different lung lobes (*arrows*). The ventral image shows the midline position occupied by the accessory (*RAcc*) lung lobe. It is flanked on either side by the right caudal and left caudal lung lobes. *LPB,* Left principal bronchus; *RPB,* right principal bronchus.

Pulmonary Vasculature

At the hilum, each principal bronchus is accompanied by a pulmonary artery, arising from the pulmonary trunk. The right and left pulmonary arteries will branch out, in a pattern similar to the airways, coursing dorsal and lateral to the lobar bronchus. The pulmonary vein occupies a medial/ventral position to the bronchus. The smaller, individually indistinguishable vessels and bronchi contribute to the normal background opacity of the lung.

THE BREATHING CYCLE APPLIED TO THORACIC RADIOGRAPHY

Exposure factors tailored to the lungs will favor a wide range of shades of gray (low mAs, high kVp) to maximize detection of lung lesions. A short exposure time (e.g., 1/60 seconds or 1/120 seconds) minimizes motion artifact associated with respiration. Full inflation of the lungs promotes the visibility of the bronchial and vascular structures, and is more likely to depict lung lesions (Fig. 36.5).[3] Overinflation results in more radiolucency than normally expected.

Exhalation is passive during quiet breathing. Relaxing muscles and diaphragm return to their normal position, allowing carbon dioxide containing air to be exhaled, and thus, generating increased pulmonary opacity and decreased contrast between bronchial and vascular structures and pulmonary parenchyma, and pulmonary lesions (see Fig. 36.5).[3]

Factors Affecting Lung Volume

A dog's or cat's ability to inflate and then deflate their lungs depends on many factors, some of which are discussed in further detail later.

- Sedated dogs and cats with shallow breathing may not achieve maximal lung inflation.
- Placing healthy, conscious dogs in left or right lateral recumbency for 10 minutes leads to lung volume loss, even faster if sedated or anesthetized (Fig. 36.6, eFig. 36.2).[4–6] Keeping patients in lateral recumbency for as little time as possible prior to and during radiography acquisition best limits the effects of recumbency on lung volume (eFig. 36.3). Mechanical ventilation and adequate species-specific airway pressure during breath-hold technique and positive end-expiratory pressure may also help maintain better lung aeration while the animal is under general anesthesia.[7–11]
- Impaired caudal displacement of the diaphragm by, for example, excess abdominal content reduces the size of the thoracic cavity and is often compensated by increasing the width and depth leading to a barrel-chested appearance.[12]
- Any mechanism preventing ventilation of the alveoli, whether as a result of airway occlusion by tissue, fluid, or solid material, or as a result of compression by an extrapulmonary mass, will result in a reduction in volume.

Airways have to remain open during exhalation to expel air out of the lung parenchyma. Abnormal closure of the airways on exhalation traps air. On imaging, abnormal air retention (i.e., dynamic air trapping) beyond the closed airway manifests as a region, segment, or lobe of the lung that fails to decrease in volume at expiration (eFig. 36.4).[13]

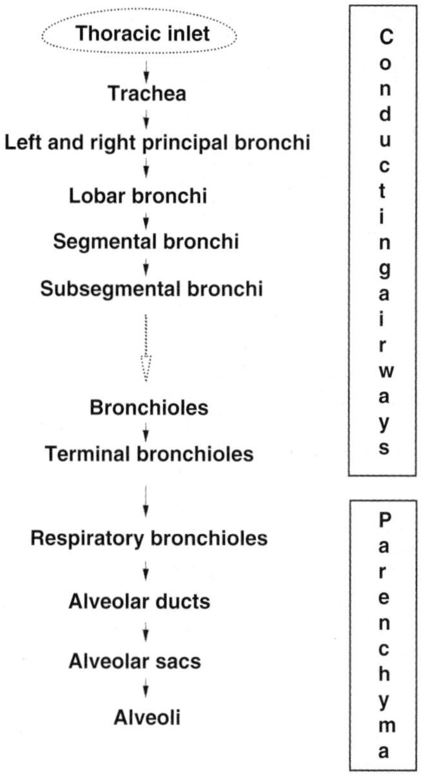

Fig. 36.3 Flowchart indicating the different structures traversed by air following its entry into the thoracic cavity. Air will flow from the nostrils through a series of upper and then lower conduits until the terminal respiratory units of the lungs are reached, where gas exchange occurs. Dogs and cats ventilate each lung through the left and right principal bronchi, also referred to as the mainstem bronchi, partitioning from the trachea. After a short course in the mediastinum, each principal bronchus, constituting the first generation of airways, enters the hilum of the right or left lungs and divides almost immediately into lobar bronchi, named after the lobe they ventilate. The lobar bronchi represent the second generation of airways and their branching pattern is fairly conserved among dogs and cats. Within each lung lobe, the lobar bronchus gives rise to segmental bronchi, also called tertiary bronchi (third generation) arising dorsally and ventrally for most lung lobes except for the right middle lung lobe, from which they emerge cranially and caudally. Segmental bronchi divide into subsegmental bronchi (fourth generation) which further subdivide into smaller subsegmental bronchi to 9 or 10 divisions. At the end, air will reach the smallest airway, the bronchiole. In contrast to bronchi, bronchioles lack cartilage in their walls. The terminal bronchioles are interposed between the conducting airways and the pulmonary parenchyma. No gas exchange occurs at this level. Air will then diffuse through the respiratory bronchioles, alveolar ducts, and alveolar sacs until they reach the pulmonary alveoli where exchange of oxygen or carbon dioxide will occur. The pulmonary parenchyma also includes small vessels <20–25 μm in diameter, predominantly capillaries, and represents the major component of lungs.

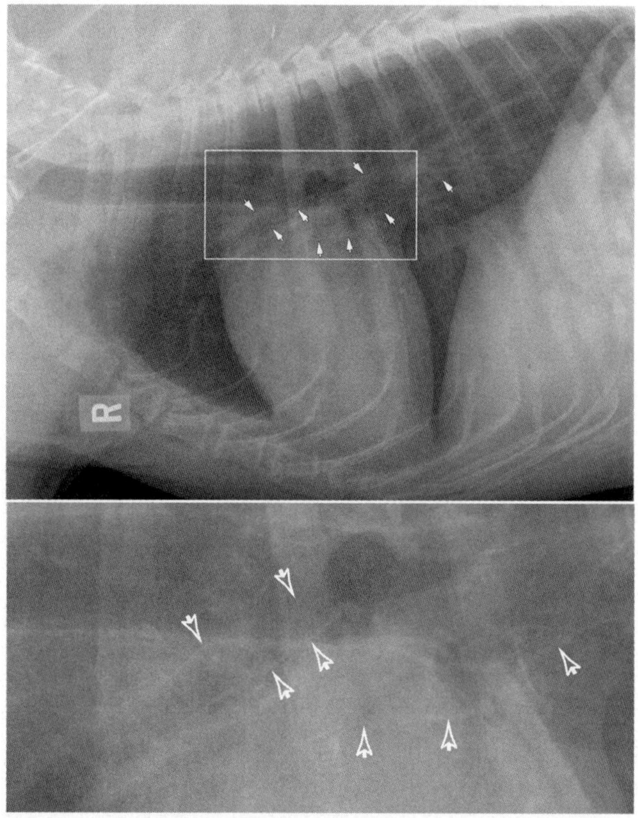

Fig. 36.4 Mineralization of the airway walls. Right lateral radiographic view showing mineralization of the bronchial walls (*arrows*) in an 8-year-old male castrated German shepherd dog without any respiratory clinical signs. *Inset,* the walls are sharply demarcated, thin, and of regular thickness. They are only detected near the hilum of the lungs.

Standard Examination: Three Recumbent View Study (R, L, and VD/DV)

Lung assessment is best performed on thoracic radiographs captured during the inspiratory phase of respiration. Acquiring additional expiratory views can be useful for highlighting dynamic airway collapse.[14–17]

Right and left lateral recumbent views are mandatory for radiographic assessment of lung disease to mitigate the negative effect of recumbency on lung volume and aeration (Fig. 36.7). Omission of one (left or right) of the lateral recumbent views may result in misdiagnosis.[18] A VD view is usually best for assessment of the accessory lung lobe, whereas a dorsoventral (DV) view may be indicated for dorsally located lesions or to evaluate the caudodorsal pulmonary vasculature.

Description of Lung Lesions

Interpretation of lung disease on thoracic radiography is challenging and there are several reasons for this.

1. The lungs are surrounded by numerous soft tissue and osseous structures that become superimposed over the lungs and add opacity on radiographs.
2. The different conformations of dog breeds challenge what is considered normal for one breed while abnormal for another.
3. The degree of lung expansion influences its radiographic appearance. Subtle lung lesions may be missed in expiratory radiographs.
4. Very few diseases, if any, have a pathognomonic radiographic appearance. It is common for diseases to share a few or even many radiographic findings.
5. A given disease may present with a wide spectrum of radiographic manifestations

RADIOGRAPHIC ASSESSMENT OF PULMONARY DISEASE

The pulmonary pattern recognition paradigm is widely used to assess the radiographic appearance of the lungs, with the intent to focus on the compartment of the lung that is abnormal (i.e., the pattern) as an organized approach to image evaluation. Certain patterns are associated with certain diseases, which can

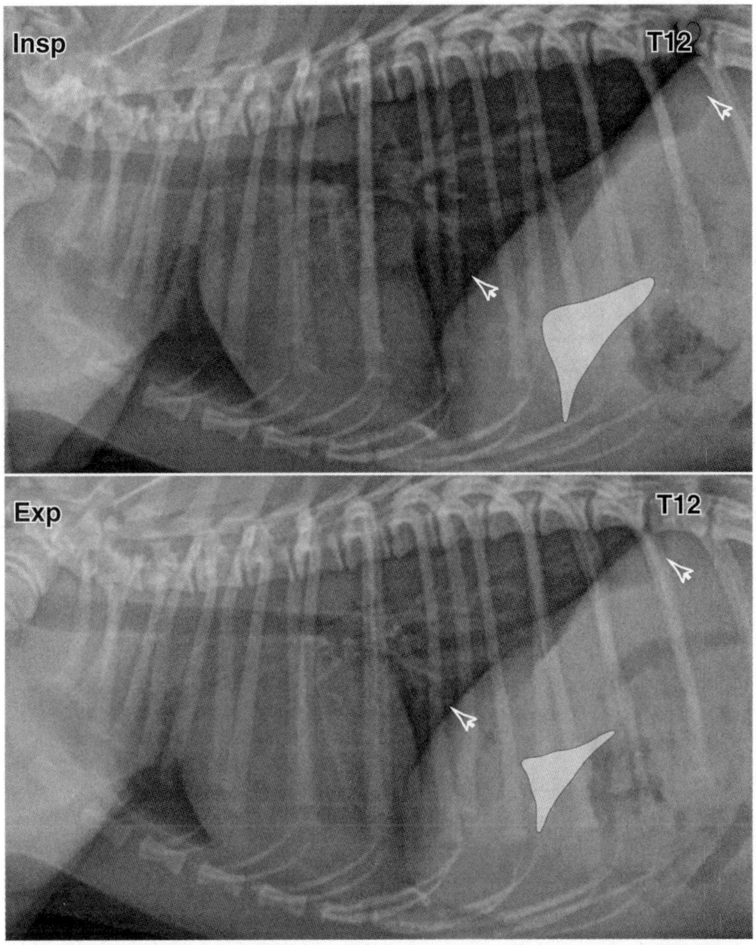

Fig. 36.5 Inspiratory and expiratory left lateral radiographic views. The lateral inspiratory view (*top, Insp*) is characterized by a slight elevation of the cranial border of the cardiac silhouette from the sternum due to inflation of the cranial lung lobes, caudal excursion of the lumbodiaphragmatic angles (*arrows*) caudal to T12, decreased diaphragmatic contact with the caudal border of the cardiac silhouette, and enlargement of the caudoventral lungs. These changes may not be visible in panting or tachypneic dogs.[4] Passive exhalation (*bottom, Exp*) is characterized by the cranial location of the diaphragmatic cupula, often superimposed the caudal border of the cardiac silhouette. A triangle-shape region (*white overlay*) outlining the borders of the cardiac silhouette, diaphragm, and caudal vena cava, represent a quick method to assess the phase of respiration. This region is larger on a view taken in inspiration compared to expiration.

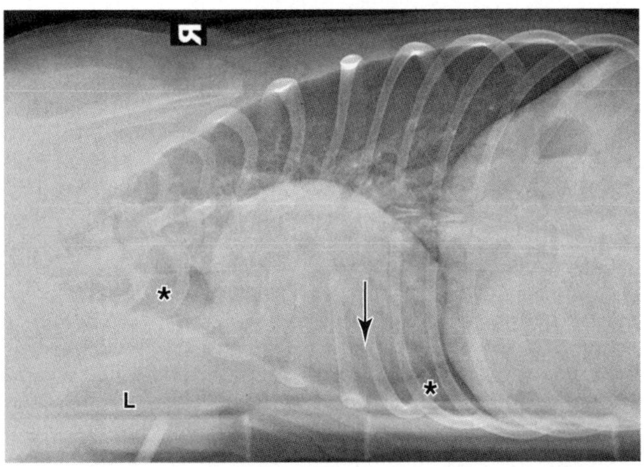

Fig. 36.6 Effect of body position on lung aeration using a horizontal x-ray beam. The patient was placed in left lateral recumbency and a horizontal x-ray beam oriented towards the sternum of the dog was used. The left lung ("bottom lung") is decreased in size (i.e., decreased lung volume) and increased in opacity (*asterisks*). The cardiac silhouette is shifted to the left (*arrow*). The nondependent lung ("top" lung), in this case the right lung, is well aerated and of normal opacity.

help in formulating differential diagnoses for a particular radiographic presentation. It is critical to understand, however, that the pulmonary patterns are not specific to any particular lung disease, with most conditions presenting at least two different pulmonary patterns or different combinations of patterns. It is therefore important to use roentgen signs (i.e., number, location/position, size, shape, opacity, contour, severity) in concert with pulmonary patterns to formulate a comprehensive description of pulmonary pathology.

The Use of Roentgen Signs

Number

A single lesion is called *focal* or *solitary*. When two or more lesions are visible surrounded by unaffected areas in the lung, the term *multifocal* is used. Multifocal lesions can be found in different lung lobes or in a single lung lobe.

Lesions involving the majority of a lung lobe/segment, with no evidence of unaffected areas, or with very little unremarkable lung, are ultimately *diffuse*. Although diffuse lesions often involve two or more lung lobes or segments, they can apply to lesions involving a single lung lobe or segment. Lesions targeting a specific anatomy, such as all intrathoracic airways, may also be termed diffuse.

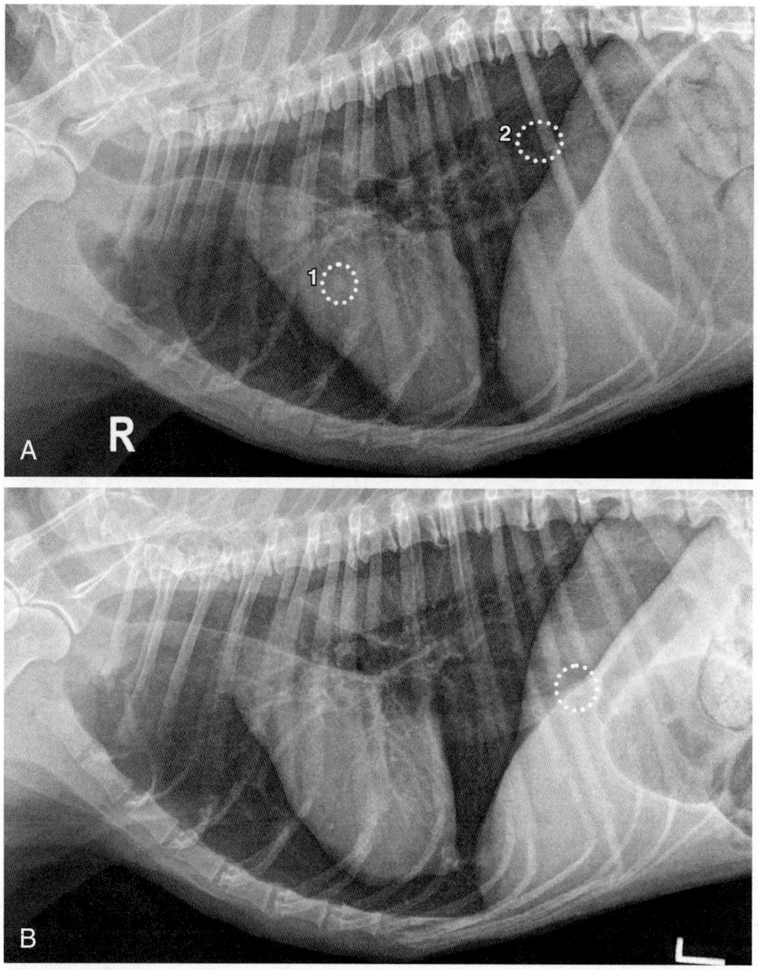

Fig. 36.7 The effect of recumbency on the detection of pulmonary nodules on radiography. **A,** Right lateral view showing an oval, well-demarcated, soft tissue opacity nodule superimposed over the cardiac silhouette (*1, dotted circle*). A second less defined soft tissue opaque nodule, is seen in the eighth intercostal space, partially superimposed over the ninth rib (*2, dotted circle*). **B,** When the dog is placed in left lateral recumbency, the nodules are no longer seen, instead a different nodule is visible superimposed over the caudal vena cava. The inflation of the dependent lung is reduced while the nondependent lung (i.e., the top lung) has better inflation. Because of this effect, small lesions in the left lung can only be seen in the right lateral view, and vice versa. The pulmonary nodules corresponded to pulmonary metastases from a transitional cell carcinoma of the urinary bladder.

Location/Position

The position of a lesion should be described based on lung lobation. Anatomical landmarks such as the heart base, caudal vena cava, and trachea can also be used to describe the position of a lesion relative to another structure. The location of lesions has also been categorized according to three concentric zones relative to the hilum of each lung, the central or perihilar, middle and peripheral regions.

There are a few diseases that tend to be more often associated with specific lung lobes or a location. Pulmonary edema of cardiogenic or noncardiogenic origin tends to have a bilateral symmetrical or asymmetrical appearance localizing first to the hilar region, and more pronounced in the caudal lung lobes, although other locations and distributions, especially in cats, are possible (Fig. 36.8).[19] Bronchopneumonia or aspiration pneumonia often localizes to the cranial or right middle lung lobes (Fig. 36.9). The caudal lung lobes are a common site for primary lung tumors (Fig. 36.10), while histiocytic sarcoma most commonly occurs in the left cranial and right middle lung lobes (Fig. 36.11).[20,21]

Size

Circular or oval lesions are commonly reported according to their diameter. Circular or oval lesions with a diameter of <3 cm are called *nodules*, while a lesion of or exceeding 3 cm is termed a *mass* (Fig. 36.12).[13,20,22] The presence of numerous small punctate soft tissue nodules throughout the lungs has been described as *miliary* nodules (Fig. 36.13).[23]

Mineral opacity lesions and metallic objects can be detected even if they are very small (~ 1 mm). Digital radiography can today reliably depict soft tissue nodules of 2 to 3 mm in diameter.[24–26] However, some nodules may be difficult to identify or completely missed on radiography compared to computed tomography (CT), even if their size exceeds the minimum detection threshold.[24–26] Pulmonary vessels can sometimes be confused with pulmonary nodules when viewed in cross-section or, in other words, end on (Fig. 36.14A). End-on vessels are superimposed over a parent vessel, usually linearly oriented, of the same or greater diameter, and located next to an end-on bronchus. End-on vessels are larger near the hilar region and smaller as they move away towards the periphery. When in doubt, oblique views can help to compensate for a possible overlap with a vascular shadow and to confirm the identification of a nodule.

Shape

Lung lesions can vary considerably in shape depending on their anatomical location and this topic is discussed further later.

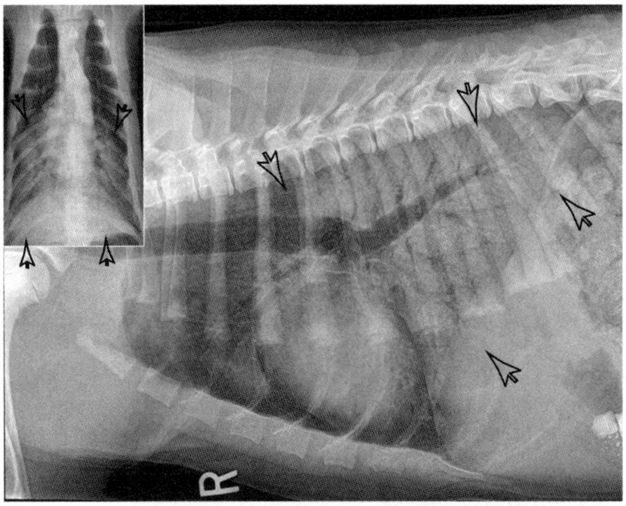

Fig. 36.8 Noncardiogenic pulmonary edema and its predominant caudal and bilateral lung distribution of lesions in 4-month-old Irish Wolfhound puppy after near-drowning. Right lateral view showing more profound lesions in the caudal lungs (*arrows*) in comparison to the cranial lungs. The marked increase in opacity associated with a loss of distinction of the pulmonary vessels, revealing only the air contained in the bronchi, corresponds to an alveolar pattern. *Inset,* Ventrodorsal view of the same dog showing lesions preferentially distributed to the left caudal, right caudal, and accessory lung lobes (*arrows*). A full-size ventrodorsal view is available on the online version (see eFig. 36.5).

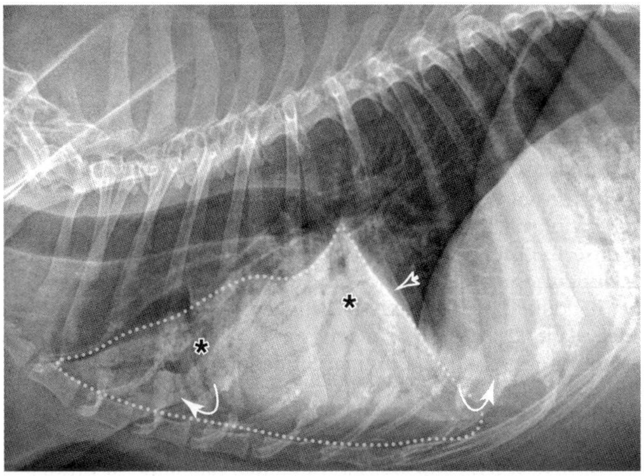

Fig. 36.9 Aspiration pneumonia in a 13-year-old female spayed mixed-breed canine. Left lateral view showing a severe increase in opacity in the region of the right cranial and right middle lung lobes (*dotted outline*) with air bronchograms (*asterisks*). There is border effacement (*curved arrows*) between the affected lung and the cardiac silhouette, and the diaphragm/liver. A lobar sign (*straight arrow*) is also noted between the affected right middle and spared right caudal lung lobes. These radiographic changes are characteristic of an alveolar pattern.

Opacity

The lung opacity is intrinsically linked to lung volume. Lung underinflation results in an overall increase in opacity with crowded pulmonary vasculature, and crowded air bronchograms. In severe cases the pulmonary vasculature may be completely obscured by the lack of aeration of a lung segment or lobe(s) belonging to the side of which the animal was lying on (see eFig. 36.2). A mediastinal shift towards the dependent lung is an indirect sign of underinflation and atelectasis associated with recumbency.

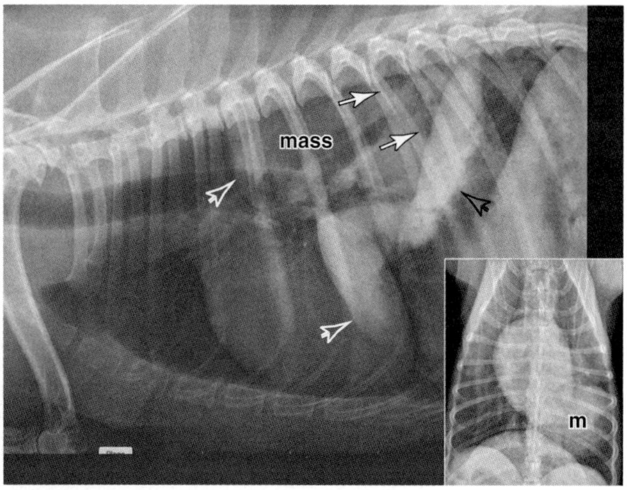

Fig. 36.10 A solitary soft tissue opaque pulmonary mass in a 12-year-old female spayed Labrador retriever. A large well-defined irregularly shaped solitary mass is seen in the left caudal lung lobe on the right lateral view. The soft tissue opaque mass has smooth margins cranially (*open white arrows*) and irregular margins caudally (*open black arrow*). Several small irregularly marginated gas bubbles are seen within the mass (*solid arrows*). No pulmonary nodules are seen in the reminder of the lung. *Inset,* The pulmonary mass (*m*) occupies the left caudal lung lobe. A full-size ventrodorsal view is available on the online version (eFig. 36.6). The dog underwent a left caudal lobectomy and recovered uneventfully. The mass was diagnosed as a grade II (moderately differentiated) pulmonary carcinoma on histopathology.

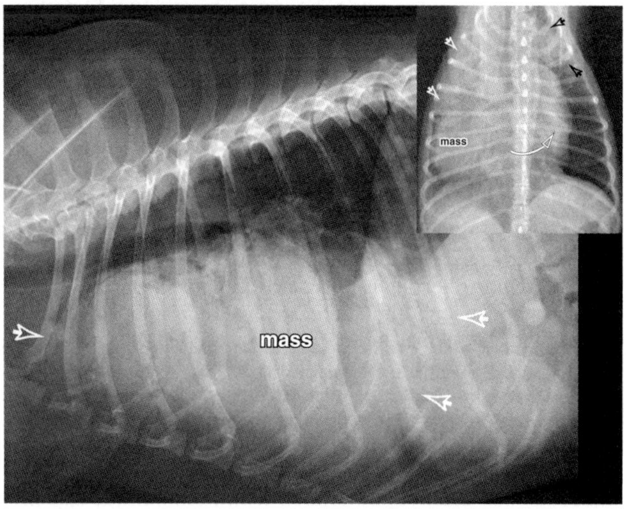

Fig. 36.11 Primary pulmonary histiocytic sarcoma in a 9-year-old female spayed miniature schnauzer. Left lateral view showing a large irregularly shaped and lobulated mass (*arrows*) occupying the entire cranioventral thorax extending caudally to silhouette with the diaphragm, and liver (*caudal arrows*). The soft tissue opaque mass also creates border effacement with the cranial mediastinum and cardiac silhouette. *Inset,* On the ventrodorsal view, the lung mass is distinguished in the region of the right middle and right caudal lung lobes with air surrounding its lateral aspect. The right cranial thorax is entirely soft tissue opaque with no distinction between the mass and the thoracic wall, cardiac silhouette, and mediastinum (*white arrows*). The left cranial thorax is occupied by an irregularly-shaped soft tissue opaque mass (*black arrows*), corresponding to enlarged mediastinal lymph nodes based on a following computed tomography (CT) study. The cardiac silhouette is slightly shifted to the left (*curved arrow*). A full-size ventrodorsal view (eFig. 36.7) and an inspiratory CT image (eFig. 36.8) are available on the online version.

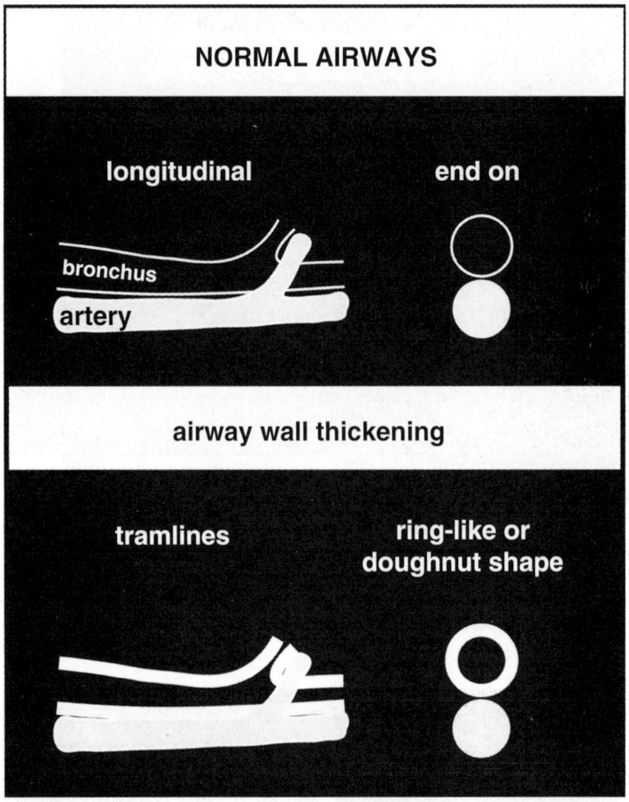

Fig. 36.16 Schematic illustration of bronchial wall thickening. The *top panel* shows a normal bronchus in longitudinal and cross-section (end-on) with its paired pulmonary artery. Normal airways should have thin walls that are not usually perceived on radiography. *Bottom panel,* thickening of the bronchial wall may result in tramlines-like appearing structures when the bronchus is cut in a longitudinal plane or in a ring-like or doughnut-shape like appearance when cut in cross-section. The thickened bronchial wall, in close proximity with the paired pulmonary artery, may become effaced, due to a silhouette sign.

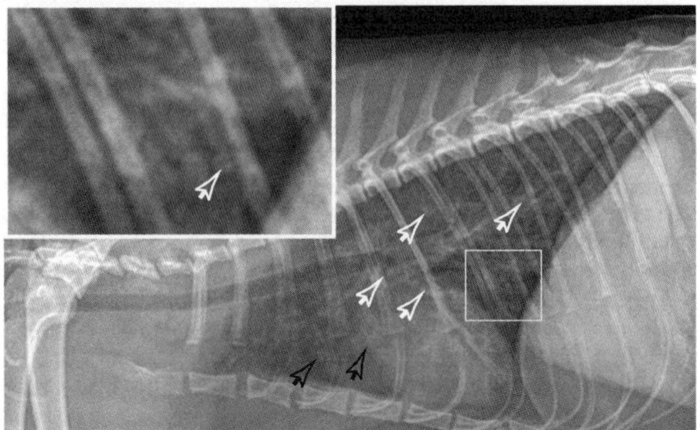

Fig. 36.17 Bronchial pattern in a 2-year-old female spayed Ocicat with allergic asthma. A large number of ring-like or doughnut-shape like (*white arrows*) and tramlines (*black arrows*) lesions are seen diffusely throughout the lung. *Inset,* Close-up on thickened airway walls viewed end on (*arrow*).

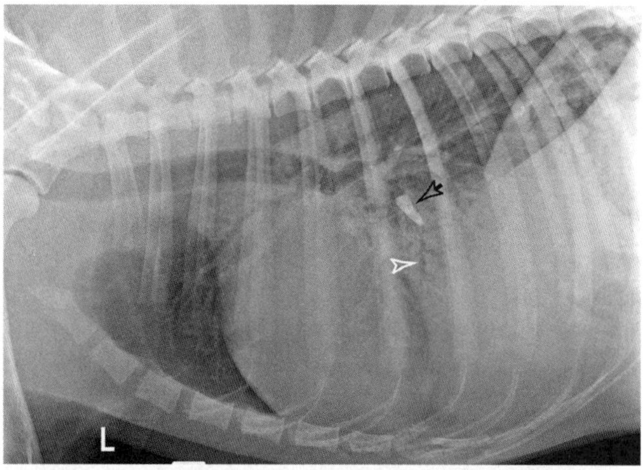

Fig. 36.18 Mineralized foreign object (a canine tooth) in the accessory lung lobe of a 2-year-old intact male German Shepherd dog. The dog was recently diagnosed with a fracture of the right maxillary canine tooth (#104). On the left lateral view, the fractured fragment of canine tooth (*black arrow*) is present in the accessory lung lobe. This lung lobe is also increased in opacity, with air bronchograms (*white triangle*) causing border effacement with the diaphragm and caudal border of the cardiac silhouette. On bronchoscopy, there was purulent exudate collected in the accessory lung lobe and the tip of the tooth could be seen in the lobar bronchus. Multiple attempts to remove the tooth with a basket retrieval device and biopsy forceps were unsuccessful. Upon recovery, the dog coughed the tooth up which was subsequently swallowed and visible in the gastrointestinal tract. The tooth was passed uneventfully. The dog was prescribed antimicrobials for bacterial pneumonia following aerobic and anaerobic bacterial growth on direct culture of isolates from collected bronchoalveolar lavage fluid.

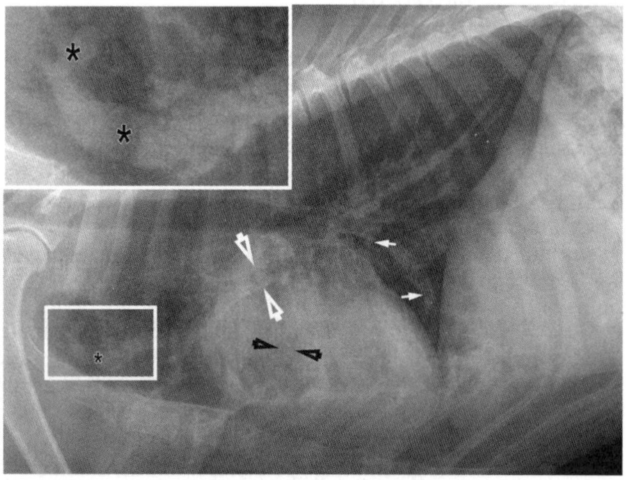

Fig. 36.19 Bronchial luminal filling in a 10-year-old female spayed Labrador retriever with bacterial pneumonia. Right lateral view showing a dilated bronchus (*large white arrows*) with intraluminal soft tissue material at its distal aspect (*asterisks*). Bronchial wall thickening is also visible in the ventral lungs as revealed by tramlines (*open black arrows*) and ring-like lesions (*solid white arrows*). *Inset,* Close-up image of the bronchial intraluminal soft tissue filling (*asterisk*).

plane (Fig. 36.19) and circular when viewed in cross-section, independently of the nature of the content. This is more easily seen if the proximal aspect of the bronchus still contains air, providing contrast at the interface with the distal content. Purulent material/cellular debris/fluid/mucus may collect in bronchi in cases of infectious bronchopneumonia or eosinophilic disease,[33] more so in dilated bronchi.[34]

Bronchial plugging refers to the collection of mucoid material in the lumen of a dilated bronchus. It has been reported in asthmatic cats with hyperplasia of the submucosal glands and proliferation of goblet cells. In this instance, resorptive atelectasis may occur in the nonventilated alveoli and airspaces beyond the occlusion (Fig. 36.20).

Bronchiectasis refers to the irreversible dilation of medium- and large-sized bronchus, a consequence of the destruction of the muscular elements of the bronchial walls. The imaging

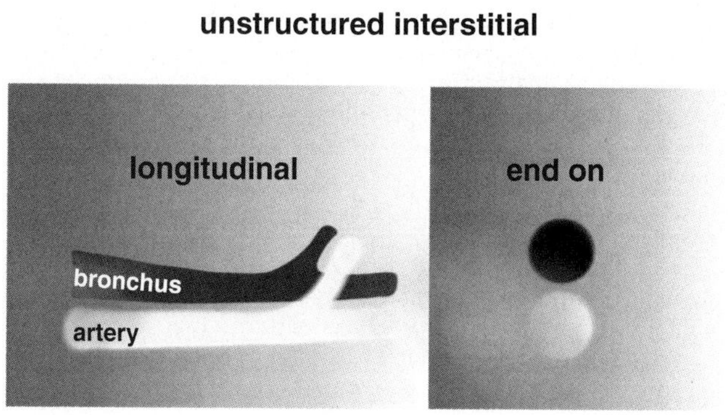

Fig. 36.25 Schematic representation of an unstructured interstitial pattern. When the opacity of the lung is increased focally, multifocally or diffusely, the affected region will show a reduction in the sharpness of the pulmonary artery margination on both longitudinal or cross-sectional planes.

It may also exhibit multiple, short indistinct nonvascular linear or reticular opacities in one or more lung lobe or segment (Fig. 36.25).[23] Overall increase in opacity associated with under inflated lungs, obesity, or motion artifact can have the appearance of an unstructured interstitial pattern and should be taken into account when interpreting lung patterns. The unstructured interstitial pattern can be detected with a variety of lung diseases such as infection, inflammation, neoplasia, edema, trauma, or toxicity (Table 36.3; Fig. 36.26, eFigs. 36.15 and 36.16).

The Paradox of Aging Lungs

Increased nonvascular linear markings in the lungs in association with pleural thickening and bronchial cartilage calcification in dogs has previously been attributed to aging.[1] At the time, the authors attributed these markings to increased connective tissue, mainly focal alveolar fibrosis, in lungs of old dogs associated with prior inflammation.[1] Two recent studies found no differences in pulmonary lesions scores between young and old dogs on radiography or CT, although older dogs were shown to have increased bronchial mucosal irregularity, prominent vessels, and bronchiectasis on bronchoscopy.[43] It remains unclear whether these discordant findings are associated with different environmental contexts, digitization of radiographic systems, or with the modality. It appears reasonable to suspect that as dogs live longer, they have a higher likelihood of accumulating structural lesions over time, possibly resulting in a subtle increase in nonvascular pulmonary markings. It may then become difficult to differentiate these structural lesions from clinically relevant active lesions. In these instances, advanced imaging (i.e., CT, bronchoscopy, positron emission tomography [PET]) and ancillary tests may be beneficial.

Alveolar Pattern

The *alveolar pattern* is characterized by increased pulmonary opacity with effacement of vascular markings, air-bronchograms, and a lobar sign. Increased opacity is of no particular shape, showing ill-defined or wispy margins in comparison to the surrounding parenchyma, rendering the pulmonary vessels within the affected area indistinct (Fig. 36.27). These areas do not appear as discrete circular or oval shaped lesions, as these would often be categorized as belonging to a structured interstitial pattern. Affected parenchymal areas silhouette (i.e., border effacement) with adjacent soft tissue lesions or structures (i.e., cardiac silhouette, diaphragm, cranial mediastinum, pleural fluid). The affected area may or may not

result is a dilated bronchus that fails to taper as it extends away from its origin (referring to the parent bronchus from which it branches).[22] Bronchiectasis should not be confused with an air bronchogram, which consists in an air-filled bronchus surrounded by collapsed (nonventilated) or soft tissue-filled alveoli. Unlike an air bronchogram, an ectatic bronchus will remain dilated on serial radiography, even in the absence of active infection. Dogs with primary ciliary dyskinesia have defective respiratory cilia that impair mucociliary clearance and predispose to recurrent infection, often resulting in bronchiectasis.[35]

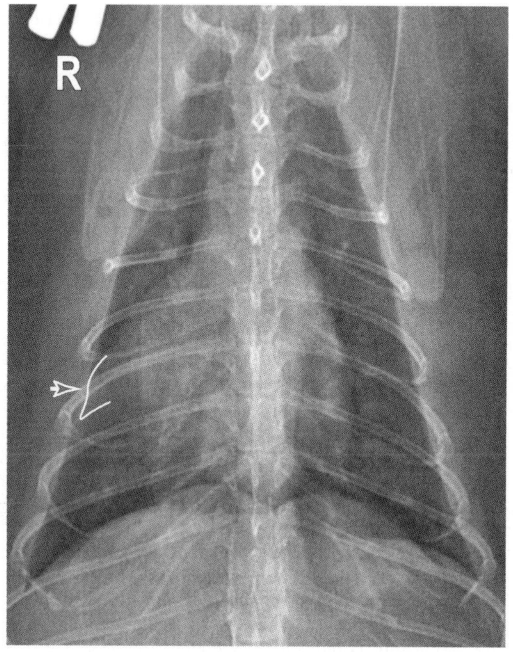

Fig. 36.20 Resorptive atelectasis of the right middle lung lobe in a 6-year-old female spayed Ocicat with allergic asthma. This is the same cat as in Fig. 36.17, but 4 years later. The right middle lung lobe (*arrow*) is collapsed, resulting in a triangular-shaped soft tissue opacity (*white outline*). A rightward mediastinal shift is visible. The right middle lobar bronchus was presumably plugged with mucus, the production of which is abnormally increased in asthma, causing a resorptive atelectasis of the right middle lung lobe.

Ectatic airways can take a cylindrical (or tubular; Fig. 36.21), saccular (sometimes also called cystic), or varicose shape, with some authors classifying saccular and cystic as two distinct forms[34] (see Fig. 36.21, eFigs. 36.13 and 36.14).[36] Bronchiectasis is often accompanied by bronchial wall thickening, which may explain accentuation of a bronchial pattern on radiography.

Lesions Localized to the Pulmonary Parenchyma

Parenchymal lesions include abnormalities of the terminal respiratory units including the alveoli (specifically the lumen of the alveoli), the interstitium (the septa bordering the alveolus), and the small vessels. Lesions affecting the pulmonary parenchyma may share a similar radiographic appearance regardless of etiology, chronicity, or anatomic structure affected. Several hypotheses can be put forward to explain this finding:

1. Radiography cannot distinguish between different types of cellular infiltration, fluid collection, fibrin and collagen deposits, formation of small thrombi, or emboli.
2. There is a close spatial relationship between the alveolar lumen and the septa.
3. Many diseases affect all three components of the parenchyma to varying degrees.

Despite their names, interstitial and alveolar patterns may not always correlate to the same histopathological location of disease.[37] Diseases affecting small airways, small pulmonary veins (e.g., pulmonary veno-occlusive disease), or pulmonary capillaries may lead to recognition of a structured or unstructured interstitial pattern on radiography.[38,39] As a precaution, it is therefore desirable to use the alveolar and interstitial patterns for descriptive terminology of lesions affecting the lung parenchyma, rather than true histological correlates.

Interstitial Pattern

Two major distinct forms characterize the *interstitial pattern* on radiography, the *structured (nodular) interstitial pattern* or the *unstructured interstitial pattern*, both of which can occur concurrently or accompanying another pattern. The nodular or structured interstitial pattern is characterized by the presence of nodules or masses in the lungs. A nonexhaustive list of differential diagnoses is provided for a structured interstitial pattern (Table 36.2). The number, size, location, and contour of nodules or masses can vary considerably within a group of diseases (e.g., neoplasia) or between diseases of different etiologies (e.g., histoplasmosis vs. neoplasia). Nodules are commonly seen with pulmonary metastatic disease

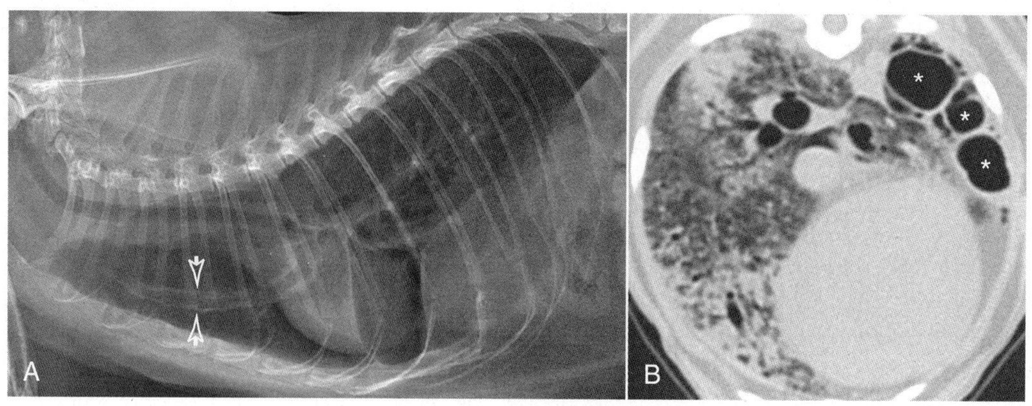

Fig. 36.21 Cylindrical and cystic bronchiectasis. **A,** Cylindrical bronchiectasis characterized by dilation of a cranial lobar bronchus *(between arrows)* in a 10-year-old male castrated Egyptian Mau cat. The bronchial walls are thickened and do not taper as they course away from their origin. On postmortem histopathologic examination, the cat was diagnosed with acute suppurative bronchopneumonia with chronic allergic asthma. **B,** Cystic bronchiectasis of the left caudal lobar bronchus (*asterisks*) on a transverse computed tomography image of an 8-year-old intact male miniature poodle canine with post-infectious bronchiolitis obliterans.

Table • 36.2

Differential Diagnoses for a Structured Interstitial Pattern (Nodule <3 cm in Diameter; Mass ≥3 cm in Diameter).

Pulmonary osteomas (synonyms: heterotopic bone formation, osseous metaplasia)*
Metastatic neoplasia
Pulmonary blastomycosis
Lymphoma
Hematogenous pneumonia
Primary lung tumor
Epithelial lung tumors (malignant > benign) such as adenocarcinoma (papillary, acinar), bronchioloalveolar carcinoma, bronchial gland carcinoma, or squamous cell carcinoma
Histiocytic sarcoma
Heartworm disease
Pulmonary histoplasmosis (active form; inactive is often associated with mineralization of the pulmonary nodules)
Eosinophilic lung disease not associated with *Dirofilaria immitis*
Hematoma
Paragonimiasis
Pulmonary coccidioidomycosis
Paenibacillus amylolyticus osteomyelitis with pulmonary granulomatous inflammation
Leptospirosis pulmonary hemorrhage syndrome
Pulmonary alveolar microlithiasis and pulmonary interstitial mineralization
Pulmonary meningotheliomatosis
Pulmonary veno-occlusive disease and pulmonary capillary hemangiomatosis
Bronchiolar disorders (CT only)

*Usually small mineralized nodules of 1–2 mm in diameter.

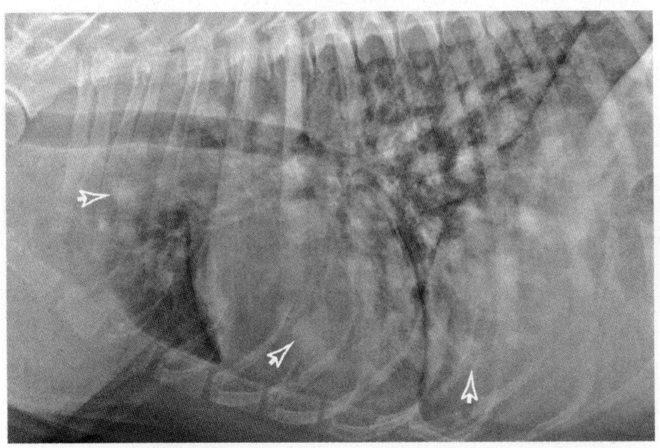

Fig. 36.22 Ill-defined nodular-shaped pulmonary lesions associated with eosinophilic lung disease in a 2-year-old male intact Rottweiler. There are numerous ill-defined soft tissue pulmonary nodules throughout the lung (*arrows*), in addition to bronchial wall thickening, an airway-centered unstructured interstitial pattern transitioning to multifocal areas of consolidation (or alveolar pattern). The dog had greatly improved after treatment with almost complete resolution of the nodular and consolidated parenchymal lesions.

be associated with the recognition of an *air-bronchogram(s)* or *lobar sign*. An air-bronchogram consists of a bronchus containing air that contrasts with the soft tissue opacity generated by the surrounding alveolar filling or alveolar collapse, making it visible (see Figs. 36.8 and 36.9). A *lobar sign* is seen when the borders of two lung lobe(s)/segment(s) become distinct from one another due to increased opacity in one lobe/segment while the other is relatively spared (Fig. 36.28, eFigs. 36.17–36.19). Diseases associated with an alveolar pattern can be of various origins (e.g., infectious, inflammatory, neoplastic, traumatic, toxic, foreign, or associated with fluid overload/congestive heart failure, fibrosis) and acute or chronic (Table 36.4).[42] Obstruction of an airway with subsequent resorptive atelectasis of the nonventilated alveoli may also result in an alveolar pattern.[23]

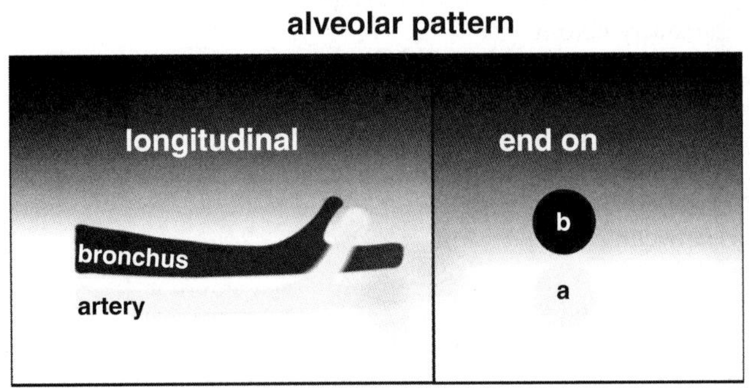

Fig. 36.27 Schematic representation of an alveolar pattern. The opacity of the lung is increased to the point where the pulmonary artery (*a*) becomes indistinct, silhouetting with the abnormal lung parenchyma. When air remains in the bronchus (*b*), an air bronchogram is visible, resulting from the contrast between the air black shadow and the surrounding alveolar filling or alveolar collapse.

An alveolar pattern does not necessarily reflect an alveolar filling disorder, and alveolar filling disorders may result in different patterns than an alveolar pattern on radiography (Table 36.5).[2]

Vascular Pattern

Enlargement of the pulmonary vasculature may disrupt the regular linear background markings of the lung, making it stand out more than normal. A vascular pattern could therefore be included in a comprehensive discussion of pulmonary patterns, but the vascular pattern is covered in Chapter 35 and not included here.

Focal, Multifocal, or Diffuse Areas of Decreased Radiographic Opacity

Cystic Air-Filled Lesions

Cystic air-filled lesions (synonym: pneumatocyst) can occur as the result of a congenital or acquired process.[44,45] Their content is typically air which is not limited by septa, airways, and capillaries, resulting in a focal radiolucency. They are usually well circumscribed, relatively circular in shape, and surrounded by a thin wall (<3 mm).[46] Malignant transformation of air-filled cystic lesions has been shown in two dogs.[47] In human medicine, cystic air-filled lesions comprise bulla, pneumatoceles, blebs, cavity or cavitating or cavitary nodule/mass/consolidation, and lung cysts. In veterinary medicine, several of these terms have been used interchangeably, the most often all-encompassing term being *bullae* for any thin-walled, relatively circular, air-filled structure, regardless of its size or presence or absence of concurrent lung diseases (Fig. 36.29).

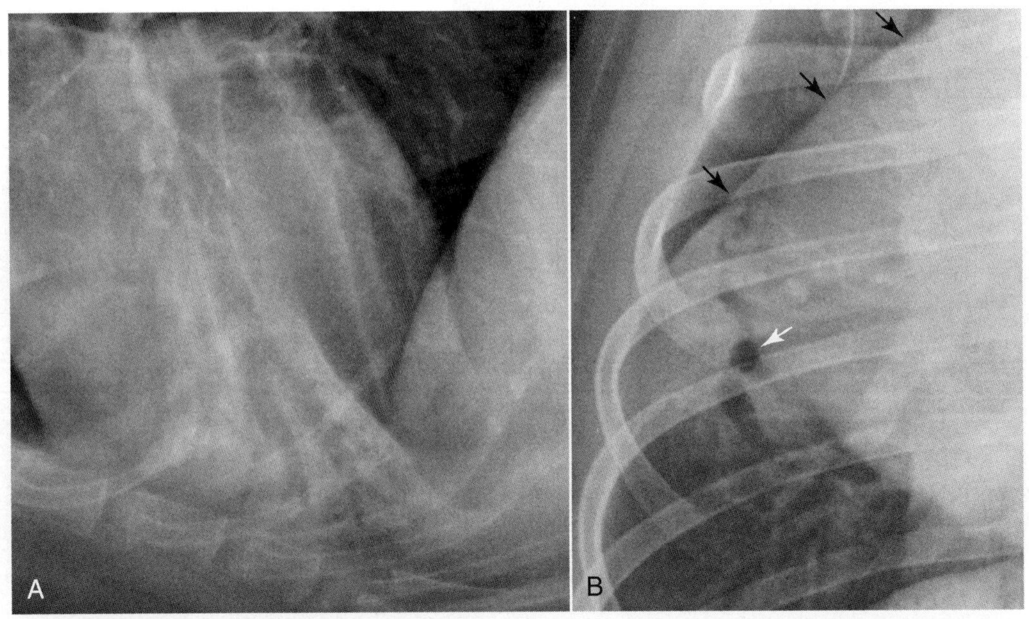

Fig. 36.28 Ventral **(A)** and right middle **(B)** regions of the thorax of a dog with an alveolar pattern. Numerous air bronchograms are seen throughout the increased lung opacity. In **A**, the branches of the air bronchogram are more crowded than normal because the lobe is also partially collapsed. In **B**, note how the increased opacity of the lung has caused border effacement, or silhouetting, of the right aspect of the cardiac silhouette. Border effacement of the heart is a common finding with an alveolar pattern when the abnormal lung and heart are in contact. The junction between the opacified right middle lobe and the normally aerated right cranial lobe creates a distinct transition, termed a *lobar sign* (*black arrows*). Also in **B**, an air bronchogram is struck end-on by the x-ray beam, creating a conspicuous circular radiolucency (*white arrow*).

Table • 36.4

Differential Diagnoses for an Alveolar Pattern on Radiography.

Aspiration pneumonia
Bacterial pneumonia (i.e., community acquired, nosocomial, or secondary infection)
Cardiogenic or noncardiogenic pulmonary edema
Pulmonary contusions or hemorrhage
Obstructive (resorptive) or nonobstructive atelectasis
Severe lung underinflation associated with exhalation
Pulmonary thromboembolic disease
Eosinophilic lung disease
Heartworm disease (*Dirofilaria immitis, Angiostrongylus vasorum*)
End-stage pulmonary fibrosis
Fungal pneumonia
Bronchiolar disorder
Parasitic lung disease (e.g., aelurostrongylosis, paragonimiasis, parasitic disease associated with *Crenosoma vulpis*)
Pulmonary veno-occlusive disease and pulmonary capillary hemangiomatosis
Pulmonary alveolar proteinosis

Table • 36.5

Differential Diagnoses for Alveolar Filling Disorders.

SUBSTANCE FILLING THE ALVEOLI	DISEASE
Serous fluid	Cardiogenic or noncardiogenic pulmonary edema
Pus	Pneumonia
Blood	Pulmonary hemorrhage
Malignant cells	Bronchioloalveolar carcinoma
Concretions (calcium)	Pulmonary alveolar microlithiasis
Proteins	Pulmonary alveolar proteinosis, amyloidosis

Hypoperfusion

Occlusion of a pulmonary artery by a thrombus, embolus, or both can result in perfusion deficits of the terminal respiratory units beyond the blockage. Radiographic findings include an area of decreased opacity, or hypovascular pattern, in a peripheral, middle, or central region, relative to the rest of the lung (Fig. 36.30).[48,49] Abrupt truncation of a pulmonary artery may occasionally be detected.[48] Other radiographic parenchymal manifestations include interstitial pattern, mixed interstitial-alveolar pattern, and an alveolar pattern, with the right lung being more affected than the left, and the caudal lung lobes being more commonly favored. Cardiomegaly, pleural effusion, and pneumothorax can also be seen.[50]

Emphysema

The term *emphysema* implies a destruction of alveolar septa with air freely escaping from alveoli, and dilated airspaces distal to the terminal bronchiole as a consequence of inflammation.[22] It has been reported histologically in lungs of dogs with interstitial fibrosis,[1] pulmonary alveolar microlithiasis,[27] and broncholithiasis. The amount of emphysema necessary for its radiographic detection is unknown. It is rarely observed in canines and felines, but more frequent in cattle and humans.[1]

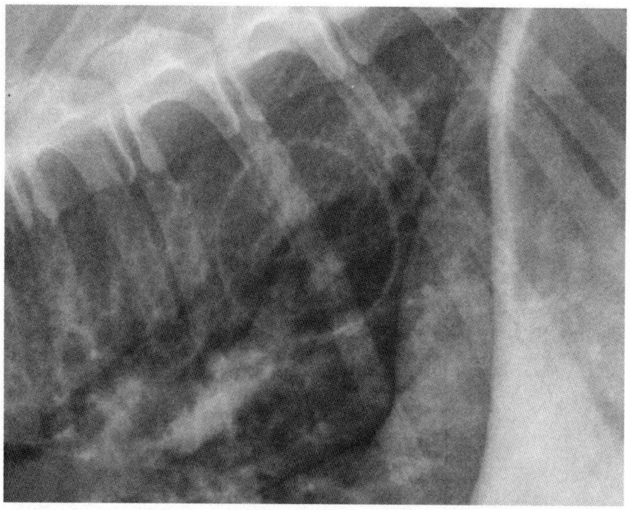

Fig. 36.29 Lateral radiograph of a dog with a bulla in the right caudal lung lobe. The lesion appears to only contain air and has a thin wall. This lesion could be congenital or secondary to previous lung trauma.

Hyperinflation and Air Trapping

Hyperinflation refers to an increase in lung volume exceeding that of a normal inspiration. In a conscious animal, it may be a fear response. In an animal under general anesthesia, increased lung volume may be a sequela of overinflation. In both instances, the opacity of the lungs is associated with a homogeneous decrease in radiopacity. Extension of the caudal boundaries of the lungs, flattening of the diaphragm, and cranial expansion of the rib cage may also be seen with hyperinflation. Hyperinflation may also occur as a compensatory mechanism when the ventilation of a lung lobe or segment is compromised or as a sequela of lobectomy.

Air trapping refers to an excessive retention of air in the airspaces (i.e., respiratory bronchioles, alveolar ducts, alveolar sacs) and alveoli without destruction of the alveolar septa (see eFig. 36.4).[13] Severe lung hyperinflation on radiography captured in inspiration and expiration in an animal showing expiratory efforts may be suggestive of air trapping (Fig. 36.31, eFig. 36.20).

DIAGNOSTIC IMAGING OF SPECIFIC LUNG DISEASES

A wide variety of airway and parenchymal diseases can affect dogs and cats. Only a limited number of conditions will be presented here.

Aspiration Pneumonia

Aspiration of fluid, food, or acidic gastric content is common in dogs with pharyngeal and esophageal dysphagia, regurgitation, or vomiting. Dogs repetitively aspirating may have an impaired cough reflex. In brachycephalic dogs, recurrent aspiration pneumonia frequently underlies a comorbid condition such as hiatal hernia. In dogs having recently been under general anesthesia, aspiration pneumonia may be the result of a single episode. Dogs with aspiration pneumonia have similar radiographic changes to those seen with nonhematogenous bacterial

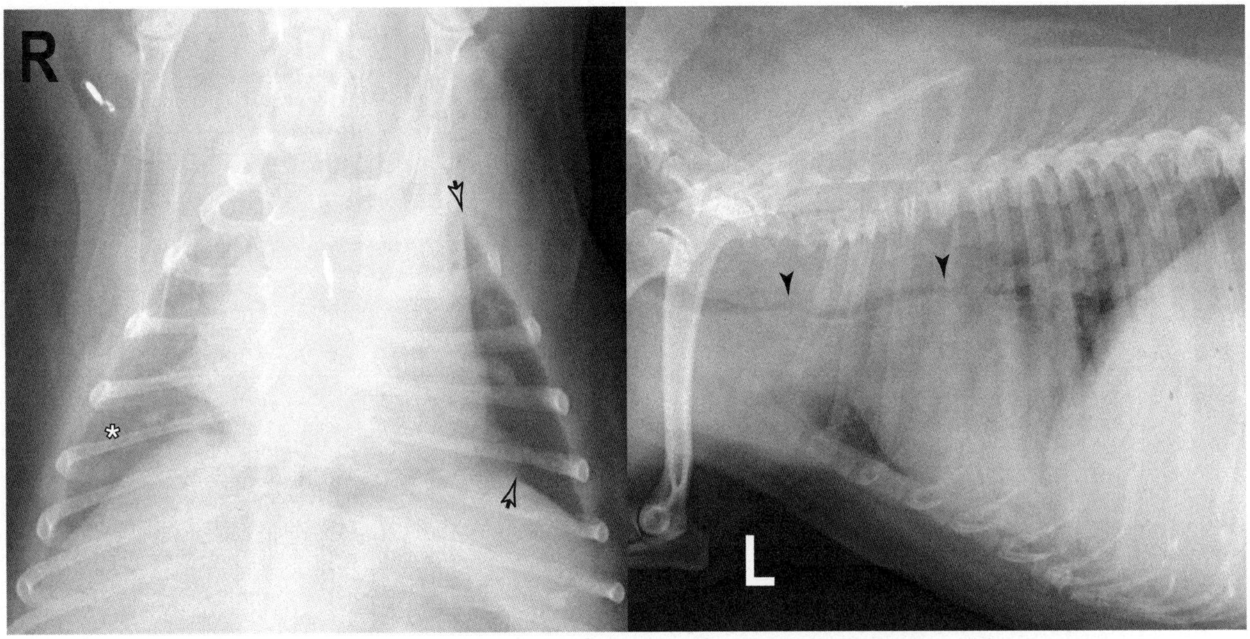

Fig. 36.30 Asymmetric lung opacity attributed to suspected pulmonary thromboembolic disease in a dog with a protein-losing nephropathy. The ventrodorsal view (*left panel*) shows the left lung (*arrows*) being less opaque than the right (*asterisk*). *Right panel,* Final diagnoses included tracheal and mainstem bronchial collapse (*black triangles*), suspect pulmonary thromboembolism secondary to a protein-losing nephropathy, and suspect mitral valve degenerative disease.

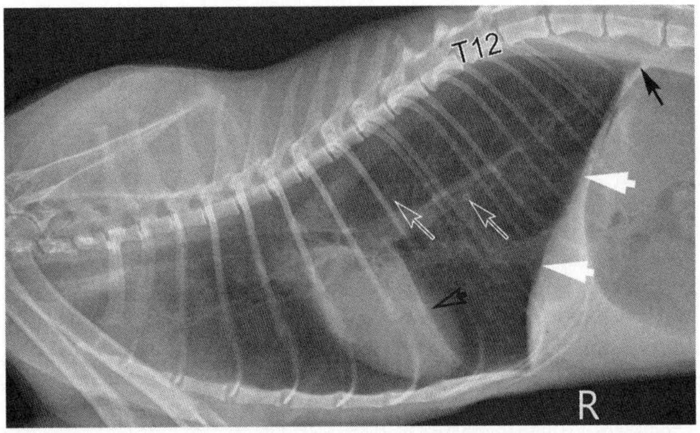

Fig. 36.31 Lung hyperinflation on a lateral radiographic view in an 8-year-old female spayed domestic shorthair cat with allergic asthma. Hyperinflation was diagnosed based on the marked caudal extension of the caudal lung beyond T12 with the lumbodiaphragmatic angles reaching the second lumbar vertebra (*solid black arrow*). Additional findings consistent with hyperinflation included flattening of the diaphragm (*solid white arrows*), marked cranial extension of the lungs cranial to the first ribs, and increased distance between the cardiac silhouette and the diaphragm. In this cat, hyperinflation was presumably attributed to air trapping secondary to allergic asthma. Additionally, a few thickened end-on bronchi are also noted (*open white arrows*). A lobar sign is seen between the atelectatic right middle (*open black arrow*) and right caudal lung lobes. The marked gas filled dilated stomach suggest aerophagia secondary to respiratory distress.

pneumonia, with the right middle and cranial lung lobes being more commonly affected. Dogs who have aspirated in other positions than standing or sternal may have a different distribution of lung lesions. An alveolar pattern with air bronchograms, a mixed interstitial-alveolar pattern, an interstitial pattern, or a mixed bronchial-interstitial-alveolar pattern is often seen with aspiration pneumonia (see Fig. 36.9, eFigs. 36.21 and 36.22). The number of lobes or segments affected is often limited, preferentially involving one or two lung lobes or segments. Aspiration pneumonia may be complicated by secondary bacterial pneumonia.

Bacterial Pneumonia

Bacterial pneumonia may occur secondary to impaired respiratory defenses, secondary to aspiration, respiratory viral infections, comorbid diseases, environmental stresses, and drug-induced immunosuppression or neutropenia. Bacterial pathogens responsible for community-acquired pneumonia in dogs are often opportunistic, whereas nosocomial pneumonia commonly involves multidrug-resistant and pathogenic bacteria. Bacterial pneumonia may be the result of canine infectious respiratory disease complex, in which multiple factors play a role. Lesions of bacterial pneumonia are often found in the cranioventral regions of the lungs, similar to aspiration pneumonia, and characterized by a multifocal or focal alveolar pattern, or less commonly a mixed patchy unstructured interstitial and bronchial pattern (Fig. 36.32). Of note, radiographic lesions may lag behind clinical and hematologic resolution of disease. Colonization of lungs by bacteria spreading from the blood circulation may have a different distribution of lesions with multifocal alveolar pattern or multifocal areas of consolidation or nodules that are not limited to the cranioventral regions of the lungs (see Fig. 36.24).

Feline Asthma

Hallmark features of asthma in cats include airway inflammation, excessive mucus production, intermittent reversible airway obstruction, nonspecific airway hyperreactivity, and airway remodeling. The lack of airway or lung parenchymal radiographic changes does not rule out asthma. Cats with asthma may show a bronchial pattern (see Fig. 36.17). Excessive mucus production can lead to bronchial luminal plugging, which can lead to lung collapse and resorptive atelectasis (see Fig. 36.20). Airway inflammation and remodeling result more commonly in an unstructured interstitial pattern on

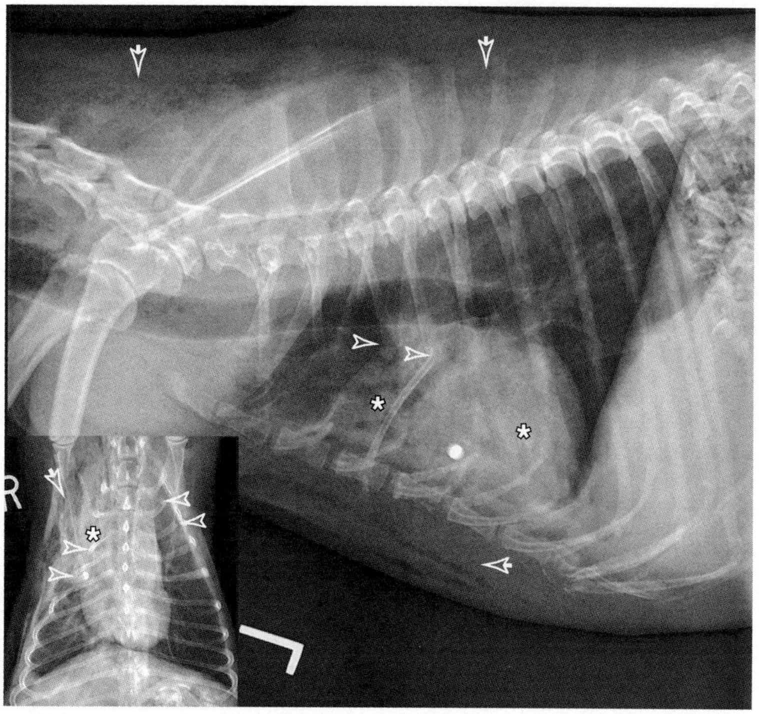

Fig. 36.38 Pulmonary contusions in a 10-year-old male castrated mixed-breed dog following a presumed encounter with a circulating motorized vehicle the evening prior to presentation. There is subcutaneous emphysema, predominantly right-sided (*open arrows*), rib fractures bilaterally (*triangles*) with intercostal tear, and increase in the opacity of the right cranial and right middle lung (*asterisks*), consistent with pulmonary contusions, although their visibility was impeded by superimposition with subcutaneous emphysema and edema/cellulitis associated with thoracic muscle injury. A circular metallic object visible in the right fourth intercostal space was believed to be incidental.

from focal, multifocal, or diffuse, ill-defined areas of interstitial to alveolar pattern on radiography (Fig. 36.38). The absence of pulmonary contusions on radiographs taken immediately after trauma or progression of pulmonary dysfunction despite mild radiographic changes on the initial study may require repeating radiography as detectable imaging changes can be delayed. Cavities which can contain gas and/or fluid can also be seen (Fig. 36.39). Radiography has a tendency to overestimate the severity of pulmonary contusions, and may not accurately reflect the severity of pulmonary dysfunction.[60] Radiographs should also be carefully examined for concurrent traumatic injuries such as pneumothorax, hemothorax, fractures, luxation and subluxation, and hemoperitoneum.

Pulmonary hemorrhage may also occur following non-traumatic causes such as bleeding disorders, rodenticide poisoning or other intoxication (e.g., copper sulfate powder), infection (e.g., leptospirosis, plague caused by *Yersinia pestis, Angiostrongylus vasorum*), drugs including anticoagulants, thrombosis, acute respiratory distress syndrome, pulmonary capillary hemangiomatosis, pulmonary veno-occlusive disease, or neoplasia. Unstructured interstitial, alveolar, and mixed interstitial-alveolar lung patterns have been described, with subtle differences in distribution according to the cause of pulmonary hemorrhage (Fig. 36.40).[61–63] Concurrent pleural effusion may occasionally be seen with pulmonary hemorrhage of various etiologies.

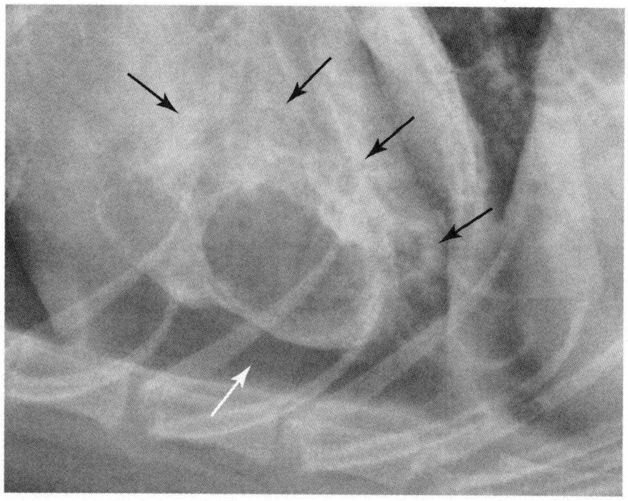

Fig. 36.39 Lateral radiograph of a dog recently hit by a car. There are multiple traumatic lacerations forming cavities filled with air in the periphery of the lung. Traumatic laceration cavities can collect air (pneumatocele), blood (hematocele), or both air and blood (hematopneumatocele). The wall of these lesions is slightly thicker and more irregular than encountered in a congenital bulla. However, the history of recent trauma and the finding of pneumothorax (*white arrow*) and an alveolar pattern consistent with hemorrhage (*black arrows*), support the occurrence of traumatic lesions.

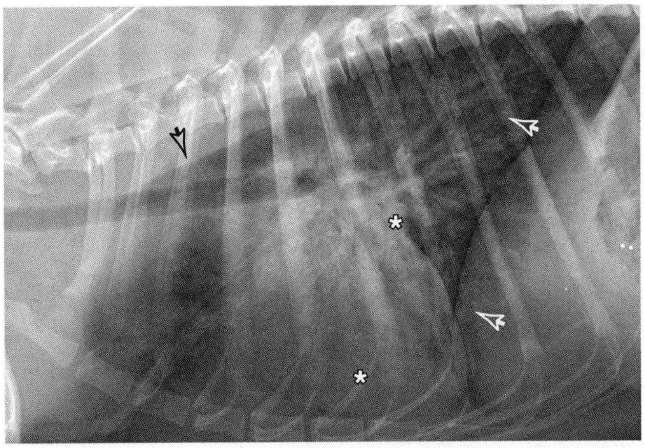

Fig. 36.40 Pulmonary hemorrhage secondary to suspected anticoagulant rodenticide exposure in a 17-month-old female spayed Labrador retriever. There is a diffuse mixed pulmonary pattern, with predominance of an unstructured interstitial pattern. Several irregularly marginated thickened end-on airways are seen (*white arrows*), although it is difficult to determine if this is the sole result of an airway-centered parenchymal infiltration or whether concurrent thickened bronchial walls also accompany the former. In the perihilar region and peripheral ventral areas, the severe unstructured interstitial pattern transitions to an alveolar pattern (*asterisks*). The cranial thoracic portion of the esophagus is gas filled (*black arrow*).

Acknowledgment

With special thanks to prior authors of this chapter for their contributions.

REFERENCES

1. Reif JS, Rhodes WH. The lungs of aged dogs: a radiographic-morphologic correlation. *Vet Radiol*. 1966;7:5–11.
2. Caswell JL, Williams KJ. Chapter 5 – respiratory system. In: Maxie MG, ed. *Jubb, Kennedy & Palmer's Pathology of Domestic Animals*. 6th ed. vol. 2. W.B. Saunders; 2016: 465–591.e464.
3. Silverman S, Suter PF. Influence of inspiration and expiration on canine thoracic radiographs. *J Am Vet Med Assoc*. 1975;166:502–510.
4. Lee SK, Park S, Cheon B, et al. Effect of position and time held in that position on ground-glass opacity in computed tomography images of dogs. *Am J Vet Res*. 2017;78: 279–288.
5. Foo TS, Pilton JL, Hall EJ, et al. Effect of body position and time on quantitative computed tomographic measurements of lung volume and attenuation in healthy anesthetized cats. *Am J Vet Res*. 2018;79:874–883.
6. Rozanski EA, Bedenice D, Lofgren J, et al. The effect of body position, sedation, and thoracic bandaging on functional residual capacity in healthy deep-chested dogs. *Can J Vet Res*. 2010;74:34–39.
7. Guarracino A, Lacitignola L, Auriemma E, et al. Which airway pressure should be applied during breath-hold in dogs undergoing thoracic computed tomography? *Vet Radiol Ultrasound*. 2016;57:475–481.
8. Allison A, Huizing X, Jolliffe C, et al. Effect of fixed value positive end expiratory pressure valves on canine thoracic volume and atelectasis. *J Small Anim Pract*. 2017;58:645–651.
9. Bernhard C, Masseau I, Dodam J, et al. Effects of positive end-expiratory pressure and 30% inspired oxygen on pulmonary mechanics and atelectasis in cats undergoing non-bronchoscopic bronchoalveolar lavage. *J Feline Med Surg*. 2017;19:665–671.
10. Martins ARC, Ambrósio AM, Fantoni DT, et al. Computed tomography assessment of tidal lung overinflation in domestic cats undergoing pressure-controlled mechanical ventilation during general anesthesia. *Front Vet Sci*. 2022;9:842528.
11. Henao-Guerrero N, Ricco C, Jones JC, et al. Comparison of four ventilatory protocols for computed tomography of the thorax in healthy cats. *Am J Vet Res*. 2012;73:646–653.
12. Morooka T, Niiyama M, Kougo A, et al. Radiographic evaluation of obesity-caused oppression of the thoracic cavity in beagles. *J Vet Med Sci*. 2004;66:489–494.
13. Masseau I, Reinero CR. Thoracic computed tomographic interpretation for clinicians to aid in the diagnosis of dogs and cats with respiratory disease. *Vet J*. 2019;253:105388.
14. Johnson LR, Singh MK, Pollard RE. Agreement among radiographs, fluoroscopy and bronchoscopy in documentation of airway collapse in dogs. *J Vet Intern Med*. 2015;29:1619–1626.
15. Lebastard M, Le Boedec K, Howes M, et al. Evaluation of bronchial narrowing in coughing dogs with heart murmurs using computed tomography. *J Vet Intern Med*. 2021;35(3):1509–1518.
16. Yoon H, Yu J, An G, et al. CT and radiographic evaluation of bronchial collapsibility at forced expiration in asymptomatic brachycephalic dogs. *Vet Radiol Ultrasound*. 2020;61:167–180.
17. Macready DM, Johnson LR, Pollard RE. Fluoroscopic and radiographic evaluation of tracheal collapse in dogs: 62 cases (2001–2006). *J Am Vet Med Assoc*. 2007;230:1870–1876.
18. Ober CP, Barber D. Comparison of two- vs. three-view thoracic radiographic studies on conspicuity of structured interstitial patterns in dogs. *Vet Radiol Ultrasound*. 2006;47:542–545.
19. Wilkins PA, Otto CM, Baumgardner JE, et al. Acute lung injury and acute respiratory distress syndromes in veterinary medicine: consensus definitions: the Dorothy Russell Havemeyer Working Group on ALI and ARDS in Veterinary Medicine. *J Vet Emerg Crit Care*. 2007;17:333–339.
20. Tsai S, Sutherland-Smith J, Burgess K, et al. Imaging characteristics of intrathoracic histiocytic sarcoma in dogs. *Vet Radiol Ultrasound*. 2012;53:21–27.
21. Barrett LE, Pollard RE, Zwingenberger A, et al. Radiographic characterization of primary lung tumors in 74 dogs. *Vet Radiol Ultrasound*. 2014;55:480–487.
22. Hansell DM, Bankier AA, MacMahon H, et al. Fleischner Society: glossary of terms for thoracic imaging. *Radiology*. 2008;246:697–722.
23. Suter PF, Chan KF. Disseminated pulmonary diseases in small animals: a radiographic approach to diagnosis. *Vet Radiol*. 1968;9:67–79.
24. Nemanic S, London CA, Wisner ER. Comparison of thoracic radiographs and single breath-hold helical CT for detection of pulmonary nodules in dogs with metastatic neoplasia. *J Vet Intern Med*. 2006;20:508–515.
25. Armbrust LJ, Biller DS, Bamford A, et al. Comparison of three-view thoracic radiography and computed tomography for detection of pulmonary nodules in dogs with neoplasia. *J Am Vet Med Assoc*. 2012;240:1088–1094.
26. Alexander K, Joly H, Blond L, et al. A comparison of computed tomography, computed radiography, and film-screen radiography for the detection of canine pulmonary nodules. *Vet Radiol Ultrasound*. 2012;53:258–265.
27. Sousa AC, Santos JC, Landolt C, et al. Clinicopathological and imaging features of pulmonary alveolar microlithiasis in a dog – a case report. *BMC Vet Res*. 2020;16:376.

28. Kubba MAG. Pulmonary ossification and microlithiasis in a bitch with multicentric mammary tumors. *Open Vet J.* 2017;7:273–276.
29. Bennett AD, Lalor S, Schwarz T, et al. Radiographic findings in cats with mycobacterial infections. *J Feline Med Surg.* 2011;13:718–724.
30. Ackerman N, Spencer CP. Radiologic aspects of mycotic diseases. *Vet Clin North Am Small Anim Pract.* 1982;12:175–189.
31. Jackson K, Boger L, Goldschmidt M, et al. Malignant pilomatricoma in a soft-coated wheaten terrier. *Vet Clin Pathol.* 2010;39:236–240.
32. Meola SD, Mazzaferro EM, Wheeler JL, et al. Medical and surgical management of severe barium aspiration in a dog. *J Vet Emerg Crit Care.* 2008;18:639–645.
33. Mesquita L, Lam R, Lamb CR, et al. Computed tomographic findings in 15 dogs with eosinophilic bronchopneumopathy. *Vet Radiol Ultrasound.* 2015;56:33–39.
34. Meler E, Pressler BM, Heng HG, et al. Diffuse cylindrical bronchiectasis due to eosinophilic bronchopneumopathy in a dog. *Can Vet J.* 2010;51:753–756.
35. Beck JA, Ard M, Howerth EW. Pathology in practice. Primary ciliary dyskinesia (PCD) with associated bronchopneumonia, bronchiectasis, and hydrocephalus in a dog. *J Am Vet Med Assoc.* 2014;244:421–423.
36. Hawkins EC, Basseches J, Berry CR, et al. Demographic, clinical, and radiographic features of bronchiectasis in dogs: 316 cases (1988–2000). *J Am Vet Med Assoc.* 2003;223:1628–1635.
37. Reinero CR, Jutkowitz LA, Nelson N, et al. Clinical features of canine pulmonary veno-occlusive disease and pulmonary capillary hemangiomatosis. *J Vet Intern Med.* 2019;33:114–123.
38. Jaffey JA, Williams KJ, Masseau I, et al. Vasoproliferative process resembling pulmonary capillary hemangiomatosis in a cat. *BMC Vet Res.* 2017;13(72).
39. Katajavuori P, Melamies M, Rajamaki MM. Eosinophilic pulmonary granulomatosis in a young dog with prolonged remission after treatment. *J Small Anim Pract.* 2013;54:40–43.
40. Confer AW, Qualls Jr CW, MacWilliams PS, et al. Four cases of pulmonary nodular eosinophilic granulomatosis in dogs. *Cornell Vet.* 1983;73:41–51.
41. Wolf AM, Green RW. The radiographic appearance of pulmonary histoplasmosis in the cat. *Vet Radiol.* 1987;28:34–37.
42. Rampacci E, Sforna M, Dentini A, et al. *Paenibacillus amylolyticus* osteomyelitis in a Poodle dog: case report and literature review. *J Vet Diagn Invest.* 2022;34:703–708.
43. Hornby NL, Lamb CR. Does the computed tomographic appearance of the lung differ between young and old dogs? *Vet Radiol Ultrasound.* 2017;58:647–652.
44. Dahl K, Rørvik AM, Lanageland M. Bronchogenic cyst in a German shepherd dog. *J Small Anim Pract.* 2002;43:456–458.
45. Pechman RD. The radiographic features of pulmonary paragonimiasis in the dog and cat. *Vet Radiol.* 1976;17:182–191.
46. Johnson VS, Corcoran BM, Wotton PR, et al. Thoracic high-resolution computed tomographic findings in dogs with canine idiopathic pulmonary fibrosis. *J Small Anim Pract.* 2005;46:381–388.
47. Bello AM, Anselmi C, Frau M, et al. Pulmonary carcinoma associated with cystic airspaces in two dogs. *J Small Anim Pract.* 2022;63:486–491.
48. Venco L, Genchi C, Genchi M, et al. Clinical evolution and radiographic findings of feline heartworm infection in asymptomatic cats. *Vet Parasitol.* 2008;158:232–237.
49. Flückiger MA, Gomez JA. Radiographic findings in dogs with spontaneous pulmonary thrombosis or embolism. *Vet Radiol.* 1984;25:124–131.
50. Johnson LR, Lappin MR, Baker DC. Pulmonary thromboembolism in 29 dogs: 1985–1995. *J Vet Intern Med.* 1999;13:338–345.
51. Mortier JR, Mesquita L, Ferrandis I, et al. Accuracy of and interobserver agreement regarding thoracic computed tomography for the diagnosis of chronic bronchitis in dogs. *J Am Vet Med Assoc.* 2018;253:757–762.
52. Hofeling AD, Jackson AH, Alsup JC, et al. Spontaneous midlobar lung lobe torsion in a 2-year-old Newfoundland. *J Am Anim Hosp Assoc.* 2004;40:220–223.
53. Seiler G, Schwarz T, Vignoli M, et al. Computed tomographic features of lung lobe torsion. *Vet Radiol Ultrasound.* 2008;49:504–508.
54. Belmudes A, Gory G, Cauvin E, et al. Lung lobe torsion in 15 dogs: peripheral band sign on ultrasound. *Vet Radiol Ultrasound.* 2021;62:116–125.
55. Ballegeer EA, Forrest LJ, Stepien RL. Radiographic appearance of bronchoalveolar carcinoma in nine cats. *Vet Radiol Ultrasound.* 2002;43:267–271.
56. Bouyssou S, Specchi S, Desquilbet L, et al. Radiographic appearance of presumed noncardiogenic pulmonary edema and correlation with the underlying cause in dogs and cats. *Vet Radiol Ultrasound.* 2017;58:259–265.
57. Johnson LR, Johnson EG, Hulsebosch SE, et al. Eosinophilic bronchitis, eosinophilic granuloma, and eosinophilic bronchopneumopathy in 75 dogs (2006–2016). *J Vet Intern Med.* 2019;33:2217–2226.
58. Fina C, Vignoli M, Terragni R, et al. Computed tomographic characteristics of eosinophilic pulmonary granulomatosis in five dogs. *Vet Radiol Ultrasound.* 2014;55:16–22.
59. Clercx C, Peeters D, Snaps F, et al. Eosinophilic bronchopneumopathy in dogs. *J Vet Intern Med.* 2000;14:282–291.
60. Campbell VL, King LG. Pulmonary function, ventilator management, and outcome of dogs with thoracic trauma and pulmonary contusions: 10 cases (1994–1998). *J Am Vet Med Assoc.* 2000;217:1505–1509.
61. Lippi I, Puccinelli C, Perondi F, et al. Predictors of fatal pulmonary haemorrhage in dogs affected by leptospirosis approaching haemodialysis. *Vet Sci.* 2021;8.
62. Schaffer PA, Hershkowitz CS, Dowers KL, et al. Delayed diagnosis of fatal pneumonic canine plague: clinical and pathologic features in two naturally infected Colorado dogs. *BMC Vet Res.* 2020;16:160.
63. Chapman PS, Boag AK, Guitian J, et al. *Angiostrongylus vasorum* infection in 23 dogs (1999–2002). *J Small Anim Pract.* 2004;45:435–440.

ELECTRONIC RESOURCES

Additional information related to the content in Chapter 36 can be found online at eBooks.Health.Elsevier.com.

- Chapter Quiz

CHAPTER 37

Equine Thorax

Stephanie G. Nykamp

RADIOGRAPHIC TECHNIQUE

Technical aspects of radiographing the equine thorax are covered in Chapter 28, but important principles are reiterated here. Radiographing the entire thorax of an adult horse requires a grid and large stationary x-ray tubes that are generally available only at referral centers. Portable radiographic tubes require an excessively long exposure time to penetrate the adult thorax; this usually results in motion artifact, rendering the images nondiagnostic. The advantages of digital imaging are covered in Chapter 2. The improved contrast of digital imaging is advantageous but the various processing algorithms from different systems can also increase the conspicuity of normal lung markings resulting in overinterpretation of the images. Digital images can have scatter correction in the processing algorithm but an antiscatter grid is still recommended for adult horses.[1]

Four overlapping 14-inch × 17-inch views are usually required to image the entire thorax of an adult horse. They are acquired in the craniodorsal, caudodorsal, caudoventral, and cranioventral aspects of the thorax (Fig. 37.1). In addition to these standard views, radiographs centered over any identified lesions may also be useful.

Lateral radiographs of the foal thorax may be made with a single 14-inch × 17-inch cassette and some portable x-ray tubes. Dorsoventral (DV) or ventrodorsal (VD) radiographs should also be acquired on foals whenever possible.

The horse should be positioned with the thoracic limbs slightly forward to reduce the amount of muscle mass superimposed on the cranial aspect of the thorax. Radiographs should be obtained during peak inspiration. In some instances, radiographs should also be obtained during expiration because a comparison of the degree of lung inflation between inspiratory and expiratory radiographs may be helpful in the diagnosis of air trapping from chronic pulmonary disease.

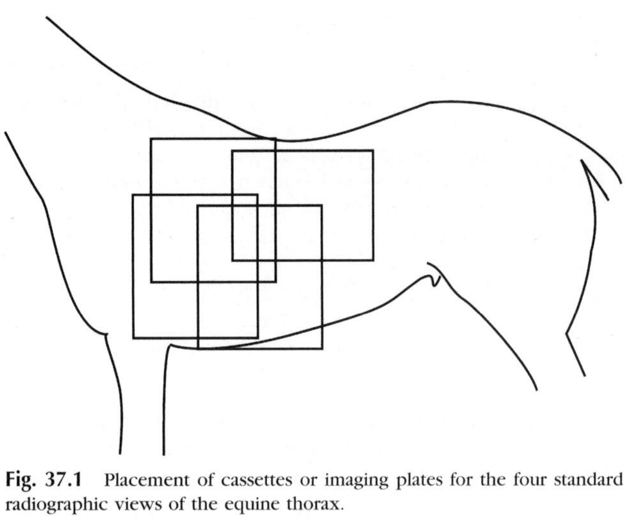

Fig. 37.1 Placement of cassettes or imaging plates for the four standard radiographic views of the equine thorax.

When thoracic radiographs are obtained in a standing horse, the lung closest to the cassette is seen most clearly. This occurs because the large width of the equine thorax results in the lung farthest from the cassette being magnified and blurred to the extent that even large lesions can be obscured. This is opposite to the situation in lateral radiographs of dogs and cats where lesions in the nondependent lung (i.e., farthest from the cassette) are seen most clearly because of the atelectasis that occurs in the dependent lung. In the horse, therefore, left-right and right-left radiographs are necessary to assess both the left and right lungs adequately in patients with pneumonia or neoplasia. Bilateral radiographs are less likely to impact the diagnosis in patients with diffuse or inflammatory disease but as this is not known prior to imaging bilateral radiographs are recommended.[2]

Radiographic exposure and degree of inspiration play an important role in the interpretation of thoracic radiographs and must be considered both for initial and serial radiographic examinations. As the quality of the radiograph improves, the amount of perceived interstitial lung pattern decreases.[3] If a radiograph is underexposed or obtained during expiration, the lungs will appear diffusely more opaque than normal, mimicking a mild diffuse interstitial lung pattern often mistaken for disease. If the radiographs are overexposed, small or mild lung lesions may be obscured.

Craniodorsal Projection

The dorsal portion of the heart, descending aorta, caudal vena cava, hilar pulmonary arteries and veins, trachea, and carina are visible (Fig. 37.2). The hilar portions of the lungs are visible but are difficult to evaluate because of the superimposition of the heart and blood vessels.

Caudodorsal Projection

This view provides the largest unobstructed view of the lungs (Fig. 37.3). The normal equine lung has a mild diffuse bronchointerstitial lung pattern when compared with canine and feline lungs. The pulmonary blood vessels should be seen clearly, tapering toward the periphery of the lung field.

Caudoventral Projection

The caudal borders of the heart, left atrium, caudal vena cava, pulmonary veins, and pulmonary arteries are evident on this view (Fig. 37.4). A small triangle of lung bounded by the caudal vena cava, caudal border of the heart, and cranioventral aspect of the diaphragm is evident. Because of the cardiac notch, no pulmonary markings are present over the central portion of the heart. The absence of pulmonary blood vessels in this region should not be mistaken for lung consolidation. The diaphragmatic reflection of the pleura follows the costochondral junctions to approximately the ninth rib and then travels dorsally,

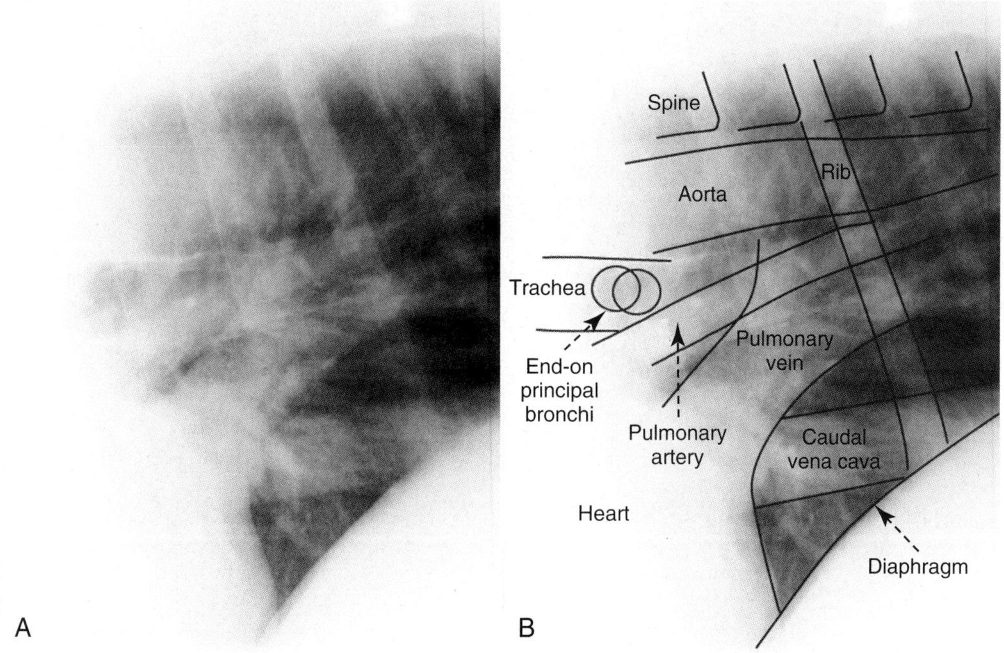

Fig. 37.2 Normal adult thoracic radiograph **(A)**, craniodorsal projection, and accompanying line drawing **(B)**.

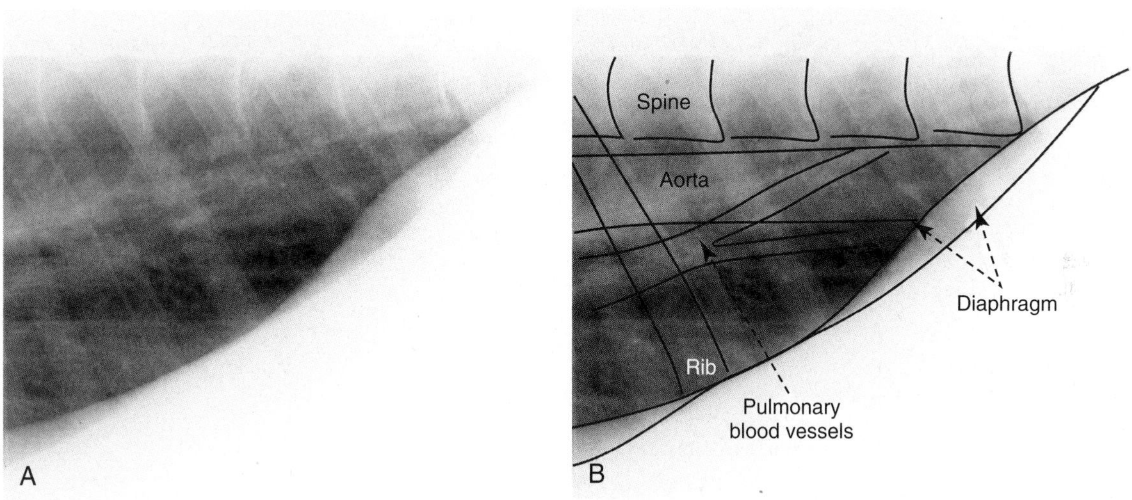

Fig. 37.3 Normal adult thoracic radiograph **(A)**, caudodorsal projection, and accompanying line drawing **(B)**.

paralleling the costal arch to the middle of the last rib. This means that the normal lung does not extend ventral to the costochondral junction and, in fact, usually ends approximately 4 inches above the costochondral junction in adult horses at rest.[4] Ventral to the costochondral junction is mediastinal fat that provides contrast between the caudal border of the heart and the diaphragm. This fat opacity should not be mistaken for pleural or pulmonary disease.

Cranioventral Projection

The cranial portions of the lung, cranial mediastinum, aortic arch, and trachea are evident on this projection (Fig. 37.5). The lung is difficult to evaluate in this region because of the superimposition of the thoracic limbs. Except for evaluating for a mediastinal mass, this is typically the least helpful of all projections.

NORMAL ANATOMY

The right and left lungs are not clearly divided by interlobar fissures. The left lung is divided into a cranial and caudal component. The right lung is divided into a cranial and caudal component and the accessory lobe. A prominent cardiac notch is present in the left and right lungs at the level of the third to the sixth ribs overlying the midventral aspect of the heart. The ventral aspect of the caudal lung lobes is visible as a triangle of lung bordered by the caudal aspect of the heart, diaphragm, and caudal vena cava. The appearance of the lungs is also influenced by the phase of respiration, age, and body condition.

Adults

Many adult horses with normal respiratory function and no clinical signs of respiratory disease have a mild, diffuse

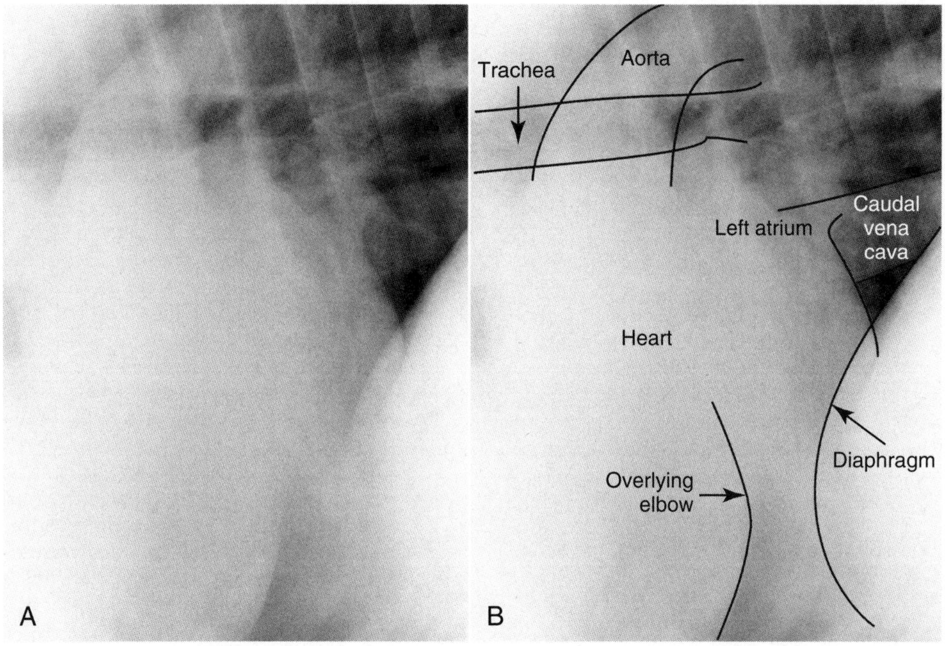

Fig. 37.4 Normal adult thoracic radiograph **(A)**, caudoventral projection, and accompanying line drawing **(B)**.

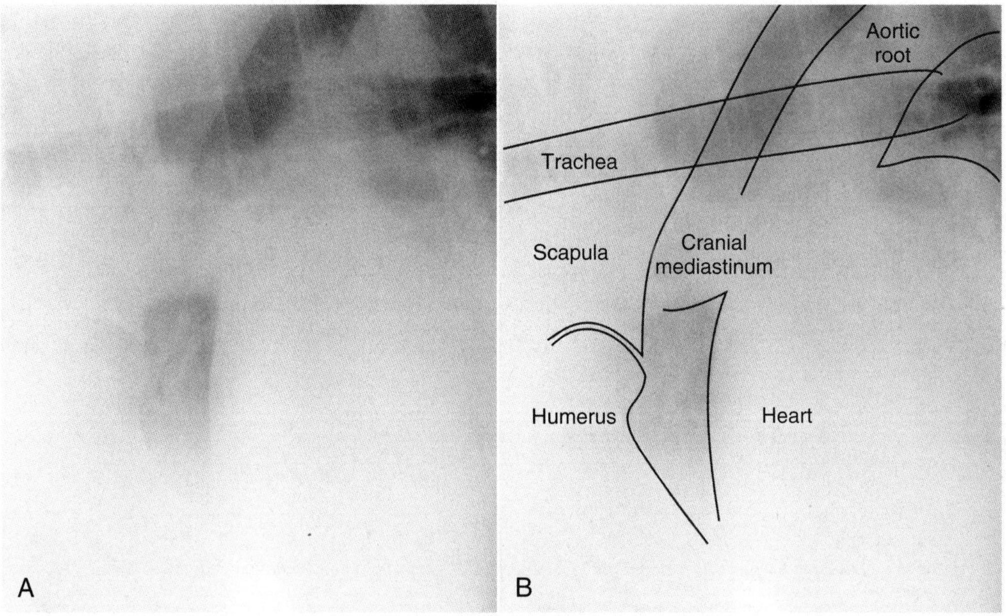

Fig. 37.5 Normal adult thoracic radiograph **(A)**, cranioventral projection, and accompanying line drawing **(B)**.

bronchointerstitial lung pattern as a normal variation which is even more prominent with digital imaging.[3,5] This opacity may be caused by the slightly more abundant lobulation and connective tissue that is present in horses or by subclinical peribronchial fibrosis.[3] The presence of this mild bronchointerstitial lung pattern means that the correlation between radiographic changes and clinical disease is often poor. Therefore, mild radiographic changes should be interpreted with caution (Fig. 37.6).[3,6,7]

Foals

When radiographed immediately after parturition, foals have a mild diffuse interstitial lung pattern because of incomplete expansion of the lungs, fluid in the small airways, and the uptake of fetal alveolar fluid in the interstitium (Fig. 37.7). This opacity should resolve within 6 hours of birth.[8–10] The thymus is large in foals and can sometimes be seen as a soft tissue opacity cranial to the heart. The thymus is largest at approximately 2 months of age and should regress as the foal ages.[9] Atelectasis occurs rapidly when foals are placed in lateral recumbency. This will result in the lungs of recumbent foals appearing more opaque than those of standing foals.[9]

Heart

Objective criteria for assessing heart size have not been established in horses.[11] The caudal border of the heart should be straight and should parallel the angle of the ribs. Elevation of the trachea and increased sternal or diaphragmatic contact are indicative of cardiomegaly.[11] Assessment of cardiac size is easiest if the entire cardiac silhouette is visible in one image acquired with the x-ray beam centered over the heart. In foals, the cardiac silhouette occupies a larger volume of the thoracic cavity than it does in adults.[9] Based on objective measurements of cardiac size in foals, the height should be 6.6 to 7.8 times the length of a midthoracic vertebral body, and the width should be 5.6 to 6.3 times the width of a midthoracic vertebral body.[8] Echocardiography is superior to radiography in assessing cardiac size and function.

ALTERNATIVE IMAGING MODALITIES

Fluoroscopy is useful to evaluate esophageal disease, tracheal collapse, and the motion of thoracic masses. Unfortunately, fluoroscopy for equine evaluation is not available readily.[12]

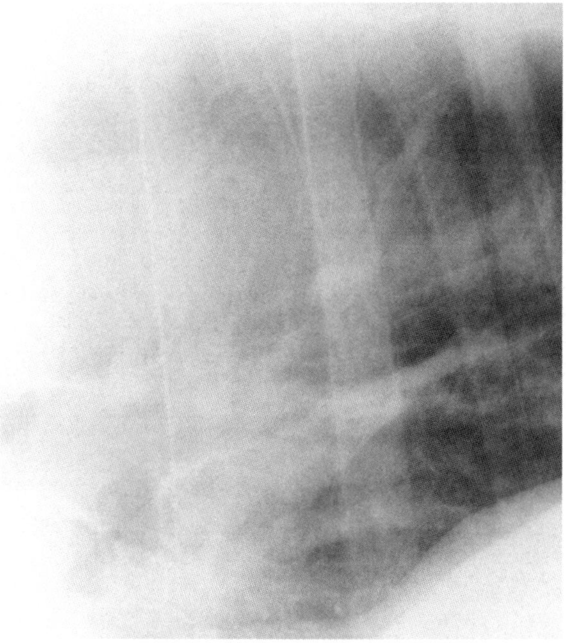

Fig. 37.6 Right lateral radiograph of the caudodorsal thorax in an adult horse with no clinical signs. Note the mild diffuse bronchial lung pattern seen in normal horses.

The use of ultrasound is common in equine practice. Air prevents the transmission of ultrasound waves, so the ultrasound appearance of the normal lung is a bright interface with reverberation artifact characterized by equally spaced lines that parallel the surface of the lung (Fig. 37.8). In real time, the normal lung slides along the body wall during respiration. Ultrasound is more sensitive than radiographs in the detection of small pulmonary lesions as long as they extend to the pleural surface.[13] Ultrasound is the diagnostic test of choice for evaluating pleural disease in the horse because it is more sensitive to the detection of small amounts of fluid and provides information on the character of the fluid. [12,14] Ultrasound can also be used to assess the surface of the lung. A few areas of rough pulmonary surfaces that create a comet tail artifact can be seen in the ventral portions of the normal lung, but more extensive lesions will be present in horses with viral pneumonia and chronic pleural fibrosis (Fig. 37.9).[15,16] Ultrasound correlates well with radiographs and postmortem in cases of diffuse pulmonary disease such as acute interstitial pneumonia in foals.[17] Ultrasound is an inexpensive and accessible diagnostic test for serial monitoring for resolution or progression of disease. Point of care ultrasound as part of the routine physical examination is valuable in horses to detect pleural, pericardial, and peripheral pulmonary disease and is more readily available than radiographs.

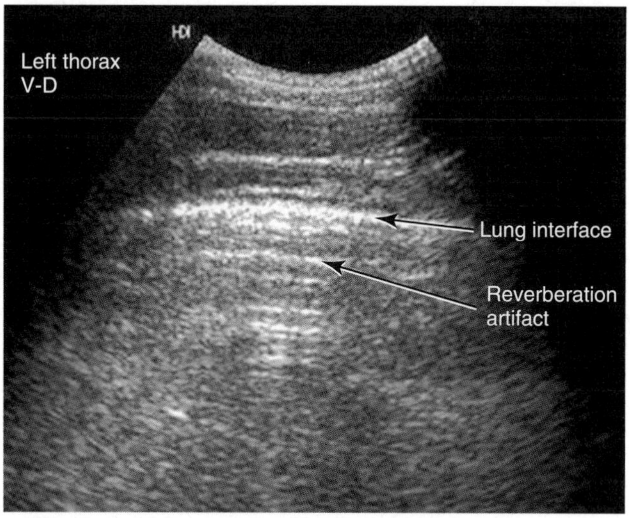

Fig. 37.8 Transverse ultrasound image of the normal left lung (ventrodorsal orientation). Note the equally spaced white lines (reverberation artifact) caused by the sound reflected at the air interface.

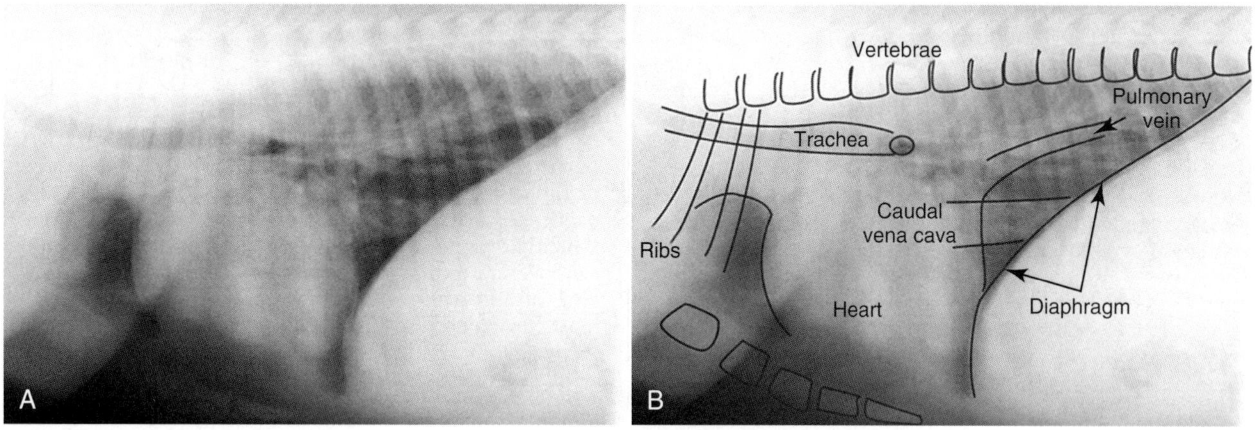

Fig. 37.7 Normal foal thoracic radiograph **(A)** and accompanying line drawing **(B)**.

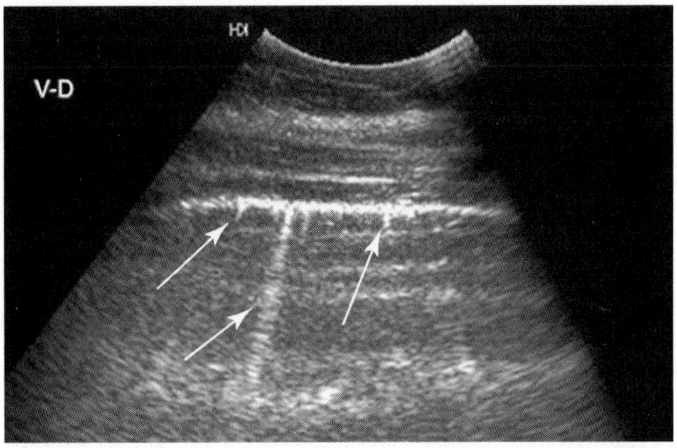

Fig. 37.9 Transverse ultrasound image of the lung. The pleural surface of the lung is rough, which results in a reverberation artifact, otherwise referred to as *comet tail artifact* (*arrows*). A few comet tails can be seen in normal horses.

Nuclear scintigraphy can provide physiologic information about perfusion and ventilation of the lungs. Ventilation studies can be useful in assessing chronic obstructive pulmonary disease and exercise-induced pulmonary hemorrhage.[18] The images are characterized by a patchy distribution with hot spots centrally caused by deposition of the injected isotope in the larger airways and cold spots peripherally from lack of ventilation. Additionally, radiopharmaceutical is cleared more rapidly from the lung of horses with chronic obstructive pulmonary disease than in normal horses.[19] Perfusion studies are used to evaluate for pulmonary thromboembolic disease, chronic obstructive pulmonary disease, and other diffuse diseases. In combination with ventilation studies, the patient can be evaluated for ventilation and perfusion mismatches. Because of the expensive equipment and the need to isolate the patient for approximately 24 hours after the study to allow for radioactive decay, these imaging studies are usually limited to referral hospitals.

Computed tomography (CT) is an excellent imaging modality for assessment of the thorax, but, because of equipment size, its use is restricted to smaller foals.[20] CT is more sensitive to the detection of pulmonary pathology and interpretation is less subjective than radiographs but is subject to positional atelectasis that occurs secondary to sedation or anesthesia (Fig. 37.10).[21] Compared to ultrasound, CT more accurately evaluates rib fractures in foals which assists in treatment planning.[22]

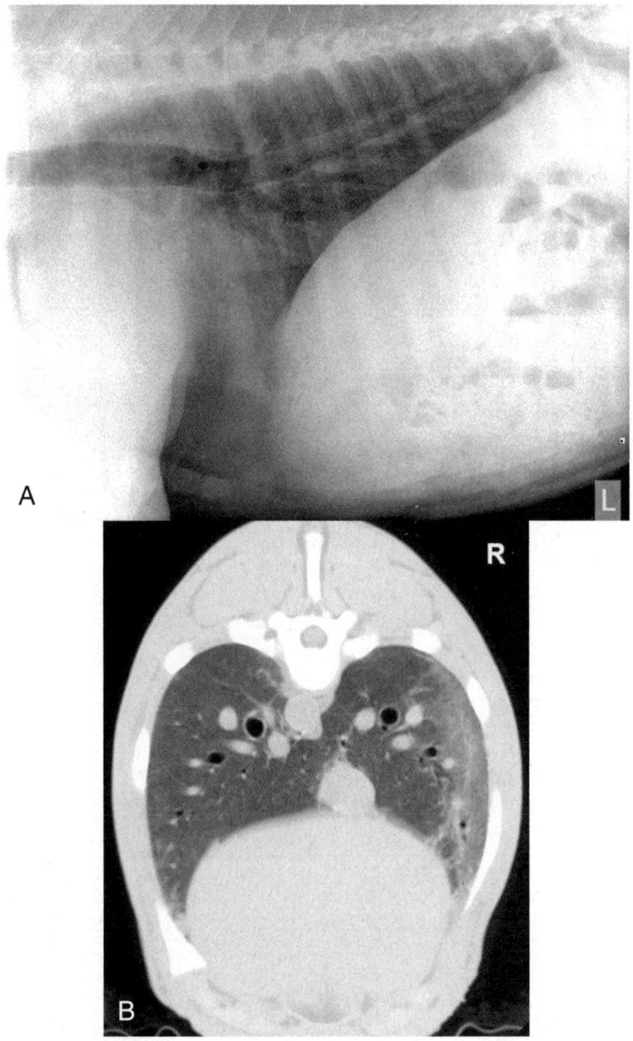

Fig. 37.10 Right-left lateral standing radiograph **(A)** and computed tomography (CT) image **(B)** of a foal that has been in right lateral recumbency. No abnormalities are noted on the radiograph. Increased attenuation is evident in the periphery of the right lung on the CT. This is due to positional atelectasis.

PULMONARY DISEASE

Radiographs complement a physical examination; they do not replace it. Physical examination can be unremarkable, and yet substantial radiographic abnormality can be present. Additionally, the radiographic resolution of disease often lags behind the clinical resolution. This should be considered when evaluating serial studies.[23] Bronchoalveolar lavage, a common diagnostic procedure in horses with respiratory disease, can cause an interstitial pulmonary pattern in the lungs and should be done following radiographs to avoid interpretation errors.[24]

The patterns of pulmonary disease have been discussed in Chapter 36. As in the dog and cat, the radiographic pulmonary pattern correlates poorly with the histologic location of the disease. For example, in equine parasitic pneumonia, the most common pulmonary pattern is interstitial, but grossly, the disease is predominantly alveolar, and horses with a diffuse interstitial lung pattern have peribronchial disease on histologic examination.[3,25] But radiographic patterns can reflect the severity of the disease, with bronchial and interstitial patterns suggesting less severe disease than an alveolar pattern.[23] The distribution of the pulmonary disease may be more useful with regard to the cause of the pulmonary disease than the pattern itself.[9,26] For example, bronchopneumonia and aspiration pneumonia tend to have a cranioventral and caudoventral distribution, whereas pulmonary edema and interstitial pneumonia are more caudodorsal to diffuse in their distribution.

Pneumonia

In adults, bronchopneumonia is usually a result of transportation or stress, whereas in foals it is usually caused by sepsis or aspiration.[27,28] In adults and foals, bronchopneumonia can occur secondary to viral pneumonia.[28] Bacterial pneumonia and aspiration pneumonia usually occur in the cranioventral and caudoventral portions of the lung. The cranial portion of the lung is difficult to evaluate radiographically, so the disease is most conspicuous when superimposed on the caudal border of the heart (Fig. 37.11, eFig. 37.1). Bacterial pneumonia can result in an interstitial or alveolar lung pattern depending on the severity (Fig. 37.12). Abscess formation presents as solid or cavitated nodules that may be poorly or well defined (eFig. 37.2).

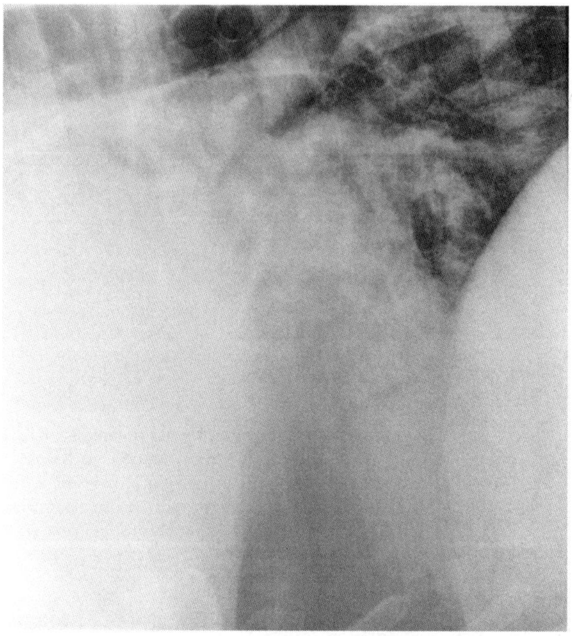

Fig. 37.11 Lateral caudoventral thoracic radiograph. A fairly intense soft tissue opacity is superimposed on the caudal aspect of the heart that partially silhouettes pulmonary blood vessels, making their margins appear indistinct. This lesion is caused by bronchopneumonia. In the pattern recognition scheme, this lesion is consistent with an interstitial pattern. The small irregular gas opacities overlying the heart are caused by small abscesses.

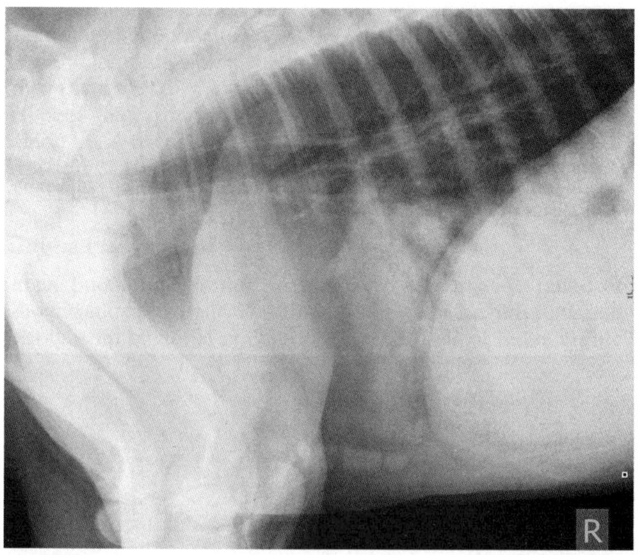

Fig. 37.12 Lateral thoracic radiograph of a foal. A soft tissue opacity that obscures the pulmonary blood vessels and faint air bronchograms is superimposed on the caudal aspect of the heart. In this foal, pneumonia developed as a result of aspiration of milk. In the pattern recognition scheme, this lesion is consistent with an alveolar pattern. A tube with a linear radiopaque marker is present in the esophagus.

The ultrasonographic appearance of pneumonic lung is a uniform echogenicity that resembles the appearance of liver (Fig. 37.13). Air-filled bronchi appear as hyperechoic, linear, branching structures that have a reverberation artifact. Fluid-filled bronchi appear as anechoic branching tubes (Fig. 37.14). Fluid-filled bronchi can be differentiated from blood vessels with Doppler interrogation.

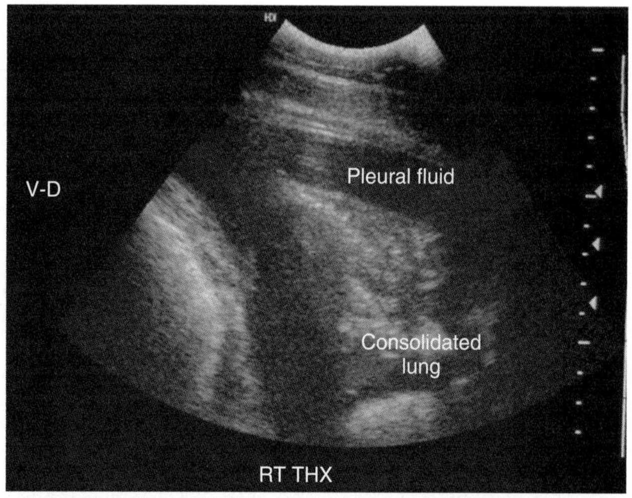

Fig. 37.13 This transverse ultrasound image is characterized by pleural fluid and consolidated lung. The lack of the normal reverberation artifact seen with aerated lung is evidence that the lung is abnormal. The lung has a relatively uniform soft tissue echogenicity similar to the appearance of normal liver and is triangular in shape. The pleural fluid is present between the lung and the body wall.

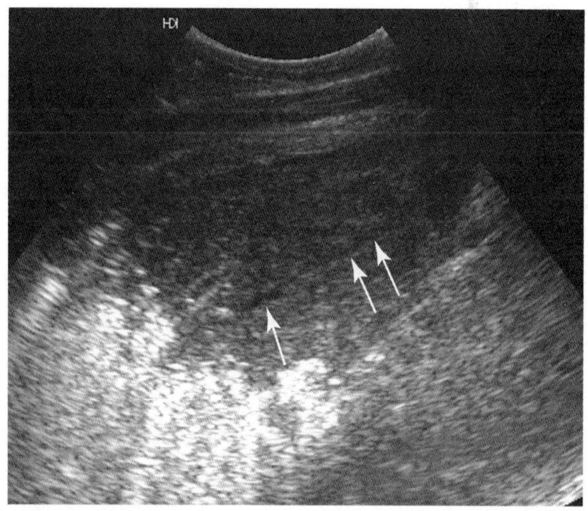

Fig. 37.14 This transverse ultrasound image shows consolidation of the lung and a fluid bronchogram (*arrows*). The deep aerated portion of the lung is the irregular hyperechoic interface.

Interstitial Pneumonia

Interstitial pneumonia occurs in foals and adults and can be acute or chronic.[29,30] The causative agent is usually not identified but may include infectious agents, toxins, systemic inflammatory response syndrome, or allergic factors.[23,27,29–31]

Interstitial pneumonia in foals is usually acute, and affected foals are typically 6 weeks to 6 months of age.[29,32] Chronic interstitial pneumonia has a more favorable prognosis, whereas acute interstitial pneumonia has a high mortality rate.[30,33] Whether the disease is acute or chronic, the radiographic changes are the same, a diffuse interstitial lung pattern.[29,32] A mild to moderate bronchial lung pattern may also be present.[30] The disease can result in increased vascular permeability and secondary pulmonary edema.[33] The severity of the changes on the initial radiographs and progression of the changes on subsequent radiographs are negative prognostic indicators.[23]

Interstitial pneumonia is rare in adults, and because the lung has a limited range of responses to injury, it usually presents as a chronic problem with secondary fibrosis, and affected horses

REFERENCES

1. Lo WY, Hornof WJ, Zwingenberger AL, Robertson ID. Multislice imaging processing and antiscatter grids in digital radiographs. *Vet Radiol Ultrasound*. 2009;50: 569–576.
2. Malek G, Leclere M, Masseau I, Linden A zur, Beauchamp G, Finck C. Bilateral thoracic radiographs increase lesion detection in horses with pneumonia or pulmonary neoplasia but do not bring any additional benefit for inflammatory or diffuse pulmonary disease. *Vet Radiol Ultrasound*. 2022.
3. Wisner ER, O'Brien TR, Lakritz J, Pascoe JR, Wilson DW, Tyler WS. Radiographic and microscopic correlation of diffuse interstitial and bronchointerstitial pulmonary patterns in the caudodorsal lung of adult thoroughbred horses in race training. *Equine Vet J*. 1993;25:293–298.
4. Singh B, Dyce KM (Keith M). *Dyce, Sack, and Wensing's Textbook of Veterinary Anatomy*. 5th ed. St. Louis, Missouri: Elsevier; n.d.
5. Sanderson GN, O'Callaghan MW. Radiographic anatomy of the equine thorax as a basis for radiological interpretation. *N Z Vet J*. 2011;31:127–130.
6. Ainsworth DM, Beck KA, Boatwright CE, Snedden KA, Rebhun WC. Lack of residual lung damage in horses in which *Rhodococcus equi*-induced pneumonia had been diagnosed. *Am J Vet Res*. 1993;54:2115–2120.
7. Lepage MFP, Gerber V, Suter MM. A case of interstitial pneumonia associated with *Pneumocystis carinii* in a foal. *Vet Pathol*. 1999;36:621–624.
8. Lamb CR, O'Callaghan MW, Paradis MR. Thoracic radiography in the neonatal foal: a preliminary report. *Vet Radiol*. 1990;31:11–16.
9. Lester GD, Lester NV. Abdominal and thoracic radiography in the neonate. *Vet Clin North Am Equine Pract*. 2001;17:19–46.
10. Kutasi O, Horvath A, Harnos A, Szenci O. Radiographic assessment of pulmonary fluid clearance in healthy neonatal foals. *Vet Radiol Ultrasound*. 2009;50:584–588.
11. Koblik PD, Hornof WJ. Diagnostic radiology and nuclear cardiology. Their use in assessment of equine cardiovascular disease. *Vet Clin North Am Equine Pract*. 1985;1:289–309.
12. Hoskinson JJ, Tucker RL, Lillich J, Bertone JJ. Advanced diagnostic imaging modalities available at the referral center. *Vet Clin North Am Equine Pract*. 1997;13: 601–612.
13. Reef VB, Boy MG, Reid CF, Elser A. Comparison between diagnostic ultrasonography and radiography in the evaluation of horses and cattle with thoracic disease: 56 cases (1984–1985). *J Am Vet Med Assoc*. 1991;198: 2112–2118.
14. Hinchcliff KW, Byrne BA. Clinical examination of the respiratory system. *Vet Clin North Am Equine Pract*. 1991;7:1–26.
15. Gross DK, Morley PS, Hinchcliff KW, Reichle JK, Slemons RD. Pulmonary ultrasonographic abnormalities associated with naturally occurring equine influenza virus infection in Standardbred racehorses. *J Vet Intern Med/ American College of Veterinary Internal Medicine*. 2004;18:718–727.
16. Rantanen NW. The diagnosis of lung consolidation in horses using linear array diagnostic ultrasound. *J Equine Vet Sci*. 1994;14:79–80.
17. Punsmann S, Hellige M, Hoppe J, Freise F, Venner M. Diagnostic imaging in acute interstitial pneumonia in foals: high variability of interpretation of chest radiographs and good conformity between ultrasonographic and postmortem findings. *Vet Radiol Ultrasound*. 2021.
18. Rush BR, Hoskinson JJ, Davis EG, Matson CJ, Hakala JE. Pulmonary distribution of aerosolized technetium Tc 99m pentetate after administration of a single dose of aerosolized albuterol sulfate in horses with recurrent airway obstruction. *Am J Vet Res*. 1999;60:764–769.
19. Votion DM, Vandenput SN, Duvivier DH, et al. Alveolar clearance in horses with chronic obstructive pulmonary disease. *Am J Vet Res*. 1999;60:495–500.
20. Wion L, Perkins G, Ainsworth DM, Dykes NL, Divers TJ. Use of computerised tomography to diagnose a *Rhodococcus equi* mediastinal abscess causing severe respiratory distress in a foal. *Equine Vet J*. 2001;33:523–526.
21. Schliewert E-C, Lascola KM, O'Brien RT, et al. Comparison of radiographic and computed tomographic images of the lungs in healthy neonatal foals. *Am J Vet Res*. 2015;76:42–52.
22. Garrett KS, Embertson RM, Hopper SA, Woodie JB, McQuerry KJ. Preoperative computed tomographic evaluation of neonatal foals with rib fractures. *Vet Surg*. 2022:1–11.
23. Bedenice D, Heuwieser W, Brawer R, Solano M, Rand W, Paradis MR. Clinical and prognostic significance of radiographic pattern, distribution, and severity of thoracic radiographic changes in neonatal foals. *J Vet Intern Med/ American College of Veterinary Internal Medicine*. 2003;17:876–886.
24. Barton AK, Schulze T, Doherr MG, Gehlen H. Influence of bronchoalveolar lavage on thoracic radiography in the horse. *J Vet Sci*. 2018;19:563–569.
25. Farrow CS. Radiographic aspects of inflammatory lung disease in the horse. *Vet Radiol*. 1981;22:107–114.
26. Nykamp SG, Scrivani P, Dykes NL. Radiographic signs of pulmonary disease: an alternative approach. *Compend Contin Educ*. 2002;24:25–36.
27. Wilkins PA. Lower respiratory problems of the neonate. *Vet Clin North Am Equine Pract*. 2003;19:19–33.
28. Wilkins PA. Lower airway diseases of the adult horse. *Vet Clin North Am Equine Pract*. 2003;19:101–121.
29. Buergelt CD. Interstitial pneumonia in the horse: a fledgling morphological entity with mysterious causes. *Equine Vet J*. 1995;27:4–5.
30. Nout YS, Hinchcliff KW, Samii VF, Kohn CW, Jose-Cunilleras E, Reed SM. Chronic pulmonary disease with radiographic interstitial opacity (interstitial pneumonia) in foals. *Equine Vet J*. 2002;34:542–548.
31. Buergelt CD, Hines SA, Cantor G, Stirk A, Wilson JH. A retrospective study of proliferative interstitial lung disease of horses in Florida. *Vet Pathol*. 1986;23:750–756.
32. Peek SF, Landolt G, Karasin AI, et al. Acute respiratory distress syndrome and fatal interstitial pneumonia associated with equine influenza in a neonatal foal. *J Vet Intern Med*. 2004;18:132–134.
33. Lakritz J, Wilson WD, Berry CR, Schrenzel MD, Carlson GP, Madigan JE. Bronchointerstitial pneumonia and respiratory distress in young horses: clinical, clinicopathologic, radiographic, and pathological findings in 23 cases (1984–1989). *J Vet Intern Med*. 1993;7:277–288.
34. Donaldson MT, Beech J, Ennulat D, Hamir AN. Interstitial pneumonia and pulmonary fibrosis in a horse. *Equine Vet J*. 1998;30:173–175.
35. Wong DM, Belgrave RL, Williams KJ, et al. Multinodular pulmonary fibrosis in five horses. *J Am Vet Med Assoc*. 2008;232:898–905.
36. Carrillo MF, Kemper D, Woods LW, Carvallo FR. Chronic interstitial pneumonia with features of organizing pneumonia in an adult horse. *J Vet Diagn Invest*. 2020;32:621–625.
37. Lavoie JP, Fiset L, Laverty S. Review of 40 cases of lung abscesses in foals and adult horses. *Equine Vet J*. 1994;26:348–352.

38. Ainsworth DM, Erb HN, Eicker SW, et al. Effects of pulmonary abscesses on racing performance of horses treated at referral veterinary medical teaching hospitals: 45 cases (1985–1997). *J Am Vet Med Assoc*. 2000;216:1282–1287.
39. Lavoie J-P, Dalle S, Breton L, Hélie P. Bronchiectasis in three adult horses with heaves. *J Vet Intern Med/American College of Veterinary Internal Medicine*. 2004;18: 757–760.
40. Ainsworth DM, Eicker SW, Yeagar AE, et al. Associations between physical examination, laboratory, and radiographic findings and outcome and subsequent racing performance of foals with *Rhodococcus equi* infection: 115 cases (1984–1992). *J Am Vet Med Assoc*. 1998;213:510–515.
41. Giguère S, Roberts GD. Association between radiographic pattern and outcome in foals with pneumonia caused by *Rhodococcus equi*. *Vet Radiol Ultrasound*. 2012;53:601–604.
42. Falcon J, Smith BP, O'Brien TR, Carlson GP, Biberstein E. Clinical and radiographic findings in *Corynebacterium equi* pneumonia of foals. *J Am Vet Med Assoc*. 1985;186:593–599.
43. Ramirez S, Lester GD, Roberts GR. Diagnostic contribution of thoracic ultrasonography in 17 foals with *Rhodococcus equi* pneumonia. *Vet Radiol Ultrasound*. 2004;45: 172–176.
44. Green SL, Hager DA, Mays MBC, Merritt AM. Acute diffuse mycotic pneumonia in a 7-month-old colt. *Vet Radiology*. 2005;28:216–219.
45. Maleski K, Magdesian KG, LaFranco-Scheuch L, Pappagianis D, Carlson GP. Pulmonary coccidioidomycosis in a neonatal foal. *Vet Rec*. 2002;151:505–508.
46. Ziemer EL, Pappagianis D, Madigan JE, Mansmann RA, Hoffman KD. Coccidioidomycosis in horses: 15 cases (1975–1984). *J Am Vet Med Assoc*. 1992;201:910–916.
47. Toribio RE, Kohn CW, Lawrence AE, Hardy J, Hutt JA. Thoracic and abdominal blastomycosis in a horse. *J Am Vet Med Assoc*. 1999;214, 1357-60–1335.
48. Mair TS, Lane JG. Pneumonia, lung abscesses and pleuritis in adult horses: a review of 51 cases. *Equine Vet J*. 1989;21:175–180.
49. Singh K, Holbrook TC, Gilliam LL, Cruz RJ, Duffy J, Confer AW. Severe pulmonary disease due to multisystemic eosinophilic epitheliotropic disease in a horse. *Vet Pathol*. 2006;43:189–193.
50. Wilkins PA. Equine multinodular pulmonary fibrosis: diagnosis and treatment. *Equine Vet Educ*. 2013;25. n/a-n/a.
51. Easton-Jones CA, Cissell DD, Mohr FC, Chigerwe M, Pusterla N. Prognostic indicators and long-term survival in 14 horses with equine multinodular pulmonary fibrosis. *Equine Vet Educ*. 2020;32:41–46.
52. Bell SA, Drew CP, Wilson WD, Pusterla N. Idiopathic chronic eosinophilic pneumonia in 7 horses. *J Vet Intern Med*. 2008;22:648–653.
53. Arens AM, Barr B, Puchalski SM, et al. Osteoporosis associated with pulmonary silicosis in an equine bone fragility syndrome. *Vet Pathol*. 2011;48:593–615.
54. Berry CR, O'Brien TR, Madigan JE, Hager DA. Thoracic radiographic features of silicosis in 19 horses. *J Vet Intern Med*. 1991;5:248–256.
55. Williams KJ, Maes R, Piero FD, et al. Equine multinodular pulmonary fibrosis: a newly recognized herpesvirus-associated fibrotic lung disease. *Vet Pathol*. 2007;44:849–862.
56. Niedermaier G, Poth T, Gehlen H. Clinical aspects of multinodular pulmonary fibrosis in two warmblood horses. *Vet Rec*. 2010;166:426–430.
57. Couëtil LL, Hoffman AM, Hodgson J, et al. *Inflammatory Airway Disease of Horses*. vol. 21. 2007:356–361.
58. Couëtil LL, Cardwell JM, Gerber V, Lavoie J-P, Léguillette R, Richard EA. Inflammatory airway disease of horses—revised consensus statement. *J Vet Intern Med*. 2016;30:503–515.
59. Léguillette R. Recurrent airway obstruction—heaves. *Vet Clin North Am Equine Pract*. 2003;19:63–86.
60. Mazan MR, Vin R, Hoffman AM. Radiographic scoring lacks predictive value in inflammatory airway disease. *Equine Vet J*. 2005;37:541–545.
61. Niedźwiedź A. Equine recurrent airway obstruction. *Macedonian Veterinary Review*. 2014.
62. Seahorn TL, Beadle RE. Summer pasture-associated obstructive pulmonary disease in horses: 21 cases (1983–1991). *J Am Vet Med Assoc*. 1993;202:779–782.
63. Sage AM, Valberg S, Hayden DW, Firshman AM, Jacob K. Echocardiography in a horse with cor pulmonale from recurrent airway obstruction. *J Vet Intern Med/American College of Veterinary Internal Medicine*. 2006;20:694.
64. Johansson AM, Gardner SY, Atkins CE, LaFevers DH, Breuhaus BA. Cardiovascular effects of acute pulmonary obstruction in horses with recurrent airway obstruction. *J Vet Intern Med/American College of Veterinary Internal Medicine*. 2007;21:302–307.
65. West JB, Mathieu-Costello O. Stress failure of pulmonary capillaries as a mechanism for exercise induced pulmonary haemorrhage in the horse. *Equine Vet Journal*. 1994;26:441–447.
66. Hinchcliff KW, Couëtil LL, Knight PK, et al. Exercise induced pulmonary hemorrhage in horses: American College of Veterinary Internal Medicine consensus statement. *J Vet Intern Med*. 2015;29:743–758.
67. Sweeney CR. Exercise-induced pulmonary hemorrhage. *Vet Clin North Am Equine Pract*. 1991;7:93–104.
68. Birks EK, Durando MM, McBride S. Exercise-induced pulmonary hemorrhage. *Vet Clin North Am Equine Pract*. 2003;19:87–100.
69. Ferrucci F, Stancari G, Zucca E, Ayalon S, Falcone C, Ferro E. Specificity and sensitivity of ultrasonography and endoscopy for the diagnosis of exercise-induced pulmonary haemorrhage (EIPH) in 157 race horses. *Vet Res Commun*. 2009;33:185–188.
70. Feudo CML, Stucchi L, Alberti E, et al. The role of thoracic ultrasonography and airway endoscopy in the diagnosis of equine asthma and exercise-induced pulmonary hemorrhage. *Vet Sci*. 2021;8:276.
71. Kollias-Baker CA, Pipers FS, Heard D, Seeherman H. Pulmonary edema associated with transient airway obstruction in three horses. *J Am Vet Med Assoc*. 1993;202:1116–1118.
72. Kaartinen MJ, Pang DSJ, Cuvelliez SG. Post-anesthetic pulmonary edema in two horses. *Veterinary Anaesthesia and Analgesia*. 2010;37:136–143.
73. Davis JL, Gardner SY, Schwabenton B, Breuhaus BA. Congestive heart failure in horses: 14 cases (1984–2001). *J Am Vet Med Assoc*. 2002;220:1512–1515.
74. Jean D, Lavoie JP, Nunez L, Lagacé A, Laverty S. Cutaneous hemangiosarcoma with pulmonary metastasis in a horse. *J Am Vet Med Assoc*. 1994;204:776–778.
75. Jorgensen JS, Geoly FJ, Berry CR, Breuhaus BA. Lameness and pleural effusion associated with an aggressive fibrosarcoma in a horse. *J Am Vet Med Assoc*. 1997;210:1328–1331.
76. Cook G, Divers TJ, Rowland PH. Hypercalcaemia and erythrocytosis in a mare associated with a metastatic carcinoma. *Equine Vet J*. 1995;27:316–318.
77. Facemire PR, Chilcoat CD, Sojka JE, et al. Treatment of granular cell tumor via complete right lung resection in a horse. *J Am Vet Med Assoc*. 2000;217:1522–1525.

78. Danton CA, Peacock PJ, May SA, Kelly DF. Anaplastic sarcoma in the caudal thigh of a horse. *Vet Rec.* 1992;131:188–190.
79. Anderson JD, Leonard JM, Zeliff JA, Garman RH. Primary pulmonary neoplasm in a horse. *J Am Vet Med Assoc.* 1992;201:1399–1401.
80. Jean D, Picandet V, Macieira S, Beauregard G, D'Anjou MA, Beauchamp G. Detection of rib trauma in newborn foals in an equine critical care unit: a comparison of ultrasonography, radiography and physical examination. *Equine Vet J.* 2007;39:158–163.
81. Schambourg MA, Laverty S, Mullim S, Fogarty UM, Halley J. Thoracic trauma in foals: post mortem findings. *Equine Vet J.* 2003;35:78–81.
82. Neil KM, Charman RE, Vasey JR. Rib osteomyelitis in three foals. *Australian Veterinary Journal.* 2010;88:96–100.
83. Punsmann S, Hoppe J, Klopfleisch R, Venner M. Acute interstitial pneumonia in foals: a severe, multifactorial syndrome with lung tissue recovery in surviving foals. *Equine Vet J.* 2021;53:718–726.
84. Dunkel B, Dolente B, Boston RC. Acute lung injury/acute respiratory distress syndrome in 15 foals. *Equine Vet J.* 2005;37:435–440.
85. Jose-Cunilleras E, Sibbons PD. Acute lung injury and acute respiratory distress syndrome: fashionable names for old conditions or new clinical entities in their own right? *Equine Vet J.* 2005;37:390–392.
86. Gough SL, Carrick J, Raidal SL, et al. *Chlamydia psittaci* infection as a cause of respiratory disease in neonatal foals. *Equine Vet J.* 2020;52:244–249.
87. Dunkel B. Acute lung injury and acute respiratory distress syndrome in foals. *Clin Techniques Equine Pract.* 2006;5:127–133.
88. Raphel CF, Beech J. Pleuritis secondary to pneumonia or lung abscessation in 90 horses. *J Am Vet Med Assoc.* 1982;181:808–810.
89. May J, Fews D, Tennant K, Mair T. Diagnostic dichotomy: a question of thoracic mesothelioma. *Equine Veterinary Education.* 2016. n/a-n/a.
90. Johns I, Marr C, DURHAM A, Mair T, McParland T. Causes of pleural effusions in horses resident in the UK. *Equine Veterinary Education.* 2016;29:144–148.
91. Prater PE, Patton CS, Held JP. Pleural effusion resulting from malignant hepatoblastoma in a horse. *J Am Vet Med Assoc.* 1989;194:383–385.
92. Boy MG, Sweeney CR. Pneumothorax in horses: 40 cases (1980–1997). *J Am Vet Med Assoc.* 2000;216:1955–1959.
93. Izing S, Kelemen Z, Bohák Z, Tóth P, Bodó G. Successful repair of diaphragmatic hernia with simultaneously performed thoracotomy and median laparotomy in a horse. *Vet Rec Case Reports.* 2021;9.
94. Everett KA, Chaffin MK, Brinsko SP. Diaphragmatic herniation as a cause of lethargy and exercise intolerance in a mare. *The Cornell Veterinarian.* 1992;82:217–223.
95. Hartzband LE, InterScience W, Kerr DV, Morris EA. Ultrasonographic diagnosis of diaphragmatic rupture in a horse. *Veterinary Radiology.* 1990:42–44.
96. Sweeney CR, Gillette DM. Thoracic neoplasia in equids: 35 cases (1967–1987). *J Am Vet Med Assoc.* 1989;195: 374–377.
97. Garber JL, Reef VB, Reimer JM. Sonographic findings in horses with mediastinal lymphosarcoma: 13 cases (1985–1992). *J Am Vet Med Assoc.* 1994;205:1432–1436.
98. Camacho-Luna P, Andrews FM, Dehghanpir SD, et al. Bicavitary effusion in a horse with multicentric lymphoma. *Equine Vet Educ.* 2021;33:e224–e230.
99. Clercq DD, Loon G van, Lefère L, Deprez P. Ultrasound-guided biopsy as a diagnostic aid in three horses with a cranial mediastinal lymphosarcoma. *Vet Rec.* 2004;154:722–726.
100. Macklin CC. Transport of air along sheaths of pulmonic blood vessels from alveoli to mediastinum: clinical implications. *Arch Intern Med.* 1939;64:913–926.
101. Carstens A, Kirberger RM, Grimbeek RJ, Donnellan CMB, Saulez MN. Radiographic quantification of tracheal dimensions of the normal thoroughbred horse. *Vet Radiol Ultrasound.* 2009;50:492–501.
102. Aleman M, Nieto JE, Benak J, Johnson LR. Tracheal collapse in American miniature horses: 13 cases (1985–2007). *J Am Vet Med Assoc.* 2008;233:1302–1306.
103. Peyrecave-Capo X, Munoz-Diaz J, Ferrer GR, Watrelot D, Desjardins I. Acute tracheal trauma and chronic tracheal collapse in an asthmatic mature pony. *Equine Vet Educ.* 2022.
104. Every LJ, Hostnik ET, Hostnik LD, et al. Radiographic tracheal lumen to vertebral ratios in the normal American Miniature Horse. *Equine Vet J.* 2020;52:428–434.
105. Feige K, Schwarzwald C, Fürst A, Hotz BK. Esophageal obstruction in horses: a retrospective study of 34 cases. *Can Vet J La Revue Vétérinaire Canadienne.* 2000;41:207–210.
106. Clabough DL, Roberts MC, Robertson I. Probable congenital esophageal stenosis in a thoroughbred foal. *J Am Vet Med Assoc.* 1991;199:483–485.
107. Baker SJ, Johnson PJ, David A, Cook CR. Idiopathic gastroesophageal reflux disease in an adult horse. *J Am Vet Med Assoc.* 2004;224, 1967-70–1931.
108. Beaulieu A, Zakia LS, Ludwig L, Kenney D, Rätsep E, Nykamp S. Oesophageal muscular hypertrophy and pulsion diverticulum in a Friesian horse. *Veterinary Record Case Reports.* 2020;8:e001093-4.
109. Wong DM, Ruby RE, Eerde EV, Miles KG. Oesophageal ectasia as a cause of dysphagia and milk regurgitation in a neonatal foal. *Equine Vet Educ.* 2020;32:O45–O49.
110. King JN, Davies JV, Gerring EL. Contrast radiography of the equine oesophagus: effect of spasmolytic agents and passage of a nasogastric tube. *Equine Vet J.* 1990;22:133–135.
111. Worth LT, Reef VB. Pericarditis in horses: 18 cases (1986–1995). *J Am Vet Med Assoc.* 1998;212:248–253.

ELECTRONIC RESOURCES

Additional information related to the content in Chapter 37 can be found online at eBooks.Health.Elsevier.com.

- Chapter Quiz

SECTION V

Abdominal Cavity: Canine and Feline

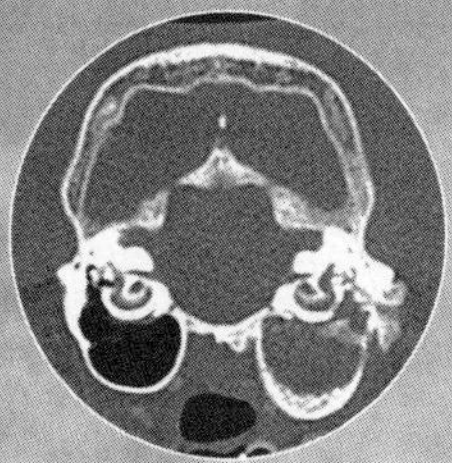

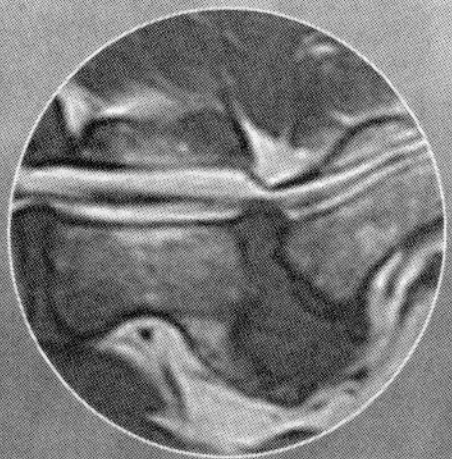

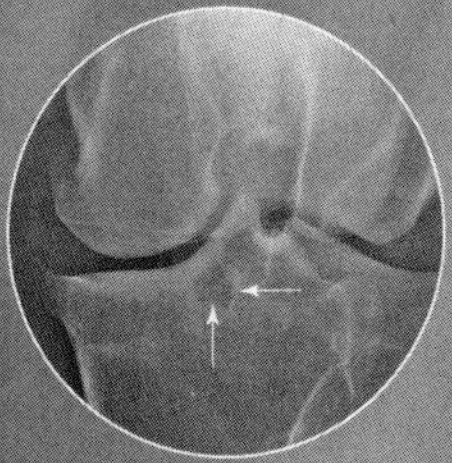

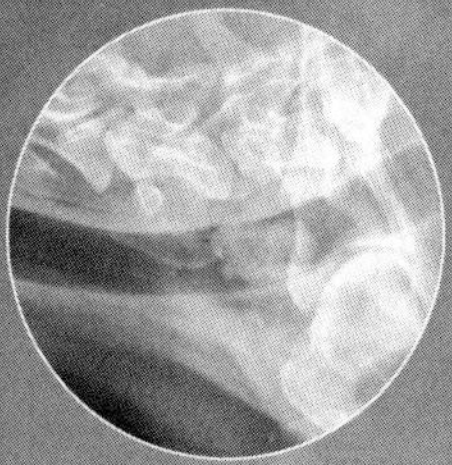

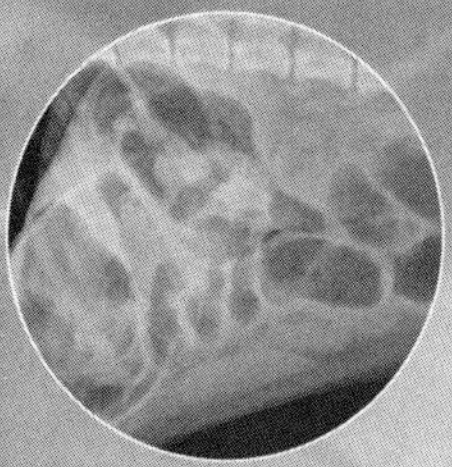

CHAPTER 38

Principles of Radiographic Interpretation of the Abdomen

Donald E. Thrall

Acquiring abdominal radiographs is common in small animal practice. Abdominal radiography is rarely performed in the adult horse, except for assessment of the cranioventral and/or ventral aspects of the abdomen for sand collections or enteroliths. The entire abdomen can be radiographed successfully in foals and miniature horses, but the conspicuity of abdominal organs is less than in dogs or cats because of the reduced abdominal fat and the larger volume of the equine gastrointestinal tract.

Sonography has many applications to assess the canine and feline abdomen but it should not be used for initial screening. Sonography is not a replacement for abdominal radiography. Sonography provides for real-time assessment of organ texture and vascular anatomy and perfusion that cannot be obtained with radiography, but sonography does not provide for a global assessment of the abdomen. Sonography is also useful for examining abdominal organs that are usually not visible radiographically, for example, gallbladder, adrenal glands, ureters, uterus, mesenteric lymph nodes, retroperitoneal lymph nodes, and the prostate gland. Because of the limited ability of radiology to examine the equine abdomen, sonography has assumed a more primary role than in small animals.

NOMENCLATURE

In daily practice, the naming of conventional lateral abdominal radiographs made with the patient lying on their side and a vertically directed x-ray beam violates the point-of-entrance to point-of-exit nomenclature system described in Chapter 6. If the patient was on the left side, for example, the correct name for this view would be a *right-left* lateral because the x-ray beam enters on the right side and exits on the left. But, in daily practice the naming of this view is abbreviated to designate the side the patient is lying on, in this case a *left lateral*. Similarly, an abdominal radiograph made with the patient lying on the right side would be a *right lateral* view. Since lateral equine abdominal radiographs are usually made with the patient standing and a horizontally directed x-ray beam, the point-to-entrance to point-of-exit system should be used. Thus, lateral radiographs should be described as either left-right or right-left views. In all species, ventrodorsal (VD) and dorsoventral (DV) radiographs of the abdomen are named according to the point-to-entrance to point-of-exit system.

PREPARATION

In the dog and cat, fasting or enema administration is not needed prior to abdominal radiography unless one is preparing the patient for a contrast study. If a bowel obstruction is being considered, enema administration is contraindicated because it will alter the native pattern of gas and fluid in the intestine, which is diagnostically important. There are no specific circumstances in the horse where fasting or enema administration is recommended before abdominal radiography.

RADIOGRAPHIC TECHNIQUE—DOG AND CAT

A relatively high-contrast image of the abdomen is preferred. This differs from the thorax where there is a large volume of air in the lung to provide contrast, making a low-contrast thoracic radiographic technique preferable. In the abdomen, it is only the interposed fat between the abdominal structures that provides contrast. Bowel gas provides contrast for assessing the lumen of the bowel, but bowel gas is not helpful for comparing parenchymal organs or for assessing the peritoneum or serosal surface of the intestines; it is the abdominal fat located in the mesentery and omentum that provides contrast between organs. As there is minimal difference in inherent radiographic opacity of fat vs. soft tissue, the contrast of an abdominal radiograph should be enhanced using radiographic technique. With analog technology, a high-contrast image is obtained using a low kilovoltage peak (kVp)—high milliampere seconds (mAs) technique, and this approach can also be used with digital systems. However, in digital imaging the contrast of the image is controlled primarily by the processing algorithm that is applied to the raw image data. Therefore, it is important that the correct processing parameters are assigned when the digital image system is set up initially. For patients thicker than 10 cm, a grid should be used to remove scattered x-rays from the beam. Exposure time is not as critical when radiographing the abdomen as when radiographing the thorax.

The respiratory pattern of the patient should be observed for a few seconds before the radiographic exposure is made so that the exposure can be coordinated with peak expiration. At expiration the diaphragm is further cranial, and there is less crowding of the abdomen. Timing the radiographic exposure to phase of respiration is not as important as in the thorax, but timing the exposure to peak expiration is a small adjustment that can be made that will add to the quality of abdominal radiographs.

RADIOGRAPHIC TECHNIQUE—HORSE

Radiographing the abdomen of all but the smallest horse requires massive exposure factors because of the sheer mass of the part. This is a major limiting factor. Also, there is relatively less fat in the equine abdomen to provide contrast, and the gastrointestinal content occupies a much greater volume of the abdomen, resulting in most organs being obscured. In adult horses, it will be difficult to assess anything but the position of large gas-containing structures or to identify large collections of radiopaque material or objects, such as ingested sand[1] or a large enterolith. A portable x-ray unit such as those used commonly to radiograph equine extremities will not be adequate for equine abdominal radiography.

POSITIONING—DOG AND CAT

The routine abdominal radiographic examination in the dog and cat should consist of left lateral, right lateral, and VD projections. DV radiographs of the abdomen should not be made routinely because the abdomen will be more crowded, organ visibility will be reduced, and portions of the pelvic limbs are often superimposed on the abdomen (Fig. 38.1). A DV view may have to suffice when a patient cannot be positioned in dorsal recumbency for a VD view.

It is important that the entire abdominal cavity be included in the image. This seems obvious, but omitting the pelvic canal and perineum from the field of view is a common error, which increases the chance of missing a lesion. The field of view should extend from just cranial to the diaphragm to the level of the anus/perineum. For lateral views, the pelvic limbs should not be pulled caudally but should be kept perpendicular to the spine. This relaxes the caudoventral aspect of the abdominal wall and reduces crowding. Likewise, in the VD view, the pelvic limbs should ideally be flexed into a so-called *frog-leg position* rather than being pulled caudally, as is usually done. If the pelvic limbs are pulled caudally for the VD view, crowding will be increased, and skin folds will be created in the lateral thigh and/or caudal abdomen region. These skin folds create noticeable opacities that interfere with assessment of the caudal aspect of the abdomen (Fig. 38.2).

Even in the largest dog, it is usually possible to include the entire abdominal cavity in one 14-inch × 17-inch image. For the occasional huge dog where this is not possible, then each projection (left lateral, right lateral, VD) should be divided into cranial and caudal portions.

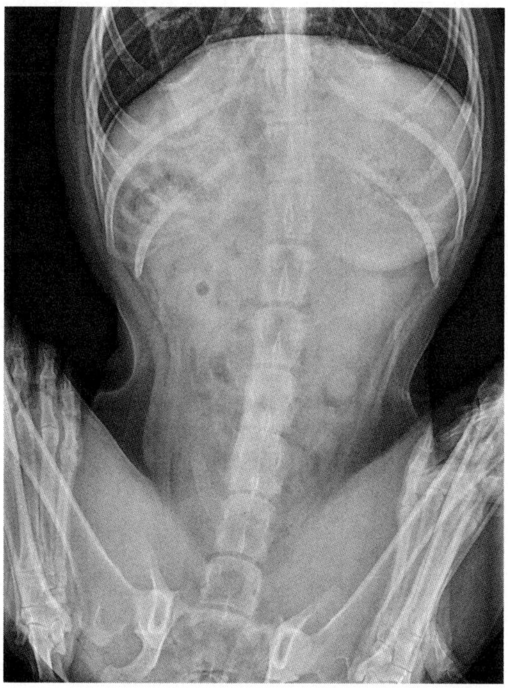

Fig. 38.1 A dorsoventral (DV) view of the abdomen. The pelvic limbs are superimposed on the caudal aspect of the abdomen and the caudal abdominal cavity is compressed and structures in this area cannot be evaluated. A DV view should not be a routine view for these reasons. This patient is also crooked, which adds to the reduced quality of this specific image.

POSITIONING—HORSE

In foals and miniature horses, it may be possible to obtain lateral abdominal radiographs by restraining a compliant animal on a conventional x-ray table and using a vertically directed x-ray beam, as in dogs and cats, but this is rarely done. Even in small horses, abdominal radiographs are usually obtained in a standing animal and using a horizontally directed x-ray beam (Fig. 38.3).

The plate should not be held by hand when radiographing the equine abdomen. The light field that corresponds to the primary x-ray beam is visible only on the side of the horse closest to the x-ray tube, meaning that no part of the light field can be seen on the plate. Therefore, aligning the x-ray beam with the plate is impossible when the plate is held by hand. This invariably results in the primary x-ray beam striking the person holding the plate. A wall-mounted plate holder, as described in Chapter 9, or a floor-mounted mobile plate holder should be used for equine abdominal radiography. When using these devices, the x-ray beam can be aligned with the plate before the horse is brought into position next to the plate.

As noted before, the overall conspicuity of abdominal organs in the horse is less than in the dog or cat because of the increased volume of the gastrointestinal tract and relatively reduced amount of abdominal fat. Some questions addressed by abdominal radiography in small horses or foals pertain to the presence of gastrointestinal foreign material, such as an enterolith or sand, or the presence of mechanical bowel obstruction, which will often be accompanied by increased bowel diameter and increased intraluminal fluid and gas.

The radiographic detail in the abdomen will be better in foals or miniature horses than in adult horses but meaningful information can sometimes be obtained in adult horses (Fig. 38.4). VD abdominal radiographs in small horses are rarely useful, or even possible to obtain, and most questions being addressed radiographically can be answered from lateral views.

Radiographic magnification has to be considered when radiographing the equine abdomen. As a result of the large diameter of the abdominal cavity of an adult horse, a lesion on the side closest to the x-ray tube could be 35 cm or more from the plate. This leads to the lesion being magnified by approximately 1.5 times. At this degree of magnification, the resultant blurring could result in the lesion being missed, especially if the lesion is small (Fig. 38.5). If a small lesion is a clinical concern, then left-right *and* right-left abdominal radiographs should be obtained.

WHY ARE BOTH LEFT AND RIGHT LATERAL ABDOMINAL VIEWS NEEDED ROUTINELY IN SMALL ANIMALS?

As in the thorax, obtaining both left lateral and right lateral views in addition to a VD view is recommended routinely but for a different reason, which is the use of bowel gas as an inherent contrast medium. The redistribution of bowel gas between the various views, and particularly between the left vs. right lateral view, can provide important information that allows the diagnosis to be made.

Of particular importance with regard to the redistribution of gastrointestinal gas as a function of position is the change in the appearance of the stomach. The stomach is an asymmetric structure with the larger fundus located in the left dorsal aspect of the abdomen, and the smaller pylorus located in the right ventral aspect of the abdomen (Fig. 38.6).[2,3] When the patient is in right recumbency, the pylorus will usually contain fluid or ingesta, and if there is gas in the

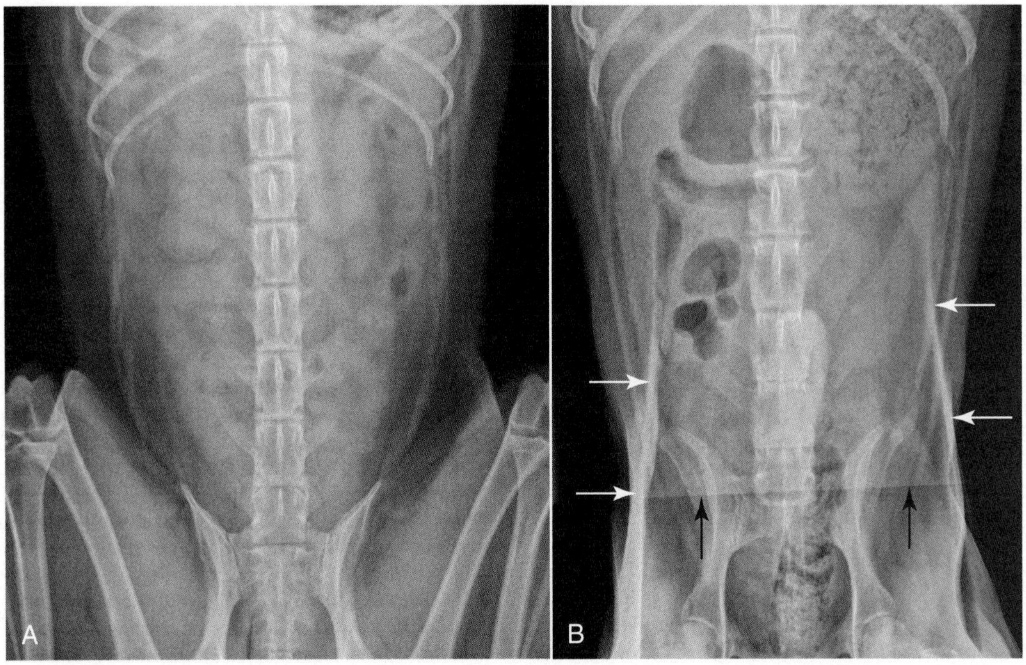

Fig. 38.2 Ventrodorsal (VD) abdominal radiographs from two dogs. In **A,** the pelvic limbs are flexed, allowing relaxation of the caudal abdominal muscles and expansion of the caudal aspect of the abdomen. In **B,** the pelvic limbs are pulled caudally, creating skin folds (*white arrows*) that can interfere with interpretation, and the caudal aspect of the abdomen is narrower and more crowded. Also in **B,** the edge of the positioning trough has created a linear opacity (*black arrows*) that can also interfere with interpretation. (Reproduced with permission from Thrall DE, Robertson IR. *Atlas of Radiographic Anatomy and Normal Anatomic Variants in the Dog and Cat.* 3rd ed. St. Louis: Elsevier/Saunders; 2023.)

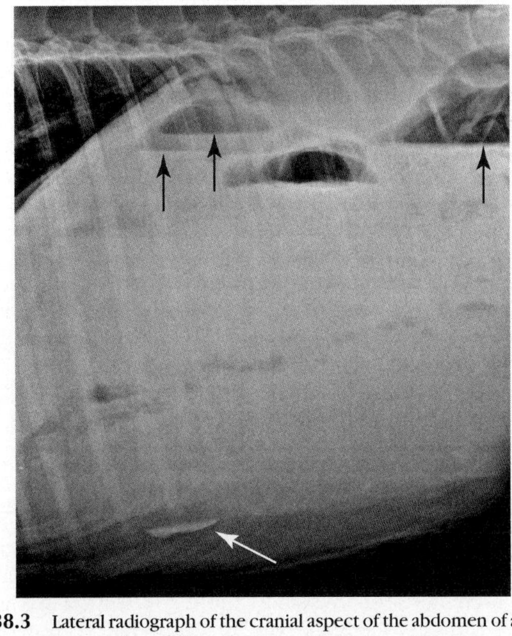

Fig. 38.3 Lateral radiograph of the cranial aspect of the abdomen of an adult American miniature horse. The small size of this horse allows for reasonable radiographic quality, but the conspicuity of organs is less than in a dog or cat because of the reduced amount of abdominal fat and the larger volume of the abdomen occupied by the gastrointestinal tract. There is a small amount of sand in the ventral aspect of the large bowel (*white arrow*); this is not significant. Horizontal gas/fluid interfaces (*black arrows*) in the bowel are seen because the radiograph was made with a horizontally directed x-ray beam. Visualization of gas/fluid interfaces to this extent is normal in the horse.

stomach, the gas will rise and collect in the body and fundus of the stomach. Alternatively, when the patient is in left recumbency, the fluid will usually gravitate to the fundus, and gas will rise and fill the pylorus. Therefore, the pylorus will be of soft tissue opacity in the right lateral view and contain gas in the left lateral view (Fig. 38.7). The difference in appearance of the stomach in left versus right lateral radiographs in an individual patient depends on the character of the gastric content and the relative amount of liquid versus solids. If there is mostly gas or mostly fluid or ingesta in the stomach, the stomach will commonly appear similar in left vs. right recumbency. The greatest difference in appearance of the stomach in the left vs. right lateral view occurs when the stomach is moderately distended and contains both gas and fluid (see Fig. 38.7).

Of particular importance is the realization that in right lateral views, especially in dogs, the pylorus can take on the appearance of a mass or foreign object because of the dependent fluid collection (see Fig. 38.7B). Also important is that ingested foreign material often becomes anchored in the pylorus. This emphasizes the importance of a left lateral radiograph to increase the chances of gas being in the pyloric antrum to provide contrast for the foreign material (Fig. 38.8). There is some evidence that it can be beneficial in dogs to obtain the left lateral projection first as it maximizes the likelihood of the duodenum being gas filled.[4]

As noted earlier, DV views of the abdomen are made rarely. Occasionally, a DV abdominal radiograph will be necessary when a VD view cannot be made (Fig. 38.9). The gravitational dependence of gas is one aspect of DV radiographs that may be useful, as illustrated in Fig. 38.9.

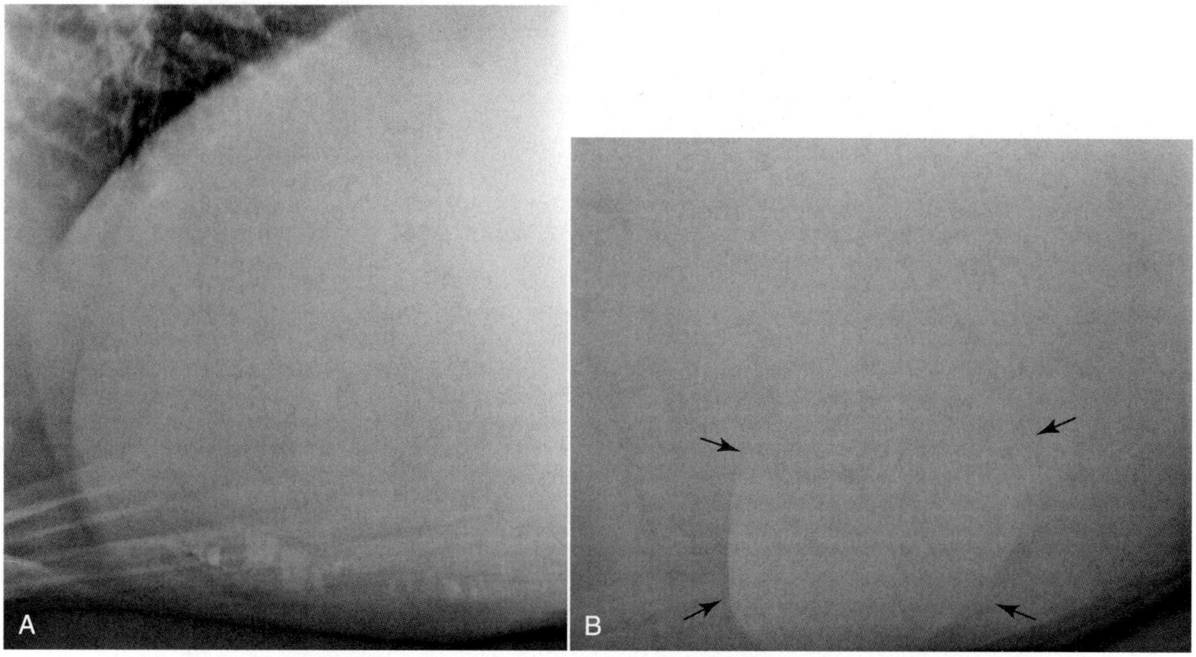

Fig. 38.4 Lateral radiographs of the cranioventral **(A)** and midventral **(B)** aspects of the abdomen of an adult Standardbred horse. The cranioventral aspect of the abdomen in **A** is devoid of any detail because of the extreme thickness of this region and the relatively homogeneous contents of the bowel; this is a normal appearance. However, this is a common location for sand to accumulate, and clinically insignificant sand accumulations are seen here. In **B,** there is a large circular radiopaque structure in the ventral aspect of the abdomen that represents an enterolith (*black arrows*).

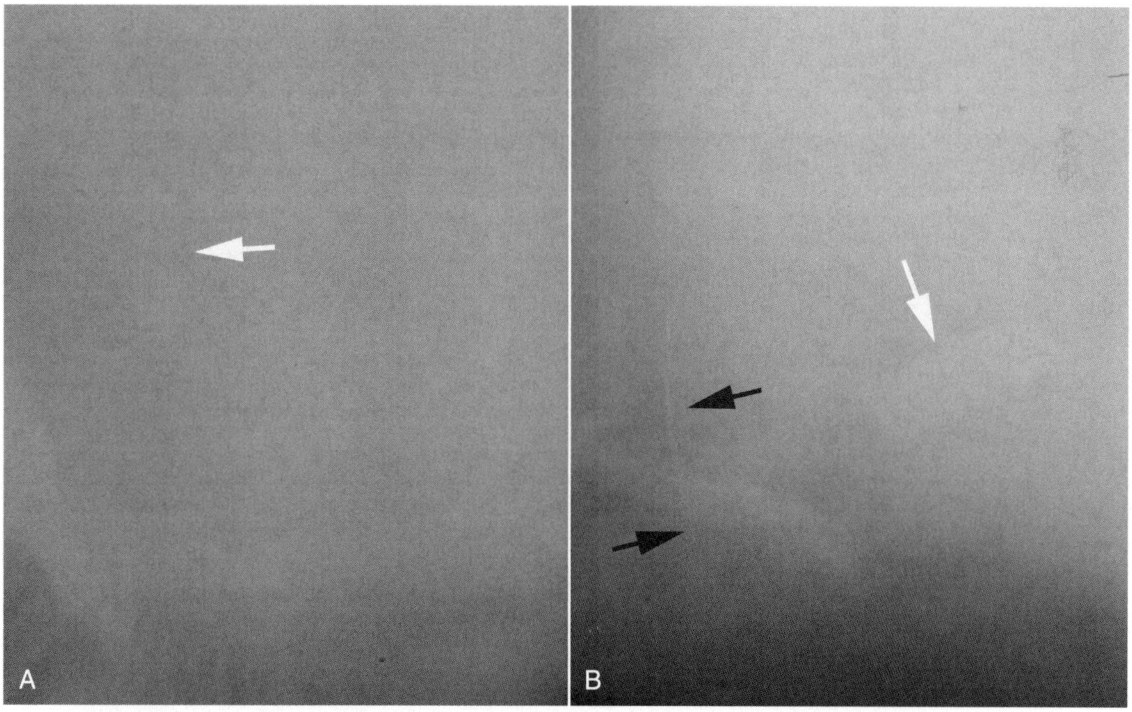

Fig. 38.5 Right-left lateral radiograph of the cranioventral aspect of the abdomen of an adult Holstein cow suspected of having traumatic reticuloperitonitis. Although this example is not in a horse, it illustrates the effect of magnification in a large patient. **(A)** There is a magnet in the reticulum (*white arrow*) but no evidence of metallic foreign material. When the opposite left-right lateral **(B)** was made, a wire (*black arrows*) is visible cranial to the reticulum confirming a penetrating foreign body from the reticulum. The magnet is also visible in **B** (***white arrow***). The wire was not visible in the right-left radiograph because of magnification related to the large distance of the wire from the plate. When radiographed from the opposite side, the wire was much closer to the plate and was not blurred by magnification.

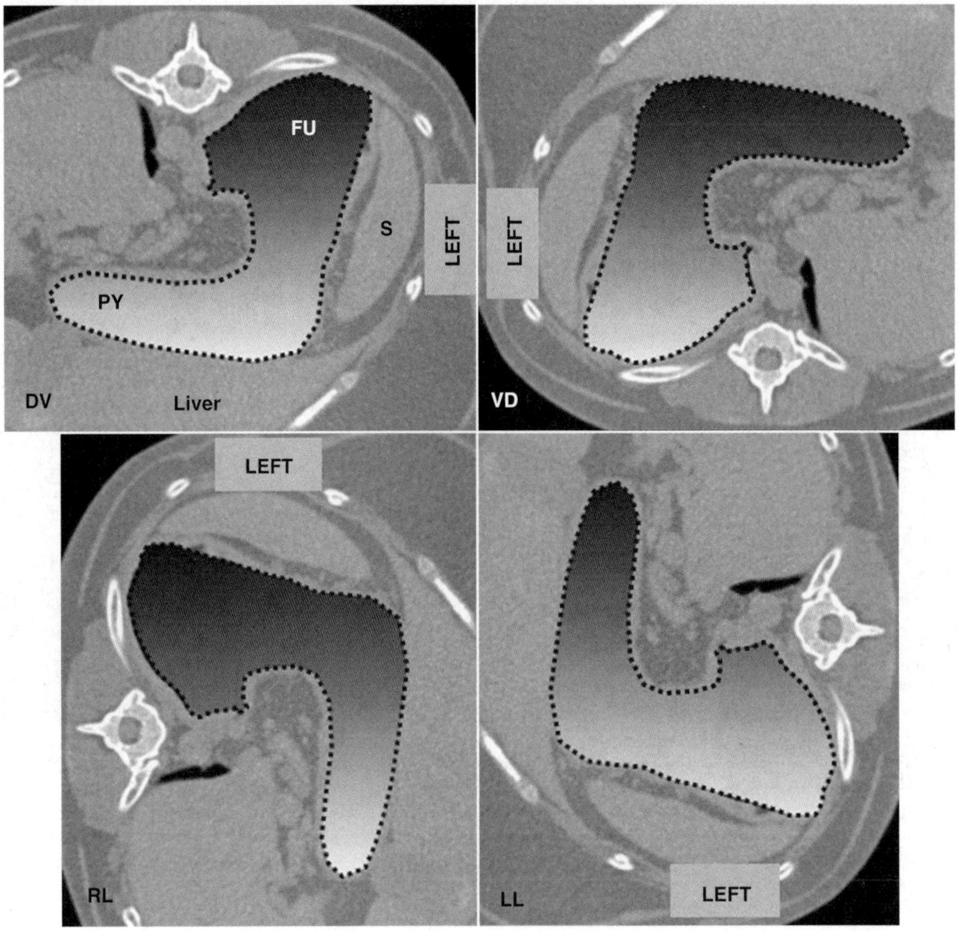

Fig. 38.6 Images depicting the normal distribution of gas vs. fluid in the stomach as a function of body position. The images are the same transverse computed tomography image of a dog rotated at 90-degree increments to illustrate sternal (*DV*), dorsal (*VD*), right (*R*), and left (*L*) recumbency. The stomach is outlined by a *dotted line.* The lumen of the stomach is shaded to illustrate the effect of gravity on redistribution of fluid (*white*) and gas (*black*) as a function of body position. The presence of gas in the pylorus in left recumbency is important clinically as the gas provides contrast for identification of foreign material that is trapped in the pylorus. *FU,* Fundus, *PY,* pylorus, *S,* spleen. (Reproduced with permission from Thrall DE, Robertson IR. *Atlas of Radiographic Anatomy and Normal Anatomic Variants in the Dog and Cat*. 3rd ed. St. Louis: Elsevier/Saunders; 2023.)

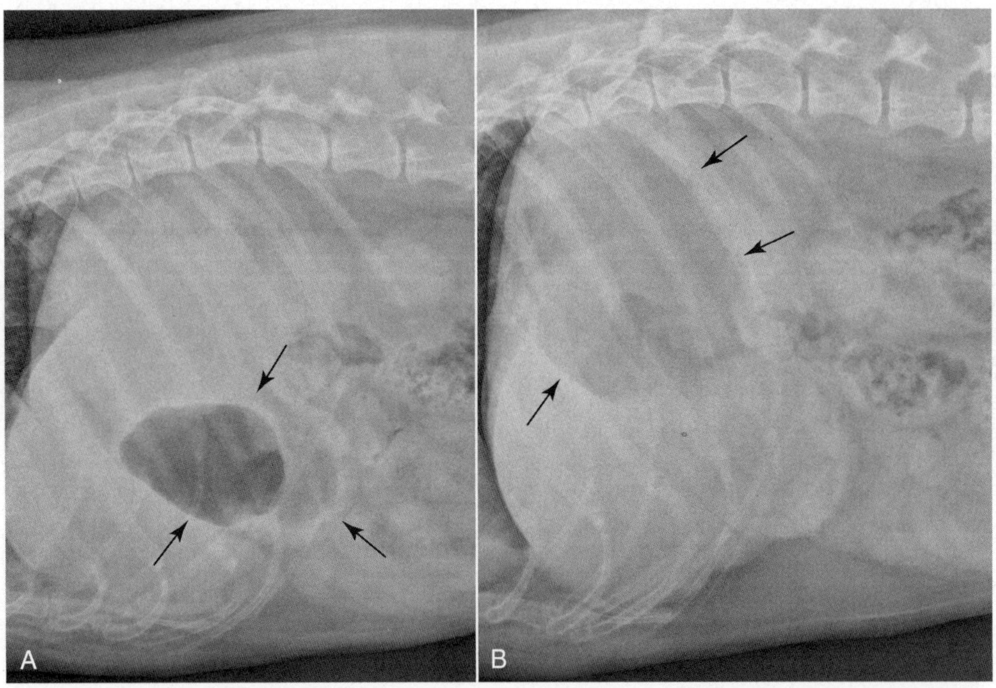

Fig. 38.7 Left **(A)** and right **(B)** lateral radiographs of the cranial aspect of the abdomen of a normal dog. In the left lateral view **(A)**, gas is present in the pylorus (*black arrows*). In right lateral recumbency, all of the gas is in the fundus (*black arrows*) and the pylorus is filled with fluid and appears as a round mass ventral to the fundus.

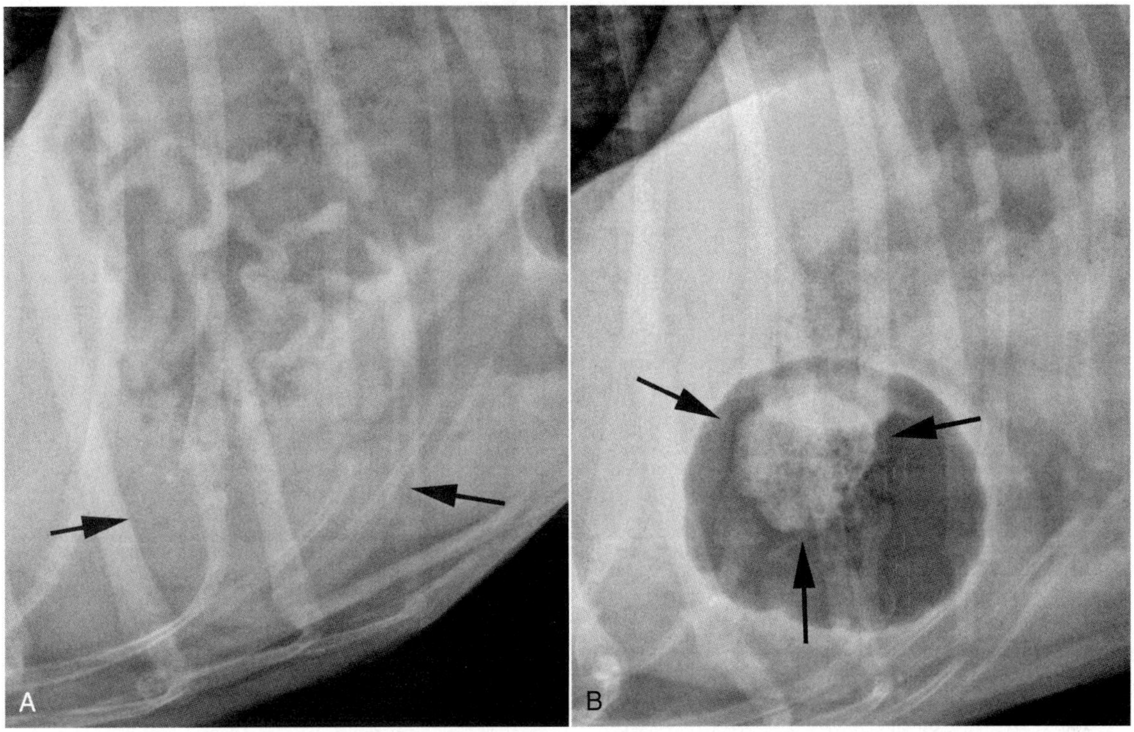

Fig. 38.8 Right lateral **(A)** radiograph of the abdomen of a dog suspected of having ingested foreign material. There is fluid in the pyloric antrum (*black arrows*) and the pylorus cannot be assessed for nonmineral foreign material due to silhouetting by the surrounding fluid. In a left lateral view **(B)**, gas in the pyloric antrum provides contrast for the foreign material anchored in the pyloric antrum (*black arrows*).

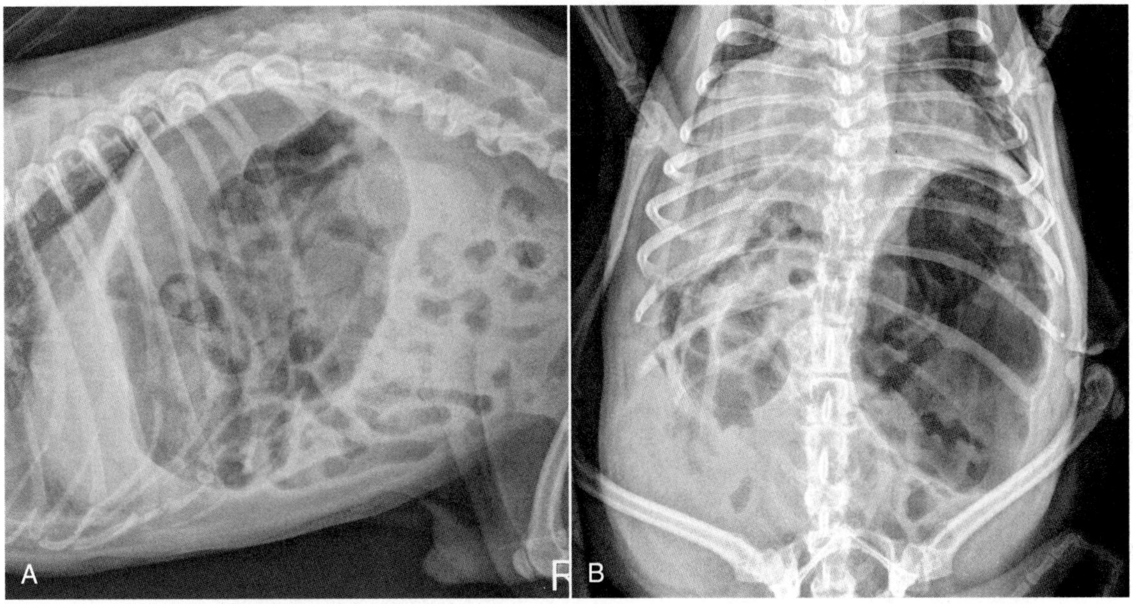

Fig. 38.9 Lateral **(A)** and dorsoventral (DV) **(B)** radiographs of the abdomen of a dog with acute abdominal distention and thoracic pain from rib fractures. In the lateral view **(A)**, there was concern whether the dilated stomach was in a normal position. Pain prevented obtaining a ventrodorsal (VD) radiograph so a DV was obtained instead. In the DV view **(B)**, gas has risen to the fundus because this part of the stomach is nondependent. There is no evidence of gastric malpositioning. This illustrates one of the few indications for obtaining a DV view of the abdomen versus a VD view. In **B,** note the increased crowding of the abdomen and superimposition of the pelvic limbs on the caudal abdomen, which are common problems with DV compared to VD abdominal radiographs.

ANCILLARY VIEWS

Right lateral, left lateral, and VD views of the abdomen will suffice for almost all canine and feline patients. If the status of the urethra in male dogs is of concern, as for assessment of urethral calculi, the right and left lateral views should be supplemented with a third lateral view made with the pelvic limbs pulled cranially. This provides an unobstructed view of the ischial arch and os penis, allowing for assessment of urethral calculi without superimposition of the pelvic limbs (Fig. 38.10).

A compression radiograph can be used to clarify a suspicious finding that cannot be confirmed because of superimposition.[5] The theory is to apply mild compression to displace superimposed organs from the field of view, leaving an unobstructed view of the region of interest. This technique can be applied in a lateral view to assess structures such as the uterine body or urinary bladder. Specialized inflatable compression paddles are available, but a wooden spatula or wooden spoon can also be used. Of course, care should be taken not to place compression on organs that are obviously diseased, and the amount of pressure placed should always be gentle (Fig. 38.11). The increased use of ultrasound for abdominal assessment has reduced the need for compression radiographs, but they remain a convenient method to increase the accuracy of radiographic interpretation in some patients where ultrasonography is not possible.

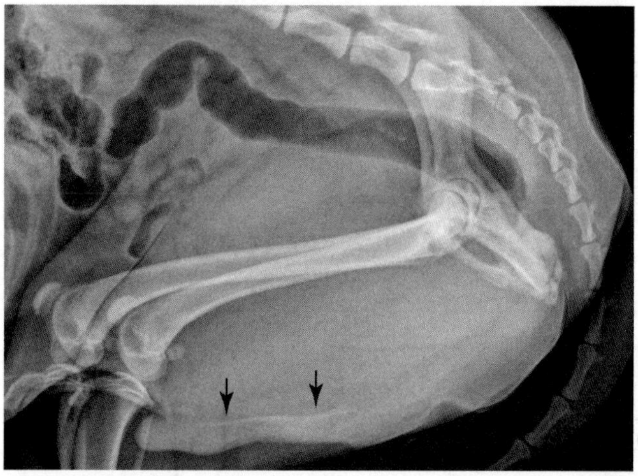

Fig. 38.10 Lateral radiograph of the caudal aspect of the abdomen with the pelvic limbs pulled cranially. This provides an unobstructed view of the urethral region and of the os penis (*black arrows*). This view is useful for assessing for urethral calculi or lesions of the os penis.

ANCILLARY FACTORS

There are no ancillary factors that affect the radiographic appearance of the equine abdomen other than body mass. However, for the dog and cat, the body habitus and presence of cutaneous structures or lesions are ancillary factors that have a significant effect on the appearance of the radiograph.

The volume of abdominal fat contained in the mesentery and omentum is directly related to the conspicuity of parenchymal organs and serosal margins in the abdomen because it is this fat that provides contrast between organs. It is absolutely critical for fat to be present if organs are going to be distinguished from one another in abdominal radiographs (Fig. 38.12). In emaciated (Fig. 38.13) or young (Fig. 38.14) animals, there is reduced fat that results in loss of conspicuity of the serosal margins.

Cutaneous lesions or superimposed superficial structures are not misinterpreted as a lesion as often in abdominal radiographs as they are in thoracic radiographs. One specific example of a superficial structure that is often misinterpreted as an abnormality in abdominal radiographs is superimposition of the prepuce and os penis on the caudal aspect of the abdomen in VD radiographs of male dogs (Fig. 38.15). The reason that cutaneous lesions create such a conspicuous opacity was discussed in Chapter 6.

SPECIFIC DIFFERENCES BETWEEN CANINE AND FELINE ABDOMINAL RADIOGRAPHS

There are several specific differences between canine and feline abdominal radiographs that are important to know to reduce the chance for an error in interpretation. These differences will all be covered in their respective section in the text, but a brief summary is also presented here.

Overconditioning results in increased intra-abdominal fat but this is disproportionate in cats compared to dogs (Fig. 38.16). The tendency for overweight cats to accumulate fat in the

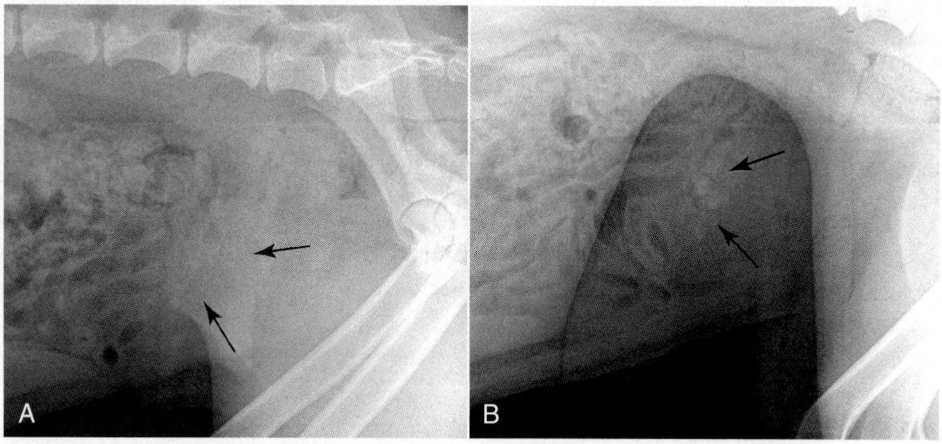

Fig. 38.11 Lateral radiograph of caudal aspect of the abdomen of a dog **(A)**. There are multiple small mineral opacities (*black arrows*) superimposed on the plane of the urinary bladder. These opacities could represent cystic calculi, but they could also represent superimposed bowel content. The caudal abdomen was compressed with a wooden spatula in a subsequent lateral radiograph **(B)** to displace the bowel, and the opacities (*black arrow*) are now clearly seen separate from the bowel, proving they are cystic calculi. The outline of the spatula is visible.

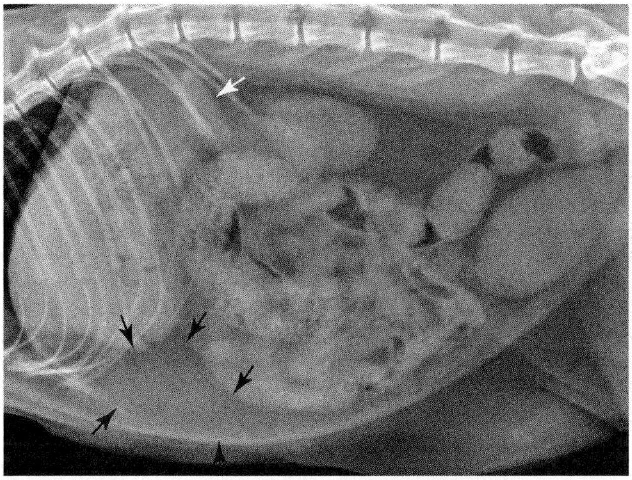

Fig. 38.12 Lateral radiograph of a cat with abundant abdominal fat. The fat provides contrast, and there is excellent discrimination between parenchymal organs. The kidneys, proximal aspect of the spleen (*white arrow*), jejunal segments, and the urinary bladder are all highly conspicuous because of the peritoneal fat. Note the large collection of falciform fat (*black arrows*).

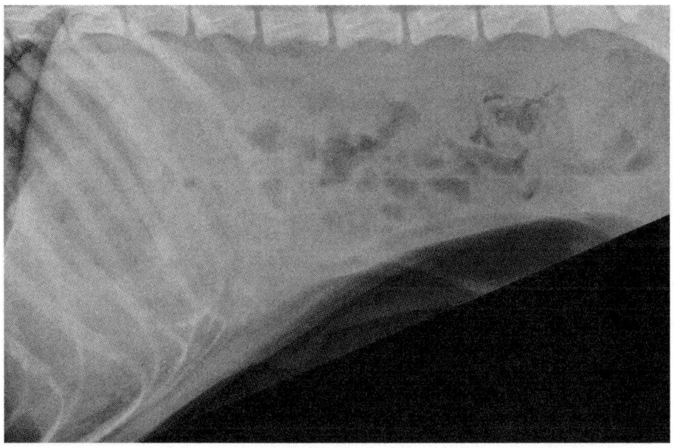

Fig. 38.13 Lateral radiograph of the abdomen of an emaciated dog. The conspicuity of the margin of abdominal organs is poor because of the lack of abdominal fat to provide contrast. With this appearance, radiographic assessment of the abdomen is compromised.

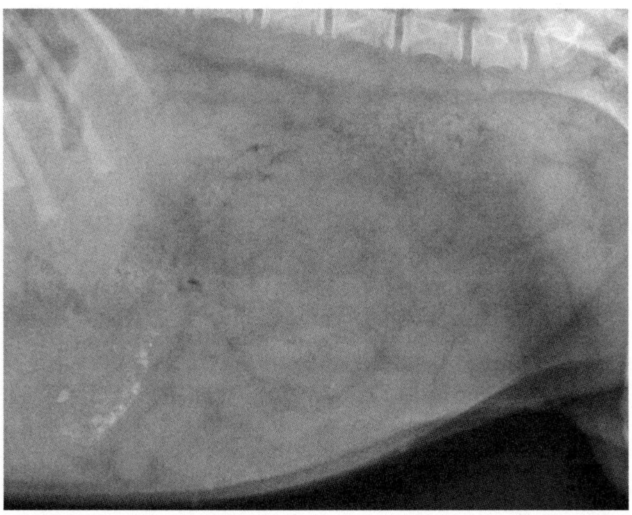

Fig. 38.14 Lateral radiograph of an 11-week-old dog. Intra-abdominal contrast is diminished because of the relative lack of abdominal fat. This is a common finding in young animals. Margin visualization is, however, better than in patients that are undernourished and emaciated (compare with Fig. 38.13).

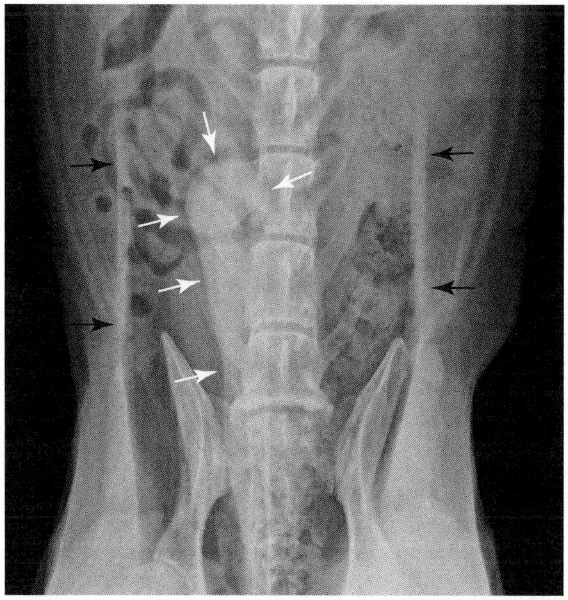

Fig. 38.15 Ventrodorsal (VD) view of the caudal aspect of the abdomen in a male dog. The superimposition opacity created by the prepuce (*white arrows*) can be misinterpreted as a mass. Note also the skin folds created by pulling the pelvic limbs caudally (*black arrows*) rather than having them flexed during radiography.

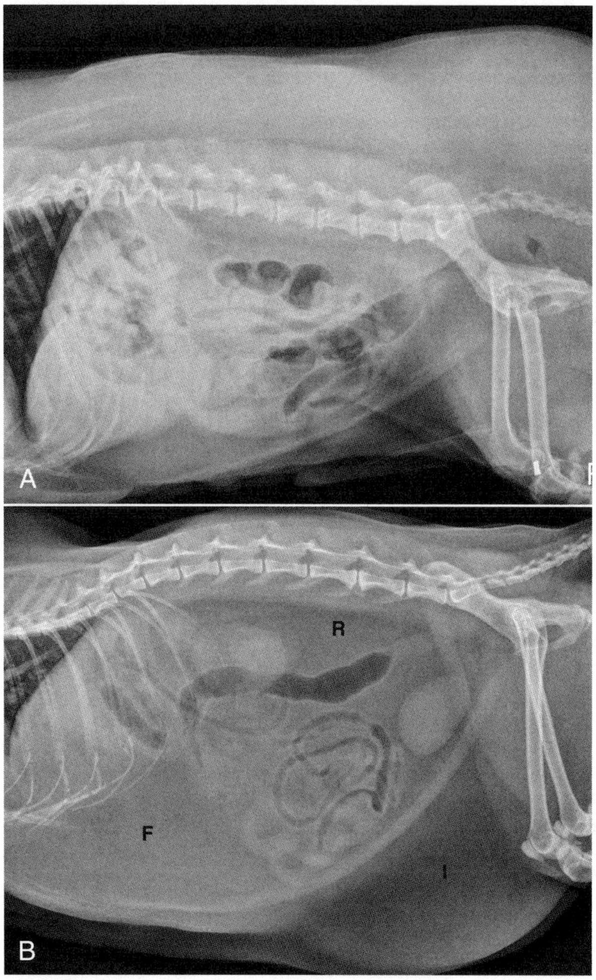

Fig. 38.16 Lateral abdominal radiographs of an overweight dog **(A)** and cat **(B)**. In the dog, there is massive subcutaneous fat accumulation. There is also marked fat deposition in the abdomen but not to the same extent as subcutaneously. In the cat, there is less subcutaneous fat deposition, but massive amounts of fat have accumulated in the abdominal cavity, retroperitoneal space (*R*), falciform region (*F*), and in the inguinal region (*I*).

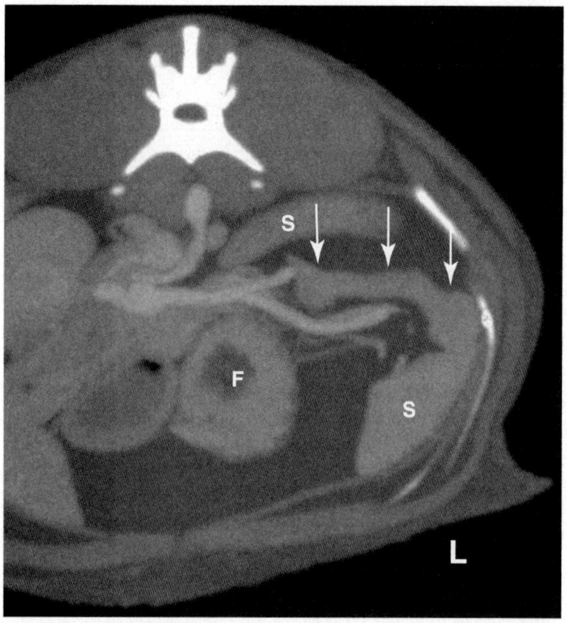

Fig. 37.17 Contrast-enhanced transverse maximum intensity projection (MIP)[a] computed tomography image of the cranial abdomen of a normal cat. The left limb of the pancreas (*white arrows*) is located between the gastric fundus (*F*) and spleen (*S*) and is surrounded by fat, which provides radiographic contrast. The lateral aspect of the left limb of the pancreas often has a nodular appearance. The right limb of the pancreas is not included in this image. The hyperattenuating tubular structures medial to the pancreas are normal splenic veins. *L*, Left. (Reproduced with permission from Thrall DE, Robertson IR. *Atlas of Radiographic Anatomy and Normal Anatomic Variants in the Dog and Cat.* 3rd ed. St. Louis: Elsevier/Saunders; 2023.)

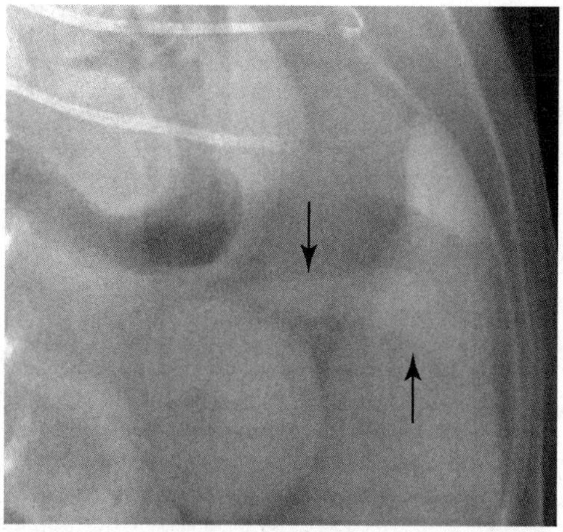

Fig. 38.18 Ventrodorsal radiograph of a 12-year-old domestic cat. The left limb of the normal pancreas is visible medial to the spleen (*black arrows*). The most lateral margin has a mildly lobular appearance. (Reproduced with permission from Thrall DE, Robertson IR. *Atlas of Radiographic Anatomy and Normal Anatomic Variants in the Dog and Cat.* 3rd ed. St. Louis: Elsevier/Saunders; 2023.)

falciform region is often misinterpreted as peritoneal fluid. Using the basic principles of radiographic opacities and the silhouette sign discussed in Chapter 6, this cannot be fluid, or the absolute opacity of the region would be greater, and there would also be silhouetting with the adjacent liver and jejunum.

In the dog, the pancreas is closely associated with the stomach, transverse colon, and descending duodenum, and as a result the normal canine pancreas is never visible radiographically. In the cat, however, the left limb of the pancreas extends lateral to the colon and resides just medial to the spleen and is surrounded by fat (Fig. 38.17). Therefore, the left limb of the pancreas can be evaluated specifically in radiographs (Fig. 38.18), and the adjacent fat can also be assessed for secondary changes as might occur with pancreatitis.

The proximal aspect of the spleen is usually visible in VD radiographs of normal dogs and normal cats, located just caudolateral to the gastric fundus. The distal aspect of the spleen is also commonly visible in dogs (Fig. 38.19A), but rarely in cats (Fig. 38.19B). This relates to the slightly different orientation of the spleen in the abdomen in dogs vs. cats. Visibility of the distal aspect of the spleen in the ventral abdomen in cats does not always mean that the spleen is enlarged, but this should be considered.

A unique feature of the feline stomach compared to the canine stomach is the presence of greater amounts of submucosal fat.[6] As fat is more radiolucent than soft tissue, the presence of fat in the gastric wall in some cats results in linear regions of decreased opacity extending radially from the lumen through the gastric wall when the stomach is empty and contracted (Fig. 38.20). This is a type of normal variation and is only found in a small fraction of cats.

Another unique feature of the feline stomach compared to the canine stomach is the relative position of the pylorus in the abdomen. In the dog, the pylorus is located to the right of midline, approximately midway between the spine and abdominal wall (Fig. 38.21A). In the cat, the pylorus is a more midline structure, being located directly on the midline, or just slightly to the right of the spine (see Fig. 38.21B). This difference is important as medial displacement of the pylorus is a sign of liver enlargement or a liver mass in dogs, whereas a medial location of the pylorus is normal in cats.

There is a marked difference in the morphology of the cecum in the dog vs. cat. In the dog, the cecum is a coiled structure that has a separate communication with the colon (Fig. 38.22). Thus, there are separate cecocolic and ileocolic valves in the dog. In the cat, the cecum is not a separate structure but is more of a small outpouching from the ascending colon and there is no unique cecocolic valve (Fig. 38.23). As a result, the cecum is a reliable landmark in the canine abdomen but not in the cat.

In many obese feline patients, the entire small intestine is lateralized into the right hemiabdomen (Fig. 38.24). It is important to recognize that this appearance is not the result of a pathologic abdominal mass.

ABDOMINAL MASS/MASS EFFECT

The location of an abdominal mass depends on its origin and the effects of gravity. Sometimes, an abdominal mass is suspected but not clearly seen. In this case, the abnormality is commonly described using the term *mass effect*. With a mass effect, displacement of multiple abdominal organs, such as the intestines, can be the only sign of the presence of a mass.

There are two anatomic compartments in the abdomen, the peritoneal and retroperitoneal spaces, and a mass can arise within either. The retroperitoneal space is in the dorsal abdomen; therefore, retroperitoneal masses are dorsal.

[a]An MIP image is a summation of several adjacent CT slices to obtain a volumetric image. The thickness of the volume depends on the number of CT images that are summed, and the thickness of each image.

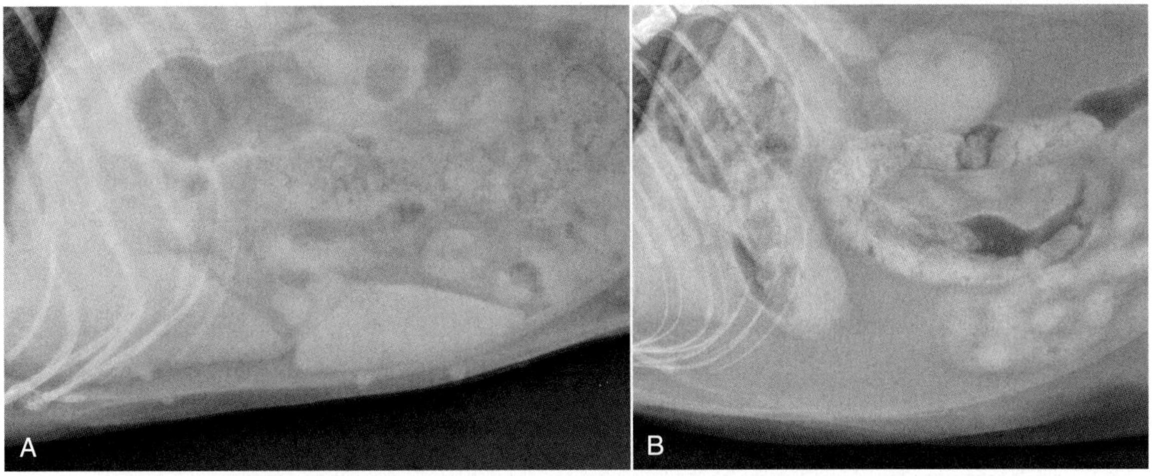

Fig. 38.19 Cranioventral aspect of the abdomen of a dog **(A)** and a cat **(B)**. In canine lateral radiographs, the distal extremity of the spleen is commonly visible, as seen here. In feline lateral radiographs, the distal aspect of the spleen is usually not seen in normal subjects, and is not present in this image.

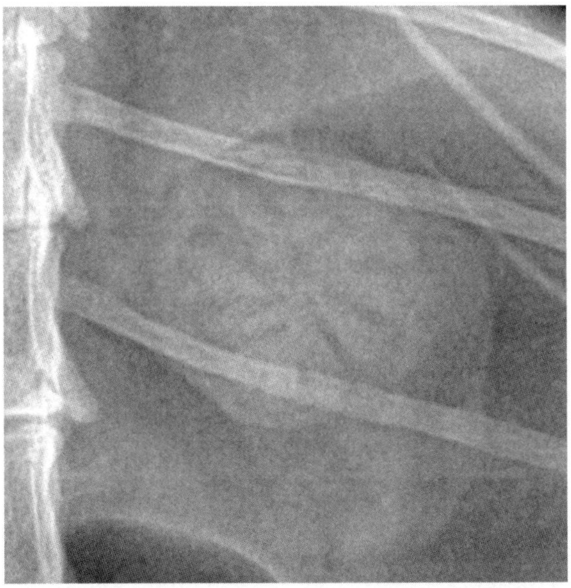

Fig. 38.20 Left cranial aspect of the abdomen of a cat having excessive fat in the gastric wall. The fat creates a striated appearance to the stomach, which is contracted. This is normal variation and is found in only a small fraction of cats.

An abdominal mass often causes displacement of the adjacent abdominal structures and the characteristics of the displacement are useful in estimating the origin of the mass; for example, cranial displacement of urinary bladder due to prostate gland enlargement, ventral displacement of colon due to renal mass, caudal displacement of stomach due to liver mass, to mention just a few (Table 38.1).

Also, the regional location of the mass within the abdomen is important in considering its origin. The origin of a mass is usually estimated in lateral views as superimposition of organs is less than in the VD view. By dividing the lateral view of the abdominal cavity into regions, the most likely origin of a mass can be estimated (Fig. 38.25, Table 38.1).

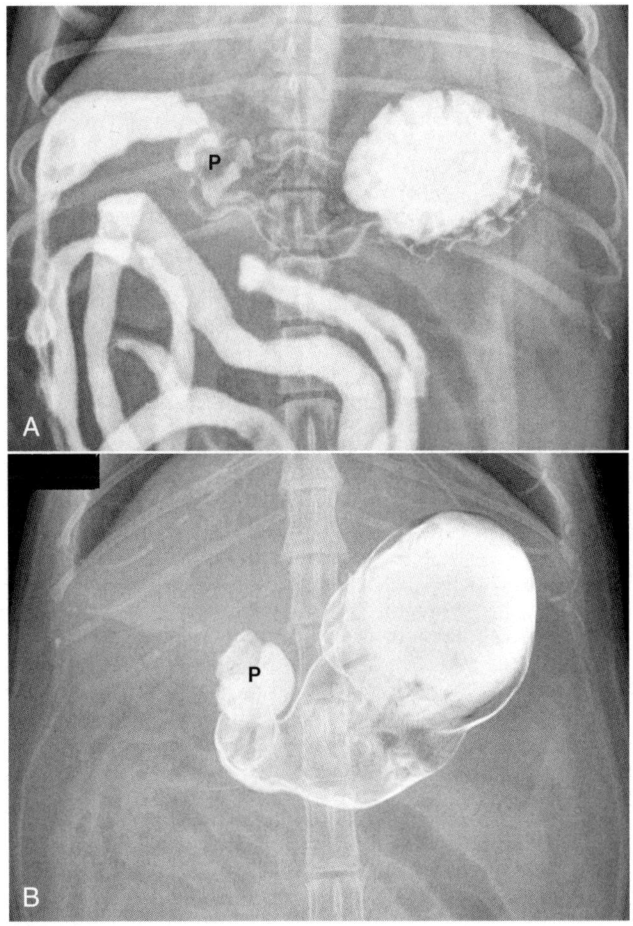

Fig. 38.21 Ventrodorsal radiographs of a 7-year-old Miniature Schnauzer **(A)** and a 12-year-old domestic cat **(B)**. In each animal, barium is present in the stomach. Note the more medial location of the pylorus (*P*) in the cat. The undulations in the pyloric antrum in **A** and **B** are due to normal peristalsis. (Reproduced with permission from Thrall DE, Robertson IR. *Atlas of Radiographic Anatomy and Normal Anatomic Variants in the Dog and Cat*. 3rd ed. St. Louis: Elsevier/Saunders; 2023.)

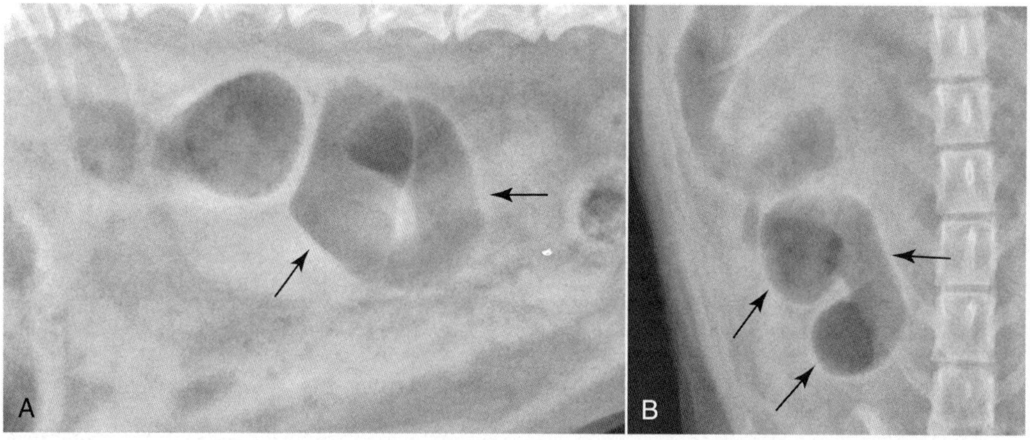

Fig. 38.22 Lateral **(A)** and ventrodorsal **(B)** radiographs of a 4-year-old Yorkshire terrier. The cecum is a gas-filled coiled structure and is visible in the central portion of the right abdomen (*black arrows*). (Reproduced with permission from Thrall DE, Robertson IR. *Atlas of Radiographic Anatomy and Normal Anatomic Variants in the Dog and Cat*. 3rd ed. St. Louis: Elsevier/Saunders; 2023.)

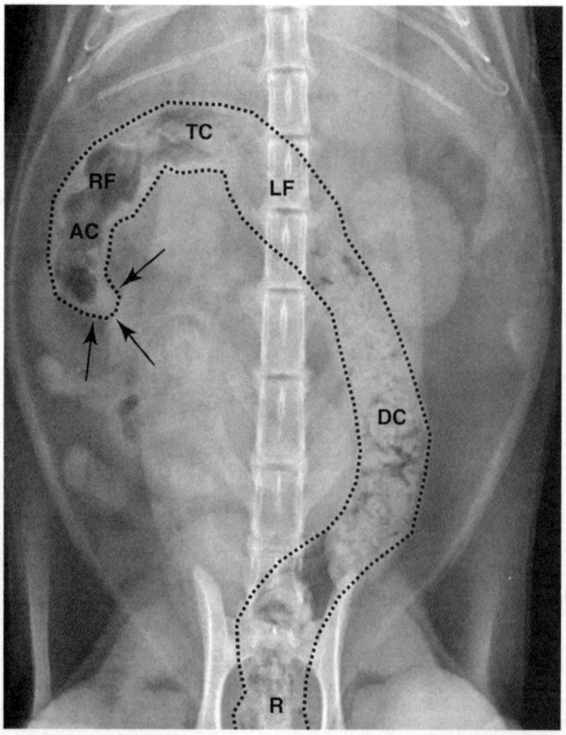

Fig. 38.23 Ventrodorsal radiograph of a 1-year-old domestic cat. The colon is outlined and various regions labeled. The feline cecum is not a distinct structure as it is in the dog, being designated as a proximal outpouching of the ascending colon (*black arrows*). *AC,* Ascending colon; *DC,* descending colon; *LF,* left colic flexure; *R,* rectum; *RF,* right colic flexure; *TC,* transverse colon. (Reproduced with permission from Thrall DE, Robertson IR. *Atlas of Radiographic Anatomy and Normal Anatomic Variants in the Dog and Cat.* 3rd ed. St. Louis: Elsevier/Saunders; 2023.)

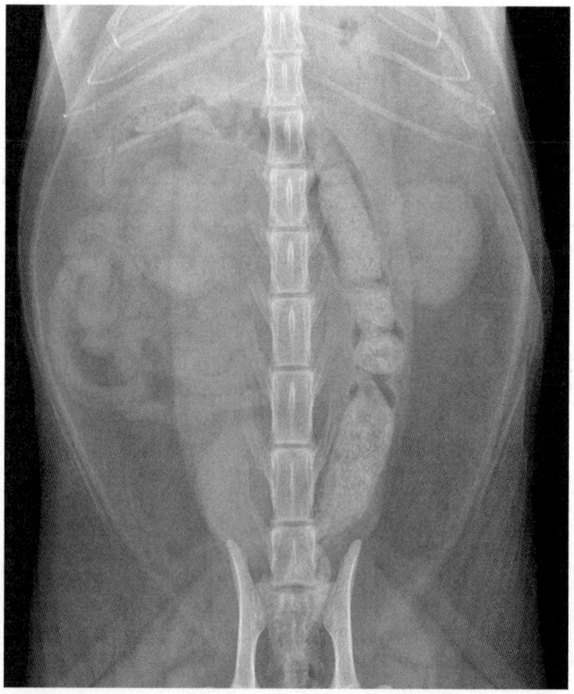

Fig. 38.24 Ventrodorsal radiograph of an overconditioned cat. The entirety of the jejunum is located in the right hemiabdomen. This is a common normal variation in overconditioned cats; there is not a pathologic mass accounting for this.

Table • 38.1

Organ Displacements Occurring as a Result of Various Abdominal Masses.

ORIGIN	COMMON SECONDARY DISPLACEMENTS
Liver	Caudal displacement of the gastric axis
Gallbladder	Caudal displacement of the pyloric antrum
Hepatic lymph nodes	Caudal displacement of the body of the stomach and/or pyloric antrum
Gastric	Often characterized by abnormal shape and gas pattern rather than a mass effect
Spleen	Location of the mass variable depending on location within the spleen
Pancreas	Widening of the gastroduodenal angle, caudal displacement of the transverse colon
Mesenteric lymph nodes	Centrally located within the intestinal convolute, peripheral displacement of intestines
Small intestines	Location varies, typically associated with abnormal gas patterns
Mesenteric mass	Peripheral enteric displacement
Urinary bladder	Naturally variable in size, a mass may be recognized by distorted shape rather than size
Prostate	Cranial displacement of the urinary bladder and dorsal displacement of the rectum
Paraprostatic cysts	May be located cranial to the prostate to intrapelvic
Uterus	Craniodorsal displacement of small intestines, medial displacement of small intestines in the VD projection
Retained testicle	Location can range from the cranial aspect of the bladder to the inguinal canal
Kidneys	Left—ventral displacement of the descending colon Right—ventral displacement of ascending colon and cecum
Adrenal glands	Caudal and lateral displacement of the kidneys if large enough
Retroperitoneal hematoma or urinoma	Diffuse mass effect, may efface contours of kidneys
Ovaries	Can cause ventral displacement of the caudal pole of the ipsilateral kidney
Sublumbar lymph center	Ventral displacement of descending colon and rectum

VD, Ventrodorsal.

Masses in the dorsal abdomen can be either peritoneal (covered on all surfaces by visceral peritoneum) or retroperitoneal (covered only ventrally by visceral peritoneum). Peritoneal masses are usually more mobile than retroperitoneal masses.

INTERPRETATION PARADIGM

Like in all body systems, an organized approach to radiographic interpretation of the abdomen is needed. This begins with an overview of technique, according to the following questions, followed by evaluation for abnormalities.

- Are the radiographic views adequate, and are all of the views needed present?
- Is the positioning adequate?
- Are the images overexposed or underexposed?
- Are the images acquired with an antiscatter grid?
- What is the body habitus of the patient, and how is this going to affect the appearance of the abdomen?
- Were the images acquired with a vertically directed x-ray beam with the cassette in an x-ray table, or was a horizontally directed x-ray beam used with the cassette in a mobile or a wall-mounted cassette holder?
- Are there morphologic aspects of the patient that are going to influence the appearance of the radiographs? These include things such as cutaneous nodules or masses.

After these variables have been considered, the images can be scrutinized for abnormalities. The roentgen sign and DAMNITV (degenerative, anomalous, metabolic, neoplastic, infectious [inflammatory, immune], traumatic, vascular) methods described in Chapter 6 should be used. Inexperienced interpreters often begin by looking at the intestine, because a suspicion of an intestinal obstruction is a common reason that abdominal radiographs are acquired. This is a mistake and will lead to other lesions being overlooked. The search pattern is also important. A random search pattern may be appropriate for experienced radiologists but beginning interpreters should develop an organized approach to searching radiographs.[6,7] Having a mental checklist to guide the order of interpretation will reduce the number of errors (Table 38.2).

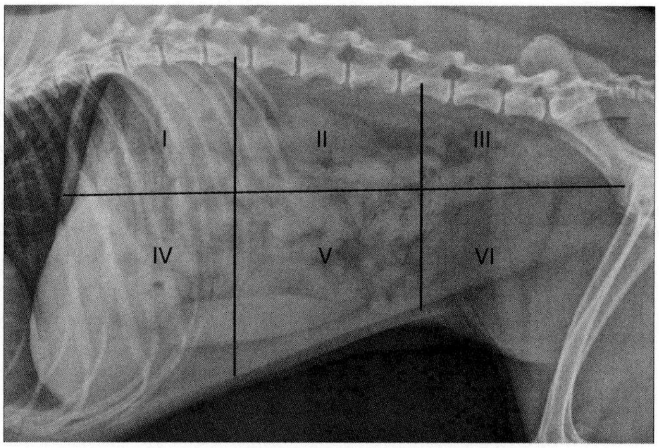

REGION	ORIGIN OF MASS WITHIN REGION
I: Masses in this region can be peritoneal or retroperitoneal	Cranial pole of right kidney Proximal extremity (head) of spleen Gastric fundus Gastric body Adrenal glands Proximal liver
II. Masses in this region are usually retroperitoneal	Caudal pole of right kidney Left kidney Ovaries Ureters Lymph nodes A dorsal jejunal mass will likely migrate ventrally into Zone V
III. Masses in this region can be peritoneal or retroperitoneal	Rectum Descending colon Sublumbar lymph nodes Ureters Cranial extension of pelvic mass
IV. Masses in this region are peritoneal	Ventral liver Pylorus Gallbladder Pancreas Proximal duodenum
V. Masses in this region are peritoneal	Pedunculated liver mass Ventral extremity (tail) of spleen Jejunum Cecum Descending colon Omentum Mesenteric lymph nodes Enlarge uterine horns
VI. Masses in this region are peritoneal	Prostate gland Urinary bladder Uterine body

Fig. 38.25 Schematic showing the abdominal cavity divided into six regions. Organs located in each region, and thus the most likely source of a mass in that region, are as shown in the following table.

Table • 38.2

Checklist for Interpretation of Abdominal Radiographs.

Stomach
Small intestine
Colon
Liver
Spleen
Kidneys/ureters
Prostate gland/uterus
Urinary bladder
Peritoneal space
Retroperitoneal space
Sublumbar lymph nodes
Bones
Penis
Abdominal wall
Included portion of the thorax

REFERENCES

1. Kendall A, Ley C, Egenvall A, et al. Radiographic parameters for diagnosing sand colic in horses. *Acta Vet Scand*. 2008;50(17).
2. Grandage J. The radiological appearance of stomach gas in the dog. *Aust Vet J*. 1974;50(12):529–532.
3. Love N. The appearance of the canine pyloric region in right versus left lateral recumbent radiographs. *Vet Radiol Ultrasound*. 1993;34:169.
4. Vander Hart D, Berry CR. Initial influence of right versus left lateral recumbency on the radiographic finding of duodenal gas on subsequent survey ventrodorsal projections of the canine abdomen. *Vet Radiol Ultrasound.* 2015;56:12–17.
5. Carrig C. The use of compression in abdominal radiography of the dog and cat. *J Am Vet Radiol Society*. 1976;17:178.
6. Heng HG, Wrigley RH, Kraft SL, Powers BE. Fat is responsible for an intramural radiolucent band in the feline stomach wall. *Vet Radiol Ultrasound.* 2005;46:54–56.
7. Halvorsen JG, Swanson D. Interpreting office radiographs. A guide to systematic evaluation. *J Fam Pract*. 1990;31(6): 602–610.

ELECTRONIC RESOURCES

Additional information related to the content in Chapter 38 can be found online at eBooks.Health.Elsevier.com

- Chapter Quiz

CHAPTER 39

Peritoneal Space

Susanne M. Stieger-Vanegas

Peritoneal disease, especially peritonitis, occurs commonly and can be life-threatening, which requires a rapid accurate diagnosis and treatment. Peritoneal disease can be primary or secondary. Imaging examinations are helpful to identify and characterize peritoneal disease. The normal peritoneal folds and ligaments are difficult to identify, regardless of the imaging modality. However, knowledge of the peritoneum and peritoneal folds is important when evaluating the presence or spread of disease processes involving the peritoneum.

NORMAL ANATOMY AND IMAGING PROCEDURES

Anatomy of the Peritoneum

The abdomen is part of the trunk extending from the diaphragm to the pelvic canal. The abdominal and pelvic cavities, in addition to the scrotum in male animals, are lined by the peritoneum. The peritoneal structure is similar to the pleura, and comprises of a single layer of meșothelium on a basement membrane. The peritoneum is a thin, serous membrane, which is divided into parietal, visceral, and connecting layers, which are all continuous.[1–3] The parietal peritoneum covers the inner surface of the abdominal, pelvic, and scrotal cavities and is closely adhered to the abdominal musculature (Fig. 39.1). The visceral peritoneum is a reflection of the parietal peritoneum onto the organs of the abdominal, pelvic, and scrotal cavities, either in whole or in part. Organs in the abdominal cavity covered by visceral peritoneum are considered intraperitoneal. This includes the liver, gallbladder, spleen, pancreas, stomach, small and large intestines, as well as the ovaries in female animals. Most of the rectum in companion animals is in the peritoneal cavity; however, a short caudal segment is retroperitoneal before it ends at the anal canal. In female animals, the cranial aspect of the vagina is covered by peritoneum, which reflects dorsal to the colon and ventral to the urinary bladder.[1] The peritoneal space or peritoneal cavity is the space between the parietal and visceral peritoneal layers, and normally contains only a small amount of fluid for lubrication. Therefore, in strict anatomic terminology, the term *intraperitoneal*, with regard to organs, does not mean within the peritoneal space but is used for organs covered by the visceral peritoneum (see Fig. 39.1). Also, in common usage, the terms *peritoneal cavity* and *abdominal cavity* are often used interchangeably, but this is incorrect because the abdominal cavity includes the intraperitoneal and retroperitoneal organs.

The connecting peritoneum includes mesenteries, omenta, and intra-abdominal ligaments. Understanding the relationship of the connecting peritoneum and especially the ligamentous structures is a crucially important aspect of image interpretation, because it helps to understand the anatomic location and relationship of organs. The liver is attached to the diaphragm craniodorsally at the level of the caudal vena cava via the coronary, triangular, and falciform ligaments. The stomach is fixed to the diaphragm and pylorus through the omentum. Additionally, the stomach and spleen are connected by the gastrosplenic ligament. Furthermore, the descending colon is connected to the spleen and therefore to the stomach. The descending duodenum, pancreas, cecum, and ascending colon are fixed in relationship to each other. Moreover, the proximal aspect of the ascending duodenum is connected to the descending colon by the duodenocolic ligament.[3] The mesenteric root is the site of the attachment of the mesentery to the dorsal abdominal wall, which commonly is located ventral to the second lumbar vertebra. The mesentery is the double layer of the visceral peritoneum suspending the intestines from the parietal peritoneum. The jejunum and ileum are not connected via ligaments to other structures in the abdomen and are therefore relatively mobile in the abdomen.

The space between the dorsal margin of the parietal peritoneum and the abdominal wall is the retroperitoneal space. The retroperitoneal space extends from the diaphragm to the

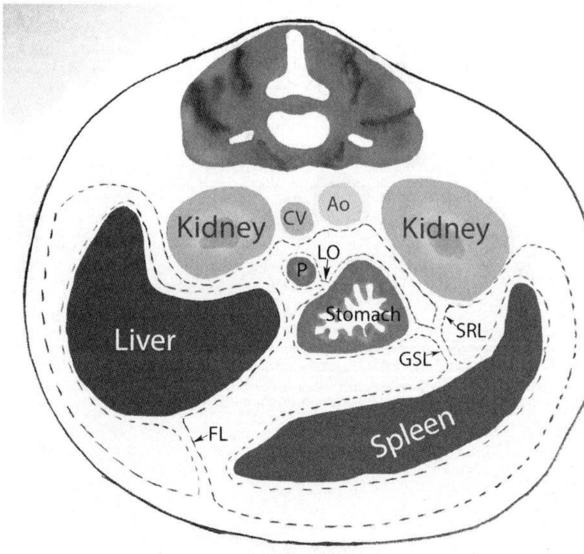

Fig. 39.1 Illustration of the anatomy of the peritoneum. The peritoneum (*dashed line*) lines the abdominal and pelvic cavities. The connecting peritoneum forms intra-abdominal ligaments including the splenorenal ligament (*SRL*), the gastrosplenic ligament (*GSL*), and falciform ligament (*FL*). The lesser omentum (*LO*) connects from the liver and diaphragm to the lesser curvature of the stomach including pylorus (*P*) and proximal aspect of the duodenum. Abdominal organs covered by the peritoneum (visceral) are considered intraperitoneal. The kidneys, aorta (*Ao*), and caudal vena (*CV*) cava are retroperitoneal. The space between parietal and visceral peritoneal layers is the peritoneal space.

anus and is outside the peritoneal cavity. Organs in part covered by visceral peritoneum and near the wall of the abdominal cavity are termed *retroperitoneal*.[4] These organs are usually covered on the ventral aspect by the peritoneum and include adrenal glands, kidneys, ureters, major blood vessels, and regional lymph nodes. Additionally, the ventral aspect of the prostate gland in male dogs is retroperitoneal. The retroperitoneal space communicates cranially with the mediastinum through the aortic hiatus and caudally with the extraperitoneal aspect of the pelvic canal.[5] The peritoneal cavity is completely closed in the male animal; in the female, it connects via the cranial aspect of the uterine horns with the exterior of the body.

Radiography of the Peritoneum

The peritoneum is typically not seen on survey radiographs, but its evaluation is an essential aspect in interpreting abdominal radiographs. It is evaluated indirectly by analyzing anatomic organ relationships and radiographic opacity variations in the abdomen.[3] Identifying the origin of peritoneal disease is based on evaluating the shape, size, location, radiopacity, and margination of organs and the radiopacity throughout the abdominal cavity. In the diseased state, connecting organs can be displaced and altered in shape and radiopacity, which can help in identifying the disease origin and the ranking of differential diagnoses.[3]

Fat is typically present throughout the abdomen, primarily in the falciform ligament, the greater omentum, the mesentery, and the retroperitoneal space. The presence of abdominal fat is important for visceral organ delineation because fat is of lesser radiographic opacity and provides contrast between the organs (Fig. 39.2). The greater omentum, which is located mainly ventral in the abdomen and is very movable, contains variable amounts of fat and therefore contributes to the areas of decreased radiopacity noted ventrally on abdominal radiographs.[3]

The amount and character of intra-abdominal fat depend on the age of the animal and the body habitus. In emaciated patients, the abdomen is often tucked up (see Fig. 39.2C); however, the possibility of coexisting small volumes of peritoneal fluid or peritonitis cannot be excluded. Larger volumes of peritoneal fluid will lead to a distended abdomen. Normal dogs and cats younger than a few months of age (approximately 2–3 months) lack sufficient fat to provide intra-abdominal contrast; thus, the abdomen appears to be of relatively uniform soft tissue opacity (see Fig. 39.2D). Another factor is that young patients have a relatively higher proportion of brown (multilocular) fat than adults. Brown fat has an opacity closer to that of soft tissue because of its higher water content. As young animals mature, the water content of the brown fat decreases.[6] As brown fat is replaced by white fat, the contrast between intra-abdominal soft tissues (organs) increases.

Ultrasound of the Peritoneum

Ultrasound is often the method of choice to evaluate the peritoneum and abdominal cavity, especially when increased peritoneal or retroperitoneal fluid is suspected. However, limited

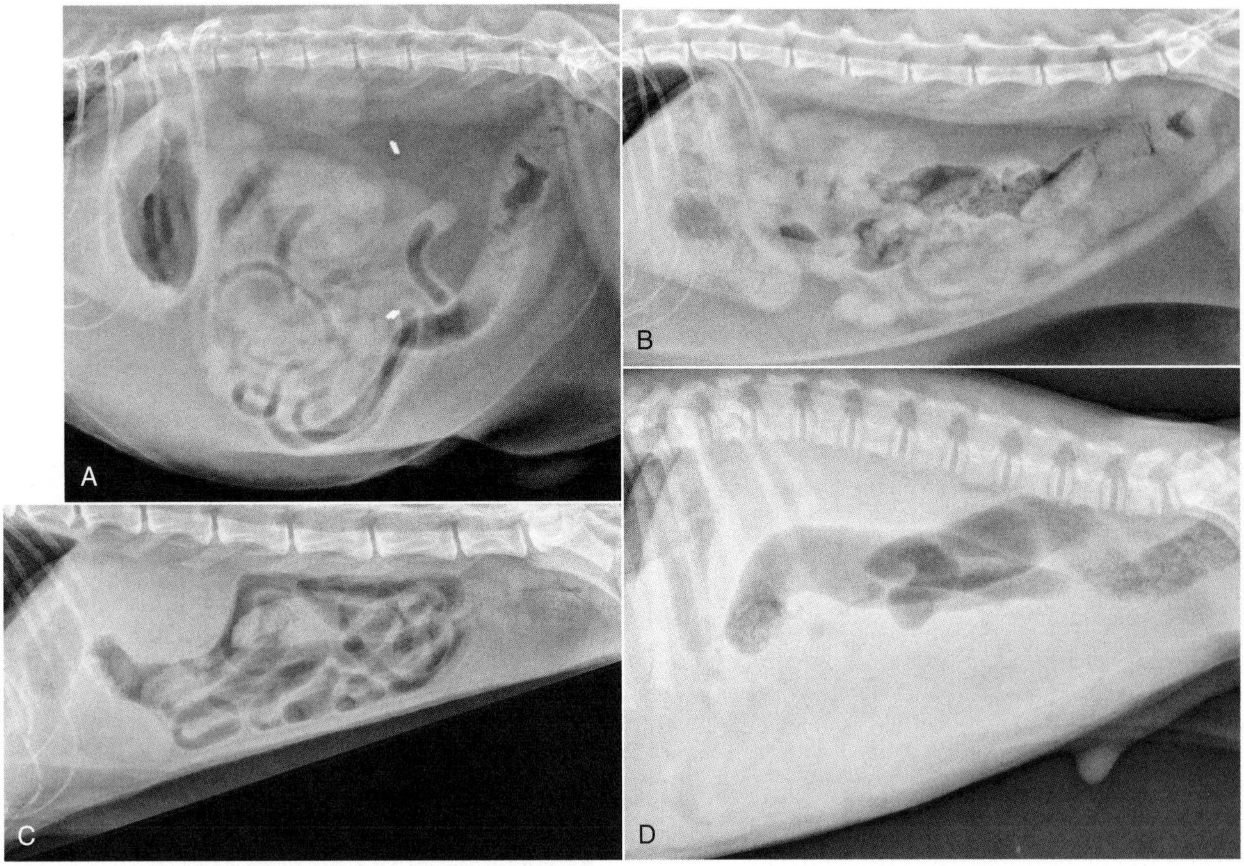

Fig. 39.2 Lateral views of the abdomen illustrating the effect of different amounts of abdominal fat. **A,** Obese cat. Extensive fat depositions in the falciform, omental, mesenteric, and retroperitoneal areas provide contrast between viscera. Metallic objects represent vascular clips from a previous ovariohysterectomy. **B,** Normal cat. Fat deposition is less than that in **A,** but it is adequate to allow visualization of viscera. **C,** Emaciated cat. Without interposed fat, border effacement of viscera is present, producing a uniform, homogeneous abdomen devoid of contrast except for gas in the bowel loops. **D,** Normal 2-month-old Golden retriever. Reduced visualization of abdominal organs and poor contrast are caused by a relative lack of fat in this young dog; this is a normal finding.

information is available regarding the ultrasound evaluation of peritoneal disease in animals, compared to the vast amount of information available regarding sonography of solid organs. In the initial ultrasound examination, an overview of the abdomen is obtained, using a medium- to high-frequency ultrasound probe. For peritoneal disease, greater attention is given to the near field and along the diaphragmatic border to evaluate for the presence of small lesions involving the peritoneum. The normal peritoneum is a smooth, thin, echogenic line in the deepest aspect of the abdominal wall. Usually, the intestinal loops can move smoothly through the abdominal cavity and motion is noted between the intestines and abdominal wall. Not only does ultrasound provide the option to assess the peritoneal surfaces, but if peritoneal disease is present, ultrasound-guided fine-needle aspiration can be performed relatively safely and can help in differentiating between normal, inflammatory, and neoplastic conditions.

Computed Tomography of the Peritoneum

Computed tomography (CT) and especially multidetector CT is suitable for the evaluation of disease of the abdominal cavity and peritoneum.[7] CT is an excellent technique to evaluate the complex anatomy of the peritoneum. Especially, the ability to perform isotropic voxel CT imaging with sagittal and dorsal reformatting provides excellent anatomic information, which is key to the understanding of peritoneal disease. Traditionally, radiography often combined with abdominal ultrasound has been the modality of choice to evaluate for peritoneal disease; however, in recent years, CT has been shown to be valuable for evaluation of the abdomen and peritoneal structures particularly in larger dogs.

PERITONEAL AND RETROPERITONEAL DISEASE

Decreased Abdominal Surface Visualization

Peritoneal Effusion

Fluid in the intraperitoneal space is termed *peritoneal fluid*, and fluid in the retroperitoneal space, *retroperitoneal fluid*. The term *abdominal fluid* should be avoided because it is nonspecific and would include peritoneal and/or retroperitoneal fluid. A small amount of peritoneal fluid is normal in the abdominal cavity of dogs and cats. Effusion is the abnormal or increased accumulation of fluid in any cavity lined by mesothelial cells. The type of fluid varies dependent on the underlying cause and can range from being acellular with low protein content (i.e., transudate) to fluid with an increased cell or protein content or fluid containing abnormal cells or substances (i.e., modified transudate or exudate). No imaging modality can provide a definitive diagnosis about the fluid characteristics, and fluid analysis is highly valuable and necessary to characterize the type of effusion.

Radiographically, increased fluid within the peritoneal cavity or retroperitoneal space causes a loss of the differential opacity interface between soft tissue and fat and therefore a loss of contrast between organs. In animals with intraperitoneal fluid, there is overall more soft tissue opacity in the peritoneal cavity. The presence of peritoneal fat normally allows us to see the serosal margins of organs. When fluid is present between abdominal viscera, this causes border effacement of viscera and results in added overall soft tissue opacity. In practice, all peritoneal fluids are of soft tissue opacity, comparable to the visceral organs. In many instances, the fluid is limited to the peritoneal space, and contrast between the kidneys and adjacent retroperitoneal fat is preserved. Causes for loss of peritoneal contrast include not only the lack of fat and peritoneal effusion, but also peritonitis, and peritoneal neoplasia. A wet hair coat, or hair coated with ultrasound gel, may create the appearance of altered peritoneal space opacity, and this should not be confused with a true loss of peritoneal detail caused by the aforementioned reasons. See Box 39.1 for causes of decreased serosal surface definition.

The idea that any volume of fluid results in complete obliteration of serosal margins on radiographs is incorrect. The degree to which serosal margin detail is obscured by fluid is determined by the relative amounts of fat versus fluid. The more fat that is present, the more fluid is needed to cause complete obliteration of serosal margins. Thus, organ margins may still be visible when free intraperitoneal fluid is present.

A large volume of peritoneal fluid appears as homogeneous soft tissue opacity uniformly distributed throughout the abdominal cavity (Fig. 39.3, eFig. 39.1). A large volume of fluid will also cause abdominal distention with outward protrusion of the contour of the abdominal wall (rounded abdomen) and may displace the diaphragm cranially. The abdomen may also be somewhat pendulous in normal immature patients. If relatively mobile segments of bowel contain gas, they often float to the highest or uppermost area within the abdominal cavity. These segments will be in the central portion of the abdomen on a lateral radiograph made with a vertical x-ray beam. Gas-filled bowel loops in a noncentral location in patients with a large amount of peritoneal fluid suggest the presence of an abdominal mass or adhesions that prevent free movement of intestinal segments (Fig. 39.4). However, this finding should be interpreted with caution, as the presence of a large amount of peritoneal fat may also cause asymmetric bowel location,

Box • 39.1

Differential Diagnoses for Decreased Serosal Surface Visualization

- Lack of intra-abdominal fat
- Young patient (brown fat)
- Peritoneal effusion (transudate, modified transudate, exudate)
- Peritonitis
- Peritoneal neoplasia (primary or metastatic)
- Mass effect caused by crowding of viscera
- Superimposed external material (wet hair, ultrasound gel, etc.)
- Underexposure

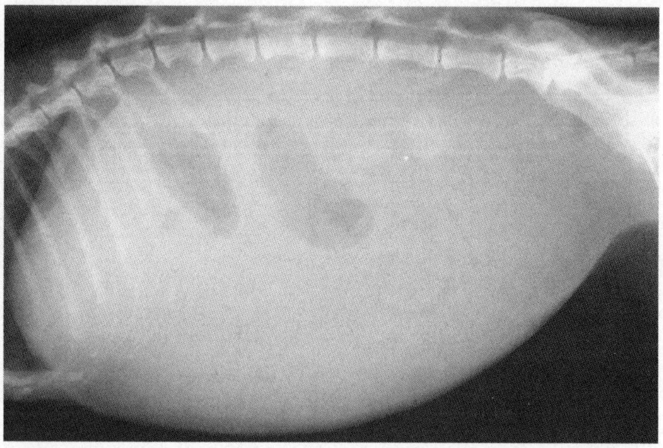

Fig. 39.3 Lateral view of the abdomen of a cat with a large volume of peritoneal fluid. Homogeneous soft tissue opacity is distributed uniformly throughout the distended abdomen, and there is a loss of contrast. No fluid is noted in the retroperitoneal space, but fascial planes and organs in the retroperitoneal space are not visible because of superimposition of the peritoneal fluid.

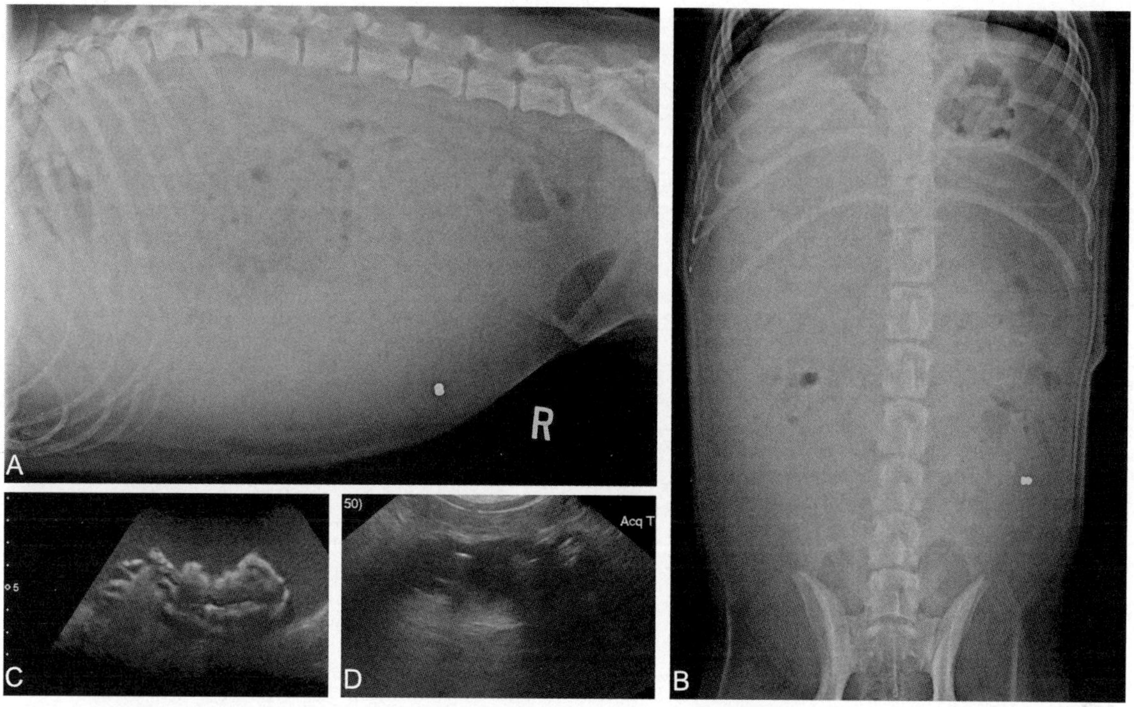

Fig. 39.4 Lateral radiograph **(A)** and ventrodorsal radiograph **(B)** of the abdomen of a 13-month-old Labrador retriever. Peritoneal fluid and gas are present. The peritoneal gas is in an unusual location for bowel gas, ventral to the urinary bladder in the lateral view, and on both views the peritoneal gas bubbles have a nonspherical shape suggesting adhesions. On transverse ultrasound images of the abdomen, multiple segments of jejunum are adhered **(C)**. Extensive echogenic peritoneal fluid is present. **D,** Additionally, peritoneal gas is present in a hypoechoic area adjacent to a segment of jejunum with severely altered wall layering suggestive of intestinal perforation.

especially in cats. Sclerosing encapsulating peritonitis, which is a rare form of chronic peritonitis, may cause soft tissue attenuating material to be asymmetrically positioned in the abdomen obscuring organ visualization and abdominal organs may be abnormally positioned. On ultrasound, large quantities of peritoneal fluid can be seen in addition to small bands of tissue covering organ surfaces.[8] The presence or absence of coexistent peritonitis cannot be ascertained in patients with a large amount of peritoneal fluid and fluid analysis is necessary for further evaluation.

Smaller amounts of peritoneal fluid, peritonitis, or carcinomatosis may produce a mottled, hazy, or irregular loss of contrast on survey radiographs (Fig. 39.5). Individual viscera may be visible, but the margins of soft tissue structures are indistinct or blurred. With small amounts of peritoneal fluid, this appearance can be the result of interdigitation of fluid within folds in the greater omentum and small bowel but without total border effacement.[3] Peritonitis may produce a similar effect. Smaller amounts of peritoneal effusion may be caused by early fluid accumulation of a generalized process or by more localized disease. Localized disease may lead to focally abnormal serosal margin detail with normal serosal margins visible elsewhere in the peritoneal space.

One method of assessing the abdominal cavity for fluid accumulation or peritoneal disease (peritonitis, carcinomatosis, steatitis) is to compare the contrast of the peritoneal versus retroperitoneal spaces. Normally, detail and contrast in the peritoneal and retroperitoneal spaces should be the same. However, because many diseases resulting in peritoneal fluid do not affect the retroperitoneal space, retroperitoneal detail is often preserved when peritoneal fluid has altered the serosal margin of bowel and other intraperitoneal organs (Fig. 39.6). It is important to remember, however, that a large volume of peritoneal fluid can obscure the retroperitoneal space because of superimposition. Loss of contrast and detail can also occur specifically in the retroperitoneal space, and is an indication of fluid or, less commonly, inflammation (Fig. 39.7).

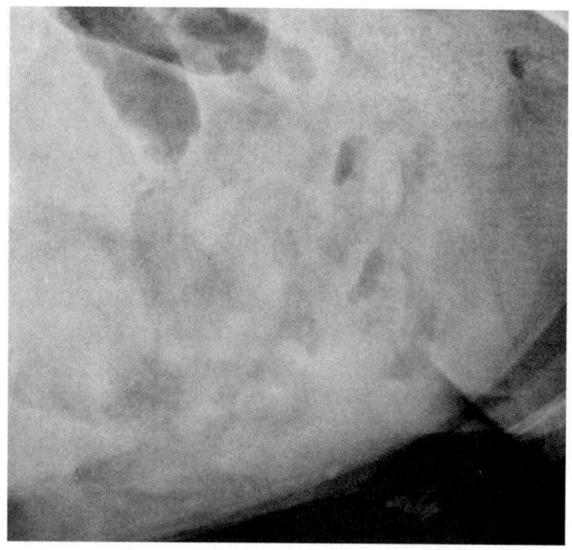

Fig. 39.5 Lateral radiograph of the midabdomen of a dog with peritoneal fluid. There is a mottled, hazy, irregular fluid opacity in the abdomen leading to blurring of the margins of soft tissue structures and a loss of contrast. This radiographic appearance could be caused by the presence of an exudate or hemorrhage; but in this dog, it was caused by hypoproteinemia.

Peritoneal fluid absorption is dependent on the properties of the fluid, as well as the peritoneal membrane.[9] Manipulation of viscera during laparotomy produces changes that may appear similar radiographically to peritonitis, and these changes may be modified by the amount of tissue trauma.[3] Solutions containing water, electrolytes, and relatively low-molecular-weight

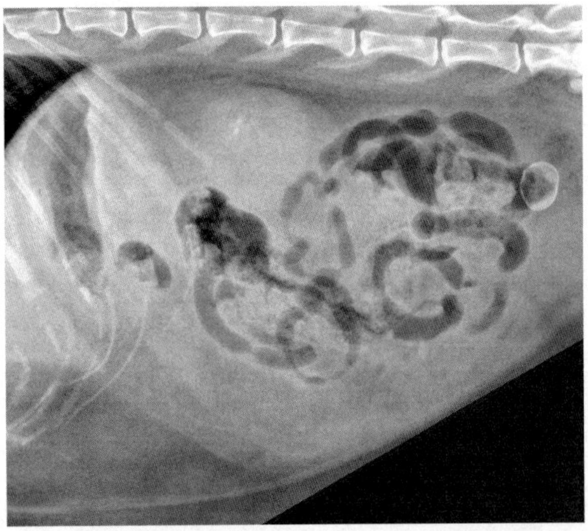

Fig. 39.6 Lateral view of the abdomen of a cat with peritoneal fluid. Serosal contrast in the peritoneal space is markedly reduced, but there is good contrast with visualization of fascial planes and fat in the retroperitoneal space. The falciform fat in the cranioventral aspect of the abdomen, which is extraperitoneal, is also normal. Comparison of the appearance of the fat in the peritoneal versus retroperitoneal spaces can assist in the radiographic detection of either retroperitoneal or peritoneal disease. There is also renal mineralization and a large calcified peritoneal body.

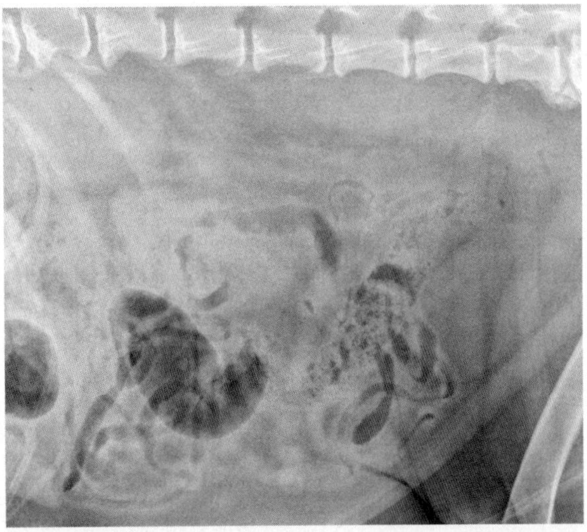

Fig. 39.7 Lateral view of the abdomen of a dog with rodenticide toxicity. There is fluid opacity in the retroperitoneal space with blurring of the margin of the lumbar musculature and a streaky appearance to the retroperitoneal fat. Note the normal sharp serosal margin detail and contrast in the peritoneal space.

components are absorbed normally by the peritoneal membrane within 24 hours. Proteinaceous fluids (such as serum, blood, and lymph) are absorbed more slowly and may be present for 1 to 2 weeks. These changes can be visible radiographically after laparotomy and should not be mistaken for complications. Static or increasing fluid accumulation in the postoperative period is abnormal. If complications are suspected, cytologic evaluation of the fluid will be necessary to differentiate between normal postsurgical fluid and fluid caused by septic peritonitis or other conditions.

Small amounts of intraperitoneal fluid may not be detected using radiography but are detected readily using ultrasound. Ultrasound guidance can be used to collect fluid samples. Using

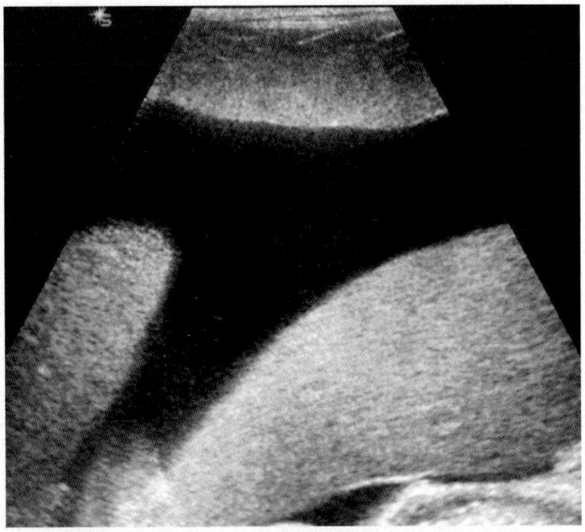

Fig. 39.8 Longitudinal ultrasound image of a dog with ascites. Anechoic fluid is present between and surrounding liver lobes. The lack of echoes in the fluid is consistent with the fluid being of low cellular content.

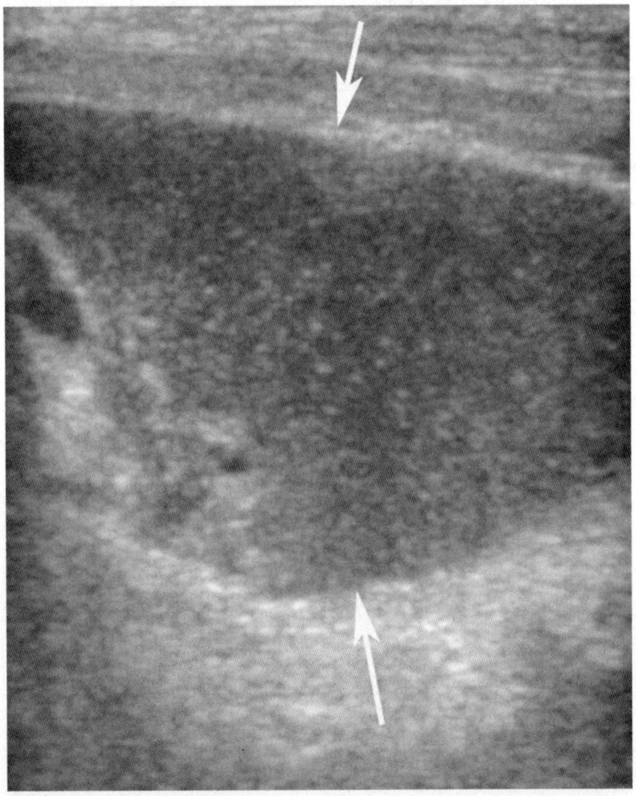

Fig. 39.9 Longitudinal ultrasound image of a 6-year-old dog with an abdominal mass and peritoneal effusion. Free peritoneal fluid (*white arrows*) with low-level echoes is compatible with highly cellular fluid.

focused assessment of the abdomen with sonography for trauma (FAST) in nontraumatized patients, it was determined that unstable patients had a higher likelihood of peritoneal fluid than stable patients.[10] Fluid can also be characterized by its echogenicity. Fluid with low cellular content, such as urine or a transudate, is anechoic (Fig. 39.8); fluid with moderate to high cellular content, such as exudate, blood, and chyle, is more echoic (Fig. 39.9; see Fig. 39.4C,D).

Peritoneal Metastasis and Steatitis

An ill-defined nodular, miliary, or granular pattern to the abdomen (Fig. 39.10, eFig. 39.2) may be caused by seeding of the peritoneum with multiple, metastatic foci, or steatitis. Examples of tumors associated with metastatic spread include hemangiosarcoma of the spleen and carcinoma of various abdominal organs. The term *carcinomatosis* in strict terms should only be used for epithelial cancers or carcinomas disseminated throughout the body. In the past, or in colloquial terms, the term *carcinomatosis* has been used to describe the spread of any cancer; however, that is not correct. Carcinoma of the liver, pancreas, and intestinal tract commonly has peritoneal metastatic seeding in dogs and cats. In cats, parietal and visceral peritoneal masses have been described with carcinomatosis, but not with other diseases, and might therefore be a strong indicator for neoplastic disease.[11] Small miliary peritoneal masses might not be seen on radiographs and can easily be missed on ultrasound (Figs. 39.11 and 39.12).

Steatitis is the inflammation of fat, commonly yellow fat, causing saponification and fat necrosis. Steatitis commonly occurs secondary to an inflammatory process (e.g., pancreas or gastrointestinal tract), abdominal neoplasia,[12] or trauma[13] or can be idiopathic.[14] Steatitis caused by pancreatitis or pancreatic neoplasia in dogs and cats can result from the escape of proteolytic enzymes causing saponification of omental and mesenteric fat.[15] Additionally, in cats, steatitis can result from vitamin E deficiency and/or an excessive amount of polyunsaturated fatty acids in their diet. Rarely steatitis is a result of

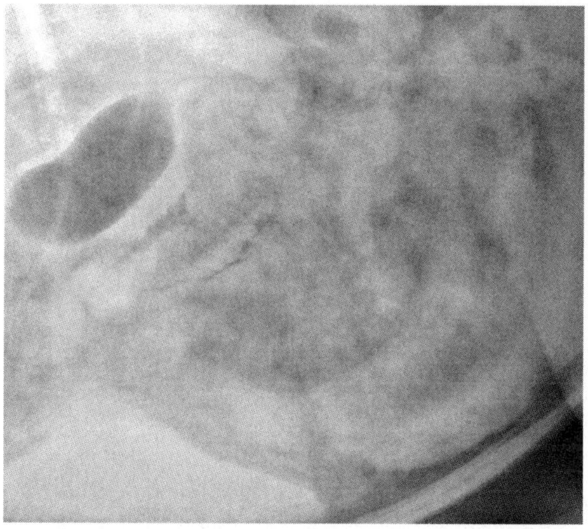

Fig. 39.10 Close-up of the cranioventral aspect of the abdomen of a dog with a ruptured splenic hemangiosarcoma leading to peritoneal metastasis. The mesenteric fat has a mottled appearance.

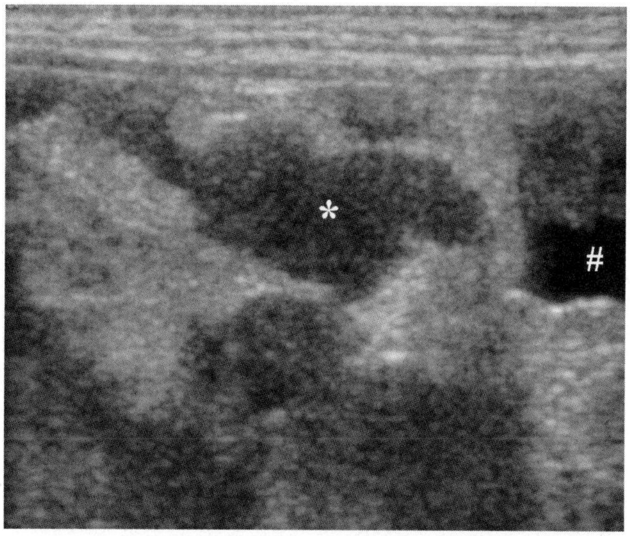

Fig. 39.12 Longitudinal ultrasound image of a 9-year-old dog with peritoneal metastasis, which is hypoechoic, irregularly shaped material (*asterisk*) interspersed through the more echogenic mesenteric fat. A small amount of anechoic peritoneal fluid is present on the right edge of the image (*number sign*).

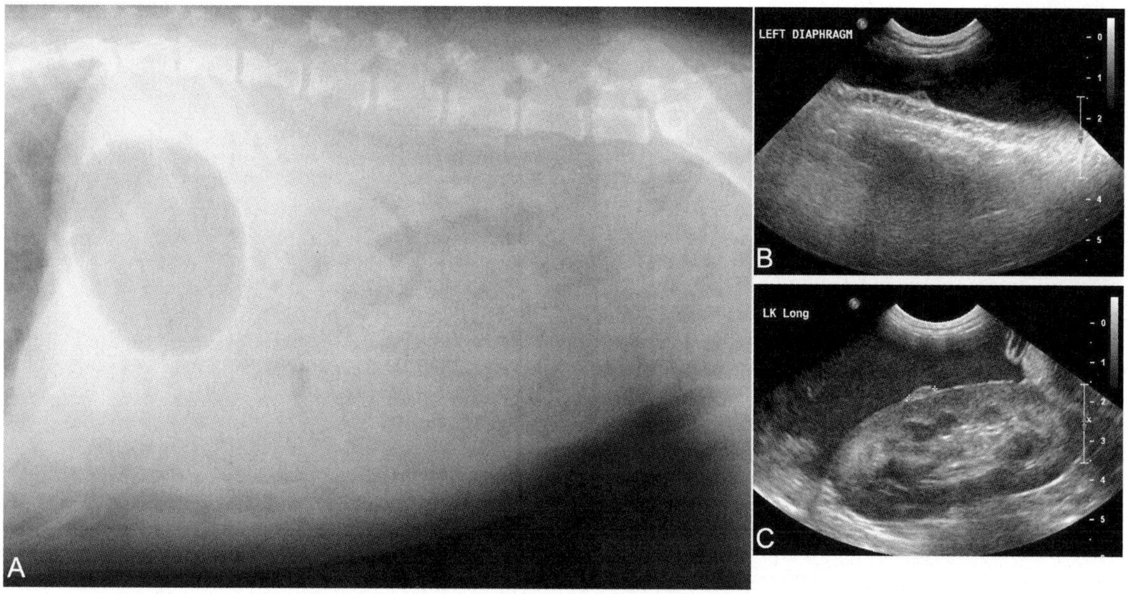

Fig. 39.11 **A,** Lateral radiograph of a dog with peritoneal fluid and lack of definition of the ventral aspect of the liver with the spleen. The gastric axis is in normal position, suggesting that the liver is of normal size. On ultrasound, a splenic tumor with rupture and echogenic peritoneal fluid, as well as multiple, small, round to ovoid, hypoechoic nodules along the peritoneal surface **(B, C)** were noted. On image **C,** no fluid is present in the retroperitoneal space, which is consistent with the lateral radiograph and the good definition of the fascial planes in the retroperitoneal area. Fine-needle aspiration confirmed peritoneal metastatic disease secondary to splenic hemangiosarcoma.

severe hypocalcemia.[16] Sonographically, hyperechoic masses, which are not part of an organ might be noted in the abdominal cavity.

Peritoneal Masses

Primary de novo peritoneal neoplasia is uncommon in companion animals. Primary peritoneal neoplasia includes mesothelioma, leiomyoma, or carcinoma where the primary origin is not identified. Other differentials for peritoneal masses include cyst, hematoma, abscess, and granuloma. In the northwestern portion of the United States and Canada, as well as portions of Europe, peritoneal infection by *Mesocestoides* species tapeworms may manifest as varying-sized, cavitary, septated structures with echogenic particles within the fluid.[17] Peritoneal masses can be solid or cavitary, and samples can be obtained for cytologic evaluation. Ultrasound sampling yielded diagnostic information in about 70% of small animal patients with peritoneal, mesenteric, and omental disease in one study. However, ultrasound criteria alone are not reliable in differentiating neoplastic from inflammatory peritoneal disease, nor for exclusion of peritoneal disease in every patient.

Retroperitoneal Fluid

Fluid in the retroperitoneal space can lead to alternating fat and soft tissue opacities, or streaking, as the fluid dissects between fascial planes in the retroperitoneal area. The most common causes of isolated retroperitoneal fluid are hemorrhage (Fig. 39.13, eFig. 39.3), as with rodenticide toxicity, trauma or neoplasia (adrenal mass, hemangiosarcoma), and urine leakage. Retroperitoneal inflammation with increased fluid can also result from a migrating grass awn, a penetrating wound, ligatures from ovariohysterectomy, and perforation of the urethra during catheterization.

Retroperitoneal Masses

Neoplastic and inflammatory masses can occur in the retroperitoneal space, and radiographically, a soft tissue mass effect may be noted. Retroperitoneal disease can result in decreased delineation of the kidneys and retroperitoneal fat. Ultrasound is often helpful for further evaluating the retroperitoneal space; however, when complex disease affecting the retroperitoneal space is suspected, contrast-enhanced CT with reformatted images in various planes likely provides the most accurate information.

Lipoma is the most common primary tumor occurring in the retroperitoneal space and is usually noted as a fat attenuating area on radiographs or CT images. Nonparenchymal hemangiosarcoma may also occur in the retroperitoneal space. Some metastatic tumors can involve the retroperitoneal space, including lymphosarcoma and neoplasia originating from the kidneys, ureters, prostate gland, anal sacs, perineum, and mammary glands. Nonneoplastic masses most commonly occur secondary to migrating foreign bodies or trauma.

Increased Abdominal Surface Visualization

Peritoneal Gas (Pneumoperitoneum)

Pneumoperitoneum is free gas or air in the peritoneal cavity. The two most common causes of pneumoperitoneum in companion animals are penetration of the abdominal wall, either during surgery or by penetrating wounds, and disruption of the wall of a hollow viscus, which most commonly involves the gastrointestinal tract.[18] It is important to realize that not all intestinal perforations lead to free peritoneal gas; in some instances, adhesions between the omentum and intestines form and seal the defect, thereby resulting in only a small volume of intestinal content leaking into the peritoneal space. After laparotomy, a moderate amount of gas may persist for days to weeks. The duration of surgically induced pneumoperitoneum depends on the amount of gas present, as well as the size and body condition of the patient. Larger quantities of gas take longer to resolve than smaller quantities. After injection of air into the peritoneal cavity, a pneumoperitoneum was noted for up to 25 days in dogs.[19] Penetrating abdominal wounds are usually diagnosed by physical findings. In patients with a penetrating wound, differentiating whether free peritoneal gas is caused solely by penetration of the abdomen or is the result of concurrent organ rupture is impossible from radiographs. However, if the penetrating wound is very small and large

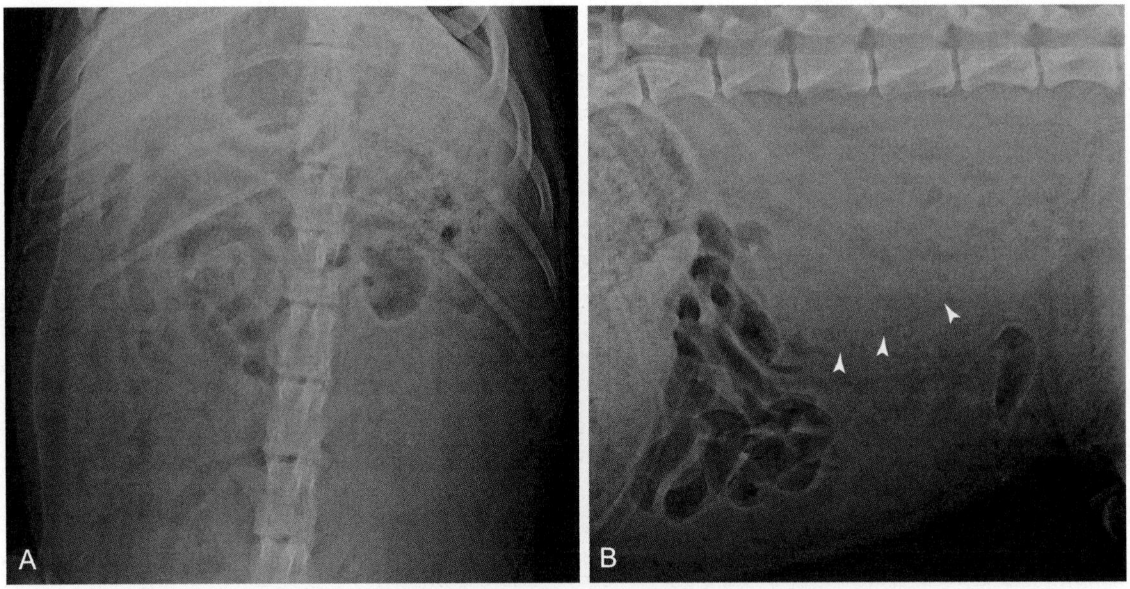

Fig. 39.13 **A,** Ventrodorsal survey radiograph of a dog with retroperitoneal hemorrhage post vehicular trauma. An area of increased soft tissue attenuation is noted in the location of the left kidney. The left kidney cannot be defined. This was caused by retroperitoneal hemorrhage due to partial rupture of the cortex of the left kidney. The ureters were intact. **B,** Lateral radiograph. A diffuse soft tissue attenuating, streaky area is noted in the retroperitoneal space (*arrowheads*), ventrally displacing the descending colon. The peritoneal serosal detail is normal.

amounts of free peritoneal gas are present, a perforation of a hollow organ secondary to injury should be highly suspected. If subcutaneous emphysema is superimposed over the abdominal cavity (such as, caused by trauma), it may be difficult to discern whether there is concurrent peritoneal gas or not.

Radiography is currently the most common technique to evaluate for the presence of free peritoneal gas. A small volume of free peritoneal gas can be difficult to recognize on conventional radiographs made with a vertically directed x-ray beam, because the gas bubbles are small and irregular in shape and may be misinterpreted as bowel gas unless they reside in a region where bowel is not found normally (Fig. 39.14, eFig. 39.4).[3] Larger gas volumes may coalesce into a larger bubble. This larger bubble may still be difficult to recognize on a radiograph made with a vertical x-ray beam, because it is superimposed over other viscera. In addition, this larger bubble may simulate a gas-containing organ, such as the stomach. Free peritoneal gas usually floats to the highest point within the abdomen. In lateral recumbency, this is usually under the caudal aspect of the ribs or in the midabdomen. The concurrent presence of peritoneal effusion may make recognition of the gas bubble easier because the fluid provides more uniform, homogeneous soft tissue background opacity (Fig. 39.15A). However, if a combination of a small volume of peritoneal gas and fluid is present, the attenuation of gas might be higher than expected as it is summating with fluid and may look more similar to peritoneal fat and might therefore be missed. Occasionally, the amount of gas will be large enough to outline serosal surfaces of viscera, such as bowel loops, the stomach, and the diaphragm (see Fig. 39.15B).

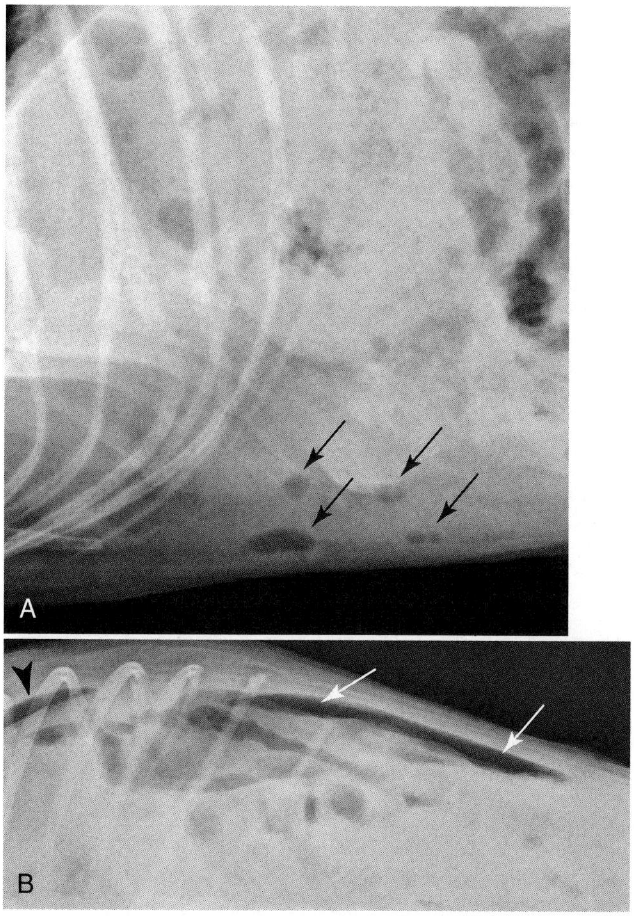

Fig. 39.14 **A,** Lateral radiograph of the cranioventral aspect of the abdomen of a dog with a ruptured bowel that has led to pneumoperitoneum. Extraluminal gas in this patient appears as small gas bubbles in a location not expected for bowel (*black arrows*). The location of this gas is a good indicator that it is extraluminal. Had these gas collections been in the mid aspect of the abdomen, they might not have been recognized as abnormal. **B,** Horizontal-beam abdominal radiograph of the same dog as in **A**. The dog was placed in left lateral recumbency and a horizontally directed x-ray beam was used to make the radiograph. The free gas has collected beneath the right abdominal wall (*white arrows*). The more cranially located gas is in the lung (*black arrowhead*). There is more free peritoneal gas than would be estimated from the conventional lateral projection in part **A**.

Because free gas rises to the highest point within the abdomen, it may be isolated visually from superimposed structures by a horizontally directed x-ray beam. With a small volume of gas, putting the patient in position for 10 minutes before radiographic exposure may be helpful to allow most of the gas to migrate and coalesce at the uppermost portion of the abdomen. The most sensitive projection for detecting a small volume of peritoneal gas is a lateral view, made with a horizontally directed x-ray beam with the patient in dorsal recumbency and with the cranial portion of the abdomen elevated slightly so small amounts of gas accumulate between the liver, diaphragm, and ventral aspect of the abdominal wall (Fig. 39.16).[20] Another projection used for documenting free peritoneal gas is a ventrodorsal (VD) view obtained with the patient in left recumbency with the use of a horizontally directed x-ray beam. Gas will usually collect under the highest portion of the right abdominal wall (see Fig. 39.14B), which is usually under the caudal aspect of the ribs. Raising or lowering either end of the animal shifts the point of gas accumulation. With film radiography, exposure factors should be lowered to intentionally underexpose the abdomen, making the gas more conspicuous. With digital images, the brightness should be increased to address the same goal. A horizontal-beam view with the animal in right recumbency is not recommended, because the gas bubble rises to the left side and gas within the fundus of the stomach may be misinterpreted as free peritoneal gas.

Horizontal-beam radiography is a useful tool for diagnosing free peritoneal gas quickly, cheaply, and with confidence; however, making radiographs with a horizontally directed x-ray beam can be technically challenging if the unit does not allow manipulation of the x-ray tube head or the imaging plate is fixed in position. The ease of performing horizontal-beam radiography should be one factor considered when purchasing a new x-ray system.

Ultrasound is a sensitive method for detection of free peritoneal gas but is dependent on the experience of the operator.[21] Additionally, it may allow the cause of pneumoperitoneum to be identified (see Fig. 39.4D). Reverberation artifacts, or dirty shadowing, are commonly noted at the soft tissue to air interface, which typically results in a high-amplitude linear echo with distal shadowing (enhanced peritoneal stripe sign/increased echogenicity of peritoneal stripe) originating at nondependent portion of the peritoneal lining (Fig. 39.17).[22] Small volumes of free peritoneal gas can also be seen as reverberation artifacts between abdominal structures, including the mesentery and omentum. Small volumes of gas may not interfere with sonographic evaluation, but large volumes of gas hinder complete evaluation of the peritoneal space. In dogs, as little as 0.4 mL air in the peritoneal space could be detected using ultrasound.[23] Additionally, movement of the free air can be noted when shifting the position of the patient.

Gas bubbles within peritoneal fluid are a strong indication for gastrointestinal perforation, especially when no prior peritoneal fluid sampling was performed.[24] As would be expected, pneumoperitoneum in conjunction with gastric dilatation or volvulus is predictive for gastric necrosis. Prior percutaneous trocarization can confound the situation by leading to pneumoperitoneum and/or pneumatosis mimicking gastric necrosis.[25]

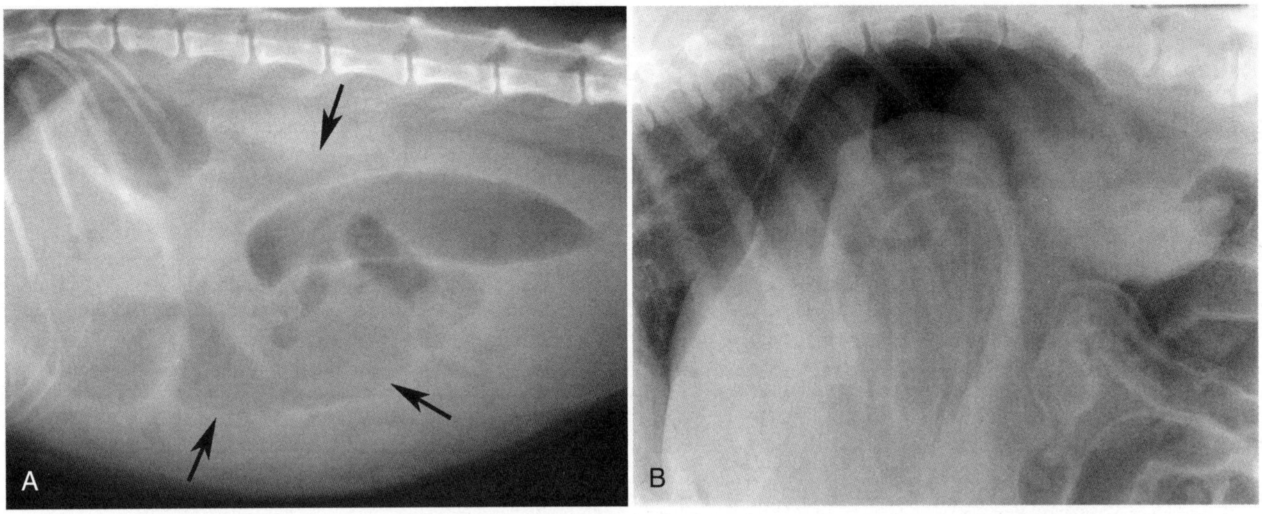

Fig. 39.15 A, Lateral survey radiograph of a cat with peritoneal effusion and a large amount of free peritoneal gas with margins of the gas pocket indicated by *black arrows*. B, Lateral survey radiograph of the abdomen of a dog immediately after laparotomy. A large volume of free peritoneal gas outlines the caudal surface of the right crus of the diaphragm, the cranial pole of the right kidney, the caudal surface of part of the liver, and the serosal surfaces of some bowel loops.

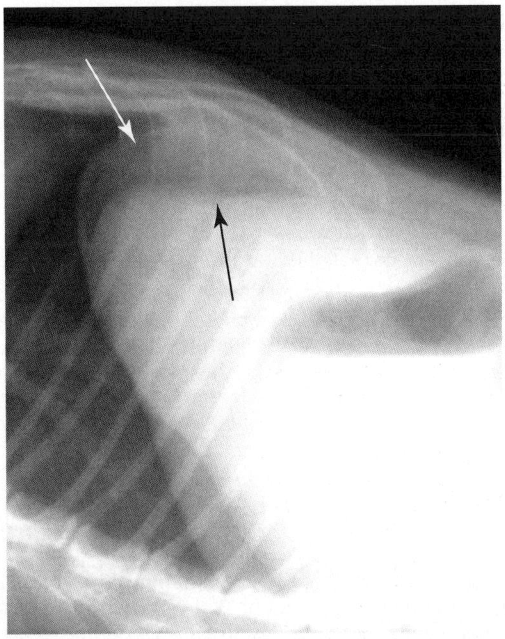

Fig. 39.16 Lateral view of the abdomen made with the patient in dorsal recumbency with the cranial abdomen slightly elevated, and the use of a horizontally directed x-ray beam. Free peritoneal gas has accumulated between the diaphragm (*white arrow*), the liver (*black arrow*), and the ventral abdominal wall. The diagnosis was ruptured stomach.

Retroperitoneal Gas (Pneumoretroperitoneum)

The term *pneumoretroperitoneum* indicates the presence of gas within the retroperitoneal space. Retroperitoneal gas is uncommon and can be caused by a perforation injury or migrating foreign body or surgical access to the retroperitoneal space, including secondary to laparoscopy or secondary to spinal surgery, perforation, or rupture of a hollow viscus, such as the rectum or the vagina in female animals. Furthermore, retroperitoneal gas can occur as a result of extension of a pneumomediastinum (see Chapter 33). Retroperitoneal gas is confined to the retroperitoneal space in the dorsal abdomen and is best seen on a lateral radiograph (Fig. 39.18).

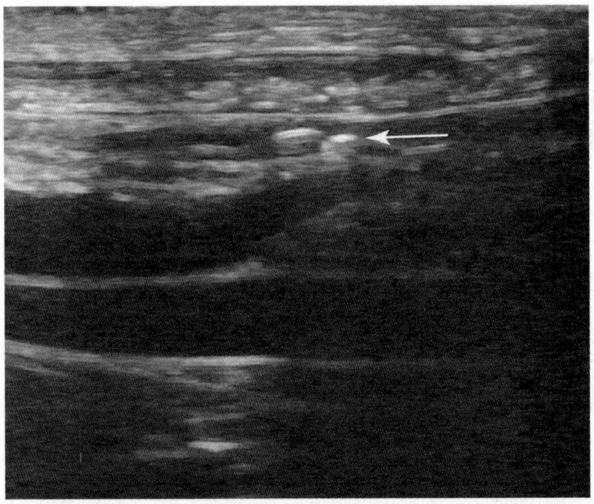

Fig. 39.17 Abdominal sonogram of a dog with a small amount of peritoneal gas. Even small gas collections create strong reflective artifacts (*white arrow*).

Intra-Abdominal Mineral Opacity

Increased mineral opacity not associated with the gastrointestinal tract is relatively uncommon in companion animals. Focal calcified bodies, usually with an opaque periphery, may be found in the peritoneal space (Fig. 39.19, eFig. 39.5; see Fig. 39.6). These are thought to be the result of dystrophic calcification of necrotic mesenteric fat and are not considered clinically significant.[26] Although not common, they are seen more often in cats than dogs. These have been referred to as *Bates bodies*.[27]

Calcification of soft tissue is divided into a metastatic and dystrophic type, and both have a wide range of causes. Metastatic calcification occurs secondary to the deposition of calcium salts in previously normal tissue secondary to abnormal calcium and phosphorus metabolism, primarily in animals with chronic renal disease,[26] hyperparathyroidism, vitamin D and possibly vitamin A intoxication, hypothyroidism, or due to paraneoplastic hypercalcemia. Metastatic calcification can occur anywhere but often involves the blood vessels, kidneys, and gastric mucosa (Fig. 39.20). It is important to remember

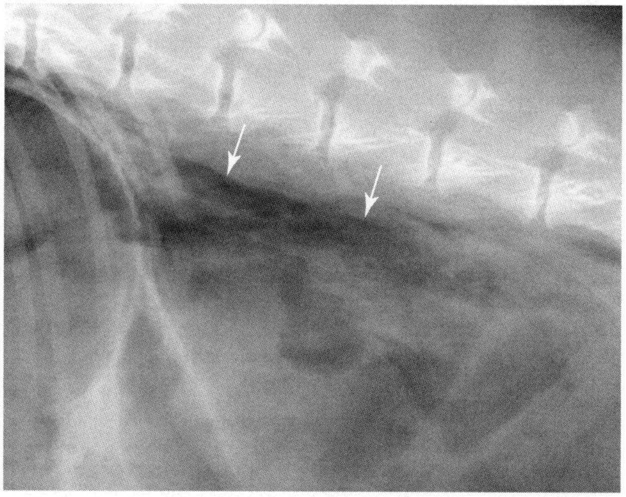

Fig. 39.18 Lateral view of a dog with pneumomediastinum. The pneumomediastinum is not visible in this image. Some of the mediastinal gas dissected along the fascial planes through the aortic hiatus into the retroperitoneal space (*white arrows*).

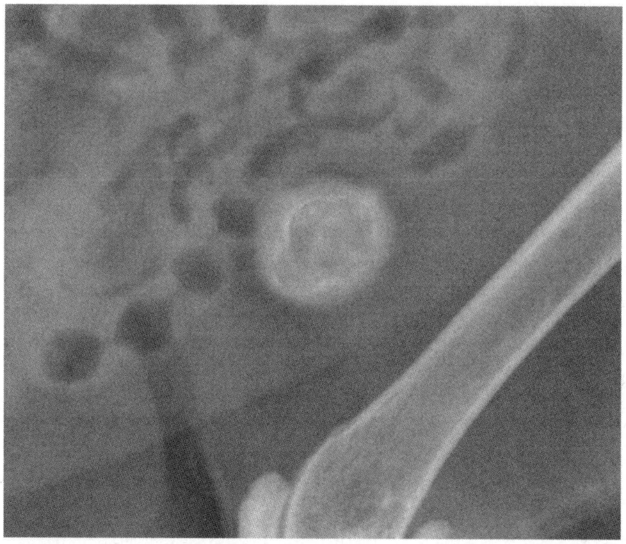

Fig. 39.19 Lateral radiograph of a cat with a focal calcified body in the peritoneal space. The calcified body was an incidental finding and thought to be a result of dystrophic calcification of necrotic fat.

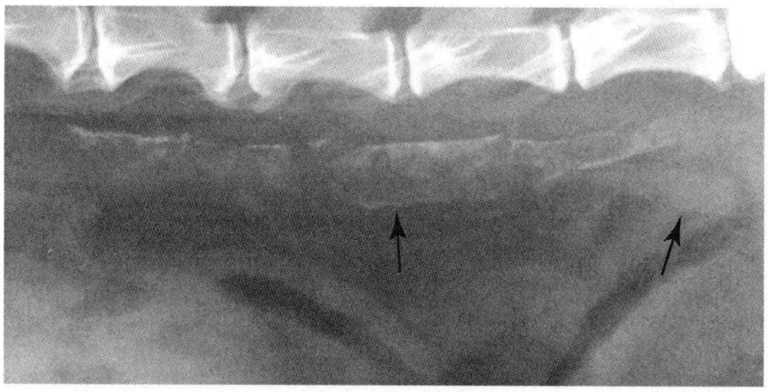

Fig. 39.20 Lateral view of the caudal abdomen of a 13-year-old Shetland sheepdog in chronic renal failure. The aorta and external iliac arteries (*black arrows*) are visible because of metastatic calcification.

that the term *metastatic* in regards to calcification does not indicate neoplasia, but indicates mineralization of normal tissue secondary to hypercalcemia. Dystrophic calcification is the deposition of calcium salts in abnormal tissue, which is injured, degenerated, or dead and causes include inflammation or infection and can in addition to the reported Bates bodies also be seen with hyperadrenocorticism or atherosclerosis.[28]

Rarely, peritoneal mineralization might be noted surrounding foreign material, such as a sponge left behind during previous surgery,[29] or a mineralized fetus may be seen in the peritoneal space with ectopic pregnancy. Clinical signs may be caused by necrosis or mechanical interference, or the condition may be an incidental finding.

NORMAL ANATOMY AND IMAGING OF THE ABDOMINAL WALL

Normal Anatomy and Imaging Techniques

The normal abdominal wall consists of the external and internal oblique abdominis and the transverse abdominis muscles. On radiographs, the external oblique muscles can be identified due to the presence of fat on either side. The internal oblique and transverse abdominis muscles are visible radiographically, because they are continuous with the rib cage. On dorsoventral (DV) or VD radiographs, the lateral abdominal wall is best visualized. On lateral radiographs, the ventral portion of the abdominal wall is best evaluated. The cranial ventral abdominal wall thins, and ventral to the liver is often difficult to evaluate. Caudally, the abdominal wall is approximately the same width as the ventral aspect of the pelvis. The internal surface of the abdominal wall should be smooth and continuous.[3] The abdominal wall muscles and lesions thereof are often best visualized when struck tangentially by the x-ray beam. Ultrasound, especially when using a high-frequency probe, allows differentiation and evaluation of the different abdominal wall layers.

Abdominal Wall Abnormalities

Primary abdominal wall lesions can be classified as nonneoplastic and neoplastic. Nonneoplastic lesions include congenital abdominal wall hernia, trauma to the abdominal wall (Fig. 39.21, eFig. 39.6), postsurgical dehiscence, inflammation, and infection (e.g., secondary to a migrating foreign body), edema, subcutaneous emphysema, or mineralization. Abdominal wall disruption may be noted on radiographs. However, the extent of abdominal wall involvement may be better evaluated using ultrasound or CT with reformatted images in various planes. Additionally, displacement of abdominal organs into the abdominal wall defect can be identified using radiography, ultrasound, and CT. Common organs displaced into abdominal wall defects include the small intestine and urinary bladder; however, any other organ can be displaced. Tubular or round gas pockets summating with the abdominal wall can indicate herniated bowel loops (Fig. 39.22, eFig. 39.7). This is important to recognize, because herniated intestinal loops can get incarcerated and necrotic due to constriction by the abdominal wall defect.

Gas from a variety of causes may be present in the soft tissues surrounding the abdomen. Abrasions with lacerations secondary to trauma often produce a mottled, irregular gas pattern.

Mineralization is occasionally present in the soft tissues surrounding the abdomen. For example, calcinosis cutis associated with Cushing syndrome may produce nodular or linear calcification of soft tissues, most often dorsally along the skin or subcutaneous tissues and sometimes in the ventral abdominal wall. Lipomas are considered one of the most common benign primary tumors of the abdominal wall, and usually appear as a fat attenuating mass in the abdominal wall on radiographs or CT images. Rarely, mineralization of lipomas occurs in animals. Diffuse amorphous mineralization may be noted summating with the abdominal cavity in an abdominal wall extra-abdominal

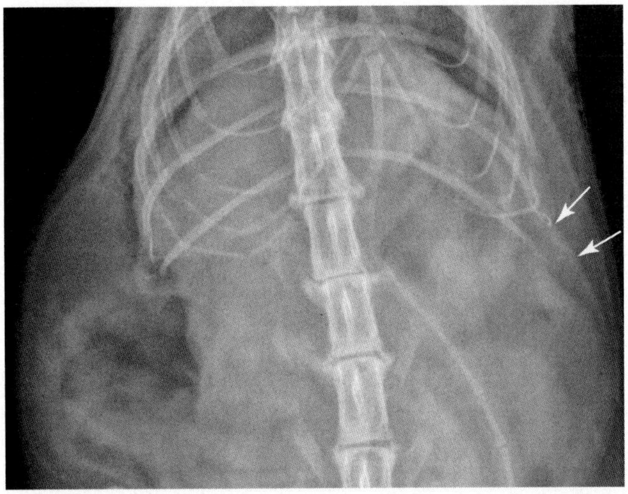

Fig. 39.21 Ventrodorsal radiograph of a cat post vehicular trauma. Extensive avulsion of the right abdominal wall is noted. The left abdominal wall is intact (*white arrows*).

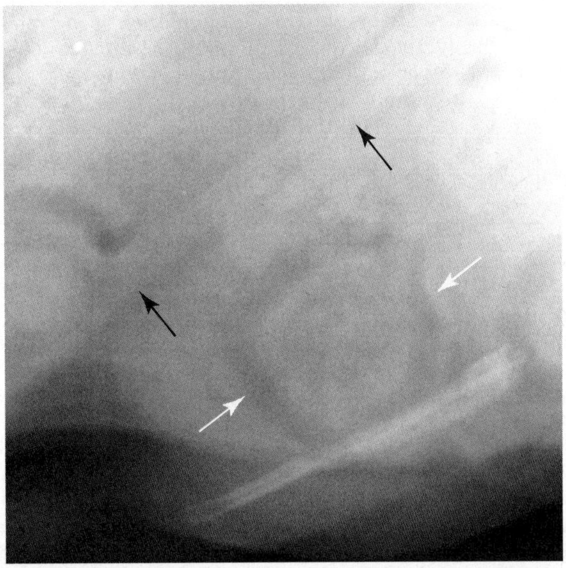

Fig. 39.22 Lateral view of the abdomen of a dog with tubular gas opacities (*white arrows*) ventral to the abdominal wall from an inguinal hernia with entrapped small intestine within the hernia. The level of the abdominal wall is indicated by the *black arrows*.

chondrolipoma, and this might be misinterpreted as a mineralized abdominal mass.[30]

Soft tissue attenuating masses of the abdominal wall such as fibrosarcoma can occur in the abdominal wall of cats, and commonly CT imaging is performed to evaluate the extent of the lesion. Transitional cell carcinoma might spread to the abdominal wall secondary to percutaneous tissue sampling or surgery and it is recommended to avoid percutaneous sampling of transitional cell carcinoma.[31]

ABDOMINAL LYMPH NODES

Normal Anatomy and Imaging Techniques

Anatomy

Abdominal lymph nodes are divided into two groups: parietal and visceral. The parietal group includes the lymph centers of the abdominal and pelvic walls, including the lumbar, iliosacral, and iliofemoral lymph centers. All parietal lymph nodes, except the iliofemoral lymph nodes, are in the retroperitoneal space and receive afferent lymphatics from the spine, adrenal glands, kidneys, genital organs, excluding part of the mammary glands, caudodorsal abdomen, pelvis, and pelvic limbs. The iliofemoral lymph center consists of only one distal femoral lymph node, which is in the deep medial femoral fascia at the distal part of the femoral triangle and only present in about 10% of dogs.[1] Efferent vessels from the parietal lymph nodes drain into the lumbar trunk, which in turn empties into the cisterna chyli. The more cranially located parietal lymph nodes may bypass the lumbar trunk and drain directly into the cisterna chyli. Many of the parietal lymph nodes are developed inconsistently and may be absent. However, the medial iliac lymph nodes, the largest lymph nodes of the iliosacral lymph center, are always present. The medial iliac lymph nodes, previously known as the *external iliac lymph nodes*,[1] are located ventral to the caudal lumbar spine between the deep circumflex iliac and external iliac arteries (aortic trifurcation). One lymph node is usually present on each side, but occasionally two lymph nodes are noted on one or both sides. The medial iliac lymph nodes are reported to lie ventral to L5 and L6[1]; however, these lymph nodes often are located ventral to L6 and L7.[3] The medial iliac lymph nodes receive afferent lymphatics from the urogenital tract, as well as from other structures in the caudal abdomen, pelvis, and pelvic limbs.

The visceral group of abdominal lymph nodes is divided into subgroups that are associated with specific organs.[1] The visceral lymph group drains the liver, spleen, pancreas, stomach, and intestine. The lymph centers of the abdominal viscera can be divided into the celiac, cranial mesenteric, and caudal mesenteric lymph centers. The celiac lymph center consists of all lymph nodes serving organs that are supplied by the celiac artery, which includes the hepatic, splenic, gastric, and pancreaticoduodenal lymph nodes. The cranial mesenteric lymph center consists of the jejunal and colic lymph nodes. The jejunal lymph nodes, which were previously called the *cranial mesenteric lymph nodes*, are the largest of the visceral lymph nodes and receive afferent lymphatics from the jejunum, ileum, and pancreas.[1] The colic lymph nodes generally are located in proximity to the ascending and transverse colon and in the dog close to the descending colon.[32] The caudal mesenteric lymph center consists of the caudal mesenteric lymph nodes and serves the caudal aspect of the descending colon to rectum.[32] The caudal mesenteric lymph nodes send lymph in part to the medial iliac lymph nodes or the lumbar trunk or like the other abdominal visceral lymph nodes to the intestinal trunk, which then empties into the cisterna chyli.[1]

Radiography of Lymph Nodes

Normal lymph nodes are usually not visible radiographically.

Ultrasound of Lymph Nodes

Ultrasound is likely the most widely used technique to assess abdominal and retroperitoneal lymph nodes in dogs and cats. Various ultrasound characteristics of normal and abnormal lymph nodes have been described. It is important to remember that normal lymph nodes can be quite variable in size, and therefore size measurements need to be treated with caution when deciding on diseased versus normal lymph nodes. When evaluating the size of lymph nodes, the maximal thickness or width of lymph nodes is more reliable than the length of lymph nodes.[33] For the medial iliac lymph nodes and other lymph nodes as well, lymph node size is directly proportional to body size. Furthermore, abdominal lymph nodes, specifically the jejunal lymph nodes, might be slightly larger in younger animals compared to older animals. Lymph nodes are often hypoechoic to isoechoic to surrounding tissue with a distinct cortex and medulla or homogeneous echotexture. Their surface is usually smooth and often clearly defined.

The medial iliac and jejunal lymph nodes are the largest and most consistent in the abdominal cavity, and can be found sonographically more often than other lymph nodes when normal.[33,34] Normal lymph nodes have an echogenicity similar to surrounding mesentery and adjacent musculature,[34] but knowledge of their location and careful identification of elongated structures of uniform echotexture and thin echogenic capsules can permit detection (Fig. 39.23). High-frequency transducers are necessary to obtain resolution adequate for imaging normal lymph nodes.

The medial iliac lymph nodes are found by following the terminal portion of the aorta and caudal vena cava carefully in long axis and transverse image planes. In some instances, finding the lymph nodes by scanning in a transverse plane and looking for subtle round structures with thin echogenic borders on either side of the aorta is easier (see Fig. 39.23B). Alternatively, the medial iliac lymph nodes may be easier to find in the dorsal plane.[35] In the sagittal plane, the lymph nodes appear fusiform (see Fig. 39.23A). The visceral lymph nodes are seen more often when abnormal and are encountered as hypoechoic nodules detected during routine scanning. They are identified as lymph nodes based on their location usually along the vascular supply of a specific organ.

Computed Tomography of Lymph Nodes

CT is an excellent technique to evaluate abdominal lymph nodes, because it allows delineation of peritoneal anatomy. Isotropic voxel scanning with reformation in sagittal, dorsal, or oblique planes helps to evaluate the size, shape, location, and contrast enhancement behavior of these lymph nodes.

The jejunal and medial iliac lymph nodes are most commonly identified in dogs[36] and cats. Colic lymph nodes are generally not identified in dogs but often seen in cats. Most abdominal lymph nodes have a homogeneous attenuation pattern before and after intravenous iodinated contrast medium injection. Some lymph nodes are peripherally hyperattenuating relative to the center.[36] Considering that the sacral lymph nodes are not routinely accessible with ultrasound, CT (or magnetic resonance imaging [MRI]) should be considered when staging dogs with apocrine gland tumors.[37]

Abnormalities of Abdominal Lymph Nodes

Imaging Findings

Abdominal lymph nodes are seen radiographically only if they are enlarged or mineralized. Abundant retroperitoneal or peritoneal fat helps provide contrast between enlarged lymph nodes and surrounding soft tissue structures. Of the parietal lymph nodes, the medial iliac nodes are most commonly the only lymph nodes that enlarge to the degree that they are seen radiographically. Care should be taken not to confuse the deep circumflex arteries and veins that are projected end-on in lateral radiographs with enlarged medial iliac lymph nodes (Fig. 39.24). Enlarged medial iliac lymph nodes appear as a soft tissue mass in the retroperitoneal space ventral to L6 and L7 (Fig. 39.25). If node enlargement is severe, the lymph nodes are

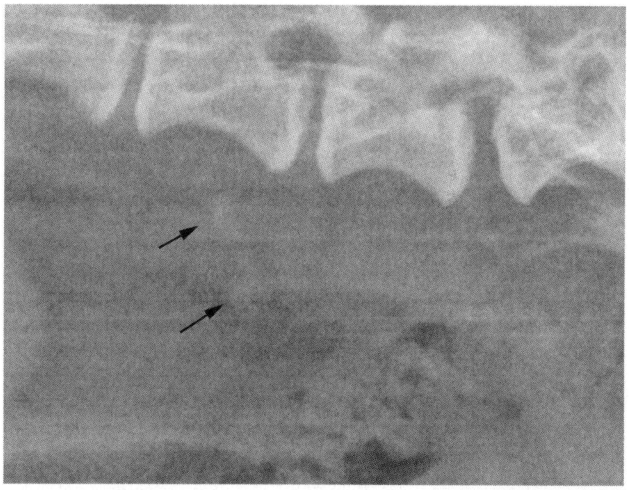

Fig. 39.24 Lateral view of the abdomen of a normal dog. Note the fat opacity within the retroperitoneal space. Ill-defined nodular soft tissue opacities in the caudal retroperitoneal space seen ventral to L6 (*black arrows*) represent end-on projections of the deep circumflex iliac arteries and veins, not lymph nodes.

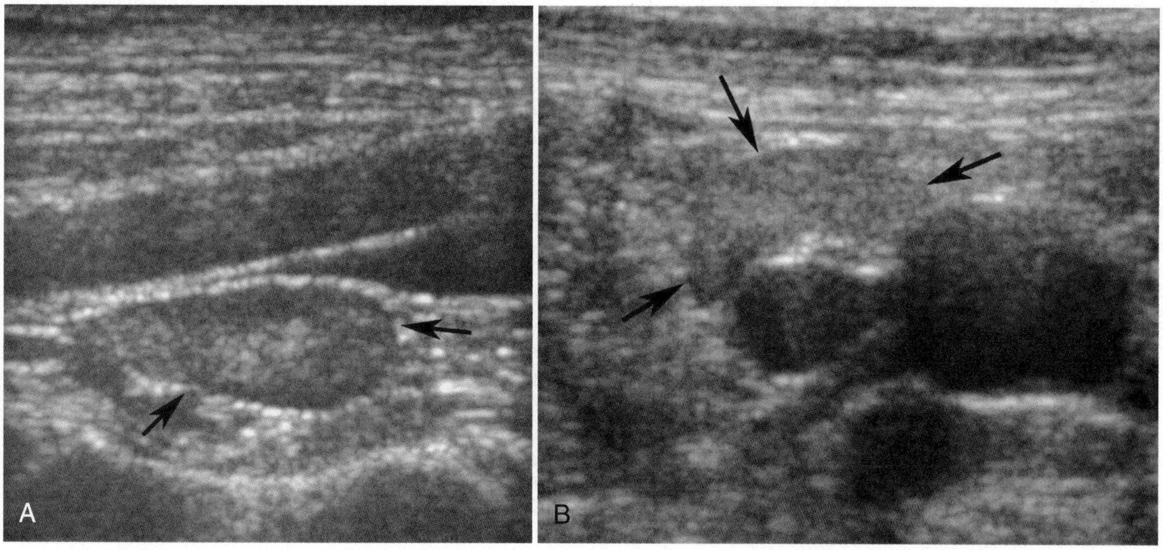

Fig. 39.23 Longitudinal (**A**) and transverse (**B**) ultrasound images of a normal medial iliac lymph node. On the longitudinal view, the lymph node (*black arrows*) is elongated and just ventral to the aorta near the aortic bifurcation. The lymph node is nearly isoechoic to surrounding structures and has a thin echogenic capsule. On the transverse image, the lymph node (*black arrows*) is a curved structure just ventrolateral to the aorta. Ventral is to the *top* (**A** and **B**), and cranial is to the *left* (**A**).

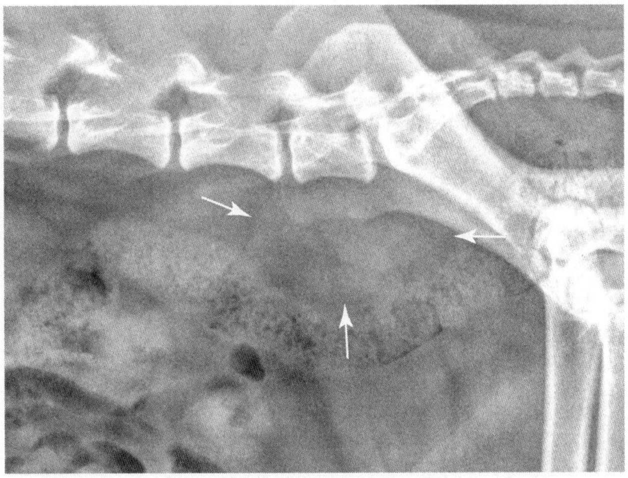

Fig. 39.25 Lateral view of the abdomen of a dog with anal gland adenocarcinoma. The medial iliac lymph nodes are mildly enlarged and appear as an ill-defined soft tissue mass (*white arrows*) in the retroperitoneal space ventral to L7. The colon is displaced ventrally.

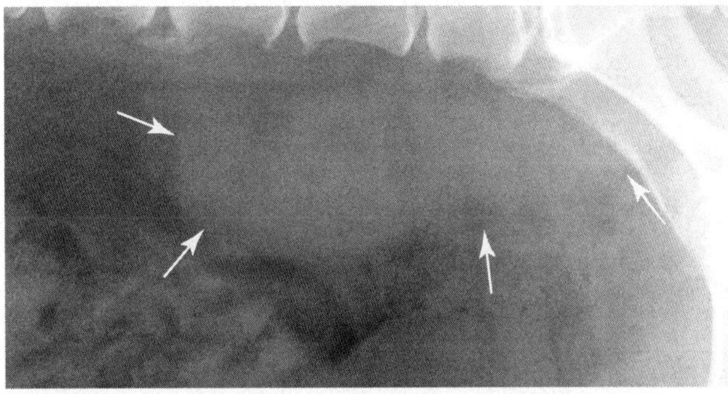

Fig. 39.26 Lateral view of the abdomen of a dog with lymphosarcoma. Medial iliac lymph node enlargement is severe and appears as a soft tissue mass in the retroperitoneal space extending caudally from L4-L5 into the pelvic canal (*white arrows*).

more conspicuous and extend more cranially (Fig. 39.26). Enlarged sublumbar lymph nodes frequently displace the descending colon and rectum ventrally (eFig. 39.8). However, a ventral course of the colon can be normal and is not an indication of medial iliac lymph node enlargement unless a soft tissue mass is present in the expected location of the lymph nodes. The most common cause of medial iliac lymphadenopathy is neoplasia. Neoplastic lymph node involvement may be primary (e.g., lymphoma) or metastatic (e.g., from caudal abdominal or pelvic neoplasms).[37] Inflammatory disease may also cause enlargement of the medial iliac lymph nodes, but this is less common. Inflammatory causes include migrating foreign bodies in the iliopsoas musculature, urogenital infection, and less commonly gastrointestinal or skeletal inflammation.

Visceral abdominal lymph nodes rarely enlarge enough to be seen radiographically, and tend to silhouette with surrounding organs. Jejunal lymph nodes may occasionally enlarge sufficiently and appear as an ill-defined central abdominal mass displacing the intestine peripherally.

Ultrasonographically, abnormal lymph nodes enlarge and become rounder and more hypoechoic (Fig. 39.27).[33,38] Neoplastic lymph nodes generally have a short-to-long axis ratio of more than 1:2, narrow or absent hilus, hypoechogenicity, sharp borders, a resistive index (RI) greater than 0.65, a pulsatility index (PI) greater than 1.45, and often distal acoustic enhancement. These findings tend to not be present in reactive lymph nodes.[38,39] Heterogeneity of enlarged lymph nodes is associated with malignancy in the dog, but lymph node heterogeneity is not predictive of malignancy in the cat.[40] Fine-needle aspirates obtained with ultrasound guidance are helpful for determining the cause of lymph node enlargement.

CT and MRI allow evaluation of abdominal and retroperitoneal lymph nodes for disease, and they may be more sensitive for detecting enlarged lymph nodes than abdominal ultrasound. Additionally, lymph nodes in the pelvic canal are not accessible with ultrasound and can easily be assessed using CT and MRI. However, similarly to ultrasound, enlargement of lymph nodes noted on CT or MRI is not an indication for metastatic disease. Currently, there are no pathognomonic imaging findings for metastatic lymphadenopathy; enlarged lymph nodes should be sampled when tumor staging is performed.[41]

PANCREAS

Normal Anatomy and Imaging Techniques

Anatomy

The body of the pancreas lies between the pylorus and the proximal descending duodenum. The right lobe of the pancreas extends caudally from the body and lies adjacent to the medial aspect of the descending duodenum. The left lobe of the pancreas lies between the stomach and transverse colon, extending from the pancreatic body toward the left kidney on the medial aspect of the spleen.[42] As opposed to dogs, the left lobe is larger than the right lobe in cats.

Radiography of the Pancreas

The normal pancreas is not visible on abdominal radiographs of dogs because of silhouetting with the adjacent tissues. Occasionally, the left limb of the pancreas can be seen on VD views in obese cats as an area of soft tissue opacity between the fundus of the stomach, the spleen, and the left kidney (Fig. 39.28).

Ultrasound of the Pancreas

Sonographic evaluation of the pancreas is standard practice for evaluating patients suspected of having pancreatitis or pancreatic masses, because the pancreas is better evaluated sonographically than radiographically. Endoscopic ultrasound shows promise evaluating the pancreas[43]; however, it is not commonly available and requires anesthesia, whereas transabdominal ultrasound can be performed in awake and sedated patients. Fasting of the patient is recommended, to reduce artifacts caused by ingesta and gas which can obscure the pancreas.[44] The normal pancreas can be difficult to identify sonographically because of its small size, usually having an echogenicity similar to surrounding fat, and absence of a well-defined capsule. Therefore, identifiable landmarks are used to scan the pancreatic area and are described in a recent consensus statement on abdominal ultrasound.[45,46]

When visible, the pancreas has a subtle echogenic capsule (Fig. 39.29), and it is somewhat hypoechoic, being less echogenic than the spleen but more echogenic than the liver.[45] Occasionally, the pancreaticoduodenal vein, which lies within the pancreas and runs parallel to the duodenum, can be identified in dogs (see Fig. 39.29).[33] The pancreas is more likely to be identified in puppies, thin dogs, and dogs with peritoneal fluid. A hyperechoic pancreas can be noted in healthy dogs and can be associated with endocrinopathies such as hyperadrenocorticism.[47] In cats, the normal pancreas is isoechoic to the liver and hypoechoic to the surrounding mesentery, findings that do not appear to change with age, sex, body weight, or body condition.[45,48] The normal width (ventral to dorsal dimension) of the left lobe and body of the pancreas is approximately 0.25 to 1.0 cm, and the right lobe is commonly reported slightly smaller at between approximately 0.3 and

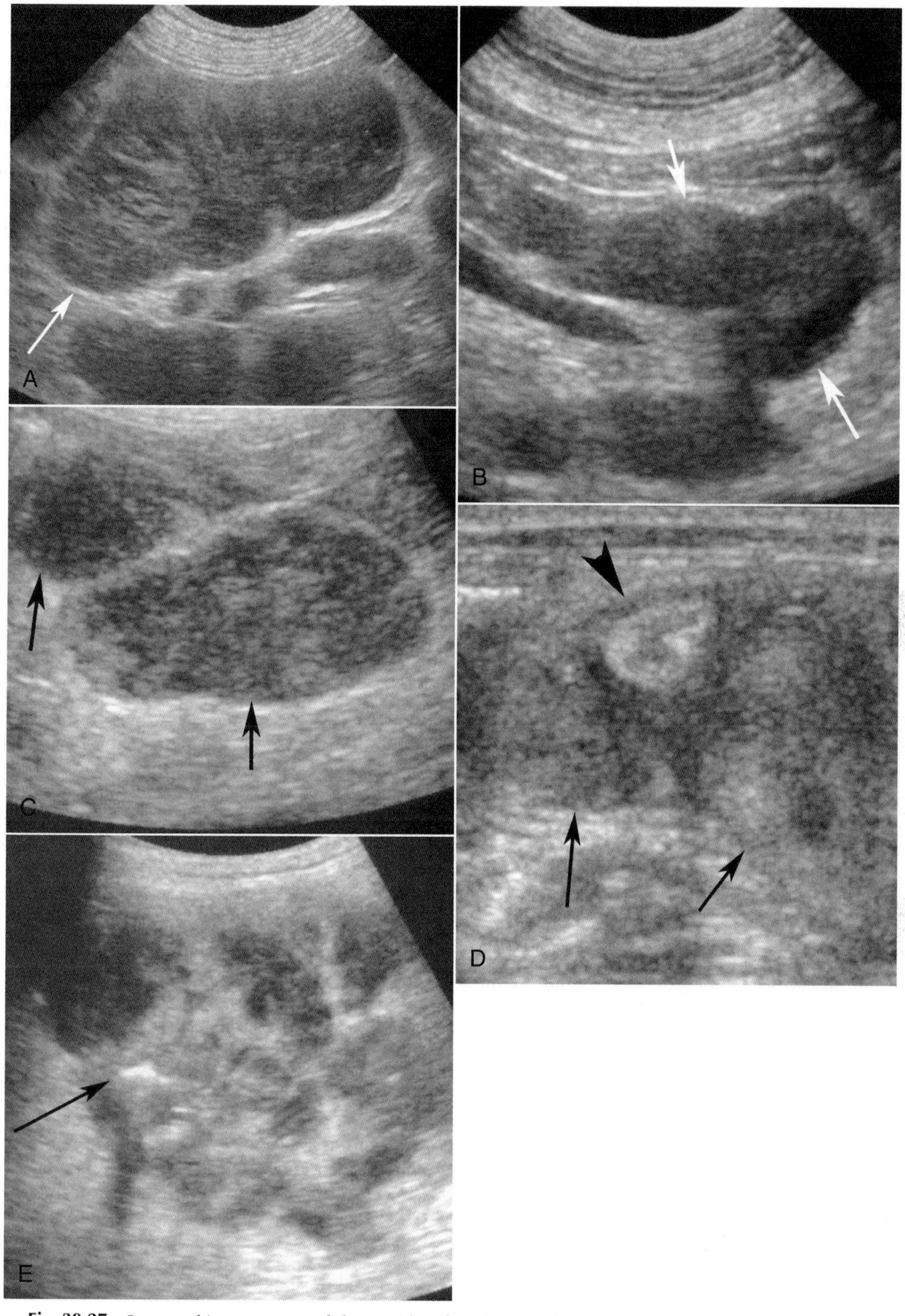

Fig. 39.27 Sonographic appearance of abnormal lymph nodes. **A,** Enlarged, hypoechoic medial iliac lymph node (*white arrow*) surrounding the aorta in a dog with lymphoma. **B,** Enlarged jejunal lymph node (*white arrows*) in a dog with lymphoma. This lymph node is hypoechoic to surrounding tissues and is irregular in shape. **C,** Enlarged jejunal lymph nodes (*black arrows*) in a dog with inflammatory bowel disease. Lymphoid hyperplasia was found on evaluation of lymph node aspirates. Both lymph nodes are hypoechoic and appear like those seen in the dog with lymphoma **(B)**. **D,** Enlarged ileocolic lymph nodes in a cat with lymphoma. The ileum (*black arrowhead*) is seen in cross-section surrounded by enlarged hypoechoic lymph nodes (*black arrows*). **E,** A large mixed echogenic mass in the mid abdomen of a dog. The mass incorporated intestinal segments. Gas (*black arrow*) within one bowel segment is seen as an echogenic focus producing acoustic shadowing. The hypoechoic to nearly anechoic areas were presumed to be enlarged mesenteric lymph nodes as lymphoma was diagnosed from aspirates of these structures.

61. Marolf AJ, Stewart JA, Dunphy TR, et al. Hepatic and pancreaticobiliary MRI and MR cholangiopancreatography with and without secretin stimulation in normal cats. *Vet Radiol Ultrasound*. 2011;52:415–421.
62. Lester NV, Newell SM, Hill RC, et al. Scintigraphic diagnosis of insulinoma in a dog. *Vet Radiol Ultrasound*. 1999;40:174–178.
63. Steiner JM, Williams DA. Feline exocrine pancreatic disorders, Vet Clin North Am small. *Anim Pract*. 1999;29:551–575.
64. Williams JM, Panciera DL, Larson MM, et al. Ultrasonographic findings of the pancreas in cats with elevated serum pancreatic lipase immunoreactivity. *J Vet Intern Med*. 2013;27:913–918.
65. Gibbs C, Denny HR, Minter HM, et al. Radiological features of inflammatory conditions of the canine pancreas. *J Small Anim Pract*. 1972;13:531–544.
66. Kleine LJ, Hornbuckle WE. Acute pancreatitis: the radiographic findings in 182 dogs. *Vet Radiol*. 1978;19: 102–106.
67. Mattoon JS, Nyland TG. *Small Animal Diagnostic Ultrasound*. ed 3. St Louis: Elsevier; 2015.
68. Hecht S, Henry G. Sonographic evaluation of the normal and abnormal pancreas. *Clin Tech Small Anim Pract*. 2007;22(3):115–121.
69. Wall M, Biller DS, Schoning P, et al. Pancreatitis in a cat demonstrating pancreatic duct dilatation ultrasonographically. *J Am Anim Hosp Assoc*. 2001;37(1):49–53.
70. Bennett PF, Hahn KA, Toal RL, et al. Ultrasonographic and cytopathological diagnosis of exocrine pancreatic carcinoma in the dog and cat. *J Am Anim Hosp Assoc*. 2001;37:466–473.
71. Saunders HM, VanWinkle TJ, Drobatz K, et al. Ultrasonographic findings in cats with clinical, gross pathologic, and histologic evidence of acute pancreatic necrosis: 20 cases (1994–2001). *J Am Vet Med Assoc*. 2002;221:1724–1730.
72. Ruaux CG. Diagnostic approaches to acute pancreatitis. *Clin Tech Small Anim Pract*. 2003;18:245–249.
73. Ferreri JA, Hardam E, Kimmel SE, et al. Clinical differentiation of acute necrotizing from chronic nonsuppurative pancreatitis in cats: 63 cases (1996–2001). *J Am Vet Med Assoc*. 2003;223:469–474.
74. Watson PJ, Archer J, Roulois AJ, et al. Observational study of 14 cases of chronic pancreatitis in dogs. *Vet Rec*. 2010;167(25):968–976.
75. VanEnkevort BA, O'Brien RT, Young KM. Pancreatic pseudocysts in 4 dogs and 2 cats: ultrasonographic and clinicopathologic findings. *J Vet Intern Med*. 1999;13: 309–313.
76. Marchevsky AM, Yovich JC, Wyatt KM. Pancreatic pseudocyst causing extrahepatic biliary obstruction in a dog. *Aust Vet J*. 2000;78(2):99–101.
77. Rutgers C, Herring DS, Orton C. Pancreatic pseudocyst associated with acute pancreatitis in a dog: ultrasonographic diagnosis. *J Am Anim Hosp Assoc*. 1985;21: 411–416.
78. Coleman MG, Robson MC, Harvey C. Pancreatic cyst in a cat, N Z. *Vet J*. 2005;53(2):157–159.
79. Branter EM, Viviano KR. Multiple recurrent pancreatic cysts with associated pancreatic inflammation and atrophy in a cat. *J Feline Med Surg*. 2010;12(10):822–827.
80. Bailiff NL, Norris CR, Seguin B, et al. Pancreatolithiasis and pancreatic pseudobladder associated with pancreatitis in a cat. *J Am Anim Hosp Assoc*. 2004;40:69–74.
81. Gerhardt A, Steiner JM, Williams DA, et al. Comparison of the sensitivity of different diagnostic tests for pancreatitis in cats. *J Vet Intern Med*. 2001;15:329–333.
82. Forman MA, Marks SL, De Cock HE, et al. Evaluation of serum feline pancreatic lipase immunoreactivity and helical computed tomography versus conventional testing for the diagnosis of feline pancreatitis. *J Vet Intern Med*. 2004;18(6):807–815.
83. Adrian AM, Twedt DC, Kraft SL, et al. Computed tomographic angiography under sedation in the diagnosis of suspected canine pancreatitis: a pilot study. *J Vet Intern Med*. 2015;29:97–103.
84. Jaeger JQ, Mattoon JS, Bateman SW, et al. Combined use of ultrasonography and contrast enhanced computed tomography to evaluate acute necrotizing pancreatitis in two dogs. *Vet Radiol Ultrasound*. 2003;44:72–79.
85. Spillmann T, Litzlbauer H, Moritz A, et al. Computed tomography and laparoscopy for the diagnosis of pancreatic diseases in dogs. In: *Proceedings of the American College of Veterinary Internal Medicine*. 2000:485–487.
86. Lamb CR, Simpson KW, Boswood A, et al. Ultrasonography of pancreatic neoplasia in the dog: a retrospective review of 16 cases. *Vet Rec*. 1995;137(3):65–68.
87. Jubb KVF, Kennedy PC, Palmer N. The pancreas. In: *Pathology of Domestic Animals*. ed 4. St Louis: Elsevier; 1985:313–327.
88. Robben JH, Pollak YWEA, Kirpensteijn J, et al. Comparison of ultrasonography, computed tomography, and single-photon emission computed tomography for the detection and localization of canine insulinoma. *J Vet Intern Med*. 2005;19(15).
89. Goutal CM, Brugmann BL, Ryan KA. Insulinoma in dogs: a review. *J Am Anim Hosp Assoc*. 2012;48:151–163.
90. Hecht S, Penninck DG, Keating JH. Imaging findings in pancreatic neoplasia and nodular hyperplasia in 19 cats. *Vet Radiol Ultrasound*. 2007;48:45–50.
91. Ramírez GA, Altimira J, García-González B, et al. Intrapancreatic ectopic splenic tissue in dogs and cats. *J Comp Pathol*. 2013;148(4):361–364.
92. Feldman EC, Nelson RW, Reusch C, et al. *Canine and Feline Endocrinology*. ed 4. St Louis: Elsevier; 2015.
93. Vanderperren K, Haers H, Van der Vekens E, et al. Description of the use of contrast-enhanced ultrasonography in four dogs with pancreatic tumours. *J Small Anim Pract*. 2014;55(3):164–169.
94. Head LL, Daniel GB, Becker TJ, et al. Use of computed tomography and radiolabeled leukocytes in a cat with pancreatitis. *Vet Radiol Ultrasound*. 2005;46:263–266.
95. Iseri T, Yamada K, Chijiwa K, et al. Dynamic computed tomography of the pancreas in normal dogs and in a dog with pancreatic insulinoma. *Vet Radiol Ultrasound*. 2007;48:328–331.
96. Lamb CR, McEvoy FJ. Comparison of ultrasonographic findings in canine pancreatitis and pancreatic neoplasia [abstract]. *Vet Radiol Ultrasound*. 1995;36.
97. Cordner AP, Armstrong PJ, Newman SJ, et al. Effect of pancreatic tissue sampling on serum pancreatic enzyme levels in clinically healthy dogs. *J Vet Diagn Invest*. 2010;22(5):702–707.
98. Newman S, Steiner J, Woosley K, et al. Localization of pancreatic inflammation and necrosis in dogs. *J Vet Intern Med*. 2004;18(4):488–493.
99. Hines BL, Salisbury SK, Jakovljevic S, et al. Pancreatic pseudocyst associated with chronic-active necrotizing pancreatitis in a cat. *J Am Anim Hosp Assoc*. 1996;32(2): 147–152.
100. VanEnkevort BA, O'Brien RT, Young KM. Pancreatic pseudocysts in 4 dogs and 2 cats: ultrasonographic and clinicopathologic findings. *J Vet Intern Med*. 1999;13: 309–313.

101. Healy DM, Cassidy JP, Martin SA. A true congenital pancreatic cyst in a dog. *BMC Vet Res*. 2022;18:304.
102. Voorhout G, Stolp R, Rijnberk A, et al. Assessment of survey radiography and comparison with x-ray computed tomography for detection of hyperfunctioning adrenocortical tumors in dogs. *J Am Vet Med Assoc*. 1990;196: 1799–1803.
103. Herbach N, Wiele K, Konietschke U, et al. Pathologic alterations of canine and feline adrenal glands. *Open J Pathol*. 2016;6:140–153.
104. Soulsby SN, Holland M, Hudson JA, et al. Ultrasonographic evaluation of adrenal gland size compared to body weight in normal dogs. *Vet Radiol Ultrasound*. 2015;56: 317–326.
105. Zimmer C, Hörauf A, Reusch C. Ultrasonographic examination of the adrenal gland and evaluation of the hypophyseal-adrenal axis in 20 cats. *J Small Anim Pract*. 2000;41:156–160.
106. Besso JG, Penninck DG, Gliatto JM. Retrospective ultrasonographic evaluation of adrenal lesions in 26 dogs. *Vet Radiol Ultrasound*. 1997;38:448–455.
107. Tidwell AS, Penninck DG, Besso JG. Imaging of adrenal gland disorders. *Vet Clin North Am Small Anim Pract*. 1997;27:237–254.
108. Hoerauf A, Reusch C. Ultrasonographic evaluation of the adrenal glands in six dogs with hypoadrenocorticism. *J Am Anim Hosp Assoc*. 1999;35:214–218.
109. Hoerauf A, Reusch C. Ultrasonographic characteristics of both adrenal glands in 15 dogs with functional adrenocortical tumors. *J Am Anim Hosp Assoc*. 1999;35:193–199.
110. Nyland TG, Mattoon JS, Herrgesell EJ, et al. Adrenal glands. In: Nyland TG, Mattoon JS, eds. *Small Animal Diagnostic Ultrasound*. St Louis: Elsevier; 2002:196.
111. de Chalus T, Combes A, Bedu AS, et al. Ultrasonographic adrenal gland measurements in healthy Yorkshire terriers and Labrador retrievers. *Anat Histol Embryol*. 2013;42: 57–64.
112. Barthez PY, Nyland TG, Feldman EC. Ultrasonographic evaluation of the adrenal glands in dogs. *J Am Vet Med Assoc*. 1995;207:1180–1183.
113. Mogicato G, Layssol-Lamour C, Conchou F, et al. Ultrasonographic evaluation of the adrenal glands in healthy dogs: repeatability, reproducibility, observer-dependent variability, and the effect of bodyweight, age and sex. *Vet Rec*. 2011;168(5):130.
114. Wenger M, Mueller C, Kook PH, et al. Ultrasonographic evaluation of adrenal glands in dogs with primary hypoadrenocorticism or mimicking diseases. *Vet Rec*. 2010;167:207–210.
115. Choi J, Kim H, Yoon J. Ultrasonographic adrenal gland measurements in clinically normal small breed dogs and comparison with pituitary-dependent hyperadrenocorticism. *J Vet Med Sci*. 2011;73:985–989.
116. Barberet V, Pey P, Duchateau L, et al. Intra- and interobserver variability of ultrasonographic measurements of the adrenal glands in healthy Beagles. *Vet Radiol Ultrasound*. 2010;51:656–660.
117. Blaser A, Dennler M, Mosing M, et al. Effects of contrast medium injection technique on attenuation values of adrenal glands in healthy dogs during contrast-enhanced computed tomography. *Am J Vet Res*. 2016;77:144–150.
118. Bertolini G, Furlanello T, De Lorenzi D, et al. Computed tomographic quantification of canine adrenal gland volume and attenuation. *Vet Radiol Ultrasound*. 2006;47: 444–448.
119. Morandi F. Adrenal glands. In: Schwarz T, Saunders J, eds. *Veterinary Computed Tomography*. Ames, IA: Wiley-Blackwell; 2011:351–355.
120. Llabres-Diaz FJ, Dennis R. Magnetic resonance imaging of the presumed normal canine adrenal glands. *Vet Radiol Ultrasound*. 2003;44:5–19.
121. Morandi F, Mays JL, Newman SJ, et al. Imaging diagnosis—bilateral adrenal adenomas and myelolipomas in a dog. *Vet Radiol Ultrasound*. 2007;48(3):246–249.
122. Tursi M, Iussich S, Prunotto M, et al. Adrenal myelolipoma in a dog. *Vet Pathol*. 2005;42(2):232–235.
123. Lee HC, Jung DI, Moon JH, et al. Clinical characteristics and outcomes of primary adrenal hemangioma in a dog. *Res Vet Sci*. 2013;95(2):572–575.
124. Barthez PY, Marks SL, Woo J, et al. Pheochromocytoma in dogs: 61 cases (1984–1995). *J Vet Intern Med*. 1997;11: 272–278.
125. Barrera JS, Bernard F, Ehrhart EJ, et al. Evaluation of risk factors for outcome associated with adrenal gland tumors with or without invasion of the caudal vena cava and treated via adrenalectomy in dogs: 86 cases (1993–2009). *J Am Vet Med Assoc*. 2013;242(12):1715–1721.
126. Myers NC. Adrenal incidentalomas. Diagnostic workup of the incidentally discovered adrenal mass. *Vet Clin North Am Small Anim Pract*. 1997;27(2):381–399.
127. Baum JI, Boston SE, Case JB. Prevalence of adrenal gland masses as incidental findings during abdominal computed tomography in dogs: 270 cases (2013–2014). *J Am Vet Med Assoc*. 2016;249:1165–1169.
128. Schaer M. Pheochromocytoma in a dog: a case report. *J Am Anim Hosp Assoc*. 1980;79:583.
129. Owens JM, Drucker WD. Hyperadrenocorticism in the dog: canine Cushing's syndrome. *Vet Clin North Am*. 1977;7(3):583–602.
130. Labelle P, Kyles AE, Farver TB, et al. Indicators of malignancy of canine adrenocortical tumors: histopathology and proliferation index. *Vet Pathol*. 2004;41:490–497.
131. Pradelli D, Quintavalla C, Domenech O, et al. Tumour thrombus: direct endoluminal 'caudal caval vein-right atrium' extension in a dog affected by adrenal neoplasia. *Vet Res Commun*. 2003;27(Suppl 1):787–789.
132. Moore LE, Biller DS, Smith TA. Use of abdominal ultrasonography in the diagnosis of primary hyperaldosteronism in a cat. *J Am Vet Med Assoc*. 2000;217:213–215.
133. Burns MG, Kelly AB, Hornof WJ, et al. Pulmonary artery thrombosis in three dogs with hyperadrenocorticism. *J Am Vet Med Assoc*. 1981;178:388–393.
134. Behrend EN, Kemppainen RJ. Diagnosis of canine hyperadrenocorticism. *Vet Clin North Am Small Anim Pract*. 2001;31:985–1003.
135. Boag AK, Neiger R, Church DB. Trilostane treatment of bilateral adrenal enlargement and excessive sex steroid hormone production in a cat. *J Small Anim Pract*. 2004;45:263–266.
136. Gould SM, Baines EA, Mannion PA, et al. Use of endogenous ACTH concentration and adrenal ultrasonography to distinguish the cause of canine hyperadrenocorticism. *J Small Anim Pract*. 2001;42(3):113–121.
137. Benchekroun G, de Fornel-Thibaud P, Rodriguez Pineiro MI, et al. Ultrasonography criteria for differentiating ACTH dependency from ACTH independency in 47 dogs with hyperadrenocorticism and equivocal adrenal asymmetry. *J Vet Intern Med*. 2010;24:1077–1085.
138. Parnell NK, Powell LL, Hohenhaus AE, et al. Hypoadrenocorticism as the primary manifestation of lymphoma in two cats. *J Am Vet Med Assoc*. 1999;214(8):1208–1211.
139. Rosenstein DS. Diagnostic imaging in canine pheochromocytoma. *Vet Radiol Ultrasound*. 2000;41:499–506.
140. Chun R, Jakovljevic S, Morrison WB, et al. Apocrine gland adenocarcinoma and pheochromocytoma in a cat. *J Am Anim Hosp Assoc*. 1997;33:33–36.

141. Whittemore JC, Preston CA, Kyles AE, et al. Nontraumatic rupture of an adrenal gland tumor causing intra-abdominal or retroperitoneal hemorrhage in four dogs. *J Am Vet Med Assoc.* 2001;219:329–333.
142. Ruckstuhl NS, Nett CS, Reusch CE. Results of clinical examinations, laboratory tests, and ultrasonography in dogs with pituitary-dependent hyperadrenocorticism treated with trilostane. *Am J Vet Res.* 2002;63:506–512.
143. Mantis P, Lamb CR, Witt AL, et al. Changes in ultrasonographic appearance of adrenal glands in dogs with pituitary-dependent hyperadrenocorticism treated with trilostane. *Vet Radiol Ultrasound.* 2003;44:682–685.
144. Chapman PS, Kelly DF, Archer J, et al. Adrenal necrosis in a dog receiving trilostane for the treatment of hyperadrenocorticism. *J Small Anim Pract.* 2004;45:307–310.
145. Horauf A, Reusch C. [Effects of mitotane therapy in dogs with pituitary dependent Cushing syndrome on the adrenal gland size—an ultrasonographic study]. *Schweiz Arch Tierheilkd.* 1999;141:239–245.
146. Gregori T, Mantis P, Benigni L, et al. Comparison of computed tomographic and pathologic findings in 17 dogs with primary adrenal neoplasia. *Vet Radiol Ultrasound.* 2015;56:153–159.
147. Schultz RM, Wisner ER, Johnson EG, et al. Contrast-enhanced computed tomography as a preoperative indicator of vascular invasion from adrenal masses in dogs. *Vet Radiol Ultrasound.* 2009;50:625–629.

ELECTRONIC RESOURCES

Additional information related to the content in Chapter 39 can be found online at eBooks.Health.Elsevier.com

Chapter Quiz

CHAPTER 40

Liver and Spleen

Martha Moon Larson

RADIOLOGY OF THE LIVER

The liver is the largest solid organ in the abdomen. Changes in hepatic size, shape, location, and opacity are used to assess the liver for possible abnormality.[1–5]

The liver is in the cranial aspect of the abdomen between the diaphragm, which delineates its cranial border, and the stomach, right kidney, and cranial portion of the duodenum, which define the caudal extent. The liver is nearly entirely within the costal arch, with the caudal ventral border, composed of the left lateral liver lobe in the dog, extending just slightly beyond the costal arch. In dogs with a deep thoracic cavity, the liver lies more completely within the costal arch, whereas greater caudal hepatic extension is present in dogs with shallow, wide thoracic conformation. Abundant falciform fat, especially in cats, can result in dorsal displacement of the ventral aspect of the liver on lateral views (Fig. 40.1). On ventrodorsal (VD) views, the liver is distributed symmetrically in dogs, but a larger portion is often right sided in cats (Fig. 40.2).

Hepatic shape may not be visible without sufficient surrounding omental and falciform fat. The caudoventral hepatic margin protruding slightly from the costal arch should be relatively sharply marginated and triangular. It may protrude farther caudally in right lateral recumbent views, where it may merge with the spleen, blurring exact definition. If lateral views are slightly oblique, the liver can appear to have round margins, which should not be confused with hepatic enlargement.

The gallbladder is located just to the right of midline, in the cranioventral portion of the liver, but is not visible normally because of silhouetting with the soft tissue of the liver (Fig. 40.3). In some cats, the gallbladder can be seen on lateral abdominal radiographs as a curved structure protruding from the ventral liver margin (see Fig. 40.3C).

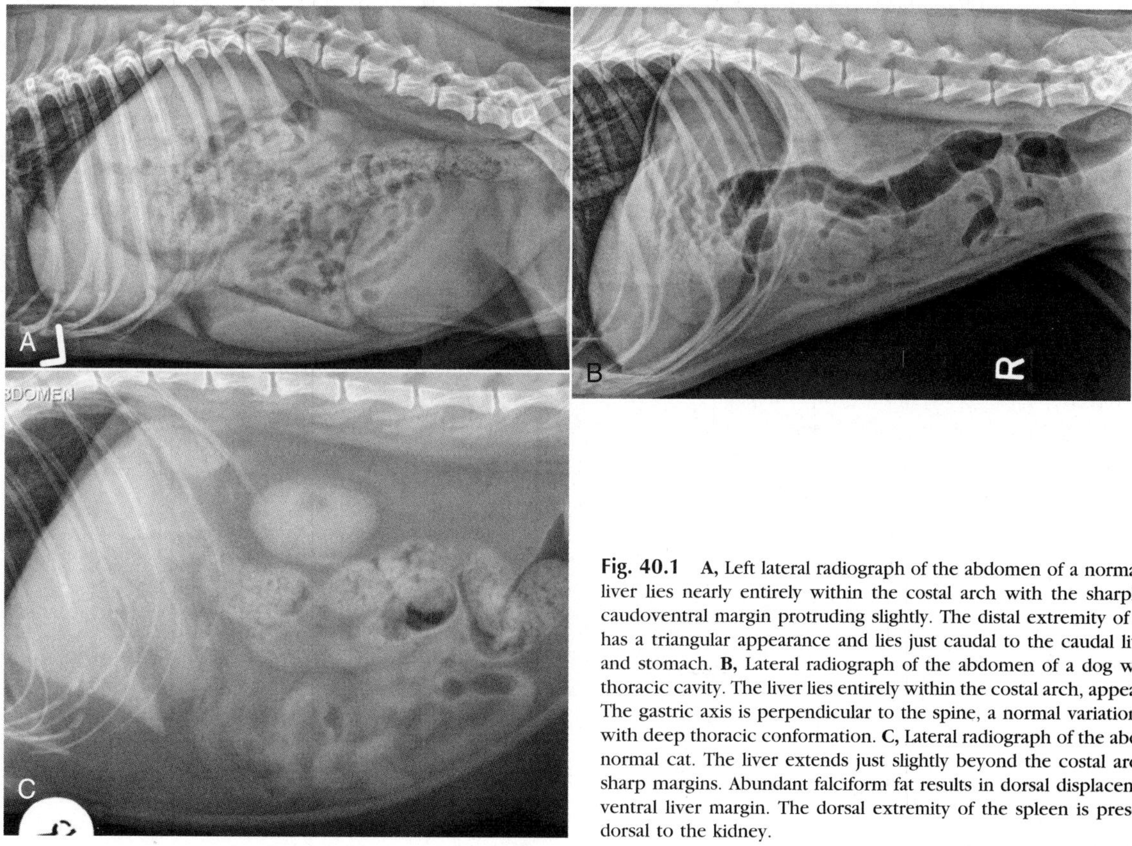

Fig. 40.1 **A,** Left lateral radiograph of the abdomen of a normal dog. The liver lies nearly entirely within the costal arch with the sharply outlined caudoventral margin protruding slightly. The distal extremity of the spleen has a triangular appearance and lies just caudal to the caudal liver margin and stomach. **B,** Lateral radiograph of the abdomen of a dog with a deep thoracic cavity. The liver lies entirely within the costal arch, appearing small. The gastric axis is perpendicular to the spine, a normal variation for a dog with deep thoracic conformation. **C,** Lateral radiograph of the abdomen of a normal cat. The liver extends just slightly beyond the costal arch and has sharp margins. Abundant falciform fat results in dorsal displacement of the ventral liver margin. The dorsal extremity of the spleen is present craniodorsal to the kidney.

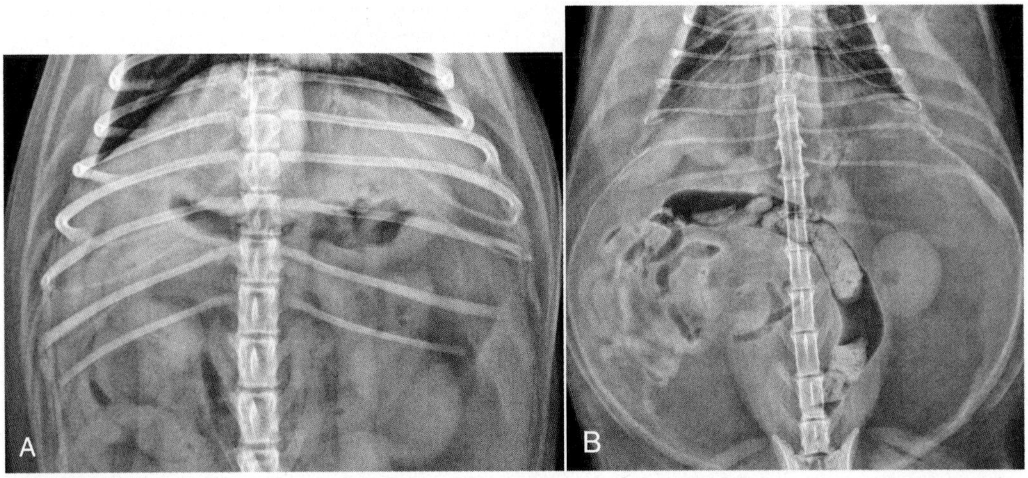

Fig. 40.2 **A,** Ventrodorsal (VD) radiograph of the cranial aspect of the abdomen of a normal dog. The liver lies cranial to and silhouettes the gastric shadow. **B,** VD radiograph of the abdomen of a normal cat. The liver is more to the right side than in a dog and is better visualized in this cat because of surrounding abundant fat.

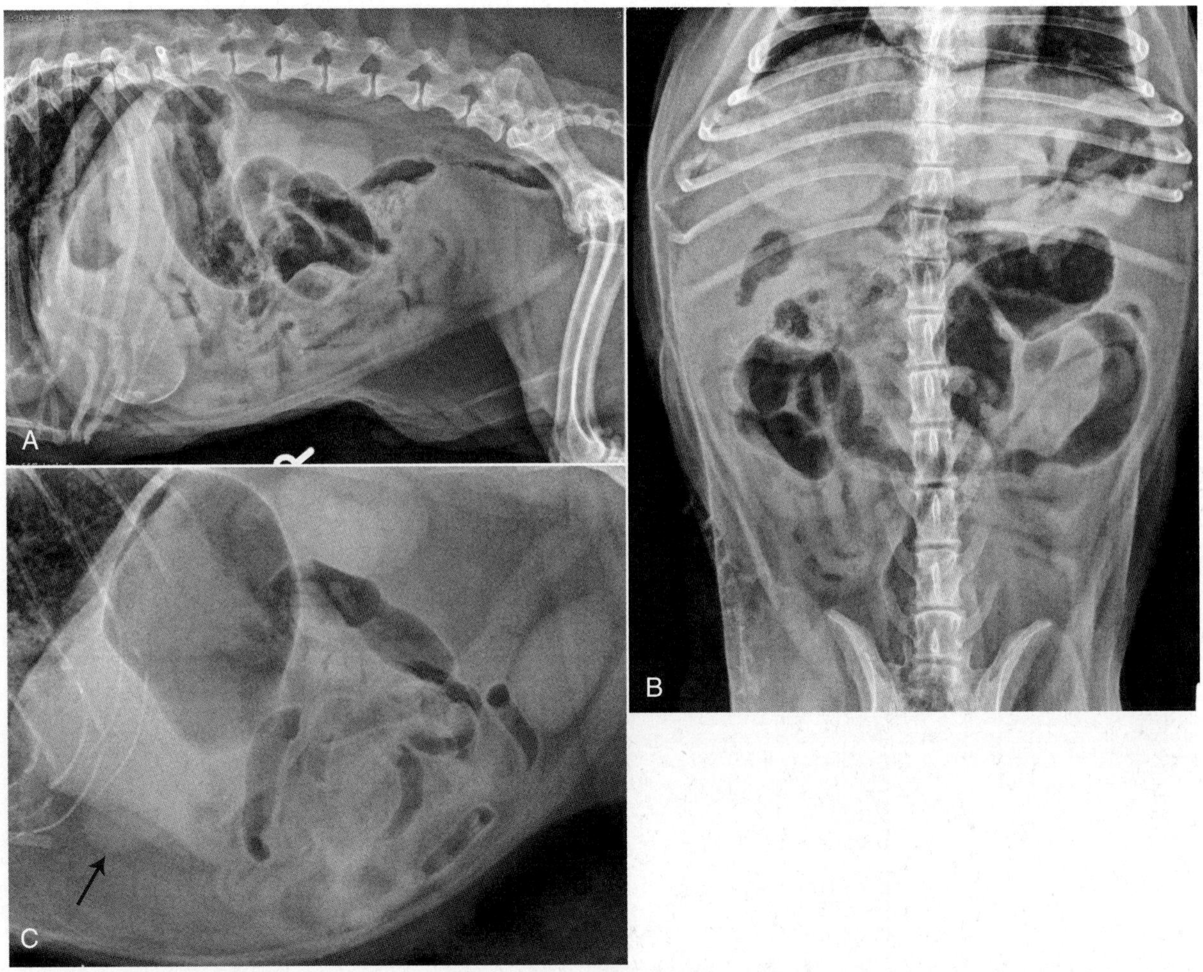

Fig. 40.3 Right lateral **(A)** and ventrodorsal (VD; **B**) radiographs of the abdomen in a dog with a history of elevated liver enzymes. The gallbladder is mineralized and is therefore conspicuous in the right cranial portion of the liver. **C,** Lateral abdomen radiograph of a cat presented for respiratory distress secondary to cardiogenic edema. The gallbladder can be seen protruding from the ventral aspect of the liver (*arrow*). This is a normal finding.

Hepatomegaly

Hepatic enlargement can be detected radiographically, although mild size changes cannot be assessed accurately. The classic radiographic signs of generalized hepatomegaly are rounding or blunting of the caudoventral liver margins, along with extension beyond the costal arch, and caudal, and perhaps medial, displacement of the gastric axis (Figs. 40.4 and 40.5).[5–7]

Several nonpathologic conditions can result in extension of hepatic margins beyond the costal arch, including overexpansion of the thorax or deep inspiration (Fig. 40.6). Older dogs and cats can have stretching or elongation of the triangular ligaments attaching the liver to the diaphragm, resulting in sagging and caudal extension of the liver. The same phenomenon can occur in obese dogs with a pendulous abdomen. In the obese dog, the liver does not extend as far dorsally. Some brachycephalic and chondrodystrophic dogs have caudal extension of the liver because of it being aligned more horizontally compared with deep-chested breeds. In addition, neonatal and young dogs and cats have a larger liver size compared with body size, creating the appearance of hepatomegaly without a true hepatic abnormality (Fig. 40.7).[1,8] Because of the numerous normal variations that can cause hepatic lobe extension beyond the costal arch, rounding or blunting of these lobes should also be present before hepatomegaly is concluded.

With generalized hepatomegaly, caudal displacement of the stomach, right kidney, transverse colon, and cranial duodenal flexure may occur, along with dorsal displacement of the

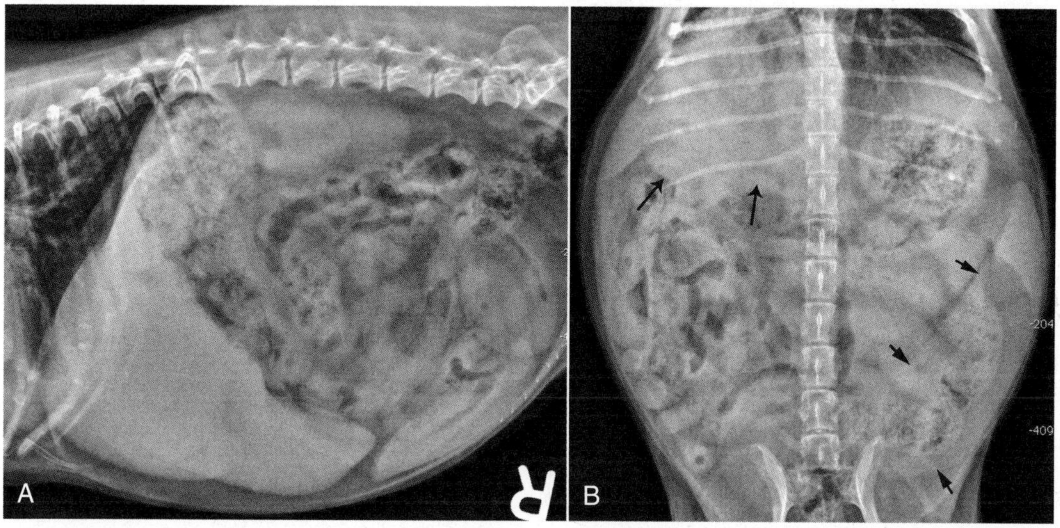

Fig. 40.4 Lateral (**A**) and ventrodorsal (VD; **B**) radiographs of a dog with generalized hepatomegaly secondary to steroid hepatopathy. The liver has rounded, blunt margins and extends well beyond the costal arch resulting in caudal displacement of adjacent viscera (*long black arrows* on VD view). On the VD view, the normal spleen is noted along the left lateral wall (*short black arrows*).

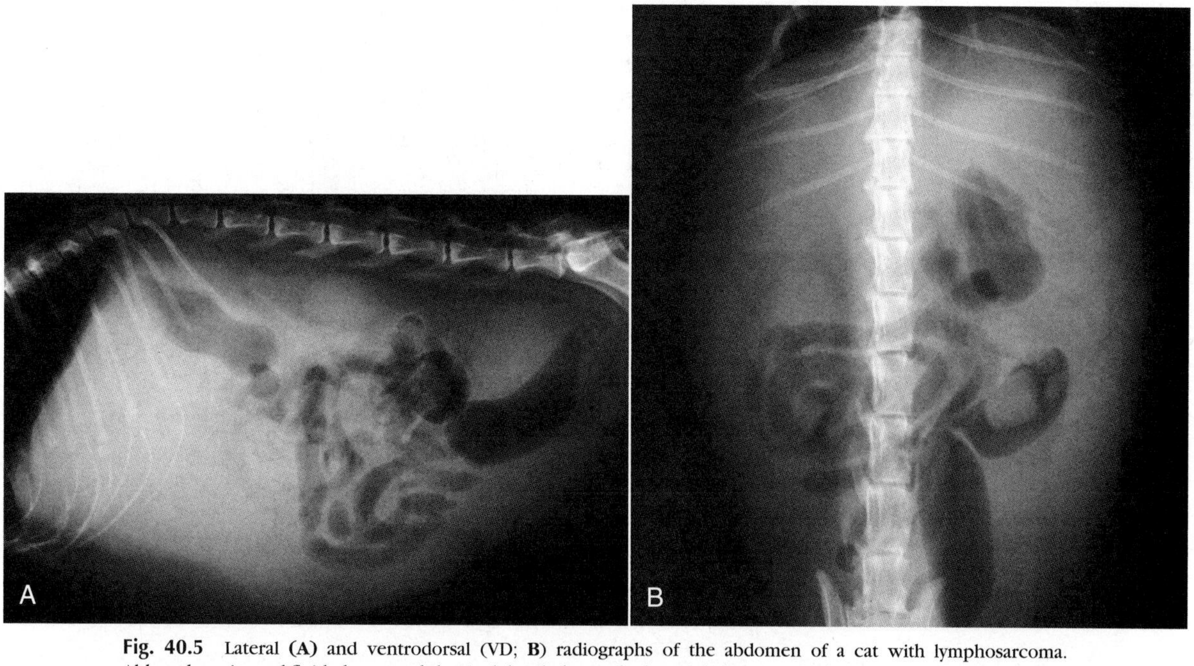

Fig. 40.5 Lateral (**A**) and ventrodorsal (VD; **B**) radiographs of the abdomen of a cat with lymphosarcoma. Although peritoneal fluid obscures abdominal detail, the marked caudal, dorsal, and left-sided gastric displacement is consistent with severe hepatomegaly.

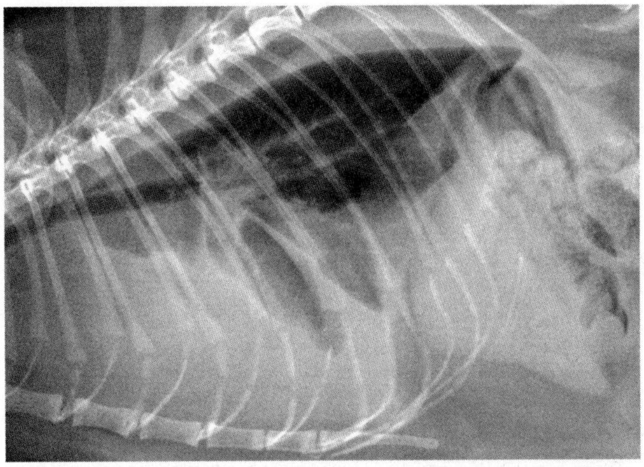

Fig. 40.6 Lateral radiograph of the thorax of a cat with pleural effusion. The overexpanded thorax results in caudal displacement of the diaphragm and liver margins with subsequent apparent hepatomegaly. The liver margins remain relatively sharp.

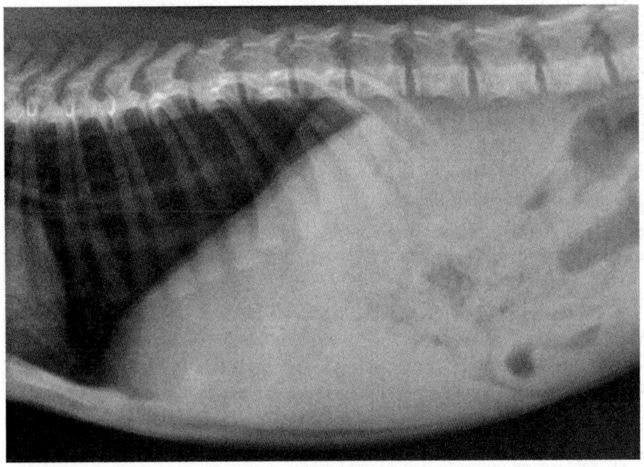

Fig. 40.7 Lateral radiograph of the abdomen of a normal puppy. The liver is large compared with overall abdominal size, which is a normal finding in young dogs and cats.

pylorus. On VD views, the enlarged liver will cause displacement of the body and pyloric portion of the stomach caudally, and to the left (see Fig. 40.4). Both lateral and VD abdominal views should be examined to evaluate liver size because hepatomegaly is sometimes obvious only on one view.

Causes of generalized hepatomegaly are numerous, and radiographs alone are insufficient in most instances to narrow the list. Hepatic congestion, vacuolar hepatopathy, inflammatory and infiltrative disease, and storage disease are all possibilities. Hepatic ultrasound can be used to determine internal architecture and is better suited than radiography for narrowing the list of considerations for hepatomegaly.

Visualization of focal hepatomegaly depends on the degree of enlargement and the lobe affected. Focal hepatic masses usually result in distortion of the hepatic outline and are continuous with the liver in at least one projection.[5–7] Left hepatic masses result in displacement of the stomach and spleen dorsally and to the right. Right-sided hepatic masses displace the stomach and duodenum to the left and dorsally and the small bowel caudally (Figs. 40.8 and 40.9, eFig. 40.1). The right kidney and distal extremity of the spleen may also be displaced caudally by a right-sided hepatic mass.

With few exceptions, masses located cranial to the ventral aspect of the stomach are hepatic in origin.[6] Although hepatic masses classically result in caudal displacement of the stomach, a focal mass can extend caudal to the stomach (Fig. 40.10, eFig. 40.2).[7] Differentiation of a caudally located, pedunculated hepatic mass from a splenic mass based on radiographs alone is difficult. Differentials for focal hepatic masses include primary and metastatic neoplasia, abscess, granuloma, and hepatic cyst.

Microhepatia

As with subtle hepatomegaly, slight decreases in hepatic size are not identified accurately radiographically. Marked microhepatia results in cranial displacement of the stomach and decreased distance between the diaphragm and gastric lumen (Fig. 40.11). Hepatic atrophy due to a congenital portosystemic shunt and chronic hepatopathy such as fibrosis or cirrhosis are the two most common causes of microhepatia. Diaphragmatic hernia with displacement of the liver cranial to the diaphragm can give the appearance of a small liver, but there will be intrathoracic abnormalities in this instance.

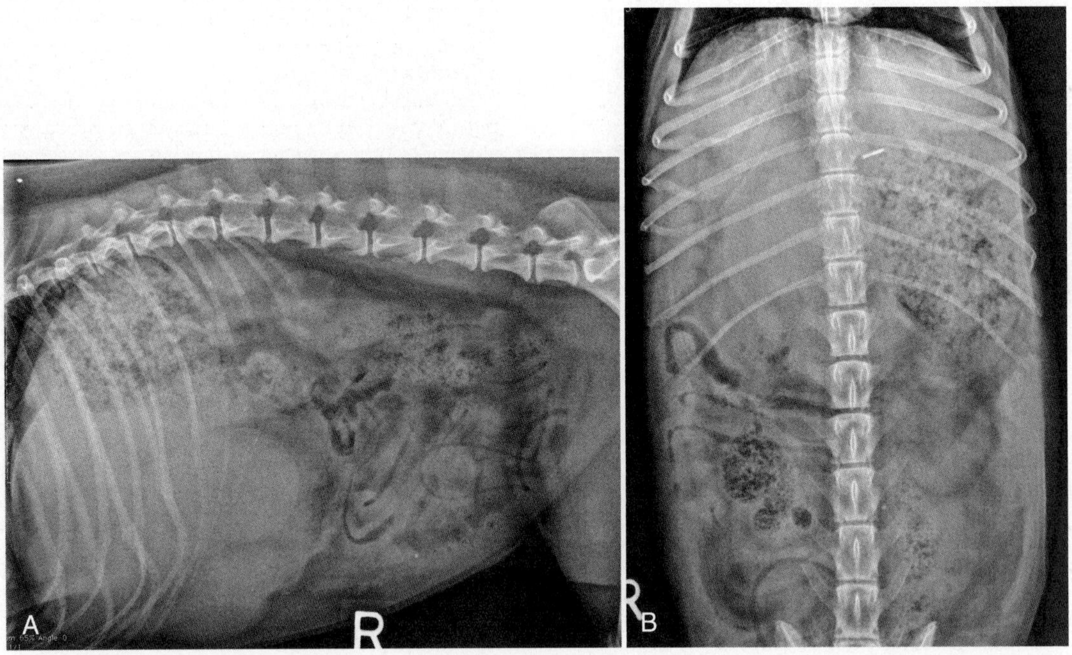

Fig. 40.8 Lateral (**A**) and ventrodorsal (VD; **B**) radiographs of the abdomen of a dog with hepatocellular carcinoma. The liver is focally enlarged with rounded margins.

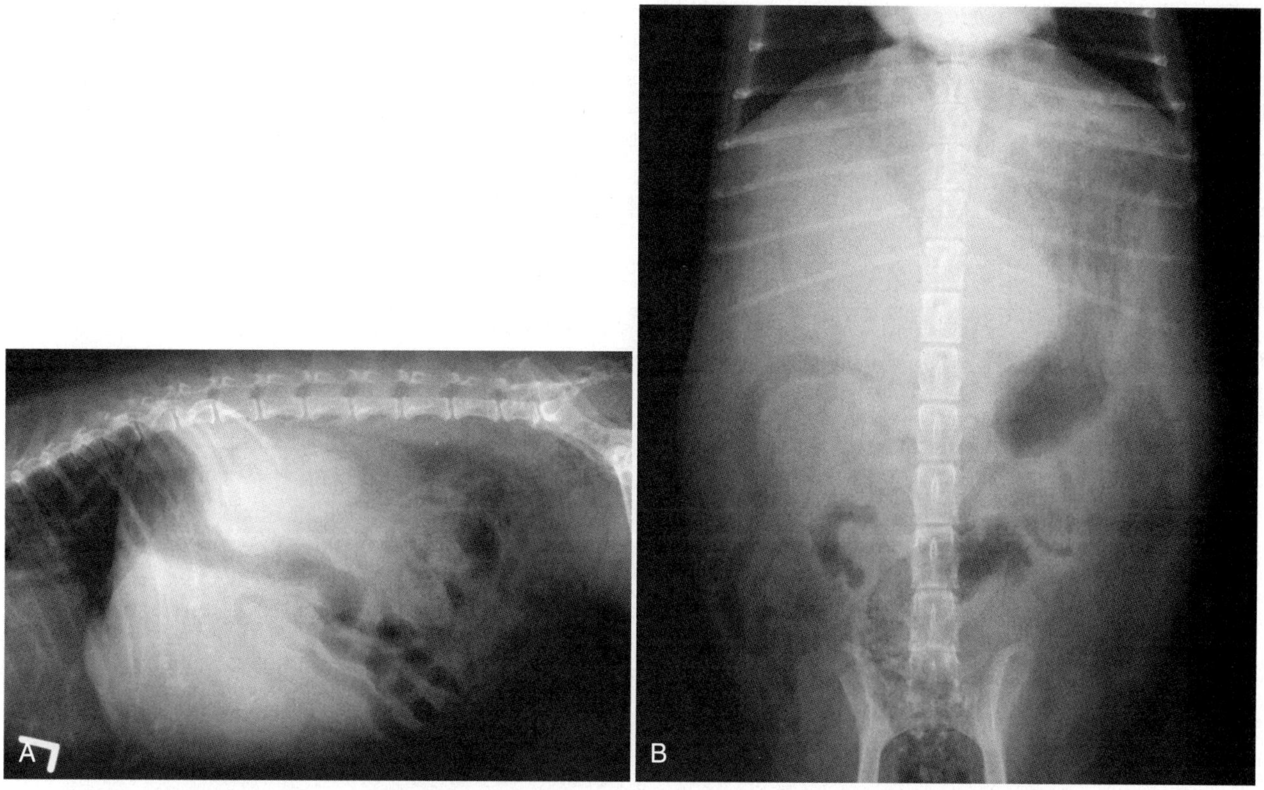

Fig. 40.9 Lateral (**A**) and ventrodorsal (VD; **B**) radiographs of the abdomen of a dog with hepatocellular carcinoma. The right side of the liver is enlarged, resulting in caudal, dorsal, and left-sided displacement of the stomach. The small bowel is displaced caudally. Faint mineralization is present in the ventral portion of the liver on the lateral view.

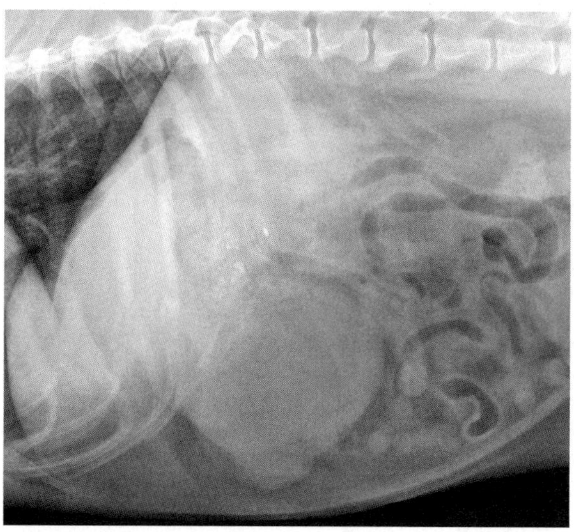

Fig. 40.10 Lateral radiograph of the abdomen of a dog with hepatic carcinoma. The hepatic mass extends caudal to the stomach, mimicking a splenic mass.

Hepatic Opacity

The normal liver is of soft tissue opacity. Mineral opacities can occur in the hepatic parenchyma or biliary system.[9] Choleliths should be considered when focal mineral opacities are visible in the area of the gallbladder (Fig. 40.12). Linear trails of mineralized opacities extending peripherally within the hepatic parenchyma are indicative of choledocholiths, or calculi within the bile ducts.[9] Biliary calculi are uncommon in dogs and cats but are visible radiographically if they contain sufficient calcium (see Fig. 40.12).[10–13] These are often incidental findings, but choledocholiths can cause biliary obstruction, especially in the cat. Mineralization of the biliary tree is seen occasionally in dogs with bile duct carcinoma.[14] Mineralization of the gallbladder wall has been associated with gallbladder carcinoma, as well as cholecystitis or cystic mucinous hyperplasia (see Fig. 40.3A,B).[13]

Dystrophic calcification of hepatic granulomas, abscesses, hematomas, neoplastic masses, or areas of hepatic necrosis have been documented (see Fig. 40.9). Echinococcosis infection can result in large hepatic soft tissue masses with mineralization of varying patterns and should be considered in endemic areas.[15]

Radiolucent areas within the liver are indicative of intrahepatic gas, either in the biliary system, portal venous system, or hepatic parenchyma. Gas within portal vessels may occur because of severe necrotizing gastritis or enteritis, which is often associated with gastric dilation and volvulus complex. Gastrointestinal ulceration, distention, trauma, or interventional procedures may allow gas to ascend into the portovenous circulation (Fig. 40.13A, eFig. 40.3).[16–18] A linear, branching radiolucent appearance, similar to air bronchograms, may be visible.

Gas in or around the gallbladder occurs with emphysematous cholecystitis, and this can be found in both diabetic and nondiabetic dogs.[19,20] Gas is seen initially in the gallbladder wall, followed by more complete filling of the lumen (see Fig. 40.13B,C). The gas eventually extends to the pericholecystic tissues. Gas bubbles conforming to the shape of the distended gallbladder can be seen within 24 to 48 hours of onset of disease. Obstruction of the cystic duct may be a common predisposing factor for emphysematous cholecystitis. Gas lucencies within the biliary system can also be seen after surgery of the duodenum or biliary system. Incidental reflux of

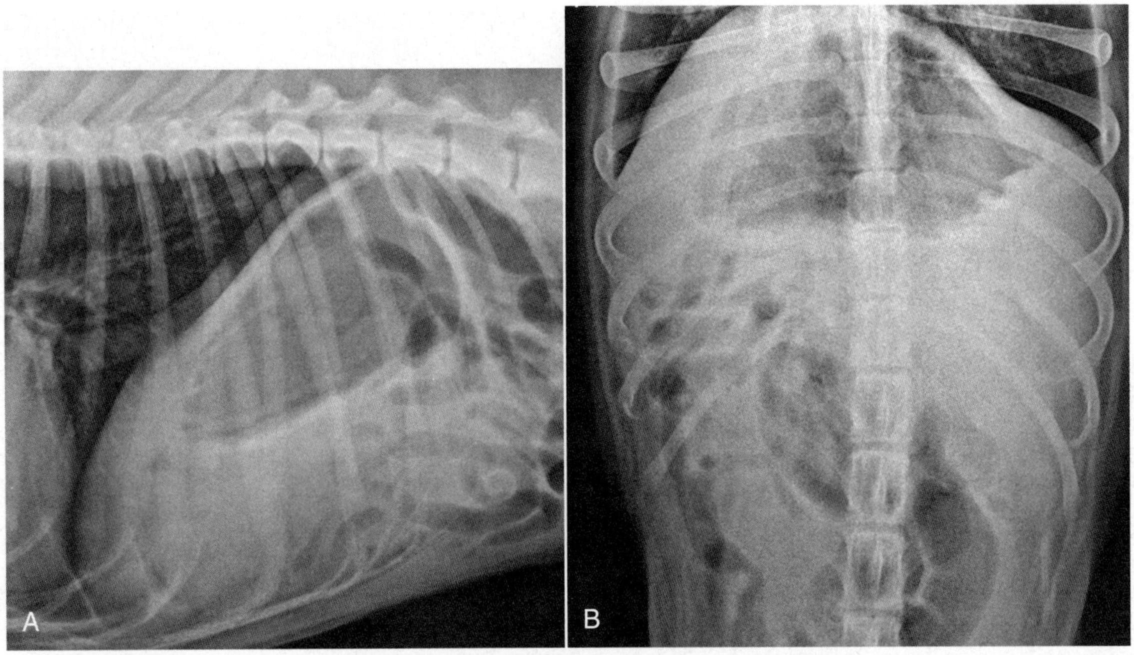

Fig. 40.11 Lateral (A) and ventrodorsal (VD; B) radiographs of the abdomen of a dog with chronic hepatitis that led to microhepatia. There is marked cranial displacement of the stomach.

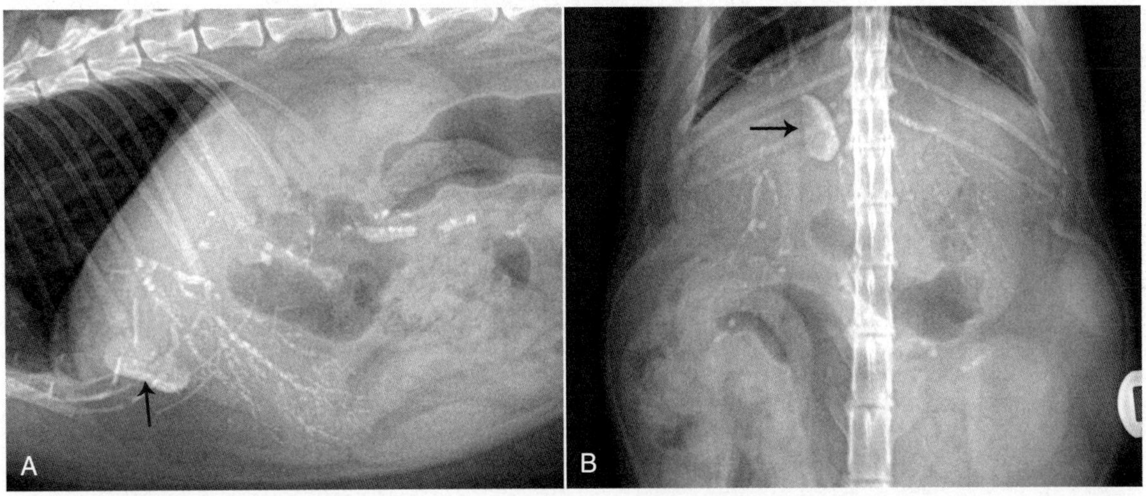

Fig. 40.12 Lateral (A) and ventrodorsal (VD; B) radiographs of a cat with a large radiopaque cholelith (*arrow*) and trails of mineralized choledocholiths and pancreatoliths.

gas into the bile duct from the duodenum is occasionally seen in cats. This may be because of incompetence of the sphincter of Oddi.[2]

Hepatic abscess with gas-forming organisms may result in gas opacities within the hepatic parenchyma.[21,22] These abscesses appear as irregularly stippled or mottled gas patterns, usually in a localized area (Fig. 40.14). Hepatomegaly or a hepatic mass is typically present with hepatic abscess with or without gas formation. Abscesses may be secondary to necrotic tumors, ascending portal infection, adjacent infection (pancreatitis), or penetrating wounds.

COMPUTED TOMOGRAPHY OF THE LIVER

Most common indications for computed tomography (CT) of the liver currently are vascular malformations and hepatic masses.

Vascular Malformations

Portosystemic shunts are congenital or acquired anomalies of the portal vasculature in which blood bypasses the liver and enters the systemic circulation directly. In the past, radiographic techniques have been used to identify and characterize the anomalous vessels, including cranial mesenteric portography, percutaneous splenoportography, and operative mesenteric portography.[23–26] CT angiography has largely replaced radiographic portography in the evaluation of portosystemic shunts.[27–32] CT is minimally invasive and provides delineation of the portal vein and portal tributaries following intravenous injection of contrast medium (Fig. 40.15, eFig. 40.4). Reformatted images in different planes or 3D renderings can be created to provide detailed evaluation of the vascular malformation, and aid in surgical planning. With dual-phase CT angiography, postcontrast images are acquired during calculated peak hepatic arterial and portal venous phases. In a survey of CT angiography studies, the most common

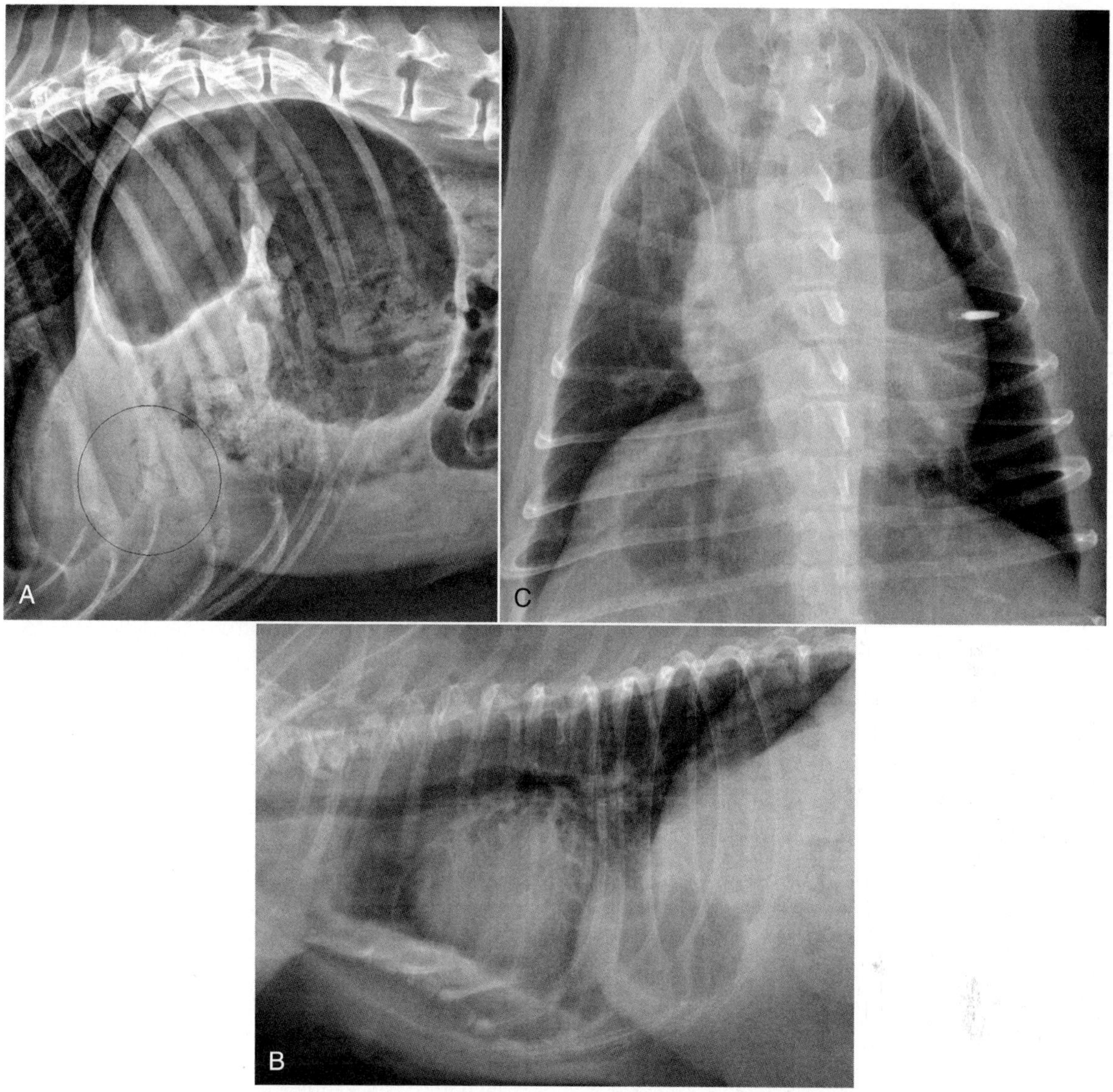

Fig. 40.13 Radiolucencies in liver. **A,** Lateral cranial abdominal radiograph of a dog with gastric dilatation and volvulus. Gas is visible in the portal vasculature of the liver (within *circle*) **(B)** lateral and **(C)** ventrodorsal thoracic radiographs of a dog with emphysematous cholecystitis. Gas completely fills the gallbladder lumen.

extrahepatic shunts identified were (named from origin to insertion) spleno-phrenic, spleno-azygous, spleno-caval, left or right gastric-caval, and right gastric-caval with caudal loop.[31,32] Arterioportal communications are rare congenital disorders where an abnormal connection between the hepatic arterial and the portal venous system is formed. CT findings include early contrast enhancement of the portal venous system in the arterial phase and typically a cluster of enlarged, tortuous vessels in a portion of the liver (eFig. 40.5).[33–35]

Hepatic Masses

CT is commonly used for evaluation of hepatic masses, helping to determine exact location in terms of lobe or lobes involved, vascular involvement, and extent of disease for surgical planning. Multiphase contrast-enhanced CT protocols have been used to evaluate patterns of contrast uptake of hepatic masses to help differentiate benign from malignant disease.[36–38] In triple-phase studies, postcontrast images are acquired at 13 to 20 seconds (hepatic arterial phase), 30 to 40 seconds (early portal venous phase), and 120 seconds (equilibrium or delayed phase) after injection.[36,37] In these studies, most hepatocellular carcinomas had heterogeneous enhancement in all phases, and were hypoattenuating compared to normal liver parenchyma in the portal and delayed phase (Fig. 40.16). Metastatic lesions within the liver were homogeneous, with hypoattenuation compared to normal liver in all postcontrast phases. Benign hepatic adenomas had more diffuse enhancement in the hepatic arterial phase, with persistent enhancement in the portal venous phase. Finally, nodular hyperplastic lesions were homogeneous, often with marked contrast enhancement in the hepatic arterial and portal venous phases, with isoattenuation compared to normal hepatic parenchyma in the delayed phase. In a similar study using dual-phase contrast imaging, with images acquired within 30 seconds and at least 60 seconds post initiation of contrast administration, no CT features were significantly associated with benign or malignant hepatic lesions.[38] There appears to be enough overlap in the contrast enhancement pattern of benign and malignant lesions, that CT findings alone are not sufficient to accurately predict the type of disease. Histopathology remains the gold standard.[38]

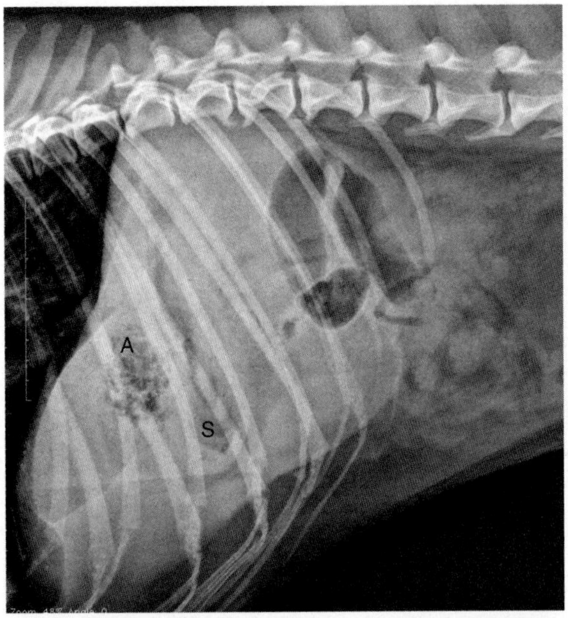

Fig. 40.14 Lateral abdominal radiograph of a dog with hepatic abscessation. Stippled radiolucencies in the cranial margin of the liver represent gas within the abscess. *A*, Abscess; *S*, stomach.

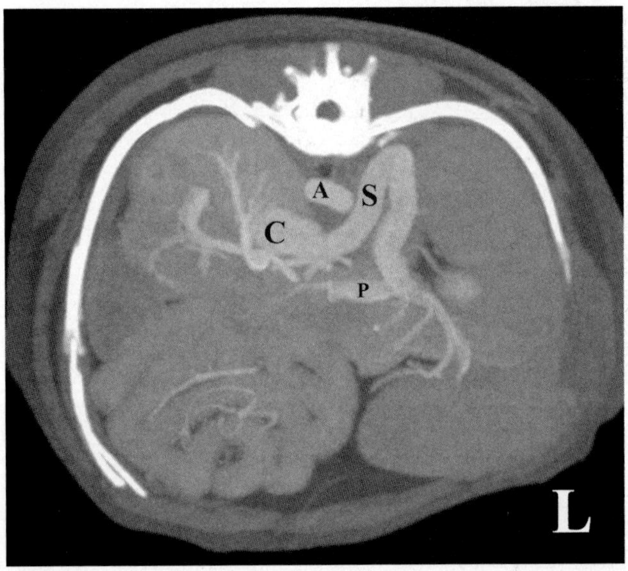

Fig. 40.15 Maximum intensity projection (MIP) reformatted transverse computed tomography angiogram of the cranial abdomen. A large tortuous extrahepatic shunting vessel (*S*) extends from the portal vein (*P*) into the caudal vena cava (*C*). *A*, Aorta; *L*, left.

ULTRASOUND OF THE LIVER

Ultrasound examination of the liver allows detailed evaluation of hepatic internal architecture, including the hepatic vasculature and biliary system. Ultrasound is also useful in guiding aspirates and biopsies for nonsurgical, less invasive diagnoses.

The liver can be imaged through a combination of subcostal, subxiphoid, and right and left intercostal windows. Intercostal windows may be the best way to evaluate the liver in a deep-chested dog, patients with gas-distended stomach, or in dogs with microhepatia. The right dorsal intercostal window allows excellent visibility of the porta hepatis, the caudate liver lobe, and the right kidney in many dogs. This window can also be used in cats but is not as often needed. Transducer frequencies ranging from 5 to 10MHz will accommodate most small animal patients. Transducers with smaller footprints are best for intercostal windows.

Based on the individual scatter pattern, each abdominal organ has a characteristic texture and appearance. The liver has a moderately coarse texture and is usually hypoechoic to the spleen and, in cats, the falciform fat (Fig. 40.17).[39–41] When using the right renal cortex for comparison to the caudate liver lobe, the liver may be isoechoic, or slightly hypoechoic or hyperechoic. The use of the renal cortex for comparison is therefore limited. The renal cortex of many normal cats is hyperechoic due to lipid deposition, and this should be considered before interpreting the liver as hypoechoic.[42] Assessment of echogenicity in any organ is subjective and any change should be correlated with the overall clinical picture.

Hepatic margins should be smooth and sharp but are better delineated ultrasonographically if adjacent peritoneal fluid is present (Fig. 40.18). The liver is bordered cranially and dorsally by an echogenic line representing the interface between the diaphragm and lung/pleura. A mirror-image artifact is frequently noted deep to the diaphragmatic interface, giving the false impression of liver on both sides of the diaphragm (see Chapter 3).

As with assessing echogenicity, the ultrasound assessment of liver size is subjective and based on operator experience, patient conformation, and adjacent organs. A small liver is difficult to evaluate sonographically, because gas from a more cranial located stomach can obscure it. The gallbladder may appear large relative to overall hepatic size (Fig. 40.19). Liver size may appear decreased in dogs with a deep thoracic cavity where liver location is more completely within the costal arch. Intercostal ultrasound windows may be needed in these patients. The enlarged liver can be examined relatively easily with ultrasound, because it extends well beyond the xiphoid cartilage and covers the right kidney more completely (Fig. 40.20). Liver margins may appear rounded and may extend beyond the left lateral margin of the stomach.

Hepatic and portal veins are visible routinely within hepatic parenchyma. Portal veins are smoothly tapering vessels characterized by bright, echogenic borders (see Fig. 40.17E).[39,40] The larger left and smaller right branches originate from the main portal vein near the porta hepatis, although they branch in different imaging planes. Portal blood flow courses normally from the hepatic hilus toward the periphery. Hepatic veins are anechoic linear structures extending through the parenchyma. Hepatic vein borders are not echogenic except at their confluence with the caudal vena cava, immediately adjacent to the diaphragm. Hepatic venous flow courses normally toward the hepatic hilus, into the caudal vena cava. In many dogs, the right lateral dorsal intercostal window provides an excellent window to the aorta, caudal vena cava, and main portal vein (Fig. 40.21). Normal hepatic arteries are not visible without Doppler examination. The caudal vena cava courses through the liver in the right lateral abdominal quadrant. The hepatic artery is located between the caudal vena cava and portal vein, coursing cranially from the celiac artery. It may not be consistently identified without Doppler ultrasound.

The gallbladder is an oval, anechoic structure in the right cranioventral portion of the liver (see Fig. 40.17A). Gallbladder size varies widely, and distention is normal in fasted or anorexic patients. Normal gallbladder volume in the dog is 1 mL/kg or less body weight, and it can be measured with the ellipsoid formula (length × width × height × 0.52).[43,44] Cats may have a more uniform gallbladder volume of 2.4 mL, with no apparent association with body weight.[43,45] Intraluminal gallbladder contents are typically anechoic, although gallbladder sludge, which is dependent echogenic material without acoustic

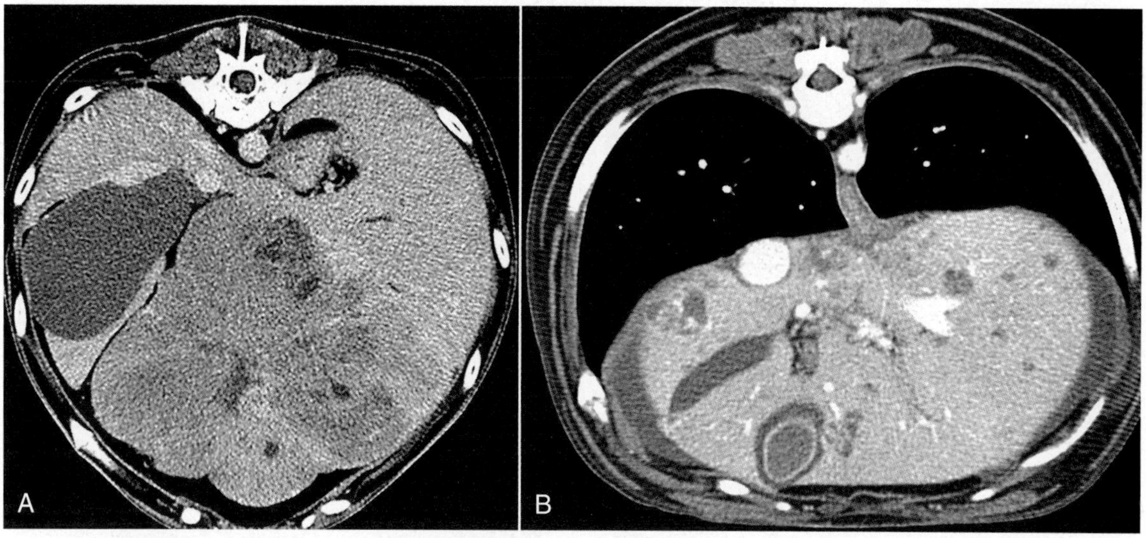

Fig. 40.16 Transverse postcontrast computed tomography images of dogs with hepatic neoplasia. In **A,** a large, hypoattenuating, lobular mass is present in the left lateral liver lobe. Hepatocellular carcinoma was diagnosed on histopathology post liver lobe resection. In **B,** multiple hypoattenuating nodules are noted throughout the hepatic parenchyma. The gallbladder wall is thickened, with a double-layered appearance. Hepatic metastasis secondary to a jejunal carcinoma was diagnosed on necropsy. Gallbladder wall edema was of undetermined etiology.

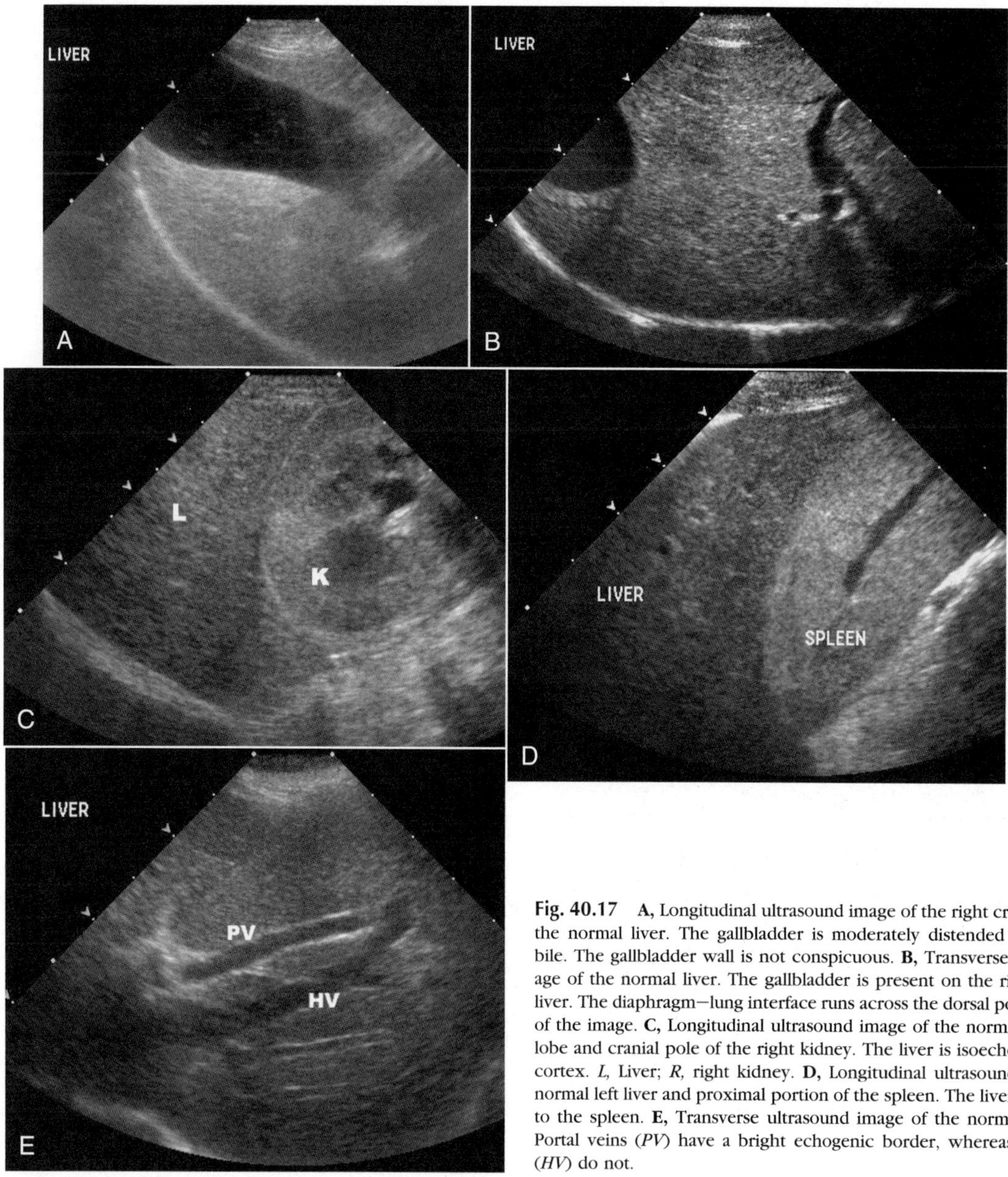

Fig. 40.17 **A,** Longitudinal ultrasound image of the right cranial portion of the normal liver. The gallbladder is moderately distended with anechoic bile. The gallbladder wall is not conspicuous. **B,** Transverse ultrasound image of the normal liver. The gallbladder is present on the right side of the liver. The diaphragm–lung interface runs across the dorsal portion (*bottom*) of the image. **C,** Longitudinal ultrasound image of the normal caudate liver lobe and cranial pole of the right kidney. The liver is isoechoic to the renal cortex. *L,* Liver; *R,* right kidney. **D,** Longitudinal ultrasound image of the normal left liver and proximal portion of the spleen. The liver is hypoechoic to the spleen. **E,** Transverse ultrasound image of the normal canine liver. Portal veins (*PV*) have a bright echogenic border, whereas hepatic veins (*HV*) do not.

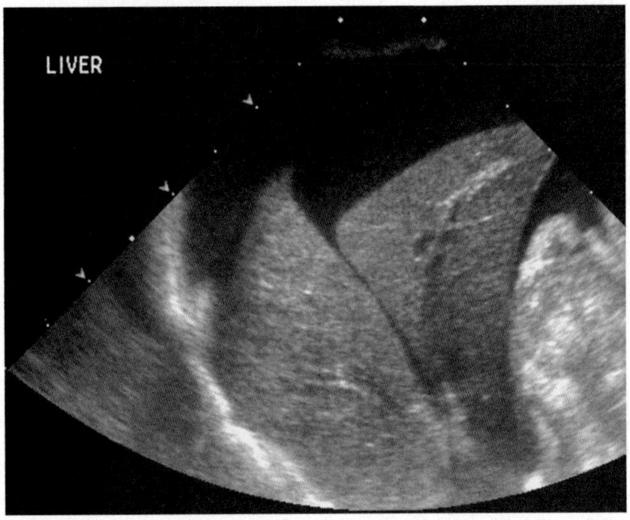

Fig. 40.18 Longitudinal ultrasound image of a dog with ascites. The normal liver lobes have a well-defined sharp, linear margin.

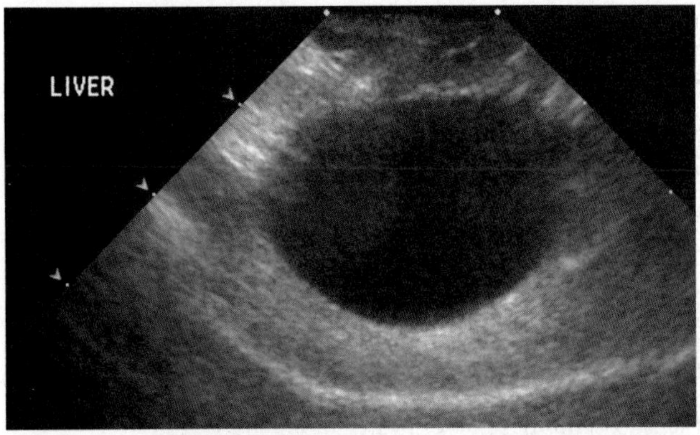

Fig. 40.19 Transverse ultrasound image of the liver in a dog with a small liver secondary to a portosystemic shunt. The liver is subjectively small with the gallbladder occupying a large portion.

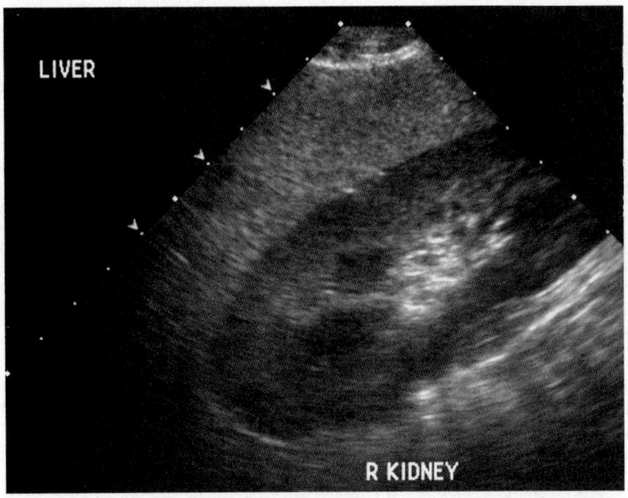

Fig. 40.20 Longitudinal ultrasound image of the caudate liver lobe and right kidney of a dog with hepatic lipidosis. The caudate lobe surrounds the right kidney completely, consistent with hepatomegaly. The liver is markedly hyperechoic to the renal cortex.

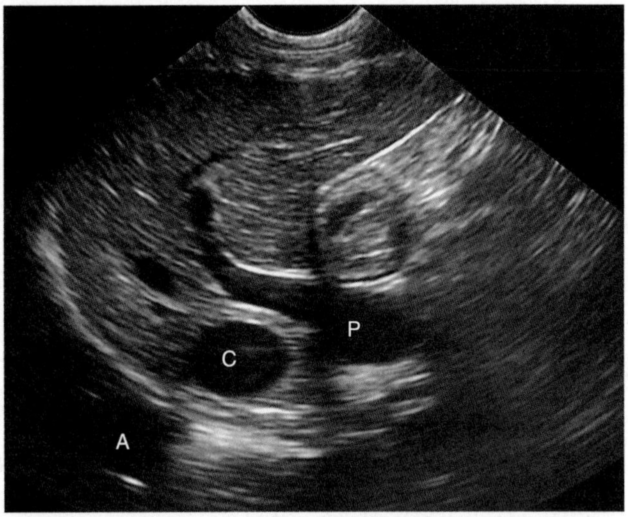

Fig. 40.21 Right lateral intercostal ultrasound image of a normal dog. Dorsal is at left and ventral is at right of the image. The top of the image represents the right abdominal wall with the left abdominal wall being at the bottom of the image. *A*, Aorta; *C*, caudal vena cava; *P*, portal vein.

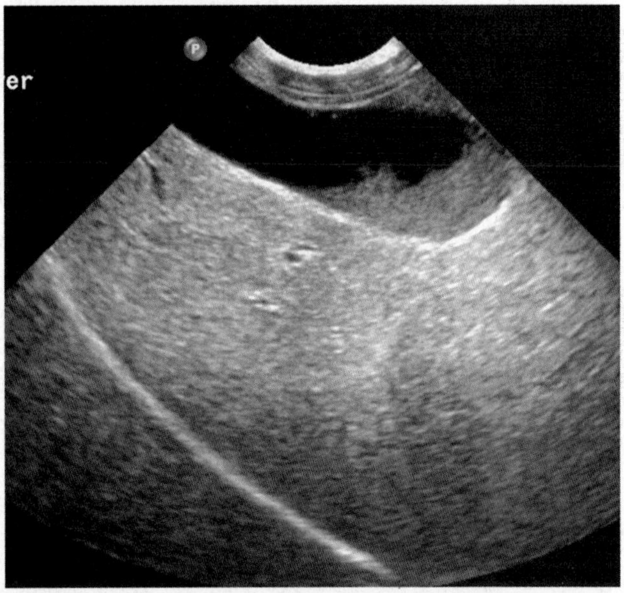

Fig. 40.22 Longitudinal ultrasound image of the liver and gallbladder of a normal dog. Echogenic biliary sludge is present in the dependent portion of the gallbladder.

shadowing, is seen frequently[46] (Fig. 40.22). Although sludge is common in dogs with no indication of biliary disease, one study suggests that it could be an indication of gallbladder dysmotility.[46–48] The normal gallbladder wall is thin and indistinct. In the cat, gallbladder wall thickness should be less than 1 mm or not visible at all.[49] The normal canine gallbladder wall typically measures 1 to 2 mm, but normal ranges have not been established.[48,50] A study of 74 normal dogs noted median gallbladder wall thickness of 1 mm.[48] A duplicate or septate gallbladder is seen occasionally as a normal variation in cats and is caused by abnormal embryonic development.[51] The common bile duct is immediately ventral to the portal vein but is visible more consistently in the cat, where it can usually be followed to the duodenal papilla (Fig. 40.23). Normal common bile duct diameter in the cat is 4 mm or less.[52] If visible, the canine bile duct should be 3 mm or less.[53] Normal intrahepatic bile ducts are not visible.

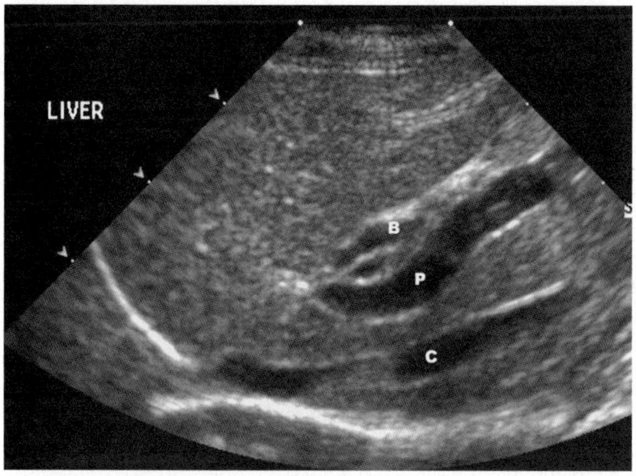

Fig. 40.23 Longitudinal ultrasound image of the liver in a normal cat. *B*, Bile duct; *C*, caudal vena cava; *P*, portal vein.

Abnormal Ultrasonographic Appearance of the Liver

Ultrasound is helpful in differentiating between diffuse and focal hepatic disease in patients with hepatomegaly and/or elevated liver enzymes. Diffuse hepatic disease may cause no change in the ultrasound appearance of the liver. However, changes in hepatic echogenicity, increase or decrease in size, and irregular or rounded margins point to diffuse hepatopathy.[39,40,54–56] A *hyperechoic* liver is identified by comparison with the echogenicity of an adjacent organ, such as being isoechoic or hyperechoic to spleen, or the in cats, the falciform fat. Loss or decreased conspicuity of the periportal echoes and abnormally increased attenuation of sound as it passes through the liver are indications of hyperechoic hepatic parenchyma (Fig. 40.24). Several diffuse hepatopathies can potentially result in either a diffusely hyperechoic liver, or a mottled appearance (i.e., hyperechoic parenchymal background with poorly defined hypoechoic nodules).[39,40,54–56] Vacuolar hepatopathies, including lipidosis and steroid hepatopathy, are likely the most frequent diagnosis when this appearance is seen (Fig. 40.25). Hepatic lipidosis in cats is a

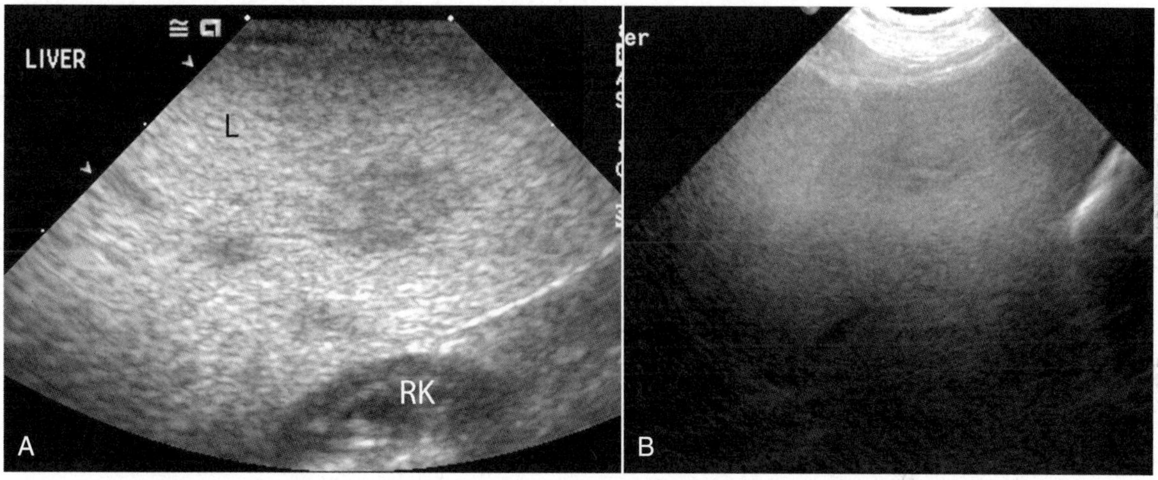

Fig. 40.24 **A,** Longitudinal ultrasound image of the caudate liver lobe and a portion of the right kidney (*RK*). The liver parenchyma is diffusely hyperechoic compared to the renal cortex, secondary to steroid hepatopathy. A few hypoechoic nodules (likely nodular hyperplasia) are present. *L*, Left. **B,** Transverse image of the liver from a dog with steroid hepatopathy. The liver is diffusely hyperechoic, with a dense texture resembling the spleen. Deeper portions of the liver are incompletely visualized due to exaggerated attenuation of the sound beam.

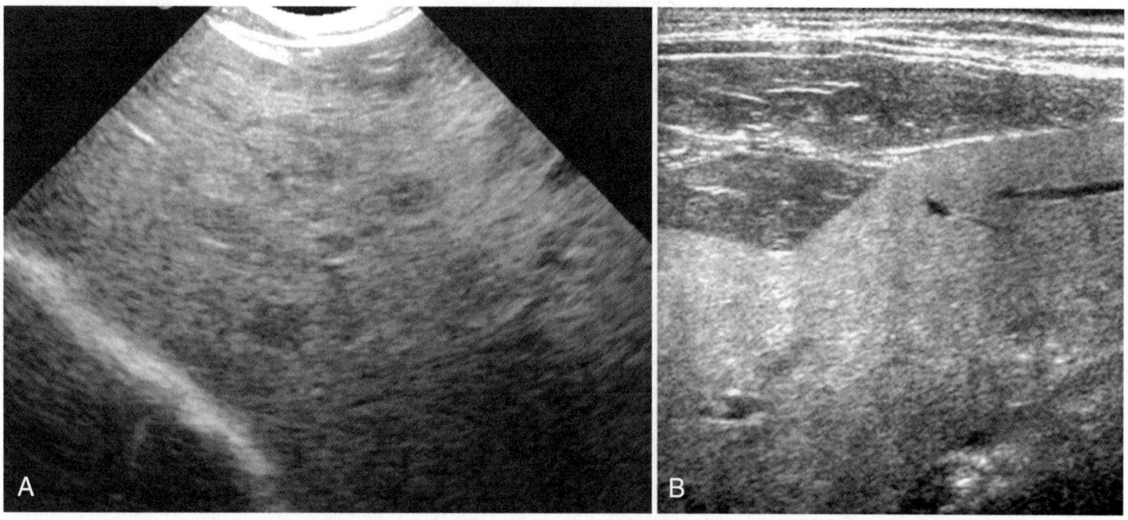

Fig. 40.25 **A,** Longitudinal ultrasound image of the liver with a mottled parenchyma (hyperechoic background with poorly defined hypoechoic nodules). Vacuolar hepatopathy was diagnosed on a fine needle aspirate. **B,** Transverse image of the liver in a cat with elevated liver enzymes. The liver parenchyma is markedly hyperechoic to adjacent falciform fat. Although this can be normal in some obese cats, hepatic lipidosis was diagnosed on cytology from a fine needle aspirate.

common diffuse feline hepatopathy, and it results in a liver parenchyma that is hyperechoic to adjacent falciform fat. However, a nonpathologic hyperechoic liver can be present in some obese cats, and ultrasound alone is likely insufficient for the diagnosis.[55,57] Chronic hepatitis with parenchymal fibrosis can also cause increased echogenicity, although liver size is variable and may be normal, increased, or decreased. Hepatic cirrhosis typically results in a small, irregular, hyperechoic liver, often with numerous hypoechoic nodules (Fig. 40.26). Ascites often accompanies cirrhosis secondary to portal hypertension. Other hepatic diseases that may result in increased/mottled parenchymal echogenicity include chronic hepatitis, lymphosarcoma, amyloidosis, and cholangiohepatitis. In cats with cholangitis/cholangiohepatitis complex, the liver can appear normal, or hyperechoic, secondary to lipidosis; hypoechoic liver may also occur.[55,57] Mast cell infiltration in the liver results in a variable appearance, from normal to increased echogenicity and size. Hypoechoic nodules may be present[58,59] (Fig. 40.27). However, the sonographic appearance of the liver (and spleen) may be a poor predictor of cytologic mast cell infiltration.[59–61]

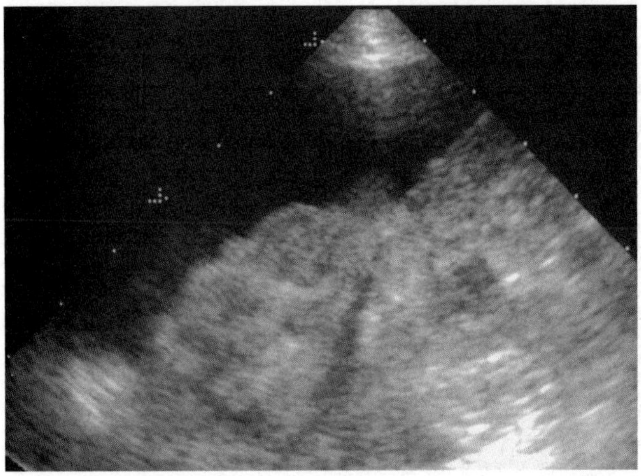

Fig. 40.26 Longitudinal ultrasound image of the liver in a dog with cirrhosis and ascites. The liver margins are irregular and rounded, and hypoechoic nodules are present within the parenchyma.

A decrease in hepatic echogenicity results in increased periportal echoes which is a somewhat subjective assessment. Decreased hepatic echogenicity may occur with hepatic congestion, lymphosarcoma, leukemia, amyloidosis, and cholangitis/cholangiohepatitis. A dilated caudal vena cava and hepatic veins will accompany hepatic congestion. Acute suppurative hepatitis such as leptospirosis can cause hypoechogenicity from inflammation and edema. However, this may be uncommon, even with severe disease.[54,62,71,83]

As noted previously, diffuse, even severe hepatic disease can appear normal ultrasonographically. Acoustic impedance of normal versus diseased tissue may simply be insufficient to permit visible change.[76,84,85] Any suspected hepatopathy should be compared with clinical signs and laboratory data, and a biopsy is necessary for definitive diagnosis.[63–66] Prebiopsy coagulation screening is a useful precaution when liver disease is suspected.

Focal hepatic disease appears as a nodule or mass that differs in texture and echogenicity from surrounding normal liver parenchyma. They may interrupt the hepatic margin, resulting in change of shape or contour. Relatively small nodules can be detected, especially when using high-frequency transducers. Although ultrasound is sensitive for detecting hepatic nodules, it is not specific, and numerous considerations are possible for focal disease. Cysts, abscesses, primary or metastatic neoplasia, hematomas, granulomas, nodular hyperplasia, and focal extramedullary hematopoiesis can all produce focal hepatic disease and may be difficult to differentiate on the basis of ultrasound appearance alone.[39,40,56,67] However, ultrasound is extremely useful in differentiating cystic versus solid masses; focal, multifocal, or diffuse distribution of masses; and the relation of the mass to adjacent structures, such as large blood vessels, diaphragm, or gallbladder.

Hepatic neoplastic masses are variable in appearance, and they can be hyperechoic, hypoechoic, or of mixed echogenicity, solid, cystic, or cavitated (Fig. 40.28).[68–80] The ultrasound appearance is not specific for a particular tumor, and as in diffuse disease, there appears to be poor correlation to cytologic and histopathologic diagnosis.[39,40,55,56,58,60,67,81–83] A positive cytological diagnosis of neoplasia is often accurate, but a negative cytologic evaluation does not rule out neoplasia.[83] Primary hepatic tumors are classified as massive (e.g., with a solitary mass affecting a single lobe), multifocal

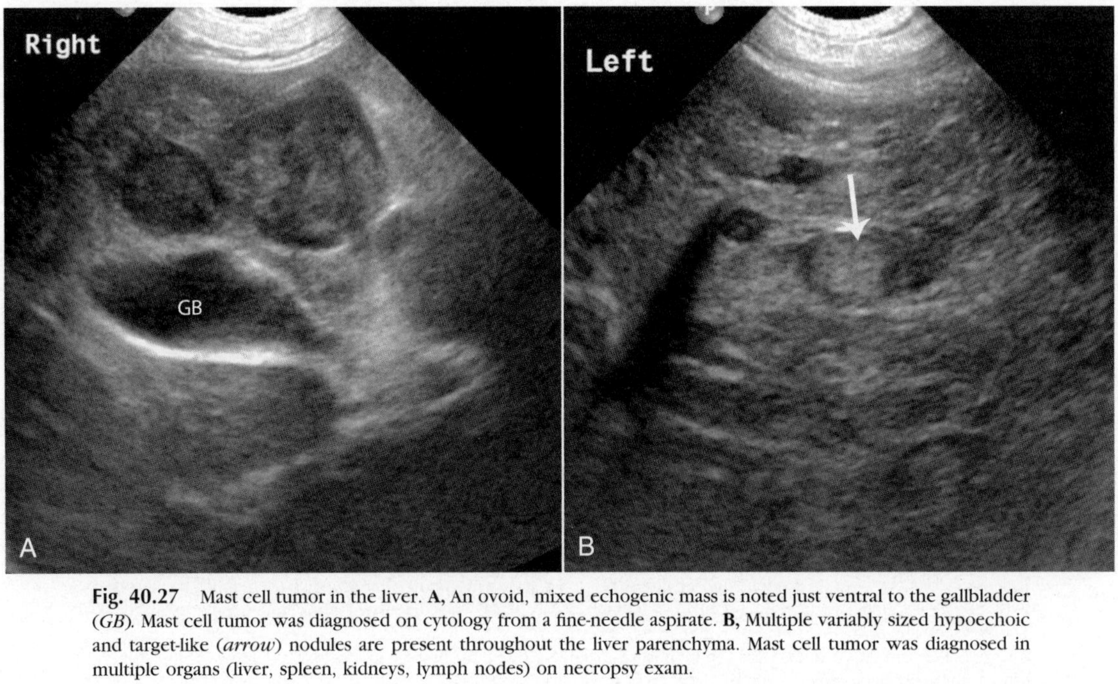

Fig. 40.27 Mast cell tumor in the liver. **A,** An ovoid, mixed echogenic mass is noted just ventral to the gallbladder (*GB*). Mast cell tumor was diagnosed on cytology from a fine-needle aspirate. **B,** Multiple variably sized hypoechoic and target-like (*arrow*) nodules are present throughout the liver parenchyma. Mast cell tumor was diagnosed in multiple organs (liver, spleen, kidneys, lymph nodes) on necropsy exam.

(e.g., with nodular disease in multiple lobes), and diffuse (e.g., multifocal coalescing nodules in all lobes).[70,73] Hepatocellular carcinoma is the most common primary tumor in the dog, and it is most often massive in classification (see Fig. 40.28A). Other primary hepatic tumors include cholangiocarcinoma, which is the second most common primary hepatic neoplasia in the dog, neuroendocrine tumor, hemangiosarcoma, and histiocytic sarcoma (see Fig. 40.28B).[70–75] Hepatic lymphosarcoma may result in a normal-appearing liver, or a diffuse increase or decrease in echogenicity; more focal changes include hypoechoic nodules/areas (see Fig. 40.28C).[64,83] Metastatic disease in the liver is the most common hepatic malignancy in the dog at 2.5 times the frequency of primary hepatic neoplasia, and most often originates from the spleen, gastrointestinal tract, and pancreas.[72] Like primary hepatic neoplasia, metastatic disease may be hyperechoic or hypoechoic, but more often it has a multifocal nodular or mass-like appearance (see Fig. 40.28D).[68,69,82] Metastatic disease cannot be differentiated from primary hepatic malignancy based solely on the ultrasound appearance.[68,69,82] Target lesions, which are focal masses with a hyperechoic center and hypoechoic periphery, are most commonly associated with malignancy, but they have been reported with benign disease processes (see Fig. 40.27B).[41,67,84] Biliary cystadenoma (bile duct adenoma) is the most common primary hepatic neoplasia in the cat, and it may be focal or multifocal.[75–80] Although variable in appearance, the presence of a cystic component somewhere in the mass is a consistent finding (Fig. 40.29). Biliary cystadenomas may appear multilocular, containing thin-walled cysts, or as hyperechoic masses with a cystic component. Most cystic portions of these masses will be characterized by acoustic enhancement. Cholangiocarcinoma is the most common feline primary hepatic malignancy.[75–80]

Hepatic nodular hyperplasia, a common benign lesion in older dogs, is usually silent clinically but may result in elevations in serum alkaline phosphatase.[71,85,86] It has a variety of sonographic appearances and cannot be differentiated from neoplasia without biopsy (Fig. 40.30). Hyperechoic,

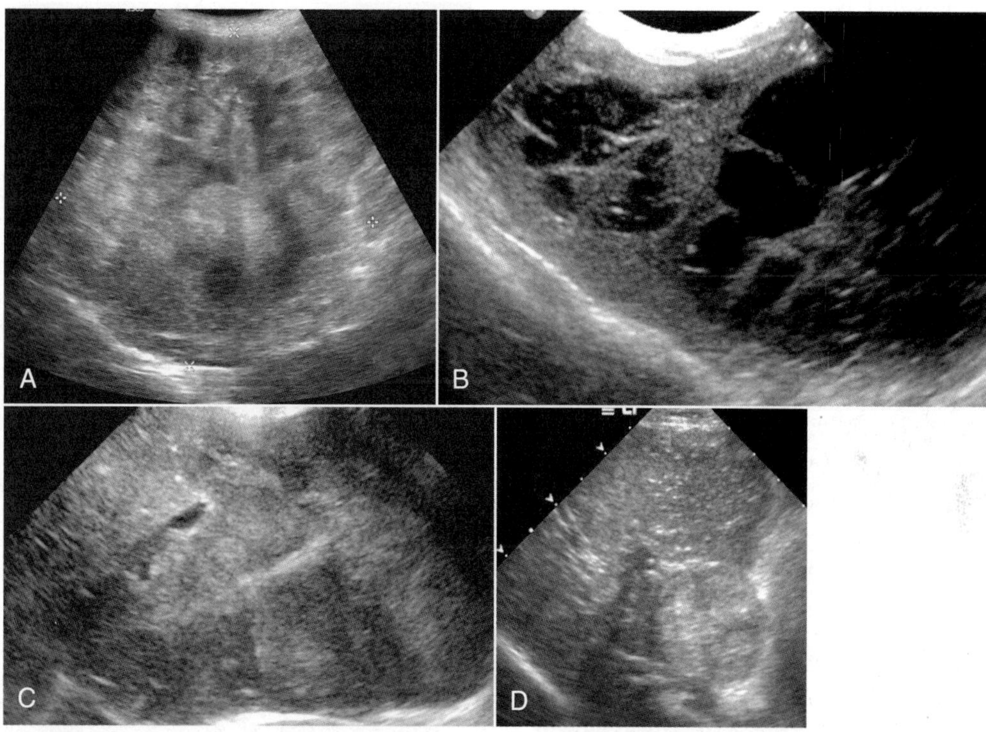

Fig. 40.28 Hepatic neoplasia. **A,** A large (approximately 10 cm) hyperechoic and hypoechoic mass (same dog as Fig. 40.8). Hepatocellular carcinoma was diagnosed on histopathology of the lobe. **B,** Multiple anechoic cavitations are present throughout the liver parenchyma. Hemangiosarcoma was diagnosed at necropsy. **C,** Longitudinal image of the left liver in a dog with lymphosarcoma. The liver is enlarged with rounded margins and a heterogeneous parenchyma. **D,** A focal hyperechoic nodule is noted distorting the liver capsule. Metastatic hemangiosarcoma was diagnosed at necropsy exam.

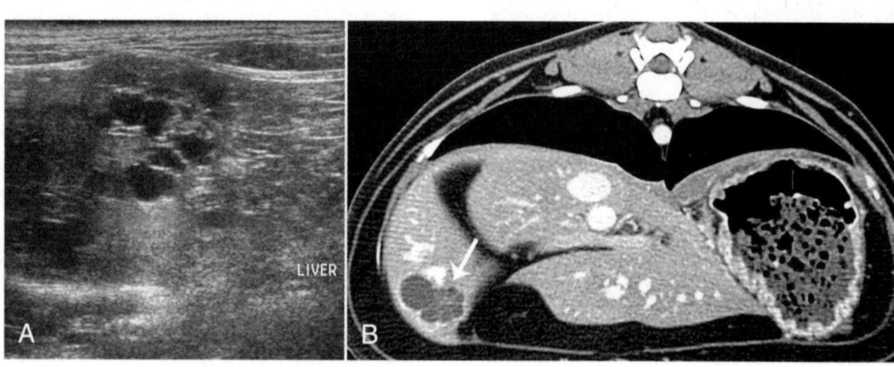

Fig. 40.29 **A,** Longitudinal ultrasound image of the liver from a cat with cystadenoma. A mass with anechoic cystic components, some with acoustic enhancement, is present. **B,** Transverse computed tomography image of a cat with cystadenoma (*arrow*). The mass is cystic in appearance and non–contrast enhancing.

accumulations of mucus, and papillary projections create the appearance of sessile or polypoid masses along an irregularly thickened gallbladder wall (see Fig. 40.35C). Edema of the gallbladder wall, with a characteristic double-layered appearance, can be present secondary to acute cholecystitis, right-sided congestive heart failure, portal hypertension, hypoproteinemia, sepsis, blood transfusions, sedation with dexmedetomidine, and anaphylaxis (see Fig. 40.35A).[40,51,97,99,101–104] Peritoneal fluid surrounding the gallbladder can result in a false impression of wall thickening. Percutaneous cholecystocentesis for culture and cytology of the intraluminal bile can be performed with care, although complications appear to be uncommon.[108,109] Gallbladder wall thickening may be permanent because of inflammation and fibrosis despite resolution of the underlying disease process.[39]

Cholecystoliths, or calculi within the gallbladder, are echogenic focal structures, often with acoustic shadowing, and they may be single or multiple.[10,12,110,111] They are typically mobile, falling to the dependent portion of the gallbladder (Fig. 40.36).

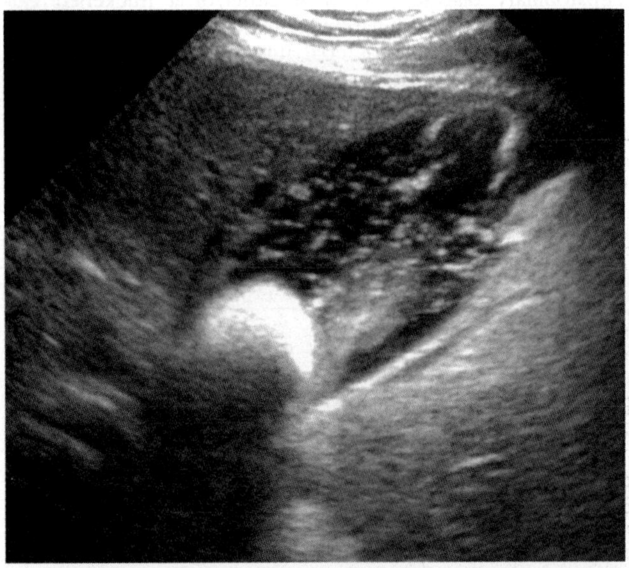

Fig. 40.36 A large, hyperechoic cholelith with acoustic shadowing is present in the dependent portion of the gallbladder lumen.

Choledocholiths are stones within the bile duct, hepatic ducts, and interlobar ducts.[9] Although cholecystoliths and choledocholiths are frequently incidental, they have the potential to cause biliary obstruction. Choledocholiths located in the distal bile duct, in or around the duodenal papilla, are one of the more common causes of biliary obstruction in cats, and they are often associated with cholangitis/cholangiohepatitis as a comorbidity.[111,112] In one study, a high prevalence of bacterial infection was noted in cats with cholelithiasis.[112]

As noted earlier, intraluminal echogenic, nonshadowing, dependent, mobile biliary sludge is present in up to 66% of dogs undergoing routine ultrasound exam, and 35% to 48% of all dogs regardless of health status.[46,48,113–115] Canine dependent biliary sludge does not appear to change significantly over time based on one study that followed asymptomatic canine patients for a 1-year period.[48] Another study noted that dogs with biliary sludge may have decreased gallbladder emptying compared to dogs without sludge.[47] It is hypothesized that decreased emptying may predispose to gallbladder mucocele formation secondary to biliary stasis, bile inspissation, and increased mucus accumulation.[47,48] Despite a high prevalence in asymptomatic dogs, biliary sludge may not be a completely benign process.[48,105–107,116] Nondependent biliary sludge may represent a risk factor for development of a biliary mucocele, particularly in predisposed breeds.[117] Prevalence of biliary sludge in cats undergoing abdominal ultrasound ranges from 14% to 44%.[118,119] While one study indicated sludge was predictive of increased liver enzymes and total bilirubin, a second study showed no increase, although gallbladder wall thickening was significantly associated with gallbladder sludge.[118,119]

Gallbladder emptying can be determined by measuring gallbladder volume pre and post feeding. After a 12-hour fast, volume is determined using the previously noted ellipsoid formula. At 60- and 120-minutes post meal or prokinetic agent, such as erythromycin, gallbladder volume is reassessed. In normal dogs, gallbladder volume post feeding should be less than 1 mL/kg, or it should be reduced by at least 25%.[44,120] Mean pre- and postprandial (2 hours post feeding) volumes of 2.47 ± 1.16 mL and 0.88 ± 0.13 mL, respectively, have been reported in normal cats.[121]

Gallbladder mucocele is an accumulation of nondependent sludge, semisolid mucin, and inspissated bile, creating an intraluminal centralized echogenicity with peripheral striations, often with a striated or stellate appearance (Fig. 40.37).[122–130]

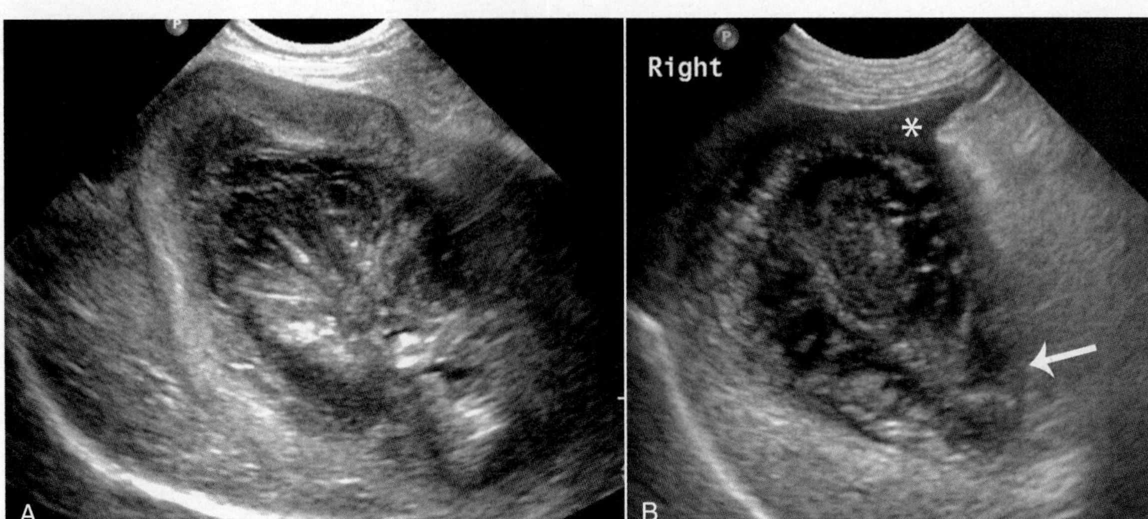

Fig. 40.37 **A,** Longitudinal ultrasound image of a gallbladder mucocele. Echogenic biliary sludge fills the gallbladder lumen, creating a striated appearance along the periphery. The gallbladder wall is markedly thickened. **B,** A gallbladder mucocele is present, with centralized, echogenic sludge and peripheral striations. The gallbladder wall is poorly defined caudally (*arrow*), and hyperechoic fat surrounds the gallbladder. Focal fluid accumulation (*asterisk*) is present. These are all consistent with gallbladder rupture.

Mucocele formation is caused by excess secretion of a gel-forming mucin by the gallbladder epithelium. Mucus granules become tethered to each other and the epithelium, resulting in abnormal physical and functional properties and inspissation of the bile.[131] Biliary obstruction by mucinous plugs within the cystic and bile duct may occur and lead to distention of the intrahepatic and/or extrahepatic biliary system. Ischemic necrosis of the gallbladder wall can lead to rupture. Gallbladder mucoceles have been associated with a 50% incidence of loss of gallbladder wall integrity and/or acute rupture.[122] The presence of discontinuity of gallbladder wall, pericholecystic hyperechoic fat, and/or pericholecystic fluid is strongly suggestive of gallbladder rupture (see Fig. 40.37B).[126] Sensitivity of ultrasound for detection of gallbladder rupture is low (56.1%), with a high specificity (91.7%) in one study.[132] Contrast-enhanced ultrasound evaluation of the gallbladder allows identification of ischemic necrosis or rupture of the gallbladder wall with a higher sensitivity and specificity than conventional sonography.[133] Predisposing factors to gallbladder mucocele include breed (Cocker Spaniel, Sheltie, Miniature Schnauzer, Border Terrier) and some endocrinopathies including hyperadrenocorticism, hypothyroidism, hyperlipidemia, and diabetes mellitus.[134–136] A biliary mucocele is identified occasionally as an incidental finding in patients without clinical signs or serum biochemical changes. Feline gallbladder mucoceles are uncommon, because cats have fewer mucus-secreting glands in the gallbladder compared to dogs.[137]

Extrahepatic biliary obstruction (EHBO) results in a retrograde dilation of the biliary system.[138] With complete obstruction, the gallbladder and cystic duct distend within 24 hours with progressive dilation of the common bile duct within 48 hours (Fig. 40.38). Gallbladder distention may be minimal in the face of chronic inflammation and fibrosis. Progressive dilation of the common bile duct and hepatic ducts occurs during the next 3 to 4 days with dilation of lobar and interlobar ducts by 7 days. This results in multiple tortuous, irregularly branching anechoic linear tracks within the liver. These can be differentiated from hepatic vessels with Doppler interrogation (see Fig. 40.38B). Pancreatitis is one of the most common causes of EHBO in the dog, with choledocholithiasis or neoplasia of the liver, bile duct, pancreas, or duodenum also capable of causing obstruction (Fig. 40.39).[139] Tumors and inflammation of the bile duct, pancreas, and duodenum, along with choledocholithiasis, are more commonly noted in the cat (see Fig. 40.39A,B,D).[111] In 30 cats with EHBO, gallbladder distension was present in only 43%, and it was not considered a reliable indicator of biliary obstruction. More reliable was dilation of the bile duct, present in 97% obstructed cats.[111] Focal sludge accumulation within the feline bile duct cannot easily be differentiated from a neoplastic mass. Incomplete or early obstruction may not cause visible biliary dilation. Bile duct dilation may be prolonged, persisting after relief of the obstruction.[39]

Cholangitis/cholangiohepatitis (inflammatory infiltrate confined to the portal region of the liver with or without involvement of the hepatic parenchyma) complex is an important biliary disease in cats. Ultrasound changes with this disease include thickened gallbladder wall, often with a palisade type irregular mucosa, intraluminal gallbladder or bile duct sludge, choleliths/choledocholiths, and thickened, tortuous, and sometimes dilated bile ducts (see Fig. 40.39A).[140,141] No ultrasound changes are present in some cats with cholangitis/cholangiohepatitis. Comorbidities include EHBO, cholecystitis, cholelithiasis, ductal plate malformations, inflammatory bowel disease, and pancreatitis.[142–144] Microcholelithiasis accumulation at the duodenal papilla may be related to pancreatitis in cats.[143] Cholangitis is now also recognized in dogs, and can be present concurrently with cholecystitis and biliary mucocele.[145,146] Ultrasound findings are variable and nonspecific, and include gallbladder wall thickening, distension of the common bile duct, cholelithiasis, and mucoceles.[145]

Vascular Disease

Venous congestion occurs with right-sided congestive heart failure or obstructive lesions in the posthepatic caudal vena cava. The hepatic caudal vena cava and hepatic veins both dilate in response to the elevated pressure (Fig. 40.40). The liver may also enlarge and become hypoechoic, although echogenicity changes may not be consistent. Dilation of the caudal vena cava and hepatic veins, along with ascites, suggests the possibility of disease cranial to the diaphragm.

Ultrasonography can be used to identify most portosystemic shunts reliably, although detection of these vascular anomalies requires a good knowledge of vascular anatomy. An abnormal shunting vessel is the most reliable indication of portosystemic shunt, but other changes, including a small liver that is uniform

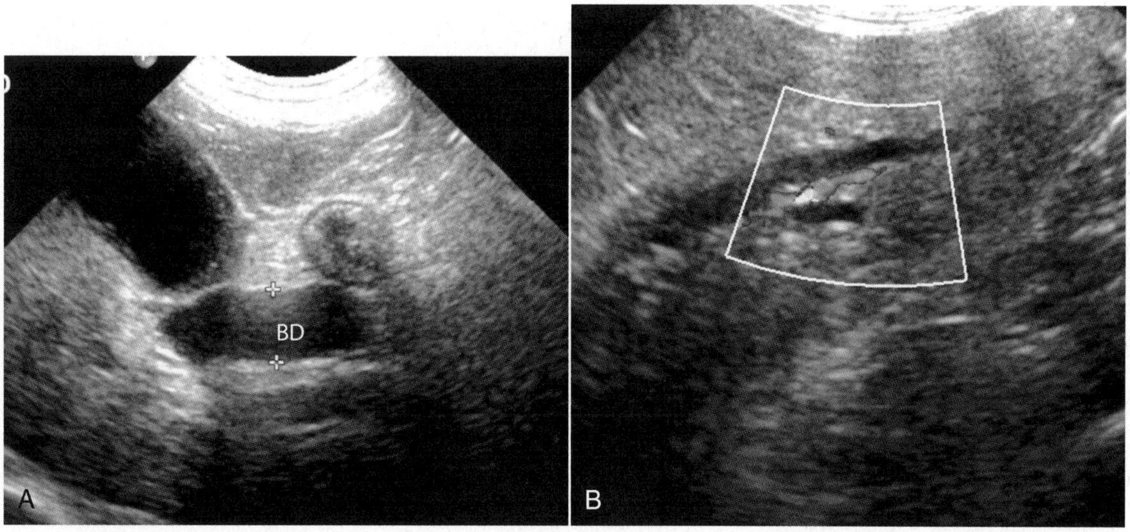

Fig. 40.38 Extrahepatic biliary obstruction. **A,** Longitudinal ultrasound image of a dog with extrahepatic biliary obstruction as a result of pancreatitis. The gallbladder and bile duct (*BD*) are moderately distended. **B,** Ultrasound image of a portion of liver in a cat with chronic biliary obstruction. Dilated intrahepatic bile ducts (with no color Doppler signal) are present.

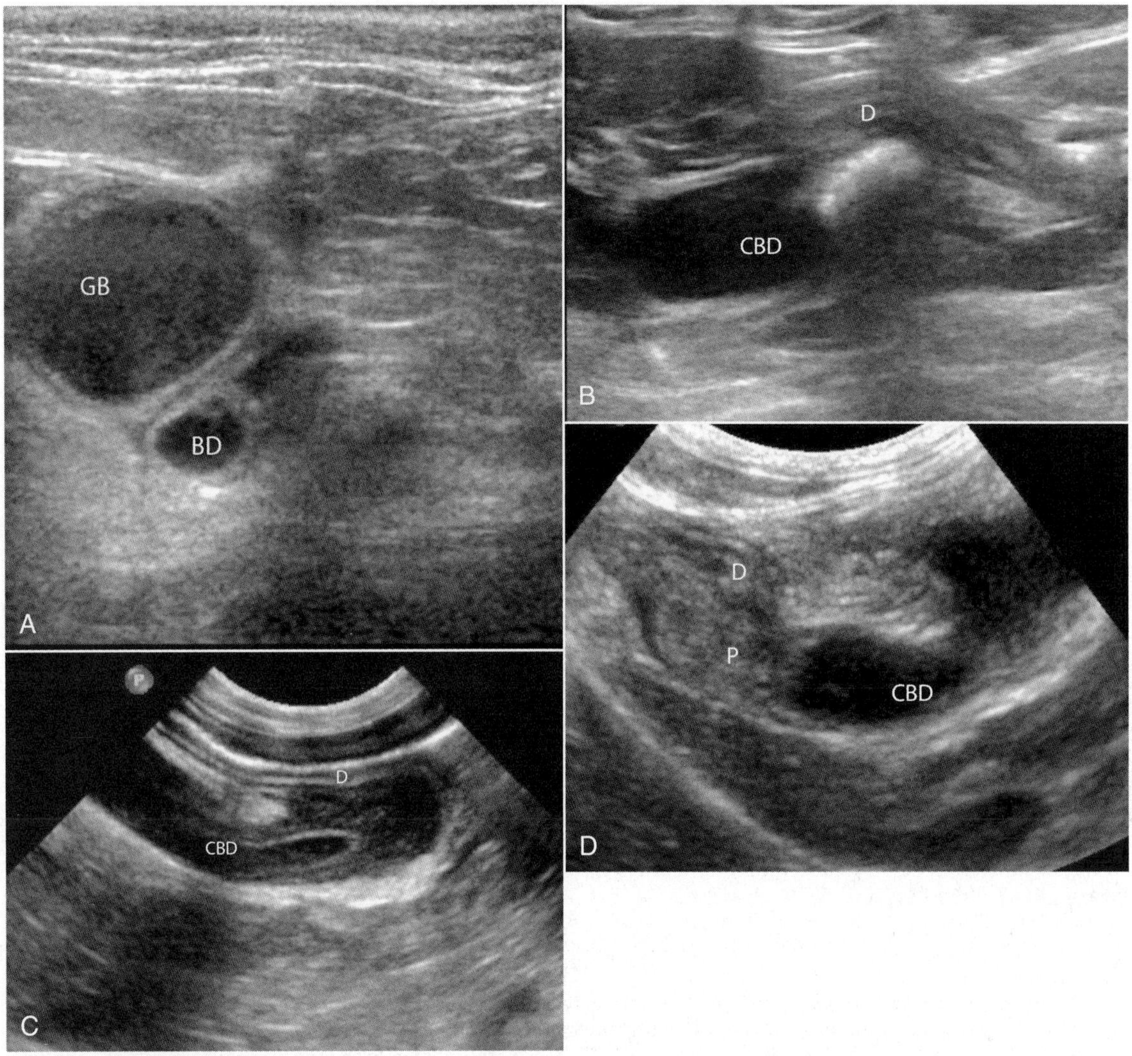

Fig. 40.39 Extrahepatic biliary obstruction. **A,** Ultrasound image of the gallbladder (*GB*) and bile duct (*BD*) in a cat with cholangitis and biliary obstruction. The bile duct is thickened and dilated. The gallbladder wall is thickened. **B,** Dilated bile duct (*CBD*) secondary to obstruction by a choledocholith at the duodenal papilla (*D*) in a cat with cholangitis. **C,** CBD secondary to obstruction by a mass at the level of the duodenal papilla (*D*) in a dog presented for elevated liver enzymes. Lymphoma was diagnosed on cytology from a fine needle aspirate of the mass. **D,** CBD secondary to a plug of inspissated bile (*P*) at the level of the duodenal papilla (*D*) in a cat with cholangitis.

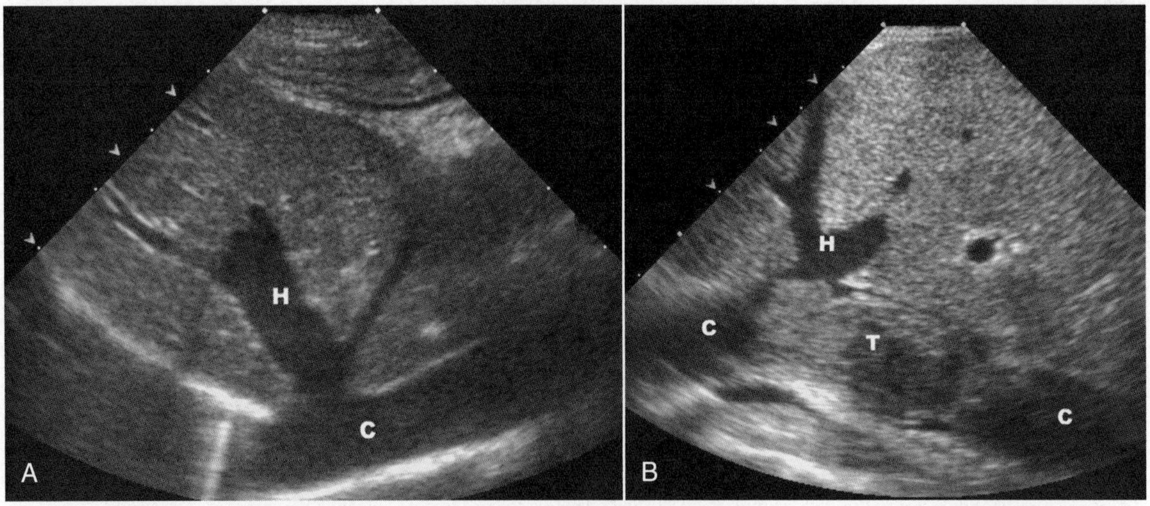

Fig. 40.40 Venous congestion. **A,** Right lateral oblique ultrasound image of the liver. The caudal vena cava (*C*) and hepatic veins (*H*) are distended as a result of right-sided congestive heart failure. **B,** An intraluminal tumor thrombus (*T*) obstructs the caudal vena cava (*C*) and hepatic veins (*H*) resulting in venous congestion.

and normal in echogenicity, decreased or absent intrahepatic portal vasculature, decreased size of extrahepatic portal veins, enlarged kidneys, and renal/ureteral/cystic and/or urethral calculi (urate calculi), are often present (Fig. 40.41; see Fig. 40.19).[147,148]

Extrahepatic shunts affect cats and small-breed dogs primarily, and the most common finding is a single shunt vessel connecting the portal vein, or more likely a major tributary of the portal vein, such as splenic, left gastric, or right gastric vein, to the caudal vena cava between the right renal vein and hepatic veins (see Fig. 40.41B,C,D).[147,148] Extrahepatic shunt vessels may be difficult to identify because of poor acoustic windows associated with the small liver or the presence of bowel gas. A right dorsal intercostal window, in addition to routine views, is helpful in detecting the anomalous shunt vessel. In this window, the portal vein and caudal vena cava are visible as they enter the porta hepatis, and abnormal shunting vessels may be identified. The portion of the portal vein cranial to the origin of the shunt is often decreased in size, with a portal vein:aortic ratio of less than 0.65, whereas the normal ratio is 0.7 to 1.25. Dogs with shunt ratio of >0.8 did not have an extrahepatic shunt.[147] Pulsed-wave or color Doppler interrogation of the caudal vena cava is helpful in assessing for abnormal turbulence where a shunting vessel enters.[147,148] Shunt vessels terminating in the azygous vein may be more difficult to follow, but they might be seen terminating in an enlarged azygous vein adjacent to the aorta or esophagus. Acquired extrahepatic shunt vessels attributable to hepatic disease and portal hypertension may appear as a grouping of multiple variably sized, tortuous vessels, often medial to the spleen and left kidney. Color Doppler imaging may be needed to find these abnormal vessels.[148]

Intrahepatic shunts affect primarily large-breed dogs. Left divisional shunts, such as a patent ductus venosus, right divisional shunts, and central-divisional shunts can be identified. A right lateral intercostal window, in addition to the standard ventral abdominal approach, is helpful in identifying the right divisional intrahepatic shunting vessel between the main portal vein and caudal vena cava (see Fig. 40.41A).[147,148,149]

Arterioportal communications are rare malformations in dogs and cats. Typically, an abnormally dilated and tortuous cluster of vessels is visible within or adjacent to the liver. Upon Doppler interrogation, hepatofugal flow and an arterial spectral Doppler signal in the portal vein confirm the presence of an arterioportal communication.[33–35] An uncommon form of splenosystemic shunt has been described in cats.[150] These splenosystemic shunts were identified as an anomalous vessel arising from the splenic vein, coursing caudal to the left kidney assuming a generally tortuous path, and continuing to the left renal vein, caudal vena cava adjacent to the renal vein, or medial to the left kidney. Neutered female cats were overrepresented. It could not be determined whether these shunts

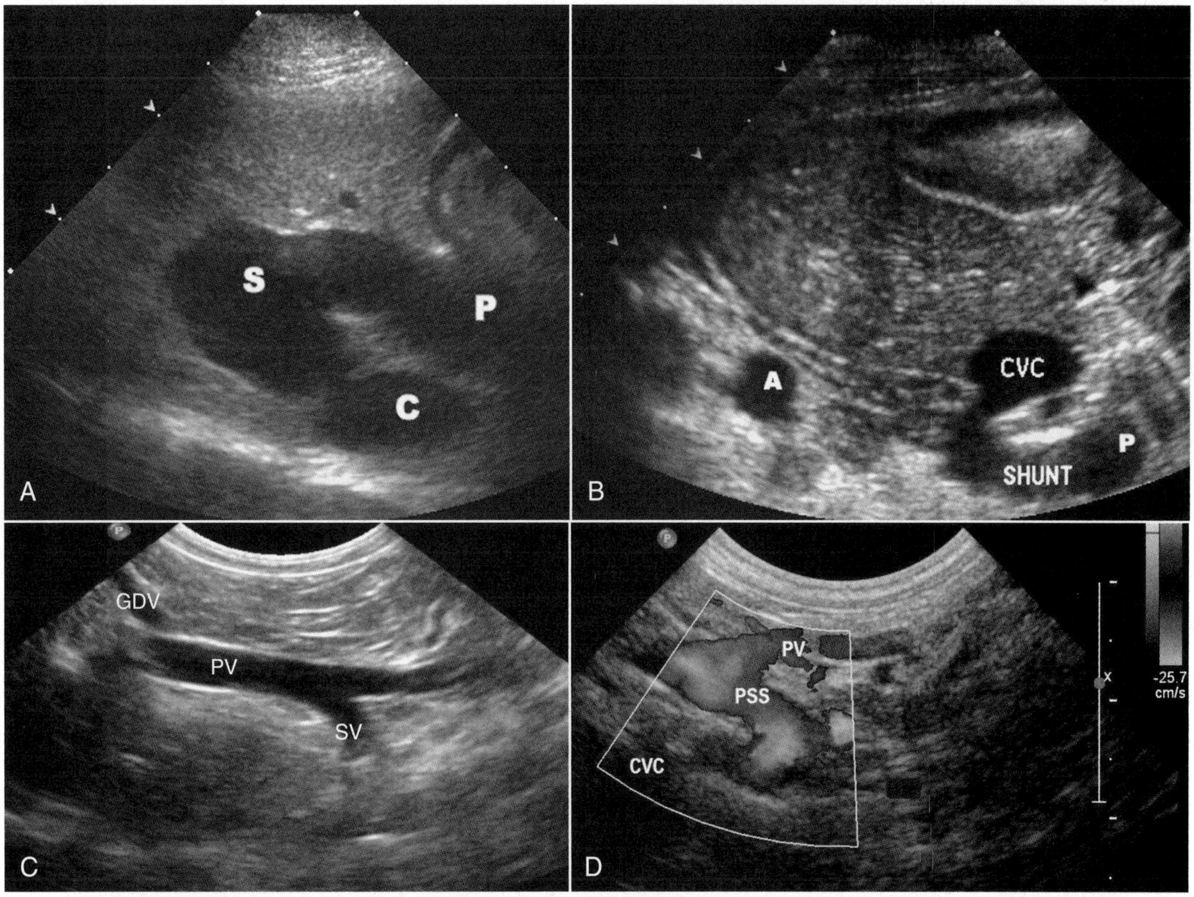

Fig. 40.41 Portosystemic shunts. **A,** Right lateral intercostal ultrasound image of a young dog with a right divisional intrahepatic portosystemic shunt. Dorsal is to the *left* of the image and right is at the *top* of the image. *C,* Caudal vena cava; *P,* portal vein; *S,* shunt. **B,** Right lateral intercostal ultrasound image of a young dog with an extrahepatic portosystemic shunt. Dorsal is to the *left* of the image, and right is at the *top* of the image. *A,* Aorta; *CVC,* caudal vena cava; *P,* portal vein. **C,** Sagittal image of the normal portal vein and tributaries. *GDV,* Gastroduodenal vein; *PV,* portal vein; *SV,* splenic vein. **D,** Same window as **C,** with color Doppler evaluation of a splenocaval shunt. Abnormal flow through the shunting vessel is blue, indicating flow away from the portal vein and towards the caudal vena cava. *CVC,* Caudal vena cava; *PSS,* portosystemic shunting vessel.

were congenital or acquired in origin. However, these shunts do not appear to share similar clinical or anatomic features with previously described congenital portosystemic shunts in cats. This type of shunt can occasionally be visible in survey abdominal radiographs as a tortuous vessel caudal to the spleen in VD radiographs (Fig. 40.42).

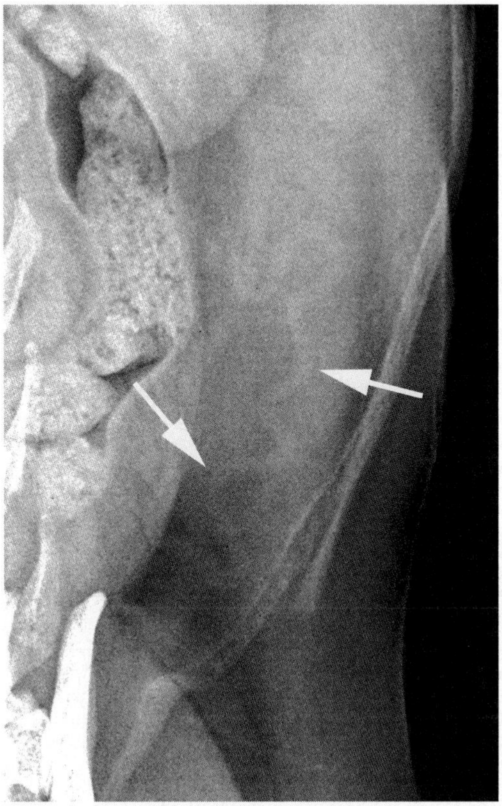

Fig. 40.42 Ventrodorsal (VD) radiograph of the abdomen of a cat in the region caudal to the spleen. A tortuous vessel, representative of a splenocaval shunt, is visible (*white arrows*).

RADIOLOGY OF THE SPLEEN

The spleen is a dynamic organ; and in the dog, the size and location of the spleen can vary widely. There are numerous variations on the radiographic appearance of the normal spleen in dogs and to a lesser extent in cats.[1–3] The spleen is divided into a dorsal extremity, termed the *head* of the spleen; a body; and a ventral extremity, termed the *tail* of the spleen. The dorsal extremity is relatively fixed in the left craniodorsal aspect of the abdomen. The ventral extremity is not fixed, and in the dog, the position of this portion of the spleen can vary considerably. On VD views of the canine abdomen, the dorsal extremity of the spleen is seen typically as a triangular soft tissue opacity caudolateral to the gastric fundus and craniolateral to the left kidney (Fig. 40.43A). The remainder of the spleen may extend caudally, adjacent to the left lateral abdominal wall, or more medially across the midline. When the spleen extends medially, the full length of the spleen is not visualized completely.

On lateral views, the triangular soft tissue opacity of the dorsal extremity of the spleen is located dorsally, caudal to the stomach. The ventral extremity typically is a triangular soft tissue opacity immediately caudal and slightly ventral to the pylorus or liver (see Fig. 40.1A). The ventral extremity of the spleen is often more conspicuous on right lateral views of the abdomen but may silhouette the caudal margin of the liver and be poorly delineated.

The feline spleen is thinner and smaller compared with the canine spleen and less variable in size and position (see Fig. 40.43B; also see Fig. 40.1C). Like the dog, the dorsal extremity of the spleen is seen on VD views in the left cranial abdomen, caudolateral to the stomach and craniolateral to the left kidney. On VD views, the ventral extremity usually extends caudally along the left lateral abdominal wall, but the amount of visible spleen varies with body fat, positioning, gastric contents, and splenic position.[151]

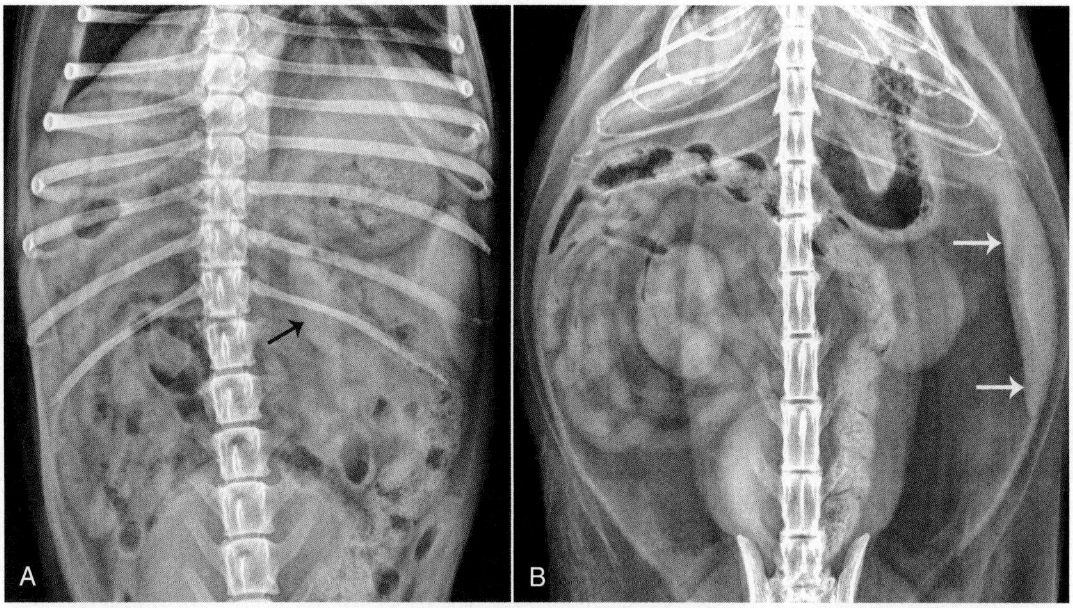

Fig. 40.43 Normal spleen. **A,** Ventrodorsal (VD) radiograph of the abdomen of a normal dog. The dorsal portion of the spleen is visible in the left cranial abdomen, caudolateral to the gastric fundus and craniolateral to the left kidney. The more ventral portion is noted by the ***black arrow***. **B,** VD radiograph of the abdomen of a normal cat. The entire spleen can be visualized extending caudally along the left lateral abdomen (*white arrows*).

On lateral abdominal views in the cat, the dorsal extremity may be visible caudal and dorsal to the gastric fundus. The ventral extremity of a normal spleen is rarely visible in the cat. In 100 cats with a presumably normal spleen, the ventral extremity was visible on a lateral radiograph in only one cat.[151]

In both dogs and cats, it is important to realize that the entire spleen is rarely visible on a single radiographic projection.

Splenic Size

Radiographic assessment of splenic size in the dog is very subjective, because normal size varies widely. Feline splenic size appears to be more consistent. Splenomegaly in the cat should be considered if the ventral extremity is visible on the lateral projection of the abdomen.[151] In the dog, and to a lesser extent in the cat, generalized splenomegaly results in thickened, rounded, blunted margins, and dorsal and caudal displacement of the jejunum on lateral views (Fig. 40.44). Organ displacement on the VD view as a result of the enlarged spleen depends on the portion of the spleen that is enlarged and the degree of enlargement. The jejunum may be displaced to the right or left, whereas an enlarged dorsal extremity results in cranial displacement of the stomach.

Considerations for diffuse splenomegaly are numerous and include inflammation caused by infection with toxoplasmosis, fungal organisms, *Mycoplasma haemofelis,* ehrlichiosis, hyperplasia (e.g., hemolytic disorders), systemic lupus erythematosus, chronic bacteremic disorders, congestion (e.g., from impaired venous drainage), portal hypertension, splenic torsion/infarction, anesthetic drugs, infiltrative disease (e.g., primary and metastatic neoplasia), and extramedullary hematopoiesis.[152–155] Lymphosarcoma, leukemia, systemic mastocytosis, multiple myeloma, and malignant histiocytosis can all result in diffuse neoplastic splenic enlargement. Splenomegaly in the cat is less likely to be benign, because the feline spleen is considered nonsinusoidal and less capable of storing large amounts of blood.[155–157] Compared with the dog, generalized splenomegaly in the cat is most commonly caused by neoplastic infiltration, primarily lymphosarcoma, and mast cell tumor (see Fig. 40.44B).[157,158]

Sedation with acepromazine resulted in significantly increased radiographic splenic size, while sedation with midazolam/butorphanol combination, and dexmedetomidine/butorphanol/ketamine combinations resulted in a trend towards increased splenic size in the cat.[159]

Splenic torsion occurs when the spleen rotates around its mesenteric axis, resulting in complete occlusion of venous drainage and eventual arterial occlusion. This results in marked splenomegaly, as well as an atypical splenic location.[160,161] The spleen may undergo torsion on its own or in association with gastric volvulus. It may acquire a reverse C-shape on the lateral view or may simply appear as a mass in the ventral abdomen

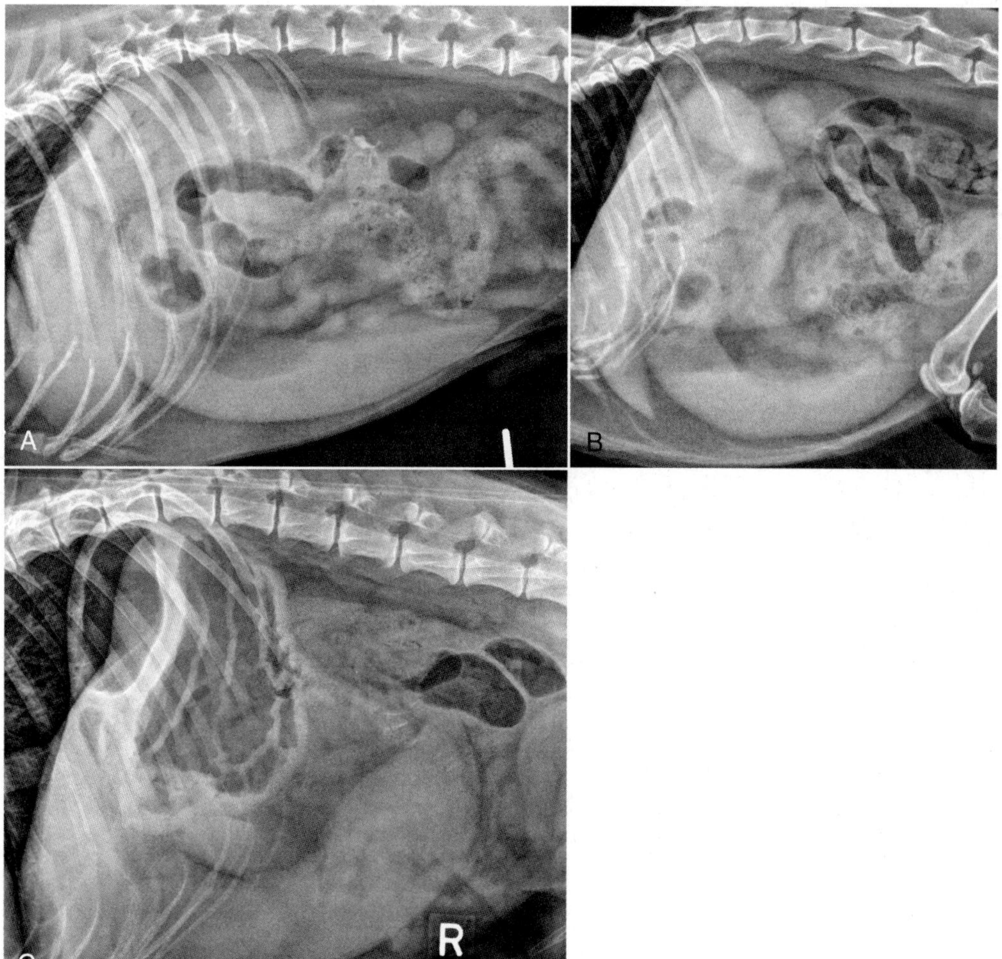

Fig. 40.44 Splenomegaly. **A,** Lateral abdominal radiograph of a sedated dog. The spleen is elongated, with rounded margins secondary to congestion. **B,** Lateral abdominal radiograph of a cat with splenic lymphosarcoma. The spleen is visible on lateral images appearing markedly elongated with rounded margins secondary to neoplastic infiltration. **C,** Lateral abdominal radiograph of a dog with gastric volvulus. The spleen is markedly enlarged, with elongation and rounding of margins secondary to splenic torsion.

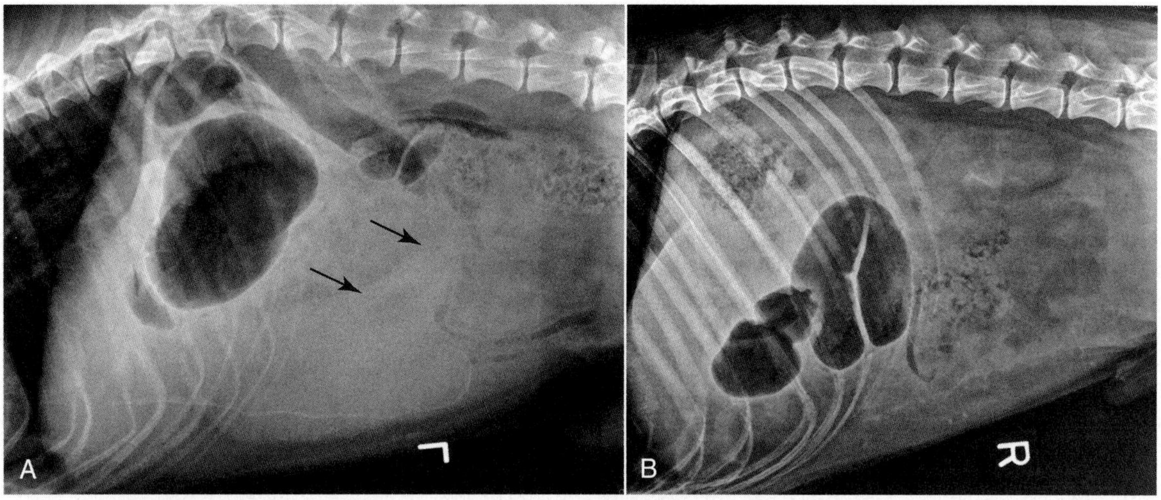

Fig. 40.45 **A,** Lateral radiograph of the abdomen of a dog with splenic torsion. The spleen is enlarged and displaced caudally and dorsally (*black arrows*). **B,** Lateral radiograph of the abdomen of a dog with a large splenic abscess. A stippled gas pattern is present within both the head and tail of the spleen.

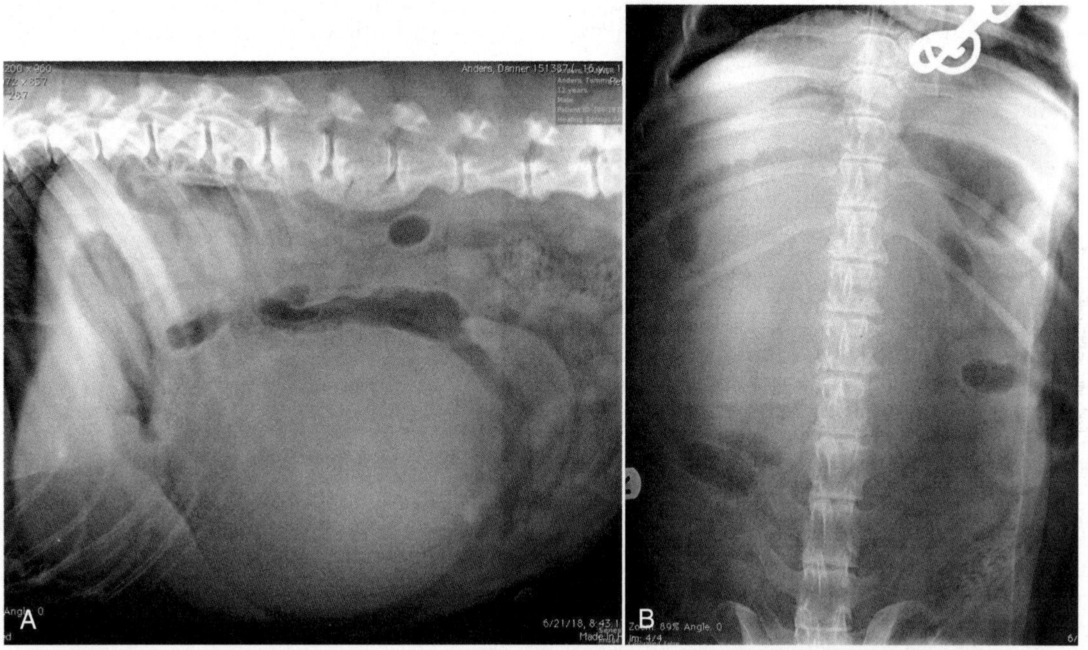

Fig. 40.46 Lateral (**A**) and ventrodorsal (VD; **B**) radiographs of the abdomen of a dog with splenic hemangiosarcoma in the ventral extremity of the spleen, seen along the ventral abdomen on the lateral view, and to the *right* of midline on the VD view.

(Fig. 40.45 and eFig. 40.6). The dorsal extremity of the spleen may not be visible in the normal left craniodorsal location because of the malposition or accompanying peritoneal fluid. If gas-producing bacteria proliferate within the ischemic parenchyma, emphysematous changes may occur and result in a mottled or foamy radiographic appearance (see Fig. 40.45B).[161] CT has been used in the diagnosis of splenic torsion, and the findings include splenomegaly, a corkscrew-like soft tissue mass representing the rotated splenic pedicle, and lack of contrast enhancement.[162]

A splenic mass results in local displacement of adjacent viscera according to the location of the mass in the spleen (Figs. 40.46 and 40.47, eFig. 40.7). Although often sharply marginated, the splenic mass may be obscured partially or completely by secondary peritoneal hemorrhage. A mass in the body or ventral extremity of the spleen is a very common cause of a ventral abdominal mass, and on the lateral view results in dorsal and caudal displacement of the jejunum. On VD views, ventral splenic masses may be midline or to the right or left of midline.

Masses of the dorsal extremity of the spleen are less common and may displace the stomach cranially with caudal, medial, and ventral displacement of the jejunum and descending colon. The left kidney may be displaced caudally as well.

Differentials for a splenic mass include benign and neoplastic conditions. Primary and metastatic neoplasia, hematoma, nodular hyperplasia, extramedullary hematopoiesis, and abscess are all considerations.[158,164–166] Hemangiosarcoma is the most common neoplasm of the canine spleen, but splenic hematoma and hyperplastic nodules are the most common

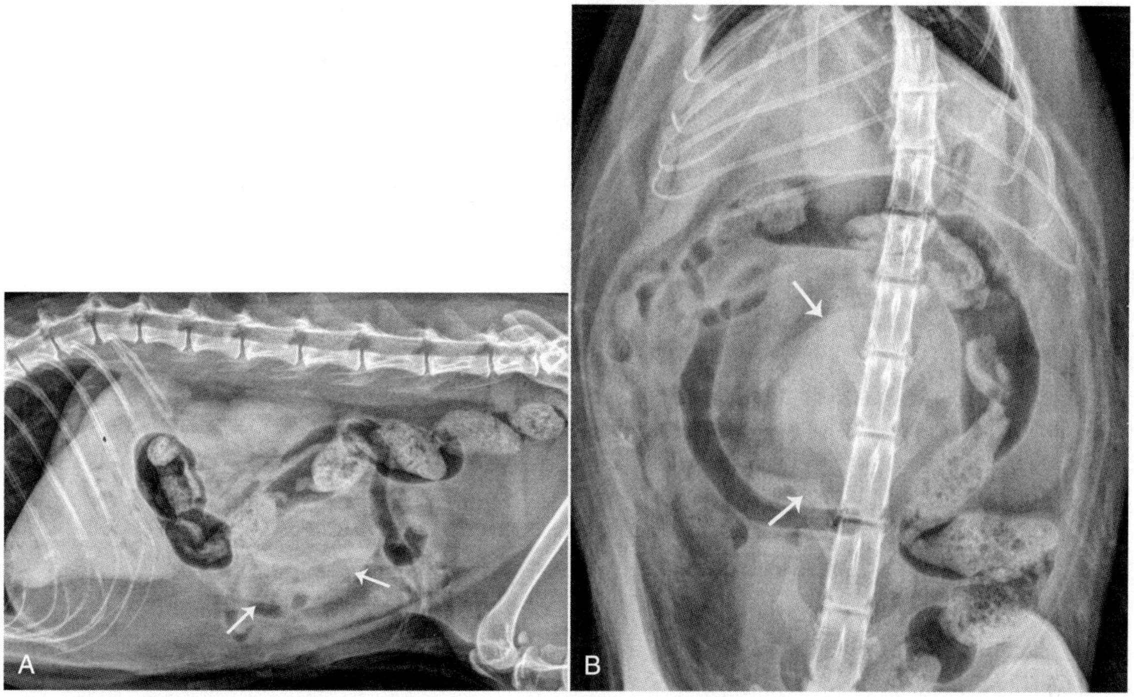

Fig. 40.47 Lateral (A) and ventrodorsal (VD; B) radiographs of the abdomen of a cat with a splenic hemangiosarcoma in the ventral extremity of the spleen, creating a poorly defined mass effect caudal to the stomach on the lateral view, and on the midline on the VD view (*arrows*). Abdominal effusion results in a partial loss of contrast and detail in the mid abdomen.

causes of splenic lesions.[166] Peritoneal effusion may accompany both benign and neoplastic diseases.

Splenic Opacity

Normal splenic opacity is that of soft tissue. Mineralization of the spleen may be the result of dystrophic calcification of abscesses, hematomas, fungal granulomas, or neoplastic masses, and can be associated with endocrine disease. Gas within the spleen may result from splenic torsion. As noted in the liver, gas may ascend into the portovenous circulation and affect the spleen.[16,17] Gas-forming organisms in splenic abscesses can create focal radiolucencies. Spontaneous emphysematous splenitis has been reported in Golden Retrievers resulting in a mass effect with coalescing vesicular-like gas pattern in the splenic region[166] (see Fig. 40.45B).

ULTRASOUND OF THE SPLEEN

The spleen is well suited to ultrasound examination because of the superficial location and lack of intervening gas-containing structures. Higher-frequency transducers may be used because of the superficial location.

Splenic location varies. The dorsal extremity of the spleen is in the left craniolateral abdominal quadrant and may be beneath the costal arch. Intercostal windows are sometimes necessary in deep-chested dogs. The canine splenic body and ventral extremity may extend caudally along the left lateral abdomen or move medially across the ventral midline. It often appears folded on itself. The feline spleen is more consistent in location, along the left lateral abdominal wall, and rarely folds on itself unless enlarged.

The splenic parenchyma has a uniform echotexture with a fine, dense pattern.[167,168] Echogenicity of the canine spleen is slightly greater than the liver (Fig. 40.48). Splenic margins are linear and smooth, with mild indentations noted along the mesenteric border where splenic veins exit. Splenic arteries are not usually seen without Doppler interrogation. Tissue surrounding splenic veins at the hilus may be highly echogenic normally because of capsular invagination and fat.[167]

When enlarged, the spleen may extend caudally or more completely cover the ventral abdomen. Splenic borders become rounded or blunted, or appear to bulge from the capsule, compared with the normal sharp, linear appearance (Fig. 40.49). The spleen has no absolute size limits in the dog. The normal feline spleen is less variable in size than the dog, and objective measurements have been determined. Mean splenic height, measured in the transverse plane, in the proximal third of the spleen, adjacent to a splenic vein, is 7.1 mm, with a range from 5.1 to 9.1 mm (see Fig. 40.48C).[169] Similar splenic measurements were determined in a second study, where normal feline splenic height was 8.2 ± 1.4 mm (range: 5.3–11.1 mm).[170]

Abnormal Splenic Ultrasonographic Findings

Diffuse Disease

As in the liver, diffuse splenic disease potentially causes changes in size, shape, or echogenicity. Splenomegaly with either normal or decreased echogenicity has numerous causes, including congestion, neoplasia, infarction, inflammation, immune-mediated disease, chronic hemolytic anemia, parasitic infection, extramedullary hematopoiesis, and bacterial or fungal infection.[157,167,168,170,175]

Extramedullary hematopoiesis often results in generalized splenomegaly, with normal echogenicity, or a coarse or mottled appearance. Lymphoid hyperplasia can also have a diffuse mottled appearance.

Splenic congestion as a result of a phenothiazine and pentobarbital drug group results in splenomegaly with no associated change in echogenicity in the dog.[170] Acepromazine has a similar appearance in the cat.[159] Congestion from portal hypertension appears similar, but dilated splenic veins may also be present. Splenic torsion, a form of splenic congestion, has a variety of appearances.[160,172] Splenomegaly may be the only

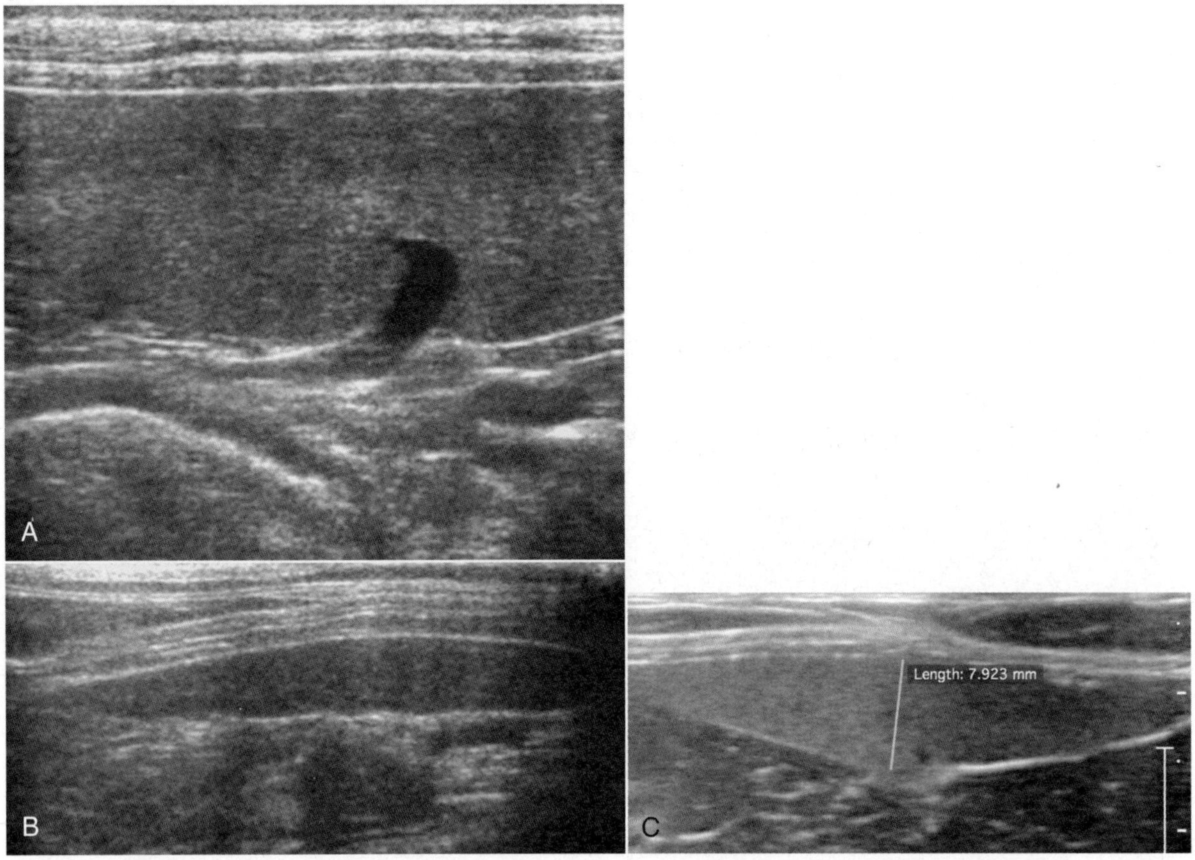

Fig. 40.48 Normal ultrasound appearance of the spleen. **A,** Longitudinal ultrasound image of the normal canine spleen. A splenic vein is visible leaving the splenic hilus. **B,** Longitudinal ultrasound image of the normal feline spleen. The feline spleen is typically a linear, thin structure, and smaller than in the dog. **C,** Transverse image of a feline spleen illustrating measurement of splenic height.

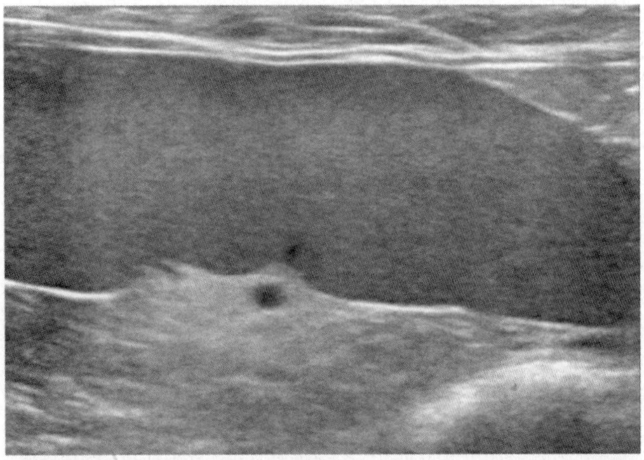

Fig. 40.49 Longitudinal ultrasound image of an enlarged feline spleen caused by lymphoma (cat from Fig. 40.43B). The spleen is rounded and thickened with undulating margins (compare with Fig. 40.48B).

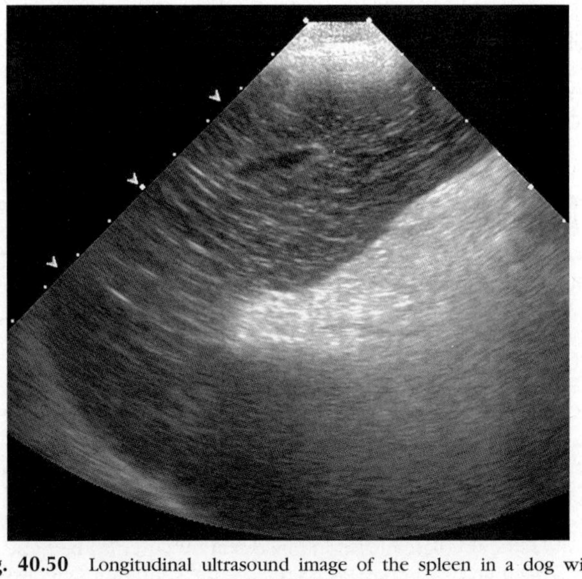

Fig. 40.50 Longitudinal ultrasound image of the spleen in a dog with splenic torsion (dog from Fig. 40.45A). The spleen is enlarged and hypoechoic with linear echogenicities representing dilated vessels.

finding. However, splenomegaly with a diffuse hypoechoic parenchyma, separated by linear echogenicities that represent dilated hyperechoic vessels, is highly suggestive of torsion (Fig. 40.50). Splenic veins may be dilated with visible intravascular echogenicities representing formed thrombi or static echogenic blood. Complete absence of flow at the splenic hilus is also common, as is accompanying peritoneal fluid. A hyperechoic triangular area surrounding the splenic veins has been associated with splenic torsion.[171] Gas within the parenchyma may indicate the presence of necrosis and gas-forming organisms. Diffuse splenic infarction as a result of other disease processes can have an identical appearance.[172]

Diffuse neoplastic infiltration of the spleen has a variety of appearances, and tumor type cannot be determined from the ultrasound appearance.[58,64,157,167,168,173,174]

Lymphosarcoma, mast cell tumor, malignant histiocytosis, leukemic infiltration, and multiple myeloma can all result in splenomegaly with normal or decreased echogenicity. The parenchyma may appear uneven or coarse. Focal or multifocal nodules of varying sizes that are usually hypoechoic may also be

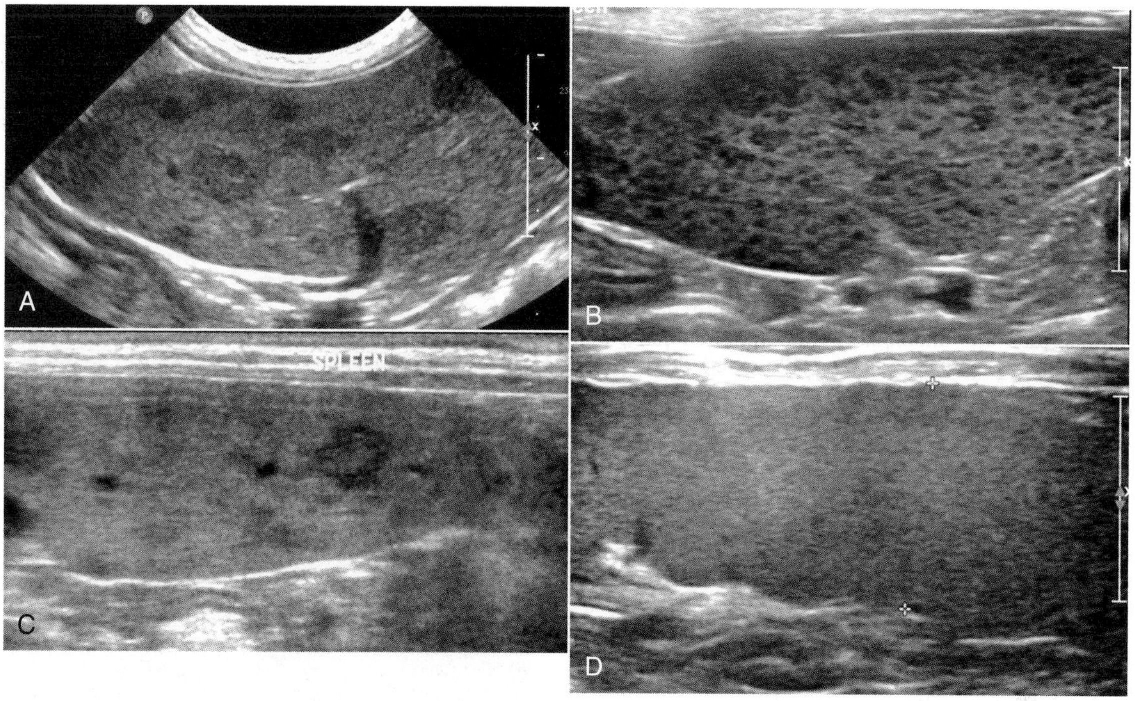

Fig. 40.51 Splenic neoplasia. **A,** Longitudinal image of the spleen in a dog with histiocytic sarcoma. Multiple variably sized hypoechoic nodules are present. **B,** Longitudinal image of the spleen in a dog with lymphoma. Multiple hypoechoic nodules create a "Swiss cheese" appearance. **C,** Longitudinal image of a dog with jejunal carcinoma. Multiple hypoechoic splenic nodules were diagnosed as metastatic carcinoma at necropsy. **D,** Longitudinal image of the spleen in a cat diagnosed with mast cell tumor. The spleen is enlarged, with rounded undulating margins.

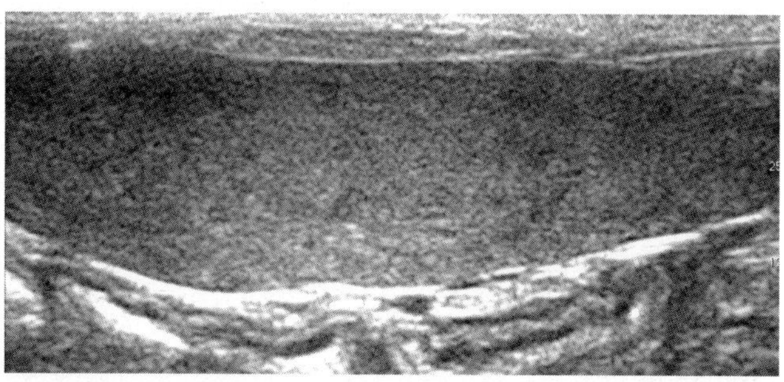

Fig. 40.52 Longitudinal image of the spleen in a cat with histoplasmosis. The spleen is mildly enlarged with a coarse and heterogeneous parenchyma.

present (Fig. 40.51; see Fig. 40.49). A diffuse nodular pattern of small hypoechoic nodules, termed a *Swiss cheese appearance*, is suggestive of lymphosarcoma, but other tumors (e.g., malignant histiocytosis and mast cell tumor) must also be considered. This appearance is normal in juvenile animals.

Splenitis due to fungal infection, such as histoplasmosis in cats, can result in irregular splenomegaly with a hypoechoic to subtle mottled or, rarely, discrete nodular appearance when imaged with a high frequency transducer (Fig. 40.52).[175]

Diffusely increased splenic echogenicity is less common but may be seen with chronic vascular compromise, peritonitis, infection, or diffuse nonneoplastic infiltrative disease, such as extramedullary hematopoiesis.[167,168]

Focal Disease

As in the liver, numerous considerations exist for focal disease, including primary and secondary neoplasia, nodular hyperplasia, hematoma, focal extramedullary hematopoiesis, abscess, cyst, and infarction (Figs. 40.53 and 40.54; see Figs. 40.51 and 40.52). Lymphosarcoma, one of the most common splenic tumors, has a variety of appearances. In addition to the diffuse changes described previously, lymphosarcoma may also produce focal hypoechoic or anechoic nodules or a single complex or cavitated mass.[64,173] Histiocytic sarcoma also creates focal hypoechoic splenic nodules/masses. Splenic masses attributable to hemangiosarcoma are typically complex with hypoechoic, hyperechoic, and anechoic areas caused by

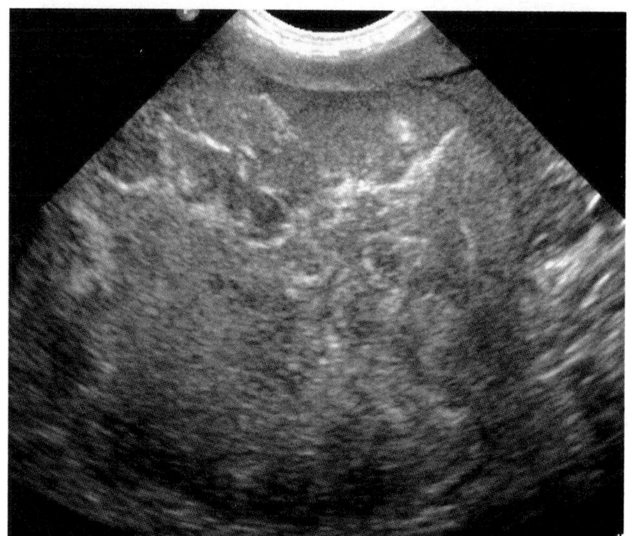

Fig. 40.53 Longitudinal image of a large, well-defined, slightly hyperechoic (to normal spleen) splenic mass with hyperechoic striations in a dog. Extramedullary hematopoiesis was diagnosed on cytology from a fine needle aspirate.

feline Hepatic emphysema: 37 cases. *Vet Radiol Ultrasound*. 2019;60:734–744.
22. Grooters AM, Sherding RG, Johnson SE. Hepatic abscesses in dogs. *Compend Cont Educ*. 1995;17:833.
23. Moon ML. Diagnostic imaging of portosystemic shunts. *Semin Vet Med Surg (Small Anim)*. 1990;5(2):120–126.
24. Hergessell EJ, Hornof WJ, Koblik PD. Percutaneous ultrasound-guided trans-splenic catheterization of the portal vein in the dog. *Vet Radiol Ultrasound*. 1999;40:509.
25. Scrivani PV, Yeager AE, Dykes NL, et al. Influence of patient positioning on sensitivity of mesenteric portography for detecting an anomalous portosystemic blood vessel in dogs: 34 cases (1997–2000). *J Am Vet Med Assoc*. 2001;219(9):1251–1253.
26. White RN, Macdonald NJ, Burton CA. Use of intraoperative mesenteric portovenography in congenital portosystemic shunt surgery. *Vet Radiol Ultrasound*. 2003;44(5): 514–521.
27. Zwingenberger AL, Schwarz T. Dual-phase angiography of the normal canine portal and hepatic vasculature. *Vet Radiol Ultrasound*. 2004;45(2):117–124.
28. Winter MK, Kinney LM, Kleine LJ. Three-dimensional helical computed tomographic angiography of the liver in five dogs. *Vet Radiol Ultrasound*. 2005;46:494.
29. Zwingenberger AL, Schwarz T, Saunders HM. Helical computed tomographic angiography of canine portosystemic shunts. *Vet Radiol Ultrasound*. 2005;46(1):27–32.
30. Bertolini G, Rolla EC, Zotti A, et al. Three-dimensional multislice helical computed tomography techniques for canine extra-hepatic portosystemic shunt assessment. *Vet Radiol Ultrasound*. 2006;47(5):439–443.
31. Nelson NC, Nelson LL. Anatomy of extrahepatic portosystemic shunts in dogs as determined by computed tomography angiography. *Vet Radiol Ultrasound*. 2011;52(5):498–506.
32. Fukushima K, Kanemoto H, Ohno K, et al. Computed tomographic morphology and clinical features of extrahepatic portosystemic shunts in 172 dogs in Japan. *The Veterinary Journal*. 2014;199:376.
33. Specchi S, Rossi F, Weisse C, et al. Canine and feline abdominal arterioportal communications can be classified based on branching patterns in computed tomographic angiography. *Vet Radiol Ultrasound*. 2018; 59(6):687–696.
34. Zwingenberger AL, McLear R, Weisse C. Diagnosis of arterioportal fistulae in four dogs using computed tomographic angiography. *Vet Radiol Ultrasound*. 2005;46(6): 472–477.
35. Bertolini G. Anomalies of the portal venous system in dogs and cats as seen on multidetector-row computed tomography: an overview and systematization proposal.
36. Fukushima K, Kanemoto H, Ohno K, et al. CT characteristics of primary hepatic mass lesions in dogs. *Vet Radiol Ultrasound*. 2012;53:252.
37. Kutara K, Seki M, Ishikawa C, et al. Triple-phase helical computed tomography in dogs with hepatic masses. *Vet Radiol Ultrasound*. 2014;55(1):7–15.
38. Jones ID, Lamb CR, Drees R, et al. Associations between dual-phase computed tomography features and histopathologic diagnoses in 52 dogs with hepatic or splenic masses. *Vet Radiol Ultrasound*. 2016;57(2):144–153.
39. Moon Larson M, Mattoon J, Lawrence Y, et al. Liver. In: Mattoon JS, Sellon RK, Berry C, eds. *Small Animal Diagnostic Ultrasound*. 4th ed. St. Louis; 2021:355–421.
40. d'Anjou MA. Liver. In: Penninck D, d'Anjou MA, eds. *Atlas of Small Animal Ultrasonography*. 2nd ed. Ames, IA: Blackwell; 2015.
41. Ivancic M, Mai W. Qualitative and quantitative comparison of renal vs. hepatic ultrasonographic intensity in healthy dogs. *Vet Radiol Ultrasound*. 2008;49(4):368–373.
42. Yabuki A, Endo Y, Sakamoto H, et al. Quantitative assessment of renal cortical echogenicity in clinically normal cats. *Anat Histol Embryol*. 2008;37(5):383–386.
43. Center SA. Diseases of the gallbladder and biliary tree. *Vet Clin North Am Small Anim Pract*. 2009;39(3):543–598.
44. Ramstedt KL, Center SA, Randolph JF, et al. Changes in gallbladder volume in healthy dogs after food was withheld for 12 hours followed by ingestion of a meal or a meal containing erythromycin. *Am J Vet Res*. 2008;69(5): 647–651.
45. Penninck DG, Brisson JO, Webster CR. Sonographic assessment of gallbladder volume in normal cats. *Vet Radiol Ultrasound*. 2010;51(6):665–666.
46. Brömel C, Barthez PY, Léveillé R, et al. Prevalence of gallbladder sludge in dogs as assessed by ultrasonography. *Vet Radiol Ultrasound*. 1998;39(3):206–210.
47. Tsukagoshi T, Ohno K, Tsukamoto A, et al. Decreased gallbladder emptying in dogs with biliary sludge or gallbladder mucocele. *Vet Radiol Ultrasound*. 2012;53(1):84–91.
48. DeMonaco SM, Grant DC, Larson MM, et al. Spontaneous course of biliary sludge over 12 months in dogs with ultrasonographically identified biliary sludge. *J Vet Intern Med*. 2016;30:771–778.
49. Hittmair KM, Vielgrader HD, Loupal G. Ultrasonographic evaluation of gallbladder wall thickness in cats. *Vet Radiol Ultrasound*. 2001;42(2):149–155.
50. Spaulding KA. Ultrasound corner: gallbladder wall thickness. *Vet Radiol Ultrasound*. 1993;34:270.
51. Moentk J, Biller DS. Bilobed gallbladder in a cat: ultrasonographic appearance. *Vet Radiol Ultrasound*. 1993;34:354.
52. Léveillé R, Biller DS, Shiroma JT. Sonographic evaluation of the common bile duct in cats. *J Vet Intern Med*. 1996;10(5):296–299.
53. Zeman RK, Taylor KJ, Rosenfield AT, et al. Acute experimental biliary obstruction in the dog. Sonographic findings and clinical implications. *Am J Roentgenol*. 1981;136(5):965–967.
54. Biller DS, Kantrowitz B, Miyabayashi T. Ultrasonography of diffuse liver disease: a review. *J Vet Intern Med*. 1992;6(2):71–76.
55. Newell SM, Selcer BA, Girard E, et al. Correlation between ultrasonographic findings and specific hepatic diseases in cats: 72 cases (1985–1997). *J Am Vet Med Assoc*. 1998;213(1):94–98.
56. Feeney DA, Anderson KL, Ziegler LE, et al. Statistical relevance of ultrasonographic criteria in the assessment of diffuse liver disease in dogs and cats. *Am J Vet Res*. 2008;69(2):212–221.
57. Marolf AJ, Leach L, Gibbons DS, et al. Ultrasonographic findings of feline cholangitis. *J Am Anim Hosp Assoc*. 2012;48(1):36–42.
58. Sato AF, Solano M. Ultrasonographic findings in abdominal mast cell disease: a retrospective study of 19 patients. *Vet Radiol Ultrasound*. 2004;45(1):51–57.
59. Finora K, Leibman NF, Fettman MJ, et al. Cytological comparison of fine-needle aspirates of liver and spleen of normal dogs and of dogs with cutaneous mast cell tumours and an ultrasonographically normal appearing liver and spleen. *Vet Comp Oncol*. 2006;4(3):178–183.
60. Stefanello D, Valenti P, Faverzani S, et al. Ultrasound-guided cytology of spleen and liver: a prognostic tool in canine cutaneous mast cell tumor. *J Vet Intern Med*. 2009;23(5):1051–1057.

61. Book AP, Fidel J, Wills T, et al. Correlation of ultrasound findings, liver and spleen cytology, and prognosis in the clinical staging of high metastatic risk canine mast cell tumors. *Vet Radiol Ultrasound*. 2011;52(5):548–554.
62. Sonet J, Barthelemy A, Goy-Thollot I. Prospective evaluation of abdominal ultrasound findings in 35 dogs with leptospirosis. *Vet Radiol Ultrasound*. 2017;59:98–106.
63. Tchelepi H, Ralls PW, Radin R, et al. Sonography of diffuse liver disease. *J Ultrasound Med*. 2002;21(9):1023–1032.
64. Lamb CR, Hartzband LE, Tidwell AS, et al. Ultrasonographic findings in hepatic and splenic lymphosarcoma in dogs and cats. *Vet Radiol*. 1991;32:117.
65. Léveillé R, Partington BP, Biller DS, et al. Complications after ultrasound-guided biopsy of abdominal structures in dogs and cats: 246 cases (1984–1991). *J Am Vet Med Assoc*. 1993;203(3):413–415.
66. de Rycke LM, van Bree HJ, Simoens PJ. Ultrasound-guided soft tissue core biopsy of liver, spleen and kidney in normal dogs. *Vet Radiol Ultrasound*. 1999;40(3):294–299.
67. Warren-Smith CM, Andrew S, Mantis P, et al. Lack of associations between ultrasonographic appearance of parenchymal lesions of the canine liver and histological diagnosis. *J Small Anim Pract*. 2012;53(3):168–173.
68. Whiteley MB, Feeney DA, Whiteley LO, et al. Ultrasonographic appearance of primary and metastatic canine hepatic tumors. *J Ultrasound Med*. 1989;8(11):621–630.
69. Nyman HT, Kristensen AT, Flagstad A, et al. A review of the sonographic assessment of tumor metastases in liver and superficial lymph nodes. *Vet Radiol Ultrasound*. 2004;45(5):438–448.
70. Liptak JM, Dernell WS, Monnet E, et al. Massive hepatocellular carcinoma in dogs: 48 cases (1992–2002). *J Am Vet Med Assoc*. 2004;225(8):1225–1230.
71. Liptak J. Hepatobiliary tumors. In: Withrow SJ, Vail DM, Page RL, eds. *Withrow and MacEwan's Small Animal Clinical Oncology*. 5th ed. St Louis: Elsevier/Saunders; 2013.
72. Cullen JM, Popp JA. Tumors of the liver and gallbladder. In: Meuten DJ, ed. *Tumors in Domestic Animals*. 4th ed. Ames, IA: Iowa State Press; 2002.
73. Patnaik AK, Hurvitz AI, Lieberman PH. Canine hepatic neoplasms: a clinicopathological study. *Vet Pathol*. 1980;17(5):553–564.
74. Affolter VK, Moore PF. Localized and disseminated histiocytic sarcoma of dendritic cell origin in dogs. *Vet Pathol*. 2002;39(1):74–83.
75. Balkman C. Hepatobiliary neoplasia in dogs and cats, vet clinic small. *Anim*. 2009;39(3):617–625.
76. Patnaik AK. A morphologic and immunohistochemical study of hepatic neoplasms in cats. *Vet Pathol*. 1992;29(5):405–415.
77. Post G, Patnaik AK. Nonhematopoietic hepatic neoplasms in cats: 21 cases (1983–1988). *J Am Vet Med Assoc*. 1992;201(7):1080–1082.
78. Lawrence HJ, Erb HN, Harvey HJ. Nonlymphomatous hepatobiliary masses in cats: 41 cases (1972 to 1991). *Vet Surg*. 1994;23(5):365–368.
79. van Sprundel R, van den Ingh T, Guscetti F, et al. Classification of primary hepatic tumours in the cat. *Vet J*. 2014;202(2):255–266.
80. Nyland TG, Koblik PD, Tellyer SE. Ultrasonographic evaluation of biliary cystadenomas in cats. *Vet Radiol Ultrasound*. 1999;40(3):300–306.
81. Bahr KL, Sharkey LC, Murakami T, et al. Accuracy of US-guided FNA of focal liver lesions in dogs: 140 cases (2005–2008). *J Am Anim Hosp Assoc*. 2013;49(3):190–196.
82. Murakami T, Feeney DA, Bahr KL. Analysis of clinical and ultrasonographic data by use of logistic regression models for prediction of malignant versus benign causes of ultrasonographically detected focal liver lesions in dogs. *Am J Vet Res*. 2012;73(6):821–829.
83. Crabtree AC, Spangler E, Beard D, et al. Diagnostic accuracy of gray-scale ultrasonography for the detection of hepatic and splenic lymphoma in dogs. *Vet Radiol Ultrasound*. 2010;51(6):661–664.
84. Cuccouillo A, Lamb CR. Cellular features of sonographic target lesions of the liver and spleen in 21 dogs and a cat. *Vet Radiol Ultrasound*. 2002;43(3):275–278.
85. Prause LC, Twedt DC. Hepatic nodular hyperplasia. In: Bonagura JD, ed. *Current Veterinary Therapy XIII: Small Animal Practice*. Philadelphia: Saunders/Elsevier; 2000:675–676.
86. Stowater JL, Lamb CR, Schelling SH. Ultrasonographic features of canine hepatic nodular hyperplasia. *Vet Radiol Ultrasound*. 1990;31:268.
87. Ziegler LE, O'Brien RT, Waller KR, et al. Quantitative contrast harmonic ultrasound imaging of the normal canine liver. *Vet Radiol Ultrasound*. 2003;44(4):451–454.
88. O'Brien RT, Iani M, Matheson J, et al. Contrast harmonic ultrasound of spontaneous liver nodules in 32 dogs. *Vet Radiol Ultrasound*. 2004;45(6):547–553.
89. Ohlerth S, O'Brien RT. Contrast ultrasound: general principles and veterinary clinical applications. *Vet J*. 2007;174(3):501–512.
90. Nyland TG, Barthez PY, Ortega TM, et al. Hepatic ultrasonography and pathologic findings in dogs with canine superficial necrolytic dermatitis. *Vet Radiol Ultrasound*. 1996;37:200.
91. Kimmel SE, Christiansen W, Byrne KP. Clinicopathological, ultrasonographic, and histopathological findings of superficial necrolytic dermatitis with hepatopathy in a cat. *J Am Anim Hosp Assoc*. 2003;39(1):23–27.
92. March PA, Hiller A, Weisbrode SE, et al. Superficial necrolytic dermatitis in 11 dogs with a history of phenobarbital administration (1995–2002). *J Vet Intern Med*. 2004;18:65.
93. Hall-Fonte DL, Center SA, McDonough SP, et al. Hepatocutaeous syndrome in Shih Tzus: 31 cases (1996–2014). *J Am Vet Med Assoc*. 2016;248(7):802–813.
94. Schwarz LA, Penninck DG, Léveillé-Webster C. Hepatic abscesses in 13 dogs: a review of the ultrasonographic findings, clinical data and therapeutic options. *Vet Radiol Ultrasound*. 1998;39(4):357–365.
95. Zatelli A, Bonfanti U, Zini E, et al. Percutaneous drainage and alcoholization of hepatic abscesses in five dogs and a cat. *J Am Anim Hosp Assoc*. 2005;41(1):34–38.
96. Sergeeff JSJ, Armstrong PJ, Bunch SE. Hepatic abscesses in cats: 14 cases (1985–2002). *J Vet Intern Med*. 2004;18(3):295–300.
97. Sonnenfield JM, Armbrust LJ, Radlinsky MA, et al. Radiographic and ultrasonographic findings of liver lobe torsion in a dog. *Vet Radiol Ultrasound*. 2001;42(4):344–346.
98. Schwartz SG, Mitchell SL, Keating JH, et al. Liver lobe torsion in dogs: 13 cases (1995–2004). *J Am Vet Med Assoc*. 2006;228(2):242–247.
99. Quantz JE, Miles MS, Reed AL, et al. Elevation of alanine transaminase and gallbladder wall abnormalities as biomarkers of anaphylaxis in canine hypersensitivity patients. *J Vet Emerg Crit Care*. 2009;19(6):536–544.
100. Gaschen L. Update on hepatobiliary imaging. *Vet Clin North Am Small Anim Pract*. 2009;39(3):439–467.
101. Van Breda Vriesman AC, Engelbrecht MR, Smithuis RH, et al. Diffuse gallbladder wall thickening: differential diagnosis. *Amer J Radiol*. 2007;188:495–501.
102. Lisciandro GR, Gambino JM, Lisciandro SC. Thirteen dogs and a cat with ultrasonographically detected gallbladder

wall edema associated with cardiac disease. *J Vet Int Med.* 2021;35:1342–1346.
103. Seitz MA, Lee AM, Woodruff KA, et al. Sedation with dexmedetomidine is associated with transient gallbladder wall thickening and peritoneal effusion in some dogs undergoing abdominal ultrasonography. *J Vet Intern Med.* 2021;35:2743–2751.
104. Bini G, Cohen EB, Chiavaccini L, et al. Intravenous dexmedetomidine, morphine, or a combination can result in gallbladder wall thickening with no significant association with plasma histamine concentrations. *Vet Radiol Ultrasound.* 2022;63:319–327.
105. O'Neill EJ, Day MJ, Hall EJ, et al. Bacterial cholangitis/cholangiohepatitis with or without concurrent cholecystitis in four dogs. *J Small Anim Pract.* 2006;47(6):325–335.
106. Mitsui I, Ohtsuki S, Uchida K. Chronic cholecystitis of dogs: clinicopathologic features and relationship with liver. *Animals.* 2021;11. https://doi.org/10.3390/ani11113324.
107. Lawrence YA, Ruaux CG, Nemanic S, et al. Characterization, treatment, and outcome of bacterial cholecystitis and bactibilia in dogs. *J Am Vet Med Assoc.* 2015;246(9):982–989.
108. Policelli Smith R, Gookin JL, Smolski W, et al. Association between gallbladder ultrasound findings and bacterial culture of bile in 70 cats and 202 dogs. *J Vet Intern Med.* 2017;31:1451–1458.
109. Schiborra F, McConnell JF, Maddox TW. Percutaneous ultrasound-guided cholecystocentesis: complications and association of ultrasonographic findings with bile culture results. *J Small Anim Pract.* 2017;58(7):389–394.
110. Aguirre A. Diseases of the gallbladder and extrahepatic biliary system. In: Ettinger S, Feldman E, eds. *Textbook of Veterinary Internal Medicine*. St Louis: Elsevier; 2010.
111. Gaillot HA, Penninck DG, Webster CR, et al. Ultrasonographic features of extrahepatic biliary obstruction in 30 cats. *Vet Radiol Ultrasound.* 2007;48(5):439–447.
112. Center SA, Randolph JF, Warner KL, et al. Bacterial culture and immunohistochemical detection of bacteria and endotoxin in cats with suppurative cholangitis-cholangiohepatitis syndrome. *JAVMA.* 2022;260(2):194–211.
113. Secchi P, Poppl AG, Ilha A, et al. Prevalence, risk factors, and biochemical markers in dogs with ultrasound-diagnosed biliary sludge. *Res Vet Sci.* 2012;93(3):1185–1189.
114. Bandyopadhyay S, Varshney JP, Hoque M, et al. Prevalence of cholecystic disease in dogs: an ultrasonographic evaluation. *Asian J Anim Vet Adv.* 2007;2(4):234–238.
115. Cook AK, Jambhekar A, Dylewski AM. Gallbladder sludge in dogs: ultrasonographic and clinical findings in 200 patients. *J Am Anim Hosp Assoc.* 2016;52:125–131.
116. Butler T, Bexfield N, Dor C. A multicenter retrospective study assessing progression of biliary sludge in dogs using ultrasonography. *J Vet Intern Med.* 2022;36(3):976–985.
117. Mizutani S, Torisu S, Kaneko Y, et al. Retrospective analysis of canine gallbladder contents in biliary sludge and gallbladder mucoceles. *J Vet Med Sci.* 2017;79(2):366–374.
118. Harran N, d'Anjou MA, Dunn M, et al. Gallbladder sludge on ultrasound is predictive of increased liver enzymes and total bilirubin in cats. *Can Vet J.* 2011;52(9):999–1003.
119. Villm J, DeMonaco S, Larson M. Prevalence of gallbladder sludge and associated abnormalities in cats undergoing abdominal ultrasound. *Vet Radiol Ultrasound.* 2022;63:601–608.
120. Viljoen AD, Tamborini A, Bexfield NH. Gall bladder ejection fractions in dogs investigated for chronic altered appetite: 14 cases (2015–2017). *J Sm Anim Pract.* 2021;62:1101–1107.
121. Diana A, Guglielmini C, Specchi S, et al. Ultrasonographic evaluation of preprandial and postprandial gallbladder volume in healthy cats. *Am J Vet Res.* 2012;73:1583–1588.
122. Besso JG, Wrigley RH, Gliatto JM, et al. Ultrasonographic appearance and clinical findings in 14 dogs with gallbladder mucocele. *Vet Radiol Ultrasound.* 2000;41(3):261–271.
123. Pike FS, Berg J, King NW, et al. Gallbladder mucocele in dogs: 30 cases (2000–2003). *J Am Vet Med Assoc.* 2004;224(10):1615–1622.
124. Worley DR, Hottinger HA, Lawrence HJ. Surgical management of gallbladder mucoceles in dogs: 22 cases (1999–2003). *J Am Vet Med Assoc.* 2004;225(9):1418–1422.
125. Walter R, Dunn ME, d'Anjou MA, et al. Nonsurgical resolution of gallbladder mucocele in two dogs. *J Am Vet Med Assoc.* 2008;232(11):1688–1693.
126. Crews LJ, Feeney DA, Jessen CR, et al. Clinical, ultrasonographic, and laboratory findings associated with gallbladder disease and rupture in dogs: 45 cases (1997–2007). *J Am Vet Med Assoc.* 2009;234(3):359–366.
127. Aguirre AL, Center SA, Randolph JF, et al. Gallbladder disease in Shetland Sheepdogs: 38 cases (1995–2005). *J Am Vet Med Assoc.* 2007;231(1):79–88.
128. Uno T, Okamoto K, Onaka T, et al. Correlation between ultrasonographic imaging of the gallbladder and gallbladder content in eleven cholecystectomised dogs and their prognoses. *J Vet Med Sci.* 2009;71(10):1295–1300.
129. Choi J, Kim A, Keh S, et al. Comparison between ultrasonographic and clinical findings in 43 dogs with gallbladder mucoceles. *Vet Radiol Ultrasound.* 2014;55(2):202–207.
130. Jaffey JA, Kreisler R, Shumway K, et al. Ultrasonographic patterns, clinical findings, and prognostic variables in dogs from Asia with gallbladder mucocele. *J Vet Intern Med.* 2022;36:566–575.
131. Gookin JL, Mathews KG, Cullen J, Seiler G. Qualitative metabolomics profiling of serum and bile from dogs with gallbladder mucocele formation. *PloS One.* 2018;13(1):e0191076.
132. Jaffey JA, Graham A, VanEerde E, et al. Gallbladder mucocele: variables associated with outcome and the utility of ultrasonography to identify gallbladder rupture in 219 dogs (2007–2016). *J Vet Intern Med.* 2018;32:195–200.
133. Bargellini P, Orlandi R, Paloni C, et al. Evaluation of contrast-enhancing ultrasonography as a method for detecting gallbladder necrosis or rupture in dogs. *Vet Radiol Ultrasound.* 2016;57(6):611–620.
134. Mesich ML, Mayhew PD, Paek M, et al. Gall bladder mucoceles and their association with endocrinopathies in dogs: a retrospective case-control study. *J Small Anim Pract.* 2009;50(12):630–635.
135. Gookin JL, Correa MT, Peters A, et al. Association of gallbladder mucocele histologic diagnosis with selected drug use in dogs: a matched case-control study. *J Vet Intern Med.* 2015;29(6):1464–1472.
136. Jaffey JA, Pavlick M, Webster CR, et al. Effect of clinical signs, endocrinopathies, timing of surgery, hyperlipidemia, and hyperbilirubinemia on outcome in dogs with gallbladder mucocele. *The Vet Journal.* 2019;251. https://doi.org/10.1016/j.tvjl.2019.105350.
137. Bennett SL, Milne M, Slocombe RF, et al. Gallbladder mucocele and concurrent hepatic lipidosis in a cat. *Aust Vet J.* 2007;85(10):397–400.

138. Nyland TG, Gillett NA. Sonographic evaluation of experimental bile duct ligation in the dog. *Vet Radiol.* 1982;23:252.
139. Wilkinson AR, DeMonaco SM, Panciera DL, et al. Bile duct obstruction associated with pancreatitis in 46 dogs. *J Vet Intern Med.* 2020;34:1794–1800.
140. Callahan JE, Haddad JL, Brown DC, et al. Feline cholangitis: a necropsy study of 44 cats (1986–2008). *J Feline Med Surg.* 2011;13(8):570–576.
141. Brain PH, Barrs VR, Martin P, et al. Feline cholecystitis and acute neutrophilic cholangitis: clinical findings, bacterial isolates, and response to treatment in six cases. *J Feline Med Surg.* 2006;8(2):91–103.
142. Jaffey JA. Feline cholangitis/cholangiohepatitis complex. *J Small Anim Pract.* 2022;63:573–589.
143. Center SA, Randolph JF, Warner KL, et al. Clinical features, concurrent disorders, and survival time in cats with suppurative cholangitis-cholangiohepatitis syndrome. *JAVMA.* 2022;260:212–227.
144. Fragkou FC, Adamamma-Moraitou K, Poutahidis T, et al. Prevalence and clinicopathological features of triaditis in a prospective case series of symptomatic and asymptomatic cats. *J Vet Intern Med.* 2016;30:1031–1045.
145. Harrison JL, Turek BJ, Brown DC, et al. Cholangitis and cholangiohepatitis in dogs: a descriptive study of 54 cases based on histopathologic diagnosis (2004–2014). *J Vet Intern Med.* 2018;32:172–180.
146. Tamborini A, Jahns H, McAllister H, et al. Bacterial cholangitis, cholecystitis, or both in dogs. *J Vet Intern Med.* 2016;30:1046–1055.
147. Anjou MA, Penninck D, Cornejo L, et al. Ultrasonographic diagnosis of portosystemic shunting in dogs and cats. *Vet Radiol Ultrasound.* 2004;45(5):424–437.
148. d'Anjou MA. The sonographic search for portosystemic shunts. *Clin Tech Small Anim Pract.* 2007;22(3):104–114.
149. Salwei RM, O'Brien RT, Mathieson JS. Use of contrast harmonic ultrasound for the diagnosis of congenital portosystemic shunts in three dogs. *Vet Radiol Ultrasound.* 2003;44:301.
150. Palerme JS, Brown JC, Marks SL, et al. Splenosystemic shunts in cats: a retrospective of 33 cases (2004–2011). *J Vet Int Med.* 2013;27:1347.
151. Johnson KL, Porter EG, Berry CB. Analysis of feline splenic radiographic measurements and their correlation to ultrasonographic measurements. *J Fel Med Surg.* 2016;1.
152. Neer TM. Clinical approach to splenomegaly in dogs and cats. *Compend Contin Educ Pract Vet Small Anim.* 1996;18(35).
153. Wilson DV, Carpenter RE, Evans AT. The effect of four anesthetic protocols on splenic size in dogs. *Vet Anaesth Analg.* 2003;30(2):100–101.
154. Baldo CF, Garcia-Pereira FL, Nelson NC, et al. Effects of anesthetic drugs on canine splenic volume determined via computed tomography. *Am J Vet Res.* 2012;73(11): 1715–1719.
155. Reese SL, Zekas LJ, Iazbik C, et al. Effect of sevoflurane anesthesia and blood donation on the sonographic appearance of the spleen in 60 healthy cats. *Vet Radiol Ultrasound.* 2013;54(2):168–175.
156. Kealy JK, McAllister H, Graham JP. *Diagnostic Radiology and Ultrasonography of the Dog and Cat.* 5th ed. Philadelphia: Saunders/Elsevier; 2011.
157. Hanson JA, Papageorges M, Girard E, et al. Ultrasonographic appearance of splenic disease in 101 cats. *Vet Radiol Ultrasound.* 2001;42(5):441–445.
158. Spangler WL, Culbertson MR. Prevalence and type of splenic disease in cats: 455 cases (1985–1991). *J Am Vet Med Assoc.* 1992;201(5):773–776.
159. Auger M, Fazio C, de Swarte M, et al. Administration of certain sedative drugs is associated with variation in sonographic and radiographic splenic size in healthy cats. *Vet Radiol Ultrasound.* 2019;60(6):717–728.
160. DeGroot W, Giuffrida MA, Rubin J, et al. Primary splenic torsion in dogs: 102 cases (1992–2014). *J Am Vet Med Assoc.* 2016;248(6):661–668.
161. Stickle RL. Radiographic signs of isolated splenic torsion in dogs: eight cases (1980–1987). *J Am Vet Med Assoc.* 1989;194(1):103–106.
162. Patsikas MN, Rallis T, Kladakis SE, et al. Computed tomography diagnosis of isolated splenic torsion in a dog. *Vet Radiol Ultrasound.* 2001;42(3):235–237.
163. Wrigley RH, Konde LJ, Park RD, et al. Clinical features and diagnosis of splenic hematomas in dogs: 10 cases (1980–1987). *J Am Anim Hosp Assoc.* 1989;25:371.
164. Weinstein MJ, Carpenter JL, Schunk CJ. Nonangiogenic and nonlymphomatous sarcomas of the canine spleen: 57 cases (1975–1987). *J Am Vet Med Assoc.* 1989;195(6):784–788.
165. Spangler WL, Culbertson MR. Prevalence, type, and importance of splenic diseases in dogs: 1,480 cases (1985–1989). *J Am Vet Med Assoc.* 1992;200(6):829–834.
166. Battiato P, Fernandez Y, Salguüero R, et al. Spontaneous emphysematous splenitis: radiographic and ultrasonographic findings in three Golden Retriever dogs. *Vet Radiol Ultrasound.* 2021;62:309–315.
167. Mattoon JS, Duffy M. Spleen. In: Mattoon JS, Sellon RK, Berry CR, eds. *Small Animal Diagnostic Ultrasound.* 4th ed. St. Louis: Elsevier; 2021.
168. Hecht S. Spleen. In: Penninck D, d'Anjou MA, eds. *Atlas of Small Animal Ultrasonography.* 2nd ed. Ames, IA: Blackwell; 2015.
169. Sayre RS, Spaulding KA. Formulation of a standardized protocol and determination of the size and appearance of the spleen in healthy cats. *J Feline Med Surg.* 2014;16(4):326–332.
170. O'Brien RT, Waller KR, Osgood TL. Sonographic features of drug-induced splenic congestion. *Vet Radiol Ultrasound.* 2004;45(3):225–227.
171. Mai W. The hilar perivenous hyperechoic triangle as a sign of acute splenic torsion in dogs. *Vet Radiol Ultrasound.* 2006;47(5):487–491.
172. Hardie EM, Vaden SL, Spaulding K, et al. Splenic infarction in 16 dogs: a retrospective study. *J Vet Intern Med.* 1995;9(3):141–148.
173. Cruz-Arámbulo R, Wrigley R, Powers B. Sonographic features of histiocytic neoplasms in the canine abdomen. *Vet Radiol Ultrasound.* 2004;45(6):554–558.
174. Ramirez S, Douglass JP, Robertson ID. Ultrasonographic features of canine abdominal malignant histiocytosis. *Vet Radiol Ultrasound.* 2002;43(2):167–170.
175. Atiee G, Kvitko-White H, Spaulding K, et al. Ultrasonographic appearance of histoplasmosis identified in the spleen in 15 cats. *Vet Radiol Ultrasound.* 2014;55(3): 310–314.
176. Hanson JA, Penninck DG. Ultrasonographic evaluation of a traumatic splenic hematoma and literature review. *Vet Radiol Ultrasound.* 1994;35:463.
177. Wrigley RH, Park RD, Konde LJ, et al. Ultrasonographic features of splenic hemangiosarcoma in dogs: 18 cases (1980–1986). *J Am Vet Med Assoc.* 1988;192(8): 1113–1117.
178. Konde LJ, Lebel JL, Park RD, et al. Sonographic application in the diagnosis of intraabdominal abscess in the dog. *Vet Radiol.* 1986;27:151.
179. Walzer C, Hittmair K, Walzer-Wagner C. Ultrasonographic identification and characterization of splenic nodular lipomatosis or myelolipomas in cheetahs *(Acinonyx jubatus). Vet Radiol Ultrasound.* 1996;37:289.

180. Schwarz LA, Penninck DG, Gliatto J. Ultrasound corner: canine splenic myelolipomas. *Vet Radiol Ultrasound*. 2001;42(4):347–348.
181. Cleveland MJ, Casale S. Incidence of malignancy and outcomes for dogs undergoing splenectomy for incidentally detected nonruptured splenic nodules or masses: 105 cases (2009–2013). *J Am Vet Med Assoc*. 2016;248(11): 1267–1273.
182. Yankin I, Nemanic S, Funes S, et al. Clinical relevance of splenic nodules or heterogeneous splenic parenchyma assessed by cytologic evaluation of fine-needle samples in 125 dogs (2011–2015). *J Vet Intern Med*. 2020;34: 125–131.
183. Ballegeer EA, Forrest LJ, Dickinson RM, et al. Correlation of ultrasonographic appearance of lesions and cytologic and histologic diagnoses in splenic aspirates from dogs and cats: 32 cases (2002–2005). *J Am Vet Med Assoc*. 2007;230(5):690–696.
184. Watson AT, Penninck D, Knoll JS, et al: Safety and correlation of test results of combined ultrasound-guided fine-needle aspiration and needle core biopsy of the canine spleen, *Vet Radiol Ultrasound* 52(3):317–322.

ELECTRONIC RESOURCES

Additional information related to the content in Chapter 40 can be found online at eBooks.Health.Elsevier.com

- Chapter Quiz

CHAPTER 41

Kidneys and Ureters

Gabriela S. Seiler • Ryan Appleby

Renal disease is common in dogs and cats, and imaging is an integral part of the diagnostic workup of these patients. Multiple imaging modalities are available to evaluate the kidneys and ureters, and the modality to select depends on the type of information desired. In this chapter, the indications, technique, and normal imaging findings, as well as the imaging appearance of diseases of the upper urinary tract, are reviewed.

NORMAL ANATOMY AND IMAGING PROCEDURES

Radiography

Indications

Radiographs are often obtained in the diagnostic workup of patients with abdominal disease, and interpretation of the radiographic appearance of the kidneys is an important skill. Radiographs are useful to identify broad changes in the roentgen signs (size, number, shape, opacity, location, margination) associated with the kidneys and ureters as well as to detect associated retroperitoneal or bone disease. Survey radiographs are indicated if there is a history of trauma to the abdomen or pelvis with possible involvement of the urinary tract or if a dorsal abdominal mass is suspected. Survey radiographs are an essential part of any abdominal radiographic procedure involving contrast medium.

Technique

A diagnostic radiographic study of the abdomen and kidneys should always include both left and right lateral as well as ventrodorsal (VD) views of the abdomen. Patient rotation should be minimized as even mild rotation may dorsally or medially displace one kidney and superimposition with the spine reduces visibility. Right lateral radiographs provide more longitudinal separation between the right and left kidney.[1] Suspected ureteral calculi can be separated from gastrointestinal content by use of oblique projections or compression techniques. Feces may have to be eliminated, by means of fasting or an enema, prior to a radiographic study to evaluate the distal ureters.

Normal Radiographic Findings

The kidneys are located in the retroperitoneal space and outlined by surrounding fat.

Canine kidneys are oval (Fig. 41.1). The cranial pole of the right kidney is often poorly visible, because it abuts and silhouettes with the caudate lobe of the liver. The left kidney is more mobile than the right, and it can be located relatively ventrally in animals with a large amount of retroperitoneal fat. In the VD projection, the right kidney is located at the level of the 13th rib but is often obscured by liver and other superimposed abdominal organs, whereas the left kidney is normally visible caudal to the gastric fundus and caudomedial to the proximal extremity of the spleen at the level of L1-L3.

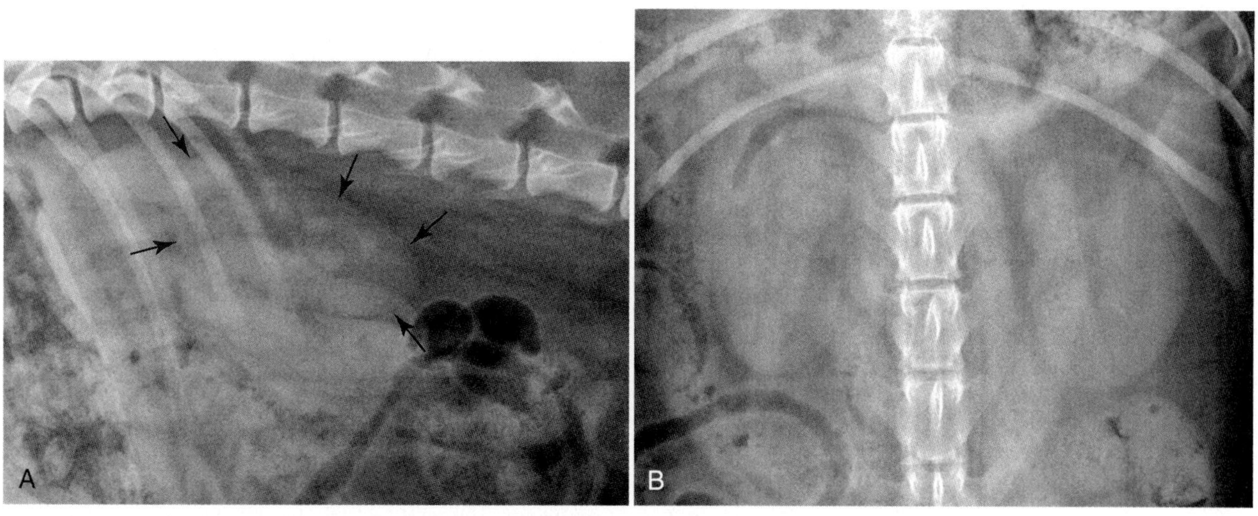

Fig. 41.1 Lateral **(A)** and ventrodorsal (VD; **B**) radiographs of the abdomen of a normal dog. The kidneys are oval and outlined by retroperitoneal fat. The right kidney (*black arrows*) is more cranial and, in this dog, slightly more dorsal to the left kidney.

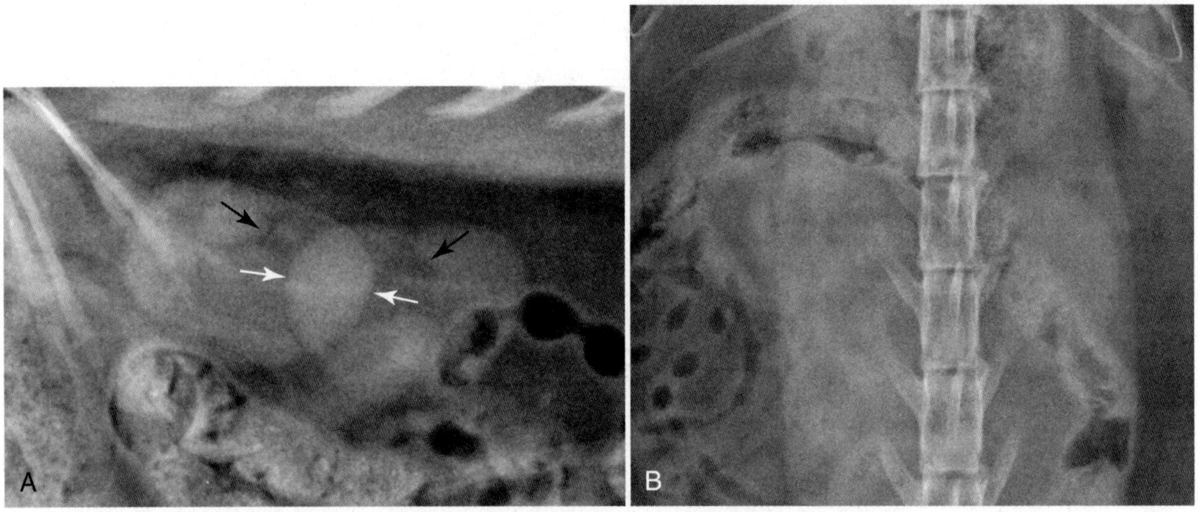

Fig. 41.2 Lateral (**A**) and ventrodorsal (VD; **B**) radiographs of the abdomen of a normal cat. Both kidneys are relatively round with a smooth surface. Fat opacity is visible at the renal hilus in the lateral view (*black arrows*); this is a normal finding in many cats. Note the summation opacity in the lateral view (*white arrows*) where the kidneys overlap. The right kidney is not readily perceptible in the VD view because of superimposed bowel.

Feline kidneys are more rounded and are located typically between L1 and L4, either at the same level or with the right kidney in a more cranial position (Fig. 41.2). In lateral radiographs, the caudal pole of the right kidney may overlap the cranial pole of the left kidney and the summation of the two poles can give the false impression of a small rounded kidney or a retroperitoneal mass (see Fig. 41.2A).

An ectopic kidney or kidneys in a very caudal location occur sporadically.[2] Normal ureters are not visible radiographically.

Small kidneys are indicative of chronic disease, whereas large kidneys are associated with more acute processes. In general, assessment of renal length is more reliable on VD projections because there is no overlap of the kidneys, and magnification of both kidneys is equal. Renal length in normal dogs ranges between 2.5 and 3.5 times the length of L2.[3] In cats, the normal renal length has been measured to be 2.4 to 3.0 times the length of L2.[4] Older cats without signs of renal disease can have smaller kidneys (1.9–2.6 times the length of L2); however, it is difficult to know whether subclinical renal disease may have been present in these cats.[4] Hormonal influence depending on reproductive status alters renal length in cats, both in males and females. Intact cats tend to have larger kidneys (range 2.1–3.2 times the length of L2) than neutered cats (1.9–2.6 times the length of L2).[5] It is important to realize that these normal relationships were determined from a relatively small number of cats and are only intended as guidelines.

Normal kidneys are of uniform soft tissue opacity and smoothly marginated, although fat deposition in the renal pelvis in cats can lead to focal central radiolucency (see Fig. 41.2A). Mineralization associated with the kidneys or ureters is always abnormal, although it may not necessarily be the cause of clinical signs.

Ultrasonography

Indications

Ultrasonographic evaluation of the renal parenchyma is indicated if there is evidence of renal dysfunction. Specific indications include clinicopathologic abnormalities (azotemia, elevated symmetric dimethylarginine [SDMA], change in urine specific gravity), abnormal renal palpation or abdominal radiographic findings, and clinical signs such as hematuria, polyuria, oliguria, or anuria. Renal ultrasound may serve as a screening tool for congenital renal diseases such as aplasia, hypoplasia, dysplasia, and polycystic kidney disease.[2,6,7]

Although ultrasound findings are usually not disease specific, they allow differentiating acute and chronic renal changes, mass lesions, cysts, mineralizations, and alterations of the collecting system and ureters. Needle aspirates or biopsies can be obtained under ultrasound guidance.[8,9] Doppler ultrasound is a useful addition to the grayscale ultrasound examination to evaluate for abnormal renal perfusion caused by infarction, transplant rejection, or mass lesions.[10] Contrast-enhanced ultrasound allows more detailed and more sensitive assessment of renal vasculature and perfusion, and normal perfusion parameters have been described in dogs and cats.[11,12] Contrast-enhanced ultrasound of the canine and feline kidney has potential for delineation of renal parenchymal lesions such as masses or infarcts.[13,14]

Technique

Renal ultrasound should be performed with the highest frequency transducer that enables adequate penetration. In most dogs and cats, 7.5 to 15 MHz is appropriate; 5 MHz or lower frequency transducers should only be used in large dogs. Subcostal or intercostal windows with the patient in lateral or dorsal recumbency allow access to the kidneys, depending on patient size and thoracic conformation. Standard image planes include dorsal (Fig. 41.3A), sagittal (see Fig. 41.3B), and transverse (see Fig. 41.3C) planes, always followed by fanning the transducer through the entire kidney. Renal length should be measured along its maximal pole-to-pole length in a sagittal or dorsal plane image, while avoiding obliquity which would result in artificial shortening of the kidney. The renal pelvis is best evaluated in dorsal and transverse planes. The ureters can be followed caudally from the renal pelvis if dilated. To verify patency and normal location of the ureterovesical junction, the bladder should be evaluated for presence of two urine jets from the dorsolateral bladder wall. If not seen with conventional grayscale imaging, Doppler ultrasound can be used to better delineate the jet. Addition of a diuretic markedly improves frequency and visibility of ureteral jets by increasing urine production and altering the specific gravity of the urine exiting the ureterovesicular junction compared with the urine already present in the bladder.[15]

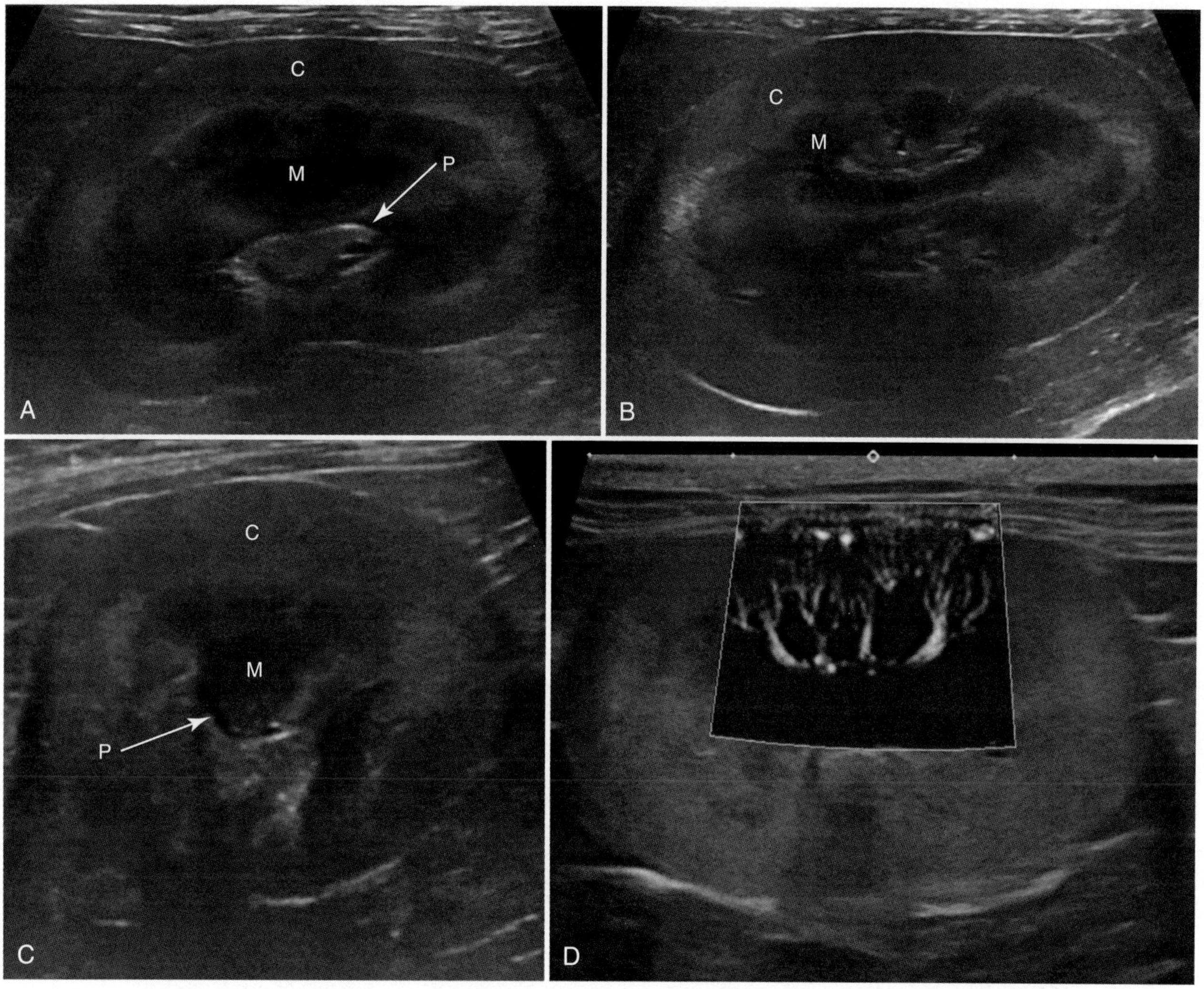

Fig. 41.3 Ultrasound images of a normal canine kidney in dorsal **(A)**, sagittal **(B)**, and transverse **(C)** planes. The renal vasculature is shown with microvascular Doppler **(D)**. The medulla (*M*) is hypoechoic relative to the cortex (*C*) and is divided by the hyperechoic interlobar vessels and pelvic diverticula. The renal pelvis (*P*) is mildly distended and is best seen in transverse and dorsal planes (*white arrows*).

Normal Ultrasonographic Findings

Normal canine and feline kidneys are outlined by a thin, smooth hyperechoic capsule and have a clear distinction between cortex and medulla (see Fig. 41.3). The renal cortex in most patients is hypoechoic to isoechoic to the liver and spleen, although dogs and cats without evidence of renal disease may have a renal cortex that is hyperechoic to liver.[16] In cats, cortical hyperechogenicity can occur with fat deposition.[17]

The normal medulla is hypoechoic, creating a well-defined transition to the cortex. The interlobar vessels and pelvic diverticula give the renal medulla a lobulated appearance. The arcuate vessels are seen at the corticomedullary junction as short, hyperechoic parallel lines that may produce a distal shadow, not to be confused with renal mineralization. The renal pelvis is normally collapsed, but a smoothly margined, thin rim of fluid of up to 2 mm in diameter can be seen in normal animals, especially when using high-resolution transducers.[18] Increased diuresis, caused by exogenous fluid administration or polyuria/polydipsia, results in mild pyelectasia.[18] The pelvic diverticula are not visible normally. The renal pelvis is surrounded by the hyperechoic sinus, which contains dense fibrous tissue and fat, particularly in overweight cats.

Normal kidney size in cats ranges between 3.0 and 4.3 cm.[19] In dogs, size is much more variable depending on body weight and conformation. As a rule of thumb, 10 mm per 10 pounds of body weight can be added within the normal range of 3 to 10 cm.[20] A ratio of 5.5 to 9.1 of the maximal renal length to the luminal diameter of the aorta at the level of the kidney is proposed to take patient size into account.[21] Even using this method, the large range of normal values makes detection of subtle size changes challenging. Renal length, therefore, is not very helpful as an isolated criterion, unless markedly abnormal, and all other ultrasonographic findings have to be taken into account to determine if a kidney is normal or not.

With Doppler ultrasound, the renal artery and vein, interlobar, arcuate, and interlobular vessels can be identified (see Fig. 41.3D). The resistive index should be less than 0.72 in dogs and 0.70 in cats, and the pulsatility index less than 1.52 in dogs and 1.29 in cats.[22] Normal ureters are visible only with high-resolution ultrasound systems and ideal patient-related conditions. Ureters are best followed from a transverse view of the renal pelvis, because they turn medially and can be tortuous until they extend caudally, lateral to the aorta and caudal vena cava. Thin hyperechoic walls and occasional waves of peristalsis with a small bolus of fluid passing through can be seen in a normal ureter.

Excretory Urography and Contrast-Enhanced Computed Tomography

Indications

Intravenous administration of iodinated contrast medium, followed by imaging either with radiography (excretory urography [EU] or intravenous pyelography) or computed tomography (CT) allows assessment of renal structure and vascularity, patency of the collecting system, and to some degree, renal function. The use of EU has decreased but it can still provide useful information. CT has the advantage of imaging the urinary tract without superimposition of other soft tissue or osseous structures, with the option of multiplanar and three-dimensional reconstructions. Indications for EU or CT include urinary tract trauma, hematuria, suspected ureteral ectopia, assessment of retroperitoneal masses, and in some instances, ureteral obstruction. Dual-phase renal angiography can be performed to assess the arterial and venous blood supply of the kidneys separately. This is used mainly for presurgical assessment of feline kidney donors.[23,24] While both methods allow a crude estimation of renal functionality, it is possible to calculate glomerular filtration rate in dogs and cats using contrast-enhanced CT imaging.[25–27]

This has to be weighed against the fact that administration of contrast medium itself poses a risk in the presence of renal disease. Adverse reactions to the intravenous administration of iodinated contrast media include nausea, vomiting, hives, hypotension, and importantly, contrast medium–induced renal failure. Renal insufficiency is a risk factor for development of contrast medium–induced nephropathy, together with the presence of hypovolemia.[10,11,28,29] Contraindications therefore include anuric renal failure, dehydration, hypotension, and known hypersensitivity to iodinated contrast media.

Technique

Patient preparation is a key to obtaining a diagnostic study. Food, but not water, should be withheld for at least 12 to 24 hours before the study. A cleansing enema can be used to evacuate the colon, preferably several hours before the study to allow fecal material and gas to pass. This is more important for EU where superimposition with a full colon may render the study nondiagnostic. The patient should be hydrated and have adequate renal function. Because iodinated contrast medium leads to increased urine-specific gravity and may also inhibit bacterial growth for at least 24 hours, urinalysis should be performed before contrast medium is administered.[30]

Sedation or general anesthesia is recommended for both studies, and an intravenous catheter should be in place throughout the study to provide venous access if complications arise. Survey radiographs or CT images prior to contrast medium administration are an essential part of both studies as small urinary calculi and parenchymal mineralizations may be obscured by the contrast medium.

Excretory urography: Iodinated contrast medium is administered intravenously as a bolus injection at a dose of 600 to 700 mg iodine (I) per kg body weight.[13,14] VD and right lateral abdominal radiographs are acquired immediately after injection and are repeated typically after 5, 20, and 40 minutes or until a diagnosis is reached. Oblique projections for better visualization of the ureters can be added at 5 minutes and later time points. To evaluate the renal arteries, a VD radiograph should be acquired 5 to 7 seconds after bolus injection of contrast medium.

Computed tomography: Iodinated contrast medium is administered intravenously as a bolus at a dose of 400 to 800 mg I/kg body weight. Image series are acquired to evaluate the different phases of contrast medium excretion as outlined later. Optimal ureteral opacification occurs 3 minutes post injection and can persist for about 1 hour.[31] Image series may have to be repeated several times to visualize the entire course of both ureters because of ureteral peristalsis. Positioning the patient in sternal recumbency with the pelvis elevated is helpful in outlining the ureterovesical junctions, because the contrast medium will accumulate in the bladder apex away from the neck, facilitating the distinction between the contrast medium–filled ureters and the bladder neck.

Normal Imaging Findings

For iodinated contrast medium to be excreted normally by the kidneys, normal arterial and venous flow, an anatomically normal kidney, functioning nephrons, and unobstructed flow of urine away from the kidneys into the urinary bladder are necessary. There are three phases of contrast medium excretion. The vascular phase starts approximately 5 to 7 seconds after intravenous bolus injection. In the nephrogram phase, contrast medium is present in the renal parenchyma through glomerular filtration into the nephrons. The nephrogram phase begins after approximately 10 seconds and lasts up to 2 minutes until the pyelogram phase starts and the nephrogram begins to fade (Fig. 41.4). Nephrogram opacity/attenuation should continue to decrease progressively; only approximately 25% of normal dogs still have a detectable nephrogram 2 hours after contrast medium injection.[32] In the pyelogram phase, contrast medium is filtered into the collecting system without tubular reabsorption or secretion.

Normal renal imaging on CT has been reported in dogs where the normal renal length–to–L2 vertebral body ratio in CT imaging was determined to be 2.7 (95% confidence interval [CI], 2.5–2.9), and the renal length–to–aortic ratio was 7.4 (95% CI, 7.07–7.74).[33,42] If renal function is normal, the collecting system is consistently more opaque/attenuating than the renal parenchyma. The normal renal pelvis is curvilinear and less than 2 mm in width. The pelvic diverticula may be seen in some dogs and most cats and appear as thin (1 mm) spikes radiating from the pelvis toward the periphery. Neither the renal pelvis nor the diverticula should have blunted, rounded edges. The ureters tend not to be filled with contrast medium uniformly throughout their length because of ureteral peristalsis. Imaging, therefore, may have to be repeated to assess the entire length of the ureters. Normal ureters are not more than 2 to 3 mm in width. They terminate at the dorsal aspect of the bladder neck, where they curve cranially for a short distance before entering the wall. The duration and intensity of the opacification of the kidney during an excretory urogram depend on the dose of contrast medium administered; renal perfusion; glomerular filtration; tubular reabsorption of water; the patient's hydration status, which is important to maintain adequate renal perfusion; and patency of the renal outflow tract.

Antegrade Ultrasound-Guided Pyelography

Indications

Ultrasound-guided injection of contrast medium into the renal pelvis leads to excellent opacification of the collecting system because the contrast medium is not diluted, and its concentration in the collecting system is not dependent on renal function. This procedure can be performed in azotemic patients without loss of image quality. In addition, each renal pelvis and ureter can be assessed individually. Other advantages include the lack of systemic contrast medium reactions and collection of urine directly from the renal pelvis for urinalysis and microbiologic testing. The main indication for this procedure is suspected ureteral obstruction. Contraindications include coagulopathies, because some hemorrhage may occur. Adverse effects may be significant and include hemorrhage, focal damage of renal tissue, and spread of infection in the presence of pyelonephritis or pyonephrosis with perirenal sepsis and abscessation. Contrast medium may also leak into the retroperitoneal space.[34] Loss of renal function secondary to the

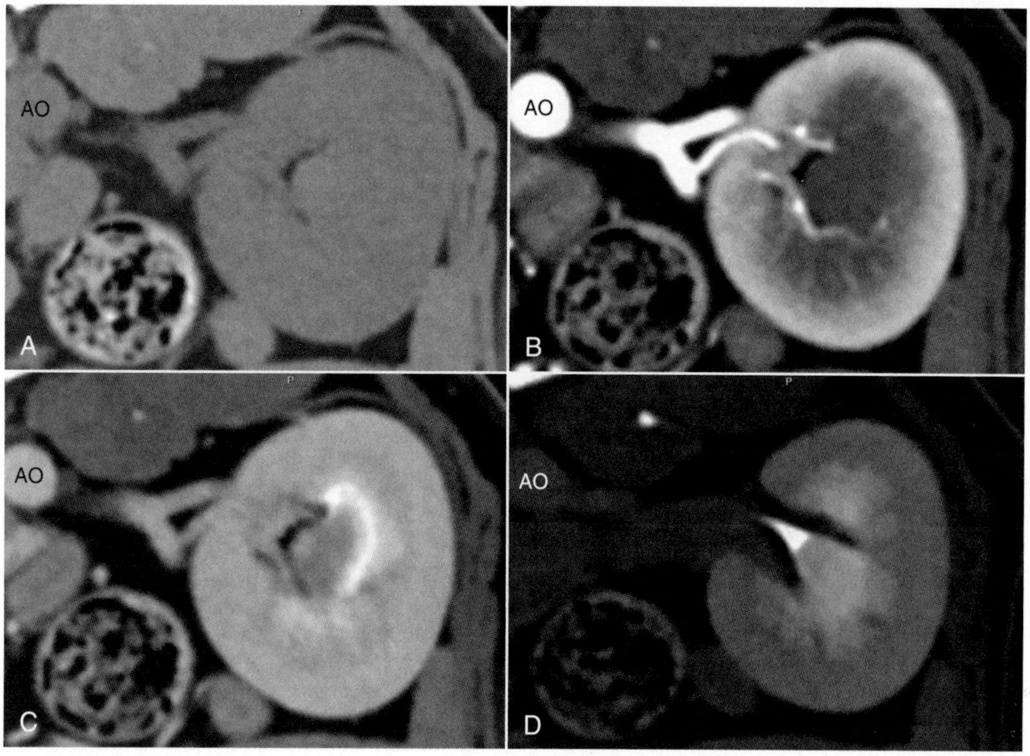

Fig. 41.4 Transverse contrast-enhanced computed tomography images of a dog with no signs of renal disease. The left kidney is shown before contrast medium administration **(A)**, during the vascular phase **(B)**, venous phase **(C)**, and pyelogram phase **(D)** after intravenous administration of iodinated contrast medium. The aorta is labeled (*AO*). In **B**, the renal vessels are enhanced; in **C**, the renal parenchyma is enhanced; and in **D**, contrast medium has reached the renal pelvis and proximal ureter.

procedure is minimal but should be a consideration in patients with already severely compromised renal function.

Technique

Heavy sedation or general anesthesia is necessary. The skin is prepared aseptically, and a 22- to 25-gauge needle connected with an extension set and three-way stopcock is introduced into the renal pelvis under ultrasound or fluoroscopic guidance. Depending on the size of the renal pelvis, 1 to 2 mL of urine is removed for laboratory testing. Nonionic iodinated contrast medium equivalent to half of the volume of urine removed is then introduced slowly, and the size of the renal pelvis is monitored with ultrasound or fluoroscopy.[34] Overdistention of the renal pelvis should be avoided, because rupture may occur. Immediately after contrast medium injection, VD, oblique, and lateral abdominal radiographs are acquired. If bilateral abnormalities are suspected, the procedure can be repeated on the contralateral side.

Normal Imaging Findings

The renal pelvis becomes distended with mild blunting of the pelvic diverticula, as contrast medium is introduced under mild pressure. If the ureter is patent, contrast medium should appear in the urinary bladder almost immediately (Fig. 41.5). Narrowing of the ureter may be observed because of peristalsis; repeat images will be needed to differentiate between peristalsis and stricture.

Magnetic Resonance Imaging

Magnetic resonance imaging (MRI) is used in people to assess renal diseases, perfusion, and function, but little work has been performed in small animals. Advantages and indications are similar to those described for CT, but use is limited by cost, availability, and duration of the imaging studies. Protocols for magnetic resonance angiography of the renal vasculature in renal transplant donors are available.[35]

Scintigraphy

Compared with other nonimaging renal function testing, renal scintigraphy using technetium-99m diethylenetriamine pentaacetic acid has the advantage of being able to determine the relative contribution of each kidney to total renal function. This is especially important in patients with impaired renal function before planned nephrectomy. Describing the technique of renal scintigraphy is beyond the scope of this chapter, and readers are referred to another source.[36]

RENAL DISEASES

Abnormal Renal Size

It is important to keep in mind that renal size and shape may be normal in the presence of renal disease. In particular, early chronic, acute toxic, inflammatory, or infectious nephropathies, as well as amyloidosis, do not always lead to alteration of renal size or shape.[37]

Small Kidneys

Reduced renal size is most commonly caused by chronic nephropathy. Chronic renal disease is also associated with other radiographic findings that may include abnormal, irregular shape due to cortical infarcts, and renal mineralizations (Fig. 41.6, eFig. 41.1). Other differentials of bilaterally reduced renal size include congenital anomalies such as dysplasia or hypoplasia.[7] Renal atrophy is seen with chronic, longstanding ureteral obstruction and is thus usually associated with hydronephrosis; the affected kidney (typically only one) can thus be reduced or relatively normal in size.

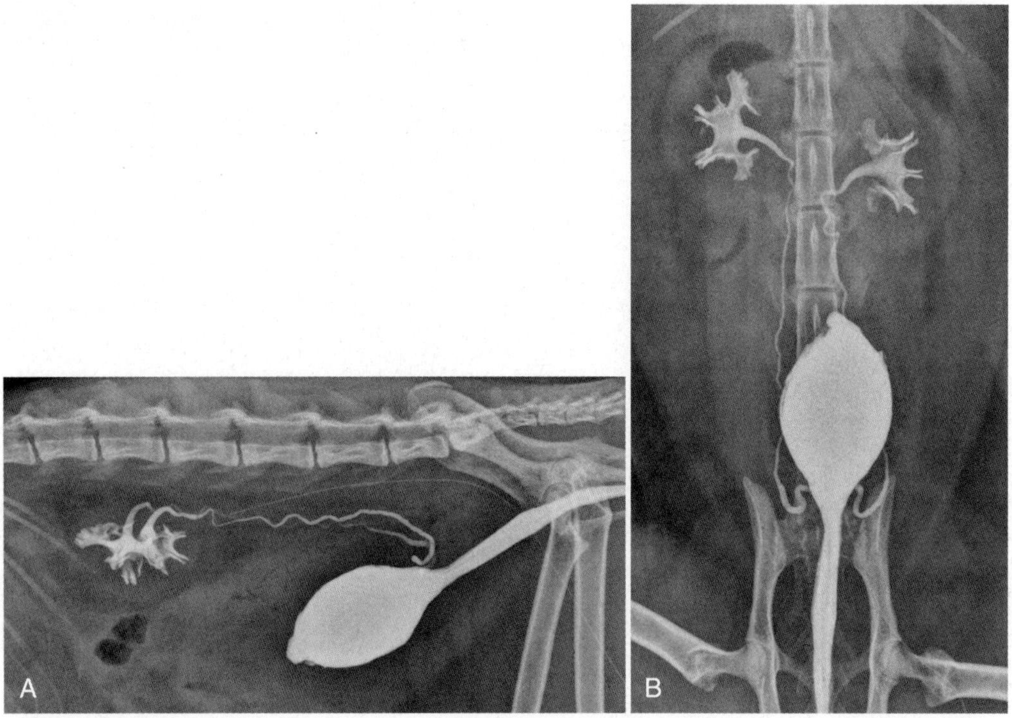

Fig. 41.5 Lateral **(A)** and ventrodorsal (VD; **B**) radiographs of a cat after an ultrasound-guided antegrade pyelogram was performed in both kidneys. The renal pelvis is mildly dilated in both kidneys because of injection pressure. Both ureters are filled with contrast medium and terminate in the dorsal aspect of the bladder neck. Ureteral obstruction is not present. Note the curved appearance of the normal distal ureter. The apex of the urinary bladder is irregular because of polypoid cystitis. A central venous catheter is present in the caudal vena cava.

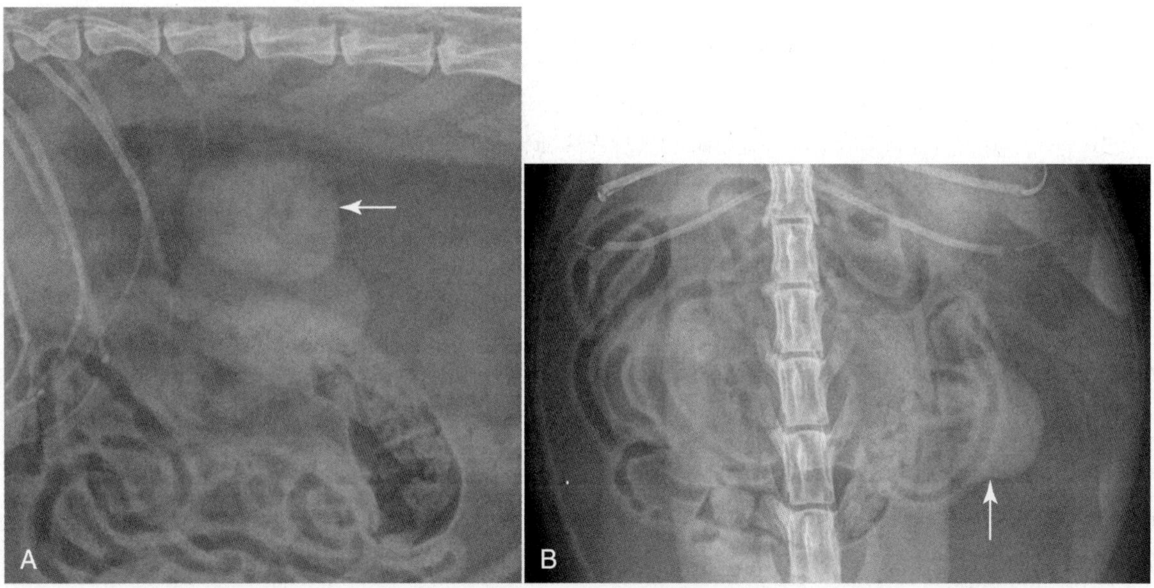

Fig. 41.6 Left lateral **(A)** and ventrodorsal **(B)** radiographs of a cat with chronic kidney disease. The left kidney is reduced in size and has a flattened caudal pole (*arrows*) due to cortical infarction.

Large Kidneys

Renomegaly causes a mass effect in the retroperitoneal space, evidenced by ventral displacement of the gastrointestinal tract and other organs (Fig. 41.7, eFig. 41.2). Left renal enlargement leads to ventral or lateral displacement of the descending colon and small intestines (Fig. 41.8, eFig. 41.3), whereas right renomegaly is associated with ventral displacement of the ascending colon and duodenum (Fig. 41.9, eFig. 41.4). Differential diagnoses for renomegaly are subdivided based on the presence of unilateral versus bilateral enlargement and alterations in margination and are listed in Table 41.1. Bilateral mild renomegaly may be seen with acute kidney injury, pyelonephritis, amyloidosis, with congenital portosystemic shunts as well as acromegaly in cats. Bilateral renomegaly in portosystemic shunts is thought to be due to hypertrophy in an attempt remove and metabolize ammonia and some gluconeogenesis.[38] Acromegalic cats have measurably larger kidneys, adrenal glands, and pancreas as well as a subjectively larger liver than

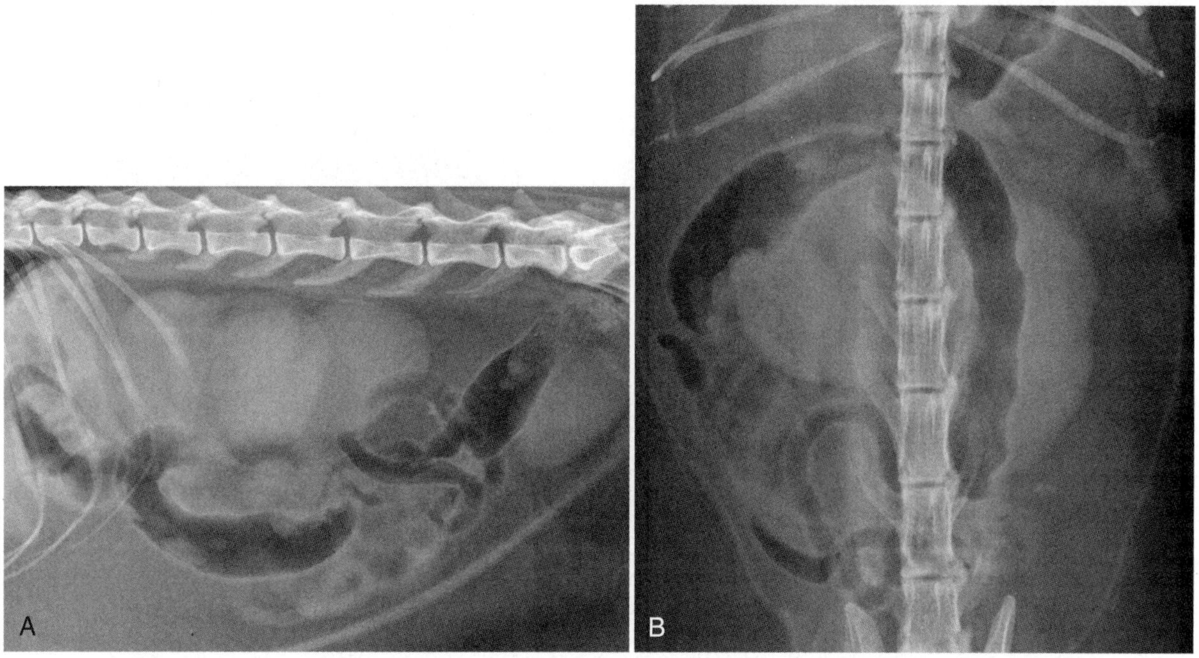

Fig. 41.7 Left lateral **(A)** and ventrodorsal (VD; **B**) radiographs of the abdomen of a cat with bilateral renomegaly caused by renal lymphoma. Both kidneys are large and have undulating margins. The gastrointestinal tract is displaced ventrally.

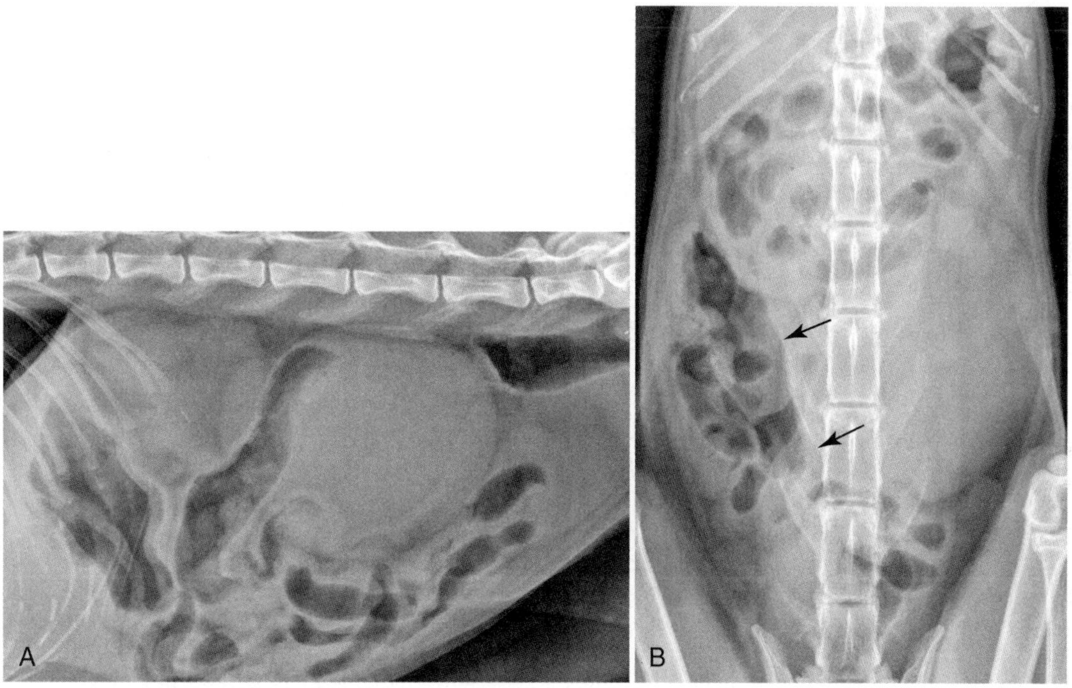

Fig. 41.8 Lateral **(A)** and ventrodorsal (VD; **B**) abdominal radiographs of a cat with left renal enlargement. The enlarged kidney displaces the small intestines ventrally and the descending colon (*black arrows*) to the right **(B)**.

nonacromegalic cats, caused by the anabolic effects of insulin-like growth factor 1 (IGF-1).[39] Unilateral mild renomegaly with a normal shape and smooth outline is most commonly seen with compensatory hypertrophy caused by contralateral chronic degenerative or obstructive disease, occasionally also due to subcapsular fluid accumulation (urine, hemorrhage or pus) or renal neoplasia, although with renal neoplasia or subcapsular changes, a change in shape is often appreciated.

Bilateral markedly enlarged kidneys with a smooth outline are seen with renal lymphoma (see Fig. 41.7), feline infectious peritonitis (FIP), bilateral hydronephrosis, or bilateral perinephric pseudocysts. Hydronephrosis and perinephric pseudocysts are often unilateral, or at least asymmetrical in appearance. Unilateral severe renomegaly with a smooth outline is most commonly seen with hydronephrosis, renal tumors and subcapsular fluid, or unilateral perinephric

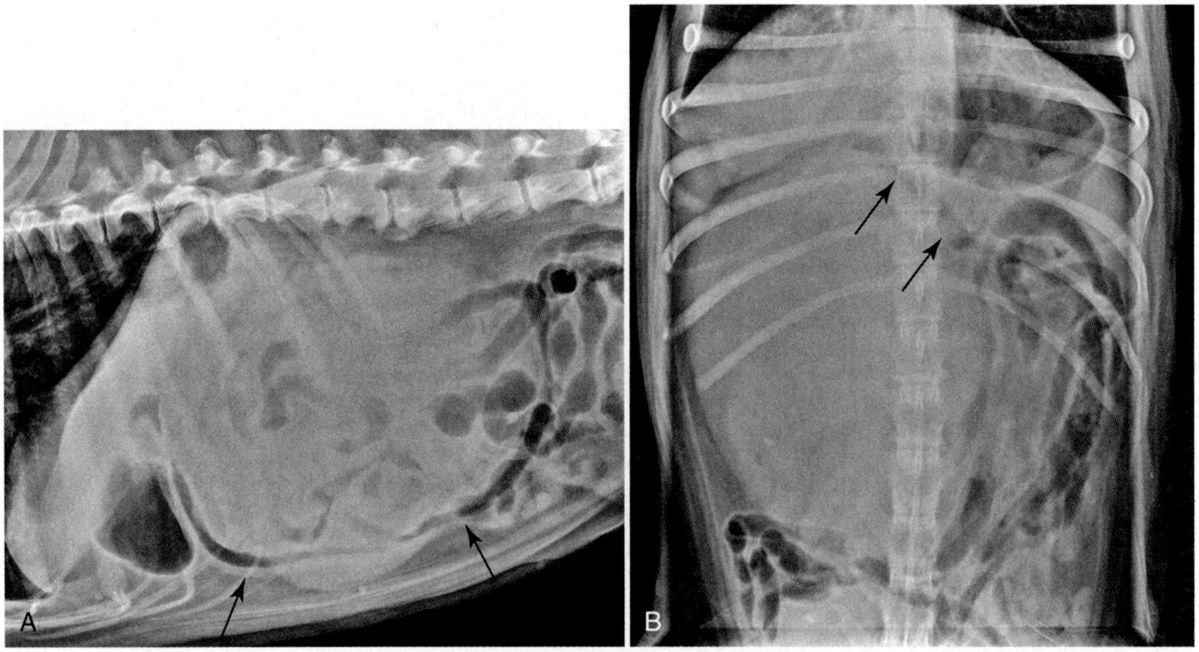

Fig. 41.9 Lateral **(A)** and ventrodorsal (VD; **B**) abdominal radiographs of a dog with right renal carcinoma. The right kidney is severely enlarged, and displaces the duodenum (*black arrows*) ventrally **(A)** and to the left **(B)**.

Table • 41.1

Differential Diagnoses for Changes in Renal Size and Shape.

BILATERAL	UNILATERAL
Mildly Enlarged Kidney, Smooth Outline	
• Acute kidney injury • Acute pyelonephritis • Congenital portosystemic shunts • Amyloidosis • Acromegaly	• Compensatory hypertrophy • Renal neoplasia (except lymphoma) • Subcapsular abscess or hemorrhage
Markedly Enlarged Kidney, Smooth Outline	
• Hydronephrosis • Renal lymphoma • Feline infectious peritonitis • Feline perinephric pseudocysts	• Hydronephrosis • Renal tumor • Subcapsular hematoma or abscess • Feline perinephric pseudocyst
Enlarged Kidney, Irregular Outline	
• Metastatic neoplasia • Polycystic kidney disease • Feline infectious peritonitis	• Primary renal tumor • Metastatic neoplasia • Renal abscess • Renal hematoma • Renal granuloma • Renal cysts
Small Kidney, Smooth or Irregular in Outline	
• Chronic renal disease • Developmental hypoplasia or dysplasia	• Chronic renal disease • Atrophy secondary to obstruction

pseudocyst. Enlarged kidneys with an abnormal shape and irregular outline increase the concern for a more severe disease process such as neoplasia, abscessation, granuloma, or hemorrhage. Renal cysts, however, can result in markedly irregular and enlarged kidneys. Bilateral enlargement is typically present with polycystic kidney disease, whereas an idiopathic renal cyst may be unilateral. Bilateral renal neoplasia is most commonly due to metastatic or multicentric disease (hemangiosarcoma, histiocytic sarcoma). Primary renal tumors such as adenocarcinoma are typically unilateral in occurrence, although they can metastasize to the contralateral side. Irregular renomegaly in a juvenile patient may be seen with nephroblastoma, which can manifest in the kidney or the spine. Presence of renomegaly should always prompt further workup of the patient to determine the source of the abnormal size, either within or outside the urinary system.

Contrast procedures (EU or CT), or ultrasound, have to be used to determine if the renal enlargement is caused by parenchymal disease or by dilation of the collecting system or renal capsule.

Abnormal Renal Structure

Diffuse Parenchymal Abnormalities

Renal structure is evaluated best with ultrasound. Because of the large variability in normal renal size, architecture, and echogenicity, subtle changes in renal structure are not always detected. In fact, it is common for patients with acute kidney injury and glomerulonephritis to have normal appearing kidneys on ultrasound.[40]

Chronic Nephropathies. Chronic tubulointerstitial inflammation and fibrosis are the predominant histopathologic findings in chronic kidney disease, regardless of the underlying cause. This results in poor corticomedullary definition caused by cortical and medullary hyperechogenicity, which is one of the most common changes associated with chronic renal disease, together with small renal size, small cortical cysts, and parenchymal mineralization (Fig. 41.10, eFig. 41.5). Renal fibrosis

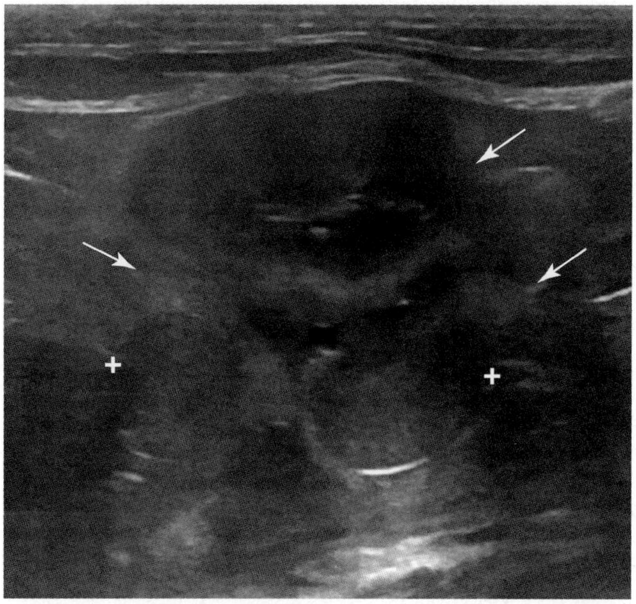

Fig. 41.10 Ultrasound image of chronic renal disease in a cat in a longitudinal plane, the length of the kidney is indicated with *cursors*. The kidney is small, rounded, and irregular with multiple wedge-shaped hyperechoic cortical indentations consistent with chronic infarction (*arrows*). The cortex and medulla are poorly delineated from each other.

may disrupt close interaction of peritubular capillaries with renal tubules resulting in ischemia and cortical infarction, which are visible as linear or triangular hyperechoic lesions in the cortex. On ultrasound, infarcts appear as wedge-shaped, hyperechoic areas in the cortex with an associated cortical defect. The appearance of infarcts has also been described on CT where they appear as a hypoattenuating region following contrast enhancement. They are often wedge shaped and are sometimes associated with flattening or depression of the adjacent cortical margin.[41] Parenchymal atrophy, infarction, and fibrosis can result in distortion of the shape of the renal pelvis. Reduced cortical thickness has been associated with reduced renal function in cats.[42] The type of underlying renal disease cannot usually be determined at this stage. Renal dysplasia is usually diagnosed late in the disease process and changes in the kidneys resemble those from any other chronic renal disease.[43,61]

Acute Nephropathies. Ultrasonographic findings associated with acute kidney injury leading to acute tubular necrosis, interstitial nephritis, or glomerulonephritis include renal enlargement, subcapsular or perirenal effusion, and cortical hyperechogenicity. In severe or advanced disease, the medullary echogenicity increases as well, leading to reduced corticomedullary distinction. Acute kidney injury in dogs and cats has many causes, including toxins (e.g., ethylene glycol, lily in cats, and grapes in dogs), bacterial, protozoal, and rickettsial infections (e.g., leptospirosis, babesiosis, Lyme disease, pyelonephritis), drugs, hypercalcemia, sepsis, ischemia, multiple organ dysfunction syndrome, pancreatitis, and hyperviscosity.[44] It is usually not possible to determine the cause of acute kidney injury by ultrasound, and biopsy may be needed. The Doppler examination of renal vasculature with calculation of the resistive index may add some information. For example, elevation of the renal resistive index is seen with active tubulointerstitial or vascular disease; however, it remains a nonspecific parameter.[45] Ethylene glycol toxicity leads to the most dramatic increase in cortical and medullary echogenicity with a hypoechoic rim at the corticomedullary junction and hypoechoic central medullary regions (Fig. 41.11).[46] The increased

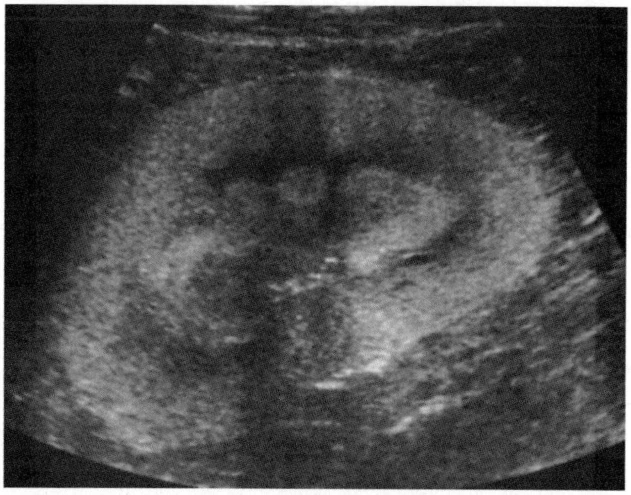

Fig. 41.11 Ultrasound image of the right kidney of a dog that ingested ethylene glycol the night before. The renal cortex and medulla are extremely hyperechoic; a thin hypoechoic rim delineates the corticomedullary junction.

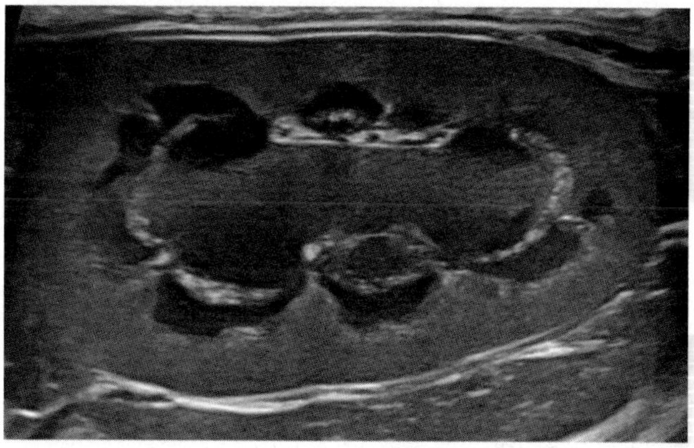

Fig. 41.12 Longitudinal ultrasound image of the left kidney of a 2-year-old cat with normal renal values and urine concentration. A thin hyperechoic medullary rim can be a normal variant.

echogenicity is attributed to deposition of calcium oxalate crystals in the kidneys.[47]

A hyperechoic medullary rim parallel to the corticomedullary junction is observed commonly and may be seen in clinically normal dogs and cats[47] (Fig. 41.12). A wide medullary band is more commonly associated with renal pathology than a thin rim.[48,49] It can be seen with mineralization, necrosis, and hemorrhage associated with many different disease processes, including acute tubular necrosis, leptospirosis, pyogranulomatous vasculitis in cats with FIP (Fig. 41.13), and in hypercalcemic nephropathy.[47–51] Hypercalcemic nephropathy is characterized by variable degrees of calcification and necrosis of renal tubules and collecting ducts. The corticomedullary rim corresponds to increased calcium deposits at this site.[52] Ring- or band-like structures with an echogenic wall in the corticomedullary region may be seen in kidneys of dogs infected with giant kidney worms *(Dioctophyme renale)* in endemic regions.[53]

Focal or Multifocal Abnormalities

Renal Mineralization. Renal mineralization, because of nephrolithiasis or dystrophic mineralization, is common, especially in older patients. All types of nephroliths are detectable ultrasonographically and are characterized by a hyperechoic

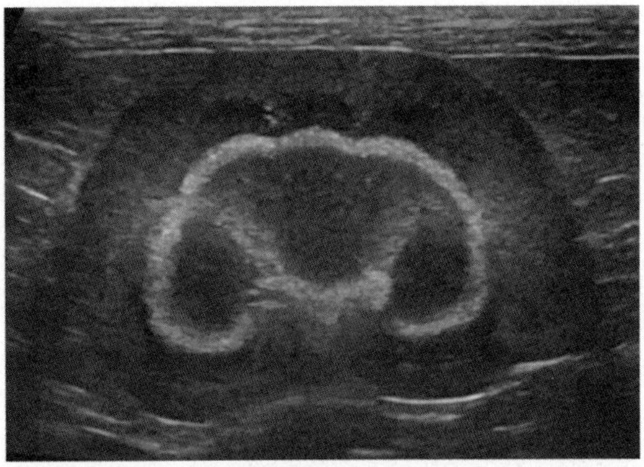

Fig. 41.13 Ultrasound image of a 7-month-old cat with feline infectious peritonitis. The kidney is overall hypoechoic, but a pronounced hyperechoic band is present parallel to the corticomedullary junction.

surface and a distal acoustic shadow. Calculi in the renal pelvis may lead to obstruction either directly in the renal pelvis or if they move into the ureter. However, it is not always possible to differentiate dystrophic mineralization from small nephroliths in the pelvic diverticula. Dystrophic mineralization tends to occur along the pelvic diverticula to form linear hyperechoic striations with a distal acoustic shadow and is usually accompanied by other chronic renal changes (Fig. 41.14). Diffuse cortical or medullary foci of mineralizations are often not detected radiographically but appear as punctate hyperechogenicities on ultrasound.

Renal Cysts. Radiographic changes due to cyst formation are seen only if cysts lead to kidney enlargement or distortion of the renal capsule (Fig. 41.15). Round filling defects may be seen in the nephrogram phase of an EU or CT, although nodules or masses could have the same appearance. Ultrasonographically, renal cysts are readily identified as anechoic round structures with distal acoustic enhancement and a thin edge artifact (Fig. 41.15, eFig. 41.6).[6,21] Internal echoes caused by hemorrhage or cellular debris may be observed. Inherited polycystic kidney disease is seen in long-haired cats (autosomal dominant), sometimes associated with hepatic and pancreatic cysts, and Cairn terriers (recessive mode of inheritance) and can be identified at a young age.[6,21,54,62] In severe instances where the renal parenchyma is almost completely obliterated by the cysts, renal function may be impaired (see Fig. 41.15). Cysts are usually located at the corticomedullary junction.[6,21] Solitary cysts can occur in any feline and canine breed and are not clinically significant if the renal architecture is otherwise normal. Small cortical cysts are observed commonly in conjunction with chronic degenerative renal disease. Nodular dermatofibrosis in German shepherd dogs is associated with renal cystadenocarcinoma. Although predominantly cystic, these lesions have a mass-like tissue component that infiltrates the renal parenchyma and may protrude into the cysts[55,63] (Fig. 41.16). Other differential diagnoses for cystic lesions with a thick wall or a solid component include renal abscess or a cavitated, necrotic tumor.

Perirenal Fluid. Perirenal or subcapsular fluid may be the result of acute renal failure, urine leakage, ureteral obstruction, hemorrhage, abscessation, perirenal pseudocysts, and neoplasia. If the fluid is subcapsular, renomegaly is seen on radiographs. EU, ultrasound, or contrast-enhanced CT is necessary to differentiate subcapsular fluid from renal parenchymal disease. Radiographically, fluid buildup outside the renal capsule leads to an increased opacity of the retroperitoneal space with a mottled or streaked appearance and loss of the outline of the kidneys or enlargement of the retroperitoneal space. Extracapsular fluid is characterized sonographically by triangular fluid accumulations adjacent to the kidney, predominantly on the dorsal aspect. Common causes include urinary tract rupture and acute renal failure (Fig. 41.17).[56,64] Proposed mechanisms for the fluid accumulation in the absence of rupture include tubular backleak of an ultrafiltrate into the renal interstitial space in excess of what the lymphatics can drain, either because of increased tubular permeability or obstructive disease.[56] Focal inflammation of the retroperitoneal fat resulting in an increased echogenicity may be seen with renal abscessation and pyelonephritis. Pseudocyst formation is caused by a transudate and has been associated with underlying renal parenchymal disease, such as interstitial nephritis. The affected kidneys are often reduced in size and have signs of chronic renal disease (Fig. 41.18).[57]

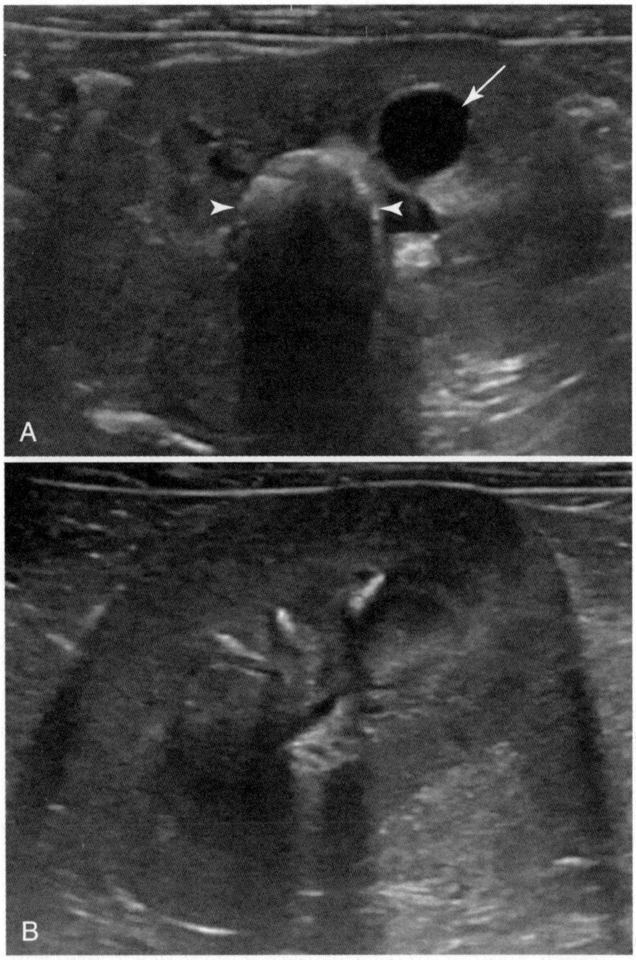

Fig. 41.14 Long-axis ultrasound images of two canine kidneys with mineralization. In image **A**, a curvilinear nephrolith is present in the renal pelvis, creating a distal shadow (*arrowheads*). A large renal cyst is seen at the corticomedullary junction of the caudal renal pole (*arrow*). In image **B**, the mineralization is dystrophic in nature and extends along the pelvic diverticula, creating a hyperechoic striated appearance.

Renal Mass Lesions. Renal mass lesions can be caused by hematoma, abscess, neoplasia, and granuloma. Primary renal tumors are usually unilateral and include renal cell carcinoma, squamous cell carcinoma, papillary carcinoma, and nephroblastoma.[58] Other tumors that may affect the kidneys are histiocytic sarcoma, plasma cell tumor, metastatic carcinoma, hemangiosarcoma, and lymphosarcoma.[59] Larger masses can be identified radiographically as asymmetric renal enlargement.

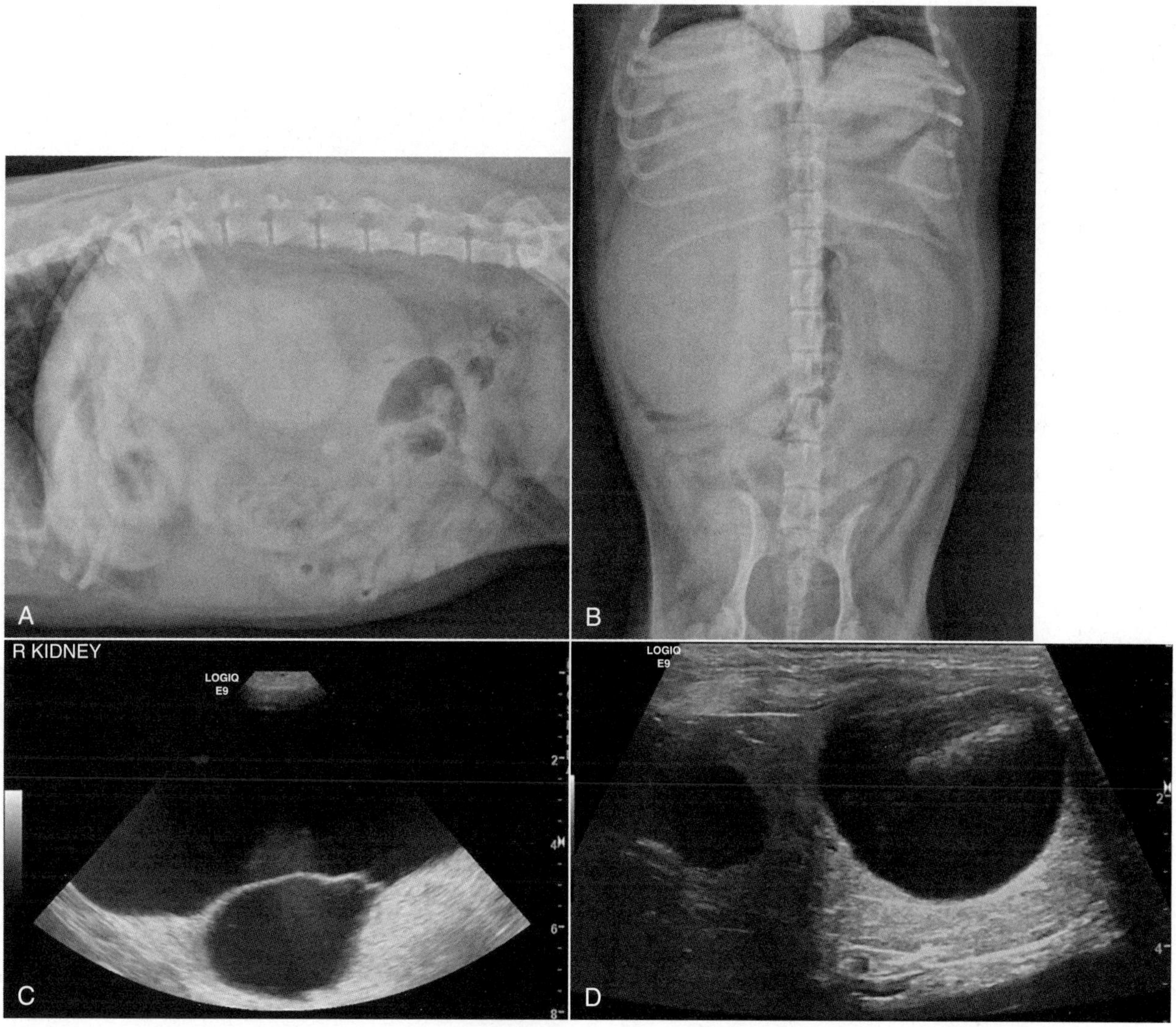

Fig. 41.15 Lateral **(A)** and ventrodorsal **(B)** radiographs and longitudinal ultrasound images of the right **(C)** and left **(D)** kidneys of a Chihuahua with polycystic kidney disease. The right renal parenchyma is almost completely effaced by large cysts **(C)** causing severe renomegaly on radiographs. Multiple cysts in the left kidney **(D)** distort the normal shape of the kidney seen both ultrasonographically and radiographically.

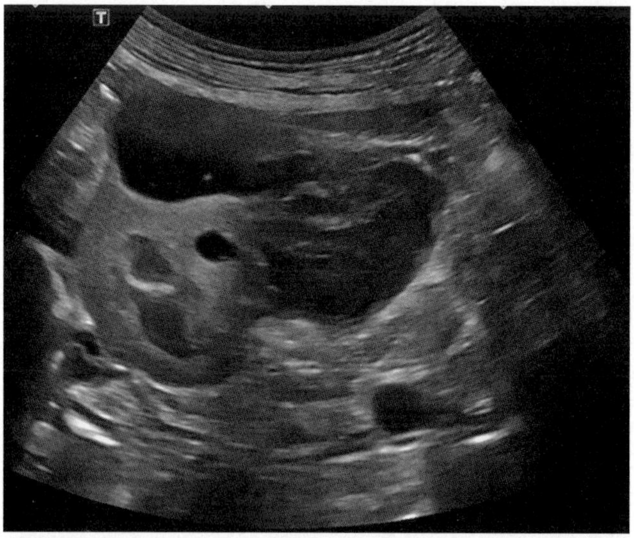

Fig. 41.16 Longitudinal ultrasound image of the left kidney of a 9-year-old German shepherd dog with nodular dermatofibrosis and renal cystadenocarcinoma. The renal parenchyma is distorted by multiple complex cystic masses.

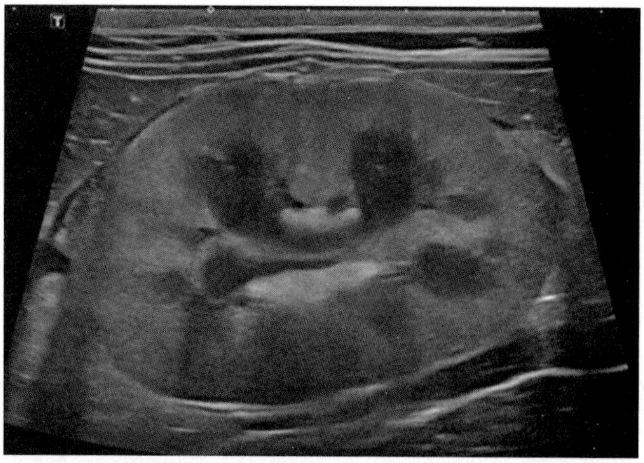

Fig. 41.17 Long-axis ultrasound image of the left kidney of a dog diagnosed with acute kidney injury due to leptospirosis infection. Anechoic fluid surrounds the renal capsule. The kidney is overall hyperechoic with mild pyelectasia.

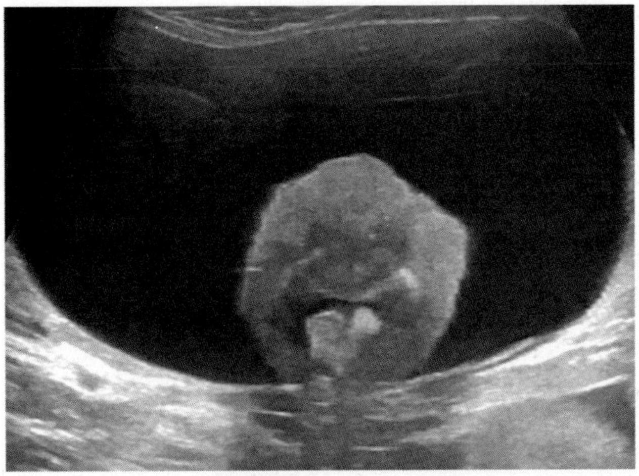

Fig. 41.18 Long-axis ultrasound image of the right kidney of a cat with a perinephric pseudocyst. The kidney is reduced in size, irregular in shape, and has poor corticomedullary distinction, parenchymal mineralizations, and pyelectasia. There is a large amount of encapsulated anechoic perirenal fluid.

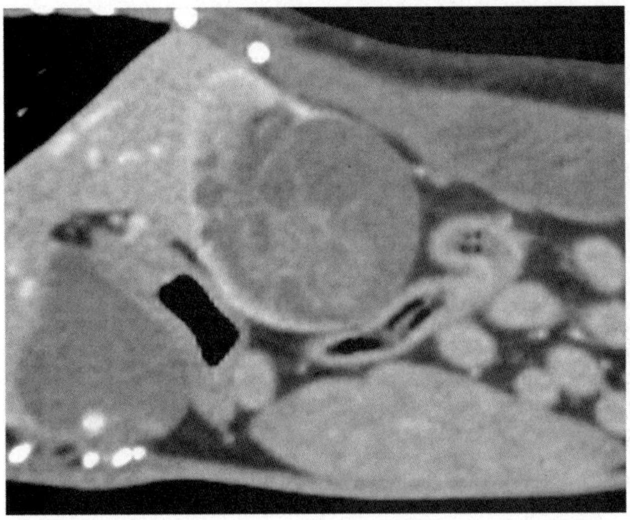

Fig. 41.19 Postcontrast sagittal computed tomography image of the right kidney of a dog with a nephroblastoma. A small portion of the cranial pole of the kidney becomes opacified with contrast medium and still resembles the original kidney, but the caudal portion is replaced by a large, heterogeneously contrast-enhancing mass.

Renal masses have less contrast medium uptake on EU or CT compared to the surrounding or contralateral renal parenchyma, because of lack of filtration and concentration of the contrast medium. Heterogeneous contrast enhancement within the mass may be seen if the mass is necrotic or cavitated (Fig. 41.19). There is a wide variability in the ultrasound appearance of renal tumors. Most primary renal tumors appear as complex or homogeneous, well-perfused masses obliterating the normal renal architecture (Fig. 41.20, eFig. 41.7). Cavitated masses are seen with renal hemangiosarcoma. Round cell tumors, such as histiocytic sarcoma, tend to be very hypoechoic.[60] Renal lymphoma occurs bilaterally and causes enlarged, irregularly shaped kidneys with a hyperechoic cortex.[61,62] Focal or multifocal nodules and masses have also been reported. A subcapsular, hypoechoic rim is associated with renal lymphoma in cats, with a positive predictive value of 80.9% and a negative predictive value or 66.7%. The subcapsular thickening is thought to represent regional subcapsular infiltrate with lymphoma rather than fluid (Fig. 41.21, eFig. 41.8).[61] Subcapsular hypoechoic rims can also be found, more rarely, with other neoplasms or with FIP. Contrast-enhanced CT may be helpful in complex renal

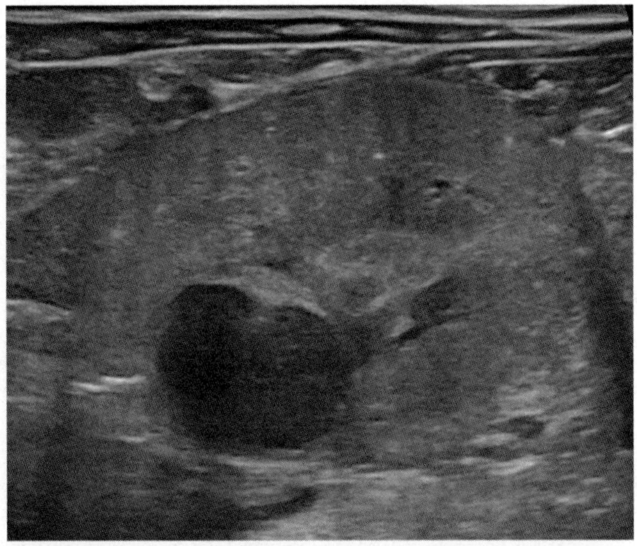

Fig. 41.20 Longitudinal ultrasound image of the right kidney of a 13-year-old Dachshund with renal carcinoma. A lobulated hypoechoic nodule is present in the cranial pole of the kidney. The renal parenchyma otherwise has signs of chronic nephropathy with poor corticomedullary definition and punctate cortical mineralizations.

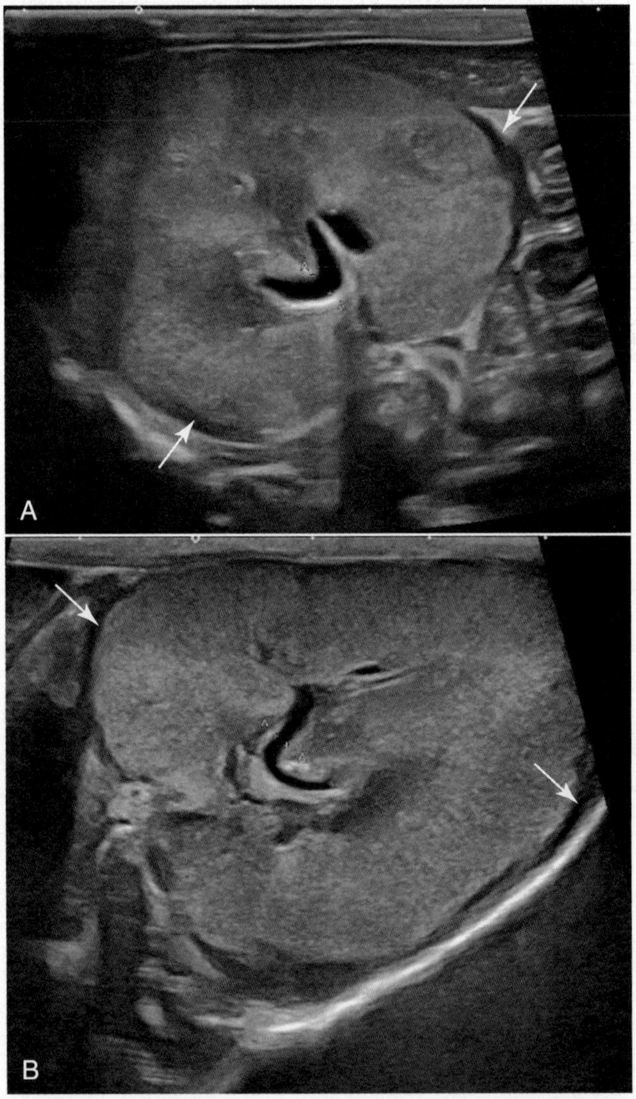

Fig. 41.21 Transverse ultrasound images of the left **(A)** and right **(B)** kidney of a cat with renal lymphoma. Both kidneys are enlarged, hyperechoic, and have a hypoechoic subcapsular rim (*arrows*). Mild pyelectasia is indicated by calipers.

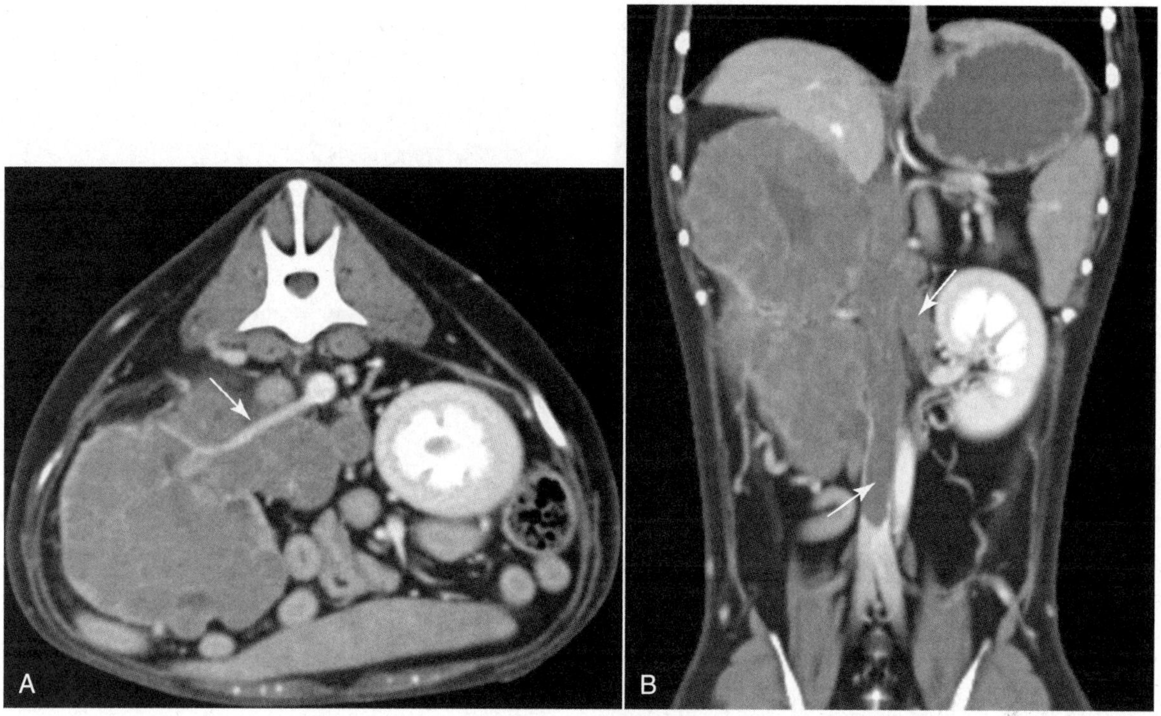

Fig. 41.22 Transverse (A) and dorsal (B) computed tomography images of a dog with a right dorsal abdominal mass. The mass is identified as right kidney by the right renal artery entering the mass (A, *arrow*). The mass is invading the left renal vein and caudal vena cava (B, *arrows*).

masses where local invasiveness and surgical resectability have to be established (Fig. 41.22).

An abscess typically has a liquid content surrounded by a thick capsule; occasionally, hyperechoic comet-tail speckles may be seen if gas is produced within the abscess (Fig. 41.23). The fluid is often very echogenic, and the cellular component tends to settle in the dependent portion.[63] Hematomas secondary to trauma or renal biopsy led to disruption of the normal kidney structure with hypoechoic or hyperechoic areas within the parenchyma and/or subcapsular fluid accumulation. However, many inflammatory lesions (such as, solid abscesses, fungal granulomas, or pyogranulomas associated with FIP) can look very similar to neoplastic masses. Needle aspirates or biopsy is required for a definitive diagnosis.

Diseases of the Collecting System

Distention of the renal pelvis can be observed in dogs and cats with increased urine production caused by diuretic therapy or renal insufficiency, or it can be associated with congenital malformations of the ureters, such as ectopic ureter or ureterocele, infection, or lower urinary tract obstruction.[18]

Pyelonephritis and Pyonephrosis

Acute pyelonephritis can lead to mild renal enlargement, whereas renal size is reduced in chronic pyelonephritis. Typically, there is mild to moderate pyelectasia.[64] The mean diameter of the renal pelvis with pyelonephritis is reported to be 3.6 mm in dogs and 4.0 mm in cats. However, this range is quite wide, with overlap with other nonobstructive or obstructive renal diseases, and even with normal animals.[18] More important, the shape of the renal pelvis is usually distorted with infection, resulting in blunted and asymmetric pelvic diverticula, seen both on EU and ultrasound (Figs. 41.24 and 41.25). Additionally, on ultrasound imaging, echogenic debris may be observed in the renal pelvis and proximal ureter rather than anechoic urine, and the renal pelvis may be surrounded by an echogenic rim caused by fibrotic change.[64–66] The echogenicity of the renal cortex may be uniformly or heterogeneously

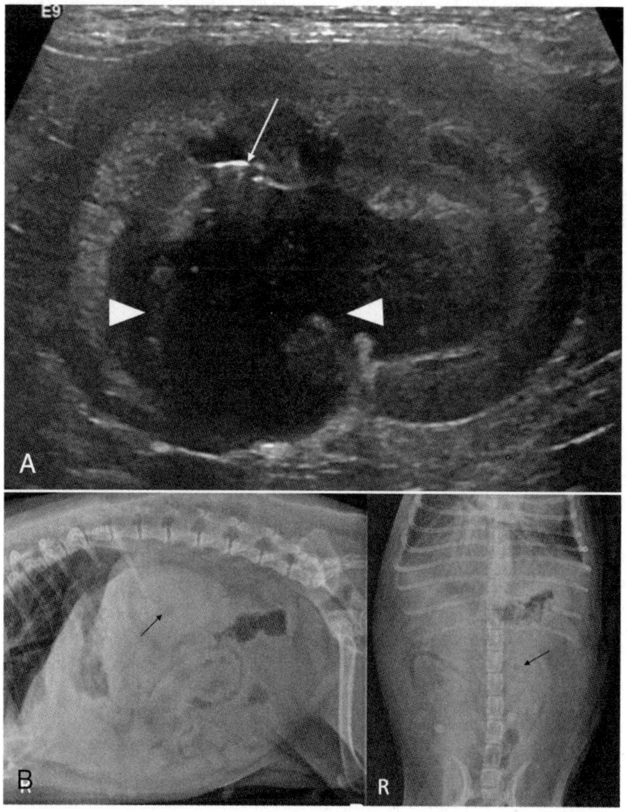

Fig. 41.23 Long-axis ultrasound image (A) and right lateral and ventrodorsal (VD) radiographs (B) of the left kidney of a dog presented for diabetic ketoacidosis and urinary tract infection that developed a renal abscess. The cranial pole of the kidney is enlarged and contains a poorly delineated hypoechoic cavity (*arrowheads*). A focus of hyperintensity with reverberation artifact, consistent with gas, is present in the dorsal portion of the cavity (*arrow*). Gas bubbles are superimposed over the cranial pole of the left renal silhouette in both radiographic projections (*arrows*).

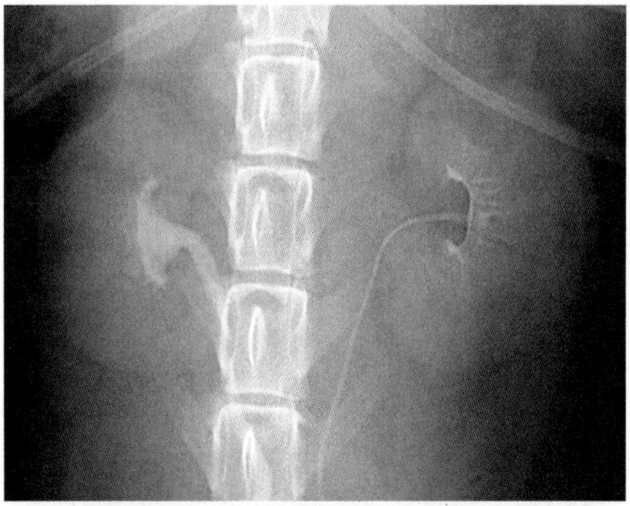

Fig. 41.24 Ventrodorsal (VD) image obtained 20 minutes after intravenous administration of iodinated contrast medium in a dog with pyelonephritis of the right kidney. The renal pelvis and proximal ureter are dilated on the right. The renal pelvis is distorted, and the pelvic diverticula are short and blunt compared with the contralateral normal left kidney.

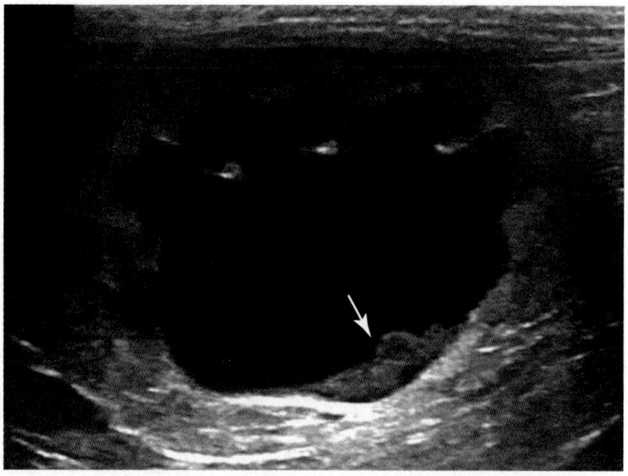

Fig. 41.26 Ultrasound image of a dog with severe hydronephrosis because of ureteral obstruction by a urinary bladder mass. The renal pelvis and pelvic diverticula are distended, and the renal cortex is thin. A small amount of cellular debris is accumulated in the dependent portion of the renal pelvis (*white arrow*).

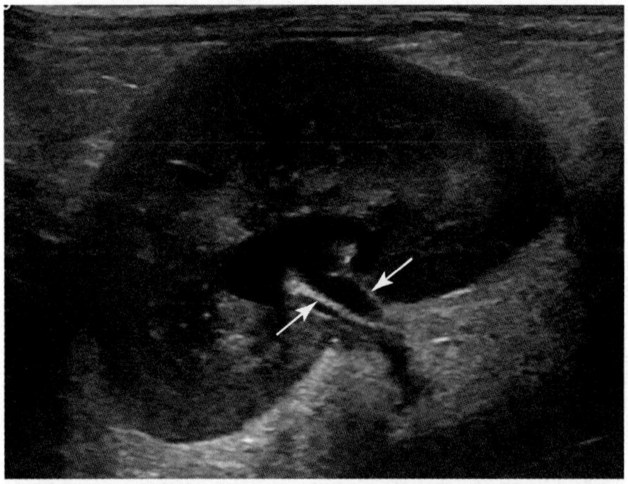

Fig. 41.25 Long-axis ultrasound image of the left kidney of a dog with acute pyelonephritis. The renal pelvis is dilated and distorted, and the pelvic diverticula are blunted. Note the hyperechoic lining of the proximal ureter (*white arrows*), which is consistent with fibrotic change. The renal medulla is hyperechoic, resulting in poor corticomedullary definition. The retroperitoneal fat surrounding the kidney is very hyperechoic and inflamed.

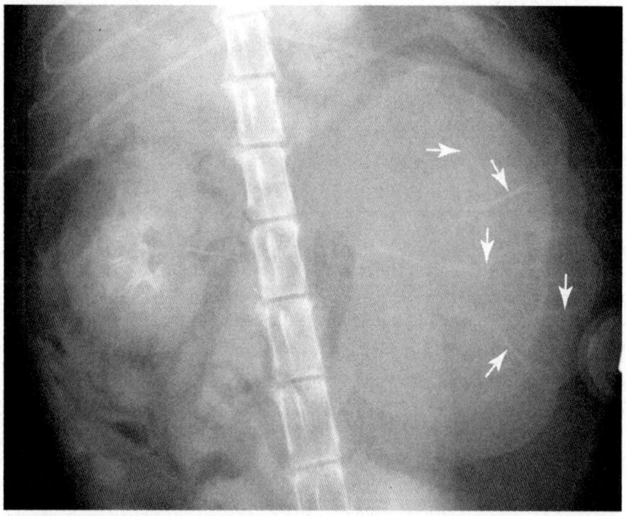

Fig. 41.27 Excretory urogram of a cat with severe left hydronephrosis. Contrast enhancement is seen only in the left kidney along the elongated renal vasculature (*white arrows*) and has not accumulated in the renal pelvis.

increased. In severe acute pyelonephritis, regional inflammation of the perirenal fat results in a hyperechoic rim around the kidney and proximal ureter (see Fig. 41.25), often with a small amount of retroperitoneal effusion. Thickening of the proximal ureteral wall and mild ureteral dilation without evidence of intraluminal obstruction are common. Chronic pyelonephritis is difficult to distinguish from other chronic renal diseases, because it is characterized by small, irregularly shaped kidneys with mild pyelectasia.[64] Pyonephrosis is characterized by echogenic fluid in the renal pelvis with sediment settling to the dependent portion (Fig. 41.26).[65]

Hydronephrosis

Hydronephrosis is defined as distention of the renal pelvis and pelvic diverticula, most commonly caused by urinary tract obstruction.[18] In severe hydronephrosis, the renal parenchyma is obliterated almost completely, and only a thin rim of cortex remains. Because renal vessels must still reach the cortex, elongated thin interlobar vessels may be seen forming radial streaks in the fluid-filled cavity in the nephrogram phase of an excretory urogram (Fig. 41.27). If the remaining renal parenchyma is functional, contrast medium will outline the dilated renal pelvis in the pyelogram phase. Anechoic fluid distention of the renal pelvis and diverticula is seen on ultrasound, until the kidney essentially becomes one cystic structure with a thin cortical rim (see Fig. 41.26). Ureteral obstruction or aberrant termination of the ureters is a primary concern if hydronephrosis is present, and a detailed investigation of the ureters should be performed (discussed later).

Abnormal Renal Function

Abnormal renal function cannot be determined radiographically or ultrasonographically. However, secondary signs of renal failure may be apparent. Acute renal failure is often associated with perirenal effusion, which is best seen with ultrasound imaging. Renal secondary hyperparathyroidism leads to

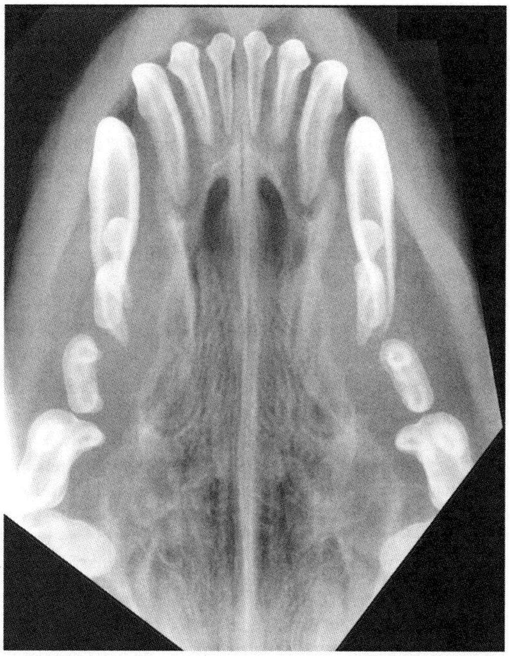

Fig. 41.28 Dorsoventral radiograph of the maxilla of a dog with renal failure and secondary hyperparathyroidism. The lamina dura and adjacent maxillary bone surrounding the teeth have been resorbed and replaced by fibrous tissue, resulting in markedly reduced opacity around the teeth.

generalized osteopenia evidenced by thinning of the bone cortex with a double cortical line. The skull is usually affected first. Bone resorption of the maxilla and mandible with fibrous replacement results in thickening with reduced radiopacity. The normally opaque lamina dura disappears, resulting in dramatically increased contrast to the teeth (Fig. 41.28).[67] Metastatic mineralization of stomach wall, blood vessels, and parenchymal organs (such as, liver and spleen) may be observed with chronic renal failure if the calcium-to-phosphate ratio is increased. Mild hyperplasia of the parathyroid glands can be detected ultrasonographically in animals with chronic, but not with acute, renal failure.[68]

Renal function can only be estimated crudely using EU or contrast-enhanced CT. However, there are instances where an estimation of renal function, such as determining whether there is any function at all in a kidney, may be adequate for surgical planning. The degree and change of renal opacification over time after contrast medium injection, as well as the relationship between nephrogram and pyelogram phase, can be used to determine problems with renal function (Fig. 41.29, eFig. 41.9).[69] The findings and their possible interpretation are listed in Box 41.1. Observation of abnormal opacification patterns after intravenous contrast medium administration is essential to recognize and treat contrast medium–associated renal dysfunction. If more precise measurement of renal function is needed, renal scintigraphy using technetium-99m diethylenetriamine pentaacetic acid can be used to calculate individual and global renal function.[36] A protocol for measurement of glomerular filtration rate using CT is also available.[26,27]

DISEASES OF THE URETERS

Most ureteral diseases result in dilatation of some or all of the ureter. Differential diagnoses for ureteral dilatation include obstruction (e.g., calculi, clots, strictures, masses), ectopic

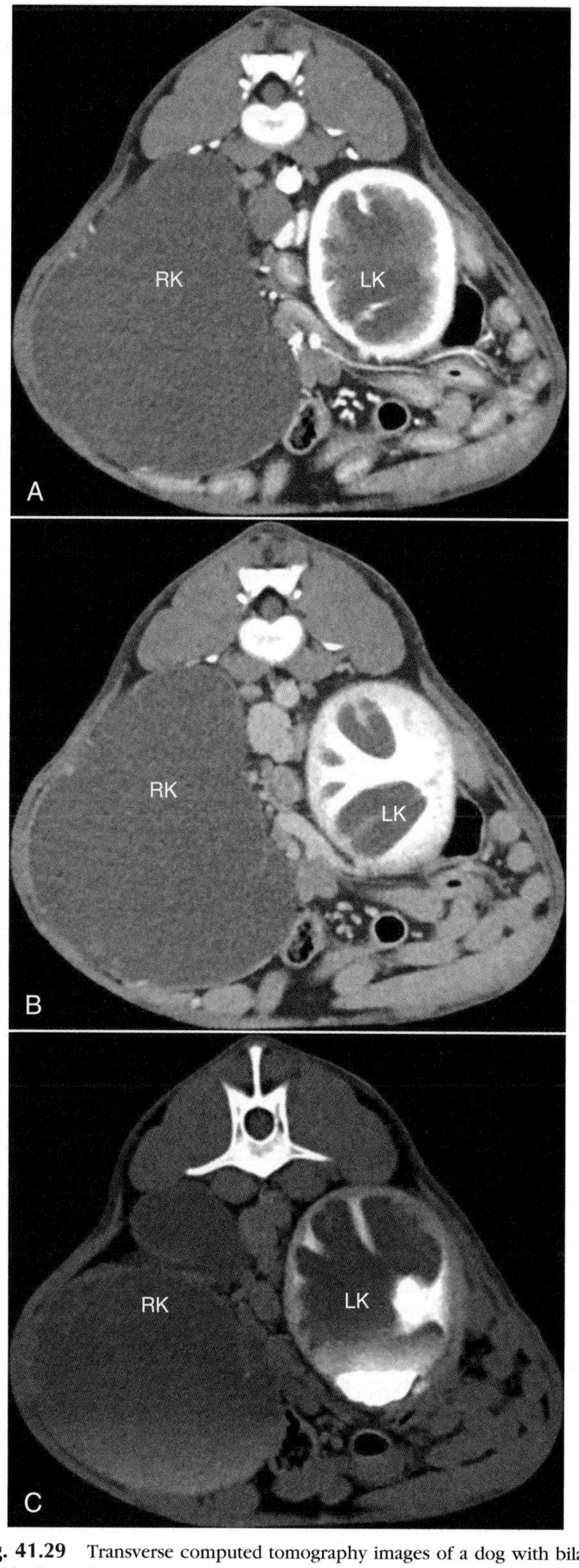

Fig. 41.29 Transverse computed tomography images of a dog with bilateral hydronephrosis, acquired immediately (**A**, vascular phase), 1 minute (**B**, nephrogram phase), and 5 minutes (**C**, pyelogram phase) after intravenous contrast medium injection. The right kidney (*RK*) is more severely affected and has almost no discernible renal tissue left and the nephrogram is almost completely absent. A small amount of contrast medium is seen in the ventral portion of the dilated renal pelvis in the pyelogram phase indicating minimal residual renal function. The left (*LK*) renal pelvis is also severely distended but there is appropriate contrast enhancement in all phases.

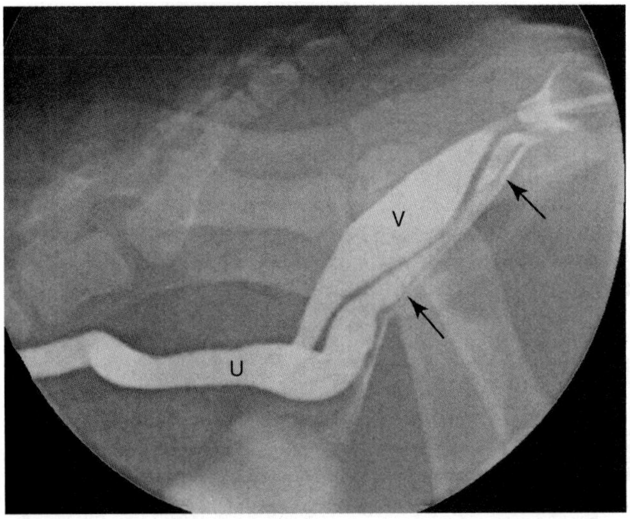

Fig. 41.34 Vaginourethrogram of a female dog with a single ectopic ureter. Contrast medium was injected into the vestibule of the vagina. The ureter (*U*) is dilated and tortuous. It extends caudally between the vagina (*V*) and urethra (*black arrows*) and enters the distal urethra.

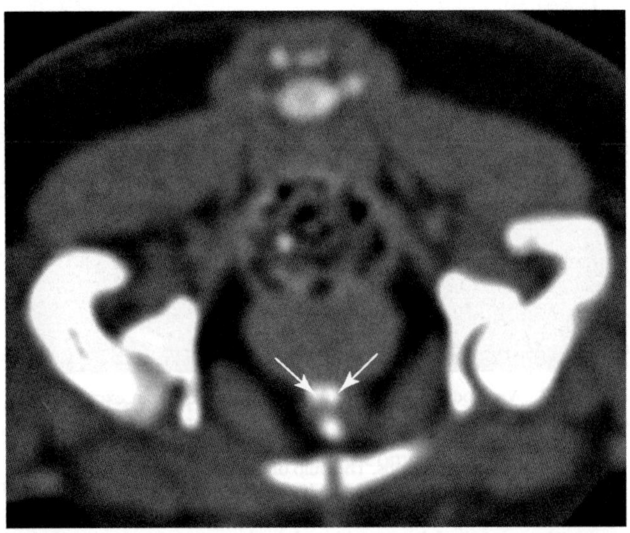

Fig. 41.35 Transverse computed tomography image of the urethra and distal ureters in a dog with bilateral ectopic ureters. The two ureters (*white arrows*) course dorsal to the urethra. They inserted into the urethra just caudal to this image plane.

Ureteroceles

Ureteroceles are cystic dilations of the terminal ureter and are classified as orthotopic or ectopic. Orthotopic ureteroceles are also called intravesicular ureteroceles and are dilatations of the submucosal portion of the distal ureter. Orthotopic ureteroceles extend into the lumen of the urinary bladder and communicate with the urinary bladder lumen through an opening. Ectopic ureteroceles on the other hand are associated with ectopic ureters and located in the bladder neck or urethra (Fig. 41.36). Ureteroceles may cause obstruction and secondary hydroureter and hydronephrosis which can be unilateral (grade 2) or bilateral (grade 3) if the ureterocele is large enough to affect the ureterovesicular junction on the contralateral side.[79,80] The appearance of ureteroceles on CT or EU depends on the timing. The ureterocele may fill with contrast medium before the urinary bladder and present as radiopaque round structure but later in the study or in a cystogram it may present as filling defect if the remainder of the urinary bladder is completely opacified. Similarly, a round, anechoic cystic structure at the ureterovesical junction, usually within the bladder lumen, is visible ultrasonographically.[79,81]

Ureteroceles are often associated with narrowing of the ureteral orifice and therefore have to be treated either surgically or with laser ablation.

Ureteral Tumors

Ureteral tumors are rare. Reported types include leiomyoma, leiomyosarcoma, and urothelial carcinoma. Extension of a transitional cell carcinoma of the urinary bladder neck into the distal ureter is common. Fibroepithelial polyps in the proximal aspect of the ureter have been described in dogs.[82] The etiology is unclear; they may be inflammatory in origin, similar to polypoid cystitis, or hamartomatous or neoplastic, but they have a good prognosis when removed.

TRAUMA TO THE URETERS AND KIDNEY

Abdominal or pelvic canal trauma may affect the kidneys and/or ureters. Renal hemorrhage, renal rupture, renal artery or vein avulsion, or ureteral or renal pelvis tears are possible consequences. Survey radiographs are always indicated if retroperitoneal trauma is suspected, and the visible portion of the retroperitoneal space should always be examined in patients with pelvic trauma. Either urine or hemorrhage in the retroperitoneal space results in decreased retroperitoneal detail as the normal fat opacity surrounding the kidneys and large vessels is replaced by heterogeneous soft tissue opacity with a streaked appearance caused by fluid traveling along fascial planes. If a

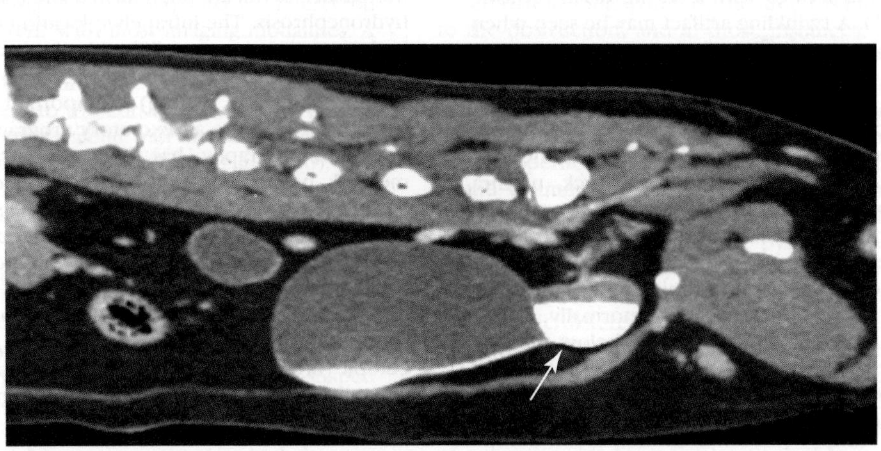

Fig. 41.36 Sagittal reconstructed computed tomography image of a dog with ectopic ureter and an ectopic ureterocele which is partially filled with contrast medium (*arrow*). A small amount of contrast medium is present in the ventral portion of the urinary bladder as well.

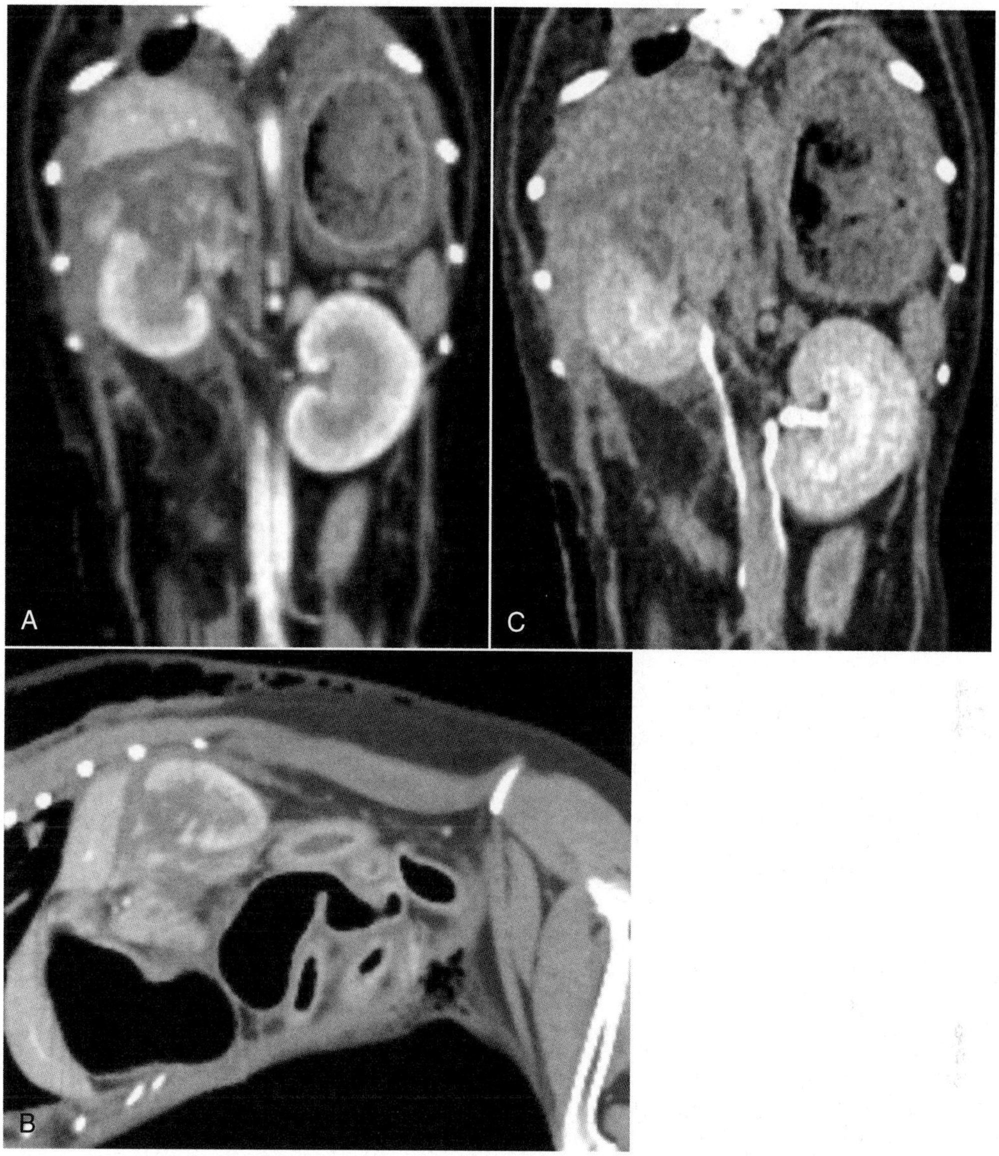

Fig. 41.37 Dorsal **(A)** and sagittal **(B)** plane reconstructed computed tomography images of the nephrogram and dorsal **(C)** plane reconstructed CT image of the pyelogram of a dog with kidney rupture after trauma (dog bite). The cranial pole of the right kidney is poorly delineated and the structure is disrupted. Contrast enhancement is reduced in the cranial pole of the right kidney. The right ureter appropriately fills with contrast medium which indicates that the remaining renal parenchyma is functional **(C)**. The surrounding retroperitoneal space is soft tissue attenuating consistent with hemorrhage and inflammation.

large volume of fluid is present, widening of the retroperitoneal space with secondary ventral displacement of large and small bowel results. Renal displacement is associated with vascular avulsion, and body wall or diaphragmatic hernias. Renal enlargement can be the result of subcapsular hemorrhage or encapsulated urine accumulation (urinoma). Urinoma formation can also be associated with ureteral injury and urine leakage.[83] All these radiographic findings need to be evaluated further with additional imaging methods. CT provides the most complete evaluation of suspected renal trauma.[84] CT allows simultaneous assessment of trauma to soft tissue and bones, as well as blood supply of injured organs (Fig. 41.37). If urinary tract rupture is suspected, a contrast study using either EU or contrast-enhanced CT is indicated unless there are contraindications to using iodinated contrast media. The site of urinary tract rupture is apparent as leakage of contrast medium (Fig. 41.38).

In clinical practice, ultrasound is often the first advanced imaging method used when urinary tract trauma is suspected and survey radiographs are not conclusive, because it is noninvasive and can be performed in the awake patient. However, information gained with regard to urinary tract trauma is often limited, except in patients with complete disruption of the renal architecture or blood supply. More subtle urinary tract tears are difficult to detect with certainty, and the use of ultrasound is limited to guide sampling of retroperitoneal fluid pockets. Complete ureteral tears of some duration can be suspected if focal dilatation of the proximal ureter is seen, in addition to retroperitoneal effusion, because the site of rupture often contracts and adhesions form, essentially leading to ureteral obstruction. Doppler ultrasound can be used to verify both arterial supply and venous drainage of the kidney.

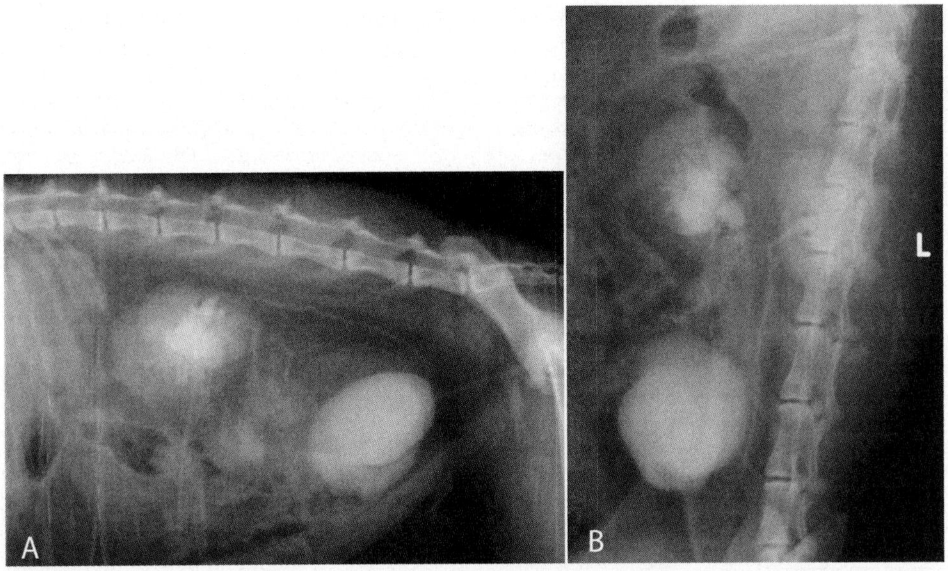

Fig. 41.38 Lateral (**A**) and oblique ventrodorsal (VD; **B**) radiographs acquired in the pyelogram phase of an excretory urogram in a cat 2 days after a ureteral calculus had been removed surgically. The left ureter is continuously filled with contrast medium and contrast medium reaches the bladder. The right ureter is dilated and tortuous and does not extend to the urinary bladder. Contrast medium has accumulated in the peritoneal space. Right ureteral rupture was confirmed surgically.

REFERENCES

1. Allen G. Radiology in the diagnosis of kidney disease. *Aust Vet Pr*. 1982;12:97.
2. Greco DS. Congenital and inherited renal disease of small animals. *Vet Clin North Am Small Anim Pract*. 2001;31(2):393–399. https://doi.org/10.1016/s0195-5616(01)50211-9. viii.
3. Finco D, Stiles N, Kneller S, Lewis R, Barrett R. Radiologic estimation of kidney size of the dog. *J Am Vet Med Assoc*. 1971;159(8):995–1002.
4. Kneller S, Barrett R. Feline kidney mensuration. *Acta Radiol*. 1972;suppl(319):279–280.
5. Shiroma JT, Gabriel JK, Carter RL, Scruggs SL, Stubbs PW. Effect of reproductive status on feline renal size. *Vet Radiol Ultrasound Off J Am Coll Vet Radiol Int Vet Radiol Assoc*. 1999;40(3):242–245. https://doi.org/10.1111/j.1740-8261.1999.tb00355.x.
6. Reichle JK, DiBartola SP, Léveillé R. Renal ultrasonographic and computed tomographic appearance, volume, and function of cats with autosomal dominant polycystic kidney disease. *Vet Radiol Ultrasound Off J Am Coll Vet Radiol Int Vet Radiol Assoc*. 2002;43(4):368–373. https://doi.org/10.1111/j.1740-8261.2002.tb01020.x.
7. Seiler GS, Rhodes J, Cianciolo R, Casal ML. Ultrasonographic findings in Cairn Terriers with preclinical renal dysplasia. *Vet Radiol Ultrasound Off J Am Coll Vet Radiol Int Vet Radiol Assoc*. 2010;51(4):453–457. https://doi.org/10.1111/j.1740-8261.2010.01674.x.
8. Vaden SL. Renal biopsy of dogs and cats. *Clin Tech Small Anim Pract*. 2005;20(1):11–22. https://doi.org/10.1053/j.ctsap.2004.12.003.
9. Vaden SL, Levine JF, Lees GE, Groman RP, Grauer GF, Forrester SD. Renal biopsy: a retrospective study of methods and complications in 283 dogs and 65 cats. *J Vet Intern Med*. 2005;19(6):794–801. https://doi.org/10.1892/0891-6640(2005)19[794:rbarso]2.0.co;2.
10. Schmiedt CW, Delaney FA, McAnulty JF. Ultrasonographic determination of resistive index and graft size for evaluating clinical feline renal allografts. *Vet Radiol Ultrasound Off J Am Coll Vet Radiol Int Vet Radiol Assoc*. 2008;49(1):73–80. https://doi.org/10.1111/j.1740-8261.2007.00321.x.
11. Choi SY, Jeong WC, Lee YW, Choi HJ. Contrast enhanced ultrasonography of kidney in conscious and anesthetized beagle dogs. *J Vet Med Sci*. 2016;78(2):239–244. https://doi.org/10.1292/jvms.15-0199.
12. Schweiger H, Ohlerth S, Gerber B. Contrast-enhanced ultrasound of both kidneys in healthy, non-anaesthetized cats. *Acta Vet Scand*. 2015;57:80. https://doi.org/10.1186/s13028-015-0172-5.
13. Haers H, Vignoli M, Paes G, et al. Contrast harmonic ultrasonographic appearance of focal space-occupying renal lesions. *Vet Radiol Ultrasound Off J Am Coll Vet Radiol Int Vet Radiol Assoc*. 2010;51(5):516–522. https://doi.org/10.1111/j.1740-8261.2010.01690.x.
14. Kinns J, Aronson L, Hauptman J, Seiler G. Contrast-enhanced ultrasound of the feline kidney. *Vet Radiol Ultrasound Off J Am Coll Vet Radiol Int Vet Radiol Assoc*. 2010;51(2):168–172. https://doi.org/10.1111/j.1740-8261.2009.01646.x.
15. Gremillion C, Cohen EB, Vaden S, Seiler G. Optimization of ultrasonographic ureteral jet detection and normal ureteral jet morphology in dogs. *Vet Radiol Ultrasound Off J Am Coll Vet Radiol Int Vet Radiol Assoc*. 2021;62(5):583–590. https://doi.org/10.1111/vru.13000.
16. Ivancić M, Mai W. Qualitative and quantitative comparison of renal vs. hepatic ultrasonographic intensity in healthy dogs. *Vet Radiol Ultrasound Off J Am Coll Vet Radiol Int Vet Radiol Assoc*. 2008;49(4):368–373. https://doi.org/10.1111/j.1740-8261.2008.00383.x.
17. Yeager AE, Anderson WI. Study of association between histologic features and echogenicity of architecturally normal cat kidneys. *Am J Vet Res*. 1989;50(6):860–863.
18. D'Anjou MA, Bédard A, Dunn ME. Clinical significance of renal pelvic dilatation on ultrasound in dogs and cats. *Vet Radiol Ultrasound Off J Am Coll Vet Radiol Int Vet Radiol Assoc*. 2011;52(1):88–94.
19. Walter PA, Feeney DA, Johnston GR, Fletcher TF. Feline renal ultrasonography: quantitative analyses of imaged anatomy. *Am J Vet Res*. 1987;48(4):596–599.

20. Barr F, Holt P, Gibbs C. Ultrasonographic measurement of normal renal parameters. *J Small Anim Pract*. 1990;31:180.
21. Mareschal A, d'Anjou MA, Moreau M, Alexander K, Beauregard G. Ultrasonographic measurement of kidney-to-aorta ratio as a method of estimating renal size in dogs. *Vet Radiol Ultrasound Off J Am Coll Vet Radiol Int Vet Radiol Assoc*. 2007;48(5):434–438. https://doi.org/10.1111/j.1740-8261.2007.00274.x.
22. Novellas R, Espada Y, Ruiz de Gopegui R. Doppler ultrasonographic estimation of renal and ocular resistive and pulsatility indices in normal dogs and cats. *Vet Radiol Ultrasound Off J Am Coll Vet Radiol Int Vet Radiol Assoc*. 2007;48(1):69–73. https://doi.org/10.1111/j.1740-8261.2007.00206.x.
23. Bouma JL, Aronson LR, Keith DG, Saunders HM. Use of computed tomography renal angiography for screening feline renal transplant donors. *Vet Radiol Ultrasound Off J Am Coll Vet Radiol Int Vet Radiol Assoc*. 2003;44(6):636–641. https://doi.org/10.1111/j.1740-8261.2003.tb00522.x.
24. Cáceres AV, Zwingenberger AL, Aronson LR, Mai W. Characterization of normal feline renal vascular anatomy with dual-phase CT angiography. *Vet Radiol Ultrasound Off J Am Coll Vet Radiol Int Vet Radiol Assoc*. 2008;49(4):350–356. https://doi.org/10.1111/j.1740-8261.2008.00378.x.
25. Alexander K, Dunn M, Carmel EN, Lavoie JP, Del Castillo JRE. Clinical application of Patlak plot CT-GFR in animals with upper urinary tract disease. *Vet Radiol Ultrasound Off J Am Coll Vet Radiol Int Vet Radiol Assoc*. 2010;51(4):421–427. https://doi.org/10.1111/j.1740-8261.2010.01670.x.
26. Granger LA, Armbrust LJ, Rankin DC, Ghering R, Bello NM, Alexander K. Estimation of glomerular filtration rate in healthy cats using single-slice dynamic CT and Patlak plot analysis. *Vet Radiol Ultrasound Off J Am Coll Vet Radiol Int Vet Radiol Assoc*. 2012;53(2):181–188. https://doi.org/10.1111/j.1740-8261.2011.01899.x.
27. O'Dell-Anderson KJ, Twardock R, Grimm JB, Grimm KA, Constable PD. Determination of glomerular filtration rate in dogs using contrast-enhanced computed tomography. *Vet Radiol Ultrasound Off J Am Coll Vet Radiol Int Vet Radiol Assoc*. 2006;47(2):127–135. https://doi.org/10.1111/j.1740-8261.2006.00118.x.
28. Rao QA, Newhouse JH. Risk of nephropathy after intravenous administration of contrast material: a critical literature analysis. *Radiology*. 2006;239(2):392–397. https://doi.org/10.1148/radiol.2392050413.
29. Thomsen HS. European Society of Urogenital Radiology (ESUR) guidelines on the safe use of iodinated contrast media. *Eur J Radiol*. 2006;60(3):307–313. https://doi.org/10.1016/j.ejrad.2006.06.020.
30. Feeney DA, Osborne CA, Jessen CR. Effect of multiple excretory urograms on glomerular filtration of normal dogs: a preliminary report. *Am J Vet Res*. 1980;41(6):960–963.
31. Barthez PY, Begon D, Delisle F. Effect of contrast medium dose and image acquisition timing on ureteral opacification in the normal dog as assessed by computed tomography. *Vet Radiol Ultrasound Off J Am Coll Vet Radiol Int Vet Radiol Assoc*. 1998;39(6):524–527. https://doi.org/10.1111/j.1740-8261.1998.tb01643.x.
32. Feeney DA, Barber DL, Culver DH, Prasse KW, Thrall DE, Lewis RE. Canine excretory urogram: correlation with baseline measurements. *Am J Vet Res*. 1980;41(2):279–283.
33. Hoey SE, Heder BL, Hetzel SJ, Waller KR. Use of computed tomography for measurement of kidneys in dogs without renal disease. *J Am Vet Med Assoc*. 2016;248(3):282–287. https://doi.org/10.2460/javma.248.3.282.
34. Adin CA, Herrgesell EJ, Nyland TG, et al. Antegrade pyelography for suspected ureteral obstruction in cats: 11 cases (1995-2001). *J Am Vet Med Assoc*. 2003;222(11):1576–1581. https://doi.org/10.2460/javma.2003.222.1576.
35. Cavrenne R, Mai W. Time-resolved renal contrast-enhanced MRA in normal dogs. *Vet Radiol Ultrasound Off J Am Coll Vet Radiol Int Vet Radiol Assoc*. 2009;50(1):58–64. https://doi.org/10.1111/j.1740-8261.2008.01490.x.
36. Daniel GB, Mitchell SK, Mawby D, Sackman JE, Schmidt D. Renal nuclear medicine: a review. *Vet Radiol Ultrasound Off J Am Coll Vet Radiol Int Vet Radiol Assoc*. 1999;40(6):572–587. https://doi.org/10.1111/j.1740-8261.1999.tb00883.x.
37. Stokes JE, Forrester SD. New and unusual causes of acute renal failure in dogs and cats. *Vet Clin North Am Small Anim Pract*. 2004;34(4):909–922. https://doi.org/10.1016/j.cvsm.2004.03.006. vi.
38. D'Anjou MA, Penninck D, Cornejo L, Pibarot P. Ultrasonographic diagnosis of portosystemic shunting in dogs and cats. *Vet Radiol Ultrasound*. 2004;45(5):424–437. https://doi.org/10.1111/j.1740-8261.2004.04076.x.
39. Lourenço BN, Randall E, Seiler G, Lunn KF. Abdominal ultrasonographic findings in acromegalic cats. *J Feline Med Surg*. 2015;17(8):698–703. https://doi.org/10.1177/1098612X14556847.
40. Rivers BJ, Johnston GR. Diagnostic imaging strategies in small animal nephrology. *Vet Clin North Am Small Anim Pract*. 1996;26(6):1505–1517. https://doi.org/10.1016/s0195-5616(96)50138-5.
41. Sutthigran S, Saisawart P, Klaengkaew A, et al. Use of contrast-enhanced computed tomography to detect kidney infarction in dogs. *J Vet Intern Med*. 2022;36(1):164–170. https://doi.org/10.1111/jvim.16343.
42. Yan GY, Chen KY, Wang HC, Ma TY, Chen KS. Relationship between ultrasonographically determined renal dimensions and International Renal Interest Society stages in cats with chronic kidney disease. *J Vet Intern Med*. 2020;34(4):1464–1475. https://doi.org/10.1111/jvim.15814.
43. Felkai C, Vörös K, Vrabély T, Vetési F, Karsai F, Papp L. Ultrasonographic findings of renal dysplasia in cocker spaniels: eight cases. *Acta Vet Hung*. 1997;45(4):397–408.
44. Ross L. Acute kidney injury in dogs and cats. *Vet Clin North Am Small Anim Pract*. 2022;52(3):659–672. https://doi.org/10.1016/j.cvsm.2022.01.005.
45. Morrow KL, Salman MD, Lappin MR, Wrigley R. Comparison of the resistive index to clinical parameters in dogs with renal disease. *Vet Radiol Ultrasound*. 1996;37(3):193–199.
46. Adams WH, Toal RL, Breider MA. Ultrasonographic findings in dogs and cats with oxalate nephrosis attributed to ethylene glycol intoxication: 15 cases (1984–1988). *J Am Vet Med Assoc*. 1991;199(4):492–496.
47. Mantis P, Lamb CR. Most dogs with medullary rim sign on ultrasonography have no demonstrable renal dysfunction. *Vet Radiol Ultrasound Off J Am Coll Vet Radiol Int Vet Radiol Assoc*. 2000;41(2):164–166. https://doi.org/10.1111/j.1740-8261.2000.tb01471.x.
48. Cordella A, Pey P, Dondi F, et al. The ultrasonographic medullary "rim sign" versus medullary "band sign" in cats and their association with renal disease. *J Vet Intern Med*. 2020;34(5):1932–1939. https://doi.org/10.1111/jvim.15878.
49. Ferreira A, Marwood R, Batchelor D, Maddox T, Mortier JR. Prevalence and clinical significance of the medullary rim sign identified on ultrasound of feline kidneys. *Vet Rec*. 2020;186(16):533. https://doi.org/10.1136/vr.105619.

50. Forrest LJ, O'Brien RT, Tremelling MS, Steinberg H, Cooley AJ, Kerlin RL. Sonographic renal findings in 20 dogs with leptospirosis. *Vet Radiol Ultrasound Off J Am Coll Vet Radiol Int Vet Radiol Assoc.* 1998;39(4):337–340. https://doi.org/10.1111/j.1740-8261.1998.tb01617.x.
51. Lewis KM, O'Brien RT. Abdominal ultrasonographic findings associated with feline infectious peritonitis: a retrospective review of 16 cases. *J Am Anim Hosp Assoc.* 2010;46(3):152–160. https://doi.org/10.5326/0460152.
52. Barr FJ. Hypercalcemic nephropathy in three dogs: sonographic appearance. *Veterinary Radiology.* 1989;30:169–173. https://onlinelibrary.wiley.com/doi/abs/10.1111/j.1740-8261.1989.tb00770.x. Accessed July 13, 2022. Accessed.
53. Rahal SC, Mamprim MJ, Oliveira HS, et al. Ultrasonographic, computed tomographic, and operative findings in dogs infested with giant kidney worms (*Dioctophyme renale*). *J Am Vet Med Assoc.* 2014;244(5):555–558. https://doi.org/10.2460/javma.244.5.555.
54. McKenna SC, Carpenter JL. Polycystic disease of the kidney and liver in the Cairn Terrier. *Vet Pathol.* 1980;17(4):436–442. https://doi.org/10.1177/030098588001700405.
55. Moe L, Lium B. Computed tomography of hereditary multifocal renal cystadenocarcinomas in German shepherd dogs. *Vet Radiol Ultrasound Off J Am Coll Vet Radiol Int Vet Radiol Assoc.* 1997;38(5):335–343. https://doi.org/10.1111/j.1740-8261.1997.tb02094.x.
56. Holloway A, O'Brien R. Perirenal effusion in dogs and cats with acute renal failure. *Vet Radiol Ultrasound Off J Am Coll Vet Radiol Int Vet Radiol Assoc.* 2007;48(6):574–579. https://doi.org/10.1111/j.1740-8261.2007.00300.x.
57. Beck JA, Bellenger CR, Lamb WA, et al. Perirenal pseudocysts in 26 cats. *Aust Vet J.* 2000;78(3):166–171. https://doi.org/10.1111/j.1751-0813.2000.tb10585.x.
58. Bryan JN, Henry CJ, Turnquist SE, et al. Primary renal neoplasia of dogs. *J Vet Intern Med.* 2006;20(5):1155–1160. https://doi.org/10.1892/0891-6640(2006)20[1155:prnod]2.0.co;2.
59. Borjesson DL. Renal cytology. *Vet Clin North Am Small Anim Pract.* 2003;33(1):119–134. https://doi.org/10.1016/s0195-5616(02)00086-4.
60. Cruz-Arámbulo R, Wrigley R, Powers B. Sonographic features of histiocytic neoplasms in the canine abdomen. *Vet Radiol Ultrasound Off J Am Coll Vet Radiol Int Vet Radiol Assoc.* 2004;45(6):554–558. https://doi.org/10.1111/j.1740-8261.2004.04095.x.
61. Valdés-Martínez A, Cianciolo R, Mai W. Association between renal hypoechoic subcapsular thickening and lymphosarcoma in cats. *Vet Radiol Ultrasound Off J Am Coll Vet Radiol Int Vet Radiol Assoc.* 2007;48(4):357–360. https://doi.org/10.1111/j.1740-8261.2007.00256.x.
62. Williams AG, Hohenhaus AE, Lamb KE. Incidence and treatment of feline renal lymphoma: 27 cases. *J Feline Med Surg.* 2021;23(10):936–944. https://doi.org/10.1177/1098612X20984363.
63. Hylands R. Veterinary diagnostic imaging. Retroperitoneal abscess and regional cellulitis secondary to a pyelonephritis within the left kidney. *Can Vet J Rev Veterinaire Can.* 2006;47(10):1033–1035.
64. Neuwirth L, Mahaffey M, Crowell W, et al. Comparison of excretory urography and ultrasonography for detection of experimentally induced pyelonephritis in dogs. *Am J Vet Res.* 1993;54(5):660–669.
65. Choi J, Jang J, Choi H, Kim H, Yoon J. Ultrasonographic features of pyonephrosis in dogs. *Vet Radiol Ultrasound Off J Am Coll Vet Radiol Int Vet Radiol Assoc.* 2010;51(5):548–553. https://doi.org/10.1111/j.1740-8261.2010.01702.x.
66. Vourganti S, Agarwal PK, Bodner DR, Dogra VS. Ultrasonographic evaluation of renal infections. *Radiol Clin North Am.* 2006;44(6):763–775. https://doi.org/10.1016/j.rcl.2006.10.001.
67. Sarkiala EM, Dambach D, Harvey CE. Jaw lesions resulting from renal hyperparathyroidism in a young dog—a case report. *J Vet Dent.* 1994;11(4):121–124.
68. Reusch CE, Tomsa K, Zimmer C, et al. Ultrasonography of the parathyroid glands as an aid in differentiation of acute and chronic renal failure in dogs. *J Am Vet Med Assoc.* 2000;217(12):1849–1852. https://doi.org/10.2460/javma.2000.217.1849.
69. Feeney DA, Barber DL, Osborne CA. Functional aspects of the nephrogram in excretory urography: a review. *Vet Radiol.* 1982;23:43.
70. Pey P, Marcon O, Drigo M, Specchi S, Bertolini G. Multidetector-row computed tomographic characteristics of presumed preureteral vena cava in cats. *Vet Radiol Ultrasound Off J Am Coll Vet Radiol Int Vet Radiol Assoc.* 2015;56(4):359–366. https://doi.org/10.1111/vru.12251.
71. Zaid MS, Berent AC, Weisse C, Caceres A. Feline ureteral strictures: 10 cases (2007–2009). *J Vet Intern Med.* 2011;25(2):222–229. https://doi.org/10.1111/j.1939-1676.2011.0679.x.
72. Kyles AE, Hardie EM, Wooden BG, et al. Clinical, clinicopathologic, radiographic, and ultrasonographic abnormalities in cats with ureteral calculi: 163 cases (1984–2002). *J Am Vet Med Assoc.* 2005;226(6):932–936. https://doi.org/10.2460/javma.2005.226.932.
73. Choi H, Won S, Chung W, et al. Effect of intravenous mannitol upon the resistive index in complete unilateral renal obstruction in dogs. *J Vet Intern Med.* 2003;17(2):158–162. https://doi.org/10.1111/j.1939-1676.2003.tb02427.x.
74. Lulich JP, Osborne CA, Albasan H, Koehler LA, Ulrich LM, Lekcharoensuk C. Recent shifts in the global proportions of canine uroliths. *Vet Rec.* 2013;172(14):363. https://doi.org/10.1136/vr.101056.
75. Shabana W, Bude RO, Rubin JM. Comparison between color Doppler twinkling artifact and acoustic shadowing for renal calculus detection: an in vitro study. *Ultrasound Med Biol.* 2009;35(2):339–350. https://doi.org/10.1016/j.ultrasmedbio.2008.09.023.
76. Berent AC, Mayhew PD, Porat-Mosenco Y. Use of cystoscopic-guided laser ablation for treatment of intramural ureteral ectopia in male dogs: four cases (2006–2007). *J Am Vet Med Assoc.* 2008;232(7):1026–1034. https://doi.org/10.2460/javma.232.7.1026.
77. Samii VF, McLoughlin MA, Mattoon JS, et al. Digital fluoroscopic excretory urography, digital fluoroscopic urethrography, helical computed tomography, and cystoscopy in 24 dogs with suspected ureteral ectopia. *J Vet Intern Med.* 2004;18(3):271–281. https://doi.org/10.1892/0891-6640(2004)18<271:dfeudf>2.0.co;2.
78. Yoon HY, Mann FA, Punke JP, Jeong SW. Bilateral ureteral ectopia with renal dysplasia and urolithiasis in a dog. *J Am Anim Hosp Assoc.* 2010;46(3):209–214. https://doi.org/10.5326/0460209.
79. Lautzenhiser SJ, Bjorling DE. Urinary incontinence in a dog with an ectopic ureterocele. *J Am Anim Hosp Assoc.* 2002;38(1):29–32. https://doi.org/10.5326/0380029.
80. Stiffler KS, Stevenson MAM, Mahaffey MB, Howerth EW, Barsanti JA. Intravesical ureterocele with concurrent renal dysfunction in a dog: a case report and proposed

classification system. *J Am Anim Hosp Assoc*. 2002;38(1): 33–39. https://doi.org/10.5326/0380033.
81. Eisele JG, Jackson J, Hager D. Ectopic ureterocele in a cat. *J Am Anim Hosp Assoc*. 2005;41(5):332–335. https://doi.org/10.5326/0410332.
82. Reichle JK, Peterson RA, Mahaffey MB, Schelling CG, Barthez PY. Ureteral fibroepithelial polyps in four dogs. *Vet Radiol Ultrasound Off J Am Coll Vet Radiol Int Vet Radiol Assoc*. 2003;44(4):433–437. https://doi.org/10.1111/j.1740-8261.2003.tb00481.x.
83. Tidwell AS, Ullman L, Schelling SH. Urinoma (para-ureteral pseudocyst) in a dog. *Vet Radiol Ultrasound*. 2005;31(4): 203–206.
84. Kawashima A, Sandler CM, Corl FM, et al. Imaging of renal trauma: a comprehensive review. *Radiogr Rev Publ Radiol Soc N Am Inc*. 2001;21(3):557–574. https://doi.org/10.1148/radiographics.21.3.g01ma11557.

ELECTRONIC RESOURCES

Additional information related to the content in Chapter 41 can be found online at eBooks.Health.Elsevier.com

- Chapter Quiz

CHAPTER 42

Urinary Bladder and Urethra

Angela Marolf

ANATOMY

The urinary bladder is divided grossly into three parts: the cranially located apex, the body in the middle, and the neck or trigone caudally (Fig. 42.1).[1,2] Three ligaments formed from peritoneal reflections hold the urinary bladder loosely in position.[2] The middle urinary bladder ligament extends along the ventral surface of the urinary bladder and two lateral ligaments extend along the lateral urinary bladder surfaces. These ligaments often contain large fat deposits, facilitating radiographic visualization of the urinary bladder neck and body. The cranial and dorsal surfaces of the urinary bladder are visible radiographically because of adjacent fat within the omentum and mesentery (Fig. 42.2).

The urinary bladder is located cranial to the pubis, dorsal to the rectus abdominis muscle, caudal to the small bowel and omentum, and ventral to the large bowel. In females, the body of the uterus lies between the urinary bladder and colon/rectum. The caudal portion of the normal urinary bladder may be cranial to the pubis or within the pelvic canal.[3,4] When distended, the caudal part of the urinary bladder is usually cranial to the pubis.[3,4] The normal urinary bladder in the cat is always intra-abdominal, being located 2 to 3 cm cranial to the pubis because of the long urinary bladder neck in this species (Fig. 42.3).[5]

Urinary bladder size varies with the amount of urine. After voiding, the urinary bladder may not be visible radiographically. With extreme distention, the apex may extend to the umbilicus. Severe distention may occur normally owing to lack of opportunity to void or because of a strange or unfamiliar environment. The urinary bladder in the dog is usually oval, but with distention, it becomes more ellipsoid. The feline urinary bladder is almost always ellipsoid (Fig. 42.4).

The normal urinary bladder has a soft tissue radiographic opacity. Any opacity greater or less than soft tissue within the urinary bladder on survey radiographs is abnormal. The musculomembranous urinary bladder wall consists of mucosal, submucosal, and muscular layers. The peritoneum is adherent to the serosal surface, providing a separate fourth layer. The thickness of the urinary bladder wall or characteristics of the mucosa cannot be evaluated on survey radiographs because of border effacement by urine in the lumen.

Radiographic visualization of the urinary bladder is reduced if there is insufficient abdominal fat, inadequate distention, and superimposed opacities. Intestinal content, pelvic limb musculature, and adjacent osseous structures may obscure all or part of the urinary bladder. Focal superimposition may be created by fluid-filled small bowel, nipples, the prepuce, and cutaneous masses. If necessary, some of these superimposition opacities can be eliminated or minimized by withholding food for 24 hours preceding the study, giving cleansing enemas, or using compression radiography, although these interventions are usually not necessary.

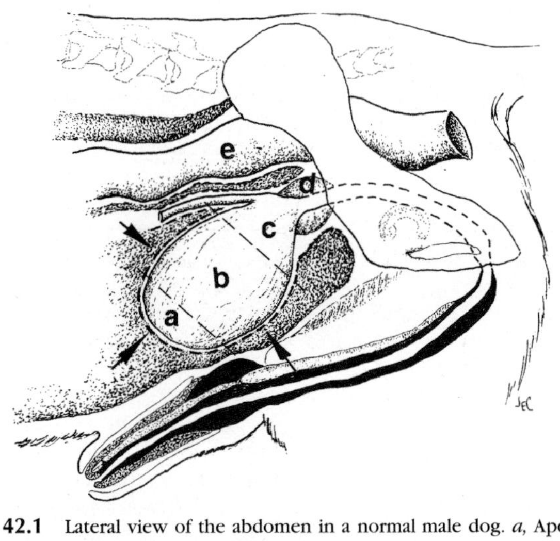

Fig. 42.1 Lateral view of the abdomen in a normal male dog. *a,* Apex of the urinary bladder; *b,* body of the urinary bladder; *c,* neck of the urinary bladder; *d,* prostate gland; *e,* descending colon. The *broken line* around the urinary bladder (*black arrows*) represents the surrounding adherent peritoneal reflection.

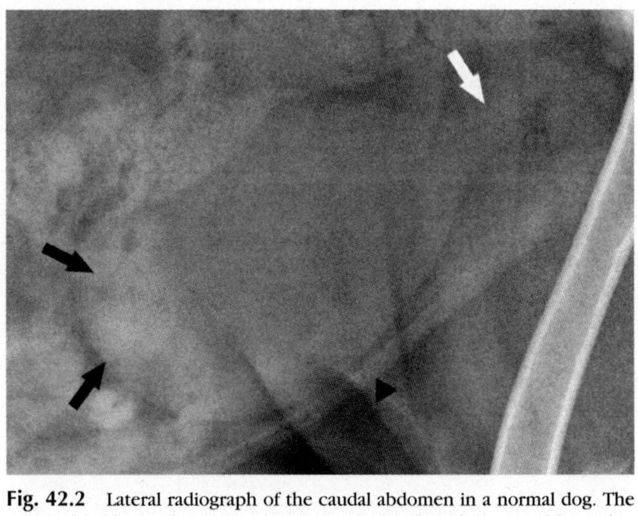

Fig. 42.2 Lateral radiograph of the caudal abdomen in a normal dog. The urinary bladder neck (*white arrow*) is well visualized because of fat within the urinary bladder ligaments. The rectus abdominis muscle (*black arrowhead*) is ventral to the urinary bladder. Bowel segments (*black arrows*) are superimposed over the apex of the urinary bladder.

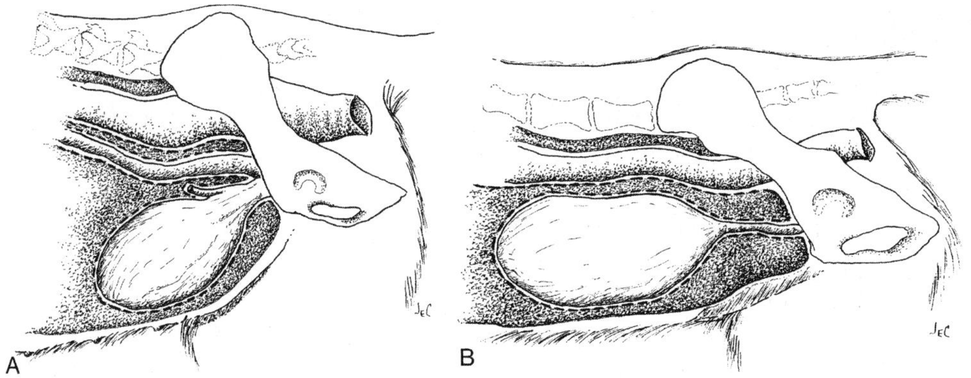

Fig. 42.3 **A,** Urinary bladder in a normal female dog. The canine urinary bladder is adjacent to the pubis and is oval. **B,** Urinary bladder in a normal cat. The feline urinary bladder is ellipsoid and has a long neck, which makes the urinary bladder appear displaced cranially from the pubis. The *broken line* around the urinary bladder in **A** and **B** denotes the peritoneal reflection. From Park RD. Radiology of the urinary bladder and urethra. In: O'Brien TR, ed. *Radiographic Diagnosis of Abdominal Disorders in the Dog and Cat.* Davis, CA: Covell Park Veterinary; 1981.

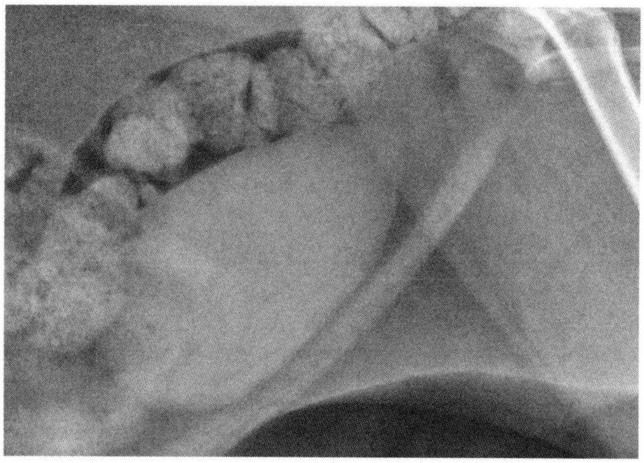

Fig. 42.4 Lateral radiograph of the caudal abdomen in a normal cat. The feline urinary bladder is ellipsoid and is located more cranially than in the dog because of a longer urinary bladder neck. Bowel segments are superimposed over the apex of the urinary bladder.

RADIOGRAPHIC SIGNS OF URINARY BLADDER DISEASE

There are few survey-radiographic signs of urinary bladder disease. Poor or nonexistent urinary bladder visualization and abnormal urinary bladder position, shape, size, and opacity indicate disease of the urinary bladder or, in many instances, disease of adjacent structures (Table 42.1).

Poor radiographic delineation of the urinary bladder may occur regardless of whether serosal contrast in the caudal abdomen is good or decreased. If serosal contrast is good and the urinary bladder is not seen, the urinary bladder is empty or has been displaced caudally or ventrally. If serosal contrast is decreased and the urinary bladder surface is not seen distinctly, free peritoneal fluid or inadequate peritoneal fat may be the cause (Fig. 42.5).

The urinary bladder may be displaced abnormally in various directions.[6] The cause of urinary bladder displacement may sometimes be determined by observation of surrounding structures or organs (Fig. 42.6). With severe urinary bladder displacement, as with a hernia, cystography or ultrasonography may be needed for its identification. Urinary bladder retroflexion was observed in 24% (10/41) of dogs with a perineal hernia.[7] A urinary bladder partially within the pelvic canal (Fig. 42.7) may be associated with congenital urinary tract anomalies.[8] A pelvic urinary bladder has also been reported as a normal variation, and this finding should be correlated with clinical signs to determine its significance.[4,9] Incontinent female dogs with a pelvic urinary bladder usually have a shorter urethra than continent dogs.[10,11]

A change in shape of the urinary bladder is not common. Abdominal masses adjacent to the serosal surface of the urinary bladder may distort its shape. Tumors originating from the urinary bladder wall occasionally protrude from the serosal surface or cause thickening of the bladder trigone to produce a discernible change in shape of the urinary bladder but this is uncommon (Fig. 42.8).[12] A pointed apex with an elongated urinary bladder may occur with a persistent urachal ligament.[13] An abnormally small or large urinary bladder is difficult to diagnose radiographically because of the wide variation in normal size. In most instances, a consistently small or large urinary bladder with associated clinical signs is an indication that a contrast study or ultrasound examination should be performed to determine the cause of the suspected size change.

Any change in radiographic opacity in the urinary bladder is abnormal and usually easy to detect. Gas in the urinary bladder may be introduced iatrogenically from catheterization or cystocentesis. Small luminal gas bubbles are usually located in the center of the urinary bladder on a recumbent lateral view (Fig. 42.9). Gas in the urinary bladder lumen, urinary bladder wall, and occasionally the urinary bladder ligaments occurs with emphysematous cystitis (Fig. 42.10, eFig. 42.1). Emphysematous cystitis is produced by glucose-fermenting organisms and may be seen in association with diabetes mellitus.[14] Emphysematous cystitis without diabetes mellitus can also occur.[15,16]

Most increased opacities associated with the urinary bladder are calculi (see Fig. 42.6B, Fig. 42.11, eFigs. 42.2 and 42.3). Opacities need to be confirmed to be in the urinary bladder based on orthogonal radiographs. If doubt exists regarding the location or presence of cystic calculi, a compression view to displace adjacent structures overlapping or surrounding the urinary bladder (Fig. 42.12) and ultrasonography are ways to confirm the presence of calculi. The entire urinary tract from the kidneys to the terminus of the urethra should be examined for additional calculi. Not all calculi are radiopaque; thus, the absence of radiopacities within the urinary bladder does not rule out the presence of cystic calculi (Table 42.2). In cats with suspected feline idiopathic cystitis, survey radiographs, cystography, or ultrasonography can be used to evaluate the urinary bladder. Often, mild urinary bladder wall thickening may be observed with cystography.[17] Additionally, a horizontal-beam radiograph can be used to diagnose sand-like material

Table • 42.1

Urinary Bladder: Survey Radiographic Signs.

RADIOGRAPHIC SIGN	GAMUT OF CONDITION(S) OR DISEASE(S)
Visualization	
Urinary bladder not seen; abdominal serosal outlines are clear	Post voiding Displaced urinary bladder Perineal hernia Inguinal hernia Pelvic urinary bladder Normal Short urethra Ectopic ureter(s) Congenital urethrorectal fistula
Urinary bladder not seen; abdominal serosal outlines are not clearly seen	Peritoneal fluid Urine secondary to urinary bladder tear/rupture Transudate Exudate Hemorrhage Lack of peritoneal fat Emaciation Young animal (<4 months of age)
Abnormal Position	
Ventral displacement	Abdominal wall hernia
Cranial displacement	Prostate gland disease Neoplasia Prostatitis Prostatic or paraprostatic cyst Benign hypertrophy Large intrapelvic mass
Cranioventral displacement	Enlarged uterus Pyometra Pregnancy Sublumbar mass Large bowel distention Uterine stump granuloma or abscess Persistent patent urachus or urachal ligament Inguinal hernia
Caudal displacement	Perineal hernia Large abdominal mass
Dorsal displacement	Abdominal mass
Abnormal shape	Adjacent abdominal mass Neoplasia Abscesses/granulomas Persistent urachal ligament
Abnormal Size	
Increased	Urethral obstruction Urinary bladder neck obstruction Neurologic deficiencies
Decreased	Congenital anomalies Ectopic ureters Fistulas Cystitis Neoplasia
Mineral opacity	Calculi Urinary bladder wall mineralization
Lucent areas	Gas Iatrogenic Emphysematous cystitis

that will collect within the dependent portion of the urinary bladder. This additional view may be helpful in cats with feline idiopathic cystitis (feline lower urinary tract disease).[18] Radiopacities in the urinary bladder can also be produced by mineralization of the urinary bladder wall associated with neoplasia, chronic or encrusted cystitis, but this is unusual.[19]

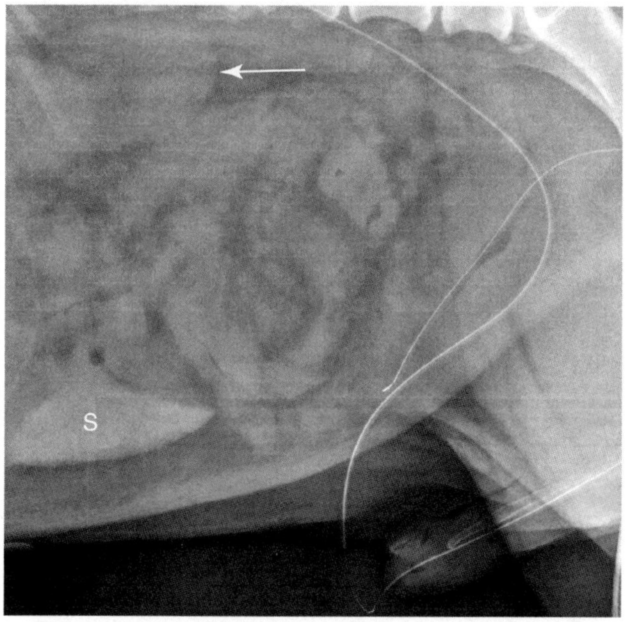

Fig. 42.5 Lateral radiograph of the abdomen of a dog. The left kidney (*white arrow*) is visible because of surrounding retroperitoneal fat. The serosal surfaces of the bowel and urinary bladder in the caudal aspect of the abdomen are indistinct because of free peritoneal fluid. The spleen (*S*) can be seen because of the focal nature of the free fluid in the caudal abdomen. A catheter is in the urinary bladder and looping over the caudal part of the abdomen.

CONTRAST CYSTOGRAPHY

Retrograde contrast cystography has largely been replaced by ultrasound but is a fast, simple, and inexpensive technique that may provide valuable diagnostic and prognostic information. Clinical indications for cystography include dysuria, pollakiuria,

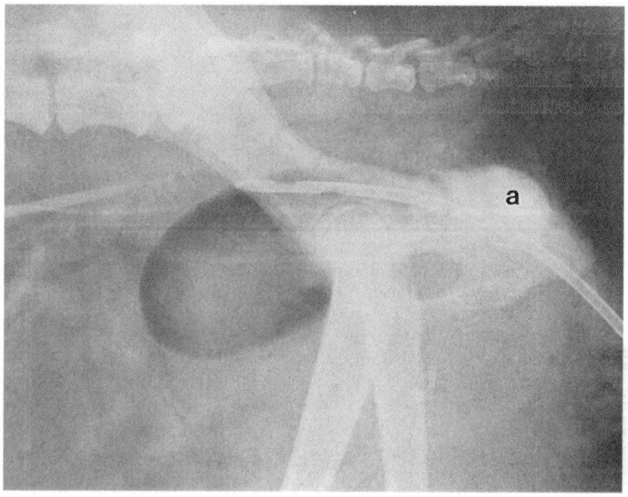

Fig. 42.7 Lateral radiograph of the caudal abdomen and pelvis after intravenous urography and double-contrast cystography. A radiopaque catheter is present in the urinary bladder, and the caudal aspect of the urinary bladder is within the pelvic canal. Contrast medium has accumulated in the vagina (*a*) because of an ectopic ureter.

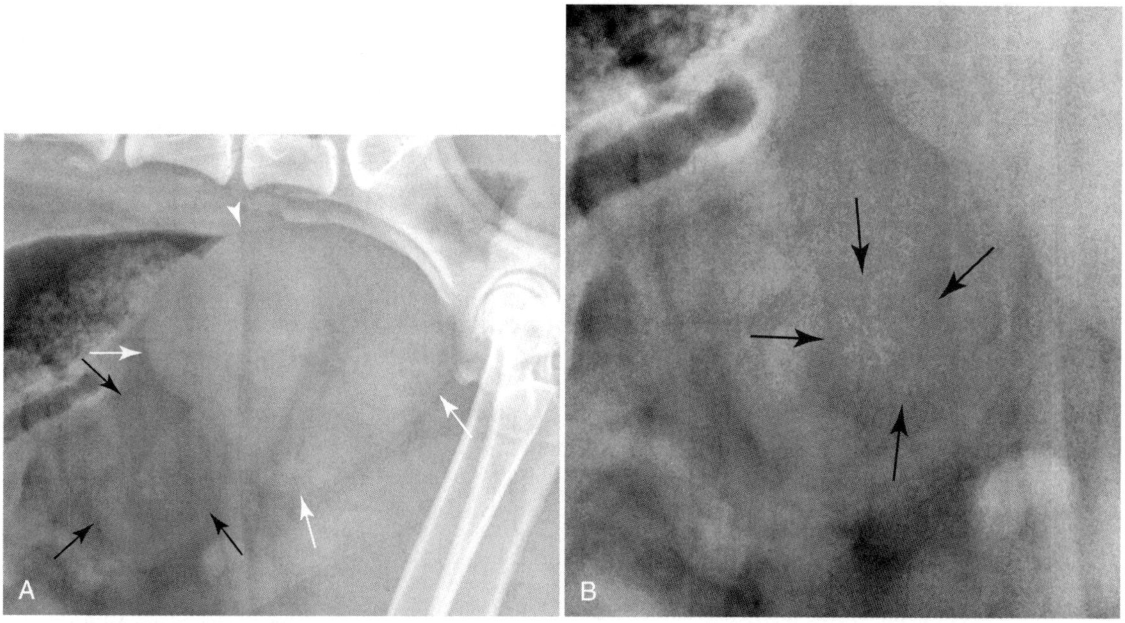

Fig. 42.6 **A,** Lateral radiograph of a dog with a large prostatic carcinoma (*white arrows*). The enlarged prostate gland displaces the urinary bladder (*black arrows*) cranially and compresses the terminal portion of the descending colon (*white arrowhead*). The prostate gland is more opaque than the urinary bladder because of its increased thickness. The enlarged prostate gland could be misinterpreted as the urinary bladder, except for the atypical shape. If there is a question whether a caudal abdominal mass is of urinary bladder origin, a positive-contrast cystogram or sonography would provide more information. **B,** Close-up of the urinary bladder from the same dog. There are numerous small radiopaque calculi in the lumen (*black arrows*).

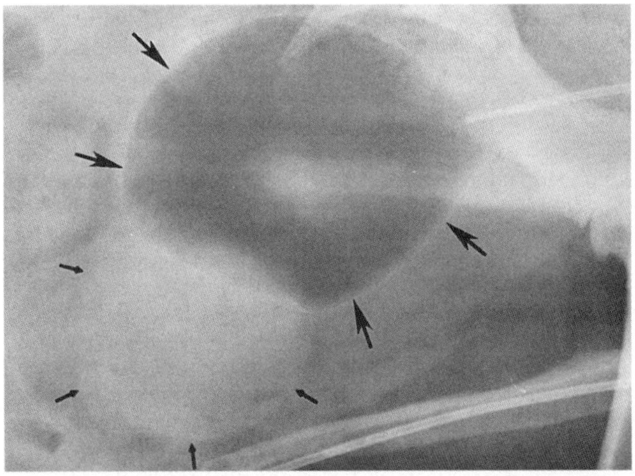

Fig. 42.8 Oblique view of the abdomen after double-contrast cystography. A mass (*small black arrows*) is present on the cranioventral aspect of the gas-filled urinary bladder (*large black arrows*). The mass is a leiomyosarcoma originating from the urinary bladder; it gave the urinary bladder a bilobed appearance on the survey radiograph. This is an unusual manifestation of tumors of the urinary bladder.

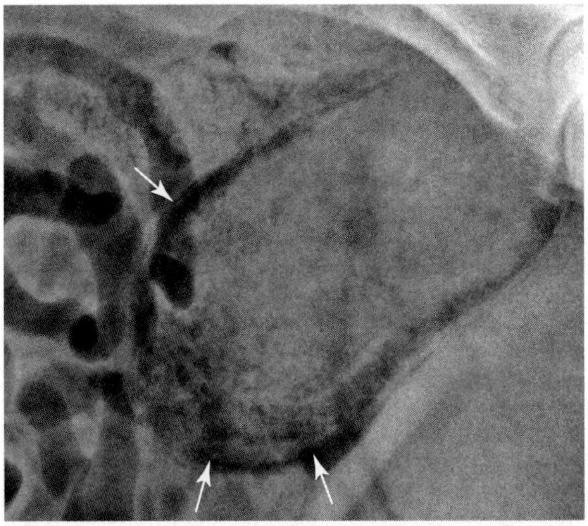

Fig. 42.10 Lateral view of the abdomen of a dog with gas (*white arrows*) in the urinary bladder wall and lumen. This appearance is typical of emphysematous cystitis, which in this dog was secondary to diabetes mellitus.

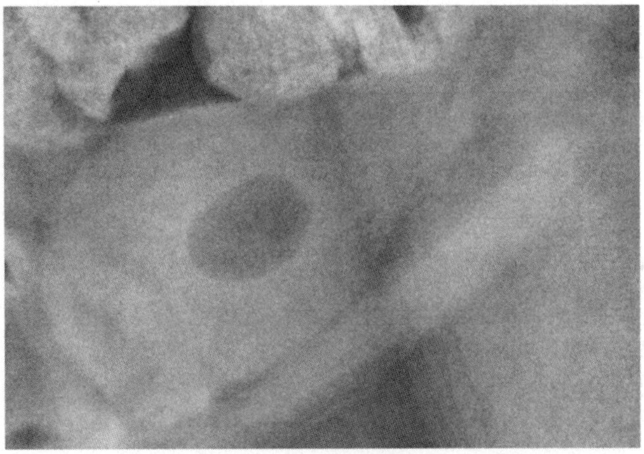

Fig. 42.9 Lateral view of the caudal abdomen of a cat. A central oblong air bubble introduced during cystocentesis is present in the urinary bladder. This radiolucency should not be misinterpreted as a calculus because positive-contrast medium has not been administered. So-called radiolucent calculi are really of soft tissue opacity and are not visible on survey radiographs. However, nonopaque calculi will appear relatively radiolucent when surrounded by positive-contrast medium is in the urinary bladder, creating a filling defect.

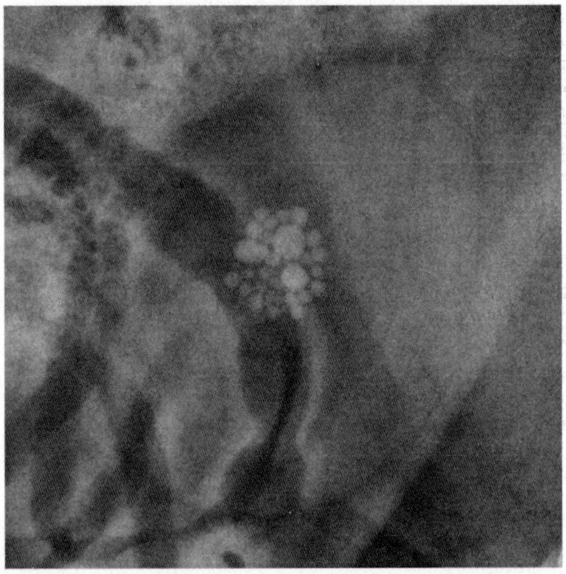

Fig. 42.11 Lateral radiograph of a dog with multiple, variably sized mineralized cystic calculi. Gas-filled bowl loops are superimposed over the apex of the urinary bladder

and intermittent or persistent chronic hematuria. Radiographic signs that suggest a need for cystography include identification of increased or decreased opacity in the urinary bladder, evaluation of caudal abdominal masses that may be associated with the urinary bladder, nonvisualization of the urinary bladder after abdominal trauma, and an abnormal shape or location of the urinary bladder. Cystography can be performed as negative-, positive-, or double-contrast procedure. Retrograde positive- and double-contrast procedures are often more useful to evaluate the urinary bladder than is negative-contrast cystography alone. Positive-contrast cystography is the method of choice for identifying urinary bladder location, tears, hernias, and abnormal communication with adjacent structures. Double-contrast cystography is better than positive-contrast cystography for assessing urinary bladder wall lesions and intraluminal filling defects. The selection of positive- or double-contrast cystography is based on clinical history, clinical signs, radiographic signs, and urinalysis findings (Table 42.3).

Cystography Technique

If possible, food should be withheld for 12 to 24 hours and an enema may need to be given preceding cystography because fecal material superimposed over the urinary bladder may mask important information.

All catheters and equipment should be sterilized, and the genitalia should be cleaned before the urinary bladder is catheterized. The equipment necessary for urinary bladder catheterization is illustrated in Fig. 42.13. Various other types of catheters are available.

Complications resulting from catheterization and cystography occur infrequently and are usually not detrimental. Iatrogenic trauma, bacterial contamination, or kinked and knotted urethral catheters may occur from improper catheterization.

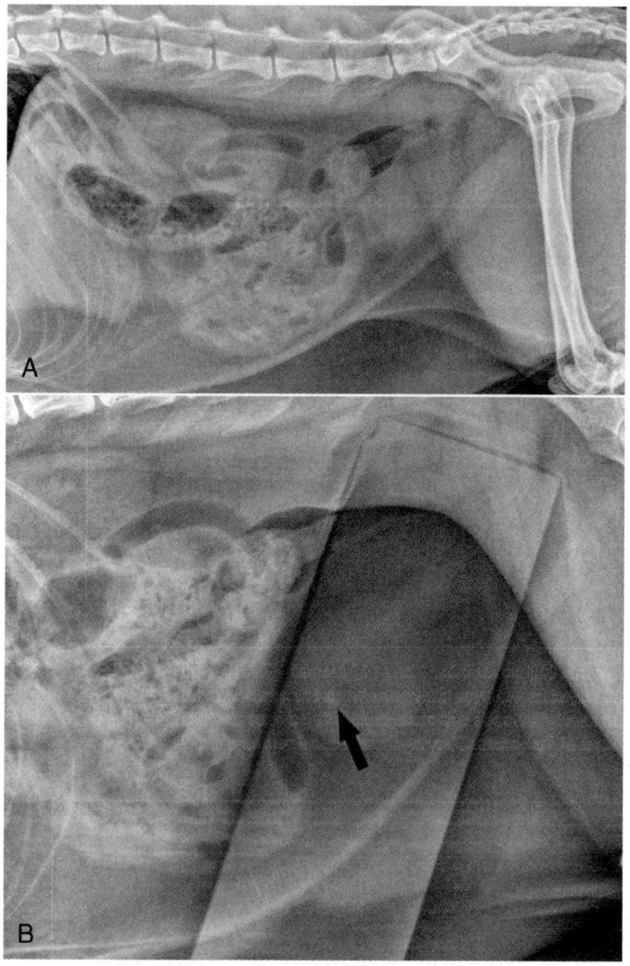

Fig. 42.12 A, Lateral radiograph of a cat with clinical signs of lower urinary tract disease. Note the superimposition of soft tissue structures and bowel over the urinary bladder. The ill-defined mineral opacity superimposed on the apex of the urinary bladder may be within the urinary bladder or in superimposed bowel. **B,** Compression view of the same animal after applying pressure with a nonradiopaque paddle. Note the displacement of bowel and radiopaque calculus in urinary bladder (*black arrow*).

Intramural and subserosal accumulation of contrast medium has occurred after maximal urinary bladder distention with a Foley catheter (Fig. 42.14).[20–22] This complication occurs more frequently in cats, often with a nondistended urinary bladder and minimal intravesicular pressure. It usually does not result in a clinical problem. Mucosal ulceration, inflammation, and granulomatous reactions may occur, but the changes are usually transitory and produce no serious clinical problems.[9] The most serious complication from negative-contrast cystography is gas embolization into the circulatory system, which may result in death.[23,24] Fortunately, such complications occur rarely. Death from gas embolism may be prevented by using more soluble nitrous oxide or carbon dioxide instead of room air.

Both negative- and positive-contrast media can be used for cystography. Negative-contrast media include room air, carbon dioxide, and nitrous oxide. Positive-contrast media are water-soluble organic iodides that should be used in an approximate 20% iodine solution. Barium should never be used for cystography.[20,24] The urinary bladder should be empty prior to administration of contrast medium. The volume of positive-contrast medium varies with body weight, the species, and the pathologic process present in the urinary bladder. An approximation of 10 mL per kilogram may be used.[24,25] The injection should be terminated before the estimated volume has

Table • 42.2

Radiopacity of Cystic Calculi on Survey Abdominal Radiographs.

CALCULUS COMPOSITION	OPACITY	SURFACE CHARACTERISTICS
Calcium oxalate	Moderately to markedly radiopaque	Sharp projections or smooth
Calcium phosphate	Moderately to markedly radiopaque	Smooth
Struvite (ammonium phosphate)	Moderately to markedly radiopaque	Usually smooth; can be spiculated
Silica	Moderately radiopaque	Jackstone appearance
Urate	Nonradiopaque to faintly radiopaque	Smooth
Cystine	Nonradiopaque to faintly radiopaque	Smooth

Table • 42.3

Indications for Type of Cystographic Procedure.

CONTRAST STUDY	INDICATIONS
Double-contrast cystogram	Suspect urinary bladder wall lesion(s), filling defects (calculi, blood clots, masses)
Positive-contrast cystogram	Suspect ruptured or abnormal urinary bladder location
Negative-contrast cystogram	Not frequently performed; can determine urinary bladder location or be used concurrently with other studies, such as CT excretory urography

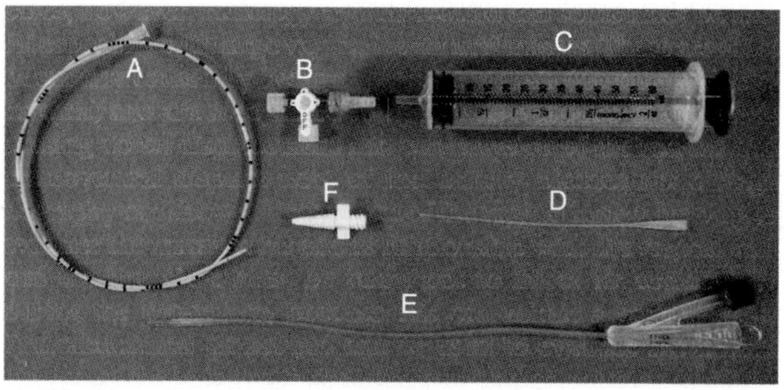

Fig. 42.13 Equipment for urinary bladder catheterization and cystography. *A,* Male urethral catheter; *B,* three-way valve; *C,* large syringe; *D,* Tomcat catheter; *E,* Foley (balloon-type) catheter; *F,* catheter connector for use with the male urethral catheter.

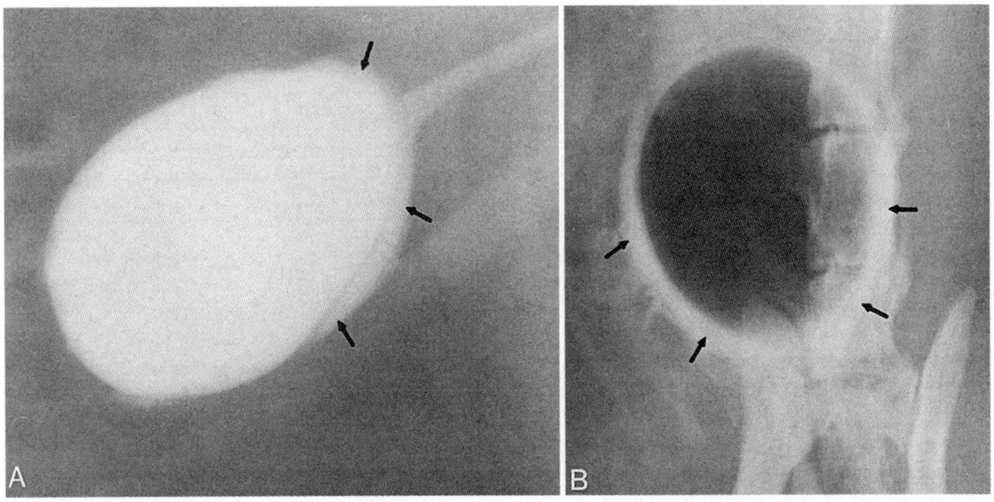

Fig. 42.14 Positive- **(A)** and double-contrast **(B)** cystogram where there has been subserosal accumulation of contrast medium (*black arrows*). This usually produces no severe or long-lasting complications. It is produced by a high intraluminal urinary bladder pressure and is predisposed by urinary bladder disease, particularly cystitis.

been administered if the urinary bladder feels adequately distended by external palpation, if reflux occurs around the catheter, or if back pressure is felt on the syringe plunger. Only moderate urinary bladder distention is recommended because maximal distention may obliterate subtle mucosal and urinary bladder wall changes and bears the risk of bladder rupture in case of chronic cystitis with reduced compliance of the bladder wall.[26] Lateral, ventrodorsal, ventral left–dorsal right, and ventral right–dorsal left radiographic views of the caudal abdomen should be made to examine the contrast medium–filled urinary bladder adequately. A double-contrast cystogram is performed by injecting a small volume of undiluted positive-contrast medium into the urinary bladder. The recommended dose of positive-contrast medium is 0.5 to 1 mL for a cat, 1 to 3 mL for a dog weighing less than 25 lb, and 3 to 6 mL for animals weighing more than 25 lb. Positive-contrast medium injection is followed by urinary bladder distention with negative-contrast medium (Fig. 42.15).

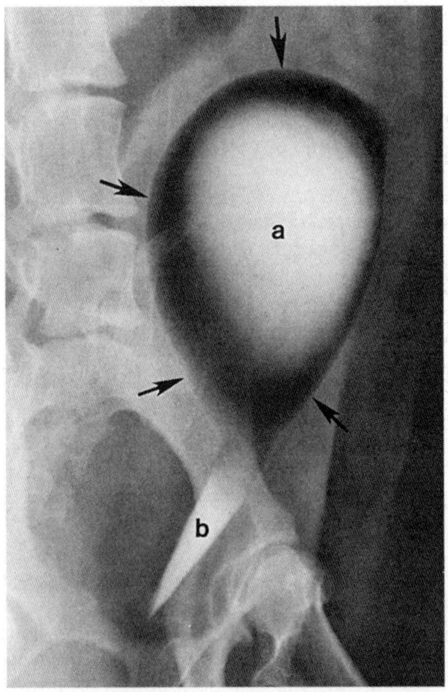

Fig. 42.15 Ventral left–dorsal right radiograph of a normal double-contrast cystogram. The urinary bladder wall (*black arrows*) is seen clearly. The contrast puddle in the dependent portion of the urinary bladder (*a*) and the contrast medium–filled urethra (*b*) are easily identified.

Radiographic Signs With Contrast Cystography

Radiographic signs observed with urinary bladder disease include intramural thickening, an irregular mucosal border, filling defects, and leakage (Table 42.4).[27] These radiographic changes must be differentiated from artifacts such as air bubbles and inadequate urinary bladder distention.

Intramural Changes (Urinary Bladder Wall Thickening)

The normal urinary bladder wall is approximately 1 mm thick regardless of the degree of distention.[9] Intramural changes are best demonstrated with double-contrast cystography and include focal or diffuse increased urinary bladder wall thickness (Fig. 42.16, eFig. 42.4). Mild urinary bladder wall thickening may be missed if the urinary bladder is distended completely.[26] Urinary bladder wall thickening may be caused by fibrous tissue proliferation or cellular infiltration from inflammation (cystitis), hemorrhage, or neoplasia. With chronic cystitis, subserosal leakage can occur due to necrosis of the urinary bladder mucosa (see Fig. 42.14). Intramural urinary bladder thickening causes decreased urinary bladder distensibility, which may be symmetric with diffuse intramural urinary bladder disease or asymmetric with focal intramural urinary bladder disease.

Mucosal Changes

The urinary bladder has a transitional epithelium, which appears smooth on a normal cystogram. Mucosal proliferation appears as an irregular outline along the inside urinary bladder surface and may be accentuated with inadequate urinary bladder distention, and can be obliterated if the urinary bladder is maximally distended.[26] The irregular mucosa is usually focally distributed but may be diffuse; it may vary in severity from a slightly irregular brush-type surface to a severe cobblestone appearance (Fig. 42.17). Ulcers may be present with mucosal

Table • 42.4

Cystographic Signs of Common Conditions of the Urinary Bladder.

	MUCOSAL CHANGES		INTRAMURAL THICKENING		FILLING DEFECT	
DISEASE	**FOCAL**	**DIFFUSE**	**FOCAL**	**DIFFUSE**	**ATTACHED**	**FREE**
Chronic cystitis	Cranioventral	Occasional	Cranioventral	Occasional (Cytoxan-induced cystitis)	Blood clots	Blood clots, calculi
Acute cystitis	—	—	—	—	—	Occasional blood clots
Cystic calculi	Cranioventral from cystitis	—	Cranioventral from cystitis	—	—	Calculi and occasional blood clots
Neoplasia	Any location within urinary bladder	Occasional	Any location within urinary bladder	Occasional	Sessile, occasionally pedunculated	Blood clots
Urinary bladder rupture or perforation	Contrast leakage into peritoneum at site of wall tear	—	—	—	—	Blood clots

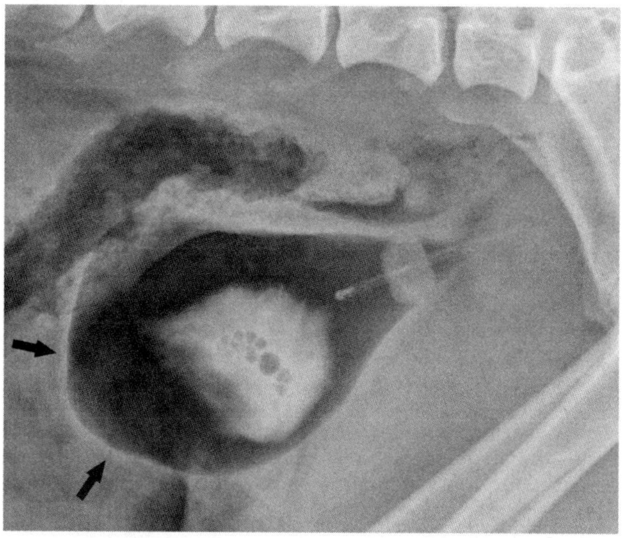

Fig. 42.16 Lateral radiograph of double-contrast cystogram. Mild diffuse urinary bladder wall thickening is present (*black arrows*). Multiple variably sized calculi appear as filling defects outlined by the contrast medium in the dependent portion of the urinary bladder.

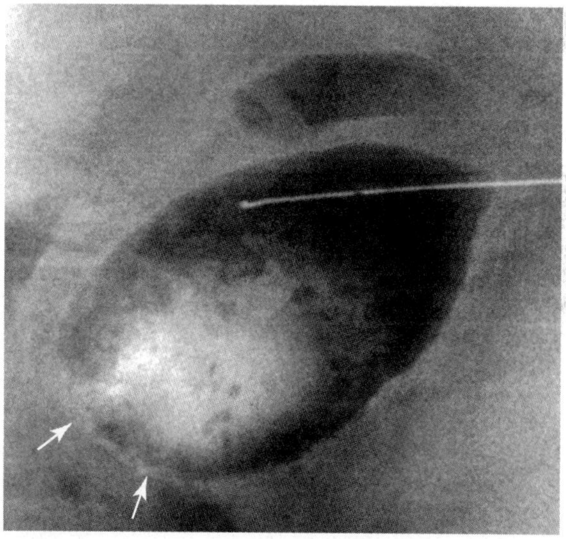

Fig. 42.17 Lateral radiograph of the urinary bladder during double-contrast cystography. Mild mucosal irregularity is present along the apex of the urinary bladder (*white arrows*) as a result of mild chronic cystitis.

proliferation and can be identified where contrast medium adheres to the mucosal surface.

Filling Defects

A urinary bladder filling defect results from anything occupying space within the urinary bladder lumen that displaces contrast medium. All filling defects appear radiolucent when surrounded with positive-contrast medium even though the opacity of the defect may not be inherently radiolucent. The size, shape, number, border contour, position within the lumen, and attachment to the urinary bladder wall help determine the nature of the filling defect (Table 42.5).

Filling defects may be *free* or *attached*. Common causes of free luminal filling defects are air bubbles, calculi, and blood clots[27] (Fig. 42.18, see eFig. 42.3). Abnormalities causing a free luminal filling defect are best demonstrated with double-contrast cystography and are located in the center of the urinary bladder on a recumbent lateral view. The concentration of the contrast medium and depth of the contrast puddle have an effect on visibility of cystic calculi.[28,29] Combining patient signalment and double-contrast cystographic findings can improve prediction of type of mineral calculus noninvasively.[30] Attached filling defects may be caused by neoplasia, inflammatory polyps, adherent calculi or blood clots, and ureteroceles.[31–33] Ureteroceles may communicate

Table • 42.5

Urinary Bladder Filling Defects.

LESION	SHAPE	ATTACHMENT	BORDER/CONTOUR	URINARY BLADDER WALL INFILTRATION (THICKENING)
Calculi	Round to slightly irregular	Free in lumen; center of contrast puddle	Indistinct	Variable; usually cranioventral if associated with cystitis
Sebaceous or mucous plug	Round or irregular	Free in lumen; center of contrast puddle	Smooth or irregular, distinct or indistinct	Variable; associated with cystitis
Polyp	Pedunculated or convex	Stalk or sessile	Smooth or irregular, often with ulceration	Variable; urinary bladder wall may be thick at attachment site
Epithelial neoplasia	Irregular or convex	Sessile	Irregular, often with ulceration	Urinary bladder wall often thick or infiltrated at base of attachment
Mesenchymal neoplasia	Convex	Sessile	Usually smooth	Originates within the urinary bladder wall
Blood clots	Irregular	Variable; may be free luminal	Irregular and indistinct	Thickened urinary bladder wall from primary disease process
Urinary bladder wall hematoma	Convex	Sessile	Smooth to slightly irregular	Originates within urinary bladder wall
Ureterocele	Convex to round	Sessile	Smooth	Originates within trigone region of the urinary bladder wall

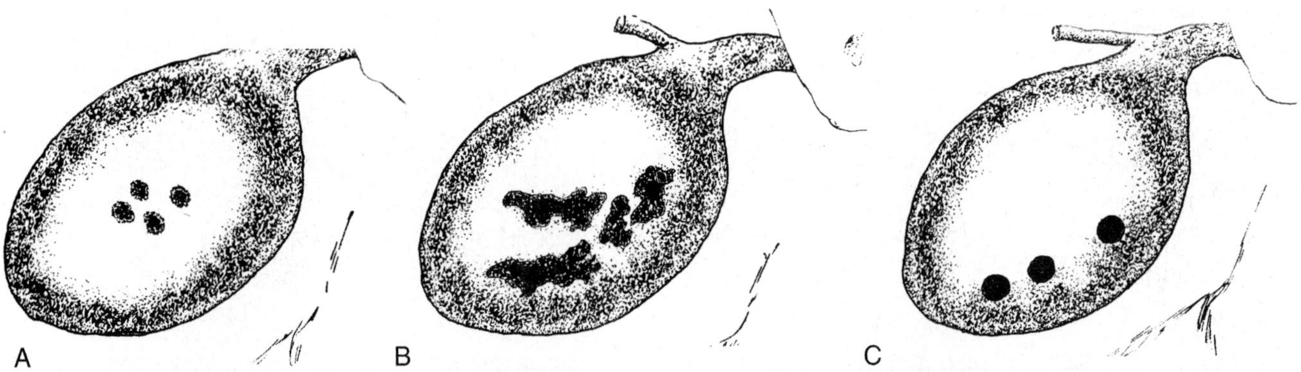

Fig. 42.18 Radiolucent luminal filling defects as might be seen in a double-contrast cystogram. **A,** Cystic calculi, in the center of the contrast puddle, are round with an indistinct border. **B,** Blood clots are irregularly shaped with irregular, indistinct borders; they may be located anywhere in the urinary bladder. **C,** Air bubbles are round with smooth, distinct borders; they are shown here at the periphery of the contrast puddle but are more often located centrally. (From Park RD. Radiology of the urinary bladder and urethra. In: O'Brien TR, ed. *Radiographic Diagnosis of Abdominal Disorders in the Dog and Cat.* Davis, CA: Covell Park Veterinary; 1981.)

partially with the urinary bladder and fill with positive-contrast medium and create what is known as the *cobra-head sign*, or they may not communicate and be a negative filling defect (see Fig. 42.19).[34] With double-contrast cystography, mural masses may be seen only when the x-ray beam is parallel to the interface between the mass and contrast medium.[35] Urinary bladder wall infiltration may be diagnosed as a thickened urinary bladder wall adjacent to the filling defect.[35] Often, a specific diagnosis of an attached filling defect cannot be made and histologic/cytologic evaluation is needed.

Contrast Leakage and Retention Patterns

Retrograde positive-contrast cystography is the best technique to assess leakage of urine from the urinary bladder. Urine leakage may occur into the urinary tract, adjacent visceral soft tissue structures, or the peritoneal cavity.

Vesicoureteral reflux can lead to contrast medium filling the ureters. Retention of urine contrast medium may occur in urachal anomalies (see Fig. 42.20), and traumatic urinary bladder diverticula (Fig. 42.21). Urachal anomalies include congenital or acquired diverticula, cysts, and persistent patent urachus or urachal ligament.[36–39] Congenital urachal anomalies are characterized by smooth contrast medium margins; they may be identified as an extension from the urinary bladder.

Contrast medium leakage from the urinary bladder to adjacent visceral structures may be seen with a congenital or acquired fistula. The organs most commonly involved are the rectum and the vagina. Such fistulas can usually be diagnosed dynamically with fluoroscopy or statically from a positive-contrast cystogram by noting contrast medium in the rectum or vagina simultaneously with or shortly after contrast medium is injected into the urinary bladder.[40]

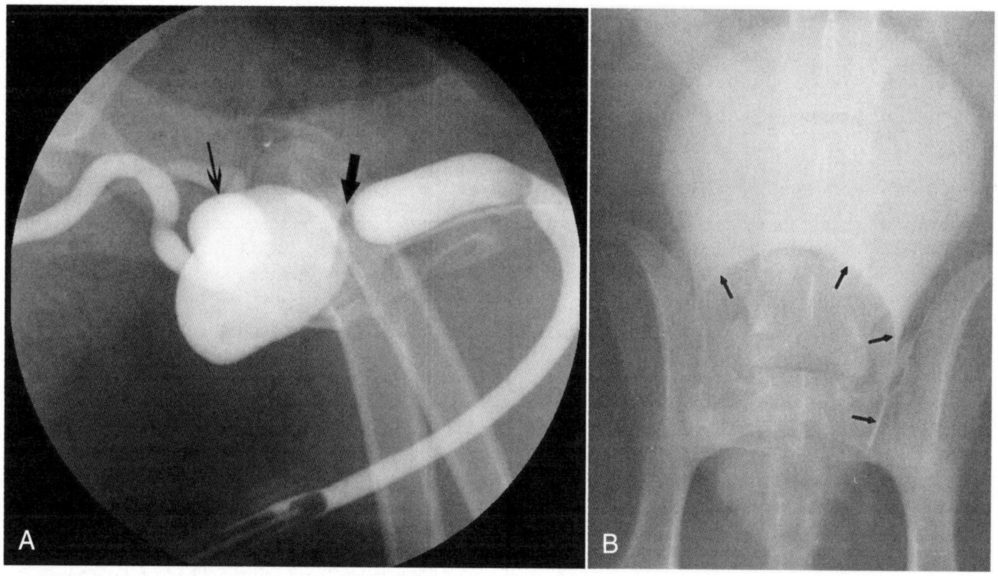

Fig. 42.19 **A,** Positive-contrast cystourethrogram. Lateral radiograph of urinary bladder and urethra. The round contrast medium–filled ureteral termination partially superimposed over the urinary bladder is a ureterocele (*thin black arrow*). Note the dilated ureter proximal to the ureterocele. A stricture of the prostatic urethra is also present (*thick black arrow*). **B,** Ventrodorsal radiograph of the urinary bladder filled with contrast medium during intravenous urography. The smooth luminal filling defect (*black arrows*) that projects into the urinary bladder neck is a ureterocele. In this patient the ureterocele is radiolucent because it does not contain contrast medium but is surrounded by contrast medium in the urinary bladder.

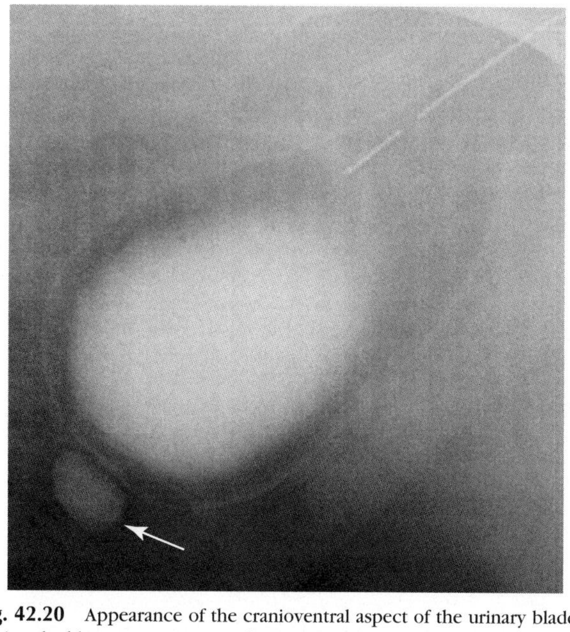

Fig. 42.20 Appearance of the cranioventral aspect of the urinary bladder during double-contrast cystography in a dog. A small oblong urachal diverticulum fills with contrast medium (*white arrow*). Contrast medium persisted in the diverticulum, evidence of urine retention that may predispose to a urinary tract infection.

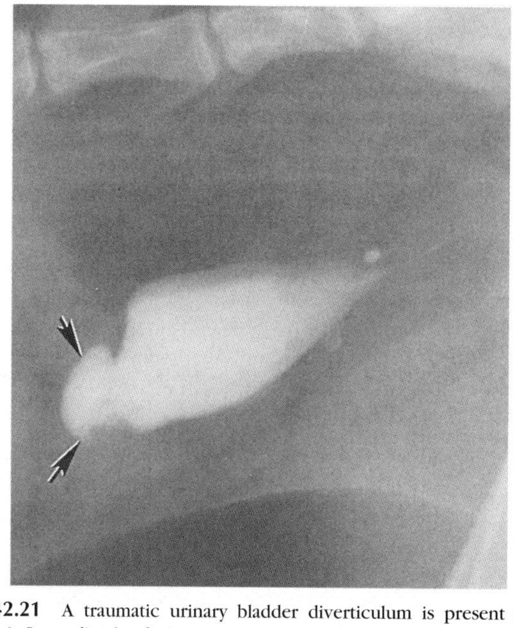

Fig. 42.21 A traumatic urinary bladder diverticulum is present (*black arrows*). Immediately after trauma, traumatic diverticula must be differentiated from a urinary bladder contusion. Contusions usually heal within 48 hours, and the urinary bladder then distends symmetrically.

Contrast medium leakage into the peritoneal cavity and surrounding soft tissues has an irregular outline and usually occurs simultaneously with injection of contrast medium into the urinary bladder (Fig. 42.22, eFig. 42.5). With small urinary bladder neck tears, leakage of contrast medium may be slow with only a small volume appearing outside the urinary bladder.[5] In these instances, a second radiograph may be required 5 to 10 minutes after injection to identify delayed leakage from the urinary bladder into the peritoneal cavity.

Pitfalls with Cystographic Interpretation

Interpretation pitfalls seen commonly with contrast cystography are air bubble artifacts and pseudofilling defects. Three types of air bubble artifacts have been recognized: small air bubbles simulating calculi or other small luminal filling defects, a large air bubble simulating urinary bladder wall thickening, and multiple air bubbles creating a honeycomb appearance (Fig. 42.23). Air bubbles are radiolucent and have smooth, distinct borders.

Pseudofilling defects may be mistaken for urinary bladder neoplasia or other attached filling defects. These defects are

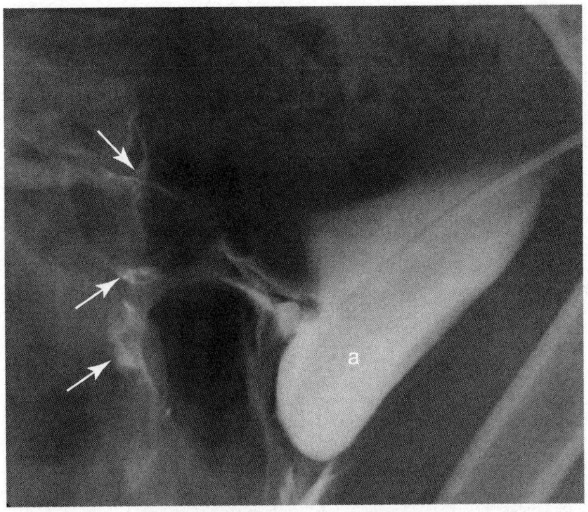

Fig. 42.22 Positive-contrast cystogram in a dog. Contrast medium fills the urinary bladder (*a*) but has also leaked into the peritoneal cavity (*white arrows*) from a dorsal urinary bladder wall tear.

created by inadequate urinary bladder distention combined with external pressure from adjacent abdominal structures. Pseudofilling defects have a smooth surface and taper on both borders; they can be obliterated with further urinary bladder distention (Fig. 42.24).

ULTRASONOGRAPHY

The fluid-filled urinary bladder is easily evaluated ultrasonographically. The superficial location of the urinary bladder enables high-resolution imaging, and urine provides high sonographic contrast, which results in good visibility of the urinary bladder wall and intraluminal abnormalities. Urolithiasis, neoplasia, cystitis, urachal, and vesicoureteral junction abnormalities can be identified by using ultrasonography.[41–43]

High-frequency transducers (7–15 MHz) are best for examination of the urinary bladder. A 5-MHz transducer may be necessary to penetrate to the far wall of a distended urinary bladder in large dogs. Linear and curved wide-aperture format transducers are particularly useful. Acoustic power and near gain should be decreased to suppress reverberation echoes generated between the transducer, the skin, and abdominal wall structures.

The ultrasonographic examination is best performed when the urinary bladder is moderately full. If a nearly empty urinary bladder is encountered, it should be reexamined when it is moderately distended after some hours of inside confinement, after administration of a diuretic, or after catheterization and sterile saline injection. The wall of a flaccid urinary bladder can be deviated inward by a distended colon, and the acoustic shadow artifacts generated by colonic contents can appear like the shadows generated by calculi.[44] A fully distended urinary bladder is also less desirable because subtle mural abnormalities may be more difficult to see. Normal urinary bladder wall thickness varies depending on the degree of urinary bladder distention and body weight, being 2.3 mm thick with minimal distention and 1.4 mm thick with moderate distention.[45] In normal adult cats, the mean urinary bladder wall thickness should not exceed 1.7 mm ± 0.6 mm.[46]

Urinary bladder ultrasonography can be performed with the patient in either dorsal or lateral recumbency. The urinary bladder should be evaluated in a transverse plane and orthogonally in either a sagittal or dorsal plane. Accurate assessment of urinary bladder wall thickness requires a perpendicular orientation of the ultrasound beam with the urinary bladder wall. Assessment of the cranial aspect of the urinary bladder wall is challenging because of the suboptimal beam alignment and the adjacent gas-filled bowel.[47] Side and grating lobe artifacts generated by the adjacent colon can give rise to an erroneous display of echogenic material in the urinary bladder lumen, and the curved urinary bladder wall can create additional echoes adjacent to the dorsal urinary bladder wall (Fig. 42.25).[48] Transducer rotation of 90 degrees over such suspicious areas is often helpful to enable recognition of the proximity of the colon and determination of the nature of the artifact. Free intraluminal abnormalities such as calculi, sediment, and blood clots gravitate to the most dependent aspect of the urinary bladder. In lateral recumbency, careful examination of the most dependent area of the urinary bladder is required so that small calculi are not overlooked. Additional imaging after the animal has been positioned in the opposite lateral recumbent or standing position allows detection of sediment swirling or gravitation of free intraluminal objects to a dependent position within the urinary bladder.

The normal urinary bladder is ovoid in shape with a slight elongation caudally at the neck. The ureters and urethra are not typically visible unless they become distended with urine. With high-resolution transducers, three distinct layers of the urinary bladder wall can be seen. The mucosa is a thin hyperechoic surface outlined against the urine, the middle muscle layer is hypoechoic, and the outer serosal layer is hyperechoic.[46] The cranioventral aspect of the wall may be slightly thinner than in other regions. Typically, normal urine is anechoic. However, suspended clumped hyperechoic foci can be identified in the urine of clinically normal cats with urine lipid.[49] The turbulence created by discharge of urine through the ureteral openings may generate transient echo jets in the urinary bladder lumen adjacent to the trigone.[50]

Intraluminal Changes

Urinary calculi, cellular and crystalline debris, gas, hemorrhage, and blood clots are detected readily by ultrasonography (Fig. 42.26A). Calculi and blood clots gravitate dependently whereas gas bubbles rise. The location of cellular and crystalline debris and fresh hemorrhage is more variable. Severe acute hemorrhage can fill the urinary bladder and give rise to a lacy hyperechoic pattern, which may change little with ballottement or animal repositioning (see Fig. 42.26B). A similar appearance can be observed with severe proteinuria and fat droplets.[51] Crystalline and cellular sediments generate a variably echogenic pattern in more dependent urine. In cats, the crystalline deposits may become thick enough to form a hyperechoic layer confluent with the urinary bladder wall that creates acoustic shadowing. Ballottement or changing patient position can differentiate the swirling sediment from calculi.

Calculi

The urine/calculus interface is intensely hyperechoic and usually appears convex. Multiple calculi often aggregate together and give rise to an irregular, somewhat continuous surface, which makes distinguishing and measuring individual calculi difficult. Distinct acoustic shadows may be observed deep to calculi (Fig. 42.27). Shadowing is related to size (height) of the calculus and transducer frequency, with increasing height of the calculus and increasing transducer frequency more likely to produce acoustic shadows.[52] The application of color Doppler to distinguish calculi based on the twinkling artifact occurring deep to the calculus can be used to discriminate mineralized from nonmineralized structures.[53] Smaller calculi may not generate the characteristic shadows if the focal zone is not optimized at the depth of the calculi. Echogenicity and acoustic shadow generation are independent of chemical composition, so radiopaque and nonradiopaque calculi can be detected by

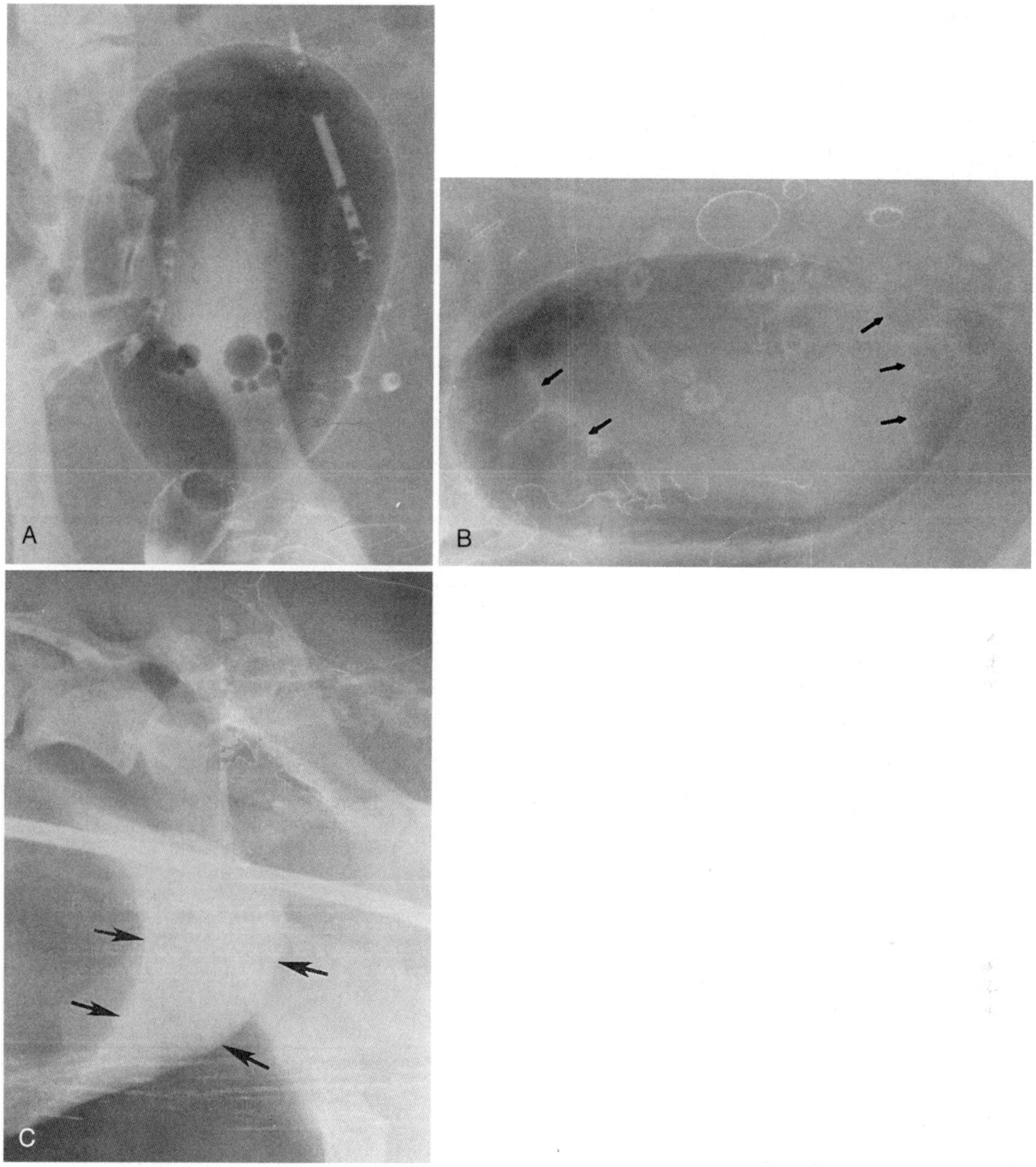

Fig. 42.23 Air bubble artifacts. **A,** Small air bubbles that cause free luminal filling defects in the urinary bladder during double-contrast cystography. Bubbles are also present in both ureters. **B,** A honeycomb appearance (*black arrows*) created by several adjacent air bubbles. **C,** A large air bubble in a mostly fluid-filled urinary bladder may produce the appearance of a thick urinary bladder wall. Here, the pseudothick wall (*black arrows*) is created by the interface between positive-contrast medium and gas. In this dog, the region between the *arrows* is more opaque than normal soft tissue because of the presence of contrast medium, and therefore this would not be confused with urinary bladder wall thickening.

sonography. Ballottement usually does not cause calculi to move, but placing the animal in a standing position allows detection of the relocated calculi into the cranioventral aspect of the urinary bladder. This action helps differentiate calculi from an adjacent colonic acoustic shadow and dystrophic mineralization in the urinary bladder wall.

Gas bubbles introduced accidentally by urinary bladder catheterization or cystocentesis are hyperechoic and can generate reverberation artifacts. Differentiation from calculi is easy because the bubble floats on top of the urine.

Blood Clots

Blood clots tend to be associated with the clinical observation of severe hematuria. Relative to normal urine, a blood clot commonly appears as a hyperechoic, nonshadowing, often layered, mobile mass.[54] Sometimes the clot may be attached to the wall, covering, or adjacent to a traumatic injury or a neoplastic mass.

Foreign Bodies

Urinary bladder foreign bodies, such as grass awns, have been reported and appear as linear to V-shaped hyperechoic structures with or without distal acoustic shadows.[55]

Mural Changes

Ultrasonography is especially useful for detecting changes from chronic cystitis and neoplasia. Contrast radiographic techniques are superior to sonography in diagnosing congenital

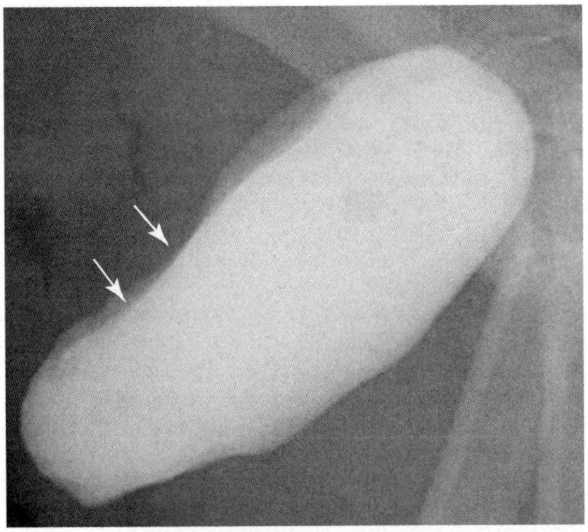

Fig. 42.24 Lateral radiograph of a positive-contrast cystogram. Pseudofilling defects or a false impression of irregularity of the urinary bladder wall (*white arrows*) can be created by pressure from adjacent abdominal structures on a partially distended urinary bladder.

abnormalities of the urachus and ureters as well as urinary bladder rupture. However, infusion of microbubbled saline into the urinary bladder during a sonographic examination has been effective for diagnosing urine leakage in some patients.[56]

Cystitis

Chronic cystitis results in focal or diffuse thickening of the urinary bladder wall and is readily detected by sonography. The urinary bladder wall becomes abnormally hypoechoic, and the normal layering becomes less parallel. The urinary bladder wall measures abnormally thick (see Fig. 42.27), and hyperechoic cellular debris frequently accumulates in the urinary bladder lumen.[57] A normal sonographic appearance of the urinary bladder does not rule out mild or acute cystitis or idiopathic lower urinary tract disease in cats. Small polypoid mucosal masses or abscesses are also occasionally observed with chronic cystitis.[58] Polypoid cystitis is uncommon in dogs and can vary in sonographic appearance ranging from pedunculated, ovoid, or nodular urinary bladder wall changes (Fig. 42.28) and can be difficult to differentiate from neoplastic proliferations.[59] Polypoid cystitis is often located in the

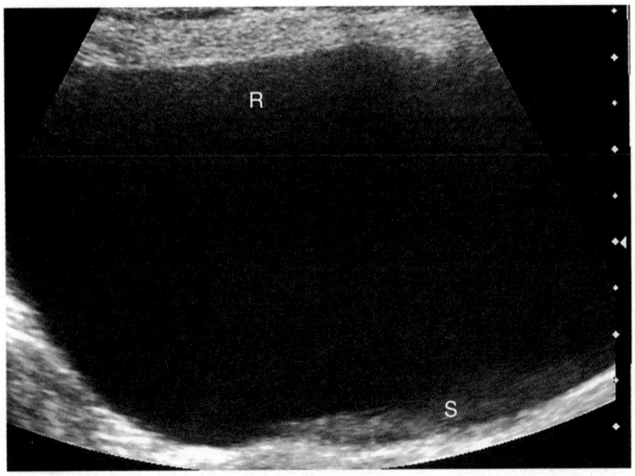

Fig. 42.25 Sonographic artifacts. Spurious echoes (*R*) are present in the ventral aspect of the lumen of the urinary bladder from reverberation artifact. Slice thickness and/or side (grating) lobe artifact (*S*) is present in the dorsal aspect of the urinary bladder, creating pseudoechogenic debris in the urine.

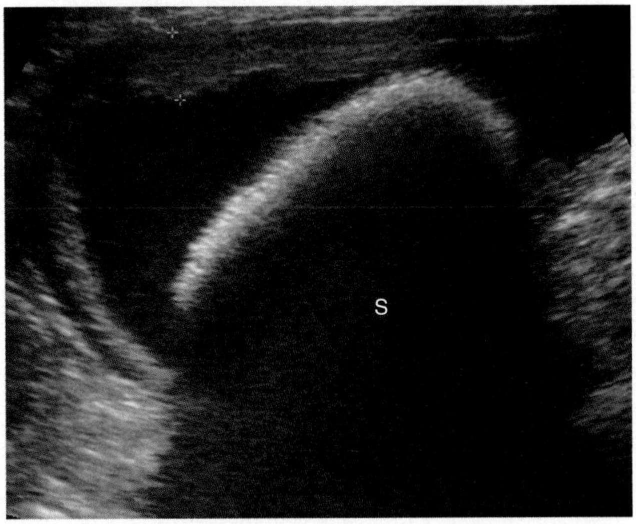

Fig. 42.27 Sagittal ultrasound image of the urinary bladder. A solitary, large calculus creates characteristic acoustic shadows (*S*) and irregular thickening of the cranioventral urinary bladder wall (calipers in image) secondary to cystitis.

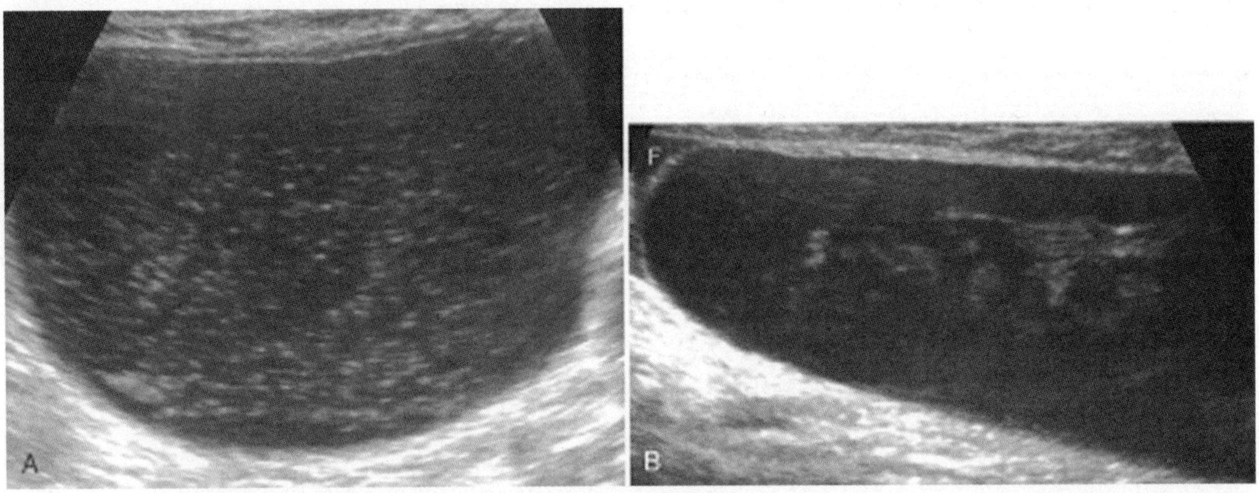

Fig. 42.26 **A,** Sagittal ultrasound image of the urinary bladder. Intraluminal, hyperechoic foci representing crystals (crystalluria) are present in the dependent portion of urinary bladder. **B,** Sagittal ultrasound image of the urinary bladder. Intraluminal, hyperechoic, lacy material is acute hemorrhage located in the mid and ventral aspects of the urinary bladder. A small amount of echogenic fluid representing free abdominal hemorrhage (*F*) is present adjacent to the cranioventral aspect of the urinary bladder.

craniovental and craniodorsal portions of the urinary bladder.[59,60] Follow-up ultrasonographic evaluations should be made after treatment of polypoid cystitis to reevaluate the masses. Biopsy is needed for definitive diagnosis. Muscular hypertrophy resulting from chronic partial lower urinary tract obstruction can also cause urinary bladder wall thickening and may simulate the ultrasonographic appearance of cystitis. Encrusted cystitis is caused by *Corynebacterium urealyticum* infection and is characterized by a thickened urinary bladder wall with mineralized mucosal plaques.[61]

Emphysematous cystitis creates a confusing sonographic appearance because the gas artifacts can alter the normal appearance of the urinary bladder (Fig. 42.29). Linear hyperechogenicities with or without reverberation artifact, trapped in the urinary bladder wall and free in the urinary bladder lumen, can be seen.[16]

Associated Conditions

Urethral obstruction commonly occurs in cats. Echogenic urine sediment, urinary bladder wall thickening, pericystic effusion, hyperechoic pericystic fat, and increased urinary bladder echoes may be present. Upper urinary tract sonographic changes can be seen as well.[62]

A rare condition called uterus masculinus can be associated with chronic cystitis and an enlarged prostate gland in male dogs.[63] The sonographic changes describing this condition include identification of hypoechoic tubular or cylindrical structures originating from the craniodorsal aspect of the prostate gland, adjacent to the urinary bladder.[63]

Mural Hemorrhage

Mural hemorrhage can occur in patients with trauma or a bleeding disorder. This is associated with diffuse thickening of the urinary bladder wall that can resolve quickly after treatment is initiated.[64]

Neoplasia

Several kinds of urinary bladder tumors have been documented, with urothelial carcinoma (also referred to as transitional cell carcinoma) being the most common.[42] Urothelial carcinoma of the urinary bladder is characterized most frequently by an irregularly shaped, broad-based, complex to hypoechoic mass protruding into the urinary bladder lumen.[42] This tumor has similar features between dogs and cats; however, location can differ between species with it typically being located in the midbody in cats compared to trigonal locations in dogs.[65] Single or multiple masses may be present (Fig. 42.30). The echo pattern can vary if internal fibrosis, mineralization, and necrosis have developed. Adjacent blood clots can occur and can

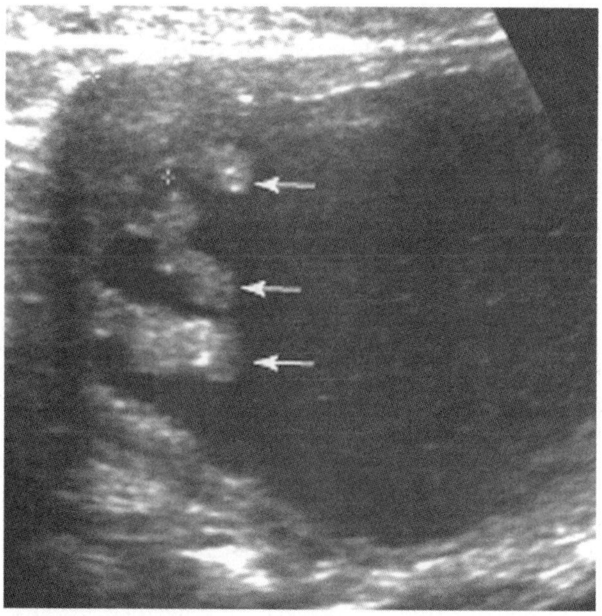

Fig. 42.28 Sagittal ultrasound image of the urinary bladder. There is focal urinary bladder wall thickening (calipers in image) with associated pedunculated, hyperechoic polyps (*white arrows*) secondary to polypoid cystitis. Echogenic intraluminal debris is present within the urine.

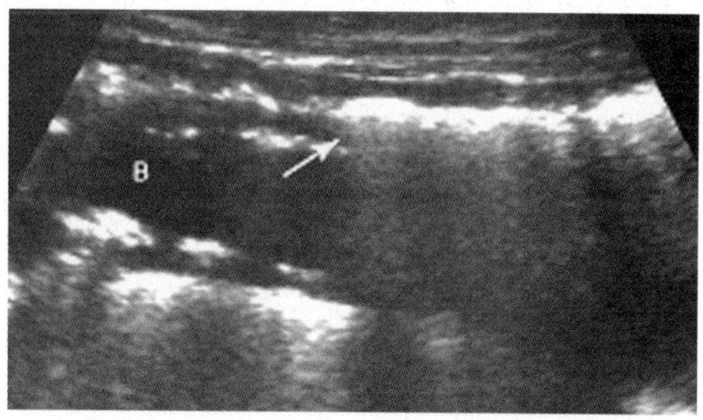

Fig. 42.29 Sagittal ultrasound image of the urinary bladder. Note the linear hyperechogenicities with and without reverberation (*white arrow*) artifact, trapped within the urinary bladder wall secondary to emphysematous cystitis. Anechoic urine is within the urinary bladder (*B*).

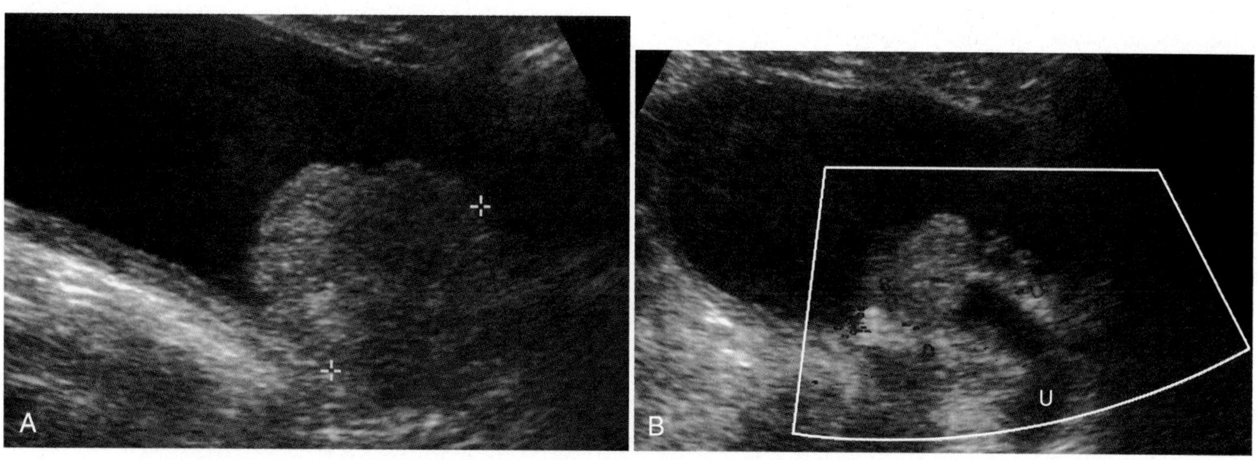

Fig. 42.30 **A,** Sagittal ultrasound image of the urinary bladder. There is a hyperechoic, broad-based mass in the urinary bladder neck from transitional cell carcinoma. **B,** This mass obstructed the adjacent ureter, causing hydroureter (*U*). Note the color Doppler box over the mass and ureter confirming no blood flow within the ureter.

contribute falsely to the size and echogenic texture of the mass. Contrast-enhanced ultrasound has been utilized to characterize transitional cell carcinoma. Features include avid enhancement of tumor tissue with a heterogeneous or homogeneous pattern with a loss of planes between the tumor and the muscular layer.[66] Regional lymph nodes can be assessed for changes in size, echogenicity, and shape which may be suspicious for metastasis. Several sonographic changes associated with canine urothelial carcinoma have been linked to a poorer prognosis; these include evidence of wall involvement by the tumor, trigone location, and heterogeneous echotexture.[42] Volume measurements of transitional cell carcinoma have been used to assess treatment response. Two-dimensional and three-dimensional ultrasound has been compared to computed tomography (CT) in assessing tumor volume in dogs with transitional cell carcinoma.[67] In this study, three-dimensional ultrasound was more accurate in assessing urinary bladder tumor volume than two-dimensional ultrasound when compared to CT.[67] A different study comparing volume measurements between ultrasound and CT utilizing different measuring techniques found that tumor volume measurements varied based on method and modality used.[68]

Smooth muscle neoplasia, such as leiomyoma or leiomyosarcoma, can appear as a single, round, well-defined intraluminal mass.[69] Urinary bladder fibrosarcomas and rhabdomyosarcomas are often located in the neck of the urinary bladder and are typically found in young dogs (eFig. 42.6).[70,71] Lymphoma has a similar sonographic appearance to other urinary bladder tumors but will usually be accompanied by lesions in other abdominal organs and lymph nodes[72] (eFig. 42.7).[71] Smooth isoechoic apex nodules have been described in Scottish terriers and were not associated with neoplasia.[73] Some highly aggressive carcinomas and mesenchymal tumors can spread through the urinary bladder wall. If a small intraluminal mass occurs, the urinary bladder can take on the appearance of severe cystitis. Unfortunately, the sonographic appearance of polypoid cystitis, adherent blood clots, and mural hematomas is similar to that of urinary bladder neoplasia. The observation of ureter dilation adjacent to the urinary bladder wall mass (see Fig. 42.30) and focal medial iliac lymphadenopathy tends to support the diagnosis of neoplasia. An aspirate, biopsy, or both are necessary to confirm the presence of urinary bladder neoplasia. The information gained from percutaneous aspiration of a urinary bladder mass must be weighed against the possibility of seeding the needle tract with tumor cells.[74]

Ureterovesicular Junction

The ureterovesicular junctions are small convex structures on the dorsal part of the urinary bladder.[50,76] However, they may not be identified if the urinary bladder is caudally located. Identifying a ureteral jet in the urinary bladder confirms a normal ureterovesicular junction.[50,76] Orthotopic and ectopic ureteroceles can be identified with ultrasound.[41,43] Ureteroceles are smooth, thin-walled cystic structures within the urinary bladder lumen, urinary bladder wall, or proximal urethra.[75,76] Ureteroceles have been described sonographically as a cyst within a cyst (Fig. 42.31).[77]

Computed Tomography and Magnetic Resonance Imaging of the Urinary Bladder

CT imaging is useful to diagnose abnormalities of the urinary bladder wall and ureterovesicular junction.[78] CT-excretory urography has also been used to definitively diagnose orthotopic ureteroceles in a dog.[79] CT imaging has been used to diagnose urinary bladder torsion noting the classic "whirl sign" often noted as a feature of torsion in other abdominal organs.[80]

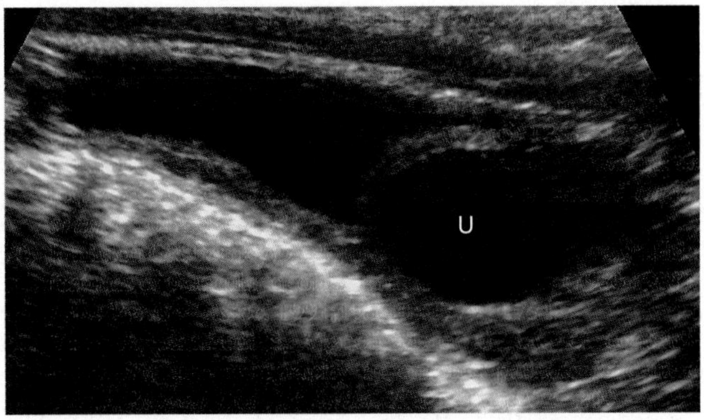

Fig. 42.31 Sagittal ultrasound image of the urinary bladder. Note the "cyst-within-a-cyst" appearance to the ureterocele (*U*) with the urinary bladder neck.

Advanced imaging of urinary bladder neoplasia in dogs and cats is more limited due to cost and decreased availability compared to ultrasound. Both modalities are excellent at evaluation of the primary lesion, ureters, adjacent lymph nodes, and other organs[81] (Fig. 42.32). Urothelial carcinoma of the urinary bladder can be evaluated with CT to determine extent of tumor size for pretreatment staging and to assess tumor response to treatment via volumetric comparison measurements (Fig. 42.33).[68,82]

URETHRA

Anatomy

The male urethra comprises three major areas: the prostatic urethra, membranous urethra, and penile urethra (Fig. 42.34).[83] Combined, the prostatic and membranous portions make up the pelvic part of the urethra.[84] The prostatic urethra is surrounded completely by the prostate gland in the dog, whereas only dorsolaterally in the cat.[85] The membranous urethra is enveloped by cavernous tissue and the urethralis muscle.[85] The penile urethra extends from the ischial arch to the tip of the penis. This part of the urethra is also known as the cavernous urethra because the majority of it is encased by erectile tissues of the penis.[84] The most distal part of the penile urethra is inserted in and protected by the ventral urethral groove of the os penis in the dog. The arrangement of urethral muscle and surrounding spongy tissues confers a diffuse sphincter mechanism to the urethra in male dogs.

The female urethra is shorter and wider than in males and entirely pelvic in location. The external urethral orifice lies caudal to the vestibulovaginal junction, where a muscular urethral sphincter is present.[84]

In the cat, the urinary bladder is typically intra-abdominal in position, and a relatively long prepelvic part of the urethra extends between the neck of the urinary bladder and the pelvic urethra.[85]

RADIOGRAPHY AND URETHROGRAPHY

Radiography of the urethra must include orthogonal caudal abdominal and/or pelvic images to ensure that the urethra is fully included in the field of view. In male dogs, lateral pelvic radiographs with the pelvic limbs both hip-extended (pulled caudally) and hip-flexed (pulled cranially) are also recommended to avoid missing lesions of the penile urethra caused by superimposition of the pelvic limbs. In a normal dog, the

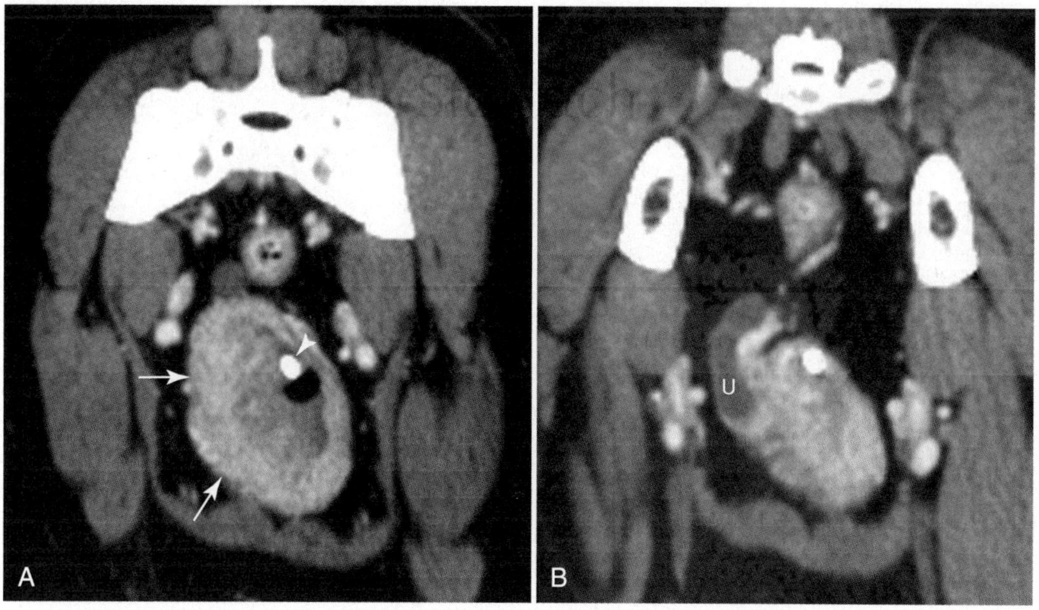

Fig. 42.32 **A,** Computed tomographic post–intravenous contrast of the urinary bladder. Note the irregularly contrast-enhancing thickened urinary bladder wall from infiltrative tumor (*white arrows*). The gas and oval hyperattenuating structure within the urinary bladder lumen is the inflated Foley bulb catheter (*white arrowhead*). **B,** Same study at level of ureterovesicular junction. Note the hydroureter (*U*) secondary to obstruction from the plaque-like mass.

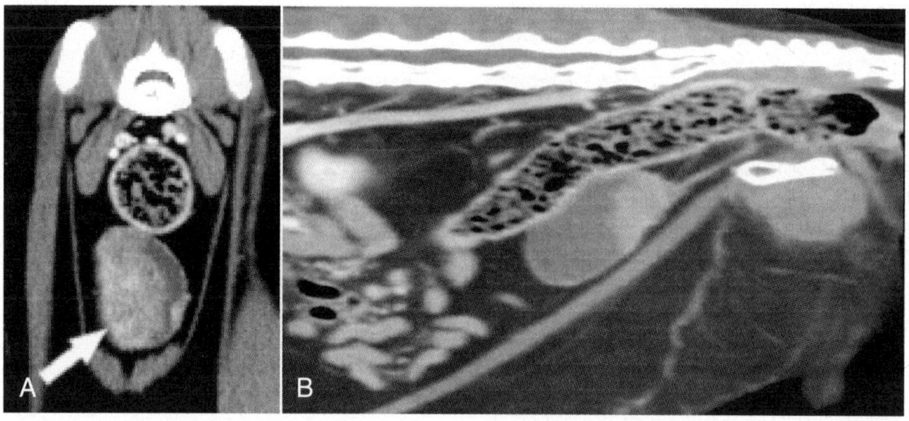

Fig. 42.33 **A,** Computed tomographic post–intravenous contrast of the urinary bladder for pretreatment radiation planning. In this transverse image there is a large contrast-enhancing mass arising from the right aspect of the urinary bladder trigone (*white arrow*). **B,** Reformatted sagittal plane image of the urinary bladder in which the contrast-enhancing mass at the trigone can be seen.

urethra is not visible on radiographs. Because of the more cranial position of the urinary bladder in cats, the prepelvic urethra may be visible if there is adequate surrounding fat to provide contrast.

Retrograde urethrography is a special radiographic technique to examine the urethra using positive-contrast medium. Only water-soluble, iodinated contrast medium should be used. The contrast medium can be diluted with sterile saline to a final concentration of approximately 150 mg iodine [I]/mL.[83,86] Patients generally require sedation, and evacuation of the colon and rectum through defecation or cleansing enemas is recommended to prevent superimposition of feces on the urethra. A fully distended urinary bladder provides counterpressure to contrast medium injection to allow maximal distention of the urethra.[87] Often cystography is performed first, and distention of the bladder with contrast medium should be maintained for urethrography. If necessary, sterile saline can be infused into an inadequately distended bladder. In addition to lateral and ventrodorsal projections, right ventral-left dorsal and left ventral-right dorsal oblique views should be included because the standard ventrodorsal projection may be less informative owing to superimposition of the pelvic and penile urethra.

In male dogs and cats, the procedure is performed by inserting a catheter into the distal penile urethra. A balloon-tipped (Foley) catheter is preferred in dogs, although a red rubber catheter may also be used.[88,86] The bulb of the Foley catheter is carefully inflated to a pressure that will not damage the urethra and left inflated no more than 15 minutes because excessive and prolonged pressure will damage the urethra.[89] In male cats, a red rubber or Tomcat catheter may be used

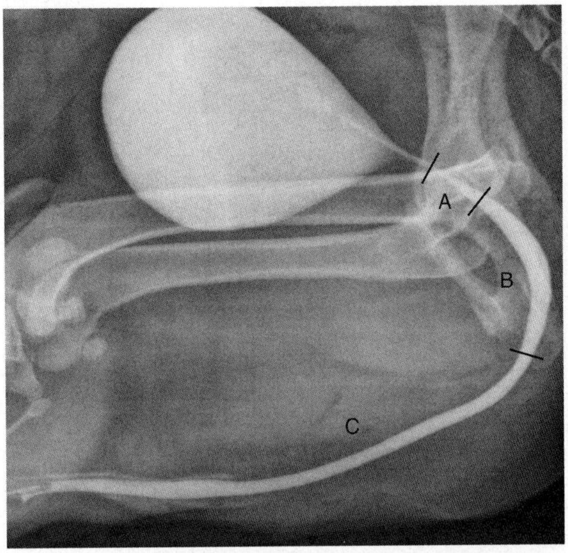

Fig. 42.34 Retrograde urethrography in a normal male dog. A Foley catheter is present in the distal penile urethra, and iodinated contrast medium was injected. The urethra comprises **(A)** the prostatic urethra, **(B)** the membranous urethra, and **(C)** the penile urethra. The normal urethra is smooth and distinctly margined with normal variation in diameter seen in the prostatic and membranous urethra.

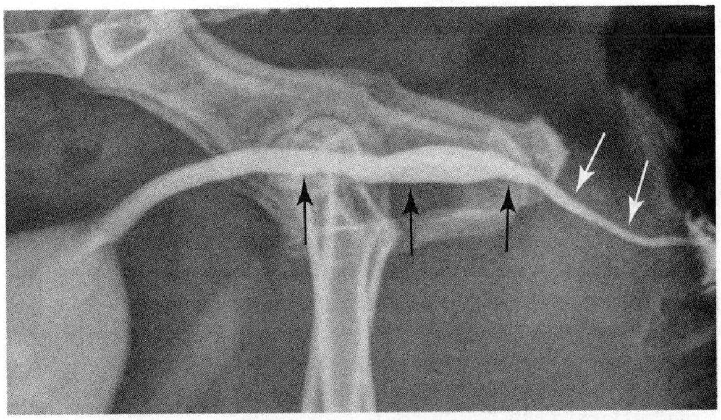

Fig. 42.35 Retrograde urethrography in a normal male cat. A Tomcat catheter is present in the distal penile urethra, and iodinated contrast medium is injected. The pelvic urethra (*black arrows*) is wide and smoothly margined. The penile urethra (*white arrows*) has a smaller diameter and does not distend as much.

(Fig. 42.35). Depending on patient size, 5 to 20 mL of contrast medium is injected and radiographs acquired during the delivery of the final 1 to 2 mL of the injection.[88] The normal urethra should be smoothly margined along its entire length. The prostatic urethra may be wider than the membranous urethra, although each can be variable in diameter depending on the degree of distention.[90] The penile urethra has a generally uniform diameter in dogs; in cats, it is relatively narrow.[91] Luminal narrowing with tapered margins may be seen normally at the ischial arch in dogs.[88]

Retrograde urethrography is challenging in female dogs and female cats because of the relatively shorter urethra. A Foley catheter is inserted into the distal urethra and inflated gently. Five to 10 mL of contrast medium is injected to distend the urethra and radiographs made at the end of injection (Fig. 42.36).[88] Vaginocystourethrography is an alternate

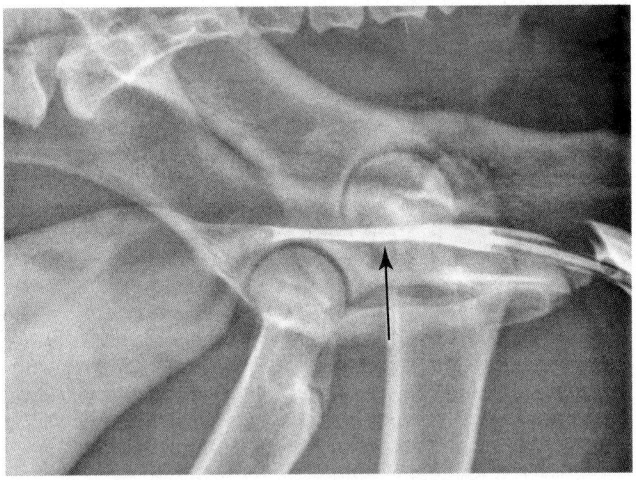

Fig. 42.36 Retrograde urethrography in a normal female dog. A Foley catheter is inserted 1 cm cranial to the external urethral sphincter and iodinated contrast medium is injected. The urethra (*black arrow*) has a smooth and distinct mucosal margin.

technique for evaluation of the female urethra and may be performed in dogs and cats (Fig. 42.37) (Video 42.1). The procedure is described in detail in Chapter 44. The normal urethra should be smoothly margined, and longitudinal striations attributable to mucosal folding may be seen depending on the degree of distention.[88]

The most significant potential complications of urethrography are iatrogenic rupture and urinary tract infection. These and other complications are uncommon when the procedure is performed correctly.[89]

ULTRASONOGRAPHY

Ultrasound examination of the urethra is generally limited to the most cranial portion of the pelvic urethra as interrogated from a ventral abdominal window.[91] Full distention of the urinary bladder promotes a more cranial position within the abdomen to allow examination of a greater length of pelvic urethra. In some patients, limited evaluation of the caudal aspect of the pelvic urethra can be performed using a sagittal perineal window. In males, the penile urethra can be traced along the penis best by using a high-frequency, linear array transducer with or without a standoff pad. Ultrasound is a complement to urethrography with the advantage of not requiring patient sedation.

The normal urethra is a smoothly margined, thin-walled, tubular structure of uniform diameter traced from the neck of the urinary bladder. Total urethral thickness is approximately 3 mm and is slightly greater in male dogs than in females.[92] The layers of the urethra usually cannot be resolved, and the normal lumen is not distended (Fig. 42.38).

Computed Tomography and CT Urethrography

CT can be used to evaluate the urethra and surrounding structures. Unlike ultrasonography, CT imaging can evaluate the portion of the urethra passing through the pelvis. The method for CT urethrography has been established in male and female dogs.[93,94] Qualitative and quantitative assessments of the urethra can be made. Urethral size differences have been noted between empty and distended urinary bladders in both male and female dogs.[93,94] Female dogs can have a normally narrowed urethra due to flexure related to an intrapelvic bladder

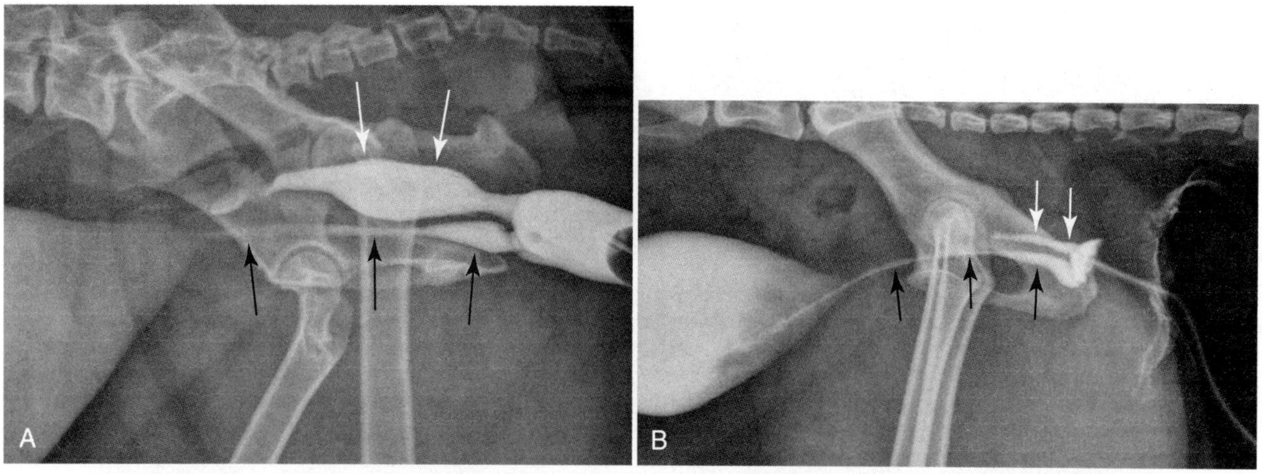

Fig. 42.37 Vaginocystourethrography in **(A)** a normal female dog and **(B)** a normal female cat. An insufflated Foley catheter is in the vestibule. As contrast medium is injected, the more cranial aspect of the vagina (*white arrows*) fills, followed by filling of the urethra (*black arrows*). Smooth, distinct mucosal margins of the urethra are seen.

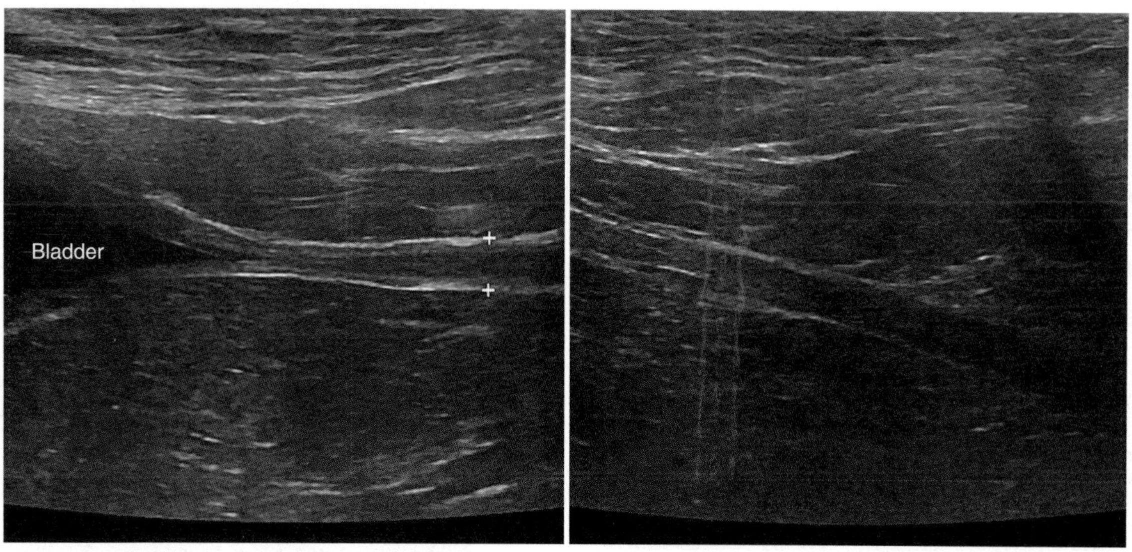

Fig. 42.38 Ultrasound image of the urethra in a normal female dog, sagittal views. The urethra (*white calipers*) is traced from the urinary bladder neck caudally in the image on the left. The more caudal aspect of the urethra is seen in the right image and is a uniform tubular structure. Visualization of the urethra becomes more difficult caudally because of the pubic bone.

location.[94] Advantages of CT urethrography over conventional radiography include lack of superimposition of pelvis and other structures and good visualization of the entire urethra.

DISEASES OF THE URETHRA

Urethral Calculi

Radiopaque urethral calculi may be seen on survey radiographs. In male dogs, calculi commonly occur at regions of luminal narrowing or restriction: the ischial arch and base of the os penis. In male cats with urethral obstruction secondary to sandy mineral calculi, a mineral plug may be seen in the penile urethra (Fig. 42.39). Because the urethra is not visible on survey radiographs, urethrography is required to confirm urethral calculi. Calculi appear as persistent, large focal or multifocal filling defects that distend the lumen of the urethra (Fig. 42.40). They are typically irregularly shaped and indistinctly margined. Air bubbles introduced into the urethra during contrast medium injection can generally be distinguished from calculi by their smoothly rounded shape, which does not distend the urethra, and inconsistent presence with subsequent injections of contrast medium (Fig. 42.41). Blood clots may be similar in appearance to calculi but may also be present inconsistently.[95,96]

On ultrasound, urethral calculi appear as focal or multifocal hyperechoic and intensely distally shadowing foci within the lumen, which may be distended proximal to the obstruction (Video 42.2) The associated urethral wall may be increased in thickness.[43,91]

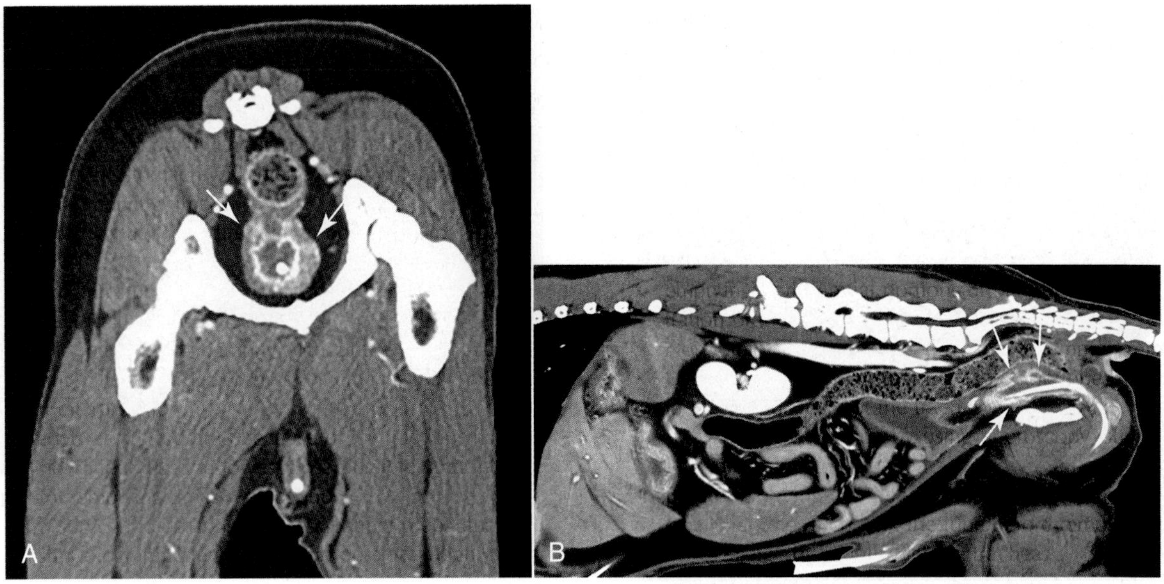

Fig. 42.45 Contrast-enhanced computed tomography images of a male dog with urethral obstruction due to prostatic carcinoma. **A,** Transverse plane image at the prostatic urethra. A hyperattenuating catheter is present in the lumen. Note the thickened urethral wall with heterogenous contrast enhancement (*white arrows*). **B,** Sagittal plane image of the prostatic urethra. Note the thickened urethral wall with heterogeneous contrast enhancement (*white arrows*).

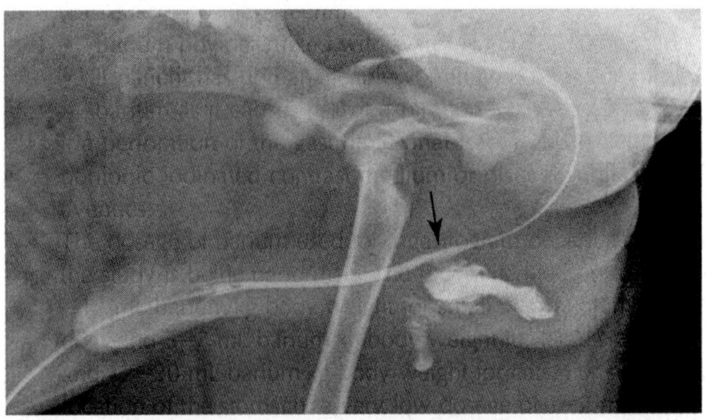

Fig. 42.46 Retrograde urethrogram in a male dog with a history of bite wounds in the region of the penile urethra. A large region of contrast medium extravasation is seen proximal to the os penis (*black arrow*) and extends through a cutaneous wound cranially, consistent with rupture of the penile urethra following puncture.

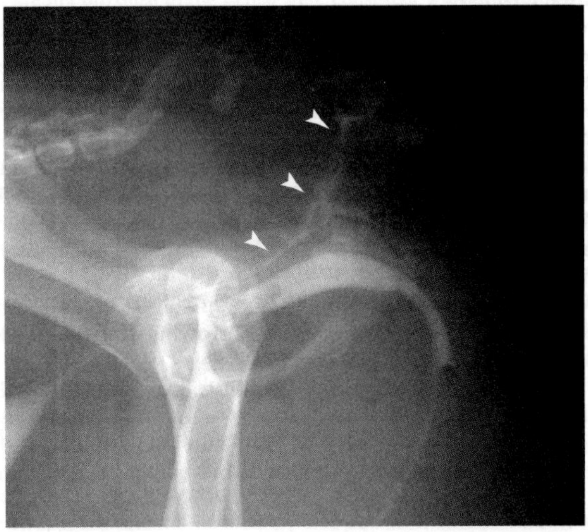

Fig. 42.47 Retrograde urethrogram in a young male English bulldog with a history of chronic urinary tract infections and urine leakage from the anus. Contrast medium extends dorsally from the membranous urethra (*white arrowheads*) to outline fecal material in the rectum. This urethrorectal fistula is likely congenital.

REFERENCES

1. International Committee on Veterinary Gross Anatomical Nomenclature (ICVGAN). *Nomina Anatomica Veterinaria*. ed 7. Hannover, Germany: Editorial Committee; 2017.
2. Hermanson JW, de Lahunta A, Evans HE. *Miller and Evan's Anatomy of the Dog*. 5th ed. Philadelphia: Saunders; 2020.
3. Mahaffey MB, Barsanti JA, Barder DL, Crowell DL. Pelvic bladder in dogs without urinary incontinence. *J Am Vet Med Assoc*. 1984;184(12):1477–1479.
4. Johnston GR, Osborne CA, Jessen CR, Feeney DA. Effects of urinary bladder distention on location of the urinary bladder and urethra of healthy dogs and cats. *Am J Vet Res*. 1986;47(2):404–415.
5. Nickel R, Schummer A, Seiferle E, et al. *The Viscera of the Domestic Mammals, (vol 184)*. 2nd ed. Berlin: Paul Parey/Springer-Verlag; 1973.
6. Neville-Towle J, Sakals S. Urinary bladder herniation through a caudoventral abdominal wall defect in a mature cat. *Can Vet J*. 2015;56(9):934–936.
7. Grand JG, Bureau S, Monnet E. Effects of urinary bladder retorflexion and surgical technique on postoperative complication rates and long-term outcome in dogs with perineal hernia: 41 cases (2002-2009). *J Am Vet Med Assoc*. 2013;243(10):1442–1447.
8. Adams WM, DiBartola SP. Radiographic and clinical features of pelvic bladder in the dog. *J Am Vet Med Assoc*. 1983;182(11):1212–1217.
9. Mahaffey M, Barber D, Basanti J. Simultaneous double-contrast cystography and cystometry in dogs. *Vet Radiol*. 1984;25:254–259.
10. Massat BJ, Gregory CR, Ling GV, Cardinet GH, Lewis EL. Cystourethropexy to correct refractory urinary incontinence due to urethral sphincter mechanism incompetence. Preliminary results in ten bitches. *Vet Surg*. 1993;22(4):260–268.
11. Applegate R, Olie S, Sabatino B. Urethral sphincter mechanism incompetence in dogs: an update. *J Am Anim Hosp Assoc*. 2018;54(1):22–29.
12. Patnaik AK, Greene RW. Intravenous leiomyoma of the bladder in a cat. *J Am Vet Med Assoc*. 1979;175(4):381–383.
13. Hansen JS. Persistent urachal ligament in the cat (report of two cases). *Vet Med Small Anim Clin*. 1972;67(10):1090.

14. Merkel LK, Lulich J, Polzin D, et al. Clinicopathologic and microbiologic findings associated with emphysematous cystitis in 27 dogs. *J Am Anim Hosp Assoc*. 2017;53(6): 313–320.
15. Lippi I, Mannucci T, Della Santa D, et al. Emphysematous cystitis: retrospective evaluation of predisposing factors and ultrasound features in 36 dogs and 2 cats. *Can Vet J*. 2019;60(5):514–518.
16. Petite A, Busoni V, Heinen MP, Billen F, Snaps F. Radiographic and ultrasonographic findings of emphysematous cystitis in four nondiabetic female dogs. *Vet Radiol Ultrasound*. 2006;47(1):90–93.
17. Buffington CA, Chew DJ, Kendall MS, et al. Clinical evaluation of cats with nonobstructive urinary tract diseases. *J Am Vet Med Assoc*. 1997;210(1):46–50.
18. Steyn P, Lowry J. Positional radiographic as an aid to diagnose sand-like uroliths in the urinary bladder of feline urologic syndrome in cats. *Feline Pract*. 1991;19:21–23.
19. Zotti A, Fant P, De Zan G, Mollo A, Busetto R. Chronic cystitis with ossification of the bladder wall in a 6-month-old German shepherd dog. *Can Vet J*. 2007;48(9):935–938.
20. Feeney DA, Johnston GR, Tomlinson MJ, Osborne CA. Effects of sterilized micropulverized barium sulfate suspension and meglumine iothalamate solution on the genitourinary tract of healthy male dogs after retrograde urethrocystography. *Am J Vet Res*. 1984;45(4):730–738.
21. Johnston GR, Stevens JB, Jessen CR, Osborne CA. Complications of retrograde contrast urethrography in dogs and cats. *Am J Vet Res*. 1983;44(7):1248–1256.
22. Barsanti JA, Crowell W, Losonsky J, Talkington FD. Complications of bladder distension during retrograde urethrography. *Am J Vet Res*. 1981;42(5):819–821.
23. Ackerman N, Wingfield WE, Corley EA. Fatal air embolism associated with pneumourethrography and pneumocystography in a dog. *J Am Vet Med Assoc*. 1972;160(12): 1616–1618.
24. Zontine W, Andrews L. Fatal air embolization as a complication of pneumocystography in two cats. *J Am Vet Med Assoc*. 1978;19:8–11.
25. Essman SC. Contrast cystography. *Clin Tech Small Anim Pract*. 2005;20:46–51.
26. Mahaffey M, Barsanti J, Browell W. Cystography: effect of technique on diagnosis of cystitis in dogs. *Vet Radiol*. 1989;30(261).
27. Johnston G, Feeney D. Radiographic evaluation of the urinary tract in dogs and cats: contemporary issues in small animal practice. *Nephrol Urol*. 1989;4:203.
28. Weichselbaum RC, Feeney DA, Jessen CR, Osborne CA, Dreytser V, Holte J. Urocystolith detection: comparison of survey, contrast radiographic and ultrasonographic techniques in an in vitro bladder phantom. *Vet Radiol Ultrasound*. 1999;40(4):386–400.
29. Weichselbaum RC, Feeney DA, Jessen CR, Osborne CA, Dunphy ED, Bartges JW. In vitro evaluation of contrast medium concentration and depth effects on the radiographic appearance of specific canine urolith mineral types. *Vet Radiol Ultrasound*. 1998;39(5):396–411.
30. Weichselbaum RC, Feeney DA, Jessen CR, Osborne CA, Holte J. An integrated epidemiologic and radiographic algorithm for canine urocystolith mineral type prediction. *Vet Radiol Ultrasound*. 2001;42(4):311–319.
31. Johnston GR, Walter PA, Feeney DA. Radiographic and ultrasonographic features of uroliths and other urinary tract filling defects. *Vet Clin North Am Small Anim Pract*. 1986;16(2):261–293.
32. Stiffler KS, McCrackin Stevenson MA, Mahaffey MB, Howerth EW, Barsanti JA. Intravesical ureterocele with concurrent renal dysfunction in a dog: a case report and proposed classification system. *J Am Anim Hosp Assoc*. 2002;38(1):33–39.
33. Colopy SA, Dennison SE, Kerwin-Lucchi LJ, Danielson KC. What is your diagnosis? Ectopic ureterocele. *J Am Vet Med Assoc*. 2011;238(3):293–294.
34. Sutherland-Smith J, Jerram RM, Walker AM, Warman CG. Ectopic ureters and ureteroceles in dogs: presentation, cause, and diagnosis. *Compend Contin Educ Pract Vet*. 2004:303–316.
35. Scrivani PV, Leveille R, Collins RL. The effect of patient positioning on mural filling defects during double contrast cystography. *Vet Radiol Ultrasound*. 1997;38(5): 355–359.
36. Remedios AM, Middleton DM, Myers SL, Outerbridge CA, Arnold PM. Diverticula of the urinary bladder in a juvenile dog. *Can Vet J*. 1994;35(10):648–650.
37. Scheepens ET. L'Eplattenier H: acquired urinary bladder diverticulum in a dog. *J Small Anim Pract*. 2005;46(12): 578–581.
38. Rahal SC, Mamprim MJ, Torelli SR. What is your diagnosis? Patent urachus. *J Am Vet Med Assoc*. 2004;225(7): 1041–1042.
39. Bartges J, Callens A. Congenital diseases of the lower urinary tract. *Vet Clin North Am Small Anim Pract*. 2015;45:703–719.
40. Osuna D, Stone E, Metcalf M. A urethrorectal fistula with concurrent urolithiasis in a dog. *J Am Anim Hosp Assoc*. 1989;25:35–39.
41. Hecht S. Diagnostic imaging of lower urinary tract disease. *Vet Clin North Am Small Anim Pract*. 2015;45(4): 639–663.
42. Hanazono K, Fukumoto S, Endo Y, et al. Ultrasonographic findings related to prognosis in canine transitional cell carcinoma. *Vet Radiol Ultrasound*. 2014;55(1):79–84.
43. Sutherland-Smith J, Penninck D. Bladder and urethra. In: *Atlas of Small Animal Ultrasonography*. 2nd ed. Ames, Iowa: Wiley & Sons Inc.; 2015.
44. Berry C. Differentiating cystic calculi from colon. *Vet Radiol*. 1992;33:283–285.
45. Geisse AL, Lowry JE, Schaeffer DJ, Smith CW. Sonographic evaluation of urinary bladder wall thickness in normal dogs. *Vet Radiol Ultrasound*. 1997;38(2):132–137.
46. Finn-Bodner S, Carter R, Gray B. *Sonographic Architecture and Morphometric Evaluation of the normal Feline Urinary Bladder wall*. Am Coll Vet Radiol; 1992.
47. Douglass J, Kremkan F. Ultrasound corner: the urinary bladder wall hypoechoic pseudolesion. *Vet Radiol Ultrasound*. 1993;34:45–46.
48. Barthez PY, Leveille R, Scrivani PV. Side lobes and grating lobes artifacts in ultrasound imaging. *Vet Radiol Ultrasound*. 1997;38(5):387–393.
49. Sislak M, Spaulding K, Zoran D, et al. Ultrasonographic characteristics of lipiduria in clinically normal cats. *Vet Radiol Ultrasound*. 2014;55(2):195–201.
50. Gremillion C, Cohen EB, Vaden S, Seiler GS. Optimization of ultrasonographic ureteral jet detection and normal ureteral jet morphology in dogs. *Vet Radiol Ultrasound*. 2021;62(5):583–590.
51. Finn-Bodem ST. The urinary bladder. In: Cartee RE, ed. *P.V. Practical Veterinary Ultrasound*. Philadelphia: Lea & Febiger; 1995:219.
52. Weichselbaum RC, Feeney DA, Jessen DA, Osborne CA, Dreytser V, Holte J. Relevance of sonographic artifacts observed during in vitro characterization of urocystolith mineral composition. *Vet Radiol Ultrasound*. 2000;41(5):438–446.
53. Louvet A. Twinkling artifact in small animal color-Doppler sonography. *Vet Radiol Ultrasound*. 2006;47(4):384–390.
54. Choi M, Kim Y. Ultrasonographic and contrast-enhanced CT imaging diagnosis of idiopathic renal hematuria with bilateral hydronephrosis and hydroureter in a dog. *Vet Radiol Ultrasound*. 2022;63(6):E21–E25.

55. Cherbinsky O, Westropp J, Tinga S, Jones B, Pollard R. Ultrasonographic features of grass awns in the urinary bladder. *Vet Radiol Ultrasound*. 2010;51(4):462–465.
56. Cote E, Carroll MC, Beck KA, Good L, Gannon K. Diagnosis of urinary bladder rupture using ultrasound contrast cystography: in vitro model and two case-history reports. *Vet Radiol Ultrasound*. 2002;43(3):281–286.
57. Finn-Bodner S, Hudson J, Brewer WG. Transabdominal sonographic evaluation of experimentally induced cystitis of the feline urinary bladder. In: *Scientific Proceedings of the ACVR*. 1993.
58. Carneiro RK, Pereira T, Brun MV, et al. Excretory urographic, ultrasonographic, and cystoscopic characteristics of urinary bladder abscesses in a dog. *Vet Radiol and Ultrasound*. 2022. https://doi.org/10.1111/vru.13095:1-4.
59. Takiguchi M, Inaba M. Diagnostic ultrasound of polypoid cystitis in dogs. *J Vet Med Sci*. 2005;67(1):57–61.
60. Martinez I, Matton JS, Easton KA, Chew DJ, DiBartola SP. Polypoid cystitis in 17 dogs (1978–2001). *J Vet Intern Med*. 2003;17(4):499–509.
61. Maurey C, Boulous HJ, Cannone-Guibert M, Benchekroun G. Clinical description of Corynebacterium urealyticum urinary tract infections in 11 dogs and 10 cats. *J Small Anim Pract*. 2019;60(4):239–246.
62. Nevins J, Mai W, Thomas E. Associations between ultrasound and clinical findings in 87 cats with urethral obstruction. *Vet Radiol Ultrasound*. 2015;56(4):439–447.
63. Lim C, Heng H, Hui T, et al. Ultrasonographic features of uterus masculinus in six dogs. *Vet Radiol Ultrasound*. 2015;56(1):77–83.
64. O'Brien RT, Wood EF. Urinary bladder mural hemorrhage associated with systemic bleeding disorders in three dogs. *Vet Radiol Ultrasound*. 1998;39(4):354–356.
65. Hamlin AN, Chadwick LE, Fox-Alvarez SA, et al. Ultrasound characteristics of feline urinary bladder transitional cell carcinoma are similar to canine urinary bladder transitional cell carcinoma. *Vet Radiol Ultrasound*. 2019;60: 552–559.
66. Macri F, Di Pietro S, Mangano C, et al. Quantitative evaluation of canine urinary bladder transitional cell carcinoma using contrast-enhanced ultrasonography. *BMC Vet Res*. 2018;14(84).
67. Naughton J, Widner W, Constable P, et al. Accuracy of three-dimensional and two-dimensional ultrasonography for measurement of tumor volume in dogs with transitional cell carcinoma of the urinary bladder. *Am J Vet Res*. 2012;73(12):1919–1924.
68. Leffler AJ, Hostnik ET, Warry EE, et al. Canine urinary bladder transitional cell carcinoma tumor volume is dependent on imaging modality and measurement technique. *Vet Radiol Ultrasound*. 2018;59:767–776.
69. Heng JG, Lowry JE, Boston S, Gabel C, Ehrhart N, Gulden SM. Smooth muscle neoplasia of the urinary bladder wall in three dogs. *Vet Radiol Ultrasound*. 2006;47(1):83–86.
70. Takiguchi M, Watanabe T, Okada H, Kudo T, Yamada K, Yasuda J, Hashimoto A. Rhabdomyosarcoma (botryoid sarcoma) of the urinary bladder in a Maltese. *J Small Anim Pract*. 2002;43(6):269–271.
71. Olausson A, Stieger SM, Loefgren S, Gillingstam M. A urinary bladder fibrosarcoma in a young dog. *Vet Radiol Ultrasound*. 2005;46(2):135–138.
72. Benigni L, Lamb CR, Corzo-Menendez N, Holloway A, Eastwood JM. Lymphoma affecting the urinary bladder in three dogs and a cat. *Vet Radiol Ultrasound*. 2006;47(6): 592–596.
73. Heng JG, Ramos-Vara JA, Fulkerson CM, et al. Ultrasonographic detection of apex nodules in the urinary bladder of Scottish Terriers. *Vet Radiol Ultrasound*. 2022;63: 234–239.
74. Nyland TG, Wallack ST, Wisner ER. Needle-tract implantation following US-guided fine-needle aspiration biopsy of transitional cell carcinoma of the bladder, urethra, and prostate. *Vet Radiol Ultrasound*. 2002;43(1):50–53.
75. Lamb CR, Gregory SP. Ultrasonographic findings in 14 dogs with ectopic ureter. *Vet Radiol Ultrasound*. 1998; 39(3):218–223.
76. Lamb CR. Ultrasonography of the ureters. *Vet Clin North Am Small Anim Pract*. 1998;28(4):823–848.
77. Takiguchi M, Yasuda J, Ochiai K, Morita Y, Hashimoto A. Ultrasonographic appearance of orthotopic ureterocele in a dog. *Vet Radiol Ultrasound*. 1997;38(5):398–399.
78. Rozear L, Tidwell A. Evaluation of the ureter and ureterovesicular junction using helical computed tomographic excretory urography in healthy dogs. *Vet Radiol Ultrasound*. 2003;44(2):155–164.
79. Secrest S, Britt L, Cook C. Imaging diagnosis—bilateral orthotopic ureteroceles in a dog. *Vet Radiol Ultrasound*. 2011;52(4):448–450.
80. Ricciardi M, Campanella A, Martino R. Computed tomographic features of urinary bladder torsion in two dogs. *J Sm Anim Pract*. 2018;59:188–195.
81. MacLeod A, Wisner E. Computed tomography and magnetic resonance imaging of the urinary tract. In: Bartges J, Polzin D, eds. *Nephrology and Urology of Small Animals*. Ames, IA: Blackwell Publishing; 2011.
82. Murphy S, Gutierrez A, Lawrence J, Bjorlin D, Mackie T, Forrest L. Laparoscopically implanted tissue expander radiotherapy in canine transitional cell carcinoma. *Vet Radiol Ultrasound*. 2008;49(4):400–405.
83. Park RD. Radiology of the urinary bladder and urethra. In: O'Brien TR, ed. *Radiographic Diagnosis of Abdominal Disorders in the Dog and Cat: Radiographic Interpretation, Clinical Signs, Pathophysiology*. Philadelphia: Saunders; 1978:605–609.
84. Evans HE, Chistensen GE. The urogenital system. In: Evans HE, Miller ME, eds. *Miller's Anatomy of the Dog*. 3rd ed. Philadelphia: Saunders; 1993:529–546.
85. Dyce KM, Sack WO, Wensing CJG. The pelvis and reproductive organs of the carnivores. In: *Textbook of Veterinary Anatomy*. 2nd ed. Philadelphia: Saunders; 1996: 438–446.
86. Johnston GR, Feeney DA, Osborne CA. Urethrography and cystography in cats. 1. Techniques, normal radiographic anatomy, and artifacts. *Compend Contin Educ Pract Vet*. 1982;4:823.
87. Johnston GR, Jessen CR, Osborne CA. Effects of bladder distension on canine and feline retrograde urethrography. *Vet Radiol Ultrasound*. 1983;24:271.
88. Ticer JW, Spencer CP, Ackerman N. Positive contrast retrograde urethrography—a useful procedure for evaluating urethral disorders in the dog. *Vet Radiol Ultrasound*. 1980;21(2).
89. Johnston GR, Stevens JB, Jessen CR, et al. Complications of retrograde contrast urethrography in dogs and cats. *Am J Vet Res*. 1983;44:1248.
90. Feeney DA, Johnston GR, Osborne CA, et al. Dimensions of the prostatic and membranous urethra in normal-male dogs during maximum distension retrograde urethrocystography. *Vet Radiol Ultrasound*. 1984;25:249.
91. Nyland TG, Mattoon JS, Herrgesell EJ, et al. Urinary tract. In: Nyland TG, Mattoon JS, eds. *Small Animal Diagnostic Ultrasound*. 2nd ed. Philadelphia: Saunders; 2002:181–191.
92. Kim G, Ji Y, Choo D, et al. Evaluation of urethral thickness using ultrasonography in healthy small-breed dogs. *Front Vet Sci*. 2022:1051898. https://doi.org/10.3389/fvets.2022.

93. Kang K, Kim K, Oh D, et al. Retrograde CT urethrography using a power injector quantitatively reveals effects of bladder distension on urethral size in healthy male Beagle dogs. *Vet Radiol Ultrasound*. 2020;61:302–311.
94. Kang K, Kim K, So J, et al. The urethra of healthy female dogs can be normally narrowed due to the urethral flexure in retrograde CT urethrography. *Vet Radiol Ultrasound*. 2021;62:61–67.
95. Pugh CR, Rhodes WH, Biery DN. Contrast studies of the urogenital system. *Vet Clin North Am Small Anim Pract*. 1993;23:281.
96. Johnston GR, Feeney DA. Comparative organ imaging—lower urinary-tract. *Vet Radiol Ultrasound*. 1984;25:146.
97. Piola V, Posch B, Aghte P, et al. Radiographic characterization of the os penis in the cat. *Vet Radiol Ultrasound*. 2011;52:270.
98. Hanson JA, Tidwell AS. Ultrasonographic appearance of urethral transitional cell carcinoma in ten dogs. *Vet Radiol Ultrasound*. 1996;37:293.
99. Moroff SD, Brown BA, Matthiesen DT, et al. Infiltrative urethral disease in female dogs—41 cases (1980–1987). *J Am Vet Med Assoc*. 1991;199:247.
100. Grant DC, Troy CG. Recurrent urethral fibroepithelial polyps in a golden retriever. *J Am Anim Hosp Assoc*. 2014;50:361–365.
101. Ticer JW, Spencer CP, Ackerman N. Transitional cell-carcinoma of the urethra in 4 female dogs—its urethrographic appearance. *Vet Radiol Ultrasound*. 1980;21(12).
102. Chandler JC, MacPhail CM. Congenital urethrorectal fistulas. *Compend Contin Educ Pract Vet*. 2001;23:995.

ELECTRONIC RESOURCES

Additional information related to the content in Chapter 42 can be found online at eBooks.Health.Elsevier.com

- Chapter Quiz
- Videos

CHAPTER 43

Prostate Gland

Jimmy C. Lattimer • Melanie Anderson

NORMAL ANATOMY AND RADIOGRAPHIC APPEARANCE

The normal prostate gland (hereafter referred to as prostate) surrounds the most proximal aspect of the male canine urethra and lies ventral to the rectum and caudal to the urinary bladder, typically within the pelvic canal. The absolute normal size of the prostate is variable in the dog and is dependent on the age, size, and neuter status.[1] In many neutered dogs, the normal prostate is small (<2 cm) and not radiographically visible (Fig. 43.1A). When visible, the prostate is recognized radiographically by its round shape, soft tissue opacity, and its relation to adjacent organs. Delineation of an enlarged prostate from the urinary bladder is evident from a triangular fat opacity ventral to and between them (see Fig. 43.1B). The normal prostate in an intact dog should not be more than 70% of the height of the pelvic inlet on lateral views, measured as the distance between the ventral aspect of S1 and the cranial border of the dorsal pubis.[2] If seen on the ventrodorsal (VD) view, the normal prostate should not be more than 80% of the width of the pelvic canal. A full rectum may obscure the prostate on the VD view. If the shape or position of the prostate is altered, the gland may not be recognizable other than as an indistinct opacity between the bladder, rectum, and pelvis.

The normal prostate gland is not visible in the cat because of its location on the dorsal lateral surfaces of the mid pelvic urethra and small size. The normal feline prostate measures up to 10 mm in diameter.[3] Prostatic diseases causing clinical signs in cats are very rare and will not be considered further in this chapter.

DISEASES OF THE PROSTATE GLAND

Intrinsic disease of the prostate usually results in enlargement. Enlargement may also occur in response to extraprostatic influences, such as an androgen-producing testicular tumor and orchitis.[1] Because of the close functional association of the prostate and testes, any animal with prostatic disease should also be examined, preferably ultrasonographically, for testicular disease.

The most common prostatic disorder is benign prostatic hyperplasia (BPH), in which the prostate enlarges as a result of increased cell number as well as enlargement of the intercellular

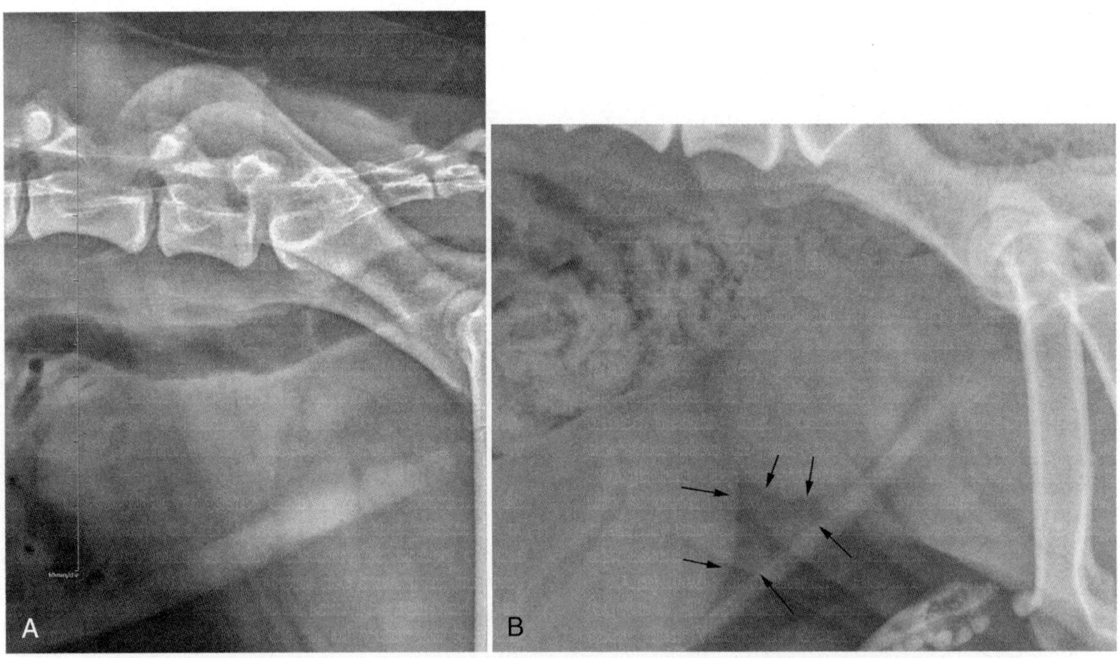

Fig. 43.1 **A,** Normal prostate in a dog neutered at a young age. The prostate is virtually indistinguishable from the urethra and the fat triangle is lost. **B,** Abdominal radiograph of a dog with benign prostatic hyperplasia. Note the cranial displacement of the urinary bladder and the triangular region of fat between the caudoventral aspect of the urinary bladder, the cranioventral aspect of the prostate gland, and the ventral abdominal wall (*black arrows*). This sign is a reliable indicator of prostate gland enlargement. There are also multiple calculi in the penile urethra.

and ductal spaces. BPH can occur in dogs are young as 2 to 3 years and affects more than 95% of intact dogs over 9 years of age.[4] This condition is considered normal in most intact dogs and may include both hyperplastic and hypertrophic processes.[1] Progressive enlargement often leads to development of dilated cystic spaces. Solid and cystic enlargements are therefore different stages of the same disease, with the latter being the advanced form.[4,5] The size of the cystic spaces varies from microscopic to large; these spaces may become so large that they distort the shape of the entire gland. Large cystic spaces predispose the gland to infection.[5]

Prostatitis is the second most common cause of prostatic enlargement and is usually bacterial in origin. The most common organisms isolated include *Escherichia coli*, *Staphylococcus* spp, *Streptococcus* spp, *Pseudomonas*, *Brucella canis*, *Proteus*, and *Mycoplasma*, among others. Usually, a mixed bacterial population is present.[6] The infection may arise within the prostate, or it may extend from other sources such as the urinary bladder or testicles. A normal prostate gland is more resistant to infection than is an enlarged or inflamed gland. Because many antibiotics do not penetrate the prostate readily, the gland may also be a reservoir for reinfection or extension to other organs.[4] There is improved penetration of antibiotics into an inflamed prostate due to disruption of the blood-prostate barrier.[6] Prostatic inflammation may vary from a mild transient process that causes minimal or no clinical signs to a fulminating hemorrhagic or emphysematous process that destroys the entire gland rapidly, resulting in severe systemic signs.[7–9] The latter may result in rupture of the capsule with secondary peritonitis and sepsis.

Chronic, recurrent prostatitis may result in a scarred, fibrotic gland that is typically normal in size or small. Chronic scarring may result in stricture of the urethra.[1,4] Such a stricture is difficult to recognize radiographically unless a urethrogram is performed.

Prostatic abscesses may form as a sequela of prostatitis or primary cystic disease. Large abscesses distort the shape of the prostate gland and may also rupture, causing peritonitis and sepsis.[10,11]

As previously stated, cysts form in advanced BPH and are usually contained within the gland. Squamous metaplasia can cause obstruction of the prostatic ducts, leading to retention cysts. Cysts protruding from the surface of the prostate or separate from the prostate are also referred to as *paraprostatic cysts* because they are no longer confined within the gland. They have been associated with cystic enlargement of the Müllerian ducts or remnants of the uterus masculinus.[12–14] Enlargement of the Müllerian ducts results in a bilateral tubular mass that resembles uterine enlargement.[15,16] These cysts may be sterile but often become infected, which may be the inciting cause for presentation to a veterinarian.[17,18] Cysts occasionally result from neoplasia, but this is rare. Formation of functional neoplastic secretory cells without an accompanying ductal system results in a cystic structure lined with neoplastic epithelium.

Prostatic tumors are rare in dogs and very rare in cats. The majority of prostatic tumors are carcinomas (adenocarcinoma, urothelial carcinomas, squamous cell carcinomas, undifferentiated carcinomas). Very rarely, mesenchymal cell tumors are identified.[19,20] Lymphoma may arise within the prostate but is more often involved secondarily and may serve as a sanctuary site for disease during treatment.[21] The incidence of all prostatic tumors is very low (0.35%).[22] Neutered male dogs have an odds ratio of approximately 2.84 in comparison to intact males.[23] Prostatic carcinoma is often advanced at presentation with metastasis to regional lymph nodes, the pelvis, lumbosacral spine, and distant sites such as the liver and lungs.[22–25] Patients may present with urinary signs as the tumor can invade or compress the urethra. Small in situ prostatic carcinomas are unusual but do occur; they are usually discovered as a result of metastasis rather than from their local effects. Large prostatic neoplasms are often infected or necrotic, and affected dogs may therefore have clinical signs of prostatitis. These tumors are often slow to be diagnosed, unless signs of metastasis are present, because of the tendency of clinical sign of cystitis or prostatitis to overshadow those of neoplasia.

Clinical Signs

The clinical signs of prostatic disease are usually localized to urinary or gastrointestinal signs. Stranguria, hematuria, and pyuria are seen commonly in cases of prostatitis and neoplasia.[1,4,5,24] In cases of marked prostatomegaly, patients may present with dyschezia and small or ribbon-like stools as the enlarged prostate gland displaces the colon and/or rectum dorsally, compressing the rectum (Fig. 43.2). Patients are often systemically ill in cases of acute prostatitis and may present with anorexia, fever, vomiting, abdominal pain, and preputial discharge, whereas patients with chronic prostatitis are often asymptomatic or display mild clinical signs. Most commonly, patients with chronic prostatitis will have a history of recurrent urinary tract infections and bloody urethral discharge. The prostate is typically normal in size and nonpainful on rectal palpation.[1,5]

A less common sign of prostatic disease is a pelvic limb gait abnormality manifesting as pelvic limb weakness and lumbar pain or myelopathy due to spinal metastasis or direct tumor extension into the vertebral canal. The animal may refuse to climb stairs and jump or may have a stiff gait. Owners often believe the animal has developed osteoarthritis, but such animals may have severe, active septic prostatitis or metastatic disease. The pain caused by the prostatic infection is exacerbated by walking, climbing, and jumping. Both pelvic limbs are usually affected. These animals are also usually sensitive to palpation of the caudal abdomen. Gait abnormalities are seen rarely in uncomplicated BPH.[22–25]

Radiographic Changes

Most common prostatic diseases cause enlargement. The enlargement may be symmetric (diffuse) or asymmetric (focal). Prostatic symmetry is usually judged by the shape of the prostate and the relative mass of the prostate gland with respect to the neck of the bladder and the pelvic inlet. Hyperplasia and

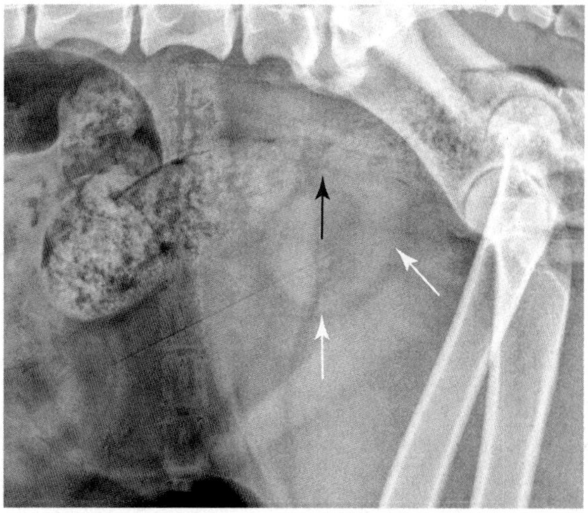

Fig. 43.2 Prostate gland enlargement in an intact dog with benign prostatic hyperplasia. The prostate gland (*white arrows*) is enlarged, and the urinary bladder is displaced cranially. The enlarged prostate is displacing the colon dorsally resulting in focal colonic narrowing (*black arrow*). The enlargement of the prostate gland is relatively symmetric in relation to the neck of the bladder.

prostatitis are examples that usually cause symmetric enlargement, whereas neoplasia and large cysts are examples that usually cause asymmetric enlargement.

Identification of prostatomegaly depends on identification of a soft tissue mass in the caudal aspect of the abdomen and on the relation of that mass to surrounding structures, principally the bladder, colon, and body wall. Prostatomegaly typically displaces the urinary bladder cranially. If prostatomegaly is uniform, bladder displacement is cranial along the floor of the abdomen. If prostatomegaly is eccentric, as often occurs with large cysts and abscesses and occasionally with tumors, the direction of bladder displacement may be variable. A cyst or abscess occasionally may extend dorsal to the bladder (Fig. 43.3). Alternatively, with ventral prostatomegaly, the bladder neck may be elevated.[1,5] Severe and irregular enlargement may also result in obliteration of the normal triangle of fat formed by junction of the caudal ventral bladder and the prostate gland.[26]

The other major radiographic sign of prostatomegaly is dorsal displacement of the colon (see Fig. 43.2). Prostatic enlargement, particularly if intrapelvic, may also cause narrowing of the lumen of the rectum and possible impaction of feces cranial to the site of rectal narrowing. This compression may be visible radiographically, or the colon may simply become confluent with the prostate mass at the pelvic inlet.

Very large prostatic lesions usually lie on the floor of the abdomen, so some dorsal displacement of the caudal abdominal contents can occur. Prostatic and paraprostatic cysts may become so large that they reach almost to the costal arch. Masses of this magnitude cause organ displacement so severe that the actual source of the mass may be difficult to determine without using special radiographic procedures, sonography, or advanced imaging such as computed tomography (CT). Prostatic disease that results in urethral stricture or urethral invasion, as in the case of neoplasia, may result in severe urinary bladder distention from obstruction, which is then secondarily responsible for the displacement of the abdominal structures cranial and dorsal to it.

A prostate that exceeds 90% of the distance from the pubis to the sacral promontory in an intact dog is considered pathologic.[2] Any enlargement (>2 cm) in a dog neutered more than a few months prior to imaging should be considered abnormal.[1,2] However, when a dog is neutered for treatment of prostatic disease, enlargement can persist for several months.[27] The actual degree of prostatic enlargement varies widely, however. For example, prostatic size may vary from slight enlargement to 10 times normal size for BPH, and the gland may actually decrease in size in chronic prostatitis due to fibrosis.[1,5] Acute prostatitis and neoplasia alone do not usually cause severe enlargement, as seen with BPH. However, a combination of pathologies may be present resulting in enlargement. Prostatic pathology may be discovered incidentally during abdominal imaging with ultrasound, CT, or magnetic resonance imaging (MRI), or on postmortem examination.

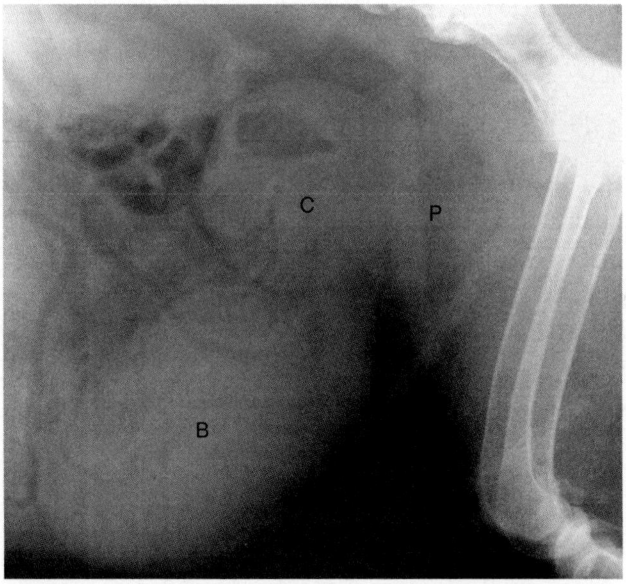

Fig. 43.3 A large, dorsally located paraprostatic cyst (*C*) arising from a prostate gland with benign prostatic hyperplasia. The cyst is seen dorsal and cranial to the enlarged prostate (*P*) and dorsal to the urinary bladder (*B*).

Paraprostatic cysts and abscesses usually have well-defined, sometimes mineralized margins that are easily seen (see Fig. 43.3, eFigs. 43.1 and 43.2).[14] Abscesses are typically poorly marginated and are often surrounded by edema or fluid, resulting poor delineation of the prostate, reduced periprostatic serosal detail, and a heterogeneous appearance of the caudal abdominal fat. A cyst or abscess may occasionally extend caudally into the pelvic canal; such lesions may not be readily visible on survey radiographs and may not produce the usual displacement of the bladder.[18] These lesions do, however, often produce marked displacement and compression of the rectum and are therefore recognized as an intrapelvic mass and on occasion can even be within the contents of a perineal hernia. Definitely distinguishing a cyst from an abscess on the basis of radiographic examination alone is impossible; however, if the margins are smooth, the structure is uniform in soft tissue opacity, and there is no evidence of regional inflammation (fluid/edema), a cyst is more likely.

Evaluation of prostatic margination is important. In the presence of emaciation, pelvic trauma, or abdominal effusion, the prostatic margins may be inconspicuous. If the prostate gland has smooth margins that are easily seen, the disease involving the gland is likely to be benign or is slowly progressing, such as BPH or low-grade or chronic prostatitis. An irregular or indistinct margin in the presence of adequate abdominal fat is more likely to be caused by an acute or aggressive process such as neoplasia or acute prostatitis.[8,9,11] Most patients with aggressive prostatic disease have some evidence of secondary inflammation affecting the surrounding tissues (Fig. 43.4, eFig. 43.3).

A change in the opacity of the prostate from its normal soft tissue opacity indicates severe or chronic disease. Areas of calcification within the gland are a sign either of longstanding prostatitis or of neoplasia. Wispy or indistinct calcification within the prostatic parenchyma has a strong positive predictive value (100%) for carcinoma in neutered dogs, whereas intact dogs are unlikely to have prostatic neoplasia if no mineralization is present (Fig. 43.5, eFig. 43.4).[28] Therefore, although unusual, indistinct calcification in the prostate gland is a serious finding that warrants biopsy. Prostate gland calcification may be more easily seen with ultrasonography or CT because of improved soft tissue contrast resolution and elimination of superimposed structures in comparison to standard radiography.

The prostate does not normally communicate with any air-containing organ, so it should not contain gas. Intraprostatic gas is evidence of gas-forming bacterial prostatitis. This is extremely rare.[9] Severe prostatitis results in hemorrhagic necrosis of the gland, potentially causing a generalized peritonitis and septic shock. Because of the rapidly fatal course of these infections, identification of noniatrogenic gas within the prostate carries an unfavorable prognosis. Rarely, the prostate may contain air because of reflux from the bladder during a negative- or double-contrast cystogram. Simple filling of the ducts with air does not necessarily indicate prostatic disease, but the

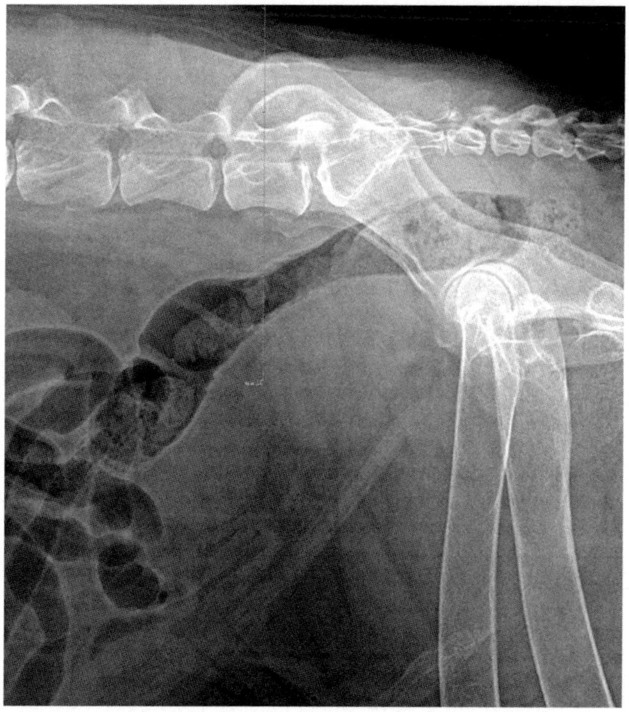

Fig. 43.4 An enlarged prostate due to bacterial prostatitis. The markedly enlarged prostate is displacing the bladder cranially and impinging on the colon causing it to narrow slightly as it passes through the pelvic inlet. Note the wispy fluid opacity along the cranioventral aspect of the prostate in the caudoventral abdomen, consistent with effusion and/or edema, commonly seen with inflammation.

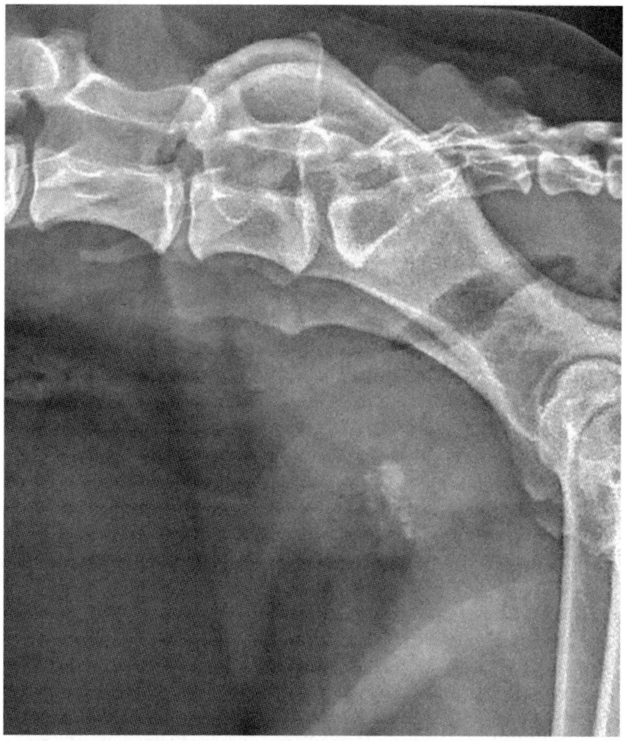

Fig. 43.5 Dense and wispy calcification in the enlarged prostate of a neutered dog. Diagnostic catheterization confirmed the radiographic diagnosis of prostatic carcinoma.

finding of air in pockets within the prostate gland following contrast administration is abnormal and most often associated with cyst formation.

Periosteal proliferation is sometimes seen on the ventral aspect of the caudal lumbar and/or sacral vertebrae (Fig. 43.6, eFig. 43.5) and pelvis because of regional metastasis from prostatic neoplasia. While this is the most common location, osseous metastasis is not limited to these regions and may also be found in the extremities and ribs.[22,24,26]

Special Radiographic Procedures for Evaluating the Prostate Gland

Although ultrasonography has enhanced the imaging of the prostatic parenchyma, retrograde urethrography is still a useful imaging procedure that should be considered in patients with suspected prostatic disease if ultrasound or other advanced imaging modalities are not available.[29]

The only special radiographic procedure that has been found to be uniformly useful in the evaluation of the prostate is the positive-contrast urethrogram. This procedure allows evaluation of the urethra itself and the position of the urethra in relation to suspected prostatic disease. Asymmetric positioning of the urethra within the prostate indicates an asymmetric disease process within the prostate such as a tumor or abscess, with abscesses being more common (Fig. 43.7). Invasion or stricture of the urethra in association with a prostatic mass, indicated by disruption of the smooth urethral margin, is a poor prognostic finding because of the danger that a urinary

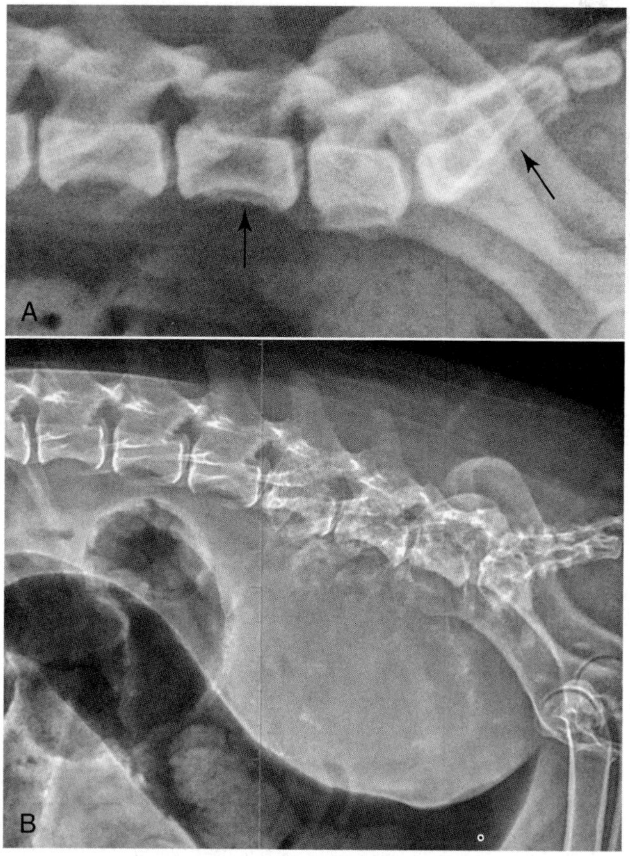

Fig. 43.6 **A**, Lateral lumbar radiographs of two dogs with metastatic prostate adenocarcinoma (early **A** and advanced **B**) to the lumbar vertebrae and the sacrum (*black arrows* in **A**). The prostate gland was not abnormal radiographically because of the small size of the tumor in both cases. A mass effect is present ventral to the lumbar spine in **B** due to the presence of metastatic lymphadenopathy.

obstruction could occur. It is also a sign that aggressive disease is present.[29,30] Evidence of either asymmetric prostatic enlargement or urethral abnormalities is an indication for prostatic cytology, which is best acquired by diagnostic urethral catheterization.

Urethrography can be performed easily in the male dog, and several methods may be used. Urethrography provides indirect evidence of prostatic disease. If the urethra is deviated around a large mass or does not pass directly through the center of the prostate gland, the disease within the prostate is asymmetric, such as a cyst, abscess, or tumor. If the urethra passes directly through the middle of an enlarged prostate, the disease is more likely to be diffuse, such as hyperplasia or prostatitis (see Fig. 43.7A).

In addition, a urethrocystogram identifies the true location of the urinary bladder. In some instances, abdominal masses, such as an omental tumor, a paraprostatic cyst, or an enlarged retained testicle, lie next to the bladder and the mass can be misinterpreted as the urinary bladder. Knowing the identity of each mass is important, and urethrocystography is useful for this, especially if ultrasound is not available.

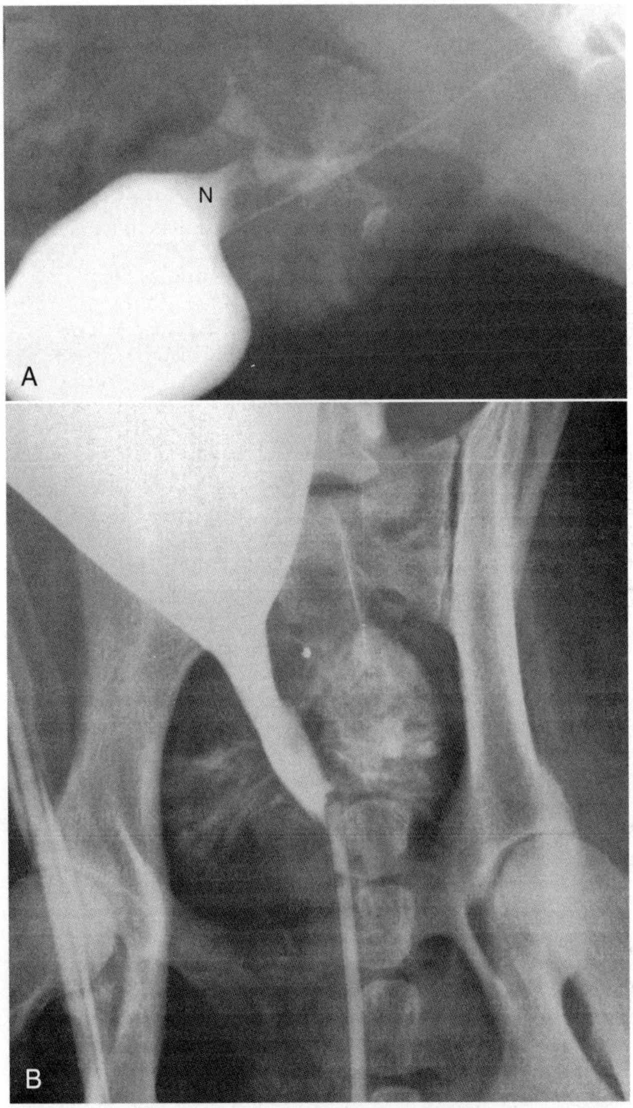

Fig. 43.7 **A,** Marked prostatic enlargement with dorsal elevation of the neck of the bladder (*N*). Note the reflux of contrast medium into the prostate gland. A catheter is present in the urethra. **B,** Filling of the prostatic ducts with contrast medium. No cavities are present. Although the prostate gland in this dog is enlarged, the filling of the prostatic ducts with contrast medium has no clinical significance.

Signs of urethral disease of prostatic origin include urethral stricture, ulceration of the mucosa, and filling defects within the urethra. Ulceration or stricture of the prostatic urethra should be regarded as highly suggestive of neoplasia.[29]

Extravasation of contrast medium into the prostate should not be interpreted as abnormal as long as only the prostatic ducts fill with contrast medium (see Fig. 43.7B).[30] This appearance is often seen in animals with a normal prostate. However, pooling of the contrast medium within the prostate is abnormal. Large cavities with irregular walls that communicate with the urethra or cavitary smooth-walled lesions containing intraluminal masses are suggestive of neoplasia; aspiration may be indicated in these instances.[13,29] Conversely, if extravasation does not occur, the prostate gland is not necessarily normal or solid. Large cavitary lesions, such as cysts and abscesses, often attain their size because they do not communicate with the urethra.[1,18] If these lesions do fill with contrast medium, they are usually ovoid with smooth walls.

The normal prostatic urethra as seen on the urethrogram has a smooth mucosal border. The urethra is usually slightly greater in diameter near the center of the prostate and tapers slightly at the cranial and caudal borders. The degree of the central dilation depends somewhat on the size of the prostate, the disease present, the degree of bladder distention, and the amount of pressure applied during injection.[31] A small, smooth filling defect in the dorsal wall of the urethra near the center of the prostate gland represents the colliculus seminalis and is a normal finding (Fig. 43.8).[30]

The point at which the prostatic urethra joins the neck of the bladder should be evaluated carefully. Small filling defects or mucosal ulcers that may be early lesions of urothelial carcinoma may be detected. These small lesions may not be detected on a cystogram or even ultrasonography because they are obscured by the internal urethral sphincter, which is actually encircled by the prostate.

Percutaneous biopsy of presumed or suspected prostatic carcinoma or any urogenital neoplasm is controversial due to risk

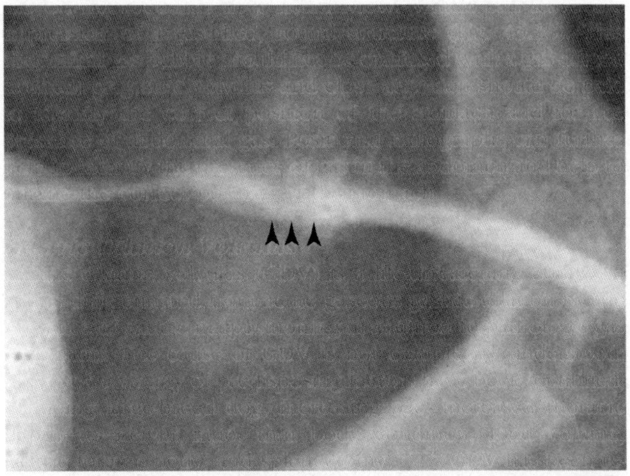

Fig. 43.8 The small filling defect (*black arrowheads*) in the dorsal wall of the prostatic urethra is a normal structure, the colliculus seminalis. It should not be mistaken for a lesion caused by prostatic or urethral disease.

of seeding the tumor cells into the peritoneum, pelvic cavity, and subcutaneous tissues. This has been seen in prostatic neoplasms as well as urinary bladder urothelial carcinoma.[32] Cytologic examination of urine sediment acquired during a urethral catheterization with flushing of the prostatic urethra should be performed before biopsy is considered as this procedure frequently is successful in confirming the presence of neoplasia.[33]

Ultrasonography for Evaluating the Prostate Gland

Diagnostic ultrasonography has largely supplanted radiography for the diagnosis of prostatic disease as it allows for evaluation of overall architecture and symmetry as well as subtle parenchymal abnormalities which are often not detected radiographically.[34]

Ultrasonographic examination of the prostate should also include the bladder and testicles, and regional lymph nodes. These associated structures may be affected secondarily in prostatic disease, or they may be the site of the primary disorder resulting in secondary prostatic changes. A very small normal gland, such as seen in a neutered dog, may not be seen if pelvic in location, but an abnormal prostate is usually visible cranial to the pubis. Images should be acquired in the transverse, sagittal, and parasagittal planes. Alternatively, a cine loop capture can be made while scanning slowly through the gland in the transverse plane. This will ensure that the entire prostate is adequately represented in captured images.[35] The prostate is typically imaged most easily from the right side of the os penis with the dog in dorsal recumbency by tracing the trigone of the urinary bladder caudally. In some dogs, angling the probe caudally is necessary to see the caudal pole of the prostate gland where it lies just dorsal to the pubic brim. Sedation is sometimes required for thorough assessment in uncooperative patients. Ultrasonographic measurement of the prostate and its lesions is performed easily with ultrasonography and has been found to be accurate.[2]

The normal prostate in a neutered male is uniformly relatively hypoechoic with a homogeneous, medium to fine echotexture relative to surrounding fat which has a coarser echotexture. The urethra is usually seen as a small hypoechoic region in the center of the gland surrounded by a narrow band of slightly hyperechoic tissue representing the urethral wall (Fig. 43.9).

BPH usually results in a uniformly enlarged gland that is hyperechoic and has smooth margins. The dorsal portion of the gland may be enlarged to a greater degree than the ventral portion, or vice versa, but the changes are generally symmetric from right to left (Fig. 43.10). This symmetry may be lost as the hyperplasia increases in severity and cysts develop. As cysts form, some invariably become larger than others and distort the shape of the prostate but typically do not extend beyond the capsule. Commonly, small anechoic cystic regions are seen within the parenchyma of dogs with BPH (Fig. 43.11).

The ultrasonographic changes seen in prostatitis vary from mild hyperechogenicity of the parenchyma with variable enlargement to severe prostatic enlargement with a mottled hyperechoic to hypoechoic pattern (Fig. 43.12). The shape of the prostate may be normal or markedly distorted. Distortion of the shape and margin is common when abscess formation is present in the gland. Some dogs may have a hypoechoic band of edema in the capsule outlining the prostate gland. Edema may also extend into the surrounding tissues, resulting in hyperechoic fat with hypoechoic striations adjacent to the prostate. In severe necrotizing prostatitis, delineation of the gland from the surrounding fat may be lost, and the prostate may appear as a dark structure with an irregular and indistinct margin. Generally speaking, the more acute and severe the inflammation is, the more hypoechoic the prostatic parenchyma becomes. In cases of chronic inflammation, the prostate is typically more hyperechoic due to fibrosis.

Cysts and abscesses within and attached to the prostate appear as thin-walled structures with variably hypoechoic centers. They vary widely in size from a couple of millimeters to several centimeters. Their contents may be anechoic, or they may have variable amounts of cellular debris within the lumen.[18] The presence of septation or large amounts of debris within the lumen is typically more indicative of abscess, whereas anechoic contents are suggestive of a cyst; however, this is not a universally accurate distinction. The presence of through transmission deep to a highly echogenic structure is indicative of a fluid-filled rather than a solid cellular mass. Color Doppler can be helpful for confirming vascularization within a prostatic lesion. Both cysts and abscesses occasionally occur in conjunction with neoplasia. Cavitary lesions with irregular internal margins or solid tissue masses within them are highly suggestive of neoplasia, whereas smooth margins are more indicative of cysts (Fig. 43.13).

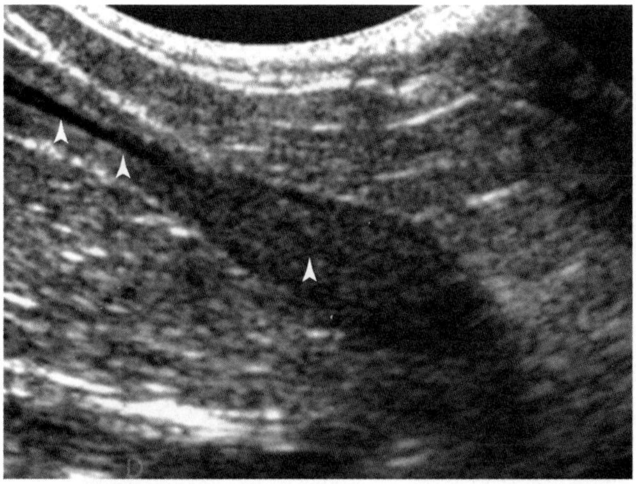

Fig. 43.9 Longitudinal ultrasonographic image of a normal prostate gland in a neutered dog. The prostate gland is small and the echogenicity is relatively homogeneous and mildly hypoechoic relative to surrounding fat. The urethra is identified a small hypoechogenicity in the center of the prostate gland (*white arrowheads*).

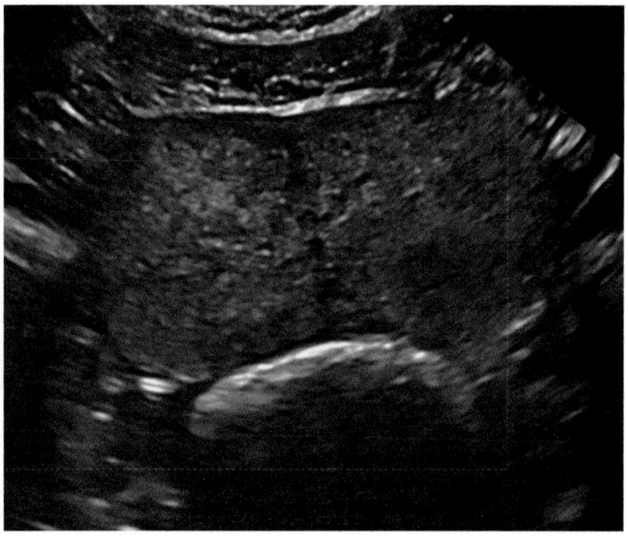

Fig. 43.10 Transverse ultrasound image of symmetric enlargement of a prostate gland in an intact male with benign prostatic hyperplasia.

easiest way to localize the uterus is to start from the body and cervix in transverse plane. With the animal in dorsal or lateral recumbency, the colon and the urinary bladder are identified cranial to the pubis, and the uterus appears as a round/oval hypoechoic structure located between the two organs, often slightly displaced to the left or right. Moving the probe cranially, the bifurcation of the body into the two uterine horns is visible.

The normal vagina is difficult to see through the abdominal approach because of the intrapelvic location. The perineal window might be useful to identify the vulva and the caudal vagina especially if enlarged by diseases like masses or if distended by fluid.

Normal Imaging Finding

Table 44.1 and associated figures summarize the ultrasound features of the normal genital tract in the different phases of the cycle.[9–12]

During anestrus, the normal ovaries are oval hypoechoic structures compared to the hyperechoic fat of the ovarian bursa. Often, they are associated with edge shadowing, which helps in their identification. The uterine horns are hypoechoic with a diameter similar to the jejunal loops but without the wall layering and peristalsis typical for intestines.

Ovaries are easier to identify in the periovulatory period because they are larger and contain small cyst-like structures representing follicles or newly formed corpora lutea. Follicles have anechoic content and a thin wall (less than 1 mm). The number and size of follicles increase during proestrus until ovulation, when they become corpora lutea with a progressively more echogenic appearance and thicker wall. Corpora lutea identification can be challenging or impossible when they become isoechoic with the surrounding ovary.[11] Since follicles and newly formed corpora lutea may have a similar appearance, B-mode ultrasound alone cannot be used to accurately determine the ovulation time but must be interpreted in combination with clinical findings and laboratory results.[9,10] Sequential (daily) scanning of the ovary during proestrus using color Doppler can accurately predict ovulation in the dog, by detecting increases of the blood flow that correlate with LH peak.[11]

Under hormonal influence during proestrus/estrus and diestrus, the uterine wall mildly thickens, and this can improve its visibility. A minimal amount of anechoic to hypoechoic fluid can be observed in the lumen in proestrus/estrus or immediately after mating. The persistence of some fluid 5 to 14 days after ovulation suggests lack of pregnancy.[13]

COMPUTED TOMOGRAPHY

Technique

Standard CT examination is performed with the animal in sternal recumbency under general anesthesia. Pre- and post-contrast series are obtained after injection of iodinated contrast medium at the dose of 400 to 700 mg I/kg body weight. Delayed sequences (3 minutes or later) may be useful to better outline the caudal ureters or the urinary bladder neck which can be affected by uterine or vaginal diseases (e.g., stump granuloma/abscess).

Similar to retrograde vaginography, CT vagino-urethrogram can be performed using the same technique as previously described, with the only difference that the contrast medium concentration can be lowered to 100 mg I/mL. This technique can be useful in the diagnosis of vaginal masses and genitourinary congenital and acquires abnormalities like clefts, fistulae, stenoses, or strictures.[14,15]

Normal Imaging Findings

In anestrus, the ovaries are small, oval, and with homogeneous soft tissue attenuation (Fig. 44.4A). Follicles and corpora lutea are visible as small round hypoattenuating structures, often protruding from the ovarian surface. The uterus is a tubular organ, the uterine horns mix with the intestinal loops as they extend into the caudal abdomen to reach the dorsal aspect of the urinary bladder.[16] The uterine horns can be distinguished from the small bowel by its smaller diameter, different wall structure, and contrast enhancement (see Fig. 44.4B).[17] The uterine body and cervix are recognized between the colon and the urinary bladder; the cervix may be thickened during estrus (see Fig. 44.4C). The vagina is located in the pelvis. In post-contrast images, the urethral wall strongly enhances; this enables its identification caudally to the bladder neck (see Fig. 44.4D). The vestibulum is oriented caudoventrally and ends caudally with the vulva.

NORMAL PREGNANCY

Radiology and ultrasonography play an essential role in the pregnancy diagnosis and follow-up. Ultrasound can be used, together with the determination of the progesterone level, to establish the gestational age and the prediction of delivery timing. Both imaging techniques allow to determine litter size; however, radiology is more accurate compared to ultrasound.

The enlargement of the uterus during pregnancy can be detected with radiology by day 33 to 41.[18] The enlarged uterus initially is soft tissue opaque as with any other uterine fluid collection. Between 30 and 40 days after ovulation, the identification of multiple ovoid bulging areas of similar size might suggest the presence of gestational sacs (Fig. 44.5). Later, the uterus becomes more tubular.[3] Fetal mineralization starts 20 to 22 days before parturition (DBP) in dogs and 25 to 29 DBP in cats. The first structures that can be identified are the spine and the skull from day 43 in the dog and day 38 in the cat.[18,19] Progression of mineralization can be followed until the parturition, when the distal extremities of the fetus and the teeth are recognized (Fig. 44.6, eFig. 44.1). Table 44.2 summarizes the mineralization timing of some fetal structures in dogs and cats, which could be useful to predict parturition. A radiographic study taken with at least two orthogonal projections at the end of pregnancy can be used to determine fetal number and position, to compare their size with the pelvic diameter, and to exclude pelvic abnormalities which could cause mechanical dystocia. Both anterior and posterior presentation with extended limbs is normal. However, radiographs are not adequate to predict fetal maturity and establish the time of Cesarean section.[20] Radiographic or CT pelvimetry has been evaluated as a tool to assess pelvic conformation in some brachycephalic breeds and correlates with dystocia.[21,22]

Early pregnancy diagnosis with ultrasound relies on the visualization of the chorionic cavity/gestational sacs, which are reported to occur on day 18 after ovulation (defined as the day when the plasma progesterone level is first >4.0 ng/mL) in the bitch and as early as 10 days after breeding in the queen.[20] In clinical practice, scanning between the 25th and 30th days in the bitch and the 20th and 25th days after breeding in the queen allows to confirm the pregnancy and obtain fetal biometry measurements. Especially in the bitch, the exact conception time is usually not known and there is a risk of a false-negative result if the ultrasound examination is performed too early. The development of the fetal organs can be followed, and the detection time of specific structures is another reliable indicator

Table • 44.1

Ultrasonographic Features of the Normal Ovary and Uterus in the Different Cyclus Phases.[9–13]

OVARY	ANESTRUS	PROESTRUS/ESTRUS	DIESTRUS
	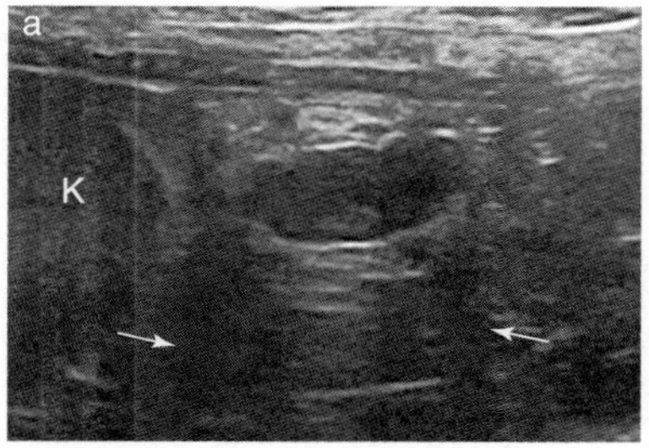 **Table Fig. 44.1a** Ovary in anestrus. *K*, Kidney	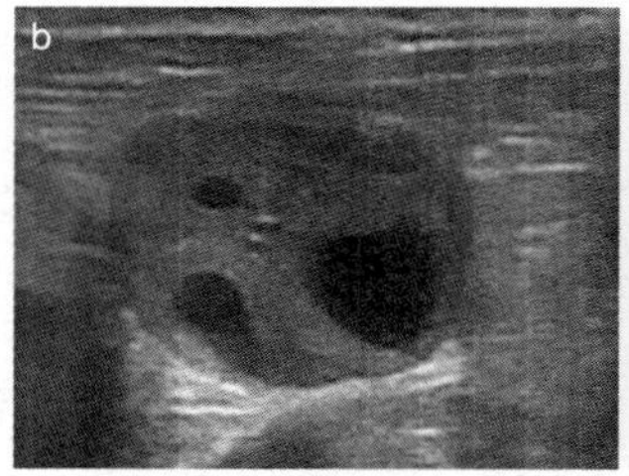 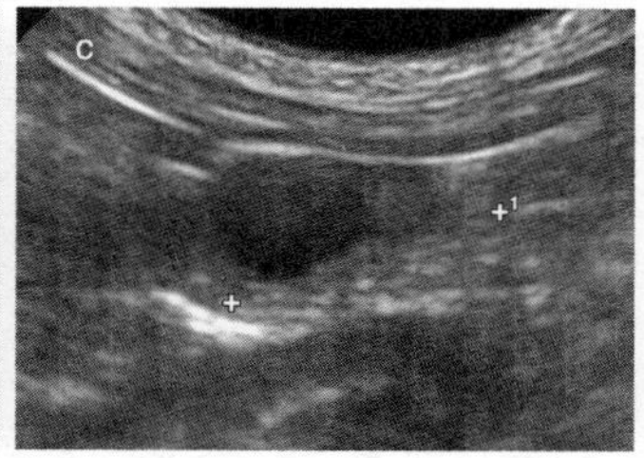 **Table Fig. 44.1b** Ovary with follicles. **Table Fig. 44.2c** Ovary (*between calipers*) with early corpus luteum	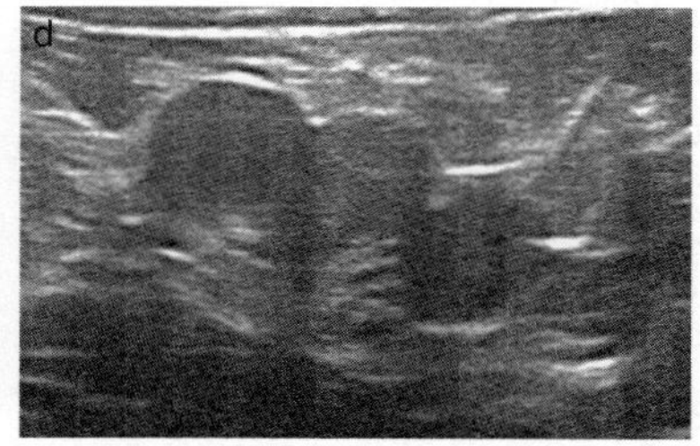 **Table Fig. 44.1d** Ovary with multiple corpora lutea.
Shape	Oval to round	Round or lumpy due to protruding follicles	Round or lumpy due to protruding corpora lutea
Size	1–2 cm of length (dog) 7.1–13.9 mm of length (cat)	Enlarges due to follicles	Enlarges due to corpora lutea
Margins	Smooth	Smooth to irregular	Smooth to irregular
Echostructure/ echogenicity	Homogeneous, hypoechoic to the surrounding fat Iso- to hypoechoic to the renal cortex Associated with edge shadowing (*arrows*)	Heterogeneous **Follicles/early corpora lutea:** - Up to 10, follicles number decreases after ovulation - 4–11 mm (dog), 1–2.3 mm (cat) in diameter - Cystic-like structures with anechoic content - **Follicula**, thin hyperechoic wall (1 mm) - **Newly formed corpora lutea**, may have thicker wall and gradual increase in echogenicity	Homogeneous Corpora lutea appear solid, hypoechoic homogeneous
Relationship with other organs	**Dorsolateral:** abdominal wall **Medial:** large vessels (aorta, caudal vena cava) **Cranial:** kidney **Caudo-ventral:** small intestinal loops and colon		
Vessels	**Ovarian arteries**—origin directly from the aorta **Ovarian veins**—drain into the caudal vena cava (*right*) or left renal vein (*left*)	A significant increase of Doppler signal of the ovary is observed after the LH peak	
Regional lymph nodes	Lumbar aortic lymph nodes		

Continued

Table • **44.1**

Ultrasonographic Features of the Normal Ovary and Uterus in the Different Cyclus Phases. [9–13]

UTERUS	UTERINE HORNS	UTERINE BODY	UTERINE CERVIX
	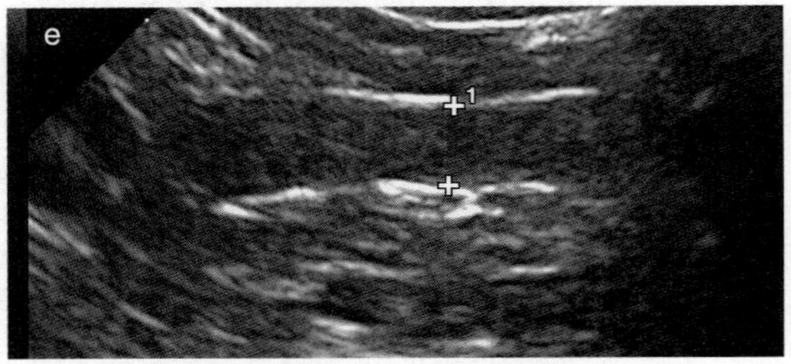 **Table Fig. 44.1e** Uterine horn in anestrus.	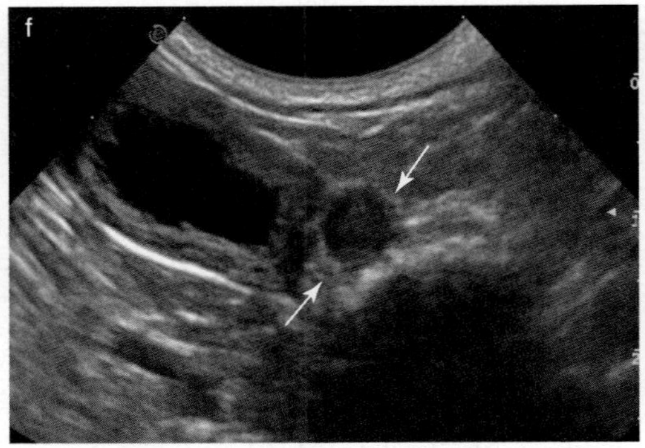 **Table Fig. 44.1f** Uterine body (*between arrows*) in anestrus.	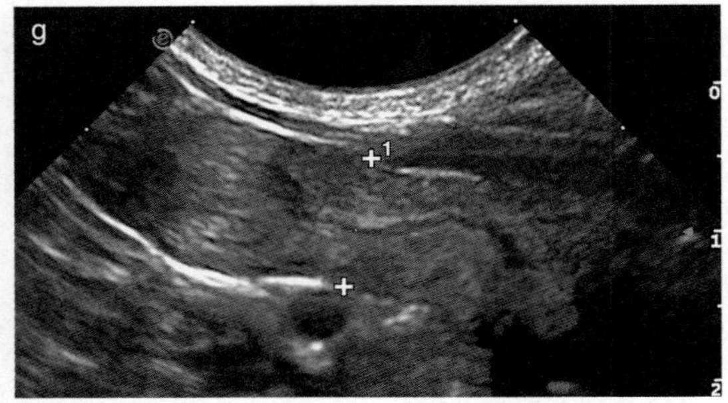 **Table Fig. 44.1g** Uterine cervix (*between calipers*) during estrus.
Shape	Tubular (longitudinal), round/oval (transverse)		
Size	Varies depending on the dog size, previous pregnancies, and cyclus Dog: 0.5–1 cm; cat: 1–5.8 mm	Dog: 0.8–1 cm; cat: 1.5–5.3 mm	Identified as a thicker area caudal to the uterine body especially in estrus Dog: 0.8–1 cm
Margins		Smooth	
Echogenicity/ echostructure	Usually homogeneous hypoechoic Outer thin hyperechoic interface between the serosa and surrounding tissue Wall layering visible with high-resolution probe (hypoechoic endometrium and hyperechoic myometrium) Central hyperechoic lumen or small fluid accumulation often visible in proestrus and estrus	Homogeneous hypoechoic Minimal intraluminal fluid accumulation often visible in proestrus and estrus	Minimal intraluminal fluid accumulation often visible in proestrus and estrus
Relationship with other organs	Cranial: ovary Dorsolateral: abdominal wall Ventral and caudal: small intestinal loops and colon, urinary bladder	Cranial: uterine horns Caudal: cervix Dorsal: colon Ventral: urinary bladder	Cranial: uterine body Caudal: vagina Dorsal: colon Ventral: urinary bladder neck
Vessels	**Ovarian arteries**—origin directly from the aorta **Ovarian veins**—drain into the caudal vena cava (right) or left renal vein (left). They supply the cranial part of the uterus and anastomize with the **uterine arteries and veins**	**Uterine arteries and veins**—arise from the vaginal arteries/veins **Vaginal arteries and veins**—branch of the iliac internal arteries/veins	**Uterine arteries and veins**—arise from the vaginal arteries/veins **Vaginal arteries and veins**—branch of the iliac internal arteries/veins
Regional lymph nodes	**Cranial half:** lumbar aortic and medial iliac **Caudal half:** Internal, medial iliac, sacral	Internal, medial iliac, sacral	Internal, medial iliac, sacral

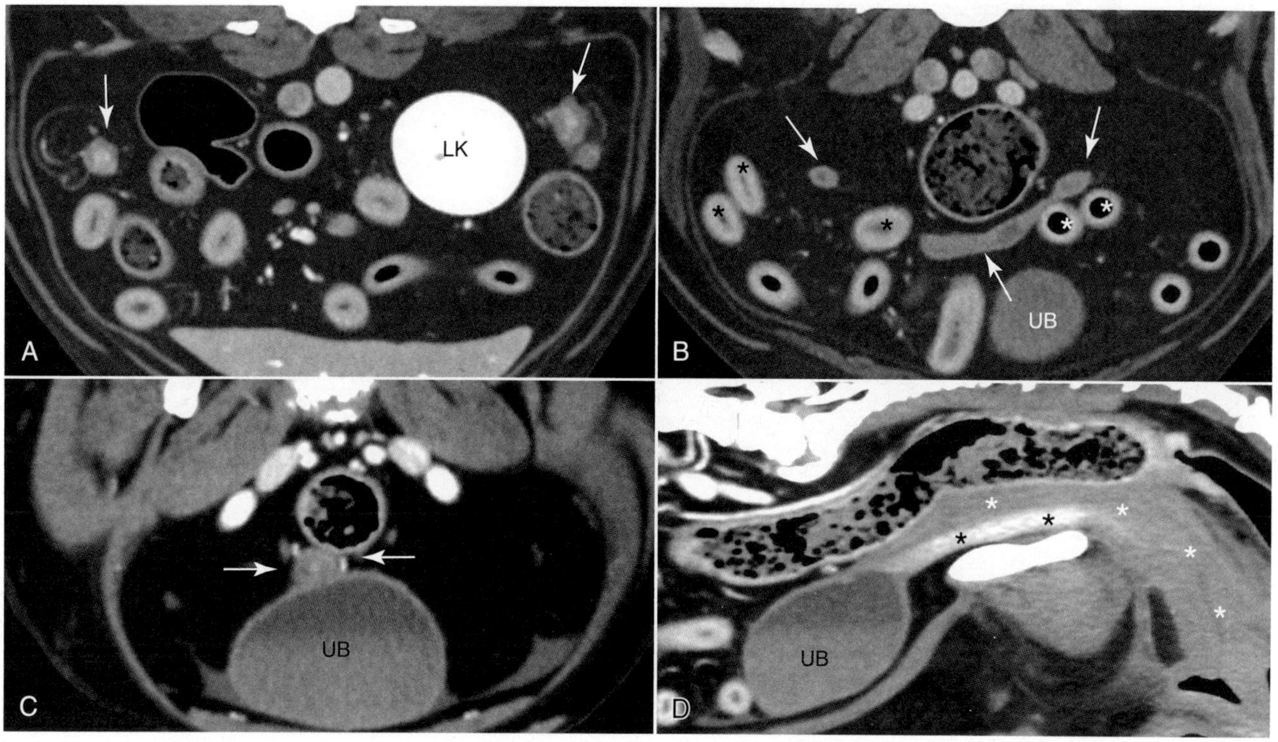

Fig. 44.4 Transverse **(A–C)** and sagittal reformatted **(D)** postcontrast computed tomography images of the normal canine female genital tract. **A**, Midabdomen. The ovaries (*white arrows)* appear as small structure with a soft tissue attenuation surrounded by the fat of the ovarian bursa. **B,** Mid-caudal abdomen. The uterine horns (*white arrows*) have a smaller diameter and different wall compared to small intestinal loops (*white asterisks*); they converge caudally dorsal to the UB and are minimally distended by fluid in this dog. **C,** Caudal abdomen. The uterine cervix (*between arrows*) is visible dorsal to the UB. **D,** The vagina (*white asterisks*) is located between the colon and the urethra (*black asterisks*). Note the strong urethra enhancement in the postcontrast study. *LK,* Left kidney; *UB,* urinary bladder.

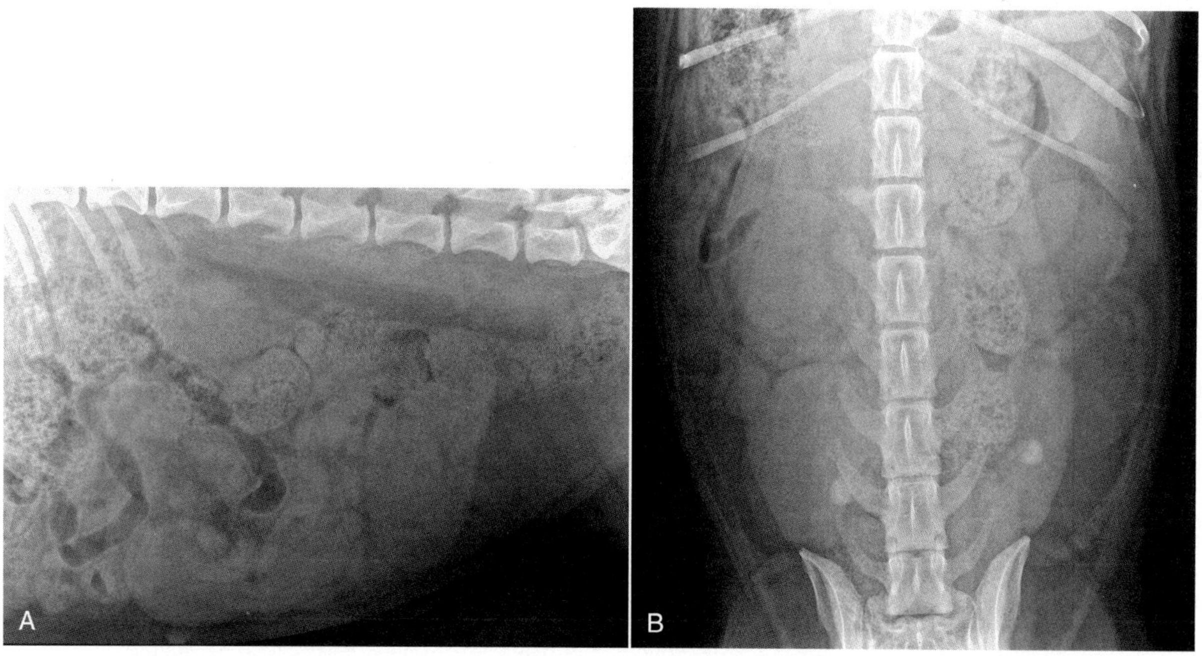

Fig. 44.5 Uterus enlargement in a pregnant bitch (35th day); the gestational chambers are seen as multiple oval soft tissue opacities located in the caudoventral abdomen in the lateral view **(A)** and close to the abdominal wall in the ventrodorsal view **(B)**.

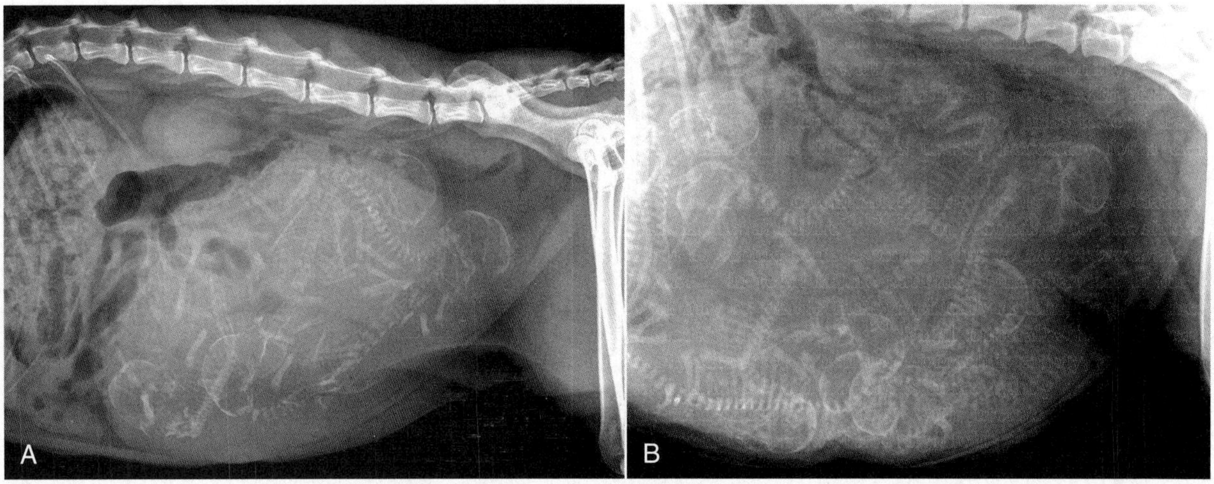

Fig. 44.6 Lateral abdominal radiograph during normal late pregnancy in a cat (A) and in a dog (B).

Table • 44.2

Approximate Timing of Mineralization of Fetal Structures in Dogs and Cats.

FETAL STRUCTURE	TIMING IN DAYS BEFORE PARTURITION[a] FELINE[21]	CANINE[20]
Uterus first seen	—	33–41
Spine	22–27	20–22
Skull	21–27	20–22
Ribs	20–25	20–22
Femur	19–23	15–18
Humerus	20–24	15–18
Radius	15–22	9–13
Tibia	15–21	9–13
Pelvis	8–20	9–13
Metacarpals/metatarsals	3–14	2–9
Phalanges	0–11	2–9
Calcaneus	0–10	2–9
Teeth	1–6	3–8

[a]The timings are given as the number of days before parturition.

of fetal age.[20,23] Table 44.3, with associated figures and videos, summarizes the timing and ultrasound features of the embryo/fetal structures during pregnancy.[23–25]

Estimation of parturition date can be performed by ultrasound. Multiple methods and formulas have been proposed with some limitations due to variation in breed and size (especially in dogs), litter size (only for cats), gestational period in which the measurement is performed, and measuring technique.[20,26–28] These formulas allow to calculate the DBP. In small- and medium-sized dogs, the internal diameter of the chorionic cavity (ICC) measured in the first half of pregnancy and the transverse biparietal skull diameter (BD) in the second half seem to be the most useful parameters, with 85% to 95% of reported accuracy in predicting DBP with an error of ±1–2 days. Accuracy is higher at week 5 of gestation and decreases after week 8. In large and giant dogs, the reported accuracy of measuring ICC is greater compared to the BD.[27]

Table 44.4 summarizes reported formulas that can be used in dogs and cats to calculate the number of DBP.

Establishing **litter size** by ultrasound is more challenging compared to radiography; this is due to technical difficulties (amount of fecal and intestinal gas content, overlapping of fetuses), limited field of view, and operator experience.[29] Embryonic or fetal resorption has an estimated incidence between 5% and 13% in bitches; this is a potential cause of litter overestimation. Reported accuracy of ultrasonography in determining litter size is 65%, increasing to 89.5% if an error of ±1 is considered.[29] To increase the success of the evaluation, scanning in transverse plane from caudal to cranial following the two uterine horns at around 30 days of gestation is recommended.[7]

ABNORMAL RADIOGRAPHIC AND ULTRASONOGRAPHIC FINDINGS DURING PREGNANCY

Combining ultrasound and radiology can be useful to detect uterine or fetal abnormalities during pregnancy.[30,31]

Early resorption of underdeveloped or malformed embryos can be documented ultrasonographically, the features depending upon the timing of the resorption. Early during pregnancy, a characteristic appearance of echogenic particles within the yolk sac, progressive loss of fluid volume, and hypoechogenicity of the adjacent uterus are observed. Gestational sacs are more irregular in shape and smaller compared to normal ones (Fig. 44.7A). Later cases are characterized by loss of the fetal heartbeat and fetal movements, blurring of the fetal margins, and more echogenic allantoic fluid.[31] Accumulation of gas in the fetal stomach or in the uterus can also be observed. Some fetal malformations can be diagnosed during pregnancy, for example, hydrocephalus and hydrops fetalis, where subcutaneous thickening due to edema, pleural, and pericardial fluid is reported.[30]

Radiographic signs of fetal death may be observed approximately 24 hours after death and are less reliable than sonographic indicators. The presence of gas within or around the fetus, overlapping or misalignment of the bones of the cranium, a tightly curled fetus, and collapse of the fetal skeleton may be evident (Fig. 44.8A,B). Care must be taken to differentiate these findings from gastrointestinal gas and projection obliquity especially in early phases. The presence of delayed development of a fetus relative to litter mates is also an indication of demise (Fig. 44.9A).

Table • 44.3

US Findings in Normal Pregnancy.[25–27]

STRUCTURE	TIME, DAYS AFTER OVULATION (PROGESTERONE RAISE)	US FEATURES	
Gestational sac **Chorionic cavity**	18th (dog) 10th (cat)	Anechoic round, thin walled	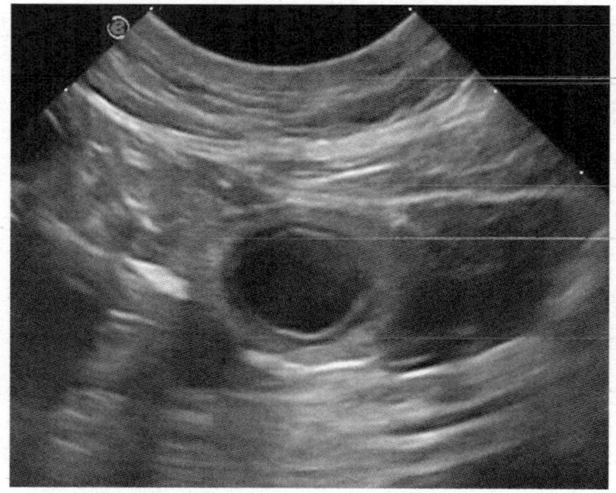 **Table Fig. 44.3a** Chorionic cavity—day 18.
Early embryo	21st–23rd (dog) 17th (cat)	**Elongated** (dog), structure in contact with the uterine wall **Hyperechoic spot** protruding into the gestational chamber **Heartbeat** appears as hyperechoic flick	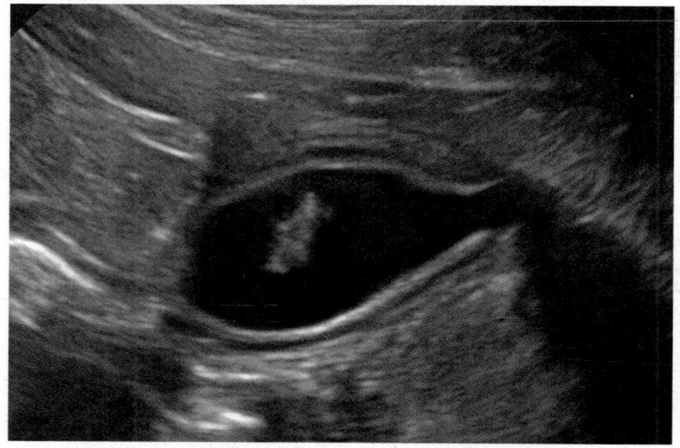 **Table Fig. 44.3b** Gestational sac with early embryo—day 21. Video 44.1 (heart flick)

Continued

Table • 44.3

US Findings in Normal Pregnancy.[25–27]*—cont'd*

STRUCTURE	TIME, DAYS AFTER OVULATION (PROGESTERONE RAISE)	US FEATURES	
Late embryo	27th–31st (dog) 18th–20th (cat)	**Bipolar** (head and trunk) with limb buds (dog) **C-shape** with head, trunk, and thoracic limb buds; moves to the center of the sac (cat) Measurement of the internal diameter of the chorionic cavity **(ICC)**	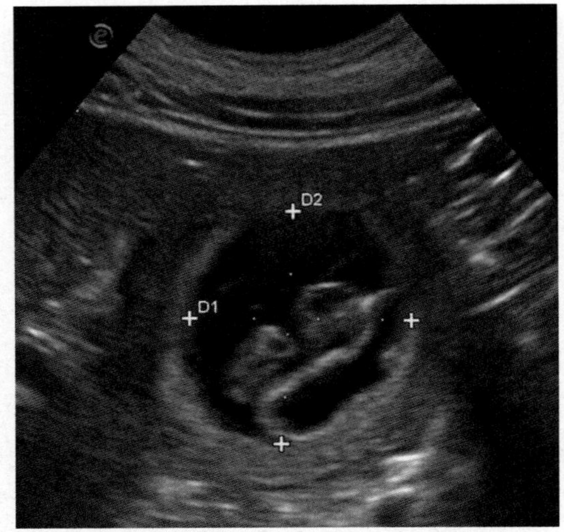 **Table Fig. 44.3c** Chorionic cavity with bipolar fetus, day 28. Measurement of the internal diameter of the chorionic cavity (ICC). 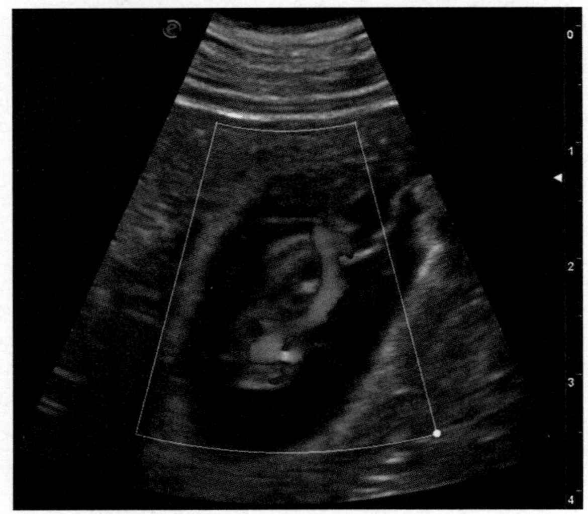 **Table Fig. 44.3d** Color Doppler of fetus—day 28.

Fetus—first organs	29th–33rd (dog) 39th (cat) 31st–35th (dog), 30th (cat) 35th–38th (dog) 40th–50th (cat) 41st–43rd (dog) 50th (cat) 50th 57th–63rd (dog), 40th (cat)	Stomach (anechoic) and skeleton (hyperechoic nonmineralized) Urinary bladder (anechoic) Lung (hyperechoic) and liver (hypoechoic) Kidneys Heart chambers and major vessels Mineralized skeleton (shadowing) Bowel—in dogs, peristalsis starts at the end Measurement of the transverse biparietal skull diameter **(BD)**	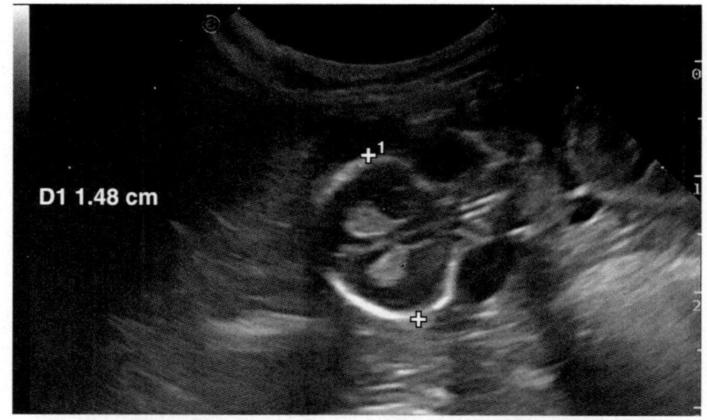 **Table Fig. 44.3e** Measurement of biparietal diameter (BD)—day 45. 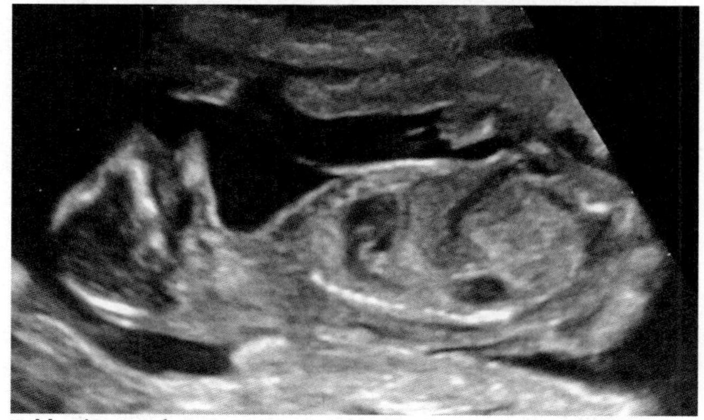 **Table Fig. 44.3f** Sagittal fetus with visible heart, lung, aorta, liver, stomach—day 45.
Fetal movements	32nd–24th (dog) 30th (cat)		Video 44.2 - fetal movements - day 45

Continued

Table • 44.3

US Findings in Normal Pregnancy.[25–27]*—cont'd*

STRUCTURE	TIME, DAYS AFTER OVULATION (PROGESTERONE RAISE)	US FEATURES	
Placenta	25th–27th (dog)	Circumferential, focal thickening of the chorionic cavity wall, protruding toward the lumen, hyperechoic, at the periphery two areas of thickening (marginal hematomas)	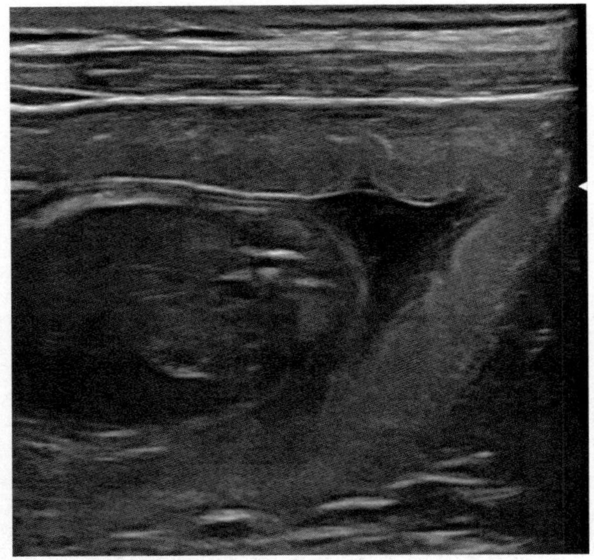 **Table Fig. 44.3g** Placenta—day 45.
Fetal membranes	18th–23rd 23rd–25th 29th–32nd 25th–29th	Anechoic content surrounds the early embryo Echogenic yolk sac membranes, folded around the embryo Collapsing yolk sac Thin hyperechoic allantoic membranes surrounding the embryo	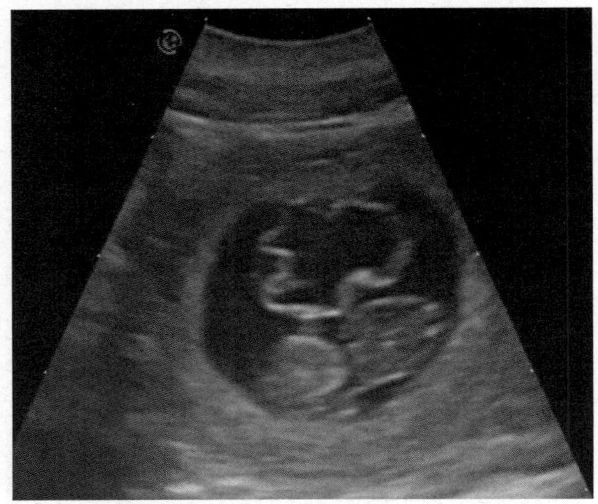 **Table Fig. 44.3h** Fetal membranes—day 33.

Uterine vessels	Early pregnancy	Utero-placental arteries seen between gestational sacs Umbilical cord arteries and veins can be distinguished with Doppler after the fourth week. Arterial resistivity index (RI) and pulsatility index (PI) decrease during pregnancy	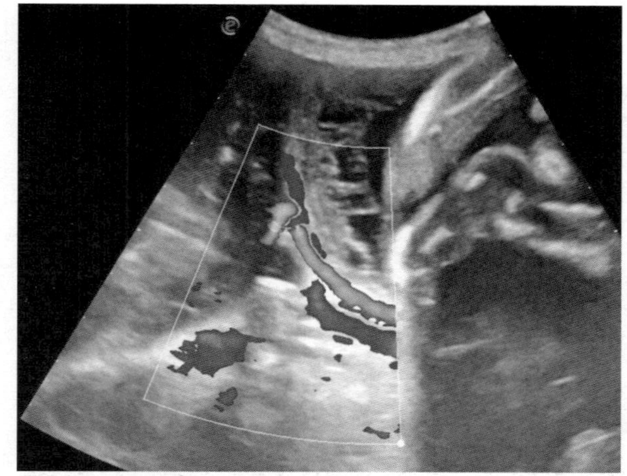 **Table Fig. 44.3i** Utero-placental vessels—day 38. 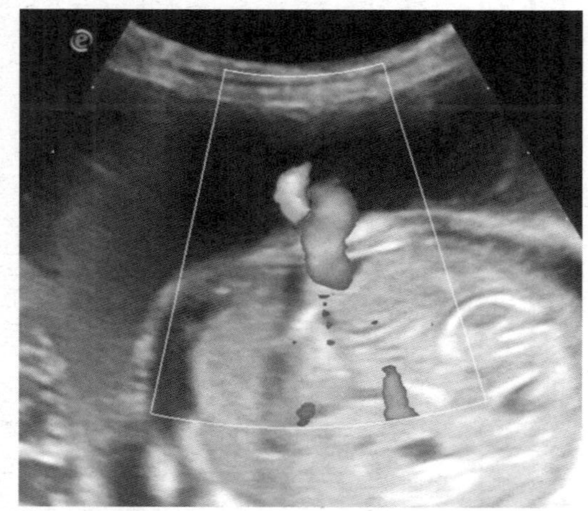 **Table Fig. 44.3j** Umbilical vessels—day 38

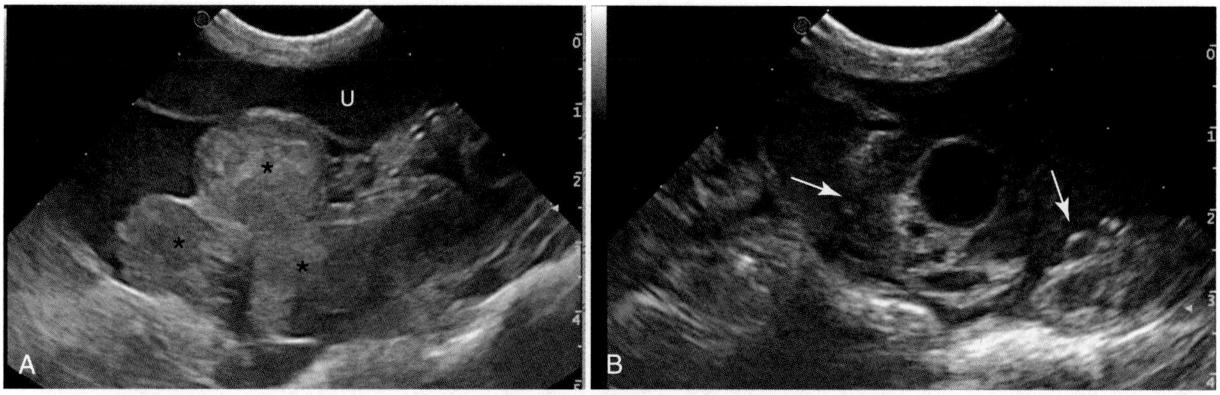

Fig. 44.20 Sonographic images of a cat with a diffuse uterine adenosquamous carcinoma, metastatic to the peritoneum. **A,** The right uterine horn (*U*) is distally distended with echogenic content, proximally multiple hyperechoic nodules are visible (*asterisks*). **B,** Free fluid, serosal thickening (*white arrows*) and cysts are visible in the adjacent peritoneum.

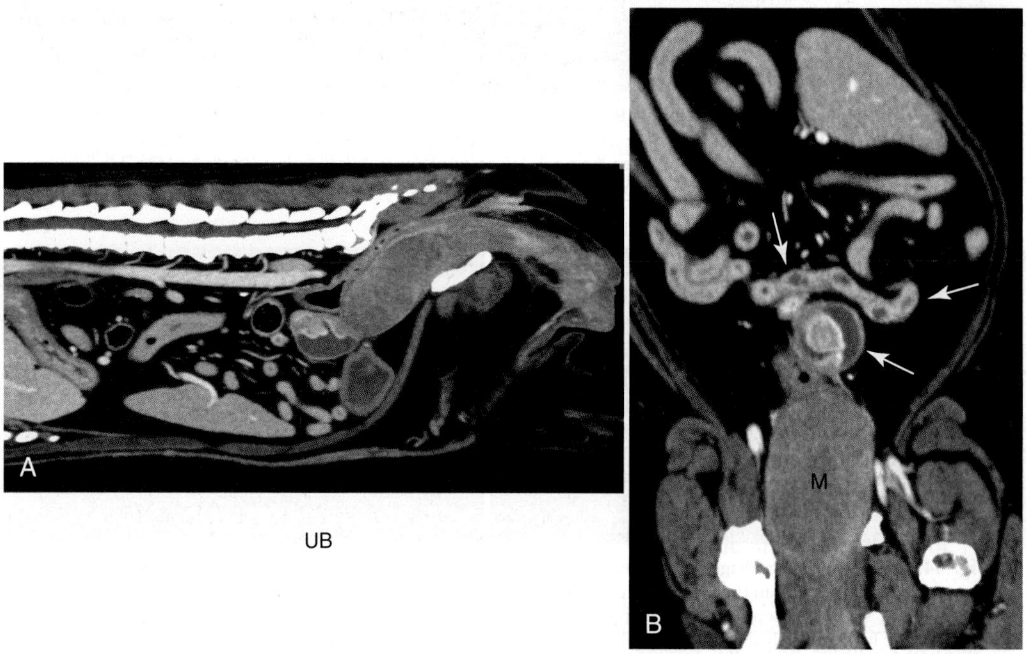

Fig. 44.21 Computed tomography images, reformatted in the sagittal **(A)** and dorsal **(B)** plane, of a dog with vaginal leiomyoma. The mass (*M*) arises from the vaginal wall and is cranially connected with the uterus. The uterine body and horns (*white arrows*) are distended with fluid-filled regions caused by concomitant endometrial cystic hyperplasia. The urinary bladder (*UB*) is compressed ventrally.

Other differential diagnoses for vaginal masses include other tumors like the transmissible venereal tumor (TVT) and some benign conditions like vaginal hyperplasia/prolapse. The clinical presentation helps the diagnosis and rarely imaging is required in these cases.

Positive urethro-vaginography may be helpful to investigate animals with genitourinary causes of dysuria. Vaginal fistula can be congenital or acquired due to trauma, surgery, or foreign bodies and can be highlighted by the passage of the contrast medium from the vagina to the urethra or to the surrounding peritoneum.

ABNORMAL CT FINDINGS IN FEMALE GENITAL TRACT DISEASES

Indications for CT include the diagnosis and staging of ovarian, uterine, and vaginal masses and challenging cases of genital tract infection or torsion. CT helps to assess the origin of genital masses and the relationship with surrounding organs and to establish surgical resectability (Fig. 44.21, eFig. 44.10).[48–50] Identification of the mass connection with an ovary or with a portion of the uterus or vagina is best performed using multiplanar reformatted images. Identifying vascular supply from an ovarian, uterine, or vaginal vessel can be used to confirm the genital origin of the mass.[51] For this reason, dual-phase CT scan, acquiring arterial and venous phases separately, can be useful (see Fig. 44.12). The vesicoureteral junction is frequently involved with uterine stump granulomas, with consequent hydroureter and/or hydronephrosis; this can be best demonstrated by scanning the animal in the delayed pyelographic/ureterographic phase (Fig. 44.22, eFig. 44.11). Placing a urinary catheter can be useful in case of large masses to assess the position and involvement of the urethra.[52] The enhancement evaluated in the postcontrast series provides information about the vascularization of the lesion. However, reliable CT criteria

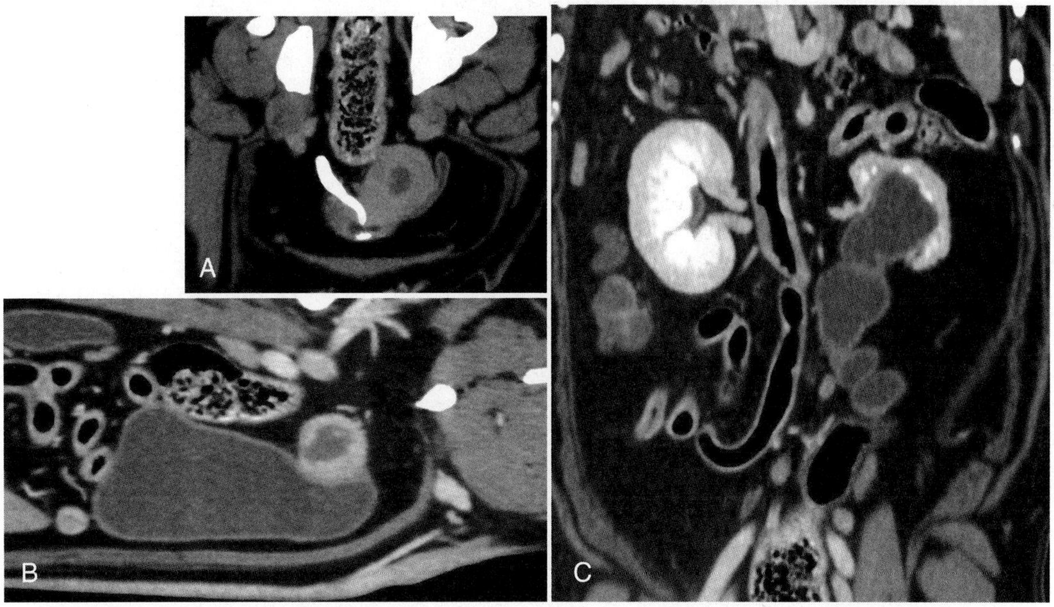

Fig. 44.22 Computed tomography images reformatted in the oblique **(A)**, sagittal **(B)**, and dorsal **(C)** plane of a dog with uterine stump granuloma, chronic hydroureter/nephrosis, and right kidney atrophy. **A, B,** The stump granuloma shows a fluid center surrounded by irregular thick wall; it compresses ventrally the bladder trigone and involves the vesicoureteral junction. Only the left ureter is functional. **C,** The right kidney is small and irregular in shape; the right ureter is severely dilated and nonfunctional.

to differentiate between benign and malignant neoplasia are not established. It has been suggested that benign mesenchymal neoplasia is associated with smaller size, homogeneous enhancement, and lack of bone involvement.[49,52] The presence of lymphadenopathy or other lesions compatible with metastatic spread indicates malignancy.

CT is an excellent image modality to diagnose complex urogenital conditions such as ureteral ectopia or urethrovaginal fistulas.[53]

IMAGING PROCEDURES AND NORMAL ANATOMY OF THE TESTICLES

Radiography is rarely used to investigate testicular diseases, with the exception of abdominal masses or torsion associated with retained testicles. Ultrasound on the other hand provides detailed information about the abnormalities of the testicular parenchyma and of the adnexa (scrotum, epididymis, distal part of the spermatic cord with the ductus deferens, vessels, and nerves).[54] Due to their superficial location, scrotal or inguinal testicles are best imaged with a high-frequency (8–13 MHz) linear probe. Longitudinal and transverse views of both testes are acquired and compared. Color, power, and pulsed-wave Doppler can be used to assess the arterial and venous flow and to investigate parenchymal vascularization.[55,56] For the search of retained abdominal testicles, which are more deeply located, a convex probe with mid to high frequency is often necessary especially in large dogs.

Color and power Doppler examination might be supportive to investigate dogs with infertility conditions.[57] CT of the normal male genital tract has been described.[58] The normal ultrasonographic anatomy of the testis and associated structures is summarized and illustrated in Table 44.5.

ABNORMAL RADIOGRAPHIC AND ULTRASONOGRAPHIC FINDINGS IN SCROTAL AND TESTICLE DISEASES

Extratesticular Diseases

Ultrasound is an accurate and rapid method to distinguish between testicular and nontesticular causes for scrotal swelling.[59,60] In case of severe scrotal skin diseases like severe edema, infection, or neoplasia, ultrasound can be used to evaluate concomitant involvement of the testicle or epididymis. Hydrocele is the most common cause of extratesticular fluid collection, and can result from trauma, neoplasia, infarction, torsion, or infection or can be idiopathic. Hydrocele may also develop secondary to peritoneal effusion, when fluid passes through the inguinal canal, and this may be associated with jejunal herniation. Hematoceles may occur with trauma, neoplasia, or diabetes mellitus. Pyoceles result from abscess rupture often within a pre-existing hydrocele. Extratesticular fluid collection is easily visualized as an anechoic to echogenic band surrounding the testicle, depending on the cellular content. Other indications for ultrasound include tunica vaginalis diseases like malformations, infections, trauma, or neoplasia.

Inflammation

Epididymitis and orchitis can occur separately or concurrently, often secondary to retrograde prostatic or urinary bacterial infections. Penetrating wounds, migrating foreign bodies, and infections caused by *Brucella canis*, Rickettsia, fungal diseases, and feline coronavirus are other rare causes of infection.[61,62] Lymphoplasmacytic/immune-mediated orchitis is also reported; unilateral or bilateral involvement is possible.[63]

Ultrasonographic findings include enlarged testicle and/or epididymis, with patchy hypoechoic appearance, eventually focal changes due to abscesses, granulomas, or necrotic/

Table • 44.5

US Feature of the Normal Testicles.

	SCROTUM/TESTICLE TUNICS (SKIN), TUNICA DARTOS (SMOOTH MUSCLE), AND ALBUGINEA (CONNECTIVE TISSUE)	TESTIS	EPIDIDYMIS	SPERMATIC CORD (DUCTUS DEFERENS AND ASSOCIATED VESSELS)
US images	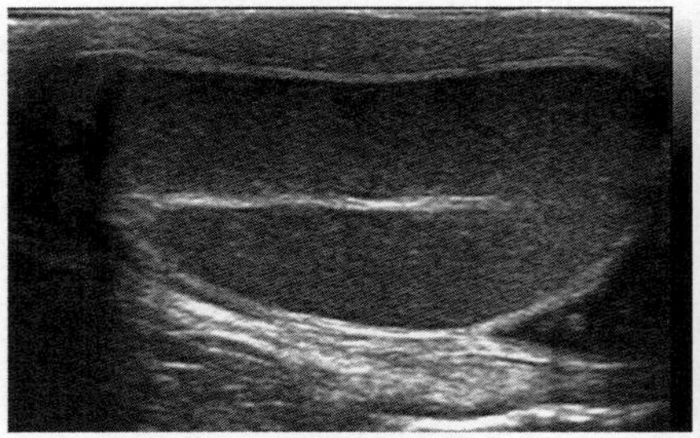 **Table Fig. 44.5a** Testicle longitudinal image.	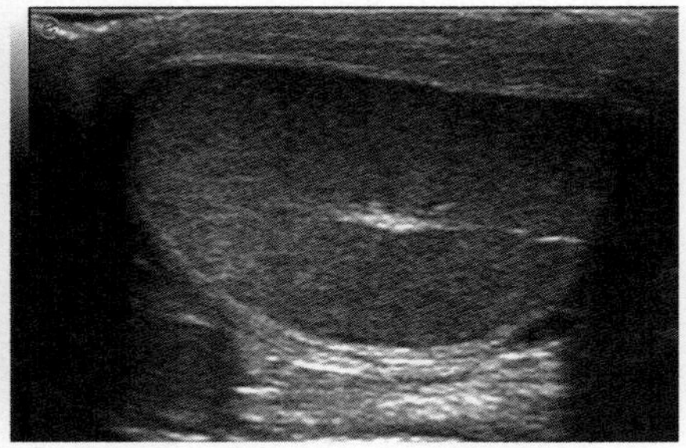 **Table Fig. 44.5b** Testicle transverse image. 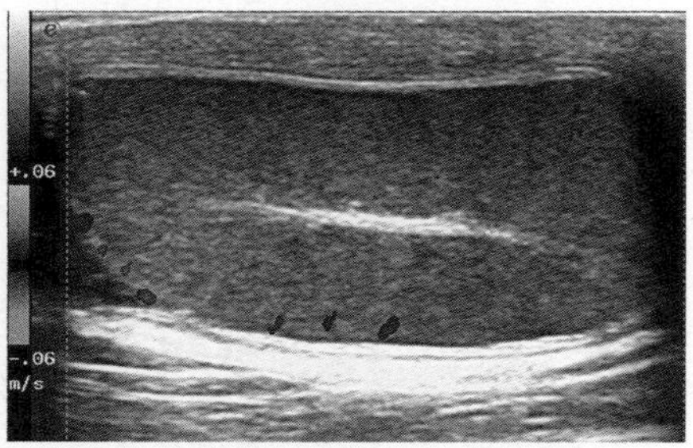 **Table Fig. 44.5c** Testicle—color Doppler.	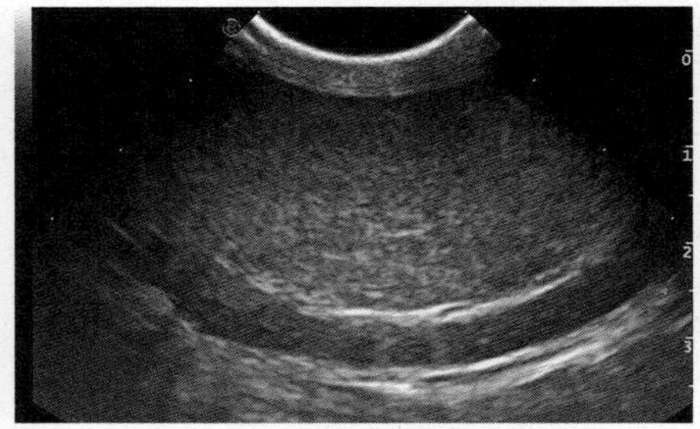 **Table Fig. 44.5d** Testicle with body of the epididymis. 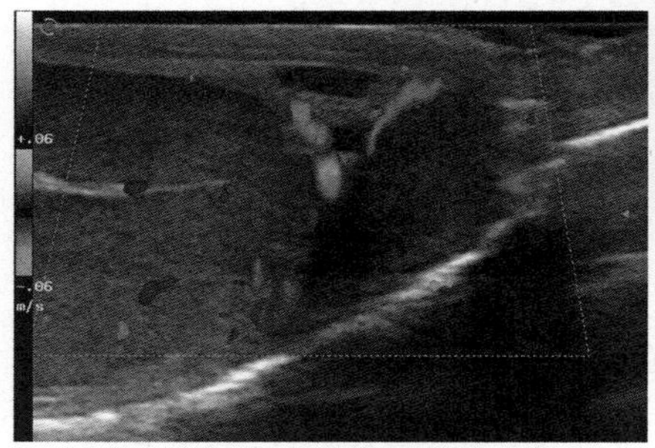 **Table Fig. 44.5e** Caudal testicle with the tail of the epididymis.	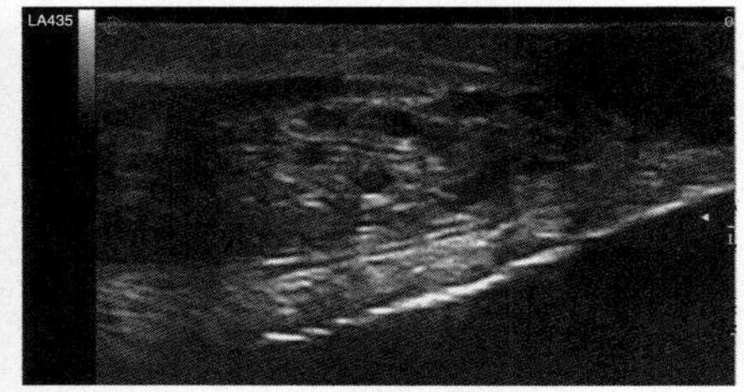 **Table Fig. 44.5f** Spermatic cord—longitudinal image. 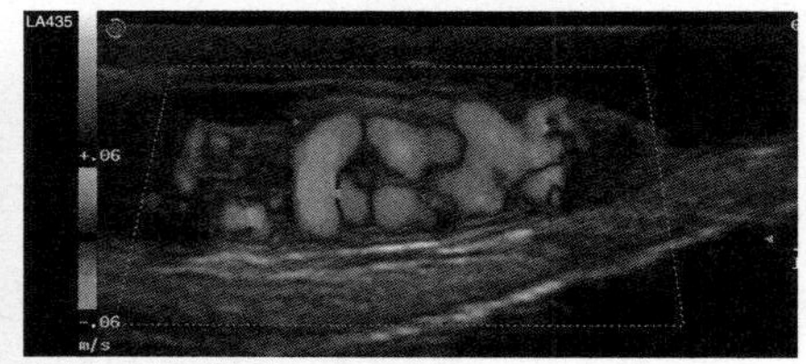 **Table Fig. 44.5g** Spermatic cord—color Doppler. *US,* Ultrasonography.
Location/ spatial orientation	Superficial, circumferential cover of the testicle	Oriented longitudinally	**Head:** at the cranial testicle pole **Body:** along the dorsolateral aspect of the testicle **Tail:** at the caudal testicle pole, continue cranially with the ductus deferens	Along the dorsomedial aspect of the testicle directed cranially to the inguinal canal, visible adjacent to the head of the epididymis

Size	Thin (few mm)	Variable depending on body weight, age, and health status Volume increases until the sixth year of age, then decreases Volume calculation (L × W × H × 0.71) accurate to predict true testicular volume	**Tail:** larger, more consistently displayed compared to the head and body	Very thin ductus deference, difficult to follow
Shape	Elongated	Oval	**Head and tail:** triangular **Body:** longitudinally elongated	
Echostructure/ echogenicity	Hyperechoic striated structure	Homogeneous, fine echotexture; echoic parenchyma interrupted by hyperechoic flecks (radiating connective septa from the albuginea) **Mediastinum testis:** central hyperechoic linear structure, longitudinally oriented	Homogeneous, hypoechoic to the testicle, might be anechoic	
Doppler exami-nation[52,53]		Small marginal arteries can be detected at the testicular membranes (low resistance flow) Parenchyma low flow detected with power Doppler	Usually, no flow detected	Arterial and venous structures visualized with color Doppler. Cranial testicular artery with high resistance flow, becomes low resistance in the distal looping part

hemorrhagic areas and extratesticular fluid collection. Abscesses may appear as focal areas of anechoic/hypoechoic content surrounded by hyperechoic wall; granulomas have a more solid appearance. In chronic cases, the testicle may be reduced in size with more irregular margins. Differential diagnoses include neoplasia and torsion. Epididymal involvement and fluid accumulation orient to the diagnosis of orchitis (Fig. 44.23). Doppler ultrasound can be useful to differentiate between acute diffuse inflammation and torsion; diffuse hypervascularity is usually present with inflammation, whereas Doppler signal is lacking with torsion.[59,60] Contrast ultrasound is another excellent method to investigate testicular perfusion and may have a role in differentiating benign and malignant testicular diseases.[61,62]

Torsion

Scrotal testicles uncommonly undergo torsion; these are usually nonneoplastic. Ultrasonographic changes are visible already between 15 and 60 minutes after torsion and include enlargement of the spermatic cord, epididymis, and testicle associated with decreased diffuse echogenicity and loss of Doppler signal of the spermatic cord.[64] Other findings are scrotal thickening and hydrocele.

Torsion of abdominal retained testicles in dogs most often occurs secondary to testicular neoplasia; however, nonneoplastic testicles can be affected.[65,66] It is thought that the increased weight of pendulous, neoplastic abdominal testes may predispose to torsion. Clinical signs are severe and acute and mimic other acute abdominal emergencies. If severely enlarged, the testicle might be identified radiographically as a soft tissue opaque mass located caudal to the kidney or cranial to the urinary bladder with or without associated abdominal fluid. Inconsistent and reduced flow with color Doppler is the only differentiation from neoplasia only in ultrasound, making the final diagnosis challenging. In these cases, the different clinical presentation may support the diagnosis. Torsion of nonneoplastic cryptorchid testicle has been reported in few cases: the testicle and epididymis are enlarged, rounded with abnormal echogenicity (Fig. 44.24). Interestingly, hyperechoic appearance of the twisted testicle has been reported.[66] Adjacent effusion and/or peritoneal hyperechogenicity can be present due to focal peritonitis. The lack of testicular blood flow can be easily demonstrated by contrast-enhanced ultrasound.[67]

Cryptorchidism

Cryptorchidism is suspected if one or both testicles are not located within the scrotum in a dog after 6 to 8 weeks and in a newborn cat. However, in puppies and kittens until 6 months of age, the small and soft testes can move from the scrotum to the inguinal canal. In dogs, a genetic basis is suspected, with a reported incidence range from 1% to 15%, higher in small-size breed, most frequently unilateral and right sided.[68] Feline cryptorchidism is less frequent compared to dogs.

Ultrasound has a high predictive value for the final, surgical location of a retained testicle.[69] The ultrasonographic search of the cryptorchid testicle is best performed with the animal in dorsal recumbency. First, the affected side is identified by palpation of the scrotal testicle; this restricts the search to 50%. The scan starts in the subcutaneous inguinal region from the scrotum to the inguinal ring, then it continues in the abdomen just lateral to the urinary bladder neck cranially to the caudal pole of the ipsilateral kidney (Fig. 44.25). The testicle must be differentiated from the inguinal or colic/jejunal lymph nodes based on the shape (oval for the testicle and more elongated for the lymph nodes), the absence of the hilus, and the presence of the testicle mediastinum. The retained testicle is usually smaller compared to the scrotal one but similar in echogenicity and structure. Even subtle changes in echogenicity or structure should be considered suspect for neoplastic transformation. Testicle agenesis is rare however possible. If a suspected testicle is not identified, CT or MRI can be useful as further diagnostic methods.

Neoplasia

Canine testicular neoplasia is common in old intact dogs, with a reported prevalence between 9% and 27%, and is mainly represented by three types of tumors: interstitial cell (Leydig cell), Sertoli cell, and seminomas. Up to 20% of dogs diagnosed with testicular cancer have more than one primary testicular tumor; most of them are characterized by local invasion but rarely metastasize, with the highest metastatic rate (less than 15%) reported for Sertoli cell tumors and seminomas.[37] The risk of developing testicular neoplasia increases with a retained testis. Hyperestrogenism and feminization syndrome are commonly associated with Sertoli cell tumors. The main clinical signs include bilateral symmetric alopecia and hyperpigmentation, pendulous prepuce, gynecomastia, galactorrhea, atrophy of the penis, and squamous metaplasia of the prostate. Severe pancytopenia can also develop. Independent of the tumor type, atrophy of the contralateral testicle is common. As in ovarian neoplasia, the mass can be located between the caudal pole of the kidney and the inguinal canal. With large or mineralized masses, abdominal radiographs can show the lesion located in the mid to caudoventral abdomen (Fig. 44.26, eFigs. 44.12 and 44.13). If caudally located, the enlarged testicle can be confused with the urinary bladder or with a large para-prostatic cyst. Positive-contrast cystogram or ultrasound is indicated for

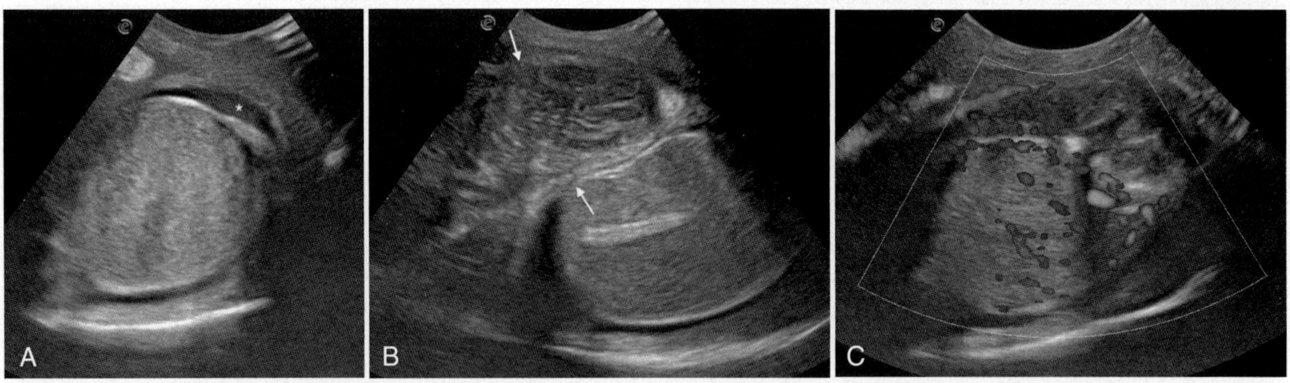

Fig. 44.23 Bacterial orchitis and epididymitis in a dog, longitudinal grey scale **(A, B)** and color Doppler **(C)** ultrasound images. **A,** The testicle is enlarged, mildly heterogeneous and surrounded by effusion (*asterisk*). **B, C,** The epididymis is severely enlarged (*between arrows*) and with increased Doppler signal.

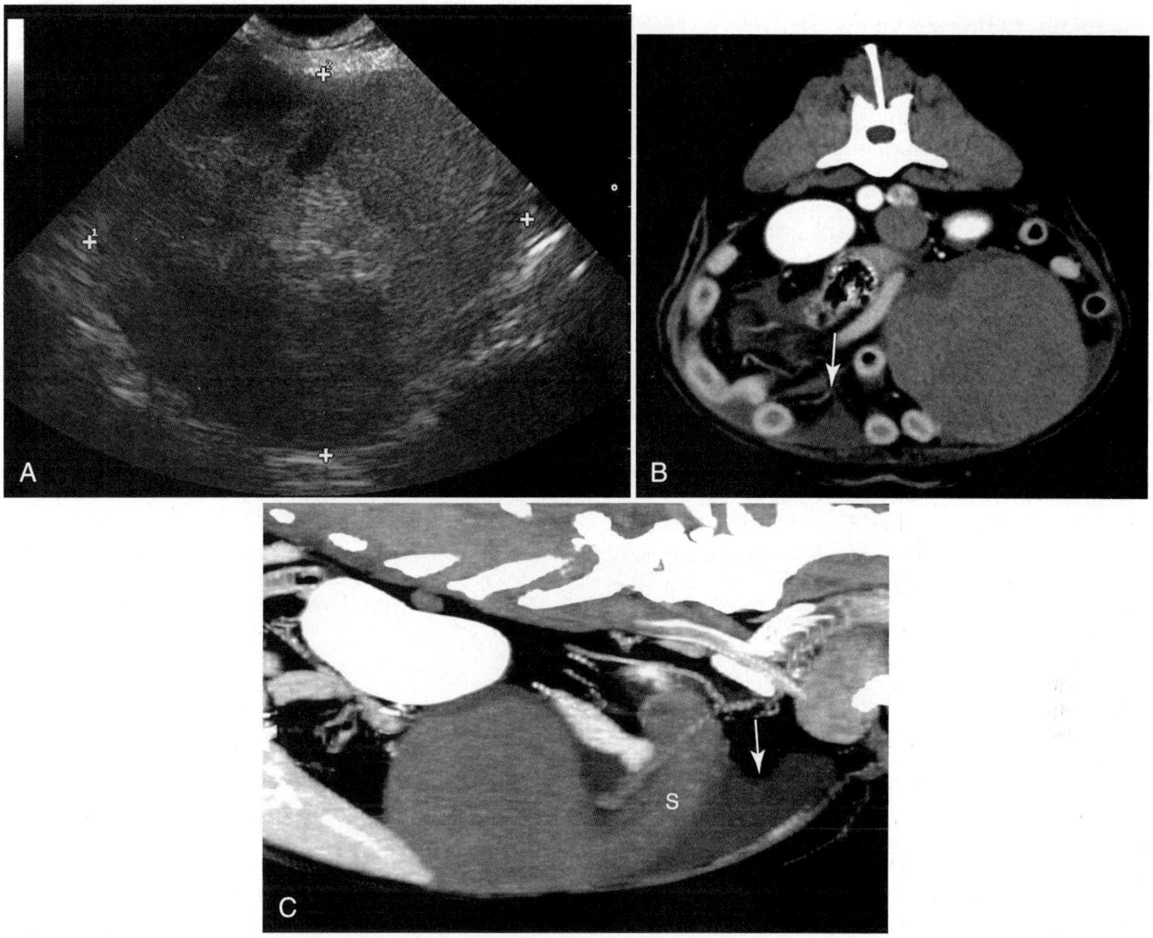

Fig. 44.24 Sonographic image **(A)**, transverse **(B)**, and oblique **(C)** reformatted computed tomography images of a dog with torsion of an abdominal testicle. The enlarged testicle (*between calipers*) has a complex echostructure in ultrasound **(A)** and appears as a nonenhancing mass in CT **(B)**. Note the enlarged spermatic cord (*S*) and some peritoneal free fluid (*white arrow*). In this case, the "whirl sign" was not detected.

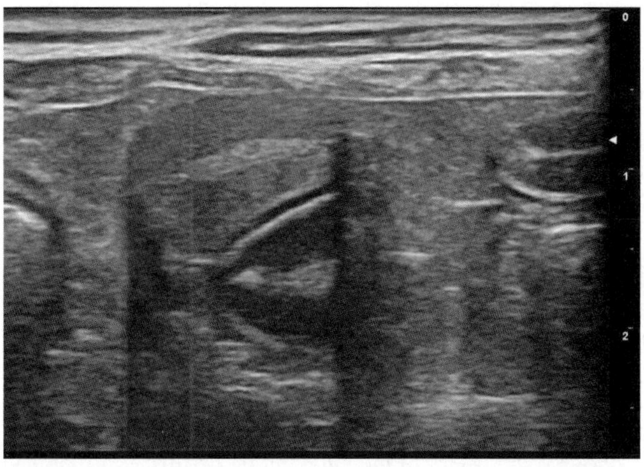

Fig. 44.25 Longitudinal sonographic image of a retained testicle. The testicle is located lateral to the urinary bladder, between a jejunal loop and the abdominal wall, and presents a normal structure, with a well-visible hyperechoic mediastinum.

identification. Thoracic radiographs complete the staging of these patients. Hypertrophic nipples can be obvious in case of Sertoli cell tumors and these must not be confused with pulmonary nodular lesions.

Ultrasound is the method of choice to image testicle nodules or masses.[70] They present with variable size, echogenicity, and structure; unfortunately, B-mode findings are not specific for the different tumor types[55,56] (see Fig. 44.26). If large, they alter the testicle architecture and may have a complex appearance with cystic, necrotic, or hemorrhagic areas and mineralization. Contralateral testicle atrophy and prostatic hyperplasia can be associated with functional neoplasia (Fig. 44.27). Color and power Doppler ultrasound can assess tumor vascularization. To improve tumor characterization, multiparameter evaluation including pulsed-wave Doppler, B-flow, and contrast ultrasound has been investigated, with some more specific pattern for Leydig cell tumors.[71,72]

ABNORMAL CT FINDINGS IN TESTICLES DISEASES

CT could be beneficial with challenging cases of retained testicles before surgery if abdominal ultrasound is not conclusive. Identification of the testicular artery and vein supplying a structure or a mass demonstrates a testicular origin. Visualization of a cord-like vascular pedicle composed by a venous plexus and tortuous arteries, consistent with the spermatic cord, is another useful CT finding.[48,73]

Testicular torsion can be also diagnosed with CT (see Fig. 44.24). The testicle is enlarged with reduced enhancement after contrast administration. Other CT findings include the

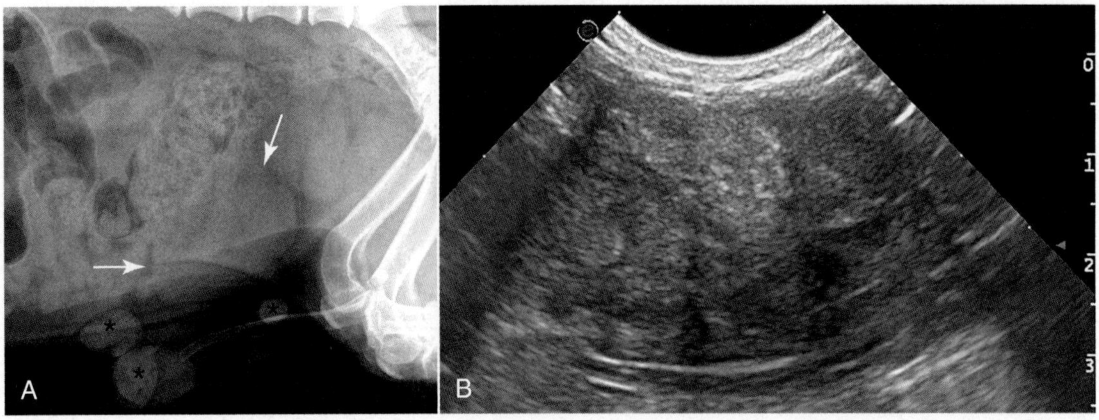

Fig. 44.26 Lateral radiograph **(A)** and sonographic image **(B)** of a Sertoli cell tumor (*arrows*) arising from a retained testicle. Note the enlarged nipples due to feminization syndrome (*asterisks*).

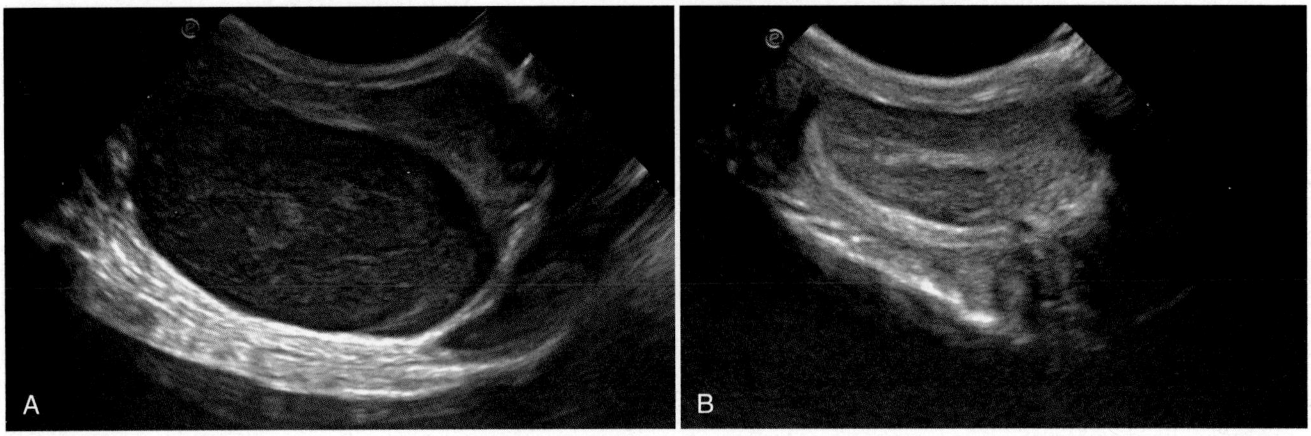

Fig. 44.27 Testicular seminoma appearing as a hypoechoic nodule **(A)** and associated contralateral testicle atrophy **(B)** in a dog.

"whirl sign," corresponding to the spermatic cord arranged in a whirl of fat and soft tissue striations, and a central testicular/spermatic cord crescentic to triangular fat pattern, described with nonneoplastic torsion.[73,74] These findings are similar to what is usually observed with splenic torsion.

Acknowledgment

With special thanks to prior authors of this chapter for their contributions.

REFERENCES

1. Armbrust LJ, Biller DS, Hoskinson JJ. Compression radiography: an old technique revisited. *J Am Anim Hosp Assoc*. 2000;36(6):537–541.
2. Woodland M, Pack L, Rist P, et al. Comparison of digital radiography, ultrasonography, and positive contrast vaginourethrography for determining reproductive status of female cats. *Vet Radiol Ultrasound*. 2014;55(4):368–373.
3. Rivers B, Johnston GR. Diagnostic imaging of the reproductive organs of the bitch. Methods and limitations. *Vet Clin North Am Small Anim Pract*. 1991;21(3):437–466.
4. Holt PE, Gibbs C, Latham J. An evaluation of positive contrast vaginourethrography as a diagnostic aid in the bitch. *J Small Anim Practice*. 1984;25:531–549.
5. Evans HE. *Miller's Anatomy of the Dog*. 3rd ed. Philadelphia: Saunders; 1993.
6. Barone R. *Anatomie Comparee des Mammiferes Domestiques*. 3rd ed. Tome 4, Splanchnologie: Baronne Edition; 2020.
7. Davidson AP, Baker TW. Reproductive ultrasound of the bitch and queen. *Top Companion Anim Med*. 2009;24(2):55–63.
8. Fulton RM. Focused ultrasound of the fetus, female and male, reproductive tracts, pregnancy and dystocia in dogs and cats. *Vet Clin Small Anim*. 2021;51(6):1249–1265.
9. Wallace SS, Mahaffey MB, Miller DM, et al. Ultrasonographic appearance of the ovaries of dogs during the follicular and luteal phases of the estrous cycle. *Am J Vet Res*. 1992;53(2):209–215.
10. England GC, Yeager AE. Ultrasonographic appearance of the ovary and uterus of the bitch during oestrus, ovulation and early pregnancy. *J Reprod Fertil Suppl*. 1993;47:107–117.
11. Bergeron LH, Nykamp SG, Brisson BA, et al. An evaluation of B-mode and color Doppler ultrasonography for detecting periovulatory events in the bitch. *Theriogenol*. 2013;79(2):274–283.
12. Gatel L, Rault DN, Chalvet-Monfray K, et al. Ultrasonography of the normal reproductive tract of the female domestic cat. *Theriogenology*. 2020;142:328–337.

13. Freeman SL, Green MJ, England GC. Prevalence and effect of uterine luminal free fluid on pregnancy and litter size in bitches. *Theriogenology*. 2013;80(2):73–76.
14. Weissmann A, Jimenez D, Torres B. Canine vaginal leiomyoma diagnosed by CT vaginourethrography. *J Am Anim Hosp Assoc*. 2013;49:394–397.
15. Agut A, Carrillo DJ, Anson A. Imaging diagnosis—urethrovaginal fistula caused by a migrating grass awn in the vagina. *Vet Radiol Ultrasound*. 2016;57(3):E30–E33.
16. Teixeira M, Francisco Gil F b, Vazquez JM, et al. Helical computed tomographic anatomy of the canine abdomen. *Veterinary J*. 2007;174:133–138.
17. Lee SK, Yoon S, Kim C, et al. Triple-phased mesenteric CT angiography using a test bolus technique for evaluation of the mesenteric vasculature and small intestinal wall contrast enhancement in dogs. *Vet Radiol Ultrasound*. 2019;60(5):493–501.
18. Rendano VT, Lein MSDH, Concannon PW. Radiographic evaluation of prenatal development in the beagle. *Vet Radiol*. 1984;25:132–141.
19. Haney DR, Levy JK, Newell SM, et al. Use of fetal skeletal mineralization for prediction of parturition date in cats. *J Am Vet Med Assoc*. 2003;223(11):1614–1616.
20. Beccaglia M, Alonge S, Trovo C, et al. Determination of gestational time and prediction of parturition in dogs and cats: an update. *Reprod Domest Anim*. 2016;51(suppl 1):12–17.
21. Eneroth A, Linde-Forsberg C, Uhlhorn M, et al. Radiographic pelvimetry for assessment of dystocia in bitches: a clinical study in two terrier breeds. *J Small Anim Pract*. 1999;40(6):257–264.
22. Dobak TP, Voorhout G, Vernooij CM, et al. Computed tomographic pelvimetry in English bulldogs. *Theriogenology*. 2018;15(118):144–149.
23. Siena G, Milani C. Usefulness of maternal and fetal parameters for the prediction of parturition date in dogs. *Animals Basel*. 2021;11(3):878.
24. Zambelli D, Prati F. Ultrasonography for pregnancy diagnosis and evaluation in queens. *Theriogenology*. 2006;66:135–144.
25. Concannon PW. Canine pregnancy: predicting parturition and timing events of gestation. In: Concannon PW, England G, Verstegen IIIJ, Linde Forsberg C, eds. *Recent Advances in Small Animal Reproduction*. United States: International Veterinary Informative Service; 2019:1–9.
26. Gatel L, Rault D, Chalvet-Monfray K, et al. Prediction of parturition time in queens using radiography and ultrasonography. *Anatomia Histologia and Embryologia*. 2015;44:241–246.
27. Alonge S, Beccaglia M, Melandri M, et al. Prediction of whelping date in large and giant canine breeds by ultrasonography foetal biometry. *J Small Anim Pract*. 2016;57(9):479–483.
28. Beccaglia M, Anastasi P, Grimaldi E, et al. Accuracy of the prediction of parturition date through ultrasonographic measurement of fetal parameters in the queen. *Vet Res Commun*. 2008;32:S99–101.
29. Lenard ZM, Hopper BJ, Lester NV, et al. Accuracy of prediction of canine litter size and gestational age with ultrasound. *Aust Vet J*. 2007;85(6):222–225.
30. England GCW. US assessment of abnormal pregnancy. *Am Vet Clin North Am Small Anim Pract*. 1998;28(4):849–868.
31. England GC, Russo M. Ultrasonographic characteristics of early pregnancy failure in bitches. *Theriogenology*. 2006;66(6–7):1694–1698.
32. Pharr W. Ultrasonography and radiography of the canine postpartum uterus. *Vet Radiol Ultrasound*. 1992;33:35–40.
33. Yeager AE, Concannon PW. Serial ultrasonographic appearance of postpartum uterine involution in beagle dogs. *Theriogenology*. 1990;34(3):523–535.
34. Ferretti LM, Newell SM, Graham JP, et al. Radiographic and ultrasonographic evaluation of the normal post-partum uterus. *Vet Radiol Ultrasound*. 2000;41:287–291.
35. Ball RL, Birchard SJ, May LR. Ovarian remnant syndrome in dogs and cats: 21 cases (2000–2007). *J Am Vet Med Assoc*. 2010;236(5):548–553.
36. Knauf Y, Bostedt H, Failing K, et al. Gross pathology and endocrinology of ovarian cysts in bitches. *Reprod Domest Anim*. 2014;49(3):463–468.
37. Vail DM, Thamm DH, Liptak JM. *Withrow & MacEven's Small Animal Clinical Oncology*. 6th ed. St Louis: Saunders; 2020.
38. Stein BS. Tumors of the feline genital tract. *J Am Anim Hosp Assoc*. 1981;17:1022–1025.
39. Diez-Bru N, Garcia-Real I, Martinez EM, et al. Ultrasonographic appearance of ovarian tumors in 10 dogs. *Vet Radiol Ultrasound*. 1998;39(3):226–233.
40. Greenlee PG, Patnaik AK. Canine ovarian tumors of germ cell origin. *Vet Pathol*. 1985;22(2):117–122.
41. Pretzer SD. Clinical presentation of canine pyometra and mucometra: a review. *Theriogenology*. 2008;70:359–363.
42. Mattei C, Fabbi M, Hansson K. Radiographic and ultrasonographic findings in a dog with emphysematous pyometra. *Acta Vet Scand*. 2018;60:67.
43. Jjeong E, Tan RM, Oh H, et al. Imaging diagnosis—endometrial mineralization in a dog. *Vet Radiol Ultrasound*. 2016;57(6):E67–E70.
44. Chambers B, Laksito M, Long F, et al. Unilateral uterine torsion secondary to an inflammatory endometrial polyp in the bitch. *Aust Vet J*. 2011;89(10):380–384.
45. Misumi K, Fujiki M, Miura N, et al. Uterine horn torsion in two non-gravid bitches. *J Small Anim Pract*. 2000;41(10):468–471.
46. Patsikas M, Papazoglou LS, Jakovljevic S, et al. Radiographic and ultrasonographic findings of uterine neoplasms in nine dogs. *J Am Anim Hosp Assoc*. 2014;50(5):330–337.
47. Ma LY, Heng HG, Chia MY, et al. Ultrasonographic appearance of pseudo-placentational endometrial hyperplasia in a dog. *Vet Radiol Ultrasound*. 2021;62(6):e58–e62.
48. Russo M, England GCW, Catone G, et al. Imaging of canine neoplastic reproductive disorders. *Animals Basel*. 2021;11(5):1213.
49. Spector DI, Fischetti AJ, Kovak-McClaran JR. Computed tomographic characteristics of intrapelvic masses in dogs. *Vet Radiol Ultrasound*. 2011;52(1):71–74.
50. Percival A, Singh A, zur Linden RA, et al. Massive uterine lipoleiomyoma and leiomyoma in a miniature poodle bitch. *Can Vet J*. 2018;59:845–850.
51. Rowan C, Cuddy L, Bryan J. Imaging diagnosis – computed tomography findings in a case of metastatic ovarian adenocarcinoma in a dog. *Vet Radiol Ultrasound*. 2017;58(6):E60–E63.
52. Barozzi MCM, Saba CF, Gendron KP. CT characteristics of uterine and vaginal mesenchymal tumours in dogs. *J Small Anim Pract*. 2021;62:293–299.
53. Schwarz T, Bommer N, Parys M, et al. Four-dimensional CT excretory urography is an accurate technique for diagnosis of canine ureteral ectopia. *Vet Radiol Ultrasound*. 2021;62(2):190–198.
54. Pugh CR, Konde LJ, Park RD. Testicular ultrasound in the normal dog. *Vet Radiol*. 1990;31(4):195–199.
55. Carrillo JD, Soler M, Lucas X, et al. Colour and pulsed Doppler ultrasonographic study of the canine testis. *Reprod Domest Anim*. 2012;47(4):655–659.

56. Gumbsch P, Gabler C, Holzmann A. Colour-coded duplex sonography of the testes of dogs. *Vet Rec.* 2002;151(5):140–144.
57. Lemos H, Dorado J, Hidalgo M, et al. Assessment of dog testis perfusion by colour and pulsed-Doppler ultrasonography and correlation with sperm oxidative DNA damage. *Top Companion Anim Med.* 2020;41:100452.
58. Dirrig H, Drees R, Lam R. Use of dual-phase contrast computed tomography for evaluation of the normal canine male genital tract. *J Small Animal Practice.* 2016.
59. Pugh CR, Konde LJ. Sonographic evaluation of canine testicular and scrotal abnormalities: a review of 26 case histories. *Vet Radiol Ultrasound.* 1991;32(5):243–250.
60. Davidson AP, Baker TW. Reproductive ultrasound of the dog and tom. *Top Companion Anim Med.* 2009;24(2):64–70.
61. Egloff S, Schneeberger M, Gobeli S, et al. *Brucella canis* infection in a young dog with epididymitis and orchitis. *Schweiz Arch Tierheilkd.* 2018;160(12):743–748.
62. Ober CP, Spaulding K, Breitschwerdt EB, et al. Orchitis in two dogs with Rocky Mountain spotted fever. *Vet Radiol Ultrasound.* 20004; 45(5):458–465.
63. Davidson AP, von Dehn BJ, Schlafer DH, et al. Adult-onset lymphoplasmacytic orchitis in a Labrador retriever stud dog. *Top Companion Anim Med.* 2015;30(1):31–34.
64. Hricak H, Lue T, Filly RA, et al. Experimental study of the sonographic diagnosis of testicular torsion. *J Ultrasound Med.* 1983;2(8):349–356.
65. Pearson H, Kelly DF. Testicular torsion in the dog: a review of 13 cases. *Vet Rec.* 1975;97(11):200–204.
66. Hecht S, King R, Tidwell AS, et al. Ultrasound diagnosis: intra-abdominal torsion of a non-neoplastic testicle in a cryptorchid dog. *Vet Radiol Ultrasound.* 2004;45(1):58–61.
67. Brown JM, Taylor KJ, Alderman JL, et al. Contrast-enhanced ultrasonographic visualization of gonadal torsion. *J Ultrasound Med.* 1997;16:309–316.
68. Khan FA, Gartley CJ, Khanam A. Canine cryptorchidism: an update. *Reprod Domest Anim.* 2018;53(6):1263–1270.
69. Felumlee AE, Reichle JK, Hecht S, et al. Use of ultrasound to locate retained testes in dogs and cats. *Vet Radiol Ultrasound.* 2012;53(5):581–585.
70. Johnston GR, Feeney DA, Johnston SD, et al. Ultrasonographic features of testicular neoplasia in dogs: 16 cases (1980-1988). *J Am Vet Med Assoc.* 1991;198(10):1779–1784.
71. Volta A, Manfredi S, Vignoli M, et al. Use of contrast-enhanced ultrasonography in chronic pathologic canine testes. *Reprod Domest Anim.* 2014;49(2):202–209.
72. Orlandi R, Vallesi E, Boiti C, et al. Characterization of testicular tumor lesions in dogs by different ultrasound techniques. *Animals (Basel).* 2022;12(2):210.
73. Stokowski S, Ruth J, Lanz O, et al. Computed tomographic features in a case of bilateral neoplastic cryptorchidism with suspected torsion in a dog. *Front Vet Sci.* 2016;27;3:33.
74. Slaughter SA, Eitzer AD, Tolliver SA, et al. Computed tomography of testicular torsion in a juvenile dog with unilateral cryptorchidism. *Can Vet J.* 2022;63(5):515–520.

ELECTRONIC RESOURCES

Additional information related to the content in Chapter 44 can be found online at eBooks.Health.Elsevier.com

- Chapter Quiz
- Videos

CHAPTER 45

Stomach

Susanne M. Stieger-Vanegas

Diagnostic imaging is an important component in the clinical evaluation of animals with gastrointestinal disease. Survey radiographs are usually the first imaging modality, often followed or sometimes replaced by an ultrasound examination. Contrast radiographic studies remain in use but they are laborious and time consuming and are often replaced by ultrasound. Nevertheless, contrast radiography remains important for evaluation of functional disorders of the stomach and obstructive processes. Computed tomography (CT) is used increasingly for evaluation of the gastrointestinal tract, especially when disease staging is required. While magnetic resonance (MR) imaging is regularly used in human patients, it is rarely used for the evaluation of the gastrointestinal tract in animals.

NORMAL ANATOMY

The stomach is the relatively large muscular, hollow aspect of the digestive system, which fulfills an important function in the transient storage and digestion of food. The stomach is caudal to the liver, and when empty normally lies cranial to the last pair of ribs or slightly caudal to the costal arch.[1,2] The empty stomach has a U shape, which disappears with filling. In the filled state, the position of the caudal aspect of the stomach is variable and can be located as far caudal as the third to fourth lumbar vertebrae. Independent of filling stage, the stomach lies primarily to the left of midline in both the dog and cat.[2]

The stomach is arbitrarily subdivided into the cardia, fundus, body, and pylorus (Fig. 45.1).[1] The cardia is a small area at the esophagogastric junction immediately caudal to the diaphragm.

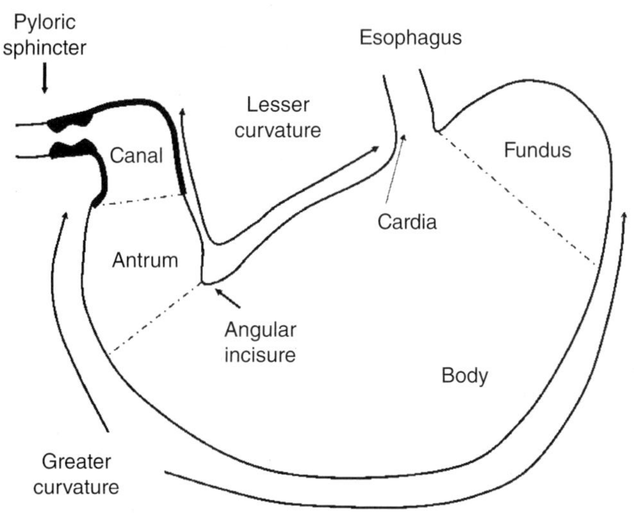

Fig. 45.1 The divisions of the stomach.

The fundus is the dome-shaped outpouching of the left dorsal aspect of the stomach. The fundus is the only portion of the stomach that normally can be in direct contact with the diaphragm. The body is the middle aspect of the stomach extending from the fundus to the pylorus and is the largest portion of the stomach. A large aspect of the body of the stomach is located to the left of midline. The distal third of the stomach is the pylorus, which is further subdivided into the pyloric antrum and the pyloric canal. The pyloric antrum includes the orad (proximal) two-thirds of the pylorus and is relatively thin walled and slightly expanded. The pyloric canal, which is the most aborad (distal) third of the pylorus, is more muscular and contains a double sphincter. The pyloric antrum is ventral to the fundus and in the dog is on or to the right of the midline, whereas in the cat, the pyloric antrum tends to be on midline. When the stomach is maximally distended, mainly the body and pyloric antrum of the stomach increase in width, whereas the pyloric canal does not change in size.[2]

Additional landmarks of the stomach include the greater and lesser curvatures and the angular incisure, or notch.[1] The greater curvature is the convex surface of the stomach extending from the cardia caudoventrally to the pylorus. The lesser curvature is the concave surface originating from the right lateral aspect of the cardia and extending cranioventrally to the pylorus. It is the shortest distance between the cardia and pylorus. The angular notch is the point of acute angulation of the lesser curvature, located approximately at the junction of the body and pyloric antrum.

The mucosal surface of the stomach is characterized by numerous folds or ridges called *rugal folds* or *rugae*, which are more distinct when the stomach is empty as they become flat when the stomach is expanded. The rugal folds are most prominent in the gastric body and fundus and flatten towards the pyloric antrum.

The greater omentum, which is a large, lacy, fat-containing double folded structure, attaches to the stomach and extends caudally to the urinary bladder, covering the intestines ventrally and laterally. The superficial aspect of the greater omentum originates from the greater curvature of the stomach and continues to the proximal part of the duodenum in alignment with the attachment of the lesser omentum to the duodenum.[1,3] The gastrosplenic ligament is part of the greater omentum and connects the hilus of the spleen to the greater curvature of the fundus and body of the stomach.[1] The lesser omentum is small and extends from the liver to lesser curvature of the stomach and the cranial part of the duodenum.[1,3] The largest aspect of the lesser omentum is the hepatogastric ligament connecting the liver with the lesser curvature of the stomach.[1]

IMAGING PROCEDURES

Radiography

Indications

Radiography is used commonly to evaluate the stomach. Survey radiographs allow evaluation of the position and content of the stomach. Sometimes, gastric wall thickening or gas within the gastric wall, called gastric pneumatosis, can be detected. Gastric dilation and volvulus (GDV), a frequently occurring life-threatening disease in dogs, can usually be diagnosed radiographically. Furthermore, mineral or metal attenuating foreign bodies are easily detected on survey radiographs. Additionally, survey radiographs are highly sensitive for evaluating the presence of peritoneal gas, if a gastric perforation is suspected. Survey radiographs are also an important baseline if a contrast radiographic study is planned.

Radiographic Technique

Three, or preferably four, views of the abdomen are required for a thorough evaluation.[4] Performing left lateral, right lateral, ventrodorsal (VD), and dorsoventral (DV) views of the abdomen is especially valuable for the evaluation of the stomach as the position of the patient affects the position of the luminal gas and fluid within the stomach.[5] Due to gravity, fluid settles dependently, and gas rises to the highest part of the lumen of the stomach. This was discussed in detail in Chapter 38. These changes in appearance of the stomach help to evaluate all aspects of the stomach. Oblique views may occasionally be of value to isolate or project certain areas of the stomach, such as the pylorus, especially when a foreign body or pyloric wall mass is suspected.

Radiographic examination of the stomach in an animal that has fasted for 12 to 24 hours may be more informative than when the stomach is in the ambient state, as ingesta within the stomach may obscure some lesions or simulate other lesions.[6–8] However, this is not done routinely due to time constraints, and in some patients fasting may be contraindicated. Also, many drugs used for treatment of gastrointestinal disorders or for sedation to facilitate radiographic positioning, alter gastric motility and may cause gas distention of the stomach.

Normal Radiographic Findings

The stomach is usually easily recognized by its location, shape, and the content of gas, ingesta, or both. The entire stomach may not be discernible on survey radiographs if it is empty or if gastric fluid silhouettes with the liver or other abdominal structures.

As a general guide, the axis of the stomach from the fundus through the body and pylorus on the lateral view is either perpendicular to the spine, parallel to the ribs, or somewhere between these angles (Figs. 45.2A,B and 45.3A). On the lateral view, the pylorus may be superimposed over the body of the

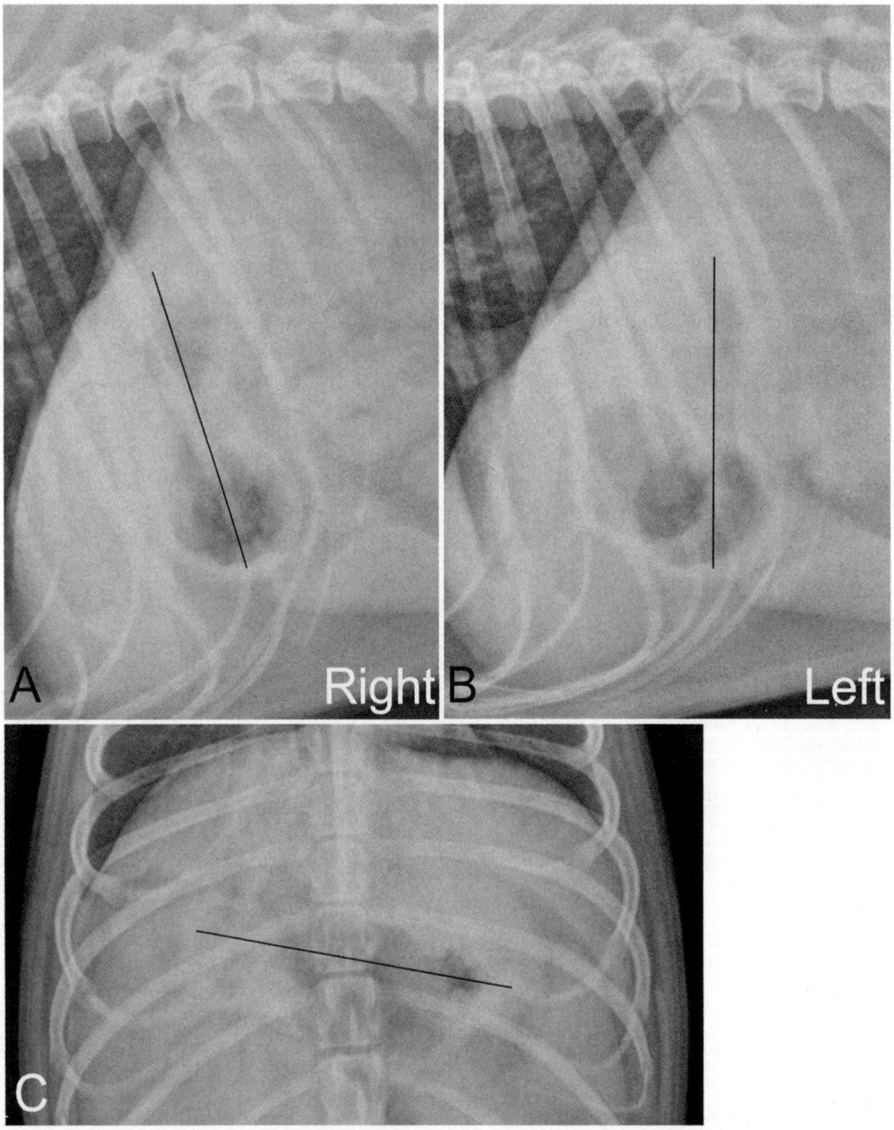

Fig. 45.2 Normal position of the gastric axis in different patient positions. **A,** Right lateral view of the abdomen of the dog. The gastric axis is parallel with the ribs. **B,** Left lateral view of the same dog. The gastric axis is perpendicular to the spine. **C,** Ventrodorsal view of the same dog. The gastric axis is mildly angled and nearly perpendicular to the spine.

stomach (see Fig. 45.2A) or located slightly cranial to the body of the stomach (see Fig. 45.2B). In VD radiographs, the long axis of the stomach is generally perpendicular to the spine with the stomach running transversely across the abdomen, making the angular notch difficult to identify (see Fig. 45.2C). On the VD view of the dog, the cardia, fundus, and body of the stomach are located to the left of midline, and the pyloric portions are located to the right of midline (Fig. 45.4A). The pyloric sphincter in the dog usually is located in the right cranial abdominal quadrant at approximately the level of the 10th or 11th rib and is usually cranial to the pyloric canal.[9] In immature dogs the pylorus may be located closer to midline than in adults.[10] Variations in the appearance of the stomach in the dog based on breed conformation have been described.[9] On the VD view of the cat, the stomach is more acutely angled compared to the dog, with the pylorus located at or near the midline (see Figs. 45.3B and 45.4B).

To understand the radiographic appearance of the stomach and movement of the gastric content when the position of the patient is altered, the stomach should be visualized as lying in a transverse plane with the fundus positioned dorsally on the left, and the pylorus ventrally on the right (eFig. 45.1). Thus, with a patient in ventral recumbency for a DV view, gas rises to the fundus, and fluid settles dependently to fill the pyloric portions and part of the gastric body (Fig. 45.5A, see eFig. 45.1A,B), whereas with a patient in dorsal recumbency for a VD view, fluid within the lumen follows gravity and settles dependently to the fundus and body of the stomach. Gas rises to the uppermost portion, which will be the pyloric antrum and the gastric body near midline (see Fig. 45.5B, eFig. 45.1C). On the left recumbent (right-left) lateral view (Figs. 45.5C and 45.6A), gas rises to the pyloric portion of the stomach, and fluid settles dependently in the fundus and body. A gas pocket may be trapped occasionally in the fundus in a left lateral view. The fundus and/or body may be difficult to see in a left lateral view because of the intraluminal fluid silhouetting with adjacent structures (see Fig. 45.6A). On the right recumbent (left-right) lateral view (see Figs. 45.5D and 45.6B), gas rises to the fundus and body, and fluid settles dependently to fill the pyloric portions and part of the body of the stomach. The fluid in the gastric body/antrum can create a round, circular, soft tissue attenuating area in the cranial abdomen (see Fig. 45.6B), which

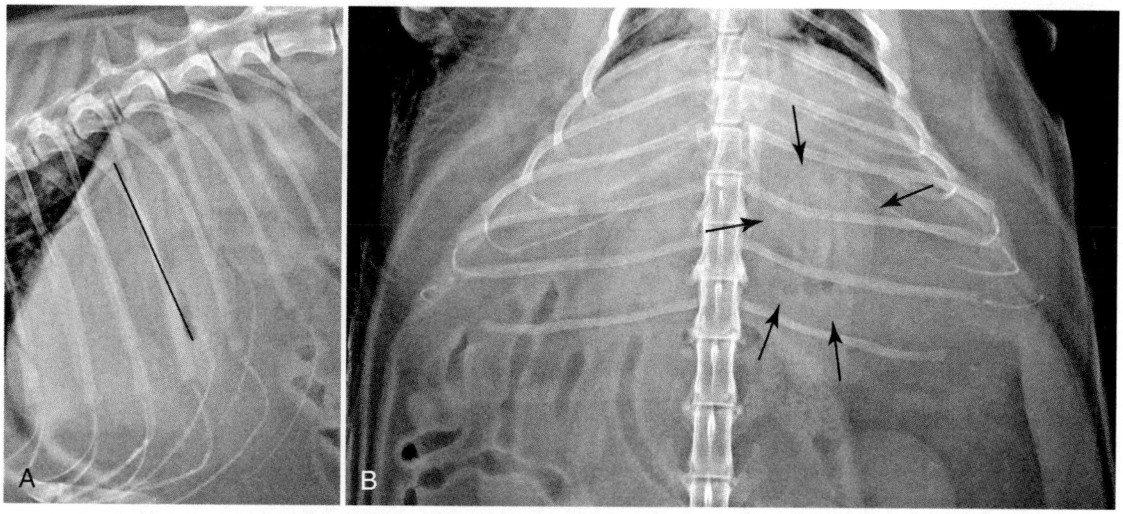

Fig. 45.3 Normal position of the stomach in a cat. **A,** Right lateral view of the abdomen of the cat. The gastric axis is parallel with the ribs. **B,** Ventrodorsal view of the same cat. The stomach (*arrows*) is acutely angled with the pylorus located on midline to slightly to the left of midline.

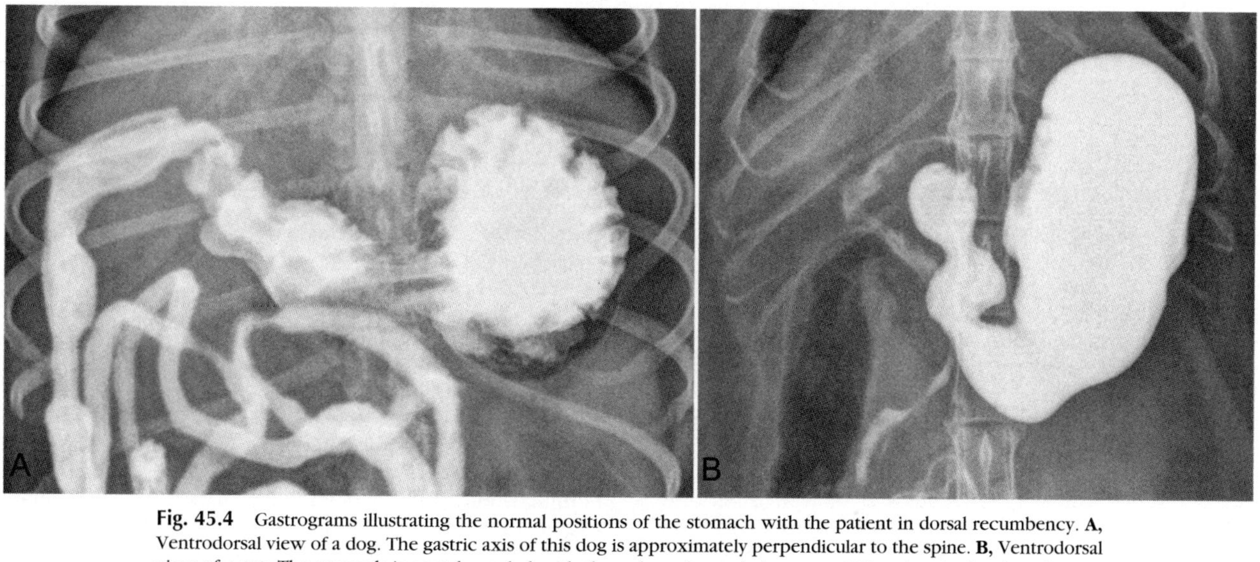

Fig. 45.4 Gastrograms illustrating the normal positions of the stomach with the patient in dorsal recumbency. **A,** Ventrodorsal view of a dog. The gastric axis of this dog is approximately perpendicular to the spine. **B,** Ventrodorsal view of a cat. The stomach is acutely angled with the pylorus located closer to midline than in the dog; this is a consistent species difference.

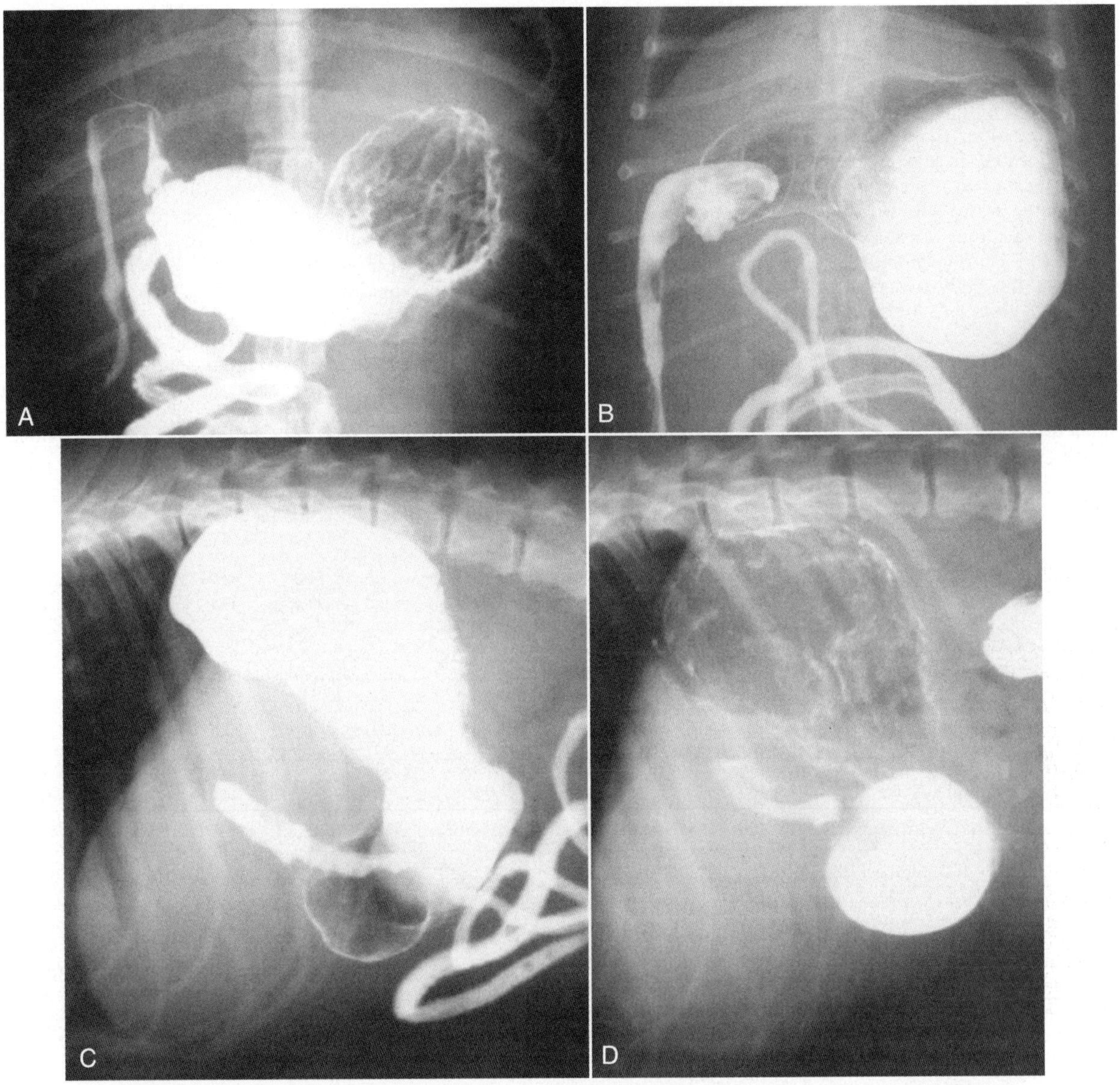

Fig. 45.5 Normal variations in fluid (barium) and gas distribution in the stomach with different patient positions. **A,** Dorsoventral view, in ventral recumbency. Gas rises to the fundus and fluid settles dependently to fill pyloric portions and part of the body. **B,** Ventrodorsal view, in dorsal recumbency. Gas is located in the body and pyloric antrum. Fluid settles dependently to fill the fundus and body. In this dog, there is a small amount of barium trapped in the pyloric antrum. **C,** Left lateral view. Gas rises to the pyloric portion, and fluid settles dependently to fill the fundus and body. **D,** Right lateral view. Gas rises to the fundus and body, when there is some barium adherent to the mucosa. Fluid settles dependently to fill the pyloric portion.

can be mistaken for a gastric foreign body or pathologic mass.[9,11] If a pyloric mass or foreign body is suspected on a right lateral view, a left lateral view should then be made to relocate gas to the pylorus to provide contrast.

Recognizing the variation in appearance of the normal stomach due to patient position and the volume and ratio of fluid to gas within the stomach is essential. The ability to take advantage of fluid and gas shifts within the stomach to highlight certain portions of the stomach more clearly is also important. Table 45.1 is a simplified summary of the expected changes in gas and fluid within the stomach due to change in patient position.

Rugal folds are seen inconsistently on survey radiographs. Radiographic assessment of rugal folds is subjective because they vary in size and number, and their appearance depends on the region of the stomach and degree of gastric distention.[8,12] Rugal folds are more tortuous in the nondistended stomach and become more uniform and parallel to the gastric curvature with increasing distention. Rugal folds may not be visible if the stomach is overdistended. Rugal folds are smaller and more spiral in the pyloric antrum.[8,13] A reference range for normal rugal fold thickness in dogs weighing 2 to 50 kg has been reported to be between 1 to 8 mm.[12] Rugal folds are smaller and fewer in number in cats than in dogs.[14] Additionally, a radiolucent line due to submucosal fat can often be seen normally in the gastric wall of the cat.[15]

Gastrography

Gastrography is often replaced by an abdominal ultrasound examination. However, due to gas in the stomach, the partial or complete intercostal location, or its large size, an ultrasound examination of the stomach might be limited and a contrast radiographic study may be needed to further evaluate the content and wall of the stomach. Furthermore, the evaluation

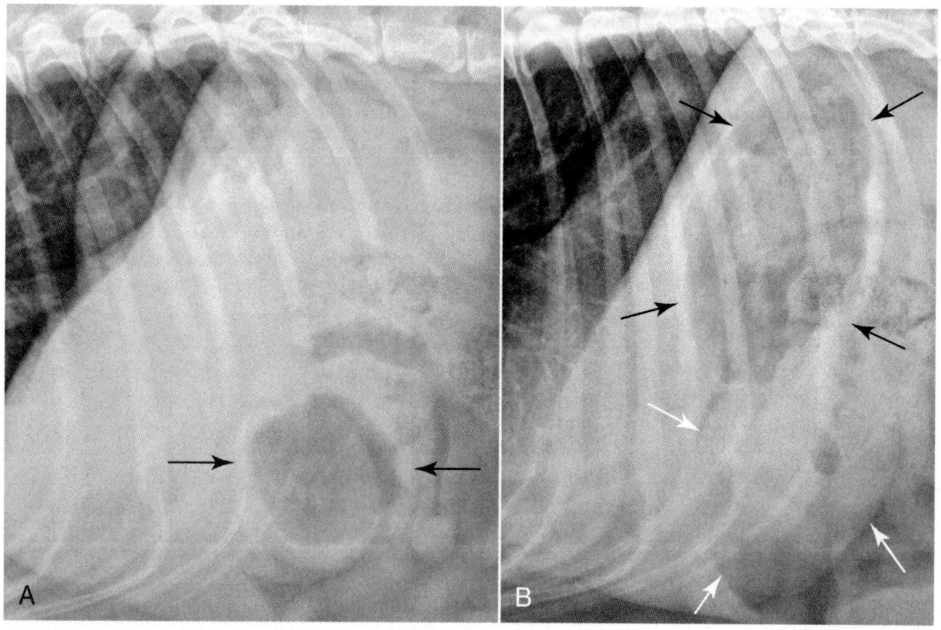

Fig. 45.6 Normal variation in fluid and gas distribution in the stomach as function of left versus right recumbency. **A,** Left lateral view. Gas rises to the pyloric portion (*black arrows*). In this dog, there is also some gas trapped in the fundus. Fluid settles dependently to the body, which is difficult to see. **B,** Right lateral view. Gas rises to fill the fundus and body (*black arrows*). Fluid settles dependently to the pyloric portion, which appears as a soft tissue mass (*white arrows*).

Table • 45.1

Distribution of Stomach Gas and Fluid as a Function of Radiographic Projection Using a Vertical X-Ray Beam.

RADIOGRAPHIC VIEW	LOCATION OF FLUID	LOCATION OF GAS
Dorsoventral	Body/pylorus	Fundus
Ventrodorsal	Fundus	Body (± pylorus)
Left recumbent lateral	Fundus	Pylorus (± body)
Right recumbent lateral	Pylorus	Fundus

of functional abnormalities of the stomach is typically performed with contrast radiography.

Survey radiographs should always be performed prior to a gastrogram. If possible, medications affecting gastric motility should be avoided or discontinued for an appropriate interval before any gastrointestinal contrast study is undertaken.[16–20] Contrast radiography of the stomach can be performed with negative- or positive-contrast media or a combination thereof. Positive-contrast radiography should not be performed or should be carried out with caution if the patient has unmanageable vomiting, suspected perforation of the gastrointestinal tract, or an evident need for surgery already noticeable on survey radiographs (Box 45.1).

Negative-Contrast Study of the Stomach (Pneumogastrography)

Negative-contrast studies of the stomach are rarely performed and are mainly used to assess for the presence of a gastric foreign body or to evaluate the position of the stomach. The benefit of negative-contrast gastrography is that endoscopy can follow immediately. However, if gastric ultrasound is planned, a pneumogastrogram is contraindicated as the air reduces the ability to evaluate the gastric wall and content.[21]

Technique for Pneumogastrography

A negative-contrast study of the stomach is performed by administering 6 to 12 mL of room air/kg body weight using an orogastric tube or by allowing the patient to drink carbonated liquid or orally administer a carbonated drink using a syringe. The stomach should palpate as moderately distended after the administration of air. The disadvantage of oral administration of carbonated liquid is that the stomach is often less distended and the additional fluid might conceal gastric lesions. Immediately after administering the gas, left lateral and VD views of the stomach should be obtained as these are usually the most diagnostic views to evaluate for pyloric outflow obstruction. These views should be followed by the other radiographic views.[21]

Positive-Contrast Gastrography

Various special contrast procedures using positive-contrast media or combinations of positive- with negative-contrast media are available to assess the stomach. They include conventional barium sulfate gastrography, low-volume gastrography, double-contrast gastrography, gastrography with iodinated contrast media, and gastric-emptying studies with barium/food or radiopaque marker/food mixtures.[6,9,10,13,14,17,22–30]

Technique for Positive-Contrast Gastrography

Patient preparation is extremely important when performing a diagnostic contrast study of the stomach. As mentioned before, food can mimic a gastric lesion and therefore the patient should be fasted for 12 to 24 hours. Orogastric intubation is recommended for all contrast studies of the stomach to reduce the risk of aspiration. Alternatively, the contrast medium can be placed in the buccal fold using a syringe or the patient can be given the opportunity to drink the contrast medium voluntarily,

Box • 45.1

Positive-Contrast Gastrogram With Barium Sulfate Suspension

- Fast for 12 to 24 hours without or with cleansing enemas.
  - Food in the stomach will interfere with interpretation of gastric emptying time.
  - Ingesta may also obscure foreign bodies or small gastric lesions.
  - Gastrograms performed with food in the stomach are difficult to interpret.
- If possible, perform radiography without the use of sedatives.
  - Motility-altering drugs such as antiemetics may interfere with interpretation.
  - If sedatives are required because of the fractious nature of the patient, use the lowest dose possible, and interpret gastric emptying times with caution.
- Perform survey radiographs to assess patient preparation, establish radiographic technique, and possibly identify the problem without gastrography.
  - If an evident need for surgery is evident on survey radiographs, do not pursue a positive-contrast study.
- Administer barium sulfate suspension by an orogastric tube with the patient on the x-ray table ready for radiography (cassette in position, technique set, etc.).
  - Barium powder mixed with water is not recommended.
  - If patient has unmanageable vomiting, do not administer barium as it causes risk of aspiration.
- If a perforation of the gastrointestinal tract is suspected, use nonionic iodinated contrast medium or discuss surgical avenues.
- The dosage of barium used for a gastrogram depends on why the study is being performed. The recommended dosage is 8 −12 mL barium/kg body weight for small and medium-sized dogs and 5−7 mL barium/kg body weight for large-sized dogs and 12−20 mL barium/kg body weight for cats. For simple location of the stomach, a very low dosage of 1−2 mL/kg can be used. If gastric emptying is of interest, the full dosage used for an upper gastrointestinal examination should be administered.
  - Feeding barium orally (i.e., without an orogastric tube) results in suboptimal distention of the stomach from emptying of the initial portions of barium before administration of the last portion.
  - Not administering enough barium is a common mistake.
  - Use caution to ensure that the orogastric tube is located in the esophagus, not the trachea.
    - Verify tube position by using fluoroscopy, survey radiograph, or palpation.
  - Before removing the tube, instill a small volume of air to clear the tube, then kink the tube before removal to prevent leakage of barium into the trachea.
- After removing the tube, immediately take radiographs centered over the stomach. All four views are recommended (right lateral, left lateral, dorsoventral, and ventrodorsal) and should be made as rapidly as possible.
- Additional radiographs (with or without obliques) should be made pending the results of the initial radiographs. If available, fluoroscopy is extremely helpful in the evaluation of gastrograms.
- Continue making radiographs (usually right lateral and ventrodorsal) until the majority of the barium is no longer seen within the stomach.
  - A small amount of residual barium coating the mucosa diffusely for several hours may be normal. Focal barium retention is suggestive of ulceration.
- The gastrogram may be combined with contrast evaluation of the small intestine.

which is easier when iodinated contrast media are used. After contrast medium administration, it has been recommended to gently turn the patient to achieve uniform coating of the gastric mucosa. Immediately after contrast medium administration, left lateral, right lateral, VD, and DV views of the stomach should be made, which are then usually followed by left recumbent lateral and VD views of the abdomen after 15 minutes, 30 minutes, 45 minutes, and 1 hour, 2 hours, 3 hours, 4 hours, or until complete emptying of the stomach content is present (Fig. 45.7A–L). See Box 45.1 for one method of performing a positive-contrast gastrogram. If an iodinated, water-soluble contrast medium is used to perform a gastrogram, it should always be remembered that these contrast media can be hyperosmolar and cause an influx of water, introducing potential for patient dehydration or, if aspirated, pulmonary edema. Therefore, when iodinated contrast media are used, an orogastric intubation should always be performed, if the patient does not voluntarily drink the iodinated contrast medium. Iodinated contrast media are used in a dose of 2 to 3 mL/kg body weight to achieve approximately 600 to 700 mg iodine (I) per kilogram body weight. If the contrast medium is diluted (1:4), the dose should be increased to 6 to 12 mL/kg body weight.[31]

Normal Positive-Contrast Gastrographic Findings

With positive-contrast gastrography, normal rugal folds are best seen at the peripheral portions of the stomach (see Fig. 45.7), where they may appear end-on as regular small filling defects at the mucosal surface. If projected en face, rugal folds are not visible with positive-contrast gastrography unless the barium is well penetrated by the x-ray beam, or there is only a small amount of barium in the stomach. Rugal folds then appear as relatively radiolucent, linear filling defects separated by barium in the interrugal spaces (eFig. 45.2).

After administration of barium, gastric emptying should start within 15 minutes in most normal patients.[9,32,33] During gastrography with barium sulfate, the stomach generally empties within 1 to 4 hours in dogs (see Fig. 45.7I–L).[12,17] Rapid emptying of the stomach has no clinical significance, whereas delayed emptying is potentially of much greater significance.

The rate of gastric emptying is a complex phenomenon that is affected by the volume of gastric content, the chemical and physical properties of chyme entering the duodenum, various reflex mechanisms, certain medications, and the type of contrast medium used. Thus, a standard approach must be used to evaluate the rate of gastric emptying radiographically. Because the stomach starts to empty faster with an increased

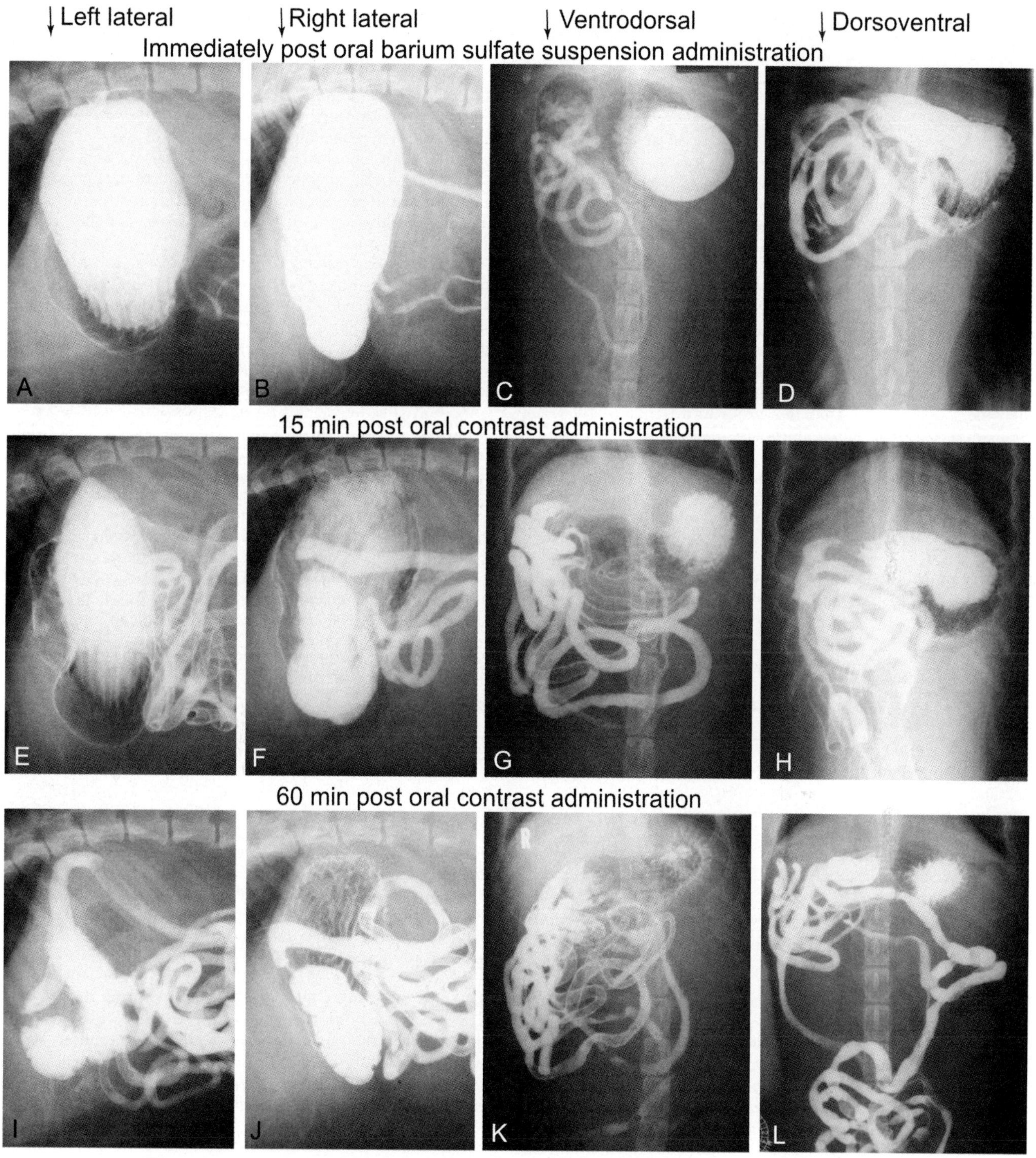

Fig. 45.7 Positive-contrast barium gastrography in a dog in different positions and with various time delays after contrast medium administration. Immediately **(A–D)**, 15 minutes **(E–H)**, and 60 minutes **(I–L)** after contrast medium administration. Continuous emptying of the stomach is noted with increasing time after contrast medium administration. **A, E, I,** Left lateral views. Most of the contrast medium is initially present in the gastric body and fundus. A small amount of gas is noted in the pylorus in the initial images, which is increasing 15 minutes after contrast medium administration and decreasing at 60 minutes with continuous emptying of the stomach. The pylorus is in part located cranial to the body of the stomach. **B, F, J,** Right lateral views. In the immediate image, the entire stomach is filled with contrast medium. In later images, gas is present in the fundus of the stomach and fluid is predominately present in the pylorus. The pylorus is summating ventrally with the body of the stomach. **C, G, F,** Ventrodorsal views. Most of the contrast medium in the stomach is in the fundus. A gas bubble is present in the body of the stomach. **D, H, L,** Dorsoventral views. Most of the contrast medium is in the body to pylorus of the stomach. Gas is present in the fundus of the stomach.

intraluminal volume, the dosage of contrast medium for a barium study must be standardized.[28] Low dosages may result in delayed gastric emptying, which leads to a false impression of pyloric obstruction or poor motility. If a standard technique has been used, and no medications that affect gastric emptying were administered, then delays in gastric emptying are likely related to psychological influences or disease at the pylorus. Emotional stress and noise may inhibit gastric movement.[34] Anxiety, fear, rage, or pain induced by physical manipulation of the patient, gastric intubation, and physical restraint may contribute to temporary delayed gastric emptying. Thus, patients with delayed gastric emptying must be allowed to calm down in a quiet environment before diagnostic significance is placed on this finding. For these reasons, minimal significance is usually placed on minor delays in gastric emptying if the stomach proceeds to empty normally after an initial delay.

Barium-food mixtures have been used to evaluate gastric function.[25,27] Emptying times for individual dogs were repeatable; however, the range of normal gastric emptying was so wide (7–15 hours) that this procedure is not useful for evaluation of gastric emptying unless gross abnormalities are present.[25] Gastric emptying times for dogs and cats can vary from 4 hours for high-moisture food to 16 hours for dry food.[8] An alternative technique for evaluating gastric emptying of solids in dogs and cats has been developed by using radiopaque barium-impregnated polyethylene spheres (BIPSs; Chemstock Animal Health Ltd., Christchurch, New Zealand) mixed with food.[23,26,30,35] The number and size of radiopaque spheres, type and amount of food, and fasting period must be standardized. An advantage of the BIPS technique is that it can be performed in most veterinary practices; however, it may require up to 10 hours to complete the study. Some controversy exists about the usefulness of BIPS for gastric emptying analysis, and these studies should be interpreted by a specialist.

Gastric peristalsis and gastric emptying may be observed directly during fluoroscopy with the use of a positive-contrast medium. Although a peristaltic contraction may be seen on a conventional radiograph during gastrography, this is a chance event depending on when the radiograph was made. A peristaltic contraction appears as an indentation of the wall of the stomach with slight dilation of the lumen immediately preceding the contraction. Peristaltic contractions are stronger and most obvious in the pyloric portion of the stomach.

Gastric Ultrasound

Indications

Ultrasound is a useful addition to radiography for evaluation of the gastrointestinal tract. It may eliminate the need for barium studies because gastric motility, wall thickness and architecture, and luminal contents may be evaluated sonographically.[36,37] In addition, ultrasound examination is quicker than an upper gastrointestinal series, not associated with electromagnetic radiation and may be equally sensitive and specific for detection of gastric disease. Ultrasound has been used to help diagnose gastric neoplasms,[38–44] inflammation or infection,[45,46] edema,[47] ulcers,[48] foreign bodies,[49,50] pyloric hypertrophy,[51] gastric mineralization,[52] gastroduodenal and gastrogastric intussusceptions,[53,54] gastric wall healing post surgery, and to evaluate gastropexy sites.[55–57] Additionally, fine needle aspirates and biopsies of the stomach can be obtained using ultrasound guidance.[42,58] Furthermore, new ultrasound techniques such as three-dimensional and endoscopic ultrasound are developing but limited in availability.[59] Endoscopic ultrasound combines the features of endoscopy with ultrasound to provide information about the gastroesophageal junction, gastric wall layers, and adjacent abdominal organs. The ability to perform the ultrasound in direct contact with the gastric wall using a high-frequency ultrasound probe allows the acquisition of high detail images.[60]

Ultrasound Technique

As a guideline for abdominal ultrasound, the highest frequency probe available and able to penetrate the area of interest should be chosen. For evaluating the stomach wall layers, 7.5 megahertz (MHz) or higher frequency transducers are preferred, but 5 MHz transducers may be needed to evaluate deeper portions of the stomach. Ideally, ultrasonography should be performed after a 12-hour fast and before barium is administered. If needed, intraluminal gas can be removed by an orogastric tube and the stomach distended with fluid to act as an acoustic window.[36,61] Technique and approaches to the stomach vary somewhat with patient conformation, position, and preference of the operator. Often, a dorsal or lateral recumbent position is chosen as a starting point. The stomach should be scanned in longitudinal and transverse planes and all aspects of the stomach from the cardia to the pylorus should be evaluated.[62] Most commonly, the ultrasound probe is positioned caudal the xiphoid and moved along the caudal aspect of ribs along the right and left abdominal wall to assess all aspects of the stomach. However, if the stomach is empty or cranially positioned, an intercostal approach to the stomach may be preferable. For the cardia a left craniodorsal and for the pylorus a right lateral intercostal approach may be chosen.[63] Gas and ingesta within the stomach may obscure the far wall and luminal content, but the lumen and far wall can be evaluated in patients in which the stomach contains fluid and little gas (Fig. 45.8A). Repositioning of the patient usually results in redistribution of luminal fluid and gas, allowing to evaluate most aspects of the stomach wall.[3,61]

Normal Ultrasonographic Findings

The appearance of the stomach varies with the amount of distention and the extent of luminal contents. When empty, the stomach may have a wagon-wheel appearance because of folding of the rugal folds (see Fig. 45.8B). This is especially noticeable in the cat. With increasing distention, rugal folds become less conspicuous. Under optimal ultrasound conditions, the five layers of the gastric wall are visible.[36] The innermost aspect of the gastric wall is hyperechoic and corresponds to the luminal surface of the mucosa, followed by the hypoechoic mucosa, the hyperechoic, thin submucosa, the hypoechoic muscularis, and the outermost hyperechoic subserosa/serosa (see Fig. 45.8). In the stomach, the mucosa and muscularis are often of similar thickness, which is different to the small intestine, where the mucosa is usually the thickest layer.[61] Sonographically, the cardia appears as a thick, tubular area at the border of the thoracic esophagus and fundus in the most left craniodorsal abdomen. All five wall layers of the cardia can be identified, with the muscularis being more prominent than the other layers.[38,64] The stomach wall thickness in dogs is 3 to 5 mm depending on the location and size of the dog, with larger dogs having a thicker stomach wall.[36] In cats, the rugal fold thickness has been reported as 2 to 5 mm, including the pylorus,[65,66] which is relatively similar to the dog. Sometimes, gastric wall thickness cannot be evaluated when the stomach is completely empty and the individual walls cannot be separated from each other. However, usually ingesta, fluid, and/or gas are present in the lumen of the stomach. Food can be difficult to differentiate from a foreign body and reevaluation of the patient may be necessary to see if the material in the stomach has changed over time. The mean number of peristaltic contractions observed in the stomach and proximal duodenum in dogs has been reported to be 4 to 5 per minute; however, with fasting of the patient (6 and 12 hours post prandial), lower mean contraction rates were observed.[36,37]

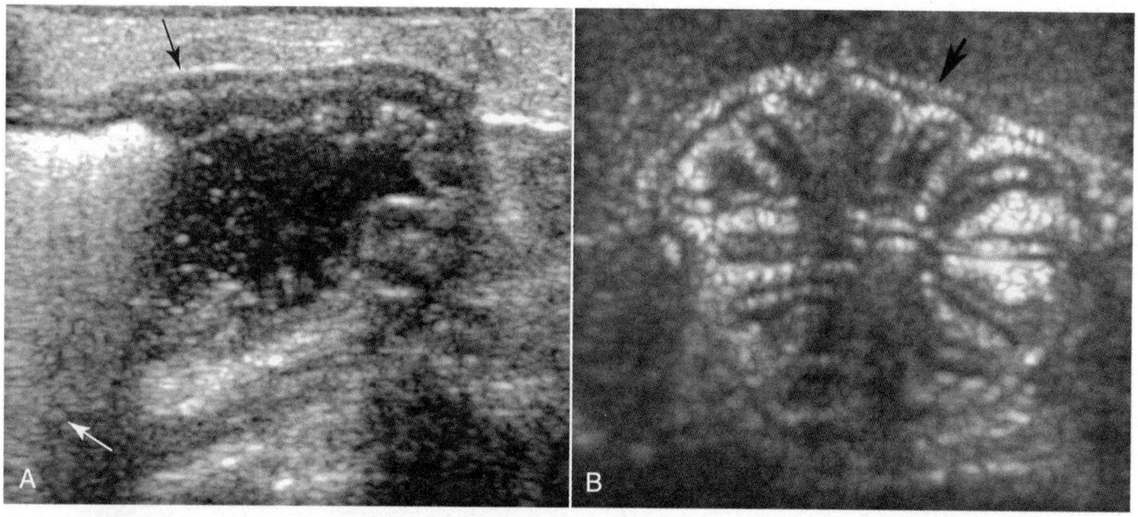

Fig. 45.8 Longitudinal ultrasound image of the stomach in a normal dog **(A)** and a normal cat **(B)**. **A,** The stomach is distended partially with gas and fluid. Gas in the lumen appears as a bright echo against the mucosal surface, producing reverberation artifact that prevents visualization of a portion of the far wall (region of *white arrow*). Fluid within the caudal half of the stomach provides a window for identification of the far wall. The five normal layers of the stomach wall can be identified as well as several rugal folds. The *black arrow* identifies the bright serosal layer. **B,** The stomach is empty and contracted, giving it a wagon-wheel appearance. The normal layered appearance of the stomach can be seen. The *black arrow* identifies the bright serosal surface. Caudal is to the *right,* and ventral is to the *top.*

Computed Tomography of the Stomach

CT is used commonly in people with gastrointestinal disease. In animals, CT is extensively used to evaluate the abdomen, but rarely used to evaluate the gastrointestinal tract. This difference is likely in part due to the difference in gas content of the gastrointestinal tract as well as the ease of intraluminal contrast medium administration in humans compared to companion animals, as well as the reduced access to CT compared with ultrasound in veterinary medicine. One of the benefits of CT is that intraluminal and extraluminal lesions of the stomach or gastrointestinal tract can be evaluated in the same procedure (Fig. 45.9A–D).

CT without intraluminal contrast medium administration has been used successfully in dogs and cats to evaluate the anatomy of the gastrointestinal tract,[67] to assess the gastrointestinal tract for the presence of wall lesions,[68,69] foreign bodies, or intestinal obstruction. However, if the stomach is collapsed or hyperattenuating intraluminal content is present, the gastric wall can appear artificially thickened or can only be incompletely evaluated. In human patients, the addition of intraluminal positive-contrast medium is considered a critical aspect of gastrointestinal CT scanning to distend the stomach and cause separation of the walls, allowing each wall to be evaluated individually. Conventional positive-contrast media such as barium sulfate and iodinated contrast medium formulations as well as neutral contrast media including water, milk, polyethylene glycol, etc., are commonly used in human patients to evaluate the gastrointestinal tract in CT studies. Hydro-CT, after orogastric tube administration of water and combining it with an intravenous iodinated contrast medium provided adequate distension of the stomach and allowed evaluation of the gastric wall in healthy dogs as well as in dogs and cats with suspected or diagnosed gastric neoplasia.[70]

Gastric Scintigraphy

Scintigraphy of the stomach is one of the least used imaging modalities in animals with gastrointestinal disease. Although nuclear medicine studies provide very limited or no information about gastric motility, they may be considered the gold standard for evaluating gastric emptying. Scintigraphy can be completed in 4 to 6 hours. However, even when using scintigraphy, there is high variability in gastric emptying or gastrointestinal transit times and this limits its clinical use.[19,71,72] Gastric emptying time is different in cats versus dogs as measured by BIPS compared with scintigraphy. Emptying times measured by BIPSs were also significantly longer relative to scintigraphy.[73,74] However, scintigraphy is of value when gastrointestinal bleeding is suspected.[75] The use of scintigraphy is limited by lack of access to scintigraphy equipment and the need for using radiopharmaceuticals, which require radiation safety precautions.[19,71,72]

GASTRIC DISEASES

Displacement

Displacement With Intact Diaphragm

The stomach is a valuable landmark in the cranial abdomen for identifying space-occupying lesions of surrounding structures such as the liver cranially, the spleen left laterally, and the pancreas caudally. If the diaphragm is intact, cranial displacement of the stomach relative to the diaphragm can occur only with a decrease in the size of the liver (Table 45.2, eFig. 45.3). It is important to realize that axial patient rotation can create the artefactual impression of microhepatia.

Because the stomach is in close apposition with the liver, changes in size or position of the liver usually cause a change in position of the stomach. Generalized hepatomegaly often produces caudal and dorsal displacement of the stomach.[76] This displacement may be asymmetric if caused by a mass.[76] However, because the cardia is relatively fixed, even generalized hepatomegaly produces a nonuniform displacement of the stomach. Thus, on the lateral view, generalized hepatomegaly often produces caudal and dorsal displacement of the pylorus and body of the stomach, but not the fundus. This displacement changes the axis of the stomach so that the axis

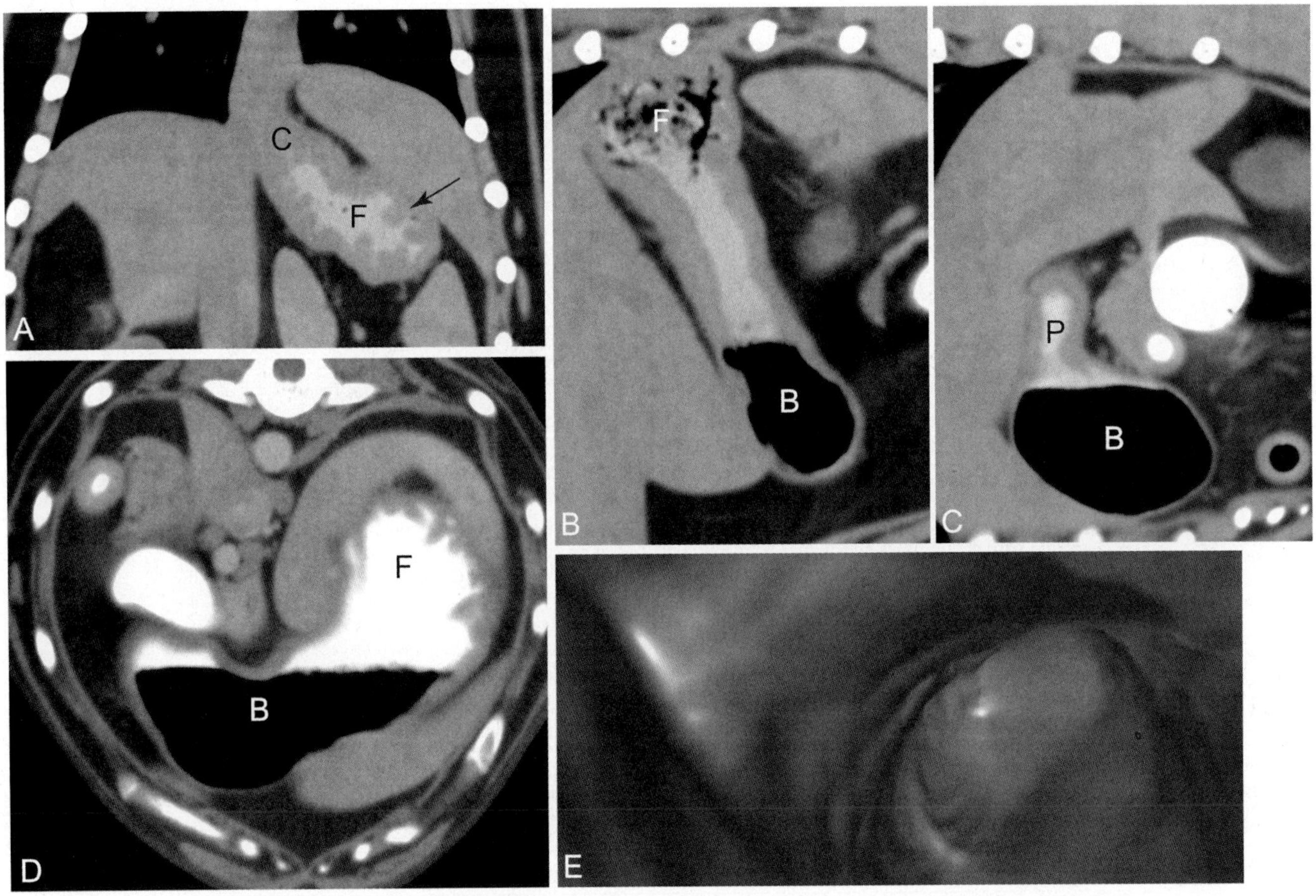

Fig. 45.9 Computed tomography (CT) images of the normal stomach of a dog after administration of iodinated contrast medium. The dog was in dorsal recumbency. **A,** Dorsally reformatted CT image of the stomach at the level of the cardia (*C*) to fundus (*F*). Normal rugal folds (*arrow*) are visible. **B,** Sagittally reformatted CT image of the stomach. The fundus (*F*) contains a small amount of contrast medium and gas. The body of the stomach (*B*) is gas filled. **C,** Sagittally reformatted CT image showing the smooth transition between the gas-filled body of the stomach and the contrast medium–filled pylorus (*P*). The gastric wall is thin and smooth, which is most noticeable in the mildly distended and gas-filled body of the stomach. **D,** Transverse CT image of the stomach. The fundus is contrast medium filled. The body of the stomach, which is the upper most aspect of the stomach with the dog in dorsal recumbency, contains a gas bubble. **E,** Virtual endoscopic image of the body of the stomach reconstructed from CT images. The wall of the body of the stomach is mildly folded and smooth outlined, similar to the CT images.

is no longer parallel with the ribs (Fig. 45.10A). On the VD or DV view, generalized hepatomegaly often causes displacement of the gastric body and pylorus caudally and toward the left (see Fig. 45.10B). This displacement changes the axis of the stomach so that it is no longer transverse. The assessment of gastric displacement as an indicator of liver size becomes especially valuable when the liver is not visible because of emaciation or abdominal effusion. In such patients, air in the stomach can often be used to define the axis of the stomach. A small volume of room air or barium may also be given to clarify the gastric axis if it cannot be assessed from the survey radiographs.

Abdominal masses that originate caudal to the stomach do not displace the stomach cranially because of the presence of the liver. Instead, such masses may distort the shape of the stomach as they press against and indent the stomach, or they may displace the stomach to the right or left. The relation of an abdominal mass to the stomach is often of value in helping define whether the mass originates in the liver, spleen, or pancreas (Fig. 45.11).

Displacement With Rupture or Hernia of the Diaphragm

Cranial displacement of the stomach may occur secondary to traumatic rupture of the diaphragm, that is, an acquired diaphragmatic hernia (Fig. 45.12), or secondary to a congenital hernia of the diaphragm and/or an abnormality of the gastroesophageal junction. These abnormalities can result in herniation of the liver, part of the liver, or the stomach into the thorax. Even if the stomach may not pass through a diaphragmatic hernia, the position of the stomach is an important consideration in patients suspected of having an acquired or congenital diaphragmatic hernia. A cranial shift of the axis of the stomach may help define whether the liver has herniated cranially through the diaphragm. Diseases of the diaphragm are discussed in more detail in Chapter 32.

Acquired Traumatic Hernia (Traumatic Diaphragmatic Rupture). Traumatic injuries to the diaphragm are commonly seen after vehicular trauma or high-rise injury in companion animals.[77] Dependent on the extent of injury to the diaphragm, gastric displacement may occur.[78] Rarely, a

Table • 45.2

Differential Diagnosis for Changes in Position of the Stomach.

NORMAL POSITION OF THE STOMACH	CRANIAL POSITION OF THE STOMACH			CAUDAL POSITION OF THE STOMACH	
Diaphragm intact	Diaphragm intact	Diaphragmatic hernia or rupture	Abnormal gastroesophageal junction	Caudal displacement of the diaphragm	Diaphragm intact, enlarged liver
Dependent on • Conformation of the patient • Gastric content • Gastric filling stage	Small liver (portosystemic shunt, cirrhosis)	Cranial displacement of the liver and/or gastrointestinal tract into the thorax • PPDH (peritoneopericardial diaphragmatic hernia) • Diaphragmatic rupture (acquired)	• Hiatal hernia	• Pneumothorax • Pleural fluid • Hyperinflation • Thoracic masses	• Generalized liver enlargement • Caudal displacement of the stomach, often asymmetric displacement
	Empty stomach	Cranial displacement of the stomach into the thorax	• Gastroesophageal intussusception		• Right liver lobe enlargement • Caudal and dorsal displacement of pylorus • Left liver lobe enlargement • Medial displacement of the fundus and body of the stomach

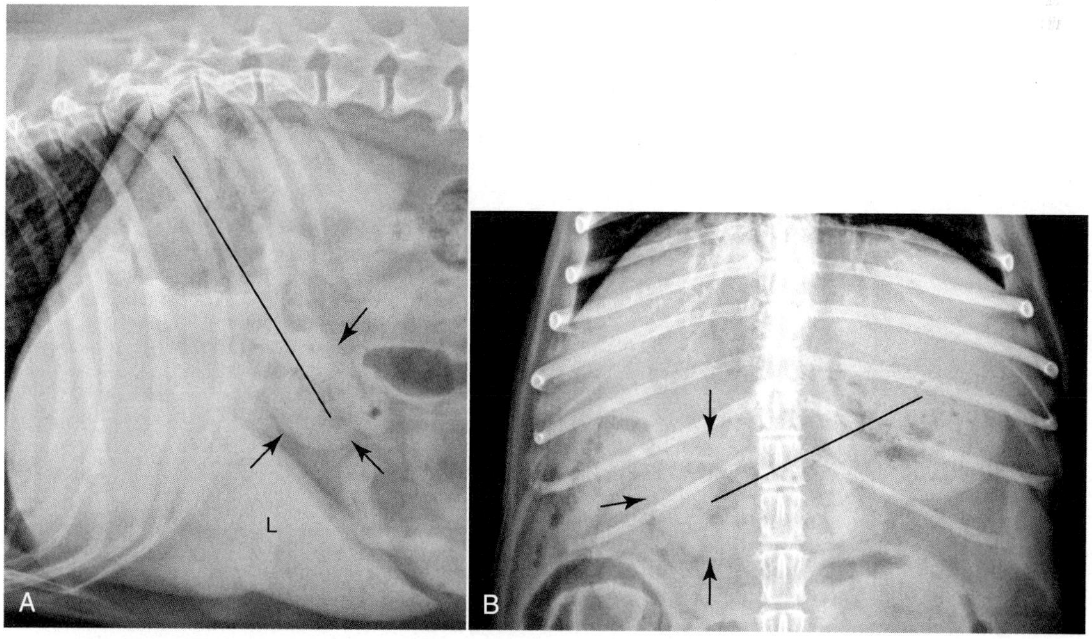

Fig. 45.10 Gastric displacement caused by hepatomegaly. **A**, Lateral view. The pylorus (*black arrows*) is displaced caudally by an enlarged liver (*L*), and the fundus-pylorus axis (*black line*) is no longer parallel with the ribs. **B**, Ventrodorsal view. The pylorus (*black arrows*) is displaced caudally and to the left, and the fundus-pylorus axis (*black line*) is no longer transverse.

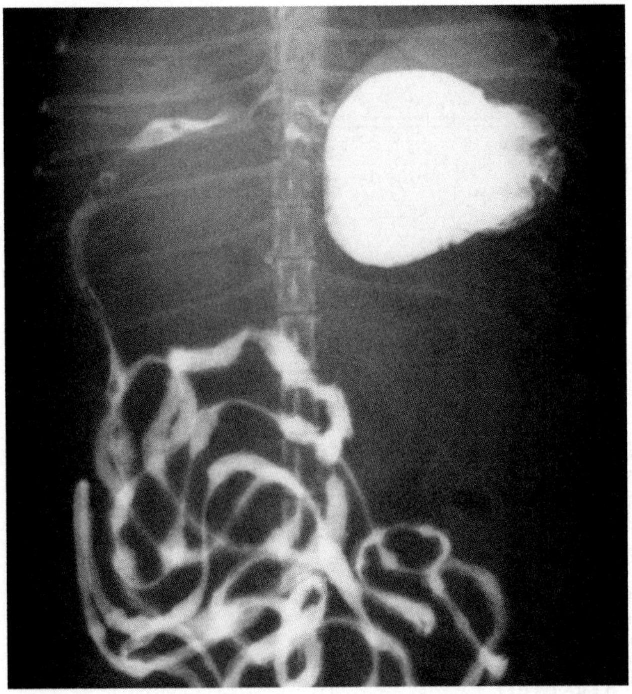

Fig. 45.11 Ventrodorsal radiograph of a dog with a large pancreatic abscess. Barium has been administered. The pylorus is displaced to the left and cranially. The cranial duodenal flexure and proximal part of the descending duodenum have a broad arc around the cranial surface of the mass, which itself is not visible.

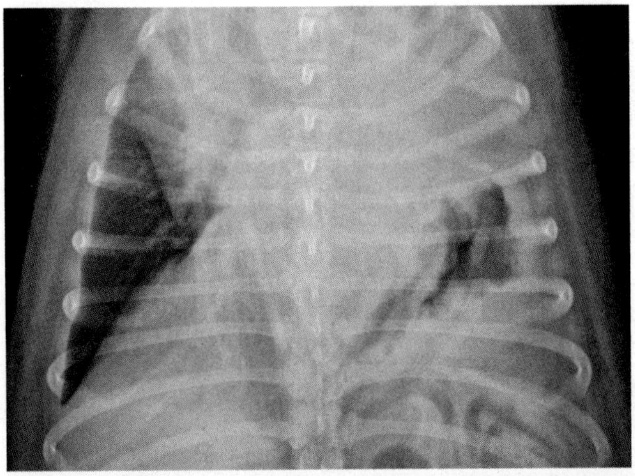

Fig. 45.12 Ventrodorsal radiograph of a dog with an acquired left-sided diaphragmatic hernia (rupture) that has allowed the fundus to shift cranially. Although there are no gas-containing bowel segments in the pleural space, the cranial position of the stomach is diagnostic for a diaphragmatic rupture.

"gastrothorax" may occur, where the stomach is displaced into the thorax and becomes markedly gas distended leading to increased pressure similar to a tension pneumothorax (Fig. 45.13). Radiography can help to differentiate between these two entities. In gastrothorax a large air-filled structure with or without an air–fluid interface is present in the thorax causing peripheral compression of the adjacent lung, obliterating the diaphragm and causing mediastinal shift. A curvilinear cranial outline is often visible. Similar radiographic features may also be noted in tension pneumothorax, but in tension pneumothorax, often the diaphragm can be outlined, while in gastrothorax, usually a left-sided loss of visualization of the diaphragm may be noted.[79] If it is unclear if the stomach is displaced cranially, a small amount of positive-contrast medium can be given to identify the location of the stomach or horizontal beam views may demonstrate a fluid–air interface in the lumen of the stomach. Alternatively, a gastric tube can be placed to release the air in the stomach and repeat radiographs should demonstrate decreased air filling of the displaced stomach.[79] It is important to remember that patients with an acquired traumatic hernia often suffer from significant other additional trauma to vital structures and stabilization of the patient before performing imaging studies is critical.

Hiatal or Peritoneopericardial Diaphragmatic Hernia. Hiatal hernia is common and results in cranial displacement of abdominal organs due to a defect in the esophageal hiatus.[80] Hiatal herniation depends on the size and location of the defect and results in cranial displacement of the gastroesophageal junction (sliding hernia or type 1 hiatal hernia) or cranial displacement of part of the stomach, usually the fundus, lateral to the esophagus with the gastroesophageal junction usually in a normal location (paraesophageal hernia or type 2 hiatal hernia) or a combination of the type 1 and 2 hiatal hernia (type 3 hiatal hernia).[81] Sliding hernias are the most common hiatal hernia in dogs and cats.[80] In patients with hiatal hernia, a cranial position of the stomach might be noted radiographically. Additionally, a soft tissue mass effect might be present in the caudodorsal thorax (Fig. 45.14). Sliding hernias can be a challenge radiographically as the stomach might not be displaced cranially at all times (see Fig. 45.14A). Obtaining radiographs after placing pressure on the abdomen or stimulating coughing to increase the abdominal pressure might help to identify the cranial position of the stomach or abdominal viscera (see Fig. 45.14C). If the stomach cannot be distinctively outlined, a low volume barium gastrogram can be performed to localize the position of the stomach.

Peritoneopericardial diaphragmatic hernia (PPDH) is an uncommon congenital malformation. A ventral communication between the abdomen and pericardial sac is present, which can result in cranial displacement of the stomach and/or other abdominal organs into the pericardial sac (Fig. 45.15).[82]

Gastroesophageal Intussusception. Gastroesophageal intussusception is uncommon and results from invagination of the stomach, with or without other abdominal organs, into the esophagus. This is only possible if a predisposing condition such as megaesophagus, dilation of the esophageal sphincter, or chronic vomiting is present. This is a surgical emergency as obstruction of vascular flow to the stomach leads to rapid decline of the patient. On radiographs a large well-defined soft tissue mass is usually present in the caudal esophagus with gas in a dilated esophagus cranial to the mass. Additionally, rugal folds might be visible at the cranial margin of the soft tissue mass due to the eversion of the gastric mucosa into the esophagus. The stomach or part of stomach is absent on abdominal radiographs.

Displacement Within the Stomach

Pylorogastric Intussusception. Pylorogastric intussusception is rarely seen in dogs and has so far not been reported in the cat. Other terms used for pylorogastric intussusception include gastrogastric or duodenogastric intussusception. Dogs with pylorogastric intussusception have ranged in age from 3 months to 15 years and there was no breed or size predilection. Radiographically, distension of the stomach and a large mass effect extending luminally into the pylorus to fundus area may be noted (Fig. 45.16). On ultrasound examination, displacement of the pylorus and duodenum into the pyloric antrum and fundus can be noted. Additionally, multiple concentric rings of hyperechogenicity and hypoechogenicity, resembling the intussuscepted gastric wall layers, thickening of

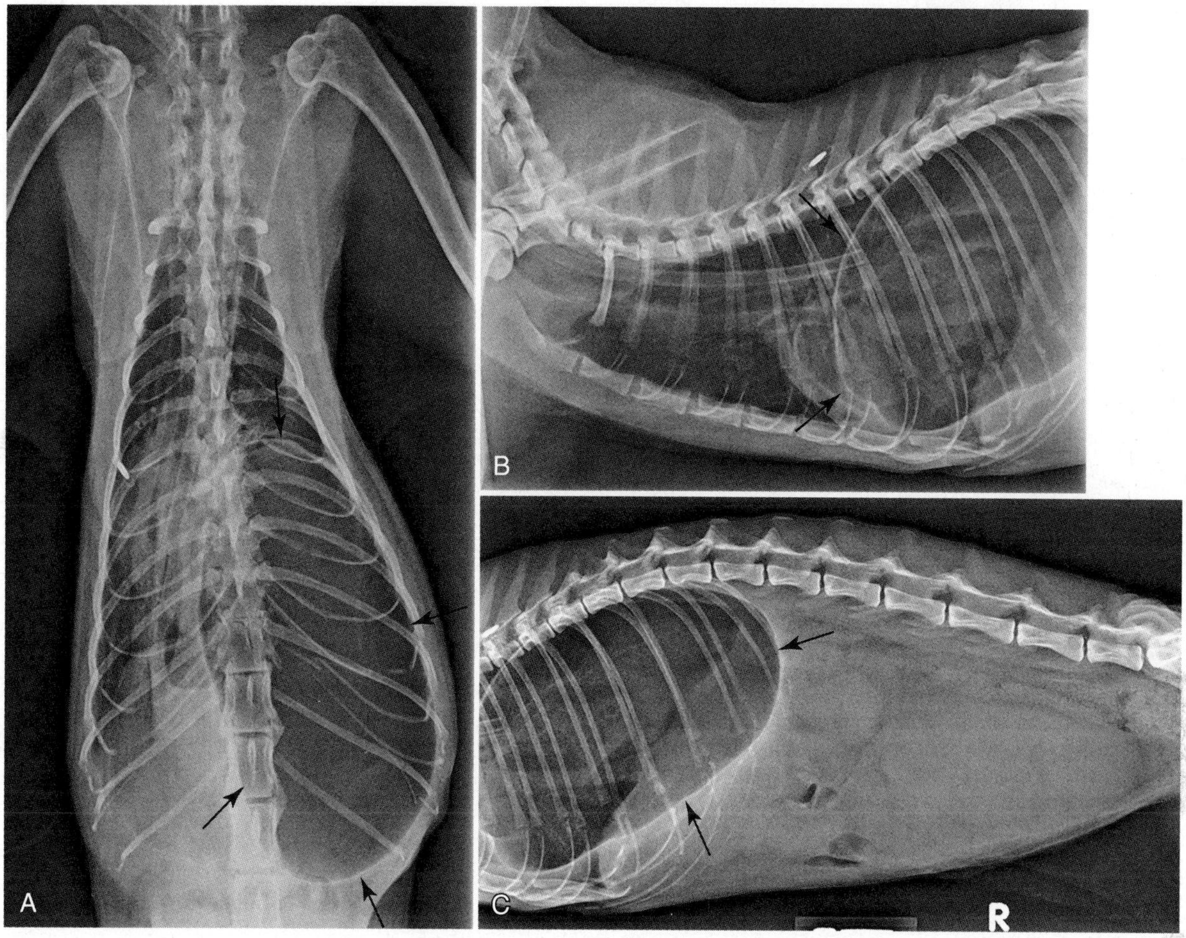

Fig. 45.13 Gastrothorax in 12-year-old cat secondary to a diaphragmatic rent which likely occurred when the cat was approximately 1-year-old and had a vehicular accident. Multiple prior thorax radiographs showed the stomach in normal position and size. Dorsoventral **(A)**, right lateral radiograph of the thorax **(B)**, and right lateral radiograph of the abdomen **(C)**. **A–C,** The stomach (*black arrows*) is severely gas distended and displaced cranially into the left hemithorax causing cranial and medial displacement of the left lung lobes. A normal left crus of the diaphragm is in the current study not seen. An esophageal feeding tube is present in thoracic esophagus. **C,** The stomach (*black arrows*) is not identified in the abdomen.

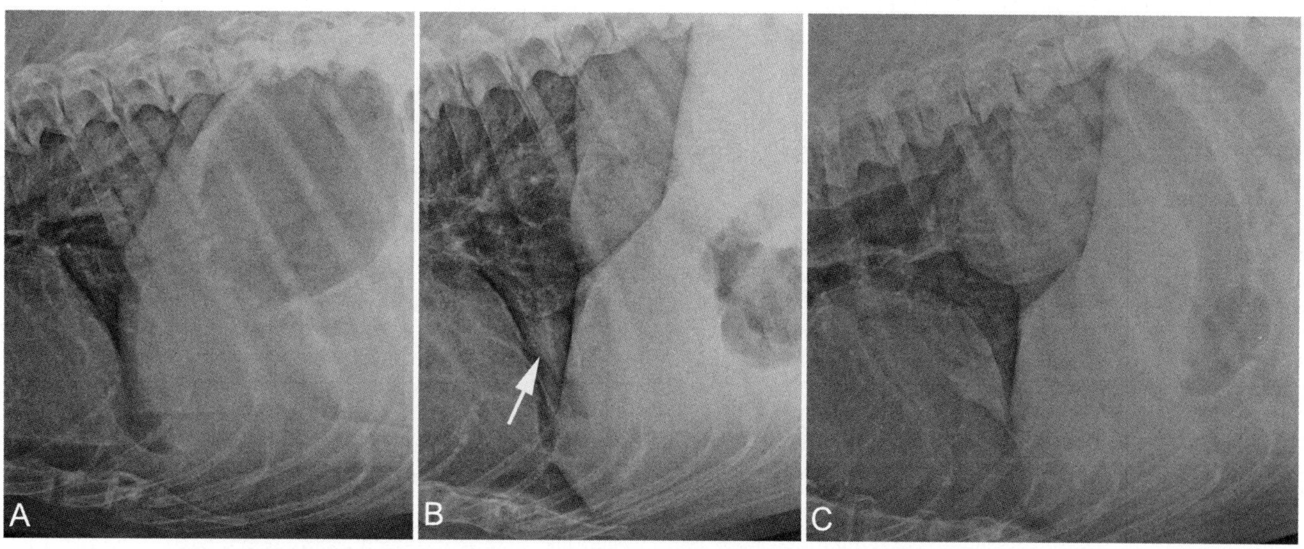

Fig. 45.14 Sliding hiatal hernia (type 1 hiatal hernia) in dog, which was presented for further evaluation of a previously detected right caudal lung mass. **A,** Right lateral radiograph. The stomach is in a normal position. **B,** Left lateral radiograph. The stomach is cranially positioned, but persistently summating mostly with the left crus of the diaphragm. The rugal folds are well visualized helping to identify the soft tissue structure as the stomach. A lung mass is noted in the ventral aspect of the right caudal lung lobe (*white arrow*). **C,** Left lateral radiograph after the dog coughed. The fundus and part of the body of the stomach are displaced cranially into dorsocaudal thorax. The esophagus and descending duodenum are dilated and gas filled.

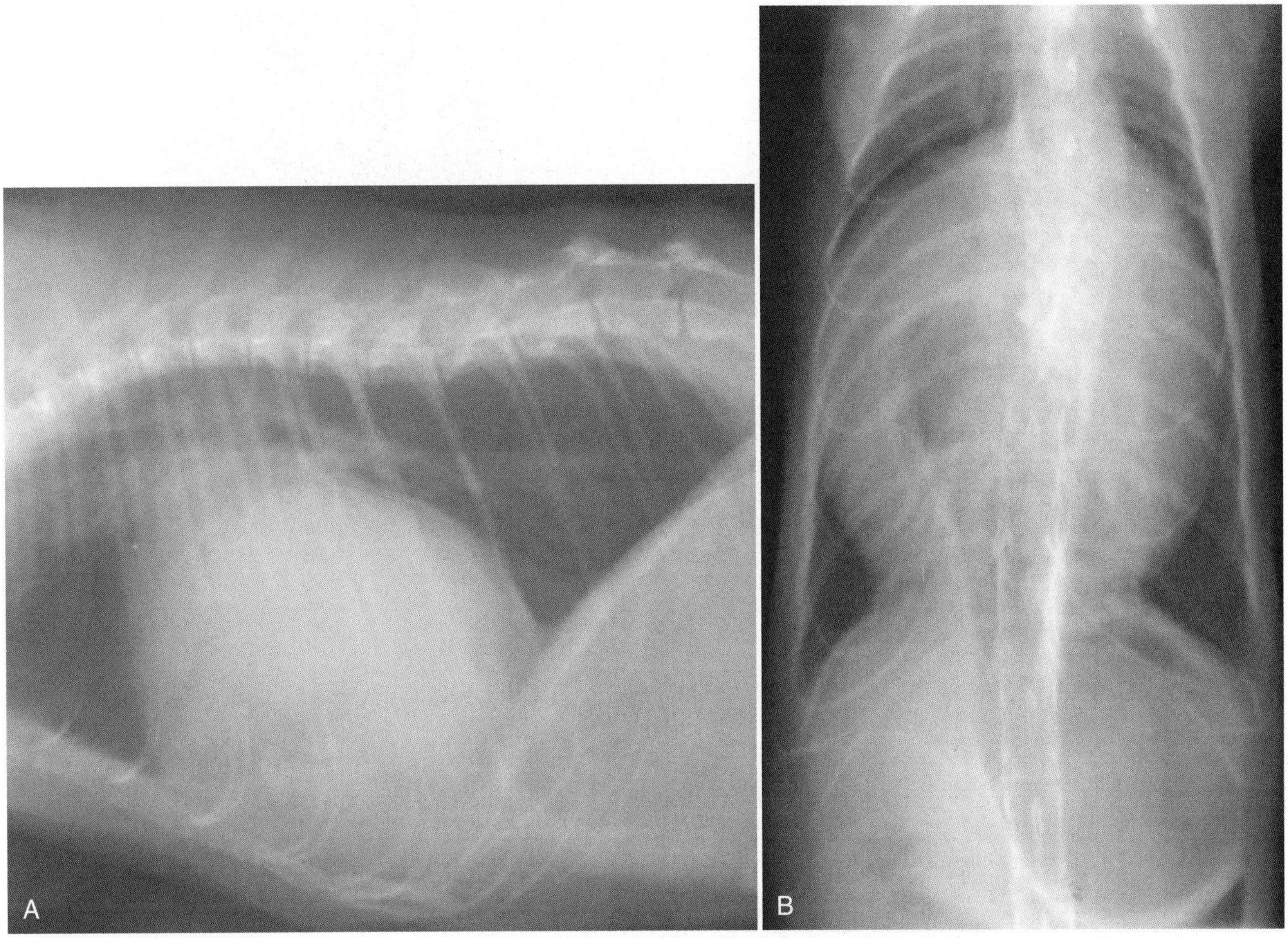

Fig. 45.15 Peritoneopericardial hernia in a cat. **A,** Right lateral radiograph. The cardiac silhouette is enlarged and has an irregular shape. Irregular gas opacities are summating with the cardiac silhouette. Effacement of the ventral diaphragmatic border is present. A large region of gas is superimposed on the liver. The thoracic spine has an undulating shape. **B,** Dorsoventral radiograph. The pylorus and part of the body of the stomach are displaced cranially and located within the pericardium.

the gastric wall with or without loss of wall layering, or a mass effect extending into the lumen of the fundus may be present.[53,83,84]

CHANGES IN GASTRIC SHAPE AND SIZE

Acute Gastric Dilation

Acute gastric dilation and gastric volvulus produce gaseous distention of the stomach. Although both fluid and gas are present in the stomach, gaseous distention is the predominant abnormality in these conditions.

Acute gaseous distention of the stomach may be attributable to a variety of causes and can be caused by aerophagia as a result of severe dyspnea (eFig. 45.4) or pain. With acute gastric dilation, the stomach is enlarged and is filled primarily with gas but retains its normal position and anatomic relations (Fig. 45.17, eFig. 45.5). Thus, the pylorus is still located ventrally on the right and the fundus dorsally on the left. The normal position of the stomach can usually be verified by comparing right vs. left lateral views, evaluating the position of the stomach in a VD view. Recognition of the pylorus of a distended stomach is usually easier on lateral views than on the VD or DV view. Contrast gastrography may help in this localization but is usually not necessary.

Large quantities of free peritoneal gas tend to accumulate in the cranial abdomen in a lateral view, which can leave the impression of a gas-filled, round structure (Fig. 45.18). This abdominal gas bubble should not be confused with a gas dilated stomach or gastric volvulus and close attention should be paid to identify the correct position of the stomach and for the presence of abdominal gas. Positional radiographs can further help to identify the presence of gas in the abdomen and help to outline the correct position of the stomach.

Gastric Dilation Volvulus

Gastric dilation volvulus (GDV) is a life-threatening condition and is differentiated from acute gaseous gastric dilation by the presence of gastric malpositioning in addition to pathologic gas distension. The cause of GDV is not completely understood; however, a variety of predisposing factors have been identified, including large-breed dog, increasing age, increased thoracic depth–to–height ratio, thin body condition, food volume, gastric foreign body, and splenectomy.[85–90] GDV has been reported in a dog as young as 5 weeks of age.[91] Although rare, a similar condition has been reported in the cat.[92] In the cat and small brachiocephalic dogs, a diaphragmatic hernia may be present as a predisposing factor.[93,94]

The radiographic appearance of the stomach varies depending on the type and degree of rotation and the amount

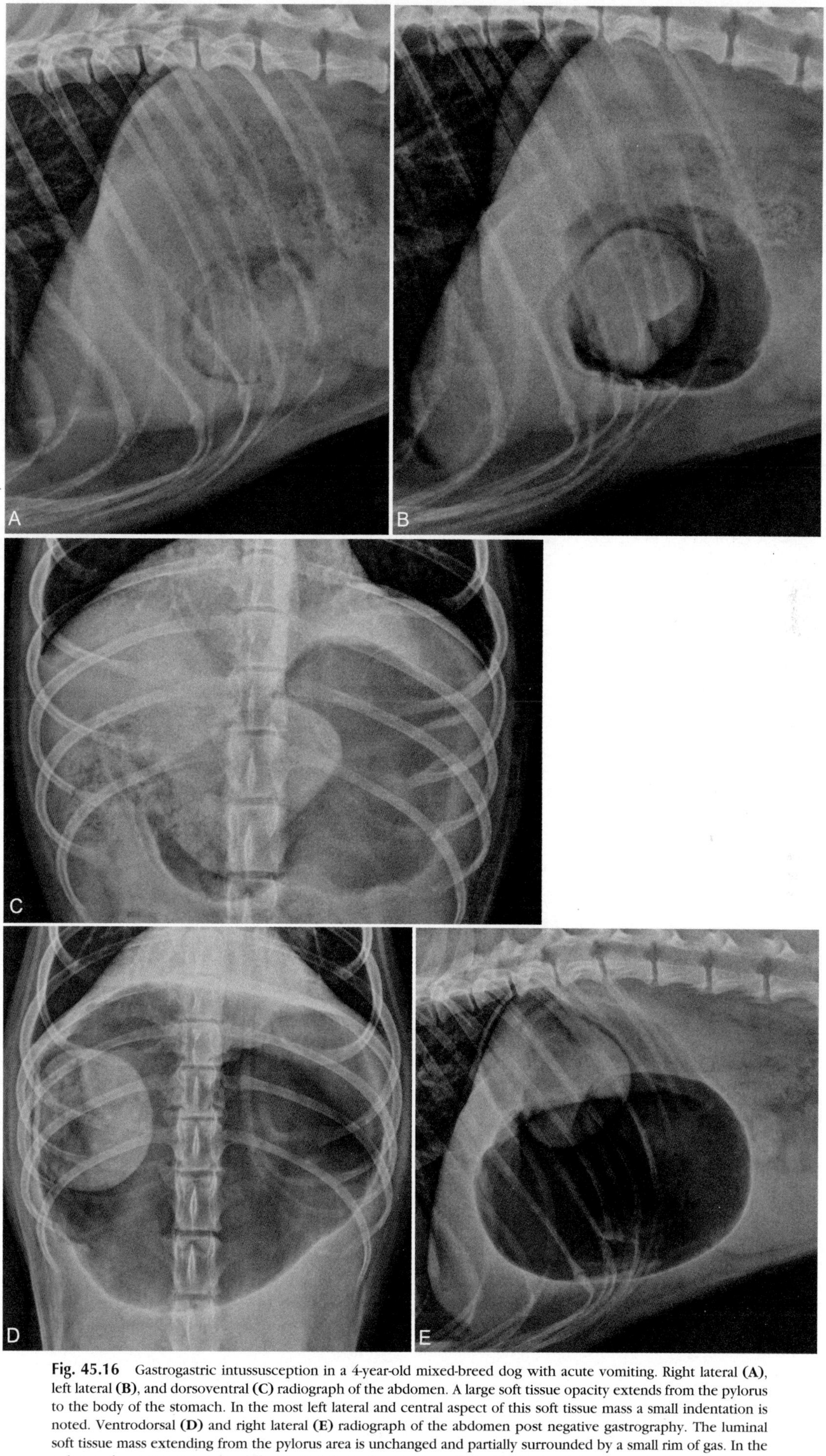

Fig. 45.16 Gastrogastric intussusception in a 4-year-old mixed-breed dog with acute vomiting. Right lateral **(A)**, left lateral **(B)**, and dorsoventral **(C)** radiograph of the abdomen. A large soft tissue opacity extends from the pylorus to the body of the stomach. In the most left lateral and central aspect of this soft tissue mass a small indentation is noted. Ventrodorsal **(D)** and right lateral **(E)** radiograph of the abdomen post negative gastrography. The luminal soft tissue mass extending from the pylorus area is unchanged and partially surrounded by a small rim of gas. In the pylorus, the mass cannot be differentiated from the gastric wall. In the body of the stomach, the mass is well differentiated from the gastric wall. Surgery confirmed a gastrogastric intussusception, in which the antrum of the stomach extended into the body of the stomach. The duodenum was not involved in the intussusception. (Courtesy DoveLewis Emergency Animal Hospital, Portland, Oregon.)

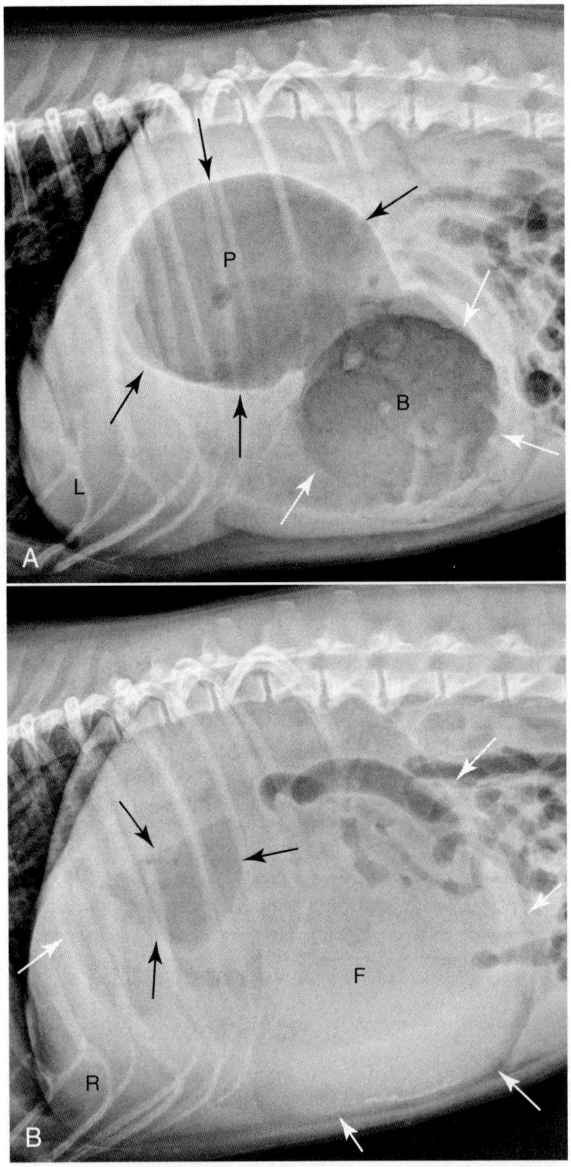

Fig. 45.17 Gastric dilation without volvulus. **A,** Left lateral view. Gas is present in the pyloric antrum (*P, black arrows*) and body (*B, white arrows*) of the stomach as expected. The narrowing between the body and pyloric antrum is a peristaltic contraction. **B,** Right lateral view. The fundus (*F, white arrows*) is extremely distended. There is a small amount of gas trapped in the pyloric antrum (*black arrows*). The distribution of gas as a function of left versus right recumbency is as expected in a normal subject, indicating that the stomach is not rotated, unless the rotation is 360 degrees, which is unusual.

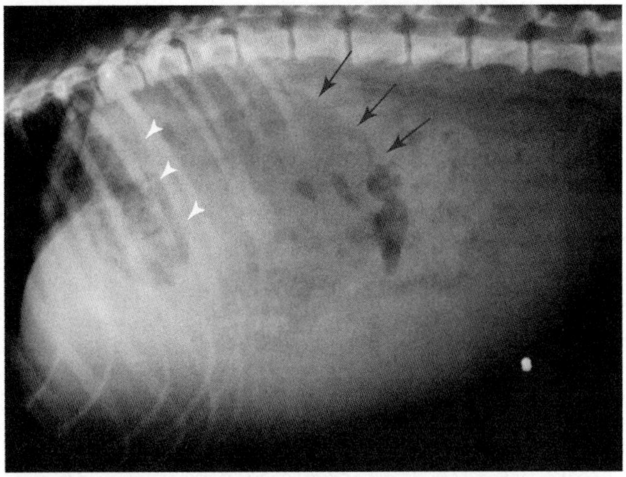

Fig. 45.18 Severe pneumoperitoneum secondary to intestinal perforations due to ballistic trauma. Left lateral radiograph. A large, round ovoid gas opacity is present in the cranial abdomen (*black arrows*). This should not be confused with acute dilation or volvulus of the stomach. The stomach is located in correct position in the cranial abdomen (*white arrowheads*), easily identified by the presence of rugal folds. The lack of serosal detail is secondary to the presence of peritoneal fluid due to severe chronic peritonitis.

of distention.[95,96] As the stomach dilates, the fundus and greater curvature rotate clockwise, when viewed from caudal to cranial, to lie along the ventral abdominal wall. The pylorus therefore shifts dorsally, cranially, and to the left, and the body of the stomach shifts toward the right. Because of the attachments of the proximal extremity of the spleen to the stomach, the spleen often follows the greater curvature toward the right.

The main radiographic features of GDV are:

- Gas and fluid distension of the stomach (more gas than fluid).
- The pylorus is displaced dorsally and to the left (unless a 360-degree torsion is present).
- With the patient in left lateral recumbency, fluid in the stomach fills the pylorus and gas fills the rest of the stomach.
- With the patient in right lateral recumbency, gas fills the pyloric portion and fluid shifts to the fundus or body of the stomach (Fig. 45.19, eFig. 45.6).
- The pylorus and duodenum are displaced to the left in the VD/DV projections.
- Compartmentalization is a term that refers to the radiographic appearance of soft tissue bands that project into or across the gas-filled lumen of the rotated stomach. These soft tissue bands result from folding of the stomach on itself as the folded wall projects into the lumen and is outlined by gas within the lumen. These bands may become more obvious with greater degrees of distention and are best seen in the right lateral view (see Fig. 45.19).
- The spleen is also often malpositioned in patients with GDV, and may be compromised because of impaired circulation (see Fig. 45.19). Outright torsion of the spleen may also occur; this further compromises the patient. The greater the gastric distention, the less likely the spleen is to be visualized radiographically because of crowding.
- Paralytic ileus of the small intestine, esophageal dilation, a reduced size of the caudal vena cava, and microcardia and small pulmonary vessels associated with shock may be present to variable degrees.
- The pylorus and fundus may be in a normal position in a 360-degree volvulus. Secondary signs of GDV as outlined earlier as well as inability to pass a tube are suggestive of a 360-degree rotation (Fig. 45.20).
- Gas within the gastric wall, termed *pneumatosis*, can occur but is infrequent (Fig. 45.21, eFig. 45.7).[9] Gastric pneumatosis in combination with GDV has a high specificity but a low sensitivity for predicting gastric wall necrosis.[97] Spontaneous pneumoperitoneum should also raise concern for the possibility of gastric necrosis. Prior trocharization of the stomach will complicate assessing the significance of pneumatosis or pneumoperitoneum. Overall, radiographs are a poor predictor of gastric wall necrosis in patients with gastric volvulus.
- Gastric volvulus may also be present without severe gastric distention. This situation may often exist for days or weeks after previous gastric decompression[98] or may be present at the time of initial presentation.[32]

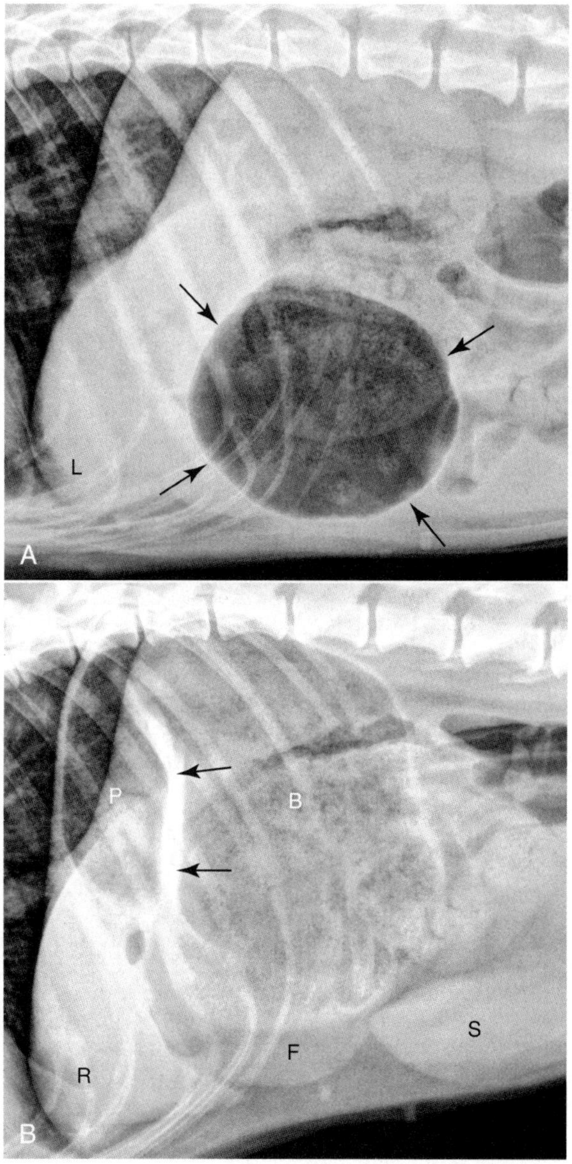

Fig. 45.19 Gastric volvulus. **A,** Left lateral view. The stomach is moderately distended with gas in the fundus (*black arrows*). This is easily misinterpreted as gas in the pylorus, as expected in the left lateral view. **B,** Right lateral view. The fluid shifts into the fundus (*F*), and gas outlines the pyloric portion (*P*) as well as the body (*B*). The compartmentalization (*black arrows*) between the pylorus and body, and the characteristic appearance of the pylorus in the dorsocranial aspect of the abdomen, indicate that the pylorus is on the *left* and the fundus is on the *right* and that there is a gastric volvulus. Note the malpositioned and slightly enlarged spleen (*S*). The spleen will follow the fundus because of anatomic connections.

The right lateral view is the most valuable radiographic projection to detect GDV as the displaced pylorus is gas-filled and compartmentalization is best visible. However, both lateral views should be acquired initially to increase the chance that the pylorus fills with gas and can be recognized. The goal is to make the diagnosis as quickly as possible because mortality is decreased if time between presentation and surgical intervention is decreased.[99] Recognizing the pyloric shift is more difficult in VD or DV radiographs; however, in unclear cases, they can be valuable. Positive-contrast gastrography may be performed to confirm the position of the stomach but usually is not needed.

Chronic Pyloric Obstruction

Pyloric outflow obstruction may be acute or chronic. Examples of causes for acute obstruction include gastric volvulus and foreign bodies. Obstructive pyloric diseases can be divided into those that encircle the pylorus, and are thus restrictive, and those that obstruct the pylorus by blocking its orifice. Restrictive diseases of the pylorus include hypertrophic pyloric stenosis, pylorospasm, inflammation or scarring, and neoplasia. Rarely, severe adhesions as caused by sclerosing encapsulating peritonitis can cause restrictive pyloric disease, where the gastric outflow tract is decreased in size and lacks normal functionality.[100] Pyloric obstructive diseases include gastric foreign bodies, mucosal inflammation or hypertrophy, and some mural lesions of the pyloric antrum.

It should also be remembered that disease of the pancreas or proximal duodenum can lead to an outflow obstruction of the stomach, which might present similar to disease occurring at the pylorus itself.

Chronic partial pyloric obstruction often manifests on survey radiographs as fluid-filled gastric distention as opposed to the acute gaseous distention of GDV (Fig. 45.22, eFig. 45.8). The stomach is commonly quite large with chronic partial pyloric obstruction. However, the enlarged stomach may be more difficult to identify on survey radiographs when it is filled with fluid. Even when distended with fluid, the stomach usually still contains some gas. In these instances, however, the gas does not totally outline or fill the entire stomach. Instead, the smaller amount of gas floats as a bubble on top of the fluid and should not be mistaken as the limits of the stomach or gastric wall thickening. Caudal displacement of the transverse colon can also be used as an indicator of gastric distension.

The major effect of pyloric obstructive diseases is to restrict gastric emptying. Survey radiographic findings may vary from normal gastric size to enlargement depending on the severity and duration of the obstruction. However, differentiation of the pyloric obstructive diseases is difficult radiographically, especially without fluoroscopy. The stomach is a dynamic organ that changes appearance rapidly because of peristaltic waves, and a radiograph is simply a snapshot of the morphologic features of the stomach. The advantage of fluoroscopy is that sequential changes of the shape of the stomach can be observed. Even with fluoroscopy, however, differentiating some pyloric obstructive diseases is not possible. For example, hypertrophic pyloric stenosis, neoplasia, and mural scarring all may produce an annular type of stricture of the pylorus that prevents the pylorus from opening adequately.

Usually, contrast radiography or ultrasound is needed to establish the cause and site of the pyloric obstruction. With contrast studies, the major radiographic abnormality is delayed gastric emptying. However, an initial delay in gastric emptying may be of no clinical significance, because of the influence of various psychogenic factors discussed previously. This point is especially important if the stomach starts to empty normally after an initial delay or after the animal is allowed to calm down. Of more significance is a pronounced delay in gastric emptying when only a small amount of contrast medium passes from the stomach in a few hours. Because the normal stomach should be empty 1 to 4 hours after administration of contrast medium, retention of most of the barium within the stomach 3 or 4 hours after administration usually indicates pyloric obstructive disease (Fig. 45.23).

An annular type of stricture narrowing the pyloric sphincter may result in characteristic radiographic abnormalities. If

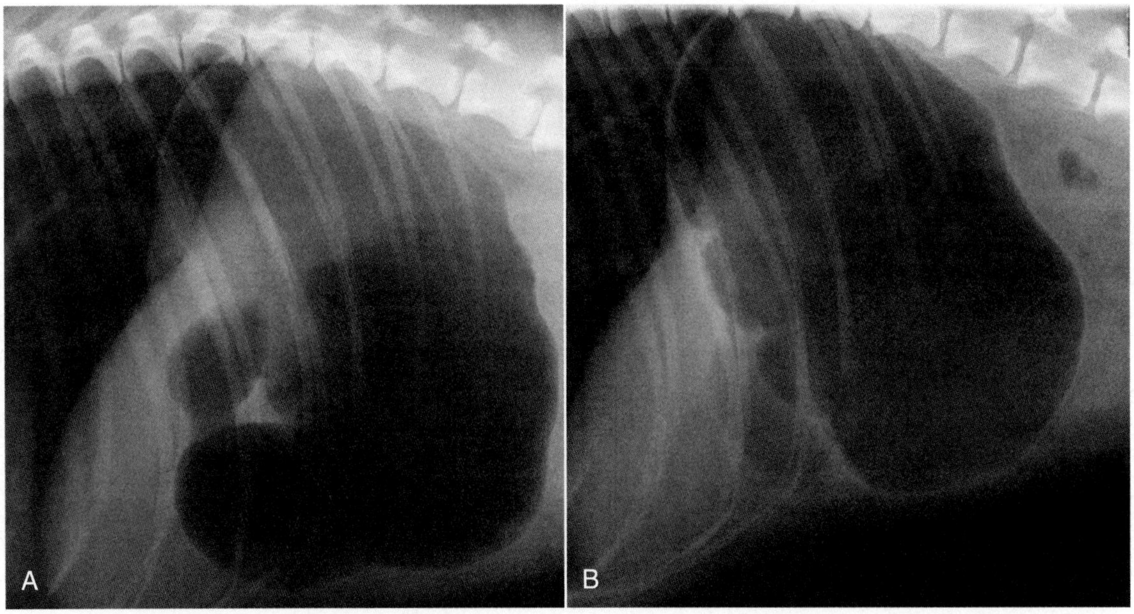

Fig. 45.20 Left **(A)** and right **(B)** lateral views of a dog with acute gastric dilatation. On the basis of these radiographic findings, the pylorus and the fundus are positioned normally. A gastric tube could not be passed into the stomach. Final diagnosis was 360-degree gastric volvulus.

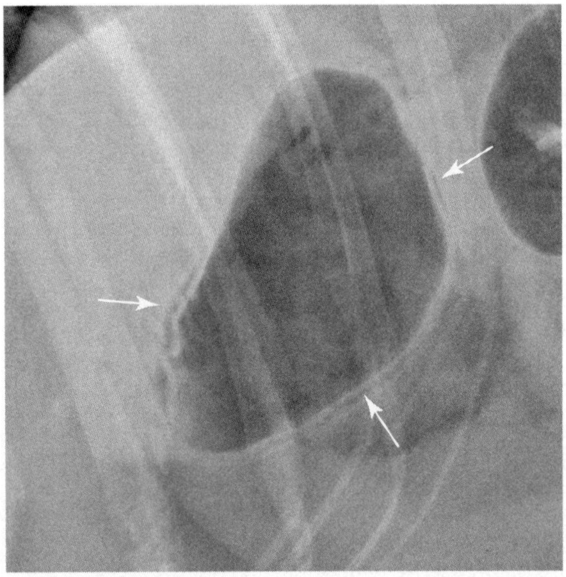

Fig. 45.21 Lateral radiograph of a dog with gas in the wall of the pyloric antrum (*white arrows*).

barium fills only the entrance of the lumen at the pyloric sphincter, the resultant radiographic appearance is referred to as the *beak sign*.[101] If barium fills the length of the narrowed lumen through the pyloric sphincter, the resultant radiographic appearance is referred to as the *string sign*.[101] A tit sign has been described as a relatively sharp, pointed outpouching of the pyloric antrum along the lesser curvature as a peristaltic wave pushes contrast medium in a peristaltic pouch up against the mass-type lesion around the pylorus[101] (Fig. 45.24, eFig. 45.9).

Sonographic thickening of the mucosa or muscular layer of the stomach wall can be noted and may help to differentiate between the various causes of pyloric obstruction. In dogs with chronic pyloric hypertrophy, the hypertrophic muscularis layer may be detected sonographically as a thick hypoechoic layer (Fig. 45.25). The thickness of the muscularis layer is greater than 3 mm in mild to moderate hypertrophy and greater than 8 mm in severely affected dogs. Vigorous, but ineffective, peristaltic contractions that fail to propel contents into the duodenum are seen in some patients.[51]

Pyloric obstructive diseases include gastric foreign bodies, mucosal inflammation or hypertrophy, and some mural lesions of the pyloric antrum. These types of lesions are more likely to produce filling defects within the lumen that occlude the orifice of the pyloric sphincter (see Fig. 45.24). Again, radiographic recognition of such a lesion is usually adequate diagnostically, and differentiation of the underlying cause may not be possible on radiographs. Ultrasound might provide additional information, including outlining of a foreign body.

ABNORMAL GASTRIC CONTENT

Gastric Foreign Bodies

Radiopaque material within the stomach is commonly identified on survey radiographs (Fig. 45.26, eFig. 45.10). These opacities are most often the result of ingested food or bone fragments and may have no clinical significance if they are small and cause no obstructive pattern. More clinically significant foreign bodies, such as fishhooks and needles, are also readily visible and present no diagnostic dilemma. The finding of discoid metallic foreign bodies is significant, because certain zinc-containing coins (U.S. pennies minted after 1982 and Euro cents) can induce intravascular hemolysis and hemolytic anemia.[102–104] Radiographs of the abdomen are indicated in the evaluation of patients with intravascular hemolysis for this reason. Other types of metallic objects may also contain zinc. Determining the denomination of suspected coins may be possible radiographically (eFig. 45.11). If projected en face, the diameter can be measured and corrected for magnification and compared to the known diameter of coins. Ingested magnets may readily be seen on survey radiographs and this can cause

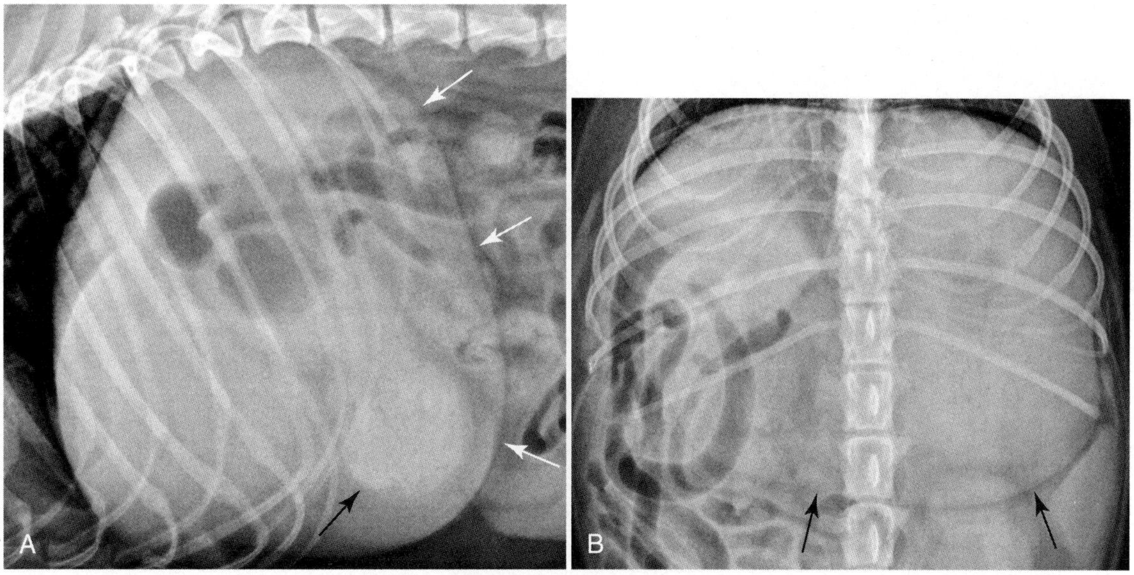

Fig. 45.22 Lateral (**A**) and dorsoventral (**B**) radiographs of a dog with fluid-filled gastric distention caused by chronic pyloric obstruction. The stomach is more difficult to identify when filled with fluid instead of gas. The caudal margin of the stomach is indicated in **A** by the *white arrows* and in **B** by the *black arrows*. In **A**, some opaque gastric contents have settled into the dependent pyloric region of the stomach (*black arrow*).

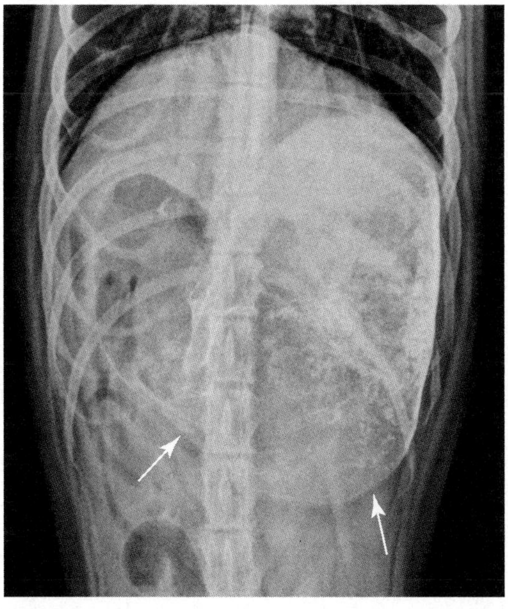

Fig. 45.23 Ventrodorsal radiograph 10 hours after barium was given. The stomach is distended (*white arrows*) with intraluminal gas and fluid and some of the barium. There should be no residual barium after 10 hours and this, along with the distention, is indicative of gastric outflow obstruction.

gastric ulceration, obstruction, and perforation secondary to pressure necrosis when more than one magnet is ingested. Early surgical intervention might help to alleviate the risk of gastric perforation or obstruction secondary to ingested magnets.[105,106] It is important to remember that certain metallic foreign bodies are not metal attenuating on radiographs; for example, aluminum is relatively radiolucent and is therefore difficult to detect on survey radiographs. It is also important to remember that dogs may swallow glue containing diphenylmethane diisocyanate, which expands extensively when exposed to moisture in the stomach filling the gastric lumen and thereby resulting in a severe outflow obstruction (eFig. 45.12).[107]

The stomach may occasionally contain nondescript radiopaque material of questionable significance (Fig. 45.27). The persistence of the abnormality is important. If the patient is stable and endoscopy is not used, repeat radiographs made after fasting for 12 to 24 hours may provide valuable information about the digestibility or potential transit of the suspicious material.

A greater problem exists with radiographic detection of nonopaque gastric foreign bodies. Such objects are usually difficult to see on survey radiographs. Several approaches exist to help in the radiographic identification of nonopaque gastric foreign bodies. The simplest is to use different patient positions. If the foreign body does not shift dependently with gastric fluid, then a different view may help outline the foreign body with gas. If a foreign body ingestion is suspected and endoscopy is not available, a contrast radiographic study, ultrasound, or CT study of the abdomen may be necessary for diagnosis. Giving a small amount of barium or gas (Fig. 45.28) may make such foreign bodies easier to see than with a standard gastrogram using a large volume of barium because the large volume may obscure the foreign body. Pneumogastrography is simple, easy to perform, cheap, and quick and requires no special equipment and can help outline gastric foreign bodies.[21]

The appearance of a foreign body on a gastrogram varies depending on the type of foreign body present. An object such as a solid ball creates a round, discrete filling defect within the barium. If the object has a nonabsorbent surface, it may not be visible after the stomach has emptied. Conversely, a rag or sock may not create an initial filling defect because the contrast medium may permeate the object. Because of absorption and retention of contrast medium, however, the foreign body may be better visible after the stomach has emptied. Gas containing radiolucent foreign bodies may be difficult to identify. Noticing a focal radiolucency with a consistent shape and often a thin peripheral soft tissue opaque rim is important to identify these foreign bodies (eFig. 45.13).

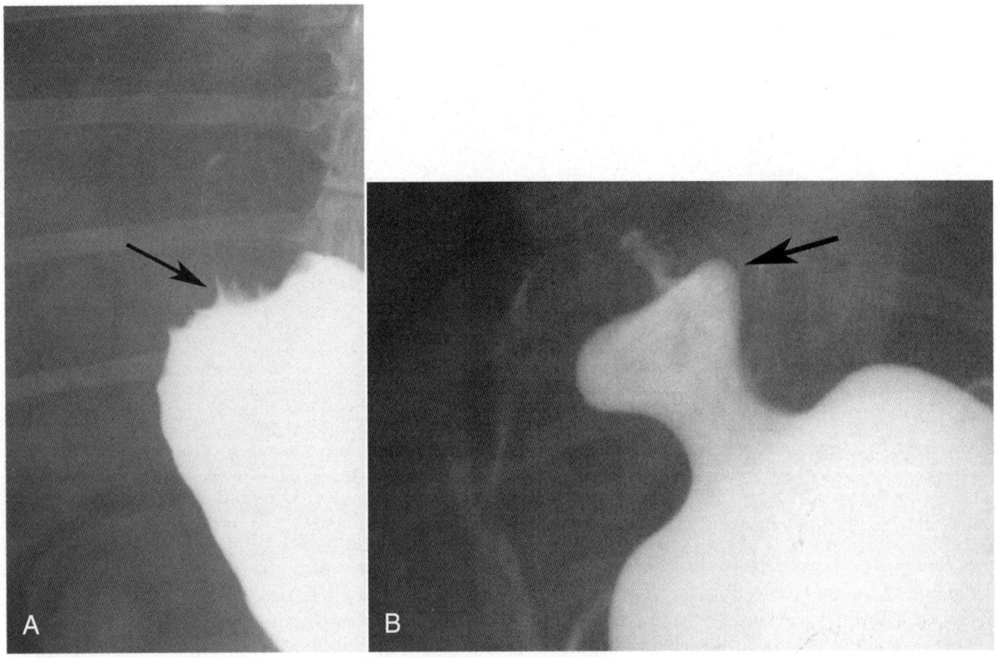

Fig. 45.24 **A,** Ventrodorsal radiograph of the pyloric region of a dog with restrictive disease of the pylorus. The string sign (*black arrow*) is caused by barium that fills the length of the lumen of the narrowed pyloric sphincter because of an annular type of stricture. **B,** Ventrodorsal radiograph of the pyloric region of another dog with restrictive disease of the pylorus. The peristaltic pouch (*black arrow*) is the outpouching of the pyloric antrum along the lesser curvature as a peristaltic wave pushes contrast medium up against the mass-type lesion encircling the pylorus. A pronounced delay in gastric emptying was also present.

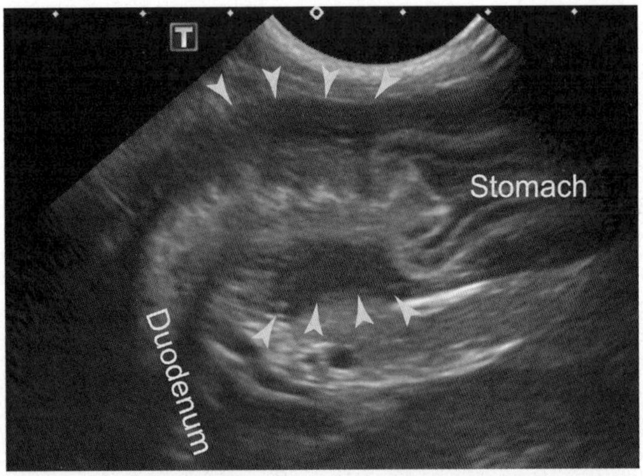

Fig. 45.25 Longitudinal ultrasound image of pyloric stenosis. The pylorus wall is moderately thickened (*white arrowheads*). The layered appearance of the pylorus wall is still present; the muscularis is markedly thickened and the luminal aspect of the pylorus wall is irregular. Caudal is to the *right*, and ventral is to the *top*.

Gastric foreign bodies may be identified ultrasonographically.[50] The ability to detect these objects depends on the presence of other gastric contents (e.g., gas, fluid, and food), the position of the object relative to the sound beam, and the object composition. Strong acoustic shadows with or without an echogenic acoustic interface are strongly suggestive of a foreign body. Linear foreign bodies are often hyperechoic, and cause plication of the stomach (Fig. 45.29); in cats the linear foreign body is often anchored around the base of the tongue; however, in dogs, they often originate from a foreign object lodged in the pylorus. Intraluminal fluid surrounding a foreign object facilitates its detection and the ability to distinguish reflective foreign body surfaces from intraluminal gas; therefore, adding water to the stomach may be beneficial in some patients. Objects that transmit sound may be seen more completely than those producing strong acoustic shadows. Repositioning of the patient while scanning might demonstrate mobility of the object in the stomach. However, like radiography, large foreign objects might not move or have only minimal movement as they might be lodged in the lumen of the stomach.

Gastric foreign bodies rarely cause perforation of the gastric wall, but when sharp objects such as wooden sticks, skewers, or metal brush bristles are swallowed, perforation may occur. Gastric perforation can result in peritoneal gas, which can be detected radiographically, sonographically, or by using CT. Sonographically, peritoneal gas as well as hyperechogenicity of the mesenteric fat and/or peritoneal fluid can be present.[108] CT may have a similar sensitivity as radiography and ultrasound in detecting peritoneal gas and may have the added benefit compared to ultrasound that no pressure to the abdomen is applied during the exam, which might be favorable in patients with acute abdominal signs.[109]

GASTRIC WALL CHANGES

Gastric Ulcers

Gastric ulceration is a multifactorial disease. Gastric ulcers may be benign or malignant. Benign gastric ulcers are also termed *peptic gastric ulcers* and result from a variety of causes.[110–112] Use of nonsteroidal anti-inflammatory drugs is a common cause of benign gastric ulcers.[113–115] Dachshunds with disc prolapse have a high prevalence of gastroduodenal ulceration.[116] This is thought to be from ulcerogenic drug administration as well as

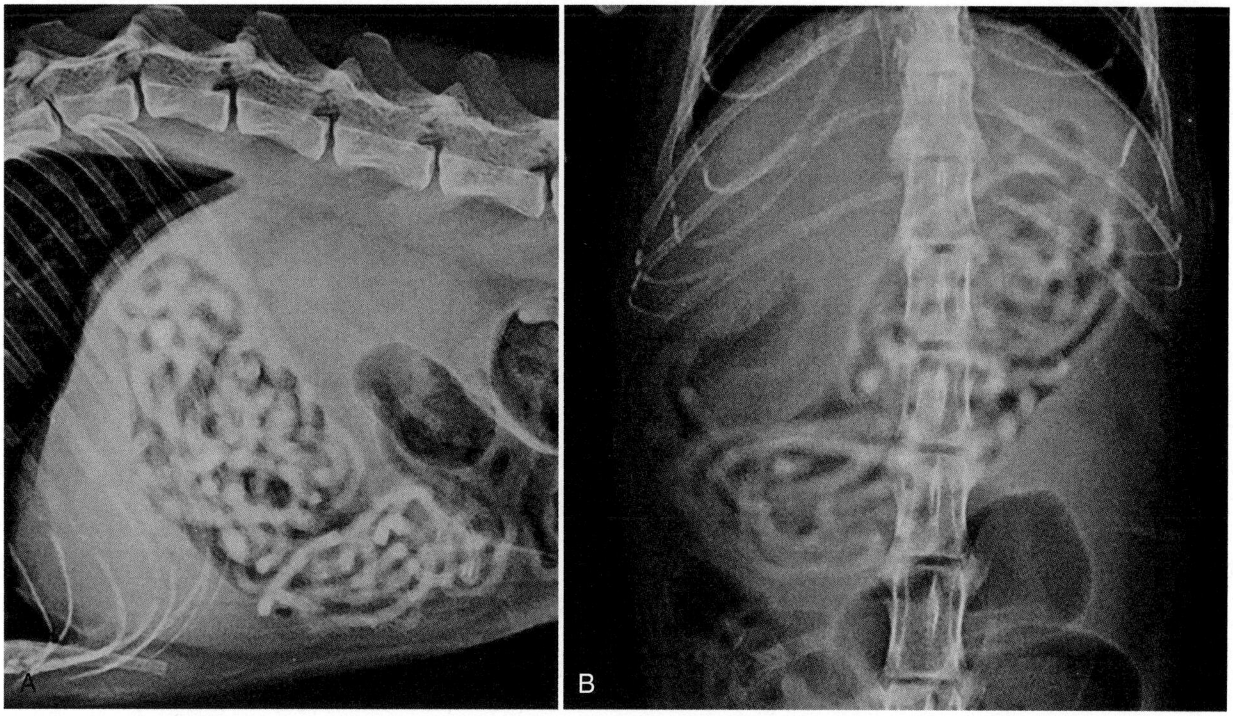

Fig. 45.26 Lateral **(A)** and ventrodorsal **(B)** radiographs of a cat with multiple linear to C-shaped foreign bodies consistent with hair ties. The hair ties are easily identified due to their attenuation and characteristic imaging appearance.

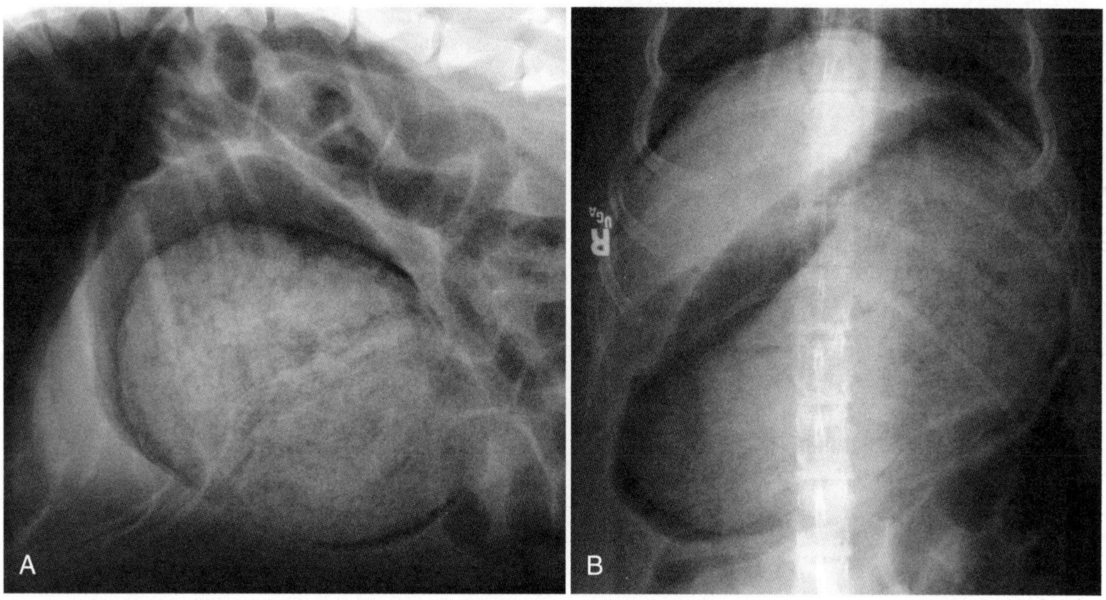

Fig. 45.27 Lateral **(A)** and ventrodorsal **(B)** radiographs of a dog with a large gastric foreign body. This radiopaque material is easy to visualize because of the large amount of gas surrounding the foreign body, which was aggregated leaves and plant material. Expansion of ingested polyurethane glue can also lead to a similar appearance.

autonomic disturbances, stress, hypovolemia, and other factors.[116] Gastric ulceration in combination with gastritis occurs frequently in working and sled dogs and its cause is not entirely understood, but might be in part caused by increased secretion of gastrin, exercise-induced hyperthermia, and damage to the gastric mucosa.[117] Malignant gastric ulcers occur in association with gastric neoplasia and may be caused by tumor necrosis.[110] The greatest risk factor for malignant ulcers in the dog is gastric adenocarcinoma.[115]

Gastric ulcers are difficult to identify on conventional radiographs. Ulcers are more conspicuous in barium studies, in which they are usually round to ovoid collections of barium. They produce craters in the wall of the stomach that appear as outpouchings from the lumen (Fig. 45.30). The contrast

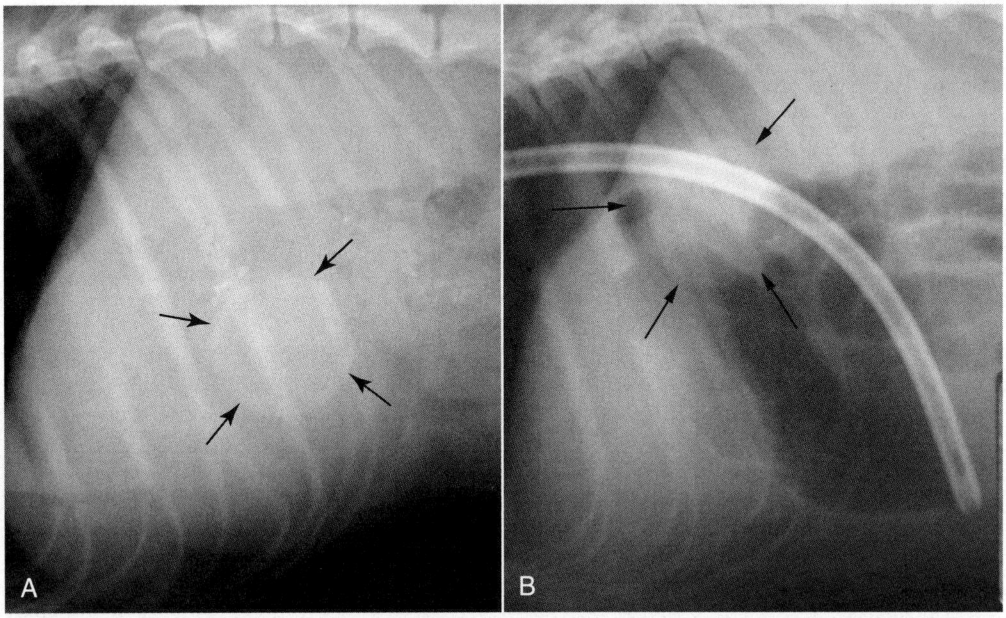

Fig. 45.28 A ball in the pyloric portion of the stomach (*black arrows*) is difficult to see on the right lateral view (**A**) because of fluid in the pylorus. In **B**, gas has been administered by a gastric tube, the ball (*black arrows*) is easier to see. Note the ball has moved to the fundus.

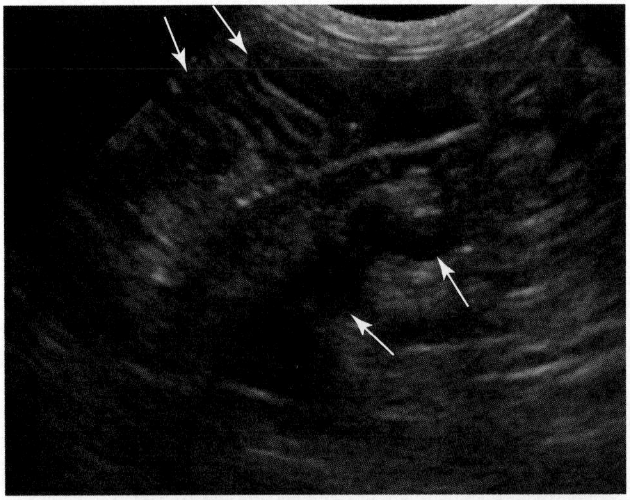

Fig. 45.29 Sagittal sonogram of the stomach of a cat with a luminal hyperechoic linear foreign object causing severe plication of the gastric wall (*white arrows*).

radiographic appearance of a gastric ulcer may vary depending on whether the ulcer is projected in profile, *en face*, or obliquely. The appearance of the ulcer may be altered further by gastric peristalsis. Manipulation of the patient during fluoroscopy allows a more complete and continuous evaluation of the margin and contour of the stomach. Double-contrast gastrography may also be of value because ulcers that are projected en face may be visible with double-contrast radiographic studies but are obscured with positive-contrast gastrography.[9]

Criteria have been established in human patients for the radiographic differentiation of benign and malignant gastric ulcers.[118–120] Thus, although contrast radiography may provide an excellent method for the recognition of gastric ulcers, infrequent use of single- and double-contrast gastrography, lack of fluoroscopy, and insufficient views all combine to limit the recognition of gastric ulcers in dogs and cats. In addition, experience is limited in differentiating benign and malignant gastric ulcers radiographically in dogs and cats. Ulceration is often associated with gastric carcinoma,[121,122] and gastric ulcers in dogs that are recognized on radiographs are often the result of neoplasia.[123] Thus, the radiographic recognition of a gastric ulcer should lead to strong consideration of neoplasia and further evaluation of the stomach with endoscopy and biopsy or by surgical exploration.

Some gastric ulcers may be detected sonographically (Fig. 45.30B) but many are not found.[48,124] Ultrasonographic features include the presence of a wall defect (crater) usually within the center of a locally thickened area of stomach wall. The thickened area may have loss of the normal layered appearance. Gastric fluid accumulation and decreased motility may also be noted. Additionally, central within the defect small hyperechogenicities with distal reverberation artifacts suggestive of gas may be noted in the gastric wall (pneumatosis) during an ultrasound examination.[125]

Gastric Bleeding

Gastrointestinal bleeding is a multifactorial disease and is suspected when the patient is vomiting blood-containing ingesta or fluid, or when digested blood is present in the feces. Survey radiographs may not demonstrate the cause of bleeding. Ultrasound or contrast radiography may demonstrate a thickening of the gastric wall[126] or a gastric ulcer as the site of the origin of bleeding; however, if no thickening or mass effect of the gastric wall is present, radiography and ultrasound may not be able to identify the precise site of bleeding and further imaging may be necessary. Gastrointestinal bleeding can be evaluated by scintigraphy using either intravenously administered ^{99m}technetium (^{99m}Tc)-labeled sulfur colloid or red blood cells. Scintigraphic studies using ^{99m}Tc-labeled red blood might be more sensitive than sulfur colloid studies as the labeled red blood cells circulate longer in the vascular system and therefore allow identification of sites of intermittent as well as acute bleeding.[127] The downside of ^{99m}Tc sulfur colloid is that it is most sensitive in patients where active bleeding occurs as the sulfur colloid is rapidly taken up by the reticuloendothelial system and therefore does not allow detection of intermittent and chronic bleeding and in addition the uptake of the colloid by the reticuloendothelial system might hinder imaging of bleeding of gastrointestinal structures at the level of the liver and spleen.[75]

Gastric Neoplasia

Primary gastric neoplasia is rare in the dog and cat and no definitive underlying etiologies have been defined. Several types of benign and malignant gastric neoplasms occur and any region of the stomach may be involved. Polyps, also called glandular hyperplasia, hyperplastic or adenomatous polyp, adenomatous hyperplasia, or adenoma, may be clinically silent and most are found incidentally.[128,129] A variety of malignant gastric tumors have been described including carcinoma, adenocarcinoma, leiomyosarcoma, histiocytic sarcoma, fibrosarcoma lymphoma, mast cell, and gastric stromal tumor.[68,130,131] Gastric stromal tumors range in classification from benign to malignant. Adenocarcinoma is the most common malignant gastric tumor in dogs.[121,132] This tumor may occur in any region of the stomach but is found most often in the pyloric portion.[132,133] Gastric neoplasia occurs less frequently in the cat than in the dog,[134] and lymphosarcoma is the most common type of feline gastric neoplasm.[135]

The imaging appearance of gastric neoplasia varies and primarily depends on the size, shape, and location of the tumor. Inflammatory lesions can also result in thickening of the gastric wall[136] and have similar imaging findings as neoplastic lesions.[137,138] Furthermore, it is important to remember that the varying types of gastric tumors are difficult to differentiate based on imaging findings and therefore cytology or more commonly histopathology is required to differentiate inflammatory from neoplastic conditions and to categorize the tumor type.

The major radiographic feature of gastric neoplasia is that of a mass lesion that projects into the gastric lumen, creating a filling defect within the contrast medium. The more nodular and pedunculated the lesion, the easier it is to recognize it as a distinct mass (see Fig. 45.31). Larger masses may also lead to outflow obstruction.[139] Smaller mass lesions may be obscured completely by a relatively large volume of barium. Oblique projections, the conformation of the stomach, and peristaltic contractions may all contribute to obscuring some mass lesions of the stomach.

Tumors that are diffuse are more difficult to identify. Diffuse infiltrative lesions of the stomach wall may not produce distinct filling defects. Instead, they may alter the shape of the stomach and produce decreased motility of the involved area. If such diffuse lesions encircle a portion of the stomach, the radiographic appearance may be that of an annular narrowing or one in which the stomach has decreased distensibility in the affected area (see Fig. 45.31B, eFig. 45.14). Because of variations in appearance of the stomach created by peristalsis, persistence of a suspected abnormality on sequential radiographs is important. As stated earlier, the recognition of a gastric ulcer should also suggest the possibility of gastric neoplasia.

Gastric masses can be found on ultrasound examination of the stomach, thus often eliminating the need for radiographic contrast studies. However, it is important to remember that patients need to be repositioned to move the ingesta, fluid, and gas in the stomach to access all aspects of the gastric wall sonographically, and that gastric wall lesions might be missed if the stomach is filled with large amounts of gas or ingesta. Common ultrasound features include thickening of the stomach wall, loss or distortion of the normal layered appearance of the wall, and altered echogenicity and motility in the affected area (Fig. 45.32).[39–42,45,122,140,142] Although such lesions are most often associated with gastric neoplasia, similar changes have

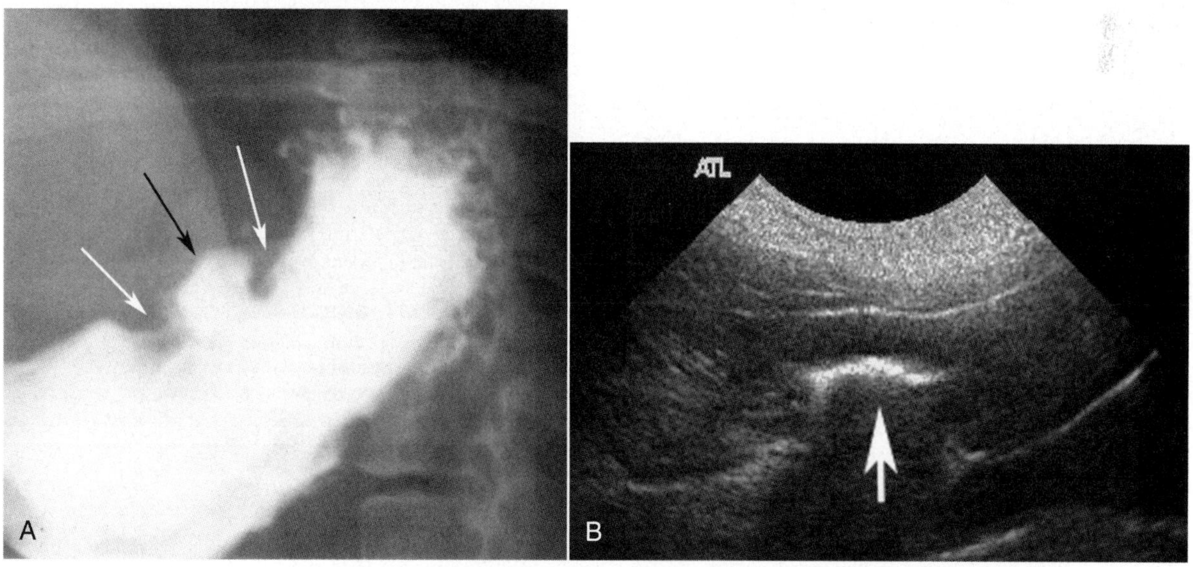

Fig. 45.30 **A,** Ventrodorsal oblique radiograph of the stomach of a dog with a gastric ulcer (*black arrow*). The filling defects protruding into the stomach (*white arrows*) represent the collar of the ulcer. **B,** Sagittal ultrasound image of the stomach of another dog. The pyloric region of the stomach is thickened, and layers are not identifiable. The *white arrow* indicates a portion of the stomach wall that is focally thinner than the remainder. The mucosal surface of this area is hyperechoic. A large ulcer was found in this area at necropsy; the diagnosis was adenocarcinoma.

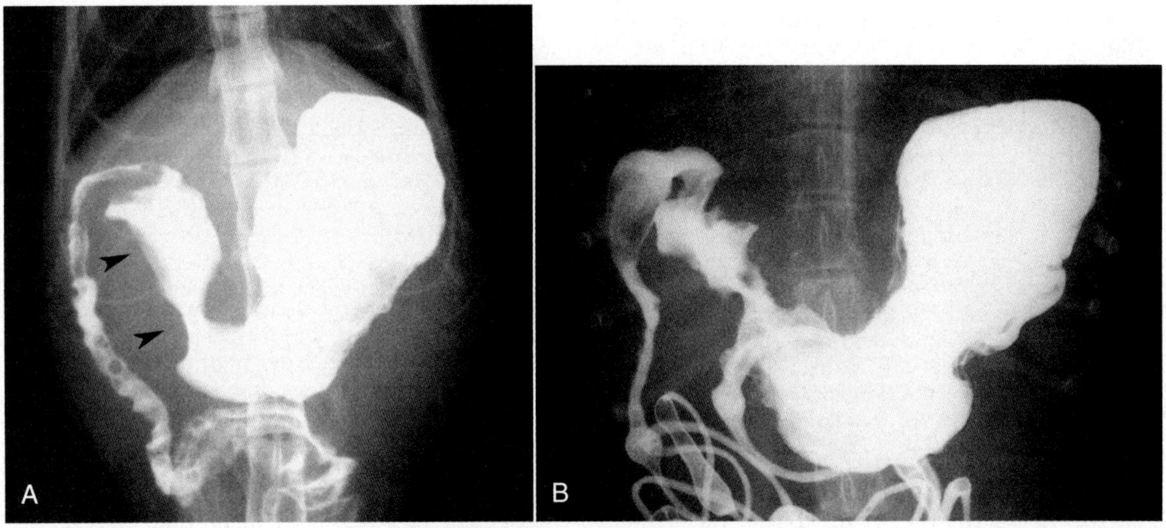

Fig. 45.31 **A,** Ventrodorsal barium gastrogram of a cat. A smooth filling defect is present from a mass along the greater curvature (*black arrowheads*). **B,** Ventrodorsal barium gastrogram of a dog. An annular mass encircles the pyloric portion and part of the body. This area failed to distend, and the abnormality persisted throughout the study. Final diagnosis was gastric adenocarcinoma.

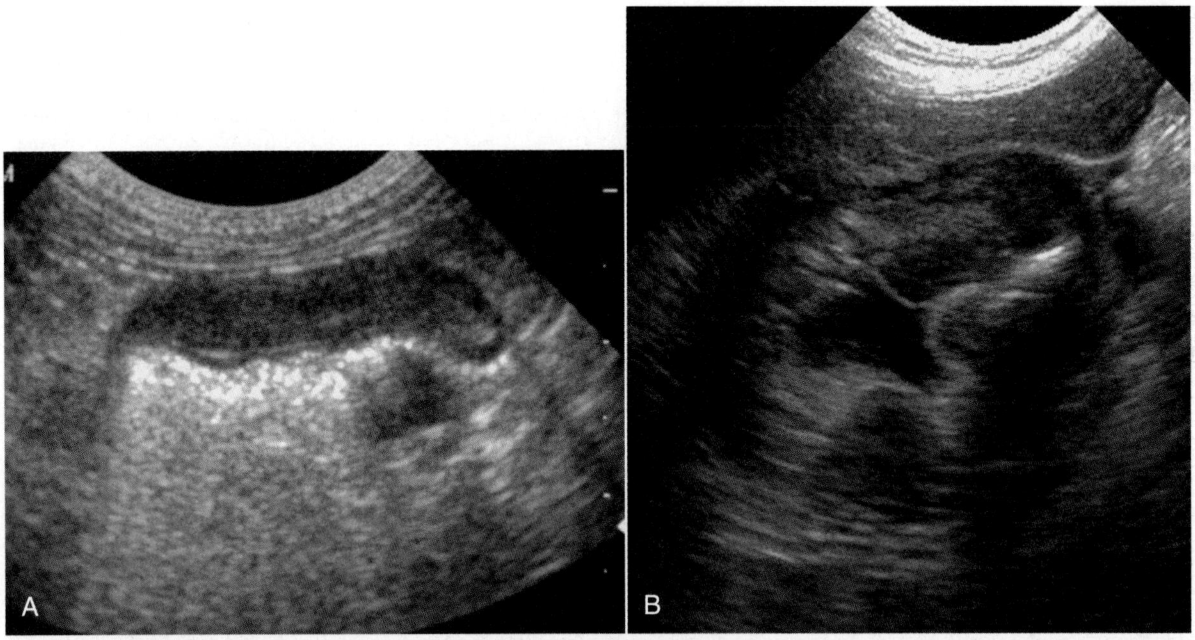

Fig. 45.32 Longitudinal ultrasound images of gastric neoplasia. **A,** Lymphosarcoma in the stomach wall of a cat. The stomach wall is thickened and hypoechoic and has lost the normal layered appearance. **B,** Suspected adenocarcinoma in the stomach wall of a dog. The wall is thickened uniformly and decreased in echogenicity. The normal layered appearance is disrupted. Caudal is to the *right,* and ventral is to the *top.*

been reported in dogs with pythiosis,[46] zygomycosis[142] and cats with eosinophilic gastritis[138] and gastritis secondary to actinomycosis.[137] Wall layering is usually preserved in gastric polyps but may have the appearance of a large sessile mass with the loss of wall layering.[143] Extension of the lesion through the serosal surface of the stomach has been reported in dogs with gastric carcinoma.[41] Another reported sonographic feature of gastric carcinoma is *pseudolayering* of the stomach wall, which is thought to be associated with uneven distribution of tumor in the layers of the stomach wall.[42,43] Instead of the five layers seen normally, a central, moderately echogenic zone between two lesser echogenic lines is seen.[43]

In dogs and cats with gastric neoplasia, maximal gastric wall thickness has been reported to range from 10 to 27 mm[40,43,52] and 8 to 25 mm, respectively,[39,44] whereas the reported normal gastric wall thickness is 3 to 5 mm in dogs and 2 to 5 mm in cats. Gastric wall measurements greater than 6 to 7 mm have been proposed as abnormal.[36] Although gastric wall thickening is an important abnormal finding, caution must be exercised when assessing wall thickness in a contracted, empty stomach because a false-positive diagnosis of gastric mass can be made.[144] Distending the stomach with water may help distinguish true- and false-positive lesions, but real-time observation of gastric motility may be an easier way to distinguish the two because a lack of motility usually is seen in an abnormal wall segment.

Ultrasound also allows the evaluation of other organs including regional lymph nodes and the remainder of the small intestinal tract. Concurrent regional lymph node enlargement and ulceration of the affected area have been reported in both gastric carcinoma and lymphosarcoma.[40] Adenocarcinoma may spread to the liver in addition to regional lymph nodes. Sonographic lesions in the small intestine in combination with the gastric wall have a high likelihood to be secondary to lymphoma.[140] Cytologic or histopathologic evaluation is necessary for a definitive diagnosis of gastric wall lesions. Specimens can be obtained by ultrasound-guided fine-needle aspiration or tissue-core biopsy.[58,145]

Diffuse Diseases of the Stomach Wall

The stomach may be involved diffusely in a variety of nonneoplastic diseases that produce inflammation, edema, hypertrophy, atrophy, or mineralization. Acute gastritis may result from a variety of causes and is rarely associated with radiographic abnormalities. One of the forms of acute gastritis called *exercise-induced gastritis* is an important condition to remember as it is associated with a high morbidity and mortality in working dogs and sled dogs.[117] Chronic gastritis is diagnosed infrequently clinically and may also result from a variety of causes. Examples include chronic atrophic gastritis, chronic hypertrophic gastritis,[146,147] eosinophilic gastritis and pythiosis,[46] and zygomycosis.[142] Gastric wall edema can cause focal or diffuse thickening of the gastric wall and can be caused by a wide range of disease including inflammation of the stomach and pancreas, peritonitis, hypoalbuminemia, or neoplasia. It is important to differentiate gastric wall edema, which is primarily considered a benign disease process from gastric wall thickening caused by neoplasia.[47]

Imaging diagnosis of diffuse gastric disease is difficult and often no definitive answer can be given based on imaging findings (Fig. 45.33). Radiographically absent or diminished rugal folds, thickened rugal folds, nodules, or a thickened gastric wall may be seen with these diseases (see Fig. 45.33). Care must be taken when evaluating stomach wall thickness on survey radiographs. Fluid within the stomach may cause border effacement with the stomach wall, creating the illusion of increased thickness (Fig. 45.34). On contrast radiography, a relatively empty or mildly distended stomach, absence of a normal gastric rugal fold pattern, and multifocal filling defects can be noted. If a contrast radiographic study is performed,

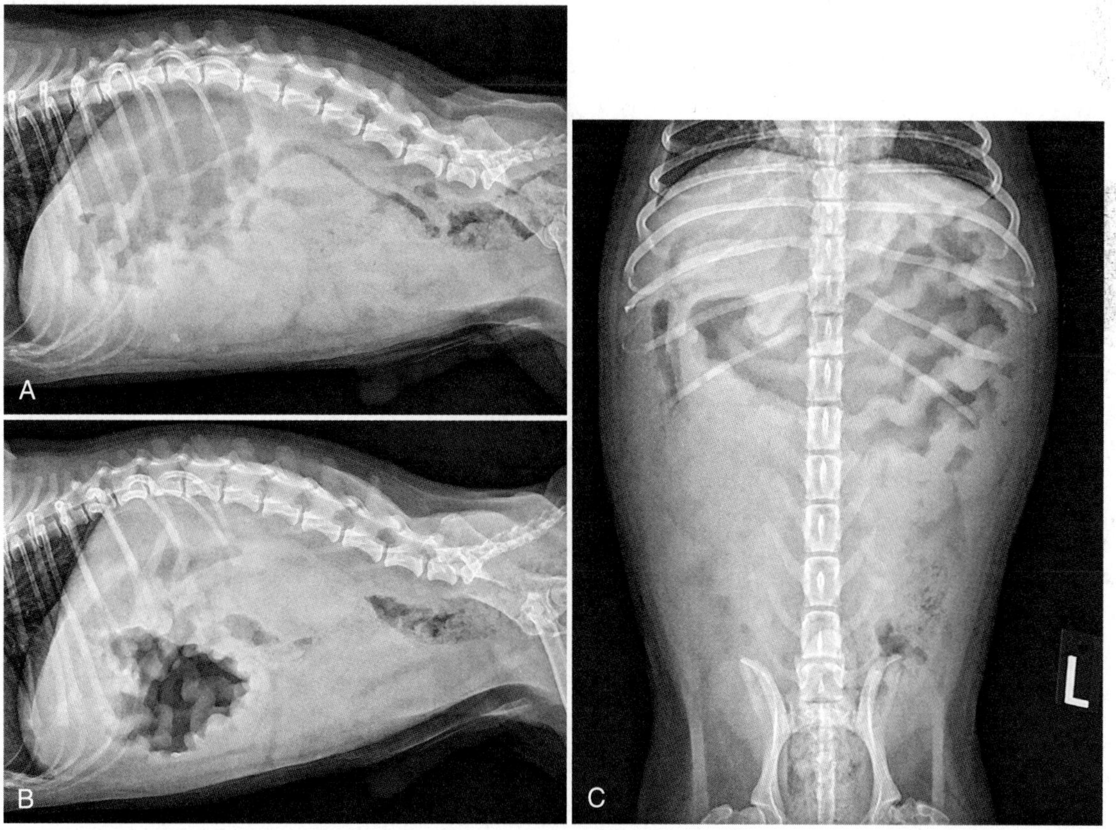

Fig. 45.33 Right and left lateral and ventrodorsal radiographs of the abdomen of a 2-year-old pug with an acute history of vomiting. The pug had previously been diagnosed with an extrahepatic shunt, portal hypoplasia, and microvascular dysplasia in all liver lobes. **A–C,** Diffuse thickening of the rugal folds is noted, which is suspected in part to be due to gastritis and gastric edema. A mildly reduced peritoneal detail is present secondary to a small volume of abdominal transudate. **C,** The rugal folds are larger in the body of the stomach and diminish in height towards the pyloric antrum, which would also be seen in normal rugal folds.

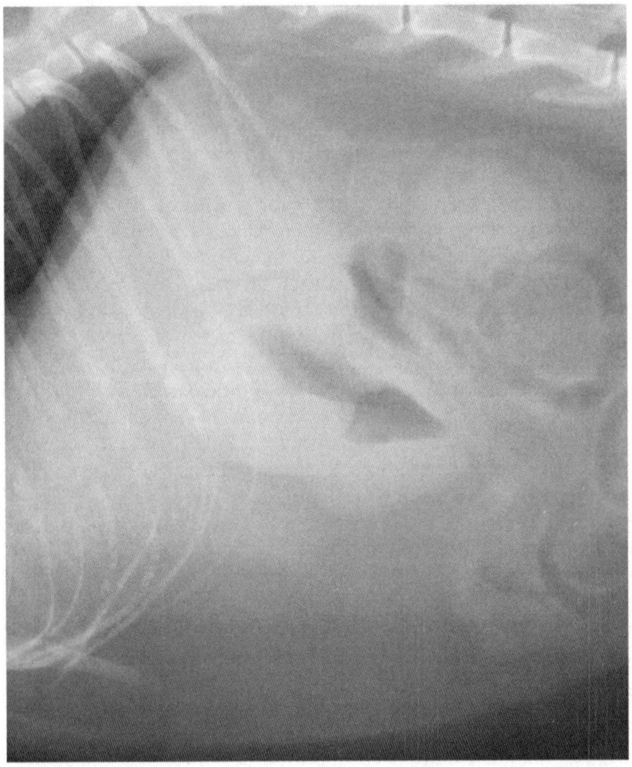

Fig. 45.34 Lateral survey radiograph of the abdomen of a cat with a thick gastric wall. The thickened wall is best visualized in the ventral midabdomen and is associated with a narrow, tubular, gas-filled lumen. Care should be taken when evaluating the stomach wall on survey radiographs because fluid in the lumen can silhouette with the wall, creating a false impression of wall thickening.

double-contrast radiography of the stomach is preferred as distension of the stomach allows to better assess the thickness of the gastric wall and rugal folds. Recent CT and ultrasound studies have described the appearance of gastric wall edema.[47,148] On ultrasound, thickening of the gastric wall, loss of wall layering, and a thickened medium echogenicity submucosal layer can be seen. On CT, a three-layer appearance of the gastric wall can be seen which is more apparent in the postcontrast images as the inner and outer layers are enhancing adjacent to the nonenhancing middle layer but can already be seen on precontrast studies (Fig. 45.35).

Gastric wall gas (pneumatosis) can sometimes be seen on radiography as well as ultrasound. A recent study suggests that similar to human patients, gastric pneumatosis can either occur secondary to life-threatening emphysematous gastritis or secondary to benign gastric emphysema. Both conditions have similar imaging features but have vastly different clinical presentations. All animals reported to have emphysematous gastritis had severe clinical signs including anorexia, hematemesis, lethargy, and leukocytosis and all animals had a poor outcome and were euthanized. All cases of gastric emphysema, which in human patients occurs secondary to mucosal rupture, had no or only mild gastrointestinal signs and resolved quickly on medical management (Fig. 45.36) without antibiotic treatment. In emphysematous gastritis and gastric emphysema, more than half of the gastric wall had gas present, which may help to differentiate these conditions from gastric ulceration.[149]

Ultrasonographic findings of inflammatory disease of the gastric wall are similar to those reported for gastric tumors and can range from increased gastric wall thickening with normal wall layering or loss of wall layer definition to altered echogenicity of the gastric wall.[39,137,138,150] Additionally, enlargement of regional lymph nodes has been noted with inflammatory disease of the stomach. As with most mass lesions discovered with ultrasound, biopsy is usually necessary for a definitive diagnosis.[151]

Soft tissue calcification may occur in association with chronic renal failure[52,150,152] or secondary to parasitic disease such as canine schistosomiasis due to *Heterobilharzia americana*.[153] In renal failure patients, mineralization of the gastric wall may be visible radiographically as thin, linear, mineralized opacities (Fig. 45.37).[150] Rugal mineralization is often more easily identified when the stomach is empty, and the mineralized mucosal fold pattern is more tightly grouped. Ultrasonographic findings of dogs with uremic gastropathy include thickened gastric wall and rugal folds and a hyperechoic zone at the mucosal/luminal interface caused by mucosal mineralization.[52] Ultrasound is likely more sensitive than radiography for detection of gastric lesions associated with uremia. *H. americana* is primarily found in the area of the Gulf Coast and south Atlantic states. Radiographically diffuse linear mineralizations can be noted throughout the small intestinal tract. On ultrasound, a thick, hyperechoic area of mineralization can be noted circumferentially through the submucosa and muscularis of the small intestinal tract.[153]

Although in many patients endoscopy is the method of choice for the diagnosis of gastric diseases, in some patients the mucosal surface of the stomach may be normal, leading to false-negative results by endoscopy.[151] Ultrasound demonstrates the morphologic features of the entire gastric wall unless the wall is hidden by gas or echogenic ingesta. In some patients, ultrasound may be more informative than endoscopy.[154]

Postoperative Stomach

Companion animals undergoing gastric surgery can have changes on postoperative imaging studies that mimic disease. It is often crucial when evaluating an imaging study to be familiar with the anatomic and physiologic changes that occur postoperatively as well as to be familiar with appropriate surgical techniques. One of the most common reasons for imaging the abdomen postoperatively include the evaluation of placed feeding tubes (gastric, gastrojejunal, etc.) or if the patient is not improving post gastric surgery as anticipated. Imaging procedures postoperatively can also be used to define a baseline appearance, allowing detection of early or late postoperative complications.

Radiography is often used as an initial technique to assess the extent of fluid and gas in the peritoneal cavity, position of the stomach, and presence and configuration of surgical clips, staples, drains, and tubes. Postoperative functional disturbances of motility of the stomach and intestinal tract, paralytic ileus, and vomiting are not uncommon.

If a subtotal gastrectomy is performed, no displacement of the stomach or stricture may be noted.[155] Similarly, if surgical gastric biopsies were performed, no displacement of the stomach would be expected. If a gastropexy was performed, which is a common procedure in dogs to prohibit GDV in the future by internally, permanently fixating the stomach to the abdominal wall in a way that gastric function is not affected, it is expected that the pylorus will be in close proximity to the right lateroventral abdominal wall. Radiographically, a caudoventral displacement of the pyloric antrum caudal to the last rib might be noted. If metallic staples were used for the gastropexy, they should be intact and the pyloric antrum should be near the staple line. The position of the stomach should remain

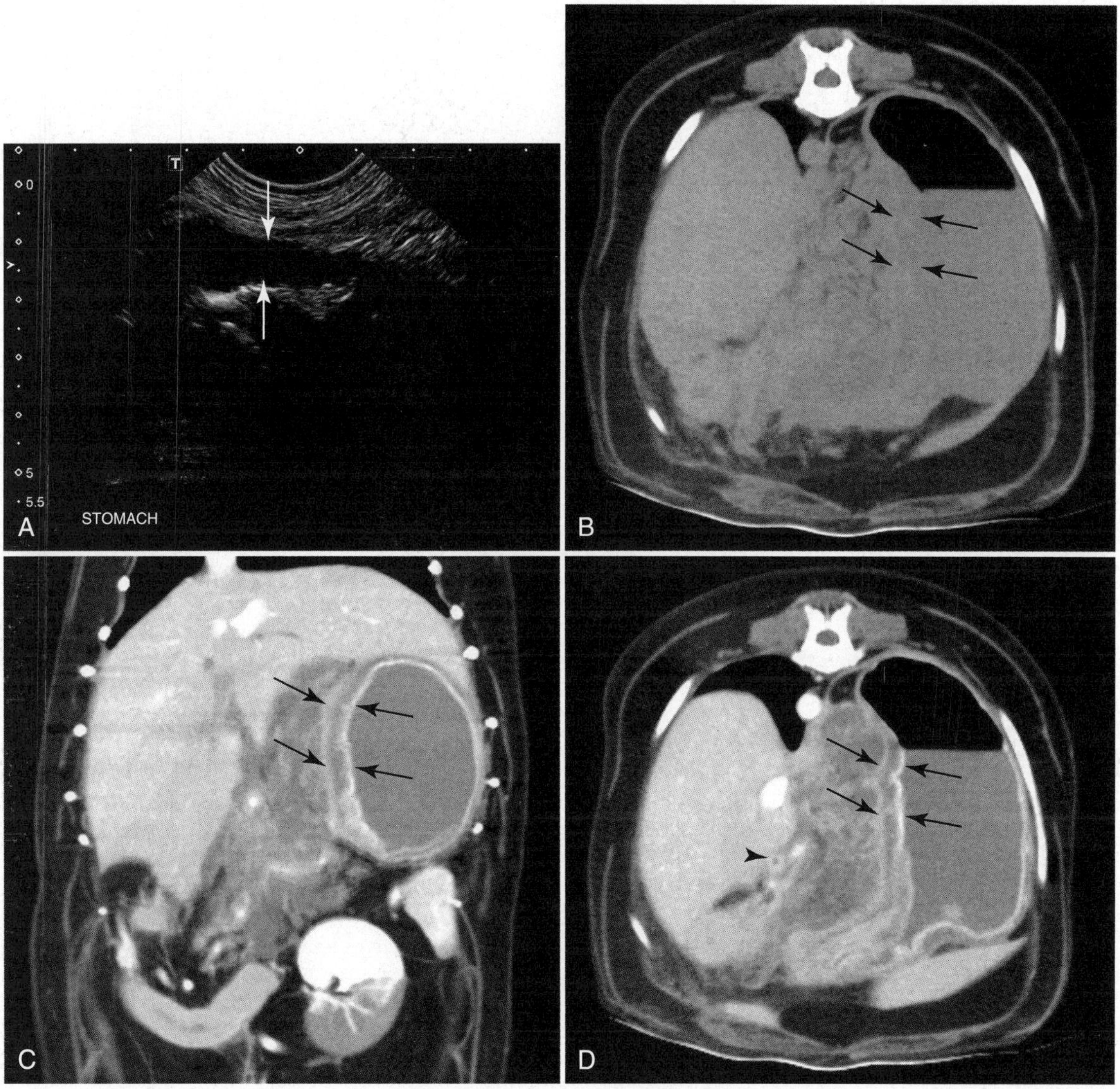

Fig. 45.35 Gastric wall edema in a dog with severe pancreatitis and portal vein thrombosis. **A,** Longitudinal ultrasonogram of the thickened hypoechoic gastric wall with loss of wall layering (*white arrows*). Computed tomography images with the dog in sternal recumbency illustrate **(B)** on precontrast administration, and **C–D,** post intravenous iodinated contrast agent injection images, the classic three-layered appearance of the gastric wall (*black arrows*). On **C–D,** the inner layer remains hypoattenuating, whereas the inner and outer layers are moderately contrast enhancing. On **B–D,** the far adjacent to the pancreas and lesser curvature of the stomach has a striated soft tissue attenuation secondary to peritonitis. **D,** A filling defect indicating thromboembolic disease is noted in the extrahepatic portal vein (*black arrowhead*) and similar lesions were seen in the intrahepatic portal veins.

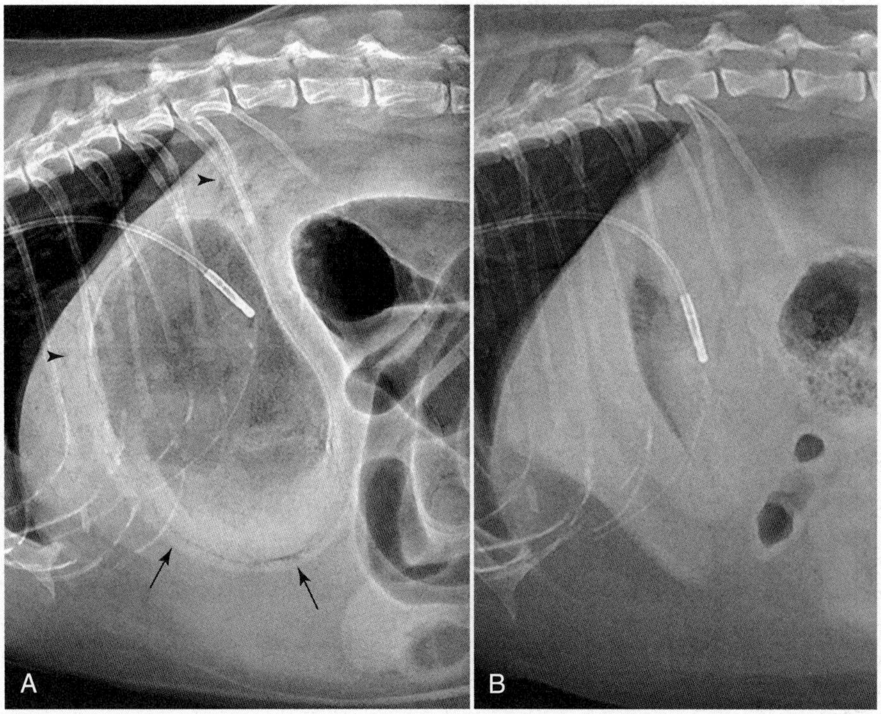

Fig. 45.36 Close-up lateral radiographs of the stomach of an 11-year-old cat, 3 days **(A)** and 4 days **(B)** after nasogastric feeding tube placement. **A,** Gas is diffusely summating with the gastric wall (*black arrows*), and as linear, branching structures with liver (*black arrowheads*). The gas in the liver was suspected to be in the portal vein branches. **B,** One day later, most of the gas in the liver and gastric wall has resolved with supportive medical management.

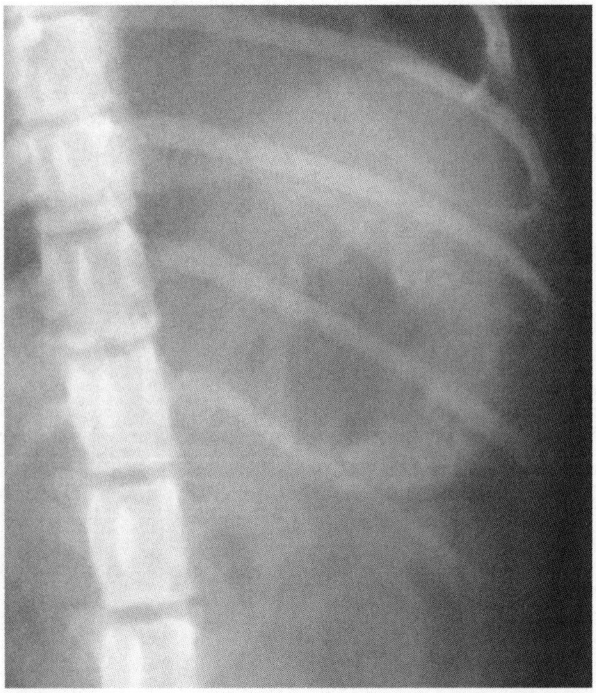

Fig. 45.37 Close-up ventrodorsal radiographs of a dog with gastric mineralization secondary to chronic renal failure. Thin, curvilinear, mineralized opacities that parallel the rugal folds of the stomach are caused by gastric calcification.

unchanged with distension of the stomach.[156] On ultrasound, gastropexy sites are easily identified, and most commonly a lack of sliding motion between the pyloric wall and the abdominal wall at the site of the gastropexy is suspected.[55,56,156]

It is also common to place gastric tubes using endoscopy and often no imaging procedures are required. However, the most common reason additional imaging might be performed is to evaluate whether the tube is misplaced submucosally, whether there is leakage at the tube site, or if inflammation at the skin surface is present and concern about extension into the peritoneal cavity exists. Submucosal placement or movement of the gastropexy tube may be noted using ultrasound. However, other imaging techniques might be chosen to further evaluate the site of the gastric tube placement. Radiography is often chosen as it provides a great overview and allows evaluation of the position of the stomach and tube relative to each other (Fig. 45.38). Additionally, iodinated contrast medium may be used to assess the patency and presence of leakage of the gastric tube (Fig. 45.39). Similarly, ultrasound might be used while a sterile saline solution is administered through the gastric tube. If leakage is present, contrast medium leakage may be noted on radiographs (see Fig. 45.39) or fluid extension outside the tube might be noted during the ultrasound examination.

Ultrasound is often chosen initially if fluid sampling is required, especially when a concern about septic peritonitis is present. If peritonitis is suspected post gastric surgery, the fat and mesentery adjacent to the stomach might be hyperechoic and additionally small to large quantities of fluid containing echogenic particles can be noted.

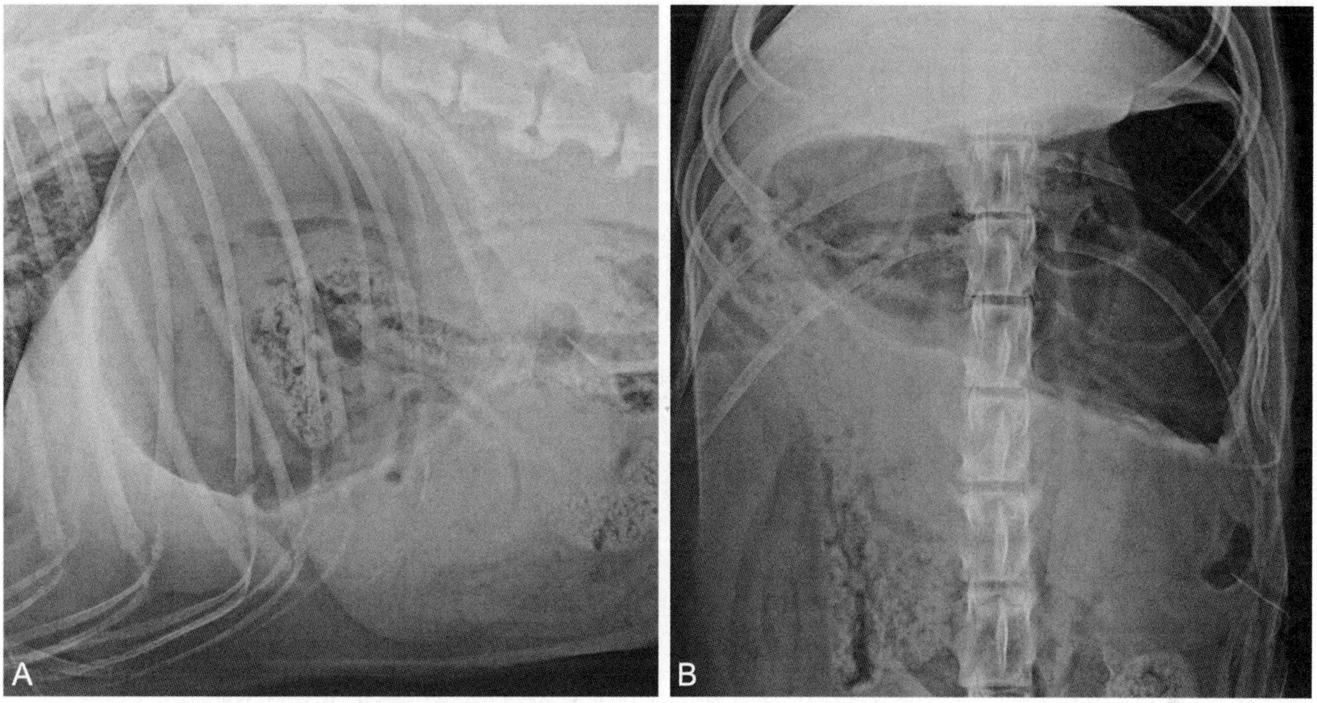

Fig. 45.38 Radiographs post gastrostomy tube placement in a dog. The dog presented with inflammation on the skin surface at the site of the tube placement and was evaluated for signs of tube leakage. **A,** Right lateral radiograph. The stomach has a pointed angle caudally toward the site of the gas-filled balloon of the gastric feeding tube. No free peritoneal gas or fluid is noted. **B,** Ventrodorsal radiograph. The stomach is altered in shape and extends along the left lateral abdominal wall further caudal and has a pointed angle. The gas-filled balloon of the gastric feeding tube is summating with the left lateral abdomen caudal of the gas dilated stomach.

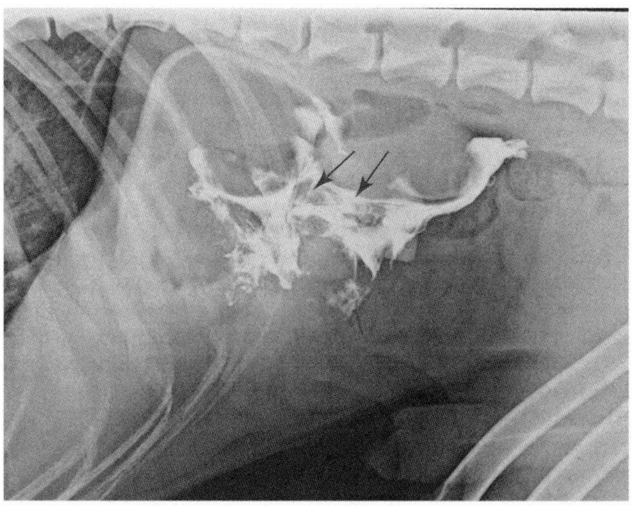

Fig. 45.39 Right lateral radiograph of a dog with leakage at the site of the placement of the percutaneous endoscopic gastrostomy (PEG) tube. The PEG tube was placed to support adequate nutrition as the patient was not gaining weight and had recurrent pneumonia due to severe megaesophagus. Iodinated contrast medium was administered through the tube and leakage of contrast medium at the level of the gastric wall was present (*arrows*). The stomach has an abnormal shape, which is commonly seen post gastric tube placement or gastropexy.

Acknowledgment

With special thanks to prior authors of this chapter for their contributions.

REFERENCES

1. Evans H, De Lahunta A. *Miller's Anatomy of the Dog*. 4th ed. St. Louis: Saunders; 2013.
2. Nickel R, Schummer A, Seiferle E. *The Viscera of the Domestic Mammals*. Berlin, Heidelberg: Springer; 1979.
3. Doom M, de Rooster H, van Bergen T, et al. Morphology of the canine omentum part 2: the omental bursa and its compartments materialized and explored by a novel technique. *Anat Histol Embryol*. 2016;45:28–36.
4. Armbrust LJ, Biller DS, Hoskinson JJ. Case examples demonstrating the clinical utility of obtaining both right and left lateral abdominal radiographs in small animals. *J Am Anim Hosp Assoc*. 2000;36:531–536.
5. Grandage J. The radiological appearance of stomach gas in the dog. *Aust Vet J*. 1974;50:529–532.
6. Brawner Jr WR, Bartels JE. Contrast radiography of the digestive tract. Indications, techniques, and complications. *Vet Clin North Am Small Anim Pract*. 1983;13: 599–626.
7. Root CR. Interpretation of abdominal survey radiographs. *Vet Clin North Am*. 1974;4:763–803.
8. Arnbjerg J. Gastric emptying time in the dog and cat. *J Am Anim Hosp Assoc*. 1992;28:77–81.
9. O'Brien TR. *Radiographic Diagnosis of Abdominal Disorders in the Dog and Cat: Radiographic Interpretation, Clinical Signs, Pathophysiology*. WB Saunders; 1978.
10. Miyabayashi T, Morgan JP. Upper gastrointestinal examinations: a radiographic study of clinically normal beagle puppies. *J Small Anim Pract*. 1991;32:83–88.
11. Love NE. The appearance of the canine pyloric region in right versus left lateral recumbent radiographs. *Vet Radiol Ultrasound*. 1993;34:169–170.

12. Jakovljevic S, Gibbs C. Radiographic assessment of gastric mucosal fold thickness in dogs. *Am J Vet Res*. 1993;54: 1827–1830.
13. Evans SM, Laufer I. Double contrast gastrography in the normal dog. *Veterinary Radiology*. 1981;22:2–9.
14. Evans SM, Biery DN. Double contrast gastrography in the cat. *Veterinary Radiology*. 1983;24:3–5.
15. Heng HG, Wrigley RH, Kraft SL, et al. Fat is responsible for an intramural radiolucent band in the feline stomach wall. *Vet Radiol Ultrasound*. 2005;46:54–56.
16. Bargai U. The effect of xylazine hydrochloride on the radiographic appearance of the stomach and intestine in the dog. *Veterinary Radiology*. 1982;23:60–63.
17. Gomez JA. The gastrointestinal contrast study. Methods and interpretation. *Vet Clin North Am*. 1974;4:805–842.
18. Hogan PM, Aronson E. Effect of sedation on transit time of feline gastrointestinal contrast studies. *Veterinary Radiology*. 1988;29:85–88.
19. Steyn PF, Twedt D, Toombs W. The effect of intravenous diazepam on solid phase gastric emptying in normal cats. *Vet Radiol Ultrasound*. 1997;38:469–473.
20. Scrivani PV, Bednarski RM, Myer CW. Effects of acepromazine and butorphanol on positive-contrast upper gastrointestinal tract examination in dogs. *Am J Vet Res*. 1998;59:1227–1233.
21. Bowlus RA, Biller DS, Armbrust LJ, et al. Clinical utility of pneumogastrography in dogs. *J Am Anim Hosp Assoc*. 2005;41:171–178.
22. Agut A, Sanchez-Valverde MA, Torrecillas FE, et al. Iohexol as a gastrointestinal contrast medium in the cat. *Vet Radiol Ultrasound*. 1994;35:164–168.
23. Allan FJ, Guilford WG, Robertson ID, et al. Gastric emptying of solid radiopaque markers in healthy dogs. *Vet Radiol Ultrasound*. 1996;37:336–344.
24. Allan GS, Rendano VT, Quick CB, et al. Gastrografin as a gastrointestinal contrast medium in the cat. *Veterinary Radiology*. 1979;20:110–116.
25. Burns J, Fox SM. The use of a barium meal to evaluate total gastric emptying time in the dog. *Veterinary Radiology*. 1986;27:169–172.
26. Chandler ML, Guilford G, Lawoko CR. Radiopaque markers to evaluate gastric emptying and small intestinal transit time in healthy cats. *J Vet Intern Med*. 1997;11:361–364.
27. Miyabayashi T, Morgan JP. Gastric emptying in the normal dog: a contrast radiographic technique. *Veterinary Radiology*. 1984;25:187–191.
28. Root CR, Morgan JP. Contrast radiography of the upper gastrointestinal tract in the dog. A comparison of micropulverized barium sulfate and U.S.P. barium sulfate suspensions in clinically normal dogs. *J Small Anim Pract*. 1969;10:279–286.
29. Williams J, Biller DS, Miyabayashi T, et al. Evaluation of iohexol as a gastrointestinal contrast medium in normal cats. *Vet Radiol Ultrasound*. 1993;34:310–314.
30. Guilford WG, Lawoko CR, Allan FJ. Accuracy of localizing radiopaque markers by abdominal radiography and correlation between their gastric emptying rate and that of a canned food in dogs. *Am J Vet Res*. 1997;58: 1359–1363.
31. Wallack ST. *The Handbook of Veterinary Contrast Radiography*. Solana Beach, CA: San Diego Veterinary Imaging, Inc.; 2003.
32. Funkquist B, Garmer L. Pathogenetic and therapeutic aspects of torsion of the canine stomach. *J Small Anim Pract*. 1967;8:523–532.
33. Gibbs C, Pearson H. The radiological diagnosis of gastrointestinal obstruction in the dog. *J Small Anim Pract*. 1973;14:61–82.
34. Gue M, Fioramonti J, Frexinos J, et al. Influence of acoustic stress by noise on gastrointestinal motility in dogs. *Dig Dis Sci*. 1987;32:1411–1417.
35. Hall JA, Willer RL, Seim 3rd HB, et al. Gastric emptying of nondigestible radiopaque markers after circumcostal gastropexy in clinically normal dogs and dogs with gastric dilatation-volvulus. *Am J Vet Res*. 1992;53:1961–1965.
36. Penninck DG, Nyland TG, Fisher PE, et al. Ultrasonography of the normal canine gastrointestinal tract. *Veterinary Radiology*. 1989;30:272–276.
37. Sanderson JJ, Boysen SR, McMurray JM, et al. The effect of fasting on gastrointestinal motility in healthy dogs as assessed by sonography. *JVECC*. 2017;27:645–650.
38. Gory G, Rault DN, Gatel L, et al. Ultrasonographic characteristics of the abdominal esophagus and cardia in dogs. *Vet Radiol Ultrasound*. 2014;55:552–560.
39. Grooters AM, Biller DS, Ward H, et al. Ultrasonographic appearance of feline alimentary lymphoma. *Vet Radiol Ultrasound*. 1994;35:468–472.
40. Kaser-Hotz B, Hauser B, Arnold P. Ultrasonographic findings in canine gastric neoplasia in 13 patients. *Vet Radiol Ultrasound*. 1996;37:51–56.
41. Lamb CR, Grierson J. Ultrasonographic appearance of primary gastric neoplasia in 21 dogs. *J Small Anim Pract*. 1996;40:211–215.
42. Penninck DG. Characterization of gastrointestinal tumors. *Vet Clin North Am Small Anim Pract*. 1998;28:777–797.
43. Penninck DG, Moore AS, Gliatto J. Ultrasonography of canine gastric epithelial neoplasia. *Vet Radiol Ultrasound*. 1998;39:342–348.
44. Penninck DG, Moore AS, Tidwell AS, et al. Ultrasonography of alimentary lymphosarcoma in the cat. *Vet Radiol Ultrasound*. 1994;35:299–306.
45. Rivers BJ, Walter PA, Johnston GR, et al. Canine gastric neoplasia: utility of ultrasonography in diagnosis. *J Am Anim Hosp Assoc*. 1997;33:144–155.
46. Graham JP, Newell SM, Roberts GD, et al. Ultrasonographic features of canine gastrointestinal pythiosis. *Vet Radiol Ultrasound*. 2000;41:273–277.
47. Murakami M, Heng HG, Lim CK, et al. Ultrasonographic features of presumed gastric wall edema in 14 dogs with pancreatitis. *J Vet Intern Med*. 2019;33:1260–1265.
48. Pennick D, Matz M, Tidwell A. Ultrasonography of gastric ulceration in the dog. *Vet Radiol Ultrasound*. 1997;38: 308–312.
49. Penninck DG, Nyland TG, Kerr LY, et al. Ultrasonographic evaluation of gastrointestinal diseases in small animals. *Veterinary Radiology*. 1990;31:134–141.
50. Tidwell AS, Penninck DG. Ultrasonography of gastrointestinal foreign bodies. *Vet Radiol Ultrasound*. 1992;33:160–169.
51. Biller DS, Partington BP, Miyabayashi T, et al. Ultrasonographic appearance of chronic hypertrophic pyloric gastropathy in the dog. *Vet Radiol Ultrasound*. 1994;35: 30–33.
52. Grooters AM, Miyabayashi T, Biller DS, et al. Sonographic appearance of uremic gastropathy in four dogs. *Vet Radiol Ultrasound*. 1994;35:35–40.
53. Huml RA, Konde LJ, Sellon RK, et al. Gastrogastric intussusception in a dog. *Vet Radiol Ultrasound*. 1992;33:150–153.
54. Watson PJ. Gastroduodenal intussusception in a young dog. *J Small Anim Pract*. 1997;38:163–167.
55. Tanno F, Weber U, Wacker C, et al. Ultrasonographic comparison of adhesions induced by two different methods of gastropexy in the dog. *J Small Anim Pract*. 1998;39:432–436.
56. Wacker CA, Weber UT, Tanno F, et al. Ultrasonographic evaluation of adhesions induced by incisional gastropexy in 16 dogs. *J Small Anim Pract*. 1998;39:379–384.

57. Mack RM, Staiger B, Langlois DK, et al. Development and characterization of a technique for percutaneous radiologic gastrojejunostomy tube placement in the dog. *J Vet Emerg Crit Care (San Antonio)*. 2016;26: 646–653.
58. Penninck DG, Crystal MA, Matz ME, et al. The technique of percutaneous ultrasound guided fine-needle aspiration biopsy and automated microcore biopsy in small animal gastrointestinal diseases. *Vet Radiol Ultrasound*. 1993;34:433–436.
59. Pal M, Singh P, Tayal R, et al. A comparative study of two-dimensional and three-dimensional ultrasonography in evaluation of gastric affections in dogs. *Vet World*. 2015;8:707–712.
60. Gaschen L, Kircher P, Wolfram K. Endoscopic ultrasound of the canine abdomen. *Vet Radiol Ultrasound*. 2007;48:338–349.
61. Lamb CR. Abdominal ultrasonography in small animals: intestinal tract and mesentery, kidneys, adrenal glands, uterus and prostate. *J Small Anim Pract*. 1990;31: 295–304.
62. Seiler GS, Cohen EB, d'Anjou MA, et al. ACVR and ECVDI consensus statement for the standardization of the abdominal ultrasound examination. *Vet Radiol Ultrasound*. 2022;63(6):661–674.
63. Larson MM, Biller DS. Ultrasound of the gastrointestinal tract. *Vet Clin North Am Small Anim Pract*. 2009;39: 747–759.
64. Couturier L, Rault D, Gatel L, et al. Ultrasonographic characterization of the feline cardia and pylorus in 34 healthy cats and three abnormal cats. *Vet Radiol Ultrasound*. 2012;53:342–347.
65. Newell SM, Graham JP, Roberts GD, et al. Sonography of the normal feline gastrointestinal tract. *Vet Radiol Ultrasound*. 1999;40:40–43.
66. Goggin JM, Biller DS, Debey BM, et al. Ultrasonographic measurement of gastrointestinal wall thickness and the ultrasonographic appearance of the ileocolic region in healthy cats. *J Am Anim Hosp Assoc*. 2000;36:224–228.
67. Hoey S, Drees R, Hetzel S. Evaluation of the gastrointestinal tract in dogs using computed tomography. *Vet Radiol Ultrasound*. 2013;54:25–30.
68. von Babo V, Eberle N, Mischke R, et al. Canine non-hematopoietic gastric neoplasia. Epidemiologic and diagnostic characteristics in 38 dogs with post-surgical outcome of five cases. *Tierarztl Prax Ausg K Kleintiere Heimtiere*. 2012;40:243–249.
69. Murakami M, Heng HG, Sola M. CT features of confirmed and presumed gastric wall edema in dogs. *Vet Radiol Ultrasound*. 2022;63:711–718.
70. Terragni R, Vignoli M, Rossi F, et al. Stomach wall evaluation using helical hydro-computed tomography. *Vet Radiol Ultrasound*. 2012;53:402–405.
71. Hornof WJ, Koblik PD, Strombeck DR, et al. Scintigraphic evaluation of solid-phase gastric emptying in the dog. *Veterinary Radiology*. 1989;30:242–248.
72. Kunze CP, Hoskinson JJ, Butine MD, et al. Evaluation of solid phase radiolabels of dog food for gastric emptying. *Vet Radiol Ultrasound*. 1999;40:169–173.
73. Goggin JM, Hoskinson JJ, Kirk CA, et al. Comparison of gastric emptying times in healthy cats simultaneously evaluated with radiopaque markers and nuclear scintigraphy. *Vet Radiol Ultrasound*. 1999;40:89–95.
74. Lester NV, Roberts GD, Newell SM, et al. Assessment of barium impregnated polyethylene spheres (Bipsr) as a measure of solid-phase gastric emptying in normal dogs—comparison to scintigraphy. *Vet Radiol Ultrasound*. 1999;40:465–471.
75. Metcalf MR. Scintigraphic gastrointestinal bleeding localization with 99mTc-labeled red blood cells. *Veterinary Radiology*. 1987;28:96–100.
76. Suter PF. Radiographic diagnosis of liver disease in dogs and cats. *Vet Clin North Am Small Anim Pract*. 1982;12:153–173.
77. Worth AJ, Machon RG. Traumatic diaphragmatic herniation: pathophysiology and management, Compendium on Continuing Education for the Practicing Veterinarian. *Compend Contin Educ Pract Vet*. 2005;27(3):178–180.
78. Hoddinott K. Traumatic diaphragmatic hernia in a 5-month-old boxer dog. *Can Vet J*. 2013;54:507–509.
79. Zarelli M, Carrillo JD, Soler M, et al. What is your diagnosis? Tension gastrothorax. *J Am Vet Med Assoc*. 2010;236:733–734.
80. Ellison GW, Lewis DD, Phillips L, et al. Esophageal hiatal hernia in small animals: literature review and a modified surgical technique. *JAAHA*. 1987;391.
81. Miles KG, Pope ER, Jergens AE. Paraesophageal hiatal hernia and pyloric obstruction in a dog. *J Am Vet Med Assoc*. 1988;193:1437–1439.
82. Burns CG, Bergh MS, McLoughlin MA. Surgical and nonsurgical treatment of peritoneopericardial diaphragmatic hernia in dogs and cats: 58 cases (1999–2008). *J Am Vet Med Assoc*. 2013;242:643–650.
83. Lee H, Yeon S, Lee H, et al. Ultrasonographic diagnosis—pylorogastric intussusception in a dog. *Vet Radiol Ultrasound*. 2005;46:317–318.
84. Choi J, Keh S, Kim T, et al. Ultrasonographic findings of pylorogastric intussusceptions in two dogs. *J Vet Sci*. 2012;13:215–217.
85. de Battisti A, Toscano MJ, Formaggini L. Gastric foreign body as a risk factor for gastric dilatation and volvulus in dogs. *J Am Vet Med Assoc*. 2012;241:1190–1193.
86. Glickman LT, Glickman NW, Schellenberg DB, et al. Non-dietary risk factors for gastric dilatation-volvulus in large and giant breed dogs. *J Am Vet Med Assoc*. 2000;217: 1492–1499.
87. Glickman LT, Glickman NW, Schellenberg DB, et al. Incidence of and breed-related risk factors for gastric dilatation-volvulus in dogs. *J Am Vet Med Assoc*. 2000;216:40–45.
88. Grange AM, Clough W, Casale SA. Evaluation of splenectomy as a risk factor for gastric dilatation-volvulus. *J Am Vet Med Assoc*. 2012;241:461–466.
89. Raghavan M, Glickman N, McCabe G, et al. Diet-related risk factors for gastric dilatation-volvulus in dogs of high-risk breeds. *J Am Anim Hosp Assoc*. 2004;40:192–203.
90. Schellenberg D, Yi Q, Glickman NW, et al. Influence of thoracic conformation and genetics on the risk of gastric dilatation-volvulus in Irish setters. *J Am Anim Hosp Assoc*. 1998;34:64–73.
91. Mazin RM, Christman A, Pasek A. Veterinary medicine today what is your diagnosis? *J Am Vet Med Assoc*. 2002;221:489–490.
92. Bredal WP, Eggertsdottir AV, Austefjord O. Acute gastric dilatation in cats: a case series. *Acta Vet Scand*. 1996;37:445–451.
93. Formaggini L, Schmidt K, De Lorenzi D. Gastric dilatation-volvulus associated with diaphragmatic hernia in three cats: clinical presentation, surgical treatment and presumptive aetiology. *J Feline Med Surg*. 2008;10:198–201.
94. Aslanian ME, Sharp CR, Garneau MS. Gastric dilatation and volvulus in a brachycephalic dog with hiatal hernia. *J Small Anim Pract*. 2014;55:535–537.
95. Funkquist B. Gastric torsion in the dog-I. Radiological picture during nonsurgical treatment related to the pathological anatomy and to the further clinical course. *J Small Anim Pract*. 1979;20:73–91.

96. Kneller SK. Radiographic interpretation of the gastric dilatation-volvulus complex in the dog. *JAAHA*. 1976;12: 154–157.
97. Mackenzie G, Barnhart M, Kennedy S, et al. A retrospective study of factors influencing survival following surgery for gastric dilatation-volvulus syndrome in 306 dogs. *J Am Anim Hosp Assoc*. 2010;46:97–102.
98. Frendin J, Funkquist B, Stavenborn M. Gastric displacement in dogs without clinical signs of acute dilatation. *J Small Anim Pract*. 1988;29:775–779.
99. Fischetti AJ, Saunders HM, Drobatz KJ. Pneumatosis in canine gastric dilatation-volvulus syndrome. *Vet Radiol Ultrasound*. 2004;45:205–209.
100. Carroll K, Wallace M, Hill T, et al. Pyloric outflow obstruction secondary to sclerosing encapsulating peritonitis in a dog. *Aust Vet J*. 2020;98:11–16.
101. Rhodes WH, Rad MMSV, Brodey RS. The differential diagnosis of pyloric obstructions in the dog. *Veterinary Radiology*. 1965;6:65–74.
102. Weingart C, Kohn B. [Zinc intoxication in a Yorkshire Terrier due to Euro cent ingestion]. *Schweiz Arch Tierheilkd*. 2009;151:75–81.
103. Meurs KM, Breitschwerdt EB, Baty CJ, et al. Postsurgical mortality secondary to zinc toxicity in dogs. *Vet Hum Toxicol*. 1991;33:579–583.
104. Torrance AG, Fulton Jr RB. Zinc-induced hemolytic anemia in a dog. *J Am Vet Med Assoc*. 1987;191:443–444.
105. Rossmeissl EM, Palmer KG, Hoelzler MG, et al. Multiple magnet ingestion as a cause of septic peritonitis in a dog. *J Am Anim Hosp Assoc*. 2011;47:56–59.
106. Hickey MC, Magee A. Gastrointestinal tract perforations caused by ingestion of multiple magnets in a dog. *J Vet Emerg Crit Care*. 2011;21:369–374.
107. Friday S, Murphy C, Lopez D, et al. Gorilla glue ingestion in dogs: 22 cases (2005–2019). *J Am Anim Hosp Assoc*. 2021;57(3):121–127.
108. Tyrrell D, Beck C. Survey of the use of radiography vs. ultrasonography in the investigation of gastrointestinal foreign bodies in small animals. *Vet Radiol Ultrasound*. 2006;47:404–408.
109. Shanaman MM, Schwarz T, Gal A, et al. Comparison between survey radiography, B-mode ultrasonography, contrast-enhanced ultrasonography and contrast-enhanced multi-detector computed tomography findings in dogs with acute abdominal signs. *Vet Radiol Ultrasound*. 2013;54:591–604.
110. Cotran RS, Robbins SL, Kumar V, et al. *Robbins Pathologic Basis of Disease*. 5th ed. Philadelphia: Saunders; 1994.
111. Howard EB, Sawa TR, Nielsen SW, et al. Mastocytoma and gastroduodenal ulceration. Gastric and duodenal ulcers in dogs with mastocytoma. *Pathol Vet*. 1969;6:146–158.
112. van der Gaag I, van Niel MH, Belshaw BE, et al. Gastric granulomatous cryptococcosis mimicking gastric carcinoma in a dog. *Vet Q*. 1991;13:185–190.
113. Stanton ME, Bright RM. Gastroduodenal ulceration in dogs. Retrospective study of 43 cases and literature review. *J Vet Intern Med*. 1989;3:238–244.
114. Jones RD, Baynes RE, Nimitz CT. Nonsteroidal anti-inflammatory drug toxicosis in dogs and cats: 240 cases (1989–1990). *J Am Vet Med Assoc*. 1992;201:475–477.
115. Jankowski M, Spużak J, Kubiak K, et al. Risk factors of gastric ulcers in dogs. *Pakistan Veterinary J*. 2015;35:93–97.
116. Dowdle SM, Joubert KE, Lambrechts NE, et al. The prevalence of subclinical gastroduodenal ulceration in Dachshunds with intervertebral disc prolapse. *J S Afr Vet Assoc*. 2003;74:77–81.
117. Davis MS, Williamson KK. Gastritis and gastric ulcers in working dogs. *Front Vet Sci*. 2016;3:30.
118. Nelson SW. The discovery of gastric ulcers and the differential diagnosis between benignancy and malignancy. *Radiol Clin North Am*. 1969;7:5–25.
119. Zboralske FF. Gastric ulcer. In: Margulis AR, Burhenne HJ, eds. *Alimentary Tract Roentgenology*. St Louis: CV Mosby; 1967:475–487.
120. Porcher P, Buffard P. Malignancy of the stomach. In: Margulis AR, Burhenne HJ, eds. *Alimentary Tract Roentgenology*. St Louis: CV Mosby; 1967:488–521.
121. Sautter JH, Hanlon GF. Gastric neoplasms in the dog: a report of 20 cases. *J Am Vet Med Assoc*. 1975;166:691–696.
122. Hayden DW, Nielsen SW. Canine alimentary neoplasia. *Zentralblatt für Veterinärmedizin Reihe A*. 2010;20: 1–22.
123. Barber DL. Radiographic aspects of gastric ulcers in dogs. *Veterinary Radiology*. 1982;23:109–116.
124. Liptak JM, Hunt GB, Barrs VR, et al. Gastroduodenal ulceration in cats: eight cases and a review of the literature. *J Feline Med Surg*. 2002;4:27–42.
125. Lang LG, Greatting HH, Spaulding KA. Imaging diagnosis—gastric pneumatosis in a cat. *Vet Radiol Ultrasound*. 2011;52:658–660.
126. Londono LA, Specht AJ, VanderHart DJ, et al. What is your diagnosis? Gastric wall hemorrhage secondary to anticoagulant rodenticide intoxication. *J Am Vet Med Assoc*. 2015;247:243–245.
127. Alavi A, Dann RW, Baum S, et al. Scintigraphic detection of acute gastrointestinal bleeding. *Radiology*. 1977;124: 753–756.
128. Gualtieri M, Monzeglio M. Gastrointestinal polyps in small animals. *European Journal of Comparative Gastroenterology*. 1996;1:1–11.
129. van der Gaag I. The histological appearance of peroral gastric biopsies in clinically healthy and vomiting dogs. *Can J Vet Res*. 1988;52:67–74.
130. Gualtieri M, Monzeglio MG, Scanziani E. Gastric neoplasia. *Vet Clin North Am Small Anim Pract*. 1999;29:415–440.
131. Willard MD. Alimentary neoplasia in geriatric dogs and cats. *Vet Clin North Am Small Anim Pract*. 2012;42:693–706.
132. Murray M, Robinson PB, McKeating FJ, et al. Primary gastric neoplasia in the dog: a clinico-pathological study. *Vet Rec*. 1972;91:474–479.
133. Patnaik AK, Hurvitz AI, Johnson GF. Canine gastric adenocarcinoma. *Vet Pathol*. 1978;15:600–607.
134. Brodey RS. Alimentary tract neoplasms in the cat: a clinicopathologic survey of 46 cases. *Zahnarztl Prax*. 1966;17:74–80.
135. Gieger T. Alimentary lymphoma in cats and dogs. *Vet Clin North Am Small Anim Pract*. 2011;41:419–432.
136. Hayden DW, Fleischman RW. Scirrhous eosinophilic gastritis in dogs with gastric arteritis. *Vet Pathol*. 1977;14: 441–448.
137. Pietra M, Zanoni RG, Peli A, et al. Gastric inflammatory pseudotumour secondary to *Actinomyces hordeovulneris* infection in a cat. *Ir Vet J*. 2015;69:12.
138. McConnell JF, Sparkes AH, Blunden AS, et al. Eosinophilic fibrosing gastritis and toxoplasmosis in a cat. *J Feline Med Surg*. 2007;9:82–88.
139. Teshima T, Matsumoto H, Michishita M, et al. Multiple inflammatory gastric polyps treated by endoscopic polypectomy with argon plasma coagulation in a dog. *J Small Anim Pract*. 2013;54:265–268.
140. Marolf AJ, Bachand AM, Sharber J, et al. Comparison of endoscopy and sonography findings in dogs and cats with histologically confirmed gastric neoplasia. *J Small Anim Pract*. 2015;56:339–344.

141. Hobbs J, Sutherland-Smith J, Penninck D, et al. Ultrasonographic features of canine gastrointestinal stromal tumors compared to other gastrointestinal spindle cell tumors. *Vet Radiol Ultrasound*. 2015;56:432–438.
142. Burke RL, Ackerman N. The abdomen. In: Burke RL, Ackerman N, eds. *Small Animal Radiology and Ultrasonography: A Diagnostic Atlas and Text*. 2nd ed. Philadelphia: Saunders; 1996:250–477.
143. Diana A, Penninck DG, Keating JH. Ultrasonographic appearance of canine gastric polyps. *Vet Radiol Ultrasound*. 2009;50:201–204.
144. Lamb CR, Forster-van Hijfte M. Ultrasound corner beware the gastric pseudomass. *Vet Radiol Ultrasound*. 1994;4;35:398–399.
145. Crystal MA, Penninck DG, Matz ME, et al. Use of ultrasound-guided fine-needle aspiration biopsy and automated core biopsy for the diagnosis of gastrointestinal diseases in small animals. *Vet Radiol Ultrasound*. 1993;34:438–444.
146. van der Gaag I, Happe RP, Wolvekamp WT. A boxer dog with chronic hypertrophic gastritis resembling Menetrier's disease in man. *Vet Pathol*. 1976;13:172–185.
147. Vaughn DP, Syrcle J, Cooley J. Canine giant hypertrophic gastritis treated successfully with partial gastrectomy. *J Am Anim Hosp Assoc*. 2014;50:62–66.
148. Murakami M, Heng HG, Sola M. CT features of confirmed and presumed gastric wall edema in dogs. *Vet Radiol Ultrasound*. 2022;63(6):711–718. https://doi.org/10.1111/vru.13123. Epub 2022 Jun 8. PMID: 35674240; PMCID: PMC9796106.
149. Thierry F, Ferreira MF, Paterson GK, et al. Canine and feline emphysematous gastritis may be differentiated from gastric emphysema based on clinical and imaging characteristics: five cases. *Vet Radiol Ultrasound*. 2019;60:136–144.
150. Barber DL, Rowland GN. Radiographically detectable soft tissue calcification in chronic renal failure. *Veterinary Radiology*. 1979;20:117–123.
151. Lidbury JA, Suchodolski JS, Steiner JM. Gastric histopathologic abnormalities in dogs: 67 cases (2002-2007). *J Am Vet Med Assoc*. 2009;234:1147–1153.
152. Parfitt AM. Soft-tissue calcification in uremia. *Arch Intern Med*. 1969;124:544–556.
153. Corapi WV, Ajithdoss DK, Snowden KF, et al. Multi-organ involvement of *Heterobilharzia americana* infection in a dog presented for systemic mineralization. *J Vet Diagn Invest*. 2011;23:826–831.
154. Beck C, O'Neill T, Holloway SA, et al. The use of ultrasound in the investigation of gastric carcinoma in a dog. *Aust Vet J*. 2001;79:332–334.
155. Bakhtiari J, Abdi M, Khalaj AR, et al. Comparative evaluation of two reconstructive methods following laparoscopic assisted subtotal gastrectomy in dogs. *BMC Res Notes*. 2012;5:1–6.
156. Belandria GA, Pavletic MM, Boulay JP, et al. Gastropexy with an automatic stapling instrument for the treatment of gastric dilatation and volvulus in 20 dogs. *Can Vet J*. 2009;50:733–740.

ELECTRONIC RESOURCES

Additional information related to the content in Chapter 45 can be found online at eBooks.Health.Elsevier.com

- Chapter Quiz

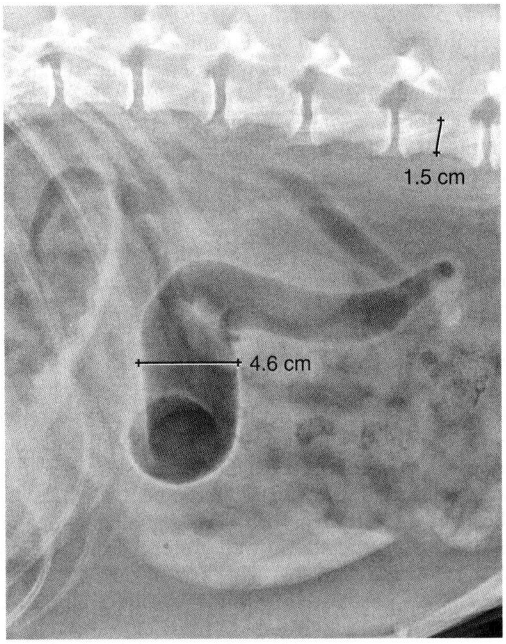

Fig. 46.14 A single severely dilated small bowel segment is present in this dog. The diameter is three times the central height of the L5 vertebral body. Several small bowel segments are seen caudal to the spleen and ventral to the fecal material in the colon. A segment of corncob, not visible, in the proximal jejunum was the cause of obstruction.

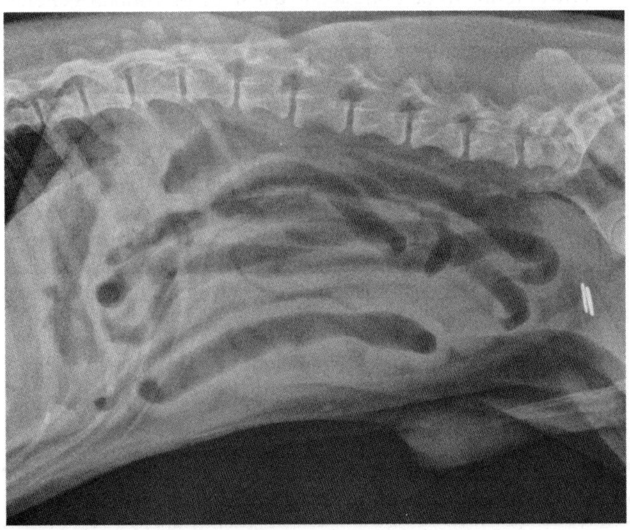

Fig. 46.15 This dog has mild generalized dilation of the small bowel. Most segments are gas filled with variable amounts of luminal gas. The bowel wall appears thick but this is likely due to silhouetting of luminal fluid with the wall. This dog had a history of mixed bowel diarrhea. The radiographic changes are supportive of but not diagnostic for enteritis.

(Fig. 46.15, eFig. 46.4); and (4) generalized/severe: all loops are involved, and luminal distention is greater than twice normal.

Mechanical Obstruction

The small intestine can be occluded by foreign objects, intussusception, mural mass, or extrinsic lesions. The radiographic features of small bowel obstruction depend on three factors: the completeness of the obstruction, the location of the obstruction in the gastrointestinal tract, and the duration. The most consistent radiographic sign of mechanical obstruction is a variable degree of dilation of bowel segments orad to the site of obstruction (Fig. 46.16, eFig. 46.5). Subjective determination that bowel is significantly dilated can be made accurately even by interpreters with a beginning level of interpretation experience.[49] However, using ratios of small intestinal diameter to vertebral measurements may increase confidence that obstructive bowel disease is present. In dogs, determining the ratio of the small intestinal diameter relative to the L5 vertebral body height can be used, but it must be remembered that this ratio is only a guideline.[5] A ratio less than 1.4 to 1.6 usually rules out mechanical obstruction. Ratios of 1.95 were associated with a 77% to 80% probability of obstruction and a ratio of 2.07 was associated with an 86% to 90% probability of obstruction (see Fig. 46.18, eFig. 46.6).[49,50] In a series of cats, when the maximum small intestinal diameter to L2 vertebral endplate height was >2.0, gastrointestinal disease was present, and at a ratio of >2.5, the most likely abnormality was intestinal obstruction.[7]

A more distal obstruction leads to a greater number of distended segments. Obstructed bowel typically contains both fluid and gas unless the obstruction is quite proximal, allowing gas and fluid to reflux into the stomach. Depending on the location of a complete obstruction, there may be two distinctly different sizes of bowel with the smaller and normal diameter bowel distal or aboral to the dilated bowel. More complete and longer duration obstruction results in greater bowel distention. As intestines become progressively more distended, the segments become crowded into a relatively smaller space, often assuming a *stacked* appearance (Fig. 46.17).

Acute duodenal obstruction is challenging to diagnose because the stomach acts as a reservoir for gas and fluid that might collect. Also, if vomiting is frequent, the accumulated fluid and gas are expelled from the stomach and duodenum. With chronic duodenal obstruction, however, gastric distention develops (Fig. 46.18) and can be pronounced. A moderate to large volume of fluid and gas in the stomach, with an otherwise empty small intestinal tract, in a vomiting patient should raise suspicion of duodenal obstruction or pyloric outflow obstruction.

Partial obstructions may also be difficult to detect. This is particularly true when the partial obstruction is of short duration and in the proximal duodenum. Longstanding partial distal obstructions result in accumulation of opaque granular material proximal to the site of obstruction. This is caused by desiccation of ingesta that becomes trapped proximal to the obstruction. The desiccated material often has the appearance of feces, and the identification of this fecal-like material in the small rather than large bowel is a reliable sign of partial distal small bowel obstruction. This appearance has been referred to as the *gravel sign*. One scenario in which chronic partial obstruction occurs is elderly cats that develop an ileal adenocarcinoma causing partial bowel obstruction (Fig. 46.19, eFig. 46.7). If a bowel obstruction is complete, the intestine distal to the obstruction is likely to be empty.

Foreign objects are a common cause of obstruction. Foreign bodies composed of mineral or metal are easily recognized. Small-sized rocks, clay litter, hard-shelled seeds, or other debris are ingested frequently by dogs and cats and opaque medicinal tablets may be administered by owners.[51] These small mineral opacities are usually incidental and pass without causing obstruction. Nonmineralized, nonmetallic foreign objects are much more difficult to identify. Fruit pits, corncobs, and other nonopaque objects may be recognized by their geometrically shaped radiolucencies on survey radiographs (see eFig. 46.6).[52] A nonopaque foreign object with irregular surfaces, especially with grooves or pockets, can entrap small, mineralized ingested debris and gas and may become more visible (Fig. 46.20, eFigs. 46.8, 46.9). Careful application of abdominal compression may enhance the conspicuity of these foreign objects (see Fig. 46.20B).

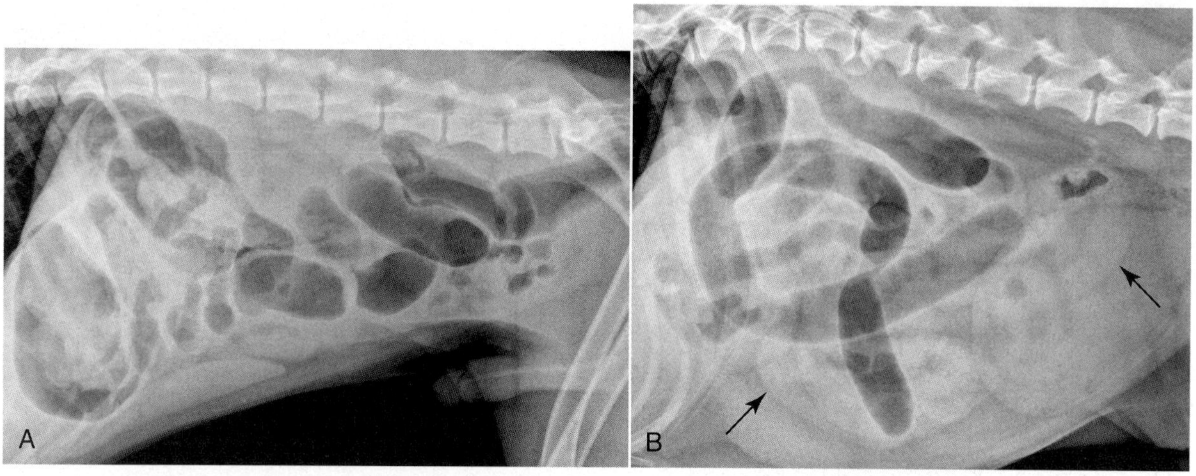

Fig. 46.16 **A,** Lateral radiograph of a dog with mechanical jejunal obstruction caused by a cloth foreign body. There are multiple small intestinal segments that are abnormally dilated. The configuration of the dilated segments indicates that they cannot all be colon. There are two populations of small bowel: large segments and normal segments. Having multiple populations of small bowel size is common in dogs with mechanical obstruction. This dog has less intraluminal fluid than most dogs with mechanical obstruction. **B,** Lateral radiograph of a dog with mechanical obstruction caused by a peach pit. There are a few gas-distended segments of jejunum, and some distended segments also contain fluid (*black arrows*).

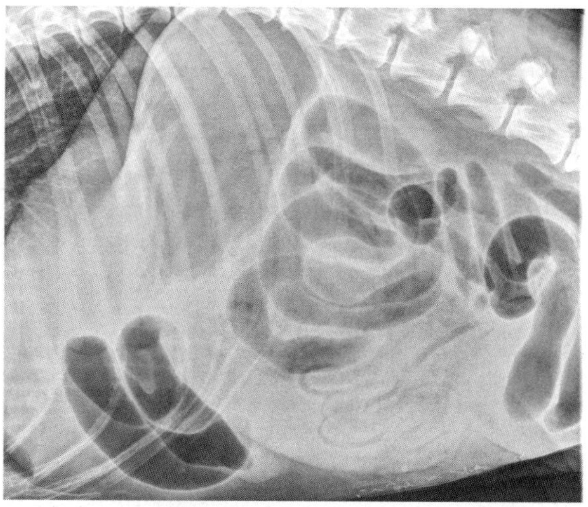

Fig. 46.17 Lateral view of a dog with a distal small bowel obstruction. The bowel is not severely dilated, and there are several segments of normal diameter. However, those segments that are gas dilated are aligned vertically and horizontally in a *stacked* pattern. Metallic abdominal wall sutures are present from a surgery 7 years prior for removal of a foreign body.

Sand impaction can also cause intestinal obstruction, and this tends to be in the distal small intestine (Fig. 46.21, eFig. 46.10).[53] Radiographically, there is segmental dilation of the bowel that contains mineral opaque material. Although sand particles are small, it is proposed that the sand coalesces and dehydrates to form the obstruction. Sequential radiographs can be used to monitor progression of the sand but if no progress is observed, a laparotomy should be considered.[53]

A pneumocolon can be used to differentiate the source of dilated bowel as small intestine versus colon and can assist in defining the location of obvious foreign material or mottled mineralized material to be in the small versus large bowel (Fig. 46.22, eFig. 46.11). The use of 24-hour serial survey radiographs, ultrasound evaluation, or a contrast study may be necessary to confirm the diagnosis of partial obstruction suggested by abnormal luminal contents. Persistence of small opaque foreign objects in the same intestinal location in serial radiographs over a 24- to 48-hour period should increase the suspicion of partial obstruction.

Two recent studies looked at the use of serial radiographs relative to mechanical bowel obstruction. One assessed the diagnostic accuracy of mechanical obstruction between initial and one follow-up radiograph between 7 and 28 hours. These dogs and cats ultimately had nonopaque foreign bodies causing partial or complete obstruction. Accuracy did not significantly increase after the follow-up radiograph, and when the repeat radiograph is inclusive, alternate diagnostic studies such as ultrasound should be considered.[54] The second study evaluated the incidence of resolution of mechanical obstruction and resolution of gastrointestinal foreign bodies as assessed by repeat radiographs after 36-hour intervals of medical management. Approximately 17% of patients with only small intestine affected and 11% of patients with gastric plus small intestinal foreign bodies and mechanical obstruction resolved after medical management.[55]

The ultrasonographic appearance of ingested foreign material varies according to the composition of the material (Fig. 46.23).[56] The acoustic pattern caused by the rigid foreign object may have a shape that can be recognized specifically. Objects that transmit the beam, such as some types of rubber balls, are more readily identified. Those that create a strong reflection with marked acoustic shadowing can be more difficult to define initially. When these objects cause incomplete obstruction, they are frequently associated with increased intestinal motility resulting from irritation. With more complete obstruction, the foreign object may be associated with accumulation of fluid in the bowel cranial to the obstruction. In vomiting dogs, ultrasound findings of a jejunal serosa-to-serosa measurement of more than 1.5 cm, with normal wall layering, and a fluid-filled or gas-filled lumen should prompt careful interrogation of the bowel for an obstructive lesion.[57] A wide range of motility, from reduced to increased, was observed in dogs with mechanical obstruction and was not found to be a useful discriminatory feature relative to nonobstructive causes of vomiting.[57]

Both dogs and cats can ingest linear foreign material. Linear types of foreign bodies accounted for 35% of foreign bodies in

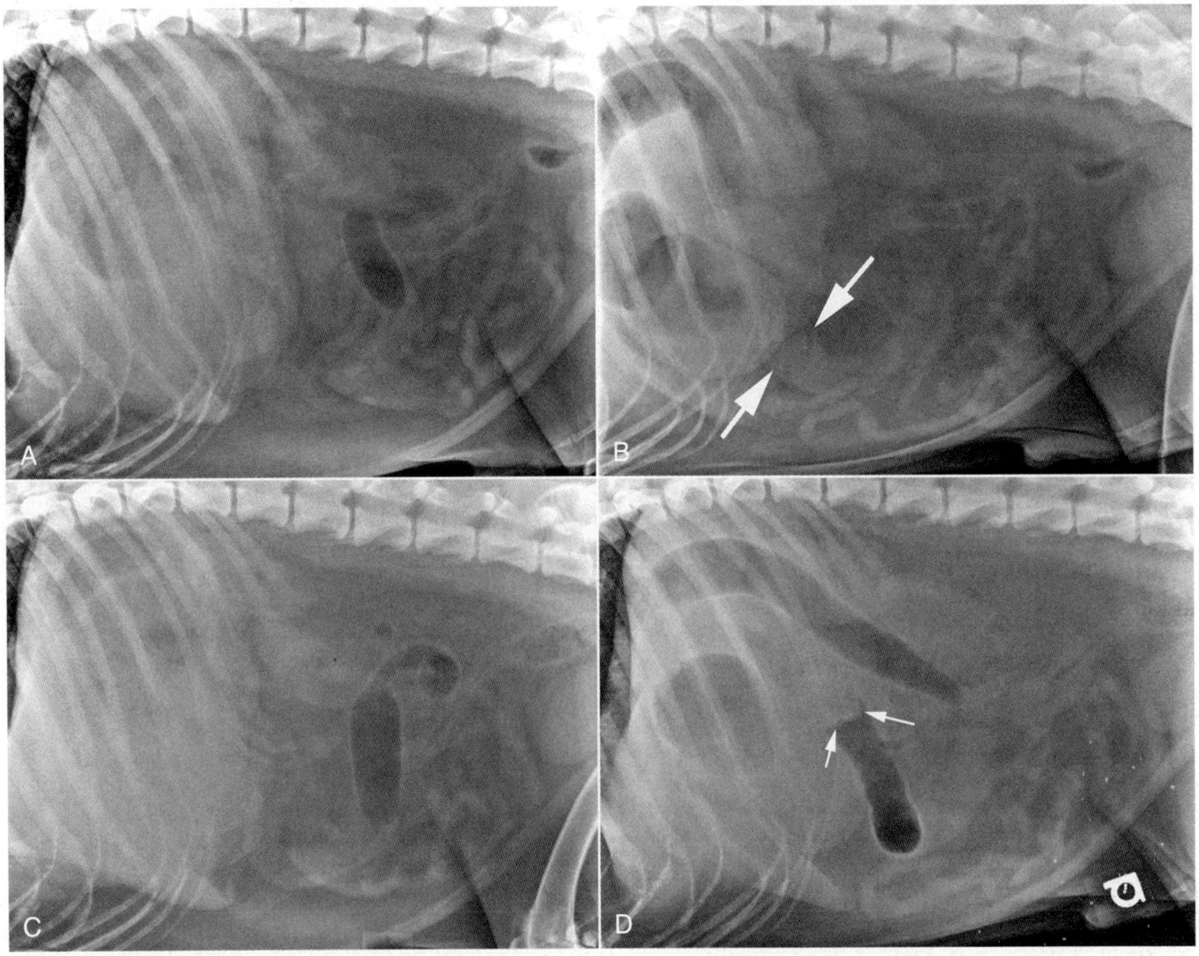

Fig. 46.18 Right and left lateral serial radiographs of a dog with acute onset of vomiting 2 days prior. Right lateral **(A)** and left lateral **(B)** views were obtained at presentation. In **A** the size of the stomach was judged to be at the upper limit of normal, containing both gas and fluid. There is also a single vertically oriented short segment of small bowel that is distended with gas, and there is a small amount of gas and granular material in the descending colon. The remainder of the bowel is gasless and of small diameter. In **B,** there is gas in the proximal duodenum, evidence that the pylorus is patent, and the duodenum is abnormally dilated. Immediately caudal and ventral to the fluid-filled pylorus is a round mottled opacity in a fluid-filled dilated segment (*white arrows*). Right **(C)** and left **(D)** lateral views were obtained several hours later. They are relatively unchanged from the earlier radiographs. However, in **D,** there is now gas in the distal duodenum outlining a soft tissue foreign body (*white arrows*). A focal mineral opacity is present in all views in the caudal ventral aspect of this foreign body that was subsequently identified as a corncob.

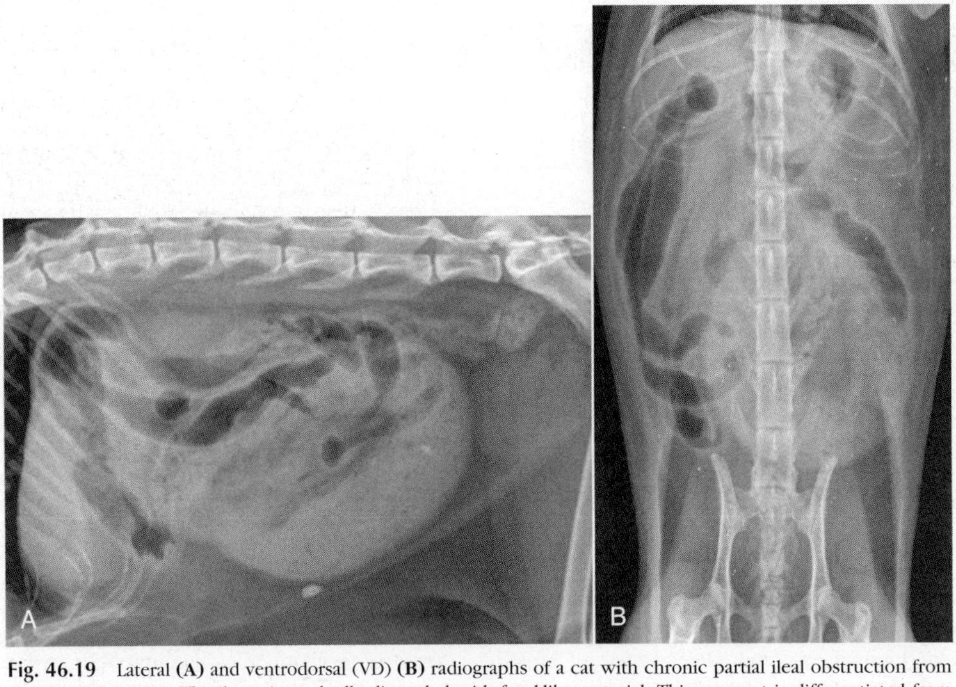

Fig. 46.19 Lateral **(A)** and ventrodorsal (VD) **(B)** radiographs of a cat with chronic partial ileal obstruction from an adenocarcinoma. The ileum is markedly distended with fecal-like material. This segment is differentiated from large bowel by its position ventral to the colon in **A** and its caudal flexure in **B**; the colon does not have a caudal flexure as seen in **B**. The opacity of the material in the bowel is caused by continued desiccation because of its inability to pass the obstruction. More proximal bowel segments may continue to remain normal.

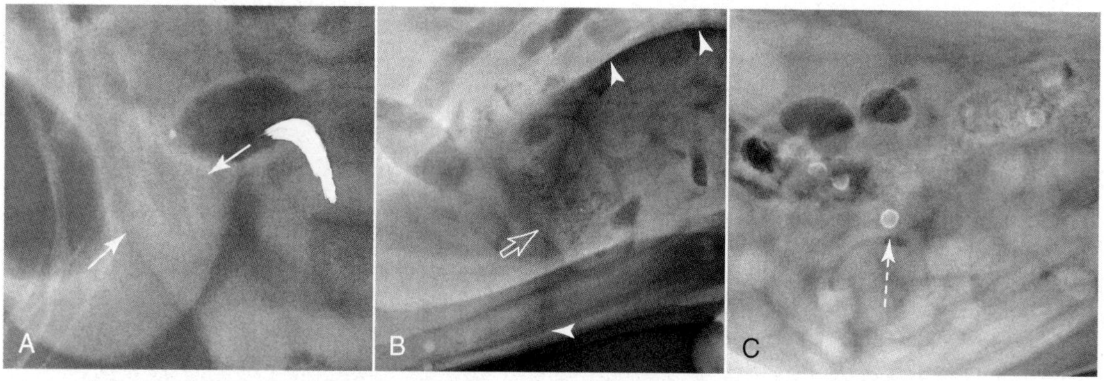

Fig. 46.20 Radiolucent and opaque foreign bodies. **A** is an obstructive peach pit (between the *white arrows*). Its subtle shape is defined best by the radiolucent oval center. A small focus of opaque debris is trapped in one of the crevasses of the outer surface. **B** is an obstructing corncob (*open arrow*). A compression paddle (border indicated by *white arrowheads*) was used to displace bowel, making the corncob more easily seen. Note the gas as well as mineral debris trapped in the kernel pockets. **C** is a dog with ingested Hackberry tree seeds (*dashed arrow*). Based on their size, they would not be expected to cause obstruction, and several are present in the colon.

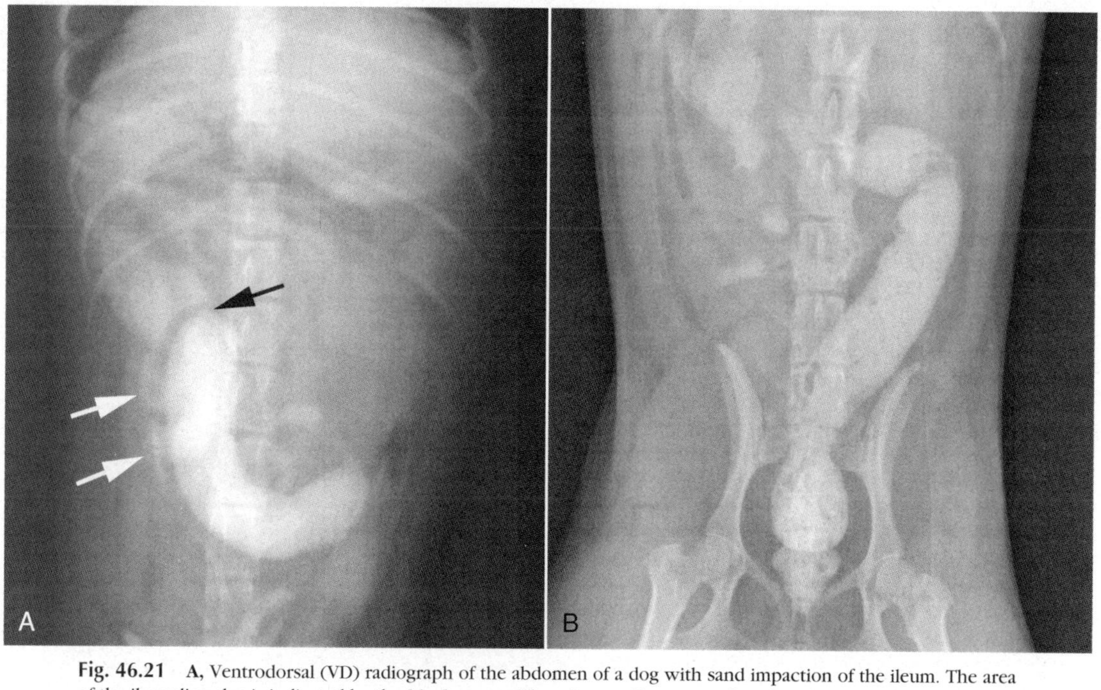

Fig. 46.21 **A,** Ventrodorsal (VD) radiograph of the abdomen of a dog with sand impaction of the ileum. The area of the ileocolic valve is indicated by the *black arrow*. There is a small amount of sand in the cecum (*white arrows*) and ascending colon. **B,** Follow-up radiograph in which the sand has moved spontaneously from the ileum into the colon, negating the need for a laparotomy. Follow-up radiographs are valuable to monitor the progression of intestinal foreign material; the clinical condition of the patient must be considered if follow-up radiographs are planned as acutely ill patients may be candidates for immediate laparotomy rather than a delay for additional images.

one population of dogs.[58] Linear foreign material that becomes trapped in the intestine usually causes both an abnormal shape and contour of the loops and an abnormal gas pattern (see Fig. 46.10).[7] Some portion of the linear material typically becomes fixed at an orad location, most commonly in the pylorus in dogs and under the tongue in cats.[58–60] The remainder of the length passes into the small intestine. The peristaltic action of the bowel causes it to climb along the linear foreign body, which results in a pleated, plicated, or bunched appearance of the affected loops. With a linear foreign body, the intestinal segments may not become markedly distended but gas commonly becomes trapped in pockets formed by the pleats. The result is an abnormal pattern of round, tapered, short-tubular, and sometimes crescent- or comma-shaped gas shapes (Fig. 46.24, eFig. 46.12). Gas bubbles of these shapes can be referred to as having a geometric shape. This pattern may be accentuated in the left lateral view as gastric gas moves into the duodenum from the stomach. The left lateral also often allows identification of foreign material anchored in the pylorus, surrounded by gas (Fig. 46.25, eFig. 46.13). The abnormal contour and plication pattern are usually obvious in a positive-contrast study (Fig. 46.26). Although barium can be used for positive-contrast studies in patients suspected of having a linear foreign body, if there is any concern for perforation of the bowel, consideration should be given to the use of low-osmolar water-soluble contrast medium to avoid barium contamination

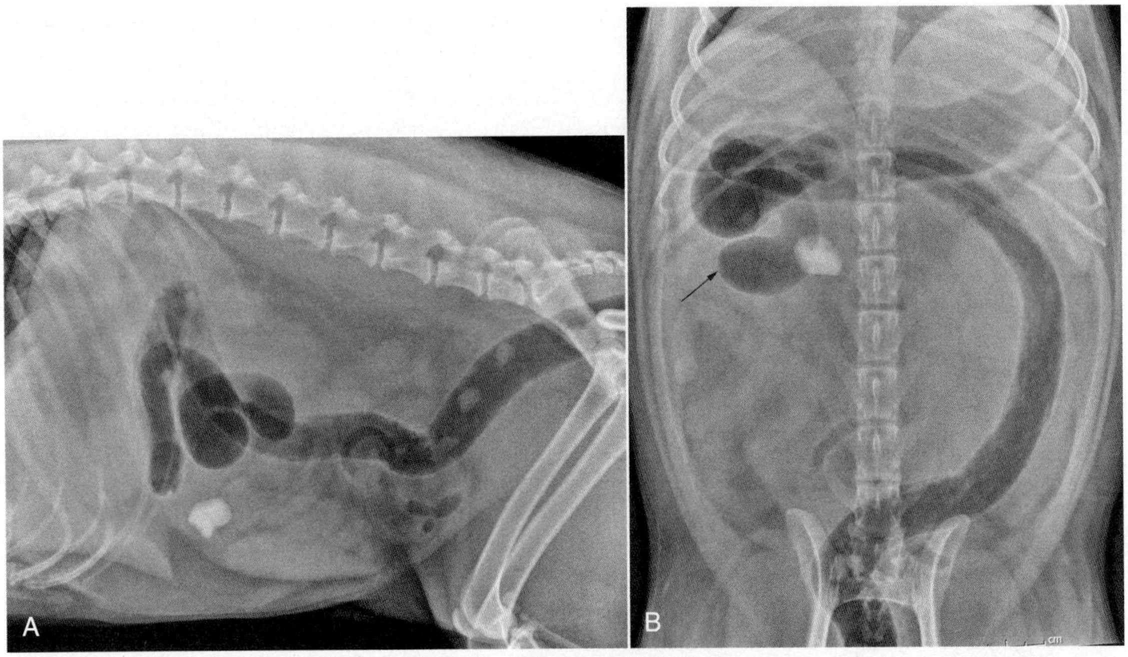

Fig. 46.22 Left lateral **(A)** and ventrodorsal (VD) **(B)** views following introduction of air into the colon (tubing evident in the distal descending colon). The pneumocolon defines that the obvious rock foreign body is not in the colon. A rock was removed from the duodenal-jejunal junction. The gas filled cecum is indicated by the *arrow*.

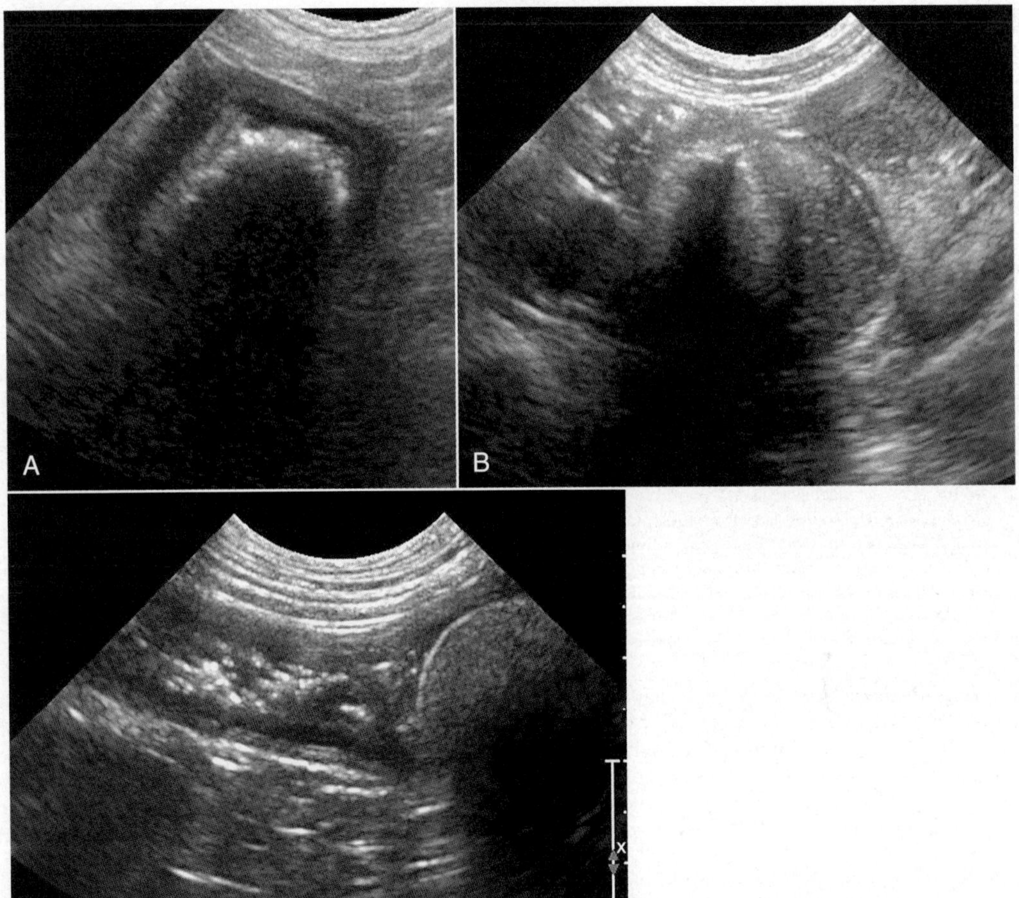

Fig. 46.23 Three ultrasound images of intestinal foreign bodies each with a different shape. All of these foreign bodies have strong acoustic shadowing. The object in **A** was undetermined, **B** was several pieces of hoof material, and **C** was a portion of a rubber ball. In **C**, there is a longitudinal section of the bowel orad to the foreign body that is filled with mucoid fluid.

of the abdomen. If the linear material is absorptive in nature, such as fabric, it can absorb fluid incompletely and have a mottled to linear, streaked gas pattern. In the cat, the plication of the bowel can cause a *clumped* or *bunched* positioning of the bowel. The displacement of the small bowel into the middle or right side of the abdomen in the obese cat should not be misinterpreted as plication caused by a linear foreign body (Fig. 46.27).

The ultrasound appearance of linear material depends on the amount of gas and fluid accumulated around the foreign material. Plication of the bowel around an echogenic line has been described most frequently (Fig. 46.28, eFig. 46.14).[56] This differs from the smooth, straight mucosa normally seen on either side of the bright linear stripe of an empty normal bowel

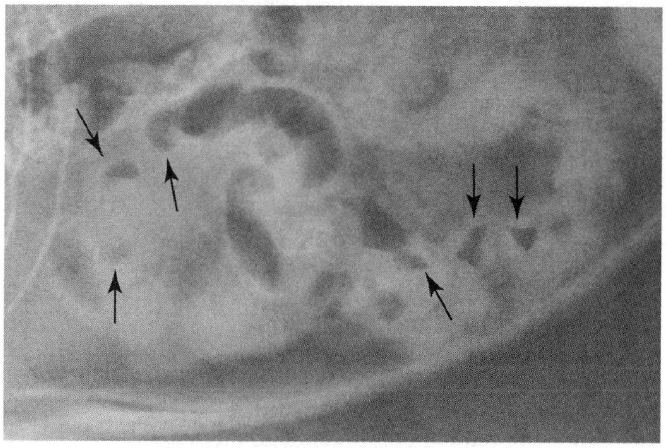

Fig. 46.24 Lateral view of a cat with a linear foreign body. The jejunum is bunched in the ventral abdomen, and gas has become trapped in the plications, creating small, irregularly shaped bubbles (*black arrows*), a pattern that is not typically present in normal bowel.

lumen. If the linear foreign material is in the duodenum, it may be traceable into the stomach.[61]

A serious complication of a chronic linear foreign body is laceration of the intestinal wall. If the laceration is small, serosal adhesion to an adjacent loop can occur, resulting in a fixed position of two or more loops. If the laceration is large, peritonitis occurs with possible free abdominal gas.

There are some differences between dogs and cats with regard to linear foreign objects: (1) affected dogs are usually older and have less irregularity in the gas pattern; (2) dogs are more prone to secondary intussusception; (3) dogs have more evidence of bowel trauma or bowel laceration and peritonitis, both radiographically and surgically; and (4) the probability of death as a result of linear foreign body is nearly twice as high in dogs as in cats.[60,61] Intestinal perforation caused by linear foreign material or other diseases should be suspected ultrasonographically when a combination of focal hyperechoic mesenteric fat, echogenic peritoneal effusion, and fluid in the bowel is identified.

Intussusception, the invagination of one portion (intussusceptum) of the gastrointestinal tract into the lumen (intussuscipiens) of an adjacent segment, can be initiated by many events, including motility disorders, inflammatory wall lesions, neoplasia, foreign bodies, or idiopathic causes.[62,63] Although an intussusception can occur anywhere along the digestive tract, the majority occur at the ileocolic or cecocolic junction. The radiographic appearance of an intussusception is influenced by the completeness of the obstruction.[8] Distal intussusceptions can result in generalized severe dilation of the small bowel, creating the typical appearance of mechanical obstruction, although many patients with an intussusception have a partial rather than a complete obstruction. The intussusceptum will occasionally create a visible soft tissue mass effect in the colon if sufficient gas is present in the intussuscipiens to provide contrast (Fig. 46.29). In most patients, however, differentiating intussusception from other causes of mechanical obstruction based solely on survey radiographs is not possible. Ultrasound

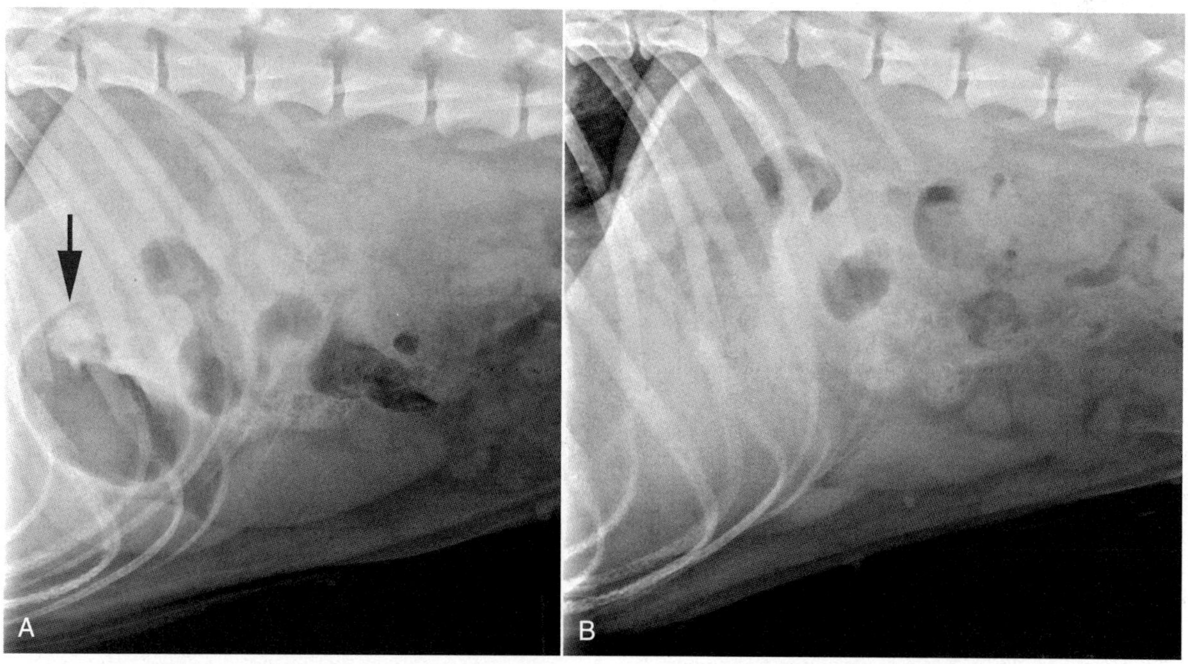

Fig. 46.25 Left **(A)** and right **(B)** lateral radiographs of a dog with a linear foreign body. The anchoring of the foreign material in the pylorus is obvious in the left lateral view (*black arrow*) due to gas being present in the pylorus. Some gas has also left the stomach in the left lateral view to enter the duodenum, and the pleated appearance of this segment of intestine is more obvious as a result compared to the right lateral.

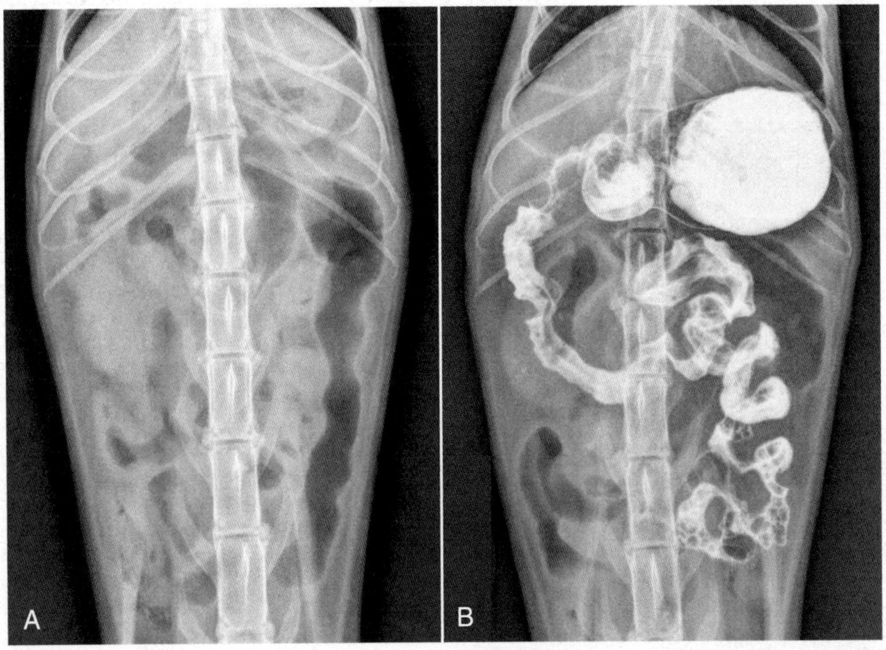

Fig. 46.26 Survey ventrodorsal (VD) and barium-contrast study of linear foreign body in a cat. In the survey image, there is an abnormally shaped gas accumulation in the right 12th intercostal space. The classic plication pattern of the bowel is visible in the barium image.

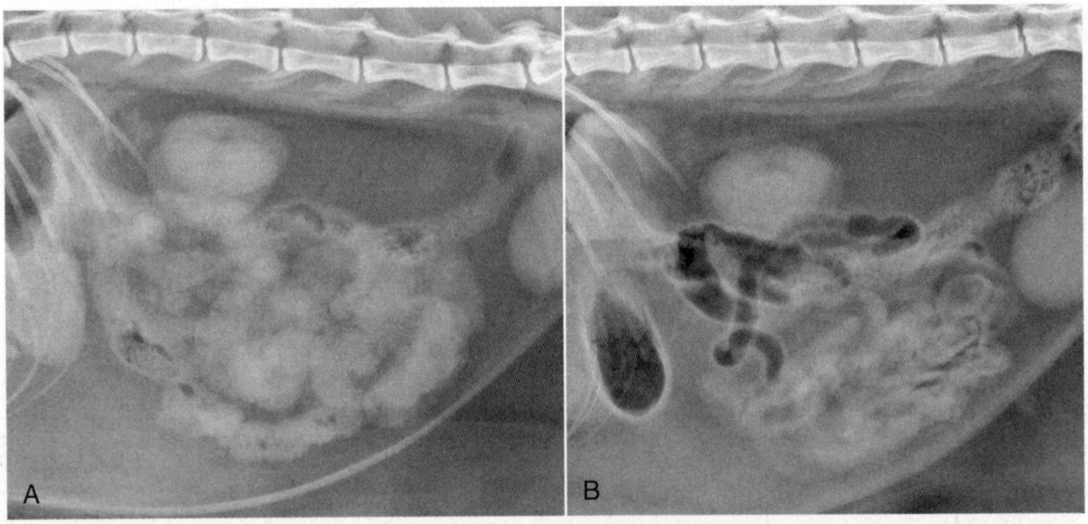

Fig. 46.27 Image **A** is an obese cat with an extensive jejunal linear foreign body. Image **B** is an obese cat without linear foreign body. Both have a relative *clumping* of the small intestine in the central abdomen. The effect of the intra-abdominal fat on the positioning of the small intestine makes differentiation of true plication difficult in the obese cat, particularly where there is minimal gas in the bowel to cause the formation of geometrically shaped gas bubbles. There is more pronounced serosal border undulation in cat **A** compared with **B** to increase suspicion of plication. Ultrasound or a contrast study can be used in such patients to confirm the linear foreign body.

evaluation is preferred to positive-contrast studies for substantiating the diagnosis.

Intussusceptions have a characteristic ultrasonographic appearance (Fig. 46.30). The telescoping effect results in a concentric ring appearance when viewed in the transverse plane and a multilinear pattern when viewed in the longitudinal plane.[64,65] A hyperechoic region is typically noted mildly eccentrically positioned within the concentric or linear pattern, caused by mesenteric fat pulled into the intussuscipiens. The shape of this hyperechoic material may be round or semilunar. If an anechoic feature is evident centrally, it most likely represents a small volume of fluid within the lumen of the intussusceptum; if evident eccentrically, it likely represents fluid between the intussusceptum and intussuscipiens. When viewed in the long axis, fluid distention is often seen in the bowel proximal to the lesion. Multiplane imaging of the suspected intussusception is important to confirm its features. Bowel loops situated immediately adjacent to each other may be misinterpreted as an intussusception.[66] Dogs with Doppler evidence of blood flow in the mesentery of the intussuscepted bowel were more likely to have successful reduction compared with those with no evidence of flow.[67]

Proliferating tissue masses originating within the intestinal wall include tumors, polyps, granulomatous infiltrates, and

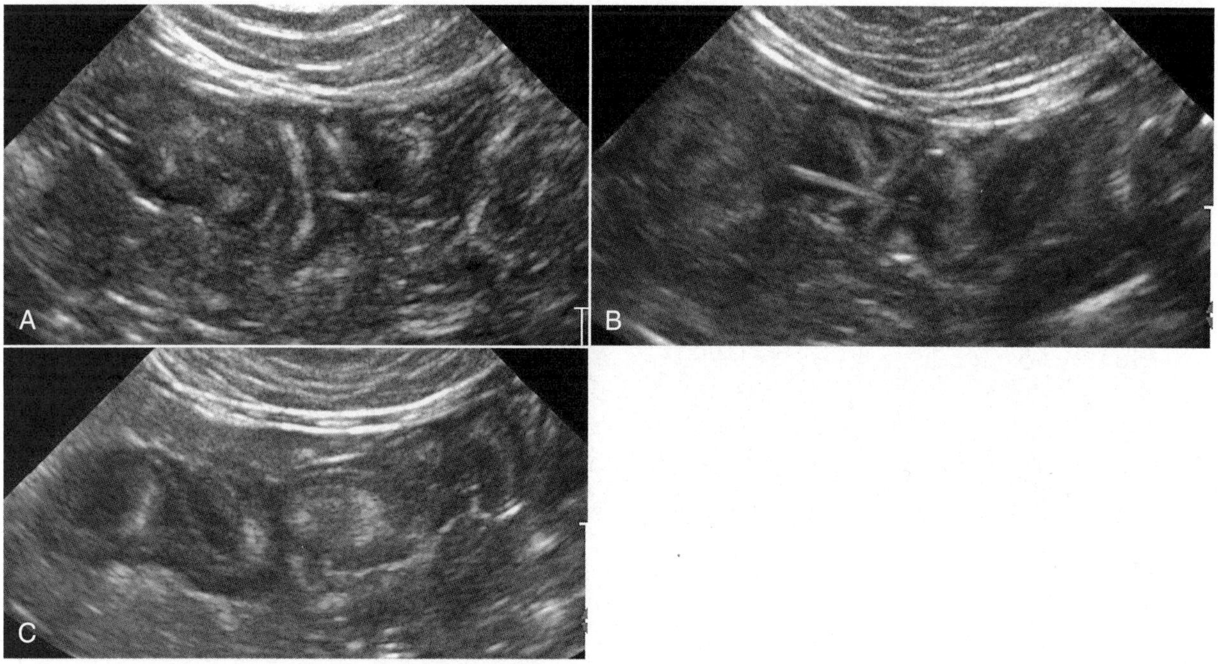

Fig. 46.28 Three ultrasound frames from a cat with a linear foreign body. The plication of the bowel is evident by the tightly undulating contour of the bowel wall and minimal distention of the lumen in all images. The linear hyperechoic streak in the central image represents the foreign material.

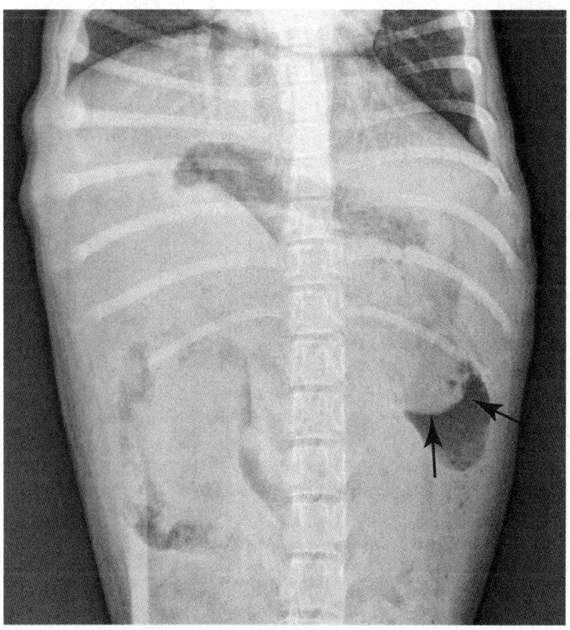

Fig. 46.29 Ventrodorsal radiograph of a dog with an ileocolic intussusception. This intussusception has not caused jejunal dilation, probably because the obstruction is not complete. The leading edge of the intussusceptum (*black arrows*) is visible in this patient as a round mass contrasted by colon gas. This appearance could be caused by a colonic foreign body but is more typical of an intussusception, and ultrasound should be performed for confirmation.

benign strictures. The development of an obstructive bowel pattern from these lesions depends on the size of the lesion and whether growth of the lesion is directed toward or away from the lumen. Progressive infiltration increases the probability of an obstruction if luminal narrowing occurs. Most patients present clinically during the phase of partial obstruction with focal mild to severe distention. Additional features of these masses are discussed later. Benign strictures in cats can occur in the duodenum, jejunum, or ileum and sonographic findings include gastric and generalized or segmental jejunal dilation consistent with mechanical obstruction. During the sonographic examination, ingesta does not propagate past the site of stricture and helps to make the diagnosis. Wall layering is typically disrupted and hypoechoic along a very short length of bowel, and wall thickening is mild to moderate (3–6 mm). Histopathology has shown fibrosis and inflammation at the stricture site.[68]

Lesions originating outside the intestinal wall can cause compression on a loop and result in partial or complete obstruction. Lesions in this category include adhesions from prior surgery, abdominal boundary hernias (congenital or traumatic), and occasionally masses originating from other abdominal organs (Fig. 46.31).

In some situations, CT may have applicability for evaluation of the patient with a clinical suspicion of mechanical bowel obstruction. Advantages include the tomographic nature of the images that eliminates superimposition of other organs on the intestinal tract, and the possibility of using reformatted images to provide a global view of the abdomen. In people, CT is used for identification of the location and level of the bowel lesion and in most instances allows the cause of obstruction to be determined. In dogs, a ratio of small intestinal diameter to L5 vertebral height of 2.5 as determined from CT images gave a sensitivity of 79% and a specificity of 72%.[69]

Functional Ileus

When peristaltic contractions of bowel cease because of vascular or neuromuscular abnormalities, the lumen dilates and remains patent. Many patients have no specific survey radiographic changes to allow discrimination between functional and mechanical ileus. As previously noted, the length of bowel affected may provide some differentiation, with localized

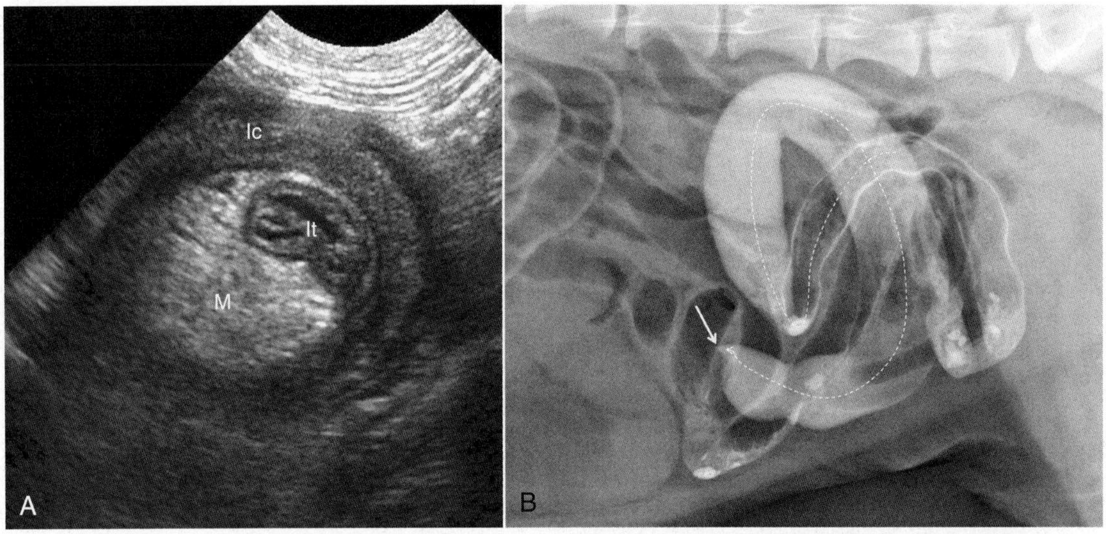

Fig. 46.30 **A,** A transverse ultrasound image of an intussusception. The wall layering pattern of the intussuscipiens in this patient is not clearly defined because of mucosal edema and dilation of mucosal lymphatics. *Ic,* Intussuscipiens; *It,* intussusceptum; *M,* hyperechoic mesenteric fat pulled in with the intussusceptum. In the radiographic study **(B)**, the narrowed lumen (*white arrow*) of the orad aspect of the intussusceptum is visible. The edema in the wall of the intussuscipiens in this patient has resulted in a stricture of the lumen, with resulting proximal dilation of small bowel. The *dashed white line* was added graphically and follows the course of the dilated bowel as it approaches the orad end of the intussusceptum. The increased opacity of the lumen of the dilated bowel was thought to be caused by medications that increased the opacity of the fluid.

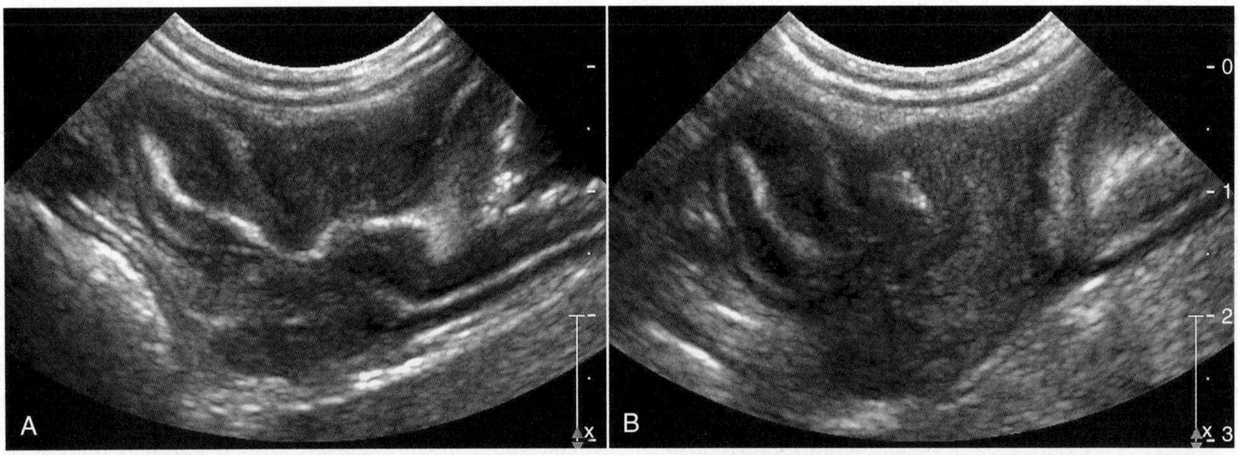

Fig. 46.31 Ultrasound images of partial bowel obstruction from an extrinsic granuloma caused by *Cryptococcus neoformans* infection. The constricting tissue does not originate from the bowel wall but focally encircles this loop. There is dilation of the orad segment on the *right* side of each image and a normal empty lumen on the aboral (*left*) side of each image.

dilation more likely from a mechanical cause and diffuse dilation more likely from functional ileus (see Fig. 46.15). However, overlap between functional and mechanical ileus occurs. Furthermore, chronic mechanical obstruction can eventually lead to functional ileus as the bowel becomes fatigued. The degree of dilation is not a specific differentiating feature.

There are no specific ultrasound or positive-contrast study features to differentiate chronic mechanical obstruction from functional ileus. The finding of peristalsis suggests exclusion of functional ileus. A thorough search of the bowel should be done to look for obvious obstructive causes such as a foreign body. The more common diseases that cause functional ileus include viral enteritis (canine parvovirus type 2 in particular), feline panleukopenia, chronic mechanical obstruction, and peritonitis.[70,71] Other less common diseases with a primary radiographic change of dilated intestinal loops include strangulation of the intestine through a hernia (vascular compromise), mesenteric volvulus (vascular compromise), spinal trauma (neurologic injury), segmental jejunal arterial thrombosis (vascular compromise), dysautonomia (autonomic nervous system disease), and intestinal pseudo-obstruction (tunica muscularis atrophy). Small intestinal segments can slip through traumatic tears or developmental hernias of the peritoneal cavity boundaries. The identification of such segments in an extra-abdominal location is usually easy because of gas within their lumen. Bowel dilation occurs if the rent becomes constrictive or if the loop twists, effectively occluding its outflow.

Mesenteric volvulus results in occlusion of the cranial mesenteric artery. The reduced blood supply leads to ischemic necrosis, gastrointestinal toxin release, shock, and subsequent paralytic ileus.[72,73] The initiating event for volvulus typically is

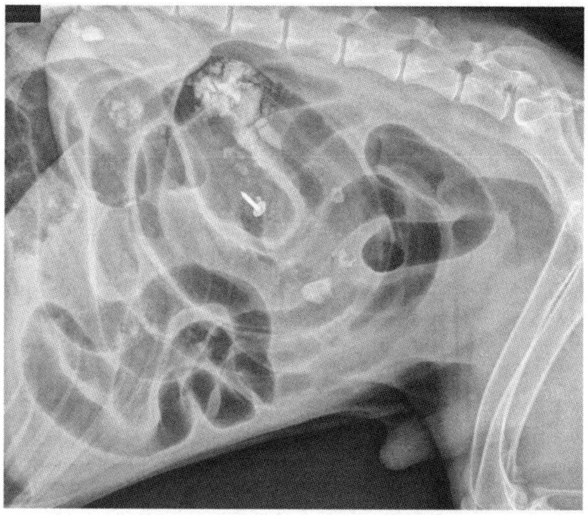

Fig. 46.32 Lateral radiograph of a dog with a jejunal volvulus. The extensive dilation of nearly all bowel segments is typical of jejunal volvulus. The metallic foreign body was incidental in this dog. A distal small bowel obstruction could cause this appearance, but more intraluminal fluid would be expected with a foreign body.

not known. Most dogs with mesenteric volvulus are large, have no distant or immediate prior history of gastrointestinal signs, and are presented for peracute or acute abdominal distention, abdominal pain, and shock. However, mesenteric volvulus has occurred after prior treatment for acute gastric dilation/ volvulus and for intussusception. One group of dogs with mesenteric volvulus had a previous clinical diagnosis of pancreatic insufficiency and clinical signs of vomiting.[74] The radiographic signs are moderate to severe dilation of the small intestine with fluid and gas (Fig. 46.32, eFig. 46.15). Peritoneal effusion may be concurrent. Mesenteric volvulus has been diagnosed using CT imaging in two dogs.[75,76] A supporting feature was the "whirl sign" due to bowel loops, blood vessels, and fat twisting around the mesenteric attachment.

Ischemic injury can also occur segmentally. A cat with jejunal thrombosis resulting in segmental bowel infarction had radiographic evidence of segmental bowel dilation and delayed gastric emptying and intestinal transit. Sonographically, over the course of 72 hours, this bowel segment underwent progressive wall thickening, loss of wall layering, and finally a generalized hypoechoic wall. Peri-enteric hyperechoic mesenteric fat also developed.[77] Intestinal leiomyositis is a cause of chronic intestinal pseudo-obstruction (CIPO) in dogs that can lead to severe generalized gastrointestinal dilation due to mononuclear inflammation, myofiber degeneration, necrosis, and fibrosis of the intestinal walls centered at the muscularis propria layer. This disease is associated with a poor prognosis and requires full-thickness biopsies to be diagnosed.[78] Pseudo-obstruction is a severe form of motility disorders and can be idiopathic or due to infectious, inflammatory, paraneoplastic, metabolic, endocrine, or toxic etiologies. Abdominal radiographs can show gastric and segmental or generalized small intestinal dilation, similar to the findings of mechanical obstruction. Ultrasonographically, there is absent peristalsis of the affected segments with segmental or generalized small intestinal dilation. Distinct wall lesions were not evident. CT findings are reported as having generalized gastrointestinal dilation similar to functional ileus.[79–82]

Dysautonomia is an autonomic nervous system disease that can include vomiting, diarrhea, and inappetence. Radiographs of the abdomen are often characterized by focal or diffuse gastrointestinal dilation. Transit of intraluminal contrast medium is markedly delayed. The most unique feature of these patients is their geographic origin, the first being reported from the United Kingdom. Both dogs and cats can be affected. Additional patients have been reported in Europe and in the United States, mainly in Missouri and Kansas.[83,84] The vaccination history (parvovirus) and geographic region of origin (Missouri, Kansas, United Kingdom, and Europe) of a patient with concomitant signs of other autonomic nervous system dysfunction (dysautonomia), history of thromboembolic disease, and a thorough current history and physical examination are the most useful factors in ranking these causes of functional ileus higher than the causes of mechanical obstruction.

Ultrasound features of parvovirus enteritis were assessed in a cohort of dogs younger than 6 months of age.[86] More than 50% exhibited fluid-filled small bowel, absent peristalsis, decreased duodenal and jejunal mucosal layer thickness despite normal total wall thickness, indistinct jejunal wall layers, hyperechoic jejunal mucosa, and normal jejunal lymph nodes. Duodenal wall corrugation, a hyperechoic duodenal mucosal layer, and an irregular duodenal mucosal border were found less frequently. The bowel diameter was not measured; however, puppies with intussusception were excluded, thus attributing the fluid distention and atony to nonobstructive ileus. Feline panleukopenia has similar intestinal wall findings as in dogs with parvovirus with thinning of the mucosal layer but also associated with a thickened muscularis layer, hyperechoic mucosa, and a hyperechoic mucosal band.[71]

Infiltrative Bowel Disease

Infiltrative bowel disease indicates generalized or segmental infiltration of the bowel wall because of nonseptic inflammation, infection, or neoplasia. The effects are a change in wall thickness and alterations in the tissue character of individual layers. Secondarily, bowel motility may be altered, resulting in a change in bowel diameter. For example, inflammation of the proximal duodenum because of pancreatitis can cause the duodenum to take on a fixed or rigid appearance demonstrated radiographically by mild gas dilation.[87] A corrugated mucosal and submucosal contour pattern has been observed to be associated with pancreatitis.[88] However, this corrugated pattern is not specific to pancreatitis and can be seen with other causes of peritonitis as well as enteritis, neoplasia, and bowel wall ischemia.[36,88] Ultrasound is the only readily available imaging modality that can differentiate bowel wall layers.

Common primary neoplasms of the small intestine include adenocarcinoma, lymphosarcoma, mastocytoma, gastrointestinal stromal tumor (GIST), leiomyoma, and leiomyosarcoma. With immunohistochemistry, many previously diagnosed leiomyomas and leiomyosarcomas have been reclassified as GIST or GIST-like tumors.[89,90] Atypical primary tumors are osteosarcoma, fibrosarcoma, carcinoid, neurilemmoma, and hemangiosarcoma.[91–96] Benign adenomatous polyps of the duodenum occur in cats, with increased frequency among Asian breeds.[97] One polypoid Brunner's gland adenoma has been described in a dog.[98] There are no unique survey radiographic findings for any of these tumors. They may create no changes, create a soft tissue mass of variable size, or cause partial to complete obstruction resulting in bowel dilation. Accumulation of radiopaque foreign material (gravel sign) may be a consequence of partial obstruction. Identification of the mural infiltration causing the partial obstruction is best diagnosed with either ultrasound, oral positive-contrast evaluation, or contrast-enhanced CT.[30]

Masses associated with intestinal wall typically cause smoothly rounded protrusions toward the lumen but may be evident as a mass deforming the serosal contour (Fig. 46.33). If the mural mass surrounds the lumen, the lumen often becomes enlarged and irregularly shaped (see Fig. 46.3). Distinguishing radiographically between a large emphysematous mural tumor and a bowel-associated abscess is not possible in most patients.

Ultrasonographically, intestinal neoplasia usually results in more extensive obliteration of the intestinal wall layering and greater wall thickness and is more likely to be focal than are inflammatory infiltrates.[10,98–106] In 150 dogs, loss of wall layering was the most predictive feature for differentiating between enteritis and neoplasia.[107] No ultrasonographic pattern is 100% specific for differentiating the type of small intestinal neoplasia.

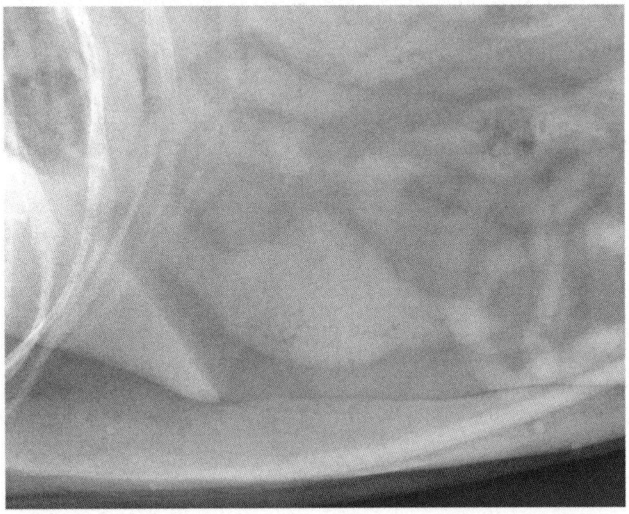

Fig. 46.33 There are bulges deforming the contour of a focal segment of small bowel. The loops entering and exiting the abnormal segment are visible. Differentials are neoplasia, granuloma, and abscess. Ultrasound imaging can further characterize the lesion and guide fine-needle aspirates and core biopsy.

Feline chronic enteropathy is common, and recognition of its causes has increased in recent years. Differentiating feline chronic inflammatory enteropathy (lymphocytic, plasmacytic, eosinophilic infiltration) from feline low-grade lymphoma poses diagnostic challenges that rely on a combination of physical examination findings, laboratory data, diagnostic imaging findings, and histopathologic, immunohistochemistry, and clonality features, which unfortunately all have overlapping findings between the two diseases.

The current nomenclature for diffuse T-cell lymphoma of the small intestines is feline low-grade intestinal T-cell lymphoma (LGITL, formerly enteropathy associated T-cell lymphoma [EATL type I or II]) due to T-cell lymphoproliferative disorder.[108]

Feline alimentary lymphoma is characterized by one of two patterns: a segmental mass or more diffuse thickening of the muscular layer (Fig. 46.34). The mass form, found in 75% of cats with alimentary lymphoma, is expressed as transmural circumferential thickening in the transverse plane (4–22 mm) with the wall layers replaced by hypoechoic or mixed echogenicity tissue and is due to high-grade alimentary lymphoma (HGAL) of small or large lymphocytes of B- or T-cell type (Fig. 46.35). About half of cats have associated enlargement of the mesenteric lymph nodes.[109,110]

The second pattern is that of LGITL that has preserved wall layers but exhibits thickening of the muscular layer

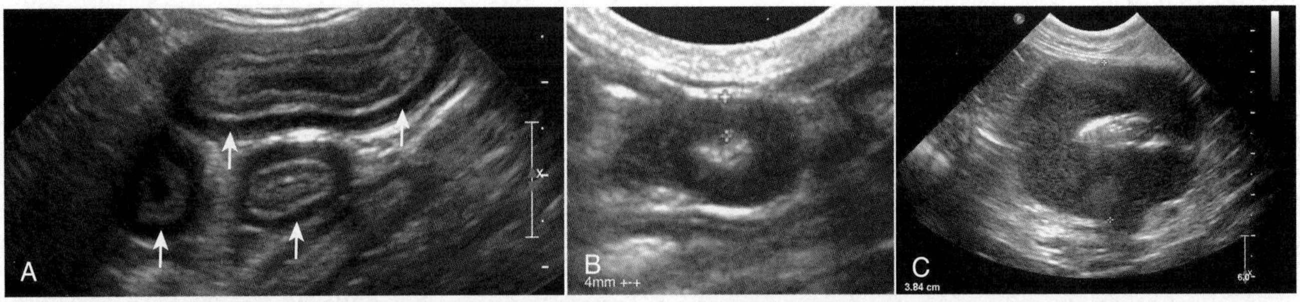

Fig. 46.34 Three examples of intestinal lymphoma in the cat. **A,** Generalized thickened muscularis due to low-grade intestinal T-cell lymphoma. **B,** Focal intestinal segment with transmural hypoechoic loss of layering. **C,** A large focal concentric wall mass with transmural hypoechoic loss of layering due to intestinal B-cell lymphoma.

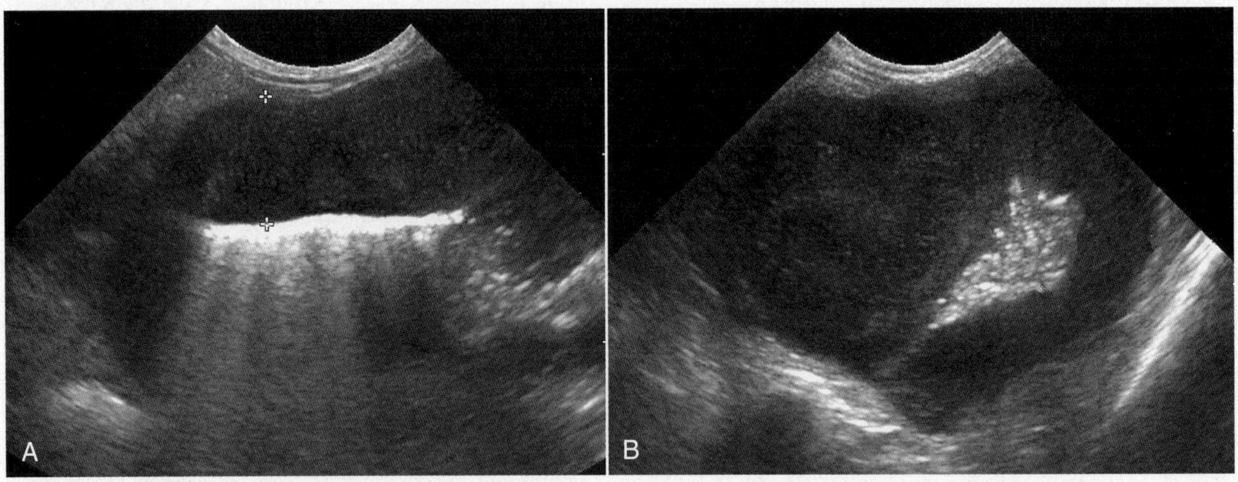

Fig. 46.35 Same cat as in Fig. 46.4. The abnormal bowel wall has transmural thickening and a loss of wall layering. The lesion is circumferential but asymmetric, and the lumen is patent, evident by gas and mucoid fluid. Although not pathognomonic, this is very characteristic of feline alimentary lymphoma.

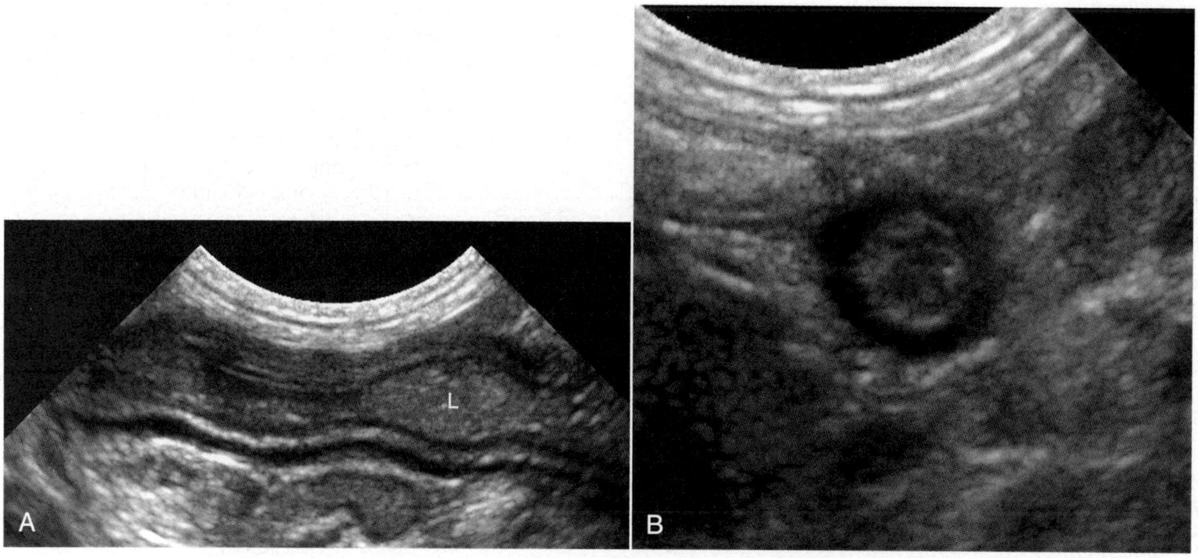

Fig. 46.36 Longitudinal section of the duodenum **(A)** and transverse section of the ileum **(B)** in a cat with muscular layer thickening associated with lymphoma. In the duodenum, the thickness of the muscular layer is best detected through the region where there is content in the lumen (*L*). At necropsy, there was extension of neoplastic cells into the submucosa and muscularis and occasionally outside of the serosa into the adjacent mesentery.

(Fig. 46.36).[108–110] Thickening of the muscular layer is characterized by it having a thickness equal to or greater than the mucosal layer. Ultrasound wall layering changes have been documented in cats with both LGITL and inflammatory enteropathy to differentiate from healthy individuals.[111]

Thickening of the muscular layer in the cat has been attributed to compensatory hypertrophy in response to a distal obstruction and idiopathic hypertrophy in the absence of obstruction.[112,113] The idiopathic form has also been associated with chronic enteritis.[113] The thickness of the muscularis of the duodenal and jejunal segments of 14 cats with small cell T-cell lymphoma and IBD and 19 healthy cats was compared. Increased (two times as thick) thickness of the muscularis propria was found in both affected groups compared to healthy cats.[109] Colic lymph nodes in this population in cats with lymphoma were increased compared to healthy cats. These findings are similar to that in a study of 300 cats with full-thickness biopsy confirmed inflammatory enteropathy (150 cats) or LGITL (124) and it was determined that the two etiologies cannot be differentiated based on wall layering and thickness.[110] In this study, it was also established that 86% of cats with a total wall thickness $\geq$2.8 mm had infiltrative disease of one or the other etiologies and suggested that segmental thickening could indicate more diffuse disease.

Fewer sonographic characteristics have been described for specific intestinal neoplasms in the dog. Differentiation of leiomyosarcoma from leiomyoma has been proposed based on leiomyosarcoma being larger (2–8 cm thick), eccentric, and having mixed echogenicity.[107] However, these patients were evaluated prior to the reclassification of many smooth muscle intestinal tumors as GISTs. In a more recent comparison of GIST and spindle cell tumors of the gastrointestinal tract, there were no specific ultrasound features that were distinguishing. Biopsy with immunohistochemical staining was needed to differentiate these tumors. The larger a bowel mass becomes, the more likely it is to have necrosis, which will appear as intralesional hypoechoic foci. Tumors that enlarge by exophytic growth can become quite large before clinical signs develop since they do not narrow the intestinal lumen. Other tumors of the canine small intestine are reported insufficiently to enable any conclusions about trends in their sonographic appearance (Fig. 46.37). Ultrasound evaluation of the intestine combined with ultrasound-guided fine-needle aspiration and microcore biopsy is an accurate method of minimally invasive diagnosis (Fig. 46.38).[109] However, depending on the sampling site, different outcomes in the same animal with both inflammatory and neoplastic infiltrative disease are possible.[30]

Metastatic bowel tumors are uncommon. Metastasis of mammary carcinoma to the jejunal muscular layer has been identified in a dog, and appeared as focal hypoechoic nodules.[114]

Infectious enteritis may be caused by viruses, bacterial, rickettsial, fungal (and fungal-like), or more rarely parasitic organisms (Fig. 46.39). Changes associated with parvovirus (canine parvovirus type 2) have been discussed earlier regarding abnormal bowel dilation. If parvoviral enteritis is suspected, imaging should be delayed until clinical testing can be performed. Other viral diseases that infect the small intestinal tract do not cause any specific radiographic or sonographic changes and thus are not discussed here. Bacterial overgrowth in the small intestine has also not been related to specific radiographic or sonographic changes.

Heterobilharzia americana (HA) or canine schistosomiasis can cause infection of the small intestines in addition to affecting other body organs.[115] Pathologically the trematode infiltrates the submucosa with oocytes and causes a granulomatous response. Radiographically, dogs with chronic enteropathy can show mineralization of the small intestinal wall. The mineralization is not consistently associated with hypercalcemia. In one report the mineralization was associated with a large number of calcified eggs in the bowel and other organs.[116] Ultrasonographically, the submucosa can be recognized as ill-defined thickening or contain variable degrees of pinpoint hyperechoic foci.[117–119] Hyperechoic foci can also be seen in the liver and mesenteric lymph nodes. In an assessment of HA-positive dogs compared to control dogs, thickening of the submucosa layer concurrent with the presence of hyperechoic foci in the liver, small intestine, and mesenteric lymph nodes provided differentiation of the infected dogs. The endemic range of HA is along the Atlantic and Gulf Coast of North America. Canine cases have also been diagnosed in Kansas, Oklahoma, Arkansas, Indiana, and Utah[120–122] (Fig. 46.40).

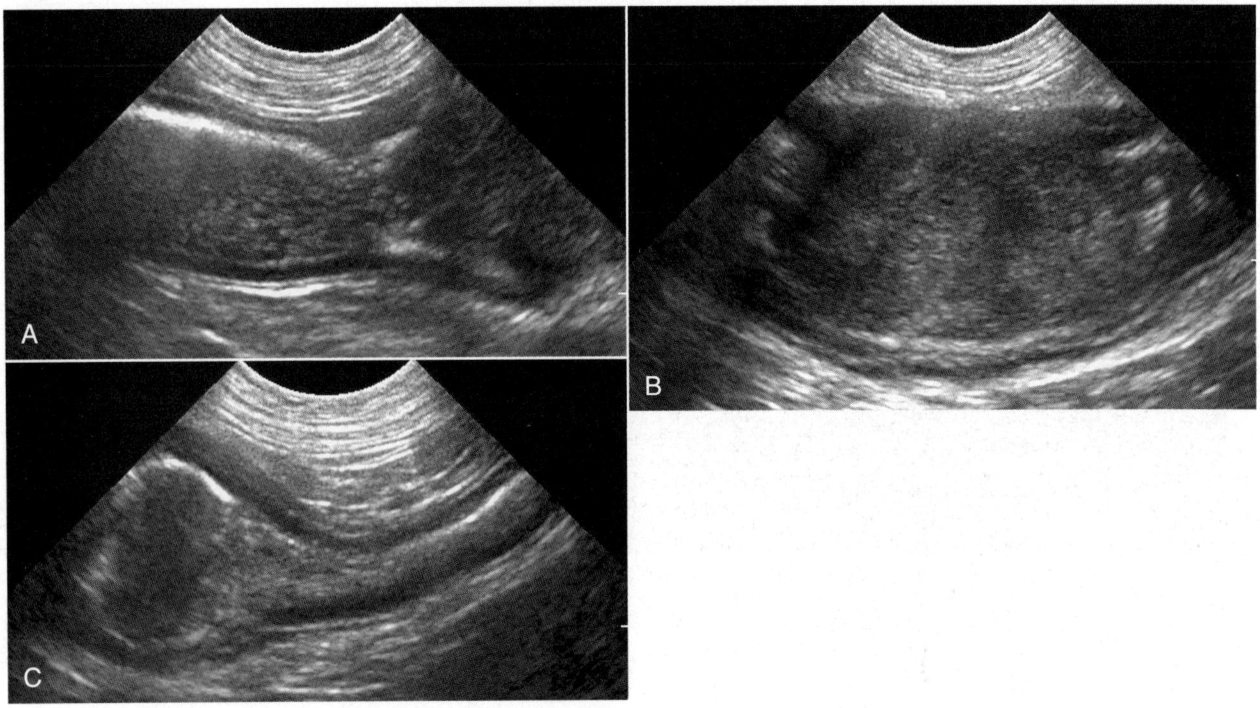

Fig. 46.37 Ultrasound images in sequence through the length of a segment of bowel with histopathologically confirmed hemangiosarcoma. **A** is orad to the mass, and there is mild dilation of the lumen filled with mucoid fluid. The mass is just evident to the *right* of the frame. **B** is at the level of the mass. The deep wall retains some evidence of wall layer pattern and the mass bulges into the lumen. **C** is aboral, and the bowel returns to normal.

When neoplasia, infection, and food-responsive disease are excluded from the broad category of infiltrative bowel disease, the general term *idiopathic IBD* is used. In both the canine and the feline patient, *IBD* refers to a group of disorders of undetermined etiology that cause chronic (>3 weeks) vomiting and/or diarrhea and have various populations of inflammatory cells in the bowel wall layers.[123–125] The most common of these is a lymphocytic-plasmacytic enteritis. Some breed-associated forms of IBD have been described—immunoproliferative enteropathy of Basenjis, familial protein-losing enteropathy (PLE) and protein-losing nephropathy in soft-coated Wheaten terriers, and gluten-sensitive enteropathy in Irish setters.[123] None of these breed-specific disorders have unique radiographic or ultrasonographic diagnostic findings. Equivocal radiographic and sonographic findings suggest additional diagnostic tests are necessary.

Inflammatory infiltrates are expected to increase bowel wall thickness or alter the character of the tissue. However, bowel wall thickness cannot be used to differentiate normal from affected dogs, although some dogs have mild thickening.[123–126] The finding of normal wall thickness may lead to a significant rate of false-negative diagnoses in animals with inflammatory infiltrates (Fig. 46.41).

Distinction of PLE from IBD and food-responsive disease in dogs is based on finding increased mucosal layer echogenicity with PLE, because of varying severity of hyperechoic vertical striations in the duodenum and jejunum (Fig. 46.42). Histologically, the vertical striations are associated with lymphangiectasia.[124,127,128] Dogs with IBD and food-responsive disease can also have increased echogenicity in the mucosal layer described as hyperechoic speckles, being oriented in a horizontal or focal dot pattern compared to the striation pattern. Total bowel wall thickening is inconsistent in PLE and, when present, is mild. Secondary findings in dogs with PLE included peritoneal effusion, edema of the pancreas, and distended bowel segments; however, these findings can also be present in dogs with IBD. Dogs with food-responsive disease do not typically have these secondary findings. Intestinal biopsy remains the definitive diagnostic test for infiltrative bowel disease.

Focal lipogranulomatous lymphangitis is a rare and severe form of canine IBD.[129,130] The etiology is undetermined, and diagnosis is made by histopathologic changes. Of the 17 dogs reported, most lesions occurred in the distal ileum and had sonographic changes of thickened wall (6–14 mm), retained layers, but with predominantly thickened muscular layer. Regional lymph nodes were enlarged but of normal echogenicity. Three dogs had an associated mass up to 4 cm in size extending from the serosa or in the adjacent mesentery. Inflammation, fibrosis, and necrosis mixed with dilated lacteals and lymphatic vessels are identified at histopathology.

Bowel-Associated Masses

Bowel-associated masses can be due to abscesses, hematomas, fungal granulomas, eosinophilic inflammation, and neoplasms. Bacterial abscesses can occur as focal lesions associated with the intestinal wall. A bowel-associated abscess can be a consequence of partial or complete intestinal perforation by foreign material with subsequent adhesions and abscess formation. The mass may result in regional loss of serosal detail or may displace adjacent bowel (Fig. 46.43). A mottled appearance may be seen in bowel-associated abscesses when exudate from the abscess drains into the lumen and is replaced by gas (see Fig. 46.43). Abscesses associated with the small intestine may originate from a source extrinsic to the wall. This may occur because of retained surgical sponges (gossypiboma) or be caused by a pancreatic abscess. Small intestinal wall hematoma has been reported with intestinal wire foreign body perforation.[131]

Although uncommon, mycotic infections of the intestinal tract include histoplasmosis, cryptococcosis,[132] and pythiosis.

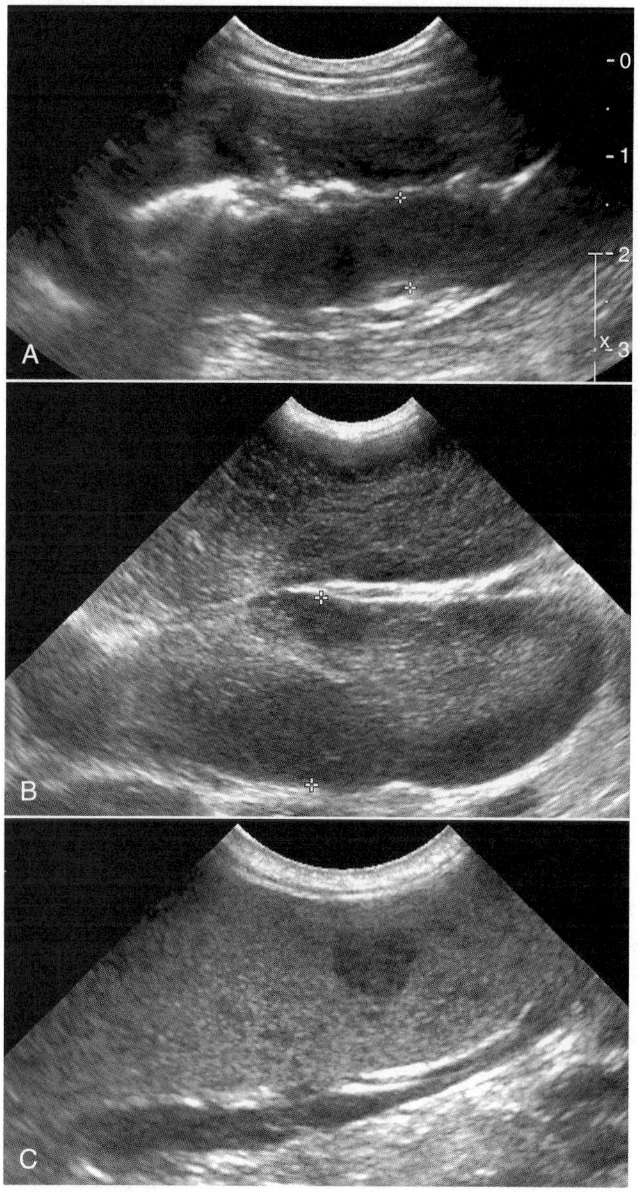

Fig. 46.38 Images of the small bowel **(A)**, mesenteric lymph node **(B)**, and spleen **(C)** in a dog with stage V lymphoma. Bowel wall layering is absent, and there is transmural thickening. The mesenteric lymph node is markedly enlarged and predominantly hypoechoic. Other abdominal lymph nodes were also abnormal. The spleen exhibits multifocal hypoechoic foci.

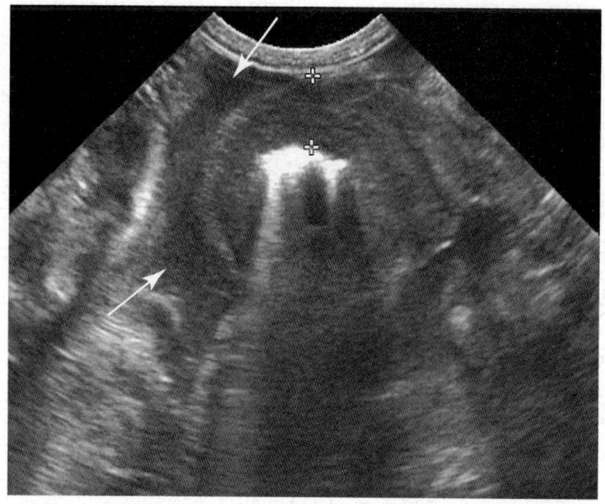

Fig. 46.39 Same dog as Fig. 46.33 at the time of initial presentation. There is echogenic peritoneal fluid (*white arrows*). A segment of jejunum was abnormal, characterized by transmural thickening (0.89 cm) with relative hyperechogenicity and no evidence of wall layering. Lymph nodes were enlarged. A diagnosis of *Cryptococcus neoformans* was made from mesenteric lymph node aspirates and confirmed when this segment of the jejunum was removed. Histopathologically, there were inflammatory cells and multiple granulomas with numerous yeasts in all layers.

Pythiosis, an opportunistic water-borne oomycete, has been diagnosed in dogs in Oklahoma, including the northern region, in addition to its more common endemic locale along the Gulf Coast of North America.[133,134] Pathologic changes are often advanced by the time of clinical presentation. Pyogranulomatous lesions cause localized thickening of the intestinal wall that frequently extends through the serosa, along the mesentery, and into the mesenteric lymph nodes. This combination results in a palpable abdominal mass. Ultrasound features in dogs with pythiosis include thickening of the intestinal wall associated with loss of the layer pattern[135] (Fig. 46.44). The sonographic features are overlapping with intestinal neoplasia. Diagnosis and differentiation from neoplasia can be performed with tissue sampling, culture, and serology.[136] Noninfectious granulomas are rare in the dog and cat. Foreign material imbedded in the bowel wall is theorized to have incited a pyogranulomatous response leading to the development of a wall mass that became obstructive. In three dogs with intestinal pyogranuloma, radiographically, there was mild to moderate focal bowel dilation and a bowel wall mass was apparent sonographically.[137] Feline gastrointestinal eosinophilic sclerosing fibroplasia (FGESF) causes a mass in the small intestine with transmural hypoechoic loss of wall layering that ultrasonographically cannot be differentiated from neoplasia[138] (Fig. 46.45). FGESF lesions are characterized by eosinophilic infiltration with reactive fibroblasts and dense collagen and affect the pyloroduodenal and ileocecocolic junctions and the small intestine. Some cats have regional lymphadenopathy.

Miscellaneous Small Intestinal Diseases

Opacity changes in the intestinal wall are rare. Diffuse mineralization of the wall can occur by metastatic calcification because of hypercalcemia. Dogs and cats poisoned by cholecalciferol-based rodenticides and having ingested human antipsoriasis ointment containing calcitriol analogues can develop vomiting, which may lead to radiography and/or ultrasonography of the abdomen.[139–142] Diffuse calcification of the gastrointestinal tract may be found in these patients. Radiographically, the degree of calcification typically creates a thin line of opacity, imparting an enhanced contrast effect. Differential diagnosis for this type of diffuse mineralization should include other causes of hypercalcemia, including severe primary renal disease. Schistosomiasis has more recently been reported as a cause for small bowel wall calcification and should be included in the differential in geographic appropriate locations.[117]

Pneumatosis intestinalis and pneumatosis coli both refer to the presence of gas in the intestinal wall and pneumotosis coli is the more common of the two and discussed in Chapter 47. Numerous underlying causes can lead to this gas accumulation, including necrotizing enterocolitis, ischemic necrosis caused by volvulus, trauma, and bacterial origin in immunocompromised patients. Pneumatosis intestinalis has been reported in a dog following trauma and was detected by ultrasound evaluation.[143]

Two rare types of congenital gastrointestinal anomalies can involve the small intestine: a duplication cyst and diverticulum. A duplication cyst requires three features: an intimate association with the gastrointestinal tract, a well-developed muscular

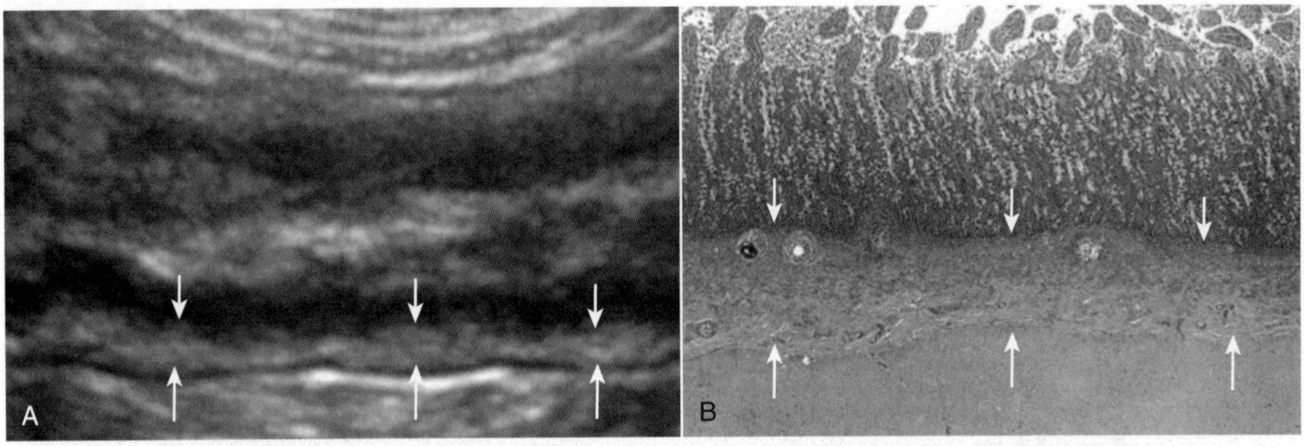

Fig. 46.40 A 4-year-old male Labrador retriever with chronic weight loss. **A,** Sagittal ultrasound image of the duodenum showing generalized disruption of the wall layering mainly due to ill-defined thickening of the submucosal layer (*white arrows*). **B,** Histologic image of the duodenum showing inflammatory infiltration and oocytes within the submucosal layer (*white arrows*) correlating to the thick submucosa in the ultrasound image. The diagnosis was *Heterobilharzia americanum* infection.

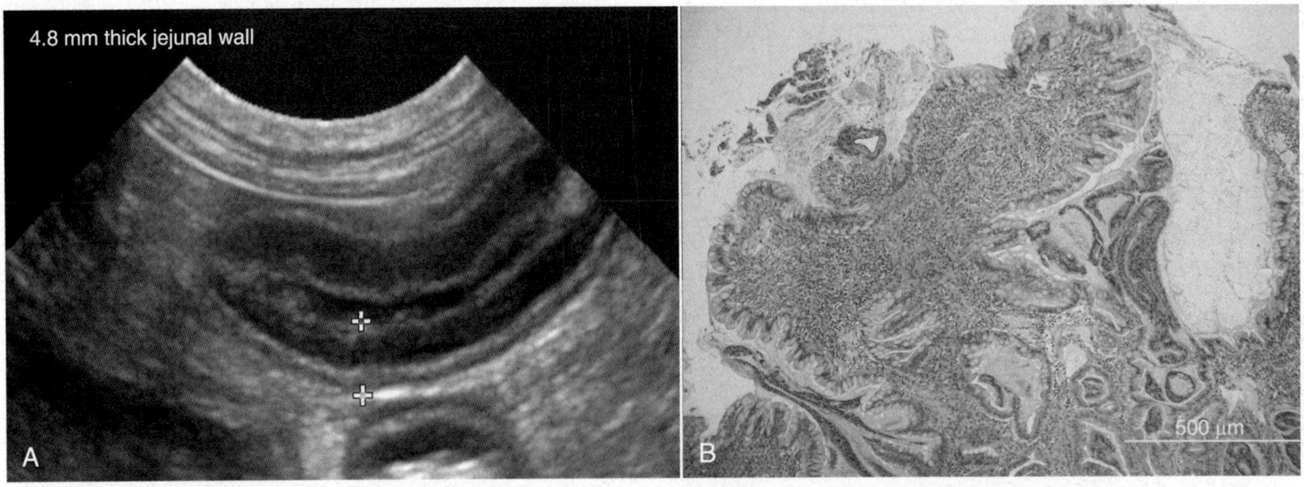

Fig. 46.41 Severe, chronic lymphocytic, plasmacytic enteritis in a 4-year-old Weimaraner with chronic small bowel diarrhea and weight loss. **A,** The intestinal wall is 4.8 mm thick (x—x), within normal limits for a large breed dog. **B,** The histopathology of mucosal biopsies shows severe chronic lymphocytic, plasmacytic enteritis which did not lead to overall wall thickening or altered wall layering. This case demonstrates that ultrasound can underestimate the presence of inflammatory bowel disease in affected dogs.

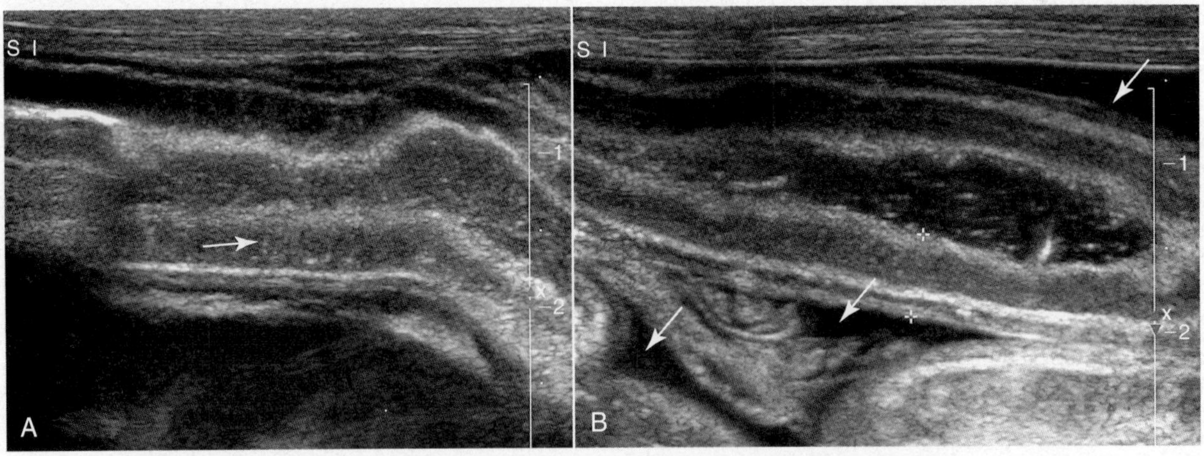

Fig. 46.42 **A,** Increased echogenicity of the mucosal layer and vertically oriented hyperechoic (*white arrow*) streaks are consistent with dilated lacteals in a patient with protein-losing enteropathy. In **B,** another patient with anechoic peritoneal fluid (*white arrows*) has a hyperechoic mucosal layer but with less evident streaking pattern. Biopsy would be needed for confirmation and identification of additional histologic abnormalities.

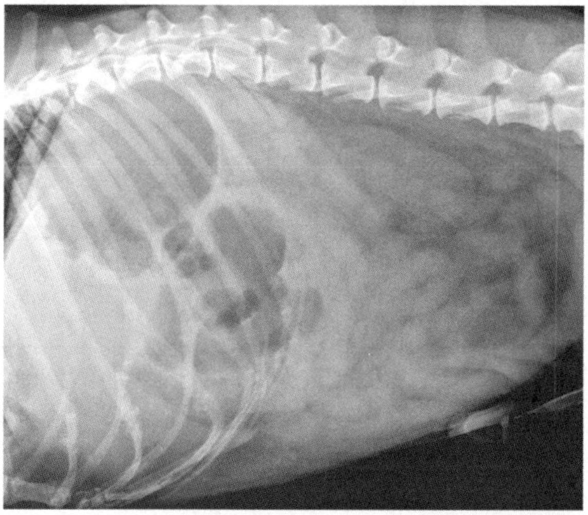

Fig. 46.43 Lateral radiograph of a dog with a large emphysematous mass caused by a jejunal abscess. The intraluminal gas arises when liquid contents of the mass drain into the bowel and the resulting cavity is filled with bowel gas. There is also a loss of serosal detail around the mass. A jejunal tumor could also have this appearance.

layer, and an epithelial lining.[145–150] They are characterized histologically by the presence of smooth muscle in their wall with an internal lining of intestinal epithelium. There may be goblet cells in the lining, which can produce mucin and fill the luminal cavity. The muscular layer of the cyst is continuous with the muscular layer of the associated bowel segment. In four dogs and three cats with a duplication cyst, the lumen of the cyst did not communicate with the lumen of the bowel. Radiographically, the cyst may be evident as an abdominal mass but may not have an obvious association with the small intestine. Sonographically, the cyst is frequently filled with fluid but may not easily be defined to be originating from the bowel. A three-layer wall character has been described with the inner and outer most layers being hyperechoic and the central layer hypoechoic.

A diverticulum is an outpouching from the wall of the gastrointestinal tract resulting in the formation of a sac.[151–153] Typically, the wall of the diverticulum contains the expected wall layering and the lumen of the diverticulum communicates with the bowel. Because of this communication, an oral positive-contrast study could be useful for demonstrating the communication. Three of the four affected dogs were young Boxers with two being littermates, and in all, the diverticulum

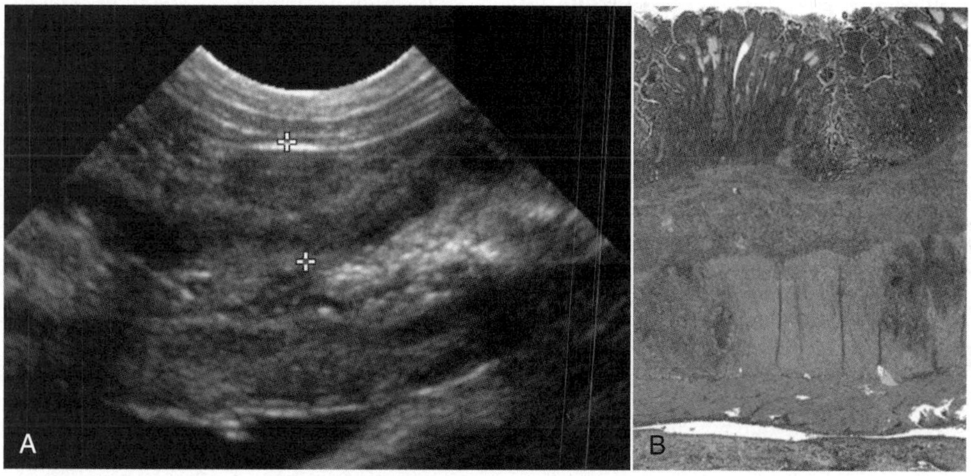

Fig. 46.44 A 1.5-year-old male neutered Labrador retriever with chronic weight loss. **A,** Sagittal ultrasound image of the duodenum showing generalized ill-defined loss of wall layering with alternating hyper- and hypoechoic bands of tissue. **B,** Histopathology image showing the diffuse inflammatory infiltration with alternating ill-defined thickened layers correlating to those identified in the ultrasound image. The diagnosis was pythiosis.

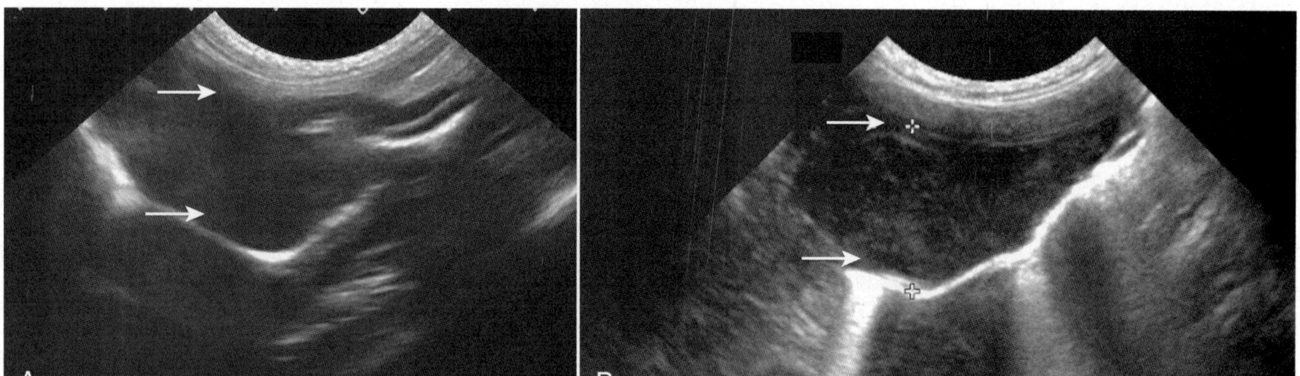

Fig. 46.45 **A,** Sagittal ultrasound image of the duodenum in a 4-year-old male neutered cat with chronic vomiting. An eccentric infiltrative wall mass is present (*white arrows*) that effaces the wall layering and displaces and distorts the hyperechoic luminal interface. **B,** A 6-year-old male neutered cat with a similar eccentric jejunal transmural hypoechoic wall mass with loss of wall layering and distortion of the hyperechoic luminal interface. Cat **A** was diagnosed with feline gastrointestinal eosinophilic sclerosing fibroplasia and cat **B** had intestinal lymphoma.

was at the distal flexure of the duodenum. Another difference between a duplication cyst and a diverticulum is that the former is more typically found on the mesenteric side of the bowel and the latter on the antimesenteric side. It is possible for the lining of the duplication cyst to be composed of heterotopic gastric mucosa.

REFERENCES

1. Armbrust LJ, Biller DS, Hoskinson JJ. Case examples demonstrating the clinical utility of obtaining both right and left lateral abdominal radiographs in small animals. *J Am Anim Hosp Assoc*. 2000;36:531.
2. Vander Hart D, Berry CR. Initial influence of right versus left lateral recumbency on the radiographic finding of duodenal gas on subsequent survey ventrodorsal projections of the canine abdomen. *Vet Radiol Ultrasound*. 2015;56(12).
3. Armbrust LJ, Biller DS, Hoskinson JJ. Compression radiography: an old technique revisited. *J Am Anim Hosp Assoc*. 2000;36:537.
4. Owens JM, Biery DN. *Radiographic interpretation for the small animal clinician*. 2nd ed. Baltimore: Williams & Wilkins; 1999.
5. Graham JP, Lord PF, Harrison JM. Quantitative estimation of intestinal dilation as a predictor of obstruction in the dog. *J Small Anim Pract*. 1998;39:521.
6. Morgan JP. The upper gastrointestinal examination in the cat: normal radiographic appearance using positive-contrast medium. *Vet Radiol*. 1981;22:159.
7. Adams WM, Sisterman LA, et al. Association of intestinal disorders in cats with findings of abdominal radiography. *J Am Vet Med Assoc*. 2010;236:880.
8. O'Brien TR. Small intestine. In: O'Brien TR, ed. *Radiographic Diagnosis of Abdominal Disorders in the Dog and Cat*. Philadelphia: Saunders; 1978:279–352.
9. Hall JA, Watrous BA. Effect of pharmaceuticals on radiographic appearance of selected examinations of the abdomen and thorax. *Vet Clin North Am Small Anim Pract*. 2000;30:349.
10. Weichselbaum RC, Feeney DA, Hayden DW. Comparison of upper gastrointestinal radiographic findings to histopathologic observations: a retrospective study of 41 dogs and cats with suspected small bowel infiltrative disease. *Vet Radiol Ultrasound*. 1994;35:418.
11. Seiler GS, Cohen EB, d'Anjou MA, et al. ACVR and ECVDI consensus statement for the standardization of the abdominal ultrasound examination. *Vet Radiol Ultrasound*. 2022;63:661–674.
12. Lamb CR. Recent developments in diagnostic imaging of the gastrointestinal tract of the dog and cat. *Vet Clin North Am Small Anim Pract*. 1999;29:307.
13. Rault DN, Besso JG, Boulouha L, et al. Significance of a common extended mucosal interface observed in transverse small intestine sonograms. *Vet Radiol Ultrasound*. 2004;45:177.
14. Le Roux AB, Granger LA, Wakamatsu N, , et alGaschen L. Ex vivo correlation of ultrasonographic small intestinal wall layering with histology in dogs. *Vet Radiol Ultrasound*. 2016;57:534.
15. Nielsen T, Lindstrom L, Ingman J, et al. High-frequency ultrasound of Peyer's patches in the small intestine of young cats. *J Feline Med Surg*. 2016;18:303.
16. Gaschen L, Granger LA, Oubre O, et al. The effects of food intake and its fat composition on intestinal echogenicity in healthy dogs. *Vet Radiol Ultrasound*. 2016; 57:546.
17. Delaney F, O'Brien RT, Waller K. Ultrasound evaluation of small bowel thickness compared to weight in normal dogs. *Vet Radiol Ultrasound*. 2003;44:577.
18. Goggin JM, Biller DS, Debey BM, et al. Ultrasonographic measurement of gastrointestinal wall thickness and the ultrasonographic appearance of the ileocolic region in healthy cats. *J Am Anim Hosp Assoc*. 2000;36:224.
19. Di Donato P, Penninck D, Pieetra M, et al. Ultrasonographic measurement of the relative thickness of intestinal wall layers in clinically healthy cats. *J Feline Med Surg*. 2014;16:333.
20. Etue SM, Pennick DG, Labatto MA, et al. Ultrasonography of the normal feline pancreas and associated anatomic landmarks: a prospective study of 20 cats. *Vet Radiol Ultrasound*. 2001;42:330.
21. Mortier JR, Maddox TW, White GM, et al. Ultrasonographic appearance of the major duodenal papilla in dogs without evidence of hepatobiliary, pancreatic, or gastrointestinal tract disease. *Am J Vet Res*. 2016;77:597.
22. An Y, Lee H, Chang D, et al. Application of pulsed Doppler ultrasound for the evaluation of small intestinal motility in dogs. *J Vet Sci*. 2001;1:71.
23. Jimenez DA, O'Brien RT, Wallace JD, et al. Intraoperative contrast-enhanced ultrasonography of normal canine jejunum. *Vet Radiol Ultrasound*. 2011;52:196.
24. Diana A, Specchi S, Toaldo MB, et al. Contrast-enhanced ultrasonography of the small bowel in healthy cats. *Vet Radiol Ultrasound*. 2011;52:555.
25. Johnson-Neitman JL, O'Brien RT, Wallace J. Quantitative perfusion analysis of the pancreas and duodenum in healthy dogs by use of contrast-enhanced ultrasonography. *Am J Vet Res*. 2012;73:385.
26. Goodall EFP: Comparative imaging of surgical small intestinal disease in dogs: evaluation of pre-operative contrast-enhanced ultrasound, intra-operative contrast enhanced ultrasound, and triple-phase contrast-enhanced computed tomography. M.S. Thesis Abstract. Dept Veterinary Clinical Sciences, University of Illinois at Urbana-Champaign. http://hdl.handle.net/2142/90791.
27. Linta N, Pey P, Toaldo MB, et al. Contrast-enhanced ultrasonography in dogs with inflammatory bowel disease. *J Vet Intern Med*. 2021;35:2167–2176.
28. Nisa K, Lim SY, Shinohara M, et al. Evaluation of duodenal perfusion by contrast-enhanced ultrasonography in dogs with chronic inflammatory enteropathy and intestinal lymphoma. *J Vet Intern Med*. 2019;33:559–568.
29. Spużak J, Kubiak K, Glińska-Suchocka K, Jankowski M, Borusewicz P, Kubiak-Nowak D. Accuracy of real-time shear wave elastography in the assessment of normal small intestine mucosa in dogs. *Pol J Vet Sci*. 2019;22(3): 457–461.
30. Hoey S, Drees R, Hetzel S. Evaluation of the gastrointestinal tract in dogs using computed tomography. *Vet Radiol Ultrasound*. 2013;554:25.
31. Siow JW, Chau J, Podadera JM, et al. Investigation of scan delays for CT evaluation of inner wall layering and peak enhancement of the canine stomach and small intestine using a 20 second fixed-injection-duration and bolus tracking technique. *Vet Radiol Ultrasound*. 2022:1–11.
32. Miniter BM, Arruda AG, Zuckerman J, et al. Use of computed tomography (CT) for the diagnosis of mechanical gastrointestinal obstruction in canines and felines. *PLoS One*. 2019. https://doi.org/10.1371/journal.pone.0219748.
33. Smelstoys JA, Davis GJ, Learn AE, et al. Outcome of and prognostic indicators for dogs and cats with pneumoperitoneum and no history of penetration trauma: 54 cases (1988–2002). *J Am Vet Med Assoc*. 2004;225:251.

34. Ko JJ, Mann FA. Barium peritonitis in small animals. *J Vet Med Sci*. 2014;76:621.
35. Renschler J, Tarigo J. What is your diagnosis? Particulate material in peritoneal fluid from a dog. *Vet Clin Pathol*. 2008;37:129.
36. Boysen SF, Tidwell AS, Pennick DG. Ultrasonographic findings in dogs and cats with gastrointestinal perforation. *Vet Radiol Ultrasound*. 2003;44:556.
37. Allan GS, Rendano VT, Quick CB, et al. Gastrografin as a gastrointestinal contrast medium in the cat. *Vet Radiol*. 1979;20(3).
38. Kang J, Oh D, Kim K, et al. Evaluation of a dual-purpose contrast medium for radiography and ultrasonography of the small intestine in dogs. *AJVR*. 2020;81(12).
39. Riedesel EA. Small bowel. In: Thrall DE, ed. *Textbook of Veterinary Diagnostic Radiology*. 5th ed. St. Louis: Elsevier-Saunders; 2007.
40. Robertson ID, Burbridge HM. Pros and cons of barium-impregnated polyethylene spheres in gastrointestinal disease. *Vet Clin North Am Small Anim Pract*. 2000;30:449.
41. Garneau MS, McCarthy RJ. Multiple magnetic gastrointestinal foreign bodies in a dog. *J Am Vet Med Assoc*. 2015;246:537.
42. Hickey MC, Magee A. Gastrointestinal tract perforations caused by ingestion of multiple magnets in a dog. *J Vet Emerg Crit Care (San Antonio)*. 2011;21:369.
43. Rossmeissl EM, Palmer KG, Hoelzler MG, et al. Multiple magnet ingestion as a cause of septic peritonitis in a dog. *J Am Anim Hosp Assoc*. 2011;47:56.
44. Creedy N, Bates N. Ingestion of multiple magnets by a dog. *Vet Rec*. 2011;169:504.
45. Kiefer K, Hottinger H, Kahn T, et al. Magnet ingestion in dogs: two cases. *J Am Anim Hosp Assoc*. 2010;46:181.
46. Luttgen PJ, Whitney MS, Wolf AM, et al. Heinz body hemolytic anemia associated with high plasma zinc concentration in a dog. *J Am Vet Med Assoc*. 1990;197:1347.
47. Clancey NP, Murphy MC. Zinc-induced hemolytic anemia in a dog caused by ingestion of a game-playing die. *Can Vet J*. 2012;53:383.
48. Pratt CL, Reineke EL, Dobratz KJ. Sewing needle foreign body ingestion in dogs and cats: 65 cases (2000–2012). *J Am Vet Med Assoc*. 2014;245:303.
49. Ciasca TC, David FH, Lamb CR. Does measurement of small intestinal diameter increase diagnostic accuracy of radiography in dogs with suspected intestinal obstruction? *Vet Radiol Ultrasound*. 2013;54:207.
50. Finck C, D'Anjou MA, Alexander K, et al. Radiographic diagnosis of mechanical obstruction in dogs based on relative small intestinal external diameters. *Vet Radiol Ultrasound*. 2014;55:472.
51. Lux DN, Hunt GB, Carr AH, et al. What is your diagnosis? An amoxicillin tablet. *J Am Vet Med Assoc*. 2013;243(45).
52. Lamb DR, Hansson K. Radiological identification on non-opaque intestinal foreign bodies. *Vet Radiol Ultrasound*. 1994;35:87.
53. Moles AD, McGhie JA, Schaaf OR, et al. Sand impaction of the small intestine in eight dogs. *J Small Anim Pract*. 2010;51(29).
54. Elser EB, Mai W, Reetz JA, et al. Serial abdominal radiographs do not significantly increase accuracy of diagnosis of gastrointestinal mechanical obstruction due to occult foreign bodies in dogs and cats. *Vet Radiol Ultrasound*. 2020;61(4):399–408.
55. Miles S, Gaschen L, Presley T, Lio C, Granger LA. Influences of repeat abdominal radiographs on the resolution of mechanical obstruction and gastrointestinal foreign material in dogs and cats. *Vet Radiol Ultrasound*. 2021;62(3):282–288.
56. Tidwell AS, Penninck DG. Ultrasonography of gastrointestinal foreign bodies. *Vet Radiol Ultrasound*. 1992;33:160.
57. Sharma A, Thompson MS, Scrivani PV, et al. Comparison of radiography and ultrasonography for diagnosing small-intestinal mechanical obstruction in vomiting dogs. *Vet Radiol Ultrasound*. 2011;52:248.
58. Hobday MM, Pachtinger GE, Drobatz KJ, et al. Linear versus non-linear gastrointestinal foreign bodies in 499 dogs: clinical presentation, management, and short-term outcome. *J Small Anim Pract*. 2014;55:560.
59. Evans KL, Smeak DD, Biller DS. Gastrointestinal linear foreign bodies in 32 dogs: a retrospective evaluation and feline comparison. *J Am Anim Hosp Assoc*. 1994;30:445.
60. Felts JF, Fox PR, Burk RL. Thread and sewing needles as gastrointestinal foreign bodies in the cat: a review of 64 cases. *J Am Vet Med Assoc*. 1984;184(56).
61. Hoffmann KL. Sonographic signs of gastroduodenal linear Foreign Body in 3 Dogs. *Vet Radiol Ultrasound*. 2003;44:466.
62. Lewis DD, Ellison GW. Intussusception in dogs and cats. *Compend Contin Educ Pract Vet*. 1987;9:523.
63. Burkitt JM, Drobatz KJ, Saunders HM, Washabau RK. Signalment, history, and outcome of cats with gastrointestinal tract intussusception: 20 cases (1986–2000). *J Am Vet Med Assoc*. 2009;234:771.
64. Lamb CR, Mantis P. Ultrasonographic features of intestinal intussusception in 10 dogs. *J Small Anim Pract*. 1998;39:437.
65. Patsikas MN, Jakovljevic S, Moustardas N, et al. Ultrasonographic signs of intestinal intussusception associated with acute enteritis or gastroenteritis in 19 young dogs. *J Am Anim Hosp Assoc*. 2003;39(57).
66. Patsikas MN, Papazoglou LG, Papaioannou NG, Dessiris AK. Normal and abnormal ultrasonographic findings that mimic small intestinal intussusception in the dog. *J Am Anim Hosp Assoc*. 2004;40:147.
67. Patsikas MN, Papazoglou LG, Jakovljevic S, Dessiris AK. Color Doppler ultrasonography in prediction of the reducibility of intussuscepted bowel in 15 young dogs. *Vet Radiol Ultrasound*. 2005;46:313.
68. Holloway A, Pivetta M, Rasotto R. Ultrasonographic and histopathological features in 8 cats with fibrotic small intestinal stricture. *Vet Radiol Ultrasound*. 2019;60:423–431.
69. Drost WT, Green EM, Zekas LJ, et al. Comparison of computed tomography and abdominal radiography for detection of canine mechanical intestinal obstruction. *Vet Radiol Ultrasound*. 2016;57:366.
70. Farrow CS. Radiographic appearance of canine parvovirus enteritis. *J Am Vet Med Assoc*. 1982;180(43).
71. Isaya R, Ciccarelli S, Enache D, et al. Gastrointestinal ultrasonographic findings in cats with feline panleukopenia: a case series. *BMC Veterinary Research*. 2021;17:20.
72. Nemzek JA, Walshaw R, Hauptman JG. Mesenteric volvulus in the dog: a retrospective study. *J Am Anim Hosp Assoc*. 1993;29:357.
73. Junius G, Appeldoorn AM, Schrauwen E. Mesenteric volvulus in the dog: a retrospective study of 12 cases. *J Small Anim Pract*. 2004;45:104.
74. Westermarck E, Rinaila-Parnanen E. Mesenteric torsion in dogs with chronic pancreatic insufficiency: 21 cases (1978–1987). *J Am Vet Med Assoc*. 1989;195:1404.
75. Chow K, Stent AW, Mile M. Imaging diagnosis – use of multiphasic contrast-enhanced computed tomography for diagnosis of mesenteric volvulus in a dog. *Vet Radiol Ultrasound*. 2014;55:74.
76. Javard R, Specchi S, Benamou J, et al. Ileocecocolic volvulus in a German shepherd dog. *Can Vet J*. 2014;55:1096.

77. Wallack ST, Hornof WJ, Herrgesell EJ. Ultrasonographic diagnosis-small bowel infarction in a cat. *Vet Radiol Ultrasound*. 2003;44:81.
78. Zacuto AC, Pesavento PA, Hill S, et al. Intestinal leiomyositis: a cause of chronic intestinal pseudo-obstruction in 6 dogs. *J Vet Intern Med*. 2016;30:132.
79. Harvey AM, Hall EJ, Day MJ, et al. Chronic intestinal pseudo-obstruction in a cat caused by visceral myopathy. *J Vet Intern Med*. 2005;19:111.
80. Couraud L, Jermyn K, Yam PS, Philbey AW. Intestinal pseudo-obstruction, lymphocytic leiomyositis and atrophy of the muscularis externa in a dog. *Vet Rec*. 2006;159(86).
81. Johnson CS, Fales-Williams AJ, Reimer SB, Lotsikas PJ, Haynes JS. Fibrosing gastrointestinal leiomyositis as a cause of chronic intestinal pseudo-obstruction in an 8-month old dog. *Vet Pathol*. 2007;44:106.
82. Eastwood JM, McInnes EF, White RN, et al. Cecal impaction and chronic intestinal pseudo-obstruction in dog. *J Vet Med A Physiol Pathol Clin Med*. 2005;52(43).
83. Detweiler DA, Biller DS, Hoskinson JJ, et al. Radiographic findings of canine dysautonomia in twenty-four dogs. *Vet Radiol Ultrasound*. 2001;42:108.
84. O'Brien DP, Johnson GC. Dysautonomia and autonomic neuropathies. *Vet Clin North Am Small Anim Pract*. 2002;32:251.
85. Novellas R, Simpson KE, Gunn-Moore DA, et al. Imaging findings in 11 cats with feline dysautonomia. *J Feline Med Surg*. 2010;12:584.
86. Stander N, Wagner WM, Goddard A, Kirberger RM. Ultrasonographic appearance of canine parvoviral enteritis in puppies. *Vet Radiol Ultrasound*. 2010;51:69.
87. O'Brien TR. Liver, spleen and pancreas. In: O'Brien TR, ed. *Radiographic Diagnosis of Abdominal Disorders in the Dog and Cat*. Philadelphia: Saunders; 1978:460–480.
88. Moon ML, Billar DS, Armbrust LJ. Ultrasonographic appearance and etiology of corrugated small intestine. *Vet Radiol Ultrasound*. 2003;44:199.
89. Maas CPHJ, Haar GT, VanDerGaag I, et al. Reclassification of small intestinal and cecal smooth muscle tumors in 72 dogs: clinical, histologic, and immunohistochemical evaluation. *Vet Surg*. 2007;36:302.
90. Hobbs J, Sutherand-Smith J, Penninck D, et al. Ultrasonographic features of canine gastrointestinal stromal tumors compared to other gastrointestinal spindle cell tumors. *Vet Radiol Ultrasound*. 2015;56:432.
91. Patniak AK, Hurvitz AI, Johnson GF. Canine gastrointestinal neoplasms. *Vet Pathol*. 1977;14:547.
92. Gibbs C, Pearson H. Localized tumors of the canine small intestine: a report of twenty cases. *J Small Anim Pract*. 1986;27:506.
93. Bruecker KA, Withrow SJ. Intestinal leiomyosarcomas in six dogs. *J Am Anim Hosp Assoc*. 1988;24:281.
94. Pardo AD, Adams WH, McCracken MD, et al. Primary jejunal osteosarcoma associated with a surgical sponge in a dog. *J Am Vet Med Assoc*. 1990;196:935.
95. Crawshaw J, Berg J, Sardinas JC, et al. Prognosis for dogs with nonlymphomatous, small intestinal tumors treated by surgical excision. *J Am Anim Hosp Assoc*. 1998;34:451.
96. Takahashi T, Kadosawa T, Nagase M, et al. Visceral mast cell tumors in dogs: 10 cases (1982–1997). *J Am Vet Med Assoc*. 2000;216:222.
97. MacDonald JM, Mullen HS, Moroff SD. Adenomatous polyps of the duodenum in cats: 18 cases (1985–1990). *J Am Vet Med Assoc*. 1993;202:647.
98. Bowen EJ, Mundy P, Tivers MS, et al. Duodenal Brunner's gland adenoma causing chronic small intestinal obstruction in a dog. *J Small Anim Pract*. 2012;53:136.
99. Hayden DW, Van Kruiningen HJ. Lymphocytic-plasmacytic enteritis in German shepherd dogs. *J Am Anim Hosp Assoc*. 1982;18(89).
100. Vest B, Margulis AR. Experimental infarction of small bowel in dogs. *AJR Am J Roentgenol*. 1964;92:1080.
101. Hendirk M. A spectrum of hypereosinophilic syndromes exemplified by six cats with eosinophilic enteritis. *Vet Pathol*. 1981;18:1888.
102. Tams TR. Chronic feline inflammatory bowel disorders: II. Feline eosinophilic enteritis and lymphosarcoma. *Compend Contin Educ Vet Pract*. 1986;8:464.
103. Rivers BJ, Walter PA, Feeney DA, et al. Ultrasonographic features of intestinal adenocarcinoma in five cats. *Vet Radiol Ultrasound*. 1997;38:300.
104. Myers NC, Penninck DG. Ultrasonographic diagnosis of gastrointestinal smooth muscle tumors in the dog. *Vet Radiol Ultrasound*. 1994;35:391.
105. Paoloni MC, Pennick DG, Moore AS. Ultrasonographic and clinicopathologic findings in 21 dogs with intestinal adenocarcinoma. *Vet Radiol Ultrasound*. 2002;43:562.
106. Crystal MA, Penninck DG, Matz ME, et al. Use of ultrasound-guided fine-needle aspiration biopsy and automated core biopsy for the diagnosis for gastrointestinal disease in small animals. *Vet Radiol Ultrasound*. 1993;34:438.
107. Penninck D, Smyers B, Webster CRL, et al. Diagnostic value of ultrasonography in differentiating enteritis from intestinal neoplasia in dogs. *Vet Radiol Ultrasound*. 2003;44:570.
108. Freiche V, Fages J, Paulin MV, et al. Clinical, laboratory and ultrasonographic findings differentiating low-grade intestinal T-cell lymphoma from lymphoplasmacytic enteritis in cats. *J Vet Intern Med*. 2021;35:2685–2696.
109. Daniaux LA, Laurenson MP, Marks SL, et al. Ultrasonographic thickening of the muscularis propria in feline small intestinal small cell T-cell lymphoma and inflammatory bowel disease. *J Feline Med Surg*. 2014;16(2):89–98.
110. Norsworthy GD. Results of histopathology, immunohistochemistry, and molecular clonality testing of small intestinal biopsy specimens from clinically healthy client-owned cats. *J Vet Intern Med*. 2019;33(4):1567–1568.
111. Chang J, Porter IR, Forman MA, Shcherban N, Basran PS. Intra- and interobserver assessments of intestinal wall thickness and segmentations from transverse sections of feline abdominal ultrasound images. *Vet Radiol Ultrasound*. 2023;64(1):131–139.
112. Bettini G, Maracchini M, Dell Salda L, et al. Hypertrophy of intestinal smooth muscle in cats. *Res Vet Sci*. 2003;75(43).
113. Diana A, Pietra M, Guglielmini C, et al. Ultrasonographic and pathologic features of intestinal smooth muscle hypertrophy in four cats. *Vet Radiol Ultrasound*. 2003;44:566.
114. Dominquez E, Anadon E, Espada E, et al. Imaging diagnosis-ultrasonographic appearance of small bowel metastasis from canine mammary carcinoma. *Vet Radiol Ultrasound*. 2014;55:208.
115. Cook AK. Schistosomiasis in the United States. *Vet Clin North Am Small Anim Pract*. 2022;52(6):1283–1303.
116. Corapi WV, Ajithdoss DK, Snowden KF, Spaulding KA. Multi-organ involvement of *Heterobilharzia americana* infection in a dog presented for systemic mineralization. *J Vet Diagn Invest*. 2011;23(4):826–831.
117. Moshnikova VS, Gilmour LJ, Cook AK, Fabiani M. Sonographic findings of pinpoint hyperechoic foci in the small intestine, liver, and mesenteric lymph nodes are indicative of canine *Heterobilharzia americana* infection. *Vet Radiol Ultrasound*. 2020;61:583–591.

118. Kvitko-White HL, Sayre RS, Corapi WV, Spaulding KA. Imaging diagnosis—*Heterobilharzia americana* infection in a dog. *Veterinary Radiology & Ultrasound.* 2011;52(5):538–541.
119. Le Roux A. What is your diagnosis? Heterobilharzia infection. *J Am Vet Med Assoc.* 2015;246(4):411–413.
120. Loker ES, Dolginow SZ, Pape S, et al. An outbreak of canine schistosomiasis in Utah: Acquisition of a new snail host (*Galba humilis*) by *Heterobilharzia americana*, a pathogenic parasite on the move. *One Health.* 17:13,
121. Rodriguez JY, Camp JW, Lenz SD, Kazacos KR, Snowden KF. Identification of *Heterobilharzia americana* infection in a dog residing in Indiana with no history of travel. *J Am Vet Med Assoc.* 2016;248(7):827–830.
122. German AJ, Hall EJ, Day MJ. Chronic intestinal inflammation and intestinal disease in dogs. *J Vet Intern Med.* 2003;17(8).
123. Gaschen L, Kircher P, Stuessi A, et al. Comparison of ultrasonographic findings with clinical activity index (CIBDAI) and diagnosis in dogs with chronic enteropathies. *Vet Radiol Ultrasound.* 2008;49(56).
124. Trepanier L. Idiopathic inflammatory bowel disease in cats—rational treatment selection. *J Feline Med Surg.* 2009;11(32).
125. Rudorf H, van Schaik G, O'Brien RT, et al. Ultrasonographic evaluation of the thickness of the small intestinal wall in dogs with inflammatory bowel disease. *J Small Anim Pract.* 2005;46:322.
126. Kull PA, Hess RS, Craig LE, et al. Clinical, clinicopathologic, radiographic and ultrasonographic characteristics of intestinal lymphangiectasia in dogs: 17 cases (1996–1998). *J Am Vet Med Assoc.* 2001;219:197.
127. Sutherland-Smith J, Penninck DG, et al. Ultrasonographic intestinal hyperechoic mucosal striations in dogs and associated lacteal dilation. *Vet Radiol Ultrasound.* 2007;48:51.
128. Watson VE, Hobday MM, Durham AC. Focal intestinal lipogranulomatous lymphangitis in 6 dogs (2008–2011). *J Vet Intern Med.* 2014;28(48).
129. Lecoindre A, Ledoindre P, Cadore JL, et al. Focal intestinal lipogranulomatous lymphangitis in 10 dogs. *J Small Anim Pract.* 2016;57:465.
130. Padalkar M, Savage M, Cohen EB. Small intestinal intramural hematoma secondary to a migrating wire foreign body in a dog. *Vet Radiol Ultrasound.* 2018;59(6):E61–E65.
131. Malik R, Hunt GB, Bellenger CR, et al. Intra-abdominal cryptococcosis in two dogs. *J Small Anim Pract.* 1999;40:387.
132. Helman RG, Oliver III J. Pythiosis of the digestive tract in dogs from Oklahoma. *J Am Anim Hosp Assoc.* 1999;35:111.
133. Miller RI. Gastrointestinal phycomycosis. *J Am Vet Med Assoc.* 1985;186:473.
134. Graham JP, Newell SM, Roberts GD, et al. Ultrasonographic features of canine gastrointestinal pythiosis. *Vet Radiol Ultrasound.* 2000;41:273.
135. Parker M, Rasche B, Mozzachio K, et al. Pathology in Practice. *J Am Vet Med Assoc.* 2022;259(S2):1–5.
136. Papazoglou LG, Tontis D, Loukopoulos P, et al. Foreign body-associated intestinal pyogranuloma resulting in intestinal obstruction in four dogs. *Vet Rec.* 2010;166:494.
137. Craig LE, Hardam EE, Hertzke DM, et al. Feline gastrointestinal eosinophilic sclerosing fibroplasia. *Vet Pathol.* 2009;46(1):63–70.
138. Gunther R, Felice LJ, Nelson RK, et al. Toxicity of a vitamin D_3 rodenticide to dogs. *J Am Vet Med Assoc.* 1988;193:211.
139. Morita T, Awakura T, Shimada A, et al. Vitamin D toxicosis in cats: natural outbreak and experimental study. *J Vet Med Sci.* 1995;57:831.
140. Fan TM, Simpson KW, Trasti S, et al. Calcipotriol toxicity in a dog. *J Small Anim Pract.* 1998;39:581.
141. Hare WR, Dobbs CE, Slaymen SA, et al. Calcipotriene poisoning in dogs. *Vet Med.* 2000;95:770.
142. Song YM, Lee JY, Lee JW, et al. Ultrasound findings of pneumatosis intestinalis in a dog. *J Vet Clin.* 2013;30:138.
143. Navas de Solis C, Palmer JE, Boston RC, et al. The importance of ultrasonographic pneumatosis intestinalis in equine neonatal gastrointestinal disease. *Equine Vet J.* 2012;44(suppl 41):64.
144. Spaulding KA, Cohn LA, Miller RT, et al. Enteric duplication in two dogs. *Vet Radiol.* 1990;31:83.
145. Radlinsky MAG, Biller DS, Nietfield J, et al. Subclinical intestinal duplication in a cat. *J Feline Med Surg.* 2005;7:223.
146. Kershaw O, Deppenmeier S, Gruber AD. Multiple cystic intestinal duplications in a cat. *Vet Pathol.* 2008;45:188.
147. Bernarde A, Forget J, Bernard F. Multiple level enteric duplication cysts in a cat. *Revue Vet Clin.* 2014;49(31).
148. Oui H, Lamm C, Stiver S, et al. Congenital lymphangiomatosis and an enteric duplication cyst in a young dog. *J Small Anim Pract.* 2014;55:379.
149. Walling BE, Arndt TM. Pathology in Practice. *J Am Vet Med Assoc.* 2015;246:1297.
150. Ablin LW, Moore FM, Shields Henney LH, et al. Intestinal diverticular malformation in dogs and cats. *Compend.* 1991;13:426.
151. van Kalveren NJ, Grinwis GCM, Brocks BAW, et al. Collapse following gastrointestinal bleeding secondary to a congenital duodenal diverticulum in two littermate boxer puppies. *J Small Anim Pract.* 2008;49:103.
152. Polf H, Poteet B. Imaging diagnosis – duodenal diverticulum in a dog. *Vet Radiol Ultrasound.* 2010;51(61).

ELECTRONIC RESOURCES

Additional information related to the content in Chapter 46 can be found online at eBooks.Health.Elsevier.com

- Chapter Quiz

CHAPTER 47

Large Bowel

Christine L. Gremillion

ANATOMY

The large intestine consists of the cecum, colon, rectum, and anal canal (Fig. 47.1). The cecum is a diverticulum arising from the proximal colon, located in the right midabdomen, at approximately the level of L3 and L4.[1] The cecum can be quite variable in shape and size depending on its luminal contents. In dogs, the cecum tends to be larger and sigmoid or c-shaped, whereas in cats the cecum is shorter in length and more cone-shaped (Fig. 47.2).[1,2] The mesentery of the colon (mesocolon) is present along its entire length, and is shorter than the mesentery of the small intestine. The mesocolon is also attached to the mesoduodenum via the duodenocolic ligament. These factors combine to make the large intestine overall less mobile than the small intestine, and thus, its normal position within the abdomen is more consistent.[1] The colon is divided into three parts: the ascending, transverse, and descending colon. The ascending colon is the most proximal portion of the colon, located in the cranial abdomen to the right of midline. The ascending colon is located near the descending duodenum, right lobe of the pancreas, and right kidney. The right colic flexure connects the ascending colon to the transverse colon. The transverse colon lives in the cranial abdomen, coursing from the right to left side, and is located adjacent to the greater curvature of the stomach and left lobe of the pancreas. The transverse colon communicates with the descending colon at the left colic flexure. The descending colon then courses caudally, parallel to the body wall, to the level of the pelvic inlet, where it transitions into the rectum without demarcation. The terminal portion of the descending colon and rectum are located dorsal to the urinary bladder, urethra, and prostate/uterus. The rectum then continues caudally to the level of the second or third caudal vertebrae, where it communicates with the anal canal.[1]

IMAGING PROCEDURES

Radiography

Normal Radiographic Findings

The colon is often readily visible on plain radiographs due to normal intraluminal gas and/or fecal contents, although areas devoid of contents may be indistinct. Fecal material often has a granular appearance with mixed soft tissue and gas opacity. The normal colon is shaped like a question mark or shepherd's crook, coursing from the ileocolic junction in the right midabdomen cranially, across midline, and then caudally along the left abdomen in the ventrodorsal view. Occasionally, the distal portion of the descending colon may partially extend to the right of midline in animals that have longer, redundant colons

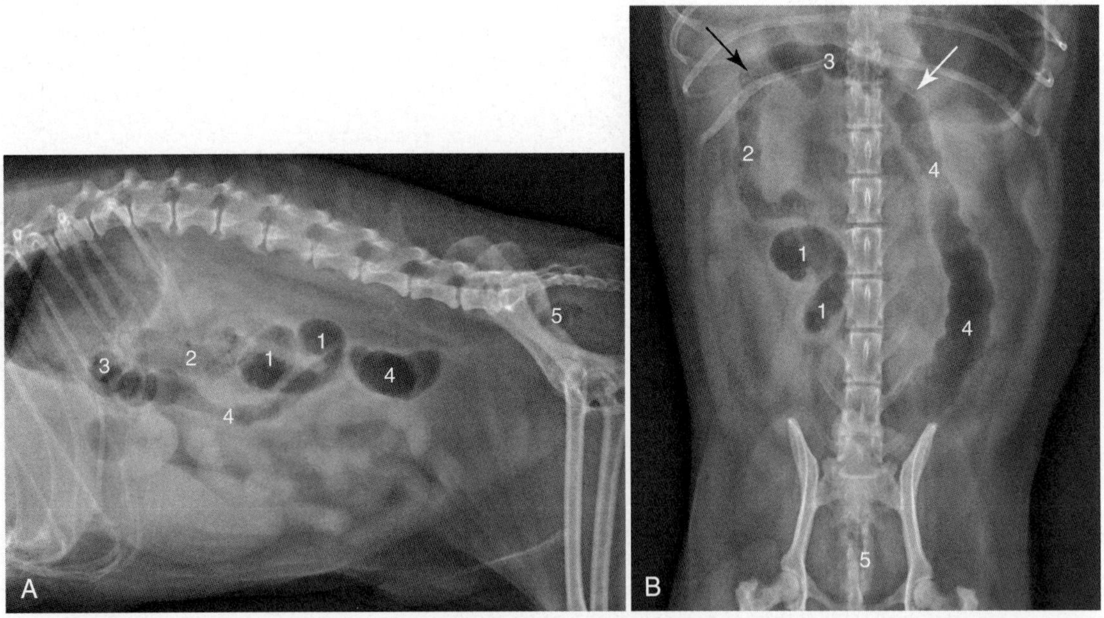

Fig. 47.1 Survey lateral **(A)** and ventrodorsal **(B)** radiographs of demonstrating normal large intestine anatomy. The large intestine is divided into the cecum *(1)*, ascending colon *(2)*, transverse colon *(3)*, descending colon *(4)*, rectum *(5)*, and anal canal. The right and left colic flexures are denoted by the *black* and *white arrows*, respectively.

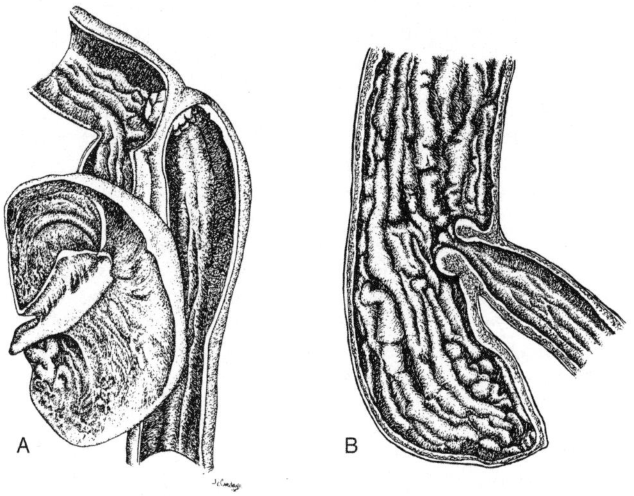

Fig. 47.2 The cecum of the dog **(A)** and cat **(B)** are anatomically and radiographically different. The canine cecum is semicircular and compartmentalized and normally contains some gas. The feline cecum is a short, cone-like structure with no compartmentalization and it rarely contains adequate gas or feces to be visualized radiographically. (Reproduced with permission from O'Brien TR. *Radiographic Diagnosis of Abdominal Disorders in the Dog and Cat.* Davis, CA: Covell Park Veterinary; 1981.)

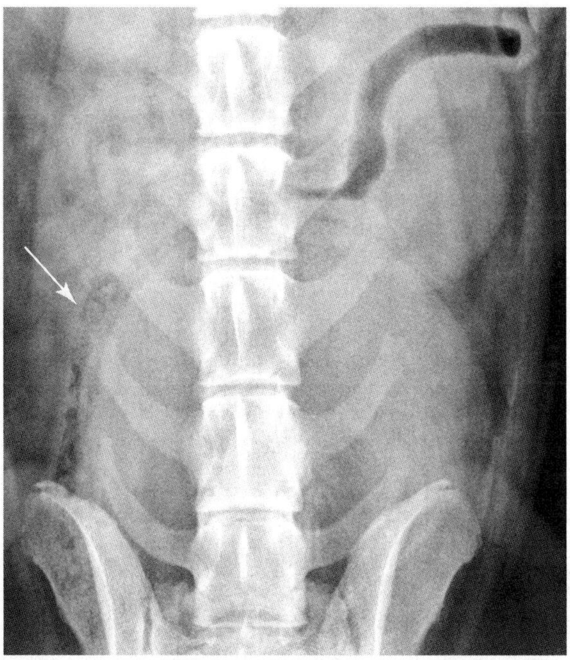

Fig. 47.3 Ventrodorsal radiograph of a dog with a distended urinary bladder that resulted in displacement of the descending colon to the right of midline (*arrow*). This is a common change in the position of the descending colon and is not clinically significant.

or distention of the urinary bladder (Fig. 47.3).[3] In the lateral views, the entirety of the colon is typically located in the dorsal third of the abdomen, running approximately parallel to the vertebral column.[3] The diameter of the normal colon can be variable depending on the luminal contents, but in dogs, a general rule of thumb is that the colon diameter should be less than the length of the L7 vertebral body.[4] In cats, normal colon diameter should be less than 1.28 times the length of the L5 vertebral body.[5] The cecum is variably visible in dogs depending on the degree of distention. Due to the smaller size of the cecum in cats, it is often not seen radiographically. Gas is occasionally present in the anal sacs, which can appear as either unilateral or bilateral well-circumscribed lucencies summating with the ischia in the ventrodorsal view (Fig. 47.4). It is important not to confuse this finding with geographic bone lysis.

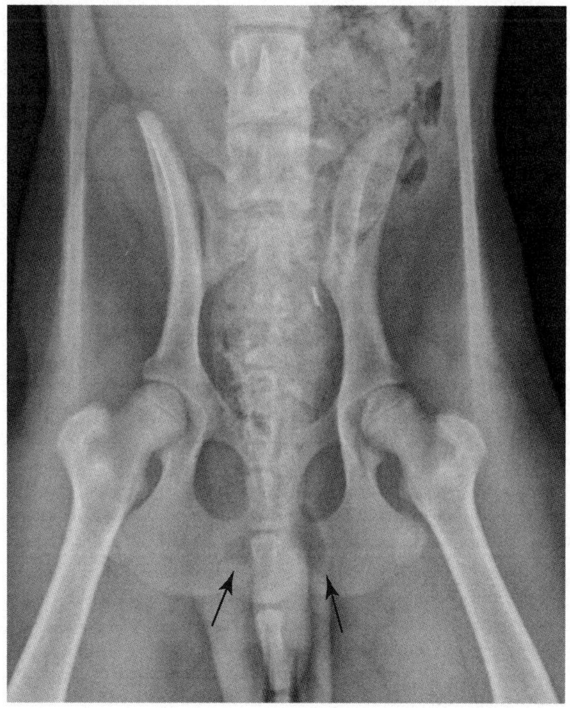

Fig. 47.4 Ventrodorsal radiograph of the pelvis. Gas is present in the anal sacs resulting in asymmetric, well-circumscribed gas opacities summating with the ischia (*arrows*). This should not be confused with bone lysis.

Contrast Radiography

Contrast radiography of the large intestine may be utilized when the diagnosis or appropriate treatment for a patient cannot be determined by survey radiographs and other imaging modalities are not available or desirable. The use of ultrasound and direct inspection of the large intestine via endoscopy have largely replaced many radiographic contrast studies of the colon[2]; however, contrast studies are still helpful for specific indications.

Pneumocolonography

Pneumocolonography, or negative contrast studies of the colon, are typically performed in patients to determine the position of the colon on radiographs and to differentiate it from distended small intestines.[3,6] Pneumocolonography has also been described in aiding the diagnosis of colonic torsion.[7] Survey radiographs should always be acquired first. With the patient positioned in lateral recumbency, approximately 1 to 3 mL/kg of air is introduced into a red-rubber catheter that is placed in the rectum and then lateral and ventrodorsal projections are obtained.[6] The final volume of air required to sufficiently fill the entirety of the colon is patient dependent, and often small increments of air are introduced, radiographs are acquired, and if there is an insufficient volume, the process is repeated. In most patients, it is desirable to fill the entirety of the colon with air to the level of the cecum.

Positive Contrast Enema

Positive contrast enemas with barium used to be the principal imaging technique for evaluation of the colon.[3,8,9] With the advancement of ultrasound and colonoscopy, barium enemas are used less frequently; however, it is still a useful, minimally invasive, and quick procedure, particularly if there is a concern for colonic torsion and survey radiographs are equivocal.[10] Barium enema can also aid in the diagnosis of intussusception and colonic strictures if ultrasound and/or endoscopy are not readily available.

Survey radiographs should always be obtained prior to initiation of the study. Unless performed as an emergency procedure, preparation including a 12- to 24-hour fast, laxatives, and cleansing enemas is preferred.[9] The volume of contrast medium utilized depends on the indication for the study. A dose of approximately 10 to 15 mL/kg of body weight of barium suspension can be expected to fill the entirety of the colon[3,9]; however, this full volume is not required for diagnosis of all disease processes. A diagnosis of colonic torsion has been made using dosages of as little as 3 mL/kg of body weight.[10] Barium is usually administered via an inflatable Foley catheter placed in the distal rectum.[4,8,9] To minimize risk of perforation, the colon should either be filled slowly by gravity or infused in small increments until the desired effect is seen radiographically. Both lateral and ventrodorsal projections should be acquired following introduction of barium. If back pressure is present on the syringe, infusion of barium should be discontinued. If colonic perforation is suspected prior to initiation of the study, iodinated contrast medium should be used instead of barium due to the risk of granulomatous peritonitis with extravasation of barium.[9]

Ultrasound of the Large Bowel

Ultrasound allows assessment of large intestinal wall thickness, layering, and evidence of mass lesions, and also provides the ability to assess the surrounding mesentery and regional lymph nodes. Ultrasound-guided tissue sampling (fine needle aspirate or biopsy) can also be performed.[11] The primary limitation of ultrasound of the large bowel is the presence of feces and gas with distal acoustic shadowing and reverberation artifacts, respectively, which result in limited visibility of the bowel wall in the far-field of the image.

The wall of the large intestine is thinner than that of the small intestine, measuring only 1 to 2 mm in thickness on ultrasound.[12] Similar to the stomach and small intestine, distinct wall layers of the large intestine are visible: a hyperechoic luminal surface, hypoechoic mucosa, hyperechoic submucosa, hypoechoic muscularis, and hyperechoic outer serosa (Fig. 47.5). When the colon is empty, the wall can have an irregular appearance due to infolding and should not be confused with wall thickening. Occasionally, a thin hyperechoic line can be seen in the muscularis layer of the colon that parallels the serosal surface. Histologically, this correlates with fibrous tissue in the myenteric plexus. As this is seen in dogs without a history of diarrhea, this finding is considered a normal variant.[13] The descending colon can be easily recognized when imaging in a transverse plane in the caudal abdomen, where it lies dorsal to the urinary bladder at the pelvic inlet. The typical appearance of the colon is a thin-walled tubular structure with a curved hyperechoic luminal interface. When identified near the urinary bladder, the descending colon can then be traced cranially through the remainder of the large bowel. The ileocolic junction (Fig. 47.6), cecum, and ascending colon are located medial to the right kidney, which can serve as a landmark as well if unable to trace the entirety of the colon from distal to proximal.

Computed Tomography of the Large Bowel

Computed tomography (CT) provides a three-dimensional view of the large bowel and surrounding structures and is particularly helpful for assessing abnormalities within the pelvic canal compared to radiographs and ultrasound (Fig. 47.7).[14] When nonionic iodinated contrast medium is administered intravenously, the colonic mucosa strongly enhances, but discrete wall layers are not visible on CT.[15] Water, barium, and air have been described as luminal contrast agents.[16,17] Bowel preparation protocols may be utilized for bowel cleansing to optimize image quality and aid in interpretation.[18]

LARGE BOWEL DISEASES

Large Intestinal Displacement From Mass Effect

Abnormalities of the organs adjacent to the large intestine can result in displacement, and sometimes compression, of the colon and rectum depending on the severity (Figs. 47.8 and 47.9). Moderate to severe enlargement of the iliosacral lymph center will result in ventral displacement of the colon and/or rectum on lateral radiographs (Fig. 47.10A). Ventral displacement of the colon will also occur secondary to renomegaly and other causes of mass effects from the retroperitoneal space such as retroperitoneal effusion. Dorsal displacement of the colon and/or rectum commonly occurs secondary to enlargement of the prostate gland, uterus, vagina, or urinary bladder (see Fig. 47.10B).

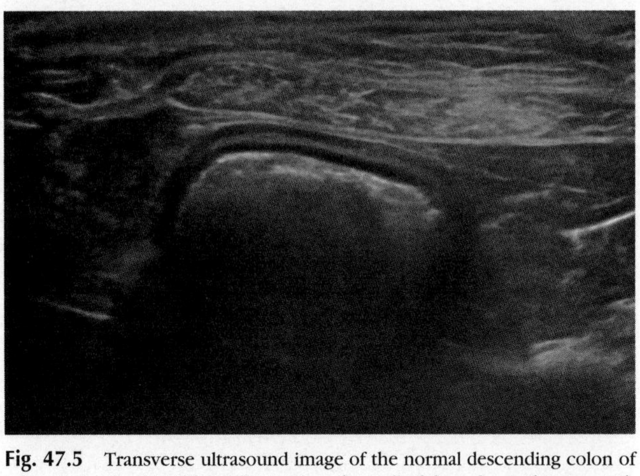

Fig. 47.5 Transverse ultrasound image of the normal descending colon of a dog. In contrast to the small intestine, the wall of the colon is thinner, with each layer contributing approximately equally to the overall wall thickness. The far wall of the colon is not visible in this image secondary to intraluminal feces and gas with associated distal shadowing and reverberation artifact.

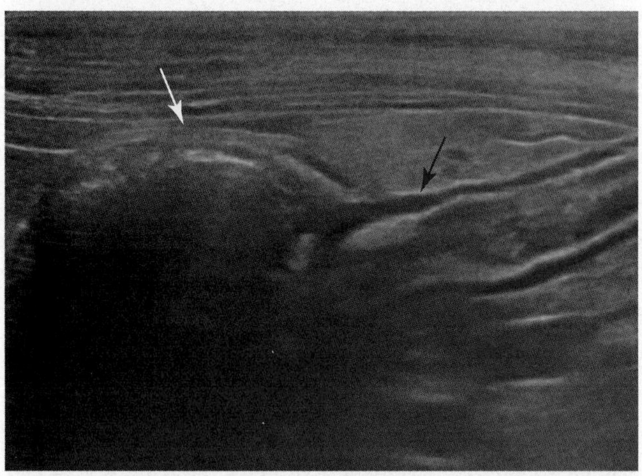

Fig. 47.6 Ultrasound image of the normal ileocolic junction in a cat. The ileum (*black arrow*), in longitudinal section, has prominent muscularis and submucosal layers. The ascending colon (*white arrow*) has a characteristic thin wall and contains internal fecal material with distal acoustic shadowing.

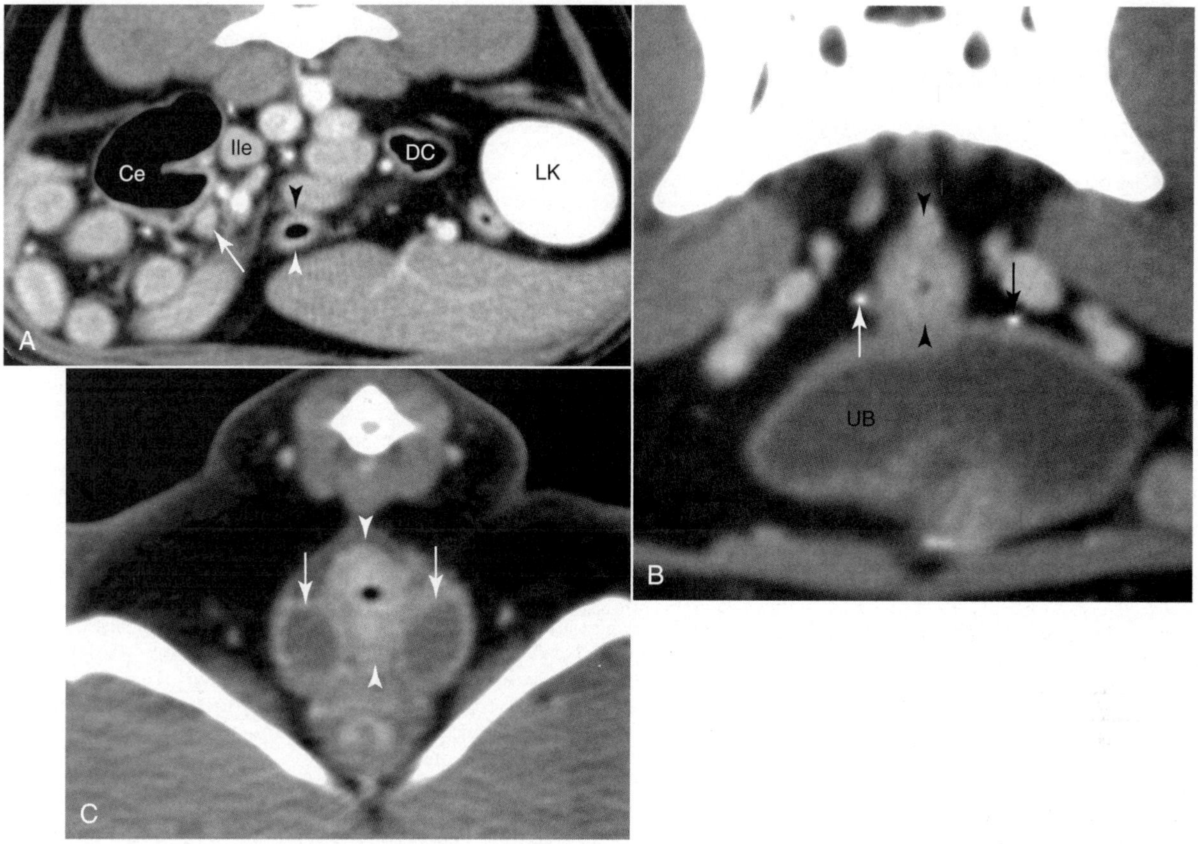

Fig. 47.7 Transverse, contrast-enhanced computed tomography images of the large intestine and adjacent organs in a normal dog. **A,** Cranial abdomen with a gas filled cecum (*Ce*), terminal ileum (*Ile*), right colic lymph node (*arrow*), transverse colon (*between arrowheads*) and descending colon (*DC*); *LK,* Left kidney. **B,** Pelvic inlet with the descending colon (*between arrowheads*), ureters (*arrows*), and urinary bladder (*UB*). The right ureter (*arrow*) is traveling toward the bladder neck in the right mesocolon directly adjacent to the colon wall. **C,** Caudal pelvis with rectum (*between arrowheads*) and adjacent anal gland sacs (*arrows*).

Displacement Within the Large Bowel

Intussusception

Intussusception occurs when a segment of intestine (the intussusceptum) telescopes or invaginates into an adjoining segment (the intussuscipiens). Intussusception is relatively common in young patients and frequently involves the ileocolic junction, although cecocolic (also referred to as "cecal inversion"; Fig. 47.11, eFig. 47.1), colocolic, and colorectal intussusceptions have also been reported.[19–22] Enteritis, parasitic infection, linear foreign bodies, and intestinal masses have been implicated as causes of intussusception, although occasionally it can be idiopathic. Radiographs in patients with intussusception can demonstrate small intestinal dilation secondary to partial or complete obstruction of the ileocolic junction, if present. Occasionally, if the lumen of the intussuscipiens contains gas, a convex soft tissue margin, representing the leading margin of the intussusceptum, can be seen (Fig. 47.12, eFig. 47.1). This is termed a *meniscus sign* and is suggestive of intussusception.[19] When the intussusceptum is outlined by barium from a positive contrast enema or gas, sometimes a "coiled-spring sign" can also be appreciated (Fig. 47.13, eFig. 47.2). On ultrasound, intussusceptions of the large intestine are similar to that seen in the small bowel, characterized by a target-like or "bullseye" appearance, consisting of multiple hyperechoic and hypoechoic concentric rings, caused by juxtaposition of the affected bowel walls, around a hyperechoic center of entrapped mesentery (Fig. 47.14).[19] Color Doppler can be helpful in assessing viability of the involved intestinal segments.[23]

Displacement Within the Abdominal Cavity

Colonic Torsion/Volvulus

Both torsion and volvulus of the colon have been described in small animals, and these terms appear to be used interchangeably in the literature. Colonic torsion/volvulus occurs primarily in young to middle-aged medium and large breed dogs, although a single case of colonic volvulus has been reported in a domestic shorthair cat.[7,10,24–26] Clinical signs of shock may or may not be present upon evaluation; when absent, this can occasionally result in treatment delays, making rapid diagnosis imperative.[10] Radiographic findings of colonic torsion include segmental dilation of the colon, focal narrowing of the descending colon, displacement of the cecum to the left of midline, and displacement of the proximal descending colon to the right of midline (Fig. 47.15).[10] Barium enema is helpful in obtaining a definitive diagnosis, with characteristic longitudinal and helical striations visible in conjunction with focal narrowing at the site of torsion (Fig. 47.16, eFigs. 47.3 and 47.4). Additional findings of colonic torsion seen with CT include presence of the "whirl sign," distention of mesenteric vasculature, peritoneal effusion, and pneumatosis coli in a subset of patients.[27]

Large Intestinal Entrapment and Strangulation

Colonic entrapment and strangulation are uncommon conditions but have been reported in dogs secondary to rupture of the duodenocolic ligament with secondary colonic entrapment, entrapment in gastropexy sites, and entrapment in omental rents and adhesions.[10,26,28,29]

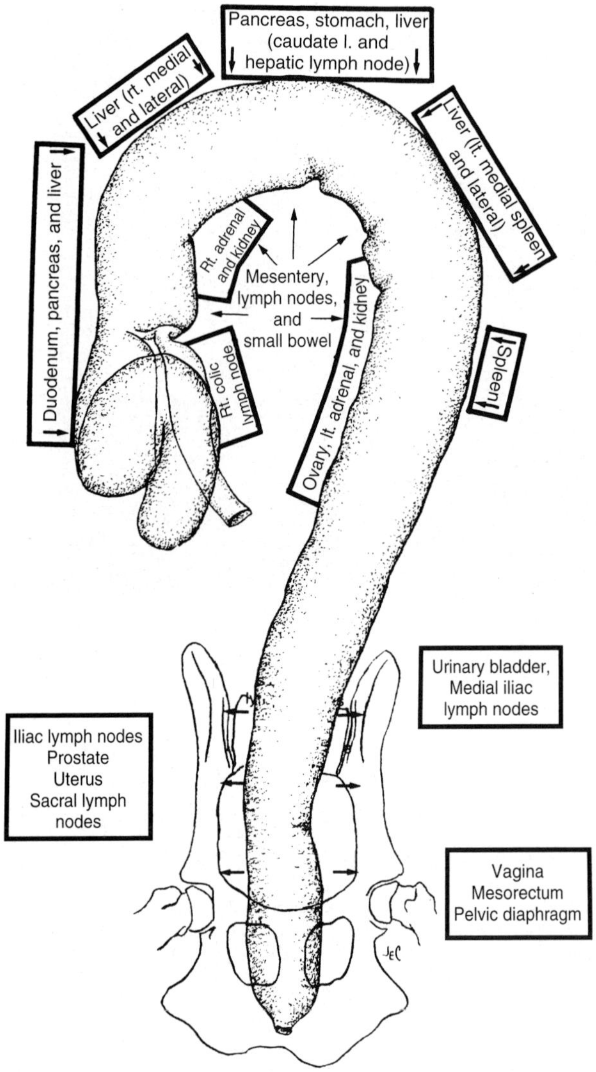

Fig. 47.8 Viscera adjacent to the large bowel may cause a change in position of a portion of the colon. This change in position may be indicative of disease or a variant of normal, depending on the cause of the deviation. The *arrows* indicate the direction of displacement of the colon that can occur when an adjacent organ enlarges. (Reproduced with permission from O'Brien TR. *Radiographic Diagnosis of Abdominal Disorders in the Dog and Cat*. Davis, CA: Covell Park Veterinary; 1981)

Displacement From Herniation

Perineal Hernia

In addition to herniation of the bladder and/or prostate into the perineal region, perineal hernias also frequently result in displacement of the rectum and/or descending colon into the perineal region (Fig. 47.17).

Alterations in Large Bowel Diameter

Constipation/Obstipation/Megacolon

Constipation is defined as reversible, infrequent, or difficult defecation with associated retention of fecal material.[2] Recurrent constipation that is refractory to treatment is termed *obstipation*, and implies a permanent loss of function.[2] Megacolon is a descriptive term, used when there is irreversible dilation of the colon, and represents end-stage colonic dysfunction in patients with obstipation.[2,5] (Fig. 47.18; eFig. 47.5A,B) Differentials for patients with chronic constipation, obstipation, and megacolon can be split into functional and mechanical causes. Functional causes include neuromuscular dysfunction; spinal cord diseases, including lumbosacral, cauda equina, and sacral spinal cord deformities (such as that seen in the Manx cat); hypogastric or pelvic nerve disorders; submucosal or myenteric plexus neuropathy; aganglionosis of the large bowel; and feline dysautonomia.[2,30–32] Metabolic and endocrine diseases can also be a functional cause of chronic constipation, with young cats with congenital hypothyroidism being particularly predisposed.[2,33,34] Mechanical causes of chronic constipation include luminal obstruction secondary to mural lesions of the large intestine (such as masses or strictures), herniation of large bowel with associated obstruction, and congenital deformities such as atresia ani and atresia coli. Extramural lesions can also result in mechanical obstruction of the large intestine, including malunion pelvic fractures with narrowing of the pelvic canal and extramural masses or neoplasia.[35] Of these differentials, the most common causes in cats are idiopathic megacolon (accounting for approximately 66% of all cases), with an additional 25% of cases being attributed to narrowing of the pelvic canal from malunion fractures.[5] To differentiate constipation from megacolon in cats, a ratio of the maximal diameter of the colon compared to the length of the L5 vertebral body can be used, with a ratio greater than 1.5 suggestive of megacolon.[5] Patients with constipation or obstipation often have fecal material that is increased in opacity compared to that of normal feces, sometimes being mineral opaque, due to excessive water resorption from colon stasis.

MURAL ABNORMALITIES OF THE LARGE BOWEL

Focal Wall Thickening

Focal wall thickening and mass lesions of the large intestine occur secondary to infiltration of the wall with cells, most commonly secondary to neoplasia, inflammation, and/or infectious disease. Mass lesions of the large intestine may be visible on radiographs if they are large in size; small lesions are better visualized with ultrasound. Ultrasound findings include focal thickening of the intestinal wall and/or discrete nodules/masses arising from the intestinal wall with alteration or loss of wall layering. While neoplasia is a common cause of these changes, these findings are not specific and there is overlap between neoplastic and inflammatory lesions. Patient signalment, history, clinical signs, and lesion location can sometimes aid in prioritizing differential diagnoses, but ultimately, tissue sampling must be performed for definitive diagnosis.

Malignant Neoplasia of the Large Intestine

The most common colonic neoplasms of dogs are adenocarcinoma and lymphoma, with adenocarcinomas of the large intestine occurring most commonly in the descending colon and rectum.[2] In dogs, gastrointestinal stromal tumors (GISTs) and leiomyosarcomas have a predilection for the cecum (Fig. 47.19, eFig. 47.6).[2] Distinguishing between GISTs and leiomyosarcomas was previously difficult until the advent of new immunohistochemistry stains, leading many historically diagnosed leiomyosarcomas to be reclassified as GISTs.[36] This reclassification may impact the incidence of smooth muscle tumors of the gastrointestinal tract reported in previous studies. In cats, the most common large intestinal neoplasm is also adenocarcinoma, followed by lymphoma (Figs. 47.20 and 47.21, and eFig. 47.7).[37,38] Other etiologies such as mast cell neoplasia and spindle cell tumors are much less common in the large intestine of cats.[37,38]

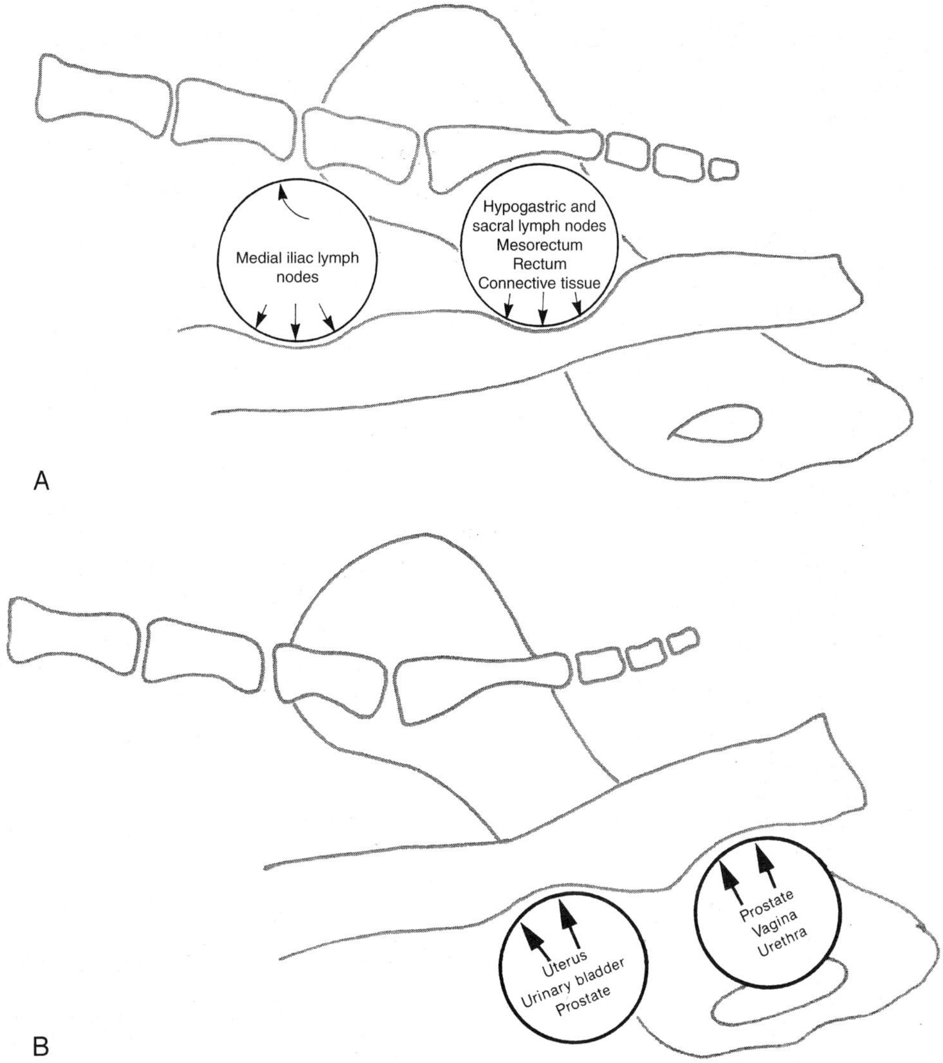

Fig. 47.9 Patterns of displacement of the descending colon and rectum by adjacent organ enlargement. **A,** Ventral displacement of the terminal descending colon and rectum commonly results from medial iliac and sacral lymph node enlargement. Although less common, a hematoma, abscess, or tumor may produce similar displacement alterations. **B,** Dorsal displacement of the rectum commonly results from enlargement of the prostate gland, the uterus, the vagina, or the intrapelvic urinary bladder. (Reproduced with permission from O'Brien TR. *Radiographic Diagnosis of Abdominal Disorders in the Dog and Cat*. Davis, CA: Covell Park Veterinary; 1981.)

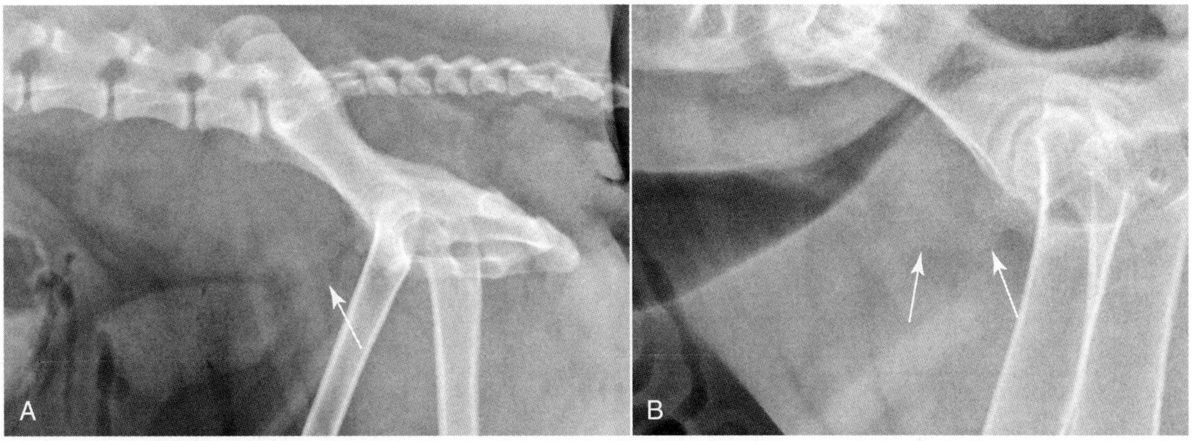

Fig. 47.10 **A,** Lateral radiograph of a dog with anal sac carcinoma metastatic to the medial iliac lymph nodes. The enlarged lymph nodes displace the colon ventrally and there is compression (*arrow*) at the pelvic inlet. **B,** Lateral radiograph of a dog with narrowing of the large bowel at the junction of the descending colon and rectum from an enlarged prostate gland (*arrows*).

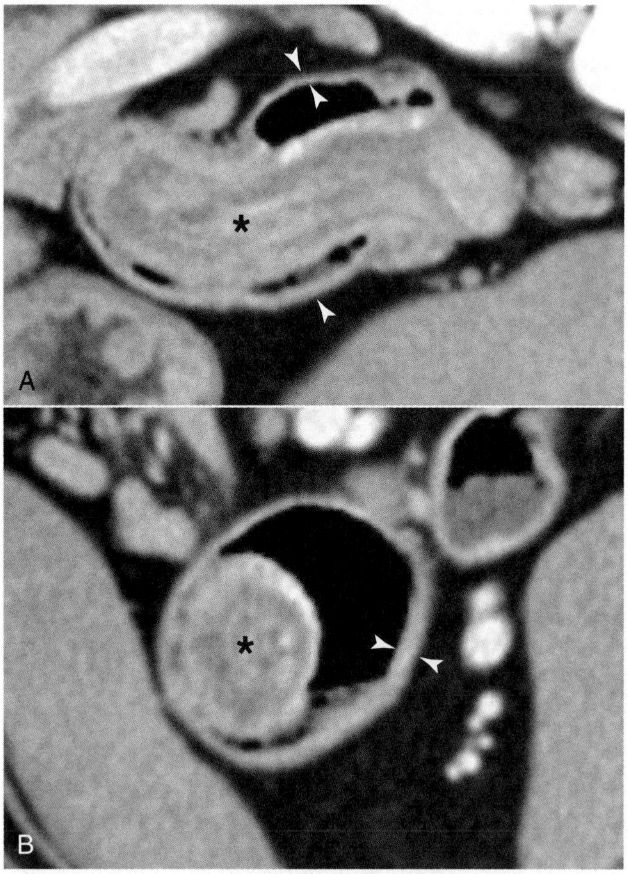

Fig. 47.11 Sagittal **(A)** and transverse **(B)** computed tomography images of a cecocolic intussusception due to large B-cell lymphoma in an older dog. Note the thickened, heterogeneously contrast enhancing cecum (*asterisk*) displaced into the lumen of the ascending colon. The ascending colonic wall is outlined by *arrowheads* and a small amount of luminal gas and fluid outlines the intussusceptum. The lymphoma most likely caused dysmotility that led to cecal inversion and intussusception.

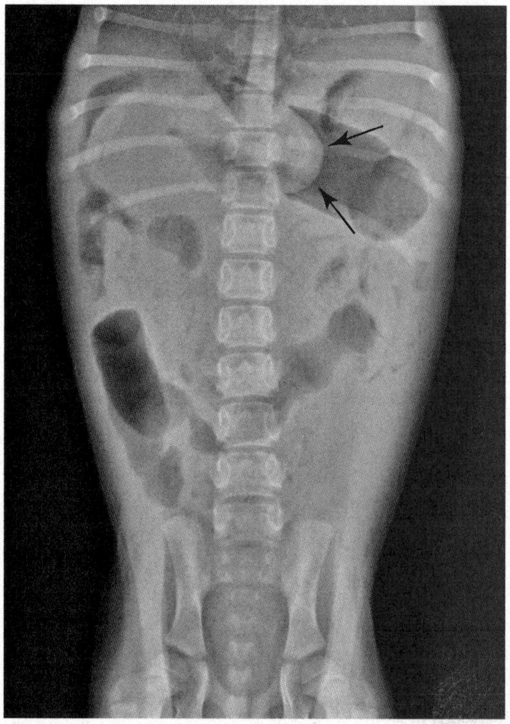

Fig. 47.12 Survey ventrodorsal abdominal radiograph of a young dog with an ileocecocolic intussusception demonstrating the meniscus sign. The transverse colon is distended by a homogeneous soft-tissue opacity with a curved gas interface caudally (*arrows*), consistent with the leading edge of the intussusceptum. A similar appearance could be seen with a soft tissue opaque foreign body or mass. Ultrasound could be used to distinguish between these differentials if indicated.

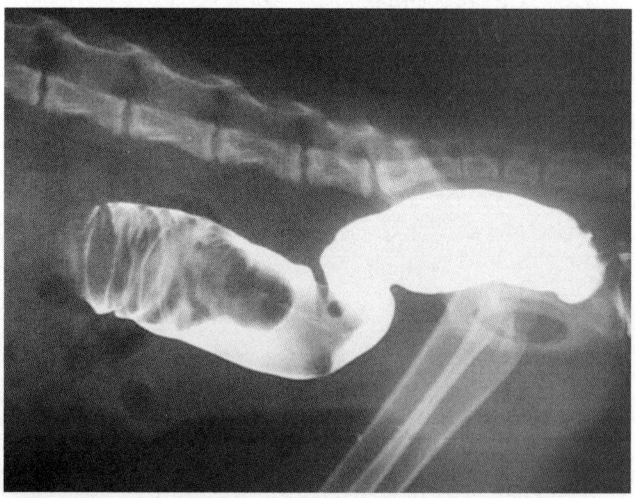

Fig. 47.13 Lateral radiograph of a barium enema of a cat with an ileocolic intussusception. The intussusceptum creates a filling defect in the barium. Edema and swelling of the intussusceptum create a coiled-spring appearance to the filling defect; this is typical of the appearance of the intussusceptum in a barium enema.

Focal Wall Thickening From Infectious/ Inflammatory Disease

A variety of infectious and inflammatory diseases can result in focal wall thickening or mass lesions of the large intestine with alteration or complete loss of wall layering. In dogs, conditions reported to cause focal masses with loss of wall layering of the colon include pythiosis, fungal disease, and protothecosis.[39–42] Granulomatous colitis can also cause focal wall thickening and masses.[43] Submucosal thickening and mineralization of the colon wall have been reported in dogs secondary to *Heterobilharzia americana* infection, although these changes are often less pronounced than that seen in the small intestine.[44,45] In cats, feline infectious peritonitis, fungal disease, and eosinophilic sclerosing fibroplasia can result in mass lesions and focal thickening of the large intestine.[46,47] In both dogs and cats, bacterial etiologies, such as disseminated mycobacteriosis, can result in focal or multifocal intestinal lesions.[48]

Benign Mass Lesions of the Large Intestine

Benign polyps have been reported in the large intestine of both dogs and cats, and have rarely been associated with intussusception.[21,38,49] Adenomas and leiomyomas are benign neoplasms that can occur within the large intestine, although these are less common than their malignant counterparts (adenocarcinoma and leiomyosarcoma, respectively). Hemorrhage and/or hematoma formation within the wall can also result in focal mass lesions of the large bowel,[50] and cecal mucoceles are a cause of intraluminal mass-like lesions which could be confused for a soft tissue mass.[51]

Diffuse Wall Thickening

Colitis/Typhlitis

With colitis, a gas- or fluid-filled colon may be seen radiographically. On ultrasound, mild diffuse thickening of the wall may be present (Fig. 47.22), usually with preservation of wall layers, in conjunction with echogenic intraluminal fluid. Corrugation of the wall may also be present, characterized by multifocal undulation of luminal margin on radiographs or as numerous small undulations of the mucosa/lumen interface

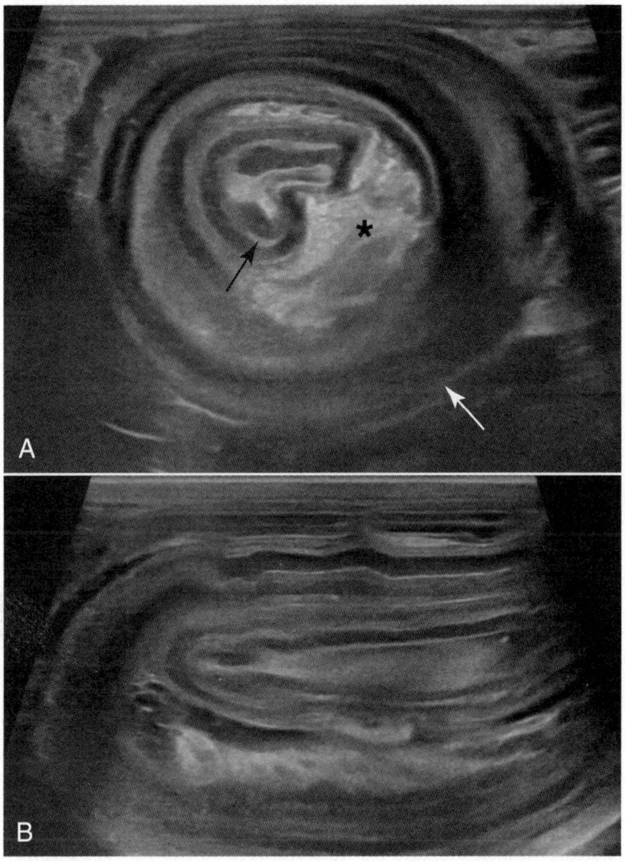

Fig. 47.14 Transverse (A) and longitudinal (B) ultrasound images of the descending colon of a dog with a jejunocolic intussusception. In **A**, note the target-like or "bullseye" appearance, consisting of multiple hyperechoic and hypoechoic concentric rings, caused by juxtaposition of the walls of the external intussuscipiens (*white arrow*) and internal intussusceptum (*black arrow*) with a hyperechoic center, representative of entrapped mesentery (*asterisk*). In **B**, the same wall layers are now parallel in orientation.

and/or submucosa on ultrasound. Occasionally, small (1–3 mm) ovoid hypoechoic nodules may be seen in the submucosal layer of the colon in patients with diarrhea, thought to represent reactive lymphoid follicles (Fig. 47.23A).[52] Lymphoid follicles can also be visible as coalescing nodules in the cecal mucosa and submucosa, termed the *follicular layer*, in cats with subclinical inflammation.[53] Typhlitis, or inflammation of the cecum, can appear as diffuse wall thickening with loss of wall layering in cats (see Fig. 47.23B).[54] In cat ceca, loss of wall layering is not a reliable predictor of the severity of inflammation or of neoplastic change. The sonographic findings of typhlitis have not been described in dogs, although wall thickening and/or fluid distention of the lumen could be suggestive.

Opacity Changes

Pneumatosis Coli

Pneumatosis coli is the presence of gas within the colon wall. This can occur secondary to a defect in the intestinal mucosa, such as an ulcer, or an increase in intraluminal pressure that allows luminal gas to pass into the bowel wall. Increased intraluminal pressure could occur secondary to large bowel obstruction, as with colonic torsion,[27] or iatrogenically from recent endoscopy.[55] Underlying gastrointestinal necrosis from ischemia or inflammatory disease can also result in introduction of luminal gas into the bowel wall.[55] Anaerobic bacterial infection of the colonic mucosa has also been implicated in the development of pneumatosis coli, namely infection with *Clostridium* species.[55] Radiographically, pneumatosis coli appears as a heterogeneous gas pattern within the wall of the colon. When a large volume of gas is present, it can present as a band of gas that follows the course of the wall (Fig. 47.24). With smaller volumes of gas, it can be difficult to distinguish between intramural gas and intraluminal gas trapped between peripherally located fecal material and the wall. Sonographically, pneumatosis coli is characterized by gas with associated reverberation artifact that originates from the submucosal or subserosal layers of the colonic wall, rather than the lumen (Fig. 47.25).[55,56] Similar to pneumatosis in other regions of the

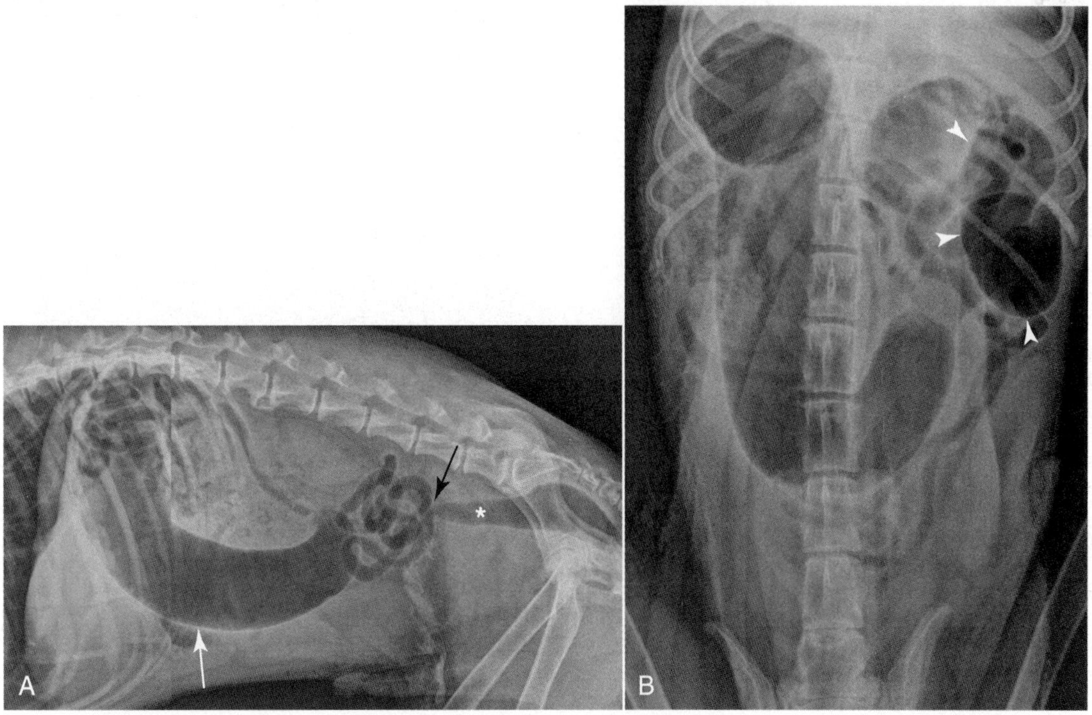

Fig. 47.15 Lateral (A) and ventrodorsal (B) views of a dog with colonic torsion. Segmental dilation and displacement of the proximal colon (*white arrow*), resulting in a C-shaped distended bowel segment in the cranial abdomen, are typical of colonic torsion. The distal descending colon (*white asterisk*) is nondistended and focally narrows in the caudal abdomen (*black arrow*). In the ventrodorsal view, the cecum (*white arrowheads*) is displaced in the left abdomen.

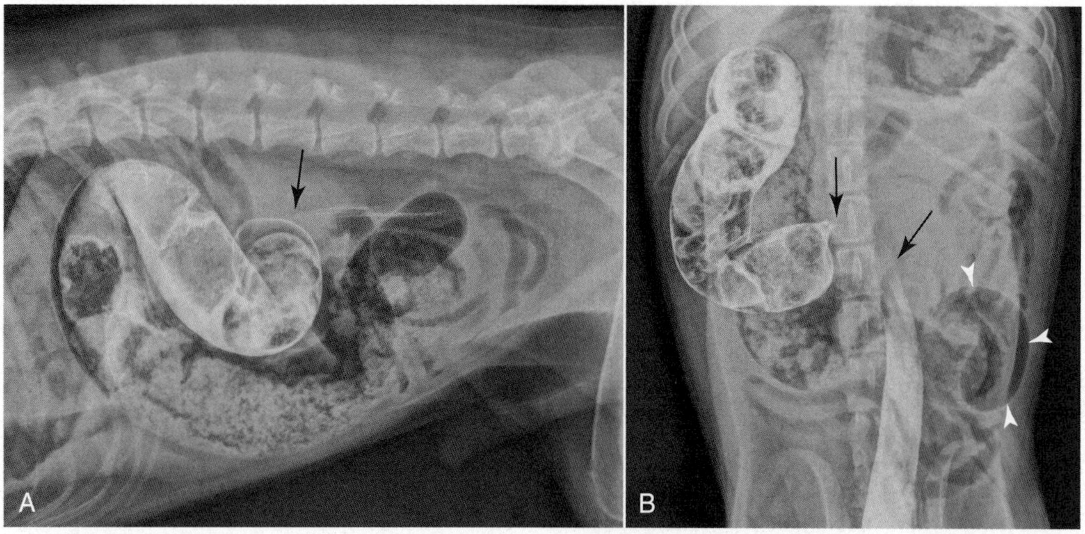

Fig. 47.16 Lateral **(A)** and ventrodorsal **(B)** views following barium enema in a dog with colonic torsion. Note the focal narrowing and longitudinal striations (*black arrows*) in the distal descending colon, which have a somewhat helical pattern in **B**. The cecum is displaced in the left abdomen in the ventrodorsal view (*white arrowheads*).

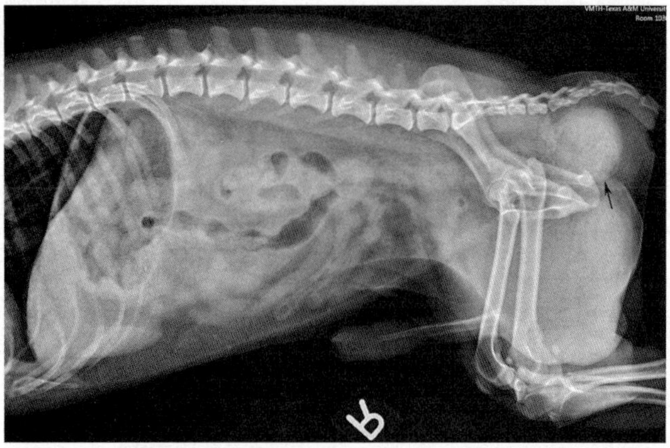

Fig. 47.17 Lateral radiograph of a dog with a perineal hernia. There is herniation of the rectum and colon into the perineal region, with accumulation of desiccated fecal material (*arrow*). Note the increased opacity of the fecal material due to inspissation.

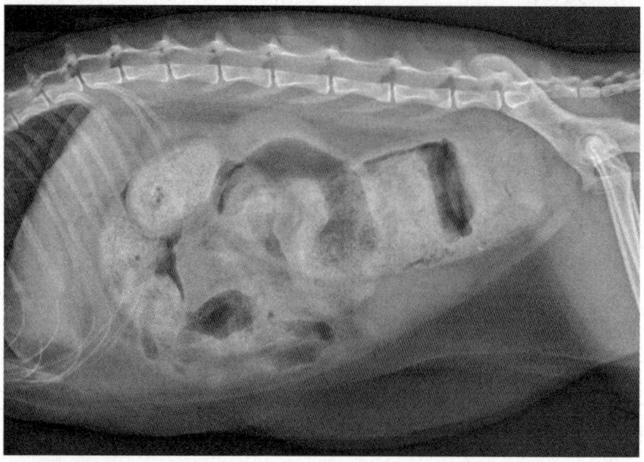

Fig. 47.18 Lateral radiograph of a cat with idiopathic megacolon. There is severe dilation of the entirety of the colon, most severely affecting the descending colon, resulting in ventral displacement of the urinary bladder. Note the increased opacity of the colonic contents, consistent with desiccated fecal material.

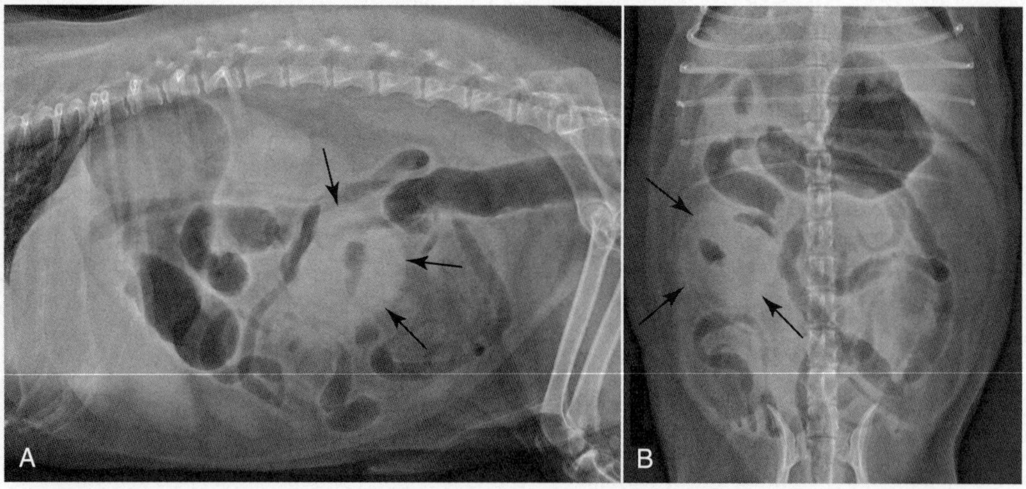

Fig. 47.19 Lateral **(A)** and ventrodorsal **(B)** views of a dog with a cecal mass. There is a round soft tissue opaque midabdominal mass with internal gas (*black arrows*) that localizes to the right of midline in the ventrodorsal projection. The location of this mass, internal gas, and lack of associated gastrointestinal mechanical obstruction are all highly suggestive of cecal origin. This was a gastrointestinal stromal tumor on histopathology.

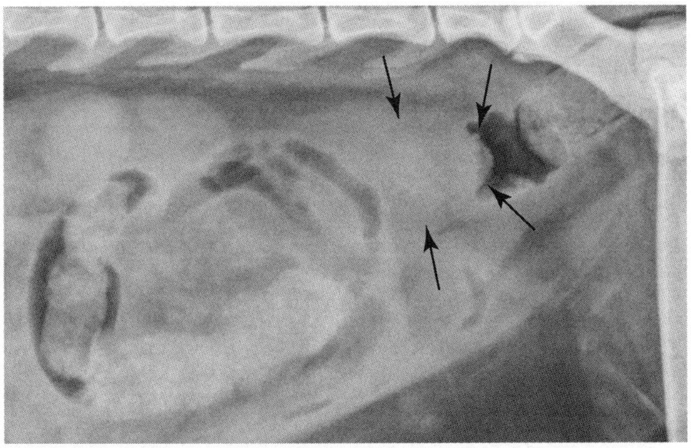

Fig. 47.20 Lateral radiograph of a cat with a descending colonic mass in a cat presented for chronic constipation. There is a large, ovoid soft tissue opaque mass in the region of the distal descending colon (*black arrows*). The caudal margin of the mass is outlined by gas, causing a meniscus sign. The colon proximal to this mass contains mineral opaque fecal material secondary to constipation. There is decreased serosal contrast throughout the ventral abdomen.

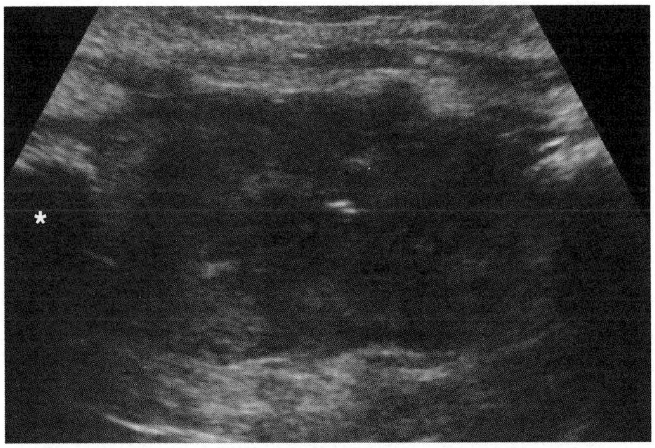

Fig. 47.21 Longitudinal ultrasound image of a cat with a descending colonic mass (same patient as Fig. 47.20). There is a large, hypoechoic, irregularly marginated mass arising from the descending colon with loss of wall layers in this region. Shadowing fecal material is present cranial to the mass (*asterisk*).

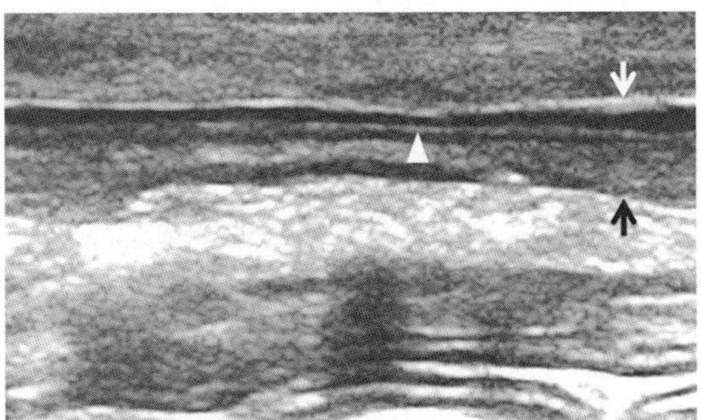

Fig. 47.22 Long-axis ultrasound image of the descending colon of a cat with short colon syndrome and *Campylobacter* colitis. The ascending and transverse colon were absent, the residual descending colon was markedly thickened (*3 mm between arrows*), with reduced wall layering. There is also a hyperechoic line within the tunica muscularis, which can be a normal finding (*arrowhead*).

gastrointestinal tract, gas within the colonic wall can drain into the portal system, resulting in portal venous gas, and sometimes pneumoperitoneum in people.[57,58] There is a wide range of diseases that can result in pneumatosis intestinalis in people, which range from innocuous to fatal.[58,59] Although this is a relatively rare condition in dogs, the veterinary literature appears to mirror this as well, with most dogs responding positively to medical therapy upon diagnosis, while others acutely deteriorated and died or were euthanized.[55–57,60,61] Due to the potential serious outcomes associated with this, investigation into the underlying cause should be performed when identified on imaging.

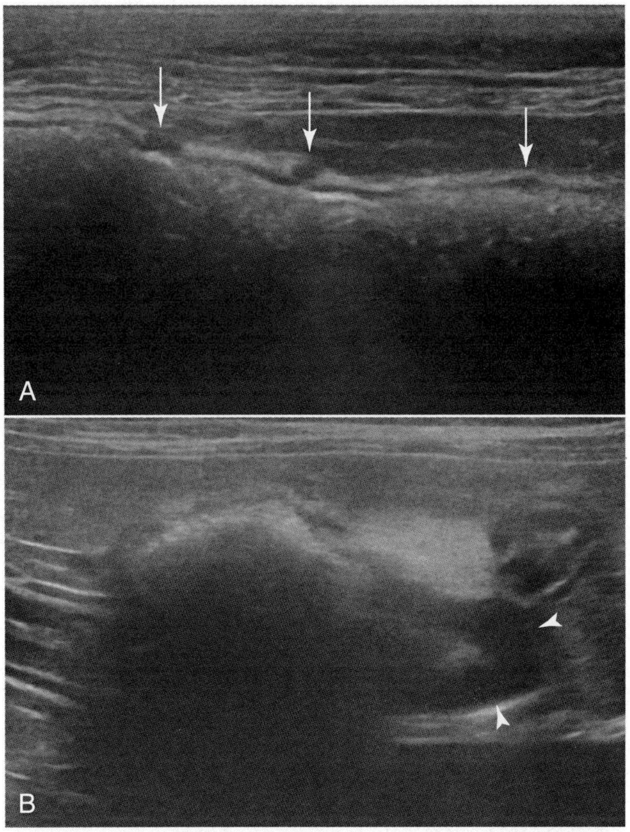

Fig. 47.23 **A,** Longitudinal ultrasound image of the descending colon. There are multifocal small, ovoid, well-defined hypoechoic nodules (*arrows*) in the submucosal layer consistent with lymphoid follicular hyperplasia. **B,** Ultrasound image of the cecum of a cat with presumed typhlitis. The cecal wall (*arrowheads*) is thickened and hypoechoic with loss of wall layering.

Large Intestinal Perforation

Neoplasia, ulceration, obstipation, trauma from enemas, endoscopic biopsy, and radiation therapy of the pelvic region can all lead to large intestinal perforation.[62–64] Colonic ulceration can occur secondary to primary large intestinal disease, but has also been reported with perforation in association with corticosteroid and nonsteroidal anti-inflammatory drugs.[65–67] Radiographic and ultrasonographic findings of large intestinal perforation are similar to that of perforation of the small intestine.[68]

CONGENITAL LARGE BOWEL DISEASES

Congenital anomalies of the large intestine are rare in dogs and cats. Atresia ani, atresia recti, and atresia coli may be a cause of large intestinal obstruction and obstipation in neonatal animals.[69] Short colon has sporadically been reported in cats and dogs and may be associated with signs of large bowel diarrhea.[70–72] Fistulae, diverticula, and duplication of large intestinal structures can also occur[73–75] (eFig. 47.8). Because of the complexity of many of these congenital anomalies, contrast studies either with radiography, fluoroscopy, and/or CT are often used in their evaluation and treatment planning.

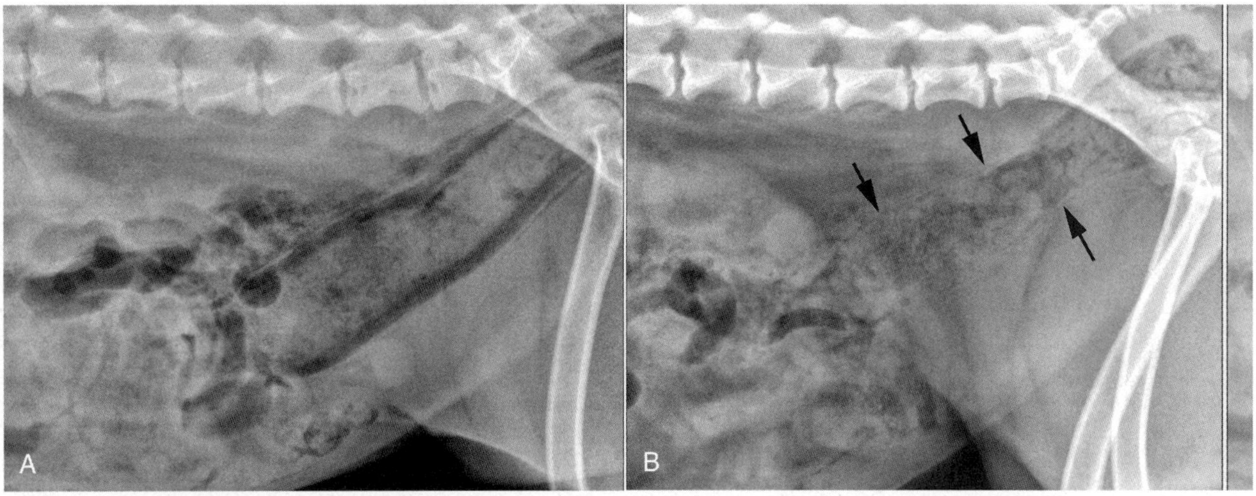

Fig. 47.24 **A,** Lateral radiograph of a dog with tenesmus and hematochezia. There is a large amount of air within the wall of the colon (i.e., pneumatosis coli). **B,** With symptomatic therapy, the clinical signs resolved and the amount of gas in the wall of the colon was markedly reduced (*arrows*) in radiographs acquired 5 days later. The cause of the pneumatosis coli in this patient was not determined but could be related to mucosal ulcerations associated with the large bowel disease.

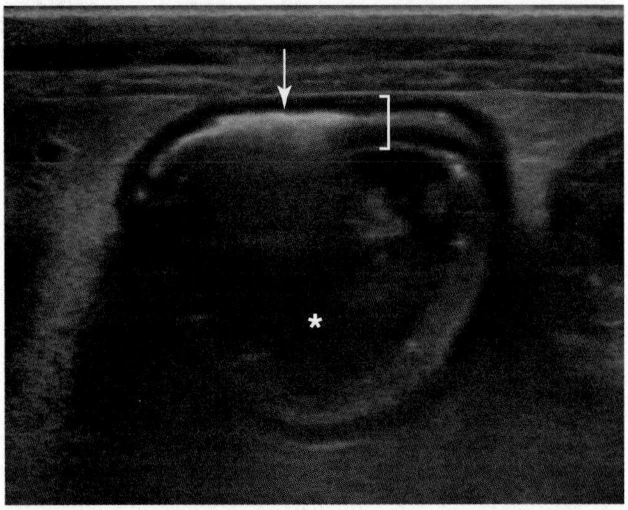

Fig. 47.25 Transverse ultrasound image of the descending colon of a different dog with pneumatosis coli. There is focal hyperechogenicity with reverberation artifact within the wall of the colon (*bracket*), consistent with gas, which obscures the mucosal layer. The colon lumen (*asterisk*) contains fluid.

Acknowledgment

With special thanks to prior authors of this chapter for their contributions.

REFERENCES

1. Evans HE, de Lahunta A. The Digestive Apparatus and Abdomen. In: *Miller and Evan's Anatomy of the Dog*. 4th ed. Philadelphia: Elsevier; 2013.
2. Hall EJ. Diseases of the Large Intestine. In: Ettinger SJ, Feldman EC, Cote E, eds. *Textbook of Veterinary Internal Medicine*. 8th ed. Philadelphia: Elsevier; 2017.
3. Kealy KJ, McAllister H. *Diagnostic Radiology and Ultrasonography of the Dog and Cat*. 5th ed. Philadelphia: WB Saunders; 2010.
4. O'Brien TR. *Radiographic Diagnosis of Abdominal Disorders in the Dog and Cat*. Davis, CA: Covell Park Veterinary; 1981.
5. Trevail T, Gunn-Moore D, Carrera I, et al. Radiographic diameter of the colon in normal and constipated cats and in cats with megacolon. *Vet Radiol Ultrasound*. 2011;52:516.
6. Nyland TG, Ackerman N. Pneumocolon: a diagnostic aid in abdominal radiography. *Vet Radiol*. 1978;19:203–209.
7. Czajkowski PS, Fryer KJ. Colonic torsion in 4 great danes. *J Vet Emerg Crit Care*. 2020;30(5):581–586.
8. Kleine LJ, Lamb CR. Comparative organ imaging: the gastrointestinal tract. *Vet Radiol*. 1989;30:133.
9. Brawner WB, Bartels JE. Contrast radiography of the digestive tract: indications, techniques, and complications. *Vet Clin North Am*. 1983;vol. 13:599.
10. Gremillion CL, Savage M, Cohen EB. Radiographic findings and clinical factors in dogs with surgically confirmed or presumed colonic torsion. *Vet Radiol Ultrasound*. 2018;59(3):272–278.
11. Neelis DA, Mattoon JS, Slovak JE, Sellon RK. Gastrointestinal Tract. In: Mattoon JS, Sellon RK, Berry CR, eds. *Small Animal Diagnostic Ultrasound*. 4th ed. St. Louis: Elsevier; 2021.
12. Gladwin NE, Penninck DG, Webster CRL. Ultrasonographic evaluation of the thickness of the wall layers in the intestinal tract of dogs. *Am J Vet Res*. 2014;75:349.
13. Heng HG, Lim CK, Miller MA, et al. Prevalence and significance of an ultrasonographic colonic muscularis hyperechoic band paralleling the serosal layer in dogs. *Vet Radiol Ultrasound*. 2015;56:666.
14. Spector DL, Fischetti AJ, Kovak-McClaran JR. Computed tomographic characteristics of intrapelvic masses in dogs. *Vet Radiol Ultrasound*. 52:71.
15. Hoey S, Drees R, Hetzel S. Evaluation of the gastrointestinal tract in dogs using computed tomography. *Vet Radiol Ultrasound*. 54:25.
16. Steffey MA, Daniel L, Taylor SL, Chen RX, Zwingenberger AL. Computed tomographic pneumocolonography in normal dogs. *Vet Radiol Ultrasound*. 56(3):278-285.
17. Cheon B, Moon S, Park S, et al. Comparison of contrast media for visualization of the colon of healthy dogs during computed tomography and ultrasonography. *Am J Vet Res*. 2016;77(11):1220–1226.

18. Steffey MA, Zwingenberger AL, Daniel L, Taylor SL. Assessment of 3 bowel preparation protocols for computed tomography pneumocolonography in normal dogs. *Vet Surg*. 2016;45(7):929–935.
19. Lamb CR, Mantis P. Ultrasonographic features of intestinal intussusception in 10 dogs. *J Small Anim Pract*. 1998;39: 437.
20. Cinti F. Caecal inversion in association with ileocolic intussusception in a dog. *J Small Anim Pract*. 2021;62(3):233.
21. Boland L, Lindsay S, Brunel L, Podadera J, Bennett P. Caecocolic intussusception associated with a caecal polyp and concurrent hepatocellular carcinoma in a cat. *JFMS Open Rep*. 2017;3(1):2055116917706652.
22. Lansdown ABG, Fox EA. Colorectal intussusception in a young cat. *Vet Record*. 1991;19:429.
23. Patsikas MN, Papazoglou LG, Jakovljevic S, et al. Color Doppler ultrasonography in prediction of the reducibility of intussuscepted bowel in 15 young dogs. *Vet Radiol Ultrasound*. 2005;46:313.
24. Plavec T, Rupp S, Kessler M. Colonic or ileocecocolic volvulus in 13 dogs (2005–2016). *Vet Surg*. 2017;46(6):851–859.
25. Drobatz KJ, Hughes D, Hill C, et al. Volvulus of the colon in a cat. *J Vet Emerg Crit Care*. 1996;6:99.
26. Gagnon D, Brisson B. Predisposing factors for colonic torsion/volvulus in dogs: a retrospective study of six cases (1992-2010). *J Am Anim Hosp Assoc*. 2013;49(3):169–174.
27. Barge P, Fina CJ, Mortier JR, Jones ID. CT findings in five dogs with surgically confirmed colonic torsion. *Vet Radiol Ultrasound*. 2020;61(2):190–196.
28. Hassinger KA. Intestinal entrapment and strangulation caused by rupture of the duodenocolic ligament in four dogs. *Vet Surg*. 1997;26:275.
29. Brand KJ, Lim CK, Cichocki BN. Radiographic and CT features of colonic entrapment due to an omental rent in a dog. *Vet Radiol Ultrasound*. 2021;62(1):E6–E10.
30. Thanaboonnipat C, Kumjumroon K, Boonkwang K, Tangsutthichai N, Sukserm W, Choisunirachon N. Radiographic lumbosacral vertebral abnormalities and constipation in cats. *Vet World*. 2021;14(2):492–498.
31. DeForest ME, Gasrur PK. Malformations and the Manx syndrome in cats. *Can Vet J*. 1979;2:304.
32. Novellas R, Simpson KE, Gunn-Moore DA, Hammond GJ. Imaging findings in 11 cats with feline dysautonomia. *J Feline Med Surg*. 2010;12(8):584–591.
33. Szabo SD, Wells KL. What is your diagnosis? Congenital hypothyroidism. *J Am Vet Med Assoc*. 2007;230(1):29–30.
34. Woodard ML, Constant CE. What is your diagnosis? Congenital hypothyroidism. *J Am Vet Med Assoc*. 2022;260(5):499–501.
35. Matthiesen DT, Scavelli TD, Whitney WO. Subtotal colectomy for the treatment of obstipation secondary to pelvic fracture malunion in cats. *Vet Surg*. 1991;20:113–117.
36. Maas CP, ter Haar G, van der Gaag I, Kirpensteijn J. Reclassification of small intestinal and cecal smooth muscle tumors in 72 dogs: clinical, histologic, and immunohistochemical evaluation. *Vet Surg*. 2007;36(4):302–313.
37. Slawienski MJ, Mauldin GE, Mauldin GN, et al. Malignant colonic neoplasia in cats: 46 cases (1990–1996). *J Am Vet Med Assoc*. 1997;211:878.
38. Kehl A, Törner K, Jordan A, et al. Pathological findings in gastrointestinal neoplasms and polyps in 860 cats and a pilot study on miRNA analyses. *Vet Sci*. 2022;9(9):477.
39. Graham JP, Newell SM, Roberts GD, et al. Ultrasonographic features of canine gastrointestinal pythiosis. *Vet Radiol Ultrasound*. 2000;41:273.
40. Schmiedt CW, Stratton-Phelps M, Torres BT, et al. Treatment of intestinal pythiosis in a dog with a combination of marginal excision, chemotherapy, and immunotherapy. *J Am Vet Med Assoc*. 2012;241(3):358–363.
41. Stenner VJ, Mackay B, King T, et al. Protothecosis in 17 Australian dogs and a review of the canine literature. *Med Mycol*. 2007;45(3):249–266.
42. Chávez-Peón Berle E, KuKanich K, Biller D. Ultrasonographic findings of gastrointestinal histoplasmosis in dogs. *Vet Radiol Ultrasound*. 2021;62(1):108–115.
43. Cordella A, Stock E, Van de Maele I, Willems A, Saunders J. Use of contrast-enhanced ultrasonography and shear-wave elastography in the diagnosis of granulomatous colitis in a French bulldog. *Vet Sci*. 2021;8(7):133.
44. Moshnikova VS, Gilmour LJ, Cook AK, Fabiani M. Sonographic findings of pinpoint hyperechoic foci in the small intestine, liver, and mesenteric lymph nodes are indicative of canine *Heterobilharzia americana* infection. *Vet Radiol Ultrasound*. 2020;61(5):583–591.
45. Corapi WV, Ajithdoss DK, Snowden KF, Spaulding KA. Multi-organ involvement of *Heterobilharzia americana* infection in a dog presented for systemic mineralization. *J Vet Diagn Invest*. 2011;23(4):826–831.
46. Harvey CJ, Lopez JW, Hendrick MJ. An uncommon intestinal manifestation of feline infectious peritonitis: 26 cases (1986-1993). *J Am Vet Med Assoc*. 1996;209(6):1117–1120.
47. Weissman A, Penninck D, Webster C, et al. Ultrasonographic and clinicopathological features of feline gastrointestinal eosinophilic sclerosing fibroplasia in four cats. *J Fel Med Surg*. 2015;15:148.
48. Kukanich KS, Vinasco J, Scott HM. Detection of *Mycobacterium avium subspecies paratuberculosis* from intestinal and nodal tissue of dogs and cats. *ISRN Vet Sci*. 2013;2013:323671.
49. Seiler RJ. Colorectal polyps of the dog: a clinicopathologic study of 17 cases. *J Am Vet Med Assoc*. 1979;174:72.
50. Hsu TC, Lin LS, Chung CS, Chiang C, Chiu HC, Huang PH. Colonic intramural hematoma in a cat: a case report. *Front Vet Sci*. 2022;9:913862.
51. McKenna M, Suárez-Bonnet A, Smith K, Stewart S. Diagnosis and treatment of a caecal mucocoele in a dog. *J Small Anim Pract*. 2021;62(4):305–309.
52. Citi S, Chimenti T, Marchetti V, et al. Micronodular ultrasound lesions in the colonic submucosa of 42 dogs and 14 cats. *Vet Radiol Ultrasound*. 54:646.
53. Hahn H, Freiche V, Baril A, et al. Ultrasonographical, endoscopic and histological appearance of the caecum in clinically healthy cats. *J Fel Med Surg*. 2017;19:85–93.
54. Hahn H, Pey P, Baril A, et al. Ultrasonographic, endoscopic and histological appearances of the caecum in cats presenting with clinical signs of caecocolic disease. *J Fel Med Surg*. 2017;19:94–104.
55. Fisk A, Allen-Durrance A. Pneumatosis coli in a dog. *J Am Anim Hosp Assoc*. 2019;55(4):e55401.
56. Azuma K, Kanemoto H, Ohno K, Fukushima K, Chambers JK, Tsujimoto H. Pneumatosis coli after partial ligation of congenital portosystemic shunt in a dog. *J Vet Med Sci*. 2018;80(10):1549–1552.
57. Cartwright JA, Breheny C, Major AC, Hill TL, Gow AG. Imaging diagnosis-a case of spontaneous hepatic portal vein gas in an 11-month-old west highland white terrier. *Vet Radiol Ultrasound*. 2016;57(5):E54–E57.
58. Lassandro F, Valente T, Rea G, et al. Imaging assessment and clinical significance of pneumatosis in adult patients. *Radiol Med (Torino)*. 2015;120:96.
59. Feczko PJ, Mezwa DG, Farah MC, et al. Clinical significance of pneumatosis of the bowel wall. *Radiographics*. 1992;12:1069.
60. Russell NJ, Tyrrell D, Irwin PJ, et al. Pneumatosis coli in a dog. *J Am Anim Hosp Assoc*. 2008;44:32.
61. Aste G, Boari A, Guglielmini C. What is your diagnosis? Pneumatosis coli. *J Am Vet Med Assoc*. 2005;227(9): 1407–1408.

62. Kim J, Yoon H, Eom K. Imaging diagnosis – radiography, ultrasonography, and computed tomography of a giant fecaloma causing stercoral perforation of the colon in a dog with a prostatic abscess. *Vet Radiol Ultrasound*. 2018;59(4):E38–E43.
63. Woolhead VL, Whittemore JC, Stewart SA. Multicenter retrospective evaluation of ileocecocolic perforations associated with diagnostic lower gastrointestinal endoscopy in dogs and cats. *J Vet Intern Med*. 2020;34(2):684–690.
64. Arthur JJ, Kleiter MM, Thrall DE, Pruitt AF. Characterization of normal tissue complications in 51 dogs undergoing definitive pelvic region irradiation. *Vet Radiol Ultrasound*. 2008;49(1):85–89.
65. Toombs JP, Caywood DD, Lipowitz AJ, et al. Colonic perforation following neurosurgical procedures and corticosteroid therapy in four dogs. *J Am Vet Med Assoc*. 1980;177:68.
66. Toombs JP, Collins LG, Graves GM, et al. Colonic perforation in corticosteroid-treated dogs. *J Am Vet Med Assoc*. 1986;188:145.
67. Longley MJ, Baines SJ, Chanoit G. Colonic perforation in 4 dogs following treatment with meloxicam. *J Vet Emerg Crit Care (San Antonio)*. 2022;32(3):413–419.
68. Boysen SR, Tidwell AS, Penninck DG. Ultrasonographic findings in dogs and cats with gastrointestinal perforation. *Vet Radiol Ultrasound*. 2003;44(5):556–564.
69. Bredal WP, Thoressen SI, Kvellestad A. Atresia coli in a nine week old kitten. *J Small Anim Pract*. 1994;35:643.
70. Fluke MH, Hawkins EC, Elliott GS, et al. Short colon in two cats and a dog. *J Am Vet Med Assoc*. 1989;195:87.
71. Schlesinger DP, Philbert D, Breur GJ. Agenesis of the cecum and the ascending and transverse colon in a twelve year old cat. *Can Vet J*. 1992;33:544.
72. Le Roux AB, Donovan T, Palma D, et al. Short colon syndrome in cats (abstract). *Vet Radiol Ultrasound*. 2016;57:651.
73. Rahal SC, Vicente CS, Mortari AC, Mamprim MJ, Caporalli EH. Rectovaginal fistula with anal atresia in 5 dogs. *Can Vet J*. 2007;48(8):827–830.
74. Longhofer SL, Jackson RK, Cooley AJ. Hindgut and bladder duplication in a dog. *J Am Anim Hosp Assoc*. 1991;27:97.
75. Shinozaki JK, Sellon RK, Tobias KM, et al. Tubular colonic duplication in a dog. *J Am Anim Hosp Assoc*. 2000;36:209.

ELECTRONIC RESOURCES

Additional information related to the content in Chapter 47 can be found online at eBooks.Health.Elsevier.com.

- Chapter Quiz

Index

Page numbers followed by "*f*" indicate figures, "*t*" indicate tables, and "*b*" indicate boxes.

D

J

K

L

N

O

T

V

W

X